KU-043-097

Tenth Edition

Caffey's Pediatric Diagnostic Imaging

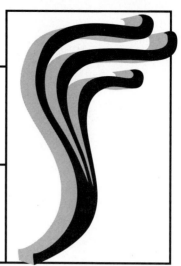

Volume 2

Edited by

Jerald P. Kuhn, M.D.
Former Radiologist and Chief, Department of Radiology
Emeritus Professor of Radiology
State University of New York at Buffalo
School of Medicine
The Children's Hospital of Buffalo
Buffalo, New York

Thomas L. Slovis, M.D.
Professor of Radiology and Pediatrics
Wayne State University School of Medicine
Chief, Pediatric Imaging
Children's Hospital of Michigan
Detroit, Michigan

Jack O. Haller, M.D.
Professor of Radiology
Albert Einstein College of Medicine
Director of Pediatric Radiology
Beth Israel Continuum Hospitals
New York, New York

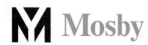

Mosby
An Affiliate of Elsevier

Section Editors

Thomas L. Slovis, M.D.
Section I: Effects of Radiation on Children
Section II: Neonatal Imaging

Eric N. Faerber, M.D.
Section III: Skull, Spine, and Central Nervous System

Charles R. Fitz, M.D.
Section III: Skull, Spine, and Central Nervous System

Jerald P. Kuhn, M.D.
Section IV: Respiratory System

Eric L. Effmann, M.D.
Section IV: Respiratory System

Virgil R. Condon, M.D.
Section V: The Heart and Great Vessels

Richard B. Jaffe, M.D.
Section V: The Heart and Great Vessels

Alan E. Schlesinger, M.D.
Section VI: Abdomen and Gastrointestinal Tract

Bruce R. Parker, M.D.
Section VI: Abdomen and Gastrointestinal Tract

Jack O. Haller, M.D.
Section VII: Urinary Tract and Retroperitoneum
Section VIII: Reproductive Organs

Barry D. Fletcher, M.D., C.M.
Section IX: Musculoskeletal System

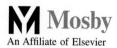
Mosby

An Affiliate of Elsevier

The Curtis Center
Independence Square West
Philadelphia, Pennsylvania 19106

CAFFEY'S PEDIATRIC DIAGNOSTIC IMAGING

Copyright © 2004, Elsevier Inc. (USA)

ISBN 0-323-01109-8
Volume 1—9997635280
Volume 2—9997635299

All rights reserved. No part of this publication may be reproduced, stored in a retrieval system, or transmitted, in any form or by any means, electronic, mechanical, photocopying, recording, or otherwise without written permisson of the publisher.

NOTICE

Medicine is an ever-changing field. Standard safety precautions must be followed, but as new research and clinical experience broaden our knowledge, changes in treatment and drug therapy may become necessary or appropriate. Readers are advised to check the most current product information currently provided by the manufacturer of each drug to be administered to verify the recommended dose, the method and duration of administration, and contraindications. It is the responsibility of the treating physician, relying on experience and knowledge of the patient, to determine dosages and the best treatment for each individual patient. Neither the Publisher nor the editor assume any liability for any injury and/or damage to persons or property arising from this publication.

The Publisher

First Edition 1945; Second Edition 1950; Third Edition 1956; Fourth Edition 1961; Fifth Edition 1967; Sixth Edition 1972; Seventh Edition 1978; Eighth Edition 1985; Ninth Edition 1993

Library of Congress Cataloging-in-Publication Data

Caffey's pediatric diagnostic imaging—10th ed./[edited by] Jerald P. Kuhn, Thomas L. Slovis, Jack O. Haller.
   p. ; cm.
  Includes bibliographical references and index.
  ISBN 0-323-01109-8
  1. Pediatric radiography. 2. Diagnostic imaging. 3. Pediatrics. I. Title: Pediatric diagnostic imaging. II. Kuhn, Jerald P. III. Slovis, Thomas L., IV. Haller, Jack O. (Jack Oliver), V. Caffey, John, VI. Caffey's pediatric X-ray diagnosis.
  [DNLM: 1. Diagnostic Imaging—Child. 2. Diagnostic Imaging—Infant. WN 240 C1292 2003]
RJ51.R3 C3 2003
618.92'007572—dc21

2002075115

BARTS & THE LONDON QMSMD

CL   WN240 CAF 2004 V.2

CL   1 WK

SL   OAW 24|v|62
     E281 (2 VOL SET)

RE

OLD

Printed in the United States of America

Last digit is the print number: 9 8 7 6 5 4 3 2

Dedication

This book is dedicated to the memory of my parents, Dr. Horace and Frances Kuhn, who gave me the drive to succeed, and to the many teachers who guided me along the way. Particular thanks are due to Drs. Mitchell Rubin and Jean Cortner from my days as a pediatrician; Dr. G. Newton Scatchard, who showed me how exciting Pediatric Radiology could be; Dr. Felix Fleischner, who kindled my interest in chest radiology; Dr. E. B. D. Neuhauser and his staff, who taught me the basics; and Dr. John Dorst, who was my mentor in Pediatric Radiology. Nothing, however, would have been achieved without the love and support of my wife of over 40 years, Tina.

Jerald P Kuhn, M. D.

To my partners (Cristie Becker, David Bloom, John Crowley, Dan Eggleston, Sam Kottamasu, Aparna Joshi, Swati Mody, Wilbur Smith, and Mike Zerin) and clinical colleagues at Children's Hospital of Michigan and Wayne State University School of Medicine, who gave their time and thoughtful suggestions.

To my mentors: in medical school (Lewis Barnes, Frank Oski, and Grant Morrow), in pediatrics (Henry Kempe, Henry Silver, Arnie Silverman, Vince Fulginiti, George Comerci, and Les Pensler), and in radiology (Walter Berdon, David Baker, Parker Allen, and Joe Reed), for giving me the skills to provide guidance to others through this text.

To the deep and wonderful friendship of my co-editors, Jack Haller and Jerry Kuhn.

To my children and their spouses (Michael and Kellie, Debbie and Michael, Max and Lisa, and Lisa and David) and grandchildren (Ryan, Kyle, Andrew, Charles, Samantha, Jeremy, Chardon, Brenon, and Kedon), for understanding why "Pop-pa" wasn't always attentive.

To my wife Ellie, for allowing me to convert her dining room table into a home of the "book"! Her patience and love allowed me to finish this massive project.

Thomas L. Slovis, M.D.

To my wife Ozie ("happiness is you") and my children, Evan, Terry, Ziva, Harry, and Kivi, who can't imagine how proud I am of them.

Jack O. Haller, M.D.

CONTRIBUTORS

E. Michel Azouz, M.D., F.R.C.P.C.
Professor of Clinical Radiology, University of Miami;
Senior Radiologist, Section of Pediatric Radiology,
Jackson Memorial Hospital, Miami, Florida

Paul S. Babyn, M.D., C.M.
Associate Professor, Department of Medical Imaging,
University of Toronto; Radiologist-in-Chief,
Department of Diagnostic Imaging, Hospital for Sick
Children, Toronto, Ontario, Canada

James W. Backstrom, M.D.
Specialist, North Pittsburgh Imaging, Lucien
Diagnostic Imaging, Pittsburgh, Pennsylvania; Former
Chief, Pediatric Radiology, Devos Children's Hospital,
Spectrum Health, Grand Rapids, Michigan

Cristie J. Becker, M.D.
Associate Professor of Radiology, Wayne State
University School of Medicine; Chief, Interventional
Radiology, Children's Hospital of Michigan, Detroit,
Michigan

Mary P. Bedard, M.D.
Associate Professor of Pediatrics, Wayne State
University; Clinical Director, Neonatal Intensive Care
Unit, Children's Hospital of Michigan, Detroit,
Michigan

Walter E. Berdon, M.D.
Professor of Radiology, Columbia University College of
Physicians and Surgeons; Director of Radiology
Emeritus, Babies Hospital, Children's Hospital of New
York, New York, New York

David A. Bloom, M.D.
Assistant Professor of Radiology, Wayne State
University School of Medicine; Director, Body CT/
MRI, Children's Hospital of Michigan, Detroit,
Michigan

Danielle K. B. Boal, M.D.
Professor of Radiology and Pediatrics, The
Pennsylvania State University College of Medicine,
Chief, Section of Pediatric Radiology, The Milton S.
Hershey Medical Center, Hershey, Pennsylvania

A'Delbert Bowen, M.D.
Professor of Radiology, University of Pittsburgh School
of Medicine; Pediatric Radiologist, Children's Hospital
of Pittsburgh, Pittsburgh, Pennsylvania

Sharon E. Byrd, M.D.
Professor of Radiology, Attending Neuroradiologist,
Department of Diagnostic Radiology and Nuclear
Medicine, Rush-Presbyterian-St. Luke's Medical
Center, Rush University School of Medicine, Chicago,
Illinois

Harry T. Chugani, M.D.
Professor of Pediatrics, Neurology, and Radiology
Wayne State University School of Medicine; Director,
PET Center, and Chief of Neurology, Children's
Hospital of Michigan, Detroit, Michigan

Harris L. Cohen, M.D., F.A.C.R.
Visiting Professor of Radiology, Johns Hopkins School
of Medicine, Baltimore, Maryland; Professor of
Radiology, and Vice Chairman (Research Affairs),
Director, Division of CT/US/MR, Director, Pediatric
Body Imaging, Department of Radiology, SUNY-Stony
Brook, Stony Brook, New York

Virgil R. Condon, M.D.
Professor Emeritus, Diagnostic Radiology, University of
Utah; Former Director, Medical Imaging, Primary
Children's Medical Center, University of Utah, Salt
Lake City, Utah

Moira L. Cooper, M.D., F.R.C.P.(C)
Associate Professor, Dalhousie University; Staff
Radiologist, I.W.K. Health Center, Halifax, Nova
Scotia, Canada

Alan Daneman, M.B.B.Ch., F.R.C.P.C., F.R.A.C.R.
Professor of Radiology, Department of Medical
Imaging, University of Toronto; Staff Radiologist,
Department of Diagnostic Imaging, Hospital for Sick
Children, Toronto, Ontario, Canada

James S. Donaldson, M.D.
Professor of Radiology, The Feinberg School of
Medicine, Northwestern University; Chairman,
Department of Medical Imaging, Children's Memorial
Hospital, Chicago, Illinois

Eric L. Effmann, M.D.
Director, Department of Radiology, Children's
Hospital and Regional Medical Center; Professor of
Radiology and Division Director of Pediatric
Radiology, University of Washington School of
Medicine, Seattle, Washington

Douglas F. Eggli, M.D.
Professor of Radiology, The Pennsylvania State
University College of Medicine; Chief, Division of
Nuclear Medicine, Department of Radiology, The
Milton S. Hershey Medical Center, Hershey,
Pennsylvania

Kathleen H. Emery, M.D.
Associate Clinical Professor of Radiology and
Pediatrics, University of Cincinnati Medical Center;
Staff Radiologist, Cincinnati Children's Hospital
Medical Center, Cincinnati, Ohio

Eric N. Faerber, M.D.
Professor of Radiology, Drexel University College of
Medicine; Director, Department of Radiology, and
Chief, Section of Neuroradiology, St. Christopher's
Hospital for Children, Philadelphia, Pennsylvania

Diana L. Farmer, M.D.
Professor of Surgery, Pediatrics and Obstetrics,
Gynecology and Reproductive Sciences; Chief, Division
of Pediatric Surgery, Department of Surgery and the
Fetal Treatment Center, University of California, San
Francisco, San Francisco, California

Kate A. Feinstein, M.D., F.A.C.R.
Associate Professor of Radiology, The University of
Chicago Pritzker School of Medicine, The University
of Chicago, Chicago, Illinois

Sandra K. Fernbach, M.D.
Professor of Radiology, Feinberg School of Medicine,
Chicago; Evanston Northwestern Healthcare,
Evanston, Illinois

Charles R. Fitz, M.D.
Professor of Radiology, University of Pittsburgh School
of Medicine; Radiologist-in-Chief, Department of
Radiology, Children's Hospital, Pittsburgh,
Pennsylvania

Barry D. Fletcher, M.D., C.M.
Former Chairman, Department of Diagnostic Imaging,
St. Jude Children's Research Hospital, Memphis;
Clinical Professor of Radiology, University of
Tennessee Health Science Center, Memphis,
Tennessee; Clinical Associate, Department of
Radiology, Duke University Medical Center, Durham,
North Carolina

Eric J. Hall, D.Phil., D.Sc.
Higgins Professor of Radiation Biophysics, and
Professor of Radiology and Radiation Oncology,
Columbia University; Director, Center for Radiological
Research; Attending Radiobiologist, New York
Presbyterian Hospital, New York, New York

Jack O. Haller, M.D.
Professor of Radiology, Albert Einstein College of
Medicine–Beth Israel Campus, and Director of
Pediatric Radiology, Beth Israel Continuum Hospitals,
New York, New York

H. Theodore Harcke, M.D., F.A.C.R.
Professor of Radiology and Pediatrics, Jefferson
Medical College, Philadelphia, Pennsylvania; Director
of Imaging Research, Alfred I. DuPont Hospital for
Children, Wilmington, Delaware

Thomas E. Herman, M.D.
Associate Professor of Radiology, Washington
University School of Medicine, Mallinckrodt Institute
of Radiology; Radiologist, St. Louis Children's
Hospital, St. Louis, Missouri

Richard B. Jaffe, M.D., F.A.C.R.
Clinical Professor of Radiology, University of Utah
School of Medicine; Staff Pediatric Radiologist,
Primary Children's Medical Center, University of Utah,
Salt Lake City, Utah

Victoria E. Judd, M.D.
Clinical Professor of Pediatrics, University of Utah
School of Medicine; Pediatric Cardiologist, Primary
Children's Medical Center, University of Utah, Salt
Lake City, Utah

Joseph J. Junewick, M.D.
Assistant Clinical Professor, Michigan State University,
East Lansing; Medical Director, Diagnostic Radiology,
Spectrum Health Hospital; Section Chief, Pediatric
Radiology, Devos Children's Hospital, Grand Rapids,
Michigan

Theodore E. Keats, M.D.
Alumni Professor of Radiology, University of Virginia
Health System, Charlottesville, Virginia

Sambasiva R. Kottamasu, M.D.
Clinical Professor of Radiology, Wayne State University School of Medicine, Detroit; Radiologist, Covenant Medical Center, Saginaw, Michigan

Keith A. Kronemer, M.D.
Assistant Professor of Radiology, Washington University School of Medicine, Mallinckrodt Institute of Radiology; Radiologist, St. Louis Children's Hospital, St. Louis, Missouri

Jerald P. Kuhn, M.D.
Former Radiologist and Chief, Department of Radiology, Emeritus Professor of Radiology, State University of New York at Buffalo School of Medicine, The Children's Hospital of Buffalo, Buffalo, New York

Ralph S. Lachman, M.D.
Professor of Radiology and Pediatrics, UCLA School of Medicine, Los Angeles; Visiting Scholar, Stanford University, Palo Alto; Co-Director, International Skeletal Dysplasia Clinic, Cedars-Sinai Medical Center, Los Angeles, California

Tal Laor, M.D.
Associate Professor of Radiology and Pediatrics, University of Cincinnati College of Medicine, Cincinnati Children's Hospital Medical Center, Cincinnati, Ohio

John C. Leonidas, M.D.
Professor of Radiology and Pediatrics, Albert Einstein College of Medicine, New York; Department of Radiology, Schneider Children's Hospital, New Hyde Park, New York

Gerald A. Mandell, M.D.
Adjunct Professor of Radiology, Hospital of University of Pennsylvania, Philadelphia; Professor of Radiology and Nuclear Medicine, Thomas Jefferson University Hospital, Philadelphia, Pennsylvania; Chief of Nuclear Medicine, Phoenix Children's Hospital, Phoenix, Arizona

Bradley A. Maxfield, M.D.
Assistant Clinical Professor of Radiology, Medical College of Wisconsin; Pediatric Radiologist, Children's Hospital, Milwaukee, Wisconsin

William H. McAlister, M.D.
Professor of Radiology and Pediatrics, Washington University School of Medicine, Mallinckrodt Institute of Radiology; Radiologist-in-Chief, St. Louis Children's Hospital, St. Louis, Missouri

Swati Mody, M.D., M.B.B.S.
Assistant Professor, Wayne State University School of Medicine; Staff Radiologist, Children's Hospital of Michigan, Detroit, Michigan

James F. Mooney III, M.D.
Associate Professor of Orthopedic Surgery, Wayne State University School of Medicine; Chief, Orthopedic Surgery; Children's Hospital of Michigan, Detroit, Michigan

Otto Muzik, Ph.D.
Associate Professor of Pediatrics and Radiology, Wayne State University School of Medicine; Physicist, PET Center, Children's Hospital of Michigan, Detroit, Michigan

Luciana T. Pagotto, M.D.
Associate Professor of Pediatrics, Division of Pediatric Cardiology, Primary Children's Medical Center, University of Utah, Salt Lake City, Utah

Bruce R. Parker, M.D.
Professor of Radiology and Pediatrics, Baylor College of Medicine, Houston; Professor of Radiology and Pediatrics Emeritus, Stanford University, Stanford, California; Chairman, Singleton Department of Diagnostic Imaging, Texas Children's Hospital, Houston, Texas

Tina Young Poussaint, M.D.
Assistant Professor of Radiology, Children's Hospital of Boston, Harvard Medical School, Boston, Massachusetts

Marilyn D. Ranson, M.D.
Assistant Professor, Department of Medical Imaging, University of Toronto; Staff Radiologist, Department of Diagnostic Imaging, The Hospital for Sick Children, Toronto, Ontario, Canada

Barbara S. Reid, M.D.
Associate Clinical Professor of Radiology, University of Utah School of Medicine; Pediatric Radiologist, Primary Children's Medical Center, University of Utah, Salt Lake City, Utah

Arlene A. Rozzelle, M.D.
Assistant Professor of Surgery, Wayne State University School of Medicine; Director, Craniofacial Anomalies Clinic; Chief, Plastic and Reconstructive Surgery, Children's Hospital of Michigan, Detroit, Michigan

Alan E. Schlesinger, M.D.
Professor of Radiology, Baylor College of Medicine; Singleton Department of Diagnostic Imaging, Texas Children's Hospital, Houston, Texas

Frederic N. Silverman, M.D.
Professor of Radiology and Pediatrics Emeritus, Stanford University, Stanford, California

Sudha P. Singh, M.D.
Assistant Professor of Radiology, Department of Radiology, Vanderbilt University Medical Center, Nashville, Tennessee

Carlos J. Sivit, M.D.
Professor of Pediatrics and Radiology, Case Western
Reserve School of Medicine; Director of Pediatric
Radiology, Rainbow Babies and Children's Hospital,
Cleveland, Ohio

Thomas L. Slovis, M.D.
Professor of Radiology and Pediatrics, Wayne State
University School of Medicine; Chief, Pediatric
Imaging, Children's Hospital of Michigan, Detroit,
Michigan

Sandeep Sood, M.D.
Assistant Professor of Neurosurgery, Wayne State
University School of Medicine; Staff Pediatric
Neurosurgeon, Children's Hospital of Michigan,
Detroit, Michigan

John R. Sty, M.D.
Clinical Professor of Radiology, Medical College of
Wisconsin, Milwaukee, and University of Wisconsin,
Madison; Chief of Radiology, Children's Hospital of
Wisconsin, Milwaukee, Wisconsin

Joel D. Swartz, M.D.
Medical Director, National Medical Imaging; Former
Clinical Professor of Radiologic Services, Medical
College of Pennsylvania, Philadelphia, Pennsylvania

Richard B. Towbin, M.D.
Professor of Radiology, University of Pennsylvania
School of Medicine; Radiologist-in-Chief, Van Alen
Chair in Pediatric Radiology, The Children's Hospital
of Philadelphia, Philadelphia, Pennsylvania

Gilbert Vezina, M.D.
Director, Program in Neuroradiology, Children's
National Medical Center; Associate Professor of
Radiology and Pediatrics, The George Washington
University School of Medicine, Washington, D.C.

FOREWORD

When I was asked to write a short foreword for the tenth edition of *Caffey's Pediatric Diagnostic Imaging*, I realized that this was a "sentinel event." For the first time, the "Bible" was in the hands of a group most of whom never were co-workers or original trainees of Dr. Caffey. The first edition, published in 1945, was the work of one man, Dr. John Caffey, a founding father of our speciality.

All of us who subsequently wrote for Caffey added to his original marvelous one-man work. Dr. Caffey's was a hard act to follow. He selected Dr. Fred Silverman to help him starting with the fifth edition in 1967. Fred added Dr. Jerald Kuhn as a co-editor for the ninth edition, but even in retirement Fred was the keeper/ benefactor and a guiding force of the "Bible" until this edition.

It is time to move on. The tenth edition includes contributions from many specialists, most of whom never knew Dr. Caffey. The new name, *Caffey's Pediatric Diagnostic Imaging,* recognizes Dr. Caffey's historic contributions and the tradition of the book while reflecting the major new emphasis on diagnostic imaging that has accelerated in the 10 years that have passed since the ninth edition was published. This new edition is the combined effort of three editors and over 60 contributors and represents a comprehensive collection of the work of experts in all the subspeciality areas of pediatric diagnostic imaging.

The book retains its heavy clinical orientation. Dr. Caffey always viewed his work as being addressed to all who care for children. I am proud to be asked to contribute this short foreword. Dr. Caffey and Silverman were pioneers and scholars. Drs. Kuhn, Slovis, and Haller are fully up to the task of bringing Caffey into the 21st century.

Walter E. Berdon, M.D.

PREFACE TO TENTH EDITION

Although the tenth edition of this classic reference text of pediatric radiology has been extensively revised, we have maintained the organ system, anatomic, and pathologic organizational approach of previous editions. Recognition of normal and normal variants remains an important part of diagnostic imaging, as does clinical correlation, two points always stressed by Dr. Caffey. These important features of earlier editions are preserved and emphasized in this tenth edition. Indeed, with the multitude of choices available as to the safest, most accurate, and most cost-effective way of reaching a diagnosis, it is more important than ever for the clinician and the imager to communicate for the benefit of the sick child. We must know what it is that the clinician needs to learn from the imaging procedure if we are to do our job optimally, and the clinician must be aware of the benefits, risks, and limitations of the procedures he or she requests. Therefore, we have started each major section with an overview of imaging procedures applicable to that organ system.

This text contains a new section on hazards of radiation exposure in childhood. The increasing importance of neonatal imaging has been recognized by nearly tripling the length of the section and moving it to its logical place in the front of the book. This section was written and edited by Dr. Slovis with cogent contributions from his medical, surgical, and radiologic colleagues. The chapters on radiography of the skull and facial bones as well as the section on normal bony variants retain much of the original text of Drs. Caffey and Silverman, but nearly all the other chapters have been extensively rewritten. The central nervous system section, co-edited by Dr. Charles Fitz and Dr. Eric Faerber with contributions from Dr. Slovis and several other authorities, has been strengthened by the addition of many new magnetic resonance images and a new chapter on hydrocephalus. Magnetic resonance imaging (MRI) and ultrasonography are emphasized in the cardiac section, written by Dr. Richard Jaffe and Dr. Virgil Condon. Dr. Eric Effmann has joined Dr. Kuhn to produce an improved and expanded discussion of diseases of the respiratory system featuring many new high-resolution computed tomography (CT) images.

The gastrointestinal section written by Dr. Bruce Parker and Dr. Alan Schlesinger, with a new chapter on abdominal trauma by Dr. Carlos Sivit, also features many new cross-sectional images. The genitourinary section, edited by Dr. Haller, contains many new chapters written by Drs. Fernbach, Feinstein, Cohen, and Sty, also emphasizing ultrasound, CT, and MRI in addition to conventional imaging studies. The musculoskeletal section was edited by Dr. Barry Fletcher and has been nearly completely rewritten, with new chapters on congenital anomalies by Dr. Tal Laor, bone dysplasias by Dr. Ralph Lachman, and syndromes by Dr. William McAlister, as well as chapters contributed by Dr. Fletcher on bone and soft tissue neoplasms, stressing the role of MRI. Other new chapters include those on infection by Dr. Michel Azouz, soft tissue diseases by Dr. Kathy Emery, joint diseases by Dr. Paul Babyn, trauma by Dr. Ted Harcke, and child abuse by Dr. Danielle Boal. Dr. Sam Kottamasu has consolidated and updated the chapters dealing with systemic and metabolic diseases of bone. Throughout the text, Dr. Doug Eggli has contributed material on nuclear medicine, and Dr. James Donaldson has added discussion of interventional procedures.

The reading lists have been extensively revised and updated. Often "old" references are still included because of their "classic" descriptions and historical value. As in past editions, the specific author is not always cited in the text, but the appropriate reference should be readily recognized from the titles listed. The reading suggestions are listed at the end of each chapter and subdivided according to the major topics discussed.

Nearly half of the illustrations in this volume are new; we have retained many of the classic conventional radiographic images from earlier volumes, although some have been replaced by better examples. Our publisher, Mosby, an imprint of Elsevier, has gone to great lengths to improve image quality, and a major emphasis has been placed on making the index more comprehensive. We have more than doubled the number of tables and have added new "teaching boxes" to emphasize important points, especially for the resident or other less experienced readers.

Special thanks are gratefully extended to the many

people whose efforts might otherwise go unrecognized. Our clinical colleagues at each of our hospitals, our colleagues in our imaging departments, and the many people who have contributed images to this book all helped to make this book possible. In particular, Dr. Ronald Cohen of Oakland provided many unique CT images for the respiratory section. We are deeply appreciative of the invaluable assistance provided to the editors by Dr. Slovis' secretary, Ms. Jennifer Handley.

During the 4 years it took to complete this book, there were many changes in the publishing industry as a series of mergers led to Yearbook being purchased by Mosby, Mosby by Saunders and ultimately by Elsevier. We were fortunate to work with Rebecca Gruliow, who provided a guiding beacon through these seas of change and without whom this work would probably never have been finished. Berta Steiner at Bermedica Production did a very thorough job of layout and production, resulting in what we believe will be a much improved version of an already outstanding reference textbook that we hope will contribute to advances in pediatric radiology and the health care of our most valuable resource, our children.

Jerald P. Kuhn, M.D.
Thomas L. Slovis, M.D.
Jack O. Haller, M.D.

PREFACE TO FIRST EDITION

Shadows are but dark holes in radiant streams, twisted rifts beyond the substance, meaningless in themselves.

He who would comprehend Röntgen's pallid shades need always to know well the solid matrix whence they spring. The physician needs to know intimately each living patient through whom the racing black light darts, and flashing the hidden depths reveals them in a glowing mirage of thin images, each cast delicately in its own halo, but all veiled and blended endlessly.

Man—warm, lively, fleshy man—and his story are both root and key to his shadows; shadows cold, silent and empty.— (JOHN CAFFEY)

Within a few weeks after Röntgen announced his now renowned discovery to the world in December, 1895, the x-ray method of examination was applied to infants and children. The Vienna letter of February 29 (M. Rec. 49:312, 1896) contained a roentgen print of the arm of an infant made of Kreidl in Vienna: this is the second reproduction of a roentgen image in the American literature. Credit for the first recorded roentgen examination of an infant in the United States undoubtedly belongs to Dr. E. P. Davis of New York City, who described the roentgen shadows cast by the trunk of a living infant and the skull of a dead fetus in March, 1896. In his remarkable article (The study of the infant body and the pregnant womb by the roentgen ray, Am. J. M. Sc. 111:263, 1896) Dr. Davis also included three drawings of shadows visualized by means of a skiascope— shadows of the feet, elbows and orbit of a living infant. Feilchenfeld's discussion of spina ventosa in May, 1896, is probably the first roentgen description of morbid anatomy in children (Berlin. Klin. Wchnschr. 33:403, 1896). There were only two roentgen pediatric publications in 1896; the number increased to 14 in 1897.

In 1898, Escherich of Graz had had sufficient experience with pediatric roentgen examinations to write a general exposition on the merits and weaknesses of the method (La valeur diagnostique de la radiographie chez les enfants, Rev. d. mal. de l'enf. 16:233, May, 1898). This is a highly interesting and illuminating discussion in which Escherich points out that roentgen examination was already not being used as commonly in young patients as in adults. He states that a roentgen laboratory was established especially for children at Graz in 1897, and it seems probable that this was the first of its kind. A single film is reproduced—a print of an infantile hand and forearm which shows rachitic changes. The uncertainties of the mediastinal shadows, which still bedevil us, were fully appreciated by Escherich, and he was quite unhappy about this baffling structure "in which so many important infantile lesions lie concealed." He was enthusiastic in regard to the possible estimation of the state of hydration of soft tissues in infantile diarrhea from their roentgen densities.

Reyher's German monograph in 1908 is the earliest review of the world literature on pediatric roentgenology which I have found (Reyher, P.: Die roentgenologische Diagnostik in der Kinderheilkunde, Ergebn. d. inn. Med. u. Kinderh. 2:613, 1908). In it there are 276 references to articles published during the first 12 years following Röntgen's discovery, and these furnish a good key for the study of the early writings in this field. The appendix contains 40 small but clear roentgen prints.

Rotch's *The Roentgen Ray in Pediatrics* appeared in 1910—the first book in any language devoted exclusively to pediatric x-ray diagnosis and still, I believe, the only one in English. Dr. Thomas Morgan Rotch was Professor of Pediatrics, Harvard University, and an outstanding pediatrist of his time.* In this pioneer treatise he stresses the importance of mastering the shadows of normal structure before attempting the recognition and interpretation of the abnormal, and he carefully correlates the clinical findings with the roentgen findings in the cases illustrated; 42 of 264 figures depict the "normal living anatomy of infants and children." This material was taken largely from the files of the Boston Children's Hospital, and the author's statement that more than 2,300 cases were available for study demonstrates that roentgen examination had long been a commonplace in his clinic. Dr. Rotch's early fostering of roentgen examination of infants and children, his appreciation of the special problems in

---

*Jacobi, A.: In memoriam Thomas Morgan Rotch, Am. J. Dis. Child. 8:245, 1914.

applying this method to the young, his careful anatomicroroentgen studies and his text, monumental for this time, all mark him as the father of pediatric roentgenology in America.

Two years later—1912—the first German book, Reyher's *Das Roentgenverfahren in der Kinderheilkunde,* was published. Later and more familiar texts are Gralka's *Roentgendiagnostik im Kindesalter* (1927), Becker's *Roentgendiagnostik und Strahlentherapie in der Kinderheilkunde* (1931) and the *Handbuch der Roentgendiagnostik und Therapie im Kindesalter* by Engel and Schall (1933). As far as I have been able to determine, no book on pediatric roentgen diagnosis has been published in English during the 35 years which have passed since Rotch's unique publication in 1910. The absence of pediatric roentgenology in the flood of medical texts which has streamed from the American and English presses during the last three decades constitutes a dereliction unmatched in other equally important fields of medical diagnosis—a literary developmental hypoplasia which it is hoped *Pediatric X-Ray Diagnosis* will remedy.

This book stems from the roentgen conferences held semimonthly at the Babies Hospital during the last 20 years. The films reproduced herein were all selected from our own roentgen files save those for which credit to others is indicated in the legends. The purpose of the author is two-fold: description of shadows cast by normal and morbid tissues, and clinical appraisal of roentgen findings in pediatric diagnosis. Roentgen physics, technic and therapy have been omitted intentionally. As references and acknowledgments testify, the writer has borrowed freely from the literature and is indebted to many contributors for subject matter and illustrations. To all of them I am sincerely grateful. In the broad and deep field of pediatric diagnosis, selection of the most appropriate material has posed many dilemmas. In the main, data have been chosen which have proved the most useful and instructive in solving the common and important diagnostic problems which have arisen during two decades in a large and busy pediatric hospital and out-patient clinic.

The limitations of space do not permit adequate recognition here of all those to whom credit is due for the making of this book. The roentgen examinations which are its foundation could not have been made without the cooperation of thousands of patients—many weak and painweary; to all of these I am profoundly thankful. Intimate clinical contacts have been maintained and essential collateral examinations have been made possible through the sustained collaboration of my colleagues—attending physicians and surgeons, resident physicians and nurses. I am under deep and solid obligation to Dr. Rustin McIntosh who read the entire manuscript; his discerning criticism and valuable suggestions are responsible for numerous corrections and improvements in the text. The sympathetic reception given to our early endeavors by Dr. Ross Golden will always be remembered gratefully, as well as his continuing wise and friendly counsel. We have benefited much and often from the discipline of the necropsy table— from the instructive dissections of Dr. Martha Wollstein, Dr. Beryl Paige and Dr. Dorothy Andersen,

To none, however do I owe more that to my loyal coworkers in the roentgen department of the Babies Hospital—Edgar Watts, Cecelia Peck, Moira Shannon, Mary Fennell and Mary Jean Cadman—for their gentle handling of patients, unfailing industry and superlative technical skill. Mrs. Cadman typed the manuscript; I am grateful to her for the speedy completion of a thorny chore. The drawings are the work of Alfred Feinberg, and they reflect his rich experience in medical illustration.

The final phase in the preparation of the manuscript was saddened by the death of Mr. H. A. Simons, President of the Year Book Publishers. His stimulating enthusiasm and generosity were indispensable to the completion of the book during these unsettled war years. His passing was a grievous loss. The task of publication has fallen to the capable and patient hands of Mr. Paul Perles and Mrs. Anabel Ireland Janssen.

John Caffey
Babies Hospital
New York 32
June 10, 1945

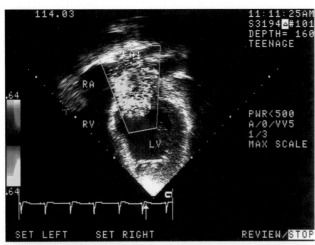

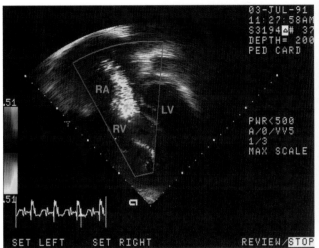

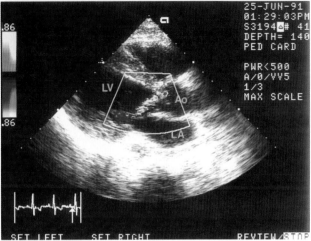

Section V, Part I, Chapter 2, Figures 17, 18, and 19, see pages 1241 and 1242.

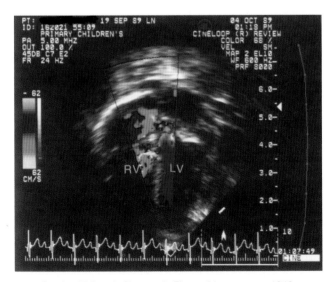

Section V, Part I, Chapter 2, Figure 21, see page 1243.

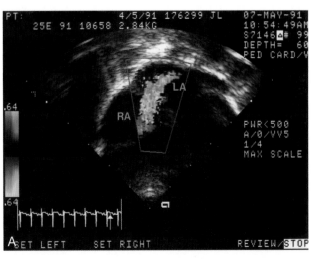

Section V, Part I, Chapter 2, Figure 20A, see page 1242.

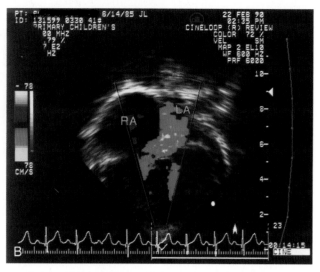

Section V, Part I, Chapter 2, Figure 20B, see page 1242.

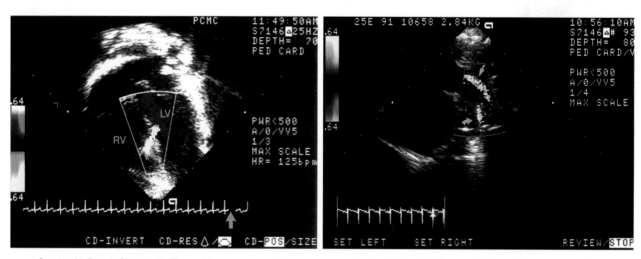

Section V, Part I, Chapter 2, Figure 22, see page 1244.

Section V, Part I, Chapter 2, Figure 23, see page 1244.

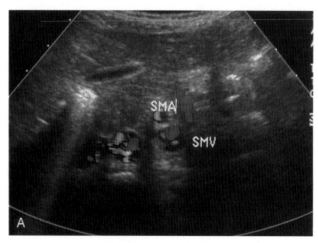

Section VI, Part VII, Figure 4A, see page 1619.

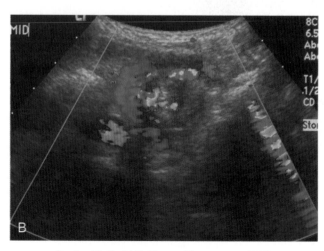

Section VI, Part VII, Figure 4B, see page 1619.

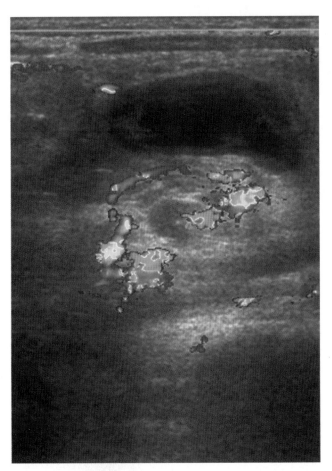

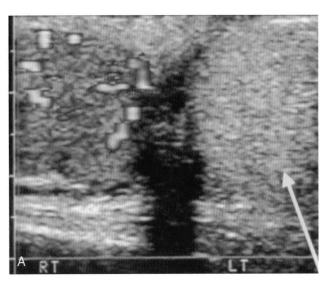

Section VIII, Part I, Figure 18A, see page 1927.

Section VI, Part VII, Figure 24, see page 1630.

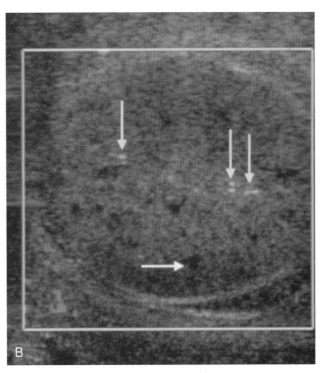

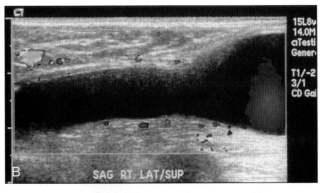

Section VIII, Part I, Figure 13B, see page 1924.

Section VIII, Part I, Figure 18B, see page 1927.

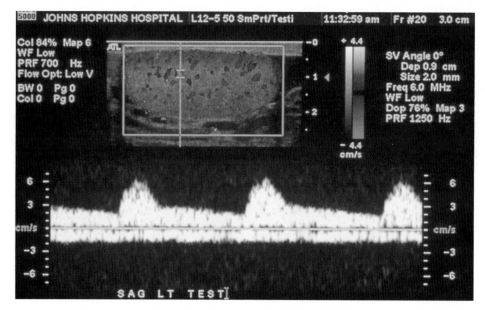

Section VIII, Part I, Figure 19, see page 1928.

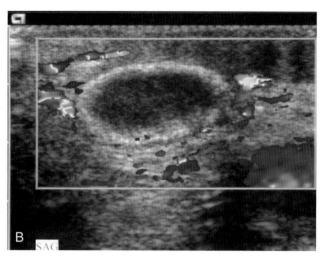

Section VIII, Part I, Figure 20B, see page 1929.

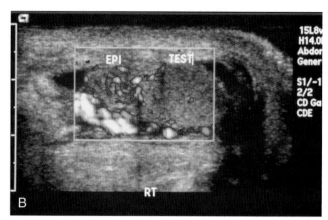

Section VIII, Part I, Figure 22B, see page 1930.

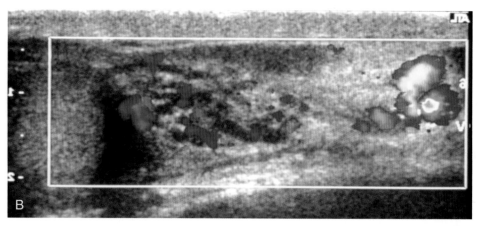

Section VIII, Part I, Figure 31B, see page 1937.

CONTENTS

SECTION V

THE HEART AND GREAT VESSELS

VIRGIL R. CONDON

RICHARD B. JAFFE

BARBARA S. REID

LUCIANA T. PAGOTTO

VICTORIA E. JUDD

PART I

INTRODUCTION

VIRGIL R. CONDON
RICHARD B. JAFFE
BARBARA S. REID
LUCIANA T. PAGOTTO
VICTORIA E. JUDD

Chapter 1

OVERVIEW OF HEART DISEASE

VIRGIL R. CONDON

Heart disease is the fifth most common cause of death in infants and children and has actually increased from 7.2 per 1000 live births to 11 per 1000 live births in the last 29 years. In spite of medical and surgical advances, total death rates have remained stable for the last two decades. Congenital cardiac lesions account for approximately 90% of these fatalities. Congenital heart disease (CHD) occurs in approximately 1% of all live births.

The exact prevalence of CHD is difficult to calculate because of differing methods of diagnosis, the inclusion or exclusion of spontaneously closing lesions, and differing patient populations (i.e., live births alone or all births and aborted fetuses). Ventricular septal defect is the most common CHD at 28% (range 19% to 42%), followed by atrial septal defect (ASD) at 10% (7% to 13%), pulmonary valvular stenosis (PVS) at 10% (5% to 14%), patent ductus arteriosus (PDA) at 10% (5% to 14%), tetralogy of Fallot (TOF) at 10% (3% to 10%), aortic stenosis (AS) at 7% (3% to 8%), coarctation at 5% (5% to 10%), transposition of the great arteries at 5% (5% to 14%), and atrioventricular septal defect (AVSD) (2% to 7%), hypoplastic left heart syndrome (2% to 7%), total anomalous pulmonary venous return (TAPVR) (1% to 3%), truncus arteriosus (1% to 3%), and miscellaneous lesions.

Many other factors play important roles in the incidence of CHD. The sex of the infant is not particularly important in relation to incidence; however, it is important in relation to the type of CHD present. Male infants are more prone to dextrotransposition of the great arteries, as well as left heart obstructive lesions, whereas PDA, PVS, ASD, and AVSD are more common in girls. Parental age is important, particularly as it relates to the increased incidence of Down syndrome with its high rate of CHD. No significant overall difference of incidence can be found in different racial groups, although some different trends of types of CHD can be demonstrated in whites, blacks, and Mexican-Americans.

Genetic factors are very important in relation to CHD. Although most cases of CHD represent isolated lesions, patients with chromosomal abnormalities, heritable syndromes, and major organ abnormalities are at a much greater risk for developing CHD. This is discussed in greater detail in Section V, Part IV, page 1364. It should be noted that 25% to 30% of patients with CHD have extracardiac abnormalities, which are particularly prevalent in the group with CHD involving genetic factors.

Other causative factors relate to environmental exposure to known teratogens but this is a relatively minor source, although outbreaks have been described related to water and ground contamination. Certain medications are well documented to relate to CHD, such as thalidomide, antimetabolites, and vitamin A cogeners. Insecticides and other garden and household chemicals may also be implicated. Ionizing radiation is a recognized causative factor. Infections acting as cardiac teratogens include rubella, herpes simplex viruses, echovirus II, mumps, and many others. All of the above factors are important in the several months prior to and after conception. Maternal diabetes (insulin dependent) significantly increase the risk of congenital cardiac lesions and cardiomyopathies.

Finally, it should be recognized that there is a significantly increased risk of CHD if older siblings or parents have CHD. Because patients now survive long enough to have children, the incidence of CHD will significantly increase in these families. The risk is particularly great if the affected parent was the mother.

Two thirds of infants who die of CHD do so within the first year of life, one third within the first month. The most common cause of death in the first year relates to hypoplastic left heart syndrome. Severe coarctation, critical AS, and transposition of the great arteries are other important causes of death in this age group (Table 1).

CLINICAL PRESENTATIONS

The primary clinical presentation of congenital and acquired heart disease is congestive heart failure (CHF)

Table 1 ■ CONGESTIVE HEART FAILURE ETIOLOGIES, BY PATIENT AGE

0–24 Hours
Intrauterine arrhythmia
Placental transfusion
Hypoplastic left heart syndrome (rare)

1–7 Days
Hypoplastic left heart syndrome—most common (usually appears within 24–48 hr)
Total anomalous pulmonary venous return with obstruction
Persistent fetal circulation
Infant of diabetic mother
Myocardial dysfunction (hypoxia, acidosis, sepsis)
Arteriovenous malformation (and other volume overload)

2–4 Weeks
Coarctation syndrome (with ventricular septal defect/patent ductus arteriosus)—most common (usually appears within 7–14 days)
Critical aortic stenosis
Tachyarrhythmia
Transposition of the great arteries
Cardiomyopathies (endocardial fibroelastosis)
Anomalous left coronary artery
Large left-to-right shunts
Complex malformation, common ventricle, etc.

1–4 Months
Left-to-right shunts
  Ventricular septal defect
  Atrial septal defect
  Patent ductus arteriosus
  Atrioventricular canal
Truncus arteriosus
Transposition of the great arteries (other forms, e.g., double-outlet right ventricle)
Cardiomyopathies (endocardial fibroelastosis)
Total anomalous pulmonary venous return without obstruction

or cyanosis, or both. CHF, particularly in infants, is frequently diagnosed late and often mistaken for infection or other pulmonary processes. Other manifestations in the neonate include failure to thrive, tachypnea, and poor feeding. CHF usually relates to (1) pressure overload from obstructive lesions; (2) volume overload (i.e., high-output states, left-to-right shunt, or valvular insufficiency); and (3) myocardial damage (i.e., hypoxia and infection). The patient's age at the time of presentation with CHF is of considerable value in predicting the cause of failure (Table 1). In the first few hours, CHF usually relates to volume overload or arrhythmia. Hypoplastic left heart syndrome (aortic valve atresia) with pressure overload is the most common etiology in the first week of life. Coarctation is the usual cause in the second and third weeks. After 1 month, as the pulmonary resistance decreases, left-to-right shunts are the primary cause for failure.

Cyanosis may relate to either CHF or CHD with right-to-left or admixture shunting (Table 2). Severe cyanosis in the first week of life is usually associated with transposition of the great arteries, hypoplastic right heart syndrome with pulmonary atresia, or TAPVR with obstruction. In the first few weeks of life, less severe cyanosis is more likely associated with TOF, truncus arteriosus, or TAPVR without obstruction.

Radiographic manifestations of CHD with CHF include cardiomegaly, diffuse haziness of vascular struc-

Table 2 ■ ETIOLOGIES OF CYANOTIC CONGENITAL HEART DISEASE, BY PATIENT AGE

0–7 Days—Severe Cyanosis
Transposition of the great arteries
Hypoplastic right heart syndrome
Hypoplastic left heart syndrome
Ebstein's anomaly and tricuspid insufficiency
Tricuspid atresia
Total anomalous pulmonary venous return with obstruction

1–4 Weeks
Tetralogy of Fallot—most common
Truncus arteriosus
Total anomalous pulmonary venous return without obstruction
Left-to-right shunts (large) with congestive heart failure (usually subclinical cyanosis)

1 Month and Older
Pulmonary hypertension with reversing shunt
Pulmonary arteriovenous malformations

tures, hyperinflation, thymic atrophy, and interstitial and minor pleural fluid (Fig. 1).

DEVELOPMENT AND GROWTH

An in-depth discussion of the development and embryology of the heart is beyond the scope of this text. Those interested in a more complete discussion are referred to Clark's paper on cardiac embryology.

The heart tube develops in the primitive embryo from fusion of a pair of vessels arising from the mesoderm that covers the ventral aspect of the foregut. Rapid growth of this tube leads to a marked ventral flexure, proceeding to a series of dilatations. The most cephalic of these, the bulbus cordis and the ventricle, lie on the ventrocephalic side of this redundant loop; the more dorsocaudal dilatation is the developing atrium. These dilatations are connected by a constricted portion to become the atrioventricular canal. The truncus arteriosus arises from the cephalic end of the bulbus cordis, while the systemic venous drainage of the embryo empties into the dorsal portion of the atrium. In the fourth embryonic week, the bulboventricular loop twists sharply to the right; the bulbus cordis now joins the ventricle at a right angle before passing up on the ventral aspect of the heart.

Before this common tubular heart can become a four-chambered structure, septation must occur at the atrial and ventricular level. Two primary septa form to develop the interatrial septum. The first, or septum primum, develops as a fold from the dorsocephalic wall of the primitive atrium and grows ventrocaudad toward a septum originating from the atrioventricular canal. The initial passage between these two developing septa will form the foramen primum of the interatrial septum. During the sixth week of embryonic life, the cephalic portion of the septum primum divides to form the ostium secundum. A second septum (septum secundum) appears in the sixth embryonic week as a fold from the ventrocephalic wall of the atrium and grows dorso-cephalad to overlap the ostium secundum and eventually form the foramen ovale. Failure of this septum to form properly produces the ostium secundum ASD. The common ventricle is divided into left and right ventricles by a crescentic ridge that appears near the apex of the common ventricle, with ridges extending on the dorsal and ventral aspect to the atrioventricular cushion. The atrioventricular cushion similarly has developed in the fifth week of intrauterine life from two cushions that have appeared and begun to grow from the dorsal and ventral aspects of the atrioventricular constriction. The fusions of these atrioventricular septa give rise to the primitive tricuspid and mitral valves. Defects in the normal growth pattern of the dorsal and ventral atrial ventricular canal septa lead to the variety of atrioventricular canal defects noted clinically. Eventual closure of the common ventricle results from the fusion of the right and left ridges of the apical ridge; this continued growth proceeds into the cavity of the bulbus cordis, dividing it into an infundibular portion and the aortic vestibule. Simultaneous with the development of the interventricular septum occurs a torsion of the bulbus cordis and ventricles. Final fusion of the interventricular septum occurs as an extension of tissue arising from the inferior atrioventricular cushion and forms the fibrous or membranous portions of the interventricular septum.

In addition to the division of the ventricular chambers, two other developing ridges continue the division of the bulbus cordis into the aortic vestibule and infundibulum. During the fifth week of embryonic life, the outlines of the pulmonary and aortic valve become evident at the apex of the infundibulum and aortic vestibule, respectively. By the eighth week, the pulmonary and aortic valves have fairly well-demarcated cusps and leaflets. Developmental failures in these areas result in the various forms of valvular and subvalvular aortic and pulmonary stenosis. Anomalous development in the bulboventricular area with abnormal torsion causes the various forms of transposition. The final stages in cardiac development are the division of the truncus arteriosus into the ascending aorta and pulmonary

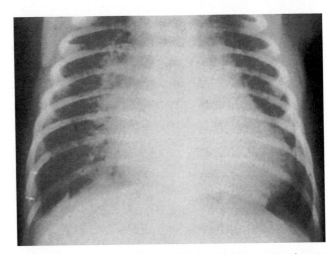

FIGURE 1. Congestive heart failure at 10 days, secondary to coarctation. Pulmonary venous congestion with interstitial fluid lines in the costophrenic angle and minor pleural fluid can be seen. Note cardiomegaly and hyperinflation.

arteries, along with the development of aortic arches, which are discussed with the various anomalies of these arches in Section V, Part III, page 1338. Separation of the truncus arteriosus into the ascending aorta and pulmonary artery results from an outgrowth of mesenchymous tissue from both sides of the truncus toward the bulbus cordis. This division takes a spiral course so that the final aortic–pulmonary septum represents a relative spiral with the base of the pulmonary artery originating to the left of the aortic root. Failure in the spiral development of this truncus arteriosus septum leads to various forms of truncus arteriosus, aortic–pulmonary windows, and transposition of the great arteries.

The mean weight of the heart in a full-term newborn is approximately 17 g, with a disproportionate prominence of the right ventricle. During the first month of life there is a 25% increase in cardiac weight, primarily as a result of an increase in left ventricular mass. Subsequently, the rate of growth is less than that of the body as a whole and of most other organs. The heart doubles in weight during the first year, and is four times its birth weight after 5 years.

Acknowledgements. The authors gratefully acknowledge the dedicated work of the Primary Children's Medical Center Medical Imaging staff and our clinical colleagues, without whose help Section V would not have been possible. Technical assistance in magnetic resonance imaging and angiography were provided by Laurie Coburn, Mickey Falkner, Nancy Broadbent, Paul Jellinich, Daren Andrews, Tina Young, Torey Jackson, and Chris Garrett. Processing and conversion of digital images for illustrations were done by Darin Day and Kristin Bernhisel-Osborn. Outstanding secretarial support for this section was provided by Valorie Kemp and Susan Rohan.

SUGGESTED READINGS

Development and Growth

Clark EB: Cardiac embryology: its relevance to congenital heart disease. Am J Dis Child 1986;140:41

Clark EB: Growth, morphogenesis, and function: the dynamics of cardiac development. *In* Moller JH, Neal WA (eds): Fetal, Neonatal, and Infant Cardiac Disease. Norwalk, CT, Appleton-Lange, 1990: 3–24

Dawes GS: Fetal and Neonatal Physiology. St Louis, Mosby–Year Book, 1968

Driscoll DJ: Left-to-right shunt lesions. Pediatr Clin North Am 1999;46:355

Du ZD, Roguin N, Barak M, et al: High prevalence of muscular septal defect in preterm neonates. Am J Cardiol 1996;78:1183

Duckworth JWA: Embryology of congenital heart disease. *In* Keth JD, Rowe RD, Vlad P (eds): Heart Disease in Infancy and Childhood. New York, Macmillan, 1978:129–152

Ferencz C, Boughman JA, Neill CA, et al: Congenital cardiovascular malformations: questions on inheritance. J Am Coll Cardiol 1989; 14:755

Ferencz C, Rubin JD, Loffredo CA, Magee C (eds): Perspectives in Pediatric Cardiology, vol 4. Epidemiology of Congenital Heart Disease: The Baltimore-Washington Infant Study, 1981–1989. Mount Kisco, NY, Futura, 1993

Gillum RF: Epidemiology of congenital heart disease in the United States. Am Heart J 1994;127:919

Grech V: Epidemiology and diagnosis of ventricular septal defect in Malta. Cardiol Young 1998;8:329

Krovetz LJ: Spontaneous closure of ventricular septal defect. Am J Cardiol 1998;81:100

Moore KL: The Developing Human. Philadelphia, WB Saunders, 1974

Olshan AF, Schnitzer PG, Baird PA: Paternal age and the risk of congenital heart defects. Teratology 1994;50:84

Patten BN: Human Embryology, 3rd ed. New York, Blakiston, 1968

Perry LW, Neill CA, Ferencz D, et al: Infants with congenital heart disease: the cases. *In* Ferencz C, Rubin JD, Loffred CA, Magee C (eds): Perspectives in Pediatric Cardiology, vol 4. Epidemiology of Congenital Heart Disease: The Baltimore-Washington Infant Study, 1981–1989. Mount Kisco, NY, Futura, 1993:33–62

Schunkert H, Brockel U, Kromer EP, et al: A large pedigree with valvuloseptal defects. Am J Cardiol 1997;80:968

Chapter 2

CARDIAC EVALUATION

RICHARD B. JAFFE, VIRGIL R. CONDON, BARBARA S. REID, LUCIANA T. PAGOTTO, and VICTORIA E. JUDD

ROUTINE CHEST RADIOGRAPHY

Although chest radiography remains routine in the initial and follow-up evaluation of infants and children with cardiovascular disease, its importance has decreased with the increased use and sophistication of echocardiography. Posteroanterior (PA) or anteroposterior (AP) and lateral chest radiographs are often the initial imaging modality for suspected cardiac disease. Critical attention to good inspiration, motion, exposure factors, and position and rotation are mandatory. Oblique views and barium swallow have little place in the evaluation of the cardiac patient except for anomalies of the aortic arch and pulmonary arteries. Chest fluoroscopy is useful for the evaluation of cardiac calcifications and prosthetic valve motion but has only limited usefulness and is not indicated in the neonate and infant.

Radiographic manifestations of congestive heart failure (CHF) and congenital heart disease (CHD) vary considerably, particularly in the neonate, and recognition is often complicated by pulmonary disease, atelectasis, and increased pulmonary blood flow. Cardiomegaly is usually present, although the configuration of the heart is frequently nonspecific. In rare situations (e.g., obstructed total anomalous pulmonary venous return), the heart size may be normal or even small. In the neonate, plain films usually show loss of sharp definition of the bronchovascular structures (see Fig. 1). Rarely is there evidence of interstitial or interlobular fluid or significant pleural effusion unless severe pulmonary venous obstruction is present, as in obstructed total anomalous pulmonary venous return. The thymus is usually atrophic, and exaggerated inspiratory effort (air hunger) produces flattening of the diaphragm. In the older child, findings may be similar to those in the adult, with pulmonary vascular redistribution into the upper lungs, interstitial septal (Kerley B) lines, fluid retention, and pleural effusion.

The differential diagnosis of the patient with CHD and CHF from an infant or child with pneumonia, cardiomyopathy, or other diffuse pulmonary process may be very difficult. Group B streptococcal sepsis in the neonate may be particularly confusing, with most of the clinical and radiographic findings quite similar. Differentiation will necessitate the use of other diagnostic methods, including blood culture (and other laboratory tests) and echocardiography. Another primary differential consideration is transient tachypnea of the newborn, in which interstitial fluid, minor pleural fluid, and mild

cardiomegaly may also present a very similar radiographic pattern. In the older infant, diffuse interstitial pulmonary disease, as frequently seen with viral infection, may produce some radiographic findings similar to CHF, including poor definition of vascular markings, hyperinflation, and thymic atrophy. Heart size and shape, however, remain normal, and Kerley's B lines or pleural effusion is rarely seen. It must be recognized that pulmonary disease frequently is present in patients with left-to-right shunts, especially those with Down syndrome.

PULMONARY VASCULATURE

Evaluating the pulmonary vasculature is the most important and difficult step in the systematic review of the chest radiograph in CHD. Difficulty is caused, in part, by the factors noted previously—overexposed, underexposed, or expiratory films—all of which may produce faulty interpretation.

Pulmonary flow may appear normal in the presence of clinical heart disease (Table 1). It should be emphasized that pulmonary flow in the presence of CHD is an age-related factor. The normally elevated pulmonary vascular resistance in the neonate may prevent the diagnosis of increased flow even in the presence of a typical left-to-right anatomic shunt lesion. It is also difficult to differentiate pulmonary arteries from veins in the neonate and young infant, whereas they become more discrete in the older child and the adult. The pulmonary vessels should be evaluated both centrally

Table 1 ■ CONGENITAL HEART DISEASE RELATED TO PULMONARY BLOOD FLOW AND CYANOSIS

CYANOSIS	INCREASED FLOW	NORMAL FLOW	DECREASED FLOW
Acyanotic	Ventricular septal defect (VSD)	Pulmonary stenosis	Cerebral arteriovenous malformation (occasionally)
	Patent ductus arteriosus	Aortic stenosis	
	Atrial septal defect (ASD)	Coarctation (interrupted aortic arch)	
	Secundum	Levotransposition of the great arteries without associated defects	
	Primum	Ebstein anomaly (without large ASD)	
	Atrioventricular canal	Neonatal high pulmonary resistance with left-to-right shunt lesions	
	Partial anomalous pulmonary venous return		
	Levotransposition of the great arteries with VSD		
Cyanotic	Admixture lesions	Pulmonary arteriovenous malformation	Severe pulmonary stenosis with VSD, tetralogy of Fallot
	Transposition of the great arteries, with or without a single ventricle	Neonatal high pulmonary resistance with admixture shunt lesions	ASD or patent foramen ovale
	Double-outlet right ventricle		Pulmonary atresia
	Truncus arteriosus		With VSD (pseudotruncus)
	Total anomalous pulmonary venous return		Without VSD (hypoplastic right heart syndrome)
	Tricuspid atresia with transposition of the great arteries		Tricuspid atresia with small VSD/pulmonary atresia
			Transposition of the great arteries with pulmonary stenosis or pulmonary atresia
			Common ventricle or double-outlet right ventricle with pulmonary stenosis
			Right-to-left atrial shunt, Ebstein's anomaly, congenital tricuspid insufficiency

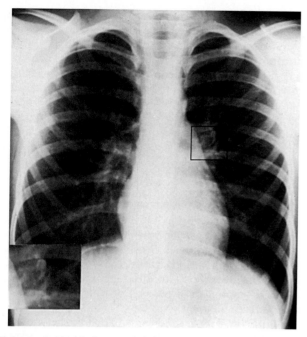

FIGURE 1. Ventricular septal defect with left-to-right shunt. Mild enlargement of the central pulmonary arteries demonstrates reversed pulmonary artery–bronchus size relationship *(box)*.

and peripherally. Centrally, the right pulmonary artery should be compared with the size of the trachea in the PA (AP) projection and normally should be of approximately equal size. In the lateral view, the left pulmonary artery should be compared with the trachea and they should be of similar size. In the end-on projection, the peripheral pulmonary vessels should be related to an accompanying bronchus (Fig. 1). The transverse diameter of the vessels should not exceed the internal diameter of the bronchus in a patient with normal pulmonary flow. An increase in vessel size indicates a left-to-right or admixture shunt (volume overload), although occasionally the vessel appears enlarged sec-

ondary to pulmonary venous hypertension and failure (pressure overload). Increased pulmonary flow with enlarged pulmonary vessels is rarely seen with lesions where the ratio of pulmonary to systemic flow is less than 2:1. In patients with a left-to-right shunt, the main pulmonary artery is characteristically enlarged. A large central pulmonary artery is common in all children, particularly in teenage females. Therefore, the size of the main pulmonary artery is probably of less diagnostic value than the size of the right and left segment or peripheral pulmonary vessels. It is important to learn to evaluate the hilar vasculature on a lateral chest film, especially in the neonate. Recognizing increased flow may be difficult on the AP film because of the overlying thymus or a large cardiac silhouette (Fig. 2).

Decreased, like increased, pulmonary vascularity is difficult to recognize with a small right-to-left shunt. In lesions with major right-to-left shunting, there is a decrease in size of the central pulmonary arteries in relation to the trachea and, in general, a decrease in the prominence of the hilar vessels on both the frontal (Fig. 3) and the lateral views. The peripheral lung appears unusually clear and hyperlucent, and one is rarely able to evaluate an end-on artery with accompanying bronchus. The diaphragm is frequently depressed as a secondary manifestation of hypoxemia. In severe disease, or in older patients with right-to-left shunting, increased bronchial artery flow may appear as a disorganized vascular pattern.

Asymmetry in pulmonary vascularity may relate to unilateral peripheral pulmonary stenosis, pulmonary aplasia-hypoplasia, surgically created systemic–pulmonary shunts, patent ductus inserting peripherally into the left or occasionally right pulmonary artery, and directional flow created by anatomic relationships of the right ventricular outflow tract, as in tetralogy of Fallot and transposition of the great vessels.

CHD is frequently complicated by the presence of CHF or pulmonary disease and may obscure the shunt vascularity until failure has been treated and the vessels

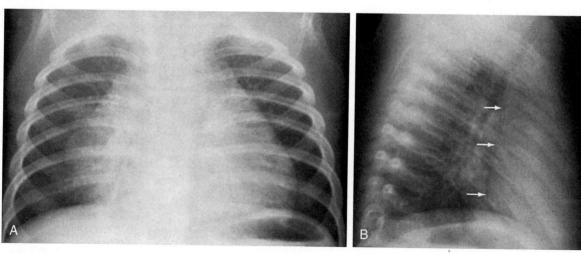

FIGURE 2. Normal thymus: frontal **(A)** and lateral **(B)** chest films demonstrate a large cardiomediastinal silhouette caused predominantly by the large thymus, which obliterates the cardiac silhouette in the frontal view and fills in the anterior mediastinal space *(arrows* in **B)** in the lateral projection. The posterior cardiac contour is not enlarged.

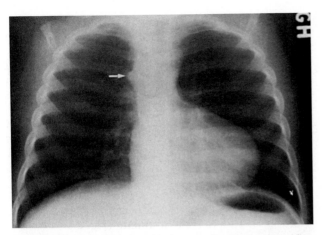

FIGURE 3. Tetralogy of Fallot with decreased pulmonary blood flow. Central pulmonary arteries are small, and the peripheral lungs are hyperlucent; the diaphragm is depressed and the thymus atrophic, which is consistent with hypoxia. The right aortic arch pushes the trachea to the left and displaces the azygos vein lateral to the aortic arch *(arrow)*.

become more discrete. Similarly, the pulmonary flow pattern may be obscured in the premature infant with respiratory distress syndrome.

CARDIOMEDIASTINAL SILHOUETTE

Evaluation of the cardiomediastinal silhouette in the infant is difficult for a variety of reasons. A large normal thymus is frequently present (see Fig. 2). Its size is exaggerated on the supine AP projection and on a less-than-optimal inspiratory film. It is usually possible to distinguish the thymus by its slightly different and more radiolucent density. The caudal margin can usually be identified as a minor indentation where it blends with the cardiac silhouette. The lateral film is also of considerable value in the differentiation of the thymus from an enlarged heart. The thymus may totally obscure the retrosternal space, and yet the posterior cardiac silhouette will be normal. Left ventricular–inferior vena caval relationships and left main stem bronchial–cardiac relations will remain normal. Failure to visualize a normal thymic silhouette in children with CHD may indicate significant stress related to CHF or hypoxemia, or both and right-to-left shunts. Absence of the thymus is also a sign in a number of syndromes (e.g., DiGeorge syndrome).

Cardiac position, of course, should be critically evaluated; a major increase in CHD is frequent in patients having dextrocardia with situs solitus or levocardia with situs inversus (see Section V, Part IV, Chapter 1, page 1360). Mesocardia is a common finding that may or may not be related to CHD. Evaluation of systemic venous return from both the inferior and superior vena cava is helpful in diagnosing congenital heart problems (asplenia, polysplenia).

The size of the heart varies considerably with the age of the patient. In the neonate, a cardiac silhouette greater than 57% of the thoracic diameter on an AP 40-inch supine film with good inspiration indicates cardiomegaly and, therefore, heart disease. The cardiothoracic ratio gradually decreases during the first year of life and after the second year should not exceed 50% in an upright 6-foot PA or AP chest film. A film obtained during good inspiration is vital when the cardiothoracic ratio is used as an index. The evaluation of specific heart chambers is particularly difficult in the infant, whereas prominence of any portion of the cardiac silhouette in the older child has the same implication for cardiac enlargement that one expects in the adult.

Although the shape or silhouette of the heart is frequently nonspecific, certain classic configurations may well be indicative of a specific lesion. Classically, the coeur en sabot or boot-shaped heart is typical of tetralogy of Fallot (see Fig. 3). The configuration results from the underlying pathologic condition, with the transversely oriented heart related to the right heart enlargement, and the concavity in the upper left heart border secondary to the small pulmonary artery resulting from the right-to-left shunt. In supracardiac total anomalous pulmonary venous return, the typical "snowman" configuration (see Section V, Part II, Chapter 3, Fig. 12, page 1313) is due to a large left vertical vein and a dilated right superior vena cava. This radiographic appearance is seen rarely today as a result of early operative intervention. A prominent convex left upper heart border may be a fairly good indicator of levotransposition of the great arteries (see Section V, Part II, Chapter 3, Fig. 9, page 1310) or a juxtaposed atrial appendage (see Section V, Part II, Chapter 4, Fig. 7, page 1329), as frequently seen with tricuspid atresia and transposition. The egg-shaped or egg-on-side configuration, while certainly nonspecific, is suggestive of transposition of the great arteries (Fig. 4) and is occasionally seen with truncus arteriosus. The triangular

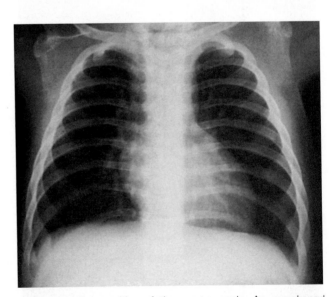

FIGURE 4. Transposition of the great vessels. An egg-shaped cardiac silhouette secondary to transposition of the great vessels can be seen. The main pulmonary artery is inconspicuous because its medial position produces a narrow base for the heart. Thymic atrophy and hyperinflation secondary to hypoxia are evident. Pulmonary flow is only mildly increased in this patient without a ventricular septal defect.

cardiac silhouette, indicative of a prominent right ventricle and right atrium with a small superior vena cava, may be quite suggestive of an ostium secundum atrial septal defect (ASD). Poststenotic dilatation of the ascending aorta is characteristic of valvular aortic stenosis (AS) (Fig. 5). The configuration seen in scimitar syndrome, showing the typical changes related to partial anomalous pulmonary venous return to the inferior vena cava (with associated pulmonary hypoplasia), is another classic cardiopulmonary silhouette (Fig. 6).

It is particularly important to define the position of the aortic arch in vascular rings and congenital cardiac lesions associated with a right aortic arch (Table 2). In the infant, the aortic arch location can usually be determined by evaluating minor deviation of the trachea at the level of the aortic arch. An overpenetrated or filtered chest film may be necessary to see the trachea optimally (Fig. 7). With these techniques, it can usually be identified adequately down to the level of the carina. Although the trachea often deviates considerably in the extrathoracic segment, the deviation in the intrathoracic segment is almost always to the side opposite that of the aortic arch. If there is no tracheal deviation in the presence of CHD, interruption of the aortic arch is an important consideration. The presence of a right-sided aortic arch is suggestive of tetralogy of Fallot (30%), truncus arteriosus (25%), tricuspid atresia, (20%), ventricular septal defect (VSD) (5%), and transposition of the great vessels with pulmonary stenosis. The visualization of a right aortic arch in the absence of intrinsic CHD usually indicates some form of double aortic arch or arch anomaly.

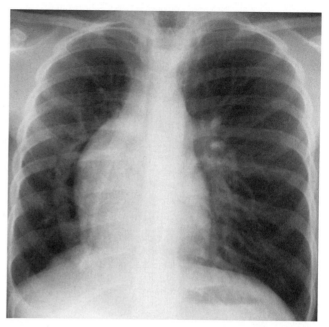

FIGURE 6. Scimitar syndrome. Frontal radiograph in a 12½–year-old child demonstrates hypoplasia of the right lung and pulmonary artery. Dextroposition of the heart is present with increased pulmonary blood flow to the left lung. Partial anomalous pulmonary venous return from the right lung to the inferior vena cava is seen adjacent to the right heart margin.

The configuration of the aorta also merits special attention in relation to coarctation of the aorta. The figure three sign is usually evident on plain films, showing an indentation resulting from the coarctation and the dilated poststenotic segment of the aorta immediately below it (Fig. 8A). The proximal segment may or may not appear dilated, depending on whether it represents an isolated discrete coarctation or is associated with a hypoplastic aortic isthmus. The converse manifestation can be seen on an esophagogram, where an E sign (reversed three sign) can be observed, with the lower portion of the E secondary to the dilatation of the poststenotic segment of the aorta (Fig. 8B). The proximal ascending aorta also should be closely examined. It has more significance in children than in adults because minor dilatation may be highly suggestive of valvular AS with poststenotic dilatation, aortic insufficiency, or systemic hypertension (see Fig. 5).

The main pulmonary artery likewise plays an important role in the cardiac silhouette and may be highly indicative of CHD (Tables 3 and 4). A large pulmonary artery secondary to poststenotic dilatation is the classic

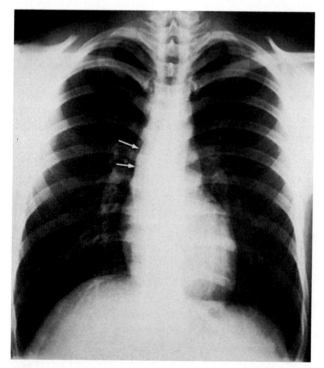

FIGURE 5. Valvular aortic stenosis. Poststenotic dilatation of the ascending aorta (arrows) secondary to valvular aortic stenosis (AS). Dilatation of the aorta produces a slight prominence of the aortic arch, but not the more striking enlargement seen in patients with combined AS and aortic insufficiency.

Table 2 ■ CONGENITAL LESIONS ASSOCIATED WITH A RIGHT AORTIC ARCH
Tetralogy of Fallot
Tricuspid atresia
Truncus arteriosus
Dextrotransposition of great arteries with pulmonary stenosis
Ventricular septal defect
Aortic arch anomalies

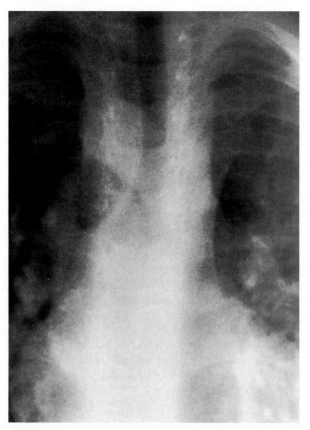

FIGURE 7. High-kilovoltage peak and added-filtration film of the mediastinal area. Note the deviation of the trachea to the left with a right aortic arch traversing behind the trachea and esophagus in a patient with a circumflex aortic arch (right ascending aorta with posterior left descending aorta).

Table 3 ■ CONGENITAL LESIONS ASSOCIATED WITH A PROMINENT MAIN PULMONARY ARTERY
Valvular pulmonary stenosis
Left-to-right shunts
Truncus arteriosus—type I
Total anomalous pulmonary venous return

Table 4 ■ CONGENITAL LESIONS ASSOCIATED WITH A CONCAVE (SMALL) MAIN PULMONARY ARTERY
Tetralogy of Fallot
Pulmonary atresia
Tricuspid atresia with pulmonary stenosis
Pulmonary artery malpositions (i.e., transposition)

finding of pulmonary valvular stenosis (PVS) (Fig. 9); the dilatation usually extends into the left pulmonary artery, as seen on the lateral chest radiograph. With tetralogy of Fallot and corrected transposition of the great arteries, the main pulmonary artery is inconspicuous but directional flow may enlarge the right pulmonary artery. The pulmonary artery is enlarged in all significant left-to-right shunts, as well as in admixture shunts (e.g., truncus arteriosus type I and double-outlet right ventricle) (see Table 3). Massive enlargement of the main or left and right pulmonary arteries is also present with congenital absence of the pulmonary valve, a variant of tetralogy of Fallot (Fig. 10). Idiopathic dilatation may be a normal variant, particularly in the teenage female. A concave left upper heart border may

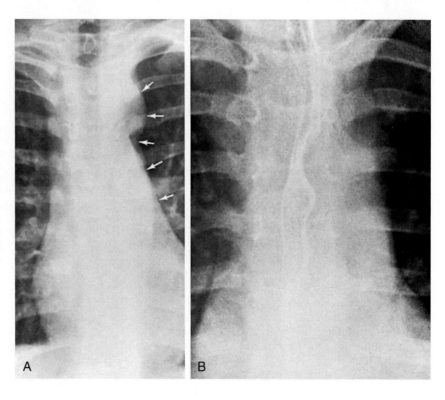

FIGURE 8. Coarctation of the aorta. **A,** A figure three sign indicates coarctation between the large proximal segment of the aorta and/or a prominent left subclavian artery above the narrowing and the poststenotic dilatation of the descending aorta below it *(arrows).* **B,** Barium esophagogram demonstrates the reversed three sign (E sign) impression on the barium-filled esophagus adjacent to the coarcted aorta that is produced by the medial aspect of the same structures described in **A.**

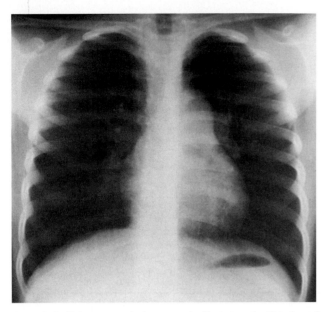

FIGURE 9. Pulmonary valvular stenosis. Poststenotic dilatation of the main and left pulmonary artery, normal pulmonary flow, and a prominent, slightly elevated apex secondary to right ventricular hypertrophy can be seen.

indicate a hypoplastic pulmonary artery, as in all patients with right-to-left shunts, or a malposition of the pulmonary artery in admixture lesions, as in transposition and truncus type II or III (see Table 4).

SKELETAL MANIFESTATIONS OF CONGENITAL HEART DISEASE

Other changes on chest radiographs that may indicate CHD include the following:

1. Eleven pairs of ribs, frequently seen in Down syndrome.
2. Variations in sternal ossification centers.
3. Metaphyseal osseous irregularities related to rubella.
4. Pectus carinatum, particularly common in Marfan syndrome.
5. Rib notching. Rib notching is evaluated best in the posterolateral inferior margin of the ribs. The posteromedial rib has a very thin cortical surface with undulation, and rib notching is difficult to differentiate from the normal subcostal groove. In children and adolescents, rib notching is often well defined (Fig. 11), but in young children it may be manifested only as cortical sclerosis. Rib notching typically involves the third through ninth ribs, and may be unilateral, right- or left-sided, or bilateral (Table 5). Rib notching is only present when there is antegrade flow in the subclavian and internal mammary artery.
6. Thin ribs, particularly in trisomies 13, 18, and 21.
7. Shoulder or arm anomalies in Holt-Oram syndrome.

Spine abnormalities may be seen in tetralogy of Fallot, truncus arteriosus, VATER syndrome (*v*ertebral defects, imperforate *a*nus, *t*racheo*e*sophageal fistula, *r*adial and *r*enal dysplasia) and storage diseases; with straight back syndrome, in which a functional venous hum or murmur of mitral prolapse may be present; and with increased vertebral body height (Marfan syndrome and homocystinuria).

ANGIOCARDIOGRAPHY

Although the noninvasive evaluation of the heart with echocardiography, cine–computed tomography (cine-CT) and magnetic resonance imaging (MRI) defines the cardiac anatomy in many cases, cardiac catherization and angiocardiography are usually necessary at some point in the evaluation of most patients. Catheterization is important in (1) determining shunts, (2) evaluating gradients, (3) measuring systemic and pulmonary artery flow, (4) evaluating cardiac output, and (5) determining pulmonary vascular resistance. Angiocardiography still provides optimal anatomic detail and is particularly important prior to attempted surgical correction of CHD, although, with improved noninvasive techniques, some simpler lesions such as ostium secundum ASD, membranous VSD, coarctations, and patent ductus arteriosus (PDA) often proceed to surgery without angiocardiography and cardiac catheterization. Biplane image-intensified fluoroscopy and biplane angiocardiography are essential if cardiac catheterization is performed. Biplane videotape or direct digital recording is mandatory for immediate review of injections in order

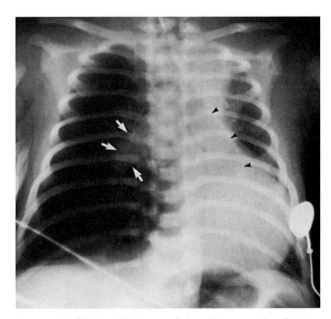

FIGURE 10. Congenital absence of the pulmonary valve. Aneurysmal dilatation of the right main pulmonary artery *(arrows)* secondary to congenital absence of the pulmonary valve (tetralogy of Fallot variant). Air trapping the right lung is caused by compression of the right main stem bronchus by the pulmonary artery and herniation of the lung across the mediastinum to the left *(arrowheads)*.

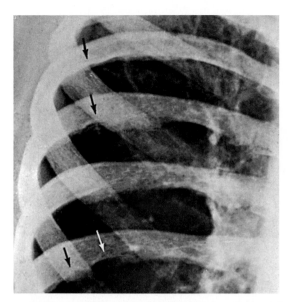

FIGURE 11. Coarctation of the aorta. Notching on the inferior aspects of the posterolateral ribs is related to collateral flow through intercostal arteries secondary to coarctation of the aorta *(arrows).* Note the characteristic, somewhat sclerotic margin, which differentiates this lesion from the normal subcostal groove.

to evaluate which further studies may be necessary. Digital angiography or cineangiography at 30 to 60 frames per second optimally visualizes shunt lesions, while obstructive malformations and chamber and great vessel relationships may be better visualized with filming at 15 to 30 frames per second. Angiocardiography is performed in differing projections, including

1. AP and lateral projections in critically ill infants assisted by respirators
2. Long-axis (Fig. 12A) or four-chambered (Fig. 12B)

Table 5 ■ CAUSES OF RIB NOTCHING

Bilateral
Coarctation
Aortic arch interruption, type A*
Neurogenic tumors†
Intercostal collateral flow to the lungs with chronic pulmonary oligemia†
Superior vena cava obstruction†

Right-sided
Right Blalock-Taussig anastomosis
Coarctation with stenotic left subclavian artery
Aortic arch interruption, types B, C*
Right thoracotomy
Vascular malformations

Left-sided
Left Blalock-Taussig anastomosis
Coarctation with aberrant right subclavian artery
Aortic arch interruption, type A with aberrant right subclavian artery*
Left thoracotomy
Vascular malformations

---

*See Section V, Part II, Chapter 2, page 1284.
†May also be unilateral.

---

projections for septal anatomy and great vessel relations
3. A 45-degree "sitting-up" AP (Fig. 13) or a steep left anterior oblique (LAO) projection with maximum cranial–caudal angulation and lateral projections for pulmonary valve, pulmonary artery, and right ventricular outflow tract disorders

Most venous cardiac catheterizations are performed from the percutaneous femoral approach utilizing a Berman-type, double-lumen balloon catheter. When the atrial septum is intact or when other indications warrant left heart evaluation, percutaneous retrograde arterial catheterization with a thin-walled pigtail catheter is usually performed. In infants, low-osmolar or nonionic contrast is usually used in a dose of 1 to 2 ml/kg injected in less than 1 second per injection, with a total volume ideally limited to 5 ml/kg. The use of low-osmolar or nonionic contrast may permit the use of larger volumes up to 6 or 7 ml/kg. If digital angiography is utilized, concentrations of contrast may be decreased to 180 to 240 mg/ml. In patients with small cardiac chambers or obstructive lesions, a dose of 1 ml/kg per injection is usually sufficient. Mortality related to heart catheterization and angiocardiography is low (less than 1%) and usually relates to cardiac perforations, severe arrhythmia, and contrast reaction. Morbidity relates to hypertonic solutions and electrolyte imbalance, renal or hepatic damage, and direct myocardial injury.

ECHOCARDIOGRAPHY

The development of real-time (two-dimensional) and Doppler echocardiography probably represents the most important advance in the noninvasive evaluation of CHD over the past two decades. Ultan et al. first described the use of echocardiography in CHD, and Meyer and Kaplan pointed out the specificity of echocardiographic findings in certain conditions (e.g., hypoplastic left heart syndrome), making a definitive diagnosis possible without further invasive procedures, except in unusual clinical situations. Specific diagnostic criteria for various CHDs have subsequently been developed with real-time echocardiography. The utilization of Doppler, and more recently two-dimensional Doppler color-flow mapping, allows the examiner to obtain both anatomic and physiologic information in real time.

TECHNICAL FACTORS

Echocardiography is performed with a pulsed ultrasound beam of less than 1-μsec duration repeated 2000 to 3000 times per second; the intervals between pulsations are used for recording the returning echo. At present, no significant reproducible harmful effects have been demonstrated with the energies and frequencies used. With the development of two-dimensional equipment utilizing either sector scanners, linear phased-array scan, or multicrystal rays, a much more

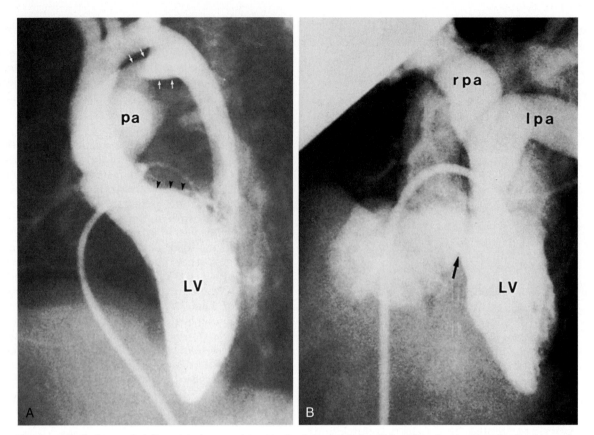

FIGURE 12. A, Long-axis left ventriculogram elongates the left ventricular *(LV)* outflow tract and optimally shows the interventricular septum as well as the subaortic and aortic areas. The left atrium projects well posterior to the outflow tract, and the mitral–aortic relationship is easily identified *(arrowheads)*. pa = pulmonary artery. Patent ductus arteriosus with a moderate left-to-right shunt *(arrows)*. **B,** Four-chamber left ventriculogram in a patient with transposition and a ventricular septal defect *(arrow)* identifies the left ventricular *(LV)* pulmonary artery relationship and ideally shows the right and left pulmonary arteries *(rpa, lpa)*.

vivid, dynamic image of intracardiac anatomy can be obtained. The two-dimensional study is commonly recorded on videotape for delayed slow-motion, or stop-action evaluation. Relations of the great vessels to cardiac chambers, as well as to the intracardiac anatomy, are easily recorded.

Currently, a combined M-mode, real-time, Doppler and color Doppler examination is performed in nearly all patients with serious CHD. In real-time echocardiography, a more complex series of maneuvers is carried out with the transducer. Initially, the heart is evaluated in a long-axis view, with the transducer scan oriented from the right shoulder toward the left hip to the left of the sternum (Fig. 14). Clockwise or counterclockwise rotations identify the tricuspid valve, aorta, and pulmonary valve. Utilizing a transverse position of the transducer, and sweeping from the apex of the heart cephalad through the level of the mitral valve into the root of the great vessels, gives a short-axis view of the heart. The great vessels can also be evaluated in this position, with both the aortic and pulmonary valve identifiable. The transducer is then placed at the apex of the heart, with the central beam parallel to the plane of the ventricular and atrial septa, producing a four-chamber configuration that shows both atrioventricular valves as well as the cardiac chambers. Next, a subxiphoid projection pro-

duces a modified four-chamber configuration demonstrating the interventricular and intra-atrial septa and, with angulation, the aortic and pulmonary root and left and right ventricular outflow tracts (Fig. 15). Pulmonary venous return is also best seen in this projection, while systemic venous return can be seen in a modified long-axis view. Finally, the aortic arch is evaluated from the suprasternal notch, where the origin of the great vessels can be seen, along with the aortic isthmus beyond the level of the left subclavian artery. The aortic arch also may be evaluated from the subxiphoid view, although, in our experience, this has been somewhat more difficult than with the suprasternal notch view.

DOPPLER ECHOCARDIOGRAPHY

According to the Doppler principle, the frequency of a sound wave that is reflected off a moving object will differ with the frequency of the incident wave. Frequency will increase or decrease depending on the object's direction and velocity relative to the incident wave. This change in frequency is called the *Doppler shift.* When an ultrasonic beam is parallel to the expected direction of flow, Doppler shift is proportional to blood

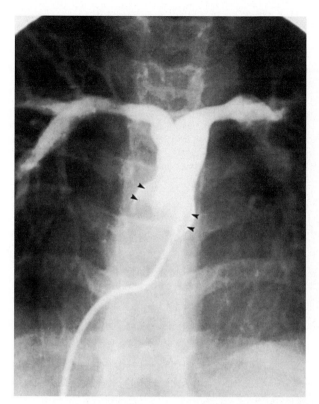

FIGURE 13. Sitting-up anteroposterior (AP) pulmonary arteriogram in a patient with peripheral pulmonary hypoplasia produces a central beam tangential to the pulmonary valve leaflets *(arrowheads)*. The main pulmonary artery is relatively elongated. The right and left pulmonary arteries are easily distinguished, and the left pulmonary artery is not obscured by the main pulmonary artery, as in the conventional AP projection.

flow velocity. This principle is the basis of Doppler echocardiography.

With this technique, a burst of ultrasonic signals is transmitted into the heart at very high frequency. The signals are reflected back by the moving erythrocytes, producing the Doppler shift signals. By convention, flow toward the transducer shifts the velocity upward above the baseline, whereas motion away from the transducer shifts the frequency downward.

Although there are several types of ultrasonic transmission and processing techniques, current Doppler echocardiography utilizes one of three techniques, each with its own advantages and disadvantages. These include pulsed, continuous-wave, and high pulse repetition frequency Doppler.

Pulsed Doppler is similar to M-mode echocardiography, in which a burst of ultrasonic waves is transmitted to the tissues and reflected back to the same transducer. However, unlike M-mode, the pulse repetition frequency is varied, depending on the depth of sampling. The pulse mode system offers a great advantage in that it permits range resolution so that flow can be characterized in any selected location in a given cardiac chamber or great vessel. Utilizing a simultaneous two-dimensional echocardiogram, the examiner can place the sample volume within a chamber or great vessel of interest, and determine its velocity and direction of flow (Fig. 16; see also Section V, Part II, Chapter 1, Fig. 18, page 1271). Its major disadvantage is that there are significant velocity measurement limitations. High velocities, particularly those encountered across stenotic valves, result in an aliasing error, which makes the determination of the true Doppler shift ambiguous.

Continuous-wave Doppler utilizes two crystals, one that continuously sends, and the other that continuously receives ultrasound. Because ultrasound is transmitted continuously, range gating is not possible. The continuous-wave Doppler receives information all along the beam and does not allow determination of the depth at which the frequency shift occurred (range ambiguity). Unlike pulsed mode, there is no limit on the maximum velocity that can be measured by this technique. Therefore, continuous-wave Doppler is excellent for the analysis of high velocities, particularly across stenotic orifices.

High pulse rate frequency Doppler represents an intermediate between continuous-wave and pulsed Doppler that has been developed to allow measurements of higher velocities than is possible for standard

FIGURE 14. Normal two-dimensional long-axis parasternal echocardiogram identifying the left atrium *(LA)*, left ventricle *(LV)*, and ascending aorta *(Ao)* with appropriate valve structures. There is normal continuity of the interventricular septum *(IS)* with the anterior annulus of the aortic valve and the anterior leaflet of the mitral valve *(MV) (arrows)* with the posterior aortic annulus (right papillary muscle *[RPM]*). Anatomic relationships are very similar to the levoangiocardiogram as seen in the long-axis left anterior oblique projection (see Fig. 12A).

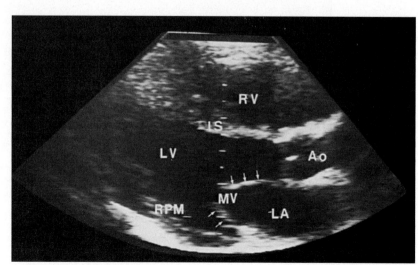

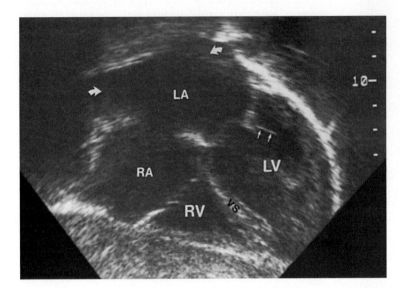

FIGURE 15. Two-dimensional subxiphoid echocardiogram produces a four-chamber cardiac silhouette visualizing both atria *(RA, LA)*, both ventricles *(RV, LV)*, atrioventricular valves, and interventricular *(VS)* and interatrial septa. Minor rotation from this view makes it possible to sweep into the aortic and pulmonary outflow tract and visualize these great vessels. Pulmonary veins enter the left atrium *(curved arrows)* and posterior papillary muscle and chordae and proceed to the mitral valve *(arrows)*. Angiography in the hepatoclavicular (four-chamber) view closely simulates this echocardiographic projection (see Fig. 12*B*).

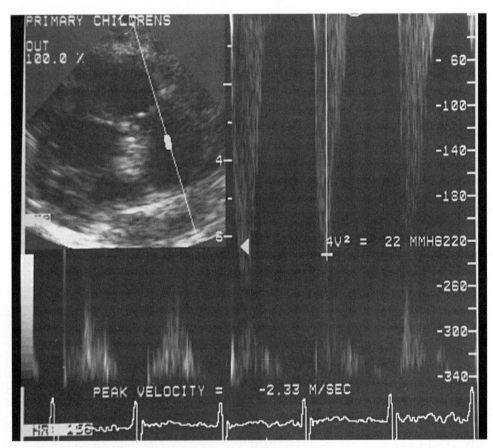

FIGURE 16. Pulmonary valvular stenosis with Doppler estimation of pulmonary valve gradient. In the short-axis projection the Doppler sample is placed in the pulmonary artery in the jet of laminar flow distal to the stenotic pulmonary valve *(upper left corner)*. The recorded peak velocity is 2.33 m/sec. The calculated pulmonary valve gradient utilizing the modified Bernoulli equation $(4V^2)$ is 22 mm Hg.

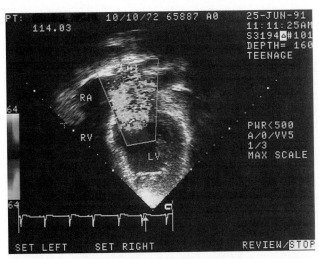

FIGURE 17. Color Doppler documentation of severe rheumatic mitral regurgitation. Utilizing the apical four-chamber projection, the color field is positioned in the region of the mitral valve and left atrium. A systolic image (*arrow* on electrocardiogram) demonstrates severe mitral regurgitation with turbulent flow producing a mosaic pattern throughout the left atrium. In this illustration, the flow toward the transducer is colored red with the highest velocities in yellow; flow away from the transducer is blue with the highest velocities in light blue. Turbulent flow produces a mosaic pattern. *RA* = right atrium; *LA* = left atrium; *RV* = right ventricle; *LV* = left ventricle. *See Color Plate*

pulsed Doppler. Multiple sample volumes can be placed simultaneously at different depths within the heart. Summation of velocities at each sample volume permits measurement of higher velocities than can be measured from a single, more distant sample volume.

In the evaluation of patients with CHD, Doppler echocardiography is most utilized in the recognition of flow disturbances, flow computation, and Doppler measurement of pressure gradients. Doppler echocardiography can distinguish normal or laminar flow from disturbed or turbulent flow. Laminar flow is characterized by a well-defined flow profile, whereas turbulent flow is incoherent, with wide spectral dispersion both positively and negatively. Flow computation is possible by Doppler echocardiography. The average velocity of blood flow multiplied by the area through which the blood passes enables determination of flow volume. Determination of aortic, pulmonary artery, tricuspid valve, and mitral valve flow permits determination of cardiac output, calculation of left-to-right shunts, and determination of regurgitant fractions. The greatest utilization of Doppler echocardiography is in the estimation of pressure gradients across areas of obstruction. The pressure gradient across an obstruction to blood flow can be estimated noninvasively by measuring the maximum velocity (V) beyond the obstruction with Doppler echocardiography, then utilizing the simplified Bernoulli equation (pressure gradient = $4V^2$). The maximal gradient obtained by utilizing the modified Bernoulli equation has an excellent correlation with the maximal instantaneous pressure gradient measured at catheterization. Recall that most catheterization laboratories report a peak-to-peak gradient, whereas Doppler

echocardiography measures instantaneous velocities and instantaneous gradients. Because of the high-velocity flows typically encountered across stenotic valves, continuous-wave Doppler is the optimal method for use in quantitation of valve gradients. With use of Doppler echocardiography, gradients can be estimated across areas of pulmonary obstruction such as PVS, infundibular pulmonic stenosis, and pulmonary artery band (see Fig. 16). The gradient can be estimated across the left ventricular outflow tract, permitting estimation of the severity of subaortic, valvular, or supravalvular AS. The severity of coarctation can be estimated by placing the sample volume distal to the site of coarctation.

The utilization of real-time two-dimensional Doppler color-flow mapping permits the rapid determination of anatomic and physiologic information. The Doppler velocities present within any particular spatial location are determined separately and rapidly by digital electronic processing using an autocollator, which estimates velocities and passes them to a digital scan convertor, where they are read out into a color convertor for display. In several systems, flow toward the transducer has been coded in increasing brightness of red to yellow and flow away from the transducer in increasing brightness of blue. Turbulent, or abnormal, flow with spectral broadening has been shown in green. This method provides excellent spatial orientation of flow. One can rapidly define the location and distribution of the area where normal or abnormal flows occur, such as regurgitant or stenotic jets. One can rapidly localize the maximal velocity area of a jet through stenotic orifices, and can quantitate valvular insufficiency (Figs. 17 through 19) rather than continually sampling with single-pulse Doppler around the cavity receiving the

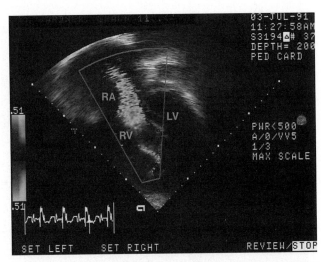

FIGURE 18. Color Doppler documentation of moderate tricuspid regurgitation. In the subcostal four-chamber projection the color field is positioned in the right ventricle and right atrium. A systolic image (*arrow* on electrocardiogram) documents turbulent blood flow through the tricuspid valve, producing a mosaic pattern of blue and yellow in the medial right atrium. In this illustration, flow toward the transducer is in shades of red with the highest velocities in yellow; flow away from the transducer is in shades of blue with the highest velocities in light blue. Turbulent flow produces a mosaic pattern. *RA* = right atrium; *RV* = right ventricle; *LV* = left ventricle. *See Color Plate*

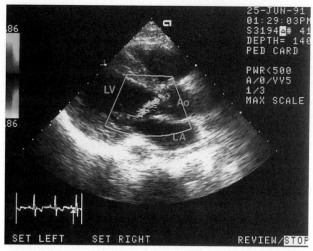

FIGURE 19. Color Doppler documentation of mild aortic regurgitation. In the long-axis projection, the color field is positioned in the region of the aortic valve and left ventricular outflow tract. This diastolic image (*arrow* on electrocardiogram) demonstrates a mosaic pattern of turbulent blood flow through the aortic valve directed against the anterior mitral valve leaflet. In this illustration, flow toward the transducer is in shades of red with the highest velocities in yellow; flow away from the transducer is in shades of blue with the highest velocities in light blue. Turbulent flow produces a mosaic pattern. *LV* = left ventricle; *Ao* = aorta; *LA* = left atrium. *See Color Plate*

regurgitant flow. Recognition of left-to-right shunts, especially ASDs (Fig. 20), membranous (Fig. 21) and muscular VSDs (Fig. 22), and PDA (Fig. 23), is also facilitated.

FETAL ECHOCARDIOGRAPHY

The incidence of congenital heart disease is 0.8% of live births, and may be higher if fetal losses are taken into account. Consequently, early detection of cardiac defects is essential for appropriate prenatal management of the fetus, counseling of the family, and planning of the delivery. Fetal echocardiography is playing an increasing role in the prenatal diagnosis and management of CHD.

Advances in high-resolution ultrasound equipment have made detailed analysis of cardiac anatomy and function possible. As early as 10 to 12 weeks in gestation, small, high-frequency transvaginal probes may be used to image the fetal heart and examine flow across the cardiac valves by Doppler. The transabdominal approach may be used as early as 14 weeks' gestation. However, optimal images are usually obtained after the fetus has reached 18+ weeks' gestation. A variety of risk factors specific to the mother and fetus are known to increase the risk of CHD and warrant a detailed fetal echocardiogram (Table 6).

The four-chamber view of the fetal heart can be obtained in 95% of fetuses between 18 and 40 weeks' gestation. This transverse thoracic view gives important information regarding abdominal situs, cardiac position in the chest, sizes of the cardiac chambers, the atrioventricular connections, and the atrial and ventricular septae (Table 7). The sonographer must first know the fetal position in order to identify the right and left sides of the fetus. Normally, the stomach and aorta lie to the left of the spine and the inferior vena cava lies to the right of the spine. Variations of this anatomy are seen

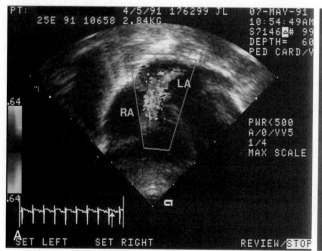
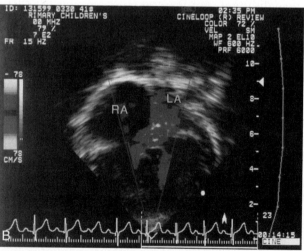

FIGURE 20. A, Color Doppler documentation of ostium secundum atrial septal defect (ASD). In the subcostal four-chamber projection, the color field is positioned in the region of the atrial septum. This image, recorded during ventricular systole (atrial diastole) (*arrow* on electrocardiogram [ECG]), documents a moderate-sized ostium secundum ASD with left-to-right shunt flow. In this illustration, flow toward the transducer is in shades of red with the highest velocities in yellow; flow away from the transducer is in shades of blue with the highest velocities in light blue. Turbulent flow produces a mosaic pattern. *RA* = right atrium; *LA* = left atrium. **B,** Color Doppler documentation of ostium primum ASD. In the apical four-chamber projection, the color field is positioned in the region of the atrial septum. This image, recorded during atrial systole (*arrow* on ECG), documents a moderate-sized ostium primum ASD with left-to-right shunt flow. Early diastolic filling of the right and left ventricles is also noted. The color legend is similar to **A.** *RA* = right atrium; *LA* = left atrium. *See Color Plate*

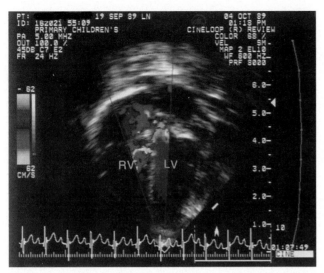

FIGURE 21. Color Doppler documentation of small membranous ventricular septal defect (VSD). In the apical four-chamber projection, the color field is positioned in the region of the membranous and anterior muscular septum. This image at end-ventricular systole (*arrow* in electrocardiogram) demonstrates high-velocity flow through a small membranous VSD into the upper medial right ventricle. In this illustration, flow toward the transducer is in shades of red with highest velocities in yellow; flow away from the transducer is in shades of blue, with the highest velocities in light blue. Turbulent flow produces a mosaic pattern. *RV* = right ventricle; *LV* = left ventricle. (From Jaffe RB: Ventricular septal defect—echocardiography. *In* Elliott LP [ed]: Cardiac Imaging in Infants, Children, and Adults. Philadelphia, JB Lippincott, 1991:575, with permission.) *See Color Plate*

with situs inversus and heterotaxy syndromes. The normal heart occupies 25% to 35% of the thoracic area, and the normal cardiac circumference : thoracic circumference ratio varies between 0.46 and 0.58, increasing with advancing gestational age (Fig. 24). Enlargement of the heart may result from atrioventricular and/or

Table 6 ■ INDICATIONS FOR A FETAL ECHOCARDIOGRAM
Fetal Suspicious level I obstetric ultrasound Extracardiac abnormality Chromosome anomaly Arrhythmia Fetal hydrops
Maternal Family history of CHD Advanced maternal age Metabolic disorders (i.e., IDDM, PKU) Connective tissue diseases (i.e., SLE) Rubella infection Exposure to teratogens
Miscellaneous Paternal history of CHD Sibling with CHD Inheritable disorders or syndromes

CHD = congenital heart disease; IDDM = insulin-dependent diabetes mellitus; PKU = phenylketonuria; SLE = systemic lupus erythematosus.

Table 7 ■ NORMAL CARDIAC EXAM

Situs
  Aorta and stomach lie to the left of spine
  IVC to the right of spine
Size
  0.25–0.35 of the thoracic area
  0.46–0.58 of the thoracic circumference
Apex
  45 degrees to the left of midline
Valves
  Tricuspid and mitral valves are proportionate in size
  Tricuspid valve lies slightly inferior to mitral valve
  Pulmonary and aortic valves are proportionate in size
Atria
  Proportionate in size
  Foramen ovale shunts right to left
Ventricles
  Proportionate in size
  Intraventricular septum intact
  Right ventricle anterior and identified by the moderator band

semilunar valve regurgitation, ventricular outflow obstruction, volume overload (i.e., twin-to-twin transfusion, chorioangioma), ventricular systolic dysfunction (i.e., CHF, myocarditis, cardiomyopathy), anemia, or arrhythmias. Cardiomegaly requires careful evaluation to determine its etiology.

The cardiac apex is then determined by drawing an imaginary line through the interventricular septum and a second imaginary line through the spine and sternum. The angle constructed by this line represents the cardiac apex and should be 45 degrees to the left of the midline. Dextrocardia is defined as rightward malposition of the cardiac apex. Isolated dextrocardia is almost always associated with intracardiac anomalies, most commonly congenitally corrected transposition of the great arteries. Levocardia is defined as a cardiac axis that is more to the left than normal. Levocardia occurring with situs inversus is almost invariably associated with major intracardiac anomalies and either asplenia or polysplenia. Mesocardia is defined as a midline position of the heart and may be associated with congenitally corrected transposition, as well as complete transposition of the great arteries.

The intracardiac anatomy is usually evaluated next. In the structurally normal heart, the atria should be proportionate in size. The right and left upper pulmonary veins can frequently be seen entering the left atrium. Asymmetry of the cardiac chambers may indicate a structural defect (Table 8). The foramen ovale allows shunting of blood from right to left during fetal life. This makes prenatal detection of a true ASD difficult. Occasionally, the atrial septum may be aneurysmal, with extension toward the lateral wall of the left atrium. There is a well-established association between fetal atrial arrhythmias and atrial septal aneurysms.

The tricuspid and mitral valves should be approximately the same size. The annulus of the tricuspid valve is situated closer to the apex than that of the mitral valve. The papillary muscles of the tricuspid valve are "septo-

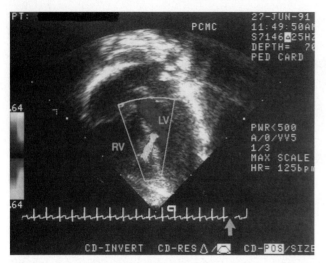

FIGURE 22. Color Doppler documentation of small mid-muscular ventricular septal defect (VSD). In the apical four-chamber projection, the color field is positioned in the region of the muscular septum. This systolic image (*arrow in electrocardiogram*) demonstrates high-velocity, left-to-right shunt flow through an oblique mid-muscular VSD. In this illustration, flow toward the transducer is in shades of red with highest velocities in yellow; flow away from the transducer is in shades of blue, with the highest velocities in light blue. Turbulent flow produces a mosaic pattern. *RV* = right ventricle; *LV* = left ventricle. *See Color Plate*

philic" in that they attach to the free wall of the right ventricle as well as to the interventricular septum. The mitral valve, in contrast, is "septophobic" in that its papillary muscles have attachments only to the free wall of the left ventricle. The right and left ventricles should be symmetric in size and both should open to the apex. The right ventricle is closest to the sternum and contains the moderator band. The ventricular septum should be intact. Frequently, "dropout" of the ventricular septum may be seen when the transducer is parallel to the long axis of the septum. In this case, care must be taken to visualize the ventricular septum in additional views and with color Doppler interrogation to rule out a ventricular septal defect (VSD).

Disproportion in size of the ventricles should prompt evaluation for an outflow tract abnormality. Right ventricular enlargement may be caused by right ventricular outflow obstruction or left ventricular obstructive lesions. Lesions associated with significant volume overload, such as pulmonary regurgitation (i.e., absent pulmonary valve syndrome, tricuspid regurgitation, or arteriovenous malformations), may cause the right ventricle to dilate. Constriction or occlusion of the ductus arteriosus may result in dilatation of the right heart secondary to increased right ventricular afterload. In some cases, intrauterine growth retardation has been associated with right ventricular enlargement caused by redistribution of blood flow to the head, rather than to the body. Left ventricular enlargement, on the other hand may be seen with isolated left-sided myocardial dysfunction. Occasionally, the left ventricle may appear dilated in cases where flow is predominantly to the left,

such as tricuspid atresia, pulmonary atresia with a hypoplastic right ventricle, and malaligned atrioventricular canal defects.

Although most cardiac anomalies can be identified by the four-chamber view of the heart, this view does not adequately assess the outflow tracts. Relying on the four-chamber view alone may allow abnormalities such as transposition of the great arteries to go undetected. Consequently, most centers recommend obtaining views of the ventricular outflow tracts as part of routine screening for congenital heart disease. The diameters of the aortic and pulmonary roots should be similar in size. The aortic outflow can be visualized from the four-chamber view by rotating the transducer a quarter turn, clockwise or counterclockwise depending on the fetal position. Scanning anteriorly, the left atrium will disappear from view and the aortic outflow will come into view. In the short-axis view of the right ventricular outflow tract, the pulmonary artery may be identified lying anterior to the aortic root (Fig. 25).

Obstruction to inflow or outflow early in gestation may be associated with hypoplasia of the ventricular chambers. A hypoplastic right ventricle may be encountered with tricuspid atresia and pulmonary atresia. In the hypoplastic left heart syndrome, a combination of severe left-sided obstructive abnormalities, including mitral and aortic atresia with aortic arch hypoplasia and

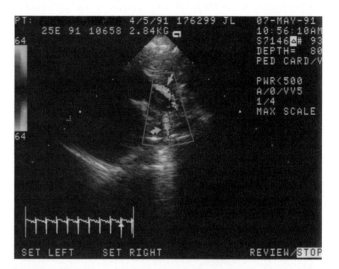

FIGURE 23. Color Doppler documentation of patent ductus arteriosus (PDA). In the short-axis projection, the color field is positioned in the region of the main pulmonary artery. This image at end-diastole (*arrow on electrocardiogram*) demonstrates a jet of turbulent flow into the main pulmonary artery at end-diastole (*arrow*) confirming the presence of a PDA with left-to-right shunt flow. Turbulent blood flow also is seen in the left pulmonary artery (*curved arrow*). Although a PDA may not be visualized directly on two-dimensional examination in some patients, the color documentation of retrograde turbulent blood flow in the main pulmonary artery during diastole confirms the presence of a PDA with left-to-right shunt flow. In this illustration, flow toward the transducer is in shades of red with highest velocities in yellow; flow away from the transducer is in shades of blue, with the highest velocities in light blue. Turbulent flow produces a mosaic pattern. *See Color Plate*

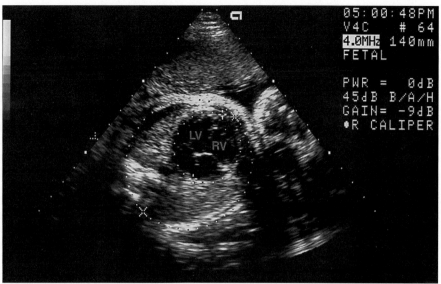

FIGURE 24. Four-chamber view of the structurally normal fetal heart. Cardiac circumference and area are represented by the smaller circle (o). Thoracic circumference and area are represented by the larger circle (O). The normal heart occupies 25% to 35% of the thoracic area, whereas the normal cardiac circumference to thoracic circumference ratio varies between 0.46 and 0.58. *RV* = right ventricle; *LV* = left ventricle.

coarctation, are seen. In this lesion, the degree of obstruction to flow is so severe that flow to the proximal arch vessels and the coronary circulation is retrograde via the ductus.

Sagittal views of the thorax are helpful in identifying the inferior and superior vena caval connections to the right atrium, as well as the ductal and aortic arches. Scanning to the right of the spine, the venae cavae and aortic arch can often be identified in the same plane.

The aortic arch resembles a "candy cane" (Fig. 26). Difficulty visualizing the arch should lead one to suspect an abnormality such as coarctation or arch interruption. Extending posteriorly toward the descending aorta, the "ductal arch" can be seen, resembling a hockey stick. Ductal constriction or occlusion may occur in mothers taking nonsteroidal anti-inflammatory medications such as aspirin, ibuprofen, or indomethacin.

In addition to two-dimensional scanning techniques, M-mode echocardiography may provide information regarding ventricular chamber dimensions, thickness of the ventricular walls, size of the aortic and pulmonary roots, and ventricular function. This technique is useful for detecting pericardial effusions and documenting atrial and ventricular activity in the evaluation of fetal arrhythmias. Doppler echocardiography is also a valuable adjunct for evaluating fetal structural and functional defects. Pulsed, continuous-wave, and color Doppler ultrasound may be used to evaluate flow patterns across the various valves, veins, and arteries. Normal flow velocities and patterns have been established for the fetus at varying stages of gestation.

Fetal echocardiography has limitations. Timing of the study, fetal position, and the progressive nature of certain cardiac lesions must be considered. Maternal factors affecting image quality include maternal obesity, the amount of amniotic fluid, and abdominal striae. Normal fetal physiology may also preclude the ability to exclude cardiac abnormalities. For example, an aneurysmal foramen ovale or widely patent ductus arteriosus may make it difficult to exclude an ASD or coarctation of the aorta. Whether the ductus arteriosus will close or remains patent after birth cannot be determined prenatally. Likewise, small to moderate-size VSDs may be missed because the ventricular pressures are nearly equal prior to birth and Doppler echocardiography may show little shunting. Smaller structures, such as the pulmonary veins, are frequently difficult to visualize,

---

Table 8 ■ DIFFERENTIAL DIAGNOSIS OF CARDIAC ABNORMALITIES

Right Atrial Enlargement
Ebstein's anomaly of the tricuspid valve
Tricuspid valve atresia
Tricuspid regurgitation

Left Atrial Enlargement
Mitral regurgitation
Severe aortic stenosis
Hypoplastic left heart with restrictive foramen ovale

Right Ventricular Enlargement
Critical pulmonic stenosis
Pulmonary atresia with intact ventricular septum
Coarctation of the aorta
Unbalanced atrioventricular canal (right ventricle dominant)
Absent pulmonary valve syndrome
Arteriovenous malformation
Constriction or occlusion of the ductus arteriosus
Intrauterine growth retardation

Left Ventricular Enlargement
Myocarditis
Endocardial fibroelastosis
Critical aortic stenosis
Unbalanced atrioventricular canal (left ventricle dominant)

Abnormal Great Artery Relationship
Transposition of the great arteries
Truncus arteriosus
Tetralogy of Fallot
Double-outlet right ventricle

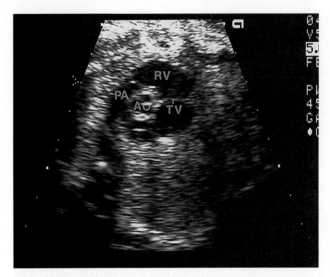

FIGURE 25. Short-axis view of the right ventricular outflow tract. The pulmonary artery may be identified lying anterior to the aortic root. *TV* = tricuspid valve; *RV* = right ventricle; *PA* = main pulmonary artery; *AO* = aorta.

making it extremely challenging to rule out anomalous pulmonary venous return. Parents should be informed of these limitations and how they may affect fetal follow-up and outcome.

The close of the 1990s brought with it new imaging techniques such as harmonic imaging, which greatly improved image quality. This method differs from fundamental imaging in that it transmits ultrasound at one frequency and receives it at twice the transmitted frequency. Compared with fundamental imaging, harmonic imaging improves resolution of the image in fetuses with suboptimal echocardiographic windows. Improvement is primarily the result of decreased artifact. Results are limited to those patients with poor echocardiographic windows. No improvement in image quality is seen in patients with adequate images. In fact, thin structures such as the atrioventricular and semilunar valves may appear thicker or less defined with harmonic imaging, than with fundamental imaging. Whether harmonic imaging improves diagnostic accuracy of the fetal echocardiogram is yet to be determined.

Another recent development, color Doppler energy (CDE), utilizes a nondirectional color map to show only fast- vs slow-moving velocities. This modality enhances visualization of thin structures, such as the membranous septum, the endocardial borders and small blood vessels. CDE improves imaging of structures with low blood flow velocities, such as the pulmonary veins, and is useful for detecting small VSDs that might otherwise be missed with conventional imaging.

Direct evaluation of myocardial velocities is possible using Doppler tissue imaging (DTI). Rather than interrogating blood flow velocity, the Doppler filtering is set so that objects with high backscattering amplitude and low velocity, such as the myocardium are shown, while low amplitude, high velocity signals from blood cells are filtered out. This technique provides important information regarding myocardial function, and there have been recent reports of its use in diagnosing fetal tachycardias.

Recent developments in three-dimensional echocardiography have allowed organized acquisition and storage of a large number of B-mode two-dimensional computer images for later reconstruction of the cardiac anatomy. The interactive nature of the three-dimensional cinegraphic display enhances visualization of structures that are sometimes difficult to see by standard two-dimensional methods. Cumbersome acquisition techniques, larger transducer assemblies, and the need for excess memory space to run processing programs have limited the use of three-dimensional imaging in the fetus.

Echocardiographic evaluation of the fetal heart is fundamental to prenatal diagnosis and perinatal management. More important than advanced technology is a keen understanding of fetal cardiac anatomy and function. Accurate detection of fetal cardiac anomalies allows for better care of the fetus, counseling and preparation for the parents, and proper selection of time and location of the delivery.

COMPUTED TOMOGRAPHY

CT, particularly helical or multidector CT with contrast enhancement, provides opportunities for cross-sectional evaluation of cardiac malformations. When this is used with a cine-loop technique, cardiac function and shunts can be evaluated. Arch anomalies with

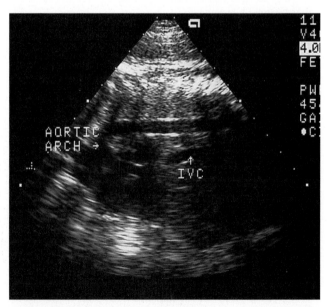

FIGURE 26. Sagittal view identifying the inferior vena cava and the aortic arch. The aortic arch resemble a "candy cane" in appearance. *IVC* = inferior vena cava.

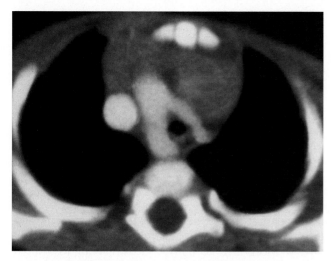

FIGURE 27. Double aortic arch with both arches patent. Axial enhanced EBCT image at the level of the aortic arches demonstrates the right arch to be the dominant arch. The smaller left arch is more anterior as it encircles the trachea. More caudad images (not shown) demonstrated the left arch to join the right arch to form the right posterior descending aorta. (Courtesy of Jerald Kuhn, Buffalo, NY.)

associated abnormalities of the tracheobronchial tree (Fig. 27). may be one of the primary uses of EBCT. These arch and tracheal anomalies are also well demonstrated with MRI.

MAGNETIC RESONANCE IMAGING

During the past several years, electrocardiographic (ECG)-gated MRI of the heart has been used to evaluate selected patients with CHD. Whereas two-dimensional, Doppler, and color-flow Doppler echocardiography provide excellent anatomic and hemodynamic informa-

tion about almost all intracardiac lesions, MRI is largely limited to imaging of extracardiac anatomy and a few intracardiac lesions.

High-quality ECG-gated MRI depends on the contrast between rapidly flowing blood, which produces little or no signal, and stationary cardiac structures and vessel walls. The major advantages of MRI are the ease with which large fields of view can be obtained, and an ability to image orthogonal planes at any angle.

CONTRAINDICATIONS TO MAGNETIC RESONANCE IMAGING

Patients with ferromagnetic foreign bodies in or around the orbit, intracranial metallic aneurysm clips, and epicardial or intracardial pacemakers must be excluded from MRI studies. Patients with prosthetic valves, sternal wires, or small metallic hemostatic clips in the thorax or abdomen can be imaged safely.

Obtaining high-quality images of the heart and great vessels requires sedation in infants and children to avoid motion artifact. Sleep deprivation is a helpful adjunct when used before sedation and in older children who are not sedated. We sleep-deprive all patients under 12 years of age and those older patients who are hyperactive, mentally retarded, or emotionally unstable. Our sedation protocol is listed in Table 9. Infants and children under the age of 6 years are routinely sedated before examination. We administer oral sodium pentobarbital (Nembutal) to infants under one year, intravenous sodium pentobarbital to small and large children, and midazolam (Versed) to older children and adolescents.

IMAGING PROTOCOL

ECG-gated images are dependent on a high-quality ECG tracing for accurate gating. Lead placement varies

Table 9 ■ SEDATION PROTOCOL FOR MAGNETIC RESONANCE IMAGING

PATIENT	DRUG	INITIAL DOSE/ ADMINISTRATION	SUPPLEMENTAL DOSE
Infants up to 1 yr of age	Sodium pentobarbital (Nembutal)	7 mg/kg PO	IV ketamine 1 mg/kg
Small and large children	Sodium pentobarbital (Nembutal)	6 mg/kg IV Administer ½ total dose, observe 30 seconds, administer ½ of the remaining dose, observe 30 seconds, administer remainder of dose	1–2 mg/kg
Older children and adolescents	Midazolam (Versed)	0.1 mg/kg Infuse IV in 1–2 min Maximum dose 5 mg	Repeat initial dose if necessary Fentanyl citrate 1 mg/kg for pain, if necessary

with each patient and with different machines. Some vendors have an optional retrospective ECG-gating program. Our standard imaging technique uses multi-section spin-echo imaging. Imaging parameters for 1.5-tesla (1.5-T) scanning are listed in Table 10. When performed as two separate sequences of interleaved images, tomographic sections at 3- or 5-mm intervals with no gap are obtained throughout the heart and great vessels at varying times during the cardiac cycle. To evaluate blood flow, turbulence, and valvular regurgitation, gated cine-MRI is utilized. Imaging parameters are listed in Table 11. Gadolinium-enhanced three-dimensional time-of-flight examination, with or without breath hold, is particularly useful for examination of the thoracic aorta, great vessels, and, in certain patients, the pulmonary arteries (see Section V, Part III, Chapter 1, Fig. 13, page 1347 and Section V, Part II, Chapter 2, Fig. 19, page 1296).

The imaging sequences described above are utilized primarily for anatomic evaluation. Functional analysis of the heart utilizes segmented fast (turbo) gradient-recalled echoes (GRE), velocity-encoded cine GRE, or echo planar imaging sequences. Utilizing these se-quences, one can determine cardiac dimensions, vol-umes, and regional and global function of the right and left ventricles. Velocity-encoded cine-GRE enables (1) quantification of valvular regurgitation; (2) estima-tion of peak valvular gradients; (3) determination of stroke volume and cardiac output of right and left ventricles; (4) shunt quantification; and (5) quantifica-tion of gradients across areas of stenosis, such as coarctation.

INDICATIONS FOR MAGNETIC RESONANCE SCANNING

Aortic Anomalies

The entire thoracic aorta, the brachiocephalic vessels, and their relationship to the airway are well visualized in patients of any age. The large fields of view obtainable in any plane make MRI the imaging modality of choice for the aorta and brachiocephalic vessels. Vascular rings and their relationship to the tracheobronchial tree are exceptionally well depicted in the coronal and axial planes (see Section V, Part III, Chapter 1, Figs. 8, page 1343, 9, page 1344, 11, page 1346, 18, page 1351, and 19, page 1352). Patients with coarctation are imaged best in the sagittal, LAO, and axial planes to visualize the dilated ascending aorta (secondary to an associated bicuspid valve), transverse arch, coarctation, and post-stenotic descending aorta (see Section V, Part II, Chap-ter 2, Fig. 18, page 1295). MRI is the modality of choice to serially follow the results and recognize associated complications and development of recoarctation follow-ing operation or balloon dilatation (see Section V, Part II, Chapter 2, Fig. 20, page 1297). In these patients, the coronal plane is also imaged after sagittal and axial images have been obtained. In patients with cystic medial necrosis, MRI in the sagittal, axial, and coronal oblique planes clearly depicts the thoracic aorta in its entirety (see Section V, Part IV, Chapter 2, Fig. 5, page 1367). It is the preferred modality for following these patients for serial changes in aortic size and for compli-cations, such as dissection. Patients with supravalvular

Table 10 ■ IMAGING PARAMETERS FOR SPIN-ECHO IMAGING (1.5 T)

PARAMETER	INFANTS	SMALL CHILDREN	LARGE CHILDREN
TE (msec)			
GE	"Min full"	"Min full"	"Min full"
Siemens	14–30	14–30	14–30
TR (msec)			
GE	Dependent on the R–R interval (R–R – 150 + TR)		
Siemens	TR = 80%–85% of the R–R interval		
Signal Average	4	4	3–4
Coil			
GE	Quadrature head	Quadrature head or Torso	Torso or Body
Siemens	CP head	Large flex/CP body array	CP body array
Field of view			
GE	180–240 min	240–320 min	320–480 min
Siemens	3/4 rectangular	3/4 rectangular	3/4 rectangular
Slice thickness			
GE	3 mm	3–4 mm	3–6 mm
Siemens	2–3 mm	3 mm	3–6 mm
Interslice gap			
GE	1 mm	1 mm	1 mm
Siemens	1–2 mm	1–2 mm	1–2 mm
Matrix	128 × 256	128 × 256	128 × 256
Imaging options			
GE	RC, GAT		
Siemens	Dark blood TSE, breath hold		

TE = echo time; TR = repetition time.

Table 11 ■ IMAGING PARAMETERS FOR GATED CINE–MAGNETIC RESONANCE IMAGING

	INFANTS	SMALL CHILDREN	LARGE CHILDREN
TE (msec)			
GE	12–16	12–16	12–16
Siemens	5–7	5–7	5–7
TR (msec)			
GE	18	18	18
Siemens	30	30	40–45 breath hold view sharing
Signal average			
GE	2–3	2–3	2–3
Siemens	3	3	1
Coil			
GE	Quadrature head	Quadrature head or Torso	Torso or Body
Siemens	CP head	Large flex/CP body array	CP body array
Field of view			
GE	200–240 mm	240–320 mm	320–480 mm
Siemens	3/4 rectangular	3/4 rectangular	3/4 rectangular
Interslice gap	0–100%	0–100%	0–100%
Matrix	128 × 256	128 × 256	128 × 256
Flip angle			
GE	30 degrees	30 degrees	30 degrees
Siemens	30 degrees[*]	30 degrees[*]	30 degrees[*]
Phases		number of phases = R–R – 100/25	
Locations			
GE	2	2	2
Siemens	2	2	1, with breath hold

[*]In plane flow, 20 degrees.
TE = echo time; TR = repetition time.

AS and associated peripheral pulmonary artery stenosis can be imaged accurately in the sagittal and coronal planes (see Section V, Part II, Chapter 2, Fig. 10, page 1290). After surgery, imaging in the sagittal, coronal, and axial planes should be obtained. In patients with dissection, spin-echo imaging (Fig. 28) should be followed by cine-MRI to best evaluate abnormalities in flow in the true and false lumina. Abnormalities involving the descending thoracic aorta, such as mycotic aneurysms, are well visualized in the sagittal, coronal, and axial planes (see Section V, Part V, Chapter 2, Fig. 4, page 1379).

Pulmonary Anomalies

Although the central pulmonary arteries and veins can be visualized well by echocardiography, they cannot be seen to the level of the pulmonary hila with a high degree of confidence. These vessels can be imaged in multiple planes with MRI and their relation to the tracheobronchial tree well depicted. The pulmonary artery origin and central confluence are evaluated best in the axial projection with 3- to 5-mm interleaved scans. Aberrant origin of the left pulmonary artery from the right pulmonary artery (pulmonary sling) is well visualized in the axial, coronal, and sagittal projections (see Section V, Part III, Chapter 2, Fig. 6, page 1357). Cine-MRI can be helpful in identifying pulmonary flow in small vessels, distinguishing them from bronchi. Evaluation of pulmonary size, before and after systemic–pulmonary artery shunts, is best performed in the axial and axial-oblique planes with interleaved 3- to 5-mm

images (Fig. 29). The main right pulmonary artery also is well visualized in the coronal plane, and the left pulmonary artery in the sagittal or sagittal oblique plane. In patients with pulmonary artery stenosis, axial and coronal oblique planes permit identification of peripheral pulmonary artery stenosis in the supravalvular region, at the pulmonary bifurcation (see Section V, Part VII, Chapter 1, Figs. 13, 14, page 1402, and 29, page 1413), and in the right and left pulmonary arteries to the level of the hila. Aneurysmal enlargement of the central pulmonary arteries, typically seen in patients with tetralogy of Fallot and absent pulmonary valve, and their relation to the tracheobronchial tree can be evaluated in all planes with 3- to 5-mm interleaved images. In other patients, aneurysmally dilated pulmonary arteries (see Section V, Part VII, Chapter 1, Fig. 11, page 1401) can be distinguished from hilar masses such as bronchogenic cysts, tumors, or adenopathy (see Section V, Part II, Chapter 1, Fig. 32, page 1280). Although most patients with anomalies in pulmonary venous return can be accurately evaluated on two-dimensional echocardiography, certain patients with partial or total anomalous pulmonary venous drainage may benefit from MRI (see Section V, Part II, Chapter 1, Fig. 32, page 1280). Because patients with complex cyanotic CHD related to asplenia invariably have anomalies in pulmonary venous return, MRI may permit evaluation of systemic and pulmonary venous return and complex intracardiac anomalies in a single study (see Section V, Part IV, Chapter 2, Fig. 1, page 1365). Patients with suspected focal pulmonary venous steno-

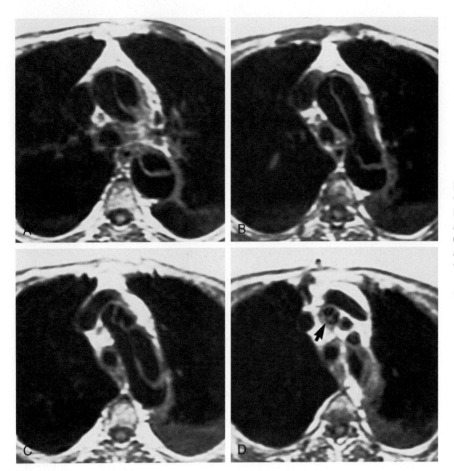

FIGURE 28. Magnetic resonance imaging of type I aortic dissection. **A,** Axial spin-echo image demonstrates the intimal flap in the ascending and descending aorta. **B** and **C,** The intimal flap is seen at the level of the aortic arch. **D,** The dissection with intimal flap extends into the right innominate artery *(arrow)*. Left pleural fluid is also noted. (Courtesy of George S. Bissell III, M.D.)

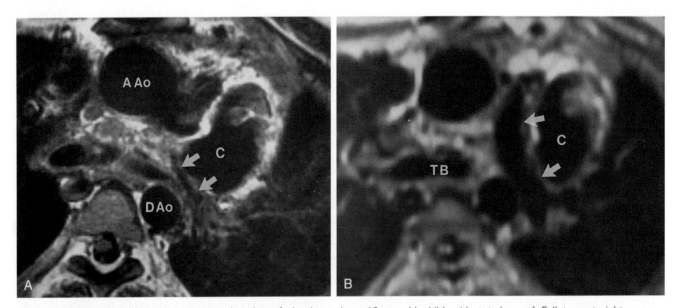

FIGURE 29. Magnetic resonance imaging of the heart in a 16-year-old child with tetralogy of Fallot, post right ventricular–right pulmonary artery conduit *(C)*. The left pulmonary artery could not be identified at angiography. **A,** Axial 5-mm spin-echo image demonstrates a 3-mm left pulmonary artery *(arrows)* passing between the conduit *(C)* and left bronchus. *AAo* = ascending aorta; *DAo* = descending aorta. **B,** Follow-up axial 3-mm image 6 months after Blalock-Taussig anastomosis demonstrates interval growth of the central left pulmonary artery, now measuring 10 to 11 mm *(arrows)*. C = right ventricular–right pulmonary artery conduit; *TB,* tracheal bifurcation.

sis should be studied in both axial and coronal planes with thin 3-mm interleaved images.

Complex Heart Disease

MRI is an excellent modality for visualizing both extra-cardiac and intracardiac anomalies in patients with complex heart disease related to abnormality in situs and those with asplenia or polysplenia syndrome (see Section V, Part IV, Chapter 2, Fig. 1, page 1365). Scans in the coronal plane allow analysis of the tracheobronchial tree for symmetry (see Section V, Part IV, Chapter 2, Fig. 1A, page 1365), and determination of abdominal situs. Coronal and sagittal images may be utilized to locate the inferior vena cava and aorta within the abdomen, and to document azygos and hemiazygos continuation of the inferior vena cava (see Section V, Part IV, Chapter 2, Fig. 1B, page 1365). Atria, unilateral or bilateral superior venae cavae, and their relation to the coronary sinus are easily identified on coronal and axial images (see Section V, Part IV, Chapter 2, Fig. 1C, page 1365). Segmental analysis of complex intracardiac anomalies can then be performed in multiple planes.

Pericardiac and Intracardiac Masses

MRI can identify primary and secondary myocardial and pericardiac masses in the axial and coronal planes. Differentiating mediastinal masses from the aorta, central pulmonary arteries, atria, and ventricles is facilitated by the contrast between flowing blood in these structures (see Section V, Part II, Chapter 1, Fig. 32, page 1280). The fibrous pericardium is of low signal intensity and provides a cleavage plane between mediastinal tissue and cardiac structures. Pericardial tumor involvement may be visualized as focal thickening of the pericardium or disruption of the low-intensity pericardial line. Pericardial effusions and vascular extension of tumor in either the inferior or superior vena cava can be recognized in any imaging plane. While most intracardiac masses can be recognized on echocardiography (see Section V, Part VI, Chapter 1, Fig. 2, page 1389), those lesions involving myocardial walls are best evaluated by MRI with its large field of view. Multiple imaging planes, including true long- and short-axis images of the ventricles, are suggested (see Section V, Part VI, Chapter 1, Fig. 3, page 1390). Cine-MRI is helpful in showing tumor motion between atria and ventricles and associated valvular regurgitation.

Postoperative Evaluation

Surgical correction of complex CHD is often accomplished by creating geometrically complex structures or by creating pathways within the mediastinum that are difficult to interrogate by ultrasound. MRI is a particularly useful modality to evaluate patients with many systemic–pulmonary artery shunts (Fig. 30), conduits between the right atrium and right ventricular outflow tract or pulmonary artery, and atrial baffles (Mustard or Senning procedure) (see Section V, Part VII, Chapter 1, Fig. 20, page 1407). MRI is also useful in evaluation of the central pulmonary arteries following pulmonary artery band (see Section V, Part VII, Chapter 1, Fig. 13, page 1402) or systemic–pulmonary artery shunt (see Fig. 30 and Section V, Part VII, Chapter 1, Fig. 11, page 1401), and for all operations involving the aorta.

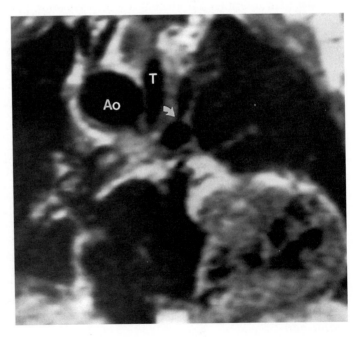

FIGURE 30. Magnetic resonance imaging of stenotic left Blalock-Taussig shunt in a 10-year-old girl with single ventricle, transposition, and pulmonic and mitral atresia. Coronal 3-mm spin-echo image demonstrates stenosis of the left Blalock-Taussig shunt *(arrow)* at the anastomosis with the left pulmonary artery. *Ao* = right aortic arch; *T* = trachea.

A: NUCLEAR CARDIOLOGY

BARBARA S. REID

Radionuclides are used in pediatric cardiovascular studies for detection of shunts, functional cardiac evaluation, evaluation of myocardial perfusion and regional metabolism, identification of myocardial necrosis, and the detection of inflammation.

SHUNT DETECTION

First-pass radionuclide scintigraphy has been used in pediatric cardiology primarily for detection and quantitation of cardiac shunts, as well as measurement of ejection fraction and determination of cardiac output. The radiation dose to the patient is negligible. However, this examination is seldom performed today, having been replaced by Doppler echocardiography and color-flow imaging.

CARDIAC FUNCTION IMAGING

Gated blood pool angiography (multiple gated acquisition blood pool scans) permit evaluation of both global and regional ventricular function. Autologous red cells are labeled with ^{99m}Tc in vitro and reinjected into the patient. The scintillation data acquisition is synchronized with the R–R interval from the ECG, which is divided into a number (usually 16 or 32) of chronologic segments. The scintillation data acquired during hundreds of cardiac angles are partitioned by the computer into these segments resulting in a single sequence spanning the entire cardiac cycle. The images may be played back sequentially at any speed to produce a cine display for evaluating wall motion. Imaging should be performed in anterior, LAO, and left lateral projections. Cardiac output, right and left ventricular ejection fractions, stroke volume, and end-diastolic and end-systolic volumes can be determined. Unlike first-pass scintigraphy, injection technique is unimportant and the counting statistics and spatial resolution are much better.

Sedation may be necessary for the uncooperative child, but, because radioactive decay is not rapid, sleep deprivation, feeding, and patience may help to achieve a diagnostic study. The gated radionuclide study is used to evaluate wall motion and ejection fractions. In many oncology centers, the left ventricular ejection fraction is studied serially in those patients on cardiotoxic drugs to help determine when these drugs should be discontinued. A value of less than 50% is abnormal, but generally the drugs are not discontinued until the ejection fraction decreases to about 30%.

Because the right ventricle can be evaluated by this method, it is better in some cases than myocardial perfusion for wall motion evaluation. It may be useful in cardiac transplants and cardiac trauma for wall motion evaluation.

MYOCARDIAL PERFUSION

Myocardial perfusion scintigraphy is used to detect myocardial ischemia and infarction caused by diseases such as anomalous left coronary artery, cardiomyopathy of glycogen storage disease, and thalassemia. It can be used to evaluate perfusion in septal hypertrophy (Fig. 31) and postoperative arterial switch for transposition.

Thallium-201 as thallous chloride is the most widely used imaging agent. Thallium acts as a potassium analog and is extracted by the myocardial cells proportionate to coronary flow. In adults, a single injection is made during exercise-induced stress. In children it is difficult to obtain adequate stress, so pharmacologic stress agents may be used. There are two types: coronary vasodilating agents such as dipyridamole and adenosine, and cardiac positive inotropic agents such as dobutamine and arbutamine. Vasodilating drugs work directly on the coronary arteries to increase blood flow. The flow in normal coronary arteries will increase from three to five times; abnormal coronary arteries will not dilate, resulting in detectable regional differences in perfusion. Inotropic drugs work indirectly by increasing myocardial work load, leading to an increase in coronary blood flow. Both drug classes are accurate for diagnosing coronary artery disease, and have excellent safety records with acceptably low occurrences of side effects.

The patient should be fasting for 3 to 4 hours to decrease flow to the splanchnic bed, and because sedation will be necessary in some children. Planar ^{201}Tl images are obtained in anterior, LAO, and left lateral projections and repeated in 3 to 4 hours or even later to evaluate redistribution of ^{201}Tl. In noninfarcted myocardium, satisfactory perfusion should be obtained. Cine playback of resting myocardial perfusion images will demonstrate specific areas of decreased ventricular contraction.

Single-photon emission computed tomography (SPECT) acquisition increases the contrast resolution of the images and increases the sensitivity of the study. Reconstruction of the images in the short axis, vertical long axis, and horizontal long axis is performed, and the coronary artery territories are well defined.

There are ^{99m}Tc-labeled compounds available, such as ^{99m}Tc sestamibi, ^{99m}Tc teboroxime, and ^{99m}Tc tetrofosmin, that are distributed to the myocardium proportionate to blood flow, like ^{201}Tl (Fig. 32). ^{99m}Tc sestamibi and ^{99m}Tc tetrofosmin do not redistribute, and, if images are obtained at rest, a repeat injection must be given at a later interval for stress imaging. Technetium-99m teboroxime redistributes quickly and is less well suited for SPECT imaging and use in pediatrics. The lack of redistribution allows for long acquisition times with sestamibi. The physical half-life is less for ^{99m}Tc than ^{201}Tl, and the radiation dose for the same activity is less. Because the photon energy of technetium (140 keV) is ideal for current scintillation cameras and the injected dose can contain more activity, there is improved count density with improved image quality and spatial resolution.

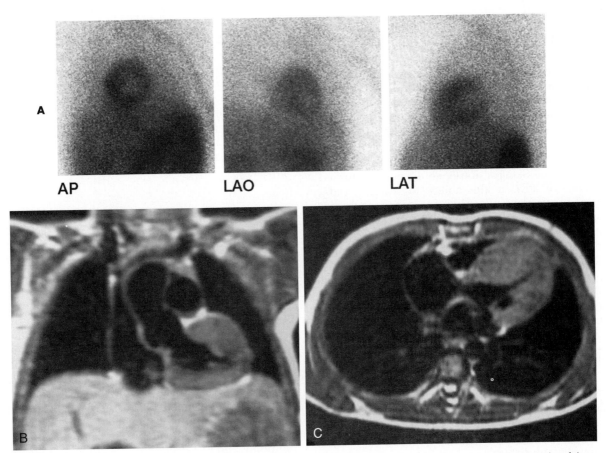

FIGURE 31. Six-year-old boy with hypertrophic cardiomyopathy. **A,** Thallium planar imaging demonstrates hypertrophy of the anterior wall of the left ventricle and ventricular septum. *AP* = anteroposterior; *LAO* = left anterior oblique; *LAT* = lateral. Coronal **(B)** and axial **(C)** T_1-weighted magnetic resonance image demonstrates marked hypertrophy of the left ventricular wall and septum.

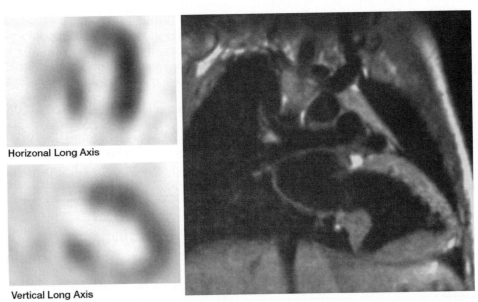

FIGURE 32. Traumatic left ventricular aneurysm in a 3-year-old boy run over by an automobile. Following an abnormal electrocardiogram, single-photon emission computed tomography imaging was performed with ^{99m}Tc sestamibi. The horizontal long-axis image shows nonperfusion of the anterior ventricular septum. The vertical long-axis image shows decreased perfusion of the posterior ventricular wall. Coronal T_1-weighted spin-echo magnetic resonance image confirms the posterior wall left ventricular aneurysm.

METABOLIC FUNCTION EVALUATION

Positron emission tomography (PET) imaging can evaluate and quantify regional metabolic rates and regional blood flow in the myocardium. The development of metabolic tracers such as [^{13}N]ammonia for perfusion, [^{11}C]hydroxyephedrine for heart neuronal studies, and [^{11}C]acetate and [^{18}F]fluorodeoxyglucose for metabolic assessment of the myocardium enables imagers to assess functions that previously could not be studied. The value of PET is the ability to identify viable myocardium on the basis of intact metabolic activity in regions of otherwise underperfused and dysfunctional myocardium. Impairment of oxidative and glucose metabolism may precede decreased blood flow. Primary metabolic impairment is considered to be dominant in hypertrophic myocardium. Although clinically useful, PET is available only at centers with a cyclotron.

Iodine-123–labeled fatty acids have been used to study myocardial metabolism. These radiolabeled fatty acids have been studied as potential markers of tissue metabolism and viability. Because myocardial fatty acid metabolism is severely impaired in patients with hypertrophic myocardiopathy, even though perfusion and contractility may be normal, this examination may be useful in the management of these patients. The longer retention of the radiolabel permits longer image acquisitions more compatible with SPECT imaging, especially with single-detector imaging systems.

MYOCARDIAL NECROSIS EVALUATION

Technetium-99m pyrophosphate is the current standard for myocardial necrosis imaging. Peak activity in an area of myocardial necrosis is seen at approximately 48 to 72 hours following chest trauma, and changes may be present for up to a week. However, this study is relatively insensitive and not often performed in children. Indium-111–labeled antimyosin Fab is a more sensitive and specific test, especially with the addition of SPECT imaging. The antimyosin antibody adheres to myosin, which is exposed to extracellular fluid only if cells die. The extent and intensity of antimyosin uptake are an indicator of necrotic myocardial tissue. A positive antimyosin test indicates myocardial cell death and not merely an ischemic episode. The limitation is that, as with pyrophosphate, there is a delay caused by the delayed blood clearance of the antibody protein macromolecules. A new agent, ^{99m}Tc glucarate, may provide an earlier imaging method. A large infarction can be seen by 1 hour and a small infarction by 3 hours.

INFLAMMATION

Indium-111–labeled autologous white blood cells or ^{67}Ga are useful to identify patients with myocarditis or Kawasaki disease. SPECT imaging identifies the tracer in the myocardium or pericardium. Technetium-99m–labeled white blood cells with hexamethylpropyleneamine oxime are a useful new technique for detecting infection in the heart. Antimyosin imaging is effective for the detection of myocyte necrosis associated with active myocarditis, and in patients with dilated cardiomyopathy. It has a negative predictive value, which may obviate the need for endomyocardial biopsy in suspected myocarditis and in post-transplant patients.

B: ELECTROCARDIOGRAPHY AND ELECTROPHYSIOLOGY

VICTORIA E. JUDD

Disturbances in cardiac rhythm are an important aspect of pediatric cardiology. In a patient with a suspected arrhythmia, palpitations, or syncope, the 12-lead ECG is a useful initial diagnostic tool. Important diagnostic clues may be present on the ECG. The presence of ventricular pre-excitation, cardiac chamber enlargement, conduction abnormalities, or Q–T prolongation may indicate the need for further diagnostic testing. Ambulatory ECG monitoring allows for the detection of episodic rhythm abnormalities and the correlation of symptoms and ECG findings. The Holter monitor allows 24 to 48 hours of continuous monitoring of cardiac rhythm, conduction, and rate. In patients with suspected arrhythmias that occur daily or more than once a day, the Holter monitor will provide ECG documentation during symptoms. In patients whose symptoms are less frequent, a cardiac event recorder allows for ECG recording only when activated by the patient or parent at the time of symptoms. Transtelephonic transmission of events has greatly improved the ability to document the etiology of symptoms. These continuous-loop recorders record the heart rhythm for 1 minute before activated and several minutes subsequent to activation. Signal-averaged ECG is used extensively in the diagnosis of heart disease in adult patients and is being utilized in pediatric patients, especially where there is a concern for clinically important ventricular arrhythmias.

Intracardiac electrophysiology studies require the insertion of electrode catheters within the heart to record local myocardial electrical activity and perform programmed stimulation of myocardial tissue. This study provides information concerning the evaluation and management of cardiac arrhythmias. Electrophysiology studies in pediatric patients are frequently performed to evaluate patients with paroxysmal tachycardias, often in conjunction with a radiofrequency catheter ablation. Radiofrequency catheter ablation allows for the application of radiofrequency energy via an electrode catheter, causing local tissue heating and thermal injury. This results in a well-circumscribed myocardial lesion. Selective application of radiofrequency lesions allows for the elimination or modification of a targeted arrhythmia substrate and is used to cure many types of tachycardia. For example, application of radiofrequency energy to an accessory atrioventricular connection results in tissue destruction, elimination of electrical conduction, and a cure for supraventricular tachycardia.

SUGGESTED READINGS

Cardiac Imaging: General

Freedom RM, Mawson JB, Yoo S-J (eds): Congenital Heart Disease. Armonk, NY, Armonk Futura Publishing Co., 1997

Garson A Jr, Bricker JT, Fisher DJ (eds): The Science and Practice of Pediatric Cardiology, 2nd ed. Baltimore, Williams & Wilkins, 1998

Hubbard AM, Fellows KE, Miller WT (eds): MRI of the heart. Semin Roentgenol 1998;33(3)

Link KM, Lesko NM (eds): Cardiac imaging. Radiol Clin North Am 1994;32(3)

Magnetic resonance imaging. Pediatr Cardiol 2000;21(1)

Rebergen SA, Niezen RA, Helbing WA, et al: Cine gradient-echo MR imaging and MR velocity mapping in the evaluation of congenital heart disease. Radiographics 1996;16:467

Reddy GP, Higgins CB: Congenital heart disease: measuring physiology with MRI. Semin Roentgenol 1998;33:228

Routine Chest Radiography

Coussement AM, Gooding CA: Objective radiographic assessment of pulmonary vascularity in children. Radiology 1973;109:649

Edwards DK, Higgins CB: Radiology of neonatal heart disease. Radiol Clin North Am 1980;18:369

Edwards DK, Higgins CB, Gilpin EA: The cardiothoracic ratio in newborn infants. AJR Am J Roentgenol 1981;136:907

Elliott LP: An angiocardiographic and plain film approach to complex congenital heart disease: classification and simplified nomenclature. Curr Probl Cardiol 1978;3:1–64

Rosario-Medina W, Strife JL, Dunbar JS: Normal left atrium: appearance in children on frontal chest radiographs. Radiology 1986;161:345

Angiocardiography

Arciniegas JG, Soto B, Coghlan HC, et al: Congenital heart malformations: sequential angiographic analysis. AJR Am J Roentgenol 1981;137:673

Bargeron LM Jr, Elliott LP: Axial cineangiocardiography in congenital heart disease. I. Concept, technical and anatomic considerations. Circulation 1977;56:1075

Ceballos R, Roto B, Bargeron LM Jr: Angiographic anatomy of the normal heart through axial angiography. Circulation 1981;64:351

Elliott LP, Bargeron LM Jr, Soto B, et al: Axial cineangiography in congenital heart disease. Radiol Clin North Am 1980;15:515

Fellows KE, Keane JF, Freed MD: Angled views in cineangiography of congenital heart disease. Radiology 1977;56:485

Garcia-Medina V, Bass J, Braunlin E, et al: A useful projection for demonstrating the bifurcation of the pulmonary artery. Pediatr Cardiol 1990;11:147–149

Mitchell SW, Kan J, White RI: Interventional techniques in congenital heart disease. Semin Roentgenol 1985;20:290

Echocardiography

Allen HD, Goldberg SJ, Sahn DJ, et al: Suprasternal notch echocardiography: assessment of its clinical utility in pediatric cardiology. Circulation 1977;55:605

Bierman FZ, Williams RG: Subxiphoid two-dimensional imaging of the interatrial septum in infants and neonates with congenital heart disease. Circulation 1979;60:80

Gramiak R, Nanda NC: New techniques in cardiac imaging with ultrasound: state of the art. Radiology 1979;133:609.

Henry WL, Maron BJ, Griffiths JM: Cross-sectional echocardiography in the diagnosis of congenital heart disease: identification of the relation of the ventricles and great arteries. Circulation 1977;56:267

Kelley MJ, Jaffe CC, Shoum SM, et al: Radiographic and echocardiographic approach to cyanotic congenital heart disease. Radiol Clin North Am 1980;18:411

Kotler MN, Mintz GS, Segal BL, et al: Clinical uses of two-dimensional echocardiography. Am J Cardiol 1980;45:1061

Lange LW, Sahn DJ, Allen HD, et al: Subxiphoid cross-sectional echocardiography in infants and children with congenital heart disease. Circulation 1979;59:513

Lee RT, Bhatia SJS, St. John Sutton MG: Assessment of valvular heart disease with Doppler echocardiography. JAMA 1989;262:2131

Ludomirsky A, Huhta JC (eds): Color Doppler of Congenital Heart Disease in the Child and Adult. Mount Kisco, NY, Futura Publishing, 1987

Maron BJ, Henry WL, Griffiths JM, et al: Identification of congenital malformations of the great arteries in infants by real-time two dimensional echocardiography. Circulation 1975;52:671

Meyer RA, Kaplan S: Non-invasive techniques in pediatric cardiovascular disease. Prog Cardiovasc Dis 1973;15:341

Miyatake K, Okamoto M, Kinoshita N, et al: Clinical applications of a new type of real-time two-dimensional Doppler flow imaging system. Am J Cardiol 1984;54:857–868

Popp RL, Fowles RE, Collart DJ, et al: Cardiac anatomy viewed systematically with two-dimensional echocardiography. Chest 1979;75:579

Sahn DJ: Real-time two-dimensional Doppler echocardiographic flow mapping. Circulation 1985;71:849

Silverman NH, Schiller NB: Apex echocardiography: two-dimensional technique for evaluating congenital heart disease. Circulation 1978;57:503

Snider AR, Silverman NH: Suprasternal notch echocardiography: a two-dimensional technique for evaluating congenital heart disease. Circulation 1981;63:165

Tajik AJ, Seward JB, Hagler DJ, et al: Two-dimensional real-time ultrasonic imaging of the heart and great vessels: technique, image orientation, structure identification and validation. Mayo Clin Proc 1978;53:271

Ultan LB, Segal BL, Likoff W: Echocardiography in congenital heart disease—preliminary observations. Am J Cardiol 1967;19:74

Fetal Echocardiography

Achiron R, Weissman A, Rotstein Z, et al: Transvaginal echocardiographic examination of the fetal heart between 13 and 5 weeks' gestation in a low-risk population. J Ultrasound Med 1994;13:783–789

Allan LD, Chita SK, Al-Ghazali W, et al: Doppler echocardiographic evaluation of the normal human fetal heart. Br Heart J 1987;57:528–533

Ayres NA: Advances in fetal echocardiography. Texas Heart Inst J 1997;24:250–259

Copel JA, Pilu G, Green J, et al: Fetal echocardiographic screening for congenital heart disease: the importance of the four-chamber view. Am J Obstet Gynecol 1987;157:648–655

Copel JA, Pilu G, Kleinman CS: Congenital heart disease and extracardiac anomalies: associations and indications for fetal echocardiography. Am J Obstet Gynecol 1986;154:1121–1132

Friedman AH, Copel JA, Kleinman CS: Fetal echocardiography and fetal cardiology: indications, diagnosis and management. Semin Perinatol 1993;17:76–88

Hornberger LK, Sanders SP, Rein AJ, et al: Left heart obstructive lesions and left ventricular growth in the midtrimester fetus: a longitudinal study. Circulation 1995;92:1531–1538

Hornberger LK, Sanders SP, Sahn DJ, et al: In utero pulmonary artery and aortic growth and potential for progression of pulmonary outflow tract obstruction in tetralogy of Fallot. J Am Coll Cardiol 1995;25:739–745

Kirk JS, Riggs TW, Comstock CH, et al: Prenatal screening for cardiac anomalies: the value of routine addition of the aortic root to the four-chamber view. Obstet Gynecol 1994;84:427–431

Kovalchin JP, Lewin MB, Bezold LI, et al: Harmonic imaging in fetal echocardiography. J Am Soc Echocardiogr 2001;14:1025–1029

Rein AJJT, Levine JC, Nir A: Use of High-frame rate imaging and Doppler tissue echocardiography in the diagnosis of fetal ventricular tachycardia. J Am Soc Echocardiogr 2001;14:149–151

Sklansky MS, Nelson TR, Pretorius D: Usefulness of gated three-dimension fetal echocardiography to reconstruct and display structures not visualized with two-dimensional imaging. Am J Cardiol 1997;80:665–668

Sohaey R, Zwiebel WJ: The fetal heart: a practical sonographic approach. Semin Ultrasound CT MR 1996;17:15–33

Toro L, Weintraub RG, Shiota T, et al: Relation between persistent atrial arrhythmias and a redundant septum primum flap (atrial septal aneurysm) in fetuses. Am J Cardiol 1994;73:711–713

Weil SR, Huhta JC: Sonographic differential diagnosis of fetal cardiac abnormalities. Semin Ultrasound CT MR 1993;14:298–317

Computed Tomography

Choi BW, Park YH, Choi JY, et al: Using electron beam CT to evaluate conotruncal anomalies in pediatric and adult patients. AJR Am J Roentgenol 2001;177:1045–1049

Farmer DW, Lipton JJ, Webb WR, et al: Computed tomography in congenital heart disease. Radiology 1985;155:284

Gilkeson RC, Ciancibello L, Zahka K: Pictorial essay. Multidetector CT evaluation of congenital heart disease in pediatric and adult patients. AJR Am J Roentgenol 2003;180:973–980

Lackener K, Thurn P: Computed tomography of the heart: ECG gated and continuous scans. Radiology 1981;140:413

Morehouse CC, Brody WR, Guthaner DF, et al: Gated cardiac computed tomography with a motion phantom. Radiology 1980;134:213

Ritman EL, Harris LD, Kinsey JH, et al: Computed tomographic imaging of the heart: the dynamic spatial reconstructor. Radiol Clin North Am 1980;18:547

Westra SJ, Hurteau J, Galindo A, et al: Cardiac electron-beam CT in children undergoing surgical repair for pulmonary atresia. Radiology 1999;213:502–512

Magnetic Resonance Imaging

Burrows PE: Magnetic resonance imaging of the aorta in children. Semin Ultrasound CT MR 1990;11:221–233

Chung T: Assessment of cardiovascular anatomy in patients with congenital heart disease by magnetic resonance imaging. Pediatr Cardiol 2000;21:18

Didier D, Higgins CB, Fisher MR, et al: Congenital heart disease: gated MR imaging in 72 patients. Radiology 1986;158:227–235

Duerinckx AJ, Wexler L, Banerjee WL, et al: Postoperative evaluation of pulmonary arteries in congenital heart surgery by magnetic resonance imaging: comparison with echocardiography. Am Heart J 1994;128:1139

Formanek AG, Witcofski RL, D'Souza VJ, et al: MR imaging of the central pulmonary arterial tree in conotruncal malformation. AJR Am J Roentgenol 1986;147:1127–1131

Gomes AS, Lois JF, Williams RG: Pulmonary arteries: MR imaging in patients with congenital obstruction of the right ventricular outflow tract. Radiology 1990;174:51–57

Gutierrez F, Mirowitz S, Canter C: Magnetic resonance imaging in the evaluation of postoperative congenital heart defects. Semin Ultrasound CT MR 1990;11:234–245

Hayes AM, Baker EJ, Parson J, et al: Evaluation of pulmonary artery anatomy using magnetic resonance: the importance of multiplanar and oblique imaging. Pediatr Cardiol 1994;15:8

Higgins CB: MR of the heart: anatomy, physiology and metabolism. AJR Am J Roentgenol 1988;151:239–248

Jaffe RB: Magnetic resonance imaging of vascular rings. Semin Ultrasound CT MR 1990;11:206–220

Julsrud PR: Magnetic resonance imaging of the pulmonary arteries and veins. Semin Ultrasound CT MR 1990;11:184–205

Reddy GP, Higgins CB: Congenital heart disease: measuring physiology with MRI. Semin Roentgenol 1998;33:228

Rienmuller R, Tiling R: Evaluation of paracardiac and intracardiac masses in children. Semin Ultrasound CT MR 1990;11:246–250

Sieverding L, Klose U, Apitz J: Morphological diagnosis of congenital and acquired heart disease by magnetic resonance imaging. Pediatr Radiol 1990;20:311

Nuclear Cardiology

Corbett JR: Fatty acids for myocardial imaging. Semin Nucl Med 1999;29:237

Jain D: Technetium-99m labeled myocardial perfusion imaging agents. Semin Nucl Med 1999;29:221

Khaw BA: The current role of infarct avid imaging. Semin Nucl Med 1999;29:259

Peng N-J, Advani R, Kopiwoda S, et al: Clinical decision making based on radionuclide determined ejection fraction in oncology patients. J Nucl Med 1997;38:702

Pretorius PH, Xia W, King MA, et al: Evaluation of right and left ventricular volume and ejection fraction: using a mathematical cardiac torso phantom. J Nucl Med 1997;38:1528

Tadamura E, Tamaki N, Matsumori A, et al: Myocardial metabolic changes in hypertrophic cardiomyopathy. J Nucl Med 1996;37:572

Travin MI, Wexler JP: Pharmacological stress testing. Semin Nucl Med 1999;29:298

Vogel M, Smallhorn JR, Gilday D, et al: Assessment of myocardial perfusion in patients after the arterial switch operation. J Nucl Med 1991;32:237–241

Wakasugi S, Shibata N, Kobayashi T, et al: Thallium-201 imaging in a patient with mid-ventricular hypertrophic obstructive cardiomyopathy. J Nucl Med 1988;29:1738–1741

Williams HT, Miller JH: Scintigraphy of major closed chest cardiac trauma in childhood. Pediatr Radiol 1988;18:74–76

Williamson SL, Williamson MR, Seibert JJ: Indium-111 leukocyte localization for detecting early myocarditis in patients with Kawasaki disease. Am J Roentgenol 1986;146:255

Electrocardiography and Electrophysiology

Goldstein MA, Hesslein P, Dunnigan A: Efficacy of transtelephonic electrocardiographic monitoring in pediatric patients. Am J Dis Child 1990;144:178

Haines DE, Watson DD: Tissue heating during radiofrequency catheter ablation: a thermodynamic model and observations in isolated perfused and superperfused canine right ventricular free wall. Pacing Clin Electrophysiol 1989;12:962

Stelling JA, Danford DA, Kugler JD: Late potentials and inducible ventricular tachycardia in surgically repaired congenital heart disease. Circulation 1990;82:1690

PART II

CONGENITAL HEART DISEASE

VIRGIL R. CONDON
RICHARD B. JAFFE

Chapter   1

ACYANOTIC CONGENITAL HEART DISEASE WITH INCREASED PULMONARY FLOW

VIRGIL R. CONDON and RICHARD B. JAFFE

VENTRICULAR SEPTAL DEFECT

Ventricular septal defect (VSD) accounts for approximately 25% of all congenital heart disease (CHD), with an incidence of between 1.3 and 2.5 per 1000 live births. This number would be significantly larger if those VSDs associated with complex CHD (tetralogy of Fallot, etc.) were included. Many small VSDs close spontaneously (33%), so the incidence varies depending upon age at evaluation.

CLASSIFICATION

A VSD may be isolated or part of a complex congenital heart malformation, such as tetralogy of Fallot, truncus arteriosus, atrioventricular canal (AVC) coarctation syndrome, tricuspid atresia, transposition of the great arteries, and double-outlet right ventricle. Although many classifications of VSDs have been proposed, a common working classification divides the septum into four components: (1) *inlet* septum separating the mitral and tricuspid valves, (2) *trabecular* septum extending from the attachment of the tricuspid valve leaflets to the apex and upward to the crista supraventricularis, (3) *outlet* septum extending from the crista supraventricularis to the pulmonary valve, and (4) the thin *membranous* septum (Fig. 1). Approximately 80% of VSDs occur in the membranous septum and may extend and involve the inlet, trabecular, or outlet septum, in which case they are called perimembranous defects. Less commonly, VSDs occur in the inlet, trabecular, or muscular septum.

These defects, their frequency, and associated malformations and complications are listed in Table 1. A VSD is the most common lesion in the chromosomal syndromes of trisomies 13, 18, and 21.

PATHOPHYSIOLOGY

The pathophysiologic effect of a VSD is a high-pressure left-to-right shunt at the ventricular level. This subjects the pulmonary vasculature to high flow and high pressure, which frequently results in obstructive pulmonary vascular disease that may be irreversible in advanced stages.

CLINICAL MANIFESTATIONS

Symptoms relate to the size of the VSD and the degree of left-to-right shunt. Failure to thrive and congestive heart failure (CHF) usually do not appear until after the first month as pulmonary vascular resistance falls. A characteristic systolic murmur is evident over the low precordium with a restricted VSD. This murmur is always holosystolic and extends to the second heart sound. A soft, low-pitched early diastolic murmur is also frequently heard in the apical area. With a large VSD, no murmur may be present, or there may be a midsystolic crescendo–decrescendo murmur. A widely split and accentuated second sound is frequently noted. With pulmonary hypertension the second sound becomes louder and fixed.

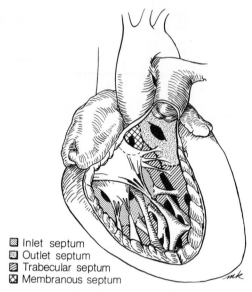

☷ Inlet septum
☶ Outlet septum
▨ Trabecular septum
☒ Membranous septum

FIGURE 1. Schematic representation of ventricular septal defect (VSD) position as seen from the right ventricle. VSDs are illustrated in *black* in the four components of the ventricular septum: inlet, outlet, trabecular, and membranous septa. Multiple VSDs are illustrated in the trabecular septum. A defect in the membranous septum may extend into the inlet, outlet, or trabecular septum and is then known as a perimembranous VSD.

CHEST RADIOGRAPHY

Radiographic findings vary depending upon the size of the VSD. A normal chest radiograph will be seen with a small VSD. Common findings with a larger defect include (1) cardiomegaly (75% under age of 2 years);

(2) increased pulmonary blood flow (Fig. 2; see also Section V, Part I, Chapter 2, Fig. 1, page 1232) with a large main pulmonary artery segment; (3) enlargement of the left atrium and displacement of the left main stem bronchus (Fig. 2*B*); and (4) right aortic arch (5%). CHF is frequent in the infant (Fig. 2*A*), whereas pulmonary hypertension becomes evident in the older child with enlarged central pulmonary arteries.

Spontaneous closure of the VSD or development of acquired infundibular pulmonary stenosis (acquired tetralogy of Fallot) results in a decrease in heart size and pulmonary blood flow. The differential diagnosis includes patent ductus arteriosus (PDA), atrioventricular septal defect (AVC), aorticopulmonary window, and atrial septal defect (ASD).

ECHOCARDIOGRAPHY

Real-time echocardiography allows direct imaging of larger membranous and muscular septal defects, particularly from the subxiphoid (subcostal) and parasternal projections (Fig. 3). Enlargement of the left atrium, membranous septum aneurysms, and other associated lesions may also be seen. Doppler interrogation along the right ventricular margin of the ventricular septum will show a positive flow pattern (see Section V, Part I, Chapter 2, Figs. 21, page 1243, and 22, page 1244). Color Doppler examination also will document directional shunting and turbulence and permit more rapid identification of muscular VSDs (see Section V, Part I, Chapter 2, Fig. 22, page 1244).

Table 1 ■ CLASSIFICATION OF VENTRICULAR SEPTAL DEFECT

TYPE	SYNONYM	FREQUENCY	ASSOCIATED WITH OR COMPLICATED BY	OPTIMAL ANGIOGRAPHIC PROJECTION(S)*
Membranous	Perimembranous Infracristal	80%	Aneurysm of the membranous septum, and spontaneous closure Adherence of tricuspid valve tissue to defect with left ventricle–right atrial shunt Extension to trabecular, outlet septum Malalignment with subaortic stenosis	Long axis (steep LAO)
Inlet	Atrioventricular canal type	8%	Straddling tricuspid valve	Long axis (shallow LAO)
Outlet	Conal Subpulmonary Subarterial Supracristal Infundibular	5%–7%	Aortic valve prolapse through defect with right ventricular outflow tract obstruction Aortic regurgitation Dilatation of the sinus of Valsalva Aortic–right ventricular fistula	AP, RAO, lateral

Trabecular	Muscular
	    Central muscular
	    Apical muscular
	    Marginal
	    "Swiss cheese" muscular
		5%–20%		Long axis and four chamber (shallow and steep LAO)

*AP = anteroposterior; LAO = left anterior oblique; RAO = right anterior oblique.

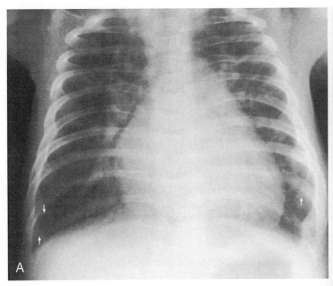
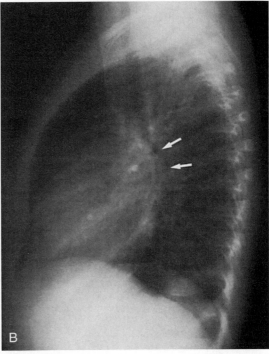

FIGURE 2. Ventricular septal defect. **A,** An 11-week-old infant with increased pulmonary flow and congestive failure, prominent central and main pulmonary arteries, cardiomegaly, and left atrial enlargement. Interstitial fluid and Kerley's lines *(arrows)*, thymic atrophy, and hyperinflation are secondary to failure in this acyanotic heart lesion. **B,** A lateral view shows left atrial enlargement displacing the left main stem bronchus posteriorly *(arrows)* and prominent central pulmonary vasculature with large vessels extending into the peripheral lungs (see Section V, Part I, Chapter 2, Fig. 1, page 1232).

ANGIOCARDIOGRAPHY

A selective left ventriculogram performed in the long-axis or four-chamber projection, or in both projections, is preferred (Figs. 4 and 5; see also Section V, Part I, Chapter 2, Fig. 12*B*, page 1238). With large defects, 2 ml/kg contrast should be injected in as short a time as possible. Catheterization can usually be performed from the venous approach, although, with a closed atrial septum, retrograde aortic catheterization will be necessary. Because of the combined presence of membranous and muscular septal defects (see Fig. 5), the entire septum must be adequately visualized. Supracristal VSDs may be visualized best in true anteroposterior (AP) and lateral projections or right anterior oblique projection of the long-axis view (Fig. 6). Appropriate injections to rule out associated lesions such as coarctation, PDA, and ASD must be made. If significant pulmonary hypertension exists, contrast angiography should be performed with caution. VSD imaging with magnetic resonance imaging (MRI) has been successful.

PROGNOSIS

The prognosis is good with an early diagnosis and operative treatment. Muscular septal defects are more difficult to close than are membranous ones. Operative correction is preferable before the age of 2 or 3 years to decrease the chance of irreversible pulmonary hypertension (Eisenmenger's syndrome). In high-risk pa-

tients or patients with a complex associated lesion, pulmonary artery banding may be performed as a palliative procedure. Early closure of all outlet defects is recommended to prevent development of aortic sinus prolapse and subsequent development of aortic regurgitation. Without surgery, endocarditis develops in 1% to 5% of patients. Catheter closure techniques are becoming more commonly employed, particularly with muscular defects (Fig. 7).

ATRIAL SEPTAL DEFECT

INCIDENCE

ASD accounts for approximately 10% of all CHD. The incidence in females is more than twice that in males. Most cases occur sporadically, but secundum defects have been reported in families as a genetic abnormality. Anomalies of the upper extremities and a secundum ASD (Holt-Oram syndrome) also occurs in families.

Secundum defects account for greater than 90% of all ASDs and are usually isolated anomalies. Important associated lesions include abnormalities of the mitral valve, particularly mitral valve prolapse with or without mitral regurgitation. A sinus venosus defect accounts for 5% to 10% of ASDs, and is located posterior to the secundum defect. This defect is commonly associated with anomalous connection of the right pulmonary veins, particularly the upper lobe veins to either the right atrium or superior vena cava (SVC). The coronary

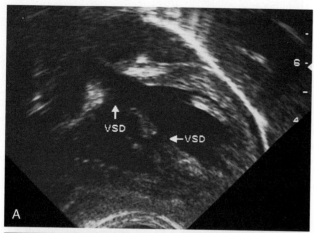

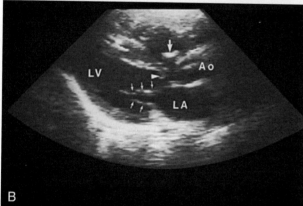

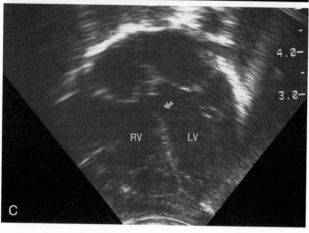

FIGURE 3. A, Subcostal four-chamber projection demonstrates a moderate-sized membranous VSD *(vertical arrow)* and a small midmuscular VSD *(horizontal arrow).* (From Jaffe RB: Ventricular septal defect—echocardiography. *In* Elliott LP [ed]: Cardiac Imaging in Infants, Children, and Adults. Philadelphia, JB Lippincott, 1991:575, with permission.) **B,** A two-dimensional long-axis echocardiogram demonstrates a VSD and aneurysm of the membranous septum *(large arrow)* projecting into the right ventricular outflow tract. Membranous subaortic stenosis is present caudad to the VSD arising from the membranous septum *(arrowhead). Small arrows* indicate the mitral valve. *LV* = left ventricle; *Ao* = aorta; *LA* = left atrium. **C,** In the apical four-chamber projection, a moderate-sized inlet VSD *(curved arrow)* is present in the posterior muscular septum in the plane of the tricuspid and mitral valves. *RV* = right ventricle; *LV* = left ventricle.

sinus ASD is a rare lesion occurring at the expected site of the coronary sinus ostium. It is usually part of a developmental complex that includes absence of the coronary sinus and persistent left SVC emptying into the left atrium.

PATHOPHYSIOLOGY

Low-pressure left-to-right shunting occurs with increased right ventricular compliance and produces right atrial and right ventricular dilatation. Shunt volume relates to the size of the defect, right heart compliance, and pulmonary resistance. Pulmonary hypertension in childhood is uncommon.

CLINICAL MANIFESTATIONS

Systolic ejection murmurs in the pulmonary region and parasternal diastolic murmurs are present. The second sound is split and does not vary with respiration. Children with a large ASD have a mild diastolic flow murmur through the tricuspid valve.

CHEST RADIOGRAPHY

In the neonate, the heart and pulmonary flow are usually within normal limits. Findings in later infancy and childhood include (1) mild cardiomegaly with right atrial and right ventricular enlargement; (2) mild increased pulmonary blood flow (particularly centrally); (3) a "triangular" cardiac silhouette related to right heart and main pulmonary artery enlargement; and (4) a relatively inconspicuous SVC (Fig. 8). Primary differential diagnoses include AVC, VSD, PDA, and other left-to-right shunts.

ECHOCARDIOGRAPHY

Two-dimensional imaging reveals an ASD, a large right atrium, and a large right ventricle (Fig. 9). M-mode and real-time evaluation demonstrate paradoxical or flat septal motion. Doppler interrogation in the right atrium demonstrates a positive flow pattern in the right atrium. Color Doppler examination permits rapid identification of left-to-right shunting at the atrial level (see Section V, Part I, Chapter 2, Fig. 20, page 1242).

ANGIOCARDIOGRAPHY

In many pediatric cardiology practices, echocardiography is thought to be adequate for the preoperative evaluation of simple secundum atrial septal defects. However, if angiocardiography is indicated, optimal visualization is achieved with a right upper lobe pulmonary vein injection in the four-chamber projection with a biplane cineangiocardiogram. The secundum ASD and associated left-to-right shunting will be well demon-

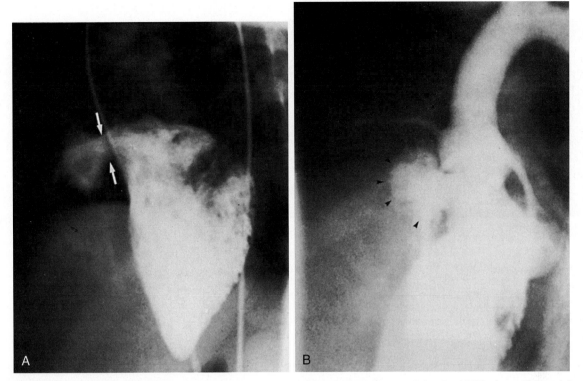

FIGURE 4. Angiocardiography of ventricular septal defect (VSD). **A,** Membranous infracristal VSD *(arrows)* in a left ventriculogram in the long-axis projection. Note the proximity of the defect to the right aortic sinus. **B,** Left ventricular long-axis angiocardiogram showing a membranous infracristal VSD with associated aneurysm of the interventricular septum *(arrowheads).* This clover-like aneurysm bulges in systole into the right ventricle beneath the tricuspid valve.

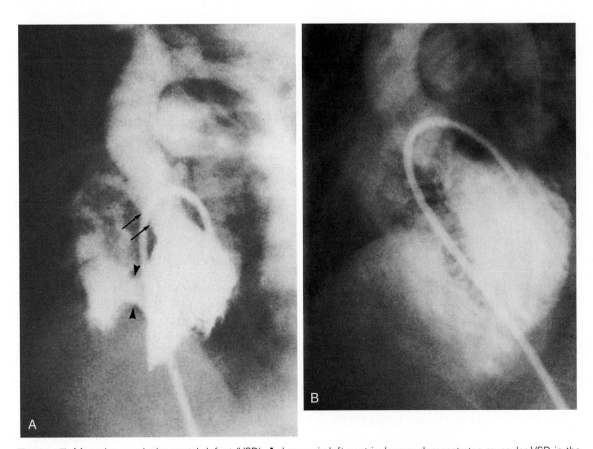

FIGURE 5. Muscular ventricular septal defect (VSD). **A,** Long-axis left ventriculogram demonstrates muscular VSD in the midportion of the septum with an associated left-to-right shunt *(arrowheads).* The membranous portion of the septum is intact *(arrows).* **B,** Left ventriculogram demonstrates multiple muscular VSDs with associated left-to-right shunting (Swiss cheese septum).

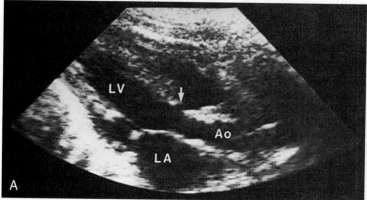

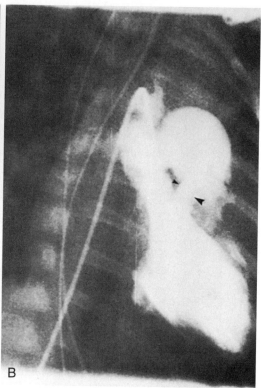

FIGURE 6. Supracristal ventricular septal defect (VSD). **A,** Long-axis echocardiogram demonstrates an oblique defect *(arrow)* extending from just beneath the aortic valve into the right ventricular outflow tract below the pulmonary valve. *LV* = left ventricle; *Ao* = aorta; *LA* = left atrium. **B,** Angiocardiogram in the frontal long-axis view demonstrates the supracristal defect extending superolaterally from the left ventricle into the right ventricular outflow tract *(arrowheads).*

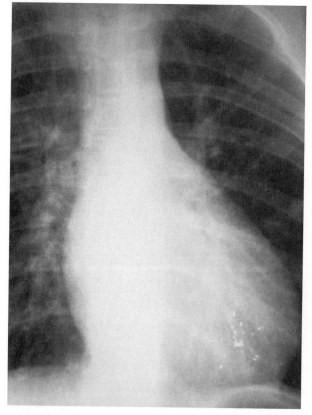

FIGURE 7. Catheter closure of muscular ventricular septal defect (VSD). Chest radiograph demonstrates clamshell occlusion device across a muscular VSD prior to complete repair of double-outlet right ventricle.

strated and differentiated from sinus venosus and ostium primum defects (Fig. 10). Long-axis left ventriculography is important to exclude associated VSD or PDA.

MAGNETIC RESONANCE IMAGING

MRI in the four-chamber projection through the atrial septum may clearly show an ASD (Fig. 11).

PROGNOSIS

The prognosis after surgical correction is excellent. Large left-to-right shunts should be closed in childhood. Closure of ASD by interventional catheter techniques is infrequently performed (Fig. 12). Closure of small defects is controversial. Complications of untreated patients mainly relate to arrhythmia, late pulmonary hypertension, and right-to-left embolization.

OSTIUM PRIMUM ATRIAL SEPTAL DEFECT AND ENDOCARDIAL CUSHION DEFECT (ATRIOVENTRICULAR CANAL)

These lesions result from abnormal development of the embryologic endocardial cushion that produces, in its milder form, a defect limited to the lower portion of the atrial septum and an associated cleft mitral valve (ostium primum ASD); the complete form produces an associ-

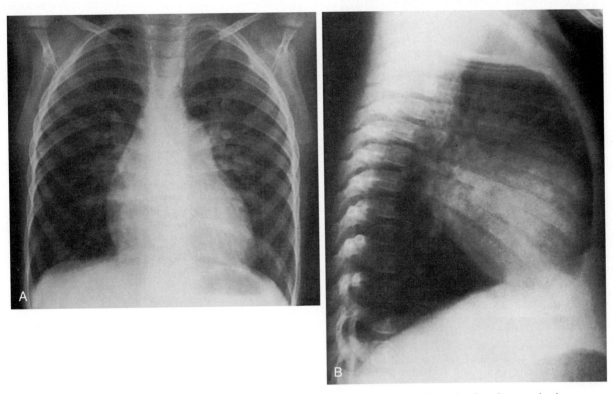

FIGURE 8. Atrial septal defect (ASD), secundum type. AP **(A)** and lateral **(B)** chest radiographs show increased pulmonary vascularity and moderate cardiomegaly. Fullness of the right heart border (right atrium) and relatively inconspicuous superior vena cava and aortic arch are common findings with this lesion. Right ventricular dilatation fills in the retrosternal space in the lateral view.

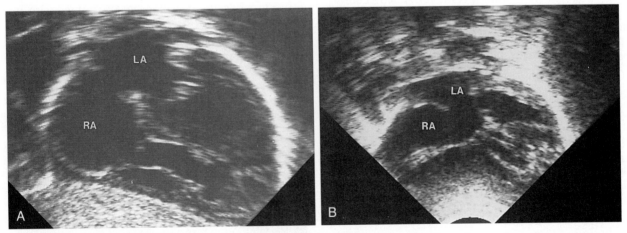

FIGURE 9. A, Ostium secundum atrial septal defect (ASD). Subxiphoid four-chamber echocardiogram demonstrates a large defect in the midportion of the atrial septum, typical of an ostium secundum defect. Enlargement of the right atrium *(RA)* is also noted. *LA* = left atrium. **B,** Ostium primum ASD. Subxiphoid four-chamber echocardiogram demonstrates a large defect in the lower portion of the atrial septum extending to the level of the mitral and tricuspid valves. Note that the mitral and tricuspid valves are at the same level, typical of an endocardial cushion defect. *RA* = right atrium; *LA* = left atrium.

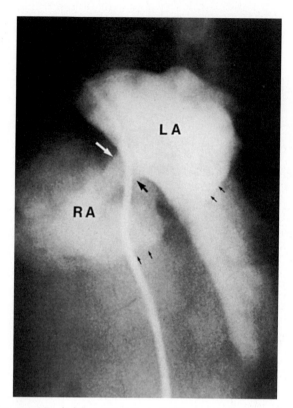

FIGURE 10. Atrial septal defect (ASD), secundum type. Four-chamber hepatoclavicular angiocardiogram with contrast injected into a right upper lobe pulmonary vein. Contrast streams along the interatrial septum and through an ostium secundum ASD *(large arrows)*. Mitral and tricuspid valves *(small arrows)* are apparent. *RA* = right atrium; *LA* = left atrium.

ated VSD and common atrioventricular (AV) valve (AVC). Associated lesions include PDA, coarctation, pulmonary valvular stenosis (PVS), pulmonary atresia, tricuspid atresia, transposition of the great arteries, tetralogy of Fallot, and total anomalous pulmonary venous return.

PATHOPHYSIOLOGY

Mild to moderate left-to-right shunting occurs predominantly at the atrial level. Pulmonary hypertension develops more commonly in patients with Down syndrome than in others.

CLINICAL MANIFESTATIONS

Clinical findings are similar to those of ostium secundum lesions, although more dramatic in the complete endocardial cushion defect and in those patients with Down syndrome (30% to 40% of patients with AVC). Failure to thrive, dyspnea, fatigue, and occasionally CHF and cyanosis may be seen.

CHEST RADIOGRAPHY

Radiographic findings include (1) mild to moderate cardiomegaly with right atrial and right ventricular enlargement, (2) occasional left atrial enlargement related to mitral insufficiency, (3) moderate increased pulmonary vascularity, (4) moderate pulmonary disease, and (5) 11 pairs of ribs and accessory sternal ossification centers, frequently added findings in Down syndrome patients (Fig. 13). The differential diagnosis includes ASD, PDA, and VSD.

ECHOCARDIOGRAPHY

Real-time evaluation demonstrates echo dropout in the lower atrial septum (see Fig. 9B). Displacement of the anterior mitral valve leaflet into the left ventricular outflow tract may be observed along with abnormal anterior excursion of the anterior mitral valve leaflet. In complete AVC, abnormal orientation and an oval or figure-8 configuration of the AV valve are frequently seen. The adjacent membranous VSD will also be evident, with anomalous chordal attachment and prominent papillary muscles frequently noted. A common leaflet bridging the VSD may be seen (Fig. 14). In partial AVC (ostium primum ASD), Doppler interrogation in the right atrium demonstrates a positive flow pattern in diastole, whereas in those patients with complete AVCs, a similar systolic positive flow pattern will be evident in the right ventricle (see Section V, Part I, Chapter 2, Fig. 20, page 1242).

ANGIOCARDIOGRAPHY

In patients with an ostium primum ASD, a biplane four-chamber angiocardiogram performed with injec-

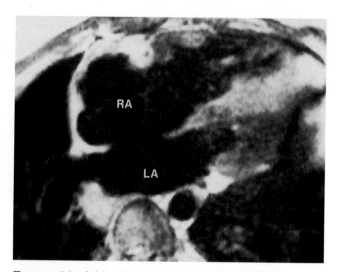

FIGURE 11. Axial oblique magnetic resonance image in the four-chamber projection demonstrates a large secundum atrial septal defect. The defect could not be visualized well by echocardiography in this 12-year-old obese patient. *RA* = right atrium; *LA* = left atrium.

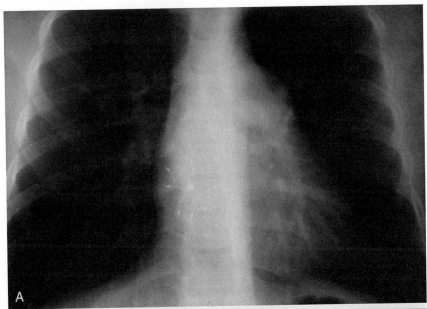

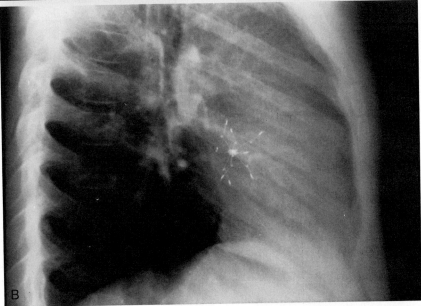

FIGURE 12. Frontal **(A)** and lateral **(B)** chest radiographs demonstrate a clamshell occlusion device utilized for catheter closure of an ostium secundum atrial septal defect.

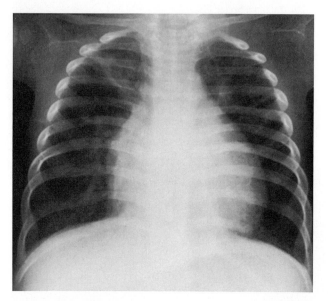

FIGURE 13. Atrioventricular canal. A chest radiograph demonstrates moderate cardiomegaly with a round (globular) cardiac silhouette having a prominent right atrium and right ventricle. There is increased pulmonary flow with a relatively narrow cardiac base. Patchy right upper lobe and left lower lobe pulmonary disease is commonly seen in patients with Down syndrome.

tion into the right upper lobe pulmonary vein identifies the ostium primum ASD and left-to-right shunt. A long-axial left ventriculogram will identify the left ventricular outflow tract abnormality ("gooseneck" deformity) related to the abnormal position of the mitral valve, and also demonstrate the mitral valve cleft and severity of mitral regurgitation. No ventricular shunting should be seen. Patients with a complete AVC will demonstrate on long-axis and four-chamber left ventriculograms a left-to-right shunt through a VSD. The common AV valve, the severity of mitral regurgitation, abnormal chordal attachments, and left ventricular size and function will be identified on these injections (Fig. 15). If pulmonary hypertension is present, a

right ventriculogram in the axial projections to evaluate the VSD may be necessary. An aortogram may be necessary to exclude a PDA and, occasionally, coarctation. Other injections may be needed to exclude other associated lesions.

PROGNOSIS

Simple ostium primum ASDs have an excellent prognosis with early surgery before the age of 5 years. Catheter closure techniques have now been developed and are in limited use. The prognosis in complete AVC defects is good. Early surgery is necessary prior to the development of significant pulmonary vascular disease. This may necessitate pulmonary artery banding in infancy. Residual AV valvular dysfunction is a common problem with complete AVC defects.

PATENT DUCTUS ARTERIOSUS

PDA represents the persistence of a vital normal embryologic structure, the sixth aortic arch, that connects the pulmonary artery and the upper descending aorta. This structure may persist on either side, but normally the right involutes while the left persists. The ductus normally closes after birth and becomes a residual fibrous cord (ligamentum arteriosum) that may calcify. PDA occurs once in 2500 to 5000 live births, constitutes approximately 10% of CHD, and is more common in females. PDA in premature infants may be as common as 21% to 35%.

PATHOPHYSIOLOGY

Closure of the ductus arteriosus begins immediately after birth with the onset of normal respiration and the fall of pulmonary vascular resistance. Ninety percent of the ductus arteriosus has closed by 2 months of age.

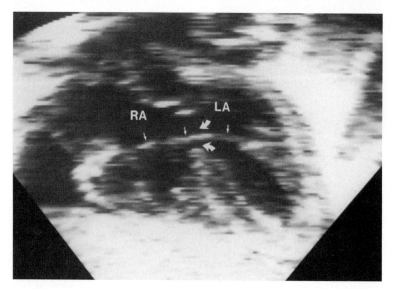

FIGURE 14. Complete atrioventricular (AV) canal. Subcostal four-chamber projection demonstrates the atrial and ventricular septal defects *(upper* and *lower curved arrows)* and the large common anterior leaflet *(small arrows)* traversing the AV orifice. *RA* = right atrium; *LA* = left atrium. (From Jaffe RB: Ventricular atrioventricular defect—echocardiography. *In* Elliott LP [ed]: Cardiac Imaging in Infants, Children, and Adults. Philadelphia, JB Lippincott, 1991, with permission.)

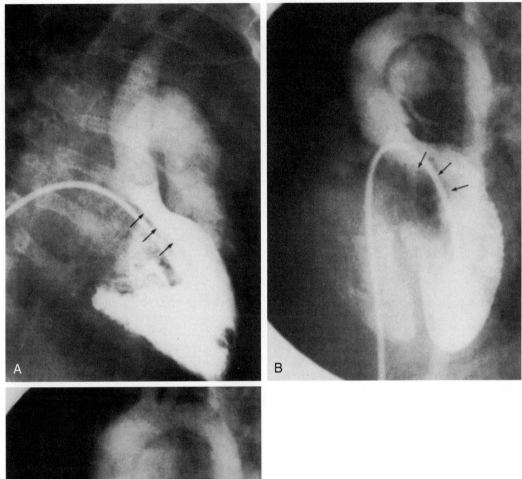

FIGURE 15. Atrioventricular (AV) canal. **A,** Long-axis left ventriculogram (frontal tube view) demonstrates malposition of the mitral valve, with the anterior leaflet projecting into the left ventricular outflow tract (gooseneck deformity) *(arrows)*. An absence or altered alignment of the normal straight segment of the proximal interventricular septum is apparent. **B,** Long-axis lateral view in diastole again shows the medial malposition of the mitral valve opening into the left ventricular outflow tract *(arrows)*. Note the ventricular septal defect (VSD) and common AV valve. **C,** Long-axis left ventriculogram in systole shows the posterior VSD component *(arrow)* and the chordae *(arrowheads)* as they attach to the interventricular septum.

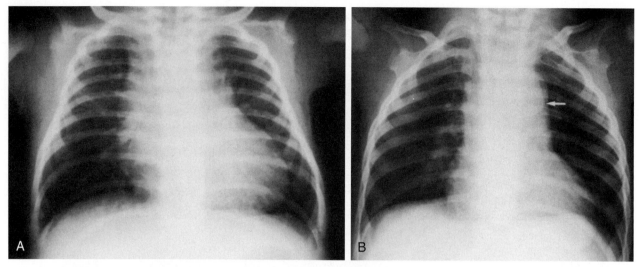

FIGURE 16. Patent ductus arteriosus. **A,** Chest radiograph in a 3-week-old infant with increased pulmonary vascularity, cardiomegaly, and a prominent right ventricle. The base of the heart is obscured by the thymus. The aortic arch pushes the trachea to the right. Enlargement of the aorta secondary to the patent ductus is not seen. **B,** Enlarged left aortic arch shows a second lateral "ductus bump" *(arrow)* and a slight prominence of the descending thoracic aorta. The mildly increased prominence of the central hilar vessels is related to the left-to-right shunt, and cardiomegaly is present.

Closure is delayed in premature infants with respiratory distress and hypoxia. Persistence of the ductus is probably multifactorial, with genetic factors and rubella being contributing factors. Blood flow is predominantly left to right from the aorta into the pulmonary artery, although right-to-left shunting (persistent fetal circulation) will occur in the presence of severe lung disease and pulmonary hypertension.

CLINICAL MANIFESTATIONS

An infant with a small patent ductus normally has no clinical manifestations except for a murmur. With a larger ductus, failure to thrive and CHF are seen in 40% of children under 2 years of age. Classically, a machinery-like murmur is heard in the pulmonic area, and the second sound is accentuated. PDA is often associated with such conditions as VSD, coarctation, aortic stenosis, PVS, and mitral regurgitation.

CHEST RADIOGRAPHY

Chest radiograms in patients with significant shunting will show (1) increased pulmonary blood flow (Fig. 16A); (2) cardiomegaly; (3) a prominent ascending aorta and aortic arch; (4) focal aortic dilatation (ductus bump) (Fig. 16B); and (5) left atrial enlargement. Primary differential diagnoses are VSD, aortico-pulmonary window, and truncus arteriosus.

ECHOCARDIOGRAPHY

Real-time echocardiography will frequently demonstrate the patent ductus from the suprasternal notch projection or modified short-axis view (Fig. 17). Dopp-

ler interrogation of the pulmonary artery, however, has proved to be a much more sensitive diagnostic modality (Fig. 18). Color Doppler rapidly identifies the left-to-right shunting through a PDA (see Section V, Part I, Chapter 2, Fig. 23, page 1244). An increased aortic:left atrial ratio is frequent.

ANGIOCARDIOGRAPHY

Again, as with ASD, echocardiography is the only preoperative examination performed in simple cases. When indicated, biplane left ventriculography or aortography, or both, are performed, preferably in the

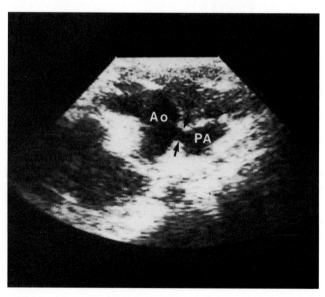

FIGURE 17. Patent ductus arteriosus. Short-axis echocardiogram shows a defect in the aortic *(Ao)* wall and continuity between the aortic arch and pulmonary artery *(PA) (arrow)*.

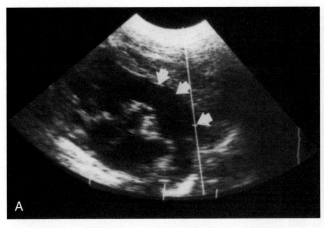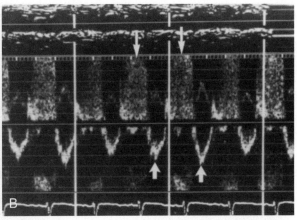

FIGURE 18. Patent ductus arteriosus (PDA). **A,** Doppler real-time parasagittal longitudinal image demonstrates a large main pulmonary artery *(top two arrows)* with a Doppler sample marker *(bottom arrow)* at the pulmonary artery junction of the PDA. **B,** Doppler image demonstrates pandiastolic retrograde pulmonary artery flow *(long arrows)*, which represents a positive Doppler signal directed toward the transducer head. *Short arrows* represent systolic forward pulmonary artery flow.

long-axis projection (Fig. 19; see also Section V, Part I, Chapter 2, Fig. 12A, page 1238). The ductus can be quantitated with respect to size and shunt in this view. Other lesions (i.e., VSD, coarctation, etc.), must be ruled out. The differential angiographic diagnosis includes aorticopulmonary window and truncus arteriosus.

PROGNOSIS

The prognosis is excellent with surgery before 24 months of age. Operative mortality is extremely low. Indomethacin is often a successful method of ductus closure in the neonate. Nonsurgical catheter closure has been successful in over 90% of patients (over 8 kg) (Fig. 20). Rarely stenosis of the left pulmonary artery may occur after coil occlusion. Complications of delayed surgical closure include pulmonary vascular occlusive disease, bacterial endocarditis and mycotic aneurysm of the left pulmonary artery, and aneurysm of the ductus arteriosus. Inadvertent ligation of the left pulmonary artery during attempted PDA closure is an uncommon but serious operative complication (Fig. 21) in neonates and infants.

ANEURYSM OF THE DUCTUS ARTERIOSUS

Aneurysm of the ductus arteriosus is relatively rare. These aneurysms are usually discovered at birth or shortly thereafter. They involve the entire length of the ductus arteriosus, although in some cases the pulmonary end is occluded when first diagnosed. At the time of diagnosis or shortly thereafter, thrombus usually forms in the aneurysm. The etiology is thought to relate to the relative weakening of the aortic end of the ductus during normal involution. In the infantile form, embolization, rupture, infection, and nerve palsy are rare complications.

The aneurysm is often first suspected on a newborn chest film because of abnormal mass or density in

the area of the main pulmonary artery and aortic arch (Fig. 22A). Sometimes the diagnosis is made during echocardiography. Confirmation of the diagnosis is possible in a noninvasive manner with MRI (Fig. 22B). This will usually show an area of increased signal on T_1-weighted spin-echo images in the region of the ductus arteriosus secondary to thrombus formation. Low-signal flow voids may be seen if the ductus is still open or with turbulence around a partial clot. Confirmation may also be obtained with contrast-enhanced spiral computed tomography or angiography.

Some controversy persists related to the significance of a ductus aneurysm. If there is evidence of good thrombus formation within several days, most cardiologists will continue to monitor the patient without operative intervention. Persistence of flow in the aneurysm, signs of infection, rupture, or embolization are indications for operation.

OTHER ACYANOTIC CONGENITAL HEART DISEASE WITH LEFT-TO-RIGHT SHUNTS

AORTICOPULMONARY WINDOW

An aorticopulmonary window represents the failure of the septa dividing the truncus arteriosus to fuse. This leaves a communication between the ascending aorta and pulmonary artery immediately above the aortic valve. The presence of this oval defect creates a major high-pressure left-to-right shunt. An aorticopulmonary window is usually an isolated lesion but may be associated with VSD and PDA. Occasionally ASD, an interrupted aortic arch, coarctation, subaortic stenosis, and an anomalous coronary artery have been noted.

Clinical Manifestations

Tachypnea, tachycardia, and cardiomegaly are common. A systolic murmur may be heard along the left sternal border; a diastolic murmur may occur when an

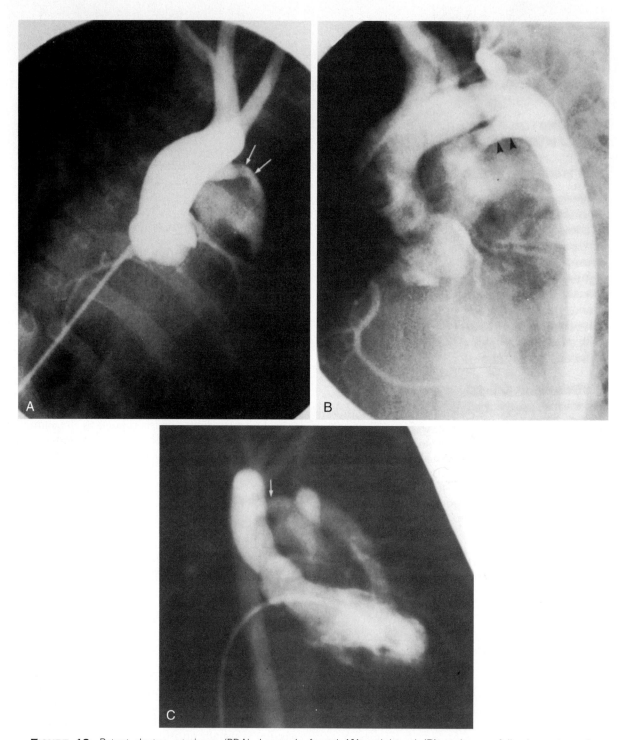

FIGURE 19. Patent ductus arteriosus (PDA). Long-axis frontal **(A)** and lateral **(B)** angiogram following retrograde catheterization demonstrate a moderately large left-to-right shunt through a PDA with a left aortic arch *(arrows)* (see also Section V, Part I, Chapter 2, Fig. 12*A*, page 1238). Minor pulmonary insufficiency can often be seen with this examination. **C,** PDA *(arrow)* originates from the right aortic arch and extends to the left to a normal main pulmonary artery with a moderate left-to-right shunt (see also Section V, Part III, Chapter 1, Fig. 14, page 1348).

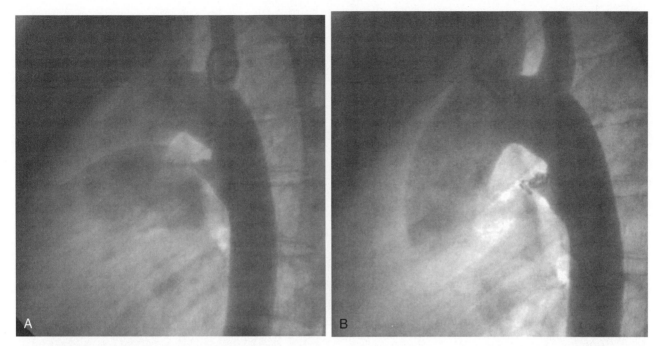

FIGURE 20. Gianturco coil closure of patent ductus arteriosus (PDA) in a 15-year-old girl. **A,** Lateral digital aortogram demonstrates a PDA with filling of the pulmonary artery. A jet of contrast is seen through the distal end of the patent ductus. **B,** Lateral digital aortogram after Gianturco coil occlusion demonstrates closure of the ductus arteriosus. The majority of the coil is in the ampulla of the ductus arteriosus, and approximately one turn of the coil is in the superior aspect of the left pulmonary artery. Significant narrowing of the left pulmonary artery is a rare complication of coil occlusion.

aorticopulmonary window is associated with pulmonary insufficiency. The pulses are frequently bounding.

Chest Radiography

Abnormal radiographic findings include (1) cardiomegaly with a nonspecific silhouette, (2) an enlarged left atrium, (3) increased pulmonary blood flow related to the left-to-right shunt, and (4) prominence of the ascending aorta and pulmonary artery. Primary differential diagnostic considerations are truncus arteriosus and PDA.

Echocardiography

Findings are similar to those in other left-to-right shunts with left atrial enlargement. The actual defect between the great vessels may be seen with real-time and color-flow Doppler studies.

Angiography

Aortic root injection with biplane AP and lateral cineangiography will demonstrate the left-to-right shunt near the aortic root (Fig. 23). Differentiation from truncus arteriosus is critical and may be accomplished by identification of two separate semilunar valves. With a large shunt, at least 2 ml/kg of contrast must be injected into the aortic root or left ventricle through a relatively large catheter in minimal time.

Prognosis

The prognosis is good with early surgery prior to the development of pulmonary vascular occlusive disease.

ANOMALOUS ORIGIN OF A PULMONARY ARTERY FROM THE AORTA (HEMITRUNCUS ARTERIOSUS)

This rare anomaly is characterized by anomalous origin of a pulmonary artery, usually the right (88%), from the ascending aorta. The other pulmonary artery, usually the left, is a continuation of the main pulmonary artery arising from the right ventricle (see Section V, Part III, Chapter 2, Table 1, page 1358). A PDA is present in up to 80% of patients. The aortic arch is usually left-sided.

Clinical Manifestations

Clinical manifestations include, in almost all patients, the rapid development in infancy of CHF from the large left-to-right shunt. If the malformation is not recognized and corrected at an early age, pulmonary vascular obstructive disease rapidly develops in both lungs.

Chest Radiography

Patients with aberrant origin of the pulmonary artery from the ascending aorta show (1) increased pulmonary blood flow to the lung supplied by the aberrant artery, unless complicated by pulmonary hypertension

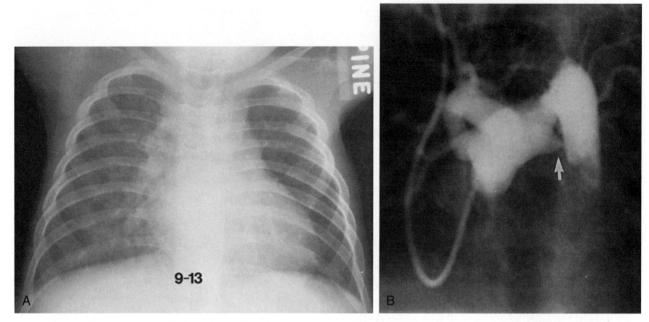

FIGURE 21. Inadvertent ligation of the left pulmonary artery during attempted patent ductus arteriosus (PDA) closure. **A,** Chest radiograph 5 months and 10 days after attempted PDA closure demonstrates asymmetric pulmonary blood flow, decreased to the left lung and increased to the right lung in this patient with Down syndrome. **B,** Left anterior oblique pulmonary cineangiocardiogram demonstrates inadvertent ligation of the left pulmonary artery at its origin (arrow), PDA, and filling of the proximal descending thoracic aorta. There was delayed collateral filling of the distal left pulmonary artery from the left intercostal collaterals (not illustrated). (From Jaffe RB, Orsmond GS, Veasy LG: Inadvertent ligation of the left pulmonary artery. Radiology 1986;161:355–357, with permission.)

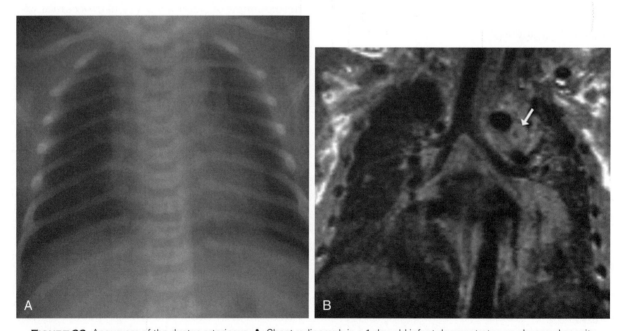

FIGURE 22. Aneurysm of the ductus arteriosus. **A,** Chest radiograph in a 1-day-old infant demonstrates an abnormal opacity in the left mediastinum in the region of the left aortic arch. The pulmonary blood flow and heart size are normal. **B,** Coronal T_1-weighted spin-echo magnetic resonance image performed at 6 days of age demonstrates abnormal increased signal intensity consistent with near-complete thrombosis of the aneurysm of the ductus arteriosus (arrow). A portion of the aortic arch is seen as a flow void superior and medial to the ductal aneurysm.

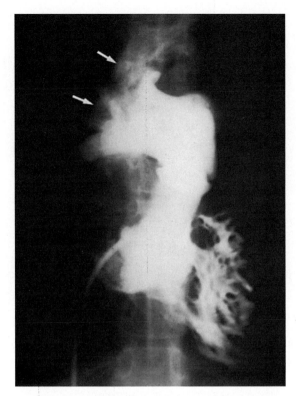

FIGURE 23. Aorticopulmonary window. A right ventriculogram demonstrates minor right-to-left shunting through an aorticopulmonary defect and opacification of the ascending aorta *(arrows)*. The left ventriculogram (not shown) showed a much larger left-to-right shunt through the defect, but the lesion itself was less well appreciated.

(Fig. 24); (2) CHF; and (3) cardiomegaly with right heart and main pulmonary artery enlargement.

Echocardiography

The diagnosis can readily be made on two-dimensional examination. In the most common form, the main pulmonary artery continues as the left pulmonary artery, best appreciated in the short-axis high parasternal projection, while the right pulmonary artery is seen to originate from the ascending aorta.

Angiocardiography

Selective right ventricular injection will demonstrate absence of the normal pulmonary artery bifurcation (Fig. 25A). Typically the left pulmonary artery is a continuation of the main pulmonary artery. An aortogram or left ventricular angiogram will demonstrate origin of the aberrant pulmonary artery from the proximal ascending aorta, and can confirm the presence of an associated PDA (Fig. 25B).

Prognosis

The prognosis is good with early recognition and operative anastomosis of the aberrant pulmonary artery to the main pulmonary artery. If diagnosis is delayed, pulmonary vascular obstructive disease rapidly develops, with an extremely poor prognosis.

ANOMALOUS ORIGIN OF THE LEFT CORONARY ARTERY

This rare congenital malformation creates a small left-to-right shunt as blood flows from a normal right coronary artery into the low-pressure system of the left coronary artery arising from the base of the pulmonary artery. As pulmonary resistance drops, the left coronary artery blood flow into the myocardium diminishes, resulting in left ventricular hypoxemia, ventricular dilatation, and dysfunction.

Clinical Manifestations

CHF, failure to thrive, irritability, and respiratory infections usually commence in the second month of life.

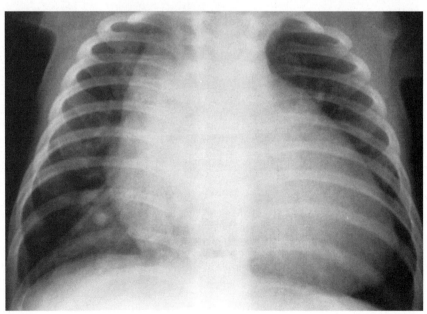

FIGURE 24. A 1-year-old infant with anomalous origin of the right pulmonary artery from the aorta. Increased pulmonary blood flow to the right lower lung is seen with moderate cardiomegaly.

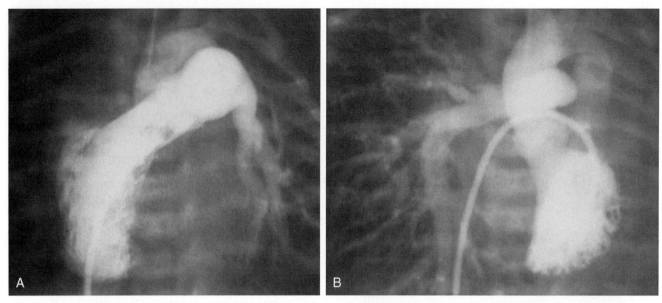

FIGURE 25. A 2-week-old infant with anomalous origin of the right pulmonary artery from the aorta and small patent ductus arteriosus. **A,** Right ventricular injection in the frontal projection demonstrates a dextroposed right ventricle with filling of the main and left pulmonary artery. Right-to-left shunt flow through a small patent ductus opacifies the aortic arch. **B,** Left ventricular injection in the frontal projection demonstrates origin of the right pulmonary artery from the ascending aorta.

Pallor, sweating, and dyspnea may also be present. The electrocardiogram is probably more helpful in this condition than with most other congenital heart lesions, showing a pattern of anterior myocardial infarction. Thallium radionuclide cardiac scanning can show decreased coronary perfusion and confirm the presence of myocardial ischemia.

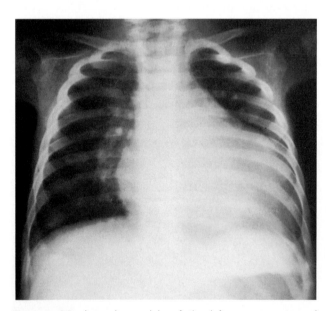

FIGURE 26. Anomalous origin of the left coronary artery. A 6-month-old infant presented with CHF, cardiomegaly, and the left coronary artery arising from the pulmonary artery. The primary differential consideration is that of cardiomyopathy. Confirmation of the diagnosis with ultrasound or aortography is usually necessary. Compression of the left main stem bronchus by the large left atrium and left ventricle produces left lower lobe atelectasis.

Chest Radiography

Marked cardiac enlargement secondary to left ventricular dilatation and left atrial enlargement is present (Fig. 26). CHF is common and frequently associated with pneumonia. Primary differential diagnoses include endocardial fibroelastosis and other cardiomyopathies.

Echocardiography

Two-dimensional echocardiography demonstrates (1) left ventricular and left atrial enlargement, (2) decreased left ventricular contractility, (3) enlargement of the right coronary artery, (4) mitral regurgitation, and (5) occasional identification of the anomalous left coronary artery arising from the base of the pulmonary artery.

Angiocardiography

Left ventriculography demonstrates (1) left ventricular dilatation, (2) diminished function, and (3) mitral regurgitation. A supravalvular aortogram demonstrates (1) enlargement of the right coronary artery, (2) an absence of a left coronary artery on early films, and (3) late visualization of the retrograde filling of the left coronary artery through collaterals emptying into the pulmonary artery (Fig. 27).

Prognosis

The prognosis is guarded depending on the severity of left ventricular dysfunction. Early surgical correction is recommended, with a bypass graft or relocation of the left coronary artery to the aorta.

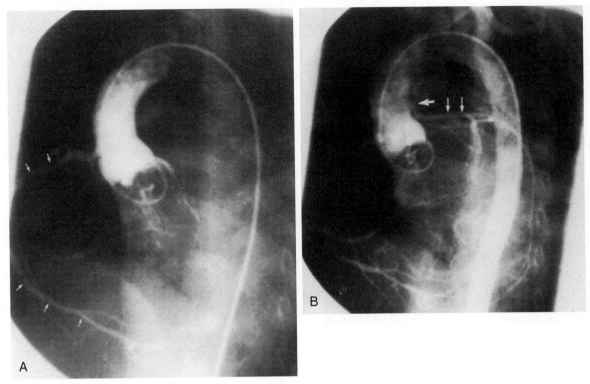

FIGURE 27. Anomalous origin of the left coronary artery. **A,** Long-axis lateral retrograde aortogram shows enlargement of the right coronary artery *(arrows)* and a failure to visualize the left coronary artery. **B,** A later film shows retrograde filling of the left coronary artery and flow into the main pulmonary artery *(arrows)*.

CORONARY ARTERY ARTERIOVENOUS FISTULA

This rare malformation relates to the anomalous development of a major branch coronary artery connecting directly to a large venous channel that drains directly into the right heart (90%) or occasionally into the left heart. When the anomaly drains into the right heart, a left-to-right shunt occurs.

Clinical Manifestation

Signs are rare except when failure results from the large left-to-right shunt. A continuous murmur may be heard over the precardium. Clinically a PDA, aorticopulmonary window, VSD with aortic insufficiency, systemic arteriovenous fistulas, and ruptured sinus of Valsalva aneurysm are differential considerations.

Chest Radiography

Radiographic findings are frequently normal. Cardiomegaly may be present because of a left-to-right shunt with associated increased pulmonary blood flow. Abnormal bulges on the cardiac silhouette may relate to the aneurysmally dilated anomalous vessels. Differential diagnoses primarily involve PDA, aorticopulmonary window, and truncus arteriosus.

Echocardiography

An echocardiogram with real-time and Doppler study easily identifies the enlarged coronary artery and left-to-right shunt. Frequently it may be followed to its point of insertion into the draining cardiac chamber. Paradoxical septal motion may occur with a large right atrial shunt.

Angiocardiography

Aortic root or selected coronary artery injections will readily demonstrate the large, dilated, and frequently tortuous coronary artery (Fig. 28). The drainage point can usually be identified with biplane angiography. The normal coronary branches may be small and difficult to visualize because of differential flow through the low-resistance fistula.

Prognosis

The prognosis is good with surgical correction.

ISOLATED PARTIAL ANOMALOUS PULMONARY VENOUS RETURN

Common sites of involvement are the right lung (two thirds) and left lung (one third). Drainage occurs to the SVC (50%), right atrium, inferior vena cava

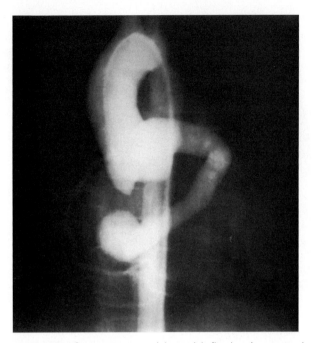

FIGURE 28. Coronary artery–right atrial fistula. A retrograde aortogram in the anteroposterior projection shows a large aneurysmally dilated left posterior circumflex coronary artery emptying into the right atrium. Other branches of the right and left coronary arteries appear uninvolved. (From Jaffe RB, Glancy DL, Epstein SE, et al: Coronary artery–right heart fistula. Circulation 1973;47:133, with permission.)

(IVC), azygos vein, and coronary sinus. The fairly common anomalous pulmonary venous drainage of the right lung to the IVC produces the so-called scimitar syndrome, with associated hypoplasia of the right lung and systemic arterial supply to the right lower lung.

Clinical Manifestations

Unless more than 50% of the pulmonary flow drains to the right heart, clinical manifestations are rare. In this instance, failure related to the left-to-right shunt may be present. Most patients with scimitar syndrome have a small right hemithorax and an increased incidence of pulmonary infection.

Chest Radiography

Patients with scimitar syndrome typically demonstrate (1) a crescent-shaped vessel paralleling the lower right heart border and enlarging in size as it approaches the cardiophrenic angle, (2) hypoplasia of the right lung, (3) varying degrees of cardiac dextroposition, (4) a small right pulmonary artery, and (5) systemic artery supply to the right lower lung from the aorta, or celiac artery (see Section V, Part I, Chapter 2, Fig. 6, page 1234).

Other forms of isolated partial anomalous pulmonary venous return (PAPVR) rarely show specific abnormalities on chest radiography. A large shunt may create cardiomegaly and right heart enlargement with increased pulmonary flow. Occasionally the horizontal anomalous course of a pulmonary vein (Fig. 29), or the

vertical course of a dilated left vertical vein, may be specifically identified.

Echocardiography

With scimitar syndrome, real-time echocardiography may demonstrate (1) the anomalous vein entering the IVC, (2) a small right pulmonary artery, and (3) an anomalous artery supplying a sequestration.

Angiography

Selective biplane AP and lateral pulmonary arteriograms will demonstrate the anomalous venous drainage of the multiple types described (Figs. 30 and 31). Thoracic and abdominal aortography should be performed to evaluate anomalous systemic pulmonary vasculature and sequestration.

Magnetic Resonance Imaging

MRI may be used to evaluate uncommon or atypical forms of PAPVR (Fig. 32).

Prognosis

Operative correction is not indicated with small isolated PAPVR. With sequestration and infection, lobectomy may be necessary. The aberrant systemic artery to the lung, typically the right lung, may be occluded by coil embolization (Fig. 33). Surgical correction of other large shunt lesions is also successful.

COMPLICATED PARTIAL ANOMALOUS PULMONARY VENOUS RETURN

PAPVR probably occurs more frequently than is suspected. It usually represents a limited left-to-right shunt and is of little clinical significance unless associated with

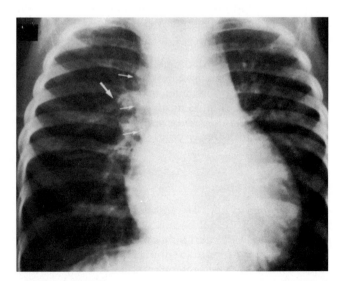

FIGURE 29. Posteroanterior chest film demonstrates anomalous pulmonary venous drainage of the right upper lobe *(large arrow)* into the dilated superior vena cava *(small arrows).*

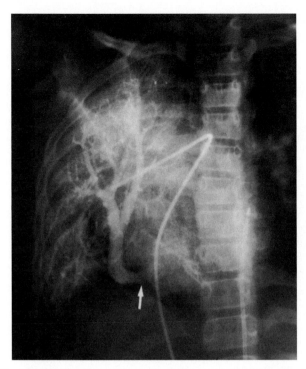

FIGURE 30. Scimitar syndrome (see Section V, Part I, Chapter 2, Fig. 6, page 1234). A late pulmonary venous-phase film after right pulmonary artery injection shows anomalous venous drainage below the diaphragm to the point of junction with the hepatic veins and inferior vena cava *(arrow)*. Hypoplasia of the right lung is present with an associated mediastinal shift to the right.

a sinus venosus ASD. Complicated PAPVR usually occurs with an ASD but may be encountered with tetralogy of Fallot, tricuspid atresia, common ventricle, VSD, and PDA. Approximately 50% of complicated PAPVR is associated with an ASD. The anomalous vein usually drains into the right atrium or SVC.

Clinical Manifestations

Signs and symptoms usually relate to the underlying lesion in this complicated variant rather than to the anomalous vein per se.

Chest Radiography

Plain film findings result from the underlying associated cardiac malformation. In the instance of sinus venosus ASD or other ASDs, they are predominantly those of (1) a left-to-right shunt, (2) right atrial dilatation, and (3) right ventricular enlargement. Differential considerations relate to the associated lesions, but most often to the ASDs.

Angiocardiography

Angiographic diagnosis is best accomplished after retrograde venous catheterization of the anomalous vein and injection into this vein with subsequent visualization of the SVC or, occasionally, direct filling of the right atrium. The latter may be difficult to differentiate from a sinus venosus defect. Four-chamber long-axis projec-

tions may be helpful in this instance. Angiography to otherwise define the other associated lesions must be appropriate for the lesions present. Selective AP and lateral pulmonary artery views may be helpful on occasion.

Prognosis

The prognosis with the associated ASD lesions is generally good. The prognosis for other variants relates primarily to the primary congenital malformation.

SINUS OF VALSALVA ANEURYSM

Sinus of Valsalva aneurysm is a rare malformation defined as localized dilatation of one of the aortic sinuses of Valsalva. The lesion may be either congenital or acquired. The incidence of this malformation has been reported as ranging from 0.1% to 3.5% of CHD.

Pathophysiology

Congenital sinus of Valsalva aneurysms are commonly associated with other congenital cardiac defects, most commonly a VSD. This is usually an outlet (supracristal) VSD (60%), with perimembranous defect significantly less frequent. Aortic insufficiency may develop in 30% to 40% of patients related to alteration in the valvular cusps secondary to prolapse of the sinus and aneurysmal expansion. Other occasionally associated congenital lesions include subaortic stenosis, ASD, infundibular pulmonary stenosis, coarctation, and Marfan syndrome. Acquired sinus of Valsalva aneurysms most often relate to inflammatory disease such as endocarditis.

The aneurysm usually involves the right coronary

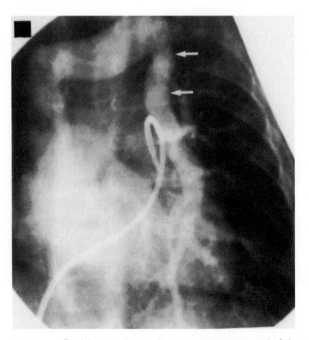

FIGURE 31. Partial anomalous pulmonary venous return. Left lung drains anomalously through a persistent left vertical vein *(arrows)* to the innominate vein and superior vena cava.

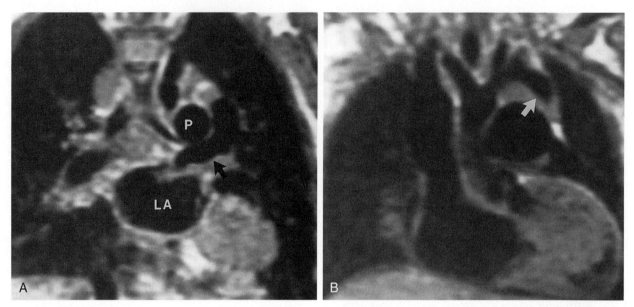

FIGURE 32. An 8-year-old boy with mitral stenosis, coarctation, and an unusual form of partial anomalous pulmonary venous return from the left lung. **A,** Coronal 3-mm magnetic resonance image demonstrates a levoatriocardinal vein *(arrow)* lateral to the pulmonary artery *(P)*. The vein communicates with the left atrium *(LA),* and then ascends vertically in the left mediastinum, receiving venous return from the left lung. Also note the paratracheal, carinal, and hilar adenopathy. **B,** The vein ascends in the left mediastinum *(arrow)* to empty into the left innominate vein.

sinus (80% to 90%), and less commonly the noncoronary sinus. The aneurysm may prolapse into and occlude the VSD, particularly an outlet VSD, and occasionally extend into the intraventricular septum. Rupture of the coronary sinus is usually into the right ventricle (70% to 80%), with almost all of the remainder extending into the right atrium.

Clinical Manifestations

Clinical manifestations of a nonruptured sinus of Valsalva aneurysm are rare. Occasionally a prolapsed aneurysm into the VSD or right ventricular outflow tracts may become symptomatic. Otherwise, symptoms primarily develop after rupture, which usually occurs

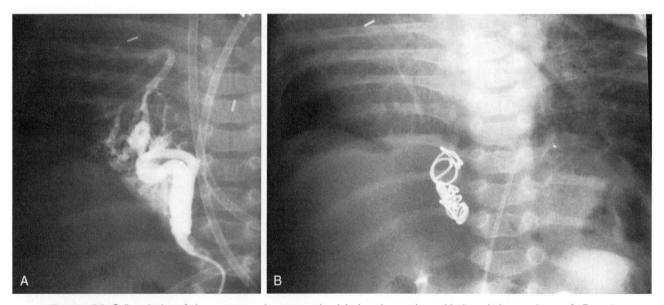

FIGURE 33. Coil occlusion of aberrant systemic artery to the right lung in a patient with the scimitar syndrome. **A,** Frontal angiogram during injection into the aberrant systemic artery after catheter passage from the abdominal aorta demonstrates opacification of the medial right lower lung and retrograde opacification of the right lower lobe pulmonary artery. **B,** Frontal radiograph of the upper abdomen and lower chest demonstrates multiple coils in the aberrant systemic artery following coil occlusion.

beyond 10 years of age. Primary symptoms relate to left-to-right shunt when the rupture is into the right ventricle or right atrium. Volume overload of the left heart may also occur in the rare instances in which rupture extends into the left ventricle and, of course, is complicated by aortic insufficiency. Clinical symptoms of shortness of breath, fatigue, tachycardia, and chest pain may develop, and auscultation usually reveals a continuous murmur.

Chest Radiography

Plain films in a nonruptured sinus of Valsalva aneurysm are usually normal. Following rupture, one identifies increasing heart size, increased pulmonary blood flow, or CHF, or any combination of these.

Echocardiography

Two-dimensional and Doppler echocardiography are sensitive in detecting sinus of Valsalva aneurysm, especially when rupture is present. Doppler manifestations are those of left-to-right shunt and aortic valvular insufficiency.

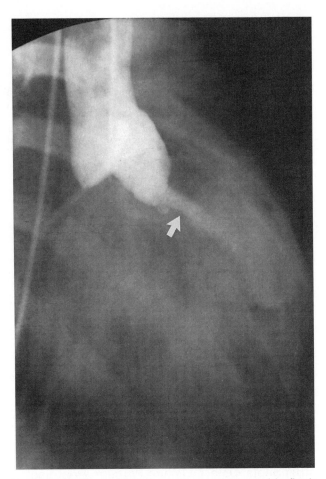

FIGURE 35. Sinus of Valsalva aneurysm–right ventricle fistula. Aortogram in the axial right anterior oblique projection demonstrates a right sinus of Valsalva aneurysm with fistulous communication *(arrow)* into the right ventricle.

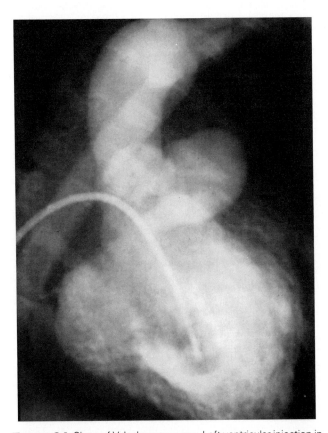

FIGURE 34. Sinus of Valsalva aneurysm. Left ventricular injection in the axial right anterior oblique projection demonstrates an enlarged left ventricle and right sinus of Valsalva aneurysm in a 6-year-old girl. An aortogram (not shown) demonstrated marked aortic regurgitation without fistulous communication to the right heart.

Angiocardiography

Angiocardiograms readily demonstrate not only the sinus of Valsalva aneurysm (Fig. 34) but also the effect of rupture and the direction of flow (Fig. 35). Injections are usually performed in the supravalvular region with long-axis biplane angiography, possibly supplemented with AP and lateral biplane angiography. The aneurysm itself is identified as a focal dilatation of the sinus of Valsalva with the direction of protrusion variable depending upon the sinus involved. Differential diagnostic considerations include aorticopulmonary window, coronary arteriovenous fistula, and aorticoatrial or aorticoventricular tunnel.

Prognosis

Treatment is operative repair, usually resecting portions of the aneurysm, then utilizing patch repair of the sinus, and the VSD, if present. On occasion, depending on the valvular anatomy, aortic valve replacement is necessary. Mortality is generally listed at 3% to 4%, although late death is a complication reported in some literature at 10% to 15%. Heart block is a significant complication.

SUGGESTED READINGS

Ventricular Septal Defect

Bremerich J, Reddy GP, Higgins CB: MRI of supracristal ventricular septal defects. J Comput Assist Tomogr 1999;23:13

Cheng CF, Wang JK, Wu MH: Morphological characterization of ventricular septal defect with posterior deviation of the outlet septum. Cardiology 1998;89:134

Didier D, Higgins CB: Identification and localization of ventricular septal defect by gated magnetic resonance imaging. Am J Cardiol 1986;57:1363

Du ZD, Roguin N, Wu XJ: Spontaneous closure of muscular ventricular septal defect identified by echocardiography in neonates. Cardiol Young 1998;8:500

Elliott LP, Bargeron LN Jr, Soto B, et al: Axial cineangiography in congenital heart disease. Radiol Clin North Am 1980;18:515

Green CE, Elliott LP, Bargeron LN Jr: Axial cineangiographic evaluation of the posterior ventricular septal defect. Am J Cardiol 1981;48:331

Helmcke F, de Souza A, Nanda NC, et al: Two-dimensional and color Doppler assessment of ventricular septal defect of congenital origin. Am J Cardiol 1989;63:1112–1116

Jaffe RB, Scherer JL: Supracristal ventricular septal defects: spectrum of associated lesions and complications. AJR Am J Roentgenol 1977;128:629

Santamaria H, Soto B, Ceballos R, at al: Differentiation of types of ventricular septal defects. AJR Am J Roentgenol 1983;141:273

Soto B, Bargeron LM Jr, Diethelm E: Ventricular septal defect. Semin Roentgenol 1985;20:200

Van Praagh R, Geva T, Kreutzer J: Ventricular septal defects: how shall we describe, name and classify them? J Am Coll Cardiol 1989;14:1298–1299

Yoo S-J, Lim T-H, Park I-S, et al: Defects of the interventricular septum of the heart: en face imaging in the oblique coronal plane. AJR Am J Roentgenol 1991;157:943–946

Atrial Septal Defect, Ostium Primum Atrial Septal Defect, and Endocardiol Cushion Defect (Atrioventricular Canal)

Diethelm L, Dery R, Lipton MJ, Higgins CB: Atrial-level shunts: sensitivity and specificity of MR in diagnosis. Radiology 1987;162:181–186

Driscoll DJ: Left-to-right shunt lesions. Pediatr Clin North Am 1999;46:355

Green CE, Gottdiener JS, Goldstein HA: Atrial septal defect. Semin Roentgenol 1985;20:214

Helgason H, Jonsdottir G: Spontaneous closure of atrial septal defects. Pediatr Cardiol 1999;20:195

Meisner H, Guenther T: Atrioventricular septal defect. Pediatr Cardiol 1998;19:276

Soto B, Bargeron LM, Pacifico AD, et al: Angiography of atrioventricular canal defect. Am J Cardiol 1981;48:492

Suzuki K, Tatsuno K, Kikuchi T, et al: Predisposing factors of valve regurgitation in complete atrioventricular septal defect. J Am Coll Cardiol 1998;32:1449

Tobin RB, Schwartz DC: Endocardial cushion defects: embryology, anatomy and angiography. AJR Am J Roentgenol 1981;136:157

Yoshida H, Funabashi T, Nakaya S, et al: Subxiphoid cross-sectional echocardiographic imaging of the "goose-neck" deformity in endocardial cushion defect. Circulation 1980;62:1319

Patent Ductus Arteriosus/Aneurysm Ductus Arteriosus

Carboni MP, Ringel RE: Ductus arteriosus in premature infants beyond the second week of life. Pediatr Cardiol 1997;18:372

Celiker A, Qureshi SA, Bilgic A: Transcatheter closure of patent arterial ducts using controlled-release coils. Eur Heart J 1997;18:359

Davis P, Turner-Gomes S, Cunningham K, et al: Precision and accuracy of clinical and radiological signs in premature infants at risk of patent ductus arteriosus. Arch Pediatr Adolesc Med 1995;149:1136

Forbes TL, Evans MG: Optimal elective management of patent ductus arteriosus in the older child. J Pediatr Surg 1996;31:765

Jaffe RB, Orsmond GS, Veasy LG: Inadvertent ligation of the left pulmonary artery. Radiology 1986;161:355–357

Laurin S, Sandstrom S, Ivancev K, et al: Ductus arteriosus aneurysm imaging using modern diagnostic methods. Acta Radiol 1992;33:285

Lee WJ, Chen SJ, Wu MH, et al: Regression of ductus arteriosus aneurysm in a neonate demonstrated by three-dimensional computed tomography. Int J Cardiol 1999;68:231

Lund JT, Hansen D, Brocks V, et al: Aneurysm of the ductus arteriosus in the neonate: three case reports with a review of the literature. Pediatr Cardiol 1992;13:222

Maisel P, Brenner J: Spontaneous closure and thrombosis of a ductal aneurysm in a neonate. Cardiol Young 1999;9:503

Newman B, Balsan M: Diagnosis of ductus arteriosus aneurysm by magnetic resonance imaging. J Perinatol 1997;17:402

Rothman A, Lucas VW, Sklansky MS, et al: Percutaneous coil occlusion of patent ductus arteriosus. J Pediatr 1997;130:447

Swischuk LE: Patent ductus arteriosus. Semin Roentgenol 1985;20:236

Verma R, Presti S, Danilowicz D: The intermittent ductus revisited: echocardiographic evidence and successful coil occlusion: a case report and review of literature. Cathet Cardiovasc Diagn 1998;45:260

Aortopulmonary Window

Bertolini A, Dalmonte P, Bava GL, et al: Aortopulmonary septal defects: a review of the literature and report of ten cases. J Cardiovasc Surg 1994;35:207

Garver KA, Hernandez RJ, Vermilion RP, et al: Images in cardiovascular medicine: Correlative imaging of aortopulmonary window: demonstration with echocardiography, angiography, and MRI. Circulation 1997;96:1036

Horimi H, Hasegawa T, Shiraishi H, et al: Detection of aortopulmonary window with ventricular septal defect by Doppler color flow imaging. Chest 1992;101:280

Incesu L, Baysal K, Kalayci AG, et al: Magnetic resonance imaging of proximal aortopulmonary window. Clin Imaging 1998;22:23

Tkebuchava T, von Segesser LK, Vogt PR, et al: Congenital aortopulmonary window: diagnosis, surgical technique and long-term results. Eur J Cardiothorac Surg 1997;11:293

Anomalous Origin of a Pulmonary Artery from the Aorta (Hemitruncus Arteriosus)

Choe YH, Kim YM, Han BK, et al: MR imaging in the morphologic diagnosis of congenital heart disease. Radiographics 1997;17:403

Duncan WJ, Freedom RM, Olley PM, et al: Two-dimensional echocardiographic identification of hemitruncus: anomalous origin of one pulmonary artery from ascending aorta with the other pulmonary artery arising normally from right ventricle. Am Heart J 1981;102:892

Fong LV, Anderson RH, Siewers RD, et al: Anomalous origin of one pulmonary artery from the ascending aorta: a review of echocardiographic, catheter, and morphological features. Br Heart J 1989;62:389

Freedom RM, Culham JAG, Moes CAF (eds): Hemitruncus arteriosus (anomalous origin of one pulmonary artery from the ascending aorta). In Angiocardiography of Congenital Heart Disease. New York, Macmillan, 1984:453

Gumbiner CH, Cheatham JP, Latson LA, et al: Radiological case of the month: anomalous origin of the right pulmonary artery from the aorta: "hemitruncus." Am J Dis Child 1989;143:1209

Kim TK, Choe YH, Kim HS, et al: Anomalous origin of the right pulmonary artery from the ascending aorta: diagnosis by magnetic resonance imaging. Cardiovasc Intervent Radiol 1995;18:118

Lin MH, Shen CT, Wang NK, et al: Magnetic resonance imaging of anomalous origin of the right pulmonary artery from the ascending aorta in association with ventricular septal defect. Am Heart J 1996;132:1073

Long WA, Perry JR, Henry GW: Radionuclide diagnosis of anomalous origin of the right pulmonary artery from the ascending aorta (so-called hemitruncus). Int J Cardiol 1985;84:492

Rosa U, Wade KC: CT findings in hemitruncus. J Comput Assist Tomogr 1987;11:698

Yoo S-J, Moes CAF, Burrows PE, et al: Pulmonary blood supply by a branch from the distal ascending aorta in pulmonary atresia with ventricular septal defect. Pediatr Cardiol 1993;14:230

Anomalous Origin of the Left Coronary Artery

Fisher EA, Sepehri B, Lendrum B, et al: Two-dimensional echocardiographic visualization of the left coronary artery in anomalous origin of the left coronary artery from the pulmonary artery. Circulation 1981;63:698

Greenberg MA, Fish BG, Spindola-Franco H: Congenital anomalies of the coronary arteries. Radiol Clin North Am 1989;23:1127

Houston AB, Pollock JC, Doig WB, et al: Anomalous origin of the left coronary artery from the pulmonary trunk: elucidation with color Doppler flow mapping. Br Heart J 1990;63:50

Karr SS, Parness IA, Spevak PJ, et al: Diagnosis of anomalous left coronary artery by Doppler color flow mapping: distinction from other causes of dilated cardiomyopathy. J Am Coll Cardiol 1992; 19:1271

Kececioglu D, Kotthoff S, Konertz W, et al: Pulmonary artery origin of the left coronary artery: diagnosis by transesophageal echocardiography in infancy. Eur Heart J 1993;14:1006

Kim SM, Park CH, Intenzo CM, et al: Thallium-201 imaging in anomalous left coronary artery originating from pulmonary trunk. Clin Nucl Med 1989;14:492

White CS, Laskey WK, Stafford JL, et al: Coronary MRA: use in assessing anomalies of coronary artery origin. J Comput Assist Tomogr 1999;23:203

Wollenek G, Domanig E, Salzer-Muhar U, et al: Anomalous origin of the left coronary artery: a review of surgical management in 13 patients. J Cardiovascular Surg 1993;34:399

Coronary Artery Arteriovenous Fistula

Barbosa MM, Katina T, Oliveira HG, et al: Doppler echocardiographic features of coronary artery fistula: report of 8 cases. J Am Soc Echocardiogr 1999;12:149

Davis JT, Allen HD, Wheller JJ, et al: Coronary artery fistula in the pediatric age group: a 19-year institutional experience. Ann Thorac Surg 1994;58:760

Farooki ZQ, Nowlen T, Hakimi M, et al: Congenital coronary artery fistulae: a review of 18 cases with special emphasis on spontaneous closure. Pediatr Cardiol 1993;14:208

Fernandes ED, Kadivar H, Hallman GL, et al: Congenital malformations of the coronary arteries: the Texas Heart Institute experience. Ann Thorac Surg 1992;54:732

Jaffe RB, Glancy DL, Epstein SE, et al: Coronary artery–right heart fistula. Circulation 1973;47:122

Nawa S, Miyachi Y, Toshino N, et al: Congenital coronary artery fistulae arising from bilateral coronary arteries and emptying into both pulmonary artery and left ventricle: a rare presentation. Cardiology 1996;87:263

Pucillo AL, Schechter AG, Moggio RA, et al: MR imaging in the definition of coronary artery anomalies. J Comput Assist Tomogr 1990;14:171

Yoshimura N, Hamada S, Takamiya M, et al: Coronary artery anomalies with a shunt: evaluation with electron-beam CT. J Comput Assist Tomogr 1998;22:682

Partial Anomalous Pulmonary Venous Return

Budorick NE, McDonald V, Flisak ME, et al: The pulmonary veins. Semin Roentgenol 1989;24:127–140

Cao Y-A, Burrows PE, Benson LN, et al: Scimitar syndrome in infancy. J Am Coll Cardiol 1993;22:873

Chang YC, Li YW, Liu HM, et al: Findings of anomalous pulmonary venous return using MRI. J Formosan Med Assoc 1994;93:462

Godwin JD, Tarver RD: Scimitar syndrome: four new cases examined with CT. Radiology 1986;159:15–20

Greene R, Miller SW: Cross-sectional imaging of silent pulmonary venous anomalies. Radiology 1986;159:279–281

Hiramatsu T, Takanashi Y, Imai Y, et al: Atrial septal displacement for repair of anomalous pulmonary venous return into the right atrium. Ann Thorac Surg 1998;65:1110

Mullen JC, Waskiewich K, Bhargava R, et al: Bilateral partial anomalous pulmonary venous return. Can J Cardiol 1997;13:567

Senocak F, Oxme S, Bilgic A, et al: Partial anomalous pulmonary venous return: evaluation of 51 cases. Jpn Heart J 1994;35:43

Thorsen MK, Erickson SJ, Mewissen MW, et al: CT and MR imaging of partial anomalous pulmonary venous return to the azygos vein. J Comput Assist Tomogr 1990;14:1007

Van Meter C Jr, LeBlanc JG, Culpepper WS 3d, et al: Partial anomalous pulmonary venous return. Circulation 1990;82:195

Woodring JR, Howard TA, Kanga JF: Congenital pulmonary venolobar syndrome revisited. Radiographics 1994;14:349

Zwetsch B, Wicky S, Meuli R, et al: Three dimensional image reconstruction of partial anomalous pulmonary venous return to the superior vena cava. Chest 1995;108:1743

Sinus of Valsalva Aneurysm

Chiang CW, Lin FC, Fang BR, et al: Doppler and two-dimensional echocardiographic features of sinus of Valsalva aneurysm. Am Heart J 1988;116:1283

Choudhary SK, Bhan A, Sharma R, et al: Sinus of Valsalva aneurysms: 20 years' experience. J Cardiac Surg 1997;12:300

Dev V, Goswami KC, Shrivastava S, et al: Echocardiographic diagnosis of aneurysm of the sinus of Valsalva. Am Heart J 1993;126:930

Goldberg N, Krasnow N: Sinus of Valsalva aneurysm. Clin Cardiol 1990;13:831

Guo DW, Cheng TO, Lin ML, et al: Aneurysm of the sinus of Valsalva: a roentgenologic study of 105 Chinese patients. Am Heart J 1987;114:1169

Keren A, Guthaner DF: Echocardiographic diagnosis of aneurysm and dissecting hematoma of the thoracic aorta. In Elliott LP (ed): Cardiac Imaging in Infants, Children, and Adults. Philadelphia, JB Lippincott, 1991:305

Liang CD, Chang JP, Kao CL: Unruptured sinus of Valsalva aneurysm with right ventricular outflow tract obstruction associated with ventricular septal defect. Cathet Cardiovasc Diagn 1996;37:158

Liang CD, Su WJ: Aneurysm of the aortic sinus of Valsalva with reversed shunt of ductus arteriosus. Cathet Cardiovasc Diagn 1995;34:333

Mayer ED, Ruffman K, Saggau W, et al: Ruptured aneurysms of the sinus of Valsalva. Ann Thorac Surg 1986;42:81

Wang KY, St. John Sutton M, Ho HY, et al: Congenital sinus of Valsalva aneurysm: a multiplane transesophageal echocardiographic experience. J Am Soc Echocardiogr 1997;10:956

Chapter 2

ACYANOTIC CONGENITAL HEART DISEASE WITH NORMAL PULMONARY FLOW

VIRGIL R. CONDON and RICHARD B. JAFFE

PULMONARY VALVULAR STENOSIS WITH INTACT VENTRICULAR SEPTUM

Pulmonary valvular stenosis (PVS) with an intact ventricular septum is the most common of the acyanotic lesions with normal flow and accounts for approximately 10% of congenital heart disease (CHD), with some familial tendencies.

PATHOPHYSIOLOGY

Fusion of the leaflets produces a dome-like pulmonary valve with a small central or eccentric opening. Residual raphes may be seen fusing with the pulmonary artery wall. In severe forms, the valve is dysplastic with a small annulus and markedly thickened cusps (15% of PVS). Additional findings include (1) right ventricular hypertrophy, (2) hypoplasia of the tricuspid valve, (3) post-stenotic dilatation of the main and left pulmonary artery, (4) tricuspid regurgitation, and (5) right atrial enlargement.

CLINICAL MANIFESTATIONS

Except with the severely stenotic and dysplastic valve, in which case dyspnea and right heart failure may develop, other children have relatively few symptoms. Physical findings include (1) a precordial bulge, (2) an ejection murmur of moderate intensity in the left second anterior intercostal space, and (3) an injection click that varies with respiration. In severe cases with right heart failure, there may be (1) cyanosis from right-to-left atrial level shunting, (2) jugular "a" waves, (3) hepatomegaly, and (4) a regurgitant systolic murmur secondary to tricuspid insufficiency.

CHEST RADIOGRAPHY

Classic plain film findings with moderate to severe PVS include (1) dilatation of the main and left pulmonary arteries (Fig. 1; see also Section V, Part I, Chapter 2,

Fig. 9, page 1236); (2) right ventricular hypertrophy with elevation and uplifting of the cardiac apex and associated filling in the upper retrosternal space; and (3) right atrial enlargement when associated with tricuspid insufficiency. Patients with mild PVS may have a normal cardiac silhouette. The pulmonary flow is normal, and the aortic arch is on the left. Differential considerations include idiopathic dilatation of the pulmonary artery (particularly in older female children), left-to-right shunts (i.e., atrial septal defect [ASD]), and pulmonary hypertension, singly or in combination.

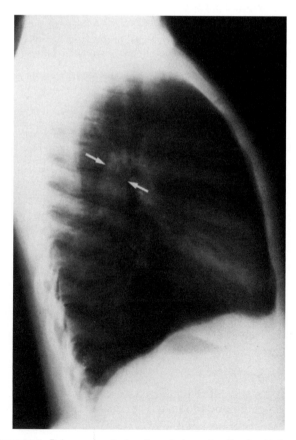

FIGURE 1. Pulmonary valvular stenosis (see also Section V, Part I, Chapter 2, Fig. 9, page 1236). A lateral chest radiograph demonstrates enlargement of the left pulmonary artery as an extension of the poststenotic dilatation from the main pulmonary artery *(arrows).*

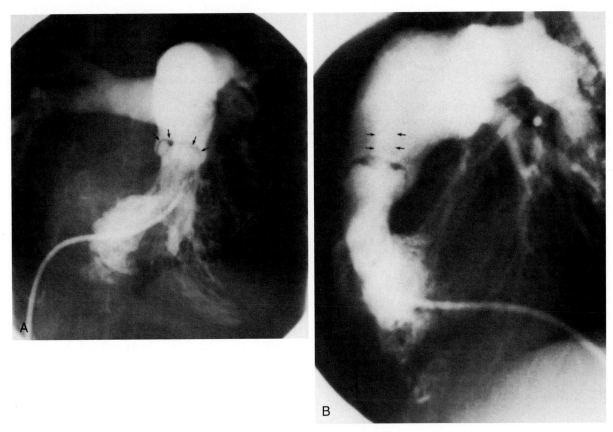

FIGURE 2. Pulmonary valvular stenosis. Anteroposterior **(A)** and lateral **(B)** sitting-up right ventriculograms show elongation of the right ventricular outflow tract with the stenotic domed pulmonary valve tangential to the central beam *(arrows)*. Characteristic thickening of the valve leaflets along with poststenotic dilatation of the main and left pulmonary arteries is apparent. A jet effect into the main pulmonary artery is evident in the lateral view *(arrows)*.

ECHOCARDIOGRAPHY

Real-time echocardiography will demonstrate (1) a thickened domed pulmonary valve, (2) a small pulmonary annulus when associated with a dysplastic valve, (3) right ventricular hypertrophy, and (4) early opening or exaggerated "a" dip of the posterior leaflet of the pulmonary valve. Doppler evaluation can accurately calculate the gradient across the valve from the modified Bernoulli equation, valve gradient = $4V^2$, where V = peak Doppler velocity beyond the obstruction (see Section V, Part I, Chapter 2, Fig. 16, page 1240).

ANGIOCARDIOGRAPHY

Biplane anteroposterior and lateral right ventriculography is preferred in the 45-degree sitting-up projection. The catheter (usually a balloon catheter) is positioned in the right ventricular outflow tract, and approximately 1 ml/kg of contrast is injected. When the left pulmonary artery cannot be adequately visualized, angled views may be a necessary supplement. Findings include (1) a thickened, domed pulmonary valve (Fig. 2); (2) poststenotic dilatation of the main and left pulmonary arteries; (3) right ventricular hypertrophy; and (4) in patients with moderate to marked PVS, dynamic in-

fundibular narrowing in systole. Right ventricular myocardial–coronary artery sinusoids may exist.

PROGNOSIS

The prognosis is good without treatment in mild cases, or with pulmonary valve balloon angioplasty (Fig. 3) or surgical intervention in the more severe cases. Correction of PVS may result in right ventricular outflow obstruction from severe infundibular hypertrophy.

VALVULAR AORTIC STENOSIS

Aortic stenosis (AS), combining valvular, subvalvular, and supravalvular types, represents the second most common form of obstructive CHD and accounts for 7% of all CHD. Congenital valvular AS accounts for 70% of all forms of AS. Valvular AS is classified according to valve types as (1) unicuspid (most severe disease), (2) bicuspid, (3) quadricuspid, and (4) tricuspid valve. The unicuspid valve usually has a central orifice and no lateral commissure. The bicuspid aortic valve with stenosis is by far the most common. A bicuspid valve is present in up to 85% of patients with coarctation, but may not be stenotic.

PATHOPHYSIOLOGY

Unicuspid valve AS presents in infancy with critical left heart obstruction and congestive heart failure (CHF). Other forms of AS progress gradually with age and lead to (1) concentric left ventricular hypertrophy, (2) elevated end-diastolic pressures, (3) elevated left atrial pressures, (4) pulmonary venous congestion, and (5) CHF. Critical AS in infancy may have associated hypoplasia of the left heart and aortic root or endocardial fibroelastosis, or both.

CLINICAL MANIFESTATIONS

Critical AS in infancy leads to failure to thrive, poor feeding, pneumonia, dyspnea, and CHF. From 1 year to 5 years of age, 70% of patients are asymptomatic. Physical finding is a characteristic systolic ejection murmur transmitted into the right side of the neck. Alarming findings in older patients requiring immediate evaluation and treatment include dyspnea, decreased exercise tolerance, angina, and syncope.

CHEST RADIOGRAPHY

Infants with critical AS present with (1) cardiomegaly, (2) pulmonary venous congestion, (3) minor pleural effusion, and (4) usually a hyperinflated inspiratory film (Fig. 4). Findings in older children (see Section V, Part I, Chapter 2, Fig. 5, page 1234) include (1) left ventricular hypertrophy with the cardiac apex depressed toward the diaphragm and posterior to the inferior vena cava, (2) poststenotic dilatation of the ascending aorta (50% of patients), and (3) left atrial enlargement. Primary differential considerations are coarctation and systemic hypertension.

ECHOCARDIOGRAPHY

Two-dimensional real-time echocardiography demonstrates (1) thickening and doming of the aortic valve (Fig. 5), (2) eccentric closure of the bicuspid valve, (3) concentric left ventricular hypertrophy, and (4) left atrial enlargement. Doppler evaluations can accurately determine the gradient across the aortic valve using the modified Bernoulli equation (see Echocardiography under Pulmonary Valvular Stenosis, above.)

ANGIOCARDIOGRAPHY

Left ventriculography is performed in the long-axis projection after retrograde aortic catheterization. In infants, the left ventricle may be entered through the foramen ovale from venous catheterization. Approximately 1 ml/kg of contrast is utilized. Angiographic findings include (1) thickened and domed aortic valve leaflets (Fig. 6), (2) poststenotic dilatation of the ascending aorta, and (3) left ventricular hypertrophy. Aortic root injection may be desirable to evaluate aortic insufficiency and rule out other frequently associated lesions such as coarctation and patent ductus arteriosus (PDA). The differential diagnosis includes subvalvular and supravalvular AS.

PROGNOSIS

The prognosis is guarded in infants with severe or critical AS. In the older child with a significant (75 mm Hg) gradient, operative valvulotomy or balloon angioplasty (Fig. 7) produces good results, although aortic insufficiency and late recurrence are common. Valve replacement may be necessary. Sudden death occurs in 4% to 18% of older patients without surgery. Balloon

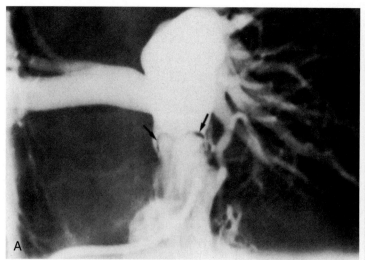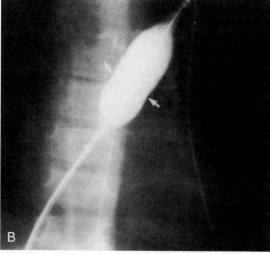

FIGURE 3. Pulmonary valvular stenosis (PVS). **A,** An anteroposterior right ventricular angiocardiogram demonstrates doming and thickening of the pulmonary valve *(arrows)* and poststenotic dilatation of the main pulmonary artery. **B,** Balloon angioplasty with the dilated balloon traversing the pulmonary valve with only a minimal waist *(arrows)* at the valve level and an excellent postangioplasty decrease in the PVS gradient.

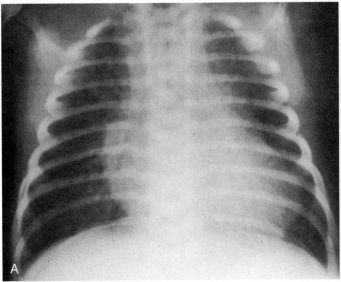

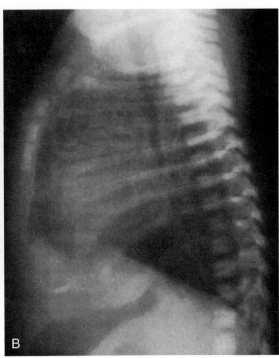

FIGURE 4. Critical aortic stenosis (AS). Anteroposterior **(A)** and lateral **(B)** chest radiographs in a 3-day-old infant show pulmonary venous congestion, moderate cardiomegaly, and hyperinflation. No abnormality of the ascending aorta is identified with AS at this age.

angioplasty and surgery have similar results with less mortality with retrograde angioplasty.

SUPRAVALVULAR AORTIC STENOSIS

Supravalvular aortic stenosis (SAS) may occur as an isolated lesion or be seen in SAS syndrome (Williams syndrome) (33%). Williams syndrome includes (1) SAS, (2) peripheral pulmonary stenosis, (3) elfin facies, (4) mental and physical retardation, (5) neonatal hypercalcemia, and (6) abnormal dentition.

PATHOPHYSIOLOGY

Types of SAS include (1) hourglass narrowing immediately above the sinuses of Valsalva (66%); (2) diffuse narrowing of the entire ascending aorta (20% to 30%); and (3) a diaphragm in the supravalvular area (10%). Additional pathologic findings include (1) thickening of the aortic valve cusps, (2) dilated tortuous coronary arteries, (3) left ventricular hypertrophy, (4) carotid artery involvement, and (5) occasionally associated coarctation.

CLINICAL MANIFESTATIONS

Findings in patients with Williams syndrome include feeding problems, failure to thrive, hypercalcemia, elfin facies, hoarse voice, strabismus, and inguinal hernia. All patients with SAS may have left heart failure, dyspnea, angina, and syncope. Physical findings include (1) an ejection systolic murmur in the aortic area, (2) increased pulses in the right arm, and (3) elevated right arm blood pressure.

FIGURE 5. Aortic stenosis. A long-axis two-dimensional echocardiogram centered at the aortic root shows doming of the aortic valve leaflet *(arrows)* and mild dilatation of the ascending aorta *(AO)*. *LV* = left ventricle; *LA* = left atrium.

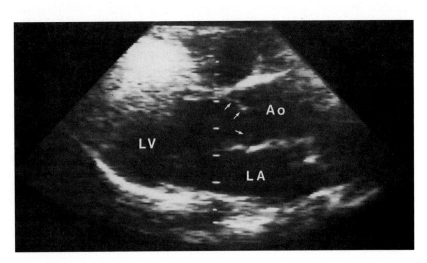

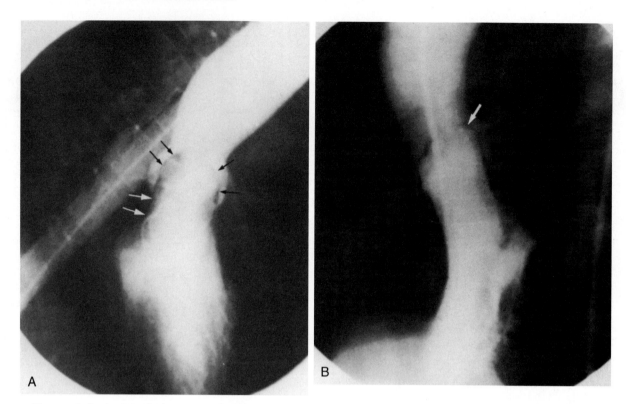

FIGURE 6. Aortic stenosis. Anteroposterior **(A)** and lateral **(B)** long-axis left ventriculograms show characteristic doming and thickening of the aortic valve leaflets *(arrows)*. Note the clear definition and elongation of the left ventricular outflow tract in these projections. The straight segment of the superior interventricular septum is nicely identified on the frontal projection *(white arrows)*.

CHEST RADIOGRAPHY

Chest radiographic findings are usually normal, although left ventricular hypertrophy and dilatation and congestive heart failure may be seen in severe cases. In the diffuse type, the ascending aorta is small and inconspicuous.

ECHOCARDIOGRAPHY

Real-time echocardiography demonstrates (1) supravalvular narrowing of the ascending aorta (Fig. 8), (2) concentric left ventricular hypertrophy, and (3) supravalvular pulmonary stenosis when it coexists. Doppler interrogation is more difficult in this lesion, although a gradient may be documented by the modified Bernoulli equation (see Echocardiography under Pulmonary Valvular Stenosis, above).

ANGIOCARDIOGRAPHY

Biplane supravalvular aortography following retrograde aortic catheterization in the long-axis projection is preferred. Angiographic findings include (1) supravalvular aortic narrowing, (2) diffuse hypoplasia of the ascending aorta (Fig. 9), (3) aortic insufficiency (15%), (4) coarctation (15%), and (5) stenosis of brachiocephalic vessels and abnormal aortic branches at their

origin. The descending thoracic and abdominal aorta may show either hypoplasia or stenotic areas and should be evaluated, as should the pulmonary artery, because of their frequent (50%) involvement (see Section V, Part IV, Chapter 2, Fig. 7, page 1369).

MAGNETIC RESONANCE IMAGING

Magnetic resonance imaging (MRI) is an excellent modality to evaluate patients with SAS syndrome, enabling recognition of SAS and peripheral pulmonary stenosis in multiple planes (Fig. 10). It is also useful in the postoperative patient.

PROGNOSIS

The prognosis is fairly poor. Surgical intervention is necessary in severe cases and may necessitate a ventriculoaortic bypass. Complications include aortic aneurysms and infective endocarditis.

MUSCULAR SUBAORTIC STENOSIS (HYPERTROPHIC OBSTRUCTIVE CARDIOMYOPATHY)

Muscular subaortic stenosis, or hypertrophic obstructive cardiomyopathy, is a form of obstructive cardiomyopa-

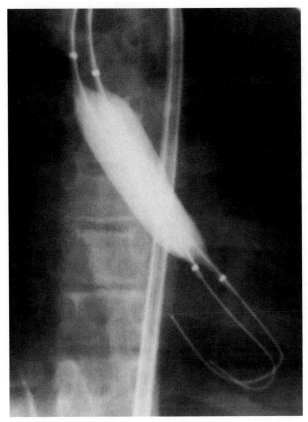

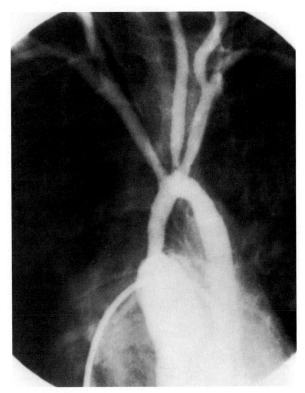

FIGURE 7. Balloon angioplasty in aortic stenosis (AS). Retrograde bifemoral artery introduction of balloon catheters passing into the left ventricle with complete obliteration of the AS waist deformity, a dramatic decrease in the aortic gradient, and only minor postangioplasty aortic insufficiency observed with an aortic root injection.

FIGURE 9. Supravalvular aortic stenosis. An anteroposterior projection of a left ventriculogram in a left anterior oblique projection shows a normal left ventricular outflow tract and sinuses of Valsalva with immediate narrowing and hypoplasia of the entire ascending aorta and aortic arch. Stenoses at the point of origins of the brachiocephalic vessel are also identified.

INCIDENCE

Familial occurrence is seen in 25% to 35% of patients. Spontaneous occurrence accounts for 65% to 75% of cases. An autosomal dominant inheritance pattern with a high degree of penetrance has been reported. Sexual incidence is equal. Hypertrophic cardiomyopathy may also be associated with Turner's and Noonan's syndromes and Friedreich's ataxia. Infants of diabetic mothers may have a reversible form of hypertrophic cardiomyopathy.

thy with asymmetric hypertrophy of the septal portion of the left ventricular outflow tract. Muscular subaortic stenosis has also been referred to as asymmetric septal hypertrophy, obstructive cardiomyopathy, and idiopathic hypertrophic subaortic stenosis (IHSS).

FIGURE 8. Supravalvular aortic stenosis. A long-axis real-time echocardiogram defines normal-sized aortic sinuses of Valsalva, with the closed aortic valve producing a linear central echo density *(arrow)* leading directly into a strikingly narrowed ascending aorta *(arrowheads)*. LV = left ventricle; *LA* = left atrium.

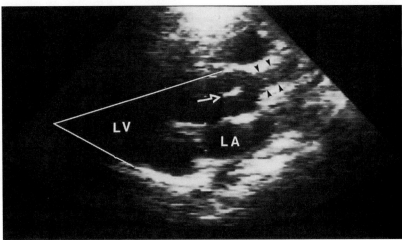

PATHOPHYSIOLOGY

Pathologic findings include (1) disproportionate hypertrophy of the interventricular septum when compared with the left ventricular free wall, (2) fibrous plaque formation in the left ventricular outflow tract, (3) left ventricular hypertrophy, and (4) thickening of the anterior leaflet of the mitral valve. Physiologic changes relate to systolic anterior motion (SAM) of the anterior mitral valve leaflet against the hypertrophied ventricular septum, producing left ventricular outflow obstruction. Failure of mitral leaflet apposition during systole may result in mitral regurgitation.

CLINICAL MANIFESTATIONS

Symptoms usually appear in the older child, but may not develop until the third or fourth decade. These include dyspnea, fatigue, angina, and occasionally, sudden death. Murmurs are difficult to hear and are of a systolic ejection type.

CHEST RADIOGRAPHY

Mild cardiomegaly of a left ventricular configuration is present in the majority of older children or adult patients. In the later stages of the disease, left atrial enlargement and pulmonary venous congestion may be seen. In severe cases in the young child, massive cardiomegaly will occasionally be present. The differential diagnosis includes cardiomyopathies and carditis.

ECHOCARDIOGRAPHY

Real-time two-dimensional echocardiography clearly defines the asymmetric thickening of the interventricular septum as well as the abnormal orientation of the anterior mitral valve leaflet into the left ventricular outflow tract in midsystole (Fig. 11). These findings are similarly documented with M-mode echocardiography showing (1) a septal–left ventricular posterior wall ratio of greater than 1.3:1, (2) premature closure of the aortic valve, and (3) anterior midsystolic motion of the anterior mitral valve leaflet.

ANGIOCARDIOGRAPHY

Biplane long-axis cineangiocardiography with biventricular injection utilizing approximately 1 ml/kg contrast optimally identifies the asymmetric septal hypertrophy. Other findings include (1) SAM of the mitral valve against the ventricular septum, producing left ventricular outflow obstruction; (2) mitral regurgitation; and (3) left ventricular hypertrophy (Fig. 12). MRI may be helpful in the differential diagnosis of intramural fibroma.

PROGNOSIS

The prognosis is poor in symptomatic patients, with a 15% 5-year mortality and 35% 10-year mortality. Surgical resection of the muscular septum in the subaortic region is indicated for patients with severe gradients not controlled medically (propranolol).

SUBVALVULAR AORTIC STENOSIS (EXCLUDING IDIOPATHIC HYPERTROPHIC SUBAORTIC STENOSIS)

Subvalvular AS (excluding IHSS) affects approximately 13% of all patients with left ventricular outflow obstruction.

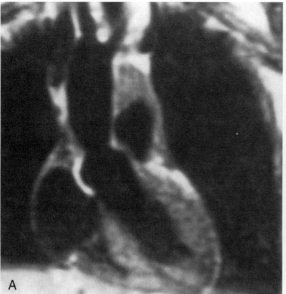 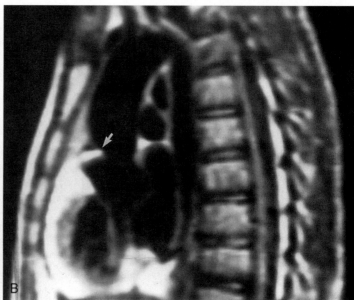

FIGURE 10. A 13-year-old with supravalvular aortic stenosis (SAS). Coronal **(A)** and sagittal **(B)** 5-mm spin-echo magnetic resonance images demonstrate SAS with a thick diaphragm *(arrow)* just above the aortic sinuses. Also noted is a right aortic arch with aberrant origin of the left subclavian artery.

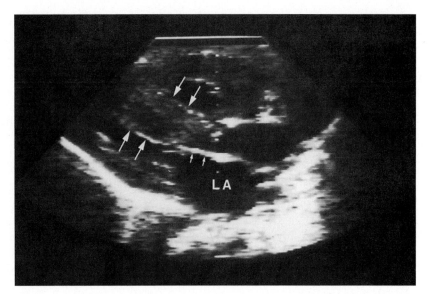

FIGURE 11. Asymmetric septal hypertrophy. A long-axis two-dimensional echocardiogram shows striking thickening of the interventricular septum *(large arrows)* that is producing significant subaortic obstruction. The anterior mitral valve leaflet *(small arrows)* comes into direct contact with this grossly enlarged septum in diastole. *LA* = left atrium.

PATHOPHYSIOLOGY

Lesions seen include (1) a thin subvalvular membrane; (2) a somewhat thicker fibromuscular ring approximately 1 cm below the valve; (3), rarely, a fibromuscular subaortic tunnel (11%). Subvalvular AS may be associated with a ventricular septal defect (VSD) and occasionally with an atrioventricular canal (AVC) or a single ventricle. Subvalvular aortic stenosis is an integral part of the Shone anomaly (parachute mitral valve, supravalvular stenosing ring of the left atrium, subaortic stenosis, and coarctation of the aorta). Other acquired effects of this lesion include (1) secondary aortic insufficiency related to thickening and deformity of the aortic valve secondary to proximal turbulent flow, (2) poststenotic dilatation of the ascending aorta when the subvalvular membrane is in immediate proximity to the aortic valve or in the presence of aortic regurgitation, and (3) concentric left ventricular hypertrophy. Some authors question whether discrete subaortic stenosis is congenital or acquired.

CLINICAL MANIFESTATIONS

Clinical symptoms are mild until a later age, when signs of left ventricular failure with dyspnea, syncope, and tachypnea may ensue. Subvalvular AS is much more common in the male, with a 6:1 male preponderance. If other congenital heart lesions are present, symptoms may occur earlier that are related to those lesions.

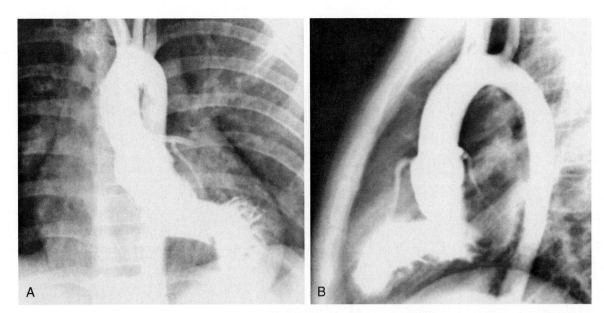

FIGURE 12. Obstructive cardiomyopathy. Selective anteroposterior **(A)** and lateral **(B)** left ventriculograms during left ventricular systole demonstrate prominence of the interventricular septum; the left ventricular outflow tract becomes narrowed and obstructed. The systolic anterior motion of the anterior leaflet of the mitral valve may be appreciated in the lateral view with cineangiography.

CHEST RADIOGRAPHY

A pattern of left ventricular hypertrophy is seen in the older child. Later manifestations, if stenosis is severe, are left ventricular dilatation and failure. Chest radiographic findings are usually normal in the infant and young child. Poststenotic dilatation of the ascending aorta usually will not be seen unless aortic regurgitation has developed. Differential diagnostic considerations are mainly those of other left heart obstruction lesions, endocardial fibroelastosis, and cardiomyopathies.

ECHOCARDIOGRAPHY

Two-dimensional real-time echocardiography readily identifies the discrete membranous (Fig. 13) as well as fibromuscular and tunnel-type subaortic lesions. Other findings include systolic preclosure of the aortic valve and systolic flutter of the leaflets.

ANGIOCARDIOGRAPHY

Biplane long-axis angiocardiography is ideal for visualization and evaluation of the various types of subvalvular AS. The thin, membranous type may be difficult to visualize unless the membrane is demonstrated tangential to the central roentgen beam (Fig. 14). Other lesions that should be evaluated with angiography include (1) mitral regurgitation and stenosis, (2) associated septal defects, and (3) aortic valve abnormality (i.e., insufficiency).

PROGNOSIS

The prognosis is good with surgical resection of the discrete membranous subvalvular lesion, although re-

stenosis occurs in approximately 25% of patients. Success with attempted correction of the fibromuscular or tunnel lesions is poor from a direct approach. Occasionally an apical left ventricular–aortic conduit (see Section V, Part VII, Chapter 1, Fig. 19, page 1406) may be necessary in these lesions with severe obstruction. Progressive hypertrophy, a continued gradient, and mitral and aortic valve dysfunction are common complications.

COARCTATION OF THE AORTA

Coarctation of the aorta is classified into (1) the juxtaductal type and its variants and (2) postductal (adult) types. The juxtaductal type, usually seen in infants and small children, typically has hypoplasia of the transverse arch and aortic isthmus. In juxtaductal coarctation, the ductus is astride the area of coarctation. In adults or children with postductal coarctation, the lesion is distal to the ductus arteriosus/ligamentum arteriosum.

INCIDENCE

Coarctation accounts for approximately 5% of CHD; males predominate 2:1 without significant familial occurrence. Associated anomalies are frequent. They include PDA (66%); VSD (33%); and other lesions, including transposition of the great vessels, ASD, mitral stenosis or regurgitation, endocardial fibroelastosis, AVC, and common ventricle. A bicuspid aortic valve is common. Other noncardiac conditions include respiratory distress syndrome, prematurity, tracheoesophageal fistula, Shone's complex, and Turner's syndrome. Coarctation also may be seen with various syndrome complexes (see Section V, Part IV, Chapter 2, page 1364 for discussion of cardiac abnormalities associated with syndromes and chromosomal aberrations).

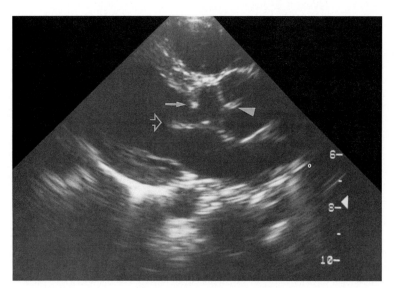

FIGURE 13. Membranous subaortic stenosis. A long-axis parasternal real-time echocardiogram demonstrates a linear echogenic structure projecting posteriorly from the superior interventricular septum that represents a discrete membranous subaortic stenosis *(arrow)*. The anterior mitral valve leaflet *(open arrow)* and closed aortic leaflets *(arrowhead)* can be seen (compare with Fig. 3*B* in Section V, Part II, Chapter 1, page 1262).

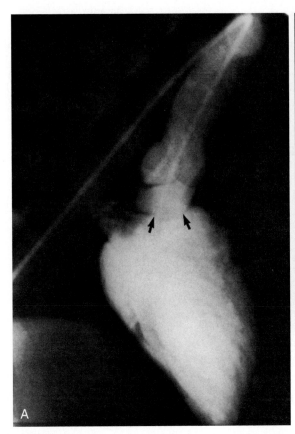

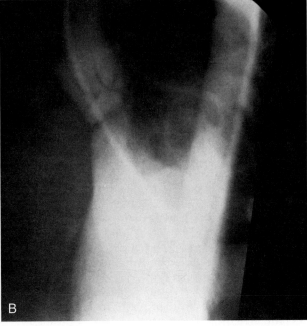

FIGURE 14. Subvalvular aortic stenosis. Anteroposterior **(A)** and lateral **(B)** long-axis left ventriculograms show a discrete subaortic membrane *(arrows)* approximately 1 cm below the aortic valve leaflets.

PATHOPHYSIOLOGY

Upper extremity hypertension is invariably present, probably relating to combined mechanical and renal factors. The mechanical process is compensated by development of collateral blood flow with enlargement of intercostal, superior epigastric, and mediastinal vessels. Intercostal artery dilatation and pulsation produce secondary rib notching. Left ventricular hypertrophy is proportionate to the degree of aortic obstruction. Some coarctations are dependent on an open ductus arteriosus and progress in severity when the ductus closes.

CLINICAL MANIFESTATIONS

Infants with coarctation, particularly when associated with left-to-right shunts (i.e., VSD or PDA), present with dramatic signs of CHF, usually in the first month of life, typically at 10 to 14 days of age. Clinical symptoms include dyspnea, poor feeding, tachycardia, and peripheral cyanosis. The murmur is variable in infants but, when heard, is similar to that in the older child. Differential blood pressures in the lower limbs are noted in two thirds of patients, but they are less dramatic when the child is in severe CHF.

Clinical signs of failure are rare in children over 1 year of age, and the diagnosis usually relates to findings of an incidental murmur, hypertension, or the recognition of abnormalities on chest radiographs. The murmur is a soft systolic ejection type that is heard best posteriorly in the left paravertebral area. Blood pressure discrepancies are readily identified. Additional murmurs related to associated lesions may be present.

CHEST RADIOGRAPHY

Infants present with (1) moderate to marked cardiomegaly with a nonspecific configuration, (2) pulmonary venous congestion and failure (see Section V, Part I, Chapter 1, Fig. 1, page 1229), and (3) poststenotic dilatation of the descending aorta of variable prominence. CHF presenting between the first and fourth weeks strongly suggests coarctation. Differentiation from an interrupted aortic arch is difficult.

Older patients (over 1 year) usually have normal heart size to mild cardiomegaly, the latter with a left ventricular configuration. Rib notching (see Section V, Part I, Chapter 2, Table 5, page 1237) is the hallmark of this condition and is usually seen after 5 years but occasionally is present in the first few years of life (see Section V, Part I, Chapter 2, Fig. 11, page 1237). The third, fourth, and fifth ribs are usually involved posteriorly, but notching may be seen in the third through ninth ribs. Poststenotic dilatation of the aorta below the coarctation will usually occur, and a figure three sign related to the dilatation of the left subclavian artery above and the poststenotic aortic segment below (see Section V, Part I, Chapter 2, Fig. 8A, page 1235), is frequently evident. The imprint of the aorta on the adjacent barium-filled esophagus is known as the E sign (see Section V, Part I,

Chapter 2, Fig. 8*B*, page 1235). Dilatation of the ascending aorta and brachiocephalic vessels is frequently observed. Retrosternal enlargement of the internal mammary arteries may be seen in the lateral chest radiograph. True coarctation must be differentiated from pseudocoarctation, where no gradient is present (see Pseudocoarctation of the Aorta, page 1296).

ECHOCARDIOGRAPHY

Two-dimensional echocardiography from the suprasternal notch or subxiphoid projection may directly visualize the area of aortic narrowing and poststenotic dilatation of the aorta (Fig. 15). Unfortunately, the adjacent lung sometimes interferes with optimal visualization. Doppler interrogation of the aorta below the coarctation may show an altered amplitude and wave pattern related to the coarctation effect. A gradient across the coarctation may be calculated by use of the modified Bernoulli equation (see Section V, Part I, Chapter 2, page 1230, under Echocardiography). Additional findings include a bicuspid aortic valve and concentric left ventricular hypertrophy.

ANGIOCARDIOGRAPHY

Long-axis biplane left ventriculography usually will not only adequately identify any intracardiac defect of significance but will also visualize the various forms of coarctation (Fig. 16). The entire arch should be closely evaluated for degrees of hypoplasia. The bicuspid aortic valve can be visualized on left ventricular or aortic root injections. Delayed films will demonstrate collateral flow to the descending aorta (Fig. 17). Occasionally, ascending aortography will be necessary to better visualize the arch and site of coarctation. In the infant, angiocardiography may be accomplished by right heart catheterization with a balloon catheter through the foramen ovale and into the left ventricle. Retrograde aortic catheterization is usually needed in older patients and may be preferable if balloon angioplasty is being considered as a therapeutic measure.

MAGNETIC RESONANCE IMAGING

MRI, particularly with cardiac and respiratory gating, will nicely identify the lesion in all children. The sagittal or sagittal oblique projection will clearly visualize the entire aortic arch, coarctation, and collateral circulation (Figs. 18 and 19).

PROGNOSIS

The prognosis is good in older patients with isolated lesions with either surgical resection or balloon angioplasty. Operative mortality in infants, especially with complex lesions, hypoplasia of the arch, or major defects, is high and ranges to 40%. Aneurysms or pseudoaneurysms may develop after either operative repair or balloon angioplasty (Fig. 20). Recurrent coarctation, more common in small children after operation, is suggested by persistence or redevelopment of rib notching (Fig. 21), and may be treated by balloon angioplasty. Mesenteric ischemia and hyperreactive hypertension may complicate operative repair of coarctation in all age groups.

AORTIC ARCH INTERRUPTION

Aortic arch interruption (AAI) is characterized by discontinuity of the arch between the proximal ascending aorta and the distal descending aorta. AAI differs from atresia of the aortic arch in that complete discontinuity exists between the aortic arch and the descending aorta. A fibrous remnant connects the ascending and descending aorta in aortic arch atresia. AAI is classified by the site of arch interruption and subclassified by the origin of the right subclavian artery: A, interruption distal to the left subclavian artery (42%); B, interruption between the left carotid artery and the left subclavian artery (53%); and C, interruption between the innominate artery and the left carotid artery (5%). The right subclavian artery may arise from the innominate artery, the descending aorta, or the right

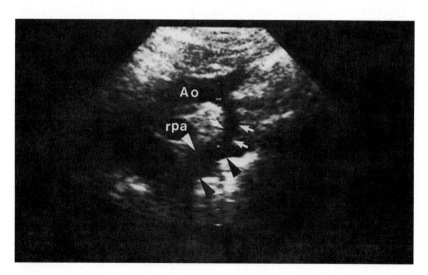

FIGURE 15. Coarctation of the aorta. Suprasternal real-time echocardiogram defining a prominent ascending aorta *(Ao)* and innominate artery, with a hypoplastic transverse aortic arch *(arrows)* extending into an area of poststenotic dilatation of the thoracic aorta *(arrowheads)*. The right pulmonary artery *(rpa)* projects centrally within the aortic arch.

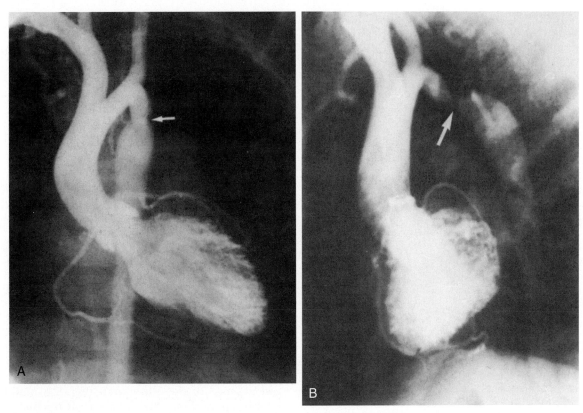

FIGURE 16. Coarctation of the aorta. Anteroposterior **(A)** and lateral **(B)** long-axis left ventriculograms demonstrate mild hypoplasia of the aortic isthmus with a focal area of coarctation *(arrow)* and moderate poststenotic dilatation distal to the coarctation site. Prominent internal mammary and collateral vessels are seen on the right. Note the absence of the left subclavian artery, which originated from the site of coarctation and filled on late films by vertebral artery steal.

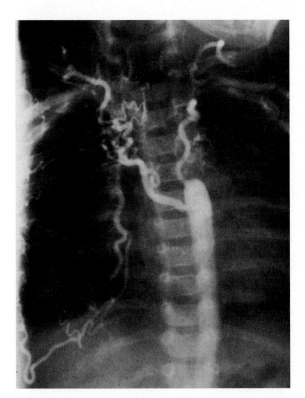

FIGURE 17. Coarctation of the aorta. Collateral blood flow through direct mediastinal collateral, internal mammary, long thoracic, and intercostal arteries into the posterior intercostal arteries, filling the thoracic aorta distal to the site of coarctation.

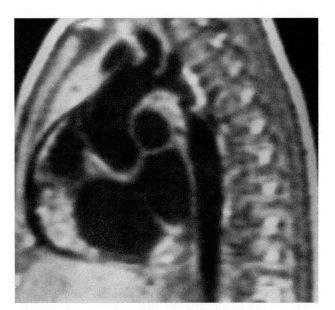

FIGURE 18. Coarctation of the aorta. Sagittal oblique 3-mm spin-echo magnetic resonance image (left anterior oblique equivalent) demonstrates the thoracic aorta in its entirety and depicts well the hypoplastic aortic isthmus and coarctation in this 1-year-old girl.

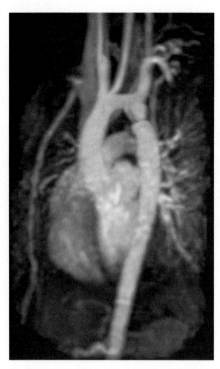

FIGURE 19. A 9½-year-old child with coarctation. Gadolinium-enhanced three-dimensional time-of-flight examination with breath hold in the left anterior oblique projection demonstrates coarctation distal to the left subclavian artery. Enlarged right and left highest intercostal arteries are seen entering the proximal descending thoracic aorta just distal to the coarctation, and serve as a source of collateral flow to the descending aorta. The ascending aorta is normal, and there is very mild hypoplasia of the transverse arch.

pulmonary artery. There is a significant familial incidence as well as association with chromosomal abnormalities, particularly DiGeorge syndrome.

PATHOPHYSIOLOGY

The pathophysiology is similar to that seen in severe coarctation. Associated defects are common, with 95% having PDA and 80% having VSDs. Other commonly associated malformations include truncus arteriosus and aorticopulmonary window.

CLINICAL MANIFESTATIONS

Clinical signs and symptoms are basically similar to those in severe infantile coarctation with early development of CHF.

CHEST RADIOGRAPHY

Chest radiographs show moderate cardiomegaly with a nonspecific silhouette and changes of pulmonary venous hypertension (Fig. 22). Increased pulmonary flow related to associated left-to-right shunt may also be evident in older infants. The trachea may show an unusual straight vertical orientation without the usual deviation related to the aortic arch. Rib notching in older children is dependent on the site of interruption: bilateral (A), right sided (B and C), or left sided (A) with aberrant right subclavian artery (see Section V, Part I, Chapter 2, Table 5, page 1237).

ECHOCARDIOGRAPHY

Real-time echocardiography demonstrates the straight ascending aorta and continuation directly into the brachiocephalic vessels without a typical rounded-arch configuration. A large patent ductus typically joins the pulmonary artery into the descending thoracic aorta and mimics an aortic arch. The frequent VSDs may also be identified in various locations.

ANGIOCARDIOGRAPHY

Biplane, long-axis, left ventriculography or ascending aortography demonstrates the straight ascending aorta with direct continuation in the brachiocephalic vessels and absence of the aortic arch (Fig. 23). Pulmonary arteriography shows the large patent ductus continuing into the descending thoracic aorta. Intracardiac defects include (1) membranous and supracristal VSDs, (2) subaortic stenosis, and (3) a bicuspid aortic valve.

PROGNOSIS

The overall prognosis is fair with operative correction related to use of a conduit across the aortic arch or use of the left subclavian artery. When associated intracardiac shunts are present, pulmonary artery banding for palliation, prior to later total repair, may be required.

PSEUDOCOARCTATION OF THE AORTA

Pseudocoarctation is characterized by elongation and kinking of the aortic arch at the ligamentum arteriosum without a focal area of narrowing or pressure gradient. A bicuspid aortic valve, PDA, and subaortic stenosis may also be present. The abnormality is often noted as an incidental finding on chest radiographs, although occasionally it may produce a soft, turbulent flow murmur. Blood pressures are equal in the arms and legs.

An abnormally prominent aortic arch projecting somewhat high and to the left may raise the question of coarctation or an aortic or ductal aneurysm. The elongated arch with kinking is often best visualized in the lateral chest radiograph. Real-time echocardiography and Doppler interrogation may be able to adequately evaluate the arch and establish a diagnosis. Otherwise, catheterization and angiography or MRI

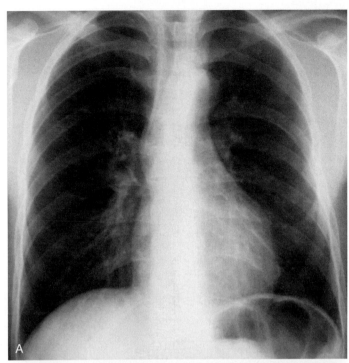

FIGURE 20. Aortic pseudoaneurysm. Frontal **(A)** and lateral **(B)** chest radiographs in a 20-year-old male, 4 years after balloon angioplasty for recoarctation, demonstrate a focal aneurysm in the region of the distal transverse arch–proximal descending aorta, best appreciated in the lateral projection. **C,** Spin-echo T_1-weighted magnetic resonance image in the sagittal oblique projection (similar to left anterior oblique projection) demonstrates the pseudoaneurysm arising from the posterolateral proximal descending thoracic aorta.

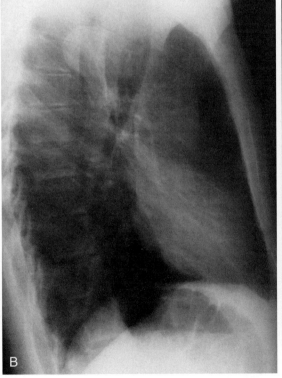

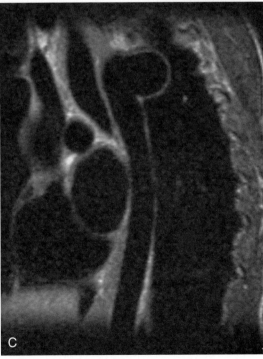

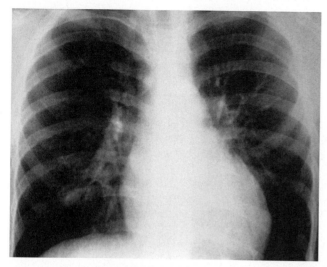

FIGURE 21. An 8½-year-old girl with recoarctation. Chest radiograph demonstrates left rib deformities from previous thoracotomy at age 2 weeks, dilatation and deformity of the left-sided descending aorta, and right lateral rib notching. Because the left subclavian artery was utilized during neonatal coarctation repair, no left-sided rib notching is seen.

(Fig. 24) is needed to rule out a true lesion with a minor gradient.

ENDOCARDIAL FIBROELASTOSIS

Endocardial fibroelastosis is classified in relation to chamber involvement, valvular involvement, and whether or not there is associated CHD.

INCIDENCE

Endocardial fibroelastosis is present in approximately 1% of all patients with CHD. Left ventricular involvement is the most common (98%), whereas right and left heart involvement is seen in approximately 16%. With left ventricular involvement, 60% have left atrial involvement. Twenty-five percent of cases are isolated, whereas 75% have associated CHD. Valvular involvement may be seen in approximately 50% of patients (aortic and mitral valve).

A fairly high incidence of familial involvement has been documented as well as the previously noted frequent association with CHD. Besides an intrinsic basic congenital etiology, other suggested etiologic factors include intrauterine infection from mumps and adenovirus and premature intrauterine closure of the foramen ovale.

PATHOPHYSIOLOGY

Because endocardial fibroelastosis is commonly associated with congenital heart defects, most physiologic manifestations relate to the primary process. Coarcta-

tion, a patent ductus, and aortic atresia are the most common associated lesions. Pathologically, the endocardium is a thickened, with a pearly-white layer covering the entire left ventricular wall, and increased stiffness of the ventricle. Increased elastic and fibrous tissues with small round-cell infiltration can also be identified on histologic examination.

CLINICAL MANIFESTATIONS

Symptoms usually develop in the first month of life that are related to CHF, with dyspnea, tachypnea, irritability, and mild cyanosis. These symptoms may relate to myocardial dysfunction or to the effects of the associated lesions (i.e., aortic atresia or stenosis and coarctation).

CHEST RADIOGRAPHY

Moderate to marked cardiomegaly with left heart dilatation and CHF are commonly seen at the time of presentation (Fig. 25). Left lower lobe atelectasis is common from left atrial enlargement compressing the left main stem bronchus. Arch abnormalities may be noted if associated with coarctation. Primary differential considerations are acute myocarditis, anomalous origin of the left coronary artery, and other forms of cardiomyopathy.

ECHOCARDIOGRAPHY

Real-time and M-mode echocardiography demonstrate dilatation of the left ventricle and outflow tract without

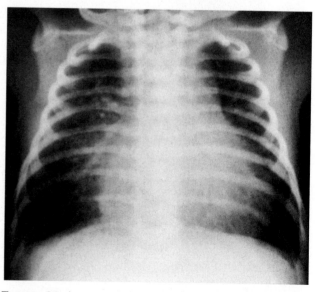

FIGURE 22. Interrupted aortic arch in a 1-week-old infant with moderate cardiomegaly and severe congestive failure. The trachea tends to be relatively midline, although difficult to identify; no aortic arch structures are evident.

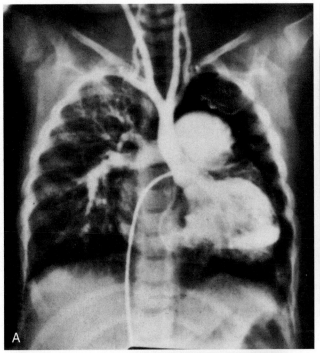

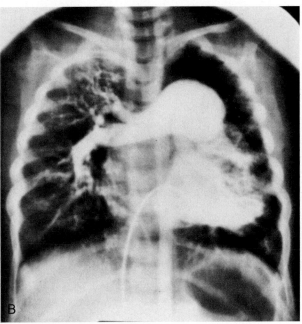

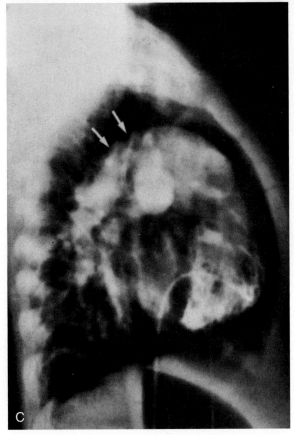

FIGURE 23. Interrupted aortic arch. **A,** Anteroposterior (AP) left ventriculogram shows a characteristic tree-like branching of the brachiocephalic vessels with an absence of the transverse aortic arch and very little visualization of the descending thoracic aorta. A left-to-right shunt through a VSD produces moderate visualization of the enlarged pulmonary vessels. AP **(B)** and lateral **(C)** right ventriculograms show the continuation of the enlarged main pulmonary artery into the descending thoracic aorta through the large PDA *(arrows)*. Some minor right-to-left shunting through the VSD produces faint opacification of the left heart and brachiocephalic vessels. (From Roberts WC, et al: Circulation 1962;26:49, with permission.)

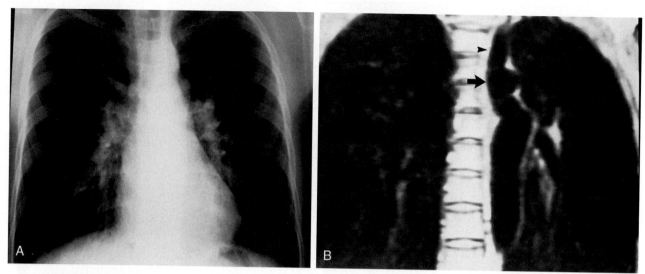

FIGURE 24. Pseudocoarctation in a 15-year-old boy after ventricular septal defect, and subaortic stenosis repair. **A,** Chest radiograph demonstrates abnormal dilatation of the proximal descending aorta. No rib notching is present. **B,** Coronal magnetic resonance image demonstrates pseudocoarctation with dilatation of the proximal descending aorta. *Arrowhead* = left subclavian artery; *arrow* = aortic arch.

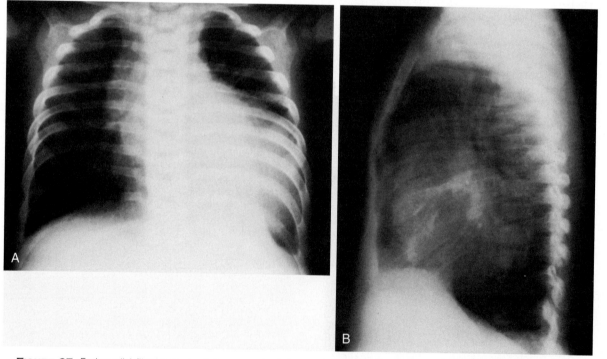

FIGURE 25. Endocardial fibroelastosis. Anteroposterior **(A)** and lateral **(B)** chest radiographs show marked cardiomegaly with striking left ventricular dilatation, congestive heart failure, and left lower lobe atelectasis. The lateral view shows displacement and narrowing of the left main stem bronchus.

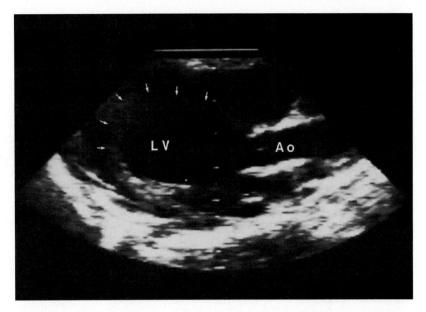

FIGURE 26. Endocardial fibroelastosis. A long-axis echocardiogram demonstrates marked left ventricular enlargement. Real-time and M-mode studies (not shown) showed markedly diminished left ventricular contractility.

hypertrophy and with poor left ventricular function (Fig. 26). Other associated cardiac lesions may also be identified.

ANGIOCARDIOGRAPHY

Left ventricular long-axis angiocardiography usually demonstrates a dilated left ventricle with poor left ventricular function, often associated with mitral regurgitation. This examination may also confirm AS, coarctation, VSD, and PDA if present. Aortic root injection or selective coronary angiography may be important in excluding an anomalous origin of the left coronary artery as a differential diagnosis.

PROGNOSIS

The prognosis is fair with aggressive digitalis treatment. Without cardiomegaly, an 80% survival rate can be expected. The survival rate is lower if marked cardiomegaly is present or there are other associated lesions.

SUGGESTED READINGS

Pulmonary Valvular Stenosis with Intact Ventricular Septum

Bonnet D, Gautier Lhermitte I, Bonhoeffer P, et al: Right ventricular myocardial sinusoidal-coronary artery connections in critical pulmonary valve stenosis. Pediatr Cardiol 1998;19:269

Elliott LP (ed): Right ventriculography in pulmonary valve stenosis. *In* Cardiac Imaging in Infants, Children, and Adults. Philadelphia, JB Lippincott, 1991:241

Elliott LP, Schiebler GL: Pathophysiology and roentgenographic findings in pulmonary valve stenosis. *In* Elliott LP (ed): Cardiac Imaging in Infants, Children, and Adults. Philadelphia, JB Lippincott, 1991:235

Fogelman R, Nykanen D, Smallhorn JF, et al: Endovascular stents in the pulmonary circulation: clinical impact on management and medium-term follow-up. Circulation 1995;92:881

Gielen H, Daniels O, van Lier H: Natural history of congenital pulmonary valvar stenosis: an echo and Doppler cardiographic study. Cardiol Young 1999;9:129

Gildein HP, Kleinert S, Goh TH, et al: Pulmonary valve annulus grows after balloon dilatation of neonatal critical pulmonary valve stenosis. Am Heart J 1998;136:276

Ino T, Kishiro M, Okubo M, et al: Balloon dilation of critical valvar pulmonary stenosis in the first month of life. Cathet Cardiovasc Diagn 1995;34:23

Jaffe RB: Pulmonary valve stenosis: echocardiography. *In* Elliott LP (ed): Cardiac Imaging in Infants, Children, and Adults. Philadelphia, JB Lippincott, 1991:239

Kovalchin JP, Forbes TJ, Nihill MR, et al: Echocardiographic determinants of clinical course in infants with critical and severe pulmonary valve stenosis. J Am Coll Cardiol 1997;29:1095

Park JH, Yoon YS, Yeon KM, et al: Percutaneous pulmonary valvuloplasty with a double-balloon technique. Radiology 1987;164:715

Schneider MB, Zartner PA, Magee AG: Images in cardiology: cutting balloon for treatment of severe peripheral pulmonary stenosis in a child. Heart 1999;82:108

Walsh KP, Abdulhamed JM, Tometzki JP: Importance of right ventricular outflow tract angiography in distinguishing critical pulmonary stenosis from pulmonary atresia. Heart 1997;77:456

White RI Jr, Mitchell SE, Kan J: Interventional procedures in congenital heart disease. Cardiovasc Intervent Radiol 1986;9:286

Valvular Aortic Stenosis

Bisset GS III, Meyer RA: Obstructive left heart lesions. Semin Roentgenol 1985;20:247

Eapen RS, Rowland DG, Franklin WH: Effect of prenatal diagnosis of critical left heart obstruction on perinatal morbidity and mortality. Am J Perinatology 1998;15:237

Hawkins JA, Minich LL, Tani LY, et al: Late results and reintervention after aortic valvotomy for critical aortic stenosis in neonates and infants. Ann Thorac Surg 1998;65:1758

Lemler MS, Valdes-Cruz LM, Shandas RS, et al: Insights into catheter/Doppler discrepancies in congenital aortic stenosis. Am J Cardiol 1999;83:1447

Magee AG, Nykanen D, McCrindle BW, et al: Balloon dilation of severe aortic stenosis in the neonate: comparison of antegrade and retrograde catheter approaches. J Am Coll Cardiol 1997;30:1061

Moore P, Etito E, Mowrey H, et al: Midterm results of balloon dilation of congenital aortic stenosis: predictors of success. J Am Coll Cardiol 1996;27:1257

O'Rourke RA: Aortic valve stenosis: a common clinical entity. Curr Probl Cardiol 2000;69:562

Simpson JM, Sharland GK: Natural history and outcome of aortic stenosis diagnosed prenatally. Heart 1997;77:205

White RI Jr, Mitchell SE, Kan J: Interventional procedures in congenital heart disease. Cardiovasc Intervent Radiol 1986;9:286

Supravalvular Aortic Stenosis

Kitchiner D, Jackson M, Walsh K, et al: Prognosis of supravalvar aortic stenosis in 81 patients in Liverpool (1960–1993). Heart 1996;75:396

McElhinney DB, Petrossian E, Tworetzky W, et al: Issues and outcomes in the management of supravalvar aortic stenosis. Ann Thorac Surg 2000;69:562

Sheikh KH, Adams DB, Kisslo J: Echo-Doppler evaluation of aortic valve stenosis. *In* Elliott LP (ed): Cardiac Imaging in Infants, Children, and Adults. Philadelphia, JB Lippincott, 1991:254

Stamm C, Kreutzer C, Zurakowski D, et al: Forty-one years of surgical experience with congenital supravalvular aortic stenosis. J Thorac Cardiovasc Surg 1999;118:874

White RD: Magnetic resonance imaging of aortic valve stenosis. *In* Elliott LP (ed): Cardiac Imaging in Infants, Children. and Adults. Philadelphia, JB Lippincott, 1991:261

Muscular Subaortic Stenosis

Maron BJ: Cardiomyopathies. *In* Adams FH, Emmanouilides GC, Riemenschneider TA (eds): Heart Disease in Infants, Children, and Adolescents. Baltimore, Williams & Wilkins, 1989

Riggs T, Hirschfeld SS, Rajai H: Pediatric spectrum of dynamic left ventricular obstruction. Am Heart J 1980;99:301

Roughneen PT, DeLeon SY, Cetta F, et al: Modified Kono-Rastan procedure for subaortic stenosis: indications, operative techniques, and results. Ann Thorac Surg 1998;65:1368

Stelzer P, Weinrauch S, Tranbaugh RF: Ten years of experience with the modified Ross procedure. J Thorac Cardiovasc Surg 1998; 115:1091

Tentolouris K, Kontozoglou T, Trikas A, et al: Fixed subaortic stenosis revisited: congenital abnormalities in 72 new cases and review of the literature. Cardiology 1999;92:4

Subvalvular Aortic Stenosis (Excluding Idiopathic Hypertrophic Subaortic Stenosis)

Bezold LI, Smith EO, Kelly K, et al: Development and validation of an echocardiographic model for predicting progression of discrete subaortic stenosis in children. Am J Cardiol 1998;81:314

Freedom RM, Culham JAG, Moes CAF: Angiocardiography of Congenital Heart Disease. New York, Macmillan, 1984:389

Rayburn ST, Netherland DE, Heath BJ: Discrete membranous subaortic stenosis: improved results after resection and myectomy. Ann Thorac Surg 1997;64:105

Serraf A, Zoghby J, Lacour-Gayet F, et al: Surgical treatment of subaortic stenosis: a seventeen-year experience. J Thorac Cardiovasc Surg 1999;117:669

Shone JD, Sellers RD, Anderson RC, et al: The developmental complex of "parachute mitral valve," supravalvular ring of the left atrium, subaortic stenosis and coarctation of the aorta. Am J Cardiol 1963;11:714

Sigfusson G, Tracy TA, Vanauker MD, et al: Abnormalities of the left ventricular outflow tract associated with discrete subaortic stenosis in children: an echocardiographic study. J Am Coll Cardiol 1997; 30:225

Silverman NH, Gerlis LM, Ho SY, et al: Fibrous obstruction within the left ventricular outflow tract associated with ventricular septal defect: a pathologic study. J Am Coll Cardiol 1995;25:475

van Son JA, Schneider P, Falk V: MR findings in Shone's complex of left heart obstructive lesions. Pediatr Radiol 1998;28:841

White RI Jr, Mitchell SE, Kan J: Interventional procedures in congenital heart disease. Cardiovasc Intervent Radiol 1986;9:286

Coarctation of the Aorta, Aortic Arch Interruption, and Pseudocoarctation of the Aorta

Babbit DB, Cassidy GE, Godard JE: Rib notching in aortic coarctation during infancy and childhood. Radiology 1974;110:169

Bailey WW: Interrupted aortic arch. Adv Card Surg 1994;5:97

Becker C, Soppa C, Fink U, et al: Spiral CT angiography and 3D reconstruction in patients with aortic coarctation. Eur Radiol 1997;7:1473

Bisset GS III, Meyer RA: Obstructive left heart lesions. Semin Roentgenol 1985;20:244

Burrows PE: Magnetic resonance imaging of the aorta in children. Semin Ultrasound CT MR 1990;11:221

Chin AJ, Jacobs ML: Morphology of the ventricular septal defect in two types of interrupted aortic arch. J Am Soc Echocardiogr 1996;9:199

Gobel JW, Pierpont ME, Moller JH, et al: Familial interruption of the aortic arch. Pediatr Cardiol 1993;14:110

Greenberg SB, Marks LA, Eshaghpour EE: Evaluation of magnetic resonance imaging in coarctation of the aorta: the importance of multiple imaging planes. Pediatr Cardiol 1997;18:345

Hamaoka K, Satou H, Sakata K, et al: Three-dimensional imaging of aortic aneurysm after balloon angioplasty for coarctation of the aorta. Circulation 1999;100:1673

Ino T, Kishiro M, Okubo M, et al: Dilatation mechanism of balloon angioplasty in children: assessment by angiography and intravascular ultrasound. Cardiovasc Intervent Radiol 1998;21:102

Jaffe RB: Complete interruption of the aortic arch. I. Characteristic radiographic findings in 21 patients. Circulation 1975;52:714

Kaulitz R, Jones RA, van der Velde ME: Echocardiographic assessment of interrupted aortic arch. Cardiol Young 1999;9:562

Magee AG, Brzezinska-Rajszys G, Qureshi SA, et al: Stent implantation for aortic coarctation and recoarctation. Heart 1999;82:600

Oshinski JN, Parks WJ, Markou CP, et al: Improved measurement of pressure gradients in aortic coarctation by magnetic resonance imaging. J Am Coll Cardiol 1996;28:1818

Pitlick PT, Anthony CL, Moore P, et al: Three-dimensional visualization of recurrent coarctation of the aorta by electron-beam tomography and MRI. Circulation 1999;99:3086

Roche KJ, Krinsky G, Lee VS, et al: Interrupted aortic arch: diagnosis with gadolinium-enhanced 3D MRA. J Comput Assist Tomogr 1999;23:197

Weber HS, Mosher T, Mahraj R, Baylen BG: Magnetic resonance imaging demonstration of "remodeling" of the aorta following balloon angioplasty of discrete native coarctation. Pediatr Cardiol 1996;17:184

White RI Jr, Mitchell SE, Kan J: Interventional procedures in congenital heart disease. Cardiovasc Intervent Radiol 1986;9:286

Endocardial Fibroelastosis

Carceller AM, Maroto E, Fouron JC: Dilated and contracted forms of primary endocardial fibroelastosis: a single fetal disease with two stages of development. Br Heart J 1990;63:311

Dinarevic S, Redington A, Rigby M, et al: Left ventricular pannus causing inflow obstruction late after mitral valve replacement for endocardial fibroelastosis. Pediatr Cardiol 1996;17:257

Mahle WT, Weinberg PM, Rychik J: Can echocardiography predict the presence or absence of endocardial fibroelastosis in infants >1 year of age with left ventricular outflow tract obstruction? Am J Cardiol 1998;82:122

Newbould MJ, Armstrong GR, Barson AJ: Endocardial fibroelastosis in infants with hydrops fetalis. J Clin Pathol 1991;44:576

Ni J, Bowles NE, Kim YH, et al: Viral infection of the myocardium in endocardial fibroelastosis: molecular evidence for the role of mumps virus as an etiologic agent. Circulation 1997;95:133

Tannouri F, Rypens F, Peny MO, et al: Fetal endocardial fibroelastosis: ultrasonographic findings in two cases. J Ultrasound Med 1998; 17:63

Ward CJ, Culham JA, Mawson J, et al: Angiographic demonstration of endocardial fibroelastosis in an infant with critical aortic stenosis. Am Heart J 1994;127:1430

■ Chapter 3

CYANOTIC CONGENITAL HEART DISEASE WITH INCREASED PULMONARY FLOW (ADMIXTURE SHUNTS)

RICHARD B. JAFFE and VIRGIL R. CONDON

COMPLETE TRANSPOSITION OF THE GREAT ARTERIES

Complete or dextrotransposition of the great arteries (d-TGA) is the most common form of cyanotic congenital heart disease (CHD) with increased pulmonary flow, and accounts for 5% to 9% of CHD. The prognosis is extremely poor without early palliation (Rashkind balloon atrial septostomy) or corrective surgery with Mustard, Senning, or great-vessel-switch procedures. Many variations of transposition are present and are more completely reviewed in works by Van Praagh and others. In isolated d-TGA, the aorta is transposed anteriorly and to the right and originates from the right ventricle, with the pulmonary artery posteriorly positioned and originating from the left ventricle.

INCIDENCE

The incidence is 1 in 4000 live births. The male:female ratio is 2:1 to 3:1. Infants of diabetic mothers have a significantly increased risk of d-TGA.

PATHOPHYSIOLOGY

A completely separate pulmonary and systemic vascular circuit is present that is incompatible with life without other associated shunts. Mixing occurs through a ventricular septal defect (VSD), patent ductus arteriosus (PDA), atrial septal defect (ASD), or patent foramen ovale. Approximately 70% of patients with d-TGA will have an intact ventricular septum and no left ventricular outflow obstruction. The two most commonly associated major lesions are VSD and left ventricular outflow tract obstruction typically coexisting with a VSD. The causes of left ventricular outflow tract obstruction in complete or d-TGA are listed in Table 1.

CLINICAL MANIFESTATIONS

Cyanosis presents at birth and is more severe in patients without VSD. Cyanosis, acidosis, and congestive heart failure (CHF) are the primary early manifestations and are exaggerated by closure of a patent ductus. Auscultation reveals no murmur or a very soft, innocent-sounding murmur. When other lesions are present, murmurs related to these lesions may be heard (i.e., VSD, pulmonary stenosis, etc.).

CHEST RADIOGRAPHY

Radiographic findings are variable and are primarily related to the presence or absence of pulmonary valvular stenosis (PVS). Findings include (1) hyperinflation of the lungs and depression of the diaphragm, (2) a narrow base of the heart, (3) an "egg-shaped" or "egg-on-side" cardiac configuration, (4) thymic atrophy, and (5) mild cardiomegaly (Fig. 1; see also Section V, Part I, Chapter 2, Fig. 4, page 1233). Pulmonary flow is

---

Table 1 ■ CAUSES OF LEFT VENTRICULAR OUTFLOW TRACT OBSTRUCTION IN COMPLETE OR DEXTROTRANSPOSITION OF THE GREAT ARTERIES

Pulmonary valvular stenosis (Fig. 4)
Subvalvular obstruction
  Fibrous diaphragm
  Fibromuscular tunnel
  Malalignment and posterior displacement of infundibular septum
  Aneurysm of the membranous septum
  Dynamic septal–mitral opposition
  Abnormal or accessory mitral valve tissue
  Abnormal mitral chordal attachments
  Herniation of tricuspid valve tissue through ventricular septal defect

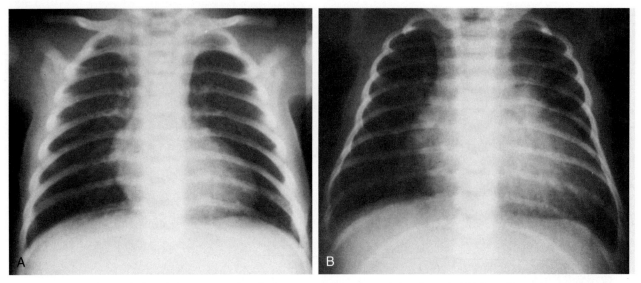

FIGURE 1. Transposition of the great arteries. **A,** Anteroposterior radiograph in a 3-week-old infant shows an egg-shaped cardiac silhouette, inconspicuous pulmonary artery segment secondary to its transposed position posterior to the aortic root, and only mild evidence of increased pulmonary vasculature and cardiomegaly. Involution of the thymus and depression of the diaphragm indicate continued hypoxia after Rashkind balloon atrial septostomy. **B,** The same patient at 1 year of age. Note the progressive cardiomegaly with an abnormal silhouette and a much greater degree of admixture shunt (see Section V, Part I, Chapter 2, Fig. 4, page 1233).

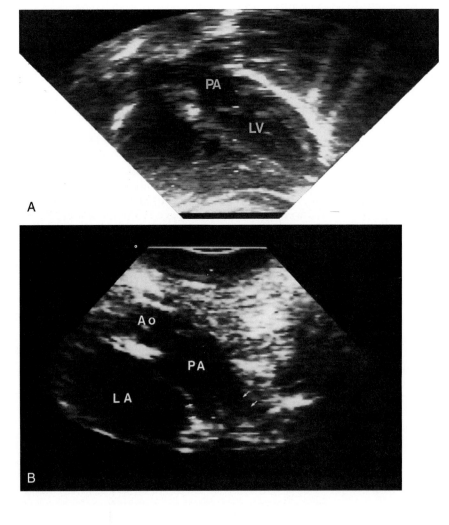

FIGURE 2. Dextrotransposition of the great arteries. **A,** Subxiphoid two-dimensional echocardiogram shows a large main pulmonary artery *(PA)* with right and left pulmonary arteries originating posteriorly from the left ventricle *(LV).* **B,** Short-axis view shows the origin of the aorta *(Ao)* anteriorly and to the right of the pulmonary artery *(PA). LA* = left atrium.

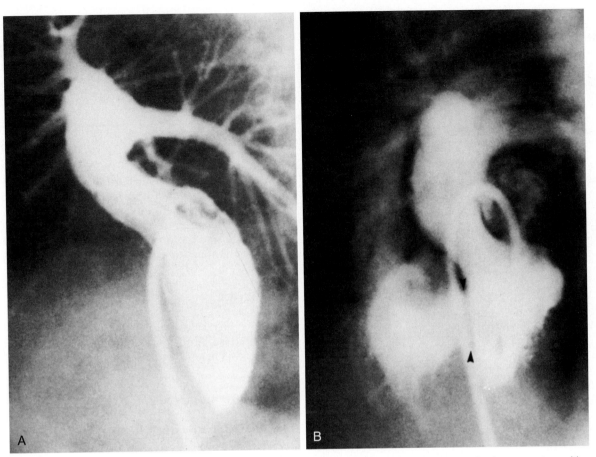

FIGURE 3. Transposition of the great arteries. **A,** Long-axis left ventriculogram shows a transposed pulmonary artery with normal mitral–pulmonary valve continuity and no evidence of pulmonary stenosis. **B,** Similar left ventriculogram shows a moderate muscular ventricular septal defect *(arrowheads)* (see Section V, Part I, Chapter 2, Fig. 12*B*, page 1238).

normal in the neonate until pulmonary vascular resistance decreases; then, pulmonary flow typically is increased unless left ventricular outflow tract obstruction or PVS is present. If pulmonary hypertension, left ventricular outflow tract obstruction, or closure of the atrial septostomy has occurred, congestive failure is frequent, particularly in patients with a VSD. Differential diagnoses include truncus arteriosus with normal or increased flow; when d-TGA is associated with PVS, tetralogy of Fallot and tricuspid atresia must be excluded.

ECHOCARDIOGRAPHY

Real-time echocardiography easily identifies the abnormal position of the aorta and pulmonary artery (Fig. 2). Other associated valvular and septal defects and arch abnormalities are readily identified. The pulmonary valve and subvalvular area should be evaluated closely because of their frequent involvement. Coronary artery origins should also be determined prior to planned arterial switch. Doppler may be helpful in identifying intracardiac and ductal shunts.

ANGIOCARDIOGRAPHY AND CATHETERIZATION

Right heart ventriculography demonstrates a large trabeculated right ventricle in a normal position giving rise to a smooth-walled infundibulum and transposed aortic valve and root. With the presence of a VSD, a right-to-left ventricular shunt will be noted. The aortic arch is on the left except when associated with PVS, in which case a right arch may be seen in 75% of patients. The right ventricle may be hypoplastic (poor prognosis).

Long-axis left ventriculography usually shows a normal-sized left ventricle, although frequently it is compressed by the large right ventricle. The left ventricle gives origin to the pulmonary artery (Fig. 3). The pulmonary valve and subvalvular area must be closely evaluated for stenosis (Fig. 4; Table 1). Pulmonary valve and anterior mitral leaflet continuity must be established to differentiate d-TGA from double-outlet right ventricle (see Section V, Part I, Chapter 2, Fig. 12*A*, page 1238). An aortogram to visualize the coronary arteries should be performed with balloon occlusion of the ascending aorta (Berman angiographic catheter) if an arterial-switch operation is planned. Filming in the anteroposte-

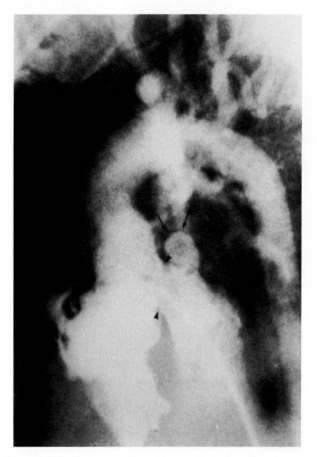

FIGURE 4. Dextrotransposition of the great arteries with pulmonary obstruction. A long-axis left ventriculogram shows transposed aorta and pulmonary artery, a large ventricular septal defect *(arrowheads)* with left-to-right shunting, and severe pulmonary valvular stenosis with doming of the thickened pulmonary leaflets *(black arrows)*.

rior (AP) projection should be performed with caudal–cranial angulation of 40 to 45 degrees ("laid-back" aortogram) supplemented with the lateral projection.

A balloon atrial septostomy must be performed early in the course of catheterization, frequently before angiography if a supporting echocardiogram is diagnostic of d-TGA. This improves atrial-level mixing and oxygenation and allows for safer, further cardiac catheterization.

PROGNOSIS

Survival rates of 70% to 80% can be expected to the age of 2 years after balloon atrial septostomy or other operative procedure (pulmonary artery banding). When utilizing a Mustard or Senning procedure, normal physiologic blood flow by intra-atrial shunting can be accomplished. An arterial switch and transplantation of the coronary arteries (Jatene procedure) is the preferred reparative operation in the absence of left ventricular outflow tract obstruction. Postoperative complications include supravalvular narrowing of the

pulmonary artery (see Section V, Part VII, Chapter 1, Fig. 14, page 1402) or aorta and left ventricular ischemia from coronary artery obstruction (see discussion of operative procedures and complications in Section V, Part VII, Chapter 1, page 1393). The prognosis is always worse when associated with a VSD and PVS.

SINGLE VENTRICLE

Single ventricle (common ventricle, univentricular heart, cor triloculare biatriatum) can be defined as a heart containing one ventricular chamber receiving blood through both the mitral and tricuspid valves or, frequently, a common atrioventricular (AV) valve. The great vessels are commonly transposed, with complications of pulmonic or systemic outflow obstructions.

INCIDENCE

A single ventricle constitutes approximately 1.5% of CHD, and is slightly more common in males. It is found in 1 in 6500 live births.

PATHOPHYSIOLOGY

A single left ventricle usually has d-TGA or corrected, or levotransposition of the great arteries (l-TGA). Other types include a single right ventricle and an undifferentiated ventricle. An outlet chamber may or may not exist and be associated with either bulboventricular or valvular stenosis, or both. Asplenia syndrome often is present.

CLINICAL MANIFESTATIONS

Early cyanosis and CHF are common, with the degree of cyanosis depending in part on the degree of pulmonary outflow obstruction. A pansystolic murmur is frequent with an associated hyperactive heart.

CHEST RADIOGRAPHY

Radiographic manifestations primarily relate to the great vessel orientation. A single ventricle with d-TGA simulates findings of conventional transposition of the great arteries (TGA). With corrected transposition, the aorta is often border-forming in the upper left heart margin. Pulmonary flow is increased in the absence of pulmonary outflow obstruction. Cardiomegaly is usually noted unless pulmonary outflow obstruction is present.

ECHOCARDIOGRAPHY

Real-time echocardiography is particularly valuable in this condition for differentiating TGA with a VSD from a single ventricle with transposition. A ventricular septum will not be evident, and two AV valves are usually seen (Fig. 5). When a common AV valve exists, this can be readily visualized. The aorta and pulmonary artery relations are easily defined and d- and l-TGA differentiated.

ANGIOCARDIOGRAPHY

Biplane long-axis angiocardiography should be performed with a large bolus injection (2 ml/kg) with a high flow rate. Ventricular chamber shape, number of AV valves, outflow chamber position, and great vessel relations all must be evaluated (Fig. 6). Pulmonary and aortic outflow obstructions may exist, along with the occasional presence of coarctation.

MAGNETIC RESONANCE IMAGING

Magnetic resonance imaging (MRI) is an ideal modality to determine the segmental anatomy and evaluate the central pulmonary arteries before the Fontan procedure. MRI may also differentiate single ventricle with d-TGA from d-TGA with large VSD (Fig. 7). MRI in the coronal plane often demonstrates well the bulboventricular foramen and outlet chamber (Fig. 8).

PROGNOSIS

Palliative surgery (i.e., pulmonary artery banding) may be helpful in the neonate when large pulmonary shunts exist. Systemic–pulmonary shunting will be needed in the presence of PVS. Reconstructive procedures include a Fontan procedure, occasionally ventricular septation, and rarely a Damus procedure to bypass subaortic or aortic valve obstruction (see Section V, Part VII, Chapter 1, page 1393).

CORRECTED TRANSPOSITION OF THE GREAT ARTERIES

Corrected TGA is characterized by ventricular inversion and levotransposition (l-TGA), resulting in discordant AV and ventriculoarterial connections (see Section V, Part IV, Chapter 1, page 1360). In the uncomplicated type, systemic venous return passes from the right atrium through the mitral valve into a morphologic left ventricle and then to the posterior and medially positioned pulmonary artery. Pulmonary venous return is to the normally positioned left atrium, and then through the tricuspid valve to the systemic morphologic right ventricle and out the levotransposed aorta. In this state, blood flows in a physiologic manner.

Unfortunately, only 1% of patients with l-TGA are without other significant intracardiac defects. Frequently associated anomalies, singly or in combination, are (1) VSD; (2) PVS or subvalvular stenosis; (3) abnormalities of the systemic AV (tricuspid) valve, including Ebstein's anomaly with regurgitation; and (4) disturbances of the AV conduction system predisposing to complete or partial heart block. Dextroversion and abnormalities in situs may be present with l-TGA (see Section V, Part IV, Chapter 1, page 1360). l-TGA of the great arteries may also be present with single ventricle (see Single Ventricle above and Fig. 8).

INCIDENCE

Corrected TGA constitutes 1% of CHD. It is slightly more common in males and occurs in 1 in 13,000 live

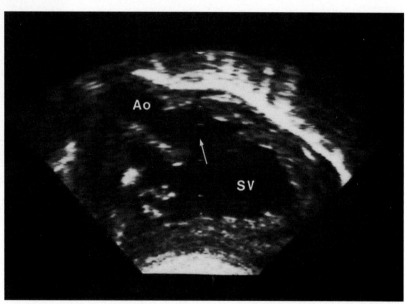

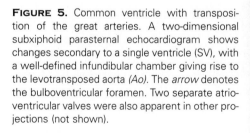

FIGURE 5. Common ventricle with transposition of the great arteries. A two-dimensional subxiphoid parasternal echocardiogram shows changes secondary to a single ventricle (SV), with a well-defined infundibular chamber giving rise to the levotransposed aorta (Ao). The *arrow* denotes the bulboventricular foramen. Two separate atrioventricular valves were also apparent in other projections (not shown).

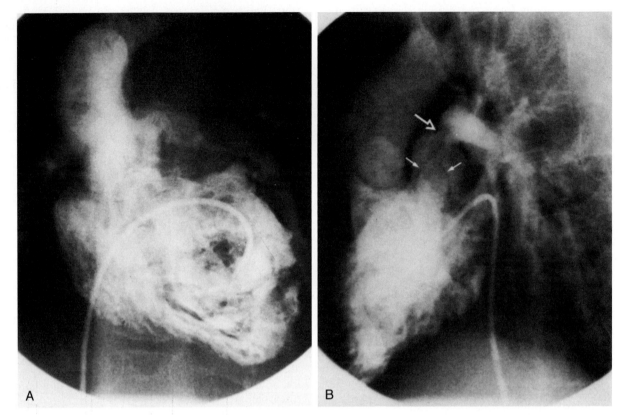

FIGURE 6. Common ventricle with transposition of the great arteries and pulmonary valvular stenosis (PVS). Anteroposterior **(A)** and lateral **(B)** ventriculograms show the large, moderately trabeculated common ventricle giving rise to transposed great arteries. PVS *(arrows)* and a pulmonary artery band *(open arrow)* are present. The right aortic arch is also evident.

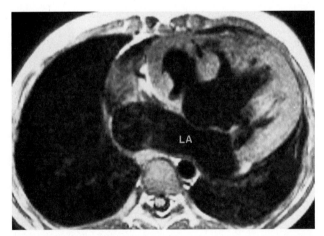

FIGURE 7. Common single ventricle. Axial spin-echo magnetic resonance image at the level of the left atrium *(LA)* demonstrates the mitral valve and single ventricle. Axial images at a lower level demonstrated a small tricuspid valve.

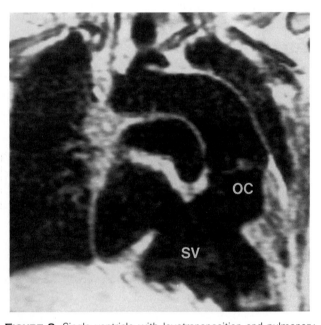

FIGURE 8. Single ventricle with levotransposition and pulmonary valve atresia. Coronal magnetic resonance image demonstrates the venous atrium, single ventricle *(SV)*, bulboventricular foramen leading to the outlet chamber *(OC)*, and levotransposed aorta. The pulmonary artery and atretic valve are seen medial to the aorta (see Section V, Part V, Chapter 2, Fig. 4, page 1379).

births. Occasionally, other variations in visceral and atrial situs occur.

PATHOPHYSIOLOGY

Ninety-five percent of patients have atrial–visceral situs solitus. The ventricles are inverted, with the morphologic right ventricle on the left and the morphologic left ventricle on the right (the levo form of ventricular loop development). This inverted ventricular relationship with atrial situs solitus produces AV discordance. The great vessels are transposed, with the aorta anteriorly to the left and the pulmonary artery arising posteriorly from the inverted, medially positioned right ventricle. There is mitral–pulmonary continuity. With the tricuspid valve related to the systemic ventricle, tricuspid incompetence may occur (20%). Inversion of the coronary arteries accompanies the ventricular inversion.

CLINICAL MANIFESTATIONS

Clinical presentation relates to the intracardiac lesions. With large intracardiac shunts, patients commonly present with CHF, whereas those patients with PVS are commonly cyanotic. Murmurs exist in 60% of patients and relate to associated intracardiac lesions.

CHEST RADIOGRAPHY

The characteristic configuration of l-TGA is abnormal fullness in the mid- and upper left heart border, which produces a gentle slope that is straight to convex in relation to the levotransposed position of the ascending aorta (Fig. 9A). Other variable findings include (1) absence of a defined main pulmonary artery segment, (2) increased pulmonary blood flow in the absence of pulmonary outflow obstruction, (3) a high position of the right pulmonary artery, and occasionally (4) dextroversion with situs solitus or levocardia with situs inversus. Primary differential diagnostic considerations are other forms of transposition, single ventricle, and truncus arteriosus.

ECHOCARDIOGRAPHY

Real-time echocardiography is particularly helpful in this condition in which definition of the great vessel relationships, ventricular septal anatomy, and orientation of the plane of the ventricular septum are critical (Fig. 9B, C). Mitral–pulmonary continuity is appreciated with either real-time or M-mode studies.

ANGIOCARDIOGRAPHY

AP and lateral biplane angiocardiography and angled projections are necessary for optimal anatomic evalua-

tion. The ventricles are usually side by side, and their morphology must be studied in detail. The morphologic left ventricle in its medial position gives rise to the pulmonary artery (Fig. 10A, B). The pulmonary valve and subvalvular area must be closely examined for stenosis, in which case right-to-left shunting through the VSD can usually be seen. A ventriculogram of the systemic ventricle shows morphologic characteristics of a trabeculated right ventricle giving rise to the levotransposed aorta, with the aortic valve in a relatively cephalic position (Fig. 10C). With associated VSD, physiologic left-to-right shunting will be apparent. Other variable findings include AV valve regurgitation, tricuspid valve dysplasia, Ebstein's anomaly, aneurysm of the membranous septum (Fig. 10), and a right aortic arch.

PROGNOSIS

The prognosis depends mainly on the severity of associated malformations. CHF and heart block are common, necessitating a pacemaker. Pulmonary artery banding is necessary when associated with a single ventricle, and systemic-to-pulmonary shunts are necessary when the pulmonary outflow obstruction is severe.

TOTAL ANOMALOUS PULMONARY VENOUS RETURN

Total anomalous pulmonary venous return (TAPVR) indicates total pulmonary venous drainage to the systemic venous circulation.

INCIDENCE

TAPVR accounts for 1% to 2% of CHD. The male:female ratio is approximately 2:1. TAPVR is of four types:

1. Supracardiac (50%)—to left vertical vein, innominate vein, azygos vein, or right superior vena cava (SVC)
2. Cardiac (30%)—to right atrium or coronary sinus
3. Infracardiac (15%)—to portal vein, ductus venosus, or gastric vein
4. Mixed (5%)—to more than one level

These types may be further subdivided into obstructed and nonobstructed categories, with 50% to 66% being obstructed. The infracardiac type is always obstructed. TAPVR is almost always present in asplenia syndrome.

PATHOPHYSIOLOGY

The pathophysiologic state depends on (1) the quantity of pulmonary flow and resistance, (2) pulmonary venous obstruction, (3) the size of the obligatory ASD, (4) the presence of a PDA, and (5) right ventricular

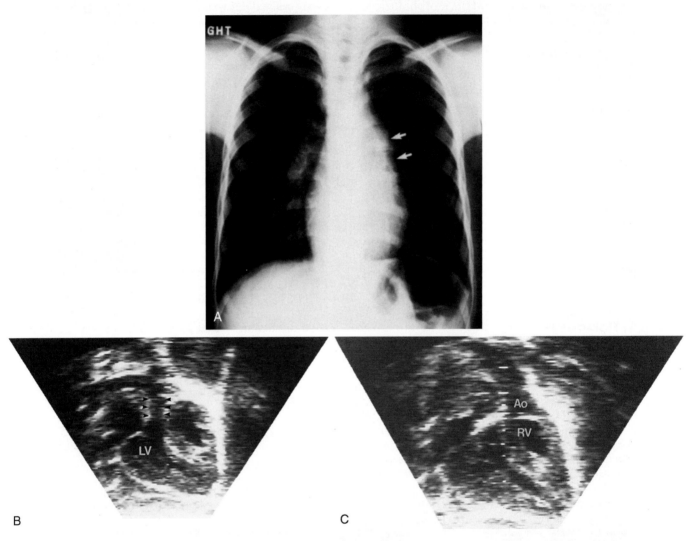

FIGURE 9. Corrected levotransposition of the great arteries. **A,** Characteristic convex mid-upper left heart border related to transposition of the ascending aorta anteriorly and to the left. This represents the relatively rare patient without intrinsic congenital malformations. Most patients have pulmonary valvular stenosis, ventricular septal defect (or a common ventricle), abnormalities of the systemic atrioventricular valve, and conduction disturbances. **B,** Two-dimensional echocardiogram in the subcostal projection demonstrates origin of the medially positioned pulmonary artery *(arrowheads)* from the right-sided morphologic left ventricle *(LV)*. **C,** Two-dimensional echocardiogram in the subcostal projection in a plane slightly anterior to **B** demonstrates origin of the levotransposed aorta *(Ao)* from the left-sided morphologic right ventricle *(RV)*. (**B** and **C** from Jaffe RB: Corrected transposition with ventricular septal defect—echocardiography. *In* Elliott LP [ed]: Cardiac Imaging in Infants, Children, and Adults. Philadelphia, JB Lippincott, 1991:634, with permission.)

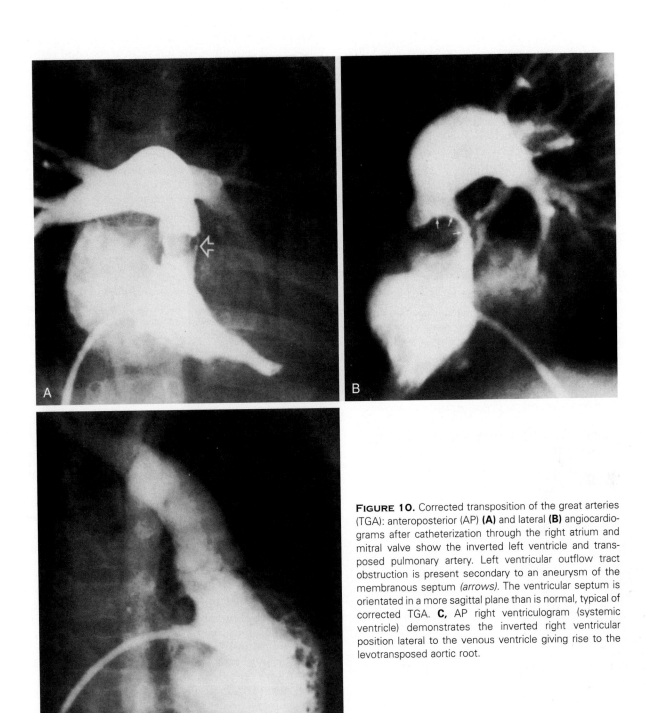

FIGURE 10. Corrected transposition of the great arteries (TGA): anteroposterior (AP) **(A)** and lateral **(B)** angiocardiograms after catheterization through the right atrium and mitral valve show the inverted left ventricle and transposed pulmonary artery. Left ventricular outflow tract obstruction is present secondary to an aneurysm of the membranous septum *(arrows)*. The ventricular septum is orientated in a more sagittal plane than is normal, typical of corrected TGA. **C,** AP right ventriculogram (systemic ventricle) demonstrates the inverted right ventricular position lateral to the venous ventricle giving rise to the levotransposed aortic root.

compliance. With high pulmonary flow and good mixing, cyanosis is mild and symptoms minimal until CHF ensues. With pulmonary venous obstruction, cyanosis is severe, and early death is common without operative correction.

CLINICAL MANIFESTATIONS

Infants with obstructed TAPVR always present with severe cyanosis, marked dyspnea, hepatomegaly, and no or insignificant-sounding murmurs. Patients without pulmonary venous obstruction show equivocal cyanosis, tachypnea, dyspnea, poor feeding, hepatomegaly, failure to thrive, and CHF. Other findings include a gallop rhythm, a loud first heart sound, and a split second heart sound.

CHEST RADIOGRAPHY

Total Anomalous Pulmonary Venous Return With Obstruction

Radiographic features are (1) normal cardiac configuration and size; (2) pulmonary venous congestion or edema, or both; (3) thymic atrophy; (4) depression of the diaphragm; and (5) occasional pleural effusion (Fig. 11). The primary differential diagnosis is diffuse interstitial pulmonary disease, including pulmonary lymphangiectasia.

Total Anomalous Pulmonary Venous Return Without Obstruction

Common roentgenographic features include (1) cardiomegaly with right atrial and right ventricular enlarge-

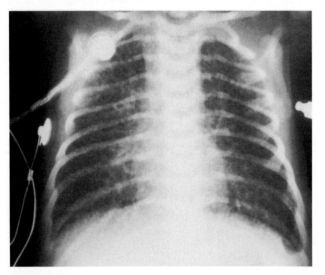

FIGURE 11. Obstructive supracardiac total anomalous pulmonary venous return (TAPVR). An anteroposterior chest radiograph in this newborn shows a characteristic pattern of pulmonary venous congestion, a small cardiac silhouette, thymic involution, and hyperinflation. An identical pattern would also be seen with the intracardiac type of TAPVR.

ment, (2) an enlarged main pulmonary artery, (3) increased pulmonary flow, and (4) occasional CHF. The primary differential diagnoses are other large left-to-right and admixture shunts.

In the older patient with a nonobstructed supracardiac-type anomalous venous return, characteristic enlargement of the left vertical vein and right SVC produces the so-called snowman or figure-8 cardiac silhouette (Fig. 12). This "snowman" appearance is rarely seen today owing to early operative intervention. Other variations in anomalous drainage may produce focal enlargement of the azygos vein, dilatation of the right SVC (Fig. 13), or visualization of abnormal veins directed toward the superior right hilum. An esophagogram, if performed, may also show an abnormal indentation of the anterior wall in the upper to midatrial level, again related to the common pulmonary vein (Fig. 14).

ECHOCARDIOGRAPHY

Real-time echocardiography can commonly track the anomalous pulmonary venous drainage to its aberrant drainage site (Fig. 15), and may be the only imaging modality needed for diagnosis. Other findings include (1) enlargement of the right atrium and tricuspid annulus and right ventricle, (2) paradoxical septal motion in the nonobstructive types, and (3) evidence of pulmonary hypertension. ASDs and PDA (when present) are similarly detected.

ANGIOCARDIOGRAPHY

Because of the large number of complex variations in cases of anomalous pulmonary venous return, angiocardiography may be necessary for complete evaluation. Biplane AP and lateral cineangiography is performed by injecting contrast material into the main pulmonary artery or, selectively, into the right or left pulmonary artery (Fig. 16). Balloon occlusion of a PDA may be necessary to improve pulmonary artery filling (Figs. 17 and 18). It is necessary to determine not only the anatomic type of anomalous venous return but also the coexistence of pulmonary venous obstruction. At times, the catheter can be introduced up the SVC to the innominate and vertical vein, with retrograde injection into the pulmonary venous confluence better demonstrating the anatomic malformation (Fig. 19). Patients with intracardiac anomalous return to the coronary sinus may show a striking aneurysmal dilatation of the distal coronary sinus.

MAGNETIC RESONANCE IMAGING

Axial and coronal MRI are useful in the evaluation of unusual forms of TAPVR, and after operation. The operative anastomosis between the common pulmonary vein and left atrium may be defined clearly by MRI. If present, areas of stenosis may be identified.

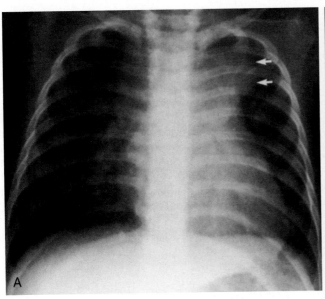

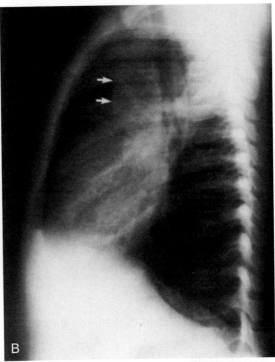

FIGURE 12. Supracardiac total anomalous pulmonary venous return to the left vertical vein (snowman) in a 5-month-old infant. The "snowman" cardiac silhouette is already evident in the anteroposterior **(A)** chest radiograph, with relative aneurysmal dilatation of the left vertical vein in **A** *(arrows)*. Increased pulmonary flow and hyperinflation of the lungs are characteristic of the cyanotic condition. On the lateral film **(B),** a band of increased density *(arrows)* anterior to the trachea represents the dilated left vertical vein and right superior vena cava. This snowman appearance is rarely seen today owing to early operative intervention.

PROGNOSIS

Symptoms may be ameliorated by Rashkind balloon septostomy, improving mixing at the atrial level. Early operation is mandatory, especially in TAPVR with obstruction and to avoid pulmonary hypertension.

COR TRIATRIATUM AND OTHER ANOMALIES OF THE PULMONARY VEINS

Cor triatriatum reflects the failure to incorporate the common pulmonary veins into the posterior left atrial wall. This produces a membrane with variable obstruction separating the accessory chamber receiving the pulmonary veins from the left atrium. Collateral flow through a persisting left vertical vein is common, bypassing the obstruction and creating pathophysiologic findings similar to supracardiac TAPVR. Varying degrees of pulmonary venous obstruction relate to the size of the orifice in the membrane.

Radiographic findings are mainly those arising from pulmonary venous congestion. The diagnosis may be established with echocardiography, angiocardiography (Fig. 20), MRI, or electron-beam or helical computed tomography. Other variations in drainage occur in this condition, including anomalous drainage into the right atrium or coronary sinus. Primary differential consider-

ations are congenital supravalvular mitral ring and congenital mitral stenosis.

Other rare forms of pulmonary venous anomalies include atresia of the common pulmonary vein and

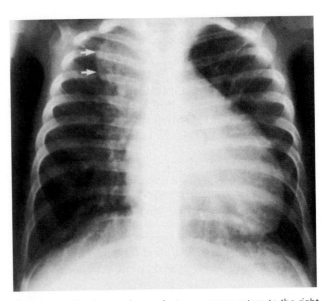

FIGURE 13. Total anomalous pulmonary venous return to the right superior vena cava (SVC): anteroposterior chest radiograph shows aneurysmal dilatation of the SVC *(arrows)*. Cardiomegaly with a right ventricular configuration and increased pulmonary blood flow is present.

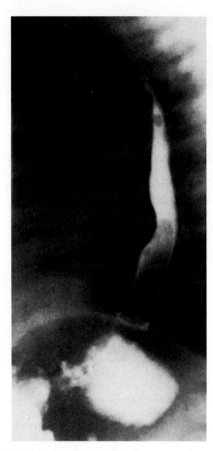

FIGURE 14. Total anomalous pulmonary venous return (TAPVR). A lateral esophagogram spot film shows a focal indentation on the anterior surface of the esophagus just below the carina at the level of the left atrium that is secondary to the anomalous pulmonary venous confluence of TAPVR. A large coronary sinus secondary to an anomalous pulmonary venous return could produce the same findings.

stenosis of the individual pulmonary veins (unilateral or bilateral) (Fig. 21).

TRUNCUS ARTERIOSUS (PERSISTENT TRUNCUS ARTERIOSUS, TRUNCUS ARTERIOSUS COMMUNIS, AND COMMON AORTICOPULMONARY TRUNK)

Truncus arteriosus is an anomaly characterized by a single vessel arising from the ventricles, overriding a VSD, and supplying the systemic, pulmonary, and coronary circulations. Only one semilunar valve is present. Embryologically, truncus arteriosus represents a failure of the truncus arteriosus to divide into a completely separate ascending aorta and pulmonary artery.

CLASSIFICATION

Many classifications have been developed, but probably the most widely utilized was that of Collette and Edwards, which categorizes truncus arteriosus as (1) type I (50%), where a single pulmonary trunk arises from the common truncal vessel, branching into right and left pulmonary arteries; (2) type II (30%), where right and left pulmonary arteries arise close together from the posterior wall of the truncal vessel; (3) type III, where the right and left pulmonary arteries arise from either side of the common trunk; and (4) type IV, where no pulmonary arteries arise from the ascending trunk but the lungs are supplied by systemic bronchial or pulmonary vessels. Some authors (Van Praagh) think that the last-named category is not a true example of truncus arteriosus and should be classified with pulmonary atresia. Many other classifications and variations have been described.

INCIDENCE

The reported incidence is approximately 1% of CHD, with an occurrence of 1 in 11,000 live births. Other associated malformations include interruption of the aortic arch, a hypoplastic aortic isthmus, coarctation, and PDA. It may occur with DiGeorge syndrome. Unilateral absence of a pulmonary artery has been reported in 12% of patients. Truncal valve stenosis and insufficiency, as well as anomalies of the coronary arteries, may also be present.

PATHOPHYSIOLOGY

The pathophysiologic process relates to increased pulmonary flow with an admixture of systemic and pulmonary blood. Complications include pulmonary hypertension, increased pulmonary vascular resistance, and truncal valve insufficiency. The truncal valve is usually tricuspid (66%), with the remainder being either bicuspid or quadricuspid valves. In rare cases, stenosis at the origin of the pulmonary arteries may be present, producing decreased pulmonary flow and exaggerating the cyanosis. Hypoxemia may lead to myocardial ischemia and poor function.

CLINICAL MANIFESTATIONS

Most patients present early in life with cyanosis, failure to thrive, dyspnea, and CHF. The heart is enlarged, with a prominent second sound that is usually single. An apical systolic ejection click and soft pansystolic or ejection murmur is heard in most patients.

CHEST RADIOGRAPHY

Common chest radiographic findings include (1) moderate cardiomegaly, (2) a narrow base of the heart, (3) a high cephalic origin of the left pulmonary artery, (4) a right aortic arch (in 25% to 33% of patients), (5) increased pulmonary blood flow, (6) a depressed dia-

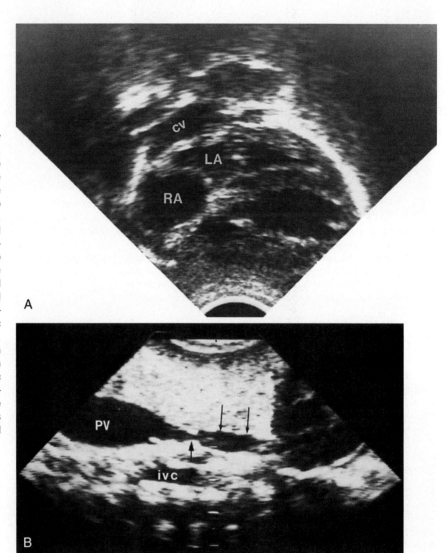

FIGURE 15. Total anomalous pulmonary venous return to the left vertical vein. **A,** Subcostal projection at the level of the right atrium *(RA)* and left atrium *(LA)*. The right and left pulmonary veins enter into the common pulmonary vein *(CV)* posterior to the left atrium rather than into the left atrium. Other imaging planes from the suprasternal notch (not illustrated) demonstrate the continuation of the common pulmonary vein into the left vertical vein and the left innominate vein. The atrial septal defect is not visualized in the image illustrated. (From Jaffe RB: Total anomalous pulmonary venous connection—echocardiography. *In* Elliott LP [ed]: Cardiac Imaging in Infants, Children, and Adults. Philadelphia, JB Lippincott, 1991:671, with permission.) **B,** Real-time echocardiogram shows changes related to infradiaphragmatic pulmonary venous return. The common venous channel *(arrows)* extends below the diaphragm, with an area of venous stenosis *(large arrow)* at its junction with the portal vein *(PV)*. *ivc* = inferior vena cava.

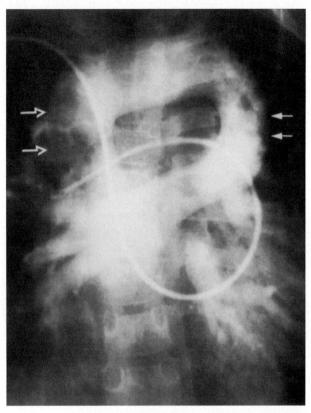

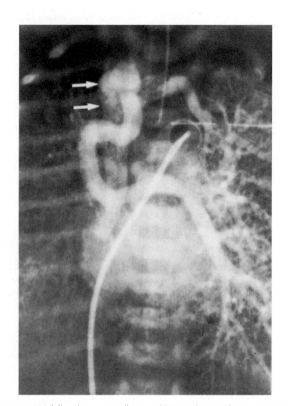

FIGURE 16. Supracardiac total anomalous pulmonary venous return (TAPVR). A late venous angiogram after a right pulmonary artery injection shows the characteristic anomalous pulmonary venous drainage secondary to nonobstructed supracardiac TAPVR. The left vertical vein is dilated and bulges laterally *(arrows)* along with the dilatation of the innominate vein and superior vena cava *(open arrows)*.

FIGURE 17. Mixed supracardiac total anomalous pulmonary venous return. A late pulmonary venous angiogram after a left pulmonary artery injection shows circuitous venous drainage predominantly to the superior vena cava *(arrows)*, with the left upper lobe draining anomalously through the innominate vein.

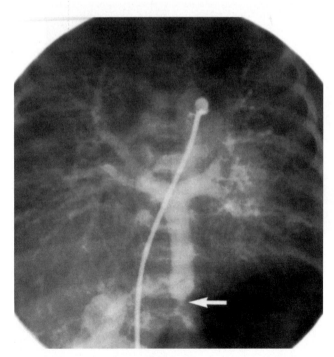

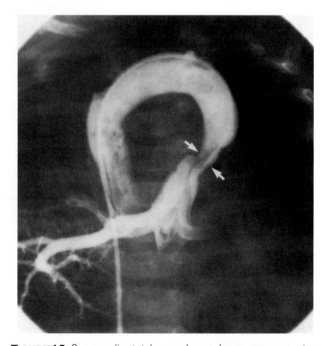

FIGURE 18. Intracardiac total anomalous pulmonary venous return (TAPVR). A late pulmonary venous angiocardiogram after main pulmonary artery injection with balloon catheter occlusion of a patent ductus arteriosus demonstrates classic findings of infracardiac TAPVR. Note the stenosis of the common pulmonary vein at its junction with the portal system *(arrow)* (see Fig. 15).

FIGURE 19. Supracardiac total anomalous pulmonary venous return with obstruction. Pulmonary venous angiogram following retrograde catheterization of the superior vena cava, innominate vein, and left vertical vein. Note the point of narrowing and obstruction *(arrows)* caused by compression of this venous channel between the left main pulmonary artery and left main stem bronchus or by intrinsic stenosis.

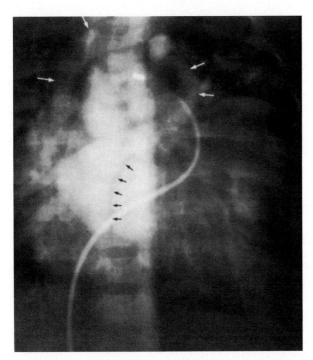

FIGURE 20. Cor triatriatum. A late pulmonary venous angiogram shows a fenestrated membrane *(black arrows)* dividing the left atrium, with collateral venous drainage to the left vertical vein *(white arrows)* and subsequent visualization of the innominate vein and superior vena cava. The radiographic patterns of cor triatriatum may resemble those of nonobstructed or obstructed total anomalous pulmonary venous return, depending upon septal defects and other patent venous collateral channels.

phragm, and (7) thymic atrophy (Fig. 22). The primary differential diagnosis is d-TGA. In a small second group of patients, pulmonary flow is decreased because of pulmonary artery stenosis or increased pulmonary resistance.

ECHOCARDIOGRAPHY

Real-time echocardiography readily identifies (1) a large single truncal vessel overriding (2) a large VSD, and (3) a large echogenic truncal valve with fibrous continuity with the anterior leaflet of the mitral valve. The main pulmonary artery in type I truncus arteriosus can usually be identified by its origin from the truncal vessel (Fig. 23).

ANGIOGRAPHY

Large-volume (2 ml/kg) biplane AP and lateral cineangiography should be performed by injecting contrast into the proximal truncal vessel or main pulmonary artery in type I lesions (Fig. 24). Supplementation with oblique views may be necessary, particularly in differentiating types II and III truncus arteriosus from type I when a short main pulmonary artery segment exists. Ventriculography, although rarely necessary, will demonstrate the conal VSD. The aortic arch, coronary

arteries, and truncal valve should be closely evaluated because of frequently associated variations. The recognition of separate pulmonary and aortic valves permit differentiation of an aorticopulmonary window from truncus arteriosus type I.

PROGNOSIS

Primary repair is usually performed in infancy with VSD closure and placement of a valved conduit between the right ventricle and pulmonary arteries (Rastelli procedure). Postoperative complications include calcification of the valve and/or conduit with obstruction (see Section V, Part VII, Chapter 1, Figs. 28 and 29, page 1413). Balloon valvuloplasty and conduit replacement may be necessary (see Section V, Part VII, Chapter 1, page 1393).

DOUBLE-OUTLET RIGHT VENTRICLE

A double-outlet right ventricle (DORV) is characterized by the origin of both great vessels predominantly from the right ventricle, and by bilateral muscular infundibula and absence of AV–semilunar valve continuity. A VSD is invariably present and may be classified as (1) subaortic, (2) subpulmonic, (3) doubly committed, or (4) noncommitted (remote). The great vessel relations are variable, but most commonly seen are side-by-side great vessels with the aorta to the right of the pulmonary artery (Taussig-Bing malformation if the VSD is subpulmonic), and the aorta anterior and to the right of the pulmonary artery. PVS is frequently present, especially when the VSD is subaortic. DORV can occur with dextro-, meso-, or levocardia, and may be associated with asplenia syndrome.

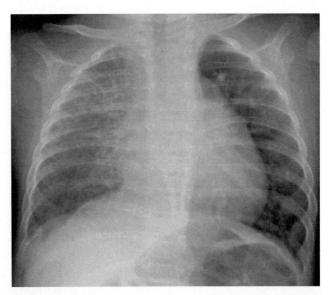

FIGURE 21. Four-month-old infant with unilateral right pulmonary venous atresia. Frontal chest radiograph demonstrates right lung interstitial edema and mild cardiomegaly with right heart enlargement.

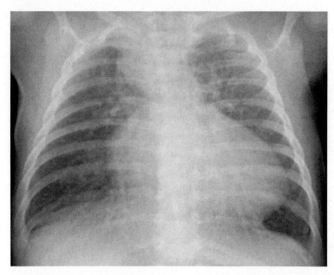

FIGURE 22. Truncus arteriosus, type I. Frontal radiograph in a 2-month-old demonstrates increased pulmonary blood flow, moderate cardiomegaly, inconspicuous main pulmonary artery, and large right aortic arch. Hyperinflation is present secondary to hypoxia.

INCIDENCE

DORV constitutes 1% to 3% of all CHD. Associated lesions include coarctation or an interrupted aortic arch. The male:female ratio is approximately 2:1.

PATHOPHYSIOLOGY

This lesion represents an admixture shunt with increased pulmonary blood flow. Patients with Taussig-Bing malformation with subpulmonic VSD have pathophysiologic findings similar to those of complete transposition.

CLINICAL MANIFESTATIONS

Symptoms depend on the type of lesion present as well as the size of the pulmonary shunt and commitment of the VSD. Mild to marked cyanosis may be present. Without PVS, clinical findings are similar to a VSD. With PVS, clinical findings simulate tetralogy of Fallot. Those patients with subpulmonic VSD without PVS present early with cyanosis and mimic transposition of the great vessels. Without PVS, CHF is frequent.

CHEST RADIOGRAPHY

Chest radiographic features correlate closely with the presence or absence of PVS or aortic arch obstruction. Without pulmonary obstruction, findings include (1) moderate cardiomegaly (right ventricular configuration); (2) large convex main pulmonary artery; (3) increased pulmonary blood flow; (4) thymic atrophy; and (5) a depressed diaphragm with hyperinflation of the lung. Early congestive failure suggests coarctation or an interrupted aortic arch.

With PVS, findings are (1) mild cardiomegaly with a right ventricular configuration, (2) a concave main pulmonary artery, (3) diminished pulmonary blood flow, and (4) a left aortic arch. If visceral heterotaxia is evident, cardiosplenic syndrome, especially asplenia, should be considered.

ECHOCARDIOGRAPHY

Real-time echocardiography demonstrates (1) side-by-side transposition of the great vessels with the aorta usually anterior and to the right, (2) overriding of the

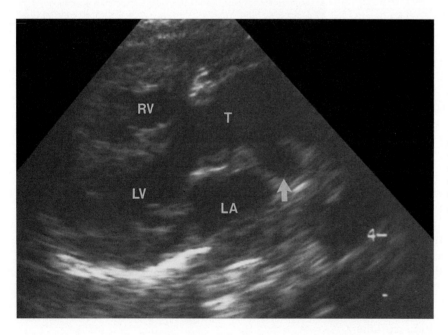

FIGURE 23. Truncus arteriosus. Two-dimensional long axis echocardiogram shows the large truncal vessel *(T)* overriding the large ventricular septal defect. A large pulmonary vessel arises posteriorly from the truncus vessel *(arrow)*. *RV* = right ventricle; *LA* = left atrium; *LV* = left ventricle.

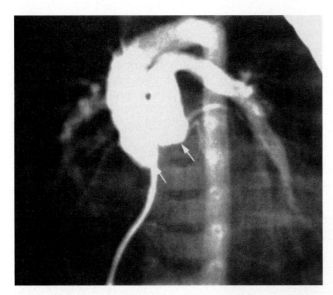

FIGURE 24. Truncus arteriosus, type I. Injection of contrast into the truncal root shows the large truncal valve *(arrows)* and simultaneous filling of a short main pulmonary artery segment and aortic arch. The origin of both pulmonary arteries is high, particularly the left, and there is symmetric flow to both lungs.

aortic root in relation to the ventricular septum, (3) a VSD, (4) subpulmonic and subaortic stenosis when present, and (5) absent fibrous continuity of the semilunar and AV valves (Fig. 25). Differential diagnoses are primarily tetralogy of Fallot and d-TGA with VSD.

ANGIOCARDIOGRAPHY

Biplane right and left ventricular injections are necessary, with filming in the AP and lateral, long-axis, and four-chamber projections to identify all anatomic abnormalities. Aortic root injections may also be needed. The VSD must be well visualized and its commitment to the great vessels adequately demonstrated (Fig. 26). The

semilunar valves, subpulmonic area, and aortic arch may all show anomalies requiring evaluation. Typically the aortic and pulmonary valves are at the same cephalocaudal position. The diagnosis of DORV is dependent on identification of more than half of each great vessel originating from the morphologic right ventricle.

MAGNETIC RESONANCE IMAGING

MRI is very helpful, especially in the axial plane and occasionally in the coronal plane, for localization and relations of the VSD to the great vessels (Fig. 27).

PROGNOSIS

Total correction is the primary goal, but early palliative procedures may be necessary, including Rashkind balloon atrial septostomy and systemic–pulmonary artery shunting when associated with pulmonary obstruction. Definitive repair requires closure of the VSD and placement of internal and external conduits to establish physiologic blood flow between the left ventricle and aorta and right ventricle and pulmonary artery (see Section V, Part VII, Chapter 1, Fig. 27, page 1412). Some patients with associated lesions may require an arterial-switch procedure, Damus procedure, or Fontan procedure; these are discussed in Section V, Part VII, Chapter 1, page 1393. Mortality remains moderate, particularly for patients with PVS and aortic arch malformations.

DOUBLE-OUTLET LEFT VENTRICLE

A double-outlet left ventricle is an extremely rare malformation characterized by both great vessels arising entirely or predominantly from the anatomic left ventricle and overriding, to a varying degree, an associated VSD. There is normal aortic–anterior mitral valve leaflet

FIGURE 25. Double-outlet right ventricle on echocardiogram. A long-axis view demonstrates an aortic root *(Ao)* overriding the interventricular septum and separated from the mitral valve *(small arrows)* by a segment of conal musculature *(curved white arrow)*. A supracristal ventricular septal defect is present *(curved black arrow)*. The discontinuity of the mitral valve from the semilunar valve is critical in this diagnosis and is better seen with the total real-time examination.

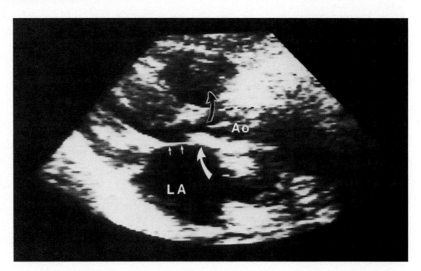

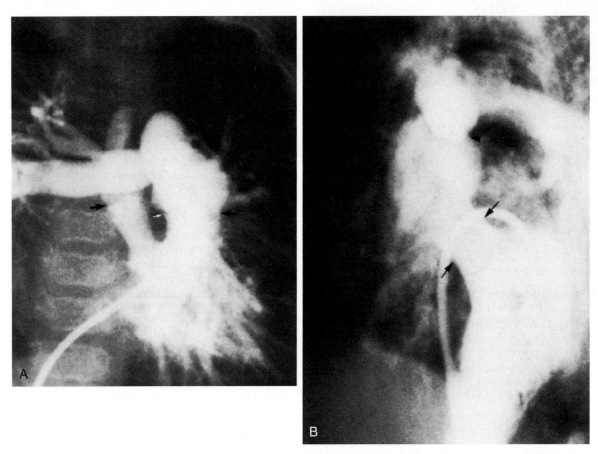

FIGURE 26. Double-outlet right ventricle (DORV). **A,** An anteroposterior right ventriculogram shows the aortic and pulmonary valves *(arrows)* at the same relative cephalocaudal position. Subaortic conal musculature narrows the aortic outflow tract. **B,** DORV, Taussig-Bing variety. A left ventriculogram (lateral long-axis) shows the supracristal ventricular septal defect *(arrows)* opening into the subpulmonic outflow tract (Taussig-Bing type). A pulmonary artery band *(arrowhead)* is present, with the aorta and pulmonary artery directly superimposed in the lateral view.

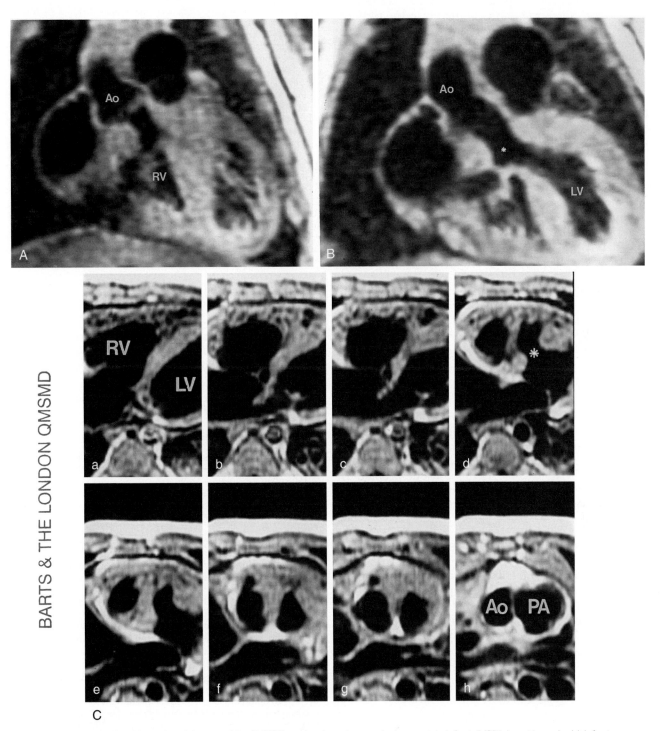

FIGURE 27. Double-outlet right ventricle (DORV) and subaortic ventricular septal defect (VSD) in a 7-week-old infant. **A,** Coronal 3-mm spin-echo magnetic resonance (MR) image demonstrates origin of the aorta *(Ao)* from the right ventricle *(RV)* with mild subaortic narrowing from conal musculature. An additional coronal image 6 mm anterior to **A** demonstrated the origin of the pulmonary artery from the right ventricle. **B,** Coronal 3-mm spin-echo MR image, 3 mm posterior to **A,** demonstrates that the only egress of blood from the left ventricle *(LV)* is through the subaortic VSD (*) into the aorta *(Ao)*. **C,** An 8-month-old infant with DORV with subpulmonic VSD (Taussig-Bing malformation): composite axial 3-mm spin-echo inferosuperior MR images demonstrate the left ventricle *(LV)* and subpulmonic VSD (*). The great vessels are side by side with the pulmonary artery *(PA)* to the right of the aorta *(Ao)*. More superior images demonstrated the bifurcation of the pulmonary artery and a pulmonary artery band in satisfactory position. *RV* = right ventricle.

continuity. Associated defects include subpulmonic and subaortic obstruction. The great vessels have a variable relation with the aorta, most commonly to the right of the pulmonary artery. Clinically and radiologically, this condition closely simulates tetralogy of Fallot and other forms of TGA, depending upon the presence or absence of pulmonary obstruction.

CHEST RADIOGRAPHY

Radiologic manifestations are nonspecific and relate predominantly to the presence or absence of PVS. In the latter case, the findings are similar to tetralogy of Fallot with a normal heart size and decreased pulmonary flow. Without PVS, moderate cardiomegaly and increased pulmonary blood flow are evident. Primary differential considerations in this setting are truncus arteriosus, TGA, and TAPVR.

ECHOCARDIOGRAPHY

Echocardiography demonstrates the abnormal origin of the pulmonary artery from the left ventricle, normal aortic–mitral continuity, and VSD.

ANGIOCARDIOGRAPHY

Biplane AP, lateral, and axial left ventricular angiocardiography demonstrates (1) the abnormal origin of the pulmonary artery from the left ventricle, (2) the VSD defect, and (3) aortic–anterior mitral valve leaflet continuity. The ventricular septum must be profiled to determine the origin of both great vessels entirely or predominantly from the left ventricle.

PROGNOSIS

Surgical correction is feasible with an external conduit from the right ventricle to the pulmonary arteries (Rastelli procedure) and closure of the VSD. A Fontan procedure may be necessary if the right ventricle is hypoplastic. See Section V, Part XII, Chapter 1, page 1393.

SUGGESTED READINGS

General

See Section V, Part I, Chapter 2, pp 1255–1256.

Complete Transposition of the Great Arteries

Carey LS, Elliott LP: Complete transposition of the great vessels: Roentgenographic findings. Am J Roentgenol Radium Ther Nucl Med 1974;91:529

Castaneda AR, Trusler GA, Paul MH, et al: The early results of treatment of simple transposition in the current era. J Thorac Cardiovasc Surg 1988;95:14–28

Chrispin A, Small P, Rutter N, et al: Echoplanar imaging of normal and abnormal connections of the heart and great arteries. Pediatr Radiol 1986;16:289

Didier D, Higgins CB, Fisher MR, et al: Congenital heart disease: gated MR imaging of 72 patients. Radiology 1986;158:227

Jaffe RB, Orsmond GS, Veasy LG: Inadvertent ligation of the left pulmonary artery. Radiology 1986;161:355–357

Mandell VS, Lock JE, Mayer JE, et al: The "laid-back" aortogram: an improved angiographic view for demonstration of coronary arteries in transposition of the great arteries. Am J Cardiol 1990;65:1379–1383

Mayer JE Jr, Sanders SP, Jonas RA, et al: Coronary artery pattern and outcome of arterial switch operation for transposition of the great arteries. Circulation 1990;82(suppl IV):IV-139–IV-145

Shapiro SR, Potter BM: Transposition of the great arteries. Semin Roentgenol 1985;20:110

Soulen RL, Donner R, Capitanio M: Postoperative evaluation of complex congenital heart disease by magnetic resonance imaging. Radiographics 1987;7:975

Tonkin LD, Sansa M, Elliott LP, et al: Recognition of developing left ventricular outflow tract obstruction in complete transposition of the great arteries. Radiology 1980;134:53

Unger FM, Cavanaugh DJ, Johnson GF, et al: Radiologic and real-time echocardiographic evaluation of the cyanotic newborn. Radiographics 1986;6:603

Van Praagh R: Transposition of the great arteries. II: Transposition clarified. Am J Cardiol 1971;28:739

Single Ventricle

Didier D, Higgins CB, Fisher MR, et al: Congenital heart disease: gated MR imaging in 72 patients. Radiology 1986;158:227

Elliott LP (ed): Angiography in single ventricle or univentricular heart. *In* Cardiac Imaging in Infants, Children, and Adults. Philadelphia, JB Lippincott, 1991:688

Elliott LP (ed): Pathophysiology and roentgenologic findings in single ventricle or univentricular heart. *In* Cardiac Imaging in Infants, Children, and Adults. Philadelphia, JB Lippincott, 1991:675

Keeton BR, Macartney FJ, Rees PG, et al: Univentricular heart of right ventricular type with double or common inlet. Circulation 1979;59:403

Kidd BSL: Single ventricle. *In* Keith JD, Rowe RD, Vlad P (eds): Heart Disease in Infancy and Childhood. New York, Macmillan, 1978:408

Macartney FJ, Partridge JB, Scott O, et al: Common or single ventricle: an angiocardiographic and hemodynamic study of 42 patients. Circulation 1976;53:543

Shinebourne EA, Lau K, Calcaterra G, et al: Univentricular heart of right ventricular type: clinical, angiographic and electrocardiographic features. Am J Cardiol 1980;46:439

Soto B, Bertranou EG, Bream PR, et al: Angiographic study of univentricular heart of the right ventricular type. Circulation 1979;60:1325

Swischuk LE: Single ventricle. Semin Roentgenol 1985;20:130

White RD, Higgins CB: Evaluation of single ventricle using magnetic resonance imaging. *In* Elliott LP (ed): Cardiac Imaging in Infants, Children, and Adults. Philadelphia, JB Lippincott, 1991:685

Corrected Transposition of the Great Arteries

Bream PR, Elliott LP, Bargeron LM: Plain film findings of anatomically corrected malposition: its association with juxtaposition of the atrial appendages and right aortic arch. Radiology 1978;126:589

Guit GL, Bluemm R, Rohmer J, et al: Levotransposition of the aorta: identification of segmental cardiac anatomy using MR imaging. Radiology 1986;161:673–679

Kidd BSL: Congenitally corrected transposition of the great arteries. *In* Keith JD, Rowe RD, Flad P (eds): Heart Disease in Infancy and Childhood, 3rd ed. New York, Macmillan, 1978:615

Krongrad E, Ellis K, Steeg CN, et al: Subpulmonic obstruction in congenitally corrected transposition of the great arteries due to ventricular membranous septal aneurysm. Circulation 1976;54:179

Ruttenberg HD: Corrected transposition of the great arteries. *In* Moss AJ, Adams FH, Emmanouilides GC (eds): Heart Disease in Infants, Children and Adolescents, 2nd ed. Baltimore, Williams & Wilkins, 1977:338

White RD: Magnetic resonance imaging of corrected transposition. *In* Elliott LP (ed): Cardiac Imaging in Infants, Children, and Adults. Philadelphia, JB Lippincott, 1991:635

Total Anomalous Pulmonary Venous Return

Budorick NE, McDonald V, Flisak ME, et al: The pulmonary veins. Semin Roentgenol 1989;24:127–140

Cathman GE, Nadas AS: Total anomalous pulmonary venous connection: clinical and physiological observations in 75 pediatric patients. Circulation 1970;42:143

Haworth SG, Reid L, Simon G: Radiologic features of the heart and lungs in total anomalous pulmonary venous return in early infancy. Clin Radiol 1977;28:561

Moes CAF, Freedom RM, Burrows PE: Anomalous pulmonary venous connections. Semin Roentgenol 1985;20:134

Cor Triatriatum and Other Anomalies of the Pulmonary Veins

Bisset GS III, Kirks DR, Strife JL, et al: Cor triatriatum: diagnosis by MR imaging. AJR Am J Roentgenol 1987;149:567

Jolles H, Henry DA, Rupp SB: General case of the day—cardiac MR of cor triatriatum. Radiographics 1988;8:1227–1231

MacMillan RM, Rees MR, Maranhao V, et al: Cinecomputed tomography of cor triatriatum. J Comput Assist Tomogr 1986;10:124

Van der Horst RL, Gotsman MS: Cor triatriatum: angiographic diagnosis by retrograde catheterization of the dorsal accessory chamber. Br J Radiol 1971;44:273

Truncus Arteriosus

Calder L, Van Praagh R, Van Praagh S, et al: Truncus arteriosus communis: clinical angiocardiographic and pathologic findings in 100 patients. Am Heart J 1976;92:23

Collett RW, Edwards JE: Persistent truncus arteriosus: classification according to anatomic types. Surg Clin North Am 1949;29:1245

Moes CAF, Freedom RM: Aortic arch interruption with truncus arteriosus or aorticopulmonary septal defect. AJR Am J Roentgenol 1980;135:1011

Nath PH, Zollikofer CL, Castaneda-Zuñiga WR, et al: Persistent truncus arteriosus associated with interruption of the aortic arch. Br J Radiol 1980;53:853

Van Praagh R: Classification of truncus arteriosus communis (TAC). Am Heart J 1976;92:129

White RD: Magnetic resonance imaging of truncus arteriosus. *In* Elliott LP (ed): Cardiac Imaging in Infants, Children, and Adults. Philadelphia, JB Lippincott, 1991:700

Double-Outlet Left Ventricle

Bharati S, Leve M, Stewart R, et al: The morphologic spectrum of double outlet left ventricle and its surgical significance. Circulation 1978;58:558

Brandt TWT, Calder AL, Barratt-Boyes BG, et al: Double outlet left ventricle: morphologic cineangiographic diagnosis and surgical treatment. Am J Cardiol 1976;38:897

Double-Outlet Right Ventricle

Adkins EW, Martin TE, Alexander JA, et al: MR in double-outlet right ventricle. AJR Am J Roentgenol 1989;152:128–130

Hallermann FJ, Kincaid OW, Ritter DG, et al: Angiocardiographic findings in origin of both great arteries from the right ventricle. Am J Roentgenol Radium Ther Nucl Med 1970;109:51–66

Lincoln C, Anderson RH, Shinebourne EA, et al: Double outlet right ventricle with malposition of the aorta. Br Heart J 1975;37:453

Mayo JR, Robertson D, Sommerhoff B, et al: MR imaging of double outlet ventricle. J Comput Assist Tomogr 1990;14:336–339

Yoo S-J, Lim T-H, Park I-S, et al: MR anatomy of ventricular septal defect in double-outlet right ventricle with situs solitus and atrioventricular concordance. Radiology 1991;181:501–505

Zamora R, Moller JH, Edwards JC: Double outlet right ventricle: anatomic types and associated anomalies. Chest 1975;68:672

Chapter 4

CYANOTIC CONGENITAL HEART DISEASE WITH DECREASED PULMONARY FLOW

RICHARD B. JAFFE and VIRGIL R. CONDON

TETRALOGY OF FALLOT

Tetralogy of Fallot (TOF) classically consists of (1) a large defect in the anterior portion of the ventricular septum, (2) obstruction of the right ventricular outflow tract, (3) overriding of the aortic root above the ventricular septal defect (VSD), and (4) right ventricular hypertrophy. Right ventricular obstruction may relate to infundibular or pulmonary valve stenosis. One must identify normal aortic–mitral valve fibrous continuity and underdevelopment or malalignment of the subpul-

monic conus. These areas are important in distinguishing other forms of cyanotic congenital heart disease (CHD) such as double-outlet right ventricle (DORV) with pulmonary valvular stenosis (PVS) and transposition of the great vessels with PVS. TOF is the most common (10%) form of cyanotic CHD.

PATHOPHYSIOLOGY

Pathophysiologic and clinical manifestations are extremely variable and related to the degree of right ventricular outflow obstruction. Infundibular and associated valvular stenosis are common (40%). Other associated anomalies include (1) a right aortic arch (25%); (2) peripheral PVS; (3) complete fibrous atresia of the main pulmonary artery (pseudotruncus); (4) fibrous atresia of the left pulmonary artery; (5) coronary artery anomalies, particularly the origin of the left anterior descending coronary artery from the right coronary artery and single coronary artery (5% to 10%); (6) bicuspid aortic valve; (7) patent ductus arteriosus (PDA); (8) partial anomalous pulmonary venous return; (9) atrial septal defect (ASD) or atrioventricular canal (AVC), or both; and (10) a persistent left superior vena cava (SVC).

CLINICAL MANIFESTATIONS

Cyanosis relates to the severity of right heart obstruction; infants are rarely cyanotic at birth, except those with pulmonary atresia. Ninety percent of patients become cyanotic by 6 months of age. Congestive heart failure (CHF) is rarely seen. Dyspnea is an early clinical manifestation, and paroxysmal dyspneic spells produce typical "blue spells." Clubbing is a late manifestation. Heart murmurs are striking, related to a loud ejection murmur along the left sternal edge caused by right ventricular obstruction. The first component of the second heart sound in the pulmonary area is loud; the second component is soft and delayed. A continuous murmur indicates (1) a persistent PDA or (2) large systemic–pulmonary artery collaterals. Complications

include thromboembolic disease and brain abscesses from right-to-left intracardiac shunting.

CHEST RADIOGRAPHY

Radiologic findings in TOF are extremely variable depending upon the degree of right heart obstruction and right-to-left shunting. In the infant with a balanced physiologic state with little right-to-left shunting, the chest radiographic findings may appear normal. A right aortic arch may be the only clue to the presence of TOF (25%) (see Section V, Part I, Chapter 2, Table 2, page 1234). In older children, the typical "boot-shaped heart" develops with (1) a prominent elevated right ventricular apex, (2) a concave main pulmonary artery segment, (3) decreased hilar and central pulmonary vessels, (4) hyperexpanded hyperlucent lungs, (5) thymic atrophy, and (6) a right aortic arch (Fig. 1; see also Fig. 4A below and Section V, Part I, Chapter 2, Fig. 3, page 1233). Other less frequent radiographic manifestations include (1) prominent systemic–pulmonary collaterals producing pulmonary vascular disorganization or abnormal indentation the esophagus on esophagrams (see Fig. 4B below); (2) unilateral absence of the pulmonary artery, usually the left one; and (3) rib notching caused by collateral vessels.

ECHOCARDIOGRAPHY

M-mode, two-dimensional (Fig. 2) and Doppler echocardiograms demonstrate (1) overriding of the aortic

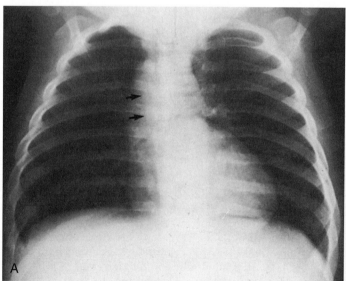
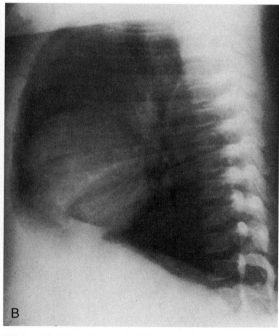

FIGURE 1. Tetralogy of Fallot. Anteroposterior (AP) **(A)** and lateral **(B)** chest radiographs show hyperlucent lungs with diminished central hilar pulmonary vessels in both the AP and lateral views. The main pulmonary artery segment is flat to concave, and a prominent right aortic arch and descending thoracic aorta *(arrows)* are evident. Thymic involution and hyperinflation are characteristic of cyanosis and stress in the 5-month-old infant (see also Section V, Part I, Chapter 2, Fig. 3, page 1233).

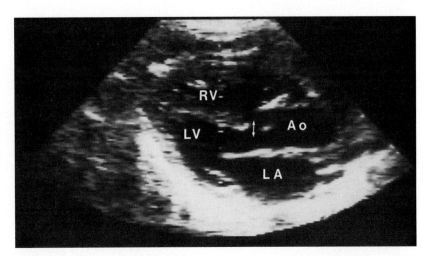

FIGURE 2. Tetralogy of Fallot. A long-axis two-dimensional echocardiogram shows the aortic root *(Ao)* overriding the ventricular septum and ventricular septal defect *(arrows)* and normal fibrous aortic–mitral continuity. *RV* = right ventricle; *LV* = left ventricle; *LA* = left atrium.

root above (2) a VSD, (3) normal aortic–mitral continuity, (4) an enlarged aortic root and right aortic arch in approximately 25% of patients, (5) small pulmonary arteries, (6) a narrowed right ventricular outflow tract, (7) valvular PVS, and (8) right ventricular hypertrophy.

ANGIOCARDIOGRAPHY

Angiocardiography is important for evaluating (1) the infundibular, valvular, and main pulmonary artery anatomy; (2) the entire ventricular septum for the possibility of multiple defects; (3) the atrioventricular (AV) valve relationships because of known associated atrioventricular canal (AVC), especially in patients with Down syndrome; (4) the coronary arteries; and (5) aortic arch and brachiocephalic vessel anatomy. A biplane right ventriculogram in the sitting-up projection or other angulated projections evaluates the outflow tract and pulmonary artery anatomy (Fig. 3). The biplane long-axis left ventriculogram evaluates the VSD and the mitral–aortic relations. A long-axis aortic root injection is important for evaluating the coronary arteries, in particular the left anterior descending branch, which frequently is anomalous, arising from the right coronary artery.

In patients with pulmonary atresia, the central pulmonary artery anatomy must be evaluated either through (1) an aortogram (Fig. 4C) or injection of systemic–pulmonary artery collaterals or a PDA, (2) a pulmonary venous wedge angiogram producing retrograde flow into the pulmonary artery confluence, or (3) magnetic resonance imaging (MRI) or helical computed tomography.

MAGNETIC RESONANCE IMAGING

Axial MRI of the central pulmonary arteries has become a common imaging procedure in patients before and after operation (see Section V, Part I, Chapter 2, page 1230 for a discussion of MRI). Thin-section axial images can depict pulmonary arteries not clearly defined by angiography (see Section V, Part I, Chapter 2, Fig. 29, page 1250).

PROGNOSIS

The long-term prognosis is good. The severely cyanotic patient needs an early modified Blalock-Taussig shunt (see Section V, Part VII, Chapter 1, page 1393). Prostaglandin E is useful in maintaining a patent ductus until operative procedures can be performed in the severely cyanotic patient with pulmonary atresia. Propranolol may ameliorate symptoms by decreasing right ventricular outflow tract obstruction. Definitive operation is postponed beyond the newborn period. Balloon angioplasty may temporarily relieve pulmonary obstruction (see Fig. 3D).

TETRALOGY OF FALLOT WITH ABSENCE OF THE PULMONARY VALVE

TOF with absent or rudimentary pulmonary valve tissue is a rare variation associated with massive dilatation of the main, right, or left pulmonary arteries, individually or severally. Besides the usual TOF anomalies, ASD, tricuspid atresia, PDA, DORV, and AVC may also be present. Rarely, congenital absence of the pulmonary valve may occur as an isolated lesion.

Patients may present with either volume overload symptoms and CHF or cyanosis related to right-to-left shunts. Pulmonary distress related to the external compression of the trachea or bronchi by the massively dilated pulmonary arteries is not uncommon and may be associated with tracheobronchomalacia. Symptoms may suggest respiratory tract obstruction as seen with arch anomalies or pulmonary artery sling.

CHEST RADIOGRAPHY

Radiographic manifestations include (1) moderate to marked cardiomegaly, (2) a striking prominence of the proximal pulmonary arteries, (3) decreased peripheral pulmonary vasculature, (4) tracheal compression, and (5) air trapping (general or unilateral) (Fig. 5A, B; see also Section V, Part I, Chapter 2, Fig. 10, page 1236).

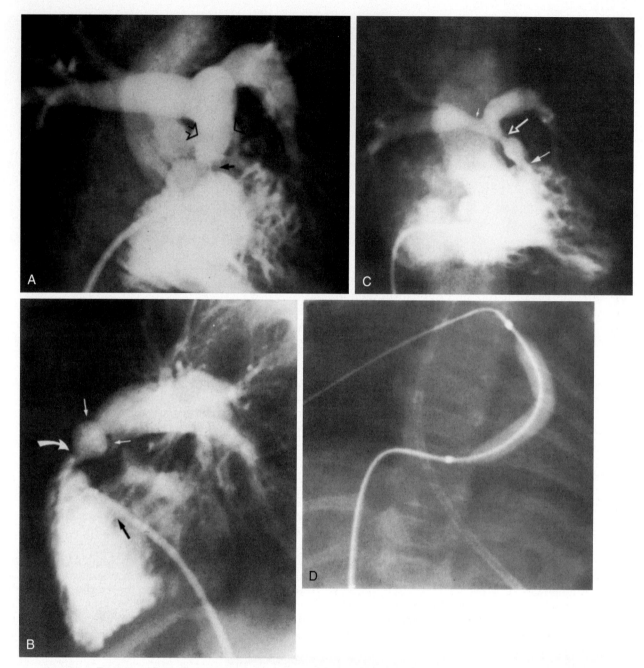

FIGURE 3. Tetralogy of Fallot. **A,** Anteroposterior sitting-up right ventriculogram demonstrates marked infundibular stenosis *(black arrow)*, pulmonary valvular stenosis *(open arrows)* with mild narrowing of the left pulmonary artery projecting behind the main pulmonary artery, right ventricular hypertrophy, and right-to-left shunting into a large aorta. **B,** Lateral view in the same patient shows the infundibular and valvular pulmonary stenoses *(white arrows)* and the ventricular septal defect with right-to-left shunting *(black arrow)*. **C,** Sitting-up right ventriculogram shows severe infundibular stenosis *(white arrow)*, a dysplastic stenotic pulmonary valve *(open arrow)*, and peripheral stenosis of the main and right pulmonary artery *(small white arrow)*. Right ventricular hypertrophy and moderate right-to-left shunting are present. **D,** Balloon angioplasty of the pulmonary valve in a 1-month-old with tetralogy of Fallot: a minimal residual waist is noted at the valve annulus with associated angulation of the balloon catheter.

ECHOCARDIOGRAPHY

Echocardiography shows some of the findings described in TOF and, in addition, the striking enlargement of the pulmonary artery; dilatation of the right ventricle and a dysplastic appearance of the pulmonary annulus are evident. Doppler studies confirm the massive pulmonary insufficiency.

ANGIOCARDIOGRAPHY

Angiographic evaluation is basically similar to that described for TOF. Right-sided ventriculography using larger amounts of contrast is necessary to adequately demonstrate the massively dilated right ventricle and pulmonary vessels. Typically the pulmonary annulus is stenotic and insufficient with rudimentary valve tissue, and there is little, if any, infundibular narrowing. The VSD may be seen with either left or right ventriculography (Fig. 5*C, D*).

TRICUSPID ATRESIA

Tricuspid atresia is characterized by (1) a complete absence of the right AV valve, (2) ASD, (3) VSD, and (4) hypoplasia of the right ventricle. Frequent associated abnormalities include (1) valvular or subvalvular PVS, (2) transposition of the great arteries (TGA), (3) a right aortic arch (see Section V, Part I, Chapter 2, Table 2, page 1234), (4) dextrocardia, (5) total anomalous

pulmonary venous return, and (6) unilateral absence of the pulmonary artery. A right aortic arch is much more common if transposition and PVS are associated anomalies. Tricuspid atresia constitutes 2% to 3% of CHD.

Pathophysiology

Tricuspid atresia produces an area of fibrosis in the floor of the right atrium, frequently with an area of depression or umbilication. An obligatory right-to-left shunt occurs through a stretched foramen ovale or ASD. The left ventricle enlarges and becomes hypertrophic. Type I tricuspid atresia (70%) has normal arterial relations and

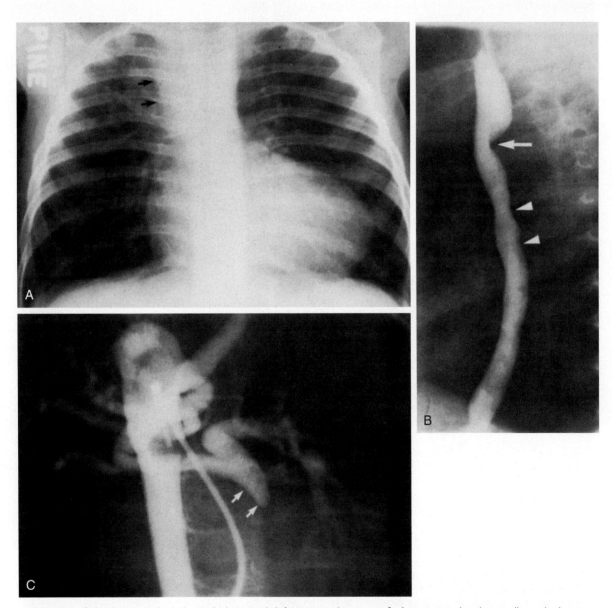

FIGURE 4. Pulmonary atresia and ventricular septal defect—pseudotruncus. **A,** Anteroposterior chest radiograph shows a prominent right aortic arch *(arrows)* and boot-shaped cardiac silhouette, with a concave pulmonary artery and disordered pulmonary vessels particularly evident in the right upper lobe. **B,** Lateral esophagogram shows abnormal retroesophageal vascular impressions. The most proximal impression *(arrow)* is an aberrant left subclavian artery from the right aortic arch, while the more caudal undulations *(arrowheads)* are pressure effects of the systemic–pulmonary artery collaterals arising from the thoracic aorta. **C,** Sitting-up thoracic aortogram shows systemic–thoracic pulmonary artery collaterals with retrograde filling of a small main pulmonary artery and annulus *(arrows)*. The demonstrated confluence and patency of these vessels make operative correction feasible.

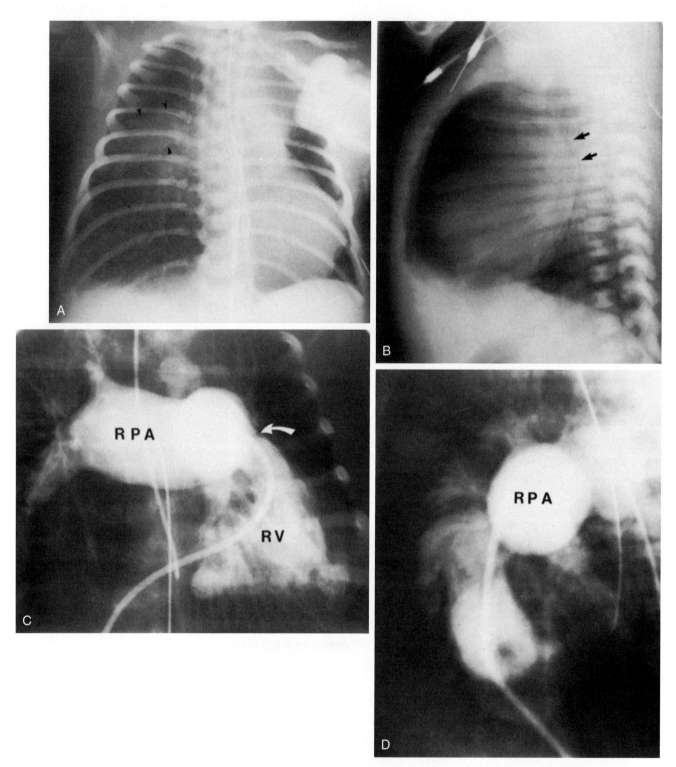

FIGURE 5. Tetralogy of Fallot with absence of the pulmonary valve. **A,** Anteroposterior (AP) chest radiograph shows a mass effect in the right hilar region secondary to aneurysmal enlargement of the right pulmonary artery *(arrowheads),* which produces right main stem bronchial obstruction, air trapping, retention of neonatal fluid in the basilar right lung, and a mediastinal shift to the left (see also Section V, Part I, Chapter 2, Fig. 10, page 1236). **B,** Lateral chest radiograph demonstrates the mass effect of the aneurysmal pulmonary artery, which produces striking narrowing of the central tracheobronchial airway *(arrows)* at the level of the carina. **C** and **D,** AP and lateral pulmonary arteriograms demonstrate the aneurysmal dilatation primarily involving the right pulmonary artery (RPA) with evidence of pulmonary regurgitation through a dysplastic pulmonary valve *(arrow).* There is a faint visualization of the aorta secondary to right-to-left shunting and a ventricular septal defect. *RV* = right ventricle.

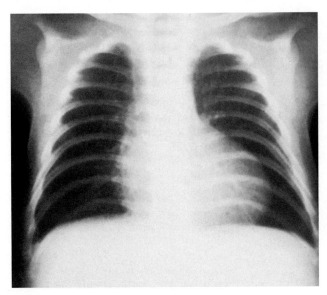

FIGURE 6. Tricuspid atresia. An anteroposterior chest radiograph shows hyperlucent lungs with deficient central pulmonary vasculature secondary to a right-to-left shunt. Mild cardiomegaly and a concave main pulmonary artery segment are present. Thymic atrophy is consistent with hypoxia and a relatively inconspicuous aortic arch. These findings closely simulate those seen in tetralogy of Fallot.

is subdivided into those with pulmonary atresia and an absent right ventricle (73%), those with a hypoplastic pulmonary artery with a small right ventricle and VSD (13%), and those with a large VSD with no PVS (13%). Type II (25%) features associated dextrotransposition of the great arteries, and is subdivided into lesions with or without pulmonary stenosis. Type III (5%) represents associated levotransposition of the great arteries (l-TGA) with ventricular inversion and atresia of the left AV (tricuspid) valve.

CLINICAL MANIFESTATIONS

Cyanosis, relative to the right-to-left shunt and the degree of right ventricular outflow obstruction, is moderate to severe in 85% to 90% of patients. The rare patient with a large VSD and no PVS exhibits mild cyanosis. Spontaneous closure of the VSD or development of PVS produces progressive cyanosis.

Other manifestations include (1) dyspnea, (2) jugular pulsations related to atrial contractions, and (3) a loud ejection murmur along the left sternal border. CHF occurs in those rare instances with a large VSD and increased pulmonary blood flow.

CHEST RADIOGRAPHY

Characteristic findings include (1) normal heart size or mild cardiomegaly, (2) decreased pulmonary vascularity, (3) hyperlucent lungs with diaphragmatic depression, (4) a concave main pulmonary artery segment (Fig. 6), and (5) a right aortic arch (9% to 25%). Five percent of patients show increased pulmonary blood flow and moderate to marked cardiomegaly with a prominent main pulmonary artery.

Other rare findings include (1) a juxtaposed atrial appendage (particularly with associated TGA) (Fig. 7) and (2) dilated venae cavae.

ECHOCARDIOGRAPHY

Two-dimensional echocardiography will demonstrate tricuspid atresia, a small right ventricle, VSD, great-vessel relations, and ASD (Fig. 8). Doppler evaluation

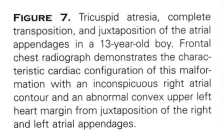

FIGURE 7. Tricuspid atresia, complete transposition, and juxtaposition of the atrial appendages in a 13-year-old boy. Frontal chest radiograph demonstrates the characteristic cardiac configuration of this malformation with an inconspicuous right atrial contour and an abnormal convex upper left heart margin from juxtaposition of the right and left atrial appendages.

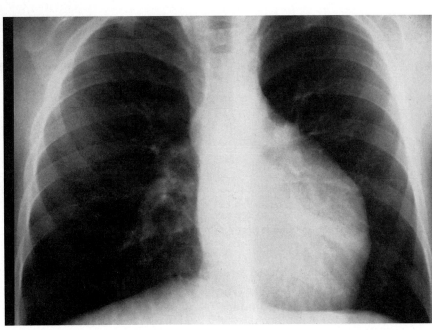

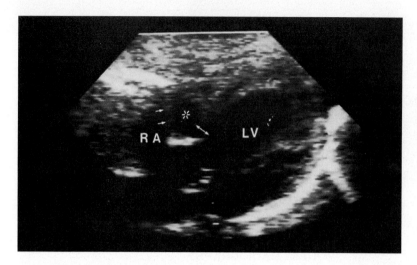

FIGURE 8. Tricuspid atresia. Subxiphoid real-time echocardiogram shows an atretic tricuspid valve *(arrows)* with a hypoplastic right ventricle (*) and ventricular septal defect *(double-headed arrow)*. *RA* = right atrium; *LV* = left ventricle.

will show a right-to-left shunt at the atrial level and a left-to-right shunt through the VSD as well as failure of flow through the tricuspid valve area.

ANGIOCARDIOGRAPHY

Injection of contrast medium into the SVC or right atrium shows sequential flow from the right atrium to the left atrium to the left ventricle. Frequently the small right ventricle and pulmonary artery will subsequently be seen along with filling of the aortic root. Early in the sequence, a triangular nonopacified area caudad to the right atrium can be seen related to the nonopacified hypoplastic right ventricle (Fig. 9). Biplane long-axis left ventriculography better defines the (1) enlarged left ventricle, (2) VSD, (3) hypoplastic right ventricle, and (4) pulmonary artery and obstructive lesions. The right aortic arch, if present, and the great-vessel relations in those patients with transposition are best seen with left ventriculography.

PROGNOSIS

A palliative measure to increase the pulmonary flow (i.e., a modified Blalock-Taussig shunt) will produce considerable palliation. Later, more long-term palliative procedures can be performed that are related to caval pulmonary (Glenn procedure) or atriopulmonary (Fontan procedure) shunting (see Section V, Part VII, Chapter 1, page 1393).

PULMONARY ATRESIA WITH AN INTACT VENTRICULAR SEPTUM (HYPOPLASTIC RIGHT HEART SYNDROME)

This malformation is characterized by (1) pulmonary atresia, (2) hypoplasia of the right ventricle, and (3) hypoplasia of the tricuspid valve annulus. Occasionally, in patients with tricuspid insufficiency (20%), there will be

marked enlargement of the right atrium and right ventricle. The incidence of hypoplastic right heart syndrome is between 1% and 2%.

PATHOPHYSIOLOGY

With complete right heart obstruction, an obligatory right-to-left shunt occurs at the atrial level through a stretched foramen ovale or true ASD. Cyanosis is present, with severity depending upon the size of the associated patent ductus. The pathophysiology is similar is that in patients with tricuspid atresia. The aortic arch is invariably on the left, and visceral atrial situs solitus is the rule.

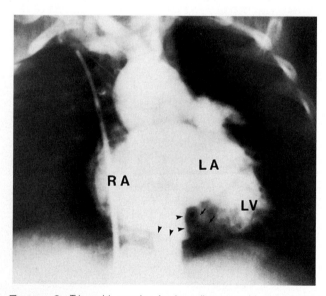

FIGURE 9. Tricuspid atresia. Angiocardiogram with right atrial–superior vena cava injection shows effects of the right-to-left shunt at the atrial level, with contrast filling the right atrium *(RA)*, left atrium *(LA)*, and left ventricle *(LV)*. The triangular lucent chamber, outlined by *arrows* and *arrowheads*, represents the incompletely opacified hypoplastic right ventricle. *Arrowheads* also demarcate the atretic tricuspid valve.

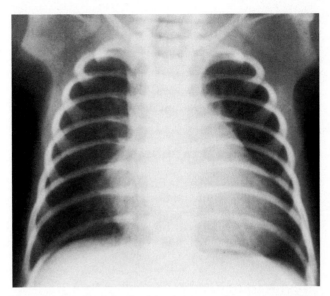

FIGURE 10. Hypoplastic right heart syndrome secondary to pulmonary atresia. Anteroposterior chest radiograph shows moderate cardiomegaly, diminished pulmonary flow with hyperlucent lungs, relatively inconspicuous pulmonary vessels, and a prominent aortic arch.

CLINICAL MANIFESTATIONS

Typical clinical findings include cyanosis, tachypnea, hepatomegaly, peripheral edema, gallop rhythm, and murmurs from tricuspid regurgitation or a PDA. CHF may occur with a large patent ductus.

CHEST RADIOGRAPHY

Radiologic manifestations correlate with the competency of the tricuspid valve. With a competent tricuspid valve, the radiographic manifestations include (1) normal heart size or mild cardiomegaly, and (2) decreased pulmonary blood flow, unless the patient is receiving prostaglandin therapy (Fig. 10). In patients with significant tricuspid insufficiency, cardiomegaly with marked enlargement of the right atrium is present. The pulmonary blood flow may be increased in those rare patients with a large patent ductus after neonatal pulmonary vascular resistance decreases.

ECHOCARDIOGRAPHY

Real-time two-dimensional echocardiography demonstrates (1) an abnormally thickened, atretic pulmonary valve; (2) a small pulmonary annulus; (3) a hypertrophic small right ventricle (Fig. 11); (4) an enlarged right atrium; and (5) an ASD or a large foramen ovale. Doppler interrogation is important and demonstrates a right-to-left atrial shunt, absence of a VSD, and no forward or retrograde flow through the pulmonary valve. With tricuspid insufficiency, Doppler evaluation similarly confirms this defect, and real-time study shows an enlarged right atrium and right ventricle.

ANGIOCARDIOGRAPHY

With a competent tricuspid valve, biplane right ventriculography with a small amount of contrast medium (Fig. 12) will demonstrate (1) right ventricular hypertrophy and hypoplasia; (2) atresia of the pulmonary valve, usually with an adequate infundibulum; (3) competency of the tricuspid valve; and (4) occasional retrograde filling of the coronary arteries from right ventricular sinusoids. If tricuspid insufficiency exists, large-volume injection will be necessary to evaluate right ventricular size and the severity of tricuspid regurgitation. Long-axis left ventriculography will visualize the normal confluence of the pulmonary vessels through either a patent ductus or, rarely, collateral systemic–pulmonary flow. The primary differential consideration is that of Ebstein's anomaly in those patients with tricuspid insufficiency. These patients with Ebstein's anomaly will have pulmonary insufficiency seen on aortography, with flow through the PDA and pulmonary artery and then into the right ventricle.

FIGURE 11. Hypoplastic right heart syndrome. A two-dimensional subxiphoid echocardiogram shows the small hypoplastic, hypertrophic right ventricle *(rv)*. Tricuspid valve motion may be limited and simulate tricuspid atresia; however, a ventricular septal defect cannot be identified. *RA* = right atrium; *LV* = left ventricle; *Ao* = aortic root.

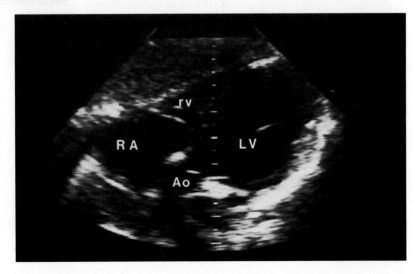

PROGNOSIS

Prostaglandin E can maintain the patency of a patent ductus and produce adequate pulmonary flow. Palliation with a modified Blalock-Taussig shunt will maintain adequate pulmonary flow. Pulmonary valvulotomy (Brock procedure) is usually performed at the same time to stimulate further development of the hypoplastic right ventricle. If the right ventricle remains hypoplastic, a Fontan procedure may be performed (see Section V, Part VII, Chapter 1, page 1393).

AORTIC ATRESIA (HYPOPLASTIC LEFT HEART SYNDROME)

Aortic atresia is characterized by hypoplasia of the entire left heart, including the ascending aorta, the aortic annuius, the left ventricle, the mitral valve, and the left atrium. Critical aortic stenosis (AS) is included in this category by some authors. Approximately 1% of all CHD involves the aortic atresia complex, although it represent approximately 9% of structural defects recognized in the newborn infant.

PATHOPHYSIOLOGY

Pathologic manifestations include (1) a hypertrophic or hypoplastic left ventricle, (2) usually small aortic sinuses of Valsalva, (3) a small aortic annulus and ascending aorta, (4) normal, but small coronary arteries, (5) a small mitral valve annulus or atresia (25%), and (6) PDA. Occasionally, a true ASD or VSD may be present.

All pulmonary and systemic circulation depends on the right ventricle, resulting in right heart enlargement and hypertrophy. Systemic flow depends on pulmonary venous blood returning to the right heart at the atrial level and subsequently flowing from right to left through the PDA, with filling of both the aortic arch and brachiocephalic vessels and descending aorta. CHF and death relate to myocardial ischemia secondary to restrictive coronary flow or poor arteriovenous mixing.

CLINICAL MANIFESTATIONS

CHF usually develops in the first few hours. Tachypnea is present from birth, and cyanosis from within the first 24 to 48 hours. Other clinical findings include tachycardia, hepatomegaly, gallop rhythm, rales, poor peripheral pulses, and murmurs in 50% of patients.

CHEST RADIOGRAPHY

Radiographic findings include (1) moderate to marked cardiomegaly, (2) a globular cardiac silhouette suggesting combined chamber enlargement, (3) pulmonary venous congestion with interstitial fluid lines or pleural fluid, (4) hyperinflation, and (5) thymic atrophy (Fig. 13).

Differential considerations include critical AS, mitral atresia, severe coarctation or interrupted aortic arch, and cardiomyopathy, such as in endocardial fibroelastosis and infants of diabetic mothers.

ECHOCARDIOGRAPHY

Real-time echocardiography shows (1) a diminutive ascending aorta with an aortic root diameter of less than

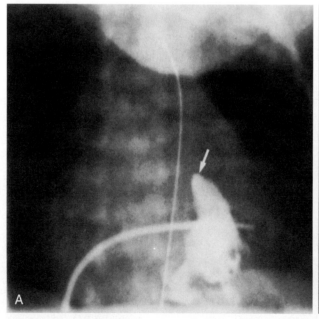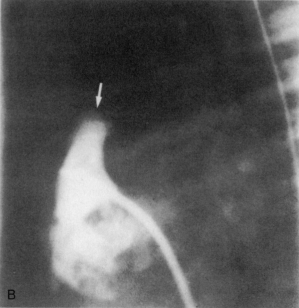

FIGURE 12. Hypoplastic right heart syndrome. Anteroposterior **(A)** and lateral **(B)** right ventriculograms demonstrate pulmonary atresia *(arrows)* with a hypoplastic right ventricle and intact ventricular septum.

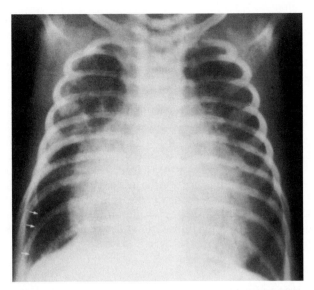

FIGURE 13. Hypoplastic left heart syndrome. Anteroposterior chest radiograph of a 2-day-old infant shows moderate cardiomegaly, severe pulmonary venous congestion with interstitial fluid, and areas of atelectasis or edema. Depression of the diaphragm is secondary to hypoxia. There is minimal fluid in the right major fissure *(arrows)*.

5 mm; (2) a small, thick-walled left ventricle; (3) a small mitral valve annulus with restricted leaflet motion; and (4) a dilated right heart, pulmonary artery, and large patent ductus (Fig. 14).

ANGIOCARDIOGRAPHY

Echocardiography usually confirms the diagnosis, although, if operative intervention is considered, angiography is necessary. Retrograde aortography, usually performed through an umbilical artery catheter, will show (1) retrograde flow into the ascending aorta, (2) a small hypoplastic ascending aorta, and (3) retrograde filling of small coronary arteries (Fig. 15). The absence of antegrade washout through the aortic valve confirms atresia. Transient left-to-right shunting through the patent ductus occasionally is observed. In the lateral view, the relative posterior position of the left anterior descending coronary artery implies the diminutive size of the left ventricle.

PROGNOSIS

This lesion is universally fatal, with 80% of patients dying within the first week. Heart transplantation or a staged Norwood procedure are alternative forms of therapy (see Section V, Part VII, Chapter 1, page 1393).

EBSTEIN'S ANOMALY OF THE TRICUSPID VALVE

Ebstein's anomaly is characterized by a malformed, redundant, and dysplastic tricuspid valve displaced downward into the right ventricle. This partitions the right ventricle into an atrialized upper segment and an apical outflow chamber. The lesion is extremely variable and is usually associated with tricuspid insufficiency. Ebstein's anomaly may occur also in patients with ventricular inversion related to l-TGA. The Ebstein malformation constitutes less than 1% of all CHD.

PATHOPHYSIOLOGY

Because of the displaced tricuspid valve, and the associated tricuspid insufficiency and relative competency of the foramen ovale, the right atrium is usually markedly enlarged. The atrialized segment of the right ventricle is thin and the pulmonary conus segment is hypertrophied. Associated anomalies include pulmonary stenosis or atresia, PDA, and VSD. Right-to-left shunting produces some degree of cyanosis and relates to the patency of the foramen ovale.

CLINICAL MANIFESTATIONS

Cyanosis occurs in 75% of patients, more often in the neonatal period or in later childhood. Other clinical findings include dyspnea, systolic murmur related to

FIGURE 14. Hypoplastic left heart syndrome. Long-axis two-dimensional echocardiogram shows a hypoplastic ascending aorta *(arrows)*, a hypoplastic left ventricle *(LV)*, and a large right ventricle *(RV)*. Arrowheads outline a hypoplastic mitral valve. *LA* = left atrium.

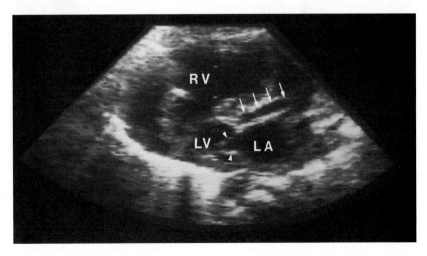

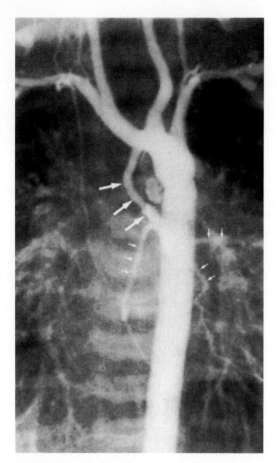

FIGURE 15. Hypoplastic left heart syndrome. A retrograde aortogram was performed after aortic catheterization through the umbilical artery. Retrograde filling of the entire ascending aorta demonstrates the severe hypoplasia *(large arrows)*, and there is retrograde filling into the coronary arteries *(small arrows)*. Left-to-right shunting also occurs through a patent ductus, with contrast visible in peripheral pulmonary artery branches.

tricuspid insufficiency, and a loud first heart sound and split second heart sound. Electrocardiographic changes may be quite helpful, including a right bundle-branch block, a large T wave, a prolonged P–R interval, and low-voltage QRS segments. Patients also may present with Wolff-Parkinson-White syndrome and tachyarrhythmias.

CHEST RADIOGRAPHY

Radiographs are extremely variable. Typically, in the cyanotic neonate, one sees (1) marked cardiomegaly, primarily related to striking right atrial enlargement, with a globular cardiac silhouette, and (2) decreased pulmonary blood flow (Fig. 16). In older children without cyanosis, marked variability exists, with (1) mild to moderate cardiomegaly related to right atrial enlargement and (2) normal pulmonary blood flow (Fig. 17).

Differential considerations include (1) primary tricuspid insufficiency, (2) tricuspid insufficiency related

to pulmonary atresia, and (3) Uhl anomaly of the right ventricle.

ECHOCARDIOGRAPHY

Two-dimensional echocardiography in the four-chamber view readily identifies (1) the displaced tricuspid valve with the septal and posterior leaflets adherent to the right ventricular wall, (2) the dysplastic nature of the tricuspid valve with a large, redundant anterior leaflet originating from the tricuspid annulus, and (3) marked enlargement of the right atrium (Fig. 18). Doppler ultrasound readily identifies tricuspid regurgitation (see Section V, Part I, Chapter 2, Fig. 18, page 1241).

ANGIOGRAPHY

Anteroposterior and lateral right ventriculograms characterize the malformation with (1) the displaced tricuspid valve in relation to the tricuspid annulus, which is localized by the position of the right coronary artery; (2) caudad bulging of the atrialized portion of the right ventricle; (3) secondary notch in the midinferior ventricular margin related to the displaced tricuspid leaflet; (4) tricuspid insufficiency; and (5) right atrial enlargement (Fig. 19). Right-to-left shunting may be seen at the atrial level. Primary differential considerations include tricuspid insufficiency as a primary lesion or secondary to pulmonary atresia. The displaced tricuspid valve will not be identified in these conditions. Pulmonary atresia can be differentiated by the demonstration of pulmonary insufficiency in patients with Ebstein's anomaly on

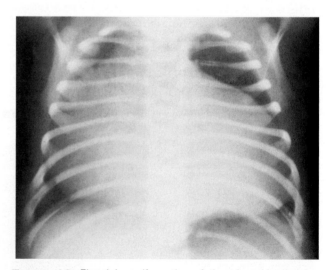

FIGURE 16. Ebstein's malformation of the tricuspid valve in a neonate with marked cardiomegaly related to massive dilatation of the right atrium. Right-to-left shunting occurs through the foramen ovale or atrial septal defect. Compression atelectasis of the left lower lobe is evident along with decreased pulmonary vasculature. Similar findings may be seen with tricuspid insufficiency associated with pulmonary atresia.

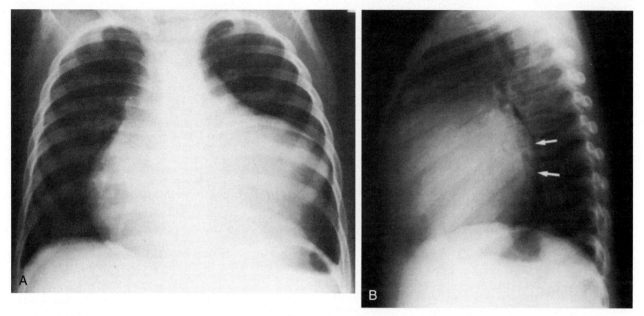

FIGURE 17. Ebstein's anomaly. Anteroposterior **(A)** and lateral **(B)** chest radiographs in a 2-year-old with moderate cardiomegaly, although the right atrial dilatation is less striking than in Figure 16. In the lateral view, the enlarged right atrium produces a prominent posterior cardiac margin *(arrows)*. The pulmonary vasculature is only mildly decreased with a limited right-to-left shunt.

FIGURE 18. Ebstein's anomaly. Two-dimensional echocardiogram in a subxiphoid projection shows massive enlargement of the right atrium *(RA)*, with the tricuspid valve *(arrows)* displaced caudad into the right ventricle *(RV)* to create a large atrialized component of the right ventricle. The *arrowhead* designates an atrial septal defect. *LA* = left atrium; *LV* = left ventricle.

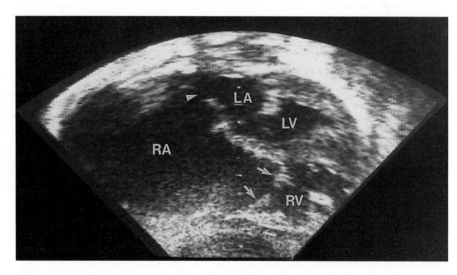

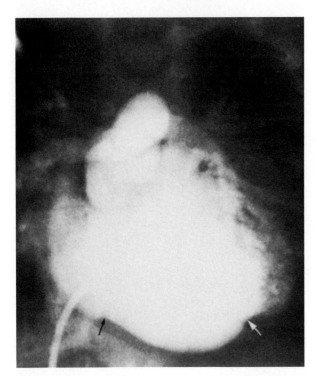

FIGURE 19. Ebstein's anomaly. Anteroposterior cine–right atriogram shows the characteristic changes of Ebstein's anomaly, with the true tricuspid annulus evident at the first notch along the lower right heart border *(black arrow)*, the displaced tricuspid leaflet producing a second notch *(white arrow)* further to the patient's left, and the smooth-walled atrialized segment of the right ventricle occupying the area between these arrows. The main pulmonary artery is displaced medially.

aortography. This occurs from retrograde filling of the pulmonary arteries through a PDA.

MAGNETIC RESONANCE IMAGING

MRI readily demonstrates the abnormal tricuspid valve and right atrial and ventricular morphology.

PROGNOSIS

The prognosis in the symptomatic neonate or infant is poor, with 50% mortality by the end of the first month. Patients presenting later usually do well for many years and may be aided by palliative procedures, including the Glenn operation or Blalock-Taussig shunting if there is associated PVS. Other procedures attempting to utilize functional components of the right ventricle have also been performed, such as plication of the tricuspid valve with associated ASD closure.

SUGGESTED READINGS
General

See Section V, Part I, Chapter 1, p 1230, and Chapter 2, pp 1255–1256.

Tetralogy of Fallot

Becker S, Hoeffel JC, Worms AM, et al: Angiographic appearance of tetralogy of Fallot: 100 cases. Ann Radiol (Paris) 1980;23:23

Calder AL, Brandt TW, Barratt-Boyes BG, et al: Variants of tetralogy of Fallot with absent pulmonary valve leaflets and origin of one pulmonary artery from the ascending aorta. Am J Cardiol 1980; 46:106

Davis GD, Fulton RE, Ritter DG, et al: Congenital pulmonary atresia with ventricular septal defect: angiographic and surgical correlates. Radiology 1978;128:133

Didier D, Higgins CB, Fisher MR, et al: Congenital heart disease: gated MR imaging in 72 patients. Radiology 1986;158:227

Diethelm E, Soto B, Nath PH, et al: Pulmonary vascularity in patients with pulmonary atresia and ventricular septal defect. Radiography 1985;5:243

Fellows KE, Freed MD, Keane JR, et al: Results of routine preoperative coronary angiography in tetralogy of Fallot. Circulation 1975;51:561

Fellows KE, Smith J, Keane JF: Preoperative angiocardiography in infants with tetralogy of Fallot. Am J Cardiol 1981;47:1279

Garcia-Medina V, Bass J, Braunlin E, et al: A useful projection for demonstrating the bifurcation of the pulmonary artery. Pediatr Cardiol 1990;11:147–149

Mirowitz SA, Gutierrez FR, Canter CE, et al: Tetralogy of Fallot: MR findings. Radiology 1989;171:207–212

Nath PH, Soto B, Bini RM, et al: Tetralogy of Fallot with atrioventricular canal: an angiographic study. J Thorac Cardiovasc Surg 1984;87:421

Singh SP, Rigby ML, Astley R: Demonstration of pulmonary arteries by contrast injection into pulmonary veins. Br Heart J 1978;40:55

Soto B, Pacifico AD, Luna RF, et al: Radiographic study of congenital pulmonary atresia with ventricular septal defect. AJR Am J Roentgenol 1977;129:1027

Soto B, Pacifico A, Seballos R, et al: Tetralogy of Fallot: an angiographic-pathologic correlative study. Circulation 1981;64:558

Soulen RL, Donner R, Capitanio M: Postoperative evaluation of complex congenital heart disease by magnetic resonance imaging. Radiographics 1987;7:975

Strife JL: Tetralogy of Fallot. Semin Roentgenol 1985;20:160

Tricuspid Atresia

Weinberg PM: Anatomy of tricuspid atresia and its relevance to current forms of surgical therapy. Ann Thorac Surg 1980;29:306

Pulmonary Atresia with an Intact Ventricular Septum (Hypoplastic Right Heart Syndrome)

Bharati S, McCallister HA, Chiemmongkoltip P, et al: Congenital pulmonary atresia with tricuspid insufficiency: morphologic study. Am J Cardiol 1977;40:70

Freedom RM, Culham JAG, Moes CAF: Differentiation of functional and structural pulmonary atresia: role of aortography. Am J Cardiol 1978;41:914

Freedom RM, Moes CAF: The hypoplastic right heart complex. Semin Roentgenol 1980;20:169

Jacobstein MD, Fletcher B, Goldstein S, Riemenschneider TA: Magnetic resonance imaging in patients with hypoplastic right heart syndrome. Am Heart J 1985;110:154–158

Patel RG, Freedom RM, Moes CAF, et al: Right ventricular volume determinations in 18 patients with pulmonary atresia and intact ventricular septum. Circulation 1980;61:428

Rowe RD, Freedom RM, Mehrizi A: The Neonate With Congenital Heart Disease. Philadelphia, WB Saunders, 1981:330

Van Praagh R, Ando M, Van Praagh S, et al: Pulmonary atresia: anatomic considerations. *In* Kidd BSL, Rowe RD (eds): The Child With Congenital Heart Disease After Surgery. Mt Kisco, NY, Futura Publishing, 1976;103

Aortic Atresia (Hypoplastic Left Heart Syndrome)

Norwood WI, Kirkin JK, Sanders SP: Hypoplastic left heart syndrome: experience with palliative surgery. Am Cardiol 1980;45:87

Roberts WC, Perry LW, Chandra RS, et al: Aortic valve atresia: new classification based on necropsy study of 73 cases. Am J Cardiol 1976;37:753

Ebstein's Anomaly of the Tricuspid Valve

Anderson KR, Lie JT: Pathologic anatomy of Ebstein's anomaly of the heart revisited. Am J Cardiol 1978;41:739

Deutsch V, Wexler L, Blieden LC, et al: Ebstein's anomaly of the tricuspid valve: critical review of roentgen features and additional angiographic signs. Am J Roentgenol Radium Ther Nucl Med 1975;125:395

Link KM, Herrera MA, D'Souza VJ, et al: MR imaging of Ebstein's anomaly: results in four cases. AJR Am J Roentgenol 1988;150:363

Tao MS, Partridge J, Radford D: The plain chest radiograph in uncomplicated Ebstein's disease. Clin Radiol 1986;37:551

PART III

VASCULAR RINGS AND GREAT VESSEL ANOMALIES

RICHARD B. JAFFE
VIRGIL R. CONDON

■ **C h a p t e r 1**

AORTIC ARCH ANOMALIES

RICHARD B. JAFFE and VIRGIL R. CONDON

Anomalies of the great vessels (e.g., an anomalous right subclavian artery) are frequently incidental findings, although other lesions tend to produce significant signs of tracheal, bronchial, or esophageal compression. Anomalies of the great vessels are frequently identified on plain films or esophagograms. The frequency of arch anomalies varies from 0.5% to 3.0%, depending on the inclusion of various anomalies.

PATHOLOGY

With use of the hypothetical double arch system described by Edwards (Fig. 1), the development of the normal aortic arch and all other anomalous malformations can be explained by the failure of different segments of the right fourth dorsal arch to regress

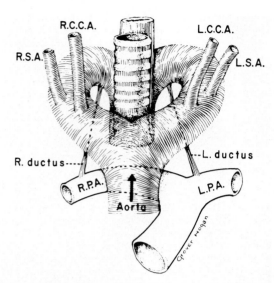

FIGURE 1. A diagram of the Edwards hypothetical double aortic arch system shows bilateral aortic arches and bilateral ductus arteriosus. *RSA*, right subclavian artery; *RCCA*, right common carotid artery; *LSA*, left subclavian artery; *LCCA*, left common carotid artery; *RPA*, right pulmonary artery; *LPA*, left pulmonary artery. (From Shuford WH, Sybers RG, Weens HS: The angiographic features of double aortic arch. Am J Roentgenol Radium Ther Nucl Med 1972;116:126, with permission.)

normally. In the normal development of the left aortic arch, complete regression of the right fourth dorsal aortic segment occurs between the origin of the right subclavian artery and the upper left descending aorta. The anomaly created by a similar regression on the left side produces the more typical right aortic arch with mirror-image branching of the brachiocephalic vessels characteristically seen in congenital heart disease (CHD) (tetralogy of Fallot). When both segments of the arch remain open, a functioning double aortic arch results.

CLINICAL MANIFESTATIONS

Important clinical manifestations, usually dating from birth, include wheezing, stridulous breathing that is constant but exacerbated by crying, tachypnea, dyspnea or cyanosis, and dysphagia. Symptoms usually become evident between 3 weeks and 2 years and are evident in 75% to 90% of patients with significant anomalies.

EVALUATION OF VASCULAR RINGS

The suggested work-up of a suspected vascular ring anomaly is described in Figure 2.

CHEST RADIOGRAPHY

Chest radiograms that penetrate the mediastinum well will frequently show the abnormal indentation or deviation of the trachea that results from a prominent right

aortic arch segment (Fig. 3). This finding, in the absence of cyanotic CHD, implies a vascular ring until proved otherwise. A high-kilovoltage anteroposterior (AP) film with added filtration of the tracheal airway (Fig. 4), or chest fluoroscopy of the trachea, and esophagography can confirm the abnormal tracheal and esophageal indentations caused by the prominent arch segments on the right of the trachea and posterior to the esophagus. Some surgeons feel comfortable when utilizing this limited evaluation to proceed with the operation, while others prefer additional evaluations with ultrasound, angiography, computed tomography (CT), and magnetic resonance imaging (MRI).

MRI or helical CT is now the preferred modality for the definitive evaluation of vascular rings. If aortography is utilized for the evaluation of arch anomalies, biplane AP and lateral or long-axis views are usually sufficient. For pulmonary sling, the sitting-up AP and lateral projections are optimal.

ECHOCARDIOGRAPHY

Two-dimensional echocardiography will usually identify a double aortic arch or right aortic arch anomaly. A complete evaluation of brachiocephalic vessels and associated fibrous bands related to interruption of the left arch component may be difficult.

LEFT AORTIC ARCH

ABERRANT ORIGIN OF THE RIGHT SUBCLAVIAN ARTERY

This anomaly, in which the right subclavian artery is the most distal brachiocephalic vessel, is a common anomaly generally thought to be an incidental finding occurring in approximately 0.5% of normal autopsies. The vessel runs a typical oblique course retroesophageally upward and to the right. Rarely, it courses between the trachea and esophagus, and it frequently coexists with CHD. If present distal to a coarctation, only unilateral left-sided rib notching is present. It may be a rare cause of tracheal

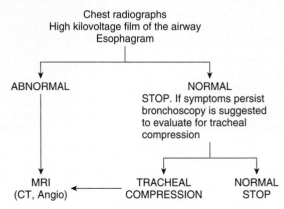

FIGURE 2. Suggested work-up for vascular ring.

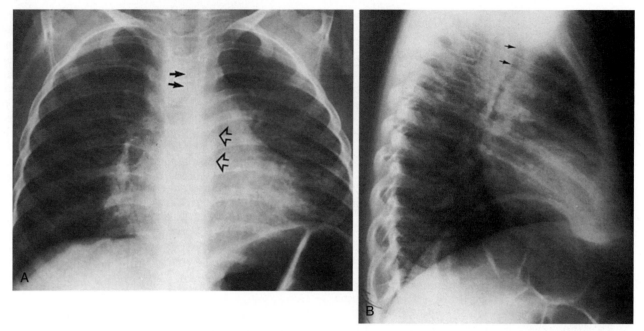

FIGURE 3. Vascular ring–double aortic arch with left arch atresia. **A,** Anteroposterior chest radiograph in 3-year-old with chronic respiratory disease demonstrates a right aortic arch displacing the trachea to the left *(arrows)* with a left-sided descending thoracic aorta *(open arrows)* (see Fig. 14). There is scattered pneumonic or atelectatic pulmonary disease in the perihilar and right middle lobe area. **B,** Lateral view shows anterior tracheal displacement *(small black arrows)* that is consistent with a large retrotracheal vascular structure or other mass.

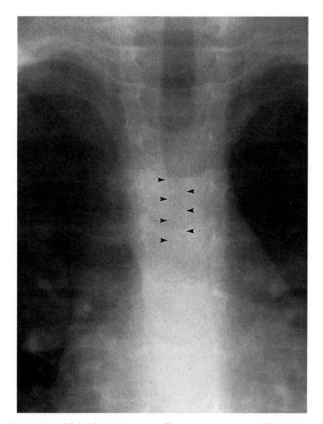

FIGURE 4. High-kilovoltage peak film made with added filtration to better define the tracheobronchial airway. A prominent right aortic arch narrows the trachea and pushes the right tracheal wall medially *(arrowheads)*. Similar findings on the left, although less evident, are related to a double aortic arch.

compression when combined with a bicarotid truncus or tortuous right common carotid artery (Fig. 5).

An esophagogram shows a typical oblique defect in the AP projection that starts on the left at the T3 to T4 level, proceeds cephalad to the right at a 60- to 70-degree angle, and terminates at T2 to T3. In the lateral view, a small posterior and oblique impression on the esophagus can be seen as the vessel passes in its oblique course (Fig. 6).

LEFT AORTIC ARCH WITH RIGHT DESCENDING AORTA

This uncommon malformation is characterized by a left aortic arch arising from the ascending aorta and passing to the left of the trachea, and a retroesophageal transverse arch passing behind the esophagus and then continuing as a right descending aorta. If associated with an aberrant right subclavian artery arising as the fourth branch of the aortic arch, and a right ligamentum arteriosum, a vascular ring may be formed. The malformation may be recognized on a chest radiograph by a left aortic arch deviating the trachea to the right, and by the right descending aorta (Fig. 7A). An esophagogram will demonstrate a large oblique posterior esophageal impression passing downward from cephalic left to caudad right. The malformation can be confirmed by angiography (Fig. 7B), MRI, or CT.

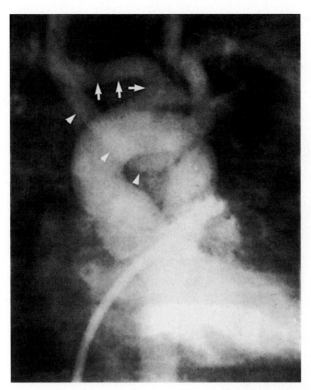

FIGURE 5. An angiocardiogram in an infant with chronic respiratory distress shows leftward origin of the right common carotid artery to the left of the trachea *(arrows)* and an aberrant retroesophageal right subclavian artery *(arrowheads)*. The pretracheal and retroesophageal course of these vessels, respectively, may be a more significant contributing cause of respiratory distress than either lesion alone.

LEFT CERVICAL AORTIC ARCH

A left cervical aortic arch is characterized by an aortic arch extending abnormally high in the upper mediastinum–low cervical region on the left side. A left cervical arch is less common than a right cervical arch. The branching of the aortic arch vessels is variable. The common carotid arteries may arise normally from the cervical arch, or there may be separate origins of the internal and external carotid arteries. Patients with a left cervical arch may present with a pulsatile left supraclavicular mass that may be mistaken for an aneurysm, or symptoms of a vascular ring. On the chest radiograph, upper mediastinal widening may be present, with the left cervical arch displacing the trachea to the right and anteriorly. As the cervical arch passes posteriorly behind the esophagus to descend on the right side, it may produce a large oblique esophageal impression passing from cephalic left to caudad right. The malformation can be confirmed by angiography, MRI, or CT.

INNOMINATE ARTERY COMPRESSION SYNDROME

Anterior tracheal compression by the innominate artery may rarely cause symptoms of respiratory obstruction.

Infants may present with frequent respiratory infections, stridor, and respiratory arrest, and are frequently misdiagnosed as having tracheomalacia. The malformation usually is recognized in symptomatic patients during bronchoscopy when a pulsatile impression is seen on the anterior wall of the trachea, approximately 1 to 2 cm above the carina. A lateral chest radiograph may show anterior tracheal compression (Fig. 8*A*), but is nondiagnostic. An esophagogram, if performed, is normal and serves only to exclude more common vascular rings. CT and preferably MRI can confirm the findings noted at bronchoscopy (Fig. 8*B–D*).

TRACHEAL COMPRESSION BY THE LEFT AORTIC ARCH WITH RIGHT LUNG AGENESIS

Anterior tracheal compression may occur by a normal left aortic arch in patients with right lung agenesis and dextroposition. As the displaced ascending aorta passes from right to left, the trachea is compressed anteriorly. This anatomic relationship produces obstruction similar to that seen with the innominate artery compression syndrome. Posterior displacement of the trachea with anterior compression may be seen on the lateral chest radiograph (Fig. 9*B*), on high-kilovoltage films of the neck with added filtration, or on fluoroscopy, and is confirmed with bronchoscopy, CT, or MRI (Fig. 9*C, D*).

DOUBLE AORTIC ARCH

This anomaly can be categorized as (1) a complete functioning double aortic arch and (2) a double aortic arch with interruption of the left arch at varying positions with fibrous continuity of the interrupted segment. A double arch is the most common cause of a symptomatic vascular ring in infants and young children.

FUNCTIONING DOUBLE AORTIC ARCH

A complete (functional) double aortic arch represents persistence of both the right and left aortic arches. Two vessels arise from the ascending aorta and course dorsally, one on each side of the trachea and esophagus, to join posteriorly, usually into a left descending aorta. The left arch is usually anterior and the right arch is posterior. Occasionally, with a descending right thoracic aorta, these arch relationships are reversed. In the usual course, the right arch is larger. This anomaly of the aortic arch is usually isolated without CHD.

Chest Radiography

Chest radiographic diagnosis is difficult in the infant. In the older child the pattern simulates a right aortic arch, although occasionally, in the lateral view, AP narrowing

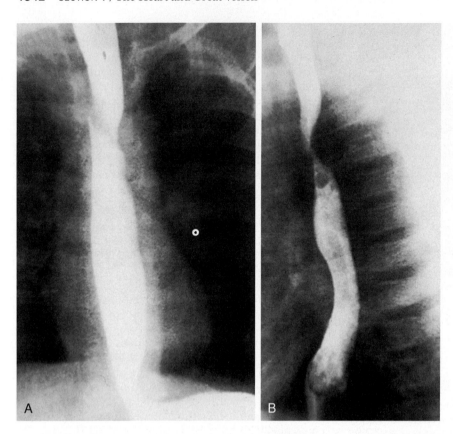

FIGURE 6. Aberrant right subclavian artery. Anteroposterior **(A)** and lateral **(B)** esophagograms show the characteristic posterior esophageal oblique defect progressing from the caudal left side to the cephalic right side. This lesion by itself is usually considered an incidental finding and not related to airway or esophageal obstruction.

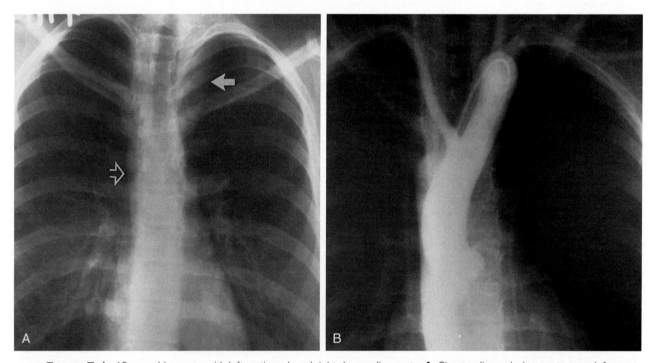

FIGURE 7. An 18-year-old woman with left aortic arch and right descending aorta. **A,** Chest radiograph demonstrates a left superior mediastinal density *(closed arrow)* representing the ascending aorta and arch, and right paraspinal density *(open arrow)* of the right descending aorta. The trachea is minimally displaced to the right. **B,** Aortogram, frontal projection, demonstrates the left ascending aorta high in the left superior mediastinum, a retroesophageal transverse arch, and right descending aorta.

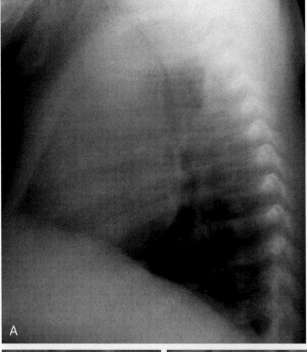

FIGURE 8. Innominate artery compression syndrome in a 5-month-old infant with respiratory distress. **A,** Lateral chest radiograph demonstrates anterior tracheal compression just below the thoracic inlet. **B–D,** Axial spin-echo T$_1$-weighted magnetic resonance image at the level of the left brachiocephalic vein and innominate artery. **B,** The right innominate artery *(shaded arrow)* is seen arising from the left transverse arch just anterior and to the right of the left carotid artery and posterior to the left brachiocephalic vein. The trachea *(arrow)* is widely patent at this level. **C** and **D,** The right innominate artery passes anterior to the trachea to ascend in the right mediastinum. Note the marked anterior–posterior tracheal compression. **E,** Sagittal T$_1$-weighted spin-echo image in the plane of the trachea demonstrates marked tracheal narrowing at the level of the innominate artery *(arrow).*

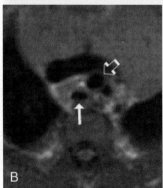
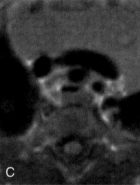
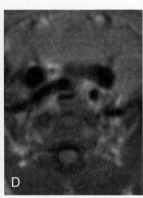
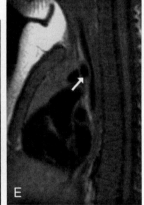

of the trachea may be observed. Pulmonary disease is frequently coexistent (see Fig. 3). A high-kilovoltage film with added filtration in the frontal projection of the tracheal airway will demonstrate the trachea to the left, and may show distal narrowing (see Fig. 4).

Esophagography provides more definitive information and shows typical indentations on the lateral and posterior aspects of the esophagus. Typically, with the larger right posterior segment, a prominent indentation is observed on the right side and posterior aspect of the esophagus. The left arch produces a less striking esophageal indentation that is usually somewhat more caudad when seen in the AP view (Fig. 10*A*). The posterior esophageal impression is frequently horizontal and more prominent (Fig. 10*B*) than is the typical aberrant right subclavian artery with a left aortic arch.

Imaging

Although some surgeons and clinicians do not believe further evaluation is necessary, MRI in the coronal and axial planes (Fig. 11), CT (see Section V, Part I, Chapter 2, Fig. 27, page 1247), or aortography (Fig. 12) does provide more definitive preoperative information concerning patency, relative size, and relations. Angiograms in the AP and lateral or long-axis projections are preferred. Three-dimensional reconstructed MRI with or without gadolinium (Fig. 13) can depict the double aortic arches in relation to the trachea and bronchi.

DOUBLE AORTIC ARCH WITH PARTIAL ATRESIA OF THE LEFT ARCH

This anomaly in arch development results from regression of varying segments of the left aortic arch with fibrous continuity of the segments completing the vascular ring (Fig. 14*A*, *C*, and *E*). Patients have many of the radiographic manifestations seen with double aortic arch. This anomaly is more common than a true simple right aortic arch except in those cases with mirror-image branching and cyanotic CHD. The most

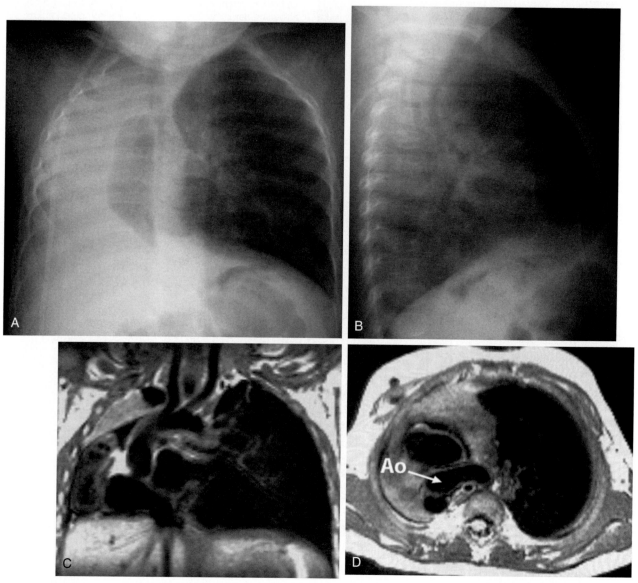

FIGURE 9. Tracheal compression by the transverse arch in a 16-month-old patient with right lung agenesis. She had multiple congenital anomalies, frequent respiratory infections, and stridorous breathing. Frontal **(A)** and lateral **(B)** chest radiographs demonstrate right lung agenesis with dextroposition of the heart, hyperinflation of the left lung, and increased pulmonary blood flow to the left lung secondary to right pulmonary artery aplasia. Note the posterior placement of the trachea in the lateral projection by the transverse aortic arch. Ventriculoperitoneal shunt tubing overlies the right chest in the frontal projection. **C,** Coronal T_1-weighted spin-echo magnetic resonance image demonstrates the aorta arising from the dextropositioned heart and passing transversely across the mediastinum to descend on the left. The descending aorta is not visualized on this image. **D,** Axial T_1-weighted spin-echo image at the level of the transverse arch *(Ao)* demonstrates marked rightward and posterior placement of the trachea. Dextroposition of the heart and hyperinflation of the left lung are also noted.

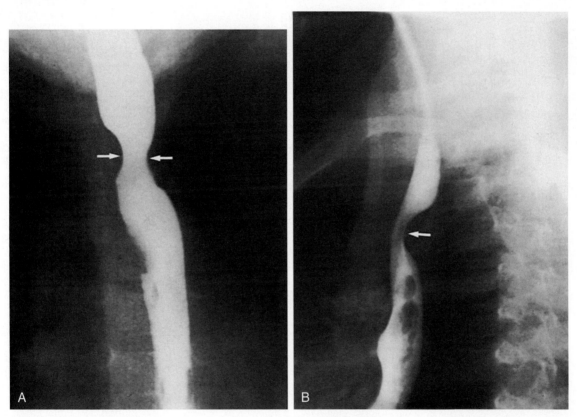

FIGURE 10. Double aortic arch. Anteroposterior (AP) **(A)** and lateral **(B)** esophagograms demonstrate prominent indentations on both the right and left sides of the esophagus in the AP projection *(arrows)* as well as a large transverse defect in the posterior portion of the esophagus *(arrow)* in the lateral view.

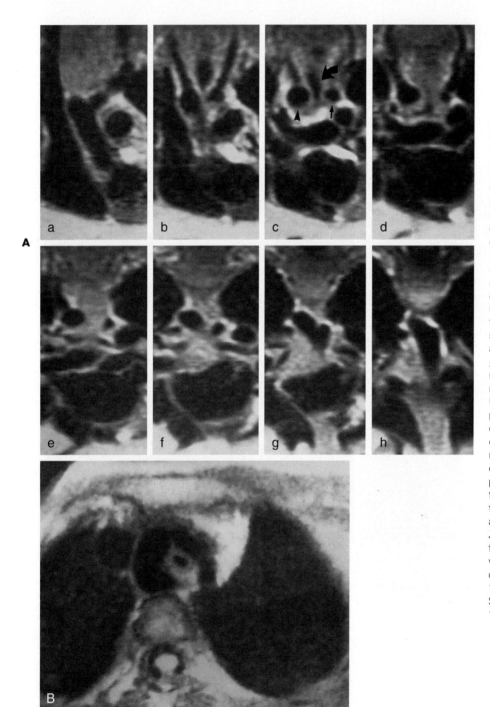

A

B

FIGURE 11. Double aortic arch with both arches patent. **A,** Composite coronal interleaved 3-mm spin-echo magnetic resonance images (anteroposterior) in a 16-month-old boy with symptoms of a vascular ring. *a,* The ascending aorta bifurcates into right and left arches. *b,* The right arch gives origin to the right common carotid, and the left arch to the left common carotid. *c,* The right arch *(arrowhead)* is larger than the left arch *(small arrow).* Note the narrowed trachea *(curved arrow)* as it passes between the two arches. *d,* The right arch gives origin to the right subclavian and vertebral arteries, and the left arch gives origin to the left subclavian and vertebral arteries. *e–g,* The arches pass posteriorly to join together in *g. h,* The aorta descends just to the left of midline. (From Jaffe RB: Magnetic resonance imaging of vascular rings. Semin Ultrasound CT MR 1990;11:208, with permission.) **B,** A 5-year-old girl with double aortic arch. This axial 5-mm spin-echo image demonstrates the dominant right arch and smaller left aortic arch encircling the trachea. As the right arch passes posteriorly to join the left arch to form a left descending thoracic aorta, there is a tendency to a right posterior arch and left anterior arch. (Courtesy of Jerald Kuhn, Children's Hospital of Buffalo, Buffalo, NY. From Cohen MD, Edwards MK: Magnetic Resonance Imaging of Children. Philadelphia, BC Decker, 1990:562, with permission.) See also Section V, Part I, Chapter 2, Fig. 27, page 1247.

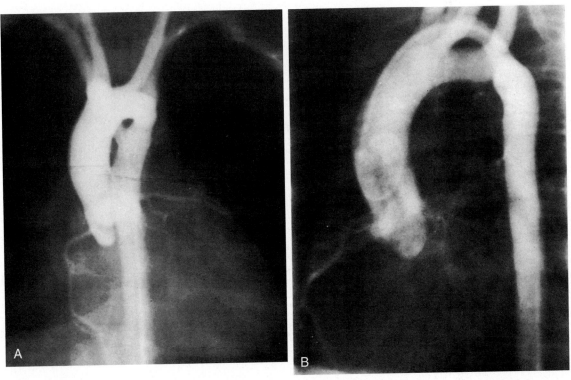

FIGURE 12. Double aortic arch. Anteroposterior **(A)** and lateral **(B)** retrograde aortograms. The catheter passes through the smaller right posterior arch into the ascending aorta; each right and left branch gives rise to the appropriate brachiocephalic vessels. At the time of the examination, the catheter was also passed through the anterior left-sided aortic arch and documented the patency of both limbs.

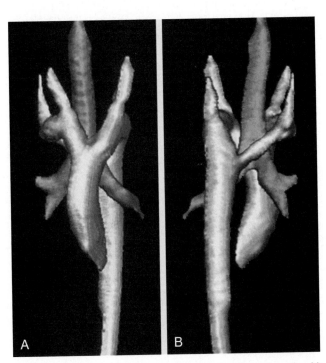

FIGURE 13. Six and one-half–year-old with double aortic arch with left arch dominance. Anterior **(A)** and posterior **(B)** projections of a three-dimensional reconstruction of T_1-weighted spin-echo magnetic resonance image demonstrate that the left arch is the dominant arch (best appreciated in **B**), with a left descending aorta. Note the absence of significant tracheal compression in this patient, who had no respiratory symptoms. (Courtesy of Marc Keller, New Haven, CT.)

common variations in this category are those with atresia between the left common carotid and left subclavian arteries (Fig. 14*E*) or distal to the left subclavian artery (Fig. 14*A* and *C*). An aortic diverticulum may be present and adds significantly to the posterior esophageal impression.

Chest Radiography

Chest radiographs show a prominent right aortic arch segment in the AP projection (Figs. 3 and 15). Esophagograms show impressions on both sides of the esophagus, although predominantly on the right, and a prominent indentation on the posterior esophageal wall (Fig. 16). The descending aorta is more often right-sided. Angiography (Fig. 17), CT, or MRI demonstrates a lack of patency of the left aortic arch distal to the left innominate artery and, frequently, an aortic diverticulum at the junction of the right arch and upper descending aorta in subtype 1 (Fig. 14*A*). Patients with atresia between the left common carotid and left subclavian arteries (subtype 3) will show separate origins of the left common carotid artery from the ascending aorta, and the left subclavian artery from the aortic diverticulum (Figs. 14*E* and 18).

RIGHT AORTIC ARCH

A right aortic arch has many similarities to a double arch with left arch atresia. The malformations result from

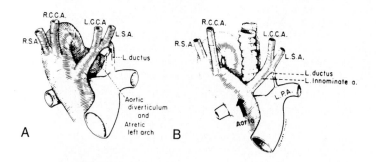

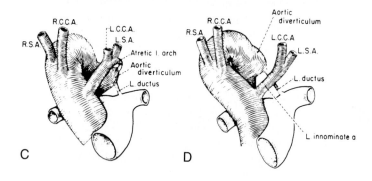

FIGURE 14. Double aortic arch with left arch atresia, subtypes 1, 2, and 3 *(left column),* and their respective right aortic arch counterparts *(right column).* **A,** Subtype 1. **B,** Mirror-image branching, no vascular ring. **C,** Subtype 2. **D,** Mirror-image branching, rare type. **E,** Subtype 3. **F,** Aberrant left subclavian artery. The anatomic difference between the double-arch malformation and its right arch counterpart is the persistence of an atretic segment in the double arch anomaly. (From Shuford WH, Sybers RG, Weens HS: The angiographic features of double aortic arch. Am J Roentgenol Radium Ther Nucl Med 1972;116:137, with permission.)

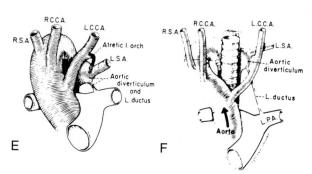

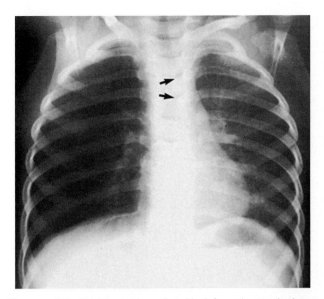

FIGURE 15. Double aortic arch with left arch atresia in an anteroposterior expiratory chest radiograph in a 2-year-old with chronic respiratory distress. Air trapping in the right lung is evident, along with a prominent right aortic arch and striking deviation of the trachea to the left *(arrows).* Air trapping is a relatively rare complication of aortic vascular rings, with right main stem bronchial obstruction secondary to a double aortic arch with atresia of the left arch, subtype 3 (see Fig. 14*E).*

interruption of the segments of the left aortic arch in relation to the great vessel origins.

RIGHT AORTIC ARCH WITH MIRROR-IMAGE BRANCHING

The most common variation of right aortic arch is mirror-image branching of the major brachiocephalic vessels. A right aortic arch with mirror-image branching is not a true vascular ring inasmuch as the ligamentum arteriosum arises from the anteriorly positioned left innominate artery and descends to the left pulmonary artery without creation of a true vascular ring (see Fig. 14*B).* This anomaly is commonly associated with cyanotic CHD: tetralogy of Fallot, truncus arteriosus, tricuspid atresia, and transposition of the great arteries with pulmonary valvular stenosis (see Section V, Part I, Chapter 2, Table 2, page 1234). Rarely, a right aortic arch with mirror-image branching may cause a vascular ring if the ligamentum arteriosum extends from the left pulmonary artery to an aortic diverticulum of the right-sided upper descending aorta (see Fig. 14*D).* A lateral esophagogram will show a large retroesophageal impression from the aortic diverticulum and ligamentum arteriosum.

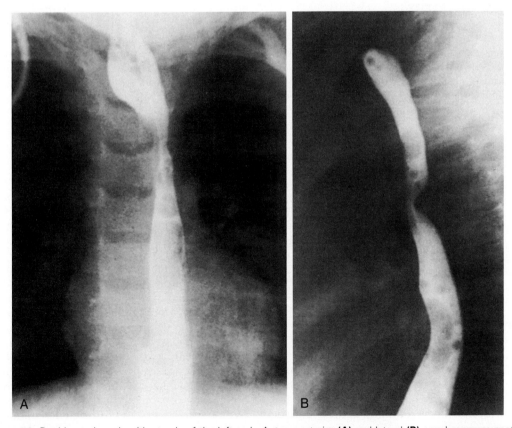

FIGURE 16. Double aortic arch with atresia of the left arch. Anteroposterior **(A)** and lateral **(B)** esophagogram spot films show a prominent impression on the right and a posterior esophageal transverse indentation in the lateral view. There is associated evidence of narrowing and compression of the trachea near the carina.

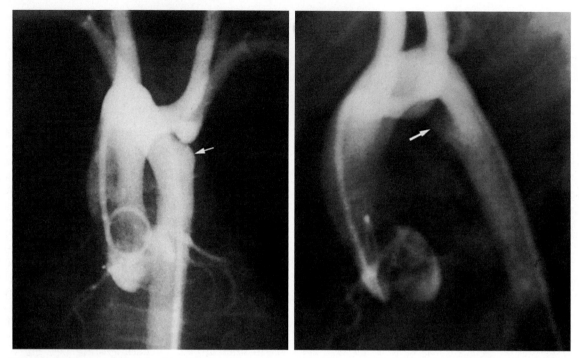

FIGURE 17. Double aortic arch with left arch atresia. Anteroposterior **(A)** and lateral **(B)** retrograde aortograms show atresia distal to the origin of both left-sided brachiocephalic vessels. The vascular ring is completed by the residual fibrous segment and the ligamentum arteriosum. Aortic diverticulum is indicated by an *arrow* (see also Fig. 14).

RIGHT AORTIC ARCH WITH ABERRANT LEFT SUBCLAVIAN ARTERY

A right aortic arch with aberrant origin of the left subclavian artery is a common cause of a vascular ring in infants and children. The distal portion of the rudimentary left arch may persist as a diverticulum giving origin to the left subclavian artery (see Fig. 14*F*). Because the ligamentum arteriosum typically attaches to the aortic diverticulum or left subclavian artery, a true vascular ring is created.

Chest radiographs show typical changes of a right aortic arch deviating the trachea to the left and the azygos vein to the right. On the esophagogram, the aortic diverticulum and aberrant left subclavian artery produce a large retroesophageal impression. The aberrant left subclavian artery may also produce an impression running obliquely from caudal right to cephalad left. MRI (Fig. 19), CT, or angiography will delineate the vascular anatomy (see Fig. 14*F*).

RIGHT AORTIC ARCH WITH LEFT DESCENDING AORTA (CIRCUMFLEX AORTA)

This malformation, considered by some to be a form of double aortic arch with left atresia, is characterized by a right aortic arch, retroesophageal segment, and left descending aorta, and is a mirror image of the left aortic arch with right descending aorta. When associated with an aberrant left subclavian artery, which frequently arises from an aortic diverticulum with stenosis at its origin, and a tight ligamentum arteriosum, a symptomatic vascular ring is formed. On radiographic study one may visualize a right aortic arch, distal tracheal displacement to the left, left descending aorta, and large posterior and oblique impressions on the esophagogram by the retroesophageal segment of the aorta. The malformation can be confirmed by aortography (Fig. 20), CT, or MRI.

RIGHT CERVICAL AORTIC ARCH

A right cervical aortic arch occurs when there is abnormal cephalic migration of the aortic arch into the supraclavicular and neck region. A right cervical arch is more common than a left cervical arch. The branching of the aortic arch vessels is variable. The common carotid arteries may arise normally from the cervical arch or there may be separate origins of both internal and external carotid arteries. The position of the brachiocephalic vessels and ligamentum arteriosum determines which patients are symptomatic from a vascular ring. Clinically a pulsatile mass may be present in the supraclavicular region, with or without symptoms of a vascular ring. Radiographic findings (Fig. 21*A*) include (1) right superior mediastinal widening, (2) tracheal displacement to the left and anteriorly, (3) a large oblique impression on the esophagogram from cephalic right to caudad left, and (4) a left descending aorta. The malformations can be confirmed by MRI, CT, or angiography (Fig. 21*B*). Operation is indicated in patients with symptoms of a vascular ring.

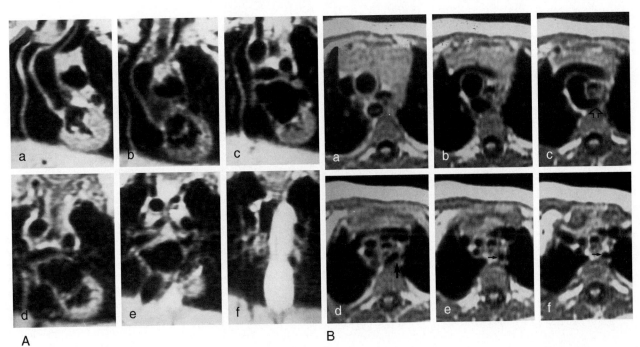

A   B

FIGURE 18. A 3-month-old infant with symptoms of a vascular ring secondary to a double aortic arch with left arch atresia between the left common carotid and left subclavian arteries (subtype 3). An esophagogram demonstrated bilateral esophageal impressions suggestive of a double aortic arch, similar to that in Figure 10A. **A,** Composite coronal interleaved 3-mm spin-echo magnetic resonance images (anteroposterior [AP]). *a* and *b,* The ascending aorta gives origin to the left common carotid artery. *c,* The right aortic arch gives origin to the right common carotid artery. *d,* The right subclavian artery arises from the right aortic arch. *e* and *f,* The origin of the left subclavian artery from the aortic diverticulum is seen; gastroesophageal reflux of formula also is noted. This branching pattern cannot be differentiated from right aortic arch with aberrant left subclavian artery. **B,** Composite axial interleaved 3-mm images (inferosuperior). *a,* Seen are the ascending aorta, right descending aorta, and tracheal bifurcation. *b* and *c,* Seen is the right aortic arch. The aortic diverticulum *(arrow)* is seen in *c. d,* As the left subclavian artery *(arrow)* arises from the aortic diverticulum, it appears tethered anteriorly. The left common carotid artery is seen anterior to the trachea and posterior to the left innominate vein. *e* and *f,* The left subclavian artery *(arrow)* then returns to its normal position. The origins of the right common carotid and right subclavian arteries are seen in *e.* Although this branching pattern cannot be differentiated from a right aortic arch with aberrant left subclavian artery, the course of the left subclavian artery as it appears tethered anteriorly, plus the AP esophagogram, suggested a double aortic arch with left arch atresia between the left common carotid and left subclavian arteries (subtype 3). This was confirmed at operation. (From Jaffe RB: Magnetic resonance imaging of vascular rings. Semin Ultrasound CT MR 1990;11:208, with permission.)

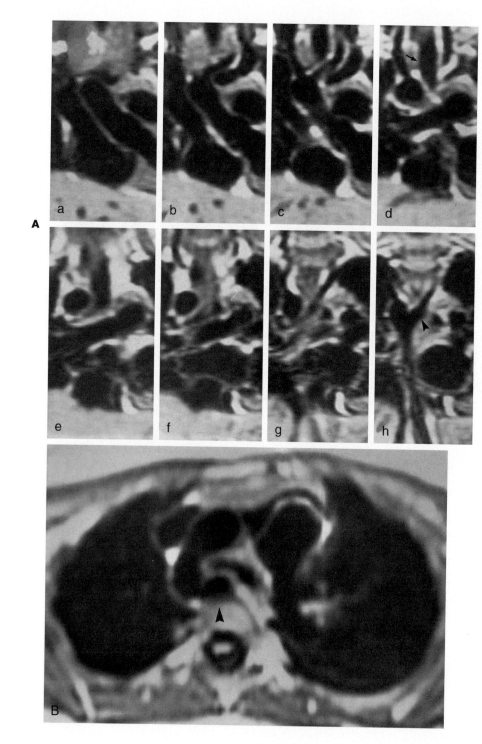

A

B

FIGURE 19. A 4-year-old boy with symptoms of vascular ring secondary to a right aortic arch with aberrant left subclavian artery. **A,** Composite coronal interleaved 3-mm spin-echo magnetic resonance images (anteroposterior). *a,* Left ventricular outflow tract and ascending aorta are seen between the superior vena cava and right atrium and pulmonary artery. *b,* Origin of the left common carotid artery is partially visualized. The left innominate vein is just lateral to the left common carotid artery. *c,* The origin of the left common carotid and right common carotid arteries is seen. *d,* The origin of the right common carotid artery from the right aortic arch is better visualized. Note that the trachea *(arrow)* is deviated to the left. *e–g,* The right aortic arch passes posteriorly and gives origin to the right subclavian and right vertebral arteries in *g.* Part of the left subclavian artery is also noted. *h,* The left subclavian artery arises from the aortic diverticulum *(arrowhead)* originating from the posterior right aortic arch. **B,** Axial 3-mm image confirms the right aortic arch with posterior aortic diverticulum *(arrowhead).* (From Jaffe RB: Magnetic resonance imaging of vascular rings. Semin Ultrasound CT MR 1990;11:211, with permission.)

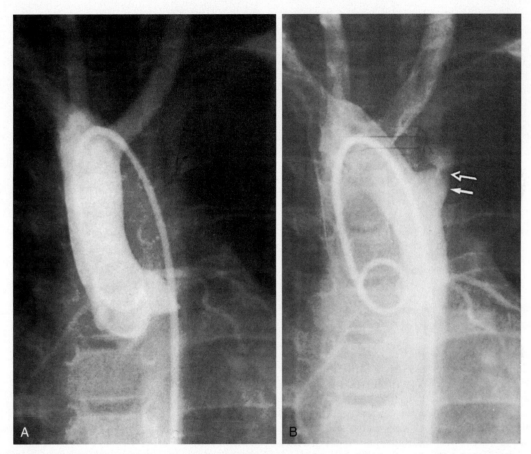

FIGURE 20. A 5-year-old girl with symptoms of a vascular ring secondary to a right aortic arch with left descending aorta (circumflex aorta). **A,** Anteroposterior aortogram demonstrates a right aortic arch with sequential origin of the left common carotid, right common carotid, and right subclavian arteries. **B,** The aorta passes behind the esophagus to descend on the left. The left subclavian artery arises from a small diverticulum *(arrow)* with stenosis at its origin *(open arrow)*. At operation, the left ligamentum arteriosum completed the vascular ring. This arch anomaly may also be considered as a form of double aortic arch with left arch atresia.

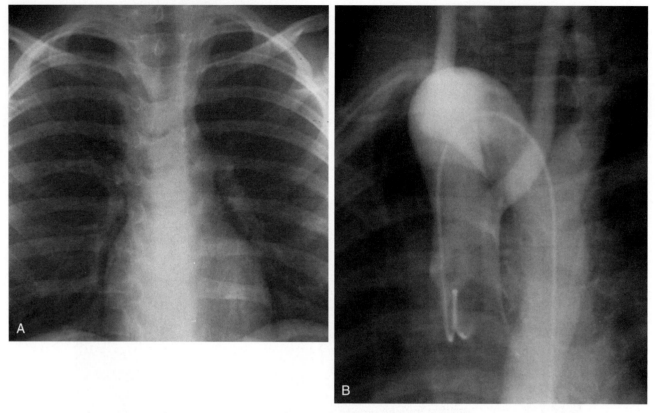

FIGURE 21. A 13-year-old boy with a pulsatile right supraclavicular mass secondary to a right cervical aortic arch. **A,** Chest radiograph demonstrates tracheal displacement to the left and a right supraclavicular mass at the upper margin of the film. The descending aorta is not visualized. **B,** Aortogram (shallow left anterior oblique projection) confirms a right cervical aortic arch.

RIGHT AORTIC ARCH WITH ISOLATION OF THE LEFT SUBCLAVIAN ARTERY

A final variation of a right aortic arch is isolation of the left subclavian artery attached by a functioning or nonfunctioning ductus arteriosus to the left pulmonary artery. This is not a true vascular ring and is of primary interest because of the clinical variation created in the brachiocephalic pulses and, occasionally, subsequent subclavian steal syndrome. The anomaly is frequently associated with CHD.

SUGGESTED READINGS

Dominiguez R, Oh KS, Dorst JP, et al: Left aortic arch with right descending aorta. Am J Roentgenol 1978;130:917

Edwards JE: Anomalies of the derivatives of the aortic arch system. Med Clin North Am 1948;32:925

Jaffe RB: Magnetic resonance imaging of vascular rings. Semin Ultrasound CT MR 1990;11:206

Jaffe RB: Radiographic manifestations of congenital anomalies of the aortic arch. Radiol Clin North Am 1991;29:319

McCormick TL, Kuhns LR: Tracheal compression by a normal aorta associated with right lung agenesis. Radiology 1979;120:659–660

Predey TA, McDonald V, Demos TC, et al: CT of congenital anomalies of the aortic arch. Semin Roentgenol 1989;24:96–111

Shuford WH, Sybers RG: The Aortic Arch and Its Malformations. Springfield, IL, Charles C Thomas, 1974

Spindolo-Franco H, Fish BG: Abnormalities of the aortic arch and pulmonary arteries—vascular rings and slings. *In* Elliott LP (ed): Cardiac Imaging in Infants, Children, and Adults. Philadelphia, JB Lippincott, 1991:344

Chapter 2

PULMONARY ARTERY ABNORMALITIES

RICHARD B. JAFFE and VIRGIL R. CONDON

ABERRANT LEFT PULMONARY ARTERY (PULMONARY SLING)

When the left sixth aortic arch fails to develop normally or becomes obliterated and the left pulmonary artery subsequently fails to develop, the left lung's arterial supply is derived from an anomalous vessel originating from the right pulmonary artery. This aberrant left pulmonary artery passes between the trachea and esophagus and produces a vascular sling or ring (Fig. 1). It is frequently accompanied by significant hypoplasia or dysplasia of the trachea and main bronchi. These structures are displaced to the left and compressed by the aberrant vessel to produce tracheobronchomalacia or intrinsic cartilaginous malformation.

CLINICAL MANIFESTATIONS

Stridor, wheezing, and dyspnea progressing to frank cyanosis develop shortly after birth. Symptoms tend to

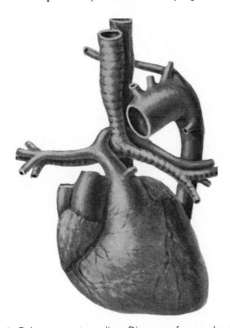

FIGURE 1. Pulmonary artery sling. Diagram of anomalous origin of the left pulmonary artery from the right pulmonary artery, showing its retrograde course between the trachea and esophagus. Note the hypoplasia of the distal trachea, often representing an intrinsic malformation with complete cartilaginous rings that may extend into the right and left main stem bronchi. This tracheal malformation is one of the most serious aspects of this anomaly.

be more severe than with other types of vascular rings. Significant unilateral bronchial obstruction of the right lung may occur.

CHEST RADIOGRAPHY

When the anomalous vessel obstructs the right main-stem bronchus, trapped fetal fluid in the right lung is seen in the newborn. In neonates and infants, a hyperlucent right lung is usually seen (Fig. 2). The left hilum is usually low, and the main stem bronchi may show a horizontal "inverted T-shaped" pattern. Branching to the upper and lower lobes tends to originate at a more peripheral level. Anterior bowing of the trachea at the carina may be seen on the lateral chest film (Fig. 3A).

Esophagography, if performed, characteristically identifies an indentation on the anterior wall of the esophagus at the level of the carina, and the trachea is anteriorly displaced from the esophagus at this level (Fig. 3B). Occasionally, the esophagogram may show normal anatomy. Bronchoscopy is recommended to evaluate the tracheobronchial tree for extrinsic pulsatile compression effects as well as underlying tracheobronchomalacia (see Section V, Part III, Chapter 1, Fig. 2, page 1339).

ECHOCARDIOGRAPHY

Real-time studies will fail to demonstrate a normal pulmonary artery bifurcation (moustache appearance). Instead, the left pulmonary artery is seen to originate from the right pulmonary artery and course back to the left lung (Fig. 4).

IMAGING

Pulmonary arteriography, thin-section computed tomography (CT), or magnetic resonance imaging (MRI) confirms the diagnosis. Biplane studies in the sitting-up position are recommended (Fig. 5) at pulmonary arteriography. Thin-section MRI in the axial plane demonstrates the aberrant course of the left pulmonary artery, tracheal compression, and hyperinflation of the right lung (Fig. 6). Thin-section CT (with three-dimensional reconstruction), MRI, or tracheobronchography (Fig. 7) can delineate the frequently associated tracheobronchial anomalies.

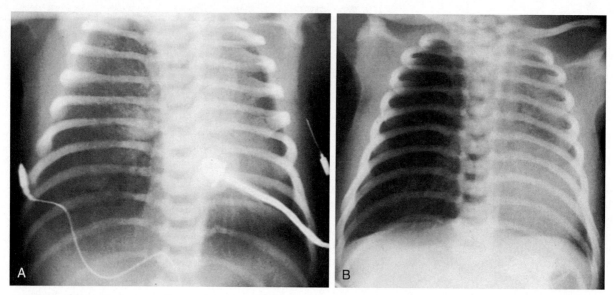

FIGURE 2. Pulmonary artery sling. **A,** Anteroposterior chest film of a neonate age 6 hours shows unilateral retained fetal fluid, increased lung volume, and hazy, ill-defined parenchymal densities secondary to right main stem bronchial obstruction. **B,** Follow-up film at the age of 6 days shows resorption of the fetal lung fluid now producing a unilateral hyperlucent lung secondary to air trapping.

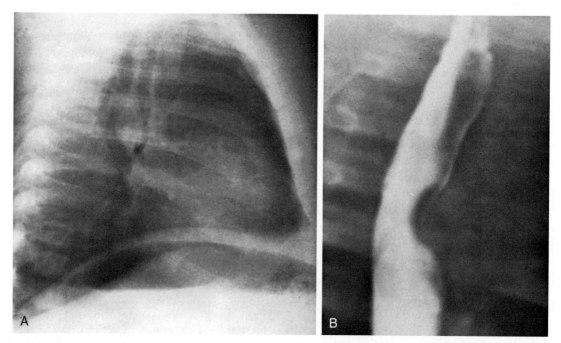

FIGURE 3. Pulmonary artery sling. A lateral chest radiograph **(A)** and lateral esophagogram **(B)** show the anomalous left pulmonary artery between the air-filled trachea and esophagus on the lateral chest film and a focal nodular indentation on the anterior portion of the esophagus at the level of the carina. This esophageal indentation is similar to that noted with total anomalous pulmonary venous return because of the venous confluence. However, the latter is usually in a more caudal position.

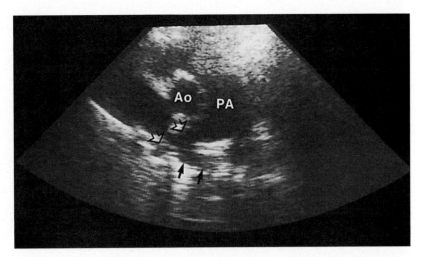

FIGURE 4. Pulmonary artery sling. Short-axis real-time echocardiogram at the level of the aortic root *(Ao)* and main pulmonary artery *(PA)* shows the large main and right pulmonary artery *(open arrows)* giving rise to the left pulmonary artery *(black arrows)*, which deviates back to the left.

PROGNOSIS

The prognosis is guarded even with surgical correction because of the underlying frequent tracheal hypoplasia or tracheobronchomalacia. At the time of vascular surgery, the surgeon should be prepared for reconstructive procedures of the tracheobronchial tree.

CONGENITAL ANOMALIES OF THE PULMONARY ARTERIES

Congenital anomalies of the pulmonary arteries are seen as isolated lesions, in many forms of congenital heart disease, and frequently in syndrome complexes.

The central pulmonary arteries develop from the sixth brachial arches, whereas the peripheral pulmonary arteries develop from the splanchnic plexus of the lungs. Table 1 presents a useful classification of congenital anomalies of the pulmonary arteries. More details

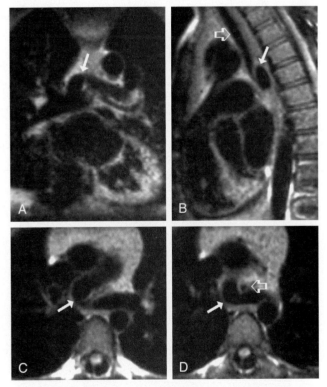

FIGURE 6. Aberrant left pulmonary artery in a child of 3 years 8 months, with frequent respiratory infections and intermittent stridor since birth, as shown on composite T_1-weighted spin-echo magnetic resonance imaging. **A,** Coronal image demonstrates aberrant origin of the left pulmonary artery *(arrow)* from the proximal right pulmonary artery. **B,** Sagittal image in the plane of the trachea *(shaded arrow)* demonstrates the aberrant left pulmonary artery *(straight arrow)* posterior to the trachea. Note the marked distal tracheal narrowing. **C** and **D,** Axial images demonstrate origin of the left pulmonary artery *(straight arrow)* from the right pulmonary artery. The left pulmonary artery passes posterior to the trachea *(shaded arrow, **D**)*. Note the marked tracheal narrowing in **C** and **D**.

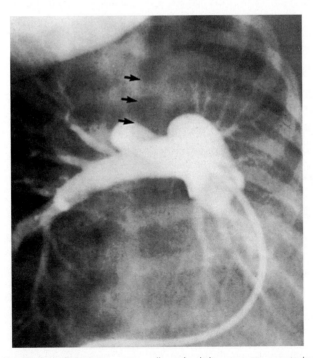

FIGURE 5. Pulmonary artery sling. A sitting-up anteroposterior pulmonary arteriogram demonstrates the left pulmonary artery ascending just to the right of the trachea *(arrows)* and then traveling posteriorly and caudad to branch normally to the left lung.

Table 1 ■ CONGENITAL ANOMALIES OF THE PULMONARY ARTERIES

Hypoplastic pulmonary artery with and without anomalous pulmonary venous return
    Scimitar syndrome—with anomalous pulmonary venous return to the inferior vena cava (Section V, Part I, Chapter 2, Fig. 6, page 1234)
    Tetralogy of Fallot—without anomalous pulmonary venous return
    Pulmonary hypoplasia
Unilateral absence of a pulmonary artery
    As an isolated lesion—pulmonary aplasia or hypoplasia
    With a patent ductus arteriosus—especially with an absent right pulmonary artery
    With tetralogy of Fallot—especially with an absent left pulmonary artery
Anomalous origin of the left pulmonary artery from the right pulmonary artery (pulmonary sling) (Figs. 1 through 6)
Direct connection of the right pulmonary artery to the left atrium
Peripheral pulmonary artery stenosis
    Idiopathic
    Rubella (Section V, Part I, Chapter 2, Fig. 13, page 1239)
    Supravalvular aortic stenosis syndrome (Section V, Part IV, Chapter 2, Fig. 7, page 1368)
    Takayasu arteritis
    Tetralogy of Fallot (Section V, Part II, Chapter 4, Fig. 3, page 1326)
    Arteriohepatic dysplasia (Alagille syndrome)
    Cutis laxa
    Ehlers-Danlos syndrome
Absence of pulmonary artery origin from the heart
    Pulmonary atresia
    Truncus arteriosus (Section V, Part II, Chapter 3, Fig. 24, page 1319)
    Ductal origin of pulmonary artery(ies)
    Systemic–pulmonary artery collaterals (Section V, Part II, Chapter 4, Fig. 4, page 1327 and Section V, Part VII, Chapter 2, Fig. 2, page 1417)
    Coronary collaterals to the lung
Anomalous origin of one pulmonary artery from the ascending aorta
    Anomalous origin of the right pulmonary artery from the ascending aorta (hemitruncus arteriosus) (Section V, Part II, Chapter 1, Fig. 25, page 1276)
    Anomalous origin of the left pulmonary artery from the ascending aorta—with tetralogy of Fallot
Pulmonary arteriovenous malformations
    Classic discrete pulmonary arteriovenous fistula
    Pulmonary telangiectasia
    Hereditary hemorrhagic telangiectasia (Rendu-Osler-Weber syndrome)

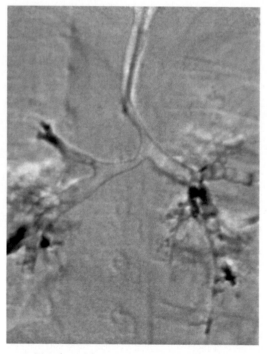

FIGURE 7. Digital subtraction tracheobronchogram in a 2½-month-old infant with aberrant left pulmonary artery. There is marked narrowing of the distal trachea and proximal bridging right bronchus from compression by the aberrant left pulmonary artery. The left bronchus and mid- and distal right bronchi are patent.

of frequent pulmonary artery anomalies are found in Section IV, Part VII, Chapters 2 and 6, and elsewhere in Section V.

SUGGESTED READINGS

General

See Section V, Part I, Chapter 1, pp 1228–1229, and Chapter 2, pp 1239–1240.

Aberrant Left Pulmonary Artery

Berdon WE, Baker DH: Vascular anomalies and the infant lung: rings, slings and other things. Semin Roentgenol 1972;7:39

Berdon WE, Baker DH, Wung JT, et al: Complete cartilage-ring tracheal stenosis associated with anomalous left pulmonary artery: the ring-sling complex. Radiology 1984;152:57–64

Jaffe RB: Magnetic resonance imaging of vascular rings. Semin Ultrasound CT MR 1990;11:206–220

Newman B, Meza MP, Towbin RB, et al: Left pulmonary artery sling: diagnosis and delineation of associated tracheobronchial anomalies with MR. Pediatr Radiol 1996;26:661

Spindolo-Franco H, Fish BG: Abnormalities of the aortic arch and pulmonary arteries—vascular rings and slings. *In* Elliott LP (ed): Cardiac Imaging in Infants, Children, and Adults. Philadelphia, JB Lippincott, 1991:34

Vogl TJ, Diebold T, Bergman C, et al: MRI in pre- and postoperative assessment of tracheal stenosis due to pulmonary artery sling. J Comput Assist Tomogr 1993;17:878

Wells TR, Gwinn JL, Landing BH, et al: Reconsideration of the anatomy of sling left pulmonary artery: the association of one form with bridging bronchus and imperforate anus: anatomic and diagnostic aspects. J Pediatr Surg 1988;23:892

Williams RG, Jaffe RB, Condon VR: Unusual features of pulmonary sling. AJR Am J Roentgenol 1979;133:1065

Congenital Anomalies of the Pulmonary Arteries

Abe T, Kuribayashi R, Sato M, et al: Direct communication of the right pulmonary artery with the left atrium. J Thorac Cardiovasc Surg 1972;62:38–44

Currarino G, Willis KW, Johnson AF Jr, et al: Pulmonary telangiectasia. Am J Roentgenol 1976;127:775–779

Ellis K: Developmental abnormalities in the systemic blood supply to the lungs. AJR Am J Roentgenol 1991;156:669–679

Gomes AS: MR imaging of congenital anomalies of the thoracic aorta and pulmonary arteries. Radiol Clin North Am 1989;27:1171

Julsrud PR: Magnetic resonance imaging of the pulmonary arteries and veins. Semin Ultrasound CT MR 1990;11:184–205

Lynch DA, Higgins CB: MR imaging of unilateral pulmonary artery anomalies. J Comput Assist Tomogr 1990;14:187

Oh KS, Bender TM, Bowen A, et al: Plain radiographic, nuclear medicine and angiographic observations of hepatogenic pulmonary angiodysplasia. Pediatr Radiol 1983;13:111

Panicek DM, Heitzman ER, Randall PA, et al: The continuum of pulmonary development anomalies. Radiographics 1987;7:747–772

Rosenfield NS, Kelley MJ, Jensen PS, et al: Arteriohepatic dysplasia: radiologic features of a new syndrome. AJR Am J Roentgenol 1980;1135:1217–1223

Spindola-Franco H, Fish BG: Abnormalities of the aortic arch and pulmonary arteries—vascular rings and slings. In Elliott LP (ed): Cardiac Imaging in Infants, Children, and Adults. Philadelphia, JB Lippincott, 1991:344

White RI Jr, Mitchell SE, Barth KH, et al: Angioarchitecture of pulmonary arteriovenous malformations. AJR Am J Roentgenol 1983;140:681–686

CARDIAC MALPOSITION, CARDIOSPLENIC (HETEROTAXY) SYNDROMES, AND CHROMOSOMAL ANOMALIES

VIRGIL R. CONDON

■
C h a p t e r   1

CARDIAC MALPOSITIONS

VIRGIL R. CONDON

The evaluation of cardiac malpositions and cardiac–visceral discordance is very complex and difficult. Approaching these conditions by utilizing a systematic, segmental approach with familiar anatomic terminology helps to simplify the evaluation of these patients. Analysis must include (1) atrial positions, (2) atrioventricular (AV) relations and connections, and (3) ventricular–great vessel relations and connections and systemic venous drainage. Segmental relations can be deduced from the knowledge of cardiac–visceral relations; the basic appearance of the chest radiograph and the cardiac silhouette; and electrocardiographic,

Table 1 ■ WORKING APPROACH TO CARDIAC AND VISCERAL MALPOSITIONS

1. Exclude cardiac malposition secondary to extracardiac abnormalities (e.g., hypoplastic lung).
2. Evaluate for visceral heterotaxia associated with asplenia or polysplenia
   a. Tracheobronchial tree for symmetry
   b. Pulmonary arteries for unilaterality or symmetry
   c. Lobation of the lung
   d. Hepatic symmetry—horizontal liver
   e. Position of the stomach
   f. Is the IVC present or is there azygos continuation of the IVC indicative of polysplenia?
3. Determine cardiac and visceral relationships. Almost always the left atrium is on the side of the stomach.
   a. Normal visceral situs
      i. Dextrocardia—high incidence of CHD, particularly l-TGA with VSD and PVS
      ii. Levocardia—no malposition; 1% incidence of CHD
   b. Visceral situs inversus
      i. Dextrocardia—3%–5% incidence of CHD
      ii. Levocardia—almost 100% incidence of CHD, particularly forms of transposition

CHD = congenital heart disease; IVC = inferior vena cava; I-TGA = corrected transposition of the great arteries; PVS = pulmonary valvular stenosis; VSD = ventricular septal defect.

echocardiographic, and angiocardiographic evaluations and gastrointestinal examination. Magnetic resonance imaging examination may be able to demonstrate cardiac and venous malformation, visceral relationships, and malformations such as gastrointestinal malrotation and biliary anomalies. Tracheobronchial anatomy, pulmonary lobation, and great vessel relationships may also be determined (Table 1).

DEFINITIONS

Dextrocardia implies a cardiac silhouette predominantly to the right of the spine (Fig. 1) without implication of intracardiac disturbance or atrial, ventricular, or great vessel relations. *Dextroversion* relates to primary visceral cardiac development, while *dextroposition* relates to thoracic or abdominal malformations.

In *levocardia*, the cardiac silhouette is on the left without implication of internal cardiac structure.

Situs solitus (totalis) indicates "normal" visceral–cardiac relations, with the cardiac apex, aortic arch, and stomach bubble on the left. The liver, inferior vena cava, and right atrial structures are on the right.

Situs inversus (totalis) indicates the mirror-image development of both the visceral and cardiac anatomy. This relation has only a slight (3% to 5%) increase in congenital heart disease (CHD).

Situs inversus viscerum (visceral situs inversus) indicates mirror-image development of the abdominal viscera and, for practical purposes, the cardiac atria. When accompanied by AV discordance (see below), a high incidence of CHD is expected.

In *visceral heterotaxia (ambiguous viscera)* numerous patients, particularly those with the asplenia or polysplenia syndrome, have an indeterminate configuration of viscera in which the liver tends to be horizontal and the stomach midline or on either the right or left side. Such cases are accompanied by multiple visceral and cardiac anomalies.

Inversion indicates the mirror-image or reversed positioning of anatomic structures. It applies to all portions of the segmental anatomy of the heart: atria, ventricles, and great vessels. A patient with a right-sided cardiac silhouette may have either inverted or noninverted ventricular anatomy just like a patient with levocardia.

AV concordance indicates that the right atrium is appropriately related to the right ventricle, with similar relations in the left heart.

AV discordance indicates that the right atrium is anatomically related to the left ventricle and, similarly, the left atrium to the right ventricle.

Ventricular inversion indicates "normal" situs solitus with normally related great vessels, viscera, atria, and a levo-loop ventricle or inverted (mirror-image) ventricular position.

Ventricular noninversion is indicative of atrial–visceral situs solitus with dextro-loop ventricular development and normally related great vessels.

SEGMENTAL CONSIDERATIONS

This approach includes the evaluation of the atrial–visceral relations, atrial–systemic venous connections, AV connections, ventricular relations, and great vessel relations and connections. Any specific segment in this normal anatomic sequence may be interrupted. A simplified approach to cardiac and visceral malpositions is summarized in Table 1.

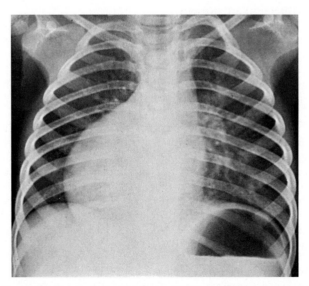

FIGURE 1. Dextrocardia with visceral situs solitus (cardiac–visceral discordance) without intrinsic organic heart disease. This is a rare combination; most patients with cardiac–visceral discordance have significant congenital heart disease.

ATRIOVISCERAL (SPLENIC) RELATIONS

Atrial situs can usually be ascertained by evaluation of the abdominal viscera. A high correlation of normal atrial situs exists when the stomach bubble can be identified on the left with a normal right liver silhouette, a right eparterial bronchus, and a normal right-sided inferior vena cava (IVC). *Atrial situs inversus* is indicated by the reversal of any or all of the aforementioned. *Indeterminate atrial situs,* or common atrium, is suggested by visceral heterotaxia, bilateral bilobed or trilobed lungs, or bilateral symmetric hyparterial or eparterial bronchi. It is also suggested by gastrointestinal malrotation, biliary malformations or atresia, and interruption of the hepatic or subhepatic segment of the IVC with azygos continuation. With the last-named group of indeterminate situs malformations, a high incidence of cardiosplenic syndromes is likely (see Section V, Part IV, Chapter 2, page 1364).

ATRIAL RELATIONS AND SYSTEMIC VENOUS CONNECTION

Normal atrial relations and systemic venous connection can be presumed with normal visceral laterality. Angiographically, the right atrium is characterized by a broad-based triangular right atrial appendage with a wide orifice. The left atrium projects to the left of the right atrium and is characterized by a large crescent-shaped atrial appendage projecting anterosuperolaterally with a small orifice. The superior vena cava (SVC) connections are less constant, and bilateral SVCs are frequent even with situs solitus. The left system usually connects with the coronary sinus. With visceral situs inversus, mirror-image positioning of the atrial chambers and venous connections is anticipated. With visceral heterotaxia (ambiguous viscera), atrial positions cannot be adequately determined, and frequently a common atrium and anomalies in systemic venous connection are present.

Asplenia syndrome exhibits bilateral right-sidedness of abdominal and pulmonary viscera with two right atrial appendages present and, frequently, two SVCs draining into the common atrium. The IVC may enter the atrium on the right or at midline. The abdominal aorta and IVC are frequently on the same side (see Section V, Part IV, Chapter 2, page 1364).

Polysplenia syndrome is characterized by bilateral left-sidedness, with a common atrium frequently demonstrating two left atrial appendages. The IVC is interrupted in the hepatic or subhepatic segment and continues to empty through the azygos system either on the right or through the left SVC. In the absence of visceral heterotaxia, visceral atrial discordance is extremely unusual (see Section V, Part IV, Chapter 2, page 1364).

VENTRICULAR RELATIONS AND LOCALIZATIONS

In normal development, as the heart tube bulges forward, it initially bends to the right (dextro-loop) and then progresses to migrate toward the left. Such development places the bulbus cordis (future right ventricle) to the right and the more distal developing bulboventricular loop (left ventricle) to the left in appropriate juxtaposition to the right and left atria. This alignment creates what is generally referred to as ventricular noninversion and AV concordance. The developing heart tube may bend to the left in its initial stage and produce a mirror-image pattern or inverted ventricular position, which produces AV discordance with the right atrium related to the left ventricle and the left atrium to the right ventricle. With ventricular inversion there is inversion of the associated AV valve. This does not have any implication with respect to the direction of the apex to the right or left in the inverted ventricular alignment. Ventricular localization can usually be determined with echocardiography or angiocardiography. Angiographically and anatomically, the right ventricle is normally triangular, with a coarse trabecular pattern, a prominent moderator band, and a septal band of the crista. A slightly elongated infundibular outflow tract with a smooth wall is characteristic. The left ventricle has a smooth wall and elongated oval configuration, fine minor sinus portion trabeculation, and a relatively short infundibular or subaortic outflow segment. There is fibrous continuity of the posterior aortic annulus with the anterior leaflet of the mitral valve.

With ventricular inversion and AV discordance, as may be seen in patients with situs solitus and corrected transposition of the great vessels, the elongated, cone-shaped left ventricle projects medially and anteriorly, with the interventricular septum fairly vertically or sagitally oriented. Mitral–semilunar (pulmonary) valve continuity may still be noted. A high recess can usually be seen in the anterosuperior aspect of the ventricle. The right ventricle then projects to the left and superiorly. It is frequently bulbous to triangular in shape. There is discontinuity of the aortic semilunar and AV valves. The infundibulum is somewhat shortened and poorly formed, and the crista presents on the posterior ventricular-infundibular wall. With a normal dextro-loop, noninversion of the coronary arteries is seen, whereas with a levo-loop, coronary arteries are inverted. With ventricular inversions and complex CHD, anomalies in the development of the subaortic and subpulmonic conus are frequently seen.

GREAT ARTERIES

Normally, the pulmonary artery connected to the right ventricle is positioned anteriorly and to the left, while the aorta connected to the left ventricle is positioned posteriorly and to the right. These vessels cross in the supracardiac area. Malposition of the great vessels is indicated whenever this anatomic relationship does not exist. *Transposition* describes the reversal of the anteroposterior relations of the great arteries. Most commonly, one considers transposition of the great vessels when the aorta arises from the right ventricle and the pulmonary artery from the left ventricle. *Dextro-* and *levo-* positions refer to the relationships of the aorta to the pulmonary artery. In the usual complete transposition, the aorta is anterior and to the right (dextrotransposition). Less commonly, the aorta is transposed anteriorly and to the left (levotransposition). This latter malposition is usually associated with ventricular inversion or single ventricle. Other forms of great vessel malposition may exist, with double-outlet right or left ventricle when both great vessels arise directly from one of the ventricular chambers. When only one great vessel or common arterial trunk is present, the vessel often arises centrally from the base of the ventricles, as in truncus arteriosus or pulmonary atresia with ventricular septal defect.

Ventricular–great vessel relationships are often suggested on conventional chest radiographs. Normal relations exist when the ascending aorta can be visualized in the right superior mediastinum, with the aortic arch evident on the left and a main pulmonary artery producing a convex configuration of the mid- and upper left heart border. Because great vessel–ventricular discordance occurs only with complex CHD, the demonstration of this normal relation tends to imply normal anatomic relations or milder forms of heart disease. Transposition is possible if the pulmonary artery segment is not visualized as a focal convexity and the ascending aorta cannot be seen. The latter is frequently difficult to see in the young infant. If there is an unusual long, convex margin of the mid- and upper left heart border, levotransposition of the great vessels and associated ventricular inversion or a single ventricle is suggested. These conclusions from plain films depend on the visualization of abnormal, decreased to increased, pulmonary flow and the presence of normal visceral situs.

DESCRIPTION METHOD BY DIRECTION OF BLOOD FLOW

With these definitions of segmental anatomy, it is possible to describe the various combined malformations regardless of whether there is dextrocardia or levocardia. Situs may be designated as solitus (s), inversus (i), or ambiguous (a). The cardiac loop and ventricular relations may be designated as d (dextro) for normal and l (levo) for left, and x may be used to indicate indeterminate. The relations of the semilunar valves and great arteries may be listed as normal solitus (s), dextrotransposition (d), and levotransposition (l). Malpositions of the great vessels with the aortic valve directed anteriorly to the pulmonary valve may be indicated as a, and the inverted relation as i. Then, listing the segments in the direction of blood flow produces a normal cardiac segmental symbolic relation-

ship of s, d, s. Complete transposition of the great arteries with situs solitus would be symbolized by s, d, d. A similar anomaly with situs inversus would be i, l, l, and so forth. With this method, it is easier to describe the segmental relations and the internal anatomy more adequately than with descriptive terminology. In some of the more common lesions, it is still simpler, because of common usage, to describe the lesions (e.g., tetralogy of Fallot, dextrotransposition of the great arteries, and so forth).

CONGENITAL HEART DISEASE WITH CARDIAC MALPOSITION

CHD with situs solitus and levocardia is relatively rare, probably less than 1% of all cases. With situs inversus totalis and dextrocardia, CHD remains rare, although its incidence may increase to 3% to 5%. The lesions are basically those seen with situs solitus. With visceral situs solitus and dextrocardia, however, the incidence of CHD increases dramatically to between 75% and 85%, and with visceral and atrial situs inversus and levocardia, CHD is almost always present. Complex CHD with some form of transposition of the great vessels is the rule in the last two categories. Mesocardia, a mild form of cardiac malrotation and malposition, may be seen with situs inversus, situs solitus, or situs ambiguous. Heart disease is also frequent with mesocardia, although indeterminate in severity and frequency.

SUGGESTED READINGS

Attie F, Soni J, Ovseyeviz J, et al: Angiographic studies of atrial ventricular discordance. Circulation 1980;62:407

Brandt PWT, Calder AL: Cardiac connections: the segmental approach to radiologic diagnosis in congenital heart disease. Curr Probl Diagn Radiol 1977;7:1

Freedom RM, Culham JAG, Moes CAF: Angiocardiography of Congenital Heart Disease. New York, Macmillan, 1984:17

Shinebourne EA, Macartney FJ, Anderson RH: Sequential chamber localization—logical approach to diagnosis in congenital heart disease. Br Heart J 1976;38:327

Van Praagh R: Terminology of congenital heart disease: glossary and commentary. Circulation 1977;56:139

Van Praagh R: Importance of segmental situs in the diagnosis of congenital heart disease. Semin Roentgenol 1985;20:254

Wang J-K, Li Y-W, Chin I-S, et al: Usefulness of magnetic resonance imaging in the assessment of venoatrial connections, atrial morphology, bronchial situs, and other anomalies of right atrial isomerism. Am J Cardiol 1994;74:701

Winer-Muram HT, Tonkin ILD: The spectrum of heterotaxic syndromes. Radiol Clin North Am 1989;27:1147

■ **C h a p t e r 2**

SYNDROMES AND CHROMOSOMAL ANOMALIES

VIRGIL R. CONDON

CARDIOSPLENIC (HETEROTAXY) SYNDROMES

The cardiosplenic (heterotaxy) syndromes are the most common congenital anomalies associated with situs problems. These anomalies are suggested when visceral heterotaxia (situs ambiguous) is present with either levocardia or dextrocardia. These syndromes are characterized by (1) asplenia or polysplenia, (2) complex congenital heart disease (CHD), and (3) visceral heterotaxia (Table 1). All abnormalities may be visualized well on magnetic resonance imaging (MRI) (Fig. 1).

Asplenia constitutes from 1% to 3% of CHD. The teratogenic insult occurs between the 28th and 40th days of gestation. The condition is characterized by asplenia, CHD, liver symmetry, gastrointestinal malformations, and bilateral trilobed lungs with eparterial bronchi (Fig. 2). Other occasional anomalies include tracheoesophageal fistula, imperforate anus, biliary atresia, and genitourinary anomalies. Cardiac abnormalities include (1) cardiac malposition (dextrocardia or mesocardia); (2) anomalous systemic venous return or bilateral superior vena cava (SVC); (3) abdominal aorta–inferior vena cava (IVC) juxtaposition; (4) total anomalous pulmonary venous return (frequently the infracardiac type) (Fig. 2); transposition of the great arteries; (6) common atrioventricular valves, (7) pulmonary or subpulmonary stenosis, and (8) common ventricle or large ventricular septal defect (VSD) (Table 1).

Polysplenia is characterized by multiple spleens (Fig. 1D), visceral heterotaxia, and CHD. Additional characteristic findings include bilateral hyparterial bronchi (Fig. 1A), bilobed lungs, and prominent azygos vein secondary to azygos continuation of the IVC (Figs. 1B and 3). Cardiac abnormalities include (1) cardiac malposition, (2) anomalous systemic venous return or interruption of the renal subhepatic segment of the IVC, (3) bilateral SVC (Fig. 1C), (4) atrial septal defect (ASD) or atrioventricular canal (AVC), (5) VSD, and (6) partial anomalous venous return (Table 1).

CHROMOSOMAL ANOMALIES AND SYNDROMES

Less than 0.5% of live births have chromosomal aberrations, and 1 in 7000 infants show some chromosomal defect. Heart disease in these patients is moderate, and approaches 100% in some of the trisomies (Table 2).

Table 1 ■ CARDIOSPLENIC SYNDROMES

ASPLENIA	POLYSPLENIA
Congenital heart disease	Renal anomalies
Dextro- or levo-transposition of the great arteries	Congenital heart disease
Common ventricles, common atria	Atrial septal defect, common atrium
Pulmonary atresia or stenosis	Interrupted inferior vena cava with azygos continuation
Total anomalous pulmonary venous return with obstruction	Other left-to-right shunts
Atrioventricular canal	Bilateral superior vena cava
Bilateral superior vena cava	Multiple spleens
Agenesis of the spleen	Bilateral bilobed lungs
Bilateral trilobed lungs	Bilateral hyparterial bronchi
Bilateral eparterial bronchi	Bilateral left pulmonary arteries
Bilateral right pulmonary arteries	Visceral heterotaxia
Visceral heterotaxia	Biliary atresia (absent gallbladder)
Gastrointestinal anomalies	Malrotation
Malrotation	
Microgastria	

TRISOMY 21 (DOWN SYNDROME)

The incidence of this disorder is 1 in 600 to 1 in 700 live births and is higher with increased maternal age. CHD occurs in 40% to 70% of patients. Common defects include AVC (see Section V, Part II, Chapter 1, Fig. 13, page 1268), ASD, VSD, and patent ductus arteriosus (PDA). Almost all forms of congenital cardiac malformations have been described. Noncardiac radiographic findings include 11 pairs of ribs, malsegmentation of the sternum, abnormal configuration of the pelvis, duodenal stenosis or atresia, and annular pancreas.

TRISOMY 18 (E SYNDROME)

The incidence is 1 in 4000 live births and increases with maternal age. CHD occurs in 90% to 100% of affected infants. Common defects include VSD, PDA, and ASD.

TRISOMY 13 (D SYNDROME)

The incidence is 1 in 7000 to 14,000 live births. CHD is found in approximately 80% of cases. Common defects include VSD and double-outlet right ventricle.

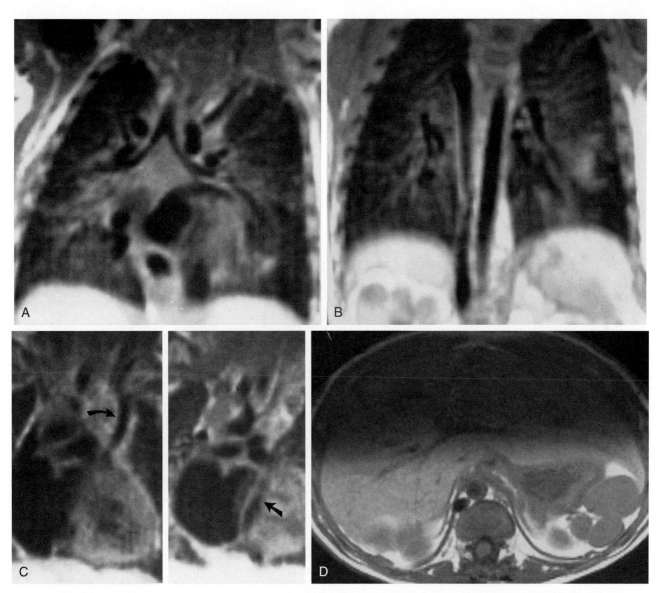

FIGURE 1.   Newborn infant with polysplenia syndrome. **A,** Coronal 3-mm spin-echo magnetic resonance image demonstrates a symmetric tracheobronchial tree with bilateral hyparterial bronchi (bilateral left-sidedness). **B,** Coronal 3-mm spin-echo image demonstrates azygos continuation of the inferior vena cava with an enlarged azygos vein to the right of the spine. A portion of the left descending thoracic aorta is also visualized. **C,** Composite axial 3-mm images demonstrate a left superior vena cava *(left, curved arrow)* emptying into the coronary sinus *(right, arrow).* **D,** Axial 5-mm spin-echo image confirms the presence of multiple spleens. There is partial visualization of the transverse liver.

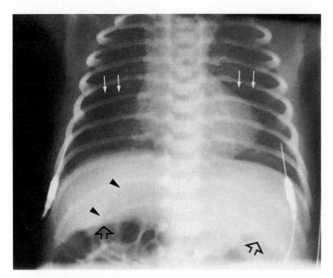

FIGURE 2. Asplenia syndrome. Characteristic changes of bilateral right-sidedness with symmetry of the tracheobronchial tree, bilateral minor fissures *(white arrows)*, visceral heterotaxia with the stomach to the right of the spine *(arrowheads)*, and a horizontal liver configuration *(open arrows)* are present.

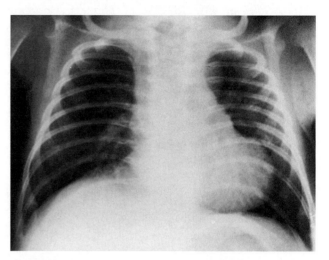

FIGURE 4. Marfan syndrome. Anteroposterior chest radiograph shows dilatation of the ascending aorta, aortic arch, and descending thoracic aorta. Mild cardiomegaly is related to aortic and mitral insufficiency. Scoliosis and pectus excavatum have not yet developed.

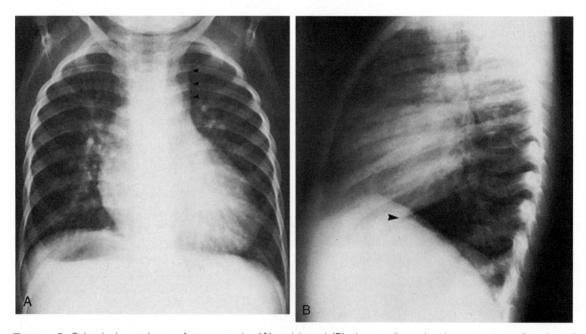

FIGURE 3. Polysplenia syndrome. Anteroposterior **(A)** and lateral **(B)** chest radiographs demonstrate cardiac–visceral discordance (right-sided stomach) and interruption of the hepatic segment of the inferior vena cava *(arrowhead)*, producing an acute angle between the cardiac silhouette and diaphragm. The dilated azygos vein is not well seen. Note the persistent left superior vena cava *(arrowheads)* and increased pulmonary vasculature related to an atrioventricular canal.

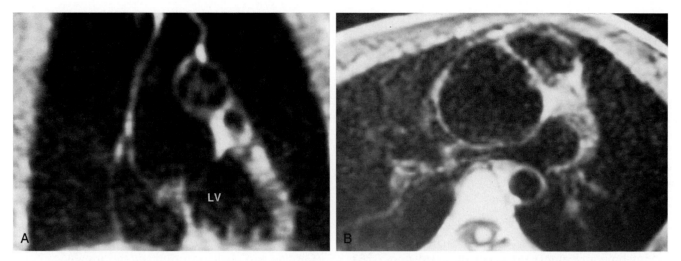

FIGURE 5. Cystic medial necrosis in a 16-year-old boy with Marfan syndrome. **A,** Coronal 10-mm spin-echo magnetic resonance image demonstrates characteristic features of the cystic medial necrosis with marked dilatation of the aortic sinuses and proximal ascending aorta. *LV* = left ventricle. **B,** Axial 10-mm spin-echo image demonstrates compression of the right pulmonary artery by the dilated aortic sinuses and ascending aorta. The left descending thoracic aorta is normal in size.

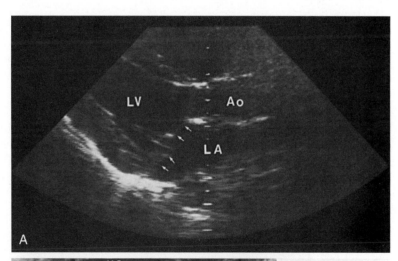

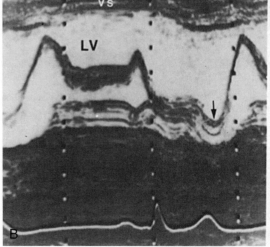

FIGURE 6. Mitral valve prolapse. **A,** Real-time long-axis echocardiogram shows the mitral valve leaflets *(arrows)* bulging cephalically into the left atrium *(LA)* instead of assuming a more cone-shaped configuration toward the left ventricular *(LV)* cavity. *Ao* = aortic root. **B,** M-mode echocardiogram shows a hammock-shaped configuration *(arrow)* of the closed mitral valve leaflets bulging posteriorly instead of assuming a straight, anteriorly sloping configuration.

TURNER'S SYNDROME (X MONOSOMY) AND NOONAN'S SYNDROME

Turner's syndrome is characterized by web neck, cubitus valgus, short stature, shield chest, and lymphedema. CHD is present in 25% to 66% of patients; coarctation is the most common lesion (70%). Coronary angiography should be performed to rule out coronary–pulmonary fistula. Noonan's syndrome has many similar clinical and cardiac findings except for a greater incidence of pulmonary valvular stenosis and hypertrophic cardiomyopathy.

KLINEFELTER'S SYNDROME (XXY ANOMALY)

This is characterized by atrophic male genitalia, a eunuchoid appearance, and mental retardation. CHD

occurs in 10%. Common defects include tetralogy of Fallot, ASD, VSD, and tricuspid atresia.

MARFAN SYNDROME (ARACHNODACTYLY, DOLICHOSTENOMELIA)

This condition is an autosomal dominant disorder of connective tissue, primarily elastic tissues. Clinical manifestations include long limbs, muscle atrophy, and hyperextendable joints. Cardiac malformations primarily relate to (1) cystic medial necrosis of the ascending aorta, which may progress to aortic dissection (Fig. 4); (2) aneurysmal dilatation of the ascending aorta and sinus of Valsalva; (3) aortic insufficiency; (4) mitral valve prolapse and insufficiency; and (5) pulmonary artery dilatation. Symptoms of heart failure, usually related to valvular insufficiencies, develop in childhood or in young adulthood.

Cardiac and aortic involvement can usually be con-

Table 2 ■ SYNDROMES WITH CARDIAC LESIONS

SYNDROME	LESION
Arteriohepatic dysplasia (Alagille syndrome)	PS, valvular/peripheral, VSD, ASD, PDA, and coarctation
Asplenia/polysplenia	See discussion under Cardiosplenic (Heterotaxy) Syndromes
Cardioauditory syndromes	PS
Cardiofacial syndrome (Cayler syndrome)	VSD, PDA, tetralogy of Fallot, right aortic arch
Carney's complex	Cardiac myxomas, cutaneous myxoma, schwannoma, testicular tumor and other lesions
Cat-eye syndrome (47 XX/XY)	TAPVR, tetralogy of Fallot, tricuspid atresia, ASD, or VSD
CHARGE association	Miscellaneous CHD
Deletion syndromes (cri du chat, Wolf, carp mouth, etc.)	Moderate incidence, various CHDs
DiGeorge syndrome	Interrupted aortic arch, truncus, tetralogy of Fallot
Ehlers-Danlos syndrome	ASD, AVC, and tetralogy of Fallot
Ellis-van Creveld syndrome	ASD (single atrium) and VSD
Fetal alcohol syndrome	VSD
Floppy valve syndrome	Mitral and aortic valve involvement with insufficiency
Holt-Oram syndrome	ASD, VSD
Kawasaki disease	See Section V, Part V, Chapter 3, page 1381
Lutembacher's syndrome	ASD with mitral valve stenosis
Mucolipidosis III	Valvular heart disease and myocardial failure
Mucopolysaccharidosis	Myocardial infiltration and failure (see Section V, Part V, Chapter 1, page 1371)
Neurofibromatosis	Abnormalities of the aorta and major branches, renovascular hypertension
Oculoauriculovertebral dysplasia (Goldenhar's syndrome)	Tetralogy of Fallot, ASD, VSD, coarctation
Osteogenesis imperfecta	Aneurysmal dilatation of the great vessels and valvular insufficiency
Rubella syndrome	PDA, peripheral pulmonary stenosis, pulmonary artery hypoplasia (see Section V, Part I, Chapter 2, Fig. 13, page 1239 and Fig. 7)
Shone syndrome	Parachute mitral valve, subaortic stenoses, coarctation, supravalvular left atrial ring
Takayasu's arteritis	Large-vessel arterial obstruction, aortic and mitral insufficiency
Thoracoabdominal wall defect (Ravitch syndrome)	Dextroposition, pericardial defects with abdominal organ herniation, VSD, ASD, PS and tetralogy of Fallot, and ventricular diverticula
Trisomy 22	Multiple forms of CHD (50%)
Uhl's anomaly	Thinning and enlargement of the right ventricle with right heart failure
VATER association	VSD, PDA, tetralogy of Fallot, single ventricle
Velocardiofacial syndrome	VSD
Williams syndrome (supravalvular aortic stenosis) (idiopathic hypercalcemia)	Supravalvular aortic stenosis and peripheral pulmonary artery stenosis (Fig. 7)

ASD = atrial septal defect; *AVC* = atrioventricular canal; *CHARGE* = coloboma, heart disease, atresia of choanae, retarded growth and development, genital hypoplasia, and ear anomalies or deafness; *CHD* = congenital heart disease; *PDA* = patent ductus arteriosus; *PS* = pulmonary stenosis; *TAPVR* = total anomalous pulmonary venous return; *VATER* = vertebral defects, imperforate anus, tracheoesophageal fistula, and radial and renal dysplasia; *VSD* = ventricular septal defect.

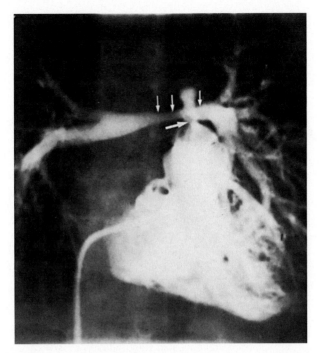

FIGURE 7. Peripheral pulmonary stenosis. An anteroposterior sitting-up right ventriculogram shows severe supravalvular pulmonary stenosis *(large arrow)* and diffuse involvement of the right and left main pulmonary arteries *(small arrows)*.

firmed with echocardiography, particularly in the evaluation of the ascending aorta and sinuses of Valsalva. MRI is the preferred modality for serial evaluation of patients with cystic medial necrosis to evaluate changes in aortic size and development of dissection (Fig. 5). Doppler ultrasound can recognize aortic and mitral insufficiency. Mitral valve prolapse also can be appreciated either with real-time or M-mode studies (Fig. 6).

OTHER SYNDROMES

Other syndromes and their most common cardiac lesions are listed in Table 2. Many other rare syndromes with associated cardiac malformations are known but are too numerous to mention here.

SUGGESTED READINGS

Cardiosplenic (Heterotaxy) Syndromes

Applegate KE, Goske MJ, Pierce G, et al: Situs revisited: imaging of the heterotaxy syndrome. Radiographics 1999;19:837
Buirski G, Jordan SC, Joffe HS, et al: Superior vena caval abnormalities: their occurrence rate, associated cardiac abnormalities and angiographic classification in a pediatric population with congenital heart disease. Clin Radiol 1986;37:131
Chen S-J, Li Y-W, Wang J-K, et al: Usefulness of electron beam computed tomography in children with heterotaxy syndrome. Am J Cardiol 1988;81:188
Freedom RM, Culham JAG, Moes CAF: Angiocardiography of Congenital Heart Disease. New York, Macmillan, 1984:643
Geva T, Vick W, Wendt RE, et al: Role of spin echo and cine magnetic resonance imaging in presurgical planning of heterotaxy syndrome. Circulation 1994;90:348
Jelinek JS, Stuart PL, Done SL, et al: MRI of polysplenia syndrome. Magn Reson Imaging 1989;7:681
Rose V, Izukawa T, Moes CAF: Syndromes of asplenia and polysplenia: a review of the cardiac and noncardiac malformations with special reference to diagnosis and prognosis. Br Heart J 1975;37:840
Van Praagh R: Importance of segmental situs in the diagnosis of congenital heart disease. Semin Roentgenol 1985;20:254
Wang J-K, Li Y-W, Chiu I-S, et al: Usefulness of magnetic resonance imaging in the assessment of venoatrial connections, atrial morphology, bronchial situs, and other anomalies of right atrial isomerism. Am J Cardiol 1994;74:701
Winer-Muram HT, Tonkin ILD: The spectrum of heterotaxic syndromes. Radiol Clin North Am 1989;27:1147

Chromosomal Anomalies and Syndromes

Cole RB: Noonan's syndrome: a historical perspective. Pediatrics 1980;66:468
Come PC, Kulkley GH, McKusick VA, et al: Echocardiographic recognition of silent aortic root dilatation in Marfan's syndrome. Chest 1977;72:789
Ferencz C, Neill CA, Boughman JA, et al: Congenital cardiovascular malformations associated with chromosome abnormalities: an epidemiologic study. J Pediatr 1989;114:79
Freedom RM, Gerald PS: Congenital heart disease and the cat eye syndrome. Am J Dis Child 1973;126:16
Gotzsche CO, Krag-Olsen B, Nielsen J, et al: Prevalence of cardiovascular malformations and association with karotypes in Turner syndrome. Arch Dis Child 1994;71:433
Lin AE, Perloff JK: Upper limb malformations associated with congenital heart disease. Am J Cardiol 1985;55:1576
Neill CA: Congenital cardiac malformations and syndromes. *In* Pierpont MEM, Moller JH (eds): Genetics of Cardiovascular Disease. Boston, Martinus Nijhoff, 1986;95
Noonan JA: Association of congenital heart disease with syndromes and other defects. Pediatr Clin North Am 1978;25:797
O'Brien KM: Congenital syndrome with congenital heart disease. Semin Roentgenol 1985;20:104
Petitalot JP, Chaix AF, Barraine R: Echocardiographic follow-up in Marfan's syndrome: mitral, tricuspid, and aortic valve prolapse with calcification of patent foramen ovale. J Clin Ultrasound 1986;14:707
Pierpont MEM, Gorlin RJ, Moller JH: Chromosomal abnormalities. *In* Pierpont MEM, Moller JH (eds): Genetics of Cardiovascular Disease. Boston, Martinus Nijhoff, 1987:69
Rosenthal A: Cardiovascular malformations in Klinefelter's syndrome: report of 3 cases. J Pediatr 1972;80:471
Sandor GGS, Smith DF, MacLeod PM: Cardiac malformations in the fetal alcohol syndrome. J Pediatr 1981;93:771
Smith DW, Jones KL: Recognizable Patterns of Human Malformation, 3rd ed. Philadelphia, WB Saunders, 1982
Torfs CP, Christianson RE: Anomalies in Down syndrome individuals in a large population-based registry. Am J Med Genet 1998; 77:431

PART V

ACQUIRED HEART DISEASE

RICHARD B. JAFFE
VIRGIL R. CONDON

Chapter 1

MYOCARDIAL DISEASES (CARDIOMYOPATHY)

VIRGIL R.CONDON and RICHARD B. JAFFE

RHEUMATIC FEVER AND RHEUMATIC HEART DISEASE

Rheumatic fever is a clinical syndrome that follows a small percentage of group A β-hemolytic streptococcal infections. It is characterized by carditis, arthritis, chorea, subcutaneous nodules, and occasionally erythema marginatum. Late complications include significant residual rheumatic valvular heart disease. It remains a common disease in Third World countries, and a recent significant resurgence of cases in the United States has been reported. Both sexes are equally affected, with the onset of disease usually between the ages of 5 and 10 years.

Rheumatic fever follows infection by 10 to 21 days and is probably related to an autoimmune reaction. Certain children are more susceptible than others, and there is a significantly increased chance of sibling involvement or involvement of closely associated children.

CLINICAL MANIFESTATIONS

Major manifestations (Jones criteria) include arthritis (75%), carditis (pericardium, myocardium, or endocardium), chorea, subcutaneous nodules, and erythema marginatum. Minor manifestations include fever, elevated erythrocyte sedimentation rate, prolonged P–R interval, and arthralgia. A positive C-reactive protein test and evidence of a preceding streptococcal infection, by antibody or culture confirmation, support the diagnosis.

CHEST RADIOGRAPHY

In the acute phase, chest radiographic findings may be normal or show pericardial or cardiac enlargement and congestive heart failure (CHF). Interstitial and alveolar edema, and pleural and occasionally pericardial effusions, may be seen on chest radiographs. In chronic rheumatic valvular disease, focal chamber enlargement, particularly involving the left ventricle and left atrium, is frequent. With aortic insufficiency, general fullness of the entire left heart that is secondary to enlargement of both the left atrium and left ventricle is seen. These chamber enlargements can also be confirmed by the relative relations of the left ventricle and atrium as projected in the lateral radiograph. Left atrial enlargement secondary to mitral valve involvement is characterized by an enlarged left atrial appendage producing a focal bulge along the mid- to upper left heart border (Fig. 1). This is unlike the more generalized left atrial enlargement seen with other causes of mitral regurgitation or generalized left heart dilatation.

ECHOCARDIOGRAPHY

Two-dimensional and color Doppler evaluation is important in the determination of atrial and ventricular size, ventricular function, and valvular abnormalities (Fig. 2). Color Doppler studies, in particular, readily evaluate aortic and mitral valve insufficiencies as well as associated stenosis (see Section V, Part I, Chapter 2, Figs. 16, page 1240, and 18, page 1241).

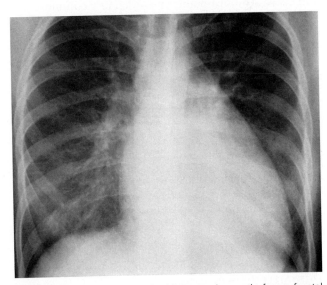

FIGURE 1. A 13-year-old girl with acute rheumatic fever: frontal chest radiograph demonstrates pulmonary venous hypertension with interstitial edema, and well-defined Kerley B lines. Cardiomegaly is present with moderate left atrial and left ventricular enlargement from mitral regurgitation. The large left atrial appendage produces an abnormal convexity along the left heart margin below the main pulmonary artery.

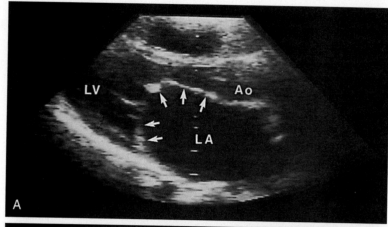

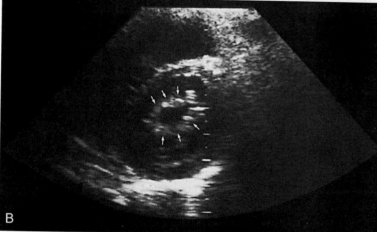

FIGURE 2. Mitral stenosis secondary to rheumatic heart disease. Real-time long-axis **(A)** and short-axis **(B)** echocardiograms show the doming and thickening of the mitral valve leaflets *(arrows)*. Note the large left atrium *(LA)* in the long-axis projection and small fish-mouthed configuration, marginal increased echogenicity *(small arrows)*, and restricted opening of the mitral valve in the short-axis view. *LV* = left ventricle; *Ao* = aortic root.

INFECTIVE CARDIOMYOPATHIES

Infective cardiomyopathies include fairly common bacterial infectious agents and coxsackievirus (Fig. 3) along with unusual infections such as that caused by *Trypanosoma cruzi* (Chagas' disease) and diphtheria. An acute illness with dyspnea, tachypnea, and CHF is characteristic.

COLLAGEN-VASCULAR DISEASE

Collagen-vascular diseases, including juvenile rheumatoid arthritis, periarteritis nodosa, systemic lupus erythematosus, dermatomyositis, and scleroderma, may all present with significant cardiac involvement. They all affect the connective tissue system, probably on an autoimmune basis, with fibrinoid degeneration and proliferation.

PERIARTERITIS NODOSA

This condition is characterized by polyarteritis involving the small- and medium-sized vessels, with clinical features of arthralgia, weakness, malaise, and pain. The kidneys are typically involved. Cardiac involvement is less common and secondary to coronary arteritis. CHF is then seen, and pericarditis may occur. Angiography of small- and medium-sized arteries, including the coronary arteries, may demonstrate small aneurysms.

SYSTEMIC LUPUS ERYTHEMATOSUS

This condition is characterized by an erythematous skin rash but otherwise has many characteristics similar to

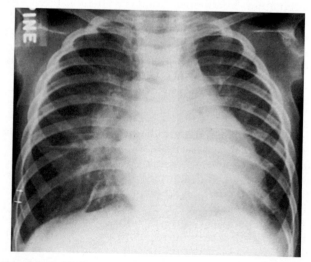

FIGURE 3. Viral myocarditis. Severe venous congestion with interstitial Kerley's lines in the bases, fissural fluid *(arrows)*, and moderate cardiomegaly are present.

periarteritis nodosa. Pericarditis is somewhat more common and frequently associated with endocarditis and valvular involvement.

DERMATOMYOSITIS

Systemic manifestations are similar to those seen in the previously discussed collagen-vascular diseases; however, involvement of muscles and cutaneous tissues is more common, while cardiac and pericardial involvement is rare (10%).

SCLERODERMA

Although exceedingly rare in childhood, when scleroderma is present, cardiac manifestations are frequent (50%). Other frequently involved areas include the cutaneous and subcutaneous tissues and, less frequently, the esophagus, musculature, and blood vessels.

CARDIOMYOPATHY SECONDARY TO METABOLIC DISEASES

GLYCOGEN STORAGE DISEASE (POMPE'S DISEASE)

This rare autosomal recessive condition is secondary to a lack of acid α-1, 4-glucosidase and produces a typical infiltrative, congestive cardiomyopathy. Clinical manifestations appear between 2 and 6 months and include anorexia, failure to thrive, dyspnea, tachypnea, weakness, hepatomegaly, macroglossia, and CHF. The Pompe type of glycogen storage disease with predominant cardiac involvement must be differentiated from von Gierke's disease and other forms of storage disease (Fig. 4). Left ventricular outflow tract obstruction and marked myocardial thickening without dilatation may be seen on echocardiography and angiocardiography.

MUCOPOLYSACCHARIDOSIS

A rare metabolic inherited disorder secondary to deficiencies in lysosomal enzymes, mucopolysaccharidosis leads to the abnormal storage of mucopolysaccharides. Cardiac involvement occurs in 50% of patients and produces primarily aortic and mitral insufficiency, although primary myocardial involvement may occur; all lead to CHF. Other manifestations include skeletal deformities, corneal opacities, and mental retardation.

THYROID DISORDERS

HYPERTHYROIDISM

Hyperthyroidism is a high-output state with tachycardia, irritability, sweating, tremors, and a bounding pulse.

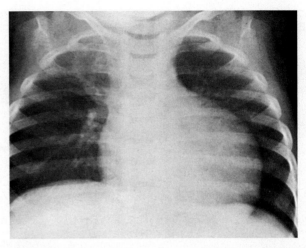

FIGURE 4. Glycogen storage disease of the heart (Pompe's disease) in a 16-month-old girl with moderate cardiomegaly and globular cardiac silhouette. A right upper lobe atelectatic–pneumonic density is also evident. The ventricular walls were grossly thickened rather than dilated.

CHF is rare, but atrial fibrillation may be present. There may be mild to moderate cardiomegaly.

HYPOTHYROIDISM

Cardiac manifestations are less likely than with hyperthyroidism. When present, they are those of nonspecific cardiac enlargement and occasionally CHF.

CARDIOMYOPATHY SECONDARY TO NEUROMUSCULAR DISEASES

FRIEDREICH'S ATAXIA

Friedreich's ataxia is a rare hereditary neurologic disorder with cardiac involvement secondary to hypertrophy of the muscle fibers of the cardiac chambers and associated round-cell infiltration. While neurologic manifestations such as gait disturbance usually precede cardiac manifestations, cardiovascular disease may be the presenting manifestation in 10% of cases. Cardiac manifestations include coronary artery stenosis, myocardial fibrosis, and hypertrophic cardiomyopathy, with left ventricular outflow tract obstruction.

PROGRESSIVE MUSCULAR DYSTROPHY

Progressive muscular dystrophy is a rare hereditary muscular disorder with relatively rare cardiac involvement. Left ventricular hypertrophy may develop early in the disease and lead to generalized cardiac enlargement and congestive failure. The Duchenne type is most commonly seen in boys in early childhood with progressive fatigability, difficulty in rising as a result of muscular weakness, and a waddling gait.

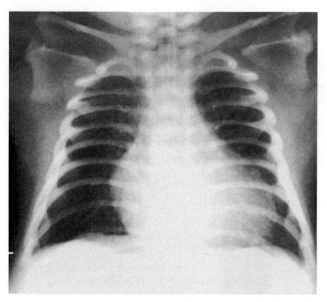

FIGURE 5. Infant of a diabetic mother. An anteroposterior chest radiograph shows characteristic increased subcutaneous fat along the lateral chest walls bilaterally with a combined right and left thickness greater than 8 mm. There is mild cardiomegaly with a nonspecific cardiac silhouette but with evidence of asymmetric septal hypertrophy on echocardiography (see Section V, Part II, Chapter 2, Fig. 11, page 1291).

HYPERTROPHIC CARDIOMYOPATHY (ASYMMETRIC SEPTAL HYPERTROPHY)

The genetic form of hypertrophic cardiomyopathy was discussed in Section V, Part II, Chapter 2, page 1284. Hypertrophic cardiomyopathy may also be seen with Turner's and Noonan's syndrome, Friedreich's ataxia, leopard syndrome, and in infants of diabetic mothers. Hypertrophy of the ventricular septum exceeds the thickness of the posterior left ventricular wall. Left ventricular outflow tract and, rarely, right ventricular outflow tract obstruction may be seen on echocardiography and angiography. Cardiac disease in infants of diabetic mothers is discussed below.

CARDIAC DISEASE IN INFANTS OF DIABETIC OR PREDIABETIC MOTHERS

Infants of diabetic or prediabetic mothers frequently exhibit cardiovascular problems, including (1) asymmetric septal hypertrophy (hypertrophic obstructive cardiomyopathy) with left ventricular outflow tract obstruction; (2) cardiomegaly with a poorly functioning heart because of intrinsic cardiomyopathy that is possibly secondary to hypoxia or hypoglycemia, or both; and (3) other intrinsic congenital cardiac malformations. Other manifestations include involvements of the genitourinary, nervous, gastrointestinal, and pulmonary

systems. Combined system involvement constitutes the VATER association (see Section V, Part IV, Chapter 2, Table 2, page 1368).

Asymmetric septal hypertrophy occurs in this condition, as in the genetic form of hypertrophic cardiomyopathy with hypertrophy of the muscle bundles involved in the upper two thirds of the ventricular septum. There may be some degree of involvement of the adjacent anterior and posterior free walls of the right and left ventricles. Unlike the genetic form of hypertrophic cardiomyopathy, the septal hypertrophy resolves within the first year of life. Intrinsic congenital heart disease (CHD) occurs in approximately 4%, with ventricular septal defect, transposition of the great vessels, and coarctation being the most common lesions.

CHEST RADIOGRAPHY

Cardiomegaly, CHF, and respiratory distress syndrome are common chest film findings. Increased subcutaneous fat, especially along the lateral chest wall, may be helpful in suggesting the diagnosis (Fig. 5).

ECHOCARDIOGRAPHY

Asymmetric septal hypertrophy shows disproportionate thickening of the mid- to upper portion of the ventricular septum and, to some extent, the free anterior and posterior left ventricular walls, with a septal–posterior wall ratio greater than 1.3:1. Narrowing of the left ventricular outflow tract may be seen, with systolic anterior motion of the mitral valve and midsystolic preclosure or flutter of the aortic valve until septal thickness resolves to normal. Other intrinsic congenital heart lesions may also be identified. Cardiac dilatation and function may also be evaluated.

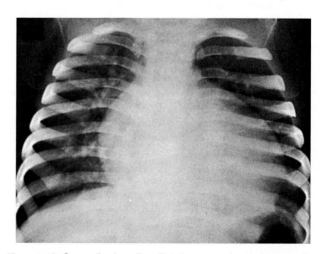

FIGURE 6. Generalized cardiac dilatation secondary to longstanding anemia with a hemoglobin level of 3.2 g/100 ml. Cardiac dilatation is slow to develop with anemia and persists for a considerable period after correction of the anemia.

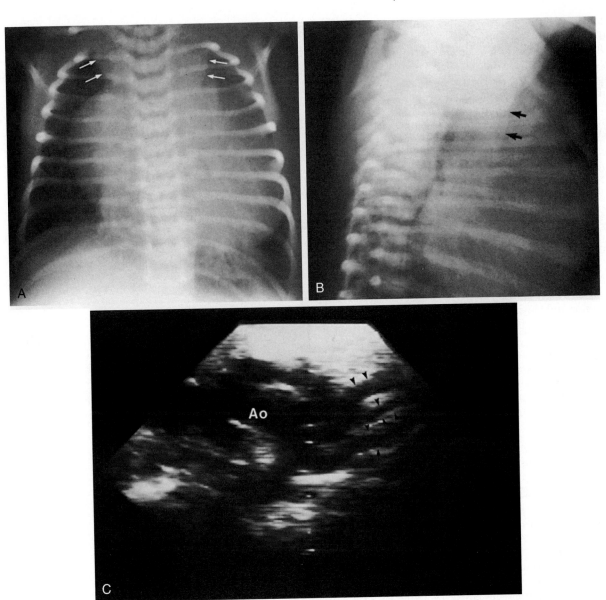

FIGURE 7. Cerebral arteriovenous malformation. Anteroposterior **(A)** and lateral **(B)** chest radiographs in a neonate show marked cardiomegaly out of proportion to the degree of congestive failure. Widening of the superior mediastinum *(arrows)* is secondary to dilatation of the ascending aorta and brachiocephalic vessels. Compression left lower lobe atelectasis is present in the retrocardiac area. **C,** Real-time echocardiogram confirms a large aorta *(Ao)* and brachiocephalic vessels *(arrowheads)*. The echoencephalogram visualized a large vein of Galen aneurysm (not shown).

ANGIOCARDIOGRAPHY

Septal thickening can be demonstrated with biventricular injection in the long-axial projection. Left ventricular and, rarely, right ventricular outflow tract obstruction also may be seen.

OTHER CARDIOMYOPATHIES

Endocardial fibroelastosis (EFE) may occur as a primary disease with a high incidence of familial involvement (25%), or secondary to CHD, particularly when associated with left ventricular outflow tract obstruction.

Ninety-five percent of patients with primary EFE have ventricular dilatation. Rarely, the left ventricle may be normal or small in size, and these patients have impaired ventricular filling on hemodynamic study, and mild to moderate reduction in left ventricular contractility.

Persistence of spongy myocardium (noncompaction cardiomyopathy) is a rare myocardial disorder characterized by the persistence of excessively prominent ventricular trabeculations and deep intertrabecular recesses. It may occur as a primary form of CHF (isolated noncompaction of left ventricular myocardium) or accompany other forms of CHD, particularly those with right or left ventricular outflow tract obstruction. Two-dimensional echocardiography and angiography demonstrate unusually fine trabeculations and multiple myocardial recesses.

Other rare forms of cardiomyopathy may include histiocytoid cardiomyopathy of infancy, characterized by intractable supraventricular or ventricular tachydysrhythmia; hypereosinophilic syndrome, with features of restrictive cardiomyopathy and mural thrombi; and right ventricular dysplasia (Uhl's anomaly), with marked right ventricular thinning and ventricular tachydysrhythmias. Uhl's anomaly must be differentiated from severe Ebstein's malformation of the tricuspid valve.

HIGH-OUTPUT STATES

ANEMIAS

Chronic severe anemia is an important cause of cardiomegaly and CHF. Most commonly observed in thalassemia major and sickle cell anemia, chronic anemia leads to high output and generalized enlargement of all cardiac chambers. Clinical features of anemia include pallor, lassitude, and specific features related to the specific anemia type. CHF relates not only to volume overload but to myocardial hypoxia secondary to an inadequate coronary oxygen content. Typical features of cardiomegaly and CHF are common (Fig. 6).

ARTERIOVENOUS MALFORMATIONS

Large arteriovenous malformations or fistulas present with high-output failure and cardiomegaly. Most commonly these malformations are cerebral, but they may occur in the liver, other viscera, or the extremities. Marked cardiomegaly is the rule. In spite of marked cardiomegaly, CHF is less conspicuous than with other forms of marked heart enlargement (Fig. 7A, B). Enlargement of the aorta may be appreciated, and, with cerebral malformations, the brachiocephalic vessels may also be enlarged (Fig. 7C). Real-time ultrasound is helpful not only in evaluating the size of the heart and vascular structures but also in actual demonstration of the arteriovenous malformation in the head, liver, or other organs. Angiography, computed tomography (CT) or cine-CT, or magnetic resonance imaging will further identify the malformation.

CHORIOANGIOMA OF THE PLACENTA

Chorioangioma is the most common benign tumor of the placenta. This hemangiomatous neoplasm results in arteriovenous shunting between the umbilical artery and vein. This may produce a syndrome of polyhydramnios, fetal hypoxia, and high-output cardiac state with cardiomegaly and CHF in the neonate. Echocardiography will demonstrate dilatation of the inferior vena cava, cardiac chambers, and thoracic and abdominal aorta secondary to the arteriovenous shunting in utero.

TWIN–TWIN TRANSFUSION SYNDROME

In twin–twin transfusion syndrome there is an intrauterine discrepancy in blood volume between twins. One twin suffers from polycythemia, and the other from anemia, at birth. The donor twin is anemic, with cardiomegaly and occasionally CHF and hydrops. The recipient twin is polycythemic and also may show cardiomegaly and congestive failure (neonatal plethora syndrome).

SUGGESTED READINGS

Rheumatic Fever and Rheumatic Heart Disease

Veasy LG, Wiedmeier SE, Orsmond GS, et al: Resurgence of rheumatic fever in the intermountain United States. N Engl J Med 1987; 316:421

Collagen-Vascular Disease

Maron BJ: Cardiomyopathies. In Adams FH, Emmanouilides GC, Riemenschneider TA (eds): Heart Disease in Infants, Children, and Adolescents. Baltimore, Williams & Wilkins, 1989.
Paget SA, Bulkley GH, Grauer LF, et al: Mitral valve disease in systemic lupus erythematosus: a cause of severe congestive heart failure reversed by valve replacement. Am J Med 1975;59:134
Steiner RE: The roentgen features of the cardiomyopathies. Semin Roentgenol 1969;4:311

Cardiomyopathy Secondary to Metabolic Diseases

Renteria VG, Ferrans VJ, Roberts WC: The heart in Hurler syndrome. Am J Cardiol 1976;38:487
Schieken RM, Kerber RE, Ionasescu VV, et al: Cardiac manifestations of the mucopolysaccharidoses. Circulation 1975;52:700

Thyroid Disorders

Farrehi C, Mitchell M, Fawcett DM: Heart failure in congenital thyrotoxicosis. Pediatrics 1968;37:640

Cardiomyopathy Secondary to Neuromuscular Diseases

Boehm TM, Dickerson RB, Glasser SP: Hypertrophic subaortic stenosis occurring in a patient with Friedreich's ataxia. Am J Med Sci 1970;260:279
Perloff JK: Cardiomyopathy associated with heredofamilial neuromyopathic disease. Mod Concepts Cardiovasc Dis 1971;40:23
Ruschhaupt DG, Thilenius OG, Cassels DE: Friedreich's ataxia associated with hypertrophic subaortic stenosis. Am Heart J 1972; 84:95
Walton JN, Gardner-Medwin D: Progressive muscular dystrophy and the myotonic disorders. In Walton JN (ed): Disorders of Voluntary Muscles, 3rd ed. London, Churchill Livingstone, 1974:561

Hypertrophic Cardiomyopathy (Asymmetric Septal Hypertrophy)

Baltaxe HA, Levin AR, Ehlers KH, et al: The appearance of the left ventricle in Noonan's syndrome. Radiology 1973;109:155–159
Ellis K: Use of angiocardiography in cardiomyopathies. In Elliott LP (ed): Cardiac Imaging in Infants, Children, and Adults. Philadelphia, JB Lippincott, 1991:477

Cardiac Disease in Infants and Diabetic or Prediabetic Mothers

Dunn V, Condon VR, Nixon GW, et al: Infants of diabetic mothers: radiographic manifestations. AJR Am J Roentgenol 1981;137:123

Gutgesell HP, Speer ME, Rosenberg HS: Characterization of the cardiomyopathy in infants of diabetic mothers. Circulation 1980;61:441

Wolfe RR, Way GL: Cardiomyopathies in infants of diabetic mothers. Johns Hopkins Med J 1977;140:177

High-Output States

Clarke CT, Geoh TH, Blackwood A, et al: Massive pulmonary arteriovenous fistula in the newborn. Br Heart J 1976;38:1092

Cubberley DA, Jaffe RB, Nixon GW: Sonographic demonstration of galenic arteriovenous malformations in the neonate. AJNR Am J Neuroradiol 1982;3:435

Lindsay J Jr, Meshel JC, Patterson RH: The cardiovascular manifestations of sickle cell disease. Arch Intern Med 1974;133:643

Sapire CW, Casta A, Donner RM, et al: Dilatation of the ascending aorta: a radiological and echocardiographic diagnostic sign in arteriovenous malformations in neonates and young infants. Am J Cardiol 1979;44:493

Swischuk LE, Crowe JE, Mewborne EG: Large vein of Galen aneurysm in the neonate: a constellation of diagnostic chest and neck radiologic findings. Pediatr Radiol 1977;6:4

Tonkin ILD: Placental chorioangioma: rare cause of congestive heart failure and hydrops fetalis in the newborn. AJR Am J Roentgenol 1980;134:181–183

C h a p t e r   2

VALVULAR DISEASES

VIRGIL R. CONDON and RICHARD B. JAFFE

BACTERIAL ENDOCARDITIS

Bacterial endocarditis is a rare but serious cardiac disease of childhood. It may be classified as acute, subacute, or chronic. In acute or subacute forms in patients under 2 years of age, the disease affects one or more normal heart valves in the absence of underlying heart disease. In patients over 2 years of age, endocarditis is usually superimposed on congenital heart disease (CHD). Streptococcal infection is the most common etiologic agent; staphylococcal infection is second, but is the prevalent organism with intravenous drug abusers and in tricuspid endocarditis.

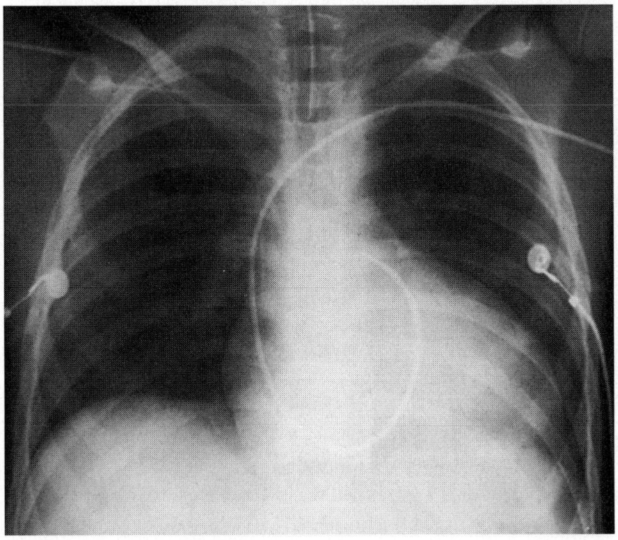

CLINICAL MANIFESTATIONS

Fever, malaise, anemia, pallor, and sepsis are common. Hematuria and petechiae indicate embolic phenomena.

CHEST RADIOGRAPHY

Cardiomegaly and congestive heart failure (CHF) are common (Fig. 1). Abnormalities in the silhouette may indicate underlying CHD. With right heart involvement, parenchymal pulmonary lesions related to septic emboli are frequent.

OTHER IMAGING

Echocardiography will demonstrate echogenic masses attached to the valves or walls of the heart (Fig. 2). Underlying cardiac disease may also be recognized, along with a degree of myocardial dysfunction. Mycotic aneurysms may develop when infections involve the great arteries or a patent ductus (Fig. 3). Prompt diagnosis by ultrasound (US), computed tomography (CT) or helical or electron-beam CT, angiography, or

FIGURE 1. Bacterial endocarditis. Anteroposterior supine chest radiograph in a patient with bacterial endocarditis superimposed upon congenital aortic valve disease. Gross cardiomegaly and left heart dilatation with mild congestive failure are present. A Swan-Ganz catheter is in the main pulmonary artery, and a central venous line is in the superior vena cava.

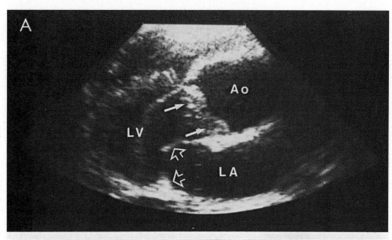

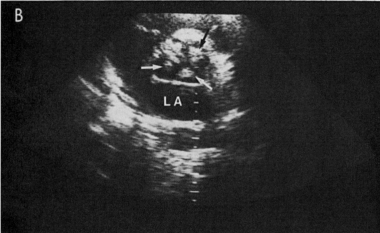

FIGURE 2. Bacterial endocarditis. Long-axis **(A)** and short-axis **(B)** echocardiograms at the level of the aortic root show the echogenic vegetations attached to all three aortic valve cusps *(arrows)*. Dilatation of the ascending aorta is related to the pre-existing valvular aortic stenosis. Echogenic mitral valves *(open arrows)* with limited opening of the anterior mitral leaflet indicate mitral stenosis.

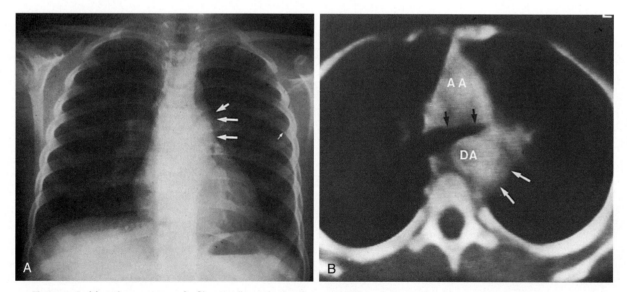

FIGURE 3. Mycotic aneurysm. **A,** Chest radiograph showing coarctation of the aorta with secondary mycotic aneurysm involving the poststenotic segment of the thoracic aorta. A fusiform paravertebral mass projects into the retrocardiac space *(arrows)*. Minor rib notching is also evident *(small arrows)* with mild cardiomegaly. **B,** Dynamic contrast-enhanced computed tomography scan at the level of the carina and left main stem bronchus *(black arrows)* demonstrates a contrast-filled mycotic aneurysm extending posteriorly into the paravertebral area with a relative fusiform configuration *(white arrows)*. *AA* = ascending aorta; *DA* = descending aorta.

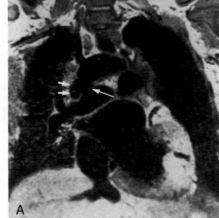
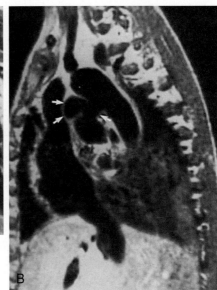

FIGURE 4. Magnetic resonance imaging of mycotic aneurysm after Potts anastomosis between the right descending aorta and right pulmonary artery. Coronal **(A)** and sagittal **(B)** cardiac-gated spin-echo images demonstrate a mycotic aneurysm *(arrows)* extending anterolaterally from the Potts anastomosis (same patient as in Section V, Part II, Chapter 3, Fig. 8, page 1308).

magnetic resonance imaging is critical in this life-threatening process (Fig. 4).

MITRAL VALVE PROLAPSE

Mitral valve prolapse refers to the posterior protrusion of mitral valve tissue beyond the boundary of the mitral annulus during systole. One or both mitral valve leaflets may be involved, and mitral insufficiency varies from minor to severe.

Mitral valve prolapse is probably a congenital malformation occurring as a familial condition and is occasionally associated with myxomatous mitral valve degeneration and CHD (ostium secundum atrial septal defect). It may occur as a complication of acquired heart disease (e.g., ischemic heart disease, bacterial endocarditis, Marfan syndrome, mucopolysaccharidosis).

CLINICAL MANIFESTATIONS

Clinical findings include apical midsystolic or late systolic murmurs and nonejection clicks, ventricular and supraventricular arrhythmia, and, occasionally, severe myocardial ischemia and CHF.

CHEST RADIOGRAPHY

Findings vary from normal to minor left atrial enlargement. On rare occasions, with severe myocardial ischemia, left ventricular dilatation is present. CHF occurs most often with complicated acquired varieties.

ECHOCARDIOGRAPHY

Anterior and posterior mitral valve leaflet prolapse may be seen with real time and M-mode studies (see Section V, Part IV, Chapter 2, Fig. 6, page 1367). Color Doppler examination may help to quantitate the severity of mitral regurgitation.

ANGIOCARDIOGRAPHY

The left ventriculogram, in the long-axis projection, demonstrates "billowing" of the leaflets posteriorly into the left atrial annulus to varying degrees. Some scalloping and irregularity of the prolapsed tissue may also be evident.

PROGNOSIS

The prognosis in isolated (congenital) mitral valve prolapse is good. In acquired or degenerative cases or with associated intrinsic cardiac malformation, progressive insufficiency and cardiac dysfunction are expected.

CONGENITAL TRICUSPID REGURGITATION

This is a rare congenital anomaly presenting in the newborn with right heart failure, marked cardiomegaly, and cyanosis. Congenital tricuspid regurgitation may be secondary to: (1) Ebstein's anomaly (see Section V, Part II, Chapter 4, Figs. 16, page 1334, and 17, page 1335), (2) tricuspid valve dysplasia, (3) pulmonary atresia with intact septum, and (4) anoxic states with myocardial ischemia.

CLINICAL MANIFESTATIONS

Tachycardia, pansystolic murmur with a gallop rhythm, and cyanosis are common.

CHEST RADIOGRAPHY

Marked cardiac enlargement (wall-to-wall heart) nearly obscures the lungs. Pulmonary blood flow appears diminished, with small central pulmonary vessels resulting from right-to-left interatrial shunting.

ECHOCARDIOGRAPHY

Echocardiogram demonstrates marked right heart enlargement. Doppler evaluation confirms the tricuspid regurgitation (see Section V, Part I, Chapter 2, Fig. 18, page 1241) as well as right-to-left shunting at the atrial level. Other intrinsic congenital heart lesions may also be demonstrated (e.g., pulmonary atresia).

ANGIOCARDIOGRAPHY

Right ventriculography demonstrates marked enlargement of the right ventricle, right atrium, tricuspid regurgitation, and right-to-left shunting at the atrial level. There is frequently no filling of the pulmonary artery, and the differential diagnosis of pulmonary atresia with tricuspid insufficiency must be resolved. Because a patent ductus is usually present, a retrograde aortogram will fill the ductus and pulmonary artery, demonstrate pulmonary regurgitation, and thus rule out pulmonary atresia. Pulmonary regurgitation may also be evaluated by Doppler ultrasound.

CONGENITAL AORTIC INSUFFICIENCY

This rare congenital lesion produces cardiomegaly with left ventricular dilatation, dilatation of the ascending and descending aorta (Fig. 5), and occasionally CHF. Doppler echocardiography will demonstrate aortic insufficiency and left ventricular dilatation. Aortography can confirm the diagnosis and differentiate other lesions simulating congenital aortic insufficiency (e.g., an aortic–left ventricular tunnel or a ruptured sinus of Valsalva aneurysm).

CONGENITAL MITRAL REGURGITATION

Congenital mitral regurgitation may be a primary malformation or part of a complex CHD. The abnormality primarily results from malformation of the valve or tensor apparatus, papillary muscle abnormality, or a ruptured chorda. It has been reported with corrected transposition of the great arteries (systemic atrioven-

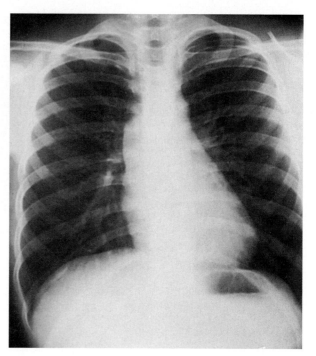

FIGURE 5. Congenital aortic stenosis and insufficiency. Chest radiograph moderate dilatation of the ascending aorta, aortic arch, and descending thoracic aorta. Mild left ventricular dilatation is present.

tricular valve), single ventricle, atrioventricular canal, Hurler's syndrome, homocystinuria, Marfan syndrome, myocarditis and myocardiopathy, mitral valve prolapse, and anomalous origin of the left coronary artery.

IMAGING

Chest radiography demonstrates marked cardiomegaly with left ventricular and left atrial enlargement. Venous congestion may be present. Doppler and real-time echocardiography demonstrate mitral regurgitation as well as some of the associated valvular defects and underlying cardiac problems. Left ventricular angiography will confirm and grade the mitral regurgitation as well as evaluate associated lesions.

SUGGESTED READINGS

Bacterial Endocarditis

Alva C, Aruguero R, Valero RG: Aneurysm of the pulmonary trunk with patent arterial duct. Cardiol Young 1999;9:70

Melvin ET, Berger M, Lutzker LG, et al: Noninvasive methods for detection of valve vegetations in infective endocarditis. Am J Cardiol 1981;47:271

Talano JV, Menlman DJ: Two-dimensional echocardiography in infective endocarditis. Semin Ultrasound CT MR 1981;2:149

Mitral Valve Prolapse

Kittredge RD, Shimonura S, Cameron A, et al: Prolapsing mitral valve leaflets: cineangiographic demonstration. Am J Roentgenol Radium Ther Nucl Med 1970;109:84

Krivokapich J, Child JS, Dadourian BJ: Reassessment of echocardiographic criteria for diagnosis of mitral valve prolapse. Am J Cardiol 1988;61:131–135

Congenital Tricuspid Regurgitation, Aortic Insufficiency, and Mitral Regurgitation

Bucciarelli RL, Nelson RN, Egan EA II: Transient tricuspid insufficiency of the newborn: a form of myocardial dysfunction in stressed newborns. Pediatrics 1977;59:330

Chan CC, Morganroth J: Tricuspid regurgitation and tricuspid prolapse demonstrated with contrast cross-section echocardiography. Am J Cardiol 1980;46:983

Freedom RM, Culham JAG, Moes CAF: Differentiation of functional and structural pulmonary atresia: role of aortography. Am J Cardiol 1978;41:914

Meltzer RS, Hoogenhuyze DV, Surruys PW, et al: Diagnosis of tricuspid regurgitation by contrast echocardiography. Circulation 1981; 63:1093

Chapter 3

CORONARY ARTERY DISEASE AND ANOMALIES

VIRGIL R. CONDON and RICHARD B. JAFFE

MUCOCUTANEOUS LYMPH NODE SYNDROME (KAWASAKI DISEASE)

Kawasaki disease is characterized by an acute illness with fever, conjunctivitis, edema of the hands and feet, and an erythematous rash on the trunk, palms, and soles. Red, dry mucous membranes, fissures about the mouth, lymphadenopathy, leukocytosis, and an elevated erythrocyte sedimentation rate are also common.

CLINICAL CARDIAC MANIFESTATIONS

In the acute phase, little evidence of cardiac involvement is identified. Later, coronary thromboarteritis leads to aneurysmal dilatation of the coronary arteries, coronary thrombosis, left ventricular ischemia and dysfunction, myocardial infarction, and rarely, death.

CHEST RADIOGRAPHY

Acutely, the heart appears normal. Later, with coronary arteritis, cardiomegaly and congestive heart failure (CHF) may be seen. Calcified coronary artery aneurysms may be seen in the course of the right and left coronary arteries (see Section IV, Part VIII, Fig. 66, page 1210).

ECHOCARDIOGRAPHY

Aneurysmal dilatation of the proximal coronary arteries may be identified (Fig. 1) in the later stages of the illness in 15% to 20% of patients. Cardiac dysfunction may also be determined.

ANGIOCARDIOGRAPHY

Aortography and coronary arteriography may occasionally be necessary to define the extent of coronary artery involvement in patients with left ventricular dysfunction (Fig. 2).

PROGNOSIS

The prognosis is good with aspirin and gamma globulin therapy. The coronary arteries may remodel with resolution or decrease in size of saccular or fusiform aneurysms.

CORONARY CALCINOSIS (IDIOPATHIC HYPERCALCEMIA OF INFANCY)

This condition indicates a rare generalized vascular abnormality with calcification of the internal elastic lamina that is associated with fibrosis and proliferation of the medium-sized arteries. Myocardial ischemia, infarction, and death may ensue. Clinical presentation is from birth to 2 years. Clinical signs include dyspnea, tachycardia, pallor, weakness, respiratory distress, and poor feeding. Chest radiography demonstrates generalized cardiomegaly and CHF. Calcification may be seen in the brachiocephalic, brachial, or subclavian arteries. Coronary calcification may be seen, particularly with chest fluoroscopy or CT.

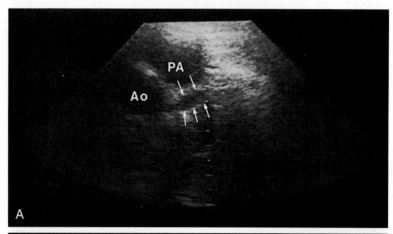

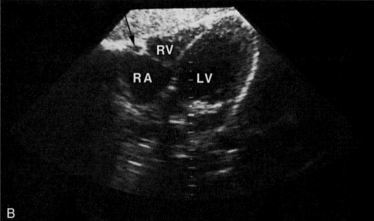

FIGURE 1. Kawasaki disease. **A,** Short-axis echocardiogram at the aortic root shows aneurysmal dilatation of the left coronary artery *(arrows)* just distal to its origin from the aorta *(Ao)*. *PA* = pulmonary artery. **B,** Subxiphoid echocardiogram shows aneurysmal dilatation of the right coronary artery as it courses in the right atrioventricular groove *(arrow)*. *RV* = right ventricle; *LV* = left ventricle; *RA* = right atrium.

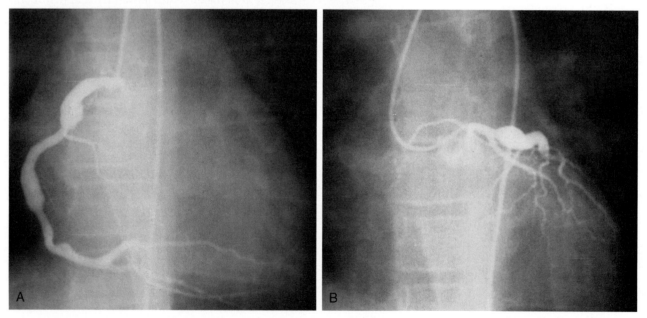

FIGURE 2. A 10-year-old girl with mucocutaneous lymph node syndrome (Kawasaki disease). Selective right **(A)** and left **(B)** coronary angiograms in the frontal projection demonstrate multiple fusiform and saccular aneurysms of the proximal and mid–right coronary artery and proximal left anterior descending coronary artery. A follow-up angiogram 1 year later was unchanged.

ATHEROSCLEROSIS

This is a relatively rare lesion of infancy and childhood and is particularly related to patients with familial hypercholesterolemia or familial type II hyperlipoproteinemia. Cardiomegaly and CHF secondary to myocardial ischemia may be seen.

POST-TRANSPLANT CORONARY ARTERY DISEASE

A late complication of cardiac transplantation is the development of coronary artery disease (cardiac allograft vasculopathy). Diffuse wall irregularities with significant areas of obstruction may be visualized on coronary angiography.

MISCELLANEOUS CONDITIONS

Many other congenital malformations of coronary arteries may be seen and are usually associated with congenital heart disease (see Section V, Part II, Chapter 1, page 1259). Coronary artery anatomy is important in surgical planning, particularly in patients with tetralogy of Fallot and in transposition where arterial-switch procedures are being contemplated. Angiography with biplane studies, either with aortic root or selective coronary arteriography, is indicated in either anteroposterior, lateral, or long-axis projections, with cranial–caudad angulation, if needed, to facilitate the planning.

SUGGESTED READINGS

Andersen GE, Friss-Hansen B: Neonatal diagnosis of familial type II hyperlipoproteinemia. Pediatrics 1976;52:2

Bisset GS III, Strife JL, McCloskey J: MR imaging of coronary artery aneurysms in a child with Kawasaki disease. AJR Am J Roentgenol 1989;152:805–807

Bloch A, Dinsmore RE, Lees RS: Coronary arteriographic findings in type II and type IV hyperlipoproteinemia. Lancet 1976;1:928

Frey EE, Matherne GP, Mahoney LT, et al: Coronary artery aneurysms due to Kawasaki disease: diagnosis with ultrafast CT. Radiology 1988;167:725–726

Fujiwara T, Fujiwara H, Ueda T, et al: Comparison of macroscopic, postmortem, angiographic and two-dimensional echocardiographic findings of coronary aneurysm in children with Kawasaki disease. Am J Cardiol 1986;57:761–764

Hewitt I, Yu JS, Kozlowski K, et al: Generalized arterial obstruction in the newborn with calcification. Aust Paediatr J 1977;13:239

Kuribayashi S, Ootaki M, Tsuji M, et al: Coronary angiographic abnormalities in mucocutaneous lymph node syndrome: acute findings and long-term follow-up. Radiology 1989;172:629–633

Lussier-Lazaroff J, Fletcher BD: Idiopathic infantile arterial calcification: roentgen diagnosis of a rare cause of coronary artery occlusion. Pediatr Radiol 1973;1:224

Onouchi Z, Simazu S, Kiyosawa N, et al: Aneurysms of the coronary arteries in Kawasaki disease: an angiographic study of 30 cases. Circulation 1982;66:1

Takahashi MT, Mason W, Lewis AB: Regression of coronary aneurysms in patients with Kawasaki syndrome. Circulation 1987;75:387–394

Chapter 4

PERICARDIAL DISEASE

VIRGIL R. CONDON and RICHARD B. JAFFE

CONGENITAL ABSENCE OF THE PERICARDIUM

Congenital absence of the pericardium is probably secondary to early atrophy of the left duct of Cuvier, which is responsible for the blood supply to the embryonic pleuropericardial membrane. In normal individuals, this membrane forms the left pericardium. The right duct of Cuvier forms the superior vena cava, almost always ensuring adequate nutrition to the right pleuropericardial membrane.

Congenital absence of the left pericardium, either partial or total, accounts for the great majority of cases (70%). Congenital isolated right-sided pericardial defects, total pericardial absence, and diaphragmatic pericardial defects are rare. Total absence of the left pericardium is the most common defect, accounting for approximately 70% of patients. Approximately 30% of patients have associated congenital anomalies of the heart and lung, including patent ductus arteriosus, atrial septal defect, tetralogy of Fallot, and pulmonary sequestration. Other associated anomalies include diaphragmatic hernia, sternal defect, omphalocele, VATER association, and split phrenic nerve.

CLINICAL MANIFESTATIONS

Patients may present with chest pain; systolic murmurs, usually heard along the left sternal border or in the pulmonary area; and an abnormal point of maximal cardiac impulse, usually seen in patients with complete absence of the left pericardium. Although usually considered a benign condition, congenital pericardial defects are potentially serious in that death may occur from herniation and strangulation of the heart.

IMAGING

Chest radiographs in patients with *partial or small left-sided pericardial defects* demonstrate the heart to be in normal position, but the configuration is abnormal except for those cases without extension of the left atrial appendage outside the confines of the defect. The abnormality consists of varying degrees of prominence or enlargement in the vicinity of the left atrial appendage along the left upper heart border (Fig. 1A). A partial pericardial defect can be confirmed by visualization of the left atrial appendage extending through the pericardial defect on computed tomography (CT) or magnetic resonance imaging (MRI) examination (Fig. 1B, C). Spontaneous pneumothorax may occur.

In patients with *complete absence of the left pericardium*, the chest radiograph demonstrates the heart to be displaced to the left with concomitant clockwise rotation so that the left border of the heart is formed by the right ventricle. Characteristically, the trachea is midline. Varying degrees of prominence of the main pulmonary artery along the left upper heart border are noted. There may be separation between the aortic arch and the pulmonary artery with interposition of a segment of lung between the aorta and pulmonary artery, and also between the inferior border of the heart and the left hemidiaphragm. Unusual prominence of the left atrial appendage may be noted along the left heart margin (Fig. 2). Fluoroscopy may demonstrate abnormal mobility of the heart during contraction, and unusually prominent pulsations of the left atrial ap-

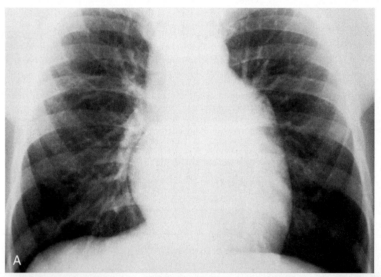

FIGURE 1. A 9-year-old boy with congenital partial absence of the left pericardium. **A,** Chest radiograph demonstrates abnormal prominence of the left atrial appendage (LAA) along the upper left heart margin. **B,** Coronal interleaved 5-mm-thick magnetic resonance (MR) images (posteroanterior) confirm herniation of the LAA through a partial defect in the left pericardium. **C,** Axial oblique MR image through the left atrium and atrial appendage demonstrates herniation of the LAA through the pericardial defect. The tricuspid aortic valve in its systolic position also is well seen.

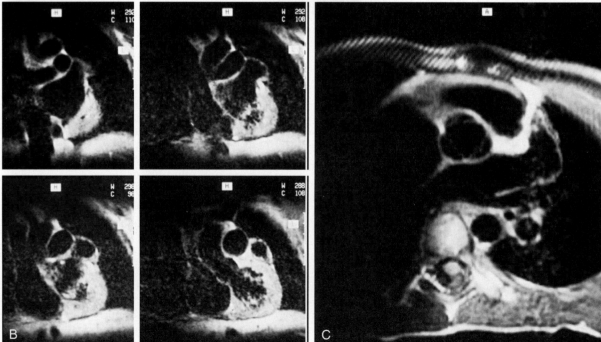

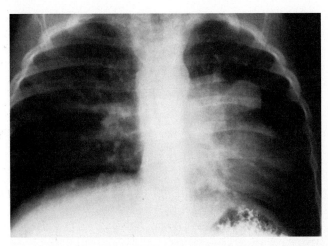

FIGURE 2. A 10-month-old boy with congenital complete absence of the left pericardium discovered incidentally at fluoroscopy. Rotation of the heart into the left chest with striking prominence of the left atrial appendage (LAA) is seen. Lung is interposed between the heart and left diaphragm. Prominent pulsations of the LAA were evident at fluoroscopy.

pendage. Confirmation again utilizes ultrasound, CT, and/or MRI.

In patients with *partial right-sided pericardial defects,* the chest radiograph may demonstrate an abnormal bulge along the right upper heart border in the vicinity of the superior vena cava from protrusion of a part of the right atrium through the defect. A part of the right upper lobe may also herniate into the pericardial sac.

The chest radiograph in patients with *surgical defects of the pericardium* may simulate the radiographic findings described above in patients with complete or partial absence of the left pericardium.

PERICARDITIS

Pericarditis represents the inflammatory response of the pericardium to a variety of insults, including acute rheumatic fever, bacterial and viral infections, trauma (Fig. 3), and rheumatoid and idiopathic factors. It is relatively rare in children.

CLINICAL MANIFESTATIONS

Fever is usually present with infectious pericarditis. Dyspnea and precordial pain may be seen with any causative factor. Physical findings include a friction rub and diminished heart tones.

CHEST RADIOGRAPHY

An enlarged pericardial-cardiac silhouette is usually evident, with differentiation of primary cardiomegaly always difficult. The classic radiographic manifestation is a globular or pear-shaped cardiomediastinal silhouette (Figs. 3 and 4A). The contour of the heart is smoother than normal; the margins are filled out, and

the cardiac chambers and great vessel contours may be obliterated. The lower cardiac margin next to the diaphragm may form a more acute angle than normal, and the cardiac silhouette changes significantly from the supine to the upright position. Fluoroscopy may demonstrate diminished cardiac pulsations, but this can be misleading and is also seen in patients with dilated hearts. Visualization of the epicardial fat as a lucent line deep to the outer border of the enlarged pericardial-cardiac silhouette may confirm the diagnosis. The line frequently appears in the retrosternal space in the lateral chest film or along the left heart border in the posteroanterior projection (Fig. 4B). Fluoroscopy may be more sensitive than chest films in demonstrating this finding.

ECHOCARDIOGRAPHY

Real-time echocardiography is the primary imaging modality in the diagnosis of pericardial effusion. A linear sonolucent area will be seen around the heart, particularly in the posterior left ventricular region. A lucent space larger than 2 mm indicates significant pericardial effusion (Fig. 5). Caution should be exercised in differentiating pericardial from pleural effusions.

OTHER FORMS OF PERICARDIAL ABNORMALITY

CONSTRICTIVE–RESTRICTIVE PERICARDITIS

This disease is usually the sequela of prior inflammatory pericarditis. With thickening of the pericardium and

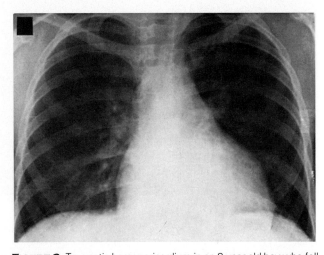

FIGURE 3. Traumatic hemopericardium in an 8-year-old boy who fell onto a metal pipe. Anteroposterior chest film shows an enlarged pericardial-cardiac silhouette with a globular water-bottle configuration. Pericardiocentesis yielded 850 ml of bloody fluid; at surgery, a 1-cm tear was found at the base of the aorta, with blood oozing directly into the pericardial cavity. (Courtesy of Dr. George Veasy, Salt Lake City, UT.)

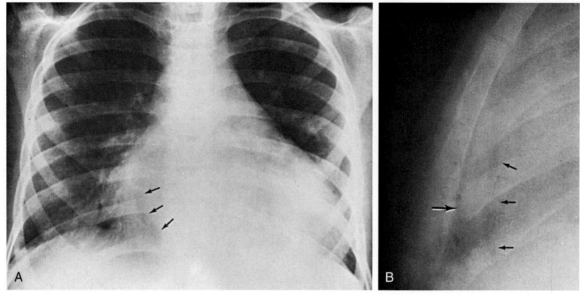

FIGURE 4. Pericardial effusion demonstrated by an epicardial fat shadow in an 11-year-old boy with acute rheumatic pancarditis. **A,** Anteroposterior chest film shows a large cardiac-pericardial silhouette with a curvilinear radiolucent line paralleling the true cardiac silhouette in the right cardiophrenic angle *(arrows)*. **B,** In a lateral radiograph, extrapericardial fat produces a linear substernal radiolucency *(large arrow)* and a second linear radiolucency *(small arrows)* indicating epicardial fat; the water density between these fat lines indicates pericardial effusion.

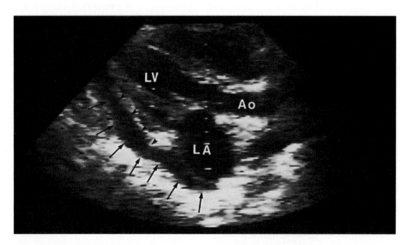

FIGURE 5. Pericardial effusion. A real-time echocardiogram demonstrates a sonolucent area between the posterior left ventricular wall *(arrowheads)* and the pericardium *(arrows)* that is characteristic of pericardial effusion. *LV* = left ventricle; *LA* = left atrium; *Ao* = aorta.

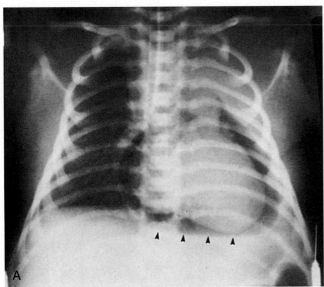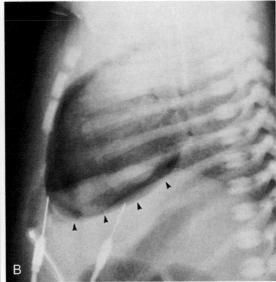

FIGURE 6. Pneumopericardium. Anteroposterior **(A)** and lateral **(B)** chest radiographs in a premature infant show a radiolucent zone around the cardiac silhouette with a characteristic well-defined continuation between the lower cardiac margin and the diaphragm *(arrowheads)*. Note the endotracheal tube in the right main stem bronchus and the left lung atelectasis.

adhesions, cardiac function is altered by restriction of diastolic filling. The cardiac silhouette may be normal with poor contractility at fluoroscopy; calcifications occasionally are noted. Dilatation of the superior and inferior venae cavae, pericardial thickening, and flattening of the right atrial contour may be seen with angiography, CT, and MRI. Chronic pericarditis may masquerade as a mass or tumor.

PNEUMOPERICARDIUM

This rare pericardial process is usually seen in the premature infant undergoing assisted ventilation. Radiographic findings are those of a continuous layer of air around the heart and particularly across the anterior mediastinal diaphragmatic surface. The air in the pericardial space will not ascend over the region of the great vessels, which differentiates this condition from a pneumomediastinum (Fig. 6).

SUGGESTED READINGS

Chen SJ, Li YW, Wu MH, et al: CT and MRI findings in a child with constrictive pericarditis. Pediatr Cardiol 1998;19:259

Cottrill CM, Tamaren J, Hall B: Sternal defects associated with congenital pericardial and cardiac defects. Cardiol Young 1998; 8:100

Furbur A, Pezard P, Jeune JJ, et al: Radionuclide angiography and magnetic resonance imaging: complementary non-invasive methods in the diagnosis of constrictive pericarditis. Eur J Nucl Med 1995;22:1292

Gassner I, Judmaier W, Fink C, et al: Diagnosis of congenital pericardial defects, including a pathognomic sign for dangerous apical ventricular herniation, on magnetic resonance imaging. Br Heart J 1995;74:60

Hartnell GG, Hughes LA, Ko JP, et al: Magnetic resonance imaging of pericardial constriction: comparison of cine MR angiography and spin-echo techniques. Clin Radiol 1996;51:268

Hoit BD: Imaging the pericardium. Cardiol Clin 1990;8:587

Jacob JL, Souza Junior AS, Parra Junior A: Absence of the left pericardium diagnosed by computed tomography. Int J Cardiol 1995;47:293

Lichtenberg GS, Meltzer RS: Echocardiography in pericardial disease. *In* Elliott LP (ed): Cardiac Imaging in Infants, Children, and Adults. Philadelphia, JB Lippincott, 1991:390

McIlhenny J, Campbell SE, Raible RJ, et al: Pediatric case of the day: Congenital absence of the pericardium. AJR Am J Roentgenol 1996;167:270

Miller SW: Imaging pericardial disease. Radiol Clin North Am 1989;27:1113

Olson MC, Posniak HV, McDonald V, et al: Computed tomography and magnetic resonance imaging of the pericardium. Radiographics 1989;9:633–649

Van Son JA, Danielson GK, Schaff HV, et al: Congenital partial and complete absence of the pericardium. Mayo Clin Proc 1993;68:743

Watanabe A, Hara Y, Hamada M, et al: A case of effusive-constrictive pericarditis: an efficacy of Gd-DTPA enhanced magnetic resonance imaging to detect a pericardial thickening. Magn Reson Imaging 1998;16:347

P A R T   V I

CARDIAC TUMORS AND ARRHYTHMIAS

VIRGIL R. CONDON
RICHARD B. JAFFE

C h a p t e r   1

CARDIAC TUMORS

Cardiac tumors in infancy and childhood are rare. They may be either (1) intrinsic to the heart and pericardium or (2) metastatic. *Intracavitary tumors* usually present with sudden dyspnea, failure, cyanosis, shock, or bizarre central nervous system manifestations from embolization. *Intramural lesions* more often produce signs related to inflow or outflow obstruction or ventricular or supraventricular arrhythmias. Pericardial tumors may be asymptomatic until they impinge upon cardiac chambers or create significant tamponade secondary to effusions.

INTRINSIC TUMORS

Eighty percent of cardiac tumors in children are intrinsic tumors, and 80% are benign. *Rhabdomyoma* is the most common and appears between 6 months and 5 years of age. It is generally a small tumor with a circumscribed mass projecting into the ventricular cavity (Fig. 1). Most patients have tuberous sclerosis (50%)

and may have multiple myocardial tumors. *Intramural fibroma* is the next most common intrinsic tumor and presents as a single large tumor mass in the myocardium, usually of the left ventricle or ventricular septum (Figs. 2 and 3); these lesions may be calcified. *Myxomas* are rare and usually occur in the left atrium and produce symptoms related to mitral valve obstruction. Almost all kinds of benign pediatric tumors have been described involving the heart and pericardium. Primary sarcomas of many types may occur and frequently metastasize.

Pericardial tumors (20% of all cardiac tumors) include teratoma, fibroma, lipoma, angioma, leiomyoma, and lymphangioma. The differential diagnosis includes other masses in the mediastinum (e.g., teratoma, lymphoma).

METASTATIC TUMORS

Metastatic tumors are rare and are usually secondary to leukemia or lymphoma, neuroblastoma, hepatoblas-

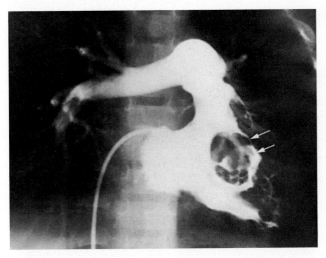

FIGURE 1. Rhabdomyoma. A right ventriculogram demonstrates a round filling defect projecting into the right ventricular cavity *(arrows)* secondary to a rhabdomyoma in a child with tuberous sclerosis.

toma, Wilms' tumor, Ewing's sarcoma, or osteosarcoma. Involvement may be by direct extension from intra-abdominal organs via the inferior vena cava or be bloodborne.

CHEST RADIOGRAPHY

Findings are markedly variable depending upon the type and location of the tumor. Cardiac dilatation related to cardiac dysfunction or obstruction is frequently present. With pericardial tumors, effusion is the rule, with the cardiac silhouette either that of effusion or an abnormal cardiac contour.

ECHOCARDIOGRAPHY

Two-dimensional echocardiography usually can define the mass and determine its intracavitary, intramural, or pericardial relations (Fig. 2). Involvement of the valves and chambers is readily appreciated, and Doppler ultrasound can evaluate valvular dysfunction.

OTHER IMAGING PROCEDURES

Magnetic resonance imaging represents the definitive imaging modality to further define pericardial, myocardial, endocardial, or intracavitary relations (see Fig. 3). Angiocardiography can adequately demonstrate the

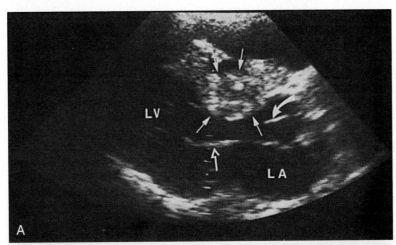

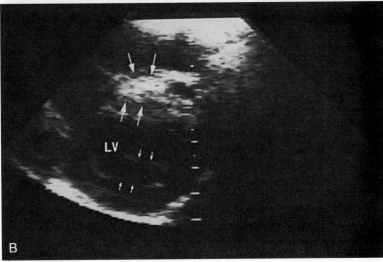

FIGURE 2. Intracardiac fibroma. Long-axis **(A)** and short-axis **(B)** real-time echocardiograms demonstrate an echogenic round mass lying within the interventricular septum *(arrows)* just below the aortic valve *(curved arrow)*. Histologically, this was a benign fibroma; however, resection was incomplete, and recurrence developed. The mitral valve is designated by the *open arrow* and *small arrows*. *LV* = left ventricle; *LA* = left atrium.

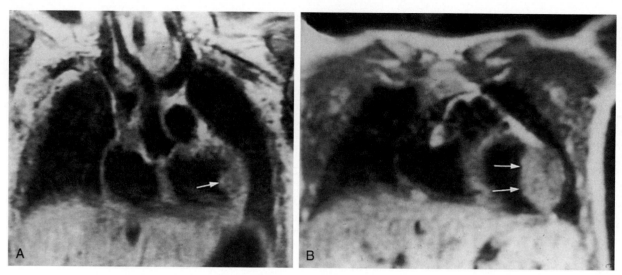

FIGURE 3. Intramural fibroma viewed by magnetic resonance imaging. Anterior **(A)** and posterior **(B)** serial coronal cardiac-gated T_1-weighted images of the left ventricle show a moderately large intramural fibroma of the left ventricular apex *(arrows).*

intracavitary and endocardial lesions (see Fig. 1). Simultaneous long-axis biventricular injections are particularly useful with septal tumors.

SUGGESTED READINGS

Araoz P, Eklund HE, Welch TJ, et al: CT and MR imaging of primary cardiac malignancies. Radiographics 1999;19:1421

Berkenblit R, Spindola-Franco H, Frater RW, et al: MRI in the evaluation and management of a newborn infant with cardiac rhabdomyoma. Ann Thorac Surg 1997;63:1475

Casolo F, Biasi S, Galzarini L, et al: MRI as an adjunct to echocardiography for the diagnostic imaging of cardiac masses. Eur J Radiol 1988;8:226

Cornalba G, Dore R: Cardiac tumor associated with tuberous sclerosis. J Comput Assist Tomogr 1985;9:809

de Ruiz M, Potter JL, Stavinoha J, et al: Real-time ultrasound diagnosis of cardiac fibroma in a neonate. J Ultrasound Med 1985;4:367

Hoadley SD, Wallace RL, Miller JF, et al: Prenatal diagnosis of cardiac tumors presenting as an arrhythmia. J Clin Ultrasound 1986;14:639

Huh J, Noh CI, Kim YW, et al: Secondary cardiac tumor in children. Pediatr Cardiol 1999;20:400

Lund JT, Ehman RL, Julsrud PR, et al: Cardiac masses: Assessment by MR imaging. AJR Am J Roentgenol 1989;152:469

McAllister HA Jr, Hall RJ, Cooley DA: Tumors of the heart and pericardium. Curr Probl Cardiol 1999;24:57

Mousseaux E, Hernigou A, Azencot M, et al: Evaluation by electron beam computed tomography of intracardiac masses suspected by transesophageal echocardiography. Heart 1996;76:256

Rienmuller R, Tiling R: Evaluation of paracardiac and intracardiac masses in children. Semin Ultrasound CT MR 1990;11:246–250

Sallee D, Spector ML, van Heeckeren DW, et al: Primary pediatric cardiac tumors: a 17 year experience. Cardiol Young 1999;9:155

Stanford W, Rooholamini SA, Galvin JR: Ultrafast computed tomography for the detection of intracardiac thrombi and tumors. *In* Elliott LP (ed): Cardiac Imaging in Infants, Children, and Adults. Philadelphia, JB Lippincott, 1991:494

Chapter 2

CARDIAC ARRHYTHMIAS

VIRGIL R. CONDON and RICHARD B. JAFFE

ARRHYTHMIAS

Rhythm disturbances are rare in infants and children, although reasonably common (1% to 2%) during late pregnancy when fetal monitoring is utilized. Supraventricular premature beats are the most common dysrhythmia. Many of the cardiac rhythm disturbances are transitory and benign. Significant recent work has shown rhythm disorders to be associated with maternal and neonatal antibodies (i.e., lupus erythematosis), infection-related antibodies (endogenous retrovirus), metabolic disorders, and other familial conditions.

Paroxysmal supraventricular tachycardia may occur in utero or in the postnatal period. In utero, it is one of the causes for neonatal hydrops and congestive failure. In the child, if this condition persists, cardiomegaly will ensue and pulmonary edema may be seen on chest radiographs (Fig. 1). The heart rate usually ranges from 140 to 240 beats per minute. In the absence of underlying congenital heart disease, the prognosis is good.

Persistent atrial tachycardia is a fairly common postnatal condition. It may occur secondary to Wolff-Parkinson-White syndrome and be associated with the Ebstein malformation of the tricuspid valve. If atrial tachycardia persists, clinical failure may occur with palpitations, shortness of breath, and development of cardiomegaly and congestive failure.

Atrial flutter, atrial fibrillation, and *paroxysmal ventricular tachycardia* are relatively rare forms of arrhythmia. Clinical findings are related to the heart rate and duration of arrhythmia. Persisting arrhythmia leads to cardiomegaly and congestive failure.

Complete heart block may be congenital and may occur as an isolated finding or accompany various forms of congenital heart disease, particularly corrected transposition of the great vessels. It is most often secondary to heart surgery. The heart rate is usually around 60 beats per minute, but, when it approaches 40, syncope, respiratory distress, dyspnea, and cyanosis may become evident. Chest radiographs show mild cardiomegaly, mild aortic dilatation and, occasionally, venous congestion related to the large stroke volume in these patients. A film made during a period of atrioventricular dyssynchrony may show a transient pattern of pulmonary congestion when the left atrium contracts simultaneously with left ventricular contraction against the closed mitral valve (Fig. 2). Primary congenital heart block rarely needs treatment. If recurrent syncopal episodes occur, epicardial or transvenous pacemaker insertion may be necessary.

ARRHYTHMOGENIC RIGHT VENTRICULAR CARDIOMYOPATHY

Arrhythmogenic right ventricular dysplasia or cardiomyopathy (ARVC) is a disease of adolescents and young adults, particularly males, in which right ventricular musculature is replaced by fatty and fibrous tissue. These patients present with recurrent ventricular tachycardia and sudden death. Although echocardiography, endomyocardial biopsy, and angiography are useful in the diagnosis of ARVC, magnetic resonance imaging (MRI) is uniquely suited to detect the structural and functional abnormalities present in ARVC. MRI uniquely can detect fatty or fibrous replacement in a right ventricular myocardium on T_1-weighted images (Fig. 3). It also can detect wall thinning, abnormal bulging, or outpouching (Fig. 3)

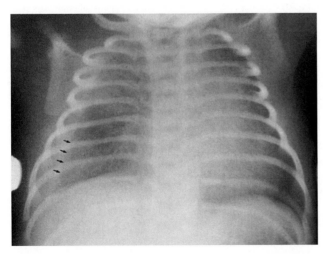

FIGURE 1. Intrauterine paroxysmal atrial tachycardia. An anteroposterior chest radiograph in a newborn with tachypnea demonstrates moderate right pleural effusion *(arrows)*, cardiomegaly, and congestive heart failure.

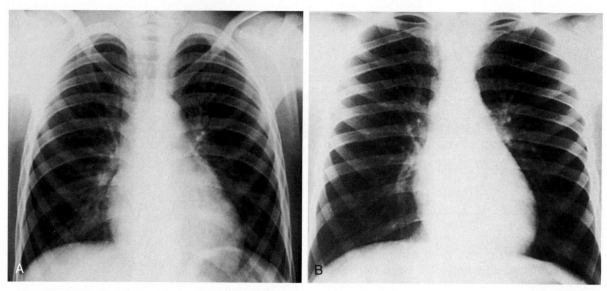

FIGURE 2. Complete congenital heart block. Posteroanterior chest radiographs (**A** and **B**) made within a few minutes of one another show a pattern of cardiomegaly and venous congestion secondary to atrioventricular dissociation and effects of a large stroke volume that changes to a totally normal appearance of the heart and lungs on the second film (**B**). (From Jaffe RB, Sherman SA, Condon VR, et al: Congenital complete heart block. Radiology 1976;121:434, with permission.)

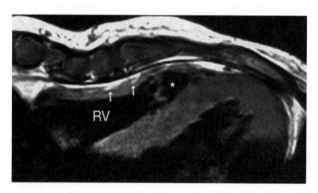

FIGURE 3. Suspected, but not proven, arrhythmogenic right ventricular cardiomyopathy. Prone axial T_1-weighted spin-echo magnetic resonance image utilizing a surface coil demonstrates fatty infiltration of the anterior right ventricular myocardium *(arrows)* and saccular dilatation of the right ventricular apex (*). (Courtesy of J. B. Mawson, Vancouver, BC.)

on spin-echo or cine imaging. Abnormalities in regional or global contractility are demonstrated by cine-MRI to include the right ventricle from the base to the pulmonary valve.

SUGGESTED READINGS

Ackerman MJ: The long QT syndrome. Pediatr Rev 1998;19:232

Auffermann W, Wichter T, Breithardt G, et al: Arrhythymogenic right ventricular disease: MR imaging vs. angiography. AJR Am J Roentgenol 1993;161:549–555

Blake LM, Scheinman MM, Higgins CB: MR feature of arrhythmogenic right ventricular dysplasia. AJR Am J Roentgenol 1994;152:809–812

Deloof E, Devlieger H, Van Hoestenberghe R, et al: Management with a staged approach of the premature hydropic fetus due to complete congenital heart block. Eur J Pediatr 1997;156:521

Etheridge SP, Judd VE: Supraventricular tachycardia in infancy: evaluation, management, and follow-up. Arch Pediatr Adolesc Med 1999;153:267

Globits S, Kreiner G, Frank H, et al: Significance of morphological abnormalities detected by MRI in patients undergoing successful ablation of right ventricular outflow tract tachycardia. Circulation 1997;96:2633–2640

Gonge HM, Wladimiroff JW, Noordam MJ, et al: Fetal cardiac arrhythmias and their effect on volume blood flow in descending aorta of human fetus. J Clin Ultrasound 1986;14:607

Higgins CB, Higgins SS, Kelley MJ, et al: Heart failure in the neonate due to extreme abnormalities of heart rate: clinical and radiographic features. AJR Am J Roentgenol 1980;134:359

Jaffe RB, Sherman SA, Condon VR, et al: Congenital complete heart block. Radiology 1976;121:434

Julkunen H, Kaaja R, Siren MK, et al: Immune-mediated congenital heart block (CHB): identifying and counseling patients at risk for having children with CHB. Semin Arthritis Rheum 1998;28:97

Kocak G, Atalay S, Tutar E, et al: Congenital complete atrioventricular block in an infant with long QT syndrome. Acta Cardiol 1998;53:153

Li JM, Fan WS, Horsfall AC, et al: The expression of human endogenous retrovirus-3 in fetal cardiac tissue and antibodies in congenital heart block. Clin Exp Immunol 1996;104:388

Marcus ML, Fontaine G: Arrhythmogenic right ventricular dysplasia/cardiomyopathy: a review. Pacing Clin Electrophysiol 1995;18:1298

Steinschneider A, Richmond C, Ramaswamy V, et al: Clinical characteristics of an apparent life-threatening event (ALTE) and the subsequent occurrence of prolonged apnea or prolonged bradycardia. Clin Pediatr 1998;37:223

Thiene G, Nava A, Corrado D, et al: Right ventricular cardiomyopathy and sudden death in young people. N Engl J Med 1988;318:129–133

PART VII

CARDIAC OPERATIONS AND INTERVENTIONAL PROCEDURES

RICHARD B. JAFFE
VIRGIL R. CONDON

Chapter 1

CARDIAC OPERATIONS

RICHARD B. JAFFE and VIRGIL R. CONDON

EVALUATION OF THE POSTOPERATIVE CHEST RADIOGRAPH

After cardiac operation, serial chest radiographs enable the pediatric radiologist to accurately monitor the patient's condition. When compared with preoperative radiographs, a small decrease in heart size is frequently seen immediately after operation, secondary to hypovolemia, but is transitory. Large increases in heart size after operation are suggestive of inadequate drainage of the pericardial space and development of pericardial effusion. Mediastinal widening typically is seen after median sternotomy, and gradually resolves in 1 to 2 weeks, but progressive widening in mediastinal contour from preoperative radiographs implies continued mediastinal hemorrhage necessitating treatment. Small pleural effusions after a thoracotomy are common, but moderate to large effusions indicate continued bleeding and inade-

quate chest drainage. Moderate to large pleural effusions are commonly seen in patients following the Fontan procedure complicated by low output. Persistent pleural effusions are suggestive of chylothorax, and may follow inadvertent severance of the thoracic duct or result from elevated superior vena cava pressures as may be seen in patients with Glenn shunts or superior vena cava obstruction after the Mustard operation (Fig. 1). They may disappear after the patient has been placed on a low-fat diet, but often clear only after ligation of the thoracic duct (Fig. 2).

Subsegmental and segmental atelectasis is seen in almost all patients following operation, particularly in the left lower lobe, especially in patients with large ventricular septal defect and others with left atrial enlargement narrowing the left main stem bronchus. Pulmonary edema may develop unilaterally or bilaterally following systemic–pulmonary artery shunts, but should resolve in several days on diuretic therapy. Persistent pulmonary edema may be indicative of pul-

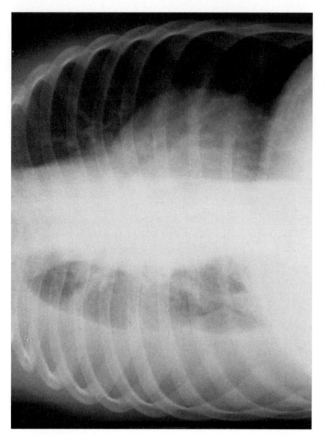

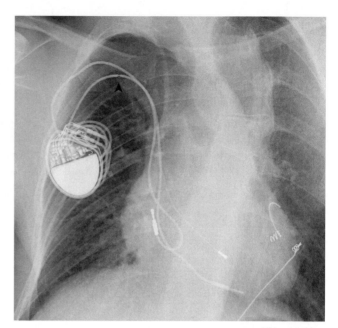

FIGURE 3. Sixteen-year-old with transvenous right atrial and right ventricular pacemaker leads. A frontal radiograph demonstrates severe thoracic scoliosis and fracture of the right atrial lead at its insertion into the right subclavian vein *(arrow)*. An older disconnected right ventricular pacemaker wire is seen in the left innominate vein and superior vena cava. Two older disconnected epicardial pacemaker levels are present over the left heart.

FIGURE 1. A 1½-year-old boy with superior vena cava obstruction 1 year after a Mustard operation for transposition. Right lateral decubitus chest radiograph demonstrates a large right chylothorax (see also Fig. 21).

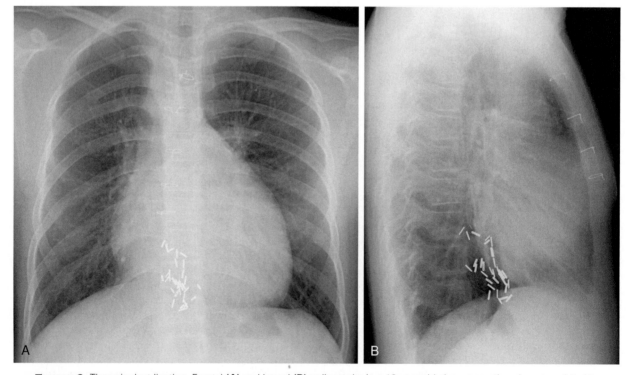

FIGURE 2. Thoracic duct ligation. Frontal **(A)** and lateral **(B)** radiographs in a 13-year-old show operative changes related to repair of tetralogy of Fallot and thoracic duct ligation. Normal pulmonary blood flow, cardiomegaly with right heart enlargement secondary to residual pulmonic regurgitation, inconspicuous main pulmonary artery segment, and right aortic arch are noted. Multiple metallic clips in the posterior mediastinum relate to thoracic duct ligation.

monary venous obstruction, as may be seen in patients after repair of total anomalous pulmonary venous drainage, or baffle obstruction of the pulmonary venous limb after the Mustard operation for transposition. It also may be an indication of persisting systemic outflow obstruction or poor myocardial function, as may be seen in patients with anoxia or sepsis. Disseminated airspace disease indicative of pulmonary hemorrhage may occur in patients with sepsis, shock, and disseminated intravascular coagulation. Elevation of a hemidiaphragm after operation is indicative of phrenic nerve injury. Fluoroscopy or ultrasonography will reveal paradoxical movement during inspiration. Patients who fail extubation should also be evaluated for phrenic nerve injury that may not be recognized with the patient intubated and ventilated.

Transvenous right atrial and right ventricular pacemaker leads, or in other patients epicardial pacemaker leads, should be evaluated closely for fracture (Fig. 3), or disconnection from the battery pack. After Mustard operation for complete transposition, transvenous pacemaker leads may be advanced into the left ventricle and systemic venous limb of the atrial baffle.

COMMON CARDIAC OPERATIONS

Table 1 describes and illustrates common cardiac operations—palliative cardiac operations and operative repair, respectively. The procedure, its description, and the radiologic findings and complications are discussed and illustrated.

Table 1 ■ CARDIAC OPERATIONS

PROCEDURE	DESCRIPTION	RADIOLOGIC FINDINGS AND COMPLICATIONS
Procedures to Increase Pulmonary Blood Flow		
Venous		
Glenn shunt	Superior vena cava (SVC)—pulmonary artery (PA) shunt. May use right SVC—right PA or left SVC—left PA. Performed as a palliative procedure in tricuspid atresia and other forms of cyanotic heart disease, usually as a staging procedure prior to a Fontan anastomosis. Performed by dividing the PA and ligating the proximal portion. The distal PA is anastomosed end to side with the SVC. The SVC is ligated on the cardiac side of the anastomosis, directing the SVC flow into the ipsilateral PA (Fig. 4). Rarely, flow can be augmented to the lung by creation of an arteriovenous fistula in the ipsilateral axilla, thus increasing SVC flow.	Late complications include anastomotic narrowing, SVC syndrome, thrombotic occlusion of the ipsilateral PAs, and pulmonary arteriovenous malformations with intrapulmonary right-to-left shunting (Fig. 5). Increased SVC pressure may result in collateral flow, particularly through the azygos vein, effectively decreasing pulmonary blood flow (Fig. 6). Operative ligation or coil occlusion of these collateral vessels may be necessary to increase SVC blood flow (see Section V, Part VII, Chapter 2, Fig. 4, page 1418).
Bidirectional Glenn shunt (Abram modification)	Right or left SVC—PA anastomosis. Similar to above, but the proximal PA is not ligated. SVC flow is directed to both pulmonary arteries (Figs. 7 and 25*B*). Similar to Fontan procedure, but only directs SVC flow to the pulmonary arteries. Inferior vena cava blood flow remains intracardiac.	Similar to Glenn shunt.
Arterial		
Blalock-Taussig shunt	Subclavian artery—PA shunt. This systemic-PA shunt is used for palliation of cyanotic heart disease, especially tetralogy of Fallot. The subclavian artery is divided, preferably on the side of the innominate artery. The proximal portion is anastomosed end to side to the ipsilateral PA. The distal stump of the subclavian is ligated. One of the advantages of this procedure is that the size and length of the subclavian artery limit flow and usually prevent development of pulmonary hypertension.	Radiologic findings may include ipsilateral elevation and enlargement of the PA, increased pulmonary blood flow on the side of the shunt, and unilateral rib notching. Complications include kinking of the subclavian artery, anastomotic narrowing (see Fig. 8 and Section V, Part I, Chapter 2, Fig. 30, page 1251), and elevation and kinking of the PA. Retrograde propagation of thrombus to involve a carotid artery may be seen. Mediastinal and intercostal collaterals supply circulation to the arm. Rarely, a withered arm may result from ligation of the subclavian artery (Fig. 9). Pulmonary hypertension is rare after the procedure.
Modified Blalock-Taussig shunt	Similar to standard Blalock-Taussig shunt, except that the subclavian artery is not divided, but rather a synthetic graft is anastomosed end to side to the subclavian and ipsilateral PA (Fig. 10).	Radiographic findings and complications are similar to the Blalock-Taussig shunt except that rib notching should not be present. If the synthetic conduit is too short, it may cause kinking of the subclavian/PA.
Central shunt	Systemic–PA shunt used for palliation of cyanotic congenital heart disease utilizing a synthetic 4-5-mm-diameter graft between the ascending aorta and the PA.	Complications include increased pulmonary blood flow and pulmonary hypertension if the shunt is too large. Anastomotic narrowing/kinking may also be seen, decreasing effective PA blood flow.

Table continued on page 1400

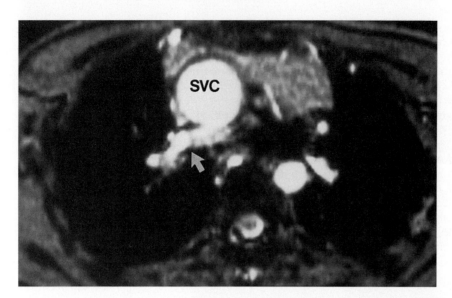

FIGURE 4. Glenn shunt in a 7-year-old girl with pulmonary atresia. Axial gradient-recalled cine–magnetic resonance image demonstrates a patent Glenn anastomosis between the superior vena cava *(SVC)* and right pulmonary artery *(arrow)*.

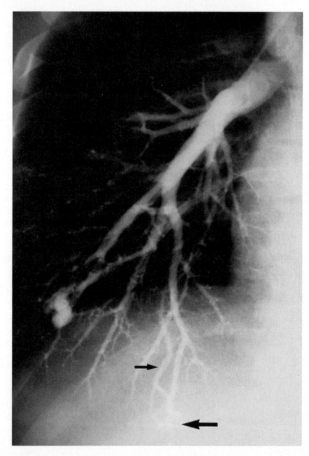

FIGURE 5. A 19-year-old boy with Glenn shunt for tricuspid atresia. Right pulmonary angiogram following catheter passage from the arm across the Glenn shunt demonstrates two small pulmonary arteriovenous malformations (AVMs) in the right lower lung. The smallest AVM, behind the diaphragm *(large arrow)*, has early venous opacification *(small arrow)* similar to the larger AVM.

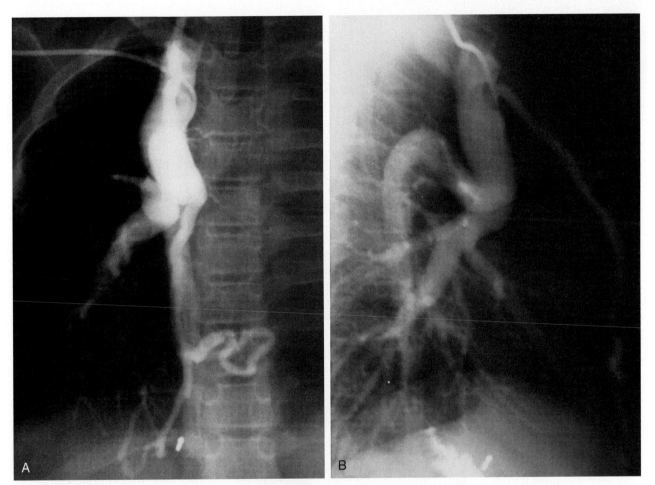

FIGURE 6. A 10-year-old girl with Glenn anastomosis for tricuspid atresia at age 5 months. Frontal **(A)** and lateral **(B)** angiograms after superior vena cava injection demonstrate a patent Glenn anastomosis, but collateral flow down the enlarged azygos vein and right internal mammary vein decreases pulmonary blood flow. The patient underwent ligation of the azygos and right internal mammary veins.

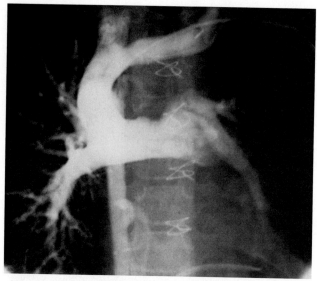

FIGURE 7. Bidirectional Glenn shunt. Superior vena cava injection in the frontal projection demonstrates a patent bidirectional Glenn shunt with opacification of both right and left pulmonary arteries. However, collateral flow down the azygos system effectively decreases pulmonary blood flow. The patient underwent coil occlusion of the azygos vein (see Section V, Part VII, Chapter 2, Fig. 4, page 1418).

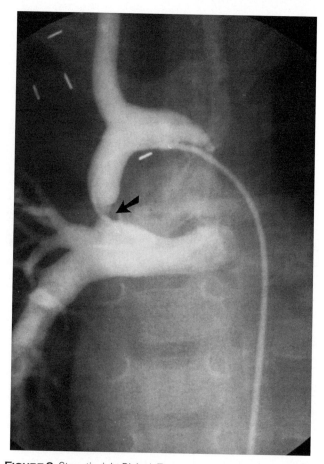

FIGURE 8. Stenotic right Blalock-Taussig shunt for tetralogy of Fallot with left aortic arch. The right subclavian artery is stenotic at the anastomosis with the right pulmonary artery *(arrow)*.

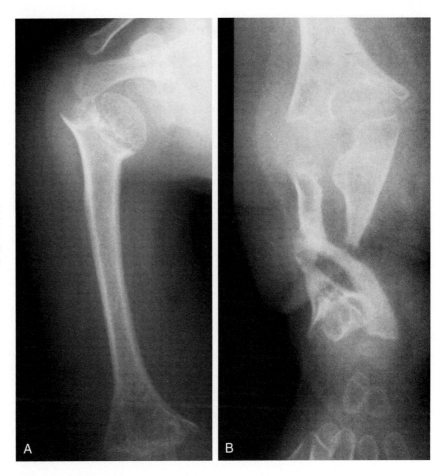

FIGURE 9. Withered right arm after right Blalock-Taussig shunt as a neonate. **A,** Right humerus: ischemic changes of the proximal and distal metaphyses are noted. **B,** Right forearm: severe ischemic changes of the radius and ulna are noted.

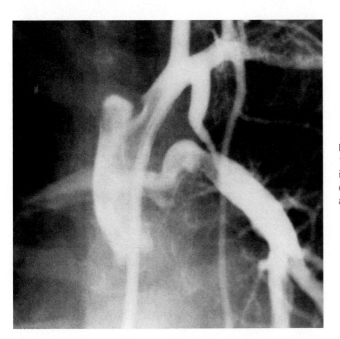

FIGURE 10. Stenotic modified left Blalock-Taussig shunt in a 1½-year-old girl with tetralogy of Fallot. Injection of contrast medium into the left innominate artery arising from the right aortic arch demonstrates the modified left Blalock-Taussig shunt with stenosis at its anastomosis with the left pulmonary artery.

Table 1 ■ CARDIAC OPERATIONS Continued

PROCEDURE	DESCRIPTION	RADIOLOGIC FINDINGS AND COMPLICATIONS
Potts anastomosis	Systemic–PA shunt created by a side-to-side anastomosis between the descending aorta and ipsilateral PA. This is an extrapericardial shunt and is rarely performed today in patients with cyanotic heart disease because of the potential development of pulmonary hypertension, and considerable difficulty in dismantling the shunt during later operative repair.	Like the Waterston-Cooley shunt, the anastomosis must be of proper size; if too large, pulmonary hypertension may develop; if too small, there will be insufficient flow to the lungs. A mycotic aneurysm at the anastomotic site is a rare complication (see Section V, Part V, Chapter 2, Fig. 4, page 1379).
Waterston-Cooley anastomosis	Systemic–PA shunt formed by side-to-side anastomosis of the ascending aorta to the right PA. This palliative procedure for cyanotic congenital heart disease is rarely performed today because of the potential development of pulmonary hypertension.	Following operation, unilateral pulmonary edema can develop, but is usually transient. The common complication of this anastomosis is the development of pulmonary hypertension, particularly in the right lung, frequently accompanied by obstruction of flow to the left PA (Fig. 11).

Procedure to Decrease Pulmonary Blood Flow

PROCEDURE	DESCRIPTION	RADIOLOGIC FINDINGS AND COMPLICATIONS
Pulmonary artery band	Palliative procedure to decrease pulmonary arterial blood flow in patients with large left-to-right shunts protecting the PAs from systemic pressures and resultant pulmonary hypertension. Synthetic material is placed around the main PA just above the pulmonary valve and the band is gradually tightened to constrict the main PA and decrease the pulmonary arterial pressures to approximately one-half systemic pressure in the newborn. When definitive operative repair is performed at a later date, the pulmonary band can be removed and, if necessary, reconstructive surgery performed on the main PA.	If metallic staples have been used to tighten the band, they are visible often as a series of parallel staples in the region of the main PA (Fig. 12). Angiography in patients with PA band typically shows thickening of the pulmonary valve leaflets, nodularity along the edges of the valve leaflets, doming of the pulmonary valve during systole, and poststenotic dilatation of the PA distal to the band. Calcification may develop in the main PA, but a calcified aneurysm of the main PA is rare. Distal migration of the PA band may produce significant obstruction of the proximal right and left pulmonary arteries (Fig. 13). Subaortic stenosis may also develop following pulmonary artery band in patients with ventricular septal defect, and in patients with single ventricle or univentricular hearts with narrowing of the bulboventricular foramen.
Arterial switch (Jatene procedure)	Definitive repair of complete transposition of the great vessels. The aorta and pulmonary arteries (PAs) are divided above the valves and the great vessels switched. The coronary arteries are removed from the aorta with a button of tissue and are reimplanted into the neoaorta.	Complications include supravalvular pulmonary stenosis (most common) (Fig. 14) at the anastomotic site, supravalvular aortic stenosis, and myocardial ischemia secondary to kinking of the coronary arteries or obstruction at the ostia. Following operation, the neoaorta may obstruct the proximal PA.
Ascending-to-descending aortic conduit	Placement of a prosthetic conduit between the ascending and descending aorta. This procedure is utilized for repair of aortic arch interruption, and severe forms of aortic coarctation when primary anastomotic repair is not possible.	The conduit is visualized usually in the left posterior superior mediastinum on chest radiographs (Fig. 15). Calcification may develop within the conduit, and indicate neointimal proliferation and obstruction. Other complications include inadequate size as the patient grows and kinking of the conduit (Fig. 16). Fistulous connection to the mediastinum or lung is a rare complication.
Blalock-Hanlon operation	Operative removal of the atrial septum. Performed as a palliative procedure to improve atrial mixing in patients with complex cyanotic congenital heart disease.	Complications are rare with this procedure.
Brock's operation	Relief of right ventricular outflow obstruction performed blindly via a right ventriculotomy. The stenotic or atretic pulmonary valve is fractured, and infundibular tissue can be excised to relieve subvalvular obstruction.	Complications include false passage and inadvertent damage to the adjacent posterior aortic valve.
Cardiac transplantation	Replacement of native heart with matched donor heart. The procedure includes anastomoses of the native and donor superior and inferior vena cavas (or alternatively a right atrial cuff from native and donor hearts), aortic anastomosis, and left atrial anastomosis to include the native pulmonary veins (unless a complete heart–lung transplant is performed)	As with all transplants, infection and rejection are the predominant complications. Anastomotic complications are rare. The donor heart may be large for the patient size. Signs of cardiac rejection include an interval increase in cardiac size, and development of congestive failure. Late complications include post-transplant coronary artery disease (cardiac allograft vasculopathy).

Table continued on page 1405

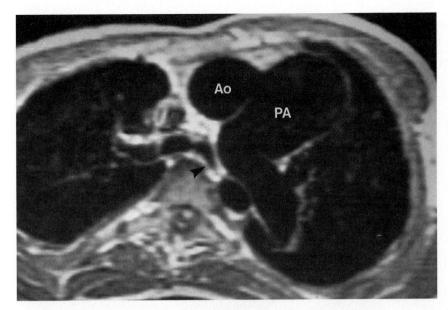

FIGURE 11. Waterston-Cooley anastomosis with pulmonary hypertension. A 20-year-old with pulmonic atresia after having a Waterston-Cooley shunt as an infant. Axial 5-mm spin-echo magnetic resonance image demonstrates the Waterston-Cooley shunt between the ascending aorta *(Ao)* and pulmonary artery *(PA)*, with aneurysmal dilatation of the central pulmonary artery and left pulmonary artery. The right pulmonary artery was not visualized. Note compression and posterior displacement of the left main-stem bronchus *(arrowhead)* and descending aorta by the aneurysmally dilated left pulmonary artery.

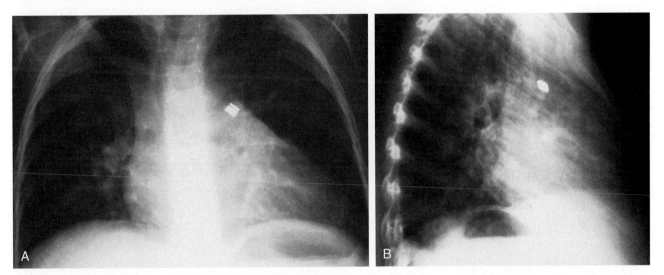

FIGURE 12. A 3-year-old girl with pulmonary artery band for membranous and muscular ventricular septal defects. Frontal **(A)** and lateral **(B)** chest radiographs demonstrate multiple parallel staples in the region of the main pulmonary artery. These staples have been placed to gradually tighten the synthetic pulmonary artery band around the pulmonary artery to decrease the pulmonary arterial pressures to approximately one-half systemic pressure.

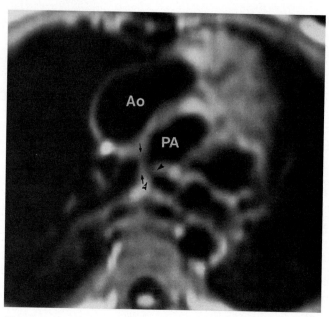

FIGURE 13. Distal migration of the pulmonary artery band (axial 3-mm spin-echo magnetic resonance image). In this 1-year-old patient with single ventricle and dextrotransposition, the pulmonary artery band has migrated distally, with marked stenosis of the proximal right *(arrows)* and proximal left *(arrowheads)* pulmonary artery. *Ao* = anterior aorta; *PA* = posterior pulmonary artery.

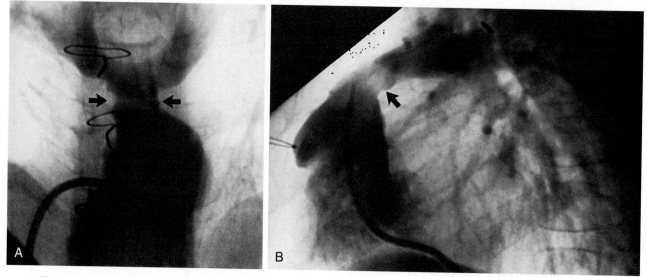

FIGURE 14. Peripheral pulmonary artery stenosis following arterial switch for transposition. Frontal **(A)** and lateral **(B)** digital angiograms following right ventricular injection demonstrate mild peripheral pulmonary artery stenosis at the anastomotic site *(arrows)* in this 7-year-old following arterial switch for transposition.

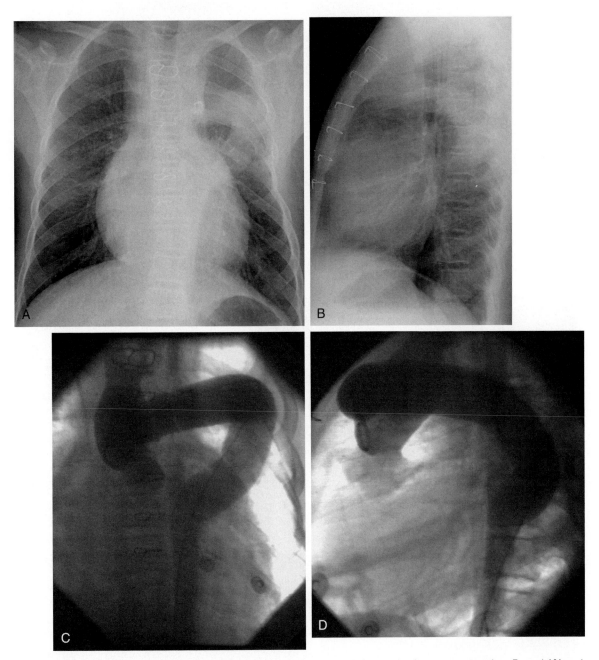

FIGURE 15. Twelve-year-old with ascending–descending aortic conduit for repair of severe coarctation. Frontal **(A)** and lateral **(B)** radiographs demonstrate the large conduit in the left mediastinum. Calcification adjacent to left T4–T5 interspace is in a nonfunctional ascending–descending aortic conduit placed in infancy. Frontal **(C)** and lateral **(D)** aortography demonstrates the large ascending–descending aortic conduit. The pigtail catheter has been passed retrograde up the descending thoracic aorta and through the conduit into the ascending aorta.

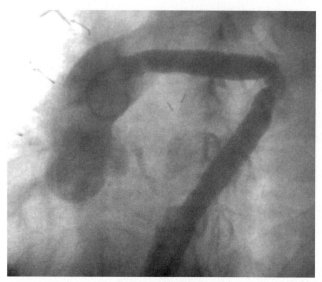

FIGURE 16. Ten-year-old with ascending–descending aortic conduit placed in infancy for repair of interrupted aortic arch. Digital aortogram in the left anterior oblique projection following catheter passage from the descending aorta through the conduit into the ascending aorta demonstrates the conduit now is of inadequate size for the patient's age and is kinked and narrowed in the midportion. This necessitated replacement of the conduit.

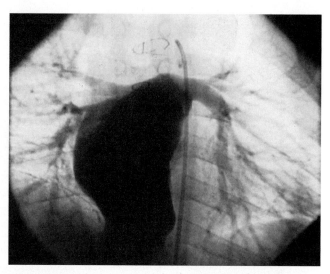

FIGURE 17. Fontan procedure in a 16-year-old boy with single ventricle and levotransposition. Frontal digital angiogram after injection of contrast medium into the inferior vena cava–right atrial junction opacifies the right atrium and its anastomosis with the pulmonary artery. A pigtail catheter is present in the left descending thoracic aorta.

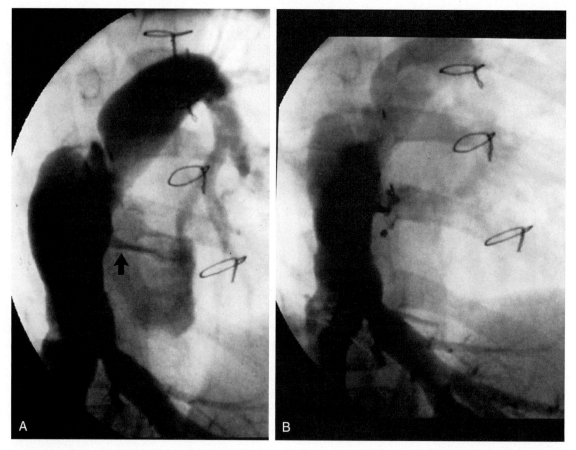

FIGURE 18. Catheter closure of a fenestrated Fontan procedure in a 4½-year-old boy with right Glenn anastomosis, and fenestrated Fontan procedure for palliation of single ventricle. **A,** Digital angiogram in the shallow right anterior oblique projection during right atrial injection demonstrates the Fontan anastomosis to the left pulmonary artery and right-to-left shunt flow *(arrow)* into the left atrium through the operatively created 4-mm fenestration. **B,** Repeat digital angiogram in the shallow right anterior oblique projection after catheter closure with a clamshell occlusion device demonstrates a very small residual shunt into the left atrium that should close spontaneously. One side of the occlusion device is in the Fontan anastomosis, the other in the left atrium.

Table 1 ■ CARDIAC OPERATIONS CONTINUED

PROCEDURES	DESCRIPTION	RADIOLOGIC FINDINGS AND COMPLICATIONS
Damus-Stansel-Kaye (Damus) procedure	Palliative procedure for certain types of complex cyanotic congenital heart disease with systemic outflow tract obstruction, particularly univentricular heart with obstructive bulboventricular foramen, forms of double-outlet right ventricle, complete transposition with subaortic stenosis, and forms of hypoplastic left heart syndrome. The procedure involves division of the PA and anastomosis of the proximal portion to the ascending aorta. This procedure effectively bypasses systemic outflow tract obstruction. Operations performed concurrently with the Damus procedure include Fontan anastomosis, Rastelli conduits, or systemic–PA shunts to provide pulmonary blood flow.	Moderately high operative mortality largely related to the serious complex cyanotic congenital heart disease. The pulmonary valve may become insufficient because of distortion.
Fontan procedure	Palliative atrial–pulmonary anastomosis for treatment of cyanotic congenital heart disease, particularly tricuspid atresia, forms of single ventricle, and hypoplastic left heart syndrome. Originally described by Fontan and Bidet for treatment of tricuspid atresia utilizing a technique of interposing a valved conduit between the right atrium (RA) and left PA, inserting a valve into the inferior vena cava, closing the atrial septal defect, and performing a superior vena cava–right PA shunt (Glenn anastomosis). Currently most commonly performed is closure of the atrial septal defect and direct placement of a valveless conduit between the RA and PA (Fig. 17). Less commonly, a valved conduit between the RA and PA is used.	Complications include atrial arrhythmias, low cardiac output, and obstruction of the prosthetic valve/conduit. Intrapulmonary arteriovenous shunting has been demonstrated with ^{99m}Tc-labeled macroaggregated albumin, but microscopic arteriovenous malformations have not been demonstrated angiographically as have been described with the Glenn procedure.
Fenestrated Fontan procedure	Similar to Fontan procedure but with creation of a small 4-mm fenestration to allow right-to-left interatrial shunting and temporary decompression of the right heart (Fig. 18A). After repeat catheterization and a trial of balloon occlusion of the fenestration, the small defect may be closed with an occlusion device (Fig. 18B) or operation.	
Konno procedure (enlargement of the left ventricular outflow tract)	Operative enlargement of the left ventricular outflow tract and aortic annulus. Necessitates placement of a prosthetic aortic valve.	Complications include inadequate relief of left ventricular outflow obstruction and ventricular septal defect (VSD).
Left ventricular apical-to-aortic conduit	Palliative procedure to bypass left ventricular outflow tract obstruction. A valved conduit is placed from the left ventricular apex to the abdominal aorta (Fig. 19).	Complications include prosthetic valve/conduit obstruction and subsequent development of left ventricular outflow obstruction and failure. Following operation, anterior or medial impression on the gastric fundus and narrowing of the distal esophagus may be seen. Rarely, dysphagia and gastric erosion may occur.
Mustard operation	Palliative repair of complete transposition of the great vessels. The atrial septum is excised and a pericardial or Dacron baffle is then sewn in place to direct superior and inferior vena cava flow through the mitral valve into the left ventricle, which supplies the pulmonary circulation (Fig. 20A, B). The pulmonary venous return is directed through the tricuspid valve into the right ventricle, which supplies the systemic circulation (Fig. 20C, D).	Common complications include systemic venous obstruction, pulmonary venous obstruction, and right ventricular (systemic) failure. Baffle obstruction may occur early as a result of compression of the left atrium by extracardiac clot, or late as a result of scarring, tethering, or incorrect positioning of the baffle. A baffle leak may result in intra-atrial shunting (Fig. 21). Systemic venous obstruction, particularly of the superior vena cava, is a late complication in 6% of cases and may cause symptoms of syncope, chylothorax (see Figs. 1 and 21), superior vena cava syndrome, and communicating hydrocephalus. Dilatation of the azygos/hemiazygos veins is an indication of systemic venous baffle obstruction (see Figs. 22A and 23). Pulmonary venous obstruction occurs as a late complication in approximately 4% of patients and is characterized by pulmonary venous hypertension and development of interstitial and alveolar pulmonary edema (Fig. 24).

Table continued on page 1411

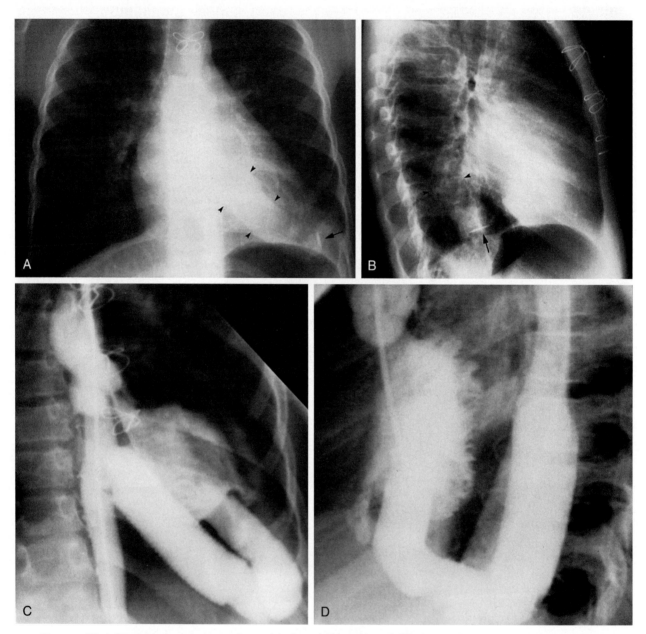

FIGURE 19. Left ventricular apical-to-aortic conduit. Frontal **(A)** and lateral **(B)** chest radiographs demonstrate a valved *(arrow)* conduit *(arrowheads)* from the left ventricular apex to the thoracic aorta in this 13-year-old girl with severe subaortic obstruction that could not be relieved with two earlier operations. Right anterior oblique **(C)** and left anterior oblique **(D)** left ventricular angiograms demonstrate the valved conduit from the left ventricular apex to the thoracic aorta. Subaortic obstruction is present.

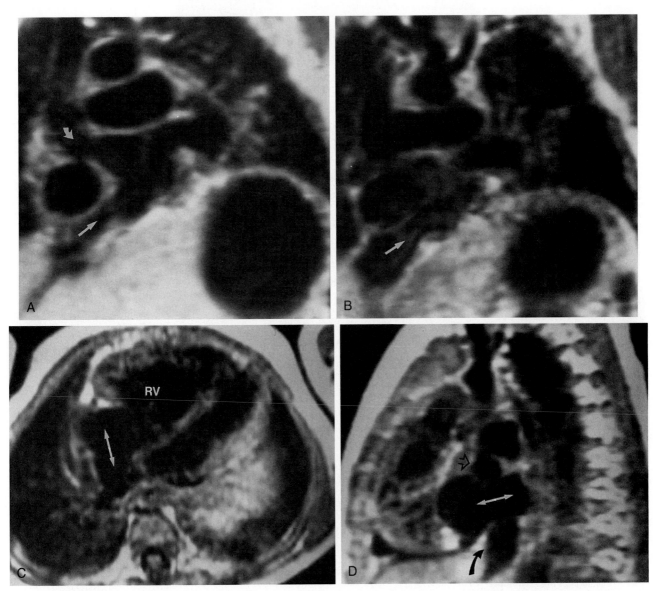

FIGURE 20. Mustard operation for complete transposition. **A,** Coronal 5-mm spin-echo magnetic resonance image (MRI) demonstrates the systemic venous limb of the atrial baffle in this 1-year-old boy. The superior vena cava *(curved arrow)* enters the superior aspect and the inferior vena cava *(straight arrow)* enters the lower aspect of the systemic venous limb. Elevation of the left hemidiaphragm secondary to phrenic nerve injury is noted above the gas-filled stomach. **B,** Coronal 5-mm spin-echo MRI of a slightly different level better demonstrates entrance of the inferior vena cava into the inferior aspect *(arrow)* of the systemic venous limb. Intraluminal echoes are consistent with slow venous flow. **C,** Axial 3-mm spin-echo MRI reveals wide patency of the pulmonary venous limb of the atrial baffle *(white double-headed arrow)*. *RV* = right ventricle. **D,** Sagittal 5-mm spin-echo MRI shows wide patency of the pulmonary venous limb of the atrial baffle *(white double-headed arrow)*. The systemic venous limb of the atrial baffle receiving the superior vena cava *(open arrow)* and inferior vena cava *(black arrow)* are also seen.

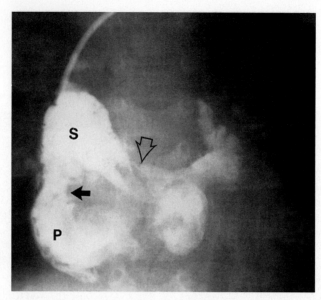

FIGURE 21. Mustard operation for complete transposition with systemic venous obstruction and chylothorax. The chest radiograph is illustrated in Figure 1. Frontal angiogram following injection of contrast into the superior aspect of the systemic venous limb of the atrial baffle *(S)* demonstrates severe obstruction of flow *(open arrow)* in this portion of the atrial baffle. A baffle leak *(closed arrow)* into the pulmonary venous limb of the atrial baffle *(P)* is also present.

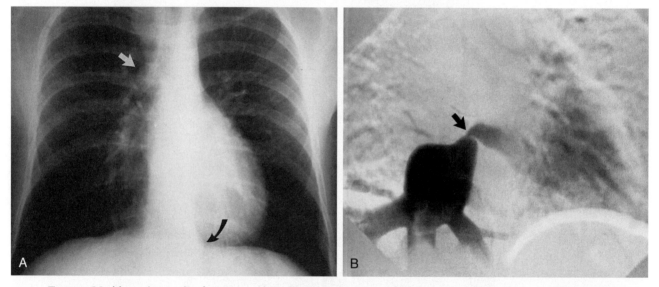

FIGURE 22. Mustard operation for transposition with systemic venous obstruction. **A,** Chest radiograph demonstrates dilatation of the azygos vein *(white arrow)* and hemiazygos vein *(black arrow)* indicating collateral flow from systemic venous obstruction. **B,** Frontal digital angiogram following injection into the inferior vena cava demonstrates severe obstruction in the inferior aspect of the systemic venous limb of the atrial baffle *(arrow)*. An injection into the superior vena cava also demonstrated obstruction of the superior aspect of the systemic venous limb of the atrial baffle similar to that in Figure 21.

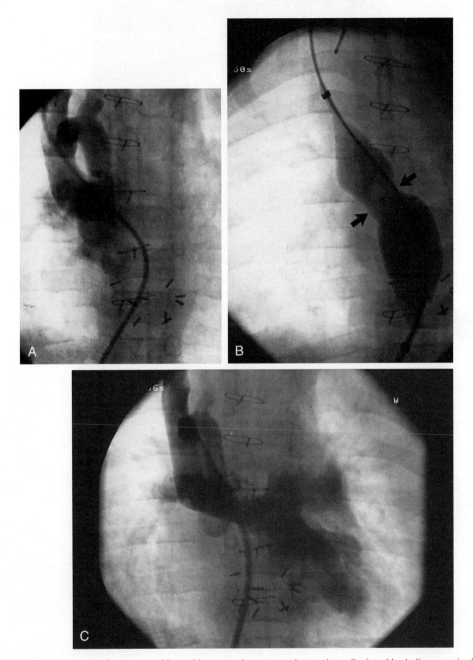

FIGURE 23. Mustard operation for transposition with systemic venous obstruction, alleviated by balloon angioplasty. **A,** In this patient with superior vena cava syndrome secondary to systemic venous obstruction following the Mustard operation, the catheter has been passed from the inferior vena cava across the inferior aspect into the superior aspect of the systemic venous limb of the atrial baffle and then into the superior vena cava. Frontal digital angiogram demonstrates complete obstruction of flow in the superior aspect of the systemic venous limb. Collateral flow through the azygos vein is seen. **B,** During balloon angioplasty of the superior aspect of the systemic venous limb, a waist is seen at the site of obstruction *(arrows)* with the balloon inflated to 20 mm. **C,** Repeat frontal digital angiogram after balloon angioplasty now demonstrates patency across the superior aspect of the systemic venous limb with filling of the left ventricle.

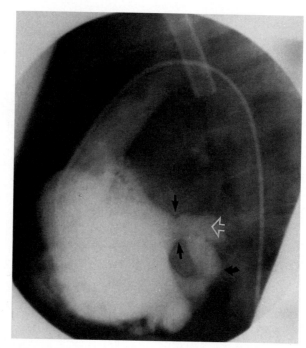

FIGURE 24. Pulmonary venous obstruction after a Mustard operation for transposition. This lateral cineangiocardiogram was made after retrograde catheter passage across the aortic valve and through the right ventricle and tricuspid valve into the distal portion of the pulmonary venous limb of the atrial baffle. Some retrograde flow of contrast into the proximal portion of the pulmonary venous limb of the atrial baffle *(open arrow)* outlines severe obstruction *(closed arrows)* in the midportion of the pulmonary venous limb. There is also retrograde opacification of the coronary sinus *(curved arrow);* this is not of significance.

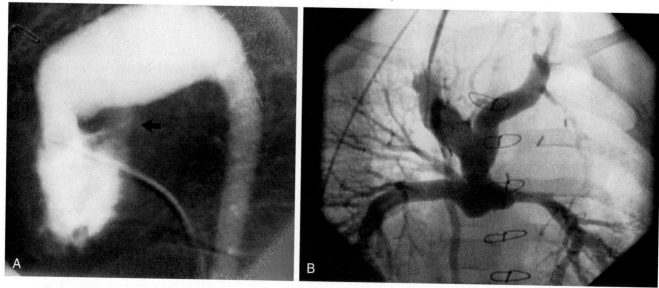

FIGURE 25. Norwood operation, stage II, in a 1-year-old boy with hypoplastic left heart syndrome. **A,** Lateral digital right ventricular angiogram opacifies the large homograft connecting the main pulmonary artery with the descending aorta. There is early opacification of the hypoplastic aorta *(arrow)* via its anastomosis with the pulmonary artery–descending aorta conduit. **B,** Anteroposterior digital angiogram after catheterization of the right internal jugular vein and injection of contrast medium into the right innominate vein opacifies the right and left innominate veins and bidirectional Glenn shunt, with opacification of the pulmonary arteries. The left pulmonary artery shows proximal narrowing, and nonfilling of the left upper lobe. Collateral flow through the right and left internal mammary veins is also seen.

Table 1 ■ CARDIAC OPERATIONS CONTINUED

PROCEDURES	DESCRIPTION	RADIOLOGIC FINDINGS AND COMPLICATIONS
Norwood operation	Palliative staged procedure for hypoplastic left heart syndrome. In stage I, the main PA is transected and an incision is made into the diminutive ascending aorta, aortic arch, and descending aorta. The hypoplastic aorta is enlarged, often with a homograft, and anastomosed to the proximal PA. The patent ductus arteriosus is ligated and an atrial septectomy performed. The distal main pulmonary artery is oversewn, and a Blalock-Taussig or central shunt placed to the pulmonary arteries. In stage II, performed around 6–12 mo, a bidirectional Glenn anastomosis or hemi-Fontan conduit is placed, and the Blalock-Taussig or central shunt ligated (Fig. 25). Stage III, performed by 2 yr, is a conversion of the Glenn anastomosis to a Fontan procedure (completion Fontan).	This procedure is associated with high morbidity and mortality. Obstruction at multiple levels, particularly the anastomosed PAs by the neoaorta and distal aorta, may be seen.
Pericardial and Dacron patch graft	Placement of pericardial and Dacron graft to operatively enlarge the right ventricular outflow tract, particularly in patients with tetralogy of Fallot. A right ventriculotomy is made, and the infundibular musculature resected. A piece of Dacron is placed across the operative incision to enlarge the right ventricular outflow tract, and if necessary can be extended across the pulmonary annulus and main PA to the PA bifurcation to enlarge a hypoplastic main PA. Currently, Dacron is placed over the right ventricular outflow tract and pericardium over the PAs.	The originally inconspicuous right ventricular outflow tract and PA become more prominent and with time show increasing convexity in this region. This prominence of the right ventricular outflow tract is normal and should not be called an aneurysm. Occasionally, calcification can be seen along the margins of the pericardial and Dacron patch graft. Rarely, postoperative aneurysms of the right ventricular outflow tract can develop, particularly in patients with persistent right ventricular outflow obstruction, residual left-to-right shunts, and significant pulmonary regurgitation (Fig. 26).
Rastelli intracardiac conduit (intracardiac baffle)	Intracardiac baffle, popularized by Rastelli, placed to establish continuity between the left ventricle and aorta (Fig. 27A) or rarely the PA. Performed usually in patients with double-outlet right ventricle and forms of transposition, particularly transposition with VSD and subpulmonic stenosis. Usually accompanied by an extracardiac conduit from the right ventricle to the PAs (Fig. 27B, C), or an arterial switch in patients with forms of transposition when the baffle has been placed to direct left ventricular blood flow to the PA.	The most common complication following this operation is residual obstruction between the left ventricle and aorta, either at the level of the VSD or from redundancy or incorrect placement of the intracardiac baffle. When the VSD must be enlarged during placement of the baffle, complete heart block may result, necessitating a pacemaker.
Rastelli extracardiac conduit	Extracardiac conduit, originally designed by Rastelli, is placement of an external conduit between the right ventricle and PAs during operative repair of patients with tetralogy of Fallot with pulmonary atresia, truncus arteriosus, and forms of double-outlet right ventricle (Fig. 27B, C). Either a homograft aortic valve with segment of ascending aorta or a Dacron conduit with porcine aortic valve is used.	Calcification of the conduit/prosthetic valve may be seen and is a clue to the development of conduit obstruction (Fig. 28). Postoperative obstruction may occur at the proximal or distal anastomotic sites (Fig. 29), at the level of the prosthetic valve, or within the conduit related to a neointimal fibrotic peel. Pseudoaneurysms may develop at the proximal or distal anastomotic site (Fig. 30).
Ross procedure	Replacement of the stenotic and/or insufficient aortic valve with the native pulmonary valve. A homograft valved conduit is then placed in the pulmonary valve position. Advantages of this procedure include native tissue in the aortic valve position, which obviates the need for anticoagulation.	Complications include stenosis and/or regurgitation of the neoaortic valve. The conduit may develop a neointimal peel and calcify.
Senning operation	Palliative repair for patients with complete transposition of the great vessels. This procedure is similar to a Mustard operation, directing superior and inferior venae cavae flow through the mitral valve into the left ventricle, and pulmonary venous flow through the right tricuspid valve into the right ventricle.	The operation has a lower incidence of systemic or pulmonary venous obstruction than the Mustard operation.
Subclavian flap	Utilization of the proximal left subclavian artery for coarctation repair. The left subclavian artery is ligated distal to the vertebral artery, and the proximal portion of the subclavian artery utilized to enlarge the aortic isthmus and site of coarctation during coarctation repair.	Anastomotic narrowing is the primary complication. The left arm is supplied by mediastinal and intercostal collaterals.

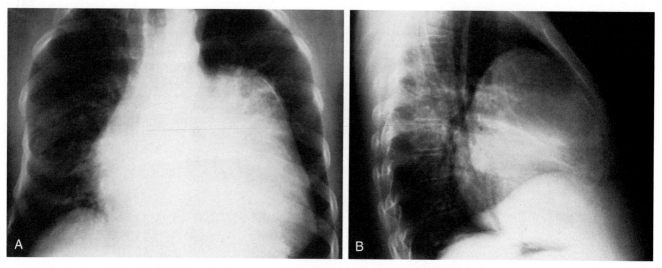

FIGURE 26. Tetralogy of Fallot repair with aneurysmal dilatation of the right ventricular outflow tract patch. Frontal **(A)** and lateral **(B)** chest radiographs demonstrate aneurysmal dilatation of the right ventricular outflow tract patch with marginal calcification. Moderate cardiomegaly is present secondary to severe pulmonary regurgitation with right ventricular dilatation.

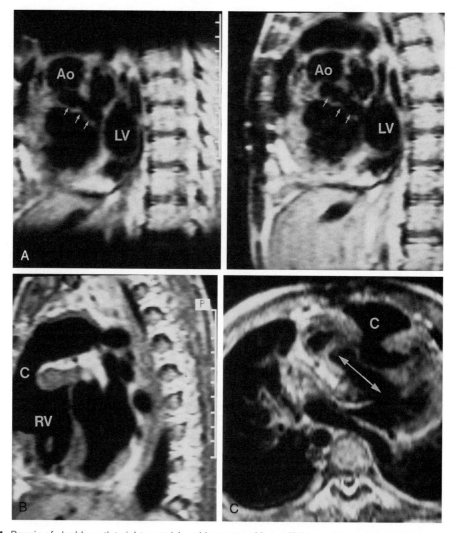

FIGURE 27. Repair of double-outlet right ventricle with transposition utilizing an intracardiac and extracardiac conduit. **A,** Sagittal 3-mm adjacent spin-echo magnetic resonance images (MRIs) demonstrate the intracardiac conduit and ventricular septal defect *(arrows)* establishing continuity between the left ventricle *(LV)* and transposed aorta *(Ao)*. Posterior to the aorta is the pulmonary artery, which has been ligated just above the valve. **B,** Sagittal 3-mm spin-echo MRI demonstrates the extracardiac conduit *(C)* establishing continuity between the right ventricle *(RV)* and pulmonary arteries. The ventricular septum and left ventricle are posterior to the right ventricle. **C,** Axial 3-mm spin-echo MRI demonstrates the patent intracardiac conduit *(arrows)* between the left ventricle and aorta, and external cardiac conduit *(C)* between the right ventricle and pulmonary artery.

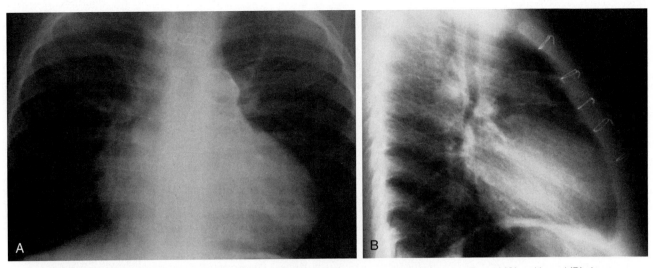

FIGURE 28. Truncus arteriosus repair in a 3-year-old patient utilizing an extracardiac conduit. Frontal **(A)** and lateral **(B)** chest radiographs demonstrate calcification of the extracardiac conduit between the right ventricle and pulmonary arteries following repair.

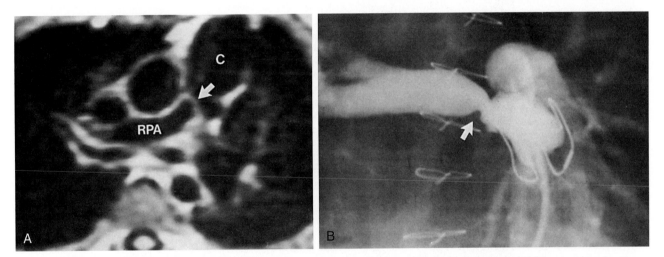

FIGURE 29. Truncus arteriosus repair utilizing an extracardiac conduit with anastomotic stenosis. **A,** Axial 3-mm spin-echo magnetic resonance image demonstrates anastomotic obstruction *(arrow)* between the extracardiac conduit *(C)* and right pulmonary artery *(RPA)*. **B,** Frontal pulmonary artery angiogram with injection of contrast into the conduit just distal to the prosthetic valve confirms the anastomotic narrowing *(arrow)* of the proximal right pulmonary artery.

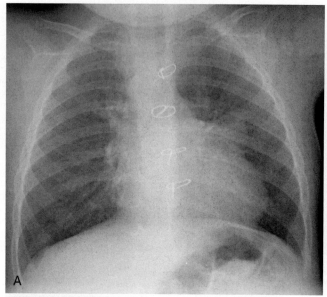
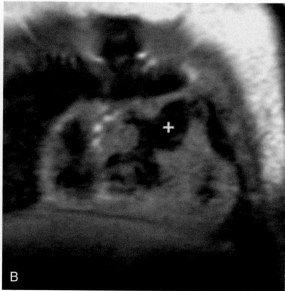
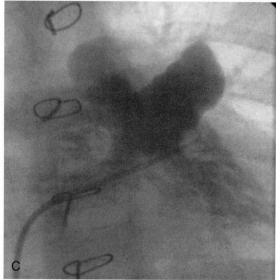

FIGURE 30. Right ventricular outflow tract pseudoaneurysm following tetralogy of Fallot repair. **A,** Frontal radiograph in a 1-year-old child, 2 months after tetralogy repair demonstrates an unusual focal density along the left heart margin. Changes related to median sternotomy, normal pulmonary blood flow, cardiomegaly with right heart enlargement, inconspicuous main pulmonary artery, and right aortic arch are also seen. **B,** Coronal T_1-weighted spin-echo magnetic resonance image demonstrates the pseudoaneurysm (+) arising from the right ventricular outflow tract. **C,** Anteroposterior digital right ventriculogram (systolic image) confirms the pseudoaneurysm arising from the right ventricular outflow tract. Mild narrowing of the proximal right pulmonary artery is present.

SUGGESTED READINGS

Ascuitto RJ, Ross-Ascuitto NT, Markowitz RI, et al: Aneurysms of the right ventricular outflow tract after tetralogy of Fallot repair: role of radiology. Radiology 1988;167:115–119

Bargeron LM Jr, Karp RB, Barcia A, et al: Late deterioration of patients after superior vena cava to right pulmonary artery anastomosis. Am J Cardiol 1972;30:211–216

Berman MA, Barash PS, Hellenbrand WE, et al: Late development of severe pulmonary venous obstruction following the Mustard operation. Cardiovasc Surg 1976;56:2-91–2-94

Bickers GH, Williams SM, Harned RK, et al: Gastroesophageal deformities of left ventricular-abdominal aortic conduit. AJR Am J Roentgenol 1982;138:867–869

Bridges ND, Jonas RA, Mayer JE, et al: Bidirectional cavopulmonary anastomosis as interim palliation for high-risk Fontan candidates. Circulation 1990;82(Suppl IV):IV-170–IV-176

Bridges ND, Lock JE, Castaneda AR: Baffle fenestration with subsequent transcatheter closure: modification of the Fontan operation for patients at increased risk. Circulation 1990;82:1681–1689

Bull C, de Leval MR, Stark J, et al: Use of subpulmonary ventricular chamber in the Fontan circulation. J Thorac Cardiovasc Surg 1983;85:21–31

Castaneda AR, Trusler GA, Paul MH, et al: The early results of treatment of simple transposition in the current era. J Thorac Cardiovasc Surg 1988;95:14–28

Ceithami EL, Puga FJ, Danielson GK, et al: Results of the Damus-Stansel-Kaye procedure for transposition of the great arteries and for double-outlet right ventricle with subpulmonary ventricular septal defect. Ann Thorac Surg 1984;38:433–437

Clouthier A, Ash JM, Smallhorn JF, et al: Abnormal distribution of pulmonary blood flow after the Glenn shunt or Fontan procedure: risk of development of arteriovenous fistulae. Circulation 1985;72:471–479

Di Donato RM, Wernovsky G, Walsh EP, et al: Results of the arterial switch operation for transposition of the great arteries with ventricular septal defect. Circulation 1989;80:1689–1705

Driscoll DJ, Nihill MR, Vargo TA, et al: Late development of pulmonary venous obstruction following Mustard's operation using a Dacron baffle. Circulation 1977;55:484–488

Ellis K: Postoperative roentgen evaluation of total correction of tetralogy of Fallot. Circulation 1973;47:1335–1348

Freedom RM, Benson LN, Smallhorn JF, et al: Subaortic stenosis, the univentricular heart, and banding of the pulmonary artery: an analysis of the courses of 43 patients with univentricular heart palliated by pulmonary artery banding. Circulation 1986;73: 758–764

Freedom RM, Culham JAG, Olley PM, et al: Anatomic correction of transposition of the great arteries: pre- and postoperative cardiac catheterization, with angiocardiography in five patients. Circulation 1981;63:905–914

Girod DA, Fontan F, Deville C, et al: Long-term results after the Fontan operation for tricuspid atresia. Circulation 1987;75:605–610

Gutierrez F, Mirowitz S, Canter C: Magnetic resonance imaging in the evaluation of postoperative congenital heart disease. Semin Ultrasound CT MR 1990;11:234–245

Kersting-Sommerhoff BA, Seelos KC, Hardy C, et al: Evaluation of surgical procedures for cyanotic congenital heart disease by using MR imaging. AJR Am J Roentgenol 1990;155:259–266

Mullins CE: Pediatric and congenital therapeutic cardiac catheterization. Circulation 1989;79:1153–1159

Norman JC, Nihill MR, Cooley DA: Valved apico-aortic composite conduits for left ventricular outflow tract obstructions. Am J Cardiol 1980;45:1265–1271

Rizk G, Moller JH, Amplatz K: The angiographic appearance of the heart following the Mustard procedure. Radiology 1973;106: 269–273

Sidi D, Planche C, Kachaner J, et al: Anatomic correction of simple transposition of the great arteries in 50 neonates. Circulation 1987;75:429–435

Trusler GA, Williams WG, Cohen AJ, et al: The cavopulmonary shunt. Circulation 1990;82(Suppl IV):IV-131–IV-138

Waldman JD, Lamberti JJ, George L, et al: Experience with Damus procedure. Circulation 1988;78(Suppl III):III-32–III-39

Welch E, Zabaleta I, Fojaco R, et al: Aneurysms of the right ventricular outflow tract: a complication of aorta-main pulmonary (central) shunt. Pediatr Cardiol 1991;12:229–232

■ C h a p t e r   2

INTERVENTIONAL CATHETERIZATION PROCEDURES

RICHARD B. JAFFE and VIRGIL R. CONDON

Since Rashkind's balloon atrial septostomy in 1966, catheters have been utilized with increasing frequency to perform therapeutic procedures within the heart. The development of balloon catheters has resulted in significant advancement in intracardiac therapeutic procedures (Table 1). Atrial septostomies can now be performed with balloon or blade catheters. Balloon catheters have been utilized to dilate valves (balloon valvuloplasty) and efficaciously treat patients with congenital pulmonary valve (see Section V, Part II, Chapter 2, Fig. 3, page 1286 and Chapter 4, Fig. 3, page 1326) or aortic valve stenosis (see Section V, Part II, Chapter 2, Fig. 7, page 1289), rheumatic mitral stenosis, and bioprosthetic valve stenosis. Balloon catheters also have been utilized to dilate vessels (balloon angioplasty) to treat coarctation (see Section V, Part II, Chapter 2, Fig. 20, page 1297), stenosis following coarctation repair, peripheral pulmonary artery stenosis (Fig. 1), pulmonary venous stenosis, and patients with baffle obstruction of the superior or inferior vena cava (see Section V, Part VII, Chapter 1, Fig. 23, page 1409). It occasionally proves efficacious in the treatment of anastomotic narrowing in patients with Blalock-Taussig shunts. In certain patients balloon catheters are indicated in the treatment of membranous subaortic stenosis. Occlusion devices are available for the closure of atrial (see Section V, Part II, Chapter 1, Fig. 12, page 1267) and ventricular (see Section V, Part II, Chapter 1, Fig. 7, page 1264) septal defects. Coil occlusion is useful for the embolic closure of systemic–pulmonary artery collaterals (Fig. 2A, B), systemic–pulmonary artery shunts (Fig. 3), venous collaterals (Fig. 4), aberrant arteries (see Section V, Part II, Chapter 1, Fig. 33, page 1280), patent ductus arteriosus closure (see Section V, Part II, Chapter 1, Fig. 20, page 1273), and pulmonary arteriovenous malformations. Rigid metallic vascular stents are utilized for long-term therapy of arterial and venous obstruction in the superior and inferior venae cavae, pulmonary arteries, and peripheral arteries. Common complications that may result from interventional procedures include "lost" occlusion coils (Fig. 2C) and "lost" balloons or balloon fragments (Fig. 5). Catheter retrieval of intravascular foreign bodies has been used to remove broken fragments of indwelling catheters that have become severed and embolized distally (Fig. 6). Many of these procedures described above are discussed further in Section V, Part II and Part VII, Chapter 1.

Table 1 ■ INTERVENTIONAL CATHETERIZATION PROCEDURES

Atrial Septostomy
Balloon
Blade

Valve Dilatation (Balloon Valvuloplasty)
Pulmonary valve stenosis (see Section V, Part II, Chapter 2, Fig. 3, page 1286 and Chapter 4, Fig. 3, page 1326)
Aortic valve stenosis (see Section V, Part II, Chapter 2, Fig. 7, page 1289)
Rheumatic mitral valve stenosis
Bioprosthetic "pulmonary" valve stenosis

Vessel Dilatation (Balloon Angioplasty)
Coarctation (see Section V, Part II, Chapter 2, Fig. 20, page 1297)
Peripheral pulmonary artery stenosis (Fig. 1)
Pulmonary venous stenosis
Atrial baffle obstruction of the superior or inferior vena cava (see Section V, Part VII, Chapter 1, Fig. 23, page 1409)
Systemic—pulmonary artery shunts

Miscellaneous
Subaortic stenosis

Vascular Stents
Venous
Arterial

Occlusion Devices
Atrial septal defect (see Section V, Part II, Chapter 1, Fig. 12, page 1267)
Ventricular septal defect (see Section V, Part II, Chapter 1, Fig. 7, page 1264)
Patent ductus arteriosus (see Section V, Part II, Chapter 1, Fig. 20, page 1273)
Systemic—pulmonary artery collaterals (Fig. 2)
Systemic—pulmonary artery shunts (Fig. 3)
Venous collaterals (Fig. 4)
Aberrant arteries (see Section V, Part II, Chapter 1, Fig. 33, page 1280)
Pulmonary arteriovenous malformations

Foreign Body Retrieval (Figs. 5 and 6)

Catheter Ablation of Cardiac Arrhythmia

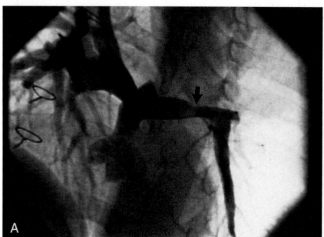 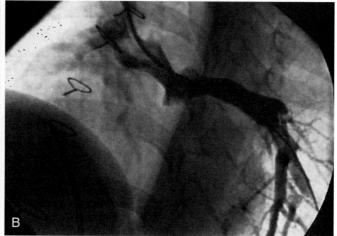

FIGURE 1. Balloon angioplasty of peripheral pulmonary artery stenosis. **A,** Digital pulmonary angiogram in the axial left anterior oblique projection following catheter passage down the superior vena cava into the pulmonary artery in this patient with bidirectional Glenn procedure demonstrates peripheral left pulmonary artery stenosis at the site of previous left pulmonary artery repair *(arrow).* **B,** Repeat digital pulmonary angiogram following balloon angioplasty with an 8-mm, then a 12-mm balloon demonstrates complete relief of the left pulmonary artery obstruction.

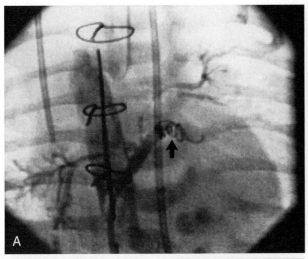

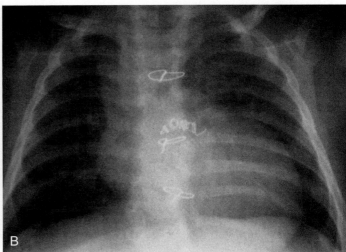

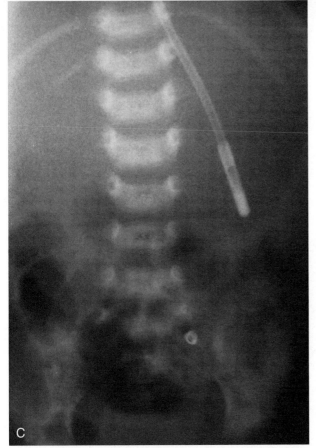

FIGURE 2. Coil occlusion of systemic–pulmonary collaterals in a neonate with pulmonary atresia. **A,** Frontal digital aortogram demonstrates coil occlusion *(arrow)* of a systemic–pulmonary artery collateral to the left lung arising from the right descending aorta. **B,** Chest radiograph demonstrates multiple vertebral anomalies, right ventricular enlargement, absence of the main pulmonary artery segment, right aortic arch, and coil occlusion of the systemic–pulmonary artery collateral to the left lung. **C,** Abdominal radiograph demonstrates a "lost" occlusion coil shown angiographically to be in the left external iliac artery.

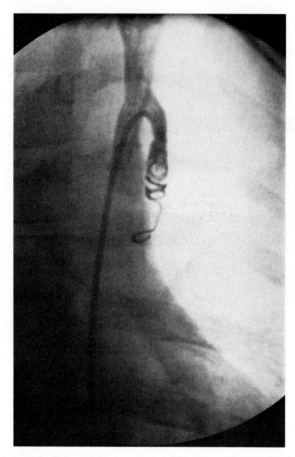

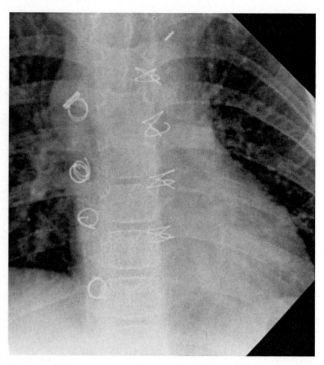

FIGURE 4. Coil occlusion of the azygos vein (same patient as in Section V, Part VII, Chapter 1, Fig. 7, page 1398). In this patient with bidirectional Glenn shunt, coil occlusion of the azygos vein has been performed at multiple levels to prevent collateral flow through the azygos system, bypassing the Glenn shunt.

FIGURE 3. Coil embolization of a left Blalock-Taussig shunt. Digital angiogram following injection in the proximal left Blalock-Taussig shunt confirms occlusion of the shunt after placement of a Gianturco coil.

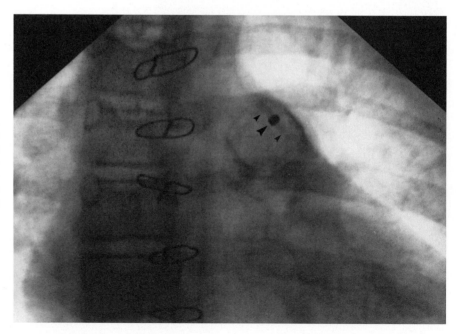

FIGURE 5. Digital spot radiograph demonstrates a broken balloon *(small arrowheads)* and catheter fragment *(large arrowhead)* lodged in the calcified extracardiac conduit following attempted balloon angioplasty of the prosthetic valve in this patient after repair of truncus arteriosus.

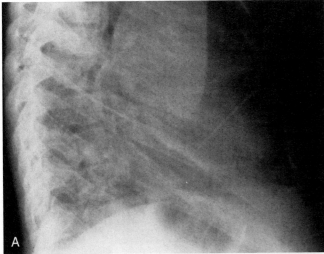

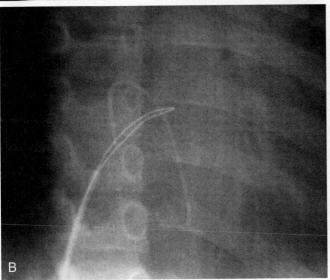

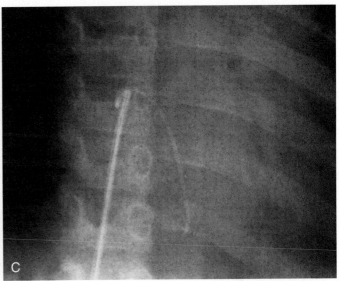

FIGURE 6. Catheter retrieval of broken right atrial line. **A,** Lateral chest radiograph demonstrates a right atrial line fractured just below the skin during attempted removal 4 days after tetralogy of Fallot repair. **B,** Fluoroscopic spot film in the frontal projection demonstrates the wire snare in position adjacent to the end of the right atrial catheter fragment. **C,** The snare has been retracted into the guiding catheter around the end of the catheter fragment. The guiding catheter, snare, and catheter fragment were withdrawn as a unit through a 6 Fr. sheath in the right femoral vein.

SUGGESTED READINGS

Lock JE, Cockerman JT, Keane JF, et al: Transcatheter umbrella closure of congenital heart defects. Circulation 1987;75:593–599

Lock JE, Block PC, McKay RG, et al: Transcatheter closure of ventricular septal defects. Circulation 1988;78:361–368

Lois JF, Gomes AS, Smith DC, et al: Systemic-to-pulmonary collateral vessels and shunts: treatment with embolization. Radiology 1988; 169:671–676

Medellin GJ, Di Sessa TG, Tonkin ILD: Interventional catheterization in congenital heart disease. Radiol Clin North Am 1989;27:1223

Mullins CE: Pediatric and congenital therapeutic cardiac catheterization. Circulation 1989;79:1153–1159

O'Laughlin MP, Perry SB, Lock JE, et al: Use of endovascular stents in congenital heart disease. Circulation 1991;83:1923–1939

Rocchini AP: Transcatheter closure of atrial septal defects. Circulation 1990;82:1044–1045

Rome JJ, Keane JF, Perry SB, et al: Double-umbrella closure of atrial defects. Circulation 1990;82:751–785

Wren C: Catheter ablation in paediatric arrhythmias. Arch Dis Child 1999;81:102

SECTION VI

Abdomen and Gastrointestinal Tract

ALAN E. SCHLESINGER

BRUCE R. PARKER

JACK O. HALLER

A'DELBERT BOWEN

CARLOS J. SIVIT

RICHARD B. TOWBIN

OVERVIEW

BRUCE R. PARKER
JACK O. HALLER

The peritoneal cavity contains the organs of digestion and absorption; the solid organs such as the liver, spleen, and pancreas; and vascular, nervous, and lymphatic structures. For this reason, abdominal imaging uses virtually every modality and type of contrast material. Each organ system within the abdomen, however, is unique and requires a different imaging approach. Each chapter within this section, therefore, covers the imaging modalities used in the specific area under discussion.

Some general comments can be made, however. Fluoroscopic and radiographic examinations continue to be the mainstay of examinations of the gastrointestinal (GI) tract. Barium continues to be the most commonly used contrast material. In specific circumstances, however, the use of other contrast materials is preferable. Water-soluble agents are of particular value when the possibility of extravasation or perforation exists. The most commonly used water-soluble agents are hyperosmolar and may lead to dehydration, especially in infants. Their use should be carefully monitored and appropriate replacement intravenous fluids given concomitantly. The use of lower osmolar water-soluble agents such as the newer intravascular contrast agents, is safer but carries a higher financial outlay. Water-soluble agents are often used when the possibility of prolonged retention of barium is present, possibly leading to inspissation, such as in aganglionosis or other forms of severe constipation. Those radiologists who prefer positive contrast agents for the reduction of intussusception also use water-soluble agents.

Although the mucosal detail of the GI tract is not as readily evaluated with water-soluble materials as it is with barium, most studies in children are done for anatomic abnormalities. The majority of children in whom mucosal lesions are of concern, such as those with suspected ulcer disease or inflammatory bowel disease, usually can tolerate barium without difficulty.

Double-contrast studies of the esophagus and upper GI tract are less commonly performed in children than in adults. Children under age 9 have difficulty swallowing the effervescent tablets or powders and frequently develop eructation. Children over that age usually are more cooperative, but the indications for the fine mucosal detail thereby obtained are infrequent in childhood.

The solid organs are amenable to study with ultrasound, computed tomography, magnetic resonance imaging, and nuclear medicine as well as angiography on occasion. The value of these studies is discussed in the respective chapters.

With interest focused on the use of advanced imaging techniques, it is not surprising that less attention is now paid to plain film evaluation of the abdomen than in prior days. Nevertheless, plain films remain a valuable tool in the assessment of abdominal abnormalities. Intestinal obstruction, free intraperitoneal air, and intra-abdominal calcifications are readily seen on plain films. With the plethora of advanced imaging modalities available to us, plain films are often an excellent guide to determining the proper imaging study to perform for a particular problem. Each chapter in this section discusses the relevant findings for the various disease entities being addressed.

PART II

ABDOMINAL WALL AND PERITONEAL CAVITY

ALAN E. SCHLESINGER

BRUCE R. PARKER

Chapter 1

ANATOMY AND EMBRYOLOGY OF THE ABDOMINAL WALL

ALAN E. SCHLESINGER and BRUCE R. PARKER

The abdomen extends from the diaphragm superiorly to the pelvis inferiorly and includes both intraperitoneal and extraperitoneal structures. The advent of cross-sectional imaging has made knowledge of abdominal anatomy and embryology even more important than previously.

■ Knowledge of the normal anatomy and embryological development of the abdominal wall and peritoneum are important for interpretation of cross-sectional imaging studies.

1424

NORMAL ANATOMY

The diaphragm forms the roof of the abdomen. Its anatomy and development are discussed in Section IV, Part V. The posterior abdominal wall comprises the spine, the paraspinous muscles, and the tissues superficial to them. The posterior wall structures are discussed in Section III, Part VIII. The remainder of the abdomen includes the abdominal wall and retroperitoneal and pelvic structures, discussed in this section, and the extraperitoneal organs, which are discussed in Section VII.

From superficial to deep, the anterior abdominal wall is composed of the skin, superficial fascia (the Camper and Scarpa layers), subcutaneous fat, muscles, transverse fascia (the Gallaudet or innominate fascia), properitoneal fat, and peritoneum. The paired rectus muscles run cephalocaudad in the midline. The paired anterolateral muscle groups include the external and internal oblique muscles and the transverse abdominal muscle (Fig. 1). The aponeuroses of the external oblique muscles carry downward and medially to cover the front of the abdomen from the xyphoid to the pubis. At the lateral margins of the rectus muscles, the aponeuroses split to form the spigelian fascia, which forms the anterior and posterior rectus sheaths. The sheaths join in the midline, forming the linea alba, which separates the two rectus muscles by up to 6 mm.

The lowermost portion of the aponeurosis of the external oblique muscle ends in a thickened free border, the inguinal ligament, which runs from the anterior superior iliac spine to the pubic tubercle. The subcutaneous (or external) inguinal ring is an opening in the aponeurosis of the external oblique muscle between the inguinal ligament inferiorly and the tendinous portion superiorly. The spermatic cord in males or the round ligament in females passes through the inguinal canal.

EMBRYOLOGY

The embryology of the abdominal wall is discussed in Section II, Part IV, Chapter 1. Congenital abnormalities are discussed in Section II, Part IV, Chapter 3.

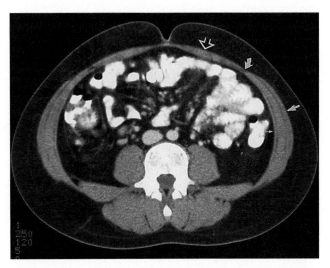

FIGURE 1. Computed tomography scan at the level of the umbilicus in an obese 11-year-old boy demonstrates the abdominal musculature to good advantage. The external oblique muscle *(solid white straight arrow)* and the transverse abdominal muscle *(small white arrow)* are seen on either side of the internal oblique muscle. The aponeurosis of the external oblique muscle becomes the spigelian fascia *(curved white arrow)*, which splits to form the anterior and posterior sheaths of the rectus abdominus muscle *(open arrow)*.

SUGGESTED READINGS

DiSantis DJ, Siegel MJ, Katz ME: Simplified approach to umbilical remnant abnormalities. Radiographics 1991;11:59

Duhamel B: Embryology of exomphalos and allied malformations. Arch Dis Child 1963;38:142

Hutchin P: Somatic anomalies of the umbilicus and anterior abdominal wall. Surg Gynecol Obstet 1965;120:1075

Moore KL, Persaud TVN (eds): Body cavities, primitive mesenteries, and the diaphragm. *In* The Developing Human, 6th ed. Philadelphia, WB Saunders, 1998:174–185

Moore KL, Persaud TVN (eds): The digestive system. *In* The Developing Human, 6th ed. Philadelphia, WB Saunders, 1998:237–264

Moore KL, Persaud TVN (eds): The urogenital system. *In* The Developing Human, 6th ed. Philadelphia, WB Saunders, 1998:265–303

Skandalakis JE, Gray SW, Rickets RR: Anterior body wall. *In* Skandalakis JE, Gray SW (eds): Embryology for Surgeons, 2nd ed. Baltimore, Williams & Wilkins, 1994:540–593

Skandalakis JE, Gray SW, Rickets RR, Richardson DD: Peritoneum. *In* Skandalakis JE, Gray SW (eds): Embryology for Surgeons, 2nd ed. Baltimore, Williams & Wilkins, 1994:113–149

Skandalakis JE, Gray SW, Rickets RR, Richardson DD: Small intestines. *In* Skandalakis JE, Gray SW (eds): Embryology for Surgeons, 2nd ed. Baltimore, Williams & Wilkins, 1994:184–241

Chapter 2

ABDOMINAL WALL ABNORMALITIES

ALAN E. SCHLESINGER and BRUCE R. PARKER

HERNIAS

DIAPHRAGMATIC HERNIAS

Herniation of abdominal contents can occur superiorly into the thorax, inferiorly through the femoral and inguinal canals, anteriorly through abdominal wall defects or the umbilical ring, and, very rarely, posteriorly through defects in the musculature. Diaphragmatic hernias are discussed more fully in Section IV, Parts IV, V, and VI; Section VI, Part V; and Section II, Part IV. Herniation of the stomach through the esophageal hiatus is the most common of these. A sliding hiatus hernia in which the esophagogastric junction is above the hiatus is the most frequently occurring type. A paraesophageal hernia occurs when the gastric fundus and proximal body herniate into the chest, leaving the esophagogastric junction in near-normal position (see Section VI, Part V, Chapter 5, Figs. 8 through 11, pages 1574 through 1576).

> ■ Hernias may occur in the diaphragm, the groin, and the anterior abdominal wall.

Diaphragmatic hernias may occur posteriorly and laterally through patent pleuroperitoneal canals, also known as the *foramina of Bochdalek*. Bochdalek's hernias usually occur during fetal development and present in the newborn (see Section II, Part IV, Chapter 3, page 111), but delayed Bochdalek hernias in older children are being reported with increasing frequency (Fig. 1). In the newborn, the hernias are more commonly left sided, but the opposite has been suggested in patients with delayed appearance. However, some studies have not confirmed the right-sided predominance of delayed Bochdalek's hernias. Berman et al. reported 26 patients with Bochdalek hernias diagnosed more than 8 weeks after birth. Twenty-two were left-sided, three were right-sided, and one was bilateral. Misdiagnosis had occurred in 16 of the patients. Only one third of the patients had pulmonary hypoplasia, consistent with a later onset of the herniation than is true of those patients diagnosed at birth. Delayed right-sided Bochdalek's hernias have been reported in neonates with group B streptococcal infection. A rare variant of Bochdalek's hernia is herniation

of abdominal contents into the pericardium through an incompletely closed pericardioperitoneal canal.

The diagnosis of congenital Bochdalek's hernia is usually made by clinical means and plain radiographs in which loops of bowel can be seen in a hemithorax with corresponding displacement of the mediastinum to the contralateral side and a paucity of intra-abdominal bowel loops. If the diagnosis is in doubt, ultrasound (US) can identify peristalsis of loops of bowel in the thorax, or contrast studies can definitively document the herniation of the intestines. Magnetic resonance imaging (MRI) can aid in the prenatal diagnosis of Bochdalek's hernia and can help to differentiate herniated bowel loops from other chest lesions. Computed tomography (CT) has been shown to be useful in the diagnosis of delayed congenital Bochdalek's hernia. In traumatic diaphragmatic hernias, CT, MRI, and oral contrast studies have been shown to play a role in imaging, but a high clinical index of suspicion of traumatic hernia is crucial.

The *foramen of Morgagni* is an anterior and medial diaphragmatic defect through which hernias occur less commonly in children than in adults. Small hernias are difficult to diagnose definitively on plain radiographs because the most common structure to herniate through the foramen is the transverse mesocolon, which appears as a solid mass in the cardiophrenic angle. The liver commonly herniates through the foramen in young children (Fig. 2). If bowel, usually transverse colon, herniates through the foramen, an air-filled structure may be seen in the same location. Morgagni's hernias are more common on the right than the left, but may be bilateral. US, CT, and MRI have all been used to identify the contents of the hernia.

GROIN AND PELVIC HERNIAS

Indirect inguinal hernias are the most common form of inferior abdominal wall herniation. If the processus vaginalis remains open, bowel can herniate through the inguinal ring into the scrotum in boys (Fig. 3A) or through the canal of Nuck into the labia majora in girls, the latter being relatively infrequent. Ovarian tissue can also herniate through the canal of Nuck (Fig. 3B). Most inguinal hernias in children are asymptomatic, but incarceration or strangulation can cause intestinal obstruction. A sliding hernia may cause sufficient bowel

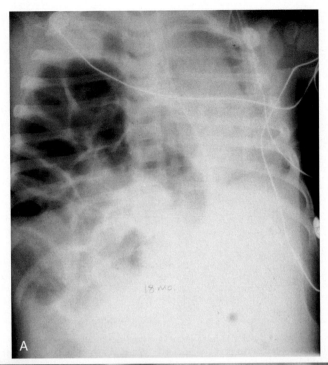

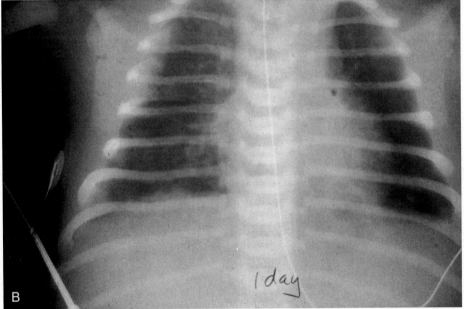

FIGURE 1. Delayed presentation of Bochdalek's hernia in an 18-month-old infant presenting with respiratory distress. **A,** Chest radiograph at presentation reveals a large right diaphragmatic hernia. **B,** Prior chest radiograph at 1 day of age (obtained because of transient tachypnea of the newborn) showed no hernia.

irritation to lead to ileus or even intermittent functional obstruction.

Inguinal hernias may be seen coincidentally on plain radiographs, usually presenting as a loop of bowel in the scrotum. In cases where the loop is persistently fluid filled, US can identify the intestinal wall surrounding the intraluminal fluid and may show small bubbles of air or peristalsis. Color Doppler US may show blood flow in the wall of the herniated bowel loop. These findings help differentiate a hernia from a hydrocele, which results from incomplete closure of the processus vagina-

lis. Contrast studies are rarely needed, but a small bowel series may demonstrate the herniated loop. Contrast enema with extensive reflux into the small intestine in infants with intestinal obstruction may show a pinched-off loop at the entrance to the inguinal canal. Contrast peritoneography (herniography) is rarely used any longer. Wechsler et al. have demonstrated the CT and MRI appearance of inguinal hernias. These studies are rarely needed for diagnostic purposes in children, but the hernias may be incidental findings when these studies are performed for other reasons.

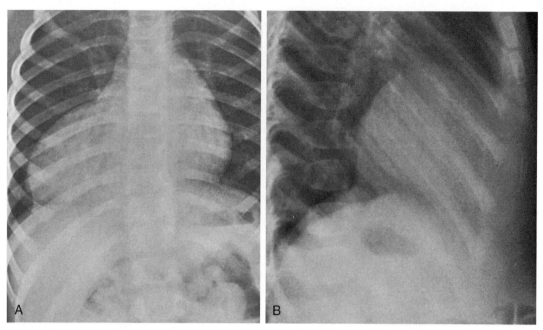

FIGURE 2. Morgagni's hernia in a 4-year-old girl in whom a chest radiograph was performed for symptoms of upper respiratory infection. Frontal **(A)** and lateral **(B)** chest radiographs reveal a right-sided anterior soft tissue mass representing the herniated portion of the liver.

Direct inguinal hernias, those in which the hernia sac is medial to the epigastric vessels, are acquired rather than congenital and are uncommon in children. *Femoral hernias* are also uncommon in the pediatric age group. The intestine herniates through the femoral ring and presents at the saphenous opening. Wechsler et al. have demonstrated the value of CT in differentiating femoral hernias from other abdominal wall masses that may have similar clinical presentations. *Hernias through the obturator foramen* typically occur in elderly women and are rarely, if ever, found in children. *Sciatic hernias* pass through the sciatic foramen into the buttock. Again,

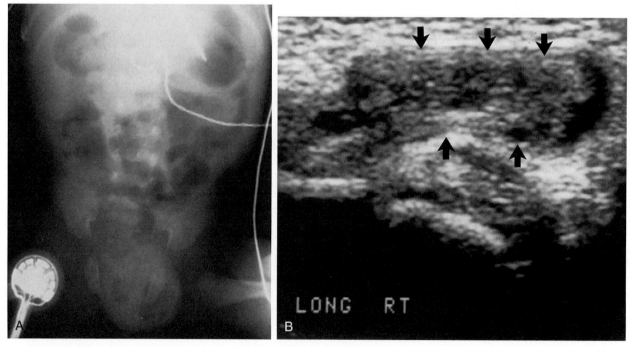

FIGURE 3. A, Anteroposterior view of the abdomen and pelvis in a newborn boy demonstrates an enlarged scrotum with multiple air-filled loops of intestine within it secondary to indirect inguinal hernia. **B,** Ultrasound in the inguinal region of an infant girl with a labial mass confirms a herniated ovary *(arrows)* in the canal of Nuck.

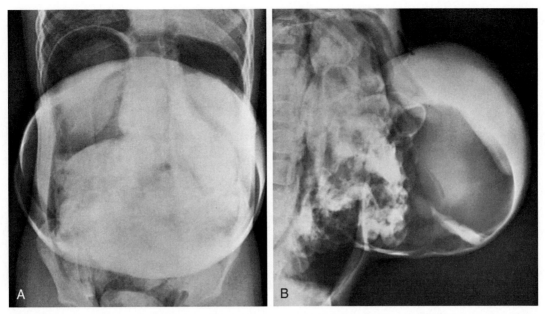

FIGURE 4. Omphalocele. Frontal **(A)** and lateral **(B)** views of the abdomen in a patient with omphalocele and pneumoperitoneum. Note that both loops of bowel and liver are included within the enclosed sac.

they are unusual in childhood but need to be included in the differential diagnosis of pelvic tumors that extend through the sciatic foramen into the buttock, such as rhabdomyosarcoma and endodermal sinus tumor.

ANTERIOR ABDOMINAL WALL DEFECTS WITH HERNIATION

The majority of patients with anterior wall defects and herniation present in the newborn period and are discussed more thoroughly in Section II, Part IV, Chapter 3, page 58. *Omphaloceles* occur in patients in whom the midgut does not return to the intraembryonic coelomic cavity by the 10th week. This leads to failure of infolding of the lateral abdominal walls. In infants, the gut appears outside the anterior abdominal wall in the base of the umbilical cord and is surrounded by a translucent sac of peritoneum and amnion (Fig. 4). With larger defects, the liver may also partially herniate into the sac. When the cephalic fold as well as the lateral folds fail to develop, the result is *ectopia cordis,* in which congenital heart disease and defects in the pericardium, diaphragm, abdominal wall, and sternum are associated (see Section IV, Parts II, IV, V, and VI). *Gastroschisis* is a paraumbilical herniation of unknown cause in newborns, half of the affected patients being prematures. Clinical differentiation from omphalocele can be made by noting the presence of a normal umbilical cord and the lack of a covering sac.

Umbilical hernias are common protrusions through the umbilical ring (Fig. 5). The majority regress as the child grows, and no diagnostic or therapeutic procedures are usually required. The hernia may rarely become incarcerated or strangulated, but the clinical diagnosis is obvious and imaging studies are not needed. The other abdominal wall hernias are rare in childhood. *Paraumbilical hernias* after infancy are unusual until adulthood. *Epigastric hernias* are defects in the linea alba between the xyphoid and umbilicus. *Spigelian hernias* are herniations through defects in the aponeurosis of the external oblique muscle and frequently are incarcerated and strangulated. CT is diagnostic in most cases, as it is with epigastric hernias. *Cloacal exstrophy* results from failure of development of the caudal fold. *Prune-belly syndrome* is the result of failure of development of the anterior wall

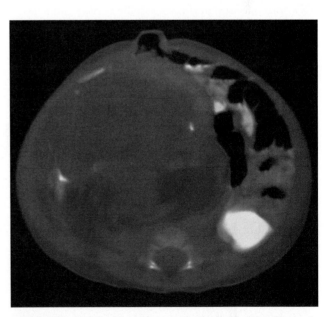

FIGURE 5. Umbilical hernia in a 3-month-old girl with cystic teratoma. Although spontaneous umbilical hernias are commonly seen, there is an increased incidence in patients with abdominal masses.

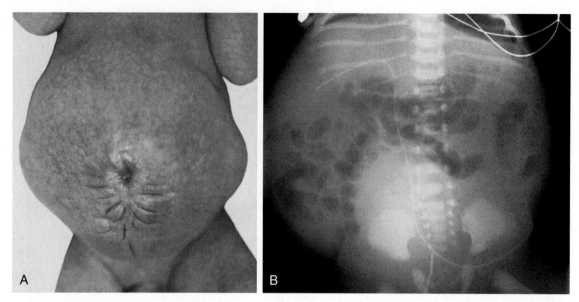

FIGURE 6. **A,** Photograph of a 5-week-old boy with prune-belly syndrome demonstrates congenital absence of the abdominal musculature. **B,** Abdominal radiograph of a different patient with prune-belly syndrome demonstrating flaccidity of the abdominal wall with marked dilatation of the bladder. An umbilical venous catheter has been misplaced in the right portal vein.

musculature (Fig. 6). These last two entities are discussed in Section II, Part IV, Chapter 3, page 111.

UMBILICAL REMNANT ABNORMALITIES

OMPHALOMESENTERIC DUCT REMNANT

The omphalomesenteric (or vitelline) duct can remain open throughout its length, at either end, or only in its midportion (Fig. 7). DiSantis et al. have defined the completely open duct as type 1, the open-ended (open either at the ilium or the umbilicus) as type 2, and the open midportion only as type 3. In type 1, fecal material can pass through the open duct from the terminal ileum to the umbilicus (Fig. 8). The opening at the umbilicus frequently can be probed and contrast material injected that passes directly into the ileum.

In type 2 open at the umbilical end, there is a sinus tract from the umbilicus to the closed portion of the omphalomesenteric duct. A nonfecal discharge may be found. Contrast injection reveals a blind-ending sinus tract. Type 2 open at the ileal end is a Meckel's diverticulum. Type 3, a vitelline duct cyst open only in the midportion of the duct, is usually asymptomatic but can lead to ileal volvulus. Vitelline duct cysts (type 3) and some Meckel's diverticula (type 2) may be large enough to be identified on US and CT as subumbilical cystic masses.

Meckel's diverticulum is not only the most commonly identified omphalomesenteric duct remnant, it is the most common congenital anomaly of the gastrointestinal tract, occurring in up to 4% of the population according to autopsy studies. As an omphalomesenteric

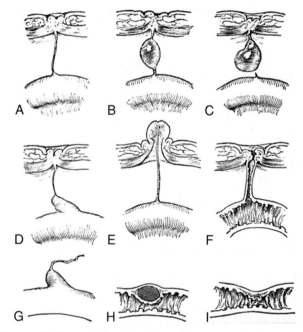

FIGURE 7. Congenital malformations that may result from persistence of the omphalomesenteric duct. *a,* Persistent cord between the ileal wall and the closed umbilicus. *b,* Cyst in the same cord. *c,* Cyst anchored at the umbilical end of the cord but free at the ileal end. *d,* Meckel's diverticulum attached to the closed umbilicus by a closed cord. *e,* Everted mucocele of the umbilicus with the cord attachment to the ileal wall. *f,* Fecal fistula open at both the umbilical and ileal ends. *g,* Meckel's diverticulum open at the ileal end but blind at the umbilical end, which is unattached. *h,* Intramural cystic diverticulum. *i,* Local stenosis of the ileum at the site of the mouth of a persistent omphalomesenteric duct. (From Cullen TS: Embryology, Anatomy and Diseases of the Umbilicus. Philadelphia, WB Saunders, 1916, with permission.)

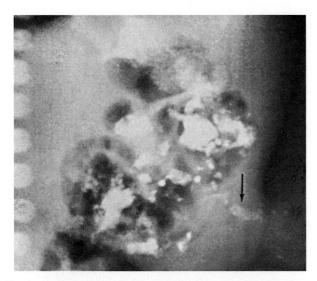

FIGURE 8. Lateral film of the abdomen from an upper gastrointestinal series demonstrates barium flowing from the ileum through a patent omphalomesenteric duct *(arrow)* to the umbilicus and the anterior abdominal wall.

the inverted Meckel's diverticulum, which acted as a lead point. Daneman, Myers, et al. described five patients with intussusception secondary to inverted Meckel's diverticula imaged with US. In four of the five children, US demonstrated the fluid-containing and/or fat-containing diverticulum at the apex of the intussusceptum.

■ Findings on plain radiographs and contrast studies in Meckel's diverticulum:
1. Common
   • Obstruction
   • Contrast studies may show point of obstruction
   • Filling defect on contrast studies if diverticulum is inverted
2. Less common
   • Enteroliths in giant diverticulum

■ Findings on ultrasound (US) and computed tomography (CT) studies in Meckel's diverticulum:
1. Common
   • Target-like mass with central echogenic fat on US if diverticulum is inverted
   • Double target sign of inverted diverticulum and associated intussusceptum on US (diverticulum may also be fluid filled)
   • Mass with fat attenuation with surrounding collar of soft tissue attenuation on CT if diverticulum is inverted
2. Less common
   • Enteroliths in giant diverticulum on CT or US

duct remnant, it projects from the antimesenteric side of the ileum anywhere from 16 to 80 cm proximal to the ileocecal valve, depending somewhat on age. Because the diverticulum represents an opening into the embryonic duct, it contains all four intestinal wall layers, making it a true diverticulum.

Most Meckel's diverticula are asymptomatic and found incidentally on imaging studies or at surgery or autopsy. Giant Meckel's diverticulum containing enteroliths may be seen on plain radiographs, CT, or US. Meckel's diverticula can lead to intestinal obstruction by acting as a lead point for intussusception (inverting into the ileal lumen) or leading to small bowel volvulus around a persistent vitelline duct remnant leading from the diverticulum to the umbilicus. Because 15% of Meckel's diverticula contain heterotopic gastric mucosa, affected patients may present with abdominal pain or gastrointestinal hemorrhage secondary to peptic ulceration. Less commonly, the diverticula may include duodenal or jejunal mucosa or pancreatic tissue.

Patients with intestinal obstruction present with typical plain radiographic findings of obstruction (see Section VI, Part VII). Contrast studies may demonstrate the point of obstruction, but the diverticulum or vitelline duct remnant is usually not seen. An inverted Meckel's diverticulum may occasionally be visualized as a filling defect on upper gastrointestinal series and small bowel follow-through. Inverted Meckel's diverticula contain invaginated mesenteric fat centrally. Therefore, they can present as a target-like mass with a central area of increased echogenicity on US and a mass of fatty attenuation with a surrounding collar of soft tissue attenuation on CT. Itagaki et al. reported an ultrasonic "double target sign" in two patients with intussusception secondary to inverted Meckel's diverticula. The two targets were adjacent to one another but of differing sizes. The larger target represented the intussusceptum and the smaller target

Patients with symptoms suspicious of peptic disease of the diverticulum are best examined initially with technetium-99m pertechnetate scintigraphy. Because the pertechnetate ion is secreted by gastric mucosa, the scan may show abnormal accumulation of radiopharmaceutical in the right midabdomen or right lower quadrant (Fig. 9). False-positive scans may result from the presence of ectopic gastric mucosa in other parts of the intestinal tract. False-negative results may occur secondary to a variety of factors. The false-negative rate may be reduced by pretreating the patient with cimetidine and glucagon. Contrast small bowel series or enema may demonstrate a Meckel's diverticulum (Figs. 10 and 11), but the sensitivity is very low, and routine barium studies are of little value. Angiography has been used to evaluate active gastrointestinal bleeding from Meckel's diverticulum and can be enhanced by the use of digital subtraction techniques. Routh et al. reported abnormal, irregular vessels supplied by an elongated, nonbranching

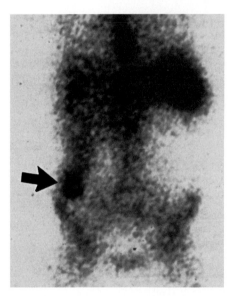

FIGURE 9. Pertechnetate nuclear medicine scan of the abdomen in a patient with chronic anemia secondary to gastrointestinal blood loss. Note the collection of radiopharmaceutical *(arrow)* in the right lower quadrant. Meckel's diverticulum was demonstrated at surgery and contained gastric mucosa at histologic examination.

ileal artery in two patients with Meckel's diverticulum who had a history of gastrointestinal bleeding but were not actively bleeding at the time of angiography. Arterial embolization in patients bleeding from Meckel's diver-

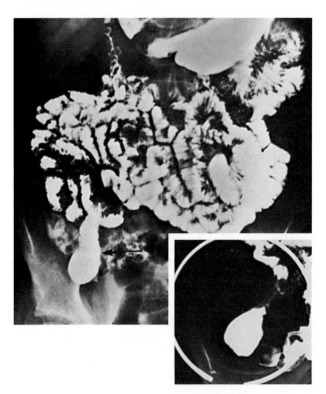

FIGURE 10. Delayed abdominal radiograph following upper gastrointestinal series in a 9-year-old child with abdominal pain demonstrates filling of a Meckel's diverticulum *(arrow)*. Inset, Pressure spot film of the involved area.

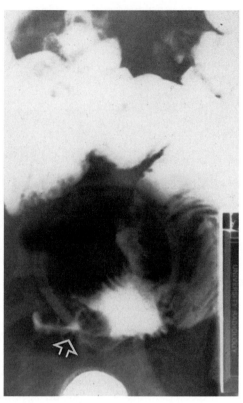

FIGURE 11. Pressure spot image of a Meckel's diverticulum from an upper gastrointestinal series in a patient with a history of gastrointestinal bleeding demonstrates a characteristic peptic ulcer with a barium-filled niche and radiating folds *(arrow)*.

ticulum has been reported. CT may show evidence of Meckel's diverticulitis, but CT diagnosis of a diverticulum is more likely to be incidental.

URACHAL REMNANT

The residuum of the embryonic allantois is known as the urachus. The urachus can be open throughout its entire course from the bladder to the skin surface at the umbilicus; a portion of the urachus can be open as a blind-ending sinus from either the dome of the bladder or the umbilical skin surface; or only the midportion may remain patent as a urachal cyst that does not communicate with the bladder or the skin surface. A fully patent urachus connects the bladder to the umbilicus, permitting urine to pass between them (Fig. 12). The umbilical opening may be difficult to catheterize because of its small size, but often the bladder can be filled in this way. Alternatively, a voiding cystourethrogram may demonstrate the connection. A urachal remnant patent only to the skin surface at the umbilicus may present with an umbilical discharge, especially when infected (Fig. 13). They are often identified by US. When open at the proximal end only, the urachal remnant appears as an extension of the bladder, most commonly at its anterosuperior portion (Fig. 12C). Cacciarelli et al. described a normal remnant of the

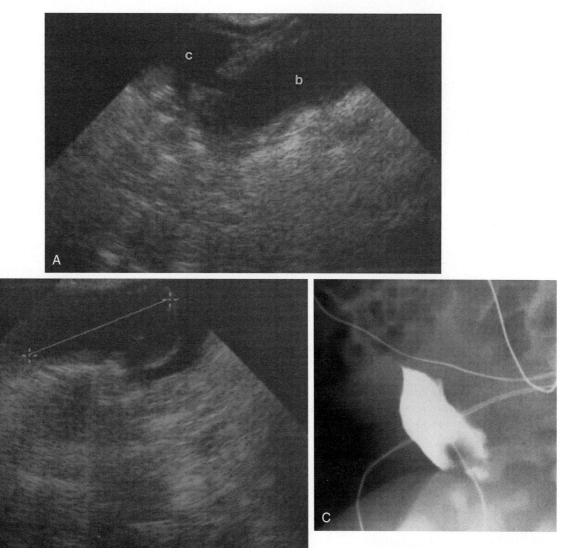

FIGURE 12. A, Longitudinal ultrasound scan demonstrates a fluid-filled tubular structure between the bladder *(b)* and a cystic structure *(c)* in the anterior abdominal wall. **B,** Transverse scan at the level of the umbilicus demonstrates a cystic structure just deep to the umbilicus. At surgery, a urachal cyst directly connecting the skin surface at the umbilicus to the bladder was excised. **C,** Cystogram in another patient demonstrates characteristic beaking of the anterosuperior aspect of the bladder caused by a patent proximal urachus. The remainder of the urachus from this point to the umbilicus is completely closed.

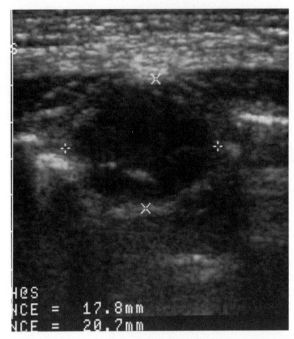

FIGURE 13. Transverse sonogram at the level of the umbilicus demonstrates a hypoechoic structure just deep to the abdominal wall. When the transducer was placed on the abdomen, purulent material was expressed from the umbilicus. An infected urachal cyst was removed at surgery.

closed urachus seen sonographically as a small, elliptical, hypoechoic structure at the anterosuperior aspect of the urinary bladder in 62 of 100 children. Urachal lesions are discussed more fully in Section VII, Part IV.

■ Incomplete involution of the umbilical structures (the omphalomesenteric duct or the urachus) can lead to a spectrum of congenital anomalies, including cysts, persistent communication between the umbilicus and either the bladder or the ileum, or blind-ending sinuses.

SUGGESTED READINGS

Hernias

Bair JH, Russ PD, Pretorius DM, et al: Fetal omphalocele and gastroschisis: a review of 24 cases. AJR Am J Roentgenol 1986; 147:1047

Balthazar EJ, Dubramanyam BR, Megibow A: Spigelian hernia: CT and ultrasonography diagnosis. Gastrointest Radiol 1984;9:81

Berman L, Stringer D, Ein SH, et al: The late-presenting pediatric Bochdalek hernia: a 20-year review. J Pediatr Surg 1988;23:735

Chou TY, Chu CC, Diau GY, et al: Inguinal hernia in children: US versus exploratory surgery and intraoperative contralateral laparoscopy. Radiology 1996;201:385

Currarino G: Incarcerated inguinal hernia in infants: plain films and barium enema. Pediatr Radiol 1974;2:247

Franken EA Jr: Anomalies of the anterior abdominal wall: classification and roentgenology. Am J Roentgenol Radium Ther Nucl Med 1971;112:58

Gayer G, Bilik R, Vardi A: CT diagnosis of delayed presentation of congenital diaphragmatic hernia simulating massive pleuropneumonia. Eur Radiol 1999;9:1672

Hubbard AM, Adzick NS, Crombleholme TM, et al: Congenital chest lesions: diagnosis and characterization with prenatal MR imaging. Radiology 1999;212:43

McCarten KM, Rosenberg HK, Borden S 4th, et al: Delayed appearance of right diaphragmatic hernia associated with group B streptococcal infections in newborns. Radiology 1981;139:385

Munden M, McEniff N, Mulvihill D: Sonographic investigation of female infants with inguinal masses. Clin Radiol 1995;50:696

Newman B, Davis PL: Sonographic and magnetic resonance imaging of an anterior diaphragmatic hernia. Pediatr Radiol 1989;20:110

Oh KS, Condon VR, Norst RP, et al: Peritoneographic demonstration of femoral hernia. Radiology 1978;127:209

Ramos CT, Koplewitz BZ, Babyn PS, et al: What have we learned about traumatic diaphragmatic hernias in children? J Pediatr Surg 2000; 35:60

Siegel MJ, Shackelford GD, McAlister WH: Left-sided diaphragmatic hernia: delayed presentation. AJR Am J Roentgenol 1981;137:43

Toyama WM: Combined congenital defects of the anterior abdominal wall, sternum, diaphragm, pericardium, and heart: a case report and review of the syndrome. Pediatrics 1972;50:778

Wechsler RJ, Kurtz AB, Needleman L, et al: Cross-sectional imaging of abdominal wall hernias. AJR Am J Roentgenol 1989;153:517

Umbilical Remnant Abnormalities

Aggarwal S, Kumar A, Nijhawan S, et al: Bleeding Meckel's diverticulum demonstrated by digital subtraction angiography. Pediatr Radiol 1989;19:438

Cacciarelli AA, Kass EJ, Yang SS: Urachal remnants: sonographic demonstration in children. Radiology 1990;174:473

Cullen TS: Embryology, Anatomy, and Diseases of the Umbilicus. Philadelphia, WB Saunders, 1916

Daneman A, Lobo E, Alton DJ, et al: The value of sonography, CT, and air enema for the detection of complicated Meckel diverticulum in children with nonspecific clinical presentation. Pediatr Radiol 1998;28:928

Daneman A, Myers M, Shuckett B, et al: Sonographic appearances of inverted Meckel diverticulum with intussusception. Pediatr Radiol 1997;27:295

Diamond RH, Rothstein RD, Aloni A: Role of cimetidine-enhanced technetium-99m pertechnetate imaging for visualizing Meckel's diverticulum. J Nucl Med 1991;32:1422

DiSantis DJ, Siegel MJ, Katz ME: Simplified approach to umbilical remnant abnormalities. Radiographics 1991;11:59

Grosfield JL, Franken EA: Intestinal obstruction in the neonate due to vitelline duct cysts. Surg Gynecol Obstet 1974;138:527

Itagaki A, Uchida M, Ueki K, et al: Double targets sign in ultrasonic diagnosis of intussuscepted Meckel diverticulum. Pediatr Radiol 1991;21:148

Okazaki M, Higashihara H, Yamasaki S, et al: Arterial embolization to control life-threatening hemorrhage from a Meckel's diverticulum. AJR Am J Roentgenol 1990;154:1257–1258

Pantongrag-Brown L, Levine MS, Elsayed AM, et al: Inverted Meckel's diverticulum: clinical, radiologic, and pathologic findings. Radiology 1996;199:693

Rossi P, Gourtsoyiannis N, Bezzi M, et al: Meckel's diverticulum: imaging diagnosis. AJR Am J Roentgenol 1996;166:567

Routh WD, Lawdahl RB, Lund E, et al: Meckel's diverticula: angiographic diagnosis in patients with non-acute hemorrhage and negative scintigraphy. Pediatr Radiol 1990;20:152

Salomonowitz E, Wittich G, Hajek P, et al: Detection of intestinal diverticula by double-contrast small bowel enema: differentiation from other intestinal diverticula. Gastrointest Radiol 1983;8:271

Sfakianakis GN, Haase GM: Abdominal scintigraphy for ectopic gastric mucosa: a retrospective analysis of 143 studies. AJR Am J Roentgenol 1982;138:7

Torii Y, Hisatsune I, Imamura K, et al: Giant Meckel diverticulum containing enteroliths diagnosed by computed tomography and sonography. Gastrointest Radiol 1989;14:167

■
Chapter   3

THE PERITONEAL CAVITY

ALAN E. SCHLESINGER and BRUCE R. PARKER

The peritoneal cavity includes the gastrointestinal viscera, the hepatobiliary structures, the spleen and pancreas, and the associated blood vessels, nerves, and supporting mesenteries. Diseases of these structures are discussed in the appropriate individual chapters.

Situs solitus refers to the intra-abdominal organs being in their normal positions, with the liver in the right upper quadrant, the spleen and stomach in the left upper quadrant, and the cecum in the right lower quadrant. Abnormalities of abdominal situs are most intimately involved with splenic abnormalities and are best understood in relationship to splenic position and anomalies, as discussed in Section VI, Part IV, page 1518.

PNEUMOPERITONEUM

Free intraperitoneal air is most commonly a consequence of perforation of a hollow viscus. In the neonate, this occurs most frequently in babies with intestinal obstruction, necrotizing enterocolitis, or spontaneous gastric perforation of unknown cause. In children beyond the neonatal period, perforated peptic ulcers and inflammatory bowel disease may produce pneumoperitoneum. Pneumoperitoneum is rarely found with appendiceal perforation. Trauma, both accidental and nonaccidental, may cause pneumoperitoneum, as discussed in Section VI, Part IX, page 1691. Tension pneumomomediastinum can dissect along the retroperitoneum and the subadventitial layer of the mesenteric vessels, rupturing freely into the peritoneal cavity. Its differentiation from perforated viscus is discussed below.

Pneumoperitoneum may be suspected clinically because of the history of an underlying disease that predisposes to bowel perforation or because of acute abdominal distention with increased tympany on physical examination, or may be a fortuitous finding on imaging examinations of the chest or abdomen. Patients typically have benign postoperative pneumoperitoneum following abdominal surgery, although the free peritoneal air clears more rapidly in children than in adults. Several studies have demonstrated clearing of free air in 68% to 90% of postoperative children by 24 hours, but free air was seen normally 6 to 7 days postoperatively in 2% to 3% of the cases of Wiot et al.

The diagnosis of pneumoperitoneum is most easily made on horizontal-beam plain radiographs obtained to evaluate for free peritoneal air or intestinal obstruction. Upright radiographs show air collecting between the diaphragm and the liver on the right and between the diaphragm and the liver, spleen, stomach, or colon on the left (Fig. 1). The intra-abdominal viscera fall away from the diaphragm in the upright position, making visualization of the free peritoneal air relatively easy.

Young children and children too ill to sit or stand can be examined in the decubitus position or supine using horizontal-beam technique. The decubitus view should be obtained with the right side up to allow the liver to fall away from the wall of the peritoneal cavity, permitting free peritoneal air to be seen between the liver and the abdominal wall. Small amounts of free air may be difficult to distinguish from intraluminal air if the left-side-up decubitus view is obtained. On the horizontal-beam supine radiograph, free peritoneal air appears between the anterior surface of the liver and the anterior abdominal wall (Fig. 2C), but small amounts of free air may be more difficult to define than on the decubitus or upright view. Seibert and Parvey described the "telltale triangle" sign of free peritoneal air on the cross-table lateral view of the abdomen; the three sides of the triangle of extraluminal air are created by the walls of the two adjacent bowel loops and the anterior abdominal wall.

Horizontal-beam films are useful in the newborn to differentiate pneumoperitoneum caused by a perforated viscus from that caused by dissecting pneumomediastinum. The latter is usually suspected because of the history of assisted ventilation and the presence of

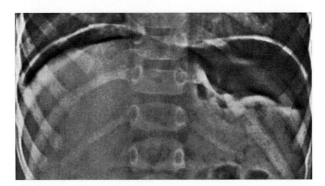

FIGURE 1. Free intraperitoneal air on an upright examination of the abdomen in a 2-year-old boy with perforated gastric ulcer. Air is easily demonstrated between the diaphragm and the liver on the right side and between the diaphragm and the spleen and stomach on the left.

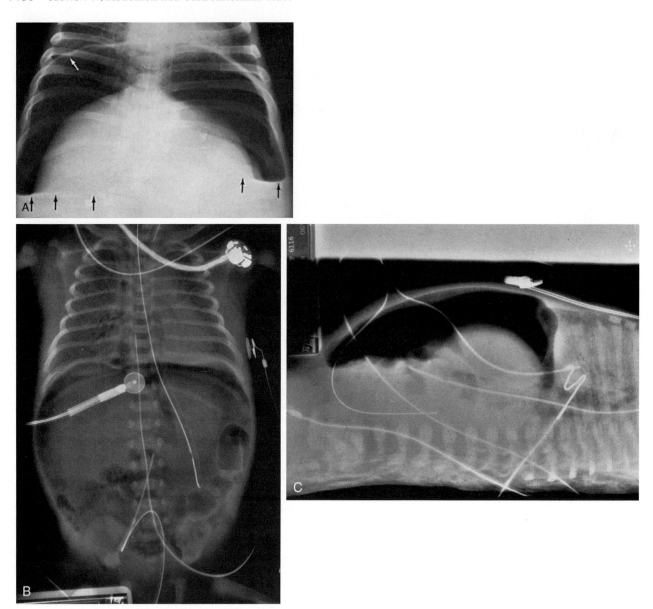

FIGURE 2. A, Massive amount of free air in the abdomen below the diaphragm *(white arrow)* with air–fluid levels *(black arrows)* on an upright film in a patient with pyopneumoperitoneum. **B,** Digitally enhanced anteroposterior view of the chest and abdomen in a newborn with pulmonary interstitial emphysea, pneumomediastinum, and pneumoperitoneum. There is a large amount of gas in the peritoneal cavity with a positive Rigler sign (see text), as well as decreased density of the liver compared with the extraperitoneal soft tissues. **C,** Digitally enhanced cross-table lateral view of the same patient demonstrates large pneumoperitoneum without air–fluid levels, suggesting that the air has dissected into the peritoneum from the chest.

pneumomediastinum on the chest radiograph. A ruptured viscus permits both air and fluid to escape into the peritoneal cavity, causing extraluminal air–fluid levels (Fig. 2A). Dissecting pneumomediastinum causes only air to dissect into the peritoneal space, so no significant air–fluid level is identified in the peritoneal space on horizontal-beam examination (Fig. 2B, C).

Pneumoperitoneum can be diagnosed on supine radiographs as well. It is imperative to recognize the signs on supine radiographs, because a single supine abdomen radiograph may be the only study requested if free peritoneal air is not clinically suspected. A sufficiently large amount of free air can be seen as a

large ovoid lucency overlying the abdominal contents (Fig. 3). This has been called the "football sign" because of the similarity of its shape to a rugby ball. This lucency caused by the free air rising to an anterior position in the abdomen is most easily appreciated where it projects over the liver. The normal liver is the same radiographic density as the abdominal wall musculature. The overlying air on a supine radiograph makes the liver (or a portion of the liver) appear more lucent than the adjacent muscles (or the remainder of the liver). Smaller amounts of free air may also cause a rounded lucent bubble to project over the midabdomen.

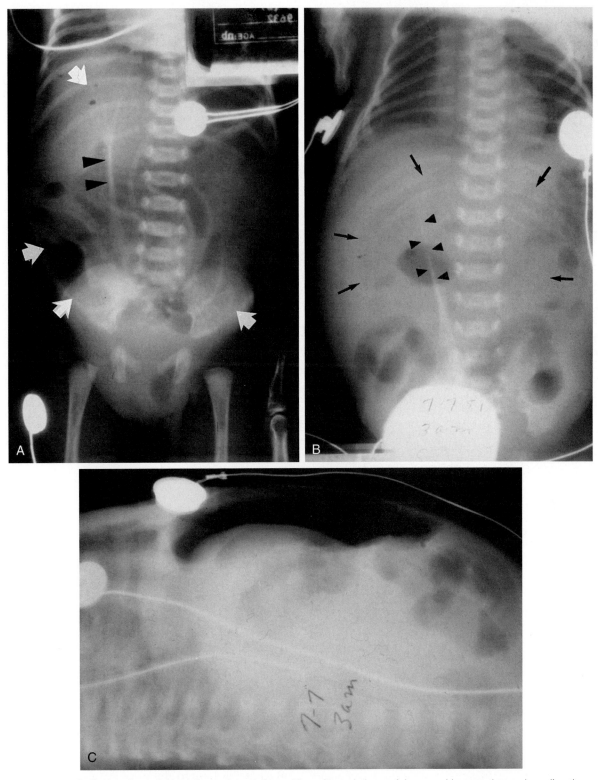

FIGURE 3. A, Supine view of the abdomen in an infant with perforated viscus. A large oval lucency *(arrows)* overlies the entire abdomen, representing the "football sign." The *arrowheads* demonstrate the very thin, dense line of the falciform ligament, which is outlined by air on both sides. **B,** Supine view of the abdomen in another infant with free peritoneal air reveals a smaller oval luceny *(arrows)* and the falciform ligament surrounded by air *(arrowheads).* **C,** Cross-table lateral view in the same infant as in **B** confirms free peritoneal air below the anterior abdominal wall.

Illustration continued on following page

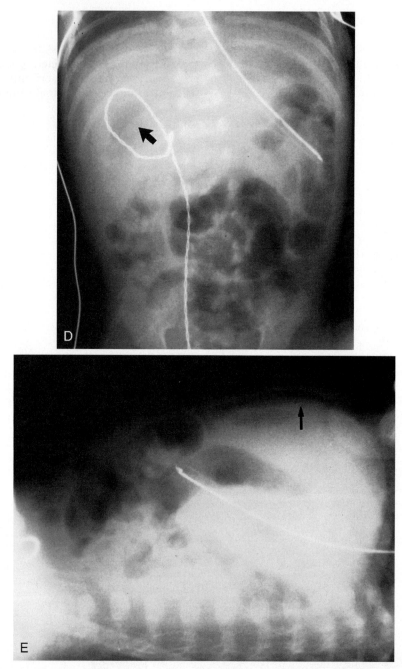

FIGURE 3. *Continued.* **D,** Supine view of the abdomen in a third infant with free air resulting from necrotizing entercolitis. A small collection of gas is noted in Morison's pouch (the hepatorenal recess) *(arrow).* **E,** Same patient as in **D** in the supine position using horizontal-beam technique. Air is demonstrated between the liver and anterior abdominal wall *(arrow).*

■ Radiographic signs of pneumoperitoneum:
  • "Telltale triangle" sign on cross-table lateral view
  • Extraluminal air–fluid levels with ruptured viscus on horizontal-beam film
  • "Football" sign on supine radiograph
  • Rigler sign with free peritoneal air
  • Linear collection in subhepatic space
  • Triangular collection in Morison's pouch

As the liver falls away from the anterior peritoneal surface in the supine position, free peritoneal air can dissect along both sides of the falciform ligament, which attaches the liver to the anterior abdominal wall. The ligament, when outlined by free peritoneal air, appears as a very thin opaque line running vertically just to the right of the spine in a nonrotated radiograph (Fig. 3*A, B*).

Pneumoperitoneum will give the adjacent bowel wall the appearance of an arciform line rather than its usual appearance of an arciform edge. This line is caused by the presence of air on both sides of the bowel wall and is known as the Rigler sign (see Fig. 2*B*). A pseudo-Rigler sign occurs when two loops of dilated air-filled bowel are adjacent to one another, but the finding is usually more focal than it is with a true Rigler sign. The line seen in the pseudo-Rigler sign is thicker than with free peritoneal air because it represents a double thickness of bowel wall (from the two adjacent bowel loops), whereas the line in patients with free peritoneal air (a true Rigler sign) represents a single bowel wall. However, this is not always a reliable differentiation, because the underlying disease causing perforation may lead to a thickened bowel wall.

Small amounts of free air may present on supine radiographs only as localized collections in the right upper quadrant. According to Levine et al., linear collections represent air in the right subhepatic space, whereas triangular collections are seen with air in Morison's pouch (the hepatorenal fossa). The linear lucency may represent air in the fissure of the ligamentum teres, as described by Cho and Baker. The collections are invariably medial in the right upper quadrant and are more likely to be seen in older children and adults than in infants, although Brill et al. described six newborns with necrotizing entercolitis in whom air in Morison's pouch was the only compelling evidence of pneumoperitoneum (Fig. 3*D, E*). A less commonly seen sign of pneumoperitoneum is the "inverted V" sign caused by air outlining the medial umbilical folds in the pelvis.

ASCITES

A small amount of fluid can normally be present in the peritoneal cavity and may be seen incidentally on cross-sectional imaging. Pathologic intraperitoneal fluid collections stem from a variety of causes and include blood, usually from trauma; urine secondary to rupture of an obstructed collecting system or the bladder; pus in cases of peritonitis; bile from biliary tract rupture; and cerebrospinal fluid (CSF) in patients with ventriculoperitoneal shunts for treatment of hydrocephalus. Transudative ascites is most commonly found in patients with hepatobiliary disease, (especially cirrhosis), heart failure, hyponatremia, renal failure, peritonitis, and Budd-Chiari syndrome. Peritoneal metastases are less common in children than adults but, when present, usually cause an exudative ascites. Exudative ascites may also be seen with certain intraperitoneal infections. Rupture of the gastrointestinal tract results in fluid as well as air escaping into the peritoneal cavity.

Fluid can be found in a variety of intraperitoneal locations that may change rapidly with changes in patient position. The greater peritoneal cavity, the lesser sac, Morison's pouch, the paracolic gutters, the pelvis, and recesses formed by many of the peritoneal ligaments are all sites where fluid can collect (Fig. 4). The larger the amount of fluid, the more likely the fluid is to be found throughout the abdomen. Typically, small amounts of ascites collect in the pelvis when the patient is supine. As the amount of fluid increases, it moves cephalad along the paracolic gutters into the subhepatic spaces and Morison's pouch. It can sometimes be identified in the fossa of the ligamentum teres (Fig. 5). A sufficient volume of ascites eventually spreads through the peritoneal cavity, separating bowel loops, and into the mesenteric recesses (Fig. 6). Loculated ascites is rare in children, although encysted collections of CSF may be seen adjacent to the tip of a ventriculoperitoneal shunt tube ("CSF peudocyst"), usually as a result of an inflammatory response around the shunt tube tip (Fig. 7).

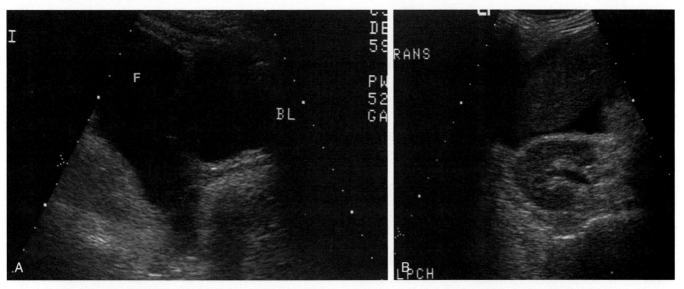

FIGURE 4. A, Transverse sonogram through the pelvis demonstrates a collection of free fluid *(F)* adjacent to the bladder *(BL)*. **B,** Transverse scan through the right upper quadrant demonstrates a small amount of free fluid between the liver and kidney in Morison's pouch.

■ Abdominal ascites:
  • Fluid can be found in a variety of intraperitoneal locations.
  • Location may change rapidly with changes in patient position.
  • The larger the amount of fluid, the more likely it will be found throughout the abdomen.

Plain radiographs are only sensitive to large amounts of intraperitoneal fluid (Fig. 8). The bowel loops may appear centrally located with widened paracolic gutters, although this appearance may be simulated by fluid-filled colon. Separation of bowel loops may also occur due to ascites, but this can be simulated by large amounts of intraluminal fluid combined with relatively small amounts of intraluminal gas (Fig. 9).

Ultrasound (US) is the most sensitive imaging modality for ascites, often visualizing even physiologic amounts of intraperitoneal fluid. Free fluid can be seen in the various peritoneal recesses and the pelvis and may cause apparent thickening of the gallbladder wall. Most tran-

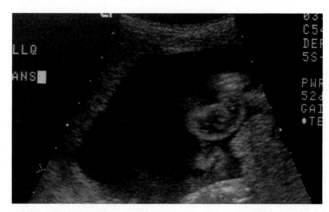

FIGURE 6. Transverse sonogram through the left lower quadrant demonstrates a massive fluid collection outlining thick-walled loops of intestine in a patient with graft-versus-host disease following bone marrow transplantation.

sudates are anechoic collections. Complex fluid collections suggest blood, chyle, inflammatory cells, or peritoneal metastases (Fig. 10). Ascites occasionally will pass through the esophageal hiatus or through patent pleuroperitoneal canals to present as intrathoracic fluid. Computed tomography (CT) is particularly useful in identifying the individual fluid-filled spaces and gives useful diagnostic information if the ascites is secondary to an intra-abdominal process. However, CT is not as sensitive as US to small volumes of fluid.

ACUTE GENERALIZED PERITONITIS

Peritonitis is a diffuse inflammatory process, usually of infectious etiology. The most common cause in children is ruptured appendix. Patients with inflammatory bowel disease may also develop peritonitis after rupture of the bowel. These entities are discussed more fully in Section VI, Parts VII and VIII. Chemical peritonitis can occur with bile leak and in patients with pancreatitis. Plain radiographs in patients with peritonitis often show a nonspecific adynamic ileus pattern with dilated bowel and multiple intraluminal air–fluid levels (Fig. 11). The signs of associated ascites may be seen. In older children, the properitoneal fat plane may be obliterated.

Because of the ease of flow of fluid within the peritoneal cavity, abscesses may develop at sites distant from the perforation as well as in the immediate area. The subhepatic and subphrenic areas are the most common distant sites for abscess formation. US will identify a focal collection of mixed echogenicity. CT shows a focal lesion, often with attenuation greater than clear fluid. The thickened walls of the abscess enhance after the intravenous injection of contrast material. CT is particularly useful as a guide for percutaneous drainage of abscesses (see Section VI, Part VII, page 1616). Both

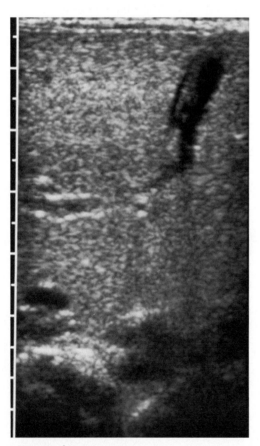

FIGURE 5. Oblique sonogram through the liver demonstrates ascitic fluid in the fissure of the ligamentum teres. The ligament, the obliterated umbilical vein, can be seen within the fluid collection.

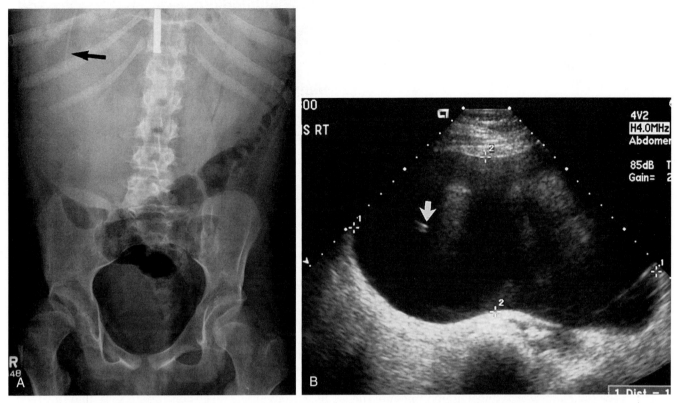

FIGURE 7. Cerebrospinal fluid pseudocyst. **A,** Abdominal radiograph demonstrates a large soft tissue mass occupying the entire upper abdomen, especially the right abdomen. The tip of a ventriculoperitoneal shunt is seen in the right upper quadrant *(arrow)*. **B,** Transverse ultrasound image through the right upper quadrant confirms a large cystic mass surrounding the tip of the shunt *(arrow)*.

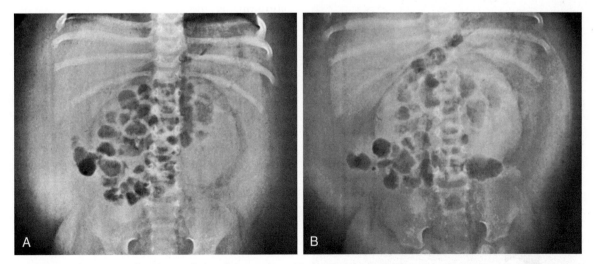

FIGURE 8. Anteroposterior views of the abdomen in a 16-month-old infant with nephrotic syndrome. **A,** Abdominal distention is noted, with numerous loops of gas-containing intestine floating in the center of the abdomen. **B,** Following the intravenous injection of contrast material, the opacified liver and kidneys can be seen, demonstrating the large amount of ascitic fluid present.

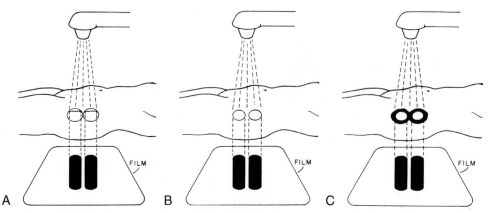

FIGURE 9. Pseudoseparation of bowel loops. **A,** Intraluminal fluid and gas simulate the appearance of bowel loop separation when there is more intraluminal fluid than gas. The x-ray beam "sees" the margin of the gas column rather than the margin of the bowel wall. **B,** True separation of bowel loops results from intraperitoneal fluid because the x-ray beam sees only the gas within the bowel. **C,** Thickened bowel wall simulates intraperitoneal fluid because the x-ray beam sees only the gas within the bowel. (From Hoffman RB, Wankmuller R, Rigler LG: Pseudoseparation of bowel loops: a fallacious sign of intraperitoneal fluid. Radiology 1966;87:845, with permission.)

gallium citrate– and indium-labeled white blood cells have been used as scintigraphic agents in the diagnosis of abscesses.

ABDOMINAL WALL AND PERITONEAL CALCIFICATION

Abdominal wall calcification is uncommon in infants and children. Calcification is commonly a consequence of

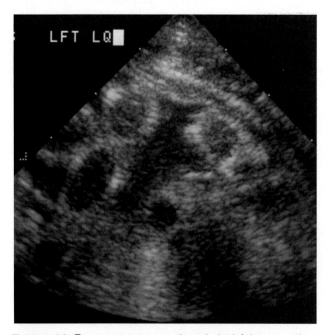

FIGURE 10. Transverse sonogram through the left lower quadrant of a 1-year-old boy with disseminated intravascular coagulation and thrombocytopenia following surgery for congenital heart disease. There is a fluid collection separating multiple loops of bowel. However, the fluid is hypoechoic rather than anechoic, which is the usual situation with ascites. Paracentesis revealed free fluid within the abdomen that had a high hematocrit.

subcutaneous fat necrosis in infants. Although some cases of fat necrosis are idiopathic, the majority are associated with neonatal sepsis. Patients with hypothermia, hepatic failure, and renal failure may also undergo subcutaneous fat necrosis. Abdominal wall calcification in infants has also been described following subcutaneous emphysema and in a case of prune-belly syndrome.

In children, abdominal wall calcification may be seen in fibrodysplasia ossificans progressiva and myositis ossificans, but these lesions are more common in the thoracic wall than the abdominal wall, where they usually are posterior and paraspinous. Calcifications secondary to dermatomyositis are more likely to be in the extremities than in the trunk, but can be found in the abdominal wall. Subcutaneous hemangiomas may contain phleboliths.

- Etiologies of calcification:
  1. Abdominal wall
     - Subcutaneous fat necrosis
     - Fibrodysplasia and myositis ossificans (more common in thoracic wall)
     - Dermatomyositis (more common in extremities)
     - Subcutaneous hemangiomas (phleboliths)
  2. Peritoneum
     - Meconium peritonitis
     - Intestinal perforation
     - Tuberculosis

The most common cause of *peritoneal calcification* in the neonate is meconium peritonitis (see Section II, Part IV, Chapter 4, page 113). This occurs secondary to intrauterine intestinal perforation with meconium-induced chemical peritonitis (Fig. 12). Meconium peritonitis is most frequently seen in association with small bowel atresia, which also occurs secondary to in utero

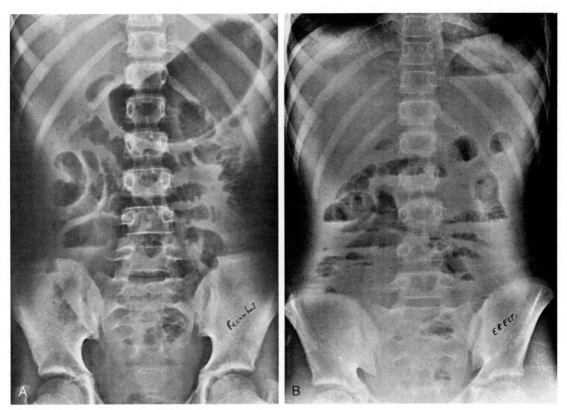

FIGURE 11. Supine **(A)** and upright **(B)** views of the abdomen in a teenage patient with purulent peritonitis. The gas-filled loops of small intestine are mildly dilated and separated from one another, and multiple air–fluid levels can be seen throughout the small intestine.

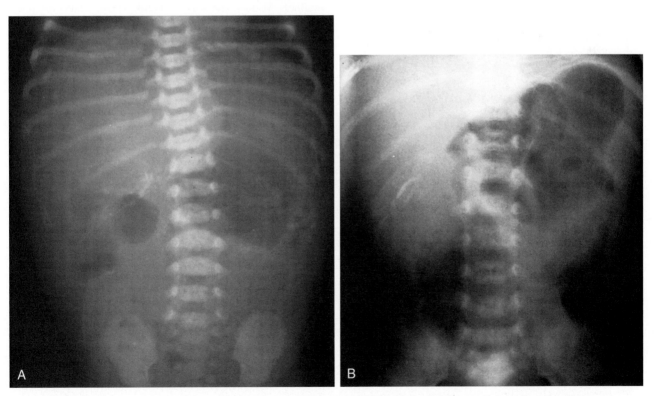

FIGURE 12. A, A newborn with meconium peritonitis. Peritoneal calcifications are demonstrated throughout the abdomen, particularly in the upper half. **B,** Meconium peritonitis in another patient. When small amounts of meconium calcify, they are usually seen along the inferior surface of the liver, as in this patient.

intestinal perforation. However, intestinal obstruction is not invariably present because the bowel may recanalize, and the perforation may heal. Meconium may migrate through the patent neonatal processus vaginalis and cause scrotal calcification in infants. Meconium peritonitis may also occur in neonates with cystic fibrosis.

Peritoneal calcification in older children is quite rare. Intestinal perforation with subsequent peritonitis may cause calcification. Tuberculous peritonitis may result in minimal to extensive calcification.

Most causes of *intra-abdominal calcification* are related to specific organs and are discussed in the appropriate chapters.

SUGGESTED READINGS

Pneumoperitoneum

Bray JF: The "inverted V" sign of pneumoperitoneum. Radiology 1984;151:45

Brill PW, Olson SR, Winchester P: Neonatal necrotizing enterocolitis: air in Morison pouch. Radiology 1990;174:469

Cho KC, Baker SR: Air in the fissure for the ligamentum teres: new sign of intraperitoneal air on plain radiographs. Radiology 1991;178:489

Levine MS, Scheiner JD, Rubesin SE, et al: Diagnosis of pneumoperitoneum on supine abdominal radiographs. AJR Am J Roentgenol 1991;156:731

Menuck L, Siemans PT: Pneumoperitoneum: importance of right upper quadrant features. AJR Am J Roentgenol 1980;127:753

Miller RE: Perforated viscus in infants: a new roentgen sign. Radiology 1960;74:65

Rigler LG: Spontaneous pneumoperitoneum: a roentgenologic sign found in the supine position. Radiology 1941;37:604

Seibert JJ, Parvey LS: The telltale triangle: use of the supine cross table lateral radiograph of the abdomen in early detection of pneumoperitoneum. Pediatr Radiol 1977;5:209

Wind ES, Pillari GP: Lucent liver in the newborn: a roentgenographic sign of pneumoperitoneum. JAMA 1977;237:2218

Wiot JF, Benton C, McAlister WH, et al: Postoperative pneumoperitoneum in children. Radiology 1967;89:285

Ascites and Acute Generalized Peritonitis

Churchill RJ: CT of intra-abdominal fluid collections. Radiol Clin North Am 1989;27:653

Colli A, Cocciolo M, Buccino G, et al: Thickening of the gallbladder wall in ascites. J Clin Ultrasound 1990;19:357

Dinkel E, Lehnart R, Troger J, et al: Sonograhic evidence of intraperitoneal fluid: an experimental study and its clinical implications. Pediatr Radiol 1984;14:299

Gruenebaum M, Ziv N, Kornreich L, et al: The sonographic signs of the peritoneal pseudocyst obstructing the ventriculo-peritoneal shunt in children. Neuroradiology 1988;30:433

Hoffman RB, Wankmuller R, Rigler LG: Pseudoseparation of bowel loops: a fallacious sign of intraperitoneal fluid. Radiology 1966; 87:845

Meyers MA, Oliphant M, Berne AS, et al: The peritoneal ligaments and mesenteries: pathways of intraabdominal spread of disease. Radiology 1987;163:593

Myers MA: Dynamic Radiology of the Abdomen: Normal and Pathologic Anatomy, 5th ed. New York, Springer Verlag, 2000

Newman B, Teele RL: Ascites in the fetus, neonate and young child: emphasis on ultrasonograhic evaluation. Semin Ultrasound CT MR 1984;5:85

Pandolfo I, Gaetta M, Scribano E, et al: Mediastinal pseudotumor due to passage of ascites through the esophageal hiatus. Gastrointest Radiol 1989;14:209

Ruess L, Frazier AA, Sivit CJ: CT of the mesentery, omentum, and peritoneum in children. Radiographics 1995;15:1995

Abdominal Wall and Peritoneal Calcification

Blane CE, White SJ, Braunstein EM, et al: Pattern of calcification in childhood dermatomyositis. AJR Am J Roentgenol 1984;142:397

Kirks DR, Taybi H: Prune-belly syndrome: an unusual cause of neonatal abdominal calcification. Am J Roentgenol Radium Ther Nucl Med 1975;123:778

Naidech HJ, Chawla HS: Soft-tissue calcification after subcutaneous emphysema in a neonate. AJR Am J Roentenol 1982;139:374

Taybi H: Thoracic and abdominal calcification in children: a review. Perspect Radiol 1989;2:135

PART III

HEPATOBILIARY SYSTEM

ALAN E. SCHLESINGER
BRUCE R. PARKER
A'DELBERT BOWEN
RICHARD B. TOWBIN

■ **Chapter 1**

INTRODUCTION TO THE HEPATOBILIARY SYSTEM

ALAN E. SCHLESINGER and BRUCE R. PARKER

NORMAL ANATOMY

The liver is the largest of the abdominal organs, occupying most of the right upper quadrant and extending across the midline. The liver is relatively larger in neonates and infants than it is in older children and adults. The right lobe is larger than the left, with the caudate and quadrate lobes being substantially smaller. The superior portion of the liver is in direct contact with the diaphragm. The posterior margin is in contact with the inferior vena cava, the right adrenal gland, and the distal esophagus. Inferiorly, the liver is in contact with the colon, the gallbladder, and the right kidney. The left lobe is in contact with the stomach. The visceral surface of the liver contains the porta hepatis with its vessels and biliary ducts. The two major intrahepatic biliary ducts join to form the common hepatic duct, which is joined by the cystic duct coming from the gallbladder to form the common bile duct. The common bile duct drains into the descending limb of the duodenum.

Cross-sectional imaging studies can identify the landmarks that divide the hepatic lobes from one another and into their respective segments. The right lobe is divided into anterior and posterior segments, while the left lobe has medial and lateral segments. The interlobar and intersegmental fissures may contain sufficient fat to be identified on ultrasound (US), computed tomography (CT), and magnetic resonance imaging (MRI). Portions of the fissures also contain readily identifiable structures. The middle hepatic vein runs in the superior portion of the main interlobar fissure, separating the left and right lobes. The fissure for the round ligament, the obliterated umbilical vein, divides the segments of the left lobe. The right hepatic vein runs in part of the fissure, separating the segments of the right lobe. US, CT, CT arterial portography, and MRI have been used to identify the hepatic segments as defined by Couinaud's nomenclature for segmental anatomy of the liver.

- The middle hepatic vein separates the right and left hepatic lobes.

- The right hepatic vein separates the segments of the right lobe.
- The fissure for the round ligament divides the segments of the left lobe.

EMBRYOLOGY OF THE LIVER

The liver and biliary duct system, including the gallbladder, arise from the most caudal part of the foregut as a ventral bud early in the fourth week of embryonic life. This bud, known as the hepatic diverticulum, extends into the septum transversum, the future diaphragm. It divides into two parts as it grows between the layers of the ventral mesentery. The larger cranial part of the hepatic diverticulum develops into the liver. As well as giving rise to the hepatocytes, some of the proliferating endodermal cells also develop into the lining epithelium of the biliary system. The reticuloendothelial portions of the liver develop from the splanchnic mesenchyme of the septum transversum. The smaller caudal part of the hepatic diverticulum expands to form the gallbladder, while its stalk becomes the cystic duct. The stalk that connects the cystic and hepatic ducts becomes the common bile duct (CBD) connecting to the duodenum, which also arises from the caudal foregut.

The liver grows very rapidly, with the right lobe becoming the larger of the two initial lobes. The caudate and quadrate lobes are thought to develop as subdivisions of the right lobe, although this has been questioned by Dodds et al., who have suggested an alternative embryologic scheme for development of the caudate lobe. By the 9th week, the liver represents 10% of the embryo's weight, primarily because of the hematopoietic function of the embryonic liver. Bile formation by hepatocytes begins during the 12th embryonic week. Bile pigments begin to develop in the 13th to 16th weeks. They enter the duodenum, giving the intraintestinal meconium its characteristic green color. The liver accounts for 5% of the newborn infant's weight.

The ventral mesentery is a double-layered membrane that gives rise to the gastrohepatic, hepatoduodenal, and falciform ligaments. The falciform ligament extends from the liver to the anterior abdominal wall. Its inferior free border contains the umbilical vein. The ventral mesentery also gives rise to the hepatic visceral peritoneum that fully covers the liver except for the bare area in contact with the diaphragm.

This synopsis of liver embryology is based on the discussion of the digestive system in the text by Moore and Persaud.

HEPATOBILIARY IMAGING

PLAIN RADIOGRAPHY

Plain radiographs play relatively little role in the evaluation of hepatobiliary diseases. Hepatomegaly is often identified on plain radiographs, but liver size can be very difficult to evaluate because one must often rely on displacement of adjacent structures such as the colon or stomach to determine the actual margins of the liver. This is especially true in neonates and infants when there is insufficient fat around the hepatic capsule for identification. Cross-sectional imaging is a much more reliable way of determining liver size. Calcifications within the liver itself (Fig. 1) or in the biliary system can be seen on plain radiographs, as can air in the portal venous system or biliary tree (Fig. 2). Profound fatty replacement of the liver may reduce its radiographic density, but cross-sectional imaging is much more sensitive to lesser degrees of fatty infiltration.

ULTRASOUND

US has been an extraordinarily useful tool in the evaluation of the liver and biliary system in children

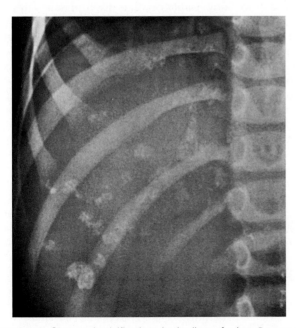

FIGURE 1. Scattered calcifications in the liver of a boy 6 years of age with chronic granulomatous disease of childhood.

because it requires no conscious sedation or anesthesia, and there is no ionizing radiation. Five-megahertz sector transducers are usually satisfactory for most children. A 3.5- or 2.0-MHz transducer may be necessary in older, larger children and adolescents. A 7.0-MHz or higher frequency transducer may be helpful in young infants. When the possibility of subcapsular disease, such as metastases, is being considered, a high-resolution linear transducer is useful.

The echogenicity of the liver should be homogeneous and uniform throughout. A complete examination requires evaluation of the hepatic parenchyma, the portal venous system, the hepatic veins, the hepatic arteries and intrahepatic bile ducts, the CBD, and the gallbladder. The upper limit for the size of the normal CBD was reported as 2 mm in the first year of life, 4 mm in older children, and 7 mm in adolescents and teenagers by Teele and Share. Hernanz-Schulman et al. studied the CBD diameter by US in 173 children ranging in age from 1 day to 13 years. The CBD diameter was less than or equal to 3.3 mm in all 173 children, was less than or equal to 1.6 in all patients 1 year or younger, and was less than or equal to 1.2 mm in all infants 3 months of age or younger.

> ■ The CBD measured 3.3 mm or less in diameter in 173 children 13 years of age or younger.

Doppler US has been especially valuable in patients with portal hypertension and other vascular disease. Color Doppler sonography is also useful in distinguishing the hepatic artery from the biliary ducts, a particular problem in neonates and infants, and has been useful in the evaluation of transplanted livers. Although the examination may be requested for suspected liver disease, full evaluation of the upper abdomen, including spleen, pancreas, and other upper abdominal organs and vascular structures, should always be performed.

NUCLEAR MEDICINE STUDIES

Nuclear medicine studies offer some physiologic as well as anatomic information. Kupffer's cells of the reticuloendothelial system of the liver and spleen take up technetium-99m sulfur colloid, permitting good anatomic definition of masses, including metastases, as well as information about the hepatic parenchyma in general. Singe-photon emission CT increases the sensitivity of the procedure as well as improving the ability to evaluate, at least grossly, hepatic function. Nevertheless, US, CT, and MRI have replaced the sulfur colloid scan in the evaluation of hepatic masses.

Biliary scanning has been especially useful in the attempt to differentiate neonatal hepatitis from congenital biliary atresia. The most commonly used agents are derivatives of iminodiacetic acid. These compounds are taken up by hepatocytes and secreted into the biliary

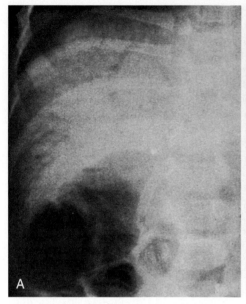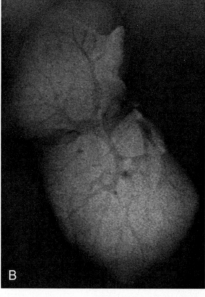

FIGURE 2. Portal venous gas. **A,** Radiolucent branching structures in the liver are best seen in the right hepatic lobe. Dilated bowel is also seen in this patient with necrotizing enterocolitis. **B,** In a postmortem radiograph of the liver, gas in the venous radicles is seen in all parts of the liver. The radicles typically taper toward the periphery of the liver. (Courtesy of Dr. Bertram Levin, Chicago, IL.)

ductules (Fig. 3). Hepatobiliary scanning in these patients should be performed after pretreatment with phenobarbitol to optimize hepatic excretion. Biliary scanning also plays a role in the evaluation of choledochal cysts and in children with cholecystitis.

COMPUTED TOMOGRAPHY

CT has added significantly to the evaluation of hepatobiliary disease. Because of the need for conscious sedation or anesthesia in young children and the exposure to ionizing radiation, CT has been most typically reserved for patients in whom a mass either is strongly suspected or has been identified on US. However, the need for sedation for CT has been dramatically reduced recently by the introduction of helical CT. Better definition of cysts, tumors, metastases, and abscesses can be obtained with CT if the initial US is not definitive. CT may also be performed if CT-guided biopsy or abscess drainage is contemplated. CT is less often used for diffuse parenchymal liver disease, although fatty liver, hemachromatosis and hemosiderosis, and changes in parenchymal attenuation secondary to cirrhosis and fibrosis can readily be identified. Dynamic CT scanning is particularly useful in the evaluation of primary and metastatic tumors of the liver. Dynamic CT with delayed images may be useful in the evaluation of vascular neoplasms such as hemangiomas or hemangio-endotheliomas.

MAGNETIC RESONANCE IMAGING

Similarly, MRI of the liver is usually reserved for patients with mass lesions that need better definition than can be obtained on US or nuclear medicine studies, evaluation of diffuse infiltrative diseases such as hemochromatosis or Gaucher's disease, and evaluation of the hepatic and extrahepatic portal vasculature (especially before and after liver transplantation in patients with portal hypertension). MRI has an advantage over CT in that it does not use ionizing radiation, has multiplanar imaging capabilities, and can better evaluate the hepatic vasculature. However, MRI is certainly more costly, the examination is significantly longer, there is more of a problem with motion artifact in young children, and sedation is more often required than in CT. In older, more cooperative children, newer breath-hold pulse sequences can significantly shorten the scan time and eliminate motion artifact caused by respiration.

Generally, the closest-fitting coil should be used to

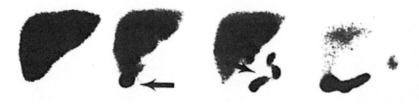

FIGURE 3. Normal biliary scintigram. **A,** Hepatobiliary scintigrams using ^{99m}Tc paraisopropyliminodiacetic acid show immediate radionuclide uptake in the liver. **B** and **C,** Scans at 20 and 30 minutes demonstrate radionuclide in the small intestine *(arrows)*. **D,** One hour after injection, radionuclide has cleared almost completely from the liver.

A #1 ANT IMMEDIATE   B #3 ANT 20 POST INJECTIO C #4 ANT 30 MIN POST INJ D #7 ANT 60 MIN POST IN

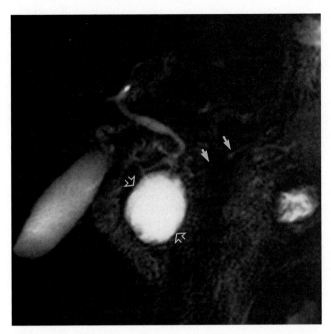

FIGURE 4. Magnetic resonance cholangiopancreatography using a two-dimensional, thick slab, heavily T_2-weighted, fast spin-echo pulse sequence demonstrates normal gallbladder, common bile duct, pancreatic duct *(arrows)*, and a large pancreatic pseudocyst *(open arrows)*.

improve signal:noise ratio and resolution. Standard spin-echo pulse sequences are most commonly used. Both T_1- and T_2-weighted sequences are useful for full evaluation. Fat-suppression techniques and chemical shift imaging may be used to evaluate masses that may contain fat. Gradient-recalled echo sequences are especially useful for evaluation of the vascular structures. Magnetic resonance (MR) angiography, both with and without intravenous contrast, can be used to better evaluate the vascular structures. MR has also recently been used in the evaluation of the biliary tree and pancreatic ducts (MR cholangiopancreatography) utilizing heavily T_2-weighted images (Fig. 4).

ENDOSCOPIC RETROGRADE CHOLANGIOPANCREATOGRAPHY

Endoscopic retrograde cholangiopancreatography (ERCP) is less frequently used in children than in adults. Nevertheless, the examination can be useful in certain congenital and acquired diseases of the biliary tree and pancreas. The examination is difficult to perform in younger children without general anesthesia. However, ERCPs can be performed even in infants, as reported by Guelrud et al. In some hands, *transhepatic cholangiography* is favored over ERCP. It has the advantage of showing the intrahepatic ducts to better advantage than is often possible with ERCP.

ARTERIOGRAPHY

Arteriography is rarely performed since the advent of cross-sectional imaging. Arteriography of the pediatric hepatobiliary system currently is essentially only performed when embolization is necessary (embolization of hemangioendotheliomas, vascular tumors prior to surgery, post-traumatic or postoperative hemorrhages, or arteriovenous fistulas) or for angioplasty of vascular stenoses (such as hepatic arterial stenosis in liver transplantation patients).

SUGGESTED READINGS

Normal Anatomy and Embryology of the Liver

Dodd GD III: An American's guide to Couinaud's numbering system. AJR Am J Roentgenol 1993;161:574

Dodds WJ, Erickson SJ, Taylor AJ, et al: Caudate lobe of the liver: anatomy, embryology, and pathology. AJR Am J Roentgenol 1990; 154:87

Kuszyk BS, Calhoun PS, Soyer PA, et al: An interactive computer-based tool for teaching the segmental anatomy of the liver: usefulness in the education of residents and fellows. AJR Am J Roentgenol 1997;169:631

Moore KL, Persaud TVN (eds): The digestive system. *In* The Developing Human: Clinically Oriented Embryology, 5th ed. Philadelphia, WB Saunders, 1993:237–264.

Hepatobiliary Imaging

Ashida K, Nagita A, Sakagichi M, et al: Endoscopic retrograde cholangiopancreatography in paediatric patients with biliary disorders. J Gastroenterol Hepatol 1998;13:598

Bonetti MG, Castriota-Scanderberg A, Criconia GM, et al: Hepatic iron overload in thalassemic patients: proposal and validation of an MRI method of assessment. Pediatr Radiol 1996;26:650

Fasel JHD, Selle D, Evertsz CJG, et al: Segmental anatomy of the liver: poor correlation with CT. Radiology 1998;206:151

Graham KS, Ingram JD, Steinberg SE, et al: ERCP in the management of pediatric pancreatitis. Gastrointest Endosc 1998;47:492

Guelrud M: Endoscopic retrograde cholangiopancreatography in children. Gastroenterologist 1996;4:81

Guelrud M, Jaen D, Mendoza S, et al: ERCP in the diagnosis of extrahepatic biliary atresia. Gastrointest Endosc 1991;37:522

Hainaux B, Christophe C, Hanquinet S, et al: Gaucher's disease: plain radiography, US, CT and MR diagnosis of lungs, bone and liver lesions. Pediatr Radiol 1992;22:78

Hernanz-Schulman M, Ambrosino MM, Freeman PC, et al: Common bile duct in children: sonographic dimensions. Radiology 1995; 195:193

Hill SC, Damaska BM, Ling A, et al: Gaucher disease: abdominal MR imaging findings in 46 patients. Radiology 1992;184:561

Irie H, Honda H, Jimi M, et al: Value of MR cholangiopancreatography in evaluating choledochal cysts. AJR Am J Roentgenol 1998;171:1381

Kornreich L, Horev G, Yaniv I, et al: Iron overload following bone marrow transplantation in children: MR findings. Pediatr Radiol 1997;27:869

Lafortune M, Madore F, Patriquin H, et al: Segmental anatomy of the liver: a sonographic approach to the Couinaud nonenclature. Radiology 1991;181:443

Matos C, Nicaise N, Deviere J, et al: Choledochal cyst: a comparison of findings at MR cholangiopancreatography and endoscopic retrograde cholangiopancreatography in eight patients. Radiology 1998; 209:443

Miyazaki T, Yamashita Y, Tang Y, et al: Single-shot MR cholangiopancreatography of neonates, infants, and young children. AJR Am J Roentgenol 1998;170:33

Mukai JK, Stack CM, Turner DA, et al: Imaging of surgically relevant hepatic vascular and segmental anatomy. Part 1: normal anatomy. AJR Am J Roentgenol 1987;149:287

Nelson RC, Chezmar JL, Sugarbaker PM, et al: Preoperative localization of focal liver lesions to specific liver segments: utility of CT during arterial portography. Radiology 1990;176:89

Norton KI, Glass RB, Kogan D, et al: MR cholangiography in children and young adults with biliary disease. AJR Am J Roentgenol 1999;172:1239

Parulekar SG: Ligaments and fissures of the liver: sonographic anatomy. Radiology 1979;130:409

Rosenthal DI, Barton NW, McKusick KA, et al: Quantitative imaging of Gaucher disease. Radiology 1992;185:841

Siegel MJ: MR imaging of the pediatric abdomen. Magn Reson Imaging North Am 1995;3:161

Smith D, Downey D, Spouge A, et al: Sonographic demonstration of Couinaud's liver segments. J Ultrasound Med 1998;17:375

Soyer P, Bluemke DA, Bliss DF, et al: Surgical segmental anatomy of the liver: demonstration with spiral CT during arterial portography and multiplanar reconstruction. AJR Am J Roentgenol 1994;163:99

Tagge EP, Tarnasky PR, Chandler J, et al: Multidisciplinary approach to the treatment of pediatric pancreatobiliary disorders. J Pediatr Surg 1997;32:158

Teele RL, Share JC: Ultrasonography of the biliary tree in infants and children. Appl Radiol 1992;21:15

Teo EL, Strouse PJ, Prince MR: Applications of magnetic resonance imaging and magnetic resonance angiography to evaluate the hepatic vasculature in the pediatric patient. Pediatr Radiol 1999;29:238

Terk MR, Esplin J, Lee K, et al: MR imaging of patients with type 1 Gaucher's disease: relationship between bone and visceral changes. AJR Am J Roentgenol 1995;165:599

Waggenspack GA, Tabb DR, Tiruchelvam V, et al: Three-dimensional localization of hepatic neoplasms with computer-generated scissurae recreated from axial CT and MR images. AJR Am J Roentgenol 1993;160:307

Yamataka A, Kuwatsuru R, Shima H, et al: Initial experience with non-breath-hold magnetic resonance cholangiopancreatography: a new noninvasive technique for the diagnosis of choledochal cyst in children. J Pediatr Surg 1997;32:1560

Chapter 2

CONGENITAL ABNORMALITIES

ALAN E. SCHLESINGER and BRUCE R. PARKER

AGENESIS OF A HEPATIC LOBE AND ANOMALIES OF THE GALLBLADDER

Agenesis or hypoplasia of a hepatic lobe is an uncommon abnormality that is being identified with higher frequency as a result of the increased use of cross-sectional imaging. Most commonly, the right lobe is absent with resulting compensatory hypertrophy of the left lobe of the liver and the caudate lobe. This anomaly can be associated with gallbladder agenesis or abnormal retrohepatic or suprahepatic positioning of the gallbladder. Associated congenital anomalies, especially those of the biliary tract, have been reported, as has portal hypertension. Most of the reported cases have been in adults, in whom the differential diagnosis should include atrophy of the right lobe secondary to cirrhosis or tumor. In children, these latter diseases are unlikely to be the cause, and agenesis is the probable diagnosis when the right lobe cannot be identified. Agenesis of the left lobe has been reported less frequently. The gallbladder may be congenitally absent (without associated biliary atresia), ectopically positioned, duplicated, or septated. Ultrasound (US) and hepatobiliary scintigraphy usually identify these rare abnormalities.

BILIARY ATRESIA AND NEONATAL HEPATITIS

There are many potential causes of neonatal jaundice (Table 1), including hemolysis, hepatic infections, metabolic abnormalities, sepsis, adrenal hemorrhage, bile plug syndrome, choledocholithiasis, spontaneous perforation of the common bile duct, and iatrogenic causes associated with various medications. Many of these causes will result in transient jaundice, and their etiology may be readily evident. Otherwise unexplained persistent neonatal jaundice is more likely to be caused by neonatal hepatitis, biliary atresia, choledochal cyst (see below), or Alagille syndrome (see below). Neonatal hepatitis and biliary atresia each account for more than a third of cases of persistent jaundice in the neonatal period and are also discussed in Section II, Part IV, Chapter 5, page 163.

■ Evaluation of patients with persistent neonatal jaundice should focus on neonatal hepatitis, biliary atresia, and choledochal cyst.

Table 1 ■ ETIOLOGY OF NEONATAL JAUNDICE

Transient
Hemolysis
Hepatic infection
Sepsis
Metabolic disease
Bile plug syndrome
Adrenal hemorrhage
Drug related

Persistent
Neonatal hepatitis
Biliary atresia
Choledochal cyst
Alagille syndrome
Spontaneous perforation of the common bile duct

Landing has suggested that biliary atresia and neonatal hepatitis may be differing manifestations of the same pathophysiologic process: fetal inflammatory cholangiopathy. In the form known as *biliary atresia,* variable parts of the biliary tree are completely obliterated. In the form known as *neonatal hepatitis,* the biliary tree remains patent, although there is substantial damage to the liver itself. Differentiating these two entities is critical because biliary atresia requires operative intervention, whereas neonatal hepatitis is treated medically. Early diagnosis of biliary atresia is particularly important because the prognosis for long-term survival is markedly reduced if surgery is performed after 3 months of age. The diseases are so closely related that in up to one third of cases the diagnosis may not be correctly made, even by liver biopsy.

Abdominal US is the recommended first imaging examination for neonates with pathologic jaundice. US may identify other anatomic causes for the patient's jaundice, such as choledochal cyst, stones, or inspissated bile in the bile plug syndrome. *Bile plug syndrome* is a rare cause of perinatal jaundice of unclear etiology (that may be related to total parenteral nutrition or cystic fibrosis) in which sludge (echogenic or hypoechoic) in the bile ducts and gallbladder forms plugs and may cause transient gallbladder hydrops and duct dilatation (see Section II, Part IV, Chapter 5, page 163).

■ Abdominal US is the first imaging examination in neonates with persistent jaundice.

Generally, the gallbladder will be visualized and appear normal in up to 90% of patients with neonatal hepatitis. About 10% of patients with this disease may be so severely affected that the gallbladder is not seen on US. In most patients with biliary atresia, the gallbladder cannot be visualized. In about one fifth of cases, however, the gallbladder may be identified, although in many of these cases it may appear smaller than expected in a fasting infant. Nevertheless, because of this overlap, US by itself has not been deemed sufficient by most authors to differentiate the two lesions, and other imaging evaluations have been required. However, a recently described sonographic sign of biliary atresia—the triangular cord sign—has been shown to be relatively specific for biliary atresia. The triangular cord sign refers to a triangular or tube-shaped echogenic density adjacent to the portal venous bifurcation on transverse or longitudinal images. In a large series of 79 infants with cholestatic jaundice, 25 were proven to have biliary atresia and 54 were diagnosed with neonatal hepatitis. Of the patients with biliary atresia, 21 of 25 had a triangular cord sign; 53 of 54 infants with neonatal hepatitis had no evidence of a triangular cord. This sonographic sign had a sensitivity of 84% and a specificity of 98%.

Ikeda et al. have reported that serial US may be useful in the differentiation of neonatal hepatitis and biliary atresia when the gallbladder is visualized. According to these authors, postprandial gallbladder contraction can be seen in patients with neonatal hepatitis but not in patients with biliary atresia. Weinberger et al., however, reported a case of biliary atresia with postprandial gallbladder contraction. Changes in the Doppler-assessed portal venous velocity have been described in patients with biliary atresia by Grunert et al. Wanek et al. have reported a correlation of decreased velocity with poor postoperative prognosis in patients with biliary atresia. Their patients with reduced portal venous velocity came to transplantation, while the patients with normal velocity did well with portoenterostomy alone. A more recent study of 30 patients with biliary atresia who underwent hepatic Doppler sonography demonstrated that those patients with diminished maximal portal venous velocities, elevated hepatic arterial resistive indices, or flattened hepatic venous Doppler waveforms had lower survival rates without liver transplantation than those patients with normal Doppler studies.

Nuclear medicine studies of the biliary tree have been the traditional definitive imaging method for the differentiation of biliary atresia from neonatal hepatitis (Figs. 1 and 2) and are typically performed after US. Evaluation of the blood pool and hepatic phases and determination of the presence or absence of radioisotope in the gastrointestinal tract on delayed images are all necessary for the proper investigation of biliary atresia. Patients should be pretreated with phenobarbital. If the early scans do not demonstrate isotopic activity in the gastrointestinal tract, delayed scans, up to 24 hours, should be obtained. The presence of radioisotope in the gastrointestinal tract essentially excludes biliary atresia. Although most patients with neonatal hepatitis have excretion of the radionuclide into the gut (although the excretion is often delayed), patients with severe hepatic injury may not have sufficient liver function to excrete detectable amounts of radiotracer into the gastrointestinal tract.

■ Hepatobiliary scintigraphy is usually required to differentiate between neonatal hepatitis and biliary atresia.

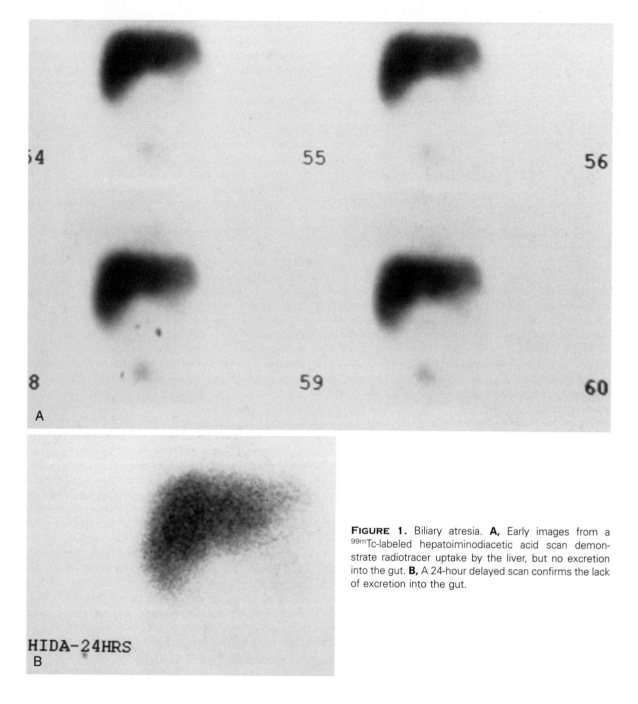

FIGURE 1. Biliary atresia. **A,** Early images from a ^{99m}Tc-labeled hepatoiminodiacetic acid scan demonstrate radiotracer uptake by the liver, but no excretion into the gut. **B,** A 24-hour delayed scan confirms the lack of excretion into the gut.

When the diagnosis remains in doubt, other imaging studies may be necessary. Percutaneous cholecystocholangiography has been used in several centers, but is not widely performed. Because biliary atresia may affect only portions of the biliary tree, opacification of hepatic ducts as well as the common bile duct is necessary to exclude the diagnosis. Some patients require exploratory laparotomy. Because biopsy can be nondiagnostic, operative cholangiograms are usually performed in an attempt to identify the intrahepatic and extrahepatic portions of the biliary system (Fig. 3). Magnetic resonance (MR) cholangiography with heavily T$_2$-weighted images has recently been utilized to identify the presence of the gallbladder and intra- and extrahepatic biliary ducts in the evaluation of neonates with jaundice in order to exclude bilary atresia. Guelrud et al. have described the use of endoscopic retrograde cholangiopancreatography (ERCP) in jaundiced neonates. Of 32 infants in whom ERCP was attempted, 30 studies were successful. These authors used their own prototypical duodenoscope for these studies.

Approximately 10% of patients with biliary atresia have a syndrome that also includes polysplenia, azygos continuation of the inferior vena cava, preduodenal portal vein, hepatic arterial anomalies, and left-sided isomerism of the lungs. US can usually identify many portions of this syndrome, not only suggesting the correct diagnosis but giving important preoperative information to the surgeon. Day et al. used computed tomography (CT) postoperatively to define associated congenital and acquired abnormalities such as polysplenia and portal hypertension. Choledochal cysts can also be seen in neonates with biliary atresia. These choledochal cysts may be distinct from those seen in older infants and children and may be caused by obstruction of the biliary tract. Imaging with US and biliary scintigraphy is typically sufficient to evaluate the biliary tree in these patients.

Treatment for neonatal hepatitis is medical unless there is such severe liver destruction that transplantation is necessary. Biliary atresia is treated by portoenterostomy (the Kasai operation). The exact form of the procedure used depends on the degree of obliteration of the biliary tree. The operation is successful in upward of 50% of patients when performed under the age of 3 months, but, because of progressive obliteration of the

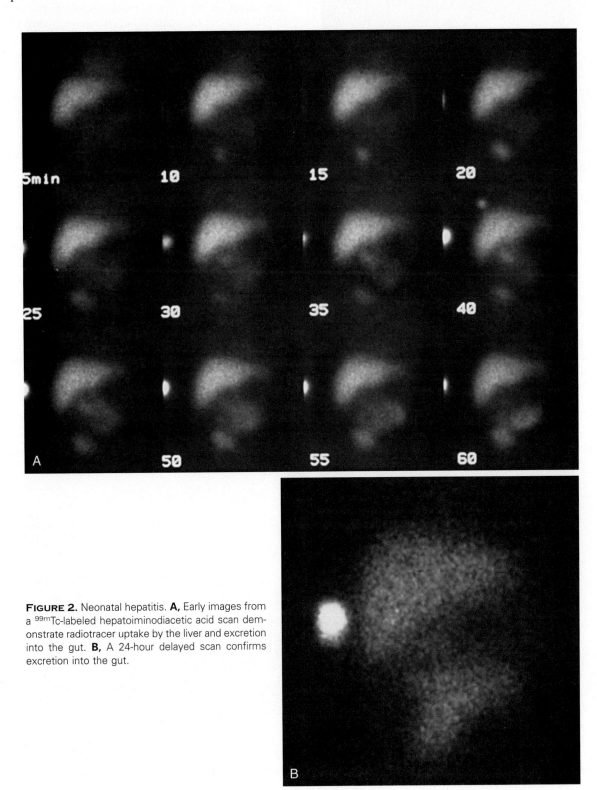

FIGURE 2. Neonatal hepatitis. **A,** Early images from a ^{99m}Tc-labeled hepatoiminodiacetic acid scan demonstrate radiotracer uptake by the liver and excretion into the gut. **B,** A 24-hour delayed scan confirms excretion into the gut.

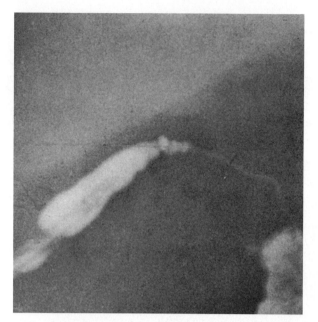

FIGURE 3. Operative cholangiogram in a 4-month-old infant with persistent jaundice since birth. Contrast material injected into the contracted gallbladder enters the duodenum via a single duct. No hepatic ducts were identified on this examination or at surgery in this infant who had extrahepatic biliary atresia.

This bowel loop, if it is fluid filled, may be seen in the region of the porta hepatis on postoperative US scans. Biliary scintigraphy can be used to evaluate the patency of the portoenterostomy. Isotopic activity should appear in the bowel by 1 hour after administration. Patients may develop ascending cholangitis with cystic dilatation of the intrahepatic bile ducts and subsequent "bile lakes" secondary to stasis. These accumulations of bile are easily seen on US, CT, and magnetic resonance imaging (MRI) and can be drained percutaneously with variable results. Percutaneous transhepatic cholangiography (PTC) has also been used to test the patency of the Kasai anastomosis.

SPONTANEOUS PERFORATION OF THE COMMON BILE DUCT

Although spontaneous peforation of the common bile duct more commonly occurs in neonates (see Section II, Part IV, Chapter 5, page 163), it can be seen in older infants and young children (Fig. 4). These patients typically present with biliary ascites, and biliary scintigraphy demonstrates radionuclide activity in the ascitic fluid.

ALAGILLE SYNDROME (ARTERIOHEPATIC DYSPLASIA)

Paucity and hypoplasia of interlobular bile ducts in association with other congenital abnormalities is known as Alagille syndrome or arteriohepatic dysplasia. Alagille, Estrada, et al. have described five major components of this syndrome: (1) abnormal facies (large forehead, small pointed chin, hypertelorism, poorly developed nasal bridge); (2) chronic cholestasis; (3) oc-

bile ducts, survival rates drop rapidly when surgery is performed after this age. Even those patients with good short-term to mid-term results may eventually develop cholangitis, cirrhosis, and portal hypertension. Ever more frequently, these patients undergo liver transplantation.

In the Kasai operation, the porta hepatis is dissected and a loop of small intestine is brought up and anastomosed to the exposed draining biliary radicles.

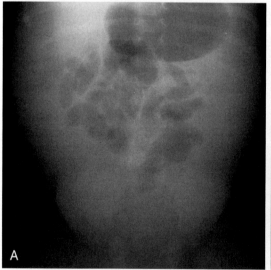
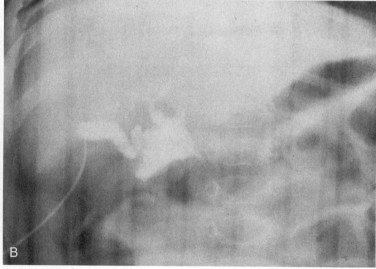

FIGURE 4. Spontaneous rupture of the common bile duct. **A,** This 9-week-old girl presented with massive ascites. Abdominal radiograph demonstrates evidence of fluid in the flanks with centrally placed loops of intestine. Paracentesis revealed biliary ascites. **B,** Operative cholangiogram with injection of contrast material into a small gallbladder demonstrates some filling of the common bile duct and intrahepatic ducts with leak of contrast material from a spontaneous perforation of the common bile duct.

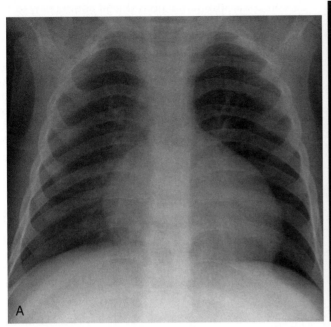
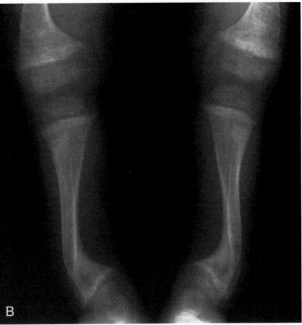

FIGURE 5. Alagille syndrome. Patient with heart murmur and abnormal liver function tests. **A,** Frontal view of the chest demonstrates cardiac enlargement. Cardiac evaluation revealed pulmonic stenosis. **B,** Rachitic changes in the metaphyses with undertubulation, osteopenia, and varus deformities of the distal femora and tibiae. Liver biopsy revealed biliary duct hypoplasia compatible with Alagille syndrome.

ular abnormalities (most typically posterior embryotoxon and pigmentary retinopathy); (4) butterfly vertebrae; and (5) pulmonary artery hypoplasia or stenosis (Fig. 5). The last may be either isolated or associated with complex cardiac anomalies. Less commonly seen vascular abnormalities suggest a broader spectrum of potential vascular anomalies in patients with Alagille syndrome. Half of the cases will have four of these abnormalities, 30% will have all five features, and 15% will have three of the abnormalities. A number of other congenital abnormalities are seen less frequently, including caudal dysplasia. The bones may show significant osteoporosis with undertubulation.

■ Major components of Alagille syndrome:
  • Abnormal facies
  • Chronic cholestasis
  • Ocular abnormalities
  • Butterfly vertebrae
  • Pulmonary artery hypoplasia or stenosis

Affected patients usually present in the neonatal period, although some present months to years later with cholestatic jaundice. The imaging characteristics in the newborn period are similar to those in biliary atresia, but the findings of other components of this syndrome should lead to the correct diagnosis. Patients presenting beyond the newborn period may have US findings suggestive of cirrhosis, with heterogeneous echogenicity within the liver and evidence of regenerating nodules. Typically, scintigraphic biliary imaging fails to show normal excretion of radioisotope into the gastrointestinal tract. The definitive diagnosis is usually made by liver biopsy, at which time the intraoperative cholangiogram usually demonstrates patency of the extrahepatic biliary tree. Most patients with Alagille syndrome die before the end of the third decade, but survival into the fifth decade has been reported. Hepatocellular carcinoma, as a complication of Alagille syndrome, has been reported in both children and adults. Liver transplantation can be performed in patients with Alagille syndrome, but results are better if surgery occurs prior to development of hepatic tumors.

Hypoplasia of the interlobular bile ducts without other associated congenital anomalies has been described as well. The differentiation from biliary atresia can be made either by later age of presentation, hepatic wedge biopsy, or demonstration of an intact extrahepatic biliary tree. Alagille, Estrada, et al. have described the characteristics of 80 patients with the syndromic form of interlobular bile duct hypoplasia and 31 cases of the nonsyndromic form.

CHOLEDOCHAL CYST

Choledochal cyst refers to dilatation of the common bile duct, which can be either saccular or fusiform. A frequently used classification is that of Alonson-Lej et al., who described four types. Todani et al. have modified the classification, describing five types with several subtypes (Fig. 6). Gastroenterologists are increasingly accepting the Todani classification. The several types differ in etiology and pathogenesis as well as in appearance and presentation. The most common form,

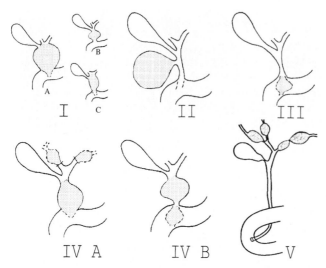

FIGURE 6. Todani's classification of choledochal cysts (see text for discussion). (Modified from Crittenden SL, McKinley MJ: Choledochal cyst—clinical features and classification. Am J Gastroenterol 1985;80:643.)

demonstrated this anomalous ductal connection to be present on ERCP in all eight of their patients, and other authors agree that the theory of Babbitt et al. is the most plausible for type I choledochal cyst. Furthermore, Han et al. have described a 6-year-old boy with documented ductal malunion who initially had normal biliary ducts but developed progressive ductal dilitation, suggesting that acquired cholecochal cyst may be a complication of pre-existing ductal malunion. Type I choledochal cyst is more common in girls than boys in Occidentals, but the gender ratio is equal in Asia. About 65% of all reported cases are from Japan.

> ■ Todani type I choledochal cyst likely is caused by either distal ductal obstruction or reflux of pancreatic enzymes due to proximal insertion of the pancreatic duct into the common bile duct.

found in 80% to 90% of cases (according to Crittenden and McKinley) is Todani's type I, consisting of dilatation of the common bile duct over a variable length and of varying degree (Fig. 7). Todani divides type I into three subtypes. Although various theories for the pathogenesis of the type I choledochal cysts exist, the leading theories invoke obstruction of the distal biliary duct and/or reflux of pancreatic enzymes into the biliary tree as a result of anomalous proximal insertion of the pancreatic duct into the common bile duct (ductal malunion), a theory originally proposed by Babbitt et al. Ductal malunion permits reflux of pancreatic enzymes into the common bile duct with subsequent inflammation and weakening of the wall (Fig. 8). According to Rosenfield and Griscom, this pathogenetic mechanism may occur in 60% of patients. Wiedmeyer et al. have

Todani's type II choledochal cyst consists of one or more diverticula of the common bile duct and is found in 2% of cases. Some theorize that this form of choledochal cyst may be caused by prenatal rupture of the common bile duct with subsequent healing. Todani's type III is a choledochocele—dilatation of the intraduodenal portion of the duct with both the common bile duct and pancreatic duct emptying into it—and is found in 1.5% to 5.0% of cases (Fig. 9). This form of cholecochal cyst may be the sequela of ampulary obstruction or may be the result of a congenital duplication of the duodenum in the region of the ampulla. Todani's type IVA is multiple intrahepatic and extrahepatic cysts and occurs in 19% of patients. Type IVB is multiple extrahepatic cysts and is rare. Todani's type V (as well as Alonson-Lej's type IV) is Caroli's disease, which is discussed below. Type IVA of Todani

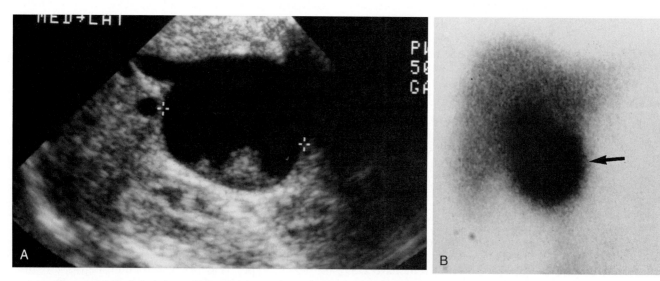

FIGURE 7. Choledochal cyst (Todani's type I). **A,** Ultrasound demonstrates a large cyst in the porta hepatis communicating with the biliary tree. **B,** ^{99m}Tc-labeled hepatoiminodiacetic acid scan confirms communication with the bilary tree as radiotracer accumulates in the cyst (arrow).

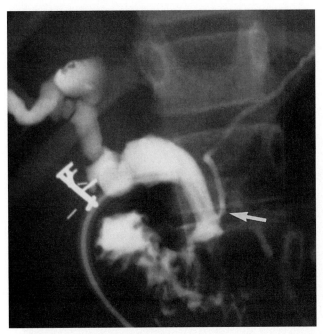

FIGURE 8. Endoscopic retrograde cholangiopancreatography in a child with choledochal cyst reveals dilatation of the common bile duct and a relatively proximal insertion of the pancreatic duct *(arrow).*

may also represent a form of Caroli's disease, but has also been called type I with intrahepatic involvement. These intrahepatic cysts seen in types IV and V may be related to reflux of pancreatic enzymes or may be the result of primary ductal ectasia.

Choledochal cyst may present in infancy with cholestatic jaundice and may be clinically inseparable from neonatal hepatitis or biliary atresia. However, US (by demonstrating the anatomy) and radionuclide studies (by demonstrating continuity with the biliary tree) usually suggest the correct diagnosis, which can be

confirmed, if necessary, by CT (Fig. 10). In older children and young adults, the clinical presentation is quite variable. A characteristic triad of abdominal pain, obstructive jaundice, and fever has been reported, but only a minority of patients present with all three findings. According to Sherman et al., abdominal pain is the most characteristic presentation, while obstructive jaundice, fever, pale stools, hepatomegaly, palpable mass, and splenomegaly represent other presenting features.

US is usually the first imaging study requested, because nearly all of the possible modes of presentation point to a hepatobiliary problem. The markedly dilated common bile duct in type I choledochal cyst is readily discernible (see Fig. 7). The gallbladder can usually be identified adjacent to the dilated common duct, and the cystic duct may also be seen. Most frequently, the intrahepatic ducts are normal, but varying degrees of dilatation have been described. Sludge or stones may be identified within the dilated duct (see Fig. 10B).

Biliary scintigraphy will show that the dilated cystic structure communicates with the biliary tree as it fills with radiotracer (see Fig. 7B). Camponovo et al. reported the findings in 12 cases of proven choledochal cyst. The dilated duct was demonstrated within 1 hour in seven patients, on delayed scans in three patients, and not at all in two patients.

If the diagnosis cannot be made definitively, PTC and ERCP have been reported useful (see Fig. 8), but rarely are required. Wiedmeyer et al. successfully performed ERCP in eight patients with type I choledochal cyst and anomalous entry of the common bile duct into the pancreatic duct, six of whom also had ectasia of the common channel. Savader et al. preferred PTC, which better delineates the intrahepatic ducts and has less chance of causing cholangitis than does ERCP. It is technically more difficult, however, especially in patients during the first few years of life.

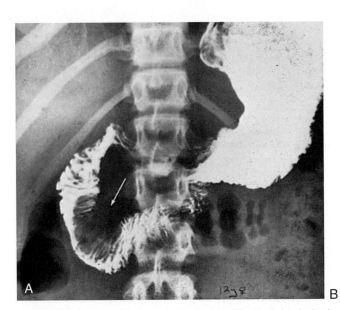

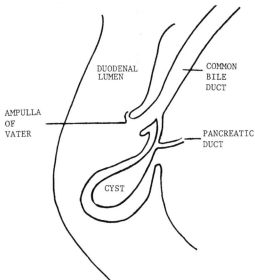

FIGURE 9. Choledochocele in a 12-year-old girl with abdominal pain. **A,** Large filling defect *(arrow)* in the duodenum caused by the choledochocele. **B,** Drawing of findings at surgery.

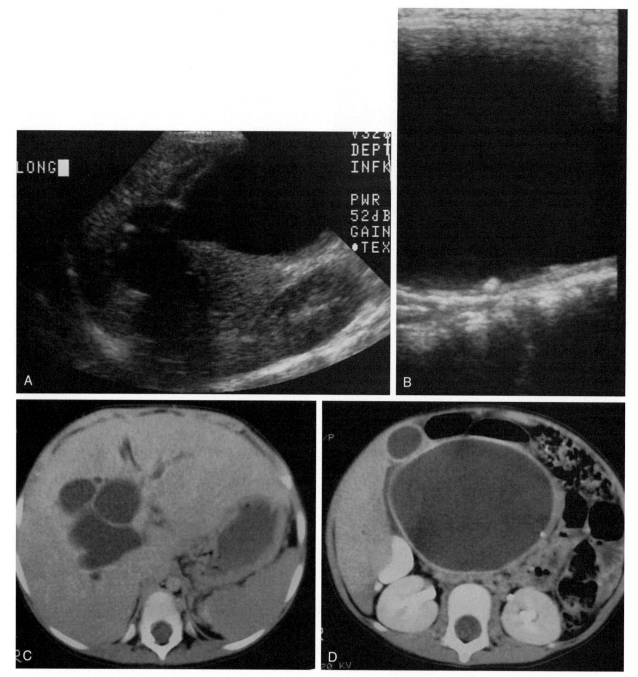

FIGURE 10. Choledochal cyst. Longitudinal **(A)** and transverse **(B)** sonograms demonstrate marked dilatation of the common bile duct. In the dependent portion of the cystic dilatation, a stone with posterior shadowing is identified. **C,** Computed tomography (CT) scan section through the liver demonstrates marked dilatation of the common bile duct and right and left hepatic ducts with lesser dilatation of the intrahepatic duct system. **D,** More caudal CT scan section demonstrates massive cystic dilatation of the common bile duct with a calcified stone on the left. The gallbladder, with a slightly thickened wall but normal-sized lumen, is seen to the right and anterior of the cystic mass.

CT may show the cyst to better advantage than US (see Fig. 10C, D), but is rarely needed to confirm the anatomic findings seen on US. Furthermore, CT does not demonstrate the ductal anatomy as well as cholangiography (Fig. 11). Because this information is important to the surgeon, CT is of less value in the routine work-up. However, it may be quite useful in evaluating intrahepatic cysts and identifying abscesses. More recently, CT cholangiography has been performed after intravenous administration of meglumine iodoxamic acid (Endobil; Bracco, Milan, Italy), which is excreted by the liver into the biliary system. MRI and MR cholangiography have also been advocated in the evaluation of children with choledochal cysts because these modalities can noninvasively provide imaging information comparable to that of ERCP, including demonstration of ductal malunion. However, CT, MR, and MR cholangiopancreatography should be reserved for isolated cases in which routine imaging with US and nuclear scintigraphy are not conclusive or cases where further evaluation of the biliary tract (such as in the evaluation of choledocholithiasis) or demonstration of postoperative complications (such as anastomotic stenoses) is necessary. An upper gastrointestinal series was commonly used for diagnosis (by demonstrating extrinsic pressure effect of the cyst on the duodenum) prior to the advent of cross-sectional imaging, but no longer plays a role in the evaluation of these patients.

■ Hepatobiliary scintigraphy and US are usually sufficient for the imaging work-up of patients with choledochal cyst. In select cases, CT, MR, MRCP, ERCP, or percutaneous transhepatic cholangiography may be necessary.

The most common complication of type I choledochal cyst is ascending cholangitis. Eventually, cirrhosis of the liver can occur with subsequent portal hypertension. Spontaneous cyst rupture has been reported. There is a 20-fold increased incidence of carcinoma of the biliary tree in patients with choledochal cyst. The risk is low in the first decade of life but increases with advancing age.

■ Complications of type I choledochal cyst:
  • Ascending cholangitis
  • Cirrhosis
  • Spontaneous cyst rupture
  • Carcinoma of the biliary tree

CAROLI'S DISEASE

Type IV (Alonson-Lej) or type V (Todani) choledochal cyst represents segmental nonobstructive dilatation of the intrahepatic bile ducts. The cause of Caroli's disease is unknown. Postulated mechanisms include occlusion of the hepatic artery in the neonatal period with associated ischemia of the bile ducts, abnormal growth rate of the biliary epithelium and supporting connective tissues, and lack of the normal involution of ductal plates surrounding the portal tracts, leading to biliary cysts surrounding the portal triads. Less commonly, only ectasia of the intrahepatic biliary ducts is present ("pure form"). This form is often associated with stone formation, cholangitis, and hepatic abscesses. More commonly, there is associated hepatic fibrosis, choledochal cyst, medullary sponge kidney, infantile polycystic renal

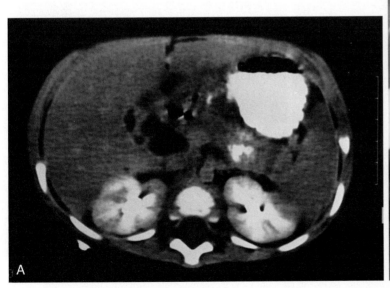

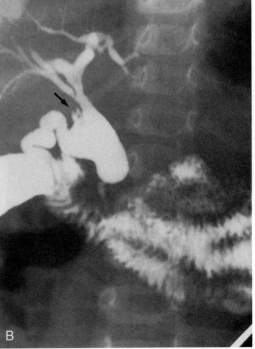

FIGURE 11. Choledochal cyst. Patient with fever, leukocytosis, and right upper quadrant pain had a choledochal cyst demonstrated on ultrasound. **A,** Computed tomography confirms the dilated extrahepatic biliary duct. **B,** Cholangiogram demonstrates an area of walled-off perforation *(arrow)* and a markedly dilated common bile duct and hepatic ducts.

disease, or nephronophthisis. This form may well represent one end of the spectrum of polycystic disease of the liver and kidneys (discussed below).

■ **Abnormalities commonly associated with Caroli's disease:**
- Hepatic fibrosis
- Choledochal cyst
- Medullary sponge kidney
- Infantile polycystic renal disease
- Nephronophthisis

Although the disease is present from birth, most patients do not present until later in life when abdominal pain secondary to cholangitis usually leads to medical attention. The abdominal pain may also be related to hepatic abscesses secondary to cholangitis or to biliary stones secondary to stasis. Patients with associated hepatic fibrosis may develop portal hypertension, whereas those without hepatic fibrosis do not. Although typically a diffuse process, monolobar Caroli's disease has been reported, with 88% of the cases involving the left lobe.

Plain radiographs are usually not revealing unless biliary stones are seen, and US is typically the first imaging study performed. In most patients, the ectatic ducts will be large enough to recognize on US (Fig. 12A, B). Recognition of the connection of the ectatic ducts with one another and with the rest of the ductal system is critical in distinguishing Caroli's disease from polycystic liver disease. The dilated ducts may give the appearance of surrounding the portal vein radicles (the "intraluminal portal vein sign") (Fig. 12C). Toma et al. believe this sign to be pathognomonic for Caroli's disease. Blood

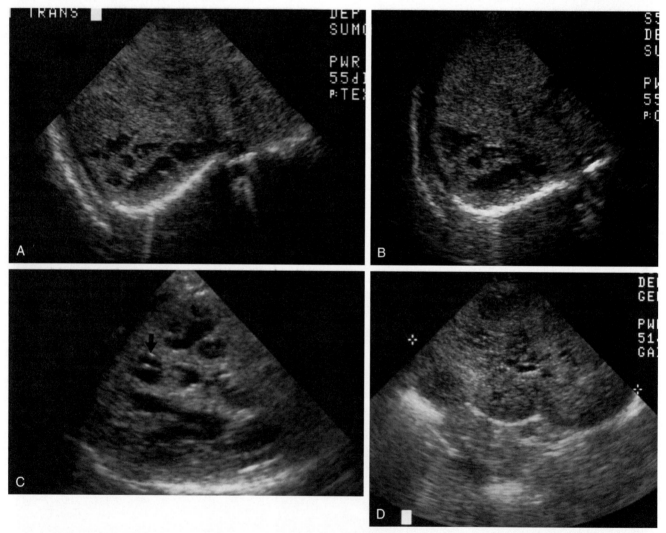

FIGURE 12. Caroli's disease in a patient with hepatic fibrosis and polycystic renal disease. **A,** Transverse ultrasound image of the liver demonstrates cystic structures in the posterior aspect of the right lobe. **B,** Slightly more cephalad, several of the cystic structures can be seen communicating. There is heterogeneous increased echogenicity of the liver parenchyma compatible with hepatic fibrosis, which was documented on liver biopsy. **C,** An "intraluminal portal vein" radicle *(straight arrow)* coursed through the dilated duct. Intraluminal protrusions of the duct wall are also identified *(curved arrow)*. **D,** An enlarged lobulated kidney shows loss of corticomedullary differentiation.

flow can be confirmed within these intraluminal portal venous branches on Doppler interogation. Biliary sludge and calculi are common findings within the anechoic dilated ducts. Both the gallbladder and the common bile duct may be enlarged. Marchal et al. have described intraluminal protrusions of the duct wall (Fig. 12C). If an abscess is present, one or more cysts will show mixed echogenicity rather than the anechoic appearance of the uncomplicated cysts. The kidneys should be examined as well. They may be normal, may be frankly polycystic, or, more commonly, may show increased echogenicity, especially in the medullary portions (Fig. 12D). Corticomedullary differentiation may be lost.

■ **Ultrasound findings in Caroli's disease:**
  1. **Common**
     - Dilated, ectatic bile ducts
     - "Intraluminal portal vein" sign with flow on Doppler
     - Biliary sludge and calculi
     - Enlarged gallbladder and common bile duct
  2. **Less common**
     - Abscesses
     - Associated renal anomalies (cysts or abnormal echogenicity)

Hepatic scintigraphy may show multiple filling defects if the ducts are sufficiently dilated. Patients with hepatic fibrosis have hepatomegaly and, frequently, splenomegaly. Biliary imaging with ^{99m}Tc iminodiacetic acid compounds shows focal defects during the hepatic phase that gradually increase in activity as the radiopharmaceutical collects in the dilated ducts, while the remainder of the liver shows decreased activity with time. Radiotracer activity in the gastrointestinal tract will be seen but is frequently delayed because of bile stasis.

CT is an excellent way to show the extent of disease, especially the intrahepatic ductal ectasia. A "central dot" may be seen that corresponds to the intraluminal portal vein seen sonographically. These structures will enhance after intravenous contrast administration. If the ducts are only minimally dilated, the connections between them and the rest of the biliary tree may be more easily seen on CT than on US. If an abscess is present, the affected cyst will typically show higher attenuation than the others. The common duct and gallbladder typically are dilated. Cystic disease of the kidneys may be identified, as will splenomegaly in those patients with hepatic fibrosis.

Cholangiography, either PTC or ERCP, demonstrates communicating cystic and tubular ductal ectasia with dilatation of the common duct and gallbladder. Stones and biliary sludge are usually identified. The relative merits of PTC and ERCP have been discussed by Savader et al. and by Wiedmeyer et al. MR cholangiopancreatography has more recently been shown to be useful in defining the anatomy of the biliary tree in children with Caroli's disease.

FIBROPOLYCYSTIC DISEASES

The hepatobiliary fibropolycystic diseases are characterized by overgrowth of the biliary epithelium and supportive connective tissues. These interrelated diseases manifest a spectrum of processes including dilatation of the extrahepatic and/or intrahepatic bile ducts, segmental dilatation of the intrahepatic bile ducts, congenital hepatic fibrosis, autosomal recessive polycystic kidney disease, and polycystic liver disease. The intriguing association of polycystic renal disease with polycystic liver disease and congenital hepatic fibrosis has been recognized for a number of years.

Several classification systems have been devised, each with its advantages and disadvantages. Summerfield et al. have suggested a new classification based on the clinical, imaging, and histologic features of 51 patients. These authors were struck by the overlap between several entities and have brought them together in a unified grouping. Of interest is that they include choledochal cysts and Caroli's disease in this classification because of the overlap. For instance, of the 51 patients, there were 12 patients with hepatic fibrosis, 8 with Caroli's disease, and 12 with both. One patient with choledochal cyst had the typical intrahepatic biliary ectasia of Caroli's disease, while another had associated congenital hepatic fibrosis. Two patients with infantile polycystic liver disease also had hepatic fibrosis and intrahepatic ductal ectasia, while 10 patients with adult polycystic liver disease did not. Further work is required to validate these authors' contentions, but they are achieving increasing acceptance. Recent genetics research has suggested that, despite the overlap of the cystic renal and hepatic diseases, there may be independent, unlinked genes for polycystic liver disease and polycystic renal disease.

CONGENITAL HEPATIC FIBROSIS

Congenital hepatic fibrosis, with or without associated biliary duct ectasia, is an autosomal recessive inherited abnormality. The associated renal abnormalities are infantile and adult polycystic disease, renal dysplasia, and medullary cystic disease. Those patients who present as newborns or infants do so because of the severity of their renal disease, which usually dictates their course and prognosis. Those patients who present later in childhood or in adulthood have less renal involvement and frequently come to attention because of hepatomegaly or portal hypertension. Patients with hepatic fibrosis have surprisingly near-normal liver function studies.

Alvarez et al. have described the US characteristics of congenital hepatic fibrosis (Fig. 13A). The liver is large. Splenomegaly may or may not be present, depending on the presence or absence of portal hypertension. The hepatic echogenicity is homogeneously or heteroge-

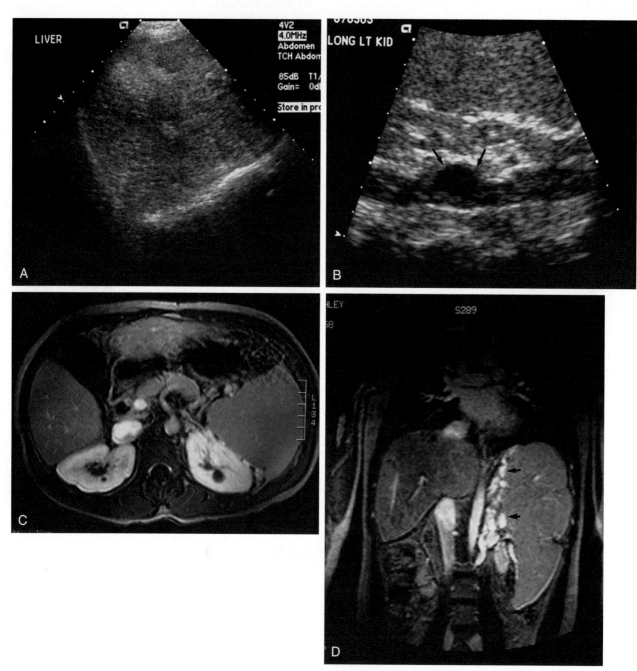

FIGURE 13. Fourteen-year-old girl with congenital hepatic fibrosis (and associated polycystic kidney disease) and secondary portal hypertension with spontaneous shunting from gastric and splenic collaterals to the left renal vein. **A,** Longitudinal ultrasound (US) image demonstrates heterogeneous echogenicity of the liver with areas of increased echogenicity resulting from hepatic fibrosis. **B,** Longitudinal US of the left kidney reveals a lower pole cyst *(arrows)*. **C,** Axial T_1-weighted magnetic resonance (MR) image demonstrates splenomegaly and bilateral renal cysts. **D** and **E,** Two coronal images from a MR angiogram (three-dimensional T_1-weighted fast gradient-echo pulse sequence) reveal collateral vessels *(arrows)* in the region of the splenic hilum and large left renal vein *(arrowheads)*. Splenomegally is again noted.

Illustration continued on opposite page

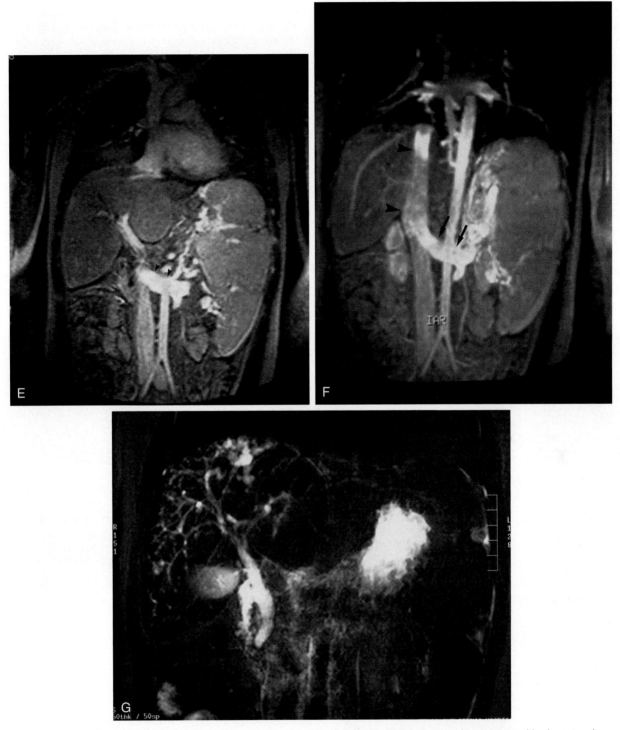

FIGURE 13. *Continued.* **F,** Maximal intensity projection reconstruction better depicts the vascular anatomy, with a large renal vein *(arrows)* secondary to spontaneous shunting of vessels from the portal venous system into the inferior vena cava *(arrowheads).* **G,** MR cholangiopancreatography demonstrates associated biliary duct ectasia and biliary cysts.

neously increased. With associated Caroli's disease, there will be intrahepatic biliary duct ectasia and dilatation of the gallbladder. If portal hypertension is present, its characteristic imaging findings (see below) will be seen. Associated renal lesions can also be identified and should always be sought (Fig. 13*B*). CT does not have a routine role in this disease but may be performed if complications are suspected or in the evaluation of patients with portal hypertension. The findings are nonspecific, with areas of heterogeneously increased and decreased attenuation on CT. MR scanning may be performed in children with portal hypertension (Fig. 13*C–G*). The liver has low signal intensity on T_1- and T_2-weighted spin-echo pulse sequences. Splenomegaly may be present. MR angiography can demonstrate vascular sequelae of portal hypertension, and MR cholangiopancreatography may reveal biliary cysts or intra- or extrahepatic biliary duct dilatation or ectasia (see Fig. 13*G*).

POLYCYSTIC LIVER DISEASE

Polycystic liver disease is divided into infantile and adult forms. The less common infantile type has an autosomal

recessive inheritance. The more common adult form is autosomal dominant. The patients with the recessive form usually present early because of the severity of the associated polycystic renal disease. Patients with the dominant form present in adulthood with nephrogenic symptoms, although the findings are often noted in asymptomatic children with a positive family history. When patients present as a result of liver disease, symptoms may result from cyst complications (infection, hemorrhage, torsion, or rupture); mass effect related to cysts (increased intra-abdominal pressure, distention, pain, biliary duct dilatation, etc.); or associated hepatobiliary abnormalities (biliary duct dilatation or hepatic fibrosis).

Hepatobiliary cysts in polycystic liver disease may be intrahepatic or peribiliary. Intrahepatic cysts tend to be peripheral in location. They are typically round but may be polygonal. Peribiliary cysts are multiple small cysts that occur in the connective tissue near larger portal triads and/or the hepatic hilum. They may appear as discrete cysts, as a string of cysts, or as a tubular cystic structure. On US, the hepatobiliary cysts are anechoic (Fig. 14). Occasionally, one may see echogenic debris if hemorrhage has occurred. On CT, the intrahepatic cysts are of lower attenuation than the surrounding paren-

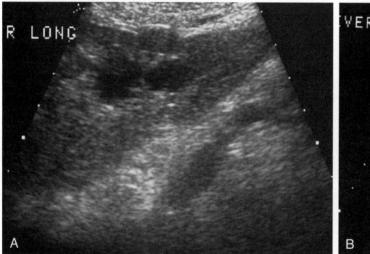

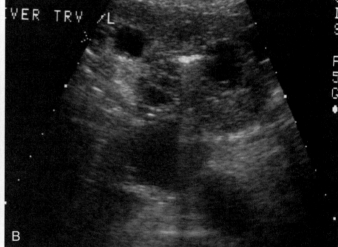

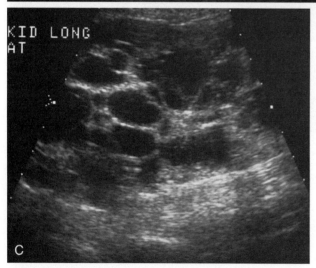

FIGURE 14. Polycystic liver disease. Longitudinal (**A**) and transverse (**B**) sonograms through the left hepatic lobe reveal multiple cysts. **C,** Longitudinal sonogram through the left kidney demonstrates nephromegaly secondary to adult-type autosomal dominant polycystic kidney disease. (Courtesy of R. Brook Jeffrey, Jr., M.D., Stanford, CA.)

chyma. They are usually of uniform attenuation, although of differing size, and are sharply demarcated from the surrounding parenchyma. On MRI, the cysts will have characteristically decreased signal on T_1-weighted and increased signal on T_2-weighted spin-echo sequences, although Davis et al. have reported heterogeneous signal intensity within the cysts, presumably because of hemorrhages of varying ages. MR cholangiography may be used to demonstrate associated Caroli's disease.

MICROHAMARTOMAS

Microhamartomas are a common incidental finding at pathologic examination of the liver. Summerfield et al. have noted an increased incidence of microhamartomas in patients with fibropolycystic disease of the liver. Although they are typically too small to see on imaging studies, a recent report described hypoechoic lesions with a micronodular pattern on sonography and multiple small low-attenuation lesions in the liver on CT in adult patient with histologically proven microhamartomatosis of the liver. Microhamartomas may give rise to hepatobiliary carcinomas.

Malignancies have also been associated with other diseases in the fibropolycystic spectrum. There is an increased incidence of biliary duct and pancreatic cancer in patients with Caroli's disease and choledochal cyst, a low incidence of hepatocellular carcinoma in congenital fibrosis, and almost no malignant complications in polycystic liver disease.

CONGENITAL SOLITARY CYSTS

Solitary cysts are uncommon in children, benign, and usually found incidentally on imaging studies or at surgery. They may be symptomatic when large, presenting as a palpable abdominal mass or with obstructive jaundice caused by mass effect on adjacent structures. Pliskin et al. have described an adult who developed a squamous cell carcinoma in a congenital cyst.

US is usually diagnostic, demonstrating an intrahepatic anechoic lesion sharply demarcated from the surrounding liver parenchyma (Fig. 15). Rarely, a cyst may be exophytic, in which case biliary scintigraphy can be useful in differentiating it from cystic dilatation of the biliary tree. The cyst will appear as a photopenic area on the hepatic phase and show no increase in activity on delayed scans during the biliary excretion phase on hepatobiliary scintigraphy. Both CT and MRI will show the characteristics of a cyst. Neither study is indicated in the work-up of a sonographically solitary cyst, but a cyst may be seen fortuitously when a patient is studied for another indication.

GLYCOGEN STORAGE DISEASE

Although numerous metabolic diseases affect the liver, the abdominal imaging findings are generally meager and nonspecific. Glycogen deposition causes hepato-

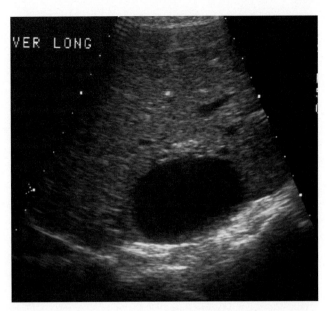

FIGURE 15. Hepatic cyst. Longitudinal ultrasound image reveals an asymptomatic simple cyst in the posterior portion of the right hepatic lobe, which was identified as an incidental finding.

megaly and increased attenuation on CT. The glycogen storage diseases, however, also cause fatty infiltration of the liver with decreased attenuation on CT, so the net effect is variable depending on the relative amounts of glycogen and fat present. US typically demonstrates increased echogenicity as a result of fatty infiltration. Patients with type I glycogen storage disease are at risk for the development of hepatic adenomas and hepatocellular carcinoma (see Section VI, Part III, Chapter 7, page 1493). One report of US findings in adults and children with glycogen storage disease demonstrated that patients with coexistent tumors tended to have more severe parenchymal sonographic changes, and suggested that the severity of parenchymal changes may therefore prove useful in predicting patients at higher risk of tumor formation. Many of the metabolic disorders lead to cirrhosis or cholelithiasis and are discussed in Section VI, Part III, Chapters 4, page 1475 and 6, page 1486, respectively.

SUGGESTED READINGS

Agenesis of a Hepatic Lobe and Anomalies of the Gallbladder

Adear H, Barki Y: Multiseptated gallbladder in a child: incidental diagnosis on sonography. Pediatr Radiol 1990;20:192

Collay R, Anne F, de Vannsay de Blavous P, et al: Agenesie du lobe hepatique droit. Ann Radiol (Paris) 1990;33:108

Coughlin JP, Rector FE, Klein MD: Agenesis of the gallbladder in duodenal atresia: two case reports. J Pediatr Surg 1992;27:1304

Demirci A, Diren HB, Selcuk MG: Computed tomography in agenesis of the right lobe of the liver. Acta Radiol 1990;31:105

Diaz MJ, Fowler W, Hnatow BJ: Congenital gallbladder duplication: preoperative diagnosis by ultrasonography. Gastrointest Radiol 1991;16:198

Inoue T, Ito Y, Okauchi Y, et al: Hypogenesis of the right hepatic lobe accompanied by portal hypertension: case report and review of 31 Japanese cases. J Gastroenterol 1997;32:836

Ishibashi T, Sato A, Hama H, et al: Liver scarring associated with congenital absence of the right hepatic lobe: CT and MR findings. J Comput Assist Tomogr 1995;19:997

Kakitsubata Y, Kakitsubata S, Watanabe K: Gallbladder abnormalities associated with hypoplasia of the right lobe of the liver. Radiat Med 1997;15:71

Kakitsubata Y, Nakamura R, Mitsuo H, et al: Absence of the left lobe of the liver: US and CT appearance. Gatrointest Radiol 1991;16:323

Maeda N, Horie Y, Shiota G, et al: Hypoplasia of the left hepatic lobe associated with floating gallbladder: a case report. Hepatogastroenterology 1998;45:1100

Pradeep VM, Ramachandran K, Sasidharan K: Anomalous position of the gallbladder: ultrasonographic and scintigraphic demonstration in four cases. J Clin Ultrasound 1992;20:593

Starinsky R, Strauss S, Vinograd I, et al: Duplication of the gallbladder in a child: sonographic appearance. J Clin Ultrasound 1991;19:575

Biliary Atresia and Neonatal Hepatitis

Abramson SJ, Berdon WE, Altman RP, et al: Biliary atresia and noncardiac polysplenic syndrome: US and surgical considerations. Radiology 1987;163:377

Betz BW, Bisset GS III, Johnson ND, et al: MR imaging of biliary cysts in children with biliary atresia: clinical associations and pathologic correlation. AJR Am J Roentgenol 1994;162:167

Brown DM: Bile plug syndrome: successful management with a mucolytic agent. J Pediatr Surg 1990;25:351

Brun P, Gauthier F, Boucher D, Brunelle F: Echographie et artesie des voies billaries l'enfant. Ann Radiol (Paris) 1985;28:259

Day DL, Mulcahy PF, Dehner LP, et al: Post-operative abdominal CT scanning in extrahepatic biliary atresia. Pediatr Radiol 1989;19:379

Grunert D, Stier B, Schoning M: The portal system and hepatic artery in children with biliary atresia. I: ultrasound and simple duplex ultrasound parameters. Klin Padiatr 1990;202:24

Guelrud M, Jaen D, Mendoza S, et al: ERCP in the diagnosis of extrahepatic biliary atresia. Gastrointest Endosc 1991;37:522

Ikeda S, Sera Y, Akagi M: Serial ultrasonic examination to differentiate biliary atresia from neonatal hepatitis—special reference to changes in size of the gallbladder. Eur J Pediatr 1989;148:396

Jaws TS, Kuo YT, Liu GC, et al: MR cholangiography in the evaluation of neonatal cholestasis. Radiology 1999;212:249

Kardoff R, Klotz M, Melter M, et al: Prediction of survival in extrahepatic biliary atresia by hepatic duplex sonography. J Pediatr Gastroenterol Nutr 1999;28:411

Kasai M, Kimura S, Asakura Y, et al: Surgical treatment of biliary atresia. J Pediatr Surg 1968;3:665

Kirks DR, Coleman RE, Filston HC, et al: An imaging approach to persistent neonatal jaundice. AJR Am J Roentgenol 1984;142:461

Landing BH: Considerations of the pathogenesis of neonatal hepatitis, biliary atresia, and choledochal cyst: the concept of infantile obstructive cholangiopathy. Prog Pediatr Surg 1974;6:113

Lilly JR, Karren FM: Contemporary surgery of biliary atresia. Pediatr Clin North Am 1985;32:1233

Majd M: (99m) Tc-IDA scintigraphy in the evaluation of neonatal jaundice. Radiographics 1983;3:88

Park WH, Choi SO, Lee HJ: The ultrasonographic "triangular cord" coupled with gallbladder images in the diagnostic prediction of biliary atresia from infantile intrahepatic cholestasis. J Pediatr Surg 1999;34:1706

Spivak W, Sarkar S, Winter D, et al: Diagnostic utility of hepatobiliary scintigraphy with ^{99m}Tc-DISIDA in neonatal cholestasis. J Pediatr 1985;106:171

Stringer DA (ed): The liver. In Pediatric Gastrointestinal Imaging. Toronto, BC Decker, 1989;471–583

Takahashi A, Tsuchida Y, Suzuki N, et al: Incidence of intrahepatic biliary cysts in biliary atresia after hepatic portoenterostomy and associated histopathologic findings in the liver and porta hepatis at diagnosis. J Pediatr Surg 1999;34:1364

Tanano H, Hasegawa T, Kawahara H, et al: Biliary atresia associated with congenital structural anomalies. J Pediatr Surg 1999;34:1687

Torrisi JM, Haller JO, Velcek FT: Choledochal cyst and biliary atresia in the neonate: imaging findings in five cases. AJR Am J Roentgenol 1990;155:1273

Treem WR, Grant EE, Barth KJ, et al: Ultrasound guided percutaneous cholesystocholangiography for early differentiation of cholestatic liver disease in infants. J Pediatr Gastroenterol Nutr 1988;7:347

Tsuchida Y, Honna T, Kawarasaki H: Cystic dilatation of the intrahepatic biliary system in biliary atresia after hepatic portoenterostomy. J Pediatr Surg 1994;29:630

Varela-Fascinetto G, Castaldo P, Fox IJ, et al: Biliary atresia-polysplenia syndrome: surgical and clinical relevance in liver transplantation. Ann Surg 1998;227:583

Wanek EA, Horgan JG, Karrer FM, et al: Portal venous velocity in biliary atresia. J Pediatr Surg 1990;25:146

Weber TR, Grosfeld JL: Contemporary management of biliary atresia. Surg Clin North Am 1984;61:1079

Weinberger E, Blumhagen JD, Odell JM: Gallbladder contraction in biliary atresia. AJR Am J Roentgenol 1987;149:401

Williamson SL, Selbert JJ, Butler HL, et al: Apparent gut excretion of Tc-99m-DISIDA in a case of extrahepatic biliary atresia. Pediatr Radiol 1986;16:245

Spontaneous Perforation of the Common Bile Duct

Haller JO, Condon VR, Berdon WE, et al: Spontaneous perforation of the bile duct in children. Radiology 1989;172:621

Kumar R, Sriram M, Bhatnagar V, et al: Spontaneous perforation of the common bile duct in infancy: role of Tc-99m mebrofenin hepatobiliary imaging. Clin Nucl Med 1999;24:847

Alagille Syndrome (Arteriohepatic Dysplasia)

Alagille D, Estrada A, Hadchouel M, et al: Syndromic paucity of interlobular bile ducts (Alagille syndrome or arteriohepatic dysplasia): review of 80 cases. J Pediatr 1987;110:195

Alagille D, Odievre M, Gautier M, et al: Hepatic ductular hypoplasia associated with characteristic facies, vertebral malformations, retarded physical, mental and sexual developmental and cardiac murmur. J Pediatr 1975:86:63

Berard E, Sarles J, Triolo V, et al: Renovascular hypertension and vascular anomalies in Alagille syndrome. Pediatr Nephrol 1998; 12:121

Brodsky MC, Cunniff C: Ocular anomalies in Alagille syndrome (atriohepatic dysplasia). Ophthalmology 1993;100:1767

Cardona J, Houssin D, Gauthier F, et al: Liver transplantation in children with Alagille syndrome—a study of twelve cases. Transplantation 1995;60:339

Kocoshis SA, Cottrill CM, O'Connor WN, et al: Congenital heart disease, butterfly vertebrae and extrahepatic biliary atresia: a variant of arteriohepatic dysplasia? J Pediatr 1981;99:436

Ong E, Wiliams SM, Anderson JC, et al: MR imaging of a hepatoma associated with Alagille syndrome. J Comput Assist Tomogr 1986; 10:1047

Rachmel A, Zeharia A, Neuman-Levin M, et al: Alagille syndrome associated with moyamoya disease. Am J Med Genet 1989;33:89

Rodriguez JI, Rivera T, Palacios J: Alagille syndrome associated with caudal dysplasia sequence. Am J Med Genet 1991;40:61

Rosenfield NS, Kelley MJ, Jensen PS, et al: Arteriohepatic dysplasia: radiologic features of a new syndrome. AJR Am J Roentgenol 1980;135:1217

Sommerville DA, Marks M, Treves T: Hepatobiliary scintigraphy in arteriohepatic dysplasia (Alagille's syndrome): a report of two cases. Pediatr Radiol 1988;18:32

Choledochal Cyst/Caroli's Disease

Alexander MC, Haaga JR: MR imaging of a choledochal cyst. J Comput Assist Tomogr 1985;9:357

Alonson-Lej F, Reven WB, Pessagno DJ: Congenital Choledochal cyst, with a report of two, and analysis of 94 cases. Int Abstr Surg 1959;108:1

Ando K, Miyano T, Kohno S, et al: Spontaneous perforation of choledochal cyst: a study of 13 cases. Eur J Pediatr Surg 1998;8:23

Babbit DP, Starshak RJ, Clemett AR: Choledochal cyst: a concept of etiology. Am J Roentgenol Radium Ther Nucl Med 1973;119:57

Boyle MJ, Doyle GD, McNulty JG: Monolobar Caroli's disease. Am J Gastroenterol 1989;84:1437

Camponovo E, Buck JL, Drane WE: Scintigraphic features of choledochal cyst. J Nucl Med 1989;30:622

Caroli J, Soupault R, Kossakowski J, et al: La dilatation polykystique congenitale des voles biliaries intrahepatiques: essai de classification. Sem Hop (Paris) 1958;34:488

Chan YL, Yeung CK, Lam WW, et al: Magnetic resonance cholangiography—feasibility and application in the pediatric population. Pediatr Radiol 1998;28:307

Crittenden SL, McKinley MJ: Choledochal cyst—clinical features and classification. Am J Gastroenterol 1985;80:643

Han SJ, Hwang EH, Chung KS, et al: Acquired choledochal cyst from anomalous pancreatobiliary duct union. J Pediatr Surg 1997;32:1735

Jequier S, Capusten B, Guttman F, et al: Childhood choledochal cyst with intrahepatic enlarged cyst-like bile ducts. J Can Assoc Radiol 1984;35:73

Johnson K, Alton HM, Chapman S: Evaluation of mebrofenin hepatoscintigraphy in neonatal-onset jaundice. Pediatr Radiol 1998;28:937

Kangarloo H, Sarti DA, Sample WF, et al: Ultrasonic spectrum of choledochal cysts in children. Pediatr Radiol 1980;9:15

Lam WW, Lam TP, Saing H, et al: MR cholangiography and CT cholangiography of pediatric patients with choledochal cysts. AJR Am J Roentgenol 1999;173:401

Marchal GJ, Desmet VJ, Proesmans WC, et al: Caroli disease: high-frequency US and pathologic findings. Radiology 1986;158:507

Matos C, Nicaise N, Deviere J, et al: Choledochal cysts: comparison of findings at MR cholangiopancreatography and endoscopic retrograde cholangiopancreatography in eight patients. Radiology 1998; 209:443

McHugh K, Daneman A: Multiple gastrointestinal atresias: sonography of associated biliary abnormalities. Pediatr Radiol 1991;21:355

Miller WJ, Sechtin AG, Campbell WL, et al: Imaging findings in Caroli's disease. AJR Am J Roentgenol 1995;165:333

Moreno AJ, Parker AL, Spicer MJ, Brown TJ: Scintigraphic and radiographic findings in Caroli's disease. Am J Gastroenterol 1984;79:299

Nakanuma Y, Terada T, Ohta G, et al: Caroli disease in congenital hepatic fibrosis and infantile polycystic disease. Liver 1982;2:348

O'Neill JA Jr: Choledochal cyst. In O'Neill JA, Rowe MI, Grosfeld JL, et al (eds): Pediatric Surgery, 5th ed. St. Louis, Mosby, 1998: 1483–1493

Padhy AK, Gopinath P, Basu AK, et al: Hepatobiliary scintigraphy in congenital cystic dilatation of biliary tract. Clin Nucl Med 1985; 10:703

Rosenfield N, Griscom NT: Choledochal cysts: roentgenographic techniques. Radiology 1975;114:113

Savader SJ, Benenati JF, Venbrux AC, et al: Choledochal cysts: classification and cholangiographic appearance. AJR Am J Roentgenol 1991;156:327

Sherman P, Kolster E, Davies C, et al: Choledochal cysts: heterogeneity of clinical presentation. J Pediatr Gastroenterol Nutr 1986;5:867

Sood GK, Mahapatra JR, Khurana A, et al: Caroli disease: computed tomographic diagnosis. Gastrointest Radiol 1991;16:243

Sty JR, Hubbard AM, Starshak RJ: Radionuclide hepatobiliary imaging in congenital biliary tract ectasia (Caroli disease). Pediatr Radiol 1982;12:111

Suarez F, Bernard O, Gauthier F, et al: Bilio-pancreatic common channel in children: Clinical, biological and radiological findings in 12 children. Pediatr Radiol 1987;17:207

Sugiyama M, Baba M, Atomi Y, et al: Diagnosis of anomalous pancreatobiliary junction: value of magnetic resonance cholangiopancreatography. Surgery 1998;123:391

Todani T, Watanabe Y, Narusue M: Congenital bile duct cyst. Am J Surg 1977;134:263

Toma P, Lucigrai G, Pelizza A: Sonographic patterns of Caroli's disease: report of 5 new cases. J Clin Ultrasound 1991;19:155

Voyles CR, Smadja C, Shands WC, et al: Carcinoma in choledochal cysts: age-related incidence. Arch Surg 1983;118:986

Wiedmeyer DA, Stewart ET, Dodds WJ, et al: Choledochal cyst: Findings on cholangiopancreatography with emphasis on ectasis of the common channel. AJR Am J Roentgenol 1989;153:969

Fibropolycystic Diseases

Alvarez F, Bernard O, Brunelle F, et al: Congenital hepatic fibrosis in children. J Pediatr 1981;99:370

Chilton SJ, Cremin BJ: The spectrum of polycystic disease in children. Pediatr Radiol 1981;11:9

Davies CH, Stringer DA, Whyte H, et al: Congenital hepatic fibrosis with saccular dilatation of intrahepatic bile ducts and infantile polycystic kidneys. Pediatr Radiol 1986;16:302

Davis PL, Kanal E, Farnum GN, et al: MR imaging of multiple hepatic cysts in a patient with polycystic liver disease. Magn Reson Imaging 1987;5:407

Ernst O, Gottrand F, Calvo M, et al: Congenital hepatic fibrosis: findings at MR cholangiopancreatography. AJR Am J Roentgenol 1998;170:409

Gupta S, Seith A, Dhiman RK, et al: CT of liver cysts in patients with autosomal dominant polycystic kidney disease. Acta Radiol 1999; 40:444

Horton KM, Bluemke DA, Hruban RH, et al: CT and MR imaging of benign hepatic and biliary tumors. Radiographics 1999;19:431

Itai Y, Ebihara R, Eguchi N, et al: Hepatobiliary cysts in patients with autosomal dominant polycystic kidney disease: prevalence and CT findings. AJR Am J Roentgenol 1995;164:339

Jung G, Benz-Bohm G, Kugel H, et al: MR cholangiography with autosomal recessive polycystic kidney disease. Pediatr Radiol 1999; 29:463

Mas A, Almirall J, Rodriguez A, et al: Microhamartomatosis of the liver associated with autosomal dominant polycystic kidney disease: CT and US appearance. J Comput Assist Tomogr 1994;18:972

Pirson Y, Lannoy N, Peters D, et al: Isolated polycystic liver disease as a distinct genetic disease, unlinked to polycystic kidney disease 1 and polycystic kidney disease 2. Hepatology 1996;23:249

Premkumar A, Berdon WE, Levy J, et al: The emergence of hepatic fibrosis and portal hypertension in infants and children with autosomal recessive polycystic kidney disease: initial and follow-up sonograhic and readiographic findings. Pediatr Radiol 1988;18:123

Summerfield JA, Nagafuchi Y, Sherlock S, et al: Hepatobiliary fibropolycystic diseases: a clinical and histological review of 51 patients. J Hepatol 1986;2:141

Torres VE: Polycystic liver disease. Contrib Nephrol 1995;115:44

Congenital Solitary Cysts/Glycogen Storage Disease

Athey PA, Lauderman JA, King DE: Case report: massive congenital solitary nonparasitic cyst of the liver in infancy. J Ultrasound Med 1986;5:585

Clinkscales NB, Trigg LP, Poklepovic J: Obstructive jaundice secondary to benign hepatic cyst. Radiology 1985;154:643

Doppman JL, Cornblath M, Dwyer AJ, et al: Computed tomography of the liver and kidneys in glycogen storage disease. J Comput Assist Tomogr 1982;6:67

Lee P, Mather S, Owens C, et al: Hepatic ultrasound findings in the glycogen storage diseases. Br J Radiol 1994;67:1062

Pliskin A, Cualing H, Stenger RJ: Primary squamous cell carcinoma originating in congenital cysts of the liver: report of a case and review of the literature. Arch Pathol Lab Med 1992;116:105

Chapter 3

INFECTIONS OF THE LIVER

ALAN E. SCHLESINGER and BRUCE R. PARKER

Viral hepatitis is the most common diffuse infection of the liver in otherwise healthy children. Parasites are more common worldwide, but typically involve the biliary tree, as in ascariasis, or produce focal infections of the liver, as in echinococcosis or amebiasis. Immunocompromised patients are susceptible to fungal infections.

VIRAL HEPATITIS

Viral hepatitis after the perinatal period is most commonly caused by the hepatitis A, hepatitis B, and hepatitis C viruses. A number of other viruses, including mumps, measles, varicella-zoster, herpes simplex, cytomegalovirus, adenovirus, coxsackievirus, and Epstein-Barr virus, have been implicated as causative agents in childhood. Most affected patients have a short-lived acute disease with complete recovery. Complications include subacute and chronic active hepatitis, cirrhosis, and hepatocellular carcinoma of the liver. Chronic active hepatitis may also be of a noninfectious etiology.

Imaging studies are rarely necessary in the acute state. Hepatomegaly will be seen on any imaging study. Ultrasound (US) most commonly demonstrates a heterogeneous increase in echogenicity, but decreased echogenicity may be noted in highly edematous areas. Periportal edema may make the normally increased echoes of the small portal veins even more prominent. The wall of the gallbladder may appear thickened, and periportal lymphadenopathy may be present (Fig. 1). Computed tomography (CT) scans may show heterogeneous changes in attenuation mirroring the sonographic changes, but more commonly are normal except for hepatomegaly. Periportal low attenuation has been described on CT in patients with acute hepatitis, but this is a nonspecific finding. Similarly, magnetic resonance imaging (MRI) may show increased signal intensity in the the periportal region on T_2-weighted images. Hepatic scintigraphy with ^{99m}Tc sulfur colloid also shows hepatomegaly and may show decreased heterogeneous uptake in the liver, with increased uptake in the spleen and bone marrow in some patients. In patients with severe necrosis of the liver and subsequent hepatic regeneration after fulminant hepatitis, Itoh et al. have demonstrated that CT and MRI can differentiate areas of necrosis from areas of nodular regeneration. Regions of necrosis have low attenuation on precontrast CT relative to regions of regeneration and enhance to an attenuation equal to or greater than areas of regeneration after intravenous contrast. Whereas the necrotic liver parenchyma has decreased signal intensity on T_1-weighted MRIs and increased signal intensity on T_2-weighted images, areas of regeneration have decreased signal on T_2 weighting and increased signal intensity on T_1 weighting.

■ US findings in acute viral hepatitis:
- Heterogeneously increased echogenicity
- Focal areas of decreased echogenicity possible in highly edematous area
- Periportal edema with increased periportal echogenicity
- Thickening of gallbladder wall
- Periportal lymphadenopathy

PYOGENIC INFECTION WITH ABSCESS FORMATION

Pyogenic infection with abscess formation after the neonatal period is most commonly found in immunocompromised patients. *Staphylococcus aureus* is the most common pathogen. Patients with chronic granulomatous disease of childhood, a syndrome of leukocyte dysfunction, or those who have had bone marrow transplantation are at high risk for pyogenic abscesses. Other susceptible patients are those on immunosuppressive chemotherapy, those with congenital or acquired immunodeficiency states, those with other intra-abdominal infection such as appendicitis, and those with inflammatory bowel disease.

■ Risk factors for pyogenic liver infection:
- Chronic granulomatous disease
- Bone marrow transplant
- Immunosuppressive chemotherapy
- Congenital or acquired immunodeficiency
- Appendicitis or other intra-abdominal infection
- Inflammatory bowel disease

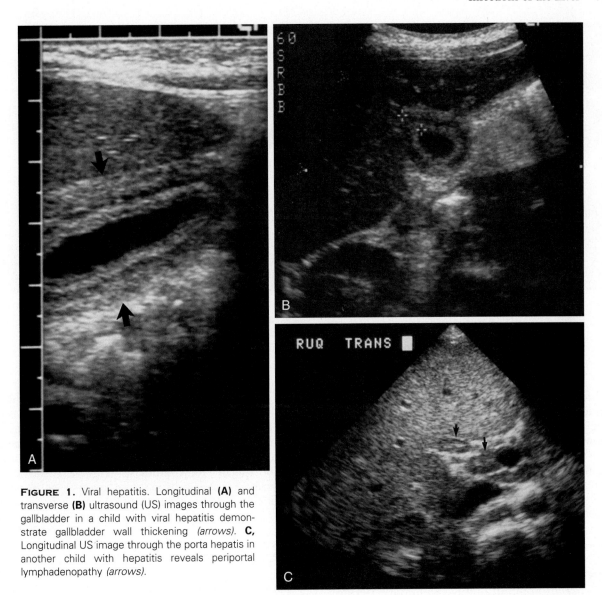

FIGURE 1. Viral hepatitis. Longitudinal **(A)** and transverse **(B)** ultrasound (US) images through the gallbladder in a child with viral hepatitis demonstrate gallbladder wall thickening *(arrows)*. **C,** Longitudinal US image through the porta hepatis in another child with hepatitis reveals periportal lymphadenopathy *(arrows)*.

Most patients develop one or more discrete masses, most frequently in the posterior right lobe, that are hypoechoic but are rarely anechoic. Increased through-transmission is usually present and confirms that the abnormality is not a solid mass. The wall is typically surrounded by a ring of hypoechoic liver edema. Rarely, there is so much internal debris that the abscess may appear hyperechoic, but there usually will still be increased through-transmission in these cases. Fluid–fluid levels have been described, and septations may be seen. Contrast-enhanced CT scans show the abscess to have lower attenuation than the surrounding liver parenchyma (Fig. 2). An enhancing high-attenuation wall is often seen surrounded by a low-attenuation ring of edema. Abscesses in patients with chronic granulomatous disease may heal with formation of granulomas, which can calcify. MRI of hepatic abscesses typically shows decreased signal intensity or nearly isointense signal on T_1-weighted images with increased signal on T_2-weighted images. Contrast enhancement may demonstrate a hyperintense ring around the abscess with

■ Ultrasound findings in pyogenic liver abscess:
  1. Common
     • Hypoechoic mass with increased through-transmission
     • Surrounding hypoechoic ring of hepatic edema
     • Internal debris
  2. Less common
     • Hyperechoic mass with increased through-transmission
     • Anechoic mass
     • Fluid–fluid levels
     • Septations

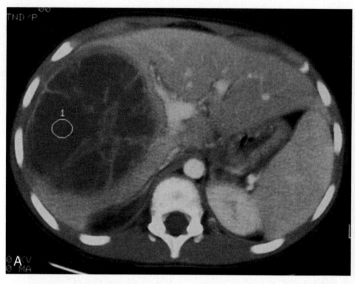
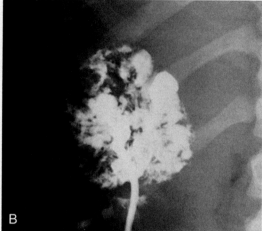

FIGURE 2. Liver abscess. **A,** Contrast-enhanced computed tomography scan demonstrates a multiloculated septated mass of decreased attenuation in the right lobe of the liver. There is increased attenuation of the septa. There is faintly seen edema between the abscess and the enhanced normal liver. **B,** Injection of contrast material following percutaneous drainage of this documented streptococcal abscess demonstrates the multilocular nature of the lesion and its irregularly marginated wall. (Courtesy of Robert Mindelzun, M.D., Stanford, CA.)

persistent low signal within the mass, differentiating it from a solid tumor. Hepatic scintigraphy shows a focal filling defect but is less sensitive than US, CT, or MRI.

Hematogenous spread of pyogenic organisms may result in small microabscesses each of which will show the imaging characteristics described above (Fig. 3). Acute tuberculous abscess cannot be differentiated on imaging studies from other pyogenic infections. Resolved tuberculosis may result in diffuse hepatic calcification.

- Common computed tomography findings in pyogenic liver abscess:
  - Low attenuation relative to hepatic parenchyma after contrast enhancement
  - Enhancing abscess wall
  - Low attenuation of hepatic edema surrounding abscess

Percutaneous abscess drainage under US or CT guidance has become a well-accepted therapeutic procedure (see Fig. 2B). The techniques used are the same as those in adults, although conscious sedation or general anesthesia may be necessary for children. Small abscesses may be drained by aspiration alone, whereas chronic drainage through a percutaneously placed indwelling catheter may be necessary for large lesions.

FUNGAL INFECTIONS

Fungal infection also occurs most frequently in immunocompromised patients. The most common offending organism is *Candida albicans,* but other ubiquitous fungi, such as the agents implicated in aspergillosis, histoplasmosis, coccidioidomycosis (in the endemic area), and

nocardiosis, have been identified in fungal hepatitis. In cases of hepatic candidiasis, multiple small hypoechoic lesions are seen on US. Occasionally these lesions look like bull's eyes, with a central hyperechoic area surrounded by an echolucent zone, an appearance thought to be specific for candidiasis (Fig. 4). Pastakia et al. described a wheel-within-wheel appearance in which a hypoechoic center is surrounded by an echogenic zone that in turn is surrounded by a hyperechogenic zone.

CAT-SCRATCH DISEASE

Cat-scratch disease may present with hepatic and splenic granulomas appearing as hypoechoic lesions (often with increased through-transmission) on US and with low attenuation on unenhanced CT (Fig. 5). The granulomas may remain low in attenuation, may remain isointense, or may demonstrate marginal enhancement after intravenous contrast administration. The granulomas either resolve or calcify.

- Cat-scratch disease may present with hypoechoic hepatic and splenic granulomas on US imaging.

PARASITIC INFESTATIONS

Parasitic infestations are common worldwide, with the offending organism varying from one endemic area to another. *Ascariasis* of the biliary tree is secondary to *Ascaris lumbricoides* infestation of the small intestine. The worms make their way into the biliary system, causing biliary dilatation and pain. On imaging studies, the characteristic vermiform defects will be seen inside the small intestine and dilated biliary ducts. The worms are echogenic on US examination. Ascaris worms have also been imaged with CT and MRI.

ECHINOCOCCOSIS

Echinococcosis (hydatid disease) is an infestation by the larval state of the *Echinococcus* tapeworm. Of the forms found in humans, *E. granulosus* is more common than *E. multilocularis*. The disease is worldwide in distribution, with the major endemic regions being the Middle East and Mediterranean nations, South America, and Australia. Beggs has reviewed the parasitologic, clinical, and radiologic aspects of *E. granulosus* infestation. The pathologic findings explain the findings on imaging studies. An echinococcal cyst has three layers surrounding clear transudative fluid. The rigid outer pericyst is formed by modified host cells. A middle laminated membrane is acellular. The inner, or germinal, layer is thin and produces the laminated membrane and scolices, which are the larval stage. The daughter cysts arise from the germinal membrane. The liver is the most involved organ, being affected in 75% of cases. The cysts may be single or multiple and may appear multilocular because of daughter cysts. The right lobe is most commonly involved. Superinfection usually occurs only after cyst rupture, because the intact middle layer is resistant to bacterial invasion.

Lewall and McCorkell have classified the sonographic findings of hepatic echinococeal cysts. Type I is a simple fluid-filled cyst that is anechoic with through-transmission. In type IR, the germinal layer is seen as an undulating membrane secondary to rupture. Movable echogenic debris in the type I cysts, "echinococcal sand" representing detached scolices, helps differentiate them from simple cysts of the liver. Type II cysts contain daughter cysts whose walls are made up of only the inner and middle layers. Type III lesions are dead cysts, usually calcified and echogenic with shadowing. Lowell and McCorkell stated that the natural progression of disease is from type I to type III.

CT can identify calcification in the cyst wall that may be too fine to see on plain radiographs. The appearance of a split wall is secondary to separation of the laminated membrane from the germinal membrane. Increased attenuation on CT (or increased echogenicity on US) of the cyst fluid suggests bacterial superinfection. In these cases, the cyst is often less well defined, and the wall may appear quite irregular and collapsed.

MRI shows anatomic findings similar to those seen on CT, with the fluid having long T_1 and T_2 relaxation times. If the lesion is multilocular, the mother cyst tends to have higher signal than the daughter cysts on T_2-weighted images. A low-signal-intensity rim may be seen, which is believed to represent fibrous tissue in the pericyst and may be specific for *Echinococcus*. High signal within the cyst on T_1-weighted images (as a result of lipid

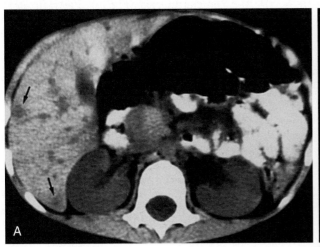

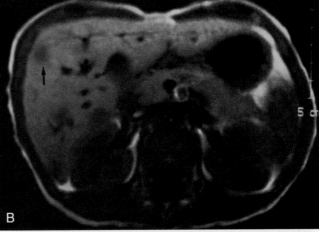

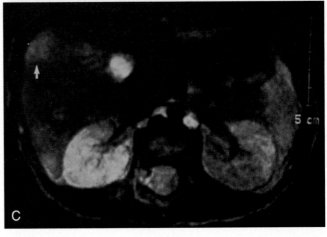

FIGURE 3. Multiple hepatic abscesses. **A,** Unenhanced computed tomography scan demonstrates multiple small low-attenuation lesions *(arrows)* in the inferior portion of the right lobe of the liver. **B** and **C,** Magnetic resonance images demonstrate the largest lesion to have low signal intensity on T_1 weighting and intermediate signal intensity with a T_2-weighted spin-echo sequence *(arrows)*. Biopsy revealed multiple *Escherichia coli* abscesses in this immunocompromised patient.

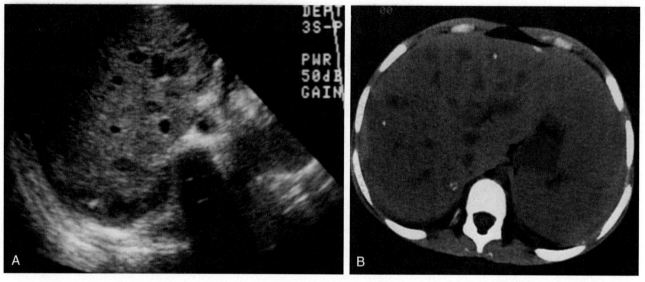

FIGURE 4. Hepatic candidiasis. Transverse sonogram **(A)** and computed tomography (CT) scan **(B)** of the upper abdomen demonstrate multiple "bull's-eye" lesions in the right lobe of the liver in an immunocompromised patient. The calcifications on the CT scan are presumed to represent sequelae of prior infection. Liver biopsy demonstrated candidiasis.

or protein macromolecules) suggests the possibility of a complication such as rupture into the biliary tree or infection. A fat–fluid level on US, CT, or MRI can be seen in hydatid cysts that have ruptured into the biliary tree.

Hydatid sand will have intermediate signal intensity on T_1- and T_2-weighted pulse sequences. Evaluation of the cyst wall is best performed on T_2-weighted images because the contrast between the low-signal wall and the high-signal cyst fluid improves visualization of both contour irregularities of the wall and membrane detachments. Percutaneous drainage of echinococcal

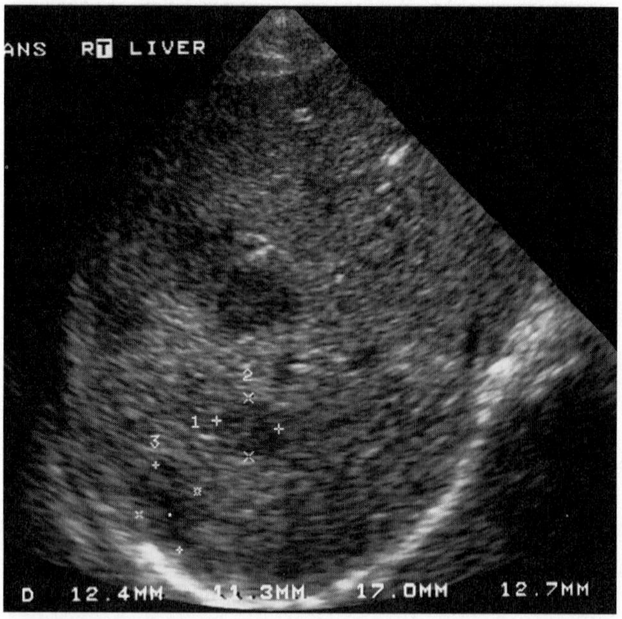

FIGURE 5. Transverse ultrasound image in a child with cat-scratch disease demonstrates multiple hypoechoic nodular lesions in the liver.

cysts has recently been successfully accomplished, although surgical extirpation is still most frequently performed. Recent trials of medical therapy seem promising.

Not only is *E. multilocularis* less common than *E. granulosus,* it shows different imaging features, which were reviewed by Didier et al. Commonly seen patterns include irregular hepatomegaly, multiple lesions with increased echogenicity on US and decreased attenuation on CT, microcalcifications, and dilatation of intrahepatic bile ducts. These authors also described involvement of parahepatic structures, portal hypertension, and involvement of the spleen, hepatic veins, and inferior vena cava.

AMEBIC ABSCESS

Amebic abscesses caused by *Entamoeba histolytica* are most commonly solitary and are most frequently found in the right lobe of the liver. The infection is primarily intestinal, with the liver involved secondary to spread via the portal vein. Amebic abscesses in children are most common under age 3 years and frequently are seen in the first year of life. On US, the lesions are seen peripherally in contact with the hepatic capsule. They are round or oval and hypoechoic, with increased through-transmission. An echogenic wall is not identified. Characteristically, homogeneous low-level echoes are seen throughout the lesion as the gain is increased. Oleszczuk-Raszbe et al. have reviewed the features differentiating pyogenic from amebic abscesses. Amebic abscesses are more likely to be better defined, with a peripheral hypoechoic "halo" (Fig. 6). Pyogenic abscesses are less well defined and have central hypoechogenicity. The wall of the amebic abscess thickens with successful therapy as the echogenicity of the contents decreases.

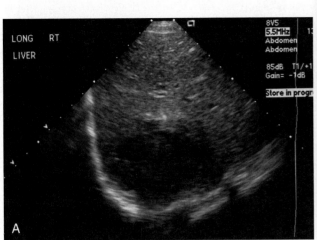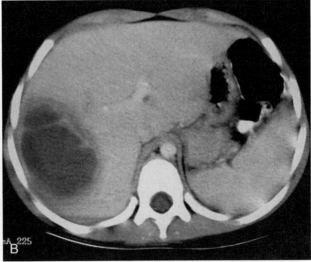

FIGURE 6. Amebic abscess. **A,** Sonogram demonstrates a hypoechogenic mass in the right lobe of the liver with a more hypoechoic surrounding rim. **B,** Computed tomography scan demonstrates a low-attenuation mass in the right lobe of the liver with a prominent "halo."

■ **US findings in amebic abscess:**
- Peripheral location in contact with liver capsule
- Round or oval hypoechoic lesions with increased through-transmission
- Often have subtle low level echoes within lesion
- Peripheral hypoechoic "halo"

CT is not generally needed for diagnosis, but if performed will have an appearance similar to those described for pyogenic abscesses but with a low-attenuation halo (see Fig. 6B). Amebic abscesses are typically unilocular, but multiple abscess may occur. MRI of amebic abscesses has demonstrated heterogeneous low signal on T_2-weighted images, with a double-layered wall. Perforation through the diaphragm may occur, as may intraperitoneal spread. Percutaneous aspiration in children is usually performed only if impending rupture is suspected clinically. Otherwise, patients generally do well with medical therapy.

SUGGESTED READINGS

General

Laurin S, Kande JV: Diagnosis of liver-spleen abscesses in children—with emphasis on ultrasound for the initial and follow up examinations. Pediatr Radiol 1984;14:187

Halvorsen RA, Korobin M, Foster WL, et al: The variable CT appearance of hepatic abscesses. AJR Am J Roentgenol 1984; 142:941

Mathieu D, Vasile N, Fagniez PL, et al: Dynamic CT features of hepatic abscesses. Radiology 1985;154:749

Okada Y, Yao YK, Yunoki M, et al: Lymph nodes in hepatoduodenal ligament: US appearances with CT and MR correlation. Clin Radiol 1996;51:160

Schmiedl U, Paajanen J, Arakawa M, et al: MR imaging of liver abscesses: application of Gd-DTPA. Magn Reson Imaging 1988;6:9

Siegel MJ (ed): Liver and biliary tract. *In* Pediatric Sonography, 2nd ed. New York, Raven Press, 1995:171–236

Siegel MJ, Herman TE: Periportal low attenuation at CT in childhood. Radiology 1992;183:685

Terrier F, Becker CD, Triller JK: Morphologic aspects of hepatic abscesses at computed tomography and ultrasound. Acta Radiol Diagn 1983;24:129

Wall SD, Fisher MR, Amparo EG, et al: Magnetic resonance imaging in the evaluation of abscesses. AJR Am J Roentgenol 1985;144:1217

Viral Hepatitis

Dietrich CF, Lee JH, Herrmann G, et al: Enlargement of perihepatic lymph nodes in relation to liver histology and viremia in patients with chronic hepatitis C. Hepatology 1997;26:1444

Giorgio A, Amoroso P, Fico P, et al: Ultrasound evaluation of uncomplicated and complicated acute viral hepatitis. J Clin Ultrasound 1986;14:675

Itoh H, Sakai T, Takahashi N, et al: Periportal high intensity on T2-weighted MR images in acute viral hepatitis. J Comput Assist Tomogr 1992;16:564

Makhene MK, Diaz PS: Clinical presentations and complications of suspected measles in hospitalized children. Pediatr Infect Dis J 1993;12:836

Murakami T, Baron RL, Peterson MS: Liver necrosis and regeneration after fulminant hepatitis: pathologic correlation with CT and MR findings. Radiology 1996;198:239

Pyogenic Infection with Abscess Formation

Bernardino ME, Berkman WA, Plemmons M, et al: Percutaneous drainage of multiseptated hepatic abscess. J Comput Assist Tomogr 1984;8:38

Callen PW, Filly RA, Marcus FS: Ultrasonography and computed tomography in the evaluation of hepatic microabscesses in the immunosuppressed patient. Radiology 1982;136:433

Francis IR, Glazer GM, Amendola MA, et al: Hepatic abscesses in the immunocompromised patient: role of CT in detection, diagnosis, management, and follow-up. Gastrointest Radiol 1986;11:257

Garel LA, Pariente DM, Nezelof C, et al: Liver involvement in chronic granulomatous disease: the role of ultrasound in diagnosis and treatment. Radiology 1984;153:117

Gerzof SG, Robbins AH, Birkett DH, et al: Percutaneous catheter drainage of abdominal abscesses guided by ultrasound and computed tomography. N Engl J Med 1981;305:653

Grumbach K, Coleman BG, Gal AA, et al: Hepatic and biliary tract abnormalities in patients with AIDS. J Ultrasound Med 1989;8:247

Pineiro-Carrero VM, Andres JM: Morbidity and mortality in children with pyogenic liver abscess. Am J Dis Child 1989;143:1424

Slovis TL, Haller JO, Cohen HL, et al: Complicated appendiceal inflammatory disease in children: pylephlebitis and liver abscess. Radiology 1989;171:823

Stricof DD, Glazer GM, Amendola MA: Chronic granulomatous disease: value of the newer imaging modalities. Pediatr Radiol 1984;14:328

Sty, JR, Starshak RJ: Comparative imaging in the evaluation of hepatic abscesses in immunocompromised children. J Clin Ultrasound 1983;11:11

Fungal Infections

Grünebaum M, Ziv N, Kaplinsky C, et al: Liver candidisasis: the various sonographic patterns in the immunocompromised child. Pediatr Radiol 1991;21:497

Miller JH, Greenfield LD, Wald BR: Candidiasis of the liver and spleen in childhood. Radiology 1982;142:375

Pastakia B, Shawker TH, Thaler M, et al: Hepatosplenic candidiasis: wheels within wheels. Radiology 1988;166:417–421

Cat-Scratch Disease

Hopkins KL, Simoneaux SF, Patrick LE, et al: Imaging manifestations of cat-scratch disease. AJR Am J Roentgenol 1996;166:435

Talenti E, Cesaro S, Scapinello A, et al: Disseminated hepatic and splenic calcifications following cat-scratch disease. Pediatr Radiol 1994;24:342

Parasitic Infestations

Ağildere AM, Aytekin C, Coşkun M, et al: MRI of hydatid disease of the liver: a variety of sequences. J Comput Assist Tomogr 1998;22:718

Beggs I: The radiology of hydatid disease. AJR Am J Roentgenol 1985;145:639

Berry M, Bazaz R, Ghargava S: Amebic liver abscess: sonographic diagnosis and management. J Clin Ultrasound 1986;14:239

Bezzi M, Teggi A, DeRosa F, et al: Abdominal hydatid disease: US findings during medical treatment. Radiology 1987;162:91

Cerri GG, Leite GJ, Simoes JB, et al: Ultrasonographic evaluation of ascaris in the biliary tract. Radiology 1983;146:753

Cremin BJ: Ultrasonic diagnosis of biliary ascariasis: "a bull's eye in the triple O." Br J Radiol 1982;55:683

Didier D, Weiler S, Rohmer P, et al: Hepatic alveolar echinococcosis: correlative US and CT study. Radiology 1985;154:179

Giovagnoni A, Gabrielli O, Coppa GV, et al: MRI appearances of amoebic granulomatous hepatitis: a case report. Pediatr Radiol 1993;23:536

Hayden CK, Toups M, Swischuk LE, et al: Sonographic features of hepatic amebiasis in childhood. J Can Assoc Radiol 1984;35:279

Katzenstein D, Rickerson V, Braude A: New concepts of amebic liver abscess derived from hepatic imaging, serodiagnosis, and hepatic enzymes in 67 consecutive cases in San Diego. Medicine (Baltimore) 1982;61:237

Khuroo MS, Zargar SA, Mahajan R, et al: Sonographic appearance in biliary ascariasis. Gastroenterology 1987;93:267

Khuroo MS, Zargar SA, Mahajan R: Echinococcus cysts in the liver: management with percutaneous drainage. Radiology 1991;180:141

Lewall DB, Bailey TM, McCorkell SJ: Echinococcal matrix: computed tomographic, sonographic and pathologic correlation. J Ultrasound Med 1986;5:33

Lewall DB, McCorkell SJ: Hepatic echinococcal cysts: sonographic appearance and classification. Radiology 1985;155:773

Lewell DB, McCorkell SJ: Rupture of echinococcal cysts: diagnosis, classification and clinical implications. AJR Am J Roentgenol 1986;146:391

Mendez Montero JV, Garcia JA, Antela Lopez, J, et al: Fat-fluid level in hepatic hydatid cyst: a new sign of rupture into the biliary tree? AJR Am J Roentgenol 1996;167:91

Merton DF, Kirks DR: Amebic liver abscess in children: the role of diagnostic imaging. AJR Am J Roentgenol 1984;143:1325

Ng KK, Wong HF, Kong MS, et al: Biliary ascariasis: CT, MR cholangiopancreatography, and navigator endoscopic appearance—report of a case of acute biliary obstruction. Abdom Imaging 1999;24:470

Oleszczuk-Raszke K, Cremin FJ, Fisher RM, et al: Ultrasonic features of pyogenic and amoebic hepatic abscesses. Pediatr Radiol 1989;19:230

Radin DR, Ralls PW, Colletti PM, et al: CT of amebic liver abscess. AJR Am J Roentgenol 1988;150:1297

Ralls PW: Sonography in the diagnosis and management of hepatic amebic abscess in children. Pediatr Radiol 1982;12:239

Ralls PW, Barnes PF, Johnson MC, et al: Treatment of hepatic amebic abscess: rare need for percutaneous drainage. Radiology 1987;165:805

Ralls PW, Barnes PF, Radin DR, et al: Sonographic features of amebic and pyogenic liver abscesses: a blinded comparison. AJR Am J Roentgenol 1987;179:499

Ralls, PW, Colletti PM, Quinn MF, et al: Sonographic findings in hepatic amebic abscess. Radiology 1982;145:123

Remedios PA, Colletti PM, Ralls PW: Hepatic amebic abscess: choles-cintigraphic rim enhancement. Radiology 1986;160:395

Schulman A, Loxton AJ, Heydenrych JJ, et al: Sonographic diagnosis of biliary ascariasis. AJR Am J Roentgenol 1982;13:485

Taourel P, Marty-Ane B, Charasset S, et al: Hydatid cyst of the liver: comparison of CT and MRI. J Comput Assist Tomogr 1993;17:80

Ustunsoz B, Akhan O, Kamiloglu MA, et al: Percutaneous treatment of hydatid cysts of the liver—long-term results. AJR Am J Roentgenol 1999;172:91

van Sonnenberg E, Mueller PR, Schiffman HR, et al: Intrahepatic amoebic abscesses: indications for and results of percutaneous catheter drainage. Radiology 1985;156:631

■ **C h a p t e r   4**

DIFFUSE PARENCHYMAL DISEASE

ALAN E. SCHLESINGER and BRUCE R. PARKER

Many diseases cause diffuse imaging abnormalities in the liver. Although some of these diseases are of congenital origin, the hepatic manifestations are acquired as complications of the disease process or its treatment.

CIRRHOSIS

Cirrhosis of the liver is a diffuse disease in which the normal hepatic parenchyma is destroyed and replaced by fibrosis. The liver tissue regenerates in a focal nodular pattern. In the micronodular form, the nodules are 1 cm in diameter or smaller, whereas the macronodular form can have nodular diameters as large as 5 cm. Portal hypertension is a common finding, as discussed in Section VII, Part III, Chapter 5, page 1814. Cirrhosis is a secondary phenomenon that has been described in children with a variety of congenital and acquired diseases, including hepatitis, hepatic fibrosis, biliary atresia, cystic fibrosis, Budd-Chiari syndrome, and chronic biliary obstruction. Cirrhosis is also seen in a number of metabolic disorders, including α_1-antitrypsin deficiency, glycogen storage disease, galactosemia, tyrosinemia, and Wilson's disease.

■ Causes of cirrhosis:
  1. Primary
  2. Secondary
     • Hepatitis
     • Hepatic fibrosis
     • Biliary atresia
     • Cystic fibrosis
     • Budd-Chiari syndrome
     • Chronic biliary obstruction
  3. Metabolic causes
     • α_1-antitrypsin deficiency
     • Glycogen storage disease
     • Galactosemia
     • Tyrosinemia
     • Wilson's disease

Ultrasound (US) examination of the cirrhotic liver shows the right lobe to be small (Fig. 1). The caudate lobe and lateral segment of the left lobe are, in compensation, enlarged. The margins of the liver are irregular rather than smooth. Both fatty infiltration of the liver and fibrosis cause increased echogenicity of the parenchyma, which may be heterogeneous. Regenerative nodules may have relatively decreased echogenicity. The intrahepatic vessels may be difficult to see because of compression by fibrosis. The gallbladder may be small, not seen, or have stones within it, depending on the primary disease leading to the cirrhosis. The findings of portal hypertension are often seen.

Hepatic scintigraphy shows a normal-sized or small liver with heterogeneous decreased uptake of the isotope-labeled colloid. Regenerating nodules show increased activity between areas of photopenic fibrosis. There is increased activity in the enlarged spleen and in the bone marrow (see Fig. 1D).

Computed tomography (CT) shows a small or normal-sized, irregularly marginated liver (Fig. 2) with decreased attenuation in areas of fatty infiltration and normal attenuation in areas of fibrosis and regenerating nodules. Contrast enhancement exaggerates the heterogeneity of attenuation. CT also may demonstrate imaging findings of portal hypertension.

Magnetic resonance imaging (MRI) of the liver shows the anatomic abnormalities seen with US and CT. The signal intensity on spin-echo images is nonspecific and variable, depending on the degree of fatty infiltration and iron deposition. Regenerating nodules may be isointense with liver or show reduced signal intensity on T_2-weighted images secondary to iron deposition. Gradient-recalled echo images are even more sensitive to the presence of iron. Hepatocellular carcinoma complicating cirrhosis is more common in adults than children. The differentiation of regenerating nodules from hepatocellular carcinoma may be difficult if the nodules are isointense with liver, but possible, because T_2-weighted signal may be decreased with nodules but increased with tumor.

• MR appearance of cirrhosis is nonspecific and variable.
• Differentiation of regenerating nodules from hepatocellular carcinoma may be difficult on MRI.

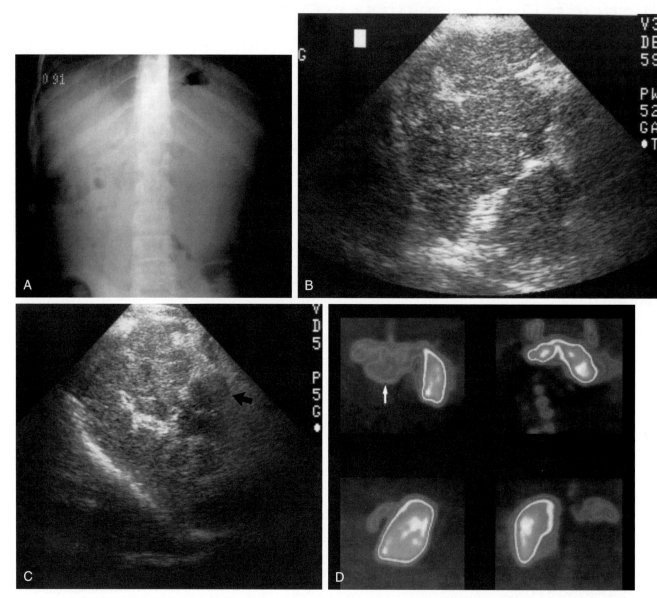

FIGURE 1. Cirrhosis in a patient with cystic fibrosis. **A,** Abdominal radiograph demonstrates a small, shrunken liver in the right upper quadrant with marked splenomegaly on the left. **B** and **C,** Transverse ultrasound images of the right lobe of the liver at two different levels demonstrate heterogeneous increased echogenicity resulting from fatty replacement, a markedly lobular configuration to the small-volume liver, and hypoechoic regenerating nodules (*arrow* in **C**). **D,** ^{99m}Tc-labeled colloid single-photon emission tomography scan in a different patient (*clockwise from the top left:* anterior, right lateral, posterior, left lateral) demonstrates reduced activity in the liver and a relatively larger caudate lobe (*arrow*). Most activity is in the greatly enlarged spleen. (Courtesy of Michael L. Goris, M.D., Stanford, CA.)

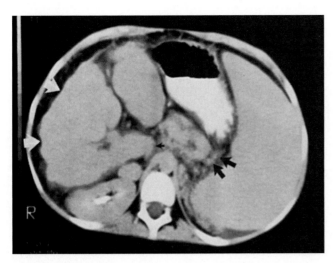

FIGURE 2. Contrast-enhanced computed tomography scan in an 11-year-old girl with cirrhosis and portal hypertension shows the small liver with nodular surface *(white arrows)* and caudate lobe hypertrophy *(small black arrow)*. Venous collateral vessels are present in the hilum of the enlarged spleen *(large black arrows)*.

FATTY INFILTRATION OF THE LIVER

Fatty infiltration of the liver is seen in diseases other than cirrhosis. Patients with endogenous Cushing's syndrome or, more commonly, those on steroid therapy may develop diffuse fatty infiltration. Metabolic disorders such as familial hyperlipoproteinemia, glycogen storage disease, Wilson's disease, and Reye's syndrome may also cause diffuse fatty infiltration. The findings may also be present in patients on combination anticancer chemotherapy, on hyperalimentation, and with extreme malnutrition. On US, there is increased echogenicity of the liver parenchyma. Usually this is diffuse, but occasionally

it may be focal. On CT, there is often dramatic decreased attenuation of the liver parenchyma that becomes more pronounced after contrast enhancement (Fig. 3). T_1-weighted spin-echo MRI demonstrates increased signal intensity in areas of fatty infiltration. The signal intensity will diminish on fat-saturated or short tau inversion recovery images. Chemical shift imaging (comparing images with water and fat opposed-phase and in-phase) can add confidence in the diagnosis of focal fatty infiltration.

■ **Causes of fatty infiltration of the liver:**
1. Cirrhosis
2. Cushing's syndrome
3. Steroid therapy
4. Metabolic disorders
   • Familial hyperlipoproteinemia
   • Glycogen storage disease
   • Wilson's disease
   • Reye's syndrome
5. Anti-cancer chemotherapy
6. Hyperalimentation
7. Extreme malnutrition

IRON DEPOSITION IN THE LIVER

Iron deposition in the liver can be seen as a result of either hepatic parenchymal iron deposition in the *hepatocytes* or iron deposition in the *reticuloendothelial (Kupffer) cells*. Parenchymal iron deposition in the hepatocytes can be seen in patients with primary hemochromatosis or cirrhosis. In primary hemochromatosis, there is excessive iron absorption by the gastrointestinal tract, and the excess iron can be deposited in the parenchyma

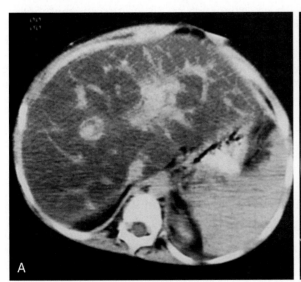

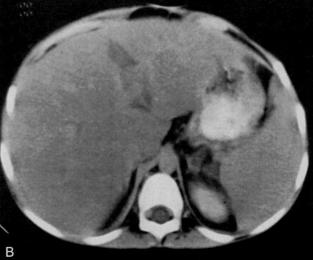

FIGURE 3. Diffuse fatty infiltration of the liver in a 5-year-old boy 2 months after liver transplantation. **A,** Enhanced computed tomography (CT) scan shows low attenuation of both hepatic lobes and relative enhancement of hyperdense blood vessels. **B,** CT scan 8 days prior to clinical deterioration shows normal attenuation of the hepatic parenchyma.

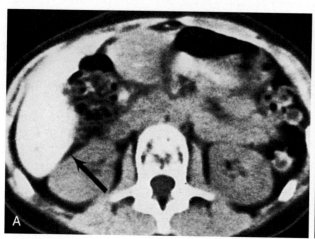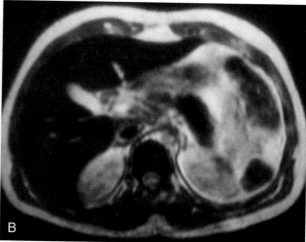

FIGURE 4. Iron overload. **A,** Unenhanced computed tomography scan of a 15-year-old girl with hemachromatosis shows the dense liver *(arrow)*. **B,** T$_1$-weighted spin-echo magnetic resonance image in a different patient with iron overload from multiple blood transfusions demonstrates dramatically decreased signal intensity of the liver.

of the liver, pancreas, heart, and other organs. In cirrhosis unrelated to hemochromatosis, there are increased iron levels in the hepatocytes from increased absorption and other obsure mechanisms. In contrast, excessive iron deposition in the reticuloendothelial system (hemosiderosis) is typically caused by hemolysis, usually from hemolytic anemia, or multiple blood transfusions, often for treatment of thalassemia or in patients undergoing bone marrow transplantation. These conditions cause accumulation of iron in the reticuloendothelial system, including the liver, spleen, and bone marrow.

■ Primary hemochromatosis causes iron deposition in hepatocytes (as well as the parenchyma of the pancreas, heart, and other organs) while hemosiderosis is associated with increased iron deposition in the reticuloendothelial (Kupffer) cells of the liver (as well as the reticuloendothelial cells of the spleen and bone marrow).

Diffuse increased attenuation of the liver on CT scan may be seen in iron overload (Fig. 4A). US is usually unrevealing, but MRI findings are dramatic, with marked decrease in signal intensity on T$_2$-weighted images and, to a lesser degree, on T$_1$-weighted images (Fig. 4B). Qualitative as well as quantitative assessment of liver signal intensity has been shown to correlate with liver iron levels on biopsy and with the number of blood transfusions. Although the MRI signal of the liver is similar in parenchymal and reticuloendothelial iron deposition, Siegelman et al. demonstrated that all of five patients with primary hemochromatosis had abnormally low signal intensity in the pancreas on T$_2$-weighted spin-echo images as well, while four of five patients had

normal splenic signal intensity. With reticuloendothelial cell iron overload, however, the spleen (a reticuloendothelial organ) showed abnormally low-intensity signal in 14 of 14 patients, while the pancreas (a nonreticuloendothelial organ) had low signal in only 3 of 16. Thus MRI appears able to discriminate between parenchymal iron deposition resulting from primary hemachromatosis and iron deposition in the reticuloendothelial cells (hemosiderosis) of the liver.

GAUCHER'S DISEASE

Gaucher's disease is a genetic disorder causing accumulation of glucocerebroside in cells of the reticuloendothelial system. Hepatomegaly alone may be seen, but focal areas of low signal intensity on T$_1$-weighted MRI with an isointense or hyperintense appearance on T$_2$-weighted images may be seen, presumably as a result of collections of Gaucher's cells or fibrosis. Treatment for this disease with enzyme replacement therapy is now available, but costly. Quantification of hepatomegaly may be important because there is a correlation between liver size and bone marrow changes and avascular necrosis. Therefore, liver volume may prove useful in treatment considerations and in enzyme dosage. MRI, US, and CT have all been used for liver volume measurement.

SUGGESTED READINGS

General

Henschke CI, Goldman H, Teele RL: The hyperechogenic liver in children: cause and sonographic appearance. AJR Am J Roentgenol 1982;138:841

Mitchell DG: Focal manifestations of diffuse liver disease at MR imaging. Radiology 1992;185:1

Weinreb JC, Cohen JM, Armstrong E, et al: Imaging the pediatric liver: MRI and CT. AJR Am J Roentgenol 1986;147:785

Cirrhosis

Agrons GA, Corse WR, Markowitz RA, et al: Gastrointestinal manifestations of cystic fibrosis: radiologic-pathologic correlation. Radiographics 1996;16:871

Daneman A, Matzinger MA, Martin DJ: Cirrhosis: an unusual pattern of enhancement on CT. Pediatr Radiol 1983;13:162

Doppman JL, Cornblath M, Dwyer AJ, et al: Computed tomography of the liver and kidneys in glycogen storage disease. J Comput Assist Tomogr 1982;6:67

Macvicar D, Dicks-Mireaux C, Leonard JV, et al: Hepatic imaging with computed tomography of chronic tyrosinaemia type 1. Br J Radiol 1990;63:605

Murakami T, Kuroda C, Marukawa T, et al: Regenerating nodules in hepatic cirrhosis: MR findings with pathologic correlation. AJR Am J Roentgenol 1990;155:1227

Ohtomo K, Itai Y, Ohtomo Y, et al: Regenerating nodules of liver cirrhosis: MR imaging with pathologic correlation. AJR Am J Roentgenol 1990;154:505

Fatty Infiltration of the Liver

Baker MK, Schauwecker DS, Wenker JC, et al: Nuclear medicine evaluation of focal fatty infiltration of the liver. Clin Nucl Med 1986;11:503

Quinn SF, Gosink BB: Characteristic sonographic signs of hepatic fatty infiltration. AJR Am J Roentgenol 1985;145:753

Iron Deposition in the Liver

Bonetti MG, Castriota-Scanderberg A, Criconia GM, et al: Hepatic iron overload in thalassemic patients: proposal and validation of an MR method of assessment. Pediatr Radiol 1996;26:650

Kornreich L, Horev G, Yaniv I, et al: Iron overload following bone marrow transplantation in children: MR findings. Pediatr Radiol 1997;27:869

Papakonstantinou O, Kostaridou S, Maris T, et al: Quantification of liver iron overload by T2 quantitative magnetic resonance imaging in thalassemia: impact of chronic hepatitis C on measurements. J Pediatr Hematol Oncol 1999;21:142

Siegelman ES, Mitchell DG, Rubin R, et al: Parenchymal versus reticuloendothelial iron overload in the liver: distinction with MR imaging. Radiology 1991;179:361

Stark DD, Moseley ME, Bacon BR, et al: Magnetic resonance imaging and spectroscopy of hepatic iron overload. Radiology 1985;154:137

Gaucher's Disease

Elstein D, Hadas-Halpern I, Azuri Y, et al: Accuracy of ultrasonography in assessing spleen and liver size in patients with Gaucher disease: comparison to computed tomographic measurements. J Ultrasound Med 1997;16:209

Glenn D, Thurston D, Garver P, et al: Comparison of magnetic resonance imaging and ultrasound in evaluating liver size in Gaucher patients. Acta Haematol 1994;92:187

Hill SC, Damaska BM, Ling A, et al: Gaucher disease: abdominal MR imaging findings in 46 patients. Radiology 1992;184:561

Terk MR, Esplin J, Lee K, et al: MR imaging of patients with type 1 Gaucher's disease: relationship between bone and visceral changes. AJR Am J Roentgenol 1995;165:599

Chapter 5

ABNORMALITIES OF HEPATIC VASCULATURE

ALAN E. SCHLESINGER and BRUCE R. PARKER

VASCULAR ANATOMY

The normal arterial blood supply to the liver is variable. In 57% of patients, there is a single common hepatic artery that arises from the celiac axis in 90% of cases, from the superior mesenteric artery in 5%, and from other visceral branches of the aorta in 5%. In the 43% of patients with multiple origins of the hepatic arterial tree, the right hepatic artery arises from the superior mesenteric artery in half and the left hepatic artery (or, more commonly, the left lateral segmental artery) from the left gastric artery in most of the others. After giving rise to the gastroduodenal artery, the common hepatic artery becomes the proper hepatic artery, which divides into right and left trunks whose branches follow a segmental distribution.

The portal vein originates from the juncture of the superior mesenteric vein with the splenic vein. In the porta hepatis, the vein divides into right and left branches. Each branch further subdivides, following the same segmental distribution as the hepatic arteries and biliary ducts. The hepatic veins, however, are interlobar and intersegmental, running in the fissures that divide the lobes, the segments, and the subsegments. The venous branches join to form the three major hepatic veins. The middle and left hepatic veins most frequently form a common trunk just before entering the suprahepatic portion of the inferior vena cava (IVC). The right hepatic vein enters the suprahepatic IVC separately. The

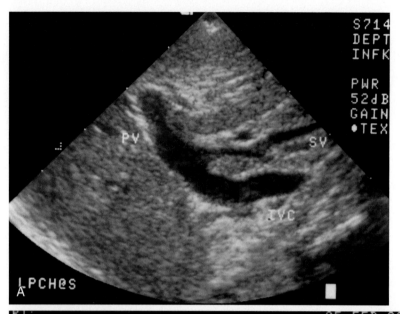

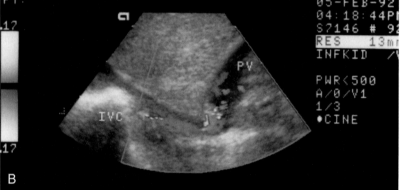

FIGURE 1. A, Transverse sonogram of the right mid-abdomen demonstrates the splenic vein draining into the portal vein, which then drains directly into the subhepatic inferior vena cava (IVC). **B,** Color Doppler examination of the portal vein and IVC demonstrates the venous flow directly from the portal vein into the IVC. No intrahepatic portal venous flow was demonstrated.

caudate lobe vein typically enters the intrahepatic portion of the IVC, as may small branches of the posterior segment of the right lobe.

Spontaneous portosystemic shunts have been described at various levels. Jabra and Taylor described an intrahepatic shunt in an infant diagnosed with color Doppler sonography. In the case of Mori et al., an enormous shunt between the portal and hepatic veins was associated with multiple coronary artery fistulas. Bellah et al. described a shunt from the portal vein to the suprahepatic vena cava, while a patient we have encountered had a shunt from the portal vein to the infrahepatic vena cava (Fig. 1). Magnetic resonance imaging (MRI) has also been used to evaluate congenital portosystemic shunts. Congenital hepatic arterial–portal venous malformations have been reported as well.

Congenital absence of the portal vein is rare, but has been documented by ultrasound (US) and MRI. Absence of the horizontal portion of the left portal vein is a rare but reported anomaly occurring in one of 507 consecutive patients in one series and in 7 of 17 patients with known portal venous anomalies in another series. Preduodenal portal vein occurs when the inferior connection between the paired embryonic vitelline veins persists instead of undergoing normal atrophy. The anomaly is associated with biliary atresia and numerous small intestinal abnormalities, as described in Section V, Part VII, page 1393. The preduodenal vein has been demonstrated by US, venography, and computed tomography (CT).

PORTAL HYPERTENSION

Portal hypertension can develop secondary to extrahepatic or intrahepatic causes.

EXTRAHEPATIC PORTAL VEIN OBSTRUCTION

Extrahepatic portal vein obstruction is more common in children. The most frequent cause is idiopathic cavernous transformation of the portal vein, in which the occluded, usually atretic, portal vein is surrounded by serpentine collateral vessels. Idiopathic cavernous transformation is probably secondary to portal vein thrombosis occurring years before clinical presentation. Neonatal omphalitis and umbilical vein catheterization have been suggested as causes of neonatal thrombosis, but the cause is usually obscure. Other causes of extrahepatic portal hypertension include acute and subacute portal vein thrombosis (in which the obstructed portal vein may still be seen even though cavernous transformation occurs), intrinsic portal vein webs, ascending mesenteric phlebitis, postoperative complications, and masses in the porta hepatis. Portal hypertension secondary to extrahepatic portal vein obstruction is usually silent until splenomegaly is noted or upper gastrointestinal bleeding occurs. Liver function tests are typically normal.

> ■ Most common cause of extrahepatic portal vein obstruction in children is cavernous transformation of the portal vein.

Plain radiographic findings are usually sparse except for splenomegaly. Paravertebral widening may be seen with large paraesophageal varices (see Section VI, Part V, Chapter 6, Fig. 1, page 1581), and the azygos vein may be dilated. Sonography shows splenomegaly and, occasionally, ascites, although the latter is more common with intrahepatic causes of portal hypertension, especially cirrhosis. The liver itself appears normal. The portal vein usually cannot be identified, but the serpentine, tortuous collaterals are easily seen in the porta hepatis (Fig. 2). Similar serpentine vessels can be identified in the splenic hilum (Fig. 3). Portosystemic collateral vessels can be identified, with the coronary vein being the most frequently seen. Collaterals are frequently identified in the gastrohepatic ligament and can be seen adjacent to the esophagogastric junction (see Section VI, Part V, Chapter 6, Fig. 1, page 1581). Other portosys-

temic pathways are more commonly seen with intrahepatic causes of portal vein obstruction, as noted below.

Brunelle, Alagille, et al. described thickening of the lesser omentum as a sign of portal venous hypertension in children. Patriquin, Tessier, et al. determined that the normal ratio of the thickness of the lesser omentum to the aortic diameter at the level of the crus of the diaphragm is less than 1.7. Ratios greater than 1.7 were seen in patients with portal hypertension, obesity, steroid therapy, and lymphadenopathy. Doppler US is useful to determine the character and direction of flow in collateral vessels. Hepatofugal flow and loss of normal respiratory pulsations in the portal vein on Doppler study are signs of portal hypertension.

On dynamic CT, the tortuous veins in the porta hepatis are easily seen, and portosystemic collaterals are often identified. If a more acute thrombus is the cause of the portal hypertension, unenhanced scans may show the high-attenuation clot within the portal vein. With contrast enhancement, the clot appears as an intravascular filling defect.

MRI and magnetic resonance angiography (MRA) have been used to evaluate the portal venous system in children with extrahepatic portal hypertension. Standard T_1- and T_2-weighted pulse sequences are used to evaluate the hepatic parenchyma. The hepatic vessels will have low signal on T_1-weighted images (black blood technique). MRA (white blood techniques) can be performed using time-of-flight, phase contrast (rarely used in evaluating the portal vessels), or gadolinium-enhanced techniques. MRI can be helpful in children with cavernous transformation because the tangled vessels in the porta can be identified (Fig. 4), but the signal characteristics will vary with the presence, ab-

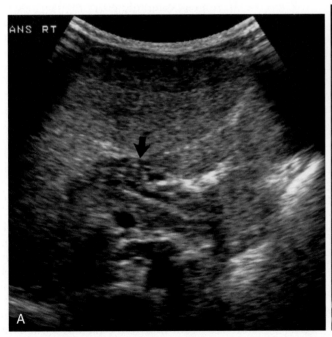
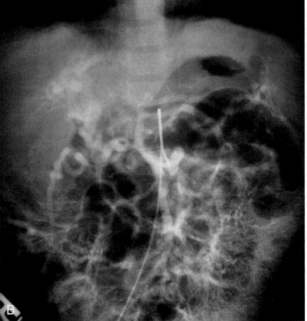

FIGURE 2. Cavernous transformation of the portal vein. **A,** Transverse ultrasound image through the region of the porta hepatis reveals a tangle of collateral vessels in the expected location of the portal vein *(arrow).* **B,** Portal venous phase of a superior mesenteric arteriogram confirms cavernous transformation of the portal vein.

sence, and velocity of blood flow. Acute and subacute thrombosis of the portal vein can be identified but may be simulated by stagnant flow. Johnson et al. compared results of time-of-flight MRA with arterial portography and endoscopy (see Section VI, Part V, Chapter 6, Fig. 1, page 1581). They concluded that MRA is a satisfactory technique for the identification of varices.

Arterial portography is less commonly utilized for diagnostic purposes than in the past. Because of the variable origin of the hepatic arteries, injection of both celiac and superior mesenteric arteries is usually necessary. In the venous phase, the existing portosystemic collaterals are well seen, particularly those arising from the left gastric artery and coursing along the esophagus. Patency of the vessels to be shunted should be demonstrated.

INTRAHEPATIC PORTAL HYPERTENSION

The most common cause of intrahepatic portal hypertension is cirrhosis of the liver. Hepatitis and congenital hepatic fibrosis have also been implicated (see Section VI, Part III, Chapter 2, Fig. 13, page 1462), as have a number of rare lesions. Portal vein thrombosis secondary to liver metastases has been described in as many as 8% of affected adults. Approximately one third of patients with hepatocellular carcinoma of the liver may also demonstrate portal thrombosis with secondary portal hypertension. Veno-occlusive disease of the liver (see below) and thrombosis of the hepatic veins or suprahepatic portion of the inferior vena cava (Budd-Chiari syndrome; see below) may also lead to secondary portal hypertension.

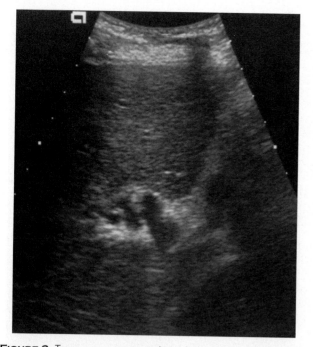

FIGURE 3. Transverse sonogram through the spleen demonstrates dilated varices in the splenic hilum with minimal dilatation of intrasplenic vascular structures and heterogeneous echogenicity of the splenic parenchyma.

The findings generally are similar to those described for extrahepatic portal hypertension, but there will also be symptoms, signs, and abnormal laboratory studies related to the underlying hepatic disease (see Cirrhosis in Section VI, Part III, Chapter 4, page 1475). In these cases, the portal vein is usually seen on imaging studies and may appear enlarged. Doppler US is particularly useful in evaluating the flow characteristics within the portal vein, as well as within collaterals. Flow may be identified in the region of the ligamentum teres. This has been demonstrated to be in paraumbilical collaterals rather than in a "recanalized umbilical vein" as originally thought. Reversed (hepatofugal) flow may be seen within the portal vein or its branches. Doppler sonography in children with portal hypertension resulting from chronic liver disease may demonstrate decrease in the normal pulsatility of the hepatic venous tracings and increased pulsatility in the portal vein. Ascites is more commonly seen in patients with portal hypertension from intrahepatic obstruction than in patients with the extrahepatic form.

> ■ **Ascites is more common in intrahepatic portal hypertension than the extrahepatic form.**

CT, in addition to the findings seen in extrahepatic portal hypertension noted above, will show the characteristics of the underlying liver disease process as well. With cirrhosis and posthepatitic states, the enlarged portal vein may also be demonstrated on CT. Varices and other collateral vessels may be more easily identified than they are in some cases of extrahepatic portal hypertension. Splenomegaly may be present.

There has been increasing interest in the use of MRI and MRA (with and without gadolinium) in the evaluation of intrahepatic portal hypertension. As discussed previously, the standard spin-echo MRI pulse sequences are used to evaluate the hepatic parenchyma as well as the vasculature, which can be complemented with MRA (white blood techniques). On MRI, the portal vein is usually well seen. However, slow or turbulent flow within the portal vein may cause increased signal intensity with T_1-weighted images, simulating thrombosis. Proton-density images or T_2-weighted spin-echo images will usually show decreased signal with turbulent flow and increased signal with a real thrombosis. MRA is better at demonstrating the flow characteristics within the portal vein and the collaterals. Rodgers et al. compared MRI (with contrast-enhanced MRA) with conventional angiography in the evaluation of the portal venous system in 18 pediatric and adult patients prior to surgery (16 prior to liver transplant, 1 prior to pancreatic resection, and 1 after liver transplant but prior to surgery to evaluate a porta hepatis mass). Of the 84 vessels evaluated by both techniques, appearances were similar in 76 (90%). Both imaging modalities confirmed that the main portal vein was patent in nine patients and occluded in five. The main portal vein was shown to be patent but abnormal in two patients by both studies. The authors concluded that

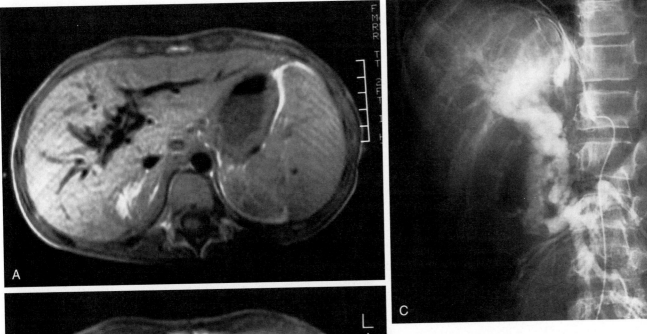

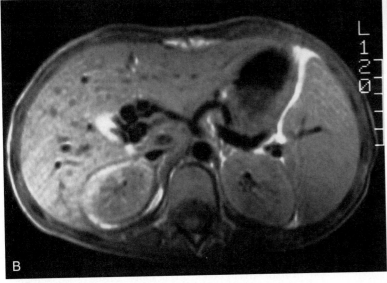

FIGURE 4. Cavernous transformation of the portal vein with portal hypertension. **A** and **B,** Axial magnetic resonance images through the porta hepatis demonstrate the portal cavernoma to excellent advantage. Note also the enlarged spleen and enlarged splenic vein. **C,** Arterial portogram demonstrates the characteristic dilated tortuous vessels of a portal cavernoma.

MRA can replace preoperative angiography in the evaluation of the portal vein in most cases. In a larger study of 102 patients evaluated for liver transplantation (adults and children), Silverman et al. performed preoperative MRA of the portal vein and compared the findings to surgical findings as well as histologic evaluation of the explanted liver. MRA identified 10 clots within portal veins, all surgically confirmed. The 92 portal veins that were patent by MRA were patent at the time of surgery. The one small chronic clot in an intrahepatic portal vein missed by MRA was also not seen at surgery, but was identified at histologic examination.

> ■ MRI (with MRA) can replace angiography in the preoperative evaluation of the portal vein in most cases.

Although conventional angiography is less commonly performed in the routine evaluation of the portal venous system, it continues to have a role in children requiring vascular intervention. Transjugular intrahepatic portosystemic shunt procedures have been performed in children with portal hypertension to treat refractory ascites and gastrointestinal bleeding.

BUDD-CHIARI SYNDROME

Budd-Chiari syndrome is a rare disorder in children, developing after obstruction of the hepatic veins or the intrahepatic or suprahepatic portions of the IVC at a point where secondary hepatic vein obstruction occurs. In most instances, the etiology is not clear. Thrombosis can occur in a variety of hypercoagulable states, with primary or secondary neoplasms, after trauma, or after liver transplantation. Obstruction secondary to congenital webs inside the hepatic veins or IVC has been reported. A rare case of Budd-Chiari syndrome in a child with Gaucher's disease has also been reported. In children, hepatomegaly is usually the presenting characteristic of the acute form of Budd-Chiarri syndrome. In chronic Budd-Chiari syndrome, the typical findings of portal hypertension are usually present.

> ■ Causes of Budd-Chiari syndrome include hypercoaguable states, primary, or secondary neoplasms, trauma, and surgery. However, most cases are idiopathic.

Sonography may demonstrate heterogeneous echogenicity of the liver. Areas of decreased echogenicity may be secondary to hemorrhagic infarction and necrosis. As these areas resolve, fibrosis and scarring may result in hyperechoic regions. The liver is generally large, with the caudate lobe being especially enlarged. Ascites may be identified. In chronic Budd-Chiari syndrome, the major hepatic veins may not be identified. More commonly, they can be seen, and color Doppler sonography is extremely useful in identifying the level of obstruction and the direction of flow in the portal venous system, hepatic veins, and IVC. With pulse Doppler evaluation, markedly reduced or reversed flow in the hepatic veins and in the IVC may be seen. These findings, if present, are the most specific and sensitive for the imaging diagnosis of Budd-Chiari syndrome.

Hepatic scintigraphy discloses heterogeneous decreased activity throughout most of the liver with normal to increased activity in the caudate lobe, which is not usually involved by the disease because of its separate venous drainage. However, Powell-Jackson et al. have shown these findings to be present in only 17% of the patients in their study.

> ■ Hepatic scintigraphy in Budd-Chiari syndrome may reveal normal to increased uptake in the caudate lobe with decreased activity in the remainder of the liver.

CT is often less specific than one might expect, but typical features include hepatomegaly with an enlarged caudate lobe, thrombus in the hepatic veins, decreased caliber of the IVC, and ascites. Following contrast infusion, there is relatively greater enhancement of the caudate lobe with decreased enhancement peripherally. Intraluminal high-attenuation filling defects within the veins are virtually diagnostic of venous thrombosis. Whereas Doppler US demonstrates the abnormal vascular anatomy better than CT, CT is superior to US in evaluating the hepatic parenchyma for cirrhosis or tumor.

MRI shows absent or narrowed hepatic veins, intrahepatic venous collaterals, IVC thrombosis or compression, or intrahepatic parenchymal abnormalities. MRA, however, can show hepatic venous obstruction and collateral circulation, possibly as well as angiography and Doppler sonography. Although inferior vena cavography and retrograde hepatic venography have been considered the only truly sensitive imaging studies in the past, the combination of Doppler US and MRA can now likely replace them.

Angiography, however, can still have a role when nonsurgical intervention is contemplated. Lois et al. described an 8-year-old girl with Budd-Chiari syndrome secondary to membranous obstruction of the hepatic veins and a web in the IVC. The vessels were recanalized and dilated percutaneously via a transhepatic approach, with prompt resolution of symptoms.

HEPATIC VENO-OCCLUSIVE DISEASE

Hepatic veno-occlusive disease (HVOD) refers to obstruction of the hepatic venous system at the level of the central and sublobular veins. Most cases are secondary to toxicity from chemotherapy, hepatic radiation, bone marrow transplantation, or certain alkaloids. Less commonly, the disease may be seen in congenital immunodeficiency states and systemic lupus erythematosus. Clinically, HVOD presents with hepatomegaly, jaundice, and ascites. Imaging can exclude Budd-Chiari syndrome by demonstrating the patency of the major hepatic veins and IVC. This can easily be accomplished by sonography. Various findings on gray-scale sonography have been described in patients with HVOD, including thickening of the gallbladder wall, ascites, hepatosplenomegaly, decreased diameter of the hepatic veins, enlargement of the portal vein, and visualization of paraumbilical venous collaterals. Doppler US can show abnormalities in the portal vein (loss of normal velocity variations with breathing, decrease in Doppler spectral density, hepatofugal or reduced hepatopedal portal venous flow, or elevation of the congestion index [cross-sectional area divided by the average velocity]); the hepatic artery (elevated resistive index); the hepatic veins (absent or monophasic flow); or the paraumbilical vein (hepatofugal flow). However, the definitive diagnosis requires biopsy and histologic examination of the liver.

SUGGESTED READINGS

Vascular Anatomy

Alpern MB, Rubin JM, Williams DM, et al: Porta hepatis: duplex Doppler US with angiographic correlation. Radiology 1987;162:53

Atri M, Bret PM, Fraser-Hill MA: Intrahepatic portal venous variations: prevalence with US. Radiology 1992;184:157

Barton JW III, Keller MS: Liver transplantation for hepatoblastoma in a child with congenital absence of the portal vein. Pediatr Radiol 1989;20:113

Bellah RD, Hayek J, Teele RL: Anomalous portal venous connection to the suprahepatic vena cava: sonographic demonstration. Pediatr Radiol 1989;20:115

Fraser-Hill MA, Atri M, Bret PM, et al: Intrahepatic portal venous system: variations demonstrated with duplex and color Doppler US. Radiology 1990;177:523

Jabra AA, Taylor GA: Ultrasound diagnosis of congenital intrahepatic portosystemic venous shunt. Pediatr Radiol 1991;21:529

McCarten KM, Teele RL: Preduodenal portal vein: venography, ultrasonography, and review of the literature. Ann Radiol (Paris) 1978;21:155

Mori K, Dohi T, Yamamoto H, et al: An enormous shunt between the portal and hepatic veins associated with multiple coronary artery fistulas. Pediatr Radiol 1990;21:66

Morse SS, Taylor KJW, Strauss EB, et al: Congenital absence of the portal vein in oculoauriculovertebral dysplasia (Goldenhar syndrome). Pediatr Radiol 1986;16:437

Routh WD, Keller FS, Cain WS, et al: Transcatheter embolization of a high-flow congenital intrahepatic arterial-portal venous malformation in an infant. J Pediatr Surg 1992;27:511

Santamaria G, Pruna X, Serres X, et al: Congenital intrahepatic portosystemic venous shunt: sonographic and magnetic resonance imaging imaging. Eur Radiol 1996;6:76

Sergent G, Gottrand F, Delemazure O, et al: Transjugular intrahepatic portosystemic shunt in an infant. Pediatr Radiol 1997;27:588

Teo EL, Strouse PJ, Prince MR: Applications of magnetic resonance imaging and magnetic resonance angiography to evaluate the hepatic vasculature in the pediatric patient. Pediatr Radiol 1999;29:238

Tsuda Y, Nishimura K, Kawakami S, et al: Preduodenal portal vein and anomalous continuation of inferior vena cava: CT findings. J Comput Assist Tomogr 1991;15:585

Portal Hypertension

Boucher D, Brunette F, Bernard O, et al: Ultrasonic demonstration of porto-caval anastomosis in portal hypertension in children. Pediatr Radiol 1985;15:307

Brunelle F, Alagille D, Pariente D, et al: Étude échographique de l'hypertension portal chez l'enfant. Ann Radiol (Paris) 1981;24:121

Colli A, Cocciolo M, Riva C, et al: Abnormalities of Doppler waveform of the hepatic veins in patients with chronic liver disease: correlation with histologic findings. AJR Am J Roentgenol 1994;162:833

Dat DL, Mulcahy PF, Dehner LP, et al: Post-operative abdominal CT scanning in extrahepatic biliary atresia. Pediatr Radiol 1989;19:379

DeGaetano AM, Lafortune M, Patriquin H, et al: Cavernous transformation of the portal vein: patterns of intrahepatic and splanchnic collateral circulation detected with Doppler sonography. AJR Am J Roentgenol 1995;165:1151

Johnson CD, Ehman RL, Rakela J, et al: MR angiography in portal hypertension: detection of varices and imaging techniques. J Comput Assist Tomogr 1991;15:578

Lafortune M, Constantis A, Breton G, et al: The recanalized umbilical vein in portal hypertension. AJR Am J Roentgenol 1985;144:549

Mathieu D, Vasile N, Dibie C, et al: Portal cavernoma: dynamic CT features and transient differences in hepatic attenuation. Radiology 1985;154:743

Mathieu D, Vasile N, Gremier P: Portal thrombosis: dynamic CT features and course. Radiology 1985;154:737

McCain AH, Bernardino ME, Sones PJ, et al: Varices from portal hypertension: correlation of CT and angiography. Radiology 1985;154:63

Mori H, Hayaski K, Uetani M, et al: High-attenuation recent thrombus of the portal vein: CT demonstration and clinical significance. Radiology 1987;163:353

Moult PJA, Waite DW, Dick R: Posterior mediastinal venous masses in patients with portal hypertension. Gut 1975;16:57

Nakao N, Miura K, Takahashi H, et al: Hepatic perfusion in cavernous transformation of the portal vein: evaluation by using CT angiography. AJR Am J Roentgenol 1989;152:985

Nelson RC, Lovett KE, Chezmar JL, et al: Comparison of pulsed Doppler sonography and angiography in patients with portal hypertension. AJR Am J Roentgenol 1987;149:77

Odievre M, Chaumont P, Montagne JP, et al: Anomalies of the intrahepatic portal venous system in congenital hepatic fibrosis. Radiology 1977;122:427

Patriquin H, Lafortune M, Burns P, et al: The duplex Doppler examination of children and adults with portal hypertension: technique and anatomy. AJR Am J Roentgenol 1987;149:71

Patriquin H, Tessier G, Grignon A, et al: Lesser omental thickness in normal children: baseline for detection of portal hypertension. AJR Am J Roentgenol 1985;145:693

Rodgers PM, Ward J, Baudouin CJ, et al: Dynamic contrast enhanced MR imaging of the portal venous system: comparison with x-ray angiography. Radiology 1994;191:741

Sassoon C, Douillet P, Gronfalt AM, et al: Ultrasonographic diagnosis of portal cavernoma in children: a study of twelve cases. Br J Radiol 1980;53:1047

Silverman JM, Podesta L, Villamil F, et al: Portal vein patency in candidates for liver transplantation: MR angiographic analysis. Radiology 1995;197:147

Westra SJ, Zaninovic AC, Vargas J, et al: The value of portal vein pulsatility on duplex sonograms as a sign of portal hypertension in children with liver disease. AJR Am J Roentgenol 1995;165:167

Widrich WC, Srinivasan M, Semine MC, et al: Collateral pathways of the left gastric vein in portal hypertension. AJR Am J Roentgenol 1984;142:375

Budd-Chiari Syndrome

Bolondi L, Gaiani S, Libassi S, et al: Diagnosis of Budd-Chiari syndrome by pulsed Doppler ultrasound. Gastroenterology 1991;100:1324

Brunelle F, Leblanc A, Chaumont P: Familial Budd-Chiari disease: angiographic study in two sisters. Pediatr Radiol 1981;11:91

Grant EG, Perrella R, Tessler FN, et al: Budd-Chiari syndrome: the results of duplex and color Doppler imaging. AJR Am J Roentgenol 1989;152:377

Haliloglu M, Hoffer FA, Haight AE, et al: Budd-Chiari syndrome caused by Gaucher's disease. Pediatr Radiol 1999;29:908

Hausdorf G: Sonography of caudal hepatic veins in children: incidence, importance and relation to cranial hepatic veins. Pediatr Radiol 1984;14:376

Kane R, Eustace S: Diagnosis of Budd-Chiari syndrome: comparison between sonography and MR angiography. Radiology 1995;195:117

Lim JH, Park JH, Auh YO: Membranous obstruction of the inferior vena cava: comparison of findings at sonography, CT, and venography. AJR Am J Roentgenol 1992;159:515

Lois JF, Hartzman S, McGlade CT, et al: Budd-Chiari syndrome: treatment with percutaneous transhepatic recanalization and dilation. Radiology 1989;170:791

Millener P, Grant EG, Rose S, et al: Color Doppler imaging findings in patients with Budd-Chiari syndrome: correlation with venographic findings. AJR Am J Roentgenol 1993;161:307

Murphy FB, Steinberg HV, Shires FT, et al: The Budd-Chiari syndrome: a review. AJR Am J Roentgenol 1986;147:9

Powell-Jackson PR, Karani J, Erde RJ, et al: Ultrasound scanning and ^{99m}Tc sulphur colloid scintigraphy in diagnosis of Budd-Chiari syndrome. Gut 1986;27:1502

Stanley P: Budd-Chiari syndrome. Radiology 1989;170:625

Stark DD, Hahn PF, Trey C, et al: MRI of the Budd-Chiari syndrome. AJR Am J Roentgenol 1986;146:1141

Vogelszang RL, Anschuetz SL, Gore RM: Budd-Chiari syndrome: CT observations. Radiology 1987;163:329

Wallace S: Primary liver tumors. In Parker BR, Castellino RA (eds): Pediatric Oncologic Radiology. St. Louis, Mosby–Year Book, 1977:301–335

Hepatic Veno-occlusive Disease

Herbetko J, Grigg AP, Buckley AR, et al: Venooclusive liver disease after bone marrow transplantation: findings at duplex sonography. AJR Am J Roentgenol 1992;158:1001

Hosoki T, Chikazumi K, Tokunaga K, et al: Hepatic venous outflow obstruction: evaluation with pulsed duplex sonography. Radiology 1989;170:733

Lassau N, Leclère J, Auperin A, et al: Hepatic veno-occlusive disease after myeloablative treatment and bone marrow transplantation: value of gray-scale and Doppler US in 100 patients. Radiology 1997;204:545

Chapter 6

ACQUIRED BILIARY TRACT DISEASE

ALAN E. SCHLESINGER and BRUCE R. PARKER

CHOLELITHIASIS

Cholelithiasis in children is uncommon. However, the diagnosis is being made with more frequency since the advent of real-time ultrasound (US). In fact, fetal gallstones have been detected sonographically. A majority of gallstones identified on prenatal sonograms resolve spontaneously.

In infants, development of gallstones has been attributed to immature physiologic regulation of bile salt secretion, because infants form bile salts at 50% the rate of adults. Chronic cholestasis probably plays a role in the pathophysiology. Bilirubinate stones are most common. Certain therapeutic regimens have been associated with the development of gallstones. Total parenteral nutrition, with its hepatoxic effects and with associated lack of oral feeding, depresses bile salt formation. Certain diuretics have also been associated with cholelithiasis (Fig. 1). Other causes of gallstones include dehydration, infection, hemolytic anemia, and short-gut syndrome. As noted previously, patients with congenital abnormal-

ities of the biliary tree have a predisposition to the development of stones (Table 1).

Although the majority of stones seen in older children (see Table 1) are idiopathic, a number of underlying states have been associated with gallstones. Prominent among these are sickle cell disease, pancreatic abnormalities, and intestinal problems that interfere with the normal enterohepatic circulation, such as inflammatory bowel disease, cystic fibrosis, and the short-gut syndrome. Cystic fibrosis can also produce cholelithiasis as a result of obstruction of the cystic duct by inspissated secretions. Patients with hemolytic anemia frequently develop bilirubinate stones. Gallstones have been reported following scoliosis surgery and cardiac surgery. Ceftriaxone, an antibiotic, may cause biliary pseudolithiasis, which typically resolves after cessation of antibiotic therapy. Gallstones in infants and young children are usually asymptomatic. In older children, the symptoms are similar to those seen in adults, with right upper quadrant colicky pain radiating to the shoulder and nausea and vomiting. However, a substantial percentage of older children with gallstones will be asymptomatic.

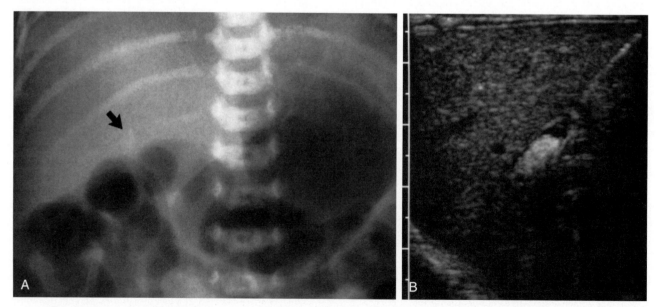

FIGURE 1. Drug-induced cholelithiasis. **A,** Coned-down view of the right upper quadrant in a 6-week-old infant treated with furosemide for chronic lung disease and congenital heart disease demonstrates calcification *(arrow)* just above the hepatic flexure. **B,** Longitudinal sonogram confirms multiple stones within the gallbladder causing prominent acoustic shadowing. The findings resolved without surgical intervention.

Table 1 ■ ETIOLOGY OF GALLSTONES

Infants and Neonates
Total parenteral nutrition
Diuretics
Dehydration
Infection
Hemolytic anemia
Short-gut syndrome
Congenital anomalies of the biliary tree

Older Children
Idiopathic
Sickle cell disease
Pancreatic disease
Inflammatory bowel disease
Cystic fibrosis
Short-gut syndrome
Hemolytic anemia
Antibiotics

■ Gallstones in infants and young children are usually asymptomatic, while older children are more likely to have symptoms similar to those seen in adults.

US is the primary imaging modality for the evaluation of cholelithiasis. Typical gallstones will be echogenic with prominent acoustic shadowing (Fig. 2). Most stones will move with changes in patient position, and the routine examination usually includes examination in the supine or decubitus position (Fig. 3). Multiple gallstones may be seen, but the number of stones identified at sonography usually underestimates the number actually found at the time of surgical exploration. Collections of very small stones may not demonstrate acoustic shadowing and may mimic the appearance of biliary sludge in the gallbladder. The lack of acoustic shadowing in these cases makes differentiation difficult. However, the sludge is more likely to have a smooth outline, whereas multiple stones may have an irregular or roughened outline. Occasionally, if the bile within the gallbladder is of high density, the stones may seem to float on the surface, giving an apparent fluid–fluid level. Tumefactive sludge (see below) may mimic gallstones, but the lack of acoustic shadowing usually leads to the correct diagnosis.

Stones are more likely to be symptomatic when they pass into the cystic duct or the common bile duct (Fig. 4). Sonography is less successful at demonstrating choledocholithiasis than it is in detecting cholelithiasis. Dilated extrahepatic bile ducts may be the only sign of an obscure, more distal obstructing stone. In such cases, hepatobiliary scintigraphy may be useful in confirming the diagnosis by demonstrating delayed excretion of radiopharmaceutical into the gastrointestinal tract. Computed tomography (CT) is occasionally used for direct imaging purposes, but biliary stones are more typically identified on CT as incidental findings. If a biliary tract stone is suspected but not seen on US, direct visualization by means of either percutaneous transhepatic cholangiography or endoscopic retrograde cholangiopancreatography (ERCP) may be considered. Stones are readily identified as nonopaque filling defects on these studies. Pariente et al. treated choledocholithiasis and the bile plug syndrome in 10 infants by percutaneous placement of an angiographic catheter and subsequent removal of the obstructing material. Generally, however, nonoperative interventional treatment of cholelithiasis is rarely performed in children. Magnetic resonance cholangiopancreatography has been used to demonstrate obstructing stones in the biliary tree in adult patients.

BILIARY SLUDGE

Biliary sludge is particulate matter within the bile, developing secondary to cholestasis. The sludge is formed predominantly of calcium bilirubinate particles and, depending on the underlying process, cholesterol crystals. On sonography, the sludge typically layers in the dependent portion of the gallbladder, and a fluid–fluid level may be seen (Fig. 5). Occasionally, the sludge coalesces sufficiently to have the sonographic appearance of a stone—so-called tumefactive sludge or "sludge ball." Tumefactive sludge moves like a stone with changes in patient position, but does not demonstrate acoustic shadowing (Fig. 6). Biliary sludge does not cause symptoms and does not need treatment; it usually resolves with therapy of the underlying condition.

CHOLECYSTITIS

Only a small percentage of children with cholelithiasis will develop cholecystitis. Acalculous cholecystitis is infrequent in children. The pathophysiology of acalcu-

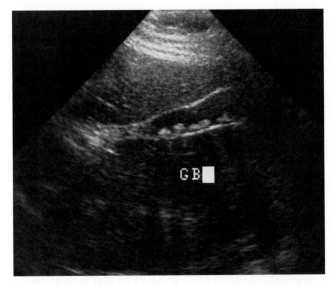

FIGURE 2. Cholelithiasis. Longitudinal sonogram with the patient in the supine position demonstrates multiple echogenic densities in the gallbladder with acoustic shadowing in this 9-year-old patient following heart transplant and treatment with several cholelithogenic drugs and prolonged hyperalimentation.

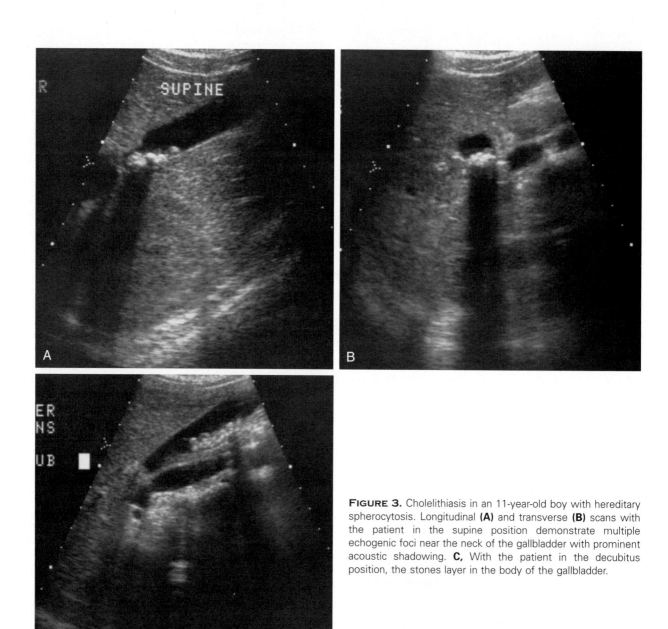

FIGURE 3. Cholelithiasis in an 11-year-old boy with hereditary spherocytosis. Longitudinal **(A)** and transverse **(B)** scans with the patient in the supine position demonstrate multiple echogenic foci near the neck of the gallbladder with prominent acoustic shadowing. **C,** With the patient in the decubitus position, the stones layer in the body of the gallbladder.

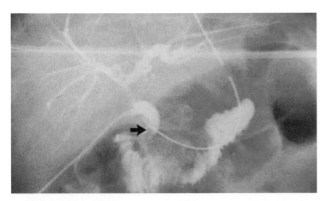

FIGURE 4. Choledocholithiasis in a 6-month-old boy who had prolonged hyperalimentation and developed obstructive jaundice. Operative cholangiogram demonstrates a stone *(arrow)* in the distal common bile duct (CBD) with dilatation of the proximal portion of the CBD.

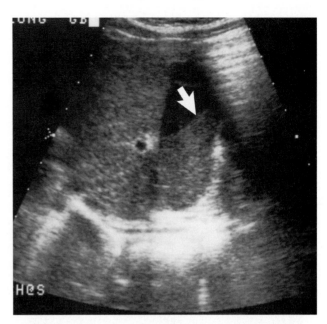

FIGURE 5. Biliary sludge. Longitudinal sonogram through the gallbladder demonstrates layering, nonshadowing, echogenic material in the gallbladder with a concave meniscus *(arrow)* typical of noncalculous biliary sludge.

lous cholecystitis is uncertain, but gallbladder ischemia, alterations in bile, and elevated ampullary pressure have been hypothesized. The sonographic findings of calculous cholecystitis and acalculous cholecystitis are similar except for the findings of gallstones in the former. Thickening of the gallbladder wall, distention of the gallbladder, pericholecystic fluid, biliary sludge, and edema of the gallbladder wall have all been described (Fig. 7). These findings are nonspecific and, except for the presence of gallstones, may be seen in a variety of other entities, especially hepatitis. Other causes of thickening of the gallbladder wall include ascites, portal hypertension, hypoproteinemia, and congestive heart failure. Irregularity of the gallbladder wall may suggest gangrenous change, and bright areas with "dirty shad-

owing" may suggest emphysema of the gallbladder wall. Coughlin and Mann suggested that hepatobiliary scintigraphy is underutilized in children with cholecystitis and reported two cases in which they made the diagnosis with a ^{99m}Tc-labeled iminodiacetic acid derivative. Perforation of the gallbladder has been described in children with acalculous cholecystitis.

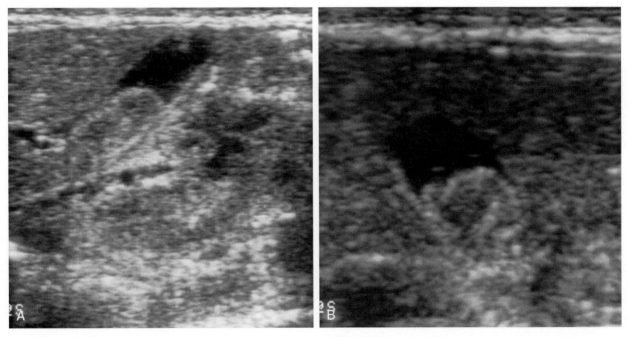

FIGURE 6. Tumefactive sludge. Longitudinal **(A)** and transverse **(B)** sonograms demonstrate echogenic material within the gallbladder that has a convex margin and moves as a unit but has no shadowing. This is the typical appearance of a "sludge ball" or tumefactive sludge.

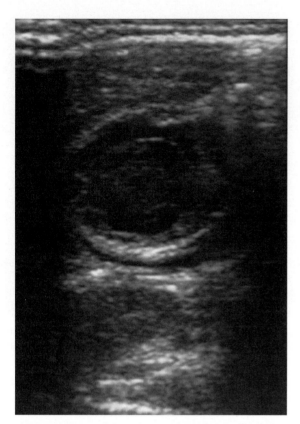

FIGURE 7. Chronic cholecystitis. Transverse sonogram through the gallbladder demonstrates a markedly thickened, edematous gallbladder wall with echogenic material in the lumen. The patient had a history of chronic recurrent abdominal pain.

- US findings in cholecystitis include:
  - Thickened gallbladder wall
  - Distention of the gallbladder
  - Pericholecystic fluid
  - Biliary sludge
  - Gallbladder wall edema
  - Irregularity of the gallbladder wall (may suggest gangrene)
  - Echogenic nonshadowing foci in gallbladder wall (may suggest emphysematous change).

CHOLANGITIS

Ascending cholangitis is associated with biliary obstruction whether congenital or acquired (Fig. 8). Although the patient may present with symptoms related to the cholangitis, appropriate therapy has to be directed to the underlying cause.

Sclerosing cholangitis is obliterative inflammatory fibrosis affecting the intrahepatic and extrahepatic biliary ducts (although the extrahepatic ducts may be normal in 40% of cases). There are features of this disease that suggest an autoimmune mechanism, but the pathophysiology of tissue damage has not been definitively determined. Sisto et al. reviewed 83 cases in childhood. Patients with inflammatory bowel disease, especially ulcerative colitis, accounted for 57% of the cases. Twenty-five percent were idiopathic, 15% were in patients with Langerhans' cell histiocytosis, and 10% were patients with disorders of the immune system. The association of sclerosing cholangitis and ulcerative colitis is not as strong in children as it is in adults. Sclerosing cholangitis has also been associated with cystic fibrosis.

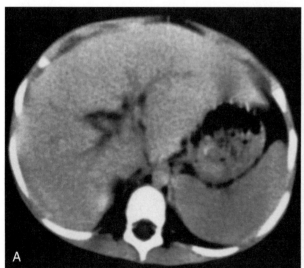
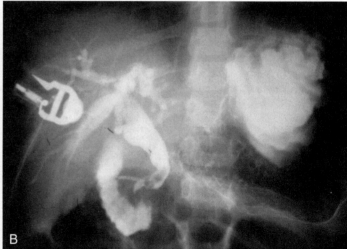

FIGURE 8. This 4-year-old girl presented with symptoms of ascending cholangitis, including fever, right upper quadrant pain, and jaundice. **A,** Computed tomography scan demonstrates dilatation of the biliary ducts and common bile duct. **B,** Cholangiogram at the time of surgical exploration following successful treatment with antibiotics demonstrates an obstructing intraductal cystic duplication of the common bile duct.

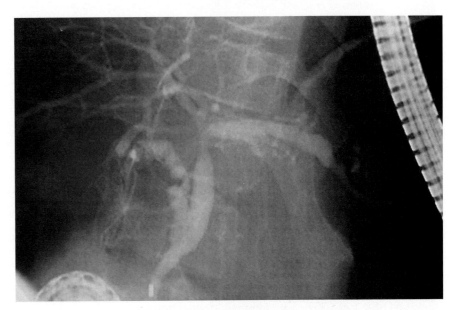

FIGURE 9. Endoscopic retrograde cholangiopancreatograph in a child with sclerosing cholangitis associated with inflammatory bowel disease shows areas of focal narrowing and areas of relative dilatation.

■ The following diagnoses have been associated with sclerosing cholangitis in children:
• Inflammatory bowel disease
• Langerhans' cell histiocytosis
• Immune disorders
• Cystic fibrosis

■ US findings in sclerosing cholangitis include:
• Dilatation of the biliary tree
• Thickened gallbladder wall
• Stones

On sonography, nonspecific dilatation of the biliary system may be seen in association with thickening of the gallbladder wall. Stones may be identified in the gallbladder. CT findings are also nonspecific, with focal dilatation of the biliary tree. With contrast enhancement, there may be increased attenuation of the ductal wall secondary to inflammatory changes. Spiral CT with administration of biliary contrast agents has been used in adults with sclerosing cholangitis. The definitive imaging study is cholangiography, via either the percutaneous transhepatic route or ERCP. The biliary tree is markedly irregular, with areas of stricture and focal dilatation proximal to the strictures (Fig. 9). Although occasionally segmental, the entire biliary tract is usually involved. Majoie et al. have developed a cholangiographic classification for primary sclerosing cholangitis that has yet to be tested for prognostic value. Magnetic resonance imaging has been used to evaluate children and adults with sclerosing cholangitis and has demonstrated peripheral wedge-shaped areas of high signal in association with dilated bile ducts.

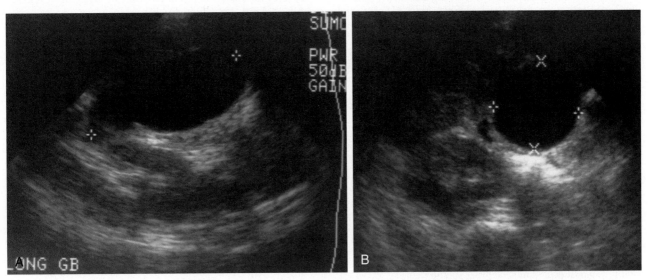

FIGURE 10. Hydrops of the gallbladder. Longitudinal **(A)** and transverse **(B)** sonograms demonstrate a markedly enlarged gallbladder in a 3-year-old girl with Kawasaki disease. The hydrops resolved spontaneously as the patient's condition improved.

Table 2 ■ ETIOLOGY OF HYDROPS OF THE GALLBLADDER

Obstruction
Mucocutaneous lymph node syndrome
Familial Mediterranean fever
Scarlet fever
Leptospirosis
Ascariasis
Typhoid fever
Sepsis
Total parenteral nutrition

HYDROPS OF THE GALLBLADDER

Hydrops of the gallbladder is thought to be secondary to transient obstruction related to cholestasis. Hydrops is also seen in the mucocutaneous lymph node syndrome (Kawasaki disease) (Fig. 10), familial Mediterranean fever, and a multiplicity of infectious diseases, including scarlet fever, leptospirosis, ascariasis, and typhoid fever (Table 2). Generalized sepsis and total parenteral nutrition have also been identified as sources of hydrops. US is striking, with marked dilatation of the gallbladder. The wall thickness is usually normal. Sludge is seen in some cases. The biliary tree is otherwise normal, and the hydrops generally responds to conservative therapy. Sty et al. reported a case of gallbladder perforation in Kawasaki disease.

SUGGESTED READINGS

General

El-Shafie M, Mah CL: Transient gallbladder distention in sick premature infants: the value of ultrasonography and radionuclide scintigraphy. Pediatr Radiol 1986;16:468

Gubernick, JA, Rosenberg HK, Ilaslan H, et al: US approach to jaundice in children. Radiographics 2000;20:173

Patriquin H, DiPietro M, Barber FE, Teele RL: Sonography of thickened gallbladder wall: causes in children. AJR Am J Roentgenol 1983;141:57

Suma V, Marini A, Bucci N, et al: Fetal gallstones: sonographic and clinical observations. Ultrasound Obstet Gynecol 1998;12:439

Cholelithiasis

Becker CD, Grossholz M, Becker M, et al: Choledocholithiasis and bile duct stenosis: diagnostic accuracy of MR cholangiopancreatography. Radiology 1997;205:523

Boraschi P, Neri E, Braccini G, et al: Choledocholithiasis: diagnostic accuracy of MR cholangiopancreatography. Three year experience. Magn Reson Imaging 1999;17:1245

Brown DL, Teele RL, Doubilet PM, et al: Echogenic material in the fetal gallbladder: sonographic and clinical observations. Radiology 1992;182:73

Callahan J, Haller JO, Cacciarelli AA, et al: Cholelithiasis in infants: association with total parenteral nutrition and furosemide. Radiology 1982;143:437

Descos B, Bernard O, Brunelle F, et al: Pigment gallstones of the common bile duct in infancy. Hepatology 1984;4:678

Garel L, Lallemand D, Montagne J-P, et al: The changing aspects of cholelithiasis in children through a sonographic study. Pediatr Radiol 1981;11:75

Keller MS, Markle BM, Laffey PA, et al: Spontaneous resolution of cholelithiasis in infants. Radiology 1985;157:345

Kirks DR: Lithiasis due to interruption of the enterohepatic circulation of bile salts. AJR Am J Roentgenol 1979;133:383

L'Heureux PR, Isenberg JN, Sharp HL, et al: Gallbladder disease in cystic fibrosis. AJR Am J Roentgenol 1977;128:953

Little JM, Avramovic J: Gallstone formation after major abdominal surgery. Lancet 1991;3375:1135

Matos C, Avni EF, van Gansbeke D, et al: Total parenteral nutrition (TPN) and gallbladder disease in neonates: sonographic assessment. J Ultrasound Med 1987;6:243

Palanduz A, Yalcin I, Tonguc E, et al: Sonographic assessment of ceftriaxone-associated biliary pseudolithiasis in children. J Clin Ultrasound 2000;28:166

Pariente D, Bernard O, Gauthier F, et al: Radiological treatment of common bile duct lithiasis in infancy. Pediatr Radiol 1989;19:104

Reif S, Sloven DG, Lebenthal E: Gallstones in children: characterization by age, etiology, and outcome. Am J Dis Child 1991;145:105

Stringer DA, Lim P, Cave M, et al: Fetal gallstones. J Pediatr Surg 1996;31:1589

Teele RL, Nussbaum AR, Wyly JB, et al: Cholelithiasis after spinal fusion for scoliosis in children. J Pediatr 1987;111:857

Williams HJ, Johnson KW: Cholelithiasis: a complication of cardiac valve surgery in children. Pediatr Radiol 1984;14:146

Cholecystitis

Chinn DH, Miller EI, Piper N: Hemorrhagic cholecystitis: sonographic and clinical presentation. J Ultrasound Med 1987;6:313

Colletti PM, Ralls PW, Siegel ME, et al: Acute cholecystitis: diagnosis with radionuclide angiography. Radiology 1987;163:615

Coughlin JR, Mann DA: Detection of acute cholecystitis in children. J Can Assoc Radiol 1990;41:213

Mirvis SE, Vainright JR, Nelson AW, et al: The diagnosis of acute acalculous cholecystitis: a comparison of sonography, scintigraphy, and CT. AJR Am J Roentgenol 1986;147:1171

Roca M, Sellier N, Mensire A, et al: Acute acalculous cholecystitis in Salmonella infection. Pediatr Radiol 1988;18:421

Samuels BI, Freitas JE, Bree RL, et al: A comparison of radionuclide hepatobiliary imaging and real time ultrasound for the detection of acute cholecystitis. Radiology 1983;147:207

Stevenson CA, Atkinson G, Ball TI: Unusual presentation of perforation of the gallbladder. Pediatr Radiol 1991;21:358

Cholangitis

Majoie CBLM, Reeders JWAJ, Sanders JB, et al: Primary sclerosing cholangitis: a modified classification of cholangiographic findings. AJR Am J Roentgenol 1991;157:495

Revelon G, Rashid A, Kawamoto S, et al: Primary sclerosing cholangitis: MR imaging findings with pathologic correlation. AJR Am J Roentgenol 1999;173:1037

Robers EA: Primary sclerosing cholangitis in children. J Gastroenterol Hepatol 1999;14:588

Sajjad Z, Oxtoby J, West D, et al: Biliary imaging by spiral CT cholangiography—a retrospective analysis. Br J Radiol 1999;72:149

Sisto A, Feldman P, Garel L, et al: Primary sclerosing cholangitis in children: study of five cases and review of the literature. Pediatrics 1987;80:918

Hydrops of the Gallbladder

Bradford BR, Reid BS, Weinstein BJ, et al: Ultrasonographic evaluation of the gallbladder in mucocutaneous lymph node syndrome. Radiology 1982;142:381

Cohen EK, Stringer DA, Smith CR, et al: Hydrops of the gallbladder in typhoid fever as demonstrated by sonography. J Clin Ultrasound 1986;14:633

Neu J, Arvin A, Ariagno L: Hydrops of the gallbladder. Am J Dis Child 1980;134:891

Sty JR, Starshak RJ, Gorenstein L: Gallbladder perforation in a case of Kawasaki disease: image correlation. J Clin Ultrasound 1987;11:381

Chapter 7

TUMORS AND TUMOR-LIKE CONDITIONS

ALAN E. SCHLESINGER and BRUCE R. PARKER

Neoplasms of the liver are relatively rare in children. They account for about 2% of all childhood tumors. The malignant hepatic tumors are the 10th most common tumors in childhood, but the third most common abdominal malignancy after Wilms' tumor and neuroblastoma. Malignancies account for 64% of primary hepatobiliary tumors. Most clinically significant hepatic neoplasms present as asymptomatic palpable masses found by the parents or at routine physical examination. Differentiating benign from malignant hepatic masses on imaging studies has been actively studied, but imaging usually is not used to definitively make this distinction. Boechat et al. showed both computed tomography (CT) and magnetic resonance imaging (MRI) to be excellent in differentiating benign from malignant tumors but less successful in discriminating between hepatocellular carcinoma, hepatoblastoma, and lymphoma.

BENIGN HEPATIC NEOPLASMS

Benign lesions account for 43% of primary liver neoplasms in children. Hemangiomas and hemangioendotheliomas, the mesenchymal vascular tumors, account for 50% of the benign tumors; mesenchymal hamartomas account for 22%, adenomas for 6%, focal nodular hyperplasia for 5%, and miscellaneous benign lesions, many of which are cystic in nature, account for 17%.

CAVERNOUS HEMANGIOMA

Cavernous hemangiomas are the most common of the benign hepatic tumors in adults. Because of occasional difficulties in distinguishing cavernous hemangiomas from other mesenchymal lesions, the overall incidence in children is not definitely known, but it may be significantly less than in adults. They are typically small and often identified in children or adults incidentally on cross-sectional imaging studies performed for other reasons. Occasionally they are large, presenting in infancy as palpable masses or with high-output congestive heart failure secondary to arteriovenous shunting through the tumor. Rarely, spontaneous rupture with massive hemoperitoneum occurs.

Much interest in definitive diagnosis of hemangiomas has resulted from the need to differentiate them from hepatic metastases in adults. Although the same problem may occur in children, metastases are much less common in the pediatric age group than in adults, in whom they are the most common hepatic malignancies. Children are also less likely than adults to have cirrhosis with regenerating nodules or focal nodular hyperplasia (FNH), other lesions that can be confused with hemangiomas. On ultrasound (US), typical small hemangiomas are well circumscribed and hyperechoic compared with surrounding liver parenchyma (Fig. 1). Acoustic shadowing may accompany larger lesions. Bree et al. believe this is secondary to hypervascularity. Very large lesions may be hyperechoic with a hypoechoic central area, possibly representing necrosis or fibrosis.

- **Ultrasound findings in hemangioma:**
  - Echogenic mass when small
  - Well circumscribed
  - Hypoechoic centrally when large
  - Acoustic shadowing when large

CT evaluation of small cavernous hemangiomas shows decreased attenuation on unenhanced scans. Calcifications may be seen. With dynamic scanning, the lesion shows enhancement, beginning peripherally and progressing centrally. Prolonged enhancement, up to 20 to 30 minutes, may occur. The rim of the lesion may appear nodular or corrugated with papillary-like projections extending toward the center. The rim is especially bright after contrast enhancement. On MRI, cavernous hemangiomas are of lower signal intensity than the adjacent liver on T_1-weighted spin-echo images and of higher signal intensity on T_2-weighted images. Both T_1-weighted spin-echo and dynamic gradient-echo images after intravenous gadopentatate administration demonstrate peripheral enhancement with central progression on delayed images. The anatomic appearance is a homogeneous, rounded mass with sharply defined margins. Sulfur colloid scans are usually unrevealing or nonspecific, but single-photon emission CT (SPECT) scans using ^{99m}Tc-labeled red blood cells show normal to decreased flow followed by delayed increased blood pool activity. In a study comparing MRI and red cell scans using SPECT, Birnbaum et al. found MRI to have a sensitivity of 91% with an accuracy of 90%, while the

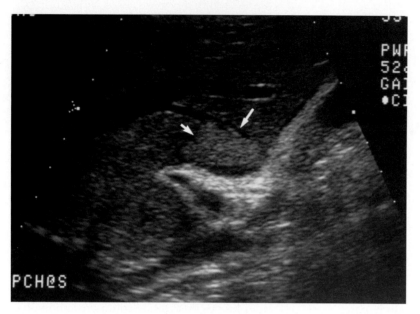

FIGURE 1. Hepatic hemangioma. Longitudinal sonogram through the liver in a patient on hyperalimentation with abdominal pain demonstrates a focal area of increased echogenicity characteristic of benign cavernous hemangioma *(arrows)*. There is sludge in the gallbladder.

nuclear medicine study had a sensitivity of 78% with 80% accuracy.

■ Computed tomography findings in hemangioma:
- Sharply demarcated mass
- Decreased attenuation precontrast
- Nodular peripheral margin postcontrast
- Peripheral-to-central progression of enhancement
- Calcification

■ Magnetic resonance imaging findings in hemangioma:
- Sharply demarcated mass
- Low signal relative to normal liver on T_1-weighted images
- High signal relative to normal liver on T_2-weighted images
- Peripheral enhancement with centripetal progression of enhancement after intravenous contrast administration

Large cavernous hemangiomas usually present in the first 6 months of life as an asymptomatic mass or with high-output congestive heart failure. On sonography, there may be enlargement of the celiac axis and hepatic artery because of the increased arterial blood supply to the tumor. Similarly, the draining hepatic veins may be enlarged. The margins are usually lobulated as opposed to the smooth margins typically seen with smaller hemangiomas. On CT, the large tumors usually have a low-attenuation central area with peripheral enhancement following intravenous contrast injection. As with the small lesions, gradually increasing enhancement of

the central portion may occur. Findings on isotope-labeled red blood cell scans and on MRI are similar to those described for the smaller lesions. Angiography is rarely performed since the advent of cross-sectional imaging. Irregular vessels arranged in an unorganized pattern and prolonged pooling of contrast material are frequently seen. The appearance is similar to that which may be found in hemangioendothelioma (see below) and even in malignancy. Embolization of the tumor can be accomplished. Fellows et al. have pointed out the importance of embolizing the frequently seen collateral vessels as well as the primary feeding vessels in order to achieve a good therapeutic effect.

INFANTILE HEMANGIOENDOTHELIOMA

Infantile hemangioendothelioma is much more likely to present as a symptomatic lesion than is cavernous hemangioma. Although there is a histologic difference between the two lesions, they may represent varying manifestations of etiologically similar entities. Hemangioendotheliomas may be isolated or may diffusely involve the liver (hemangioendotheliomatosis). The most common presentation is a palpable abdominal mass, hepatomegaly, or diffuse abdominal distention. Congestive heart failure secondary to arteriovenous shunting has been reported, but is less common than with giant hemangioma or arteriovenous malformations. In the series of Dachman, Lichtenstein, et al., almost 20% of patients had associated hemangiomas of the skin.

■ Clinical findings in children with hemangioendothelioma include:
- Palpable mass
- Hepatomegaly
- Diffuse abdominal distention
- Congestive heart failure (less common)

The sonographic appearance of infantile hemangio-endotheliomas is variable and nonspecific (Fig. 2A). The lesions may be either hyperechoic or hypoechoic. Dachman, Lichtenstein, et al. described one case that was cystic in appearance with no internal echoes. Most of the tumors are discrete on sonography, but a small percentage will be poorly delineated from the surrounding liver parenchyma. The caliber of the aorta may abruptly decrease below the level of the celiac axis as a result of the marked increase in hepatic arterial flow secondary to intrahepatic arteriovenous shunting.

On CT, hemangioendotheliomas demonstrate decreased attenuation compared with the normal liver parenchyma. The pattern may be homogeneous or heterogeneous. On unenhanced scans, as many as 40% of patients may demonstrate tumoral calcification. With intravenous contrast enhancement, many lesions demonstrate a sharp increase in attenuation around the periphery of the mass, with irregular increased enhancement throughout the lesion. With delayed scans, there is washout of the increased enhancement from the periphery of the lesion with progressive increase of enhancement in the central portion (Fig. 2B, C). Areas within the lesion that show no contrast enhancement may represent areas of necrosis or hemorrhage. In other cases, there may be rapid and homogeneous enhancement of the lesions (Fig. 3).

On T_1-weighted spin-echo MRI, the central portion of the lesion is either isointense with the surrounding hepatic parenchyma or shows somewhat decreased signal intensity. The rim may show minimally increased signal intensity. On T_2-weighted images, the central portion of the lesion shows markedly increased signal intensity. The periphery also increases in signal intensity on T_2-weighted images, but less so than the central portion (Fig. 2D, E). With magnetic resonance angiography (MRA), enlarged feeding vessels may be identified. Peripheral-to-central enhancement has been reported after intravenous gadolinium administration.

Radionuclide studies are nonspecific, but an early blush may be seen, and the blood pool studies may show increased activity corresponding with the large, high-flow feeding vessels.

Angiography is less commonly used since the advent of enhanced CT and MRI, but demonstrates large major feeding vessels with decreased caliber of the aorta distal to their origin. Characteristically, there is prolonged pooling of contrast material within the mass. Internal arteriovenous shunting with large draining veins may be seen. Typically, angiography is presently used only when embolization is considered. In patients with failed medical therapy, segmental hepatic resection (if the process is local) or embolization of the hemangioendotheliomas should be considered, either as definitive therapy or as a temporizing method prior to transplantation.

MESENCHYMAL HAMARTOMA

Mesenchymal hamartomas account for 22% of the benign liver tumors in childhood. They generally present in patients less than 2 years of age and have been diagnosed on prenatal US. As with most of the other tumors, an asymptomatic abdominal mass is usually the presenting complaint. There are documented cases of transformation of benign mesenchymal hamartomas into their malignant counterpart, undifferentiated embryonal sarcoma (UES) (also called malignant mesenchymoma and mesenchymal sarcoma), including a case of UES with structural alterations in chromosome 19, which has been postulated as a possible genetic marker for mesenchymal hamartoma. Despite this evidence suggesting possible malignant transformation of mesenchymal hamartomas, some authors have advocated conservative, nonoperative treatment in selected cases. There has recently been a report of a patient with mesenchymal hamartoma of the liver whose mother's placenta was enlarged and histologically demonstrated mesenchymal stem villous hyperplasia, an entity that has previously also been associated with Beckwith-Wiedemann syndrome.

■ Although there has been documented transformation from benign mesenchymal hamartomas to its malignant counterpart (undifferentiated embryonal sarcoma), some have advocated conservative treatment for mesenchymal hamartoma.

On US, mesenchymal hamartomas most typically demonstrate a multiseptated cystic mass (Fig. 4A). The cyst may be quite variable in size. Quite frequently, a single dominant cyst is seen. Occasionally, some echogenic material is seen within the cyst fluid secondary to blood. Less commonly, the hamartomas may appear solid on US with vascular findings like those of the other mesenchymally derived masses, hemangioma and hemangioendothelioma.

■ Ultrasound findings in cystic mesenchymal hamartoma:
  1. Common
     • Cystic mass
     • Multiple septae
     • Variable size cysts (may have a dominant cyst)
  2. Uncommon
     • Echogenic material in cyst fluid as a result of hemorrhage
     • Solid-appearing mass

CT typically shows a multilocular cystic mass with sepatations of varying thickness. The noncystic components of the mass demonstrate enhancement with intravenous contrast material (Fig. 4B).

MRI demonstrates the cystic nature of the mass well; the cystic spaces are high in signal on proton-density and T_2-weighted images and low in signal on T_1 weighted images. The signal intensity varies depending

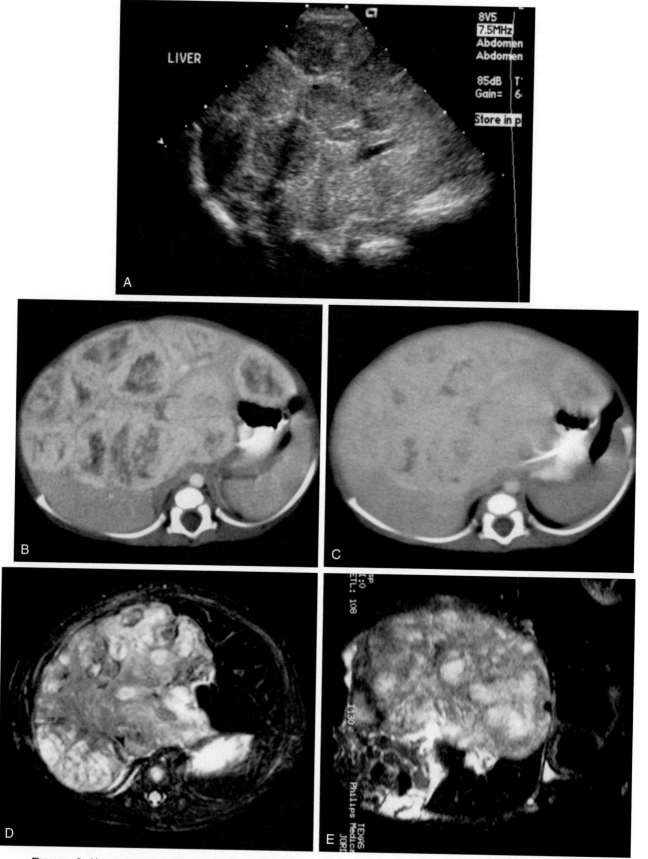

FIGURE 2. Hemangioendotheliomatosis. **A,** Longitudinal ultrasound image demonstrates multiple hypoechoic lesions. **B,** Early postcontrast computed tomography scan shows peripheral enhancement in these lesions. **C,** Delayed enhanced image confirms peripheral-to-central progression of enhancement. Axial T$_2$-weighted **(D)** and coronal T$_2$-weighted **(E)** spin-echo magnetic resonance images in another patient with hemangioendotheliomatosis reveal increased signal intensity in multiple lesions.

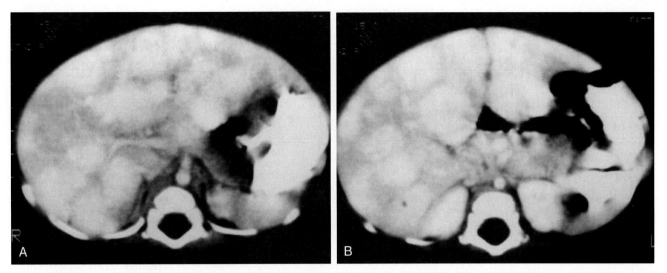

FIGURE 3. Hemangioendotheliomatosis. **A,** Early computed tomography (CT) scan at the level of the celiac axis after intravenous contrast demonstrates early complete enhancement of multiple masses in a neonate with infantile hemangioendotheliomatosis. Note the relatively large aorta and celiac axis. **B,** CT scan section just below the celiac axis demonstrates other hemangioendotheliomas and a marked decrease in aortic caliber as a result of a large amount of hepatic arterial flow.

on the stromal content of the mass, the protein content of the cyst fluid, and the presence of hemorrhage within the cysts. Gradient echo-images demonstrate the vessels and their relationship to the mass.

FOCAL NODULAR HYPERPLASIA

Benign tumors of epithelial origin are less common in children than those of mesenchymal origin. FNH is unusual in children compared with adults. Occasionally, FNH may be found in patients with type I glycogen storage disease and has been reported following the Kasai operation for biliary atresia. The lesion consists of hyperplastic hepatocytes with small bile ducts and lymphocytic infiltration. In most patients, the disease is

asymptomatic, and patients usually present with hepatomegaly.

Sonographic evaluation demonstrates one or more masses that can be hypoechoic, hyperechoic, or isoechoic with the surrounding liver parenchyma. In about one third of cases, a small central scar may be seen. This corresponds with the histologically identifiable central collection of connective tissue, bile ducts, and blood vessels. Hepatic imaging with ^{99m}Tc-labeled sulfur colloid is extremely valuable in that one half to three fourths of all cases will show uptake of the radionuclide by Kupffer's cells within the nodules.

On CT, the lesions are discrete and demonstrate early enhancement with relatively rapid washout of contrast material. The central scar will be seen in up to 60% of lesions. With dynamic CT, the central scars may become

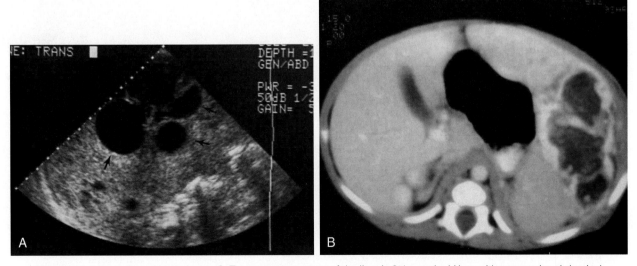

FIGURE 4. Mesenchymal hamartoma. **A,** Transverse sonogram of the liver in 3½-month-old boy with progressive abdominal distention shows the large hypoechoic mass in the right lobe (arrows). **B,** Enhanced computed tomography scan in another patient shows a large, exophytic, hypovascular mass in the left hepatic lobe with enhancing septations.

especially enhanced because of the relatively rapid contrast washout of the surrounding mass, a characteristic of FNH. On MRI, FNH may have a typical appearance. The lesions are homogeneous and isointense with the adjacent liver on all spin-echo sequences (Fig. 5). The central scar, however, is usually hypointense on T_1-weighted images and hyperintense on T_2-weighted images. The lesions of FNH appear poorly marginated on MRI.

> ■ Magnetic resonance imaging findings in focal nodular hyperplasia:
> - Homogeneous, poorly marginated mass
> - Isointense with normal liver on all spin-echo pulse sequences
> - Central scar hypointense on T_1-weighted images and hyperintense on T_2-weighted images

HEPATIC ADENOMA

Hepatic adenomas are also more common in adults than in children, but may be found in patients with type I and, less commonly, type VI glycogen storage disease. Hepatic adenomatosis is defined as the presence of four or more adenomas in the liver and is usually associated with oral contraceptives or anabolic steroids. Like FNH, the US appearance may be hypoechoic, isoechoic, or hyperechoic. The hyperechoic lesions may appear to have a rim of lower echogenicity, but the hypoechoic lesions have no well-defined wall. The adenomas do not take up labeled sulfur colloid and appear as photopenic defects on radioisotope liver scans.

CT demonstrates discrete lesions with low attenuation prior to contrast administration. The surrounding cap-sule usually creates a well-defined border. The lesions may be heterogeneous as a result of hemorrhage. Homogeneous enhancement after contrast administration may be transient because of the hepatic arterial supply of the lesion, and the mass may be isoattenuating on delayed images (Fig. 6A, B). Some lesions will show lack of enhancement secondary to intratumoral hemorrhage.

On MRI, the adenomas are usually hypointense or isointense with the surrounding liver on T_1-weighted spin-echo images and may have a hypointense rim (Fig. 6C). Increased signal intensity may be present as a result of contained fat. On T_2-weighted spin-echo images, the adenomas are usually of increased signal intensity compared with the liver parenchyma (Fig. 6D). However, the appearance is variable because of the possibility of hemorrhage. Even less commonly, the lesions may be isointense with surrounding liver, simulating the MRI appearance of FNH. The adenomas have a prolonged bright tumor stain on angiography (Fig. 6E).

NODULAR REGENERATIVE HYPERPLASIA OF THE LIVER

Nodular regenerative hyperplasia (NRH) of the liver is a regenerative nodular lesion that develops in noncirrhotic livers and is often confused with FNH, regenerating nodules in cirrhosis, adenomas, or metastases. In the series reported by Dachman, Ros, et al., 2 of 21 patients were children. The cause is unknown, but this entity has been associated with other diseases (vasculitis, collagen-vascular diseases, hematologic diseases, cardiovascular diseases, neoplasms, and metabolic diseases) and certain drugs. It has been classified as a multiacinar regenerative lesion of the liver. The nodules are composed of cells resembling hepatocytes and are not

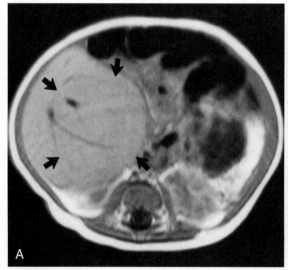
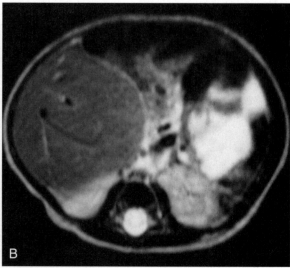

FIGURE 5. Focal nodular hyperplasia. Axial T_1-weighted **(A)** and T_2-weighted **(B)** magnetic resonance images in an infant with focal nodular hyperplasia demonstrate a mass that has isointense signal on both pulse sequences. The mass *(arrows)* is discernible only by the overall increased size of the liver in this region and mass effect on adjacent intrahepatic vessels.

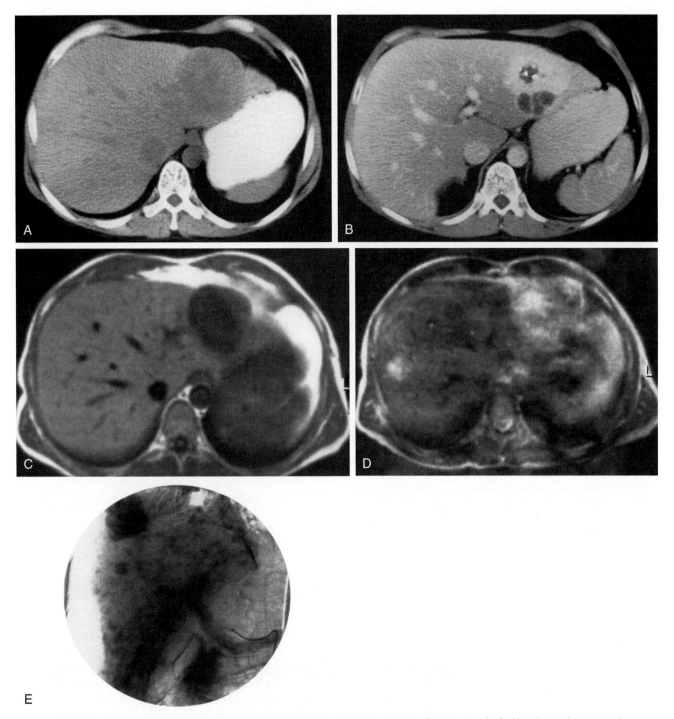

FIGURE 6. Multiple hepatic adenomas in a patient with glycogen storage disease type I. **A,** Unenhanced computed tomography scan demonstrates a low-attenuation mass in the left lobe of the liver. The overall liver attenuation is higher than normal, compatible with glycogen storage disease type I. **B,** Enhanced scan demonstrates increased attenuation of the lesion with low-attenuation areas within it, suggesting hemorrhage or necrosis. **C,** Axial T_1-weighted spin-echo magnetic resonance image demonstrates low signal intensity within the large adenoma in the left lobe. **D,** Axial T_2-weighted scan demonstrates another lesion in the right lobe (with increased signal intensity) that was not appreciated on the prior imaging studies. **E,** Digital subtraction angiography reveals multiple, highly vascular adenomas throughout the liver. (Courtesy of Roger Jackman, M.D., Palo Alto, CA.)

associated with focal fibrosis. The nodules may bleed or cause portal hypertension from pressure on portal radicles. The liver may or may not be enlarged. On sonography, the nodules may be hyperechoic, isoechoic, or hypoechoic. Sulfur colloid scintigraphy shows patchy uptake or areas of photopenia. On CT, the lesions are of lower attenuation than normal liver and do not enhance appreciably with intravenous contrast infusion. Arteriography may show vascular masses, but in most cases hepatic flow is poor because of associated portal hypertension. The MRI appearance is nonspecific and variable. The association of NRH of the liver and hepatocellular carcinoma (HCC) has recently been observed, but there is insufficient evidence to conclude that NRH is a precursor to HCC.

PELIOSIS HEPATIS

Peliosis hepatis is a rare entity characterized by multiple small, blood-filled spaces in the hepatic parenchyma. It has been associated with a variety of underlying diseases. In children, it has been most commonly found in association with the intake of androgens, type I glycogen storage disease, human immunodeficiency virus infection, and oral contraceptives. Sonography has shown a variable appearance, including a heterogeneous echo texture, scattered areas of decreased or increased echogenicity, and cystic lesions. CT demonstrates low attenuation with variable contrast enhancement. The described MRI appearances have been nonspecific, with increased signal intensity on T_2-weighted images and variable signal on T_1-weighting. The variability of the appearance may be attributed to blood of differing ages in portions of the lesions. Angiography demonstrates delayed pooling of contrast without evidence of tumor vessels.

PRIMARY MALIGNANT HEPATOBILIARY TUMORS

The most common primary malignant tumor of the liver in children is hepatoblastoma, which accounts for 54% of cases. HCC accounts for 35%, and carcinomas arising either from the liver or from the biliary tree account for 11%.

HEPATOBLASTOMA

Hepatoblastoma usually presents as an asymptomatic abdominal mass in a young child. The majority of these tumors present under 3 years of age, with the peak incidence between 18 and 24 months. Patients with advanced tumors may present with anorexia, weight loss, vomiting, or abdominal pain. In rare cases of tumor rupture, the patient may present with an acute abdomen. There is a well-known relationship between hepatoblastoma and the Beckwith-Wiedemann syndrome and with hemihypertrophy. Hepatoblastoma has also been reported in patients born of mothers taking oral contraceptives and gonadotropins and in patients with the fetal alcohol syndrome, Gardner's syndrome, and glycogen storage disease. The tumor is most commonly found in the right hepatic lobe. Serum α-fetoprotein is usually elevated. The most common sites of metastatic disease are the lungs, the local lymph nodes, and the brain.

On plain radiographs, hepatomegaly is identified, and calcification is frequently seen. On sonography, the tumor demonstrates minimal increased echogenicity

that is usually heterogeneous (Fig. 7A). Occasionally, hypoechoic or even anechoic areas can be seen with necrosis or hemorrhage. At times, the calcifications are large enough to cause shadowing on US examination. Tumor infiltration and compression of the hepatic vessels can occur. Taylor et al. have demonstrated high-velocity flow with a frequency shift over 5 kHz using duplex Doppler sonography. The angiographic phase of sulfur colloid hepatic scintigraphy demonstrates initial elevated activity in the tumor. On delayed scans, the area is typically photopenic, although Diament et al. have described a case of increased uptake of radiopharmaceutical, simulating the findings of FNH. On CT, the unenhanced scan demonstrates the tumor to have decreased attenuation with respect to the surrounding liver parenchyma. Rarely, the tumor is isodense and may not be well seen. Calcifications will be identified by CT in half of the patients (Fig. 7D, E). With intravenous contrast infusion, the tumor typically shows heterogeneous enhancement, but the normal liver parenchyma shows enhancement to a greater degree than the tumor in most cases (Fig. 7D). Occasionally, tumors will show isointense enhancement with the normal liver parenchyma and sometimes will have increased enhancement.

■ Ultrasound findings in hepatoblastoma
  1. Common
     • Hyperechoic mass
     • Calcifications
  2. Uncommon
     • Isoechoic or hypoechoic mass
     • Infiltration and/or compression of hepatic vessels

■ Computed tomography findings in hepatoblastoma:
  1. Common
     • Mass with decreased attenuation relative to normal liver on unenhanced scan
     • Mass enhances (but less than normal liver) after intravenous contrast
     • Calcifications
  2. Uncommon
     • Mass with attenuation equal to normal liver on unenhanced scan
     • Mass enhances equally or more than liver after intravenous contrast

On spin-echo MRI, the T_1-weighted scans demonstrate decreased signal intensity of the tumor relative to surrounding liver parenchyma (Fig. 7B). Occasionally, small hemorrhages are seen as increased signal intensity on T_1-weighted images. On T_2-weighted images, the tumors show increased signal intensity that is usually heterogeneous (Fig. 7C). Areas of fibrosis will appear as

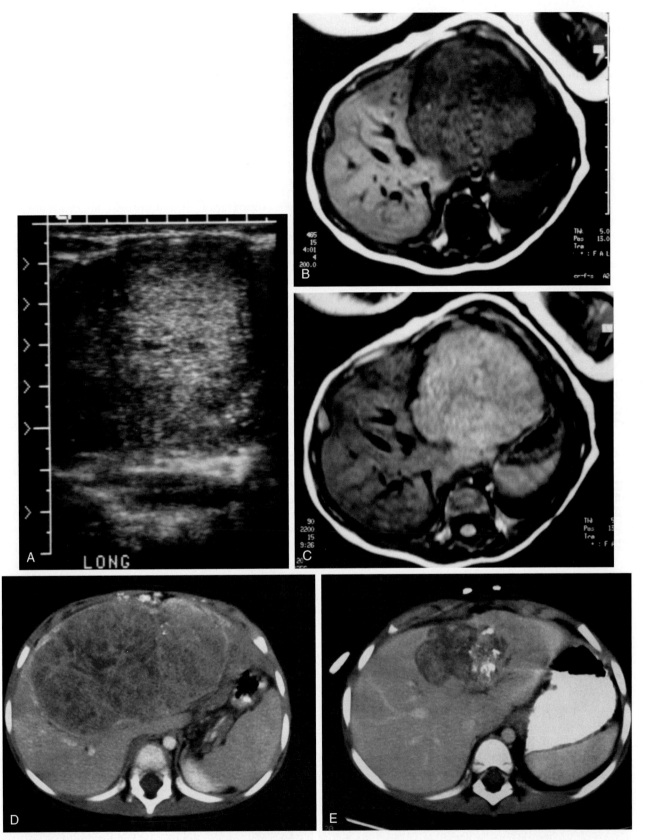

FIGURE 7. Hepatoblastoma. **A,** Longitudinal sonographic image demonstrates a large heterogeneous echogenic mass. **B,** Compared to the normal liver, there is decreased signal intensity on this axial T_1-weighted spin-echo magnetic resonance (MR) image. **C,** Axial proton-density MR image demonstrates increased signal intensity in the mass relative to normal hepatic parenchyma. **D,** Contrast-enhanced computed tomography (CT) scan through a mass in a different patient with hepatoblastoma demonstrates marked heterogeneity of attenuation with several areas of calcification identified. **E,** Repeat CT (in same patient as **D**) 1 month following initiation of chemotherapy shows that the mass has markedly shrunk, with increasing areas of calcification. Following another month of chemotherapy, the mass was successfully removed surgically.

hypointense bands on T_1- and T_2-weighted images. Gradient-echo pulse sequences or MRA are useful in demonstrating the relationship of the tumor to vessels and vascular invasion. Generally, MRI gives sufficient information for preoperative evaluation. Angiography is now rarely performed. The angiographic findings are characteristic of malignancy but nonspecific, with tumor vessels and contrast pooling frequently seen.

■ Magnetic resonance imaging findings in hepatoblastoma:
1. Common
   • Decreased signal intensity on T_1-weighted images
   • Heterogeneously increased signal intensity on T_2-weighted images
   • Decreased signal intensity on T_1 and T_2-weighted images in regions of fibrosis
2. Uncommon
   • Increased signal intensity on T_1-weighted images in regions of hemorrhage

---

HEPATOCELLULAR CARCINOMA

HCC has two age peaks in childhood: 2 to 4 years and 12 to 14 years. The association with cirrhosis is less common than it is in adults, but approximately 50% of patients with HCC have underlying liver disease, often associated with hereditary tyrosinemia, biliary atresia, Alagille syndrome (Fig. 8), and chronic hepatitis. α-Fetoprotein will be elevated in 40% to 50% of patients with HCC.

■ Although the association of hepatocellular carcinoma (HCC) and cirrhosis is less common in children than in adults, approximately 50% of children with HCC have underlying liver disease, often associated with:
• Hereditary tyrosinemia
• Biliary atresia
• Alagille syndrome
• Chronic hepatitis

The sonographic findings of HCC are much like those of hepatoblastoma described above, except that calcification is less common (see Fig. 8A). As with hepatoblastoma, tumor infiltration of adjacent vessels can be readily identified. Doppler studies demonstrate increased size of the portal vein and increased velocity of blood flow.

On CT examination, the tumor may be a solitary mass or a large mass with smaller satellite lesions, or may diffusely involve the liver. On unenhanced scans, the tumor is typically of lower attenuation than the surrounding liver but may be isodense. There is usually a well-defined circumferential zone of decreased attenuation. Calcification is seen in up to 10% of cases. Following intravenous contrast injection, enhancement can be quite intense but heterogeneous (see Fig. 8B). Vascular channels are identified on dynamic scanning, and invasion of the portal vein, inferior vena cava, hepatic veins, and hepatic arteries may be seen. Intrinsic arterial–portal shunting may lead to transiently increased attenuation of the uninvolved lobes and prolonged portal vein enhancement. Although the margins are typically well defined, this is not a universal finding. If the tumor arises in a patient with underlying

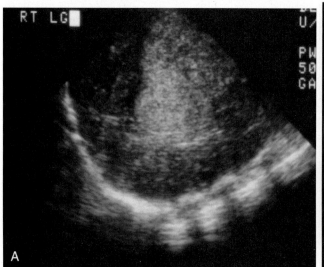
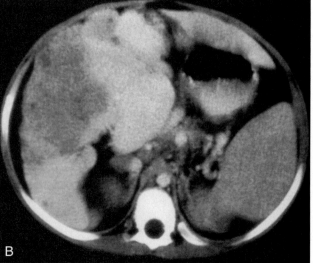

FIGURE 8. Hepatocellular carcinoma in a patient with Alagille syndrome. **A,** Longitudinal ultrasound image demonstrates a hyperechoic, ill-defined mass. **B,** Contrast-enhanced computed tomography scan confirms a mass with heterogeneous enhancement, but with lower overall attenuation than the normal liver parenchyma.

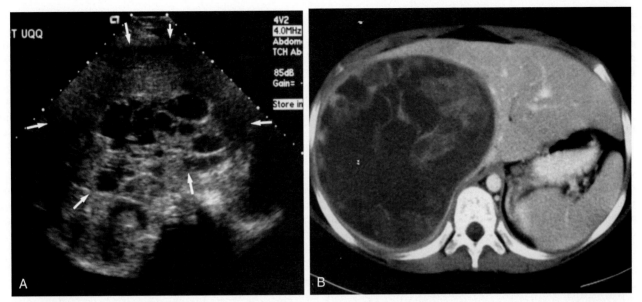

FIGURE 9. Undifferentiated embryonal sarcoma. **A,** Transverse ultrasound image demonstrates a heterogeneous, but predominantly solid-appearing intrahepatic mass *(arrows)* with anechoic regions secondary to tumor necrosis. **B,** Contrast-enhanced computed tomography scan in another patient with the same tumor demonstrates marked decrease in attenuation within the mass.

cirrhotic change, the differentiation from regenerating nodules may be difficult, as is differentiation from hepatoblastoma.

On spin-echo MRI, HCC is typically of lower signal intensity than normal liver tissue on T_1-weighted images and of higher signal intensity on T_2-weighted images. Areas of increased signal may be seen on T_1-weighted images because of fat or hemorrhage. If a fibrous pseudocapsule is present, low signal will be seen around the tumor on both pulse sequences. Displacement and invasion of the hepatic vessels can be seen to good advantage. Gradient-echo pulse sequences and MRA are useful in evaluating the relationship of the tumor to the adjacent vessels.

A histologic variation of HCC is the fibrolamellar subtype, which is typically seen in adolescents and young women. A central scar and fibrous septa may be present, similar to FNH. US typically reveals a lobulated mass with well-defined borders and a variable echotexture. If a central scar is present, it tends to be hyperechoic. In a large series of 31 patients imaged by CT, the tumor had smooth margins in 24 cases, calcifications in 21, a central scar in 22, and abdominal lymphadenopathy in 20 cases. In 20 of 25 cases with CT scans obtained during the hepatic arterial phase of enhancement, there was heterogeneous enhancement with areas of hypervascularity. Images from the portal venous phase of enhancement showed the tumor to be isoattenuating in 12, hyperattenuating in 4, and hypoattenuating in 9 cases. On MRI, the mass tends to be isointense to liver on T_1-weighted images. On T_2 weighting, the lesion typically remains isointense but may have increased or decreased signal. The fibrous scar has low signal on both pulse sequences, a feature that helps to distinguish this

lesion from FNH, in which the central scar tends to have high signal on T_2 weighting.

> ■ Signal intensity of the central scar is typically decreased on T_2-weighted images in fibrolamellar hepatocellular carcinoma, a feature that helps to differentiate it from focal nodular hyperplasia.

UNDIFFERENTIATED EMBRYONAL SARCOMA

Undifferentiated embryonal sarcoma is a rare tumor of mesenchymal origin occurring in older children and young adults that represents the malignant form of mesenchymal hamartoma. Pathologically, they are predominantly solid. A discrepancy between the appearance of the mass on US and its appearance on CT and MRI is an imaging hallmark of this tumor (Fig. 9). US confirms the solid nature of this tumor, which typically is iso- or hyperechoic. CT and MRI usually have a misleading cystic appearance, with water attenuation on CT and low signal on T_1-weighted and high signal on T_2-weighted MRI. This misleading appearance suggesting fluid on CT and MRI may be caused by water attracted by the hydrophilic acid mucopolysaccharides in the myxoid components of the tumor. Although the lesions tend to be predominantly solid on US, small fluid containing spaces may be seen. Areas of high attenuation on CT and high signal on T_1-weighted MRI may represent hemorrhage. Peripheral enhancement, corresponding to a pseudocapsule, and enhancement of solid-appearing "septa" within the lesion may be seen after intravenous contrast administration on CT. Metastases usually occur in the lungs and skeleton.

RHABDOMYOSARCOMA

Rhabdomyosarcoma of the bile ducts is one of the rarest forms of this tumor of mesenchymal origin. This tumor tends to occur in young children, with a median age at presentation of 3 years. Patients typically present with jaundice and abdominal distention or, less likely, pain, nausea, vomiting, or fever. The tumor can arise in the intrahepatic bile ducts, the gallbladder, the cystic duct, the extrahepatic biliary tree, or the ampulla, or within a choledochal cyst. When the tumor arises in one of the large bile ducts, it is usually has the gross appearance of an intraductal sarcoma botryoides (Fig. 10). US typically reveals biliary duct dilatation and a hyperechoic intraductal mass. Larger masses may have areas of cystic necrosis. CT also shows an intraductal mass with variable contrast enhancement. MRI usually demonstrates low signal on T_1-weighted images and high signal on T_2 weighting with intense but heterogeneous enhancement. Magnetic resonance cholangiopancreatography may prove useful in the evaluation of this tumor. When the tumor arises in an intrahepatic duct, it is often indistinguishable from other intrahepatic malignancies on imaging studies (Fig. 11).

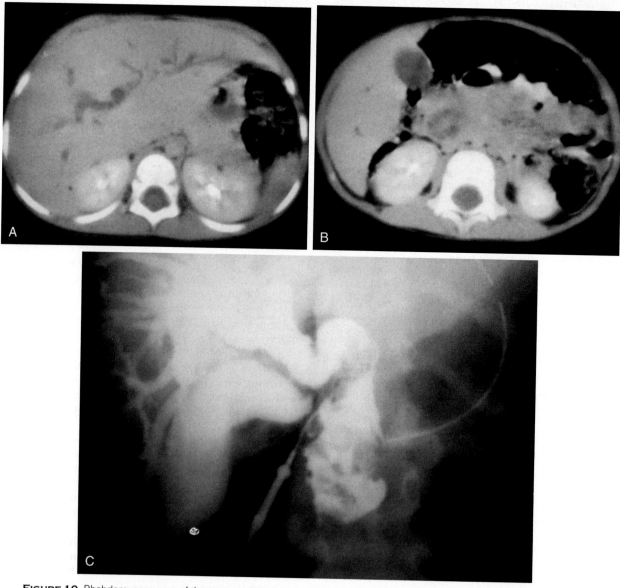

FIGURE 10. Rhabdomyosarcoma of the common bile duct. **A,** Contrast-enhanced computed tomography (CT) demonstrates dilated intrahepatic biliary ducts. **B,** A more inferior CT scan section reveals a lobulated mass in the region of the porta hepatis. **C,** Operative cholangiogram confirms that the lobulated mass originates in the dilated common bile duct.

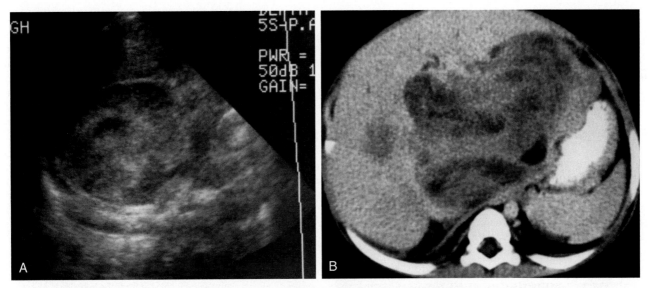

FIGURE 11. Rhabdomyosarcoma arising from the intrahepatic biliary ducts. **A,** Sonogram demonstrates a heterogeneous echogenic mass in the left lobe of the liver. **B,** Computed tomography scan demonstrates a diffuse lesion throughout the left lobe and portions of the right lobe of the liver that does not undergo contrast enhancement as much as the surrounding normal parenchyma.

CHOLANGIOCARCINOMA

Cholangiocarcinoma may arise in pre-existing chole-dochal cysts, but usually in adults.

HEPATIC METASTASES

Metastatic disease to the liver is most commonly from primary tumors arising in other abdominal organs. Wilms' tumor and neuroblastoma are the two most common tumors metastasizing to the liver in children. Virtually any other solid tumor, other than those arising in the central nervous system, can metastasize to the liver. Lymphoma and leukemia are often considered metastatic lesions, but generally represent infiltration of the liver by systemic disease of multifocal origin.

■ Wilms' tumor and neuroblastoma are the two most common tumors to metastasize to the liver in children.

Metastatic disease from neuroblastoma in infancy can simulate a primary liver tumor (Fig. 12). Careful evaluation of the sites of origin of neuroblastoma should always be performed when a solid liver tumor is first discovered. Even though metastases to the liver from infantile neuroblastoma can be massive, the prognosis in children under the age of 1 year is still remarkably good. Beyond infancy, metastases are more likely to occur during the course of neoplastic disease rather than at presentation.

Imaging studies of metastatic disease to the liver in

children show results similar to those found in adults, depending to some degree on the nature of the primary tumor. Sonography typically identifies multiple discrete lesions, but numerous metastases, especially from neuroblastoma, may simulate a large heterogeneous mass. Most metastatic lesions are hypoechoic. Neuroblastoma lesions may calcify and have acoustic shadowing. Large metastases from any tumor may undergo central necrosis or hemorrhage and show even lower areas of echogenicity within the center.

On CT, metastases are quite variable in appearance. The attenuation of metastases is usually lower than that of the surrounding liver, and the difference is exaggerated with intravenous contrast enhancement. However, some tumors will cause metastatic lesions that are isodense with the surrounding liver parenchyma, and some hypervascular metastases may have increased attenuation compared to the surrounding normal liver after intravenous contrast administration. Target-like concentric bands of variable attenuation may be seen, with the lowest density being in the center in cases of tumor necrosis. Peripheral ring enhancement is frequent following contrast injection. The MRI characteristics of liver metastases will depend to a large degree on the origin of the tumor. In general, there is lower signal intensity on T_1 weighting and higher signal intensity on T_2 weighting with respect to the normal liver parenchyma. Metastatic disease can be seen on radionuclide liver scans with multiple discrete photopenic areas or generalized decrease in activity. However, this modality is now rarely used in the evaluation of hepatic metastases. In general, the sensitivity of nuclear medicine studies is less than that of US, which is less than that of either CT or MRI.

The distinction between metastatic disease and other hepatic masses is not always easy. Brody et al. reported a

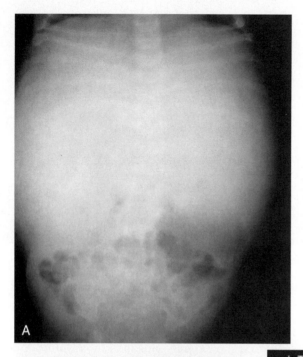

FIGURE 12. Metastatic neuroblastoma. **A,** Plain radiograph of the abdomen in a 6-week-old girl with massive abdominal distention demonstrates a very large upper abdominal mass depressing the air-filled bowel inferiorly. **B** and **C,** Longitudinal and transverse sonograms through the liver demonstrate a nodular liver with heterogeneous echogenicity. T_1-weighted **(D)** and T_2-weighted **(E)** spin-echo magnetic resonance images, demonstrate marked hepatomegaly, with heterogeneous decreased signal intensity on T_1-weighted and heterogeneous increased signal on T_2-weighted image. The patient had no extra-abdominal metastatic lesions, and the tumor had regressed almost completely 6 months after the initial studies.

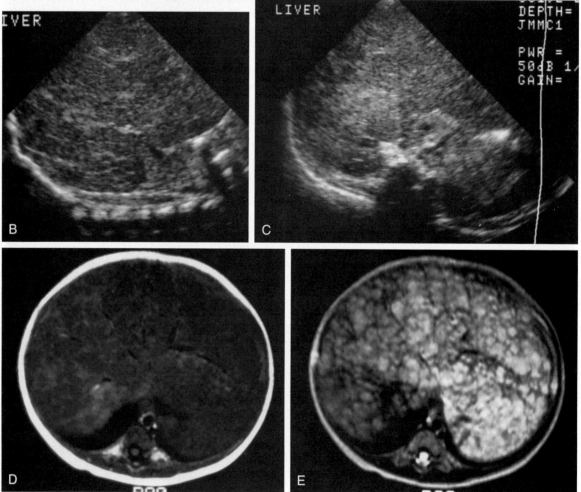

case of Wilms' tumor in which hepatic metastases had the MRI characteristics of cysts on spin-echo images. Brick et al. demonstrated small benign hepatic cysts on screening CT (in patients with known underlying malignancies) that had the appearance of solid lesions because of volume averaging. In some cases, this mistakenly raised the concern of metastatic disease. US was useful in differentiating these lesions from metastases and is a useful adjunct if the CT or MRI appearance is not diagnostic.

SUGGESTED READINGS

General

Boechat MI, Kangarloo H, Ortega J, et al: Primary liver tumors in children: comparison of CT and MR imaging. Radiology 1988; 169:727

Brunelle F, Chaumont P: Hepatic tumors in children: ultrasonic differentiation of malignant from benign lesions. Radiology 1984; 150:695

Ferrucci JT: MR imaging of the liver: Leo G. Rigler Lecture. AJR Am J Roentgenol 1986;147:1103

Greenberg M, Filler RM: Hepatic tumors. In Pizzo PA, Poplack DG (eds): Principles and Practice of Pediatric Oncology. Philadelphia, JB Lippincott, 1989;565–582

Ohtomo K, Itai Y, Yoshikawa K, et al: Hepatic tumours: dynamic MR imaging. Radiology 1987;163:27

Pobiel RS, Bissett III GS: Pictorial essay: imaging of liver tumors in the infant and child. Pediatr Radiol 1995;25:495

Rummeny E, Saini S, Wittenberg J, et al: MR imaging of liver neoplasms. AJR Am J Roentgenol 1989;152:493

Tonkin IL, Wrenn EL Jr, Hollabaugh RS: The continued value of angiography in planning surgical resection of benign and malignant hepatic tumors in children. Pediatr Radiol 1988;18:35

Benign Hepatic Neoplasms

Abramson SJ, Lack EE, Teele RL: Benign vascular tumors of the liver in infants: sonographic appearance. AJR Am J Roentgenol 1982; 138:629

Alwaidh MH, Woodhall CR, Carty HT: Mesenchymal hamartoma of the liver: a case report. Pediatr Radiol 1997;27:247

Barnhart DC, Hirschl RB, Garver KA, et al: Conservative management of mesenchymal hamartoma of the liver. J Pediatr Surg 1997;32:1495

Birnbaum BA, Weinreb JC, Megibow AJ, et al: Definitive diagnosis of hepatic hemangiomas: MR imaging versus Tc-99m-labeled red blood cell SPECT. Radiology 1990;176:95

Bree RL, Schwab RE, Glazer GM, et al: The varied appearances of hepatic cavernous hemangiomas with sonography, computed tomography, magnetic resonance imaging and scintigraphy. Radiographics 1987;7:1153

Brodsky RI, Friedman AC, Maurer AM, et al: Hepatic cavernous hemangioma: diagnosis with ^{99m}Tc-labelled red cells and single photon emission CT. AJR Am J Roentgenol 1987;148:125

Brummett D, Burton EM, Sabio H: Hepatic adenomatosis: rapid sequence MR imaging following gadolinium enhancement—a case report. Pediatr Radiol 1999;29:231

Brunelle F, Tammam S, Odievre M, et al: Liver adenomas in glycogen storage disease in children: ultrasound and angiographic study. Pediatr Radiol 1984;14:94

Dachman AH, Lichtenstein JE, Friedman AC, et al: Infantile hemangioendothelioma of the liver: a radiologic-pathologic-clinical correlation. AJR Am J Roentgenol 1983;140:1091

Dachman AH, Ros PR, Goodman ZD, et al: Nodular regenerative hyperplasia of the liver: Clinical and radiologic observations. AJR Am J Roentgenol 1987;148:717

Daller JA, Bueno J, Gutierrez J, et al: Hepatic hemangioendothelioma: clinical experience and management strategy. J Pediatr Surg 1999;34:98

Donovan AT, Wolverson MK, de Mello D, et al: Multicystic mesenchymal hamartoma of childhood: computerized tomography and ultrasound characteristics. Pediatr Radiol 1981;11:163

Fellows KE, Hoffer FA, Markowitz RI, et al: Multiple collaterals to hepatic infantile hemangioendotheliomas and arteriovenous malformations: effect on embolization. Radiology 1991;181:813

Freeny PC, Marks WM: Hepatic hemangioma: dynamic bolus CT. AJR Am J Roentgenol 1986;147:711

Gibney RG, Hendin AP, Cooperberg PL: Sonographically detected hepatic hemangiomas: absence of change over time. AJR Am J Roentgenol 1987;149:93

Giyanani VL, Meyers PC, Wolfson JJ: Mesenchymal hamartoma of the liver: computed tomography and ultrasonography. J Comput Assist Tomogr 1986;10:51

Goldberg MA, Saini S, Hahn PF, et al: Differentiation between hemangiomas and metastases of the liver with ultrafast MR imaging: preliminary results with T_2 calculations. AJR Am J Roentgenol 1991;154:727

Haliloglu M, Hoffer FA, Gronemeyer SA, et al: 3-D gadolinium-enhanced MRA: evaluation of hepatic vasculature in children with hepatoblastoma. J Magn Reson Imaging 2000;11:65

Horton KM, Bluemke DA, Hruban RH, et al: CT and MR imaging of benign hepatic and biliary tumors. Radiographics 1999;19:431

Itai Y, Ohtomo K, Araki T, et al: Computed tomography and sonography of cavernous hemangioma of the liver. AJR Am J Roentgenol 1983;141:315

Jennings CM, Merrill CR, Slater DN: Case report: the computed tomographic appearances of benign hepatic hamartoma. Clin Radiol 1987;38:103

Leary DL, Weiskittel DA, Blane CE, et al: Follow-up imaging of benign pediatric liver tumors. Pediatr Radiol 1989;19:234

Li KC, Glazer GM, Quint LE, et al: Distinction of hepatic cavernous hemangioma from hepatic metastases with MR imaging. Radiology 1988;169:409

Lucaya J, Enriquez G, Amat L, et al: Computed tomography of infantile hepatic hemangioendothelioma. AJR Am J Roentgenol 1985;144:821

Mathieu D, Bruneton JN, Drouillard J, et al: Hepatic adenomas and local nodular hyperplasia: dynamic CT study. Radiology 1986;160:53

Maves CK, Caron KH, Bissett GS III, et al: Splenic and hepatic peliosis: MR findings. AJR Am J Roentgenol 1992;158:75

Mortele KJ, Mergo PJ, Urrutia M, et al: Dynamic gadolinium-enhanced MR findings in infantile hepatic hemangioendothelioma. J Comput Assist Tomogr 1998;22:714

Ohtomo K, Itai Y, Hasizume K, et al: CT and MR appearance of focal nodular hyperplasia of the liver in children with biliary atresia. Clin Radiol 1991;43:88

Park CH, Hwang HS, Hong J, et al: Giant infantile hemangioendothelioma of the liver: scintigraphic diagnosis. Clin Nucl Med 1996; 21:293

Quillin SP, Atilla S, Brown JJ, et al: Characterization of focal hepatic masses by dynamic contrast-enhanced MR imaging: findings in 311 lesions. Magn Reson Imaging 1997;15:275

Radin DR, Kanel GC: Peliosis hepatis in a patient with human immunodeficiency virus infection. AJR Am J Roentgenol 1991; 156:91

Ramanujam TM, Ramesh JC, Goh DW, et al: Malignant transformation of mesenchymal hamartoma of the liver: case report and review of the literature. J Pediatr Surg 1999;34:1684

Ros PR, Goodman ZD, Ishak K, et al: Mesenchymal hamartoma of the liver: radiologic-pathologic correlation. Radiology 1986;158:619

Ros PR, Lubbers PR, Olmsted WW, et al: Hemangioma of the liver: heterogeneous appearance of T_2-weighted images. AJR Am J Roentgenol 1987;149:1167

Rummeny E, Weissleder R, Stark DD, et al: Primary liver tumors: diagnosis by MR imaging. AJR Am J Roentgenol 1989;152:63

Saatci I, Coskun M, Boyvat F, et al: MR findings in peliosis hepatis. Pediatr Radiol 1995;25:31

Schmidt H, Ullrich K, von Lenglerke HJ, et al: Peliosis hepatis with type I glycogen storage disease. J Inherited Metab Dis 1991;14:831

Semelka RC, Brown ED, Ascher SM, et al: Hepatic hemangiomas: a multi-institutional study of appearance on T_2-weighted and serial gadolinium-enhanced gradient-echo MR images. Radiology 1994; 192:401

Stanley P, Hall TR, Woolley MM, et al: Mesenchymal hamartomas of the liver in childhood: sonographic and CT findings. AJR Am J Roentgenol 1986;147:1035

Toma P, Taccone A, Martinoli C, et al: MRI of hepatic focal nodular hyperplasia: a report of two new cases in the pediatric age group. Pediatr Radiol 1990;20:267

Tovbin J, Segal M, Tavori I, et al: Hepatic mesenchymal hamartoma: a pediatric tumor that may be diagnosed prenatally. Ultrasound Obstet Gynecol 1997;10:63

Trenchel GM, Schubert A, Dries V, et al: Nodular regenerative hyperplasia of the liver: case report of a 13-year-old girl and review of the literature. Pediatr Radiol 2000;30:64

Tsukamoto Y, Nakata H, Kimoto T, et al: CT and angiography of peliosis hepatis. AJR Am J Roentgenol 1984;142:539

Welch TJ, Sheedy PF II, Johnson CM, et al: Focal nodular hyperplasia and hepatic adenoma: comparison of angiography, CT, US, and scintigraphy. Radiology 1985;156:593

Welch TJ, Sheedy PF II, Johnson CM, et al: Radiographic characteristics of benign liver tumours: focal nodular hyperplasia and hepatic adenoma. Radiographics 1985;5:673

Wholey MH, Wojno KJ: Pediatric hepatic mesenchymal hamartoma demonstrated on plain film, ultrasound and MRI, and correlated with pathology. Pediatr Radiol 1994;24:143

Primary Malignant Hepatobiliary Tumors

Bates SM, Keller MS, Ramos IM, et al: Hepatoblastoma: detection of tumor vascularity with duplex Doppler US. Radiology 1990;176:505

Bova JG, Dempsher CJ, Sepulveda G: Cholangiocarcinoma associated with type 2 choledochal cysts. Gastrointest Radiol 1983;8:41

Buetow PC, Buck JL, Pantongrag-Brown L, et al: Undifferentiated (embryonal) sarcoma of the liver: pathologic basis of imaging findings in 28 cases. Raiology 1997;203:779

Dachman AH, Parker RL, Ros PR, et al: Hepatoblastoma: radiologic-pathologic correlation in 50 cases. Radiology 1987;164:15

deCampo M, deCampo JR: Ultrasound of primary hepatic tumours in childhood. Pediatr Radiol 1988;19:19

Diament MJ, Parvey LS, Tonkin ILD, et al: Hepatoblastomas: technetium sulfur colloid uptake simulating focal nodular hyperplasia. AJR Am J Roentgenol 1982;139:168

Exelby PR, Filler RM, Grosfeld JL: Liver tumors in children in particular reference to hepatoblastoma and hepatocellular carcinoma: American Academy of Pediatrics Surgical Survey—1974. J Pediatr Surg 1975;10:329

Finn JP, Hall-Craggs MA, Dicks-Mireaux C, et al: Primary liver tumors in childhood: assessment of resectability with high-field MR and comparison with CT. Pediatr Radiol 1990;21:34

Friedman AC, Lichtenstein JE, Goodman Z, et al: Fibrolamellar hepatocellular carcinoma. Radiology 1985;157:583

Ichikawa T, Federle MP, Grazioli L, et al: Fibrolamellar hepatocellular carcinoma: imaging and pathologic findings in 31 recent cases. Radiology 1999;213:352

Ito E, Sato Y, Kawauchi K, et al: Type Ia glycogen storage disease with hepatoblastoma in siblings. Cancer 1987;59:1776

Lauwers GY, Grant LD, Donnelly WH, et al: Hepatic undifferentiated (embryonal) sarcoma arising in a mesenchymal hamartoma. Am J Surg Pathol 1997;21:1248

McLarney JK, Rucker PT, Bender GN, et al: Fibrolamellar carcinoma of the liver: radiology-pathologic correlation. Radiographics 1999; 19:453

Moon WK, Kim WS, Kim IO, et al: Undifferentiated embyonal sarcoma of the liver: US and CT fidings. Pediatr Radiol 1994;24:500

Nzeako UC, Goodman ZD, Ishak HG: Hepatocellular carcinoma and nodular regenerative hyperplasia: possible pathogenic relationship. Am J Gastroenterol 1996;91:879

Patil KK, Omojola MF, Khurana P, et al: Embryonal rhabdomyosarcoma within a choledochal cyst. Can Assoc Radiol J 1992;43:145

Powers C, Ros PR, Stoupis C, et al: Primary liver neoplasms: MR imaging with pathologic correlation. Radiographics 1994;14:459

Roebuck DJ, Yang WT, Lam WWM, et al: Hepatobiliary rhabdomyosarcoma in children: diagnostic radiology. Pediatr Radiol 1998; 28:101

Ros PR, Olmsted WW, Dachman AH, et al: Undifferentiated (embryonal) sarcoma of the liver: radiologic-pathologic correlation. Radiology 1986;161:141

Stoupis C, Ros PR: Imaging findings in hepatoblastoma associated with Gardner's syndrome. AJR Am J Roentgenol 1993;161:593

Taylor KJW, Ramos I, Morse SS, et al: Focal liver masses: differential diagnosis with pulsed Doppler US. Radiology 1987;164:643

Hepatic Metastases

Abramson SJ, Barash FS, Seldin DW, et al: Transient focal liver scan defects in children receiving chemotherapy (pseudometastases). Radiology 1984;150:701

Brick SH, Hill MC, Lande IM: The mistaken or indeterminate CT diagnosis of hepatic metastases: the value of sonography. AJR Am J Roentgenol 1987;148:723

Brody AS, Seidel FG, Kuhn JP: Metastatic Wilms tumor to the liver with MR findings simulating need for integrated imaging. Pediatr Radiol 1989;19:337

Reinig JW, Dwyer AJ, Miller DL, et al: Liver metastases: detection with MR imaging at 0.5 and 1.5 T. Radiology 1989;170:149

Stark DD, Wittenberg J, Butch RJ, et al: Hepatic mestastases: randomized controlled comparison of detection with MR imaging and CT. Radiology 1987;165:399

Weinreb JC, Brateman L, Maravilla KR: Magnetic resonance imaging of hepatic lymphoma. AJR Am J Roentgenol 1984;143:1211

Chapter 8

LIVER TRANSPLANTATION

A'DELBERT BOWEN and RICHARD B. TOWBIN

Liver replacement is a well-established treatment for end-stage liver disease, for certain liver-based metabolic disorders, and for selected children with primary liver tumors. With immunosuppression using tacrolimus (FK-506, Prograf) and prednisone, actuarial 6-year survival of pediatric liver recipients exceeds 85%, with graft survival rates slightly lower because of graft failure and retransplantation. This chapter focuses on imaging aspects of isolated orthotopic liver transplantation. Multivisceral transplantation, operative techniques, immunosuppression, and other clinical issues have been addressed elsewhere.

PREOPERATIVE ASSESSMENT

Preoperative imaging is tailored to the child's individual circumstances, including the underlying liver disease, coexisting clinical conditions, and the potential need for multivisceral transplantation. Virtually every candidate has chest radiographs and abdominal ultrasound (US) with Doppler. The critical items in the US examination are patency and diameter of the extrahepatic portal vein. If the portal vein is less than 4 mm in diameter, or if the portal vein is occluded or replaced by cavernous transformation, it must be established that the superior mesentery vein remains patent in order for liver transplantation to be feasible. If US cannot make this determination, conventional angiography or magnetic resonance angiography is performed. Catheter angiography entails selective injections of the celiac axis and superior mesenteric artery with the goals of demonstrating vascular anatomy, identifying normal variants, and documenting size and patency of the portal vein. The portal vein usually is best shown with a long (5-second) injection of contrast medium into the superior mesenteric artery after vasodilation with papaverine (12 to 45 mg). Filming over 20 to 30 seconds may be necessary. Alternative techniques include selective injection into the splenic artery or direct splenoportography.

■ The critical information in the preoperative ultrasound examination is the patency and diameter of the extrahepatic portal vein.

For the standard liver transplant operation, in which a segment of the recipient's inferior vena cava (IVC) is replaced by a corresponding length of donor IVC, patency of the recipient IVC is essential. The caval-sparing "piggyback" operation, now routine in children, renders IVC patency moot; however, if the primary liver disease is hepatic malignancy or Budd-Chiari syndrome, the surgeon must know if there is thrombus in the IVC. Because the anatomy of the *donor* graft dictates the type of arterial reconstruction that must be done, the *recipient's* hepatic arterial anatomy is immaterial.

A sonographic survey is made of the abdomen to document such findings as splenomegaly; venous collaterals associated with portal hypertension; and renal abnormalities, such as hydronephrosis, that may need correction prior to liver transplantation. Anomalies of visceral situs do not preclude transplantation. In some circumstances, such as living-related transplants, calculation of liver volume by computed tomography (CT) may be requested. Other imaging examinations are obtained as clinically indicated. Discovery of an unsuspected liver tumor triggers evaluation for metastases and may place the child in the urgent transplant category.

Catastrophic ruptures of unsuspected splenic artery aneurysms after liver transplantation have prompted various proposals for preoperative screening. These aneurysms are liable to escape sonographic detection, but we have found some with CT angiography with three-dimensional reconstruction.

PERIOPERATIVE IMAGING

Intraoperative Doppler US of the hepatic artery and portal vein may be requested prior to closing the abdomen, especially if the vascular reconstruction has been troublesome. US also is the mainstay of early postoperative imaging, the timing of postoperative examinations being determined by local preference—typically, an US survey of the graft and vessels is made daily for the first several days and thereafter as need arises. Particular attention is given to portal venous flow and hepatic arterial resistive index on Doppler US. A whole-liver graft requires evaluation of the main, right, and left branches of the portal vein and hepatic artery, all three hepatic veins, and the IVC. A reduced-sized graft—usually the left lobe or its lateral segment—ordinarily will have a single hepatic artery and portal vein. If arterial reconstruction employs a donor aortic conduit, it should be traced to its anastomosis with the recipient aorta, but, as a practical matter, vascular anastomoses often cannot be identified with certainty by US.

Other findings to document include hepatic parenchymal defects, biliary ductal dilatation, perihepatic fluid collections, pleural effusions, and splenic infarcts, which may occur after splenic artery ligation. Right adrenal hemorrhage and right phrenic nerve injury, complications seen after the standard transplant operation, rarely occur after the caval-sparing operation.

The normal liver graft typically exhibits transient periportal increased echogenicity as a result of lymphatic engorgement on US, with corresponding findings on CT or magnetic resonance imaging (MRI). Other transient, and usually innocuous, postoperative findings include right pleural effusion, small subhepatic liquid collections, and biliary air in recipients with choledochojejunostomies. Transient vascular abnormalities may include reduced caliber of the portal vein in the porta hepatis because of surrounding edema and a relatively high hepatic arterial resistive index. Of greater concern is a low resistive index (<0.50), which warrants close follow-up until normalization, or investigation with angiography if hepatic arterial stenosis is suspected (see below). Discrepancies in caliber of recipient and donor portal veins—the donor vein typically the larger—may produce turbulence and flow vortices downstream from the anastomosis on color Doppler, but these flow alterations have not proven to be clinically important. In the caval-sparing operation, which can be done either with whole or reduced-size grafts, the segment of donor IVC accompanying the graft often is visible "piggybacked" onto the anterior wall of the recipient IVC and may continue to receive drainage from inferior accessory hepatic veins.

The reduced-sized liver graft is placed in orthotopic position, the cut surface of the graft directed toward the patient's right side. Bowel ascends to occupy the space vacated by the excised right hepatic lobe. On postoperative imaging, the single portal vein and hepatic artery typically make an abrupt turn to the left as they enter the graft, and the stump of the amputated right portal vein may be visible. One or two hepatic veins drain the graft. A small and usually benign collection of liquid may accumulate along the cut surface of the liver.

POSTOPERATIVE COMPLICATIONS

A host of vascular, infectious, and immunosuppression-related complications (Table 1) may befall the liver recipient both early and late in the postoperative course. Essential to effective management are awareness of these possible complications; good communication between radiologist and surgeon; ready availability of all diagnostic imaging modalities; and a well-organized, skilled interventional radiology service. A dedicated radiologic nursing service is invaluable, particularly with

Table 1 ■ LIVER TRANSPLANT COMPLICATIONS

Vascular
Thrombosis/stenosis
  Hepatic artery
  Portal-vein
  Inferior vena cava/hepatic veins
Mycotic aneurysms

Biliary Tract
Bile duct stenosis
Bile leak

Hemorrhage
Postoperative/technical
Biopsy complications

Infection

Post-transplantation Lymphoproliferative Disease

Miscellaneous
Primary graft nonfunction
Rejection
Enteric complications
Neurologic complications
Renal complications
Recurrent primary liver tumor
Graft-versus-host disease
Thoracic/pulmonary complications

regard to sedation, preparation for and monitoring during interventional procedures, and postprocedure follow-up.

The most common complication of liver transplantation is infection, but vascular thrombosis and primary graft nonfunction account for most cases of graft loss leading to retransplantation. Most pediatric liver recipient deaths are caused by infection, neurologic complications, or multisystem organ failure. The mainstays of imaging for postoperative complications are US, CT, conventional radiography, and interventional techniques. Magnetic resonance cholangiopancreatography (MRCP) is gaining favor as an alternative to percutaneous transhepatic cholangiography (PTC) for assessing biliary tract complications. MRI also has a role in evaluating neurologic and some vascular complications. Radionuclide scintigraphy has selected applications. The interventional armamentarium includes angiography, PTC, imaging-guided biopsies, and therapeutic procedures, including biliary drainage, dilatation, and stenting.

■ Infection is the most common complication of liver transplantation, but vascular thrombosis and primary graft nonfunction are the most common causes of graft loss leading to retransplantation.

VASCULAR COMPLICATIONS

Hepatic arterial thrombosis (HAT), usually occurring within the first month after transplantation, is a major cause of graft loss. On Doppler US, an arterial resistive index of less than 0.50 and systolic acceleration time prolongation to greater than 0.08 seconds are strongly predictive for thrombosis or significant stenosis. Doppler US typically detects HAT by absence of arterial flow, confirmed by angiography (Fig. 1). However, severe rejection, massive hepatic necrosis, or systemic hypotension may produce false-positive ultrasound findings of undetectable arterial flow in the presence of a patent artery. Urgent reoperation to repair an acutely occluded artery may salvage the graft. Thrombolytic therapy is a temporizing measure with a substantial risk for hemorrage in the face of anticoagulation or coagulopathy. Scanty experience with balloon angioplasty for hepatic arterial stenosis in pediatric liver recipients permits no generalization. In some instances, spontaneous development of arterial collateral circulation sustains graft function indefinitely.

■ US findings in hepatic arterial thrombosis or significant stenosis include:
• Absent arterial flow
• Resistive index less than 0.50
• Systolic acceleration time prolongation to greater than 0.08 seconds

Venous complications in the liver graft are relatively uncommon but can contribute to graft loss and death. If US detects acute portal venous thrombosis early, thrombectomy and anastomotic revision may salvage the vein. Portal venous stenosis is more problematic for US, because mild anastomotic narrowing and associated flow disturbances are commonplace and usually of no

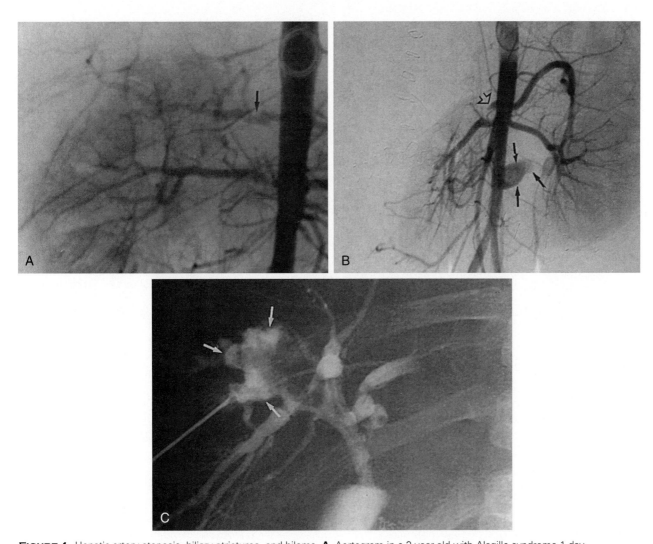

FIGURE 1. Hepatic artery stenosis, biliary strictures, and biloma. **A,** Aortogram in a 3-year-old with Alagille syndrome 1 day after transplantation shows anastomotic stenosis of hepatic artery *(arrow)*. The patient underwent operative revascularization using iliac arterial graft. Liver enzymes were elevated 1 week later; no hepatic arterial flow was seen on ultrasound (not shown). **B,** Repeat arteriogram confirms thrombosis of iliac arterial graft conduit *(arrows)* and hepatic artery stump remnant *(open arrow)*. **C,** Percutaneous transhepatic cholangiography 6 weeks after hepatic arterial thrombosis (HAT) demonstrates that the roux-en-Y choledochojejunal anastomosis is patent; right and left ductal strictures and a lobulated, central, contrast-filled biloma *(arrows)* resulting from the HAT-induced bile duct necrosis is identified. (From Bowen A, Hungate RG, Kaye RD, et al: Imaging in liver transplantation. Radiol Clin North Am 1996;34:757–778, with permission.)

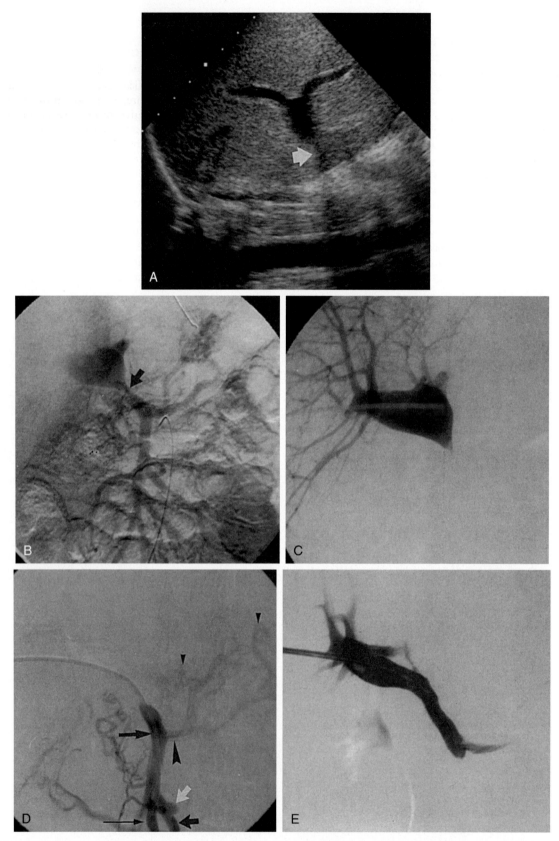

FIGURE 2. Portal vein stenosis in a 7-year-old, transplanted 8 months earlier for α_1-antitrypsin deficiency, now with elevated liver enzymes. **A,** Ultrasound shows narrowed segment of main portal vein *(arrow)* entering the porta hepatis, with abruptly increased portal vein caliber distally. **B,** Venous phase from a selective superior mesenteric arteriogram shows anastomotic stenosis *(arrow)*. **C,** Transhepatic portogram shows portal venous opacification distal to stenosis. Note apparent poststenotic dilatation. **D,** Catheter across stenosis with contrast opacification of proximal portal vein *(large arrow)*, superior mesenteric vein *(thin arrow)*, inferior mesenteric vein *(short thick arrow)*, splenic vein *(white arrow)*, coronary vein *(large arrowhead)*, and varices *(short arrowheads)*. **E,** Venogram after percutaneous transluminal angioplasty shows no residual stenosis and less dilated distal portal vein. (From Bowen A, Hungate RG, Kaye RD, et al: Imaging in liver transplantation. Radiol Clin North Am 1996;34:757–778, with permission.)

hemodynamic importance. Significant portal venous stenosis (Fig. 2) may produce clinical signs of portal hypertension and can be investigated by a variety of angiographic techniques. Rare thrombosis or anastomotic stenosis of the inferior vena cava can be detected by US, and stenosis can be treated with high-pressure balloon dilatation (Fig. 3).

BILIARY TRACT COMPLICATIONS

Bile duct stenosis or leak may result from ischemia caused by hepatic arterial occlusion or from improper graft preservation. Anastomotic strictures may result from operative technical error, and nonanastomotic strictures (Fig. 4) may ensue after ischemia, rejection, or infection. US, CT, or scintigraphy may detect biliary complications, but PTC or MRCP (Fig. 5) often is needed for definitive assessment. Biliary ductal strictures usually require repeated dilatation and long-term (>3 months) stenting. Best results seem to be obtained by using high-pressure angioplasty balloons kept inflated across strictures for 5 to 30 minutes. Operative reconstruction often becomes necessary eventually. Biliary complications seldom are directly responsible for retransplantation.

HEMORRHAGE

Early postoperative bleeding from leaking anastomoses or inadequate hemostasis occurs in as many as 15% of recipients and up to half of those undergo operative exploration. Postoperative blood loss is monitored by clinical observation and drain output. Small hematomas or other fluid collections around the liver are common and need no intervention unless there is evidence for bile leak, ongoing bleeding, or supervening infection. Mycotic arterial pseudoaneurysms at anastomoses may rupture to produce abrupt exsanguination. Any collection of fluid near an artery should be interrogated with Doppler US (Fig. 6). In selected instances, pseudoaneurysms can be treated with embolization of the affected artery or by direct injection of thrombin into the pseudoaneurysm.

INFECTION

The majority of liver recipients develop postoperative infections at some time, although consequent mortality is under 10%. Bacterial and fungal infections are most common during the first postoperative month; risk factors include technical complications (e.g., HAT),

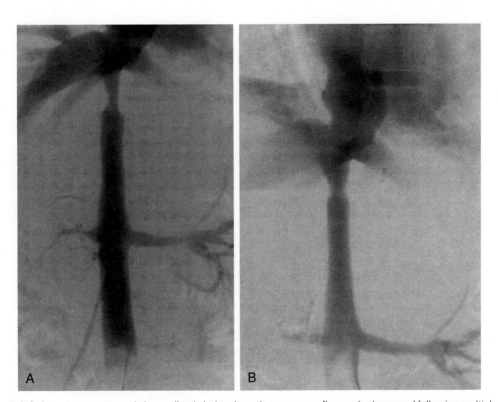

FIGURE 3. Inferior vena cava stenosis immediately below hepatic venous confluence had recurred following multiple balloon dilatations in this 8-year-old who received liver transplant for primary oxalosis. **A,** Inferior venacavogram prior to most recent angioplasty depicts stenosis. **B,** Following angioplasty using a high-pressure (17-atm) angioplasty balloon, cavogram shows increased lumen size. (From Bowen A, Hungate RG, Kaye RD, et al: Imaging in liver transplantation. Radiol Clin North Am 1996;34:757–778, with permission.)

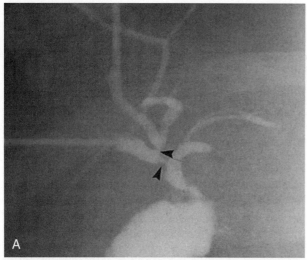

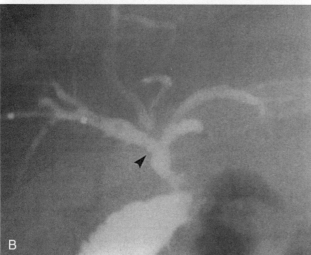

FIGURE 4. Biliary ductal stenosis in an asymptomatic 15-year-old boy with elevated liver enzymes 12 years after transplantation for α_1-antitrypsin deficiency. Liver biopsy showed proliferating bile ducts. **A,** Percutaneous transhepatic cholangiography (PTC) demonstrates biliary strictures *(arrowheads)*. **B,** PTC after three sessions of balloon dilatation demonstrates near-complete resolution of one stricture *(arrowhead)*. Second stricture was not treated at this time. Liver enzymes became normal. (From Bowen A, Hungate RG, Kaye RD, et al: Imaging in liver transplantation. Radiol Clin North Am 1996;34:757–778, with permission.)

immunosuppression, central venous catheters, and nosocomial exposures. Viral and opportunistic infections most often occur between 30 and 180 postoperative days. Standard imaging techniques are used to evaluate suspected infections. Cholangitis may prompt MRCP or PTC. CT is the mainstay of imaging for intra-abdominal infections, particularly abscesses. The interventionalist may perform percutaneous diagnostic aspiration and drainage; small abscesses (<3 cm in diameter) may be treated by aspiration alone, but larger ones require drain placement.

POST-TRANSPLANT LYMPHOPROLIFERATIVE DISORDER

Post-transplant lymphoproliferative disorder (PTLD), a lymphoma-like proliferation of B cells induced by Epstein-Barr viral infection in the face of immunosuppression, usually develops within the first year after transplantation. Disseminated or multiple-organ involvement, having up to 50% mortality, entails a much worse prognosis than the lymphadenopathic presentation in the head and neck, or involvement of a single organ, which often regresses after simply reducing immunosuppression. CT is used to follow the extent of the disease in the neck, chest, and abdomen (Fig. 7). Imaging-guided biopsy plays a major role in management.

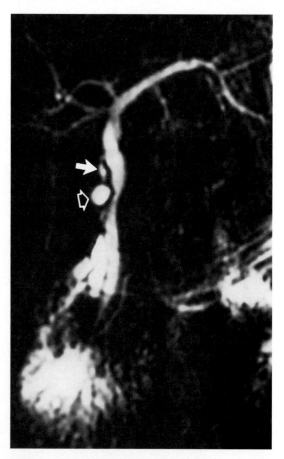

FIGURE 5. Mucocele of cystic duct remnant in a 19-year-old female with Wilson's disease, 15 months after liver transplantation with duct-to-duct biliary anastomosis. The patient was found to have dilated bile ducts following treatment for post-transplant lymphoproliferative disorder. Magnetic resonance cholangiogram (single-shot fast spin-echo, single acquisition, TE 1004/Ef) shows cystic duct stump *(solid arrow)* and mucocele *(open arrow)* that compresses adjacent common bile duct. The mucocele was resected and the biliary reconstruction converted to roux-en-Y choledochojejunostomy.

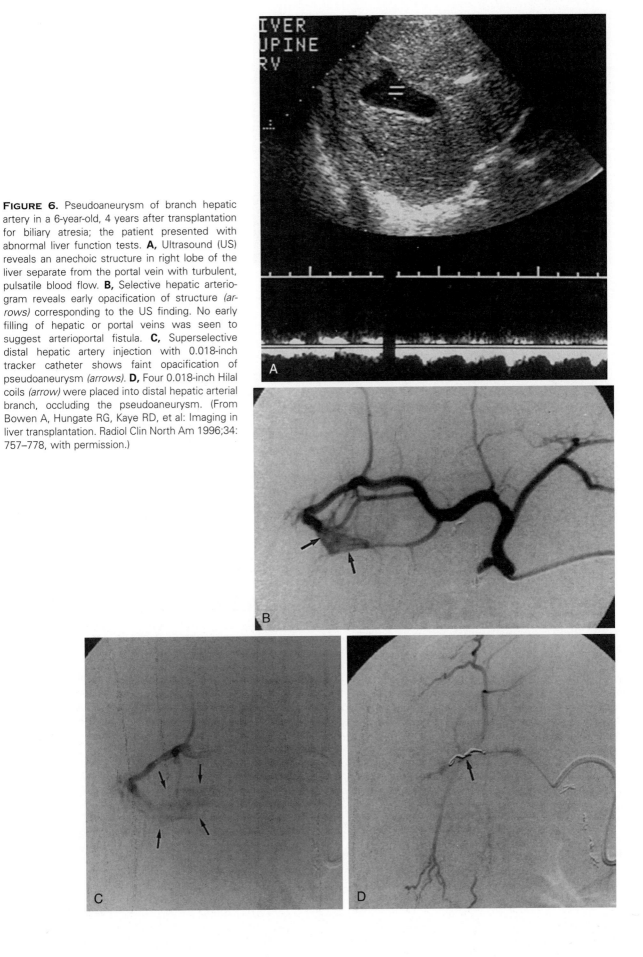

FIGURE 6. Pseudoaneurysm of branch hepatic artery in a 6-year-old, 4 years after transplantation for biliary atresia; the patient presented with abnormal liver function tests. **A,** Ultrasound (US) reveals an anechoic structure in right lobe of the liver separate from the portal vein with turbulent, pulsatile blood flow. **B,** Selective hepatic arteriogram reveals early opacification of structure *(arrows)* corresponding to the US finding. No early filling of hepatic or portal veins was seen to suggest arterioportal fistula. **C,** Superselective distal hepatic artery injection with 0.018-inch tracker catheter shows faint opacification of pseudoaneurysm *(arrows)*. **D,** Four 0.018-inch Hilal coils *(arrow)* were placed into distal hepatic arterial branch, occluding the pseudoaneurysm. (From Bowen A, Hungate RG, Kaye RD, et al: Imaging in liver transplantation. Radiol Clin North Am 1996;34: 757–778, with permission.)

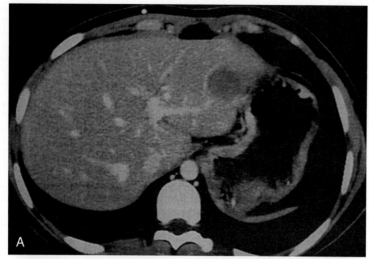

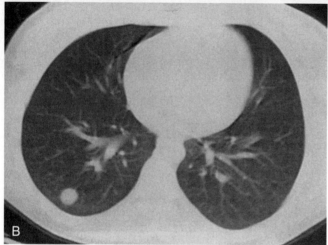

FIGURE 7. Post-transplant lymphoproliferative disorder after 6 months of FK-506 and prednisone immunosuppression in a 14-year-old girl with vomiting and abdominal pain. **A,** Abdominal computed tomography (CT) demonstrates a low-attenuation mass displacing a vessel in left lobe of liver. **B,** Chest CT reveals a pulmonary nodule. (From Bowen A, Meza MP, Ledesma-Medina J, et al: Pediatric case of the day. Radiographics 1992;12:393, with permission.)

OTHER COMPLICATIONS

Among the remaining complications, primary graft nonfunction is a leading cause of graft loss resulting in retransplantation; biliary scintigraphy may have prognostic value in the face of marginal graft function. Beyond offering biopsy guidance, imaging has no specific role in diagnosing rejection, which has become a diminished problem under tacrolimus immunosuppression and now rarely causes graft loss in children. Enteric complications include bowel perforation and obstruction, gastrointestinal hemorrhage, infectious enteritis, or bowel involvement by PTLD. Neurologic complications include cerebral hemorrhage and infarction, occasionally PTLD or infection affecting the central nervous system, and drug toxicity. Immunosuppressive drug-induced nephrotoxicity is common but has no specific imaging features. The remaining complications listed in Table 1 are rare or affect small, select subsets of recipients.

SUGGESTED READINGS

General

Reyes J, Mazariegos GV: Pediatric transplantation. Surg Clin North Am 1999;79:163

Shah AN, Dodson F, Fung J: Role of nuclear medicine in liver transplantation. Semin Nucl Med 1995;25:36

Preoperative Assessment and Perioperative Imaging

Arcement CM, Meza MP, Arumanla S, et al: MRCP in the evaluation of pancreaticobiliary disease in children. Pediatr Radiol 2001;31:92

Caron KH, Strife JL, Babcock DS, et al: Left-lobe hepatic transplants: spectrum of normal imaging findings. AJR Am J Roentgenol 1992;159:497

Jain A, Reyes J, Kashyap R, et al: What have we learned about primary liver transplantation under tacrolimus immunosuppression? Long-term follow-up of the first 1000 patients. Ann Surg 1999;230:441

Kok T, Peters PMJG, Hew JM, et al: Doppler ultrasound and angiography of the vasculature of the liver in children after orthotopic liver transplantation: a prospective study. Pediatr Radiol 1995;25:517

Lang P, Schnarkowski P, Grampp S, et al: Liver transplantation: significance of the periportal collar on MRI. J Comput Assist Tomogr 1995;19:580

Mattei P, Wise B, Schwarz K, et al: Orthotopic liver transplantation in patients with biliary atresia and situs inversus. Pediatr Surg Int 1998;14:104

McDiarmid SV, Millis MJ, Olthoff KM, et al: Indications for pediatric liver transplantation. Pediatr Transplant 1998;2:106

Reyes JD, Carr B, Dvorchik I, et al: Liver transplantation and chemotherapy for hepatoblastoma and hepatocellular cancer in childhood and adolescence. J Pediatr 2000;136:795

Postoperative Complications

Bowen A, Hungate RG, Kaye RD, et al: Imaging in liver transplantation. Radiol Clin North Am 1996;34:757

Cao S, Cox KL, Berquist W, et al: Long-term outcomes in pediatric liver recipients: comparison between cyclosporin A and tacrolimus. Pediatr Transplant 1999;3:22

Dodd GD III, Memel DS, Zajko AB, et al: Hepatic artery stenosis and thrombosis in transplant recipients: Doppler diagnosis with resistive index and systolic acceleration time. Radiology 1994;192:657

Green M, Michaels MG: Infections in solid organ transplant recipients. *In* Long SS, Pickering LK, Prober CG (eds): Principles and Practice of Pediatric Infectious Diseases. New York, Churchill Livingstone, 1997:626–634

Green M, Michaels MG, Webber SA, et al: The management of Epstein-Barr virus associated post-transplant lymphoproliferative disorders in pediatric solid-organ transplant recipients. Pediatr Transplant 1999;3:271

Jovine E, Mazziotti A, Grazi GL, et al: Rupture of splenic artery aneurysm after liver transplantation. Clin Transplant 1996;10:451

Mazariegos GV, Molmenti EP, Kramer DJ: Early complications after orthotopic liver transplantation. Surg Clin North Am 1999;79:109

Millis MJ, Seaman DS, Piper JB, et al: Portal vein thombosis and stenosis in pediatric liver transplantation. Transplantation 1996; 62:748

Noble-Jamieson G, Barnes N: Diagnosis and management of late complications after liver transplantation. Arch Dis Child 1999; 81:446

Rollins NK, Timmons C, Superina RA, et al: Hepatic artery thrombosis in children with liver transplants: false-positive findings at Doppler sonography and arteriography in four patients. AJR Am J Roentgenol 1993;160:291

Part IV

SPLEEN AND PANCREAS

BRUCE R. PARKER

Chapter 1

THE SPLEEN

BRUCE R. PARKER

The spleen is more properly considered a lymphatic organ than an organ of digestion. In fact, the spleen is the largest of the body's lymphatic structures.

ANATOMY AND EMBRYOLOGY

Situated in the left upper quadrant, the spleen normally lies between the stomach and the diaphragm. It has two surfaces. The superolateral surface approximates the diaphragm, which separates it from the ninth, tenth, and eleventh ribs and the inferior left lung and pleura. The visceral surface has a renal portion in relation to the superior pole of the left kidney and to the left adrenal gland. The gastric portion is in contact with the posterior wall of the stomach and the tail of the pancreas. The splenic hilum is a depression along the medial surface through which pass the splenic artery and vein and the splenic nerves. The inferior pole of the spleen abuts the splenic flexure of the colon. The spleen is maintained in its normal position by two ligaments formed by peritoneal folds. The phrenicosplenic ligament contains the major splenic vessels. The gastrosplenic ligament runs between the spleen and stomach and contains the short gastric and gastroepiploic arteries. The splenic vein courses rightward from the portal vein. In the adult, the spleen is comparable in length to the kidney.

The spleen appears in the fifth week of embryonic life as a localized thickening of the mesoderm in the dorsal mesogastrium above the pancreatic tail. As the stomach rotates its greater curvature to the left, the spleen is carried with it into the left upper quadrant. The gastrosplenic ligament is derived from the residuum of the dorsal mesogastrium. The primary function of the embryonic spleen is erythropoiesis, which is maximal in the mid-second trimester and subsequently diminishes.

IMAGING THE SPLEEN

Plain radiographs may demonstrate the spleen in the left upper quadrant, displacing the stomach laterally and colon inferiorly. The spleen may be obscured when large amounts of gas are present in the gastrointestinal tract. Paterson et al. have described a pattern-oriented approach to splenic imaging in children, summarizing findings using advanced techniques.

The spleen is easily identified on abdominal ultrasound (US) scans. It has a homogeneous sonographic texture. The splenic hilar vessels are usually well seen, but intrasplenic vessels typically are not. Rosenberg et al. measured normal spleen length in children during quiet respiration. Using coronal scans, they measured the spleen and correlated the results with age, height, and weight. The upper limit of normal was 6.0 cm at 3 months, 6.5 cm at 6 months, 7.0 cm at 12 months, 8.0 cm at 2 years, 9.0 cm at 4 years, 9.5 cm at 6 years, 10.0 cm at 8 years, 11.0 cm at 10 years, and 11.5 cm at 12 years. The upper limit of normal at 15 years of age and older was 12.0 cm for girls and 13.0 cm for boys (Fig. 1). As a general rule, the tip of the spleen should not extend below the inferior pole of the left kidney (Fig. 2).

The normal spleen on computed tomography (CT) has a higher attenuation than the liver. Uniform increase in attenuation occurs following the administration of intravenous contrast agents. The splenic vein is well demonstrated on dynamic scans and can usually be followed across the abdomen to its juncture with the superior mesenteric vein, forming the portal vein (Fig. 3). The splenic artery can also be seen on dynamic scans. Because the artery is less tortuous in children than in adults, it frequently can be identified throughout much of its course. Computed tomographic angiography (CTA) demonstrates the splenic vessels remarkably well, but this technique is uncommonly employed in children.

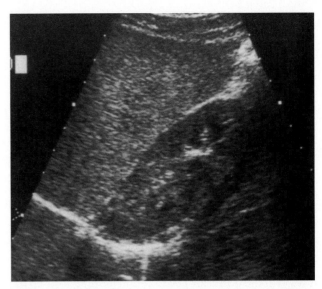

FIGURE 2. Splenomegaly in a 9-year-old boy with hereditary spherocytosis. The inferior tip of the spleen projects below the lower pole of the left kidney.

The spleen on T_1-weighted spin-echo magnetic resonance imaging (MRI) sections has lower signal intensity than does the liver and slightly greater signal intensity than muscle. On T_2-weighted images, the spleen has higher signal intensity than the liver. The major splenic vessels are well demonstrated because of the characteristic signal void of flowing blood. Magnetic resonance angiography (MRA) demonstrates the splenic vessels to excellent advantage.

Technetium-99m–labeled sulfur colloid is picked up by the spleen's reticuloendothelial system, permitting its visualization. Isotopic splenic scanning is useful for the identification of splenic ectopia, polysplenia, and asplenia, as well as numerous disease states as described below. Angiography is rarely used for intrasplenic disease, but arterial portography for the evaluation of the portal venous system offers excellent visualization of the spleen and its vessels. This technique has been largely superseded by CTA and MRA.

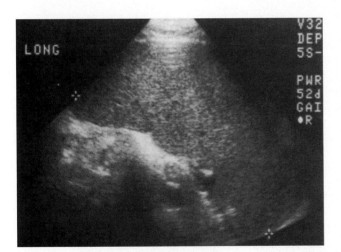

FIGURE 1. Splenomegaly in a 14-year-old boy with acute myelogenous leukemia. Longitudinal ultrasound scan demonstrates the splenic length to be 185 mm. Upper limit of normal at this age is 130 mm. (From Rosenberg HK, Markowitz RI, Kolbert H, et al: Normal splenic size in infants and children: sonographic measurement. AJR Am J Roentgenol 1994;157:119, with permission.)

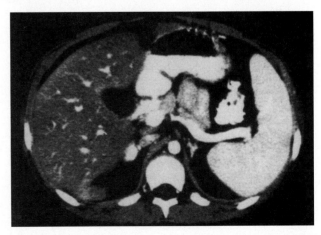

FIGURE 3. Normal spleen in an obese 11-year-old boy on computed tomography scan photographed at narrow window settings after intravenous contrast enhancement. There is uniform enhancement of the spleen and excellent visualization of the splenic vein.

CONGENITAL ANOMALIES

The most common congenital anomaly of the spleen is the presence of one or more *accessory spleens,* or spleniculi. These occur in 10% to 15% of the normal population and usually are found incidentally at autopsy or on imaging studies. They are six or less in number and most commonly are located in the splenic hilum, in association with the splenic vessels, or in the gastrosplenic ligament. They can be found, however, virtually anywhere in the abdomen. They rarely exceed 2 cm in diameter and are most frequently confused with splenic hilar or parapancreatic lymph nodes. They can be identified frequently on US or CT scans, but the definitive imaging study is ^{99m}Tc sulfur colloid liver–spleen scans.

Normally, the residuum of the dorsal mesogastrium fuses with the posterior peritoneum, helping to keep the spleen in its normal position. When this fusion does not take place, the dorsal mesogastrium may persist as a long mesentery, allowing the spleen to be displaced, the so-called *wandering spleen* (Fig. 4). The most common location for these ectopic spleens is the left lower quadrant. They may present as symptomatic masses and can be readily identified by US, CT, or sulfur colloid scan. Typically, no splenic tissue can be identified in the left upper quadrant, but a small accessory spleen may remain in the normal anatomic location. The wandering spleen may undergo torsion, causing severe pain secondary to ischemia. The twisted spleen has no uptake on radionuclide scan and no contrast enhancement on CT, and shows no flow on duplex Doppler sonography. A "whorled" appearance of the splenic artery in the splenic pedicle has been described as a characteristic CT sign of torsion. Several cases of gastric volvulus have been associated with wandering spleen.

The *splenogonadal syndrome* is a rare anomaly in which a portion of the splenic anlage fuses with primitive left gonadal tissue in the first trimester. A normal spleen develops in the left upper quadrant. When a persistent cord of splenic or fibrous tissue connects the spleen with

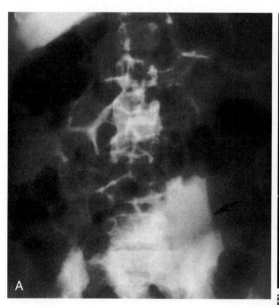

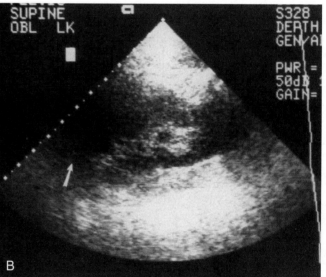

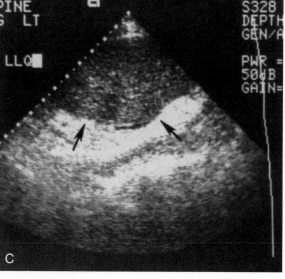

FIGURE 4. Wandering spleen in a 10-year-old girl with a left lower quadrant mass and abdominal pain. **A,** Abdominal radiograph demonstrates a left lower quadrant mass *(arrow)*. **B,** Ultrasound scan of the left upper quadrant demonstrates lack of splenic tissue *(arrow)* adjacent to the upper pole of the left kidney. **C,** Ultrasound scan of the mass in the left lower quadrant demonstrates echogenic splenic tissue *(arrows)*. Torsion of the spleen was found at surgery.

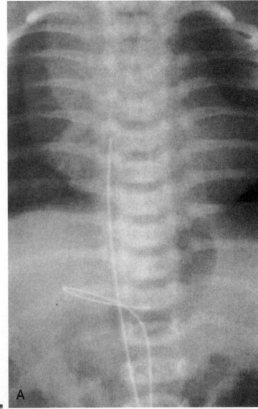

FIGURE 5. Asplenia syndrome in a newborn with double-outlet ventricle. **A,** Plain radiograph demonstrates symmetric main stem bronchi, midline liver, left-sided stomach, and a right-sided aorta containing an umbilical artery catheter. The umbilical venous catheter is coiled in the portal vein. **B,** Transverse ultrasound scan demonstrates the aorta *(A)* to be right-sided with the inferior vena cava (IVC) *(C)* to its right. *KID* = kidney. **C,** Transverse ultrasound scan at a more cephalad level demonstrates the midline liver and the IVC *(C)* crossing anterior to the aorta *(A).* No splenic tissue could be identified.

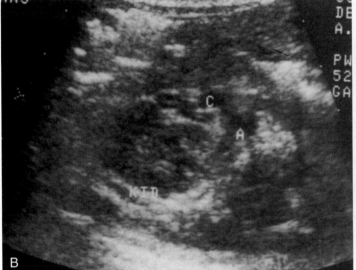

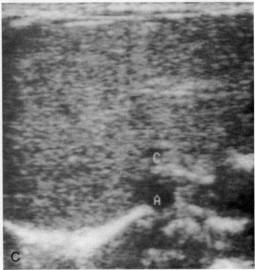

the left testis or epididymis, cryptorchidism usually results. Connection to the left ovary or mesovarium does not result in ovarian ectopia.

Abnormal visceroatrial situs is an intriguing set of entities in which the spleen plays a prominent role. The normal visceroatrial anatomy is known as situs solitus. Situs inversus refers to mirror-image visceroatrial anatomy. Patients with situs inversus are frequently asymptomatic, although there is a slightly higher incidence of congenital heart disease. Another group of patients with interesting combinations of congenital anomalies have situs ambiguous (visceral heterotaxia). This last population is divided into two major groups, one with asplenia

and one with polysplenia. Applegate et al. have recently reviewed the imaging findings in the heterotaxy syndromes and the significant correlation with congenital heart disease.

Patient with *asplenia* have right-sided isomerism (Fig. 5). The spleen is absent, the liver appears to have two mirror-image right lobes with a midline gallbladder, and two trilobed lungs with eparterial (right-sided) main stem bronchi are present in the thorax. Midgut malrotation is usually present, and the stomach may be either right or left sided. The inferior vena cava (IVC) and aorta may lie on the same side of the spine. The IVC then crosses the midline anterior to the aorta to enter the

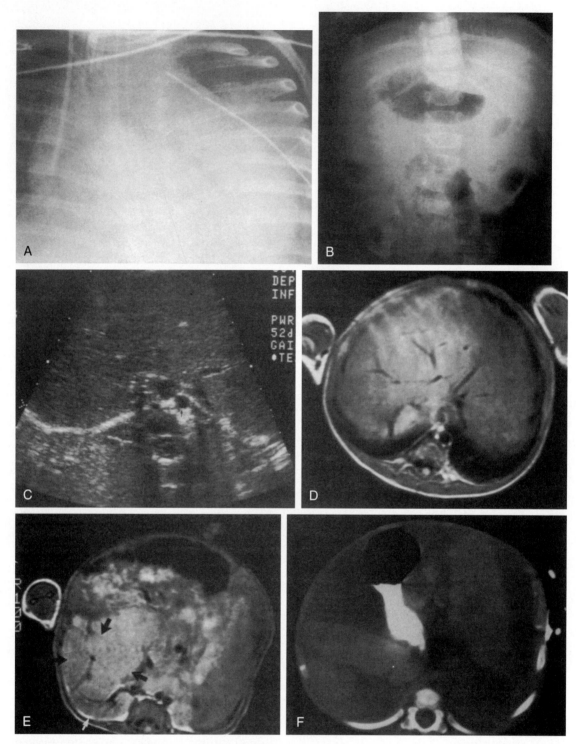

FIGURE 6. Polysplenia syndrome in a 3-month-old girl with biliary atresia and no evidence of heart disease. **A,** Chest radiograph performed following liver transplantation demonstrates the symmetric bronchi to good advantage because of the patient's postoperative pulmonary edema. **B,** Preoperative kidney, ureter, bladder film demonstrates a right-sided stomach and near-symmetric liver. **C,** Transverse ultrasound scan through the upper abdomen demonstrates a midline liver. The azygos vein *(arrow)* is enlarged because of azygos continuation of an interrupted inferior vena cava. **D,** Magnetic resonance imaging (MRI) section through the upper abdomen, performed to map out vascular anatomy, demonstrates the midline liver. The gallbladder was not identified. **E,** MRI section through the midabdomen demonstrates multiple splenules *(black arrows)* and the lower pole of the right kidney *(white arrow)*. **F,** Postoperative computed tomography scan after development of ascites demonstrates multiple splenules on the right and the transplanted liver on the left. Five splenules were identified at surgery.

atrium. Variable congenital cardiac lesions are present, the most common being a persistent atrioventricular canal. The portal vein may pass anterior to the pancreas and duodenum.

Patients with *polysplenia* have left-sided isomerism (Fig. 6). Multiple splenules are present. The liver is again midline, but the gallbladder may be hypoplastic or absent. Bilateral bilobed lungs with hyparterial (left-sided) bronchi are present, as is complex congenital heart disease, often with common atrium and anomalous pulmonary venous return below the diaphragm. Interruption of the IVC with azygos continuation is common. The aorta and IVC may be on the same side. Preduodenal portal vein is common, especially in those patients with biliary atresia. Midgut malrotation and variable stomach position may be seen. Commonly associated congenital anomalies include biliary atresia, duodenal atresia, anal atresia, and tracheoesophageal fistula. A short pancreas has been described secondary to failure of development of the dorsal pancreatic bud (see below). Rare anomalies include central nervous system malformations, palatal abnormalities, and a congenitally absent left adrenal gland.

Noninvasive imaging has been demonstrated to be useful in correctly identifying the major anomalies of asplenia and polysplenia syndromes. Combinations of US, CT, MRI, and radionuclide liver–spleen scans are sufficiently sensitive to demonstrate the above-described anomalies to preclude the need for angiography.

SPLENOMEGALY IN CONGENITAL DISORDERS

An enlarged spleen is a common concomitant of a variety of congenital diseases in childhood (Table 1). Patients with portal hypertension from a number of causes, including biliary atresia (see Section VI, Part III, Chapter 2, page 1450) have congestive splenomegaly. The hemolytic anemias frequently cause splenomegaly, with hereditary spherocytosis, hereditary elliptocytosis, and thalassemia being the most common. The imaging findings are nonspecific unless there is evidence of extramedullary hematopoiesis or infarcts, both of which

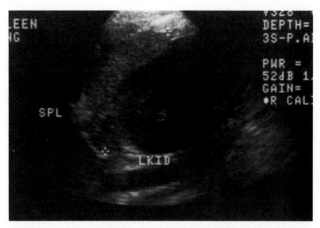

FIGURE 7. Splenic atrophy in an 8-year-old girl with sickle cell anemia. The spleen *(SPL)* measured 6 cm in length. *LKID* = left kidney.

are more common in affected adults than in children. The former causes focal areas of increased echogenicity in the spleen, while the latter present as focal areas of decreased echogenicity. Sickle cell anemia initially leads to splenomegaly followed by splenic atrophy secondary to multiple infarcts (Fig. 7). In some cases, iron deposition will result in increased attenuation of the spleen on CT examination and decreased signal intensity on MRI. The storage diseases generally cause nonspecific splenomegaly, but Gaucher's disease may lead to splenic abnormalities on US. Hill et al. described focal hypoechoic collections of Gaucher's cells as the most commonly seen pattern. The focal collections may occasionally be hyperechoic secondary to fibrosis.

ACQUIRED ABNORMALITIES

Splenomegaly can be found in a variety of acquired disorders, including infection and neoplasms, as discussed below. Acquired causes of portal hypertension, such a cavernous transformation of the portal vein and secondary cirrhosis of the liver in patients with cystic fibrosis, may present with splenomegaly, as may patients with extramedullary hematopoiesis (Fig. 8). Imaging studies of the spleen are nonspecific, but other findings, such as varices, may lead to the correct diagnosis.

INFECTIOUS DISEASES

Infectious disease involving the spleen is most commonly seen in immunocompromised patients. Serial CT scans have been shown to be of value in patients undergoing anticancer chemotherapy. Microabscesses are most commonly seen, especially with fungal infection such as candidiasis (Fig. 9). If large enough, the microabscesses may be seen on sonograms, but CT may be necessary when the lesions are very small. Larger, solitary abscesses may also occur with candidiasis. They may be seen as hypoechoic areas on US and as low-attenuation areas on CT. In rare circumstances,

Table 1 ■ DIFFERENTIAL DIAGNOSIS OF SPLENOMEGALY
Portal hypertension
Extramedullary hematopoiesis
Hemolytic anemias
Cysts
Congenital
Acquired (usually infectious)
Benign neoplasms
Hemangiomas
Lymphangiomas
Hamartomas
Malignant neoplasms
Leukemia
Lymphoma
Metastases

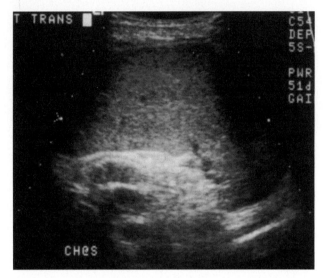

FIGURE 8. Splenomegaly in a 9-year-old girl with cavernous transformation of the portal vein. Compared with Figures 1 and 2, the spleen has a heterogeneous echo pattern with enlarged intrasplenic vessels secondary to portal hypertension.

calcification may be seen on unenhanced CT examination. In cat-scratch fever, US shows multiple small, poorly defined nodules that coalesce into an abscess with mixed echogenicity, finally resolving into a calcified granuloma. Viral infections, including infectious mononucleosis, are more likely to cause nonspecific splenomegaly because of the diffuse infiltrative nature of the disease process or because of reactive hyperplasia of the spleen's reticuloendothelial tissue. Von Sinner and Stridbeck have described the imaging findings in splenic hydatid disease. Plain films may show calcifi-

cation of the cyst wall. The cysts are generally anechoic, although one echogenic lesion was identified by Franquet et al. CT shows a focal lesion of lower attenuation than the surrounding splenic tissue that does not enhance after contrast administration. Tuberculosis, histoplasmosis, and coccidioidomycosis may produce multiple splenic granulomas, almost always associated with diffuse organ involvement secondary to hematogenous spread. Splenic granulomas may be found in patients with chronic granulomatous disease of childhood, appearing as calcifications on plain film and ill-defined hypoechogenic nodules on US (Fig. 10).

BENIGN NEOPLASMS

Benign neoplasms of the spleen are most commonly cystic in nature. Primary splenic cysts may be of epithelial lines, such as epidermoid, dermoid, or transitional cell cysts; or of endothelial lines, such as lymphangiomas and hemangiomas. Ramani et al. have described the imaging findings in splenic hemangiomas and hamartomas. Splenic lymphangiomatosis is usually associated with lymphangiomas found elsewhere. Acquired cysts may be infectious, usually caused by *Echinococcus*, or post-traumatic. Epidermoid cysts are the most common noninfectious focal space-occupying lesions of the spleen (Fig. 11). They are frequently large enough to appear on plain films as a left upper quadrant mass displacing the stomach and colon. A rim of calcification may be seen. On US scans, the cysts are characteristically anechoic and sharply demarcated from the surrounding normal splenic tissue. Internal fat droplets may cause the cyst to be hypoechoic rather than anechoic (Fig.

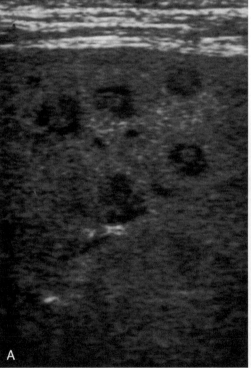

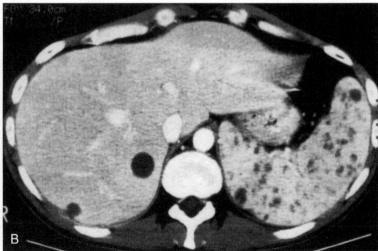

FIGURE 9. Splenic candidiasis in a teen-aged boy following bone marrow transplantation. **A,** Transverse ultrasound scan of the enlarged spleen demonstrates the characteristic "target lesions" of *Candida* microabscesses. **B,** Computed tomography scan demonstrates numerous microabscesses in the spleen as well as larger abscesses in both spleen and liver.

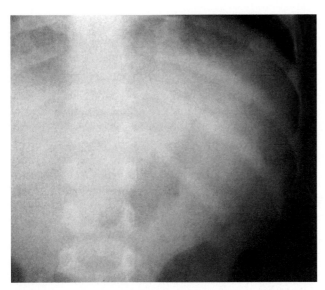

FIGURE 10. Splenic calcifications in an 18-month-old boy with chronic granulomatous disease of childhood.

11*D*). Liver–spleen scintigraphy demonstrates a focal photopenic defect. Familial occurrence of an epidermoid cyst has been reported. Lymphangiomas are rare in children. They may cause multiple splenic cystic lesions. On US, they are most commonly septated and anechoic but may occasionally be hypoechoic because of floating debris. Acquired non-neoplastic cysts may occur after trauma or intrasplenic hemorrhage.

The most common solid benign tumor of the spleen in children is *hamartoma*. Hamartomas are most commonly echogenic, although cystic hamartomas have been reported. They may have a radiopharmaceutical uptake at scintigraphic examination greater than that in the surrounding normal spleen. *Splenic hemangiomas* are usually small and associated with hemangiomas elsewhere. They may occasionally be large and associated with hypersplenism, thrombocytopenia, and consumption coagulopathy—the Kasabach-Merritt syndrome. The lesions are predominantly echogenic but may contain cystic spaces that suggest the correct diagnosis.

MALIGNANT NEOPLASMS

Malignant neoplasms of the spleen are usually metastatic or related to multifocal neoplastic disorders such as leukemia and lymphoma. Acute *lymphocytic leukemia* is the most common neoplastic disease in children, and patients usually have splenomegaly secondary to diffuse infiltration of the spleen. The other childhood leukemias also result in splenomegaly (see Fig. 1). Chronic myelogenous leukemia is rare in children but is frequently accompanied by massive splenomegaly. Imaging

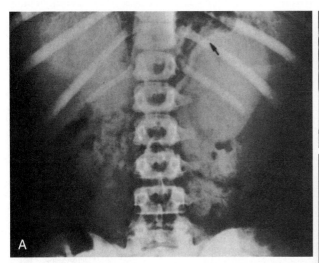

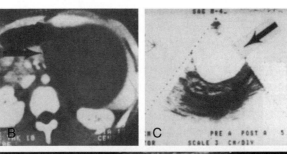

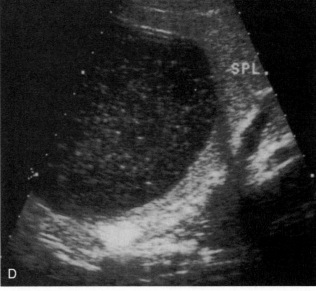

FIGURE 11. Epidermoid cyst of the spleen in an asymptomatic 12-year-old girl. **A,** Plain radiograph shows a left upper quadrant mass displacing the stomach *(arrow)*. **B,** Computed tomography scan shows the mass to be homogeneous, with attenuation values equal to water. **C,** Transverse ultrasound scan demonstrates the mass to be anechoic *(arrow)*. (**C** courtesy of Dr. E. Afshani, Buffalo, NY.) **D,** Ultrasound scan in another patient demonstrates echogenic lipid droplets within an epidermoid cyst. *SPL* = spleen.

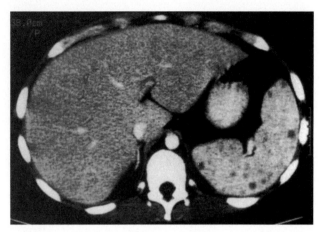

FIGURE 12. Splenic Hodgkin's disease in a 14-year-old boy. Computed tomography scan performed as part of staging evaluation demonstrates numerous low-attenuation lesions throughout the spleen. Splenic body revealed typical lesions of Hodgkin's disease.

studies of the spleen are rarely performed in children with leukemia because the diagnosis is made by other means, and the results of splenic imaging have no impact on the staging or prognosis. US scans demonstrate an enlarged spleen with heterogeneous echogenicity. Non-Hodgkin's lymphoma often has a similar appearance but may also have focal lesions large enough to be seen on US scans as ill-defined hypoechogenic areas, especially in patient with high-grade malignancy at histologic examination. On CT, they are low-attenuation lesions that do not show enhancement appreciably with intravenous contrast administration. Hodgkin's disease may also cause diffuse splenic infiltration that may not be detectable on imaging studies, but is more likely than non-Hodgkin's lymphoma to result in focal splenic masses (Fig. 12). Because splenic involvement may be the only subdiaphragmatic site, its detection is important for staging and prognosis. False-negative US, CT, and MRI examinations are common because the imaging tissue characteristics of the Hodgkin's disease lesions are similar to those of normal spleen when the organ is diffusely infiltrated with disease that is only microscopically detectable. Focal lesions may appear on US and CT scans that are similar to those of non-Hodgkin's lymphoma as described above.

Splenic metastases from solid tumors are less common with childhood tumors than they are with those in adults. They may be single or multiple and frequently do not cause splenomegaly. US may show hypoechogenicity, hyperechogenicity, or a mixed pattern. Target lesions have been described in adults.

SUGGESTED READINGS

Imaging the Spleen

Adler DD, Glazer GM, Aisen AM: MRI of the spleen: normal appearance and finding in sickle-cell anemia. AJR Am J Roentgenol Am J Roentgenol 1986;147:843

Dittrich M, Milde S, Dinkel E, et al: Sonographic biometry of liver and spleen size in childhood. Pediatr Radiol 1983;13:206

Koga T, Morikawa Y: Ultrasonographic determination of the splenic size and its clinical usefulness in various liver diseases. Radiology 1975;115:157

Markisz JA, Treves ST, Davis RT: Normal hepatic and splenic size in children: scintigraphic determination. Pediatr Radiol 1987;17:273

Mirowitz SA, Brown JJ, Lee JKT, et al: Dynamic gadolinium-enhanced MR imaging of the spleen: normal enhancement patterns and evaluation of splenic lesions. Radiology 1991;179:681

Paterson A, Frush DP, Donnelly LF, et al: A pattern-oriented approach to splenic imaging in infants and children. Radiographics 1999;19: 1465

Rosenberg HK, Markowitz RI, Kolbert H, et al: Normal splenic size in infants and children: sonographic measurement. AJR Am J Roentgenol 1994;157:119

Vick CS, Hartenberg MA, Allen HA, et al: Abdominal pseudotumor caused by gastric displacement of the spleen: sonographic demonstration. Pediatr Radiol 1985;15:253

Congenital Anomalies

Abramson SJ, Berdon WE, Altman RP, et al: Biliary atresia and noncardiac polysplenic syndrome: US and surgical considerations. Radiology 1987;163:377

Applegate KE, Goske MJ, Pierce G, Murphy D: Situs revisited: imaging of the heterotaxy syndrome. Radiographics 1999;19:837

Bollinger B, Lorentzen T: Torsion of a wandering spleen: ultrasonographic findings. J Clin Ultrasound 1990;18:510

Dodds WJ, Taylor AJ, Erickson SJ, et al: Radiologic imaging of splenic anomalies. AJR Am J Roentgenol 1990;155:805

Fujiwara T, Takehara Y, Isoda H, et al: Torsion of the wandering spleen: CT and angiographic appearance. J Comput Assist Tomogr 1995; 19:84

Groshar D, Israel A, Barzilai A, et al: The value of scintigraphy in evaluation of a wandering spleen. Clin Nucl Med 1986;11:42

Hadar H, Gadoth N, Herskovitz P, et al: Short pancreas in polysplenia syndrome. Acta Radiol 1991;32:299

Herman TE, Siegel MJ: CT of acute spleen torsion in children with wandering spleen. AJR Am J Roentgenol 1991;156:151

Herman TC, Siegel MJ: Polysplenia syndrome with congenital short pancreas. AJR Am J Roentgenol 1991;156:799

Hernanz-Schulman M, Ambrosino MM, Genieser NG, et al: Current evaluation of the patient with abnormal visceroatrial situs. AJR Am J Roentgenol 1990;154:797

Hill SC, Reinig JW, Barranger JA, et al: Gaucher disease: sonographic appearance of the spleen. Radiology 1986;160:631

Mandell GA, Heyman S, Alavi A, et al: A case of microgastria in association with splenic-gonadal fusion. Pediatr Radiol 1983; 13:95

McLean GK, Alavi A, Ziegler MM, et al: Splenic-gonadal fusion: identification by radionuclide scanning. J Pediatr Surg 1981;16(4 Suppl 1):649

Nemcek AA, Miller FH, Fitzgerald SW: Acute torsion of a wandering spleen: diagnosis by CT and duplex Doppler and color flow sonography. AJR Am J Roentgenol 1991;157:307

Phillips GWL, Hemingway AP: Wandering spleen. Br J Radiol 1987; 60:188

Setiawan H, Harrell RS, Perret RS: Ectopic spleen: a sonographic diagnosis. Pediatr Radiol 1982;12:152

Shiels WE II, Johnson JF, Stephenson SR, et al: Chronic torsion of the wandering spleen. Pediatr Radiol 1989;19:465

Spector JM, Chappell J: Gastric volvulus associated with wandering spleen in a child. J Pediatr Surg 2000;35:641

Subraanyam BR, Balthazar EJ, Horii SC: Sonography of the accessory spleen. AJR Am J Roentgenol 1984;143:47

Swischuk LE, Williams JB, John SD: Torsion of wandering spleen: the whorled appearance of the splenic pedicle on CT. Pediatr Radiol 1993;23:476

Tonkin ILD, Tonkin AK: Visceroatrial situs abnormalities: sonographic and computed tomographic appearance. AJR Am J Roentgenol 1984;138:509

Walther MM, Trulock TC, Finnerty DP, et al: Splenic gonadal fusion. Urology 1988;32:521

Winer-Muram HT, Tonkin IL: The spectrum of heterotaxic syndromes. Radiol Clin North Am 1989;27:1147

Acquired Abnormalities

Balthazar EJ, Hilton S, Naidich D, et al: CT of splenic and perisplenic abnormalities in septic patients. AJR Am J Roentgenol 1985;144:53

Bartley DL, Hughes WT, Parvey LS, et al: Computed tomography of hepatic and splenic fungal abscesses in leukemic children. Pediatr Infect Dis 1982;1:317

Bradley MJ, Metreweli C: Ultrasound appearances of extramedullary hematopoiesis in the liver and spleen. Br J Radiol 1990;63:816

Cornaglia-Ferraris P, Perlino GF, Barabino A, et al: Cystic lymphangioma of the spleen: report of CT scan findings. Pediatr Radiol 1982;12:94

Cox F, Perlman S, Sathyanarayana: Splenic abscesses in cat scratch disease: sonographic diagnosis and follow-up. J Clin Ultrasound 1989;17:511

Dachman AH, Ros PR, Murari JP, et al: Nonparasitic splenic cysts: a report of 52 cases with radiologic-pathologic correlation. AJR Am J Roentgenol 1986;147:37

Daneman A, Martin DJ: Congenital epithelial splenic cysts in children: emphasis on sonographic appearances and some unusual features. Pediagtr Radiol 1986;12:119

Duddy MJ, Calder CJ: Cystic hemangioma of the spleen: findings on ultrasound and computed tomography. Br J Radiol 1989;62:180

Ferrozzi F, Bova D, Campodonico F, et al: Cystic fibrosis: MR assessment of pancreatic damage. Radiology 1996;198:875

Flynn PM, Shenep JL, Crawford R, et al: Use of abdominal computed tomography for identifying disseminated fungal infection in pediatric cancer patients. Clin Infect Dis 1995;4:964

Franquet T, Montes M, Lecumberri FJ: Hydatid disease of the spleen: imaging findings in nine patients. AJR Am J Roentgenol 1990;154:525

Fulcher AS, Turner MA, Yelon JA, et al: Magnetic resonance cholaniopancreatography (MRCP) in the assessment of pancreatic duct trauma and its sequelae: preliminary findings. J Trauma 2000;48:1001

Goerg C, Schwerk WB, Goerg K: Sonography of focal lesions of the spleen. AJR Am J Roentgenol 1991;156:949

Goerg C, Schwerk WB, Goerg K, et al: Sonographic patterns of the affected spleen in malignant lymphoma. J Clin Ultrasound 1990;18:569

Gore RM, Shkolnik A: Abdominal manifestations of pediatric leukemias: sonographic assessment. Radiology 1982;143:207

Hahn PF, Weissleder R, Stark DD, et al: MR imaging of focal splenic tumors. AJR Am J Roentgenol 1988;150:823

Harris RD, Simpson W: MRI of splenic hemangioma associated with thrombocytopenia. Gastrointest Radiol 1989;14:308

Johnson MA, Cooperberg PL, Boisvert J, et al: Spontaneous splenic rupture in infectious mononucleosis: sonographic diagnosis and follow-up. AJR Am J Roentgenol 1981;136:111

Keidl CM, Chusid MJ: Splenic abscesses in childhood. Pediatr Infect Dis J 1989;8:368

King DJ, Dawson AA, Bayliss AP: The value of ultrasonic scanning of the spleen in lymphoma. Clin Radiol 1985;36:473

Kuykendall JD, Shanser JD, Sumner TE, et al: Multimodal approach to diagnosis of hamartoma of the spleen. Pediatr Radiol 1977;5:239

Magid D, Fishman EK, Siegelman SS: Computed tomography of the spleen and liver in sickle cell disease. AJR Am J Roentgenol 1984;143:245

Miller JH, Greenfield LD, Wald BR: Candidiasis of the liver and spleen in childhood. Radiology 1982;142:375

Okada J, Yoshikawa K, Uno K, et al: Increased activity on radiocolloid scintigraphy in splenic hamartoma. Clin Nucl Med 1990;15:112

Orduna M, Gonzalez de Orbe G, Gordillo MI, et al: Chronic granulomatous disease of childhood: report of two cases with unusual involvement of the gastric antrum and spleen. Eur J Radiol 1989;9:67

Pastakia B, Shawker TH, Thaler M, et al: Hepatosplenic candidiasis: wheels within wheels. Radiology 1988;166:417

Pawar S, Kay CJ, Gonzalez R, et al: Sonography of splenic abscess. AJR Am J Roentgenol 1982;138:259

Ramani M, Reinhold C, Semelka RC, et al: Splenitc hemangiomas and hamartomas: MR imaging characteristics of 28 lesions. Radiology 1997;202:166

Rao BK, AuBuchon J, Lieberman LM, et al: Cystic lymphangioma of the spleen: a radiologic-pathologic correlation. Radiology 1981;141:781

Rose SC, Kumpe DA, Manco-Johnson ML: Radiographic appearance of diffuse splenic hemangiomatosis. Gastrointest Radiol 1986;11:342

Siniluto T, Paivansalo M, Lahde S: Ultrasonography of splenic metastases. Acta Radiol 1989;30:463

Strijk SP, Wagener DJ, Bogman MJ, et al: The spleen in Hodgkin disease: diagnostic value of CT. Radiology 1985;154:753

Von Sinner WN, Stridbeck H: Hydatid disease of the spleen: ultrasonography, CT and MR imaging. Acta Radiol 1992;33:459

Wadsworth DT, Newman B, Abramson SJ, et al: Splenic lymphangiomatosis in children. Radiology 1997;202:173

Younger KA, Hall CM: Epidermoid cyst of the spleen: a case report and review of the literature. Br J Radiol 1990;63:652

Chapter 2

THE PANCREAS

BRUCE R. PARKER

The pancreas contains both exocrine and endocrine glandular tissue. The exocrine functions are directed toward digestion, with secretions exiting through the pancreatic duct into the duodenum. The islets of Langerhans are the endocrine tissue containing several types of hormone-producing cells.

ANATOMY AND EMBRYOLOGY

The pancreas lies transversely in the midabdomen. It is divided into head, body, and tail (Fig. 1). The head is in the right midabdomen, situated in the curve of the duodenum. At the junction of the inferior and left borders of the pancreatic head is a prolongation called the uncinate process. The anterior surface of the head is in contact with the transverse colon, the gastroduodenal artery, and several loops of small intestine. The anterior surface of the uncinate process is in contact with the superior mesenteric artery and vein. The posterior surface of the head is adjacent to the inferior vena cava, the common bile duct, the renal veins, and the aorta.

The body of the pancreas is in contact with the stomach anterosuperiorly. Its posterior portion abuts the aorta, splenic vein, left kidney, and adrenal gland and the origin of the superior mesenteric artery. The small intestine lies inferior to the body. The tail is narrower in adults than the head or body and lies in the phrenicolienal ligament in contact with the gastric surface of the spleen and the splenic flexure of the colon.

The pancreas arises from two anlagen. The dorsal part develops from a diverticulum to the dorsal aspect of the duodenum caudal to the hepatic diverticulum. It grows upward and backward into the dorsal mesogas-trium, forming part of the head and the entire body and tail. The ventral pancreatic bud is a diverticulum from the primitive bile duct and forms part of the head and the uncinate process. The two portions fuse at about the sixth week of embryonic life. The duct from the dorsal bud becomes the accessory pancreatic duct while that from the ventral bud enlarges to become the main duct after it fuses with the distal two thirds of the dorsal duct. The opening of the accessory duct is often obliterated.

IMAGING THE PANCREAS

The pancreas itself is not seen on plain radiographs. Calcifications present in patients with chronic pancreatitis or cystic fibrosis may be identified on plain films of the abdomen (Fig. 2). A pancreatic mass may be sufficiently large to displace adjacent gas-filled portions of the gastrointestinal tract.

Ultrasound (US) usually provides good visualization of the pancreas in children because the relatively large left lobe of the liver can be used as an acoustic window. The

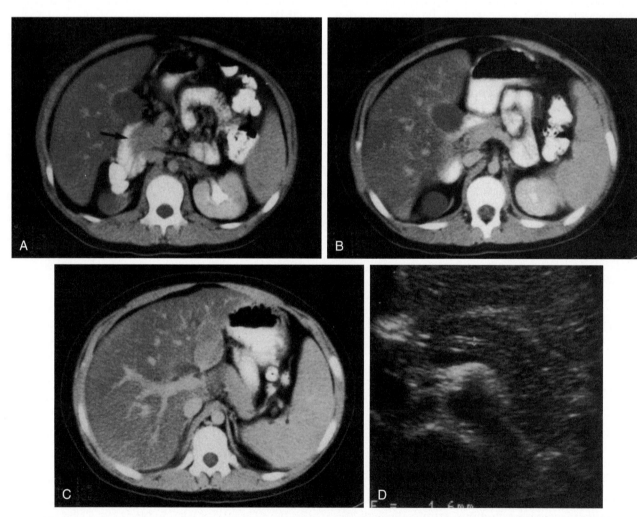

FIGURE 1. Normal pancreas in an 11-year-old boy. **A–C,** Computed tomography scan sections of the pancreas. **A,** The head of the pancreas *(arrow)* is slightly bulbous and is in contact with the contrast-filled duodenal sweep. **B,** The body of the pancreas is narrower than the head or tail and is seen anterior to the aorta, from which the superior mesenteric artery is arising. **C,** The tail of the pancreas is thicker in children than in adults and extends to the spleen. **D,** Transverse ultrasound scan demonstrates the double track of a normal pancreatic duct.

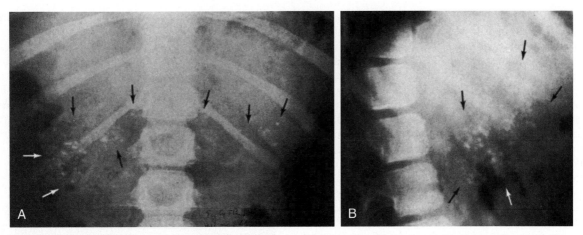

FIGURE 2. Cystic fibrosis in a 9-year-old girl with multiple pancreatic calcifications *(arrows)*, seen radiographically in anteroposterior **(A)** and lateral **(B)** projections.

pancreas is most easily seen if the stomach and duodenum are not dilated with gas. Several hours of fasting or decompression by nasogastric tube give optimal results. The body of the pancreas can be located anterior to the splenic vein. The tail is relatively larger in children than in adults and usually larger than the body. Siegel et al. have developed normal measurements of the pancreas according to age (Table 1). Pancreatic size has been found to correlate best with body height, but there is sufficient individual variation that caution must be used in determining pancreaticomegaly. Teele and Share concluded that enlargement of the pancreas should be diagnosed when the anteroposterior dimension of the body is greater than 1.5 cm. The normal duct may be seen as a single- or double-track echogenic line anterior to the junction of the splenic and mesenteric veins (see Fig. 1*D*). There is a spectrum of pancreatic echogenicity relative to that of the liver, but in most children the pancreas is nearly isoechogenic with the liver. Normally increased pancreatic echogenicity has been reported in neonates, especially prematures.

Computed tomography (CT) of the pancreas is much less frequently indicated than US but has value in certain diseases, especially tumors and pseudocysts with uncommon features. The pancreas is best visualized on CT during bolus injection of intravenous contrast material, which readily identifies the adjacent vessels, and with good gastrointestinal contrast to opacify the adjacent stomach and duodenum. The pancreas has lower atten-

uation than the liver both with and without intravenous contrast use. Because the pancreas in children is oblique to axial planes, multiple thin sections may be necessary for optimal visualization on CT.

Magnetic resonance imaging (MRI) of the pancreas in children is more difficult than in adults because of adjacent gas-filled loops of intestine and motion artifact from peristalsis and respiration. The pancreas normally has signal intensity equal to that of liver on T_1- and T_2-weighted spin-echo images with mid–field strength magnets. Pancreatic images produced with high field strength magnets may have greater signal intensity than liver. To some degree, the signal will vary with age. Although normal children do not have as much intrapancreatic fat as adults, there is more fat in the pancreatic septa of postadolescent children than is found in preadolescents. The value of MRI of the pancreas is enhanced by the use of breath-holding techniques (generally not possible in younger children), fat suppression sequences, and contrast enhancement. Relatively few studies of these techniques are available in children, however.

Endoscopic retrograde cholangiopancreatography (ERCP) is useful in directly identifying the pancreatic duct. It is much less commonly performed in children than in adults. When ERCP is performed for evaluation of the common bile duct, a more common indication in children than pancreatic disease, the pancreatic duct is also visualized, and related or incidental abnormalities can be identified.

Magnetic resonance cholangiopancreatography (MRCP) may prove more useful than ERCP in children because of its noninvasive nature. Arcement et al. have described the use of MRCP in the evaluation of ductal disease. The procedure is also useful in certain congenital abnormalities such as pancreas divisum and after pancreatic trauma.

DEVELOPMENTAL AND HEREDITARY ABNORMALITIES

Pancreas divisum occurs when the dorsal and ventral ducts fail to fuse, although the pancreas is otherwise

---

Table 1 ■ NORMAL SONOGRAPHIC DIMENSIONS OF THE PANCREAS IN CHILDHOOD

AGE	HEAD*	BODY*	TAIL*
<1 mo	1.0 ± 0.4	0.6 ± 0.2	1.0 ± 0.4
1 mo–1 yr	1.5 ± 0.5	0.8 ± 0.3	1.2 ± 0.4
1–5 yr	1.7 ± 0.3	1.0 ± 0.2	1.8 ± 0.4
5–10 yr	1.6 ± 0.4	1.0 ± 0.3	1.8 ± 0.4
10–19 yr	2.0 ± 0.5	1.1 ± 0.3	2.0 ± 0.4

*Maximum anteroposterior dimension (cm) ± SD.
Modified from Siegel MJ, Martin KW, Worthington JL: Normal and abnormal pancreas in children: US studies. Radiology 1987;165:15.

anatomically normal. This anomaly has been described in 6% to 10% of adults undergoing ERCP; its true incidence is probably at the high end of this range. There may be a higher incidence of pancreatitis in patients with pancreas divisum, although the most recent literature refutes this claim. Reports of CT examination in adults with pancreas divisum and pancreatitis demonstrate enlargement of both ducts in addition to the characteristic findings of pancreatitis (see below). Further enlargement of the duct can be provoked with pre-CT secretin stimulation, a technique that has been used in association with MRCP. Increased thickness of the pancreatic head has been described. Zeman et al. reported that thin-section CT demonstrated the unfused ducts in 5 of 12 patients, while two distinct pancreatic moieties separated by a fat cleft could be seen in 4 patients.

Congenital short pancreas occurs when the portion of the pancreas derived from the dorsal embryonic bud is absent and only that smaller portion derived from the ventral anlage is present. The anomaly has been described in patients with the polysplenia syndrome. Only a globular pancreatic head can be identified on CT.

Ectopic pancreatic tissue is found most commonly in the stomach, duodenum, and appendix and in Meckel's diverticulum. A noncommunicating gastric duplication cyst has been described that contained ectopic pancreatic ducts and islets without acini.

Annular pancreas in children is most frequently diagnosed at birth because of associated duodenal obstruction (see Section II, Part IV, Chapter 4, page 113). However, in 50% of cases, the diagnosis is made beyond infancy. Several theories of embryonic dysgenesis have been put forth. Most suggest some form of rotational anomaly of the ventral bud, which may be bifid. The pancreatic annulus, the portion surrounding the duodenum, frequently has a separate duct entering the duodenum opposite the ampulla of Vater. Duodenal contents may reflux through this duct into the annulus. Forty percent of affected patients have associated duodenal stenosis or atresia; this is the group presenting in infancy. Many other associated abnormalities have been described, the most common being intestinal malrotation, tracheoesophageal fistulas, cardiac abnormalities, and anal atresia. These associated lesions are most common in patients who also have trisomy 21. Annular pancreas has also been described in de Lange's syndrome, with partial situs inversus, and as a cause of extrahepatic biliary obstruction. Pancreatitis affecting solely the annulus has been reported in adults.

Cystic fibrosis causes exocrine pancreatic insufficiency in 80% of affected patients. As is the case with biliary ductules, the pancreatic ductules contain goblet cells that produce thickened mucus leading to obstruction. In young patients with CF, US shows pancreatic enlargement, but chronic obstruction ultimately results in shrinkage of the gland with increased echogenicity secondary to fatty infiltration and fibrosis (Fig. 3). CT shows a shrunken pancreas with reduced attenuation secondary to fatty infiltration. Fibrosis without fatty infiltration is found infrequently. Unenhanced scans may show pancreatic calcifications. Ductal dilatation

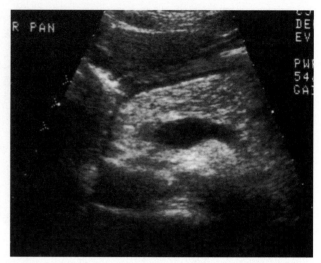

FIGURE 3. Markedly echogenic pancreas on ultrasound in an 18-year-old woman with fatty infiltration of the pancreas secondary to cystic fibrosis.

may be present, and pancreatic cysts may be identified (Fig. 4). In the MRI study by Tham et al., 9 of 17 patients had an enlarged, lobulated pancreas with fatty infiltration, 5 had an atrophic pancreas with fatty infiltration, 1 had atrophy without fatty replacement, and 2 were normal. In a series of 18 patients who underwent MRI, Murayama et al. found 12 with high signal intensity on T_1-weighted spin-echo images indicative of fatty replacement, 3 with low signal intensity, and 3 normals. Their results corresponded well with the clinical stage. Ferrozzi et al., have described several patterns on MRI of pancreatic changes of CF.

Shwachman syndrome is an autosomal recessive disorder resulting in short stature, exocrine pancreatic insufficiency, a metaphyseal chondrodysplasia (see Section IX, Part V, page 2122), and bone marrow dysfunction. Sonographic and CT evaluation of the pancreas demonstrate the same changes described above in patients with CF.

Von Hippel-Lindau disease is an autosomal dominant disorder characterized by hemangioblastomas of multiple organs, especially the retina and central nervous system, skin lesions, and cysts of numerous organs, including the pancreas. The pancreatic lesions are usually multiple (Fig. 5). Mucinous cystadenomas of the pancreas have also been reported. The cysts are typically anechoic on US and have reduced attenuation on CT compared with the surrounding pancreatic tissue. Pancreatic calcifications can be seen on unenhanced CT scans. Adenocarcinoma occurs in affected adults. *Hereditary pancreatitis* is an autosomal dominant disease in which patients have recurrent episodes of pancreatitis. The findings are described below. *Beckwith-Wiedemann syndrome* is probably an autosomal dominant disorder and is characterized by visceromegaly hemihypertrophy, and the development of malignant tumors in 10% to 15% of affected patients. Cross-sectional imaging studies may show nonspecific pancreatic enlargement. Patients may develop pancreatoblastoma or nesidioblastoma as discussed below under Pancreatic Neoplasms. *Congenital cysts* of the pancreas are rare and often

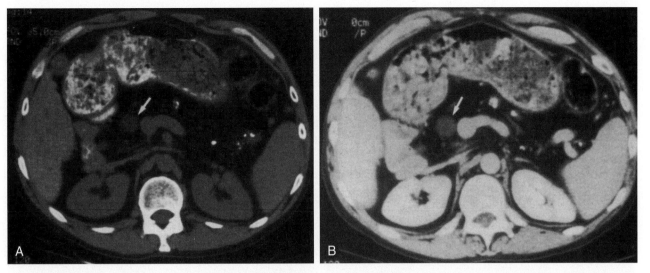

FIGURE 4. Cystic fibrosis in a 19-year-old man with marked atrophy and fatty replacement of the pancreas. A large cyst *(arrow)* is present in the pancreatic head as seen on unenhanced **(A)** and enhanced **(B)** computed tomography scans. Extensive mesenteric fat is seen secondary to steroid therapy in this patient who had a heart–lung transplant 6 months before this examination.

confused with omental or mesenteric cysts when large (Fig. 6).

ACUTE PANCREATITIS

Acute pancreatitis is uncommon in childhood, possibly because the most frequent seen predisposing factors in adults, alcoholism and cholelithiasis, are rarely found in children. Weizman and Durie reported their experience in 61 children with acute pancreatitis. The most common etiology was multisystem disease, including Reye's syndrome, sepsis, shock, hemolytic uremic syndrome, and viral infections. Mumps has been specifically implicated as an etiologic viral agent. Other causes included blunt trauma in 15%, congenital anatomic abnormali-

ties in 10%, metabolic diseases in 10%, and drug toxicity in 3% of patients. No cause was identified in 25% of patients. MRCP has been found to be useful in identifying unsuspected abnormal ductal anatomy in patients with idiopathic pancreatitis.

Anatomic abnormalities associated with pancreatitis include pancreas divisum (see above) and choledochal cyst. The latter may cause pancreatitis because of the abnormal insertion of the common bile duct into the pancreatic duct (see Section VI, Part III, Chapter 2, page 1450), which may permit reflux of bile into the pancreas. Associated metabolic disorders include hypercalcemia, hyperlipidemia, and CF, while drugs implicated most frequently in the etiology are L-asparaginase, steroids, and acetaminophen. Lee et al. reported an increased incidence of biliary sludge in their adult patients with pancreatitis. They implicated the sludge as a

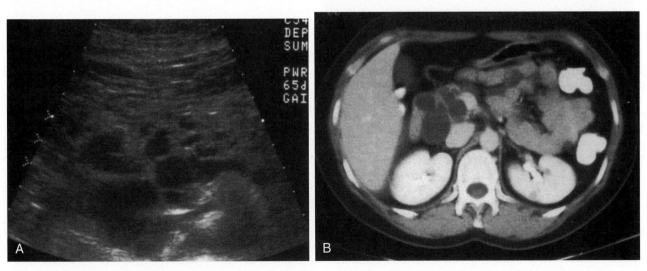

FIGURE 5. Von Hippel-Lindau syndrome in a young woman caused multiple pancreatic cysts well demonstrated on ultrasound **(A)** and computed tomography **(B)**.

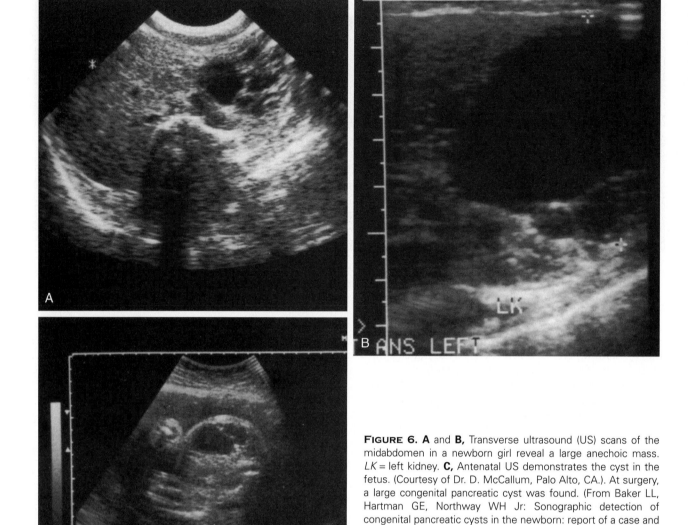

FIGURE 6. A and **B,** Transverse ultrasound (US) scans of the midabdomen in a newborn girl reveal a large anechoic mass. *LK* = left kidney. **C,** Antenatal US demonstrates the cyst in the fetus. (Courtesy of Dr. D. McCallum, Palo Alto, CA.). At surgery, a large congenital pancreatic cyst was found. (From Baker LL, Hartman GE, Northway WH Jr: Sonographic detection of congenital pancreatic cysts in the newborn: report of a case and review of the literature. Pediatr Radiol 1990;20:488, with permission.)

probable cause of idiopathic acute pancreatitis in as many as 70% of affected patients.

Patients with nontraumatic acute pancreatitis typically present with abdominal pain, most frequently in the epigastrium. Nausea and vomiting are frequent companion symptoms. Elevation of serum concentrations of pancreatic enzymes (amylase, lipase, trypsinogen) is common, but not invariable, so imaging studies may be useful in confirming the diagnosis.

Plain radiographic findings are nonspecific, but certain findings are suggestive. Reactive ileus of nearby gastrointestinal structures may lead to air–fluid levels in the stomach and duodenum, focal dilatation of the duodenal sweep, and dilatation of the transverse colon ending abruptly at the splenic flexure. Left pleural effusion may occur. Although ascites is common, rarely is there an amount sufficient to appreciate on plain abdominal radiographs.

US is the imaging procedure of choice for initial evaluation of possible pancreatitis. Jeffrey has emphasized the value of semierect and coronal scans as well as the standard scanning planes for optimal evaluation of the diseased pancreas. The edema that accompanies acute pancreatitis often results in a hypoechoic gland that is diffusely enlarged (Fig. 7). A minority of affected patients will have an increased pancreatic echogenicity (Fig. 8A), while some will have a normal-appearing pancreas. The pancreatic duct may be dilated, but this is an inconstant finding, especially when the gland is markedly swollen, causing compression of the duct. When the duct is dilated, however, there is a correlation with serum lipase in the acute and healing phases of the

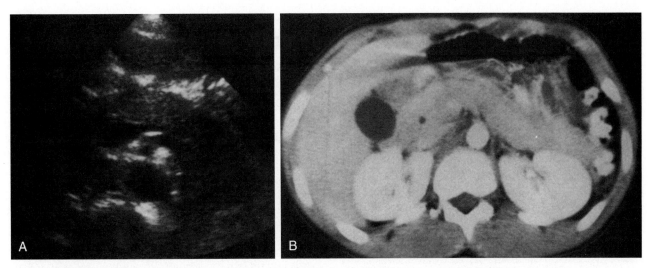

FIGURE 7. A, Transverse ultrasound scan in an 11-year-old boy with idiopathic acute pancreatitis. The body of the pancreas is enlarged and mildly hypoechoic, consistent with edema. **B,** Computed tomography scan confirms the swelling of the pancreas and demonstrates mild ductal dilatation in the pancreatic head.

disease. Masses may be identified in the pancreas representing focal areas of fluid, hemorrhage, or phlegmon formation. The last is a focal inflammatory mass that is hypoechoic. Ascites is usually identified.

The presence of acute fluid collections in the peripancreatic areas is useful evidence of acute pancreatitis. The most commonly involved areas are the lesser sac, anterior pararenal space, transverse mesocolon, and perirenal space. US is excellent in demonstrating these fluid collections. Fluid collections may be found as distant from the pancreas as the mediastinum and the inguinal regions. Fluid and inflammation may involve the adjacent splenic vein. Doppler examination is useful to rule out splenic vein thrombosis.

CT is not usually necessary for diagnosis, although it may show pancreatic abnormalities to better advantage than US in difficult cases. The findings mirror those seen with US and include pancreatic swelling, ductal dilatation, mass effect from phlegmon or hemorrhage,

peripancreatic fluid collections, thickening of adjacent fascial planes, and ascites. Abscesses are particularly well delineated on CT. Balthazar et al. used dynamic CT scanning to evaluate necrosis in adults with acute pancreatitis. Necrosis was diagnosed when all or part of the gland did not show enhancement. Patients with necrosis had a higher range of morbidity, mortality, and complications than did those without necrosis. ERCP is excellent for examination of the pancreatic duct but is infrequently needed in children. It is a useful examination for evaluation of complicated or recurent pancreatitis or in cases of unusual pseudocyst formation. The findings range from mild irregularity of the duct to ductal narrowing with acinar enlargement, which has been likened to a string of beads. Marked ductal ectasis is usually not seen in acute pancreatitis. MRCP may replace ERCP in the evaluation of childhood pancreatitis because of its noninvasive nature.

Pseudocyst formation is a potential complication of

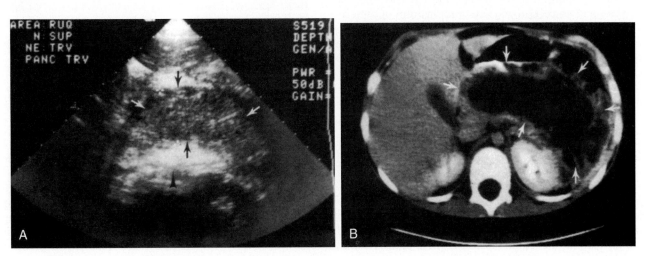

FIGURE 8. Acute pancreatitis in a 7-year-old girl. **A,** Transverse ultrasound scan reveals a thickened pancreas *(arrows)* with a coarse hyperechoic pattern. **B,** Computed tomography scan 3 weeks later shows the large pseudocyst *(arrows)* that developed in the interim.

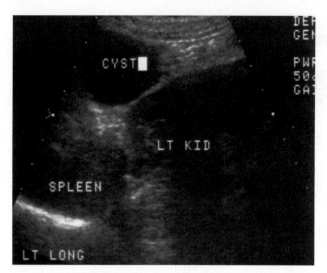

FIGURE 9. Ultrasound scan of a pancreatic pseudocyst in an adolescent girl demonstrates its intrapancreatic location adjacent to spleen and left kidney *(LT KID)*.

pancreatitis regardless of etiology (Fig. 8*B*). Although most pseudocysts are in the region of the pancreas itself (Fig. 9), they may appear nearly anywhere in the abdomen and in the mediastinum (Figs. 10 and 11). In adults, approximately 5% of patients with acute pancreatitis will develop pseudocysts. Although most pseudocysts resolve spontaneously, some will persist and require surgical intervention. Pseudocysts may be large enough to identify on plain films. They frequently cause a mass effect on adjacent structures, especially the stomach and duodenum, that may be identified on upper gastrointestinal studies performed for unexplained abdominal pain. US is indicated when a pseudocyst is suspected. Pseudocysts are typically anechoic, although some may contain debris. Their effect on adjacent organs may be identified on US scans but is seen to better advantage with CT. ERCP usually shows the irregular ductal dilatation of chronic inflammation. Successful percutaneous drainage of pseudocysts has been achieved.

Skeletal changes, particularly bone marrow infarcts, have long been recognized as a complication of pancreatitis, possibly related to increased levels of circulating lipase and to generalized enzymatic dysfunction of the pancreas. Plain films generally show late changes with characteristic medullary calcification. Haller et al. described MRI findings that preceded radiographic findings in an adult.

CHRONIC PANCREATITIS

Chronic pancreatitis in children is even rarer than acute pancreatitis. Although it occurs as a sequela of the acute form, chronic pancreatitis can be found in association with other diseases. The findings in CF are discussed above. Familial hereditary pancreatitis is an autosomal dominant disease in which most patients present in childhood or during their teenage years. Ductal dilatation (Fig. 11*G*), pseudocysts, and calcifications are the

most commonly identified imaging abnormalities in chronic pancreatitis. Spencer et al. described a 2-year-old boy with abdominal pain and a large pancreatic hemorrhagic mass who was found to have chronic pancreatitis at surgery. Subsequent abdominal US of the patient's mother revealed pancreatic ductal dilatation and calcifications. Chronic fibrosing pancreatitis is characterized by bands of collagen enclosing normal acini. The result is a mass effect that simulates a tumor. Chronic pancreatitis may result in jaundice secondary to biliary duct stricture.

PANCREATIC NEOPLASMS

Pancreatic tumors, both benign and malignant, are very rare in childhood. Hormonally active tumors arise from the islet cells and may be benign or malignant. The B cells produce insulin; A cells produce glucagon; G cells, gastrin; D cells, somatostatin; and D_1 cells, vasoactive intestinal peptide (VIP) as well as secretin. Islet cell tumors are named after the hormone produced. Insulinoma is the most commonly found islet cell tumor in children. Gastrinomas may be found in children with Zollinger-Ellison syndrome. According to Grosfeld et al., 2 of 56 reported cases of VIP-producing tumors in

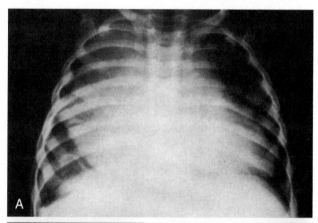
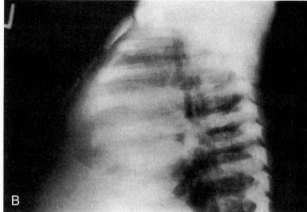

FIGURE 10. Mediastinal pancreatic pseudocyst on frontal **(A)** and lateral **(B)** radiographs in a 10-month-old girl who presented with wheezing and tachypnea. (Courtesy of Dr. S. Kirchner, Nashville, TN.)

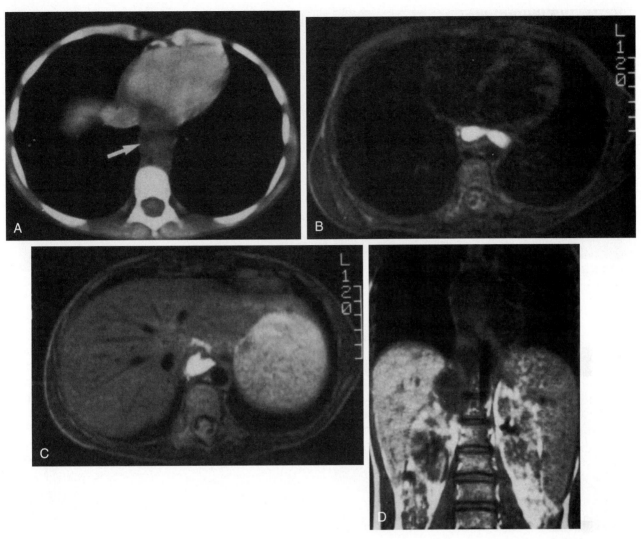

FIGURE 11. Mediastinal infiltration of a pancreatic pseudocyst. **A,** Computed tomography scan section through the lower chest demonstrates a fluid-filled mass *(arrow)* anterior to the descending aorta. Axial T_2-weighted magnetic resonance imaging sections through the lower mediastinum **(B)** and thoracolumbar junction **(C)** demonstrate the fluid content of the mass. **D,** Coronal T_1-weighted MRI section demonstrates the low-signal-intensity mass extending from a position superior to the right kidney into the posterior mediastinum. *Illustration continued on following page*

children were islet cell tumors. Neurogenic tumors generated the hormone in the other patients. Glucagonomas and somatostatinomas have not been reported in children. Islet cell tumors may be found in association with tumors in other organs as part of the several multiple endocrine neoplasia syndromes. McClain et al. reported a case of inflammatory pseudotumor of the pancreas in an 11-year-old child.

Patients with insulinoma present with hypoglycemia, typically manifested in children by erratic behavior and seizures. The symptoms are relieved by intravenous glucose administration and reproduced with fasting under controlled circumstances. In Synn et al.'s series, only 3 of 12 pediatric patients with profound hypoglycemia had identifiable islet cell tumors. The others had islet cell hyperplasia or nesidioblastosis on histologic examination of specimens resulting from partial pancreatectomy. Islet cell tumors are round or oval and well circumscribed on US. They are hypoechoic but may

have a hyperechoic rim. Isoechoic and hyperechoic lesions have been described in children and young adults. They may be superficial or deep in the pancreas. CT can be useful because contrast enhancement may cause markedly increased attenuation in the tumors. Because the tumors are hypervascular, arteriography may be necessary in high-risk patients in whom US and CT are nondiagnostic, although magnetic resonance angiography may replace this invasive technique. Intraoperative US has been used successfully to locate functioning islet cell tumors in children. Brunelle et al. have performed transhepatic venous sampling in children with hyperinsulinism. Fifteen of 19 patients had elevated insulin levels when sampling of the portal, splenic, superior mesenteric, inferior mesenteric, and pancreatic collateral veins was accomplished.

The exocrine tissues of the pancreas give rise to benign and malignant tumors that are hormonally inactive. Cystadenomas and adenocarcinoma of the

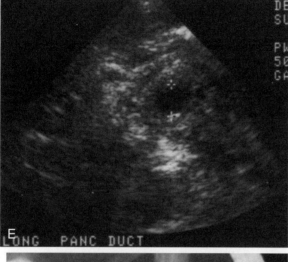

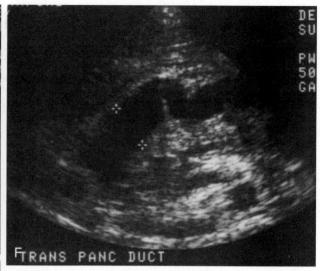

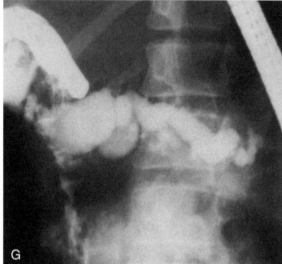

FIGURE 11. *Continued.* Longitudinal **(E)** and transverse **(F)** ultrasound scans of the midabdomen demonstrate marked dilatation of the pancreatic duct. **G,** Endoscopic retrograde cholangiopancreatography demonstrates the dilated pancreatic duct characteristic of chronic pancreatitis.

pancreas occur in children and have even been described in infants. Pancreatic adenosarcoma has been described in an adolescent male with Peutz-Jeghers syndrome. Giardiello et al. described a 100-fold increased risk of pancreatic adenocarcinoma in patients with this syndrome. The solid tumors are typically hyperechoic while the cystic lesions are anechoic or hypoechoic. Adenocarcinomas may have cystic or hemorrhagic areas resulting in mixed echogenicity. CT usually identifies a pancreatic mass of variable size often causing obstruction of the bile duct. Because the diagnosis of pancreatic carcinoma is so rare in children (only about 50 cases have been reported), imaging evaluation is often delayed, and metastases to lymph nodes and liver may be noted on CT. Rhabdomyosarcoma may arise primarily in the pancreas, as may lymphoma. Neuroblastoma has been reported in the pancreas secondary to direct extension.

Pancreatoblastoma arises from the pancreatic acinar cells, usually in the head or tail of the gland. These cells represent persistence of the fetal anlage of the acinar cells. Pancreatoblastomas are often large at presentation (up to 12 cm), with areas of central necrosis. US and CT findings are indistinguishable from those with adenocarcinoma. Montemarano et al. described the MRI findings in 10 patients with pancreatoblastoma. T_1-weighted spin-echo images showed low to intermediate signal intensity, while T_2-weighted images had very high signal intensity. Although the findings were nonspecific, they suggested the malignant nature of the tumor and clearly excluded the kidney and adrenal glands as organs of origin.

SUGGESTED READINGS

Imaging the Pancreas

Allendorph M, Werlin SL, Geenen JE, et al: Endoscopic retrograde cholangiopancreatography in children. J Pediatr 1987;110:206

Arcement CM, Meza MP, Arumania S, et al: MRCP in the evaluation of pancreaticobiliary disease in children. Pediatr Radiol 2001;31:92

Herman TE, Siegel MJ: CT of the pancreas in children. AJR Am J Roentgenol 1991;1547:375

Lawson TL, Berland LL, Foley WD, et al: Ultrasonic visualization of the pancreatic duct. Radiology 1982;144:865

Siegel MJ, Martin KW, Worthington JL: Normal and abnormal pancreas in children: US studies. Radiology 1987;165:15

Teele RL, Share JC: Ultrasonography of Infants and Children. Philadelphia, WB Saunders, 1990:389–404

Ueda D: Sonographic measurement of the pancreas in children. J Clin Ultrasound 1989;17:417

Walsh E, Cramer B, Pushpanthan C: Pancreatic echogenicity in premature and newborn infants. Pediatr Radiol 1990;20:323

Developmental and Hereditary Abnormalities

Baggott BB, Long WB: Annular pancreas as a cause of extrahepatic biliary obstruction. Am J Gastroenterol 1991;86:224

Baker LL, Hartman GE, Northway WH Jr: Sonographic detection of congenital pancreatic cysts in the newborn: report of a case and review of the literature. Pediatr Radiol 1990;20:488

Choyke PL, Filling-Katz MR, Shawker TH, et al: Von Hippel-Lindau disease: radiologic screening for visceral manifestations. Radiology 1990;174:815

Clavon M. Verain AL, Bigard MA: Cyst formation in gastroheterotopic pancreas: report of two cases. Radiology 1988;169:659

Daneman A, Gaskin K, Martin DJ, et al: Pancreatic changes in cystic fibrosis: CT and sonographic appearances. AJR Am J Roentgenol 1983;141:653

Hernanz-Schulman M, Teele RL, Perez-Atayde A, et al: Pancreatic cystosis in cystic fibrosis. Radiology 1986;158:629

Itoh Y, Hada T, Terano A, et al: Pancreatitis in the annulus of annular pancreas demonstrated by the combined use of computed tomography and endoscopic retrograde cholangiopancreatography. Am J Gastroenterol 1989;84:961

Kilman WJ, Berk RN: The spectrum of radiographic features of aberrant pancreatic rests involving the stomach. Radiology 1977;123:291

Lindstrom E, Ihse I: Dynamic CT scanning of pancreatic duct after secretin provocation in pancreas divisum. Dig Dis Sci 1990;35:1371

Liu P, Daneman A, Stringer DA, et al: Pancreatic cysts and calcification in cystic fibrosis. J Can Assoc Radiol 1986;37:279

Manfredi R, Costamagna G, Brizi MG, et al: Pancreas divisum and "satorincele": diagnosis with dynamic MR cholangiopancreatography with secretin stimulation. Radiology 2000;217:403

Marsh TD, Farach L, Wood BP: Radiological case of the month: Obstructing annular pancreas. Am J Dis Child 1990;144:505

Matos C, Metens T, Deviere J, et al: Pancreas divisum: evaluation with secretin-enhanced magnetic resonance cholangiopancreatography. Gastrointest Endosc 2001;53:728

McHugo JM, McKeown C, Brown MT, et al: Ultrasound findings in children with cystic fibrosis. Pediatr Radiol 1990;20:536

Murayama S, Robinson AE, Mulvihill DM, et al: MR imaging of pancreas in cystic fibrosis. Pediatr Radiol 1990;20:536

Nguyen KT, Pace R, Groll A: CT appearance of annular pancreas: a case report. J Can Assoc Radiol 1989;40:322

Soulen MC, Aerhouni EA, Fishman EK, et al: Enlargement of the pancreatic head in patients with pancreas divisum. Clin Imaging 1989;13:51

Tham RTOT, Heyerman HGM, Falke THM, et al: Cystic fibrosis: MR imaging of the pancreas. Radiology 1991;179:813

Ueda D, Taketazu M, Itoh S, et al: A case of gastric duplication cyst with aberrant pancreas. Pediatr Radiol 1991;21:379

Willi UV, Reddish JM, Teele RL: Cystic fibrosis: its characteristic appearance on abdominal sonography. AJR Am J Roentgenol 1980;134:1005

Zeman RK, McVay LV, Silverman PM, et al: Pancreas divisum: thin-section CT. Radiology 1988;169:395

Acute and Chronic Pancreatitis

Albu E, Buiumsohn A, Lopez R, et al: Gallstone pancreatitis in adolescents. J Pediatr Surg 1987;22:960

Amundson GM, Towbin RB, Mueller DL, et al: Percutaneous transgastric drainage of the lesser sac in children. Pediatr Radiol 1990;20:590

Atkinson GO Jr, Wyly JB, Gay BB Jr, et al: Idopathic fibrosing pancreatitis: a cause of obstructive jaundice in childhood. Pediatr Radiol 1988;18:28

Balthazar EJ, Robinson DL, Megabow AJ, et al: Acute pancreatitis: value of CT in establishing prognosis. Radiology 1990;174:331

Chao HC, Lin SJ, Kong MS, et al: Sonographic evaluation of the pancreatic duct in normal children and children with pancreatitis. J Ultrasound Med 2000;19:757

Crombleholme TM, deLorimier AA, Adzick NS, et al: Mediastinal pancreatic pseudocysts in children. J Pediatr Surg 1990;25:843

Crombleholme TM, deLorimier AA, Way LW, et al: The modified Puestow procedure for chronic relapsing pancreatitis in children. J Pediatr Surg 1990;25:749

Fleischer AC, Parker P, Kirchner SG: Sonographic findings of pancreatitis in children. Radiology 1986;146:151

Ford EG, Hardin WD Jr, Mahour GH, et al: Pseudocysts of the pancreas in children. Am Surg 1990;56:384

Garel L, Burnelle F, Lallemand D, et al: Pseudocysts of the pancreas in children: which cases require surgery? Pediatr Radiol 1983;13:120

Haller J, Greenway G, Resnick D, et al: Intraosseous fat necrosis associated with acute pancreatitis: MR imaging. Radiology 1989;173:193

Huntington DK, Hill MC, Steinberg W: Biliary tract dilatation in chronic pancreatitis: CT and sonographic findings. Radiology 1989;172:47

Jeffrey RB Jr: Sonography in acute pancreatitis. Radiol Clin North Am 1989;27:5

Jeffrey RB Jr, Laing FC, Wing VW: Extrapancreatic spread of acute pancreatitis: new observations with real-time US. Radiology 1986;159:707

Lee SP, Nicholls JF, Park HZ: Biliary sludge as a cause of acute pancreatitis. N Engl J Med 1992;326:589

Millward SF, Breatnach E, Simpkins KC, et al: Do plain films of the chest and abdomen have a role in the diagnosis of acute pancreatitis? Clin Radiol 1983;34:133

Sadry F, Hausen H: Fatal pancreatitis secondary to iatrogenic intramural hematoma: a case report and review of the literature. Gastrointest Radiol 1990;15:296

Shimizu T, Suzuki R, Yamashiro Y, et al: Magnetic resonance cholangiopancreatography in assessing the cause of acute pancreatitis in children. Pancreas 2001;2:196

Slovis TL, von Berg VJ, Mikelic V: Sonography in the diagnosis and management of pancreatic pseudocysts and effusions in childhood. Radiology 1980;135:153

Sonnenberg E, Wittich GR, Casola G, et al: Percutaneous drainage of infected and noninfected pancreatic pseudocysts: experience in 101 cases. Radiology 1980;170:757

Spencer JA, Lindsell DRM, Isaacs D: Hereditary pancreatitis: early ultrasound appearances. Pediatr Radiol 1990;20:293

Stoler J, Biller JA, Grand RJ: Pancreatitis in Kawasaki disease. Am J Dis Child 1987;141:306

Suarez F, Bernard O, Gauthier F, et al: Bilio-pancreatic common channel in children: clinical, biological and radiological findings in 12 children. Pediatr Radiol 1987;17:206

Swischuk LE, Hayden CK Jr: Pararenal space hyperechogenicity in childhood pancreatitis. AJR Am J Roentgenol 1985;145:1085

Weizman Z, Durie PR: Acute pancreatitis in childhood. J Pediatr 1988;113:24

Wheatley MJ, Coran AG: Obstructive jaundice secondary to chronic pancreatitis in children: report of two cases and review of the literature. Surgery 1988;104:863

Ziegler DW, Long JA, Philippart AI, et al: Pancreatitis in childhood. Ann Surg 1988;207:257

Pancreatic Neoplasms

Bowlby LS: Pancreatic adenocarcinoma in an adolescent male with Peutz-Jeghers syndrome. Hum Pathol 1986;17:97

Brenner RW, Sank LI, Kerner MB, et al: Resection of a VIPoma of the pancreas in a 15-year-old girl. J Pediatr Surg 1986;21:983

Brunelle F, Negre V, Barth MO, et al: Pancreatic venous samplings in infants and children with primary hyperinsulinism. Pediatr Radiol 1989;19:100

Galiber AK, Reading CC, Charboneau JW: Localization of pancreatic insulinoma: comparison of pre- and intraoperative ultrasound with CT and angiography. Radiology 1988;166:405

Giardiello FM, Welsh SB, Hamilton SR, et al: Increased risk of cancer in the Peutz-Jeghers syndrome. N Engl J Med 1987;316:1151

Grant CS, Heerden J, Charboneau W: Insulinoma: the value of intraoperative ultrasonography. Arch Surg 1988;123:843

Grosfeld JL, Vane DW, Rescorla FJ, et al: Pancreatic tumors in childhood: analysis of 13 cases. J Pediatr Surg 1990;25:1057

Hecht ST, Barsch RC, Styne DM: CT localization of occult secretory tumors in children. Pediatr Radiol 1982;12:67

McClain MB, Burton EM, Day DS: Pancreatic pseudotumor in an 11-year-old child: imaging findings. Pediatr Radiol 2000;30:610

Montemarano H, Lonergan GJ, Bulas DI, et al: Pancreatoblastoma: imaging findings in 10 patients and review of the literature. Radiology 2000;214:476

Moynan RW, Neehout RC, Johnson TS: Pancreatic carcinoma in childhood: case report and review. J Pediatr 1964;65:711

Robey G, Daneman A, Martin DJ: Pancreatic carcinoma in a neonate. Pediatr Radiol 1983;13:284

Rossi P, Allison DJ, Bezzi M: Endocrine tumors of the pancreas. Radiol Clin North Am 1989;27:129

Stephenson CA, Kletzel M, Seibert JJ, et al: Pancreatoblastoma: MR appearance. J Comput Assist Tomogr 1990;14:492

Sty JR, Wells RG: Other abdominal and pelvic masses in children. Semin Roentgenol 1988;23:216

Synn AY, Mulvihill SJ, Fonkalsrud EW: Surgical disorders of the pancreas in infancy and childhood. Am J Surg 1988;156:201

Telander Rl, Charboneau JW, Haymond MW: Intraoperative ultrasonography of the pancreas in children. J Pediatr Surg 1986;21:262

Yakovac WC, Baker L, Hummeler K: Beta cell nesidioblastosis in idiopathic hypoglycemia of infancy. J Pediatr 1971;79:226

PART V

ESOPHAGUS

ALAN E. SCHLESINGER
BRUCE R. PARKER

Chapter 1

NORMAL ESOPHAGUS

ALAN E. SCHLESINGER and BRUCE R. PARKER

NORMAL ANATOMY

The esophagus is a musculomembranous tubular structure extending from the distal hypopharynx at the level of the 7th cervical vertebra to the esophagogastric junction, normally at the level of the 10th thoracic vertebra. The caliber of the esophagus varies with peristaltic activity but is usually slightly narrower at both ends than during most of its intrathoracic course. Normal extrinsic impressions on the esophagus are caused by the aorta and the left main stem bronchus. The esophagus frequently deviates slightly to the right at the level of the left atrium just before entering the esophageal hiatus of the diaphragm. The course and topographic relationships of the esophagus are shown in Figures 1 and 2.

1539

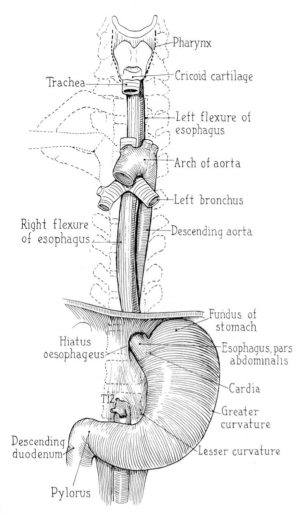

FIGURE 1. Semischematic drawing of the normal esophagus shows its relation to the trachea, aorta, diaphragm, and stomach. (Modified from Morris's Human Anatomy, 10th ed. New York, McGraw-Hill, 1943.)

METHODS OF EXAMINATION

Standard fluoroscopy and radiographic examination using opaque contrast media continue to be the primary imaging modalities used in evaluation of the esophagus. Radiation dose has been reduced by the use of video fluoroscopy instead of cinefluoroscopy and by the use of 100-mm and 105-mm spot-film cameras in place of standard spot-film devices and conventional film–screen combinations. Further dose reduction during the acquisition of fluoroscopic spot images is achieved with relatively insignificant image degradation by the use of digital fluoroscopy. In addition, pulsed fluoroscopy also can lower fluoroscopic dose. "Last image hold" features on fluoroscopic monitors can further lower dose by decreasing fluoroscopic time.

■ Techniques for fluoroscopy dose reduction:
  • Videofluoroscopy
  • Spot film cameras or digital spot images
  • Pulsed fluoroscopy
  • "Last image held" on fluoroscopy monitor

Infants and small children generally require immobilization for optimal results. Various commercial devices are available, but they may make patient rotation under the fluoroscope difficult. We have achieved excellent results by immobilizing the arms above the head with a soft towel and using a similar restraint for the lower extremities. Gonadal shielding is mandatory. A large lead shield on the fluoroscopic table also helps shield parents or personnel who may help in restraining the patient's lower extremities.

Barium suspensions are still the contrast medium of choice unless esophageal perforation or tracheoesophageal fistula is suspected, or if there is a high probability of aspiration. The typically small amounts of contrast medium aspirated secondary to unexpected swallowing dysfunction, reflux, and tracheoesophageal fistulas are usually cleared naturally from the normal airway with coughing. Nevertheless, careful fluoroscopic monitoring and small doses of oral contrast should be used at the initiation of the examination to preclude aspiration of significant amounts of contrast material. When barium is contraindicated, low-osmolar nonionic contrast media are safer than ionic media, although substantially more expensive.

Evaluation of swallowing function should always be

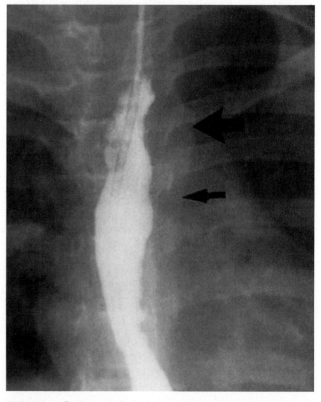

FIGURE 2. Barium swallow demonstrates the impression of the aortic knob *(large arrow)* and the left main stem bronchus *(small arrow)* on the barium-filled esophagus. These are normal impressions and are not to be confused with mediastinal abnormalities.

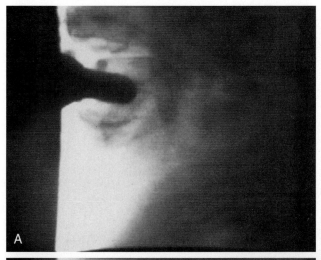

FIGURE 3. Normal swallowing. **A,** As the nipple is inserted into the infant's mouth, the tongue and soft palate are relaxed and the nasopharynx opens. **B,** At the initiation of suck, the tongue elevates, pushing the nipple to the roof of the mouth, and the soft palate elevates, closing off the nasopharynx. **C,** The initial swallow shows barium outlining the underside of the hard palate and soft palate and the posterior aspect of the base of the tongue, and entering the vallecula.

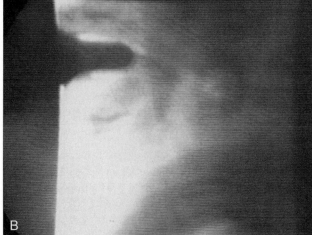

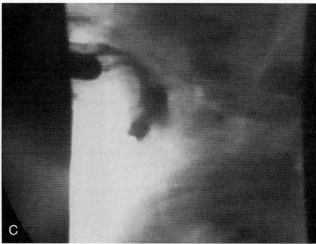

part of an esophageal imaging study. The infant should be fed by a bottle and nipple for this part of the study, while swallowing is evaluated fluoroscopically. Videotape and spot-film images can be obtained in lateral projection if necessary (Fig. 3). If the infant will not take

barium from the nipple, contrast can be carefully injected into the baby's mouth (between the cheek and the lateral aspect of the teeth or gums) or a feeding tube can be inserted through the nipple into the baby's mouth and controlled injections made on the back of

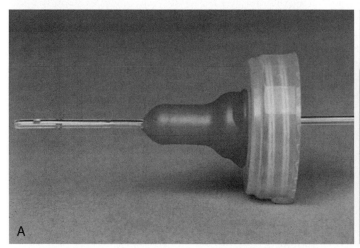

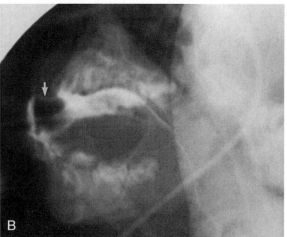

FIGURE 4. A, A No. 8 Silastic feeding tube is placed through a nipple so that a controlled injection can be made into the mouth and swallowing mechanism observed. **B,** Barium outlines the nipple *(arrow)* and the tube. (Modified from Poznanski A: A simple device for administering barium to infants. Radiology 1969;93:1106.)

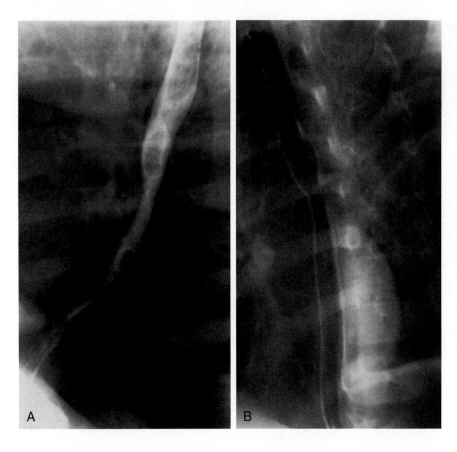

FIGURE 5. Single- **(A)** and double-contrast **(B)** esophagogram in a 5-year-old boy 6 months after lye ingestion demonstrates narrowing of the midesophagus with distal aperistalsis. The mucosa is intact.

the tongue to initiate swallowing (Fig. 4). If the patient does not ingest sufficient contrast material for evaluation of the esophagus distal to the base of the tongue, the remainder of the examination may be performed through a nasoesophageal tube. Generally, an 8 Fr. feeding tube is satisfactory. Smaller caliber tubes do not permit rapid injection of sufficient volume.

Fluoroscopic spot images of the esophagus in antero-posterior and lateral projections should be obtained. Double-contrast esophagography is difficult to perform in patients less than 8 years of age. Younger patients, even those who are otherwise cooperative, will usually let the gas escape by eructation before satisfactory images can be obtained. However, as demonstrated by Levine et al., the double-contrast examination is most useful in patients with mucosal lesions, such as infectious esophagitis, which occur more commonly in older children (Fig. 5). Unplanned double-contrast esophagus studies frequently are obtained in infants who cry, swallow air, and eructate during the examination. Nuclear medicine and ultrasound studies can be used to identify gastroesophageal reflux and are described in Section VI, Part V, Chapter 5, page 1569.

NORMAL ROENTGENOGRAPHIC APPEARANCE

Although radiologists have historically paid primary attention to anatomy, physiology, and pathologic conditions of the esophagus itself, the importance of pharyngeal and esophageal motility disorders requires an

understanding of the anatomy and physiology of the pharynx as well. The three components of the pharynx are the nasopharynx, the oropharynx, and the hypopharynx (see Section IV, Part II, Figs. 1 and 2, page 778). The nasopharynx and oropharynx communicate through the velopharyngeal portal. Through a highly

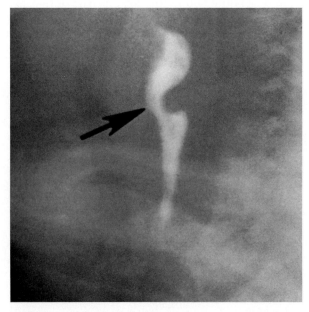

FIGURE 6. Lateral view of a barium swallow demonstrates a normal posterior impression by the contracted cricopharyngeus muscle. This is a normal variant in a patient who had no swallowing difficulties.

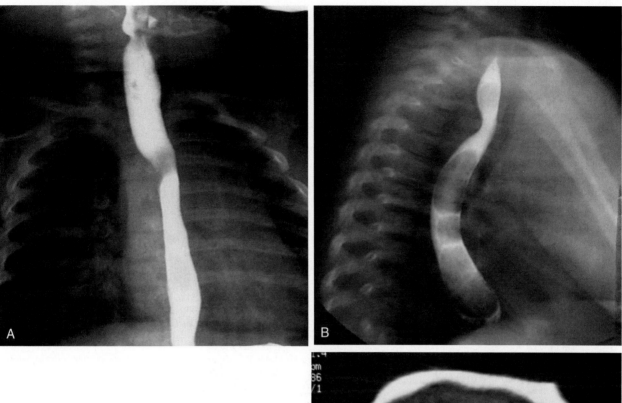

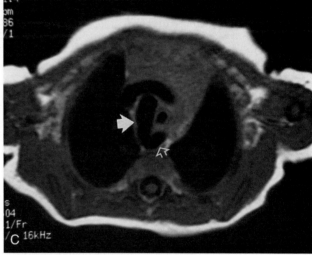

FIGURE 7. Frontal **(A)** and lateral **(B)** views from an esophagram in a patient with a right aortic arch with aberrant left subclavian artery demonstrate right-sided and posterior impressions on the barium-filled esophagus. **C,** Axial T₁-weighted magnetic resonance image reveals the right-sided aortic arch *(arrow)* and the origin of the aberrant left subclavian artery posteriorly *(open arrow).*

complex, coordinated neuromuscular mechanism, the portal closes during both speech and swallowing, although the specific neurologic pathways are different during these two physiologic functions. The hypopharynx extends from the velopharyngeal portal to the level of the larynx, including the epiglottis.

The oral phase of swallowing occurs when the patient chews and mixes food with saliva. This phase is very rapid during the injection of liquid contrast material, but the thrust of the tongue forward and superiorly can be seen. The bolus is transported quickly to the pharyngeal inlet along the dorsum of the tongue by extremely complicated peristaltic-like activity of the tongue muscles (see Fig. 3*C*).

During the pharyngeal phase of swallowing, numerous muscles contract in rapid progression to propel the bolus and elevate the soft palate, protecting the nasopharynx from reflux. The larynx and hyoid bone can be seen elevating secondary to the action of muscles that contract to seal off the oropharynx as the bolus is propelled into the cervical esophagus. The epiglottis concurrently seals off the trachea.

Over 50 different muscle groups contract during the oral and pharyngeal phases, but the esophageal phase of swallowing is relatively simpler. Distention of the cervical esophagus elicits peristalsis. The upper third of the esophagus has a striated muscle layer, and effective peristalsis here is most dependent on medullary neural reflexes and the vagus nerve. Peristalsis in the lower esophagus, with its smooth muscle layer, is independent of the central nervous system and relies predominantly on an intrinsic peristaltic mechanism that is modulated by vagus activity. Although this description is oversimplified, it does explain the variability of peristaltic activity in the upper and lower esophagus that can be seen in a variety of disease states.

The normal thoracic portion of the esophagus shows smooth primary striping by peristaltic waves during the passage of a single large bolus. Because each swallow elicits a new peristaltic wave, the normal peristaltic mechanism will appear interrupted during repetitive swallowing. Tertiary contractions are not seen in the normal infant and child. When older children are studied in the erect position, gravity plays an important role in the passage of contrast material.

On lateral view, the impression of the contracted cricopharyngeus muscle may be seen indenting the cervical esophagus posteriorly (Fig. 6). Deviation by the aorta and the left atrium, as well as the impression by the left main stem bronchus, is usually seen (see Fig. 2).

The course of the esophagus may be affected by spinal and aortic abnormalities such as severe kyphoscoliosis and aortic ectasia. Aortic arch anomalies (Fig. 7) such as aberrant vessels, double aortic arch, and right aortic arch will cause extrinsic effects on the lateral and posterior aspects of the esophagus and are discussed more fully in Section V, Part III. Aberrant left pulmonary artery typically causes an anterior extrinsic compression defect (see Section II, Part IV).

SUGGESTED READINGS

Belt T, Cohen MD: Metrizamide evaluation of the esophagus in infants. Am J Roentgenol 1984;143:367

Cohen MD: Choosing contrast media for the evaluation of the gastrointestinal tract of neonates and infants. Radiology 1987;162:447

Dodds WJ: The physiology of swallowing. Dysphagia 1989;3:171

Donner MW, Bosma JF, Robertson DL: Anatomy and physiology of the pharynx. Gastrointest Radiol 1985;10:196

Ginai AZ, Tenkate FJW, Ten Berg RGM, et al: Experimental evaluation of various available contrast agents for use in the upper gastrointestinal tract in case of suspected leakage: effects on lungs. Br J Radiol 1984a;57:895

Ginai AZ, Tenkate FJW, Ten Berg RGM, et al: Experimental evaluation of various available contrast agents for use in the upper gastrointestinal tract in case of suspected leakage: effects on mediastinum. Br J Radiol 1985b;58:585

Girdany BR: The esophagus in infancy: congenital and acquired diseases. Radiol Clin North Am 1963;1:557

Girdany BR, Lee FA: X-ray examination of the gastrointestinal tract. Pediatr Clin North Am 1967;14:3

Hernandez RJ, Goodsitt MM: Reduction of radiation dose in pediatric patients using pulsed fluoroscopy. AJR Am J Roentgenol 1996;167:1247

Jones B, Gayler BW, Donner MW: Pharynx and cervical esophagus. In Levine MS (ed): Radiology of the Esophagus. Philadelphia, WB Saunders, 1989:311–336

Kramer SS: Swallowing in children. In Jones B, Donner MW (eds): Normal and Abnormal Swallowing: Imaging in Diagnosis and Therapy. New York, Springer-Verlag, 1991:173–188

Levine MS, Rubesin SE, Ott DJ: Update on esophageal radiology. AJR Am J Roentgenol 1990;155:933

McAlister WH, Askin FB: The effect of some contrast agents in the lung: an experimental study in the rat and dog. AJR Am J Roentgenol 1983;140:245

McAlister WH, Siegel MJ: Fatal aspirations in infancy during gastrointestinal series. Pediatr Radiol 1984;14:81

Sauvegrain J: The technique of upper gastro-intestinal investigation in infants and children. In Kaufman HJ (ed): Progress in Pediatric Radiology. Basel, S. Karger, 1969:26–51

■ **C h a p t e r   2**

DISORDERS OF DEGLUTITION, THE VELOPHARYNGEAL PORTAL, AND PERISTALSIS

ALAN E. SCHLESINGER and BRUCE R. PARKER

DISORDERS OF DEGLUTITION

Most swallowing disorders in children are secondary to neurologic abnormalities, of which cerebral palsy is the most common. Other neuromuscular disorders to be considered are brainstem dysfunction, cranial nerve abnormalities, intracranial neoplasms, meningomyelocele, muscular dystrophy, and myasthenia gravis. Familial dysautonomia (Riley-Day syndrome) leads to autonomic dysfunction with esophageal dysmotility and frequent aspiration pneumonia. Disorders of the mouth and jaw such as micrognathia and macroglossia may also cause abnormal swallowing. Bulbar polio may be seen in patients who have not been properly immunized.

Depending on the specific neurologic defect, any or all components of the swallowing mechanism may be affected. Some severely damaged infants cannot suck,

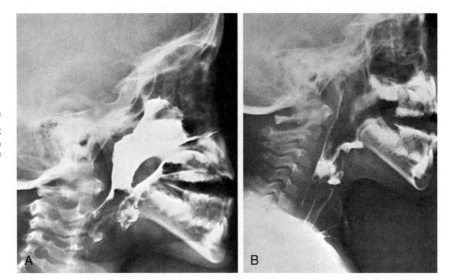

FIGURE 1. A and **B,** Marked reflux of swallowed barium into the nasopharynx secondary to neurogenic dysfunction of the muscles controlling the normal elevation of the soft palate.

and most of the barium drools out of the mouth. The tongue may not elevate to help initiate the swallowing mechanism. Abnormality of the neuromuscular mechanism elevating the soft palate may lead to reflux of contrast material into the nasopharynx, with subsequent drooling and potential aspiration into the airway (Fig. 1). Abnormalities of other muscle groups lead to defective function of the epiglottis and upper esophageal sphincter, with aspiration into the airway being common.

Defective peristalsis may be found in patients with the above-mentioned neurologic disorders as well as in patients with connective tissue disorders and esophagi-

tis. Patients with a history of repaired esophageal atresia frequently show abnormal peristalsis in the portion of the esophagus distal to the repair. Staiano et al. performed a manometric study demonstrating disordered esophageal motility in patients with colonic aganglionosis. Patients with disordered esophageal motility may show aperistalsis or hypoperistalsis with or without tertiary contractions (Fig. 2). Hypoperistalsis is more common in cases of esophagitis, including those secondary to gastroesophageal reflux.

Specialized radiographic studies of deglutition in association with occupational therapists and/or speech pathologists have been popularized by the Johns

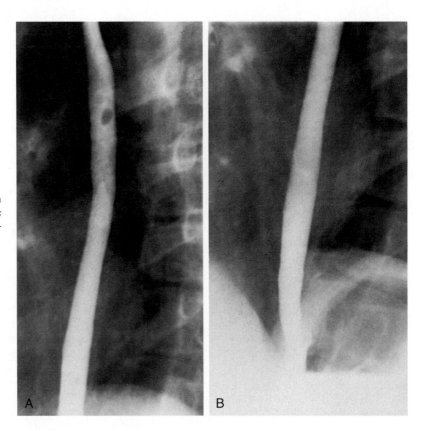

FIGURE 2. A and **B,** "Standing column" of barium in the esophagus of a patient who was aperistaltic following repair for esophageal atresia and tracheoesophageal fistula.

Hopkins Swallowing Center. The patient is placed in the position in which he or she is usually fed. Contrast medium is mixed with increasingly thicker food mixtures from liquid barium to solid food mixed with barium (if age appropriate). Videotaping in the lateral projections allows evaluation of the patient's ability to handle differently textured foods and is of enormous value in planning appropriate diet and therapy.

Cricopharyngeal achalasia, or failure of relaxation of the cricopharyngeus muscle, has been thought to be a primary cause of dysphagia. Most experts now agree that primary cricopharyngeal achalasia is probably uncommon. Secondary cricopharyngeal achalasia has been reported following trauma and in patients with autoimmune collagen disorders such as scleroderma and dermatomyositis. The results of studies from the Johns Hopkins Swallowing Center suggest that most cases of cricopharyngeal achalasia are secondary to gastroesophageal reflux (Fig. 3).

■ Causes of cricopharyngeal achalasia:
1. Primary (rare)
2. Secondary
   • Gastroesophageal reflux
   • Trauma
   • Autoimmune disorders

Direct pharyngeal trauma is an uncommon cause of disordered swallowing but may be seen after instrumentation, especially the passage of endotracheal, naso-gastric, or orogastric tubes (Fig. 4; see also Section II, Part II, Chapter 2, Fig. 12, page 34). Disordered peristalsis may be seen in patients with obstructive lesions such as strictures and achalasia. Dysphagia with disordered esophageal motility may be seen in psychogenic disorders (globus hystericus), but many of these patients eventually have an organic lesion found. The diagnosis of psychogenic dysphagia should be made only after an exhaustive investigation, especially of the central nervous system, fails to make a diagnosis of an underlying organic disorder.

Retropharyngeal masses are rare causes of dysphagia. Hemangiomas, teratomas, lymphangiomas (cystic hygromas), and lymphomas may occur at different ages. Retropharyngeal abscesses (Fig. 5) cause other symptoms that usually lead to the correct diagnosis. Congenital pharyngeal diverticula are quite rare. Spinal anomalies may rarely cause dysphagia in children.

■ Retropharyngeal masses
   • Hemangioma
   • Teratoma
   • Lymphangioma
   • Lymphoma

Scleroderma and mixed collagen disorders are rare in childhood, most frequently occurring in older adolescents and teenagers. Pharyngeal and cervical esophageal function is usually normal. Esophageal dysmotility typically begins at the level of the aortic arch, where the esophageal muscle layer begins to change from striated to smooth muscle. Poor to absent primary peristalsis occurs in the distal two thirds of the esophagus. Resulting esophageal reflux, with or without esophagitis, may occur. Levine and Ilowite described abnormal motility, diagnosed by esophageal manometry and esophageal endoscopy with biopsy, with a pattern similar to that seen in scleroderma in breast-fed children of mothers with silicone breast implants.

Dermatomyositis, in contrast, primarily affects the striated muscle of the pharynx and upper esophagus. Dilatation of these structures frequently occurs, as does reflux into the nasopharynx. The associated vasculitis may result in esophageal ulceration and perforation.

VELOPHARYNGEAL INCOMPETENCE

Disorders of the velopharyngeal portal are most commonly seen during evaluation of speech disorders. Although technically simple to perform, these studies are not part of the repertoire of most radiologists. They are most useful in patients being considered for cleft palate surgery and in those with speech disorders secondary to neurologic abnormalities. Because the muscles used in speech and swallowing are largely similar, useful information can be obtained from speech studies. The studies are feasible in most patients age 5

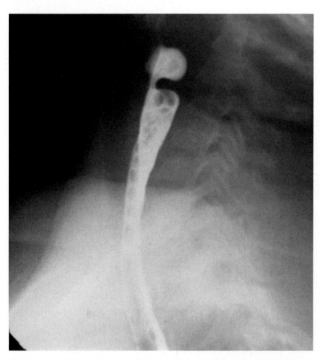

FIGURE 3. Posterior impression on the esophagus secondary to persistent contraction of the cricopharyngeal muscle in a patient with cricopharyngeal achalasia and symptoms of dysphagia. This patient had associated gastroesophageal reflux.

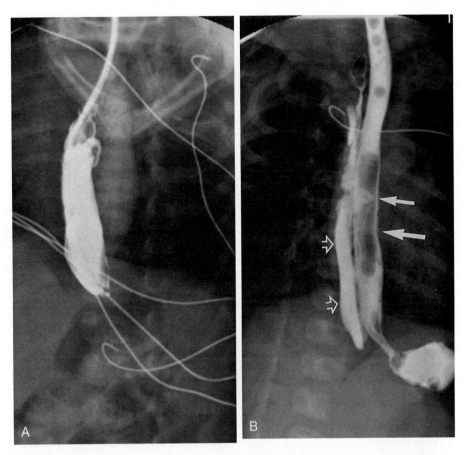

FIGURE 4. A, Frontal view of an esophagram performed through a feeding tube demonstrates a tubular collection of contrast, but lack of passage of this contrast into the stomach. **B,** Frontal image obtained after feeding the patient orally by nipple (after removing the feeding tube) demonstrates the true esophagus *(arrows)* and reveals that the original collection of contrast *(open arrows)* was within an extraluminal false passage created by the feeding tube.

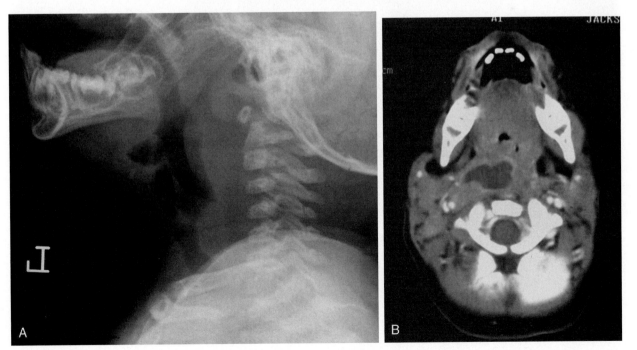

FIGURE 5. A, Lateral airway radiograph in a young infant demonstrates thickened retropharyngeal soft tissues. **B,** Axial section from a contrast-enhanced computed tomography scan confirms a retropharyngeal abscess with an enhancing rim.

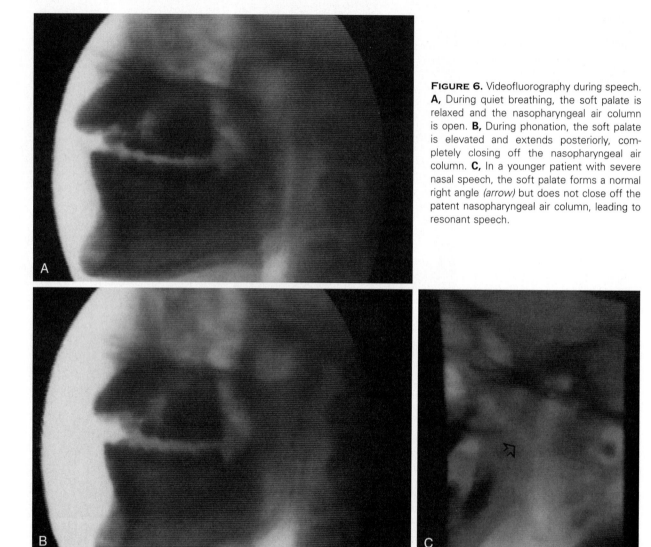

FIGURE 6. Videofluorography during speech. **A,** During quiet breathing, the soft palate is relaxed and the nasopharyngeal air column is open. **B,** During phonation, the soft palate is elevated and extends posteriorly, completely closing off the nasopharyngeal air column. **C,** In a younger patient with severe nasal speech, the soft palate forms a normal right angle *(arrow)* but does not close off the patent nasopharyngeal air column, leading to resonant speech.

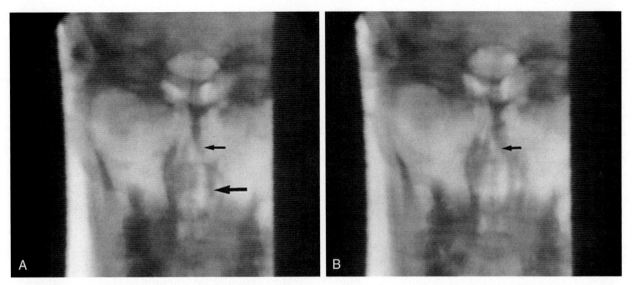

FIGURE 7. Videofluorography in the modified Towne projection. **A,** During quiet breathing, the nasopharyngeal air column *(small arrow)* and the oropharyngeal air column *(large arrow)* are well demonstrated. **B,** During speech, the nasopharyngeal air column *(arrow)* is reduced in diameter but does not close completely in this patient with nasal speech.

years or older and can be performed in cooperative children as young as 3 years. The patient is placed in an upright lateral position. A small amount of barium is injected into the nose to coat the soft palate for easier visualization. Combined audio-video recording is obtained while the patient repeats a series of words and phrases designed to maximize function of the pharyngeal muscles. During speech, the soft palate should elevate, becoming nearly horizontal in its proximal two thirds (Fig. 6). The distal one third remains roughly vertical and should make contact with the posterior pharyngeal wall throughout its course. The motion of the tongue can also be evaluated.

The procedure is then repeated with the patient's head in a modified Towne projection, allowing direct visualization of the oropharynx and nasopharynx (Fig. 7). Skolnick and Cohn recommended doing this portion of the study with the patient prone, but we have found younger patients more tolerant of the procedure if kept in a sitting or standing position. The nasopharyngeal walls are seen to function during speech like the iris of a camera. In patients with velopharyngeal incompetence, failure of normal excursion of the soft palate and the muscular pharyngeal side walls is identified. A barium swallow completes the examination and evaluates for nasopharyngeal reflux and fistulous communication between the oropharynx and nasopharynx. Speech studies have also proved quite valuable in the evaluation of patients following surgical repair of cleft palate. The study is quite useful in differentiating primary neuromuscular lesions, such as those seen in central nervous system disorders, from structural lesions, such as those in patients with craniofacial anomalies.

SUGGESTED READINGS

Fisher SE, Painter M, Milmoe G: Swallowing disorders in infancy. Pediatr Clin North Am 1981;28:845

Gyepes MT, Linde LM: Familial dysautonomia: the mechanism of aspiration. Radiology 1968;91:471

Kramer SS: Special swallowing problems in children. Gastrointest Radiol 1985;10:241

Kramer SS: Radiologic examination of the swallowing impaired child. Dysphagia 1989;3:117

La Rossa D, Brown A, Cohen M, et al: Video-radiography of the velopharyngeal portal using the Towne's view. J Maxillofac Surg 1980;8:203

Levine JJ, Ilowite NT: Sclerodermalike esophageal disease in children breast-fed by mothers with silicone breast implants. JAMA 1994;271:213

Mihailovic T, Perisic VN: Balloon dilatation of cricopharyngeal achalasia. Pediatr Radiol 1992;22:522

Skinner MA, Shorter NA: Primary neonatal achalasia: a case report and review of the literature. J Pediatr Surg 1992;27:1509

Skolnick ML: Video velopharyngography in patients with nasal speech, with emphasis on lateral pharyngeal motion in velopharyngeal closure. Radiology 1969;93:747

Skolnick ML, Cohn ER: Videofluoroscopic Studies of Speech in Patients with Cleft Palate. New York, Springer-Verlag, 1989

Staiano A, Corazziari E, Andreotti MR, et al: Esophageal motility in children with Hirschsprung's disease. Am J Dis Child 1991;145:310

Stringer DA, Witzer MA: Velopharyngeal insufficiency on multiview videofluoroscopy: a comparison of projections. AJR Am J Roentgenol 1986;146:15

Tuchman DN: Cough, choke, sputter: the evaluation of the child with dysfunctional swallowing. Dysphagia 1989;3:111

■ C h a p t e r   3

CONGENITAL ESOPHAGEAL MALFORMATIONS

ALAN E. SCHLESINGER and BRUCE R. PARKER

ESOPHAGEAL ATRESIA

Esophageal atresia, with or without tracheoesophageal fistula, is the most important congenital malformation of the esophagus. The varieties of esophageal atresia and tracheoesophageal fistula with their relative incidences are shown in Figure 1. The routine preoperative imaging evaluation of esophageal atresia and tracheoesophageal fistula is discussed in depth in Section II, Part IV, Chapter 2, page 22. In this chapter we emphasize more complicated cases, including "long-gap" esophageal atresia, complications of repaired esophageal atresia, and other associated congenital anomalies.

The preferred surgical repair of esophageal atresia is primary anastomosis of the proximal and distal pouches. When the atretic segment is too long, other approaches have been taken, including delayed repair (either delayed primary repair or staged repair) or esophageal replacement (colonic interposition, gastric tube reconstruction, or gastric pull-up). The gap between the proximal esophageal pouch and the distal esophagus spontaneously decreases during the first few months of life. Therefore, if feasible, placement of a feeding gastrostomy and delayed primary repair is the treatment of choice for "long-gap" esophageal atresia. There have been several preoperative and operative mechanical techniques described to lengthen the esophageal segments, and thereby lessen the gap, including bougienage, circular myotomies, and creation of surgical flaps. Kleinman et al. described transgastrostomy balloon dilatation of the distal pouch under fluoroscopic control in three patients that enabled a delayed primary anastomosis to be accomplished successfully that otherwise would not have been possible.

Most patients with isolated esophageal atresia and tracheoesophageal fistula do well following surgical repair. Nevertheless, complications following surgical treatment of esophageal atresia do occur. Early complications include early leaking at the site of anastomosis, esophageal diverticula, esophageal stricture, and recurrent fistula. In addition, some patients have associated congenital malformations, which often impact the ultimate prognosis of the patient. The VACTERL association is a mnemonic used to reflect the common association of *v*ertebral anomalies, *a*nal atresia, *c*ardiac anomalies, *t*racheo*e*sophageal fistula, *r*enal anomalies, and *l*imb anomalies.

Most typically no attempt is made at oral feedings until 1 to 2 weeks following surgery, when edema has subsided and the esophagus is presumably patent. Prior to the institution of oral feedings, a contrast study of the esophagus should be performed. The site of anastomosis is readily identified (Fig. 2). Although there is typically anatomic narrowing or a transition from a dilated proximal esophagus to a normal-caliber distal esophagus at the anastomotic site, contrast material normally flows readily past this area, and the infants generally have no difficulty in tolerating oral liquid feedings.

The most commonly identified early complication of surgical repair is leakage at the site of anastomosis, occurring in approximately 14% to 16% of cases. Therefore, low-osmolar nonionic contrast should be considered for esophagography in the immediate postoperative period. Although these leaks typically heal spontaneously, further surgical intervention may be necessary. Anastomotic leakage increases the risk of future esophageal stricture formation. Donnelly et al. have shown that the appearance of an extrapleural fluid collection after esophageal atresia repair performed via an extrapleural approach is associated with a high incidence of anastomotic leakage. Untreated anastomotic leakage may eventually lead to diverticulum formation (Fig. 3).

■ Early complications of esophageal atresia repair:
  • Anastomotic leak
  • Stricture
  • Recurrent fistula

Esophageal stricture is another relatively common complication after esophageal atresia repair. However, the incidence reported varies with the strictness of the criteria employed to diagnose a stricture. An apparent slight narrowing at the site of surgical anastomosis may persist for years, even though the patient has no functional problem. Similarly, the caliber change from a

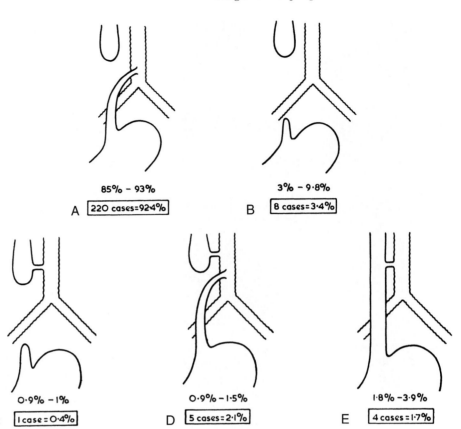

FIGURE 1. Morphologic varieties of congenital esophageal atresia. (From Rehbein P: The blood supply of the oesophagus in relation to oesophageal atresia. Arch Dis Child 1964;39:131, with permission.)

dilated proximal esophagus (resulting from in utero obstruction) to a relatively narrower distal esophagus may cause an alarming appearance in the absence of a stricture at the anastomosis. True stricture at the site of anastomosis usually leads to symptoms in the weeks following surgery. Overfilling of the upper esophagus may lead to aspiration. Most patients respond to bougienage, and reoperation is infrequently necessary. However, if the stricture is associated with gastroesophageal reflux, the stricture may not respond to dilatation if it continues to be exposed to acidic gastric contents. Therefore, patients with postoperative strictures should be evaluated for reflux by upper gastrointestinal series or pH monitoring. If an actual stricture occurs at the site of surgical repair, solid food may become impacted (Fig. 4). This is particularly true if the patient is fed hot dogs or similar foods that are difficult to chew completely. Certain dietary restrictions may be required for several years following surgical repair of esophageal atresia.

Recurrent tracheoesophageal fistula may occur following surgery (Fig. 5). This will typically be seen at the surgical site and is presumed to be related to anastomotic leakage with erosion into the trachea caused by local inflammation. Despite fistula formation in the perioperative period, symptoms may be delayed. In addition to these recurrent fistulas, postoperative studies may also show a previously undiagnosed congenital tracheoesophageal fistula that was not identified at the time of surgery. Typically these are proximal to the site of the anastomosis and originate from the proximal esophageal segment. Therefore, some have advocated

the routine performance of a preoperative "pouchogram" by carefully instilling a small amount of contrast (preferably low-osmolar nonionic contrast) into the proximal esophageal pouch via a small-caliber feeding tube under fluoroscopic control. However, this study is not routinely requested by pediatric surgeons.

Common late complications after esophageal atresia repair include dysmotility, gastroesophageal reflux, tracheomalacia, rib fusion, and scoliosis. The most commonly identified abnormality following surgical repair of the esophagus is dysmotility. This finding is present in nearly all patients who have had esophageal atresia. Associated gastroesophageal reflux is very common in these patients and has been reported in 40% to 70% of cases. Reflux likely is related to shortening of the intra-abdominal portion of the esophagus, as a result of the congenital deformity itself and/or the reparative surgery. Reflux may lead to peptic esophagitis. This is likely the cause of the more distal esophageal strictures that can be seen in patients who have had a history of repaired esophageal atresia. Although hiatal hernia resulting from surgical traction on the lower esophageal segment following anastomosis has been reported, this is an unusual complication following surgery by trained pediatric surgeons. In utero impingement of the trachea by the dilated, fluid-filled proximal segment of the esophagus may narrow the tracheal lumen, leading to cough, stridor, and cyanosis. Griscom and Martin demonstrated a decrease in cross-sectional area of the trachea in patients with persistent respiratory symptoms 2 to 21 years after repair of esophageal atresia. Gilsanz et al. reported the occurrence of rib fusion and scoliosis

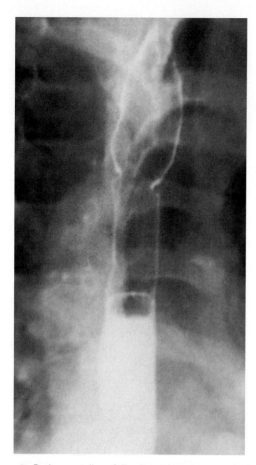

FIGURE 2. Barium swallow following primary anastomosis of an esophageal atresia demonstrates slight narrowing of the anastomotic site. The patient was asymptomatic and had no difficulty swallowing either fluids or soft solid foods.

as a long-term complication of thoracotomy for esophageal atresia. They suggested that this resulted from undiagnosed anastomotic leakage and mediastinitis.

> ■ **Late complications of esophageal atresia repair:**
> - Dysmotility
> - Gastroesophageal reflux
> - Tracheomalacia
> - Rib fusions
> - Scoliosis

Congenital stenoses at the junction of the middle and distal thirds of the esophagus can be seen in association with esophageal atresia/tracheoesophageal fistula (Fig. 6). Isolated stenoses in the esophagus (without esophageal atresia/tracheoesophageal fistula) may also occur rarely. Stenoses and lower esophageal webs probably represent variable manifestations of the same lesion. These congenital stenotic lesions are unlikely to be secondary to failure of proper vacuolization of the embryonically solid esophagus. They are often secondary to tracheobronchial or gastric remnants (Fig. 7). Fibromuscular thickening of the esophageal wall has been implicated in a number of cases of congenital stenosis. However, the question as to whether this could be a reaction to previous gastroesophageal reflux, no longer present, still needs to be considered. Anderson et al. reported a case of congenital esophageal stenosis secondary to a cartilage ring. Congenital esophageal stenoses in children can be treated by balloon dilatation. Upper cervical esophageal webs are quite rare in

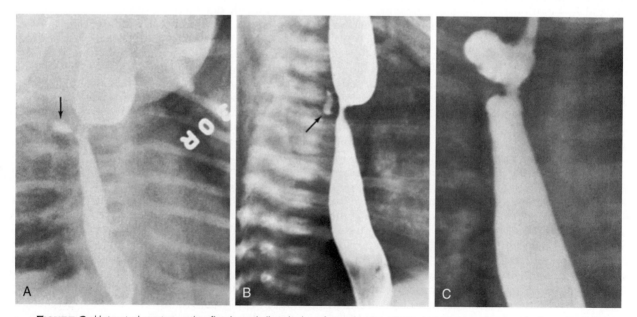

FIGURE 3. Untreated postoperative fistula and diverticulum formation in a 3-week-old infant who has had repair of an esophageal atresia and tracheoesophageal fistula. Anteroposterior **(A)** and lateral **(B)** spot films during fluoroscopy demonstrate a small leak of contrast material into the mediastinum *(arrow)*. **C,** Esophagogram 3 months later demonstrates a diverticulum at the level of the previously demonstrated mediastinal leakage.

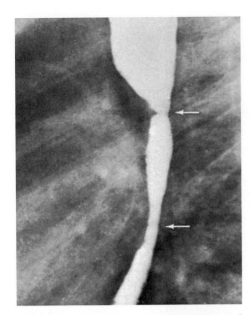

FIGURE 4. Postoperative stricture in a patient 5 years of age who had had successful primary repair of esophageal atresia and tracheoesophageal fistula. The esophagus is narrow at the site of primary anastomosis *(upper arrow)*. At the junction of its middle and lower thirds *(lower arrow)*, the esophagus is narrow and does not distend normally. Boluses of food had become impacted at this level.

children compared with the incidence in adults and are probably congenital in origin.

ISOLATED TRACHEOESOPHAGEAL FISTULAS

Congenital tracheoesophageal fistula without atresia is difficult to identify, both clinically and radiographically. These patients typically present with recurrent pneumonias either in infancy or later in childhood. Patients with unexplained chronic respiratory distress and recurrent pneumonia should always be considered at risk for the presence of a tracheoesophageal fistula, and radiographic examination is warranted.

Congenital tracheoesophageal fistula without atresia has commonly been called an H-fistula because of its appearance on an esophagogram, connecting the trachea and esophagus. However, the fistula typically runs cephalad from the esophagus to the trachea and looks more like an N (Fig. 8). Large fistulas usually present very early in life and are relatively easy to see on an esophagogram (Fig. 9). More commonly, the fistulas are small and inconstantly patent, and may require repeated examinations to identify.

Horizontal-beam fluoroscopy, with the patient lying prone on the footboard with the fluoroscopic table in the upright position, is probably not necessary in most cases. Certainly, such positioning is possible only in infancy. The examination, however, should be performed following passage of a nasoesophageal catheter. A major reason for inconstant patency of the fistula is that the normal esophageal mucosa is quite redundant and usually occludes the esophageal side of the fistula. Normal active swallowing may not distend the esophagus sufficiently to allow passage of contrast material into the fistula. The patient should be kept in the lateral recumbent position (with the right side down). The examiner withdraws the catheter from the distal esophagus cephalad, forcefully injecting contrast material to distend the esophagus maximally under constant fluoroscopic monitoring. If a fistula is present, it will be seen in the lateral projection extending anteriorly and cephalad from the esophagus to the trachea. Slightly oblique views may be necessary to see its full course. Unless a fistula is seen, the injection should continue until the catheter is withdrawn into the hypopharynx, but care must be taken not to allow contrast material to spill over into the trachea. The examination should be terminated as soon as a fistula is identified in order to minimize the amount of contrast material leaking into the airway.

FIGURE 5. Recurrent tracheoesophageal fistula. **A,** The proximal esophageal pouch is distended with contrast material, and overflow aspiration fills the trachea. The trachea is compressed from behind by the dilated proximal portion of the esophagus, and its lumen is narrowed. The fistula from trachea to distal esophagus is apparent. **B,** Lateral esophagogram demonstrates a recurrent tracheoesophageal fistula *(arrow)* at the site of the original fistula. The fistula had been ligated but not divided.

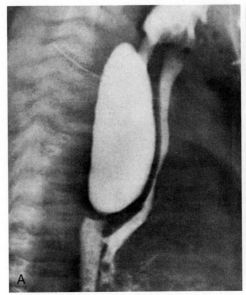
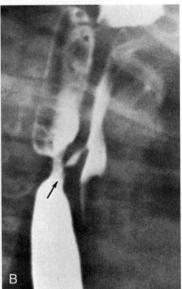

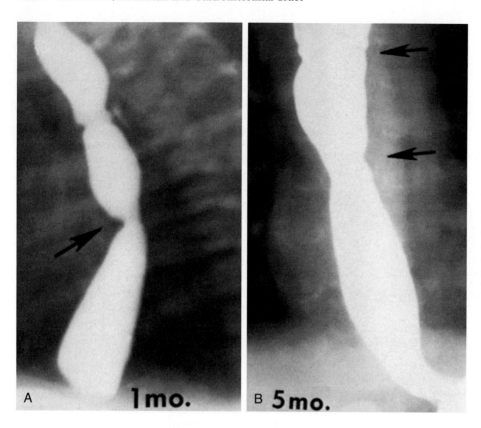

FIGURE 6. Congenital esophageal stenosis in an infant with surgical repair of esophageal atresia and tracheoesophageal fistula. **A,** A small esophageal mediastinal leak at the anastomotic site is seen posteriorly. The *arrow* demonstrates a fixed stenotic lesion distal to the site of the repair. **B,** Persistent narrowing is seen 5 months later at the same site *(lower arrow)* distal to the anastomosis *(upper arrow)*.

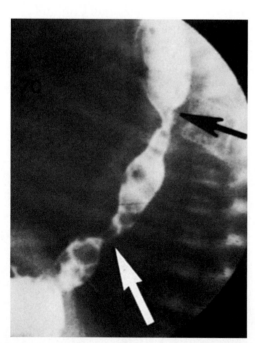

FIGURE 7. Esophagogram demonstrates stenosis in the distal portion of the esophagus *(lower arrow)* secondary to tracheal remnants. The *upper arrow* identifies narrowing at the level of the primary esophageal anastomosis following repair of esophageal atresia. (Courtesy of Dr. E. Afshani, Buffalo, NY.)

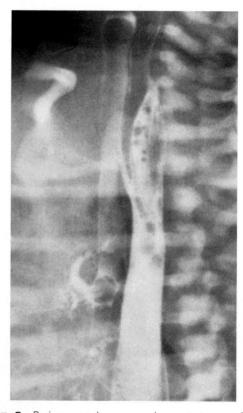

FIGURE 8. Barium esophagogram demonstrates an N-fistula between the esophagus and trachea. Note that the fistula runs cephalad and obliquely anteriorly from the esophagus to the trachea.

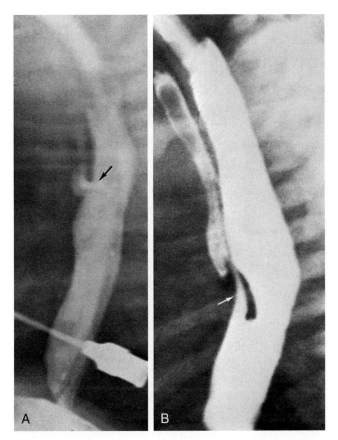

FIGURE 9. Large congenital tracheoesophageal fistula without esophageal atresia. **A,** The *arrow* points to the fistulous tract extending anteriorly and cephalad toward the tracheal lumen. **B,** A lower tracheoesophageal fistula *(arrow)* in a 7-day-old boy with imperforate anus.

Although there is a danger of spilling contrast material over into the airway with injection high in the cervical esophagus, it is important to examine this area because many of the fistulas will occur at the level of the lower cervical or upper thoracic spine. Slow retraction of the catheter and careful fluoroscopic monitoring will prevent overflow into the trachea. Multiple fistulas without atresia have been reported, but are extraordinarily rare. Filston et al. have catheterized tracheoesophageal fistulas per ora, but this method is little used by others. Bronchoscopy can play a complementary role to esophagography. Fistulas can be extremely difficult to identify, and repetitive examinations should be considered if the index of suspicion for the presence of a fistula is high. We have done as many as four esophagograms on patients before finally demonstrating a congenital tracheoesophageal fistula.

Rarely, a bronchus originates from the esophagus, resulting in an anomaly called esophagotrachea or esophageal bronchus (Fig. 10). This anomaly leads to severe respiratory distress with feeding and may be associated with esophageal atresia, tracheoesophageal fistula, or both. A bronchoesophageal fistula between the esophagus and a normal bronchial tree has also been described.

LARYNGOTRACHEOESOPHAGEAL CLEFTS

Laryngotracheoesophageal clefts are high fistulous communications between the hypopharynx and larynx. The cleft varies from a small communication between the larynx and esophagus to complete absence of the wall between esophagus and trachea—"persistent esophagotrachea." Patients with clefts typically present in infancy with respiratory distress during feeding. Stridor has been reported. Diagnosis is usually made by endoscopy or by contrast esophagogram (Fig. 11). Wilkinson et al. reported a case of a complete cleft in which the diagnosis was made by demonstration of a common tracheal and esophageal lumen on computed tomography (CT). The lumen persisted inferiorly to the carina, and hypoplasia of the right lung and cardiac dextroposition were also identified.

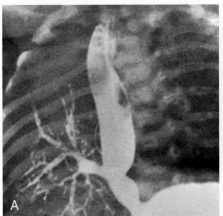
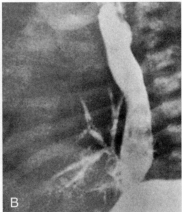
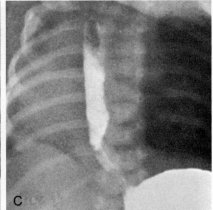

FIGURE 10. Esophageal bronchus (esophageal lung). Frontal **(A)** and oblique **(B)** views from an esophagogram in an infant 9 days of age show the right main bronchus originating from the distal end of the esophagus. **C,** The esophagus following right pneumonectomy.

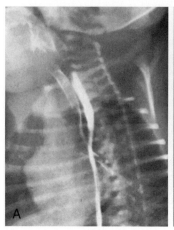
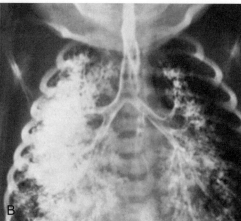

FIGURE 11. Laryngoesophageal cleft in a 2-week-old infant. **A,** Oblique projection shows barium in the esophagus and in the trachea. **B,** At fluoroscopy, persistent flow of barium into the trachea and bronchi was seen at the level of the larynx. No neuromuscular abnormalities were identified. A small laryngoesophageal cleft was identified endoscopically.

ESOPHAGEAL DUPLICATION CYSTS

Duplication cysts usually do not cause symptoms and are often identified incidentally on chest radiographs. Occasionally patients will present with symptoms of dysphasia as a result of esophageal compression. The differential diagnosis is listed in Table 1.

Duplication cysts associated with the esophagus can occur by three distinct embryologic processes leading to three varieties of duplications and/or cysts: esophageal duplication cysts with respiratory epithelium, neurenteric cysts, and true tubular duplications of the esophagus. *Esophageal duplication cysts with respiratory epithelium* represent bronchopulmonary foregut malformations that occur earlier in embryonic life than paratracheal, hilar, or carinal "bronchogenic" cysts (which are dis-

cussed in Section IV, Part VIII, page 1160 and Section V, Part I, page 1227). These cysts arise from the posterior portion of the foregut and contain mucosa that, by histologic examination, is usually gastric or, occasionally, intestinal (Fig. 12).

Table 1 ■ DIFFERENTIAL DIAGNOSIS OF ESOPHAGEAL DUPLICATION CYST
Bronchogenic cyst
Neurogenic tumors
Neuroblastoma
Ganglioneuroblastoma
Ganglioglioma
Hiatal hernia
Aortic arch congenital anomaly
Aortic aneurysm

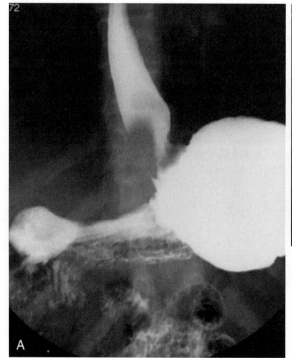
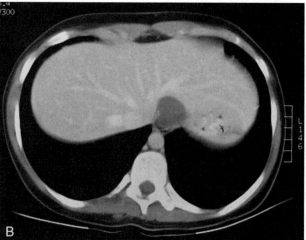

FIGURE 12. Distal esophageal duplication cyst incidentally found in a 15-year-old girl without symptoms of dysphagia. **A,** Anteroposterior view of the esophagus from an upper gastrointestinal series reveals an impression on the esophagus. **B,** Axial computed tomography section confirms the intramural esophageal cyst.

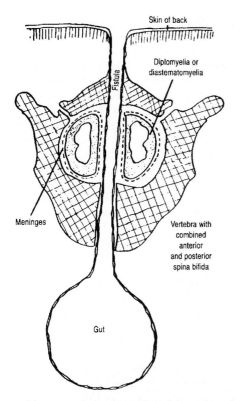

FIGURE 13. Diagrammatic representation of the archetypical dorsal enteric fistula. (From Naidich TP, McLone DG, Harwood-Nash DC: Spinal dysraphism. *In* Newton TH, Potts DG [eds]: Computed Tomography of the Spine and Spinal Cord. San Anselmo, CA, Clavadel Press, 1983:299–353, with permission.)

By contrast, *neurenteric cysts* have a distinct embryologic origin that is part of the "split notochord syndrome." The notochord forms during the third embryonic week and separates the ectoderm from the endoderm. If this separation is incomplete and leaves an adhesion between the endoderm and ectoderm, the notochord either splits to encircle the adhesion or deviates to the left or right of the adhesion. The archetype of this spectrum of anomalies is the dorsal enteric fistula, a patent communication between the gut and the dorsal midline skin surface that traverses the vertebral body (or interspace), the spinal canal and its contents, and the posterior vertebral elements (Fig. 13). As in the analogous urachal or vitelline duct remnants, some or all of the patent communication in the dorsal enteric fistula can become obliterated, leading to residual diverticula, cysts, and fibrous cords that give rise to a spectrum of anomalies, including

- A dorsal enteric sinus (a blind-ending, enteric-lined tract from the dorsal skin surface)
- An isolated dorsal enteric cyst (enteric-lined cyst derived from the intermediate portion of the tract with obliteration of the communication with the gut and skin surface), which can be prevertebral, intraspinal (Fig. 14), or postvertebral
- A dorsal enteric diverticulum (a blind-ending diverticulum from the gut), which may be intrathoracic or intra-abdominal or may cross the diaphragm

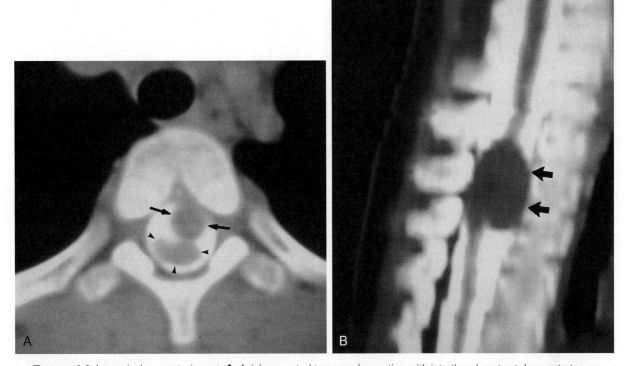

FIGURE 14. Intraspinal neurenteric cyst. **A,** Axial computed tomography section with intrathecal contrast demonstrates an intraspinal mass *(arrows)* anterior to the compressed spinal cord *(arrowheads)* surgically proven to represent an intraspinal neurenteric cyst. Note the associated congenital cleft in the vertebral body. **B,** Sagittal reformation confirms the anterior cyst *(arrows)* compressing the cord posteriorly.

Neurenteric cysts may be associated with congenital vertebral anomalies (which can help differentiate these congenital anomalies from other posterior mediastinal masses such as neuroblastoma) as well as spinal cord and meningeal anomalies. These cysts are more common in the right hemithorax.

True tubular duplications (Fig. 15) of the esophagus are even more rare than enteric cysts. These cysts may extend below the diaphragm to involve the stomach as well. They may communicate with the stomach or esophagus and be demonstrable on esophagogram. These duplications likely develop from faulty recanalization of the esophageal lumen.

The choice of imaging modalities for the evaluation of esophageal duplication cysts and neurenteric cysts will be influenced by the patient's presentation. Plain radio-graphs may demonstrate a sharply demarcated posterior mediastinal mass or congenital vertebral anomalies associated with neurenteric cysts. Esophagograms will show an intramural mass or displacement of the esophagus by the mass, but typically no connection between the two structures. Ultrasound can confirm the cystic nature of the mass, but is rarely utilized. CT and magnetic resonance imaging (MRI) are the modalities of choice to confirm the cystic nature of the mass and to best delineate the abnormality (see Figs. 12, 14, and 15). The cyst fluid typically has attenuation of water on CT (H.U. = 0 to 20) and signal characteristics of water on MRI (low signal on T_1 weighting and high signal on T_2 weighting). However, attenuation on CT and signal intensity on T_1-weighted MRI may be increased as a result of hemorrhage, infection, or increased protein.

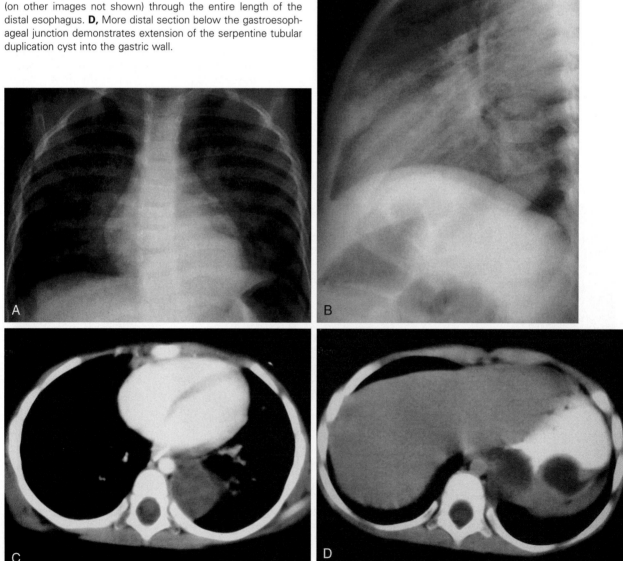

FIGURE 15. Tubular esophageal duplication cyst in a 5-year-old girl. Anteroposterior **(A)** and lateral **(B)** chest radiographs reveal a retrocardiac soft tissue mass. **C,** Axial computed tomography confirms a cystic mass in the posterior mediastinum that extends (on other images not shown) through the entire length of the distal esophagus. **D,** More distal section below the gastroesophageal junction demonstrates extension of the serpentine tubular duplication cyst into the gastric wall.

Furthermore, CT and MRI may be helpful in evaluating vertebral or intraspinal abnormalities associated with neurenteric cysts. Those enteric cysts that contain gastric mucosa with acid and pepsin secretion can be identified by nuclear imaging. They may ulcerate or hemorrhage, leading to draining sinuses in the thoracic wall, esophageal necrosis and perforation, and communication with other intrathoracic structures. Massive hemorrhage from ulceration has been reported.

■ Chest radiograph/esophagogram findings with esophageal duplication cyst include the following:
- Common
  1. Posterior mediastinal mass
  2. Sharp margins
  3. Displacement of esophagus on esophagogram
  4. Intramural esophageal mass
- Less common
  1. Congenital vertebral anomalies (neurenteric cyst)
  2. Communication with esophagus on esophagogram

■ Computed tomography (CT)/magnetic resonance imaging (MRI) findings with esophageal duplication cyst include the following:
- Common
  1. Cystic posterior mediastinal mass
  2. Sharp margins
  3. Avascular following intravenous contrast
- Less common
  1. Higher attenuation (CT), elevated signal (T_1-weighted MRI) associated with hemorrhage, infection, or elevated protein
  2. Tubular duplications extending below diaphragm to include stomach
  3. Associated vertebral anomalies in neurenteric cysts
  4. Intraspinal neurenteric cysts
  5. Dorsal enteric diverticula (thoracic and/or abdominal diverticula communicating with gastrointestinal tract)

SUGGESTED READINGS

Esophageal Atresia

Anderson LS, Shackelford GD, Mancilla-Jimenez R, et al: Cartilaginous esophageal ring: a cause of esophageal stenosis in infants and children. Radiology 1973;108:665

Briceno LI, Grases PJ, Gallego S: Tracheobronchial and pancreatic remnants causing esophageal stenosis. J Pediatr Surg 1981;16:731

Burge DM: Gastric tube interposition: a new technique for the management of long-gap oesophageal atresia. Pediatr Surg Int 1995;10:279

Chittmittrapap S, Spitz L, Kiely EM, et al: Anastomotic leakage following surgery for esophageal atresia. J Pediatr Surg 1992;27:29

Dominguez R, Zarabi M, Oh KS, et al: Congenital oesophageal stenosis. Clin Radiol 1985;36:263

Donnelly LF, Frush DP, Bisset GS: The appearance and significance of extrapleural fluid after esophageal atresia repair. AJR Am J Roentgenol 1999;172:231

Dudley NE, Phelan PD: Respiratory complications in long-term survivors of oesophageal atresia. Arch Dis Child 1976;51:279

Ein SH, Handling B: Pure esophageal atresia: a 50-year review. J Pediatr Surg 1994;29:1208

Freeman NV, Cass DT: Colon interposition: a modification of the Waterston technique using the normal esophageal route. J Pediatr Surg 1982;17:17

Garau P, Orenstein SR: Congenital esophageal stenosis treated by balloon dilatation. J Pediatr Gastroenterol Nutr 1993;16:98

Gilsanz V, Boechat IM, Birnbert FA, et al: Scoliosis after thoracotomy for esophageal atresia. AJR Am J Roentgenol 1983;141:457

Grabowski ST, Andrews DA: Upper esophageal stenosis: two case reports. J Pediatr Surg 1996;31:1438

Griscom NT, Martin TR: Trachea and esophagus after repair of esophageal atresia and distal fistula. Pediatr Radiol 1990;20:447

Harmon CM, Coran AG: Congenital anomalies of the esophagus. In O'Neill JA, Rowe MI, Grosfeld JL, et al (eds): Pediatric Surgery, 5th ed. St. Louis, Mosby, 1998:941–967

Jolley SG, Herbst JJ, Johnson DG, et al: Patterns of gastroesophageal reflux in children following repair of esophageal atresia and distal tracheoesophageal fistula. J Pediatr Surg 1980;15:857

Kirkpatrick JA, Cresson SL, Pilling GP IV: The motor activity of the esophagus in association with esophageal atresia and tracheoesophageal fistula. Am J Roentgenol Radium Ther Nucl Med 1961;86:884

Kirks DR, Filston HC: The association of esophageal duplication cyst with esophageal atresia. Pediatr Radiol 1981;11:214

Kleinman PK, Waite RJ, Cohen IT, et al: Atretic esophagus: transgastric balloon-assisted hydrostatic dilatation. Radiology 1989;171:831

Montedonico S, Diez-Pardo JA, Possogel AK, et al: Effects of esophageal shortening on the gastroesophageal barrier: an experimental study on the causes of reflux in esophageal atresia. J Pediatr Surg 1999;34:300

Murphy SB, Yazbeck S, Russo P: Isolated congenital esophageal stenosis. J Pediatr Surg 1995;30:1238

Nakazato Y, Landing BH, Wells TR: Abnormal Auerbach plexus in the esophagus and stomach of patients with esophageal atresia and tracheoesophageal fistula. J Pediatr Surg 1986;21:831

Nakazato Y, Wells TR, Landing BH: Abnormal tracheal innervation in patients with esophageal atresia and tracheoesophageal fistula: study of the intrinsic tracheal nerve plexuses by a microdissection technique. J Pediatr Surg 1986;21:838

Newman B, Bender TM: Esophageal atresia/tracheoesophageal fistula and associated congenital esophageal stenosis. Pediatr Radiol 1997;27:530

Nishina T, Tsuchida Y, Saito S: Congenital esophageal stenosis due to tracheobronchial remnants and its associated anomalies. J Pediatr Surg 1981;16:190

Osman MZ, Girdany BR: Traumatic pseudodiverticulums of the pharynx in infants and children. Ann Radiol 1973;16:143

Poznanski AK: The uppergastrointestinal tract. In Practical Approaches to Pediatric Radiology. Chicago, Year Book Medical Publishers, 1976:93–124

Rescorla FJ, West KW Scherer LR, et al: The complex nature of type A (long-gap) esophageal atresia. Surgery 1994;116:658

Skandalakis JE, Gray SW, Ricketts RR: Esophagus. In Skandalakis JE, Gray SW (eds): Embryology for Surgeons, 2nd ed. Baltimore, Williams & Wilkins, 1994:64–112

Sheridan J, Hyde I: Oesophageal stenosis distal to oesophageal atresia. Clin Radiol 1990;42:274

Spitz L: Esophageal atresia and tracheoesophageal fistula in children. Curr Opin Pediatr 1993;5:347

Stringer DA, Ein SH: Recurrent tracheo-esophageal fistula: a protocol for investigation. Radiology 1984;151:637

Stringer DA, Pablot SM, Mancer K: Grüntzig angioplasty dilatation of an esophageal stricture in an infant. Pediatr Radiol 1985;15:424

Thomason MA, Gay BB: Esophageal stenosis with esophageal atresia. Pediatr Radiol 1987;17:197

Tsai JY, Berkery L, Wesson DE, et al: Esophageal atresia and tracheoesophageal fistula: surgical experience over two decades. Ann Thorac Surg 1997;64:778

Yeung CK, Spitz L, Brereton RJ: Congenital esophageal stenosis due to tracheobronchial remnants: a rare but important association with esophageal atresia. J Pediatr Surg 1992;27:852

Isolated Tracheoesophageal Fistulas

Filston HC, Rankin JS, Kirks DR: The diagnosis of primary and recurrent tracheosophageal fistulas: value of selective catheterization. J Pediatr Surg 1982;17:144

Harmon CM, Coran AG: Congenital anomalies of the esophagus. *In* O'Neill JA, Rowe MI, Grosfeld JL, et al (eds): Pediatric Surgery, 5th ed. St. Louis, Mosby, 1998:941–967

Johnson JF, Sueoka BL, Mulligan ME, et al: Tracheo-esophageal fistula: diagnosis with CT. Pediatr Radiol 1985;15:134

Karnack I, Senocak ME, Hicsonmez A, et al: The diagnosis and treatment of H-type tracheoesophageal fistula. J Pediatr Surg 1997;32:1670

Kemp JL, Sullivan LM: Bronchoesophageal fistula in an 11-month-old boy. Pediatr Radiol 1997;27:811

Lacasse JE, Reilly BJ, Mancer K: Segmental esophageal trachea: a potentially fatal type of tracheal stenosis. AJR Am J Roentgenol 1980;134:829

Lallemand D, Quignodon JF, Courtel JV: The anomalous origin of bronchus from the esophagus: report of three cases. Pediatr Radiol 1996;26:179

Sieber WK, Girdany BR: Tracheo-esophageal fistula without esophageal atresia, congenital and recurrent. Pediatrics 1956;18:935

Laryngotracheal Cleft

Burroughs N, Leape LL: Laryngotracheoesophageal cleft: report of a case successfully treated and review of the literature. Pediatrics 1974;53:516

Griscom NT: Persistent esophagotrachea: the most severe degree of laryngotracheo-esophageal cleft. Am J Roentgenol Radium Ther Nucl Med 1966;97:211

Morgan CL, Grossman H, Leonidas J: Roentgenographic findings in a spectrum of uncommon tracheoesophageal anomalies. Clin Radiol 1979;30:353

Wilkinson AG, Mackenzie S, Hendry GMA: Complete laryngotracheoesophageal cleft: CT diagnosis and associated abnormalities. Clin Radiol 1990;41:437

Esophageal Duplication Cysts

Aoki S, Machida T, Sasaki Y, et al: Enterogenous cyst of cervical spine: clinical and radiological aspects (including CT and MR). Neuroradiology 1987;29:291

Chang SH, Morrison L, Shaffner L, et al: Intrathoracic gastrogenic cysts and hemoptysis. J Pediatr 1976;88:594

Chitale AR: Gastric cysts of the mediastinum. J Pediatr 1969;75:104

Fitch SJ, Tonkin ILD, Tonkin AK: Imaging of foregut duplication cysts. Radiographics 1986;6:189

Hemalatha V, Batcup G, Brereton RJ, et al: Intrathoracic foregut cyst (foregut duplication) associated with esophageal atresia. J Pediatr Surg 1980;15:178

Hernandez RJ: Role of CT in the evaluation of children with foregut cysts. Pediatr Radiol 1987;17:265

Kamoi I, Nishitani H, Oshiumi Y, et al: Intrathoracic gastric cyst demonstrated by ^{99m}Tc pertechnetate scintigraphy. AJR Am J Roentgenol 1980;134:1081

Kantrowitz LR, Pais MJ, Burnett K, et al: Intraspinal neurenteric cyst containing gastric mucosa: CT and MR findings. Pediatr Radiol 1986;16:324

Naidich TP, McLone DG, Harwood-Nash DC: Spinal dysraphism. *In* Newton TH, Potts DG (eds): Computed Tomography of the Spine and Spinal Cord. San Anselmo, CA, Clavadel Press, 1983:299–353

Rafal RB, Markisz JA: Magnetic resonance imaging of an esophageal duplication cyst. Am J Gastroenterol 1991;86:1809

Rhee RS, Ray CG, Kravetz MH, et al: Cervical esophageal duplication cyst: MR imaging. J Comput Assist Tomogr 1988;12:693

Skandalakis JE, Gray SW, Ricketts RR: Esophagus. *In* Skandalakis JE, Gray SW (eds): Embryology for Surgeons, 2nd ed. Baltimore, Williams & Wilkins, 1994:64–112

Snyder ME, Luck SR, Hernandez R, et al: Diagnostic dilemmas of mediastinal cysts. J Pediatr Surg 1985;20:810

Sumner TE, Auringer ST, Cox TD: A complex communicating bronchopulmonary foregut malformation: diagnostic imaging and pathogenesis. Pediatr Radiol 1997;27:799

Superina RA, Ein SH, Humphreys RP: Cystic duplications of the esophagus and neurenteric cysts. J Pediatr Surg 1984;19:527

Chapter   4

ACQUIRED ESOPHAGEAL LESIONS

ALAN E. SCHLESINGER and BRUCE R. PARKER

NONINFECTIVE ESOPHAGITIS

The most common cause of noninfective esophagitis in children is gastroesophageal reflux. This entity is discussed separately in Section VI, Part V, Chapter 5, page 1569.

CAUSTIC INGESTION

Ingestion of caustic agents is becoming less common as parents and other caregivers have become more cognizant of the dangers to children of careless storage of household agents. Nevertheless, the effects of caustic ingestion are still commonly seen and can be devastating. Acidic compounds typically affect the stomach, while caustic esophagitis is usually secondary to alkalis, most commonly household lye compounds, which are a mixture of sodium and potassium hydroxide. Burns of the mouth may not be seen or may be superficial because the time of contact is short. The upper esophagus is less likely to be affected than the middle or lower portions because transient cardiospasm may increase the time of contact between the agent and the lower esophageal mucosa. However, granules may stick to the proximal

esophageal mucosa and are more likely to affect this portion of the esophagus than liquid caustic alkalis.

> ■ Caustic ingestion with acidic compounds typically affect the stomach while alkali ingestion usually causes caustic esophagitis.

Swelling of the epiglottis (Fig. 1A) indicates that the caustic agent has reached the hypopharynx and likely has been swallowed into the esophagus. In fact, with decreasing incidence of bacterial epiglottitis caused by the *Haemophilus influenzae* type B vaccine, more "unusual" causes of epiglottic enlargement, such as caustic ingestion, should be considered when a young child with epiglottic enlargement is seen. Initial chest radiographs may reveal evidence of mediastinitis with mediastinal widening and a dilated, gas-filled esophagus. Inflammation of the pharynx may cause disordered swallowing (Fig. 1B) with subsequent aspiration. Contrast esophagography is preferable to endoscopy because traumatic perforation may occur when an endoscope is used. Spontaneous perforation may occur, as may deep ulceration and tracheoesophageal fistulas.

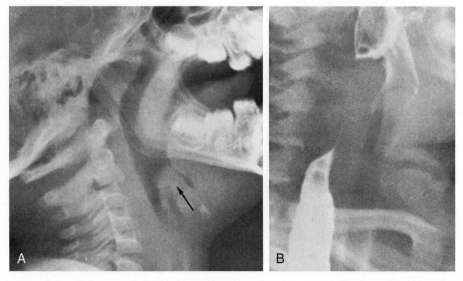

FIGURE 1. A, Lateral view of the nasopharynx demonstrates the epiglottis to be swollen *(arrow)* 20 hours after the injection of caustic material. **B,** Barium swallow 2 weeks later demonstrates the proximal segment of the cervical esophagus to be narrow, with aspiration of contrast material into the trachea.

Therefore, the initial examination is preferably performed with low-osmolar, nonionic contrast material. If no perforation or fistula is seen, barium will provide better coating for thorough evaluation of the mucosa.

> ■ Swelling of the epiglottis indicates that the ingested agent has reached the hypopharynx and likely the esophagus.

Mucosal irregularity, esophageal dysmotility, and ulceration may all be seen in the acute or subacute phase (Fig. 2). Reactive fibrosis of the esophageal wall may cause the appearance of a stenotic, rigid tube on fluoroscopy (Fig. 3). Ultimately, esophageal stricture develops (Fig. 4), necessitating esophagectomy and esophageal replacement (typically with ileum and/or colon) in the worst cases. Epithelial metaplasia (Barrett's esophagus) may occur, as may development of esophageal carcinoma in adulthood.

EPIDERMOLYSIS BULLOSA DYSTROPHICA

Epidermolysis bullosa dystrophica is a congenital disease affecting squamous epithelium and causing esophagitis. The skin has numerous bullous lesions that are friable and easily abraded, with sloughing of the skin even after the most minimal contact. These patients should not be restrained unless supervised by a derma-

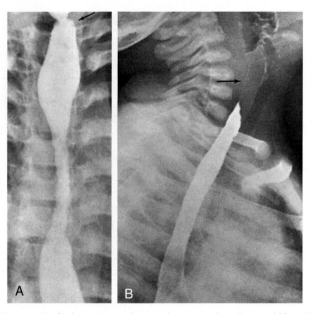

FIGURE 3. **A,** Anteroposterior esophagogram in a 7-year-old boy 5 years following ingestion of lye demonstrates narrowing of the midportion of the esophagus. The *arrow* indicates traumatic stricture of the esophagus secondary to multiple attempts at dilatation. **B,** Lateral esophagogram of the same patient shortly after ingestion of lye. Aspiration of barium into the proximal portion of the trachea and narrowing of the proximal portion of the esophagus are identified *(arrow)*.

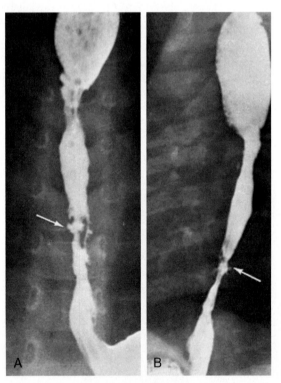

FIGURE 2. Esophagograms in anteroposterior **(A)** and lateral **(B)** projections demonstrate multiple levels of narrowing, irregularity, and marginal ulcerations *(arrows)* in a patient 6 weeks following ingestion of lye.

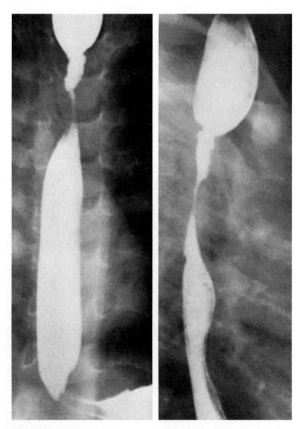

FIGURE 4. Stricture of the esophagus in a 4-year-old boy 3 weeks after he had swallowed several tablets that contained anhydrous sodium hydroxide and copper sulfite.

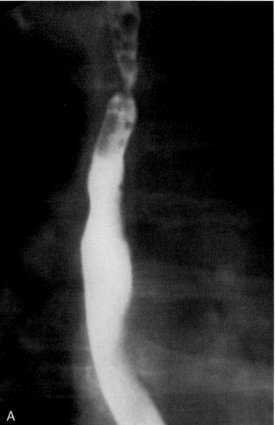
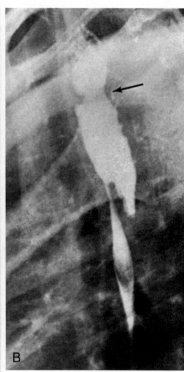

FIGURE 5. Epidermolysis bullosa dystrophica. **A,** Anteroposterior view of esophagogram demonstrates focal stricture formation in a 3-year-old girl. **B,** Esophagogram in a different patient showing an annular stenosis just below the thoracic inlet *(arrow).* Below this and posteriorly, a barium-filled pocket suggests an ulcer and submucosal abscess. (**B** courtesy of Dr. Melvin Becker, New York, NY.)

tologist. Every effort must be made to have the child drink spontaneously during esophagography because even the minimal trauma caused by a Silastic feeding tube may damage the esophageal epithelium. Loss of motility, mucosal irregularity, ulceration, and stenosis may be found in these unfortunate children (Fig. 5). Esophageal replacement may be necessary in children with severe strictures.

MISCELLANEOUS CAUSES

Crohn's disease of the esophagus is rarely seen on imaging studies but is being described with increasing frequency by endoscopists. Studies comparing endoscopy with esophagography confirm increased sensitivity of endoscopic evaluation. When abnormalities are identified on esophagograms, ulceration and stricture are the most common findings. The same finding may be seen in *Behçet's syndrome,* which also may cause an ileocolitis resembling Crohn's disease. The additional multisystem findings of Behçet's syndrome affecting skin, mucous membranes, uvea, and central nervous system can differentiate these two entities, although they are not always present in children. Focal areas of esophageal narrowing can be seen as a rare finding in *chronic granulomatous disease* of childhood, with esophageal stricture caused by the primary disease (presumably granulomatous infiltration) rather than by opportunistic infection. McDonald et al. have described the

esophageal lesions of *graft-versus-host disease* in patients who underwent bone marrow transplantation. Webs, ring-like narrowing, and smoothly tapering strictures may be seen on barium studies. *Radiation esophagitis* from low-dose radiation therapy may be manifested by esophageal inflammation with resultant dysmotility, but rarely produces long-term effects. High-dose (above 25 Gy) radiation therapy is uncommonly used in young children but may lead to dysmotility, mucosal edema, superficial and deep ulceration, and stricture at any age. Similar findings have been described in patients exposed to a variety of chemotherapeutic agents, including antibiotics and quinidine as well as anticancer agents. The combined effects of radiation therapy and doxorubicin (Adriamycin) are especially likely to lead to esophagitis, as well as cardiac and other complications, because of their synergistic actions.

INFECTIVE ESOPHAGITIS

Although occasionally reported in immune-competent children, these lesions are usually secondary to opportunistic organisms and are seen in children who are immunocompromised as a result of congenital or acquired immunodeficiency syndromes or from immunosuppressive drugs. The most common infective agent is *Candida albicans (Monilia),* but viral agents such as cytomegalovirus (CMV) and herpes simplex virus may cause esophagitis. In adult patients with acquired immunodeficiency syndrome, esophageal infection from human immunodeficiency virus and from mycobacteria has also been reported. Although some have advocated routine use of endoscopy in immune-compromised children with symptoms of esophagitis, this position is controversial and esophagography is frequently performed.

Double-contrast examinations of the esophagus are more likely to be diagnostic than single-contrast studies, but these may be difficult to perform in young or uncooperative children. In children with candidal esophagitis, dysmotility, elevated focal lesions (nodules or plaques), and mucosal edema are the common findings (Fig. 6). A "shaggy mucosa" or "cobblestone" appearance may result from barium filling the interstices between plaques and/or necrotic debris. However, the characteristic "shaggy mucosa" of candidiasis is actually nonspecific and may be seen in the viral esophagitides as well. Eventually deep ulcerations may develop, but frank ulcers are more common with herpes and CMV esophagitis. Even if cultures are positive for *Monilia,* concomitant viral infection should be suspected if ulcers are seen (Fig. 7). Pseudodiverticula may form as well.

CMV causes a vasculitis by invading the capillary endothelial cells and eventually leads to ischemic necrosis and ulceration. In addition to the classical large ulcers, linear ulcers, nodular thickening, "cobblestone" appearance, pseudodiverticula, and strictures may occur. Herpes simplex virus typically causes shallow ulcers that are stellate or diamond shaped and rarely causes linear or longitudinal ulcers. *Mycobacterium tuberculosis*

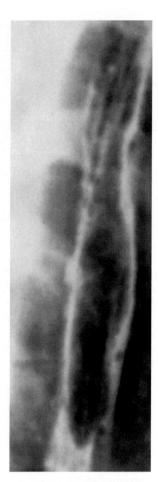

FIGURE 7. Double-contrast esophagogram in a leukemic patient severely immunocompromised by chemotherapy. Dysmotility, irregularity, inflammation, and small ulcers are seen. Esophagitis was due to combined candidiasis and cytomegalovirus infection in this patient.

can invade the esophagus by direct spread from adjacent mediastinal lymph nodes and may cause fistulas or sinus tracts.

DIVERTICULA

Diverticula of the esophagus proper are rare in children. Pulsion or pressure diverticula are herniations of the mucosa and submucosa through congenitally weak sites of the esophageal wall; little or none of the muscular layer is incorporated into the walls of such diverticula. Simple pressure diverticula are usually located above the clavicles and extend from a lateral wall of the esophagus posteriorly, where, after enlargement, they may displace the esophageal channel anteriorly and compress it. They are best seen in lateral and oblique projections, in which they appear as rounded pouches filled with barium; they fill quickly and empty relatively slowly. Traction diverticula are anterior or, less commonly, lateral projections of the esophageal lumen. Their walls may be made up of mucosa alone. However, more typically, all of the esophageal mural layers are present. They usually occur just below the tracheal bifurcation. The traction is caused by the fibrous

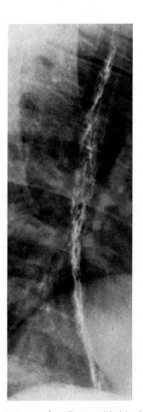

FIGURE 6. Esophagogram of a 15-year-old girl with aplastic anemia demonstrates marginal mucosal irregularities. The patient had documented moniliasis.

contraction of fibrotic lymph nodes and paraesophageal areolar tissue. Roentgenographically, they appear as triangular pouches that empty quickly. They are usually of little clinical importance except that they may be the sites of impaction and perforation of foreign bodies.

FOREIGN BODIES AND TRAUMA

Foreign bodies may be swallowed at any age. Even the youngest infants may be fed unusual articles by an obliging older sibling. Although the older child or parent may give a history of foreign body ingestion, young children often present with unexplained drooling, inability to swallow solids, or, less commonly, chest pain. Radiopaque foreign bodies are easily identified on plain radiographs. Smooth objects, such as coins, the most commonly ingested foreign bodies, usually are seen at the thoracic inlet. Less commonly, they will stop at the level of the left main stem bronchus or just above the esophagogastric junction. If coins are seen at other levels, underlying esophageal abnormalities should be considered. Sharp objects, pins being the most common, may present anywhere along the course of the esophagus if they penetrate mucosa (Fig. 8). Food, plastic and aluminum articles, and buttons are the most common nonopaque esophageal foreign bodies.

Plain radiographs of the chest and neck (including a lateral view of the upper airway that includes the nasopharynx, because foreign bodies can be placed in the nose or can reflux into the nasopharynx once placed in the mouth) should be the first imaging examination. Coins in the esophagus lie in the coronal plane (Fig. 9), while those in the trachea lie in the sagittal plane, presumably because of the anatomy of the tracheal rings. Fernbach and Tucker described development of erosions in a penny lodged in the esophagus in a child. In vitro experimentation revealed that the rapid development of erosions occurred only in pennies made after 1982, when the penny was changed to a copper-plated zinc-based coin (Fig. 10). Longstanding foreign bodies may have perforated, leading to pneumomediastinum or mediastinal mass (Fig. 11). A foreign body such as incompletely chewed food may cause high-grade obstruction with air–fluid levels in the esophagus or a frothy appearance from mixed air and fluid. Impacted food most often occurs in patients who have underlying esophageal abnormalities.

Nonopaque foreign bodies may require esophagograms for diagnosis. Because the degree of potential obstruction is unknown before the examination, only a small amount of opaque material should be given initially. Spot images should be obtained in anteroposterior and lateral views. Contrast studies generally are not performed when an opaque foreign body is identified; however, they may be useful if there is concern about edema, stricture, or perforation. Low-osmolarity contrast should be used in such cases. Currarino and Nikaidoh reported four cases of foreign bodies in patients with vascular rings and suggested that esophagograms be performed if there is clinical suspicion of such an anomaly. Herman and McAlister reported two cases of traumatic diverticula in patients with unsuspected foreign bodies.

The removal of radiopaque esophageal foreign bodies by radiologists using Foley catheters is a highly contentious subject. The procedure was initially popularized by Campbell and colleagues, who reported high success rates with no significant complications. Using their patient selection criteria and methods, many pediatric radiologists enjoyed great success with the procedure, which reduced hospital time and financial cost to the patient manyfold. More recent reports, especially in the surgical literature, have raised doubts in the minds of many radiologists as to the wisdom of continuing to remove foreign bodies by this method because of the risk of complications. Furthermore, the higher success rate of esophagoscopy relative to this technique has led some radiologists to recommend esophagoscopy as the primary method for esophageal foreign body extraction. Others have continued to report a high degree of success and few complications with the Foley catheter technique. This procedure typically is contraindicated if an underlying esophageal

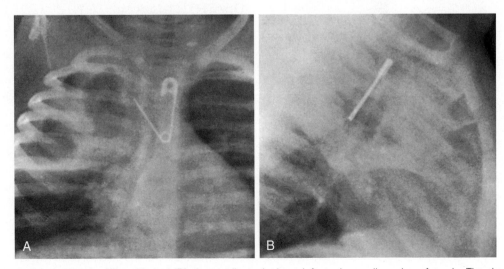

FIGURE 8. Anteroposterior **(A)** and lateral **(B)** chest radiographs in an infant who swallowed a safety pin. The sharp point of the pin projects through the wall of the esophagus and produces inflammatory changes in the adjacent lung and pleura.

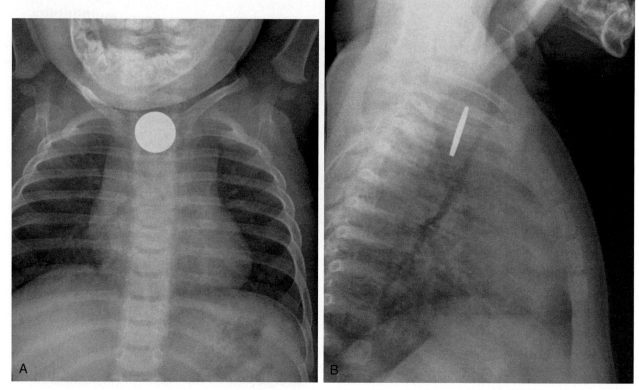

FIGURE 9. Anteroposterior **(A)** and lateral **(B)** chest radiographs demonstrate a coin lodged in the esophagus at the level of the thoracic inlet. Soft tissue thickening between the coin in the esophagus and the air within the trachea, as well as focal narrowing of the tracheal air column, suggest edema of the esophageal wall and paraesophageal soft tissues, implying that the coin has been in the esophagus for a prolonged period of time.

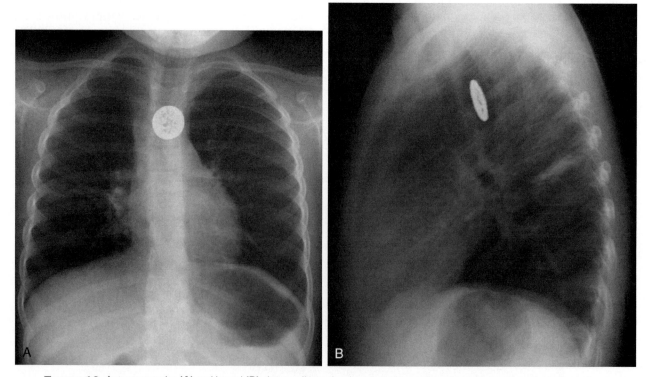

FIGURE 10. Anteroposterior **(A)** and lateral **(B)** chest radiographs demonstrate a coin with multiple areas of erosion lodged in the esophagus.

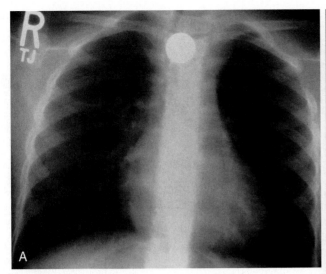

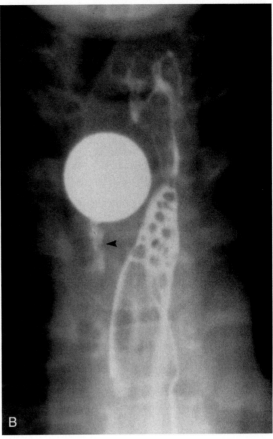

FIGURE 11. A, Anteroposterior chest radiograph demonstrates a coin overlying the mediastinum. The trachea is effaced and displaced to the right. **B,** Anteroposterior view from an esophagogram demonstrates that the coin is extraluminal in location. Surgery confirmed that the esophagus was perforated, and the coin was in a walled-off chronic abscess. A small amount of contrast entered the abscess cavity *(arrowhead).*

abnormality is present or if edema is identified on a lateral chest or airway radiograph (as evidenced by increased soft tissue between the esophageal foreign body and the air-filled adjacent trachea) (see Fig. 9B). In general, balloon-catheter removal is not recommended if the foreign body has been present for 24 hours or longer. Nonopaque foreign bodies, identified on esophagogram, can also be removed by this method.

■ Edema of the esophageal wall on lateral chest radiograph suggests that foreign body extraction with Foley catheter likely will be unsuccessful and complications may be more likely.

The other common cause of esophageal trauma is placement of tubes and catheters, which may perforate the pharynx or esophagus. Abrupt onset of new respiratory symptoms; unusual catheter position; air in the soft tissues of the neck, chest, or mediastinum; and unexplained malfunction of the tube or catheter should lead one to suspect possible perforation. Uncomplicated perforations usually resolve, but strictures may occur. A traumatic pseudodiverticulum may result (see Section VI, Part V, Chapter 2, Fig. 4, page 1547). If a contrast study is necessary after inconclusive plain film examination, low-osmolar, nonionic water-soluble contrast material should be used. In patients with prior esophageal

strictures, perforation may also occur as a result of dilatation therapy.

Severe vomiting may lead to hematemesis as a result of tears in the esophageal mucosa (the Mallory-Weiss syndrome). Spontaneous esophageal rupture (Boerhaave's syndrome) may occur in infants, presumably secondary to increased esophageal pressure from any one of several causes and typically presents with hydropneumothorax. Both syndromes are extraordinarily rare in childhood.

SUGGESTED READINGS

Noninfective Esophagitis

Amoury RA, Hrabovsky EE, Leonidas JC, et al: Tracheo-esophageal fistula after lye ingestion. J Pediatr Surg 1975;10:273–276

Appelvist P, Salmo M: Lye corrosion carcinoma of the esophagus. Cancer 1980;45:2655

Becker MH, Swinyard CA: Epidermolysis bullosa dystrophica in children: radiologic manifestations. Radiology 1968;90:124

Canty TG, LoSasso BE: One-stage esophagectomy and in situ colon interposition for esophageal replacement in children. J Pediatr Surg 1997;32:334

Creteur V, Laufer I, Kressel HY, et al: Drug-induced esophagitis detected by double-contrast radiography. Radiology 1983;147:365

Daunt N, Brodribb TR, Dickey JD: Oesophageal ulceration due to doxycycline. Br J Radiol 1985;58:1209

Franken EA Jr: Caustic damage of the gastrointestinal tract: roentgen features. Am J Roentgenol Radium Ther Nucl Med 1973;118:77

Hillemeier C, Touloukian R, McCallum R, et al: Esophageal web: a previously unrecognized complication of epidermolysis bullosa dystrophica. Pediatrics 1981;67:678

Hiller N, Fisher D, Abrahamov A: Esophageal involvement in chronic granulomatous disease: a case report and review. Pediatr Radiol 1995;25:308

Lenaerts C, Roy CC, Vaillancourt M, et al: High incidence of upper gastrointestinal tract involvement in children with Crohn disease. Pediatrics 1989;83:777

Lepke RA, Libshitz HI: Radiation-induced injury of the esophagus. Radiology 1983;148:375

Matziner MA, Daneman A: Esophageal involvement in eosinophilic gastroenteritis. Pediatr Radiol 1983;13:35

Mauro MA, Paker LA, Hartley WS, et al: Epidermolysis bullosa: radiographic findings in 16 cases. AJR Am J Roentgenol 1987;149:925

McDonald GB, Sullivan KM, Plumley TF: Radiographic features of esophageal involvement in chronic graft-vs-host disease. AJR Am J Roentgenol 1984;142:501

Parsons DS, Smith RB, Mair EA, et al: Unique case presentations of acute epiglottic swelling and a protocol for acute airway compromise. Laryngoscope 1996;106:1287

Raffensperger JC, Luck SR, Reynolds M, et al: Intestinal bypass of the esophagus. J Pediatr Surg 1996;31:38

Renner WR, Johnson JF, Lichtenstein JE, et al: Esophageal inflammation and stricture: complication of chronic granulomatous disease of childhood. Radiology 1991;178:189

Ruuska T, Vaajalahti P, Arajarvi P, et al: Prospective evaluation of upper gastrointestinal mucosal lesions in children with ulcerative colitis and Crohn's disease. J Pediatr Gastroenterol Nutr 1994;19:181

Schmidt-Sommerfield E, Kirschner BS, Stephens JK: Endoscopic and histologic findings in the upper gastrointestinal tract of children with Crohn's disease. J Pediatr Gastroenterol Nutr 1990;11:448

Tischler JM, Helman CA: Crohn's disease of the esophagus. J Can Assoc Radiol 1984;35:28

Toulokian RJ, Schonholz SM, Gryboski JD, et al: Perioperative considerations in esophageal replacement for epidermolysis bullosa: report of two cases successfully treated by colon interposition. Am J Gastroenterol 1988;83:857

Vlymen WJ, Moskowitz PS: Roentgenographic manifestations of esophageal and intestinal involvement in Behcet's disease in children. Pediatr Radiol 1981;10:193

Infective Esophagitis

Ashenburg C, Rothstein FC, Dahms BB: Herpes esophagitis in the immunocompetent child. J Pediatr 1986;108:584

Bathazar EJ, Megibow AJ, Hulnick D, et al: Cytomegalovirus esophagitis in AIDS: radiographic features in 16 patients. AJR Am J Roentgenol 1987;149:919

Chusid MJ, Oechler HW, Werlin SL: Herpetic esophagitis in an immunocompetent boy. Wisc Med J 1992;91:71

Goodman P, Pinero SS, Rance RM, et al: Mycobacterial esophagitis in AIDS. Gastrointest Radiol 1989;14:103

Grattan-Smith D, Harrison LF, Singleton EB: Radiology of AIDS in the pediatric patient. Curr Prob Diagn Radiol 1992;21:79

Haller JO, Cohen HL: Gastrointestinal manifestations of AIDS in children. AJR Am J Roentgenol 1994;162:387

Isaac DW, Parham DM, Patrick CC: The role of esophagoscopy in diagnosis and management of esophagitis in children with cancer. Med Pediatr Oncol 1997;28:229

Lallemand D, Huault G, Laboureau JP, et al: Laryngeal and oesophageal lesions in patients with herpetic disease. Ann Radiol 1974;17:317

Levine MS: Radiology of esophagitis: a pattern approach. Radiology 1991;179:1

Levine MS, Laufer I, Kressel HY, et al: Herpes esophagitis. AJR Am J Roentgenol 1981;136:863

Levine MS, Macones AJ Jr, Laufer I: *Candida* esophagitis: accuracy of radiographic diagnosis. Radiology 1985;154:581

Lewicki AM, Moore JP: Esophageal moniliasis. Am J Roentgenol Radium Ther Nucl Med 1975;125:218

Diverticula

Meadows JA Jr: Esophageal diverticula in infants and children. South Med J 1970;63:691

Foreign Bodies and Trauma

Beer S, Avidan G, Viure E, et al: A foreign body in the oesophagus as a cause of respiratory distress. Pediatr Radiol 1982;12:41

Berdon WE: Editorial commentary on the manuscript entitled: Potential hazards of esophageal foreign body extraction, by CM Myer. Pediatr Radiol 1991;21:99

Campbell JB, Condon VR: Catheter removal of blunt esophageal foreign bodies in children: survey of the Society for Pediatric Radiology. Pediatr Radiol 1989;19:361

Campbell JB, Davis WS: Catheter technique for extraction of blunt esophageal foreign bodies. Radiology 1973;108:438

Campbell JB, Quattromani FL, Foley LC: Foley catheter removal of blunt esophageal foreign bodies: experience with 100 consecutive children. Pediatr Radiol 1983;13:116

Currarino G, Nikaidoh H: Esophageal foreign bodies in children with vascular ring or aberrant right subclavian artery: coincidence or causation? Pediatr Radiol 1991;21:406

Dubos JP, Bouchez MC, Kacet N, et al: Spontaneous rupture of the esophagus in the newborn. Pediatr Radiol 1986;16:317

Fernbach SK, Tucker GF: Coin ingestion: unusual appearance of the penny in a child. Radiology 1986;158:512

Harell GS, Friedland GW, Daily WJ, et al: Neonatal Boerhaave's syndrome. Radiology 1970;95:665

Harned RK, Strain JD, Hay TC, et al: Esophageal foreign bodies: safety and efficacy of Foley catheter extraction of coins. AJR Am J Roentgenol 1997;168:443

Herman TE, McAlister WH: Esophageal diverticula in childhood associated with strictures from unsuspected foreign bodies of the esophagus. Pediatr Radiol 1991;21:410

MacPherson RI, Hill JC, Othersen HB, et al: Esophageal foreign bodies in children: diagnosis, treatment, and complications. AJR Am J Roentgenol 1996;199:919

Myer CM: Potential hazards of esophageal foreign body extraction. Pediatr Radiol 1991;21:97

Toulokian RJ, Beardsley GP, Ablow RC, et al: Traumatic perforation of the pharynx in the newborn. Pediatrics 1977;59:1019

Towbin R, Lederman JS, Dunbar JS, et al: Esophageal edema as a predictor of unsuccessful balloon extraction of esophageal foreign body. Pediatr Radiol 1989;19:359

Chapter 5

DISORDERS OF THE ESOPHAGOGASTRIC JUNCTION

ALAN E. SCHLESINGER and BRUCE R. PARKER

ANATOMY AND PHYSIOLOGY

Although the anatomy and physiology of the esophagogastric junction have been studied for decades, the mechanisms of normal and abnormal function, especially with respect to gastroesophageal reflux (GER), are still incompletely understood. There is general agreement that the lower esophageal sphincter represents the true distal end of the esophagus, and its most distal point is the true esophagogastric junction. This point may be radiographically identifiable on mucosal relief studies of the stomach (Fig. 1), but may be difficult to identify during active swallowing studies. The lower esophageal sphincter is 3 to 4 cm long in adults and shorter in infants, and progresses toward its adult length throughout childhood.

The resting lower esophageal sphincter pressure is about 15 to 30 mm Hg higher than the resting pressure in the gastric fundus. During the initiation of swallowing, the intrasphincteric pressure drops rapidly, apparently mediated by the vagus nerve, to a level equal to fundal pressure. Thus the pressure gradient between

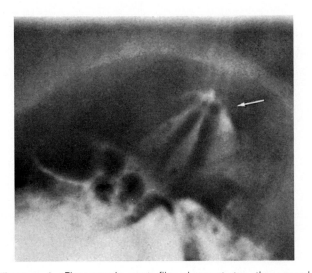

FIGURE 1. Fluoroscopic spot film demonstrates the normal esophagogastric junction. The *arrow* points to the convex margin of the "umbrella." The gastric folds diverge below. The parallel longitudinal esophagus folds are seen through the fundus above the margin of the umbrella.

lower esophagus and stomach disappears during "dry swallowing," as occurs with a pacifier or thumb sucking, as well as during true feedings. Additional antireflux activity is provided by the muscle of the esophageal hiatus of the diaphragm and by the membranous attachments of the lower esophagus to the diaphragm.

The intra-abdominal portion of the esophagus is probably relatively shorter in infants than in adults, but this varies with phases of respiration and swallowing and probably is not related to the pathophysiology of GER. The angle between the esophagus and stomach is less acute in infants than in adults. This may be a factor in permitting GER to occur even in normal infants.

GASTROESOPHAGEAL REFLUX

Anyone who has ever fed and burped an infant recognizes that GER occurs in virtually all normal babies. As with any physiologic mechanism, a wide range of normal can be seen. With GER, this varies from eructation with no vomiting of gastric contents to persistent "spitting up" during and after feedings (Fig. 2). Although sometimes alarming to parents, even persistent GER in otherwise healthy babies with normal weight gain and without chronic respiratory disease is usually physiologic. If extreme, physiologic GER often responds to thickened feedings and maintenance of the semi-upright posture, as in an infant seat. Spontaneous resolution of excessive spitting up usually occurs by 9 months of age.

Pathologic GER may be difficult to differentiate from physiologic GER in the first weeks to months of life. However, progressively severe GER after 6 weeks of age may be the first sign of a truly abnormal state. Lack of response to simple dietary and postural therapy, especially if accompanied by weight loss or deceleration of weight gain, may require evaluation for abnormal GER. Pathologic GER has been associated with failure to thrive, hematemesis, a variety of postural and neurologic disorders, torticollis, rumination, acute life-threatening events, and sudden infant death syndrome. Chronic respiratory symptoms from aspiration into the upper airway and even into the lungs may occur. GER, with or without aspiration, can often trigger bronchospasm. Therefore, evaluation for GER in children with reactive

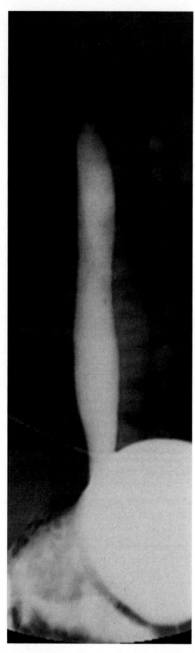

FIGURE 2. Gastroesophageal reflux demonstrated during an upper gastrointestinal series. Note the patulous esophagogastric junction, an appearance not seen on views of the esophagus obtained during antegrade flow of contrast while drinking.

airway disease is indicated because many of these children's pulmonary symptoms will improve when their reflux is treated. Recurrent pneumonia can be seen in patients with reflux and aspiration. The incidence of pathologic GER is higher in patients with trisomy 21, cystic fibrosis, and organic brain disease, especially cerebral palsy.

■ Indicators of pathologic GER include:
  • Progressively severe reflux after 6 weeks of age
  • Lack of response to dietary and postural therapy
  • Weight loss or deceleration of weight gain
  • Failure to thrive
  • Hematemesis
  • Postural or neurologic disorders
  • Torticollis
  • Rumination
  • Acute life-threatening event
  • Sudden infant death syndrome
  • Chronic respiratory symptoms
  • Bronchospasm

IMAGING STUDIES

The traditional imaging study for identification of GER has been the barium esophagogram. The examination should be a complete one, with evaluation of swallowing, esophageal peristalsis, and other causes of vomiting, such as gastric outlet obstruction resulting from hypertrophic pyloric stenosis or other causes. The total amount of barium given should be equivalent to a normal feeding volume. Because reflux is best identified with the patient in the supine position, sufficient barium must be given to reach the esophagogastric junction, which is anterior to most of the fundus. Insufficient barium may fill the dependent fundus and lead to reflux of air rather than contrast material (Fig. 3). The examination should include intermittent fluoroscopy for 5 minutes. If a nasogastric tube is present, the tip should be repositioned well above the esophagogastric junction during this evaluation period to avoid reflux possibly related to the tube crossing the junction. Some pediatric radiologists have suggested that the presence of three episodes of reflux to the level of the aortic arch

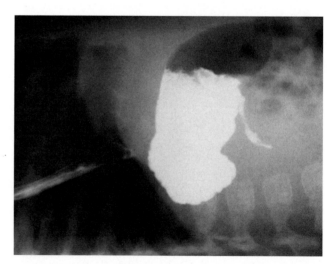

FIGURE 3. Lateral cross-table view of the stomach demonstrates barium in the dependent fundus, in the body, and in the distal esophagus. Note that insufficient barium would pool in the fundus below the esophagogastric junction and might lead to a false-negative reflux study.

within 5 minutes is pathologic. However, we have seen this much reflux in babies who are growing normally and are asymptomatic. The suggestion has been made that the only significant findings on barium swallow are continuous reflux, so-called chalasia, or signs of esophagitis.

Some radiologists advocate rolling the infant from side to side or increasing intra-abdominal pressure by external means. These maneuvers are nonphysiologic, however, and reflux elicited by them is of questionable significance. A pacifier may elicit reflux by simulating constant swallowing. Although not strictly physiologic, the use of a pacifier simulates real-life conditions in a majority of infants. Furthermore, because crying has been shown to decrease GER, the pacifier has an additional advantage.

Staging systems for GER have been developed. Typically, they differentiate between insignificant reflux, to the level of the aortic arch, and significant reflux above that level. However, because there is virtually no correlation between staging and clinical prognosis, few radiologists find staging useful. In fact, normal infants may fill the entire esophagus and pharynx without showing clinical evidence of abnormalities. If GER is seen, careful evaluation for aspiration into the airway is important. Hiatal hernias are uncommonly identified.

Comparison with 24-hour intraesophageal pH probe monitoring, the standard against which all other tests for GER must be measured, shows disappointingly high rates of false-negative barium esophagograms. The one advantage that all imaging studies have over pH probe studies is that the latter may not record immediate postprandial GER because the milk or formula may partially neutralize the refluxing gastric acid. One advantage of esophagography (compared to pH probe and many other imaging modalities used to evaluate for GER) is the demonstration of anatomic information that may identify complications of GER (such as esophagitis or strictures) or an alternative explanation for reflux-like symptoms such as esophageal obstruction, gastric outlet obstruction (including hypertrophic pyloric stenosis), or malrotation. A chest radiograph is frequently obtained at the initiation of a pH probe study to document the level of the probe, which should be at the level of the mid-left atrium.

Radionuclide studies for evaluation of GER are more sensitive than barium esophagograms, but they are commonly used in only a few centers with extensive experience. Lack of anatomic information is a limitation of scintigraphy compared with an upper gastrointestinal (GI) series. Food, milk, or formula containing the radionuclide is given orally, following which immediate and delayed images are obtained (Fig. 4A). Semiquantitation is possible in addition to the imaging studies. Concomitant gastric emptying studies (see Section VI, Part VI, page 1583) can also be performed, and aspiration into the lungs can be identified. Although highly sensitive for GER, the reflux episodes detected by nuclear scintigraphy do not tend to correlate with pH drops on pH probe studies. An investigation by Vandenplas et al. of 65 children studied with pH probe and scintigraphy found 123 episodes of reflux identified by one or both studies. However, only six of these occurred simultaneously, suggesting that these two methods measure different phenomena in the pathophysiology of GER and may play a complementary role.

■ Radionuclide studies for evaluation of GER are more sensitive than esophagrams.

Ultrasound (US) is the imaging examination that shows the highest correlation with pH probe studies. Westra et al. reported 81% to 84% agreement between the two studies. Riccabona et al. found that sonography identified GER with a sensitivity of 100% and specificity of 87.5% compared with pH monitoring and/or manometry. Gomes and Menanteau described a US scoring system for GER that correlated well with results of pH probe studies and endoscopy. For US evaluation, the infant is supine, and the area of the gastroesophageal junction identified. Water or dextrose solution is given orally or by tube in an amount equal to a normal feeding. Longitudinal imaging can identify fluid mixed with air bubbles refluxing into the distal esophagus (Fig. 4B). US, as well as being more sensitive than barium esophagograms, has the additional advantage of not using ionizing radiation. This permits longer continuous monitoring than is possible with fluoroscopy. The disadvantages are that it is time consuming and that the esophagus may be difficult to identify in some children.

The most common complications of significant GER are failure to thrive, chronic and recurrent respiratory symptoms, and esophagitis. The imaging characteristics of reflux esophagitis are nonspecific, with dysmotility being the most common finding. This may vary from mild loss of normal primary stripping waves to tertiary contractions or aperistalsis. Frank ulceration can occur, but is more common in adults with peptic esophagitis than in children. If ulcers are present, they are typically in the lower third of the esophagus near the esophagogastric junction. Reflux esophagitis may lead to strictures, most commonly in the midesophagus or lower third (Fig. 5). Barrett's esophagus, with metaplasia of the esophageal epithelium, is less common than in adults and in some cases is premalignant.

Pseudodiverticula are small intramural collections of barium that do not communicate with the lumen as do mucosal ulcers. Less commonly seen in children than in adults, they represent dilated excretory ducts of intramural mucous glands in patients with reflux or peptic esophagitis.

TREATMENT

Although medical therapy may be satisfactory for most cases of significant infantile GER, surgery may be necessary for some infants with severe symptoms, especially respiratory symptoms or profound failure to thrive. The most commonly performed procedure is the Nissen fundoplication, in which the upper fundus is wrapped around the distal esophagus (Fig. 6). Partial wraps (such as the Thal and Toupet) may also be performed. Fundoplication (with or without gastrostomy) can now be performed laparoscopically. The results of fundoplication are variable, but long-term cessation of GER can be accomplished in 60% to 70% of patients. In one large multi-institutional study of 7467 patients from seven children's hospitals, Fonkalsrud et al. reported good to excellent results in 95% of neurologically normal children and 85% of neurologically impaired children.

Complications of fundoplication may be encountered. If the wrap is too tight, distal esophageal obstruction occurs; if too loose, reflux may persist. On follow-up upper GI series, if the wrap loosens, contrast may enter the potential space between the walls of the stomach used to form the wrap (Fig. 7). This may or may not result in recurrent reflux. In a small percentage of patients, a hiatal hernia (Fig. 8) or paraesophageal hernia (Fig. 9) may develop. If a patient with a fundoplication develops distal bowel obstruction, a closed-loop obstruction may be created by the loss of ability to decompress the obstruction by eructation. A relatively high rate of postoperative small bowel intussusception has been described after Nissen fundoplication in one study. The etiology of small bowel intussusception in these patients is unclear, but may be related to abnormal bowel peristalsis in a patient population already at risk for altered foregut motility.

Although surgical antireflux procedures were commonly performed routinely in all neurologically impaired children referred for feeding gastrostomy, recent evidence suggests that the potential complications may not justify this approach. Therefore, antireflux surgery

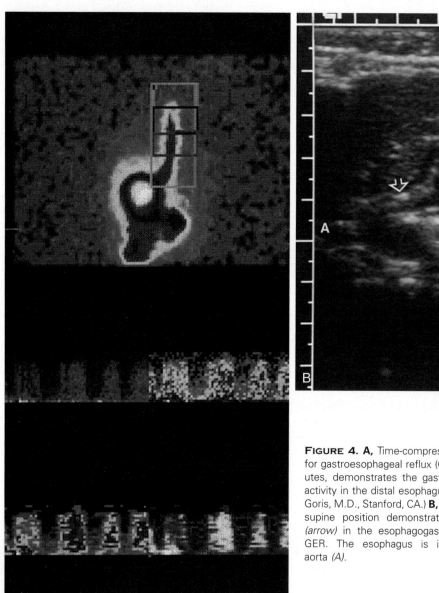

FIGURE 4. A, Time-compressed image of ^{99m}Tc study for gastroesophageal reflux (GER), obtained over 5 minutes, demonstrates the gastric fundus and prominent activity in the distal esophagus. (Courtesy of Michael L. Goris, M.D., Stanford, CA.) **B,** Ultrasound of patient in the supine position demonstrates air bubbles and fluid *(arrow)* in the esophagogastric junction during active GER. The esophagus is identified anterior to the aorta *(A).*

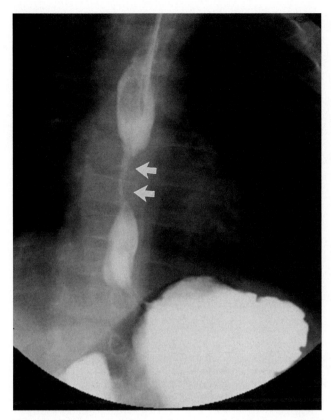

FIGURE 5. Anteroposterior esophagogram demonstrates a distal esophageal stricture *(arrows)* in a patient with chronic reflux esophagitis.

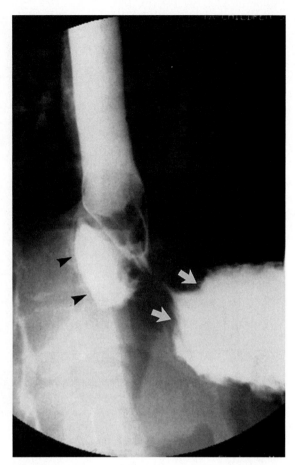

FIGURE 7. Anteroposterior view of the esophagogastric junction in a patient with a prior fundoplication. Note the fundoplication defect *(arrows)*. A small amount of barium *(arrowheads)* has entered the wrap adjacent to the distal esophagus.

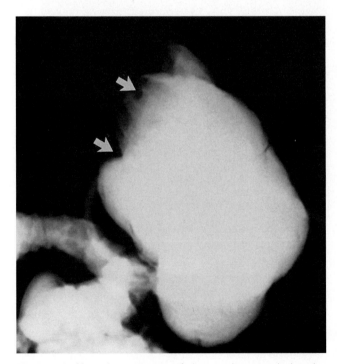

FIGURE 6. Normal appearance of the esophagogastric junction following Nissen fundoplication. Note the defect in the fundus *(arrows)* caused by the wrap.

in these children at the time of gastrostomy is reserved for those with documented reflux.

In extreme cases of esophagitis and stricture, esophagectomy with colonic interposition may be required. Marked GER may be seen in patients who survive congenital diaphragmatic hernia repair, especially of large defects, often requiring extracorporeal membrane oxygenation therapy in the newborn period. These infants may require more aggressive treatment with fundoplication and pyloroplasty.

HIATAL HERNIA

Small hiatal hernias may be seen with or without GER, may be transient, and may be of no clinical significance in the absence of GER (Fig. 10). Larger hernias may be associated with symptoms, but are uncommon. Partial or complete intrathoracic stomach is rare, but the findings on upper GI series are dramatic (Fig. 11*A, B*). Paraesophageal hernias are very uncommon in children without prior gastroesophageal surgery (Fig. 11*C*).

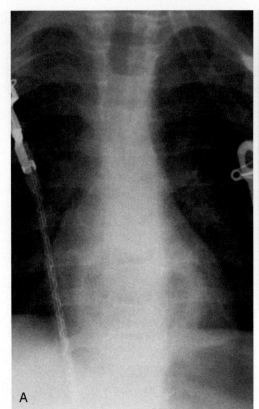

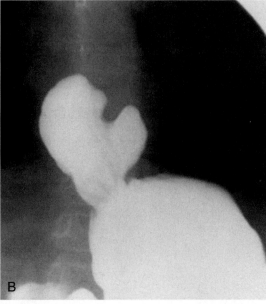

FIGURE 8. Status post–Nissen fundoplication. **A,** Anteroposterior view of the chest demonstrates a large air-filled structure projected over the cardiac silhouette. **B,** Esophagogram demonstrates herniation of the gastric fundus through the esophageal hiatus. The fundoplication is intact, and no gastroesophageal reflux was seen.

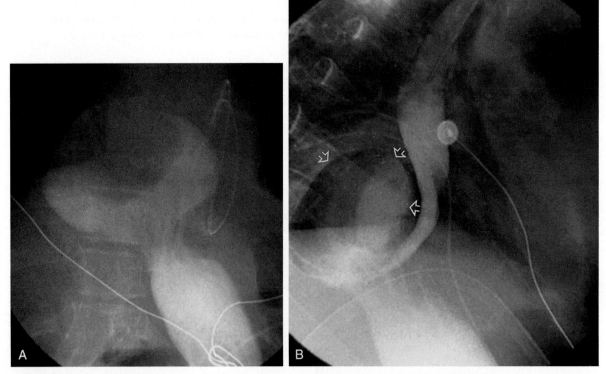

FIGURE 9. A, Anteroposterior view of the stomach (filled via a gastrostomy tube) demonstrates a portion of stomach herniated above the diaphragm. **B,** The patient was given a small amount of contrast to drink, and an oblique image of the distal esophagus shows that the herniated stomach *(arrows)* is adjacent to the distal esophagus, and therefore indicates a paraesophageal hernia.

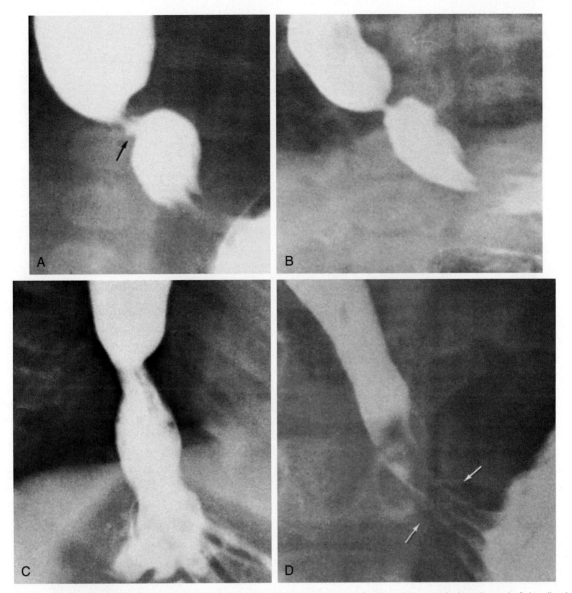

FIGURE 10. Serial films of the esophagogastric junction. **A,** At 32 months of age, stricture and ulcer *(arrow)* of the distal segment of the esophagus and a small hiatal hernia are seen. **B,** At 52 months, the ulcer is no longer present; the stricture persists. Gastrostomy had been performed. **C,** At 11 months, the hiatal hernia persists but the esophageal narrowing has diminished quite significantly. **D,** At 9 years, a small hiatal hernia remains *(arrows)*, but the patient was asymptomatic.

ACHALASIA

Failure of relaxation of the lower esophageal sphincter (achalasia or cardiospasm) is rare in children, although described even during infancy. There is often a deficiency of cells in Auerbach's plexus. Defective vagus nerve function or innervation is the most common pathophysiologic mechanism. Patients usually complain of dysphagia, chest pain, and symptoms related to lower esophageal obstruction. In severe cases, regurgitation of undigested food is virtually diagnostic. The differential diagnosis is listed in Table 1.

Although the definitive diagnosis is made by esophageal manometry, characteristic radiographic findings

Table 1 ■ DIFFERENTIAL DIAGNOSIS OF ACHALASIA
When presenting as a mediastinal mass:
Neurogenic tumors
Neuroblastoma
Ganglioneuroblastoma
Ganglioglioma
Tubular esophageal duplication cyst
Hiatal hernia
When presenting with dysphagia
Esophageal stricture
Gastroesophageal reflux
Caustic ingestion
Crohn's disease
Chronic granulomatous disease
Epidermolysis bullosa

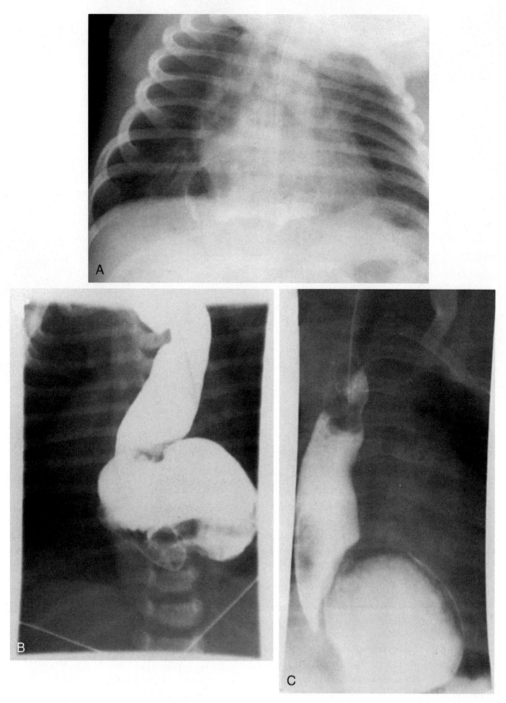

FIGURE 11. Anteroposterior view of the chest **(A)** and esophagogram **(B)** demonstrate a large intrathoracic stomach in a boy with marked symptoms of reflux and eructation. **C,** Esophagogram on a different patient demonstrates a large para-esophageal hiatal hernia.

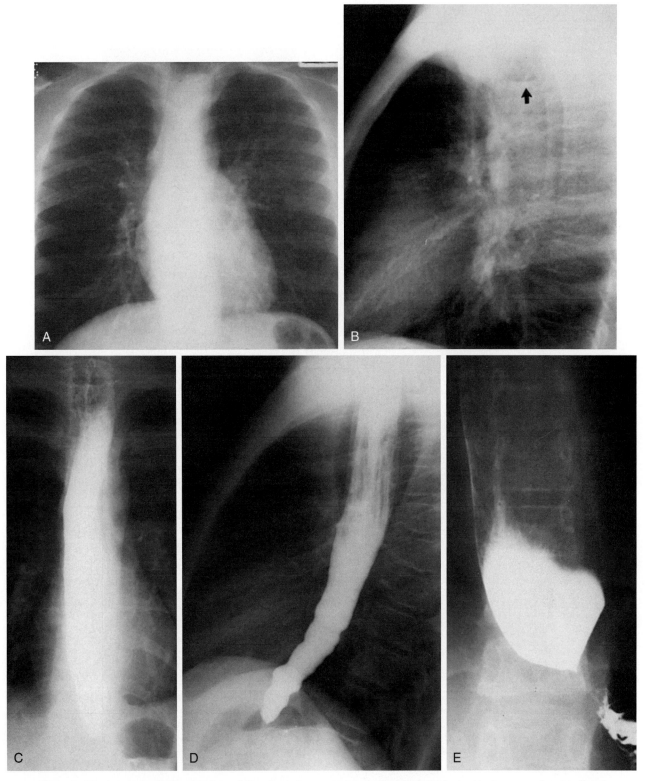

FIGURE 12. Achalasia. **A,** Frontal view of the chest demonstrates marked paravertebral widening secondary to dilated esophagus. **B,** Lateral view of the chest demonstrates air–fluid level in the dilated esophagus *(arrow)*. Frontal **(C)** and lateral **(D)** views of the esophagogram demonstrate marked dilatation with abrupt narrowing to a "beak" at the esophagogastric junction. **E,** Spot film of the esophagogastric junction demonstrates the beak to better advantage.

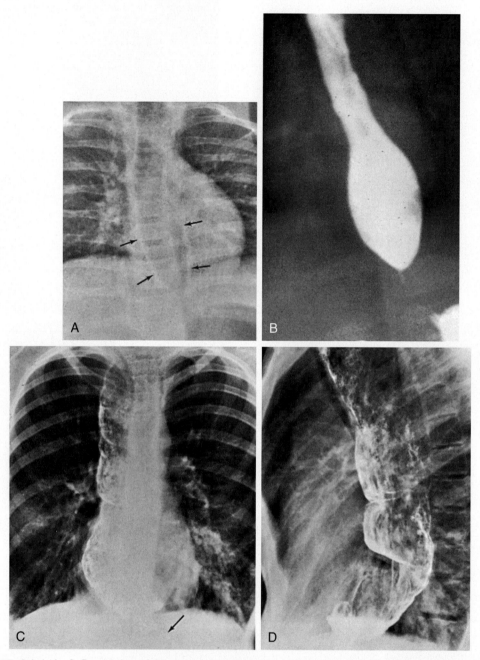

FIGURE 13. Achalasia. **A,** Frontal view of the chest demonstrates marked gaseous distention of the esophagus. **B,** Esophagogram on the same patient demonstrates markedly dilated esophagus with beak-like deformity at the esophagogastric junction. Endoscopy and manometry confirmed the diagnosis of achalasia. Anteroposterior **(C)** and lateral **(D)** views of the chest of a 15-year-old girl with achalasia and symptoms for at least 5 years. Chronic lung disease is identified, and the markedly dilated esophagus is filled with retained swallowed material.

are typically seen. Upright chest radiographs may show an air-filled esophagus, often containing an air–fluid level (Fig. 12). Esophagograms show normal swallowing and, frequently, normal peristalsis to the level of the aortic arch. Early cases may show vigorous but discoordinated peristaltic activity in the esophagus. A characteristic "beaking of the distal esophagus" (Figs. 12 and 13) has been described. Ultimately, the esophagus may become completely atonic and remain markedly dilated, almost continuously filled with ingested material.

■ Chest radiograph findings in achalasia commonly include
  • Mediastinal mass secondary to esophageal dilatation
  • Air–fluid level in dilated esophagus

■ Esophagogram findings in achalasia include the following:
  • Common
    1. Dilated esophagus
    2. Beaking of distal esophagus
    3. Normal peristalsis above aortic arch with abnormal peristalsis below aortic arch
  • Uncommon: completely atonic esophagus in severe cases

Thoracoscopic or laparoscopic repair can be performed as an alternative to standard surgical repair (with or without fundoplication). Alternative therapies have been used, including balloon dilatation and endoscopically guided injection of botulinum toxin into the lower esophageal sphincter.

SUGGESTED READINGS

Gastroesophageal Reflux

Balson BM, Kravitz EK, McGeady SJ: Diagnosis and treatment of gastroesophageal reflux in children and adolescents with severe asthma. Ann Allergy Asthma Immunol 1998;81:159

Blane CE, Turnage RH, Oldham KT, et al: Long-term radiographic follow-up of the Nissen fundoplication in children. Pediatr Radiol 1989;19:523

Boix-Ochoa J, Lafuente JM, Gilvernet JM: Twenty-four hour esophageal pH monitoring in gastroesophageal reflux. J Pediatr Surg 1980;15:74

Bowen A'D: The vomiting infant: recent advances and unsettled issues in imaging. Radiol Clin North Am 1988;26:377

Braun P, Nussie D, Roy CC, et al: Intramural diverticulosis of the esophagus in an eight-year-old boy. Pediatr Radiol 1978;6:235

Chung DH, Georgeson KE: Fundoplication and gastrostomy. Semin Pediatr Surg 1998;7:213

Cleveland RH, Kushner DC, Schwartz AN: Gastroesophageal reflux in children: results of a standardized fluoroscopic approach. AJR Am J Roentgenol 1983;141:53

Darling DB, McCauley RGK, Leape LL, et al: The child with peptic

esophagitis: a correlation of radiographic signs with esophageal pathology. Radiology 1982;145:673

Davies RP, Morris LL, Savage JP, et al: Gastroesophageal reflux: the role of imaging in diagnosis and management. Australas Radiol 1987;31:157

Eid NS, Shepherd RW, Thomson MA: Persistent wheezing and gastroesophageal reflux in infants. Pediatr Pulmonol 1994;18:39

Euler AR, Ament ME: Detection of gastroesophageal reflux in the pediatric-age patient by esophageal intraluminal pH probe measurement (Tuttle test). Pediatrics 1977;60:65

Festen C: Paraesophageal hernia: a major complication of Nissen's fundoplication. J Pediatr Surg 1981;16:496

Fonkalsrud EW, Ashcraft KW, Coran AG: Surgical treatment of gastroesophageal reflux in children: a combined hospital study of 7467 patients. Pediatrics 1998;101:419

Frantzides CT, Richards C: A study of 362 consecutive laproscopic Nissen fundoplications. Surgery 1998;124:651

Gomes H, Menanteau B: Gastro-esophageal reflux: comparative study between sonography and pH monitoring. Pediatr Radiol 1991; 21:168

Guill MF: Respiratory manifestations of gastroesophageal reflux in children. J Asthma 1995;32:173

Harnsberger JK, Corey JJ, Johnson DG: Long-term follow-up of surgery for gastroesophageal reflux in infants and children. J Pediatr 1983;102:505

Hayden CK: Ultrasonography of the gastrointestinal tract in infants and children. Abdom Imaging 1996;21:9

Heyman S: Esophageal scintigraphy (milk scans) in infants and children with esophageal reflux. Radiology 1982;144:891

Koot VC, Bergmeijer JH, Bos AP, et al: Incidence and management of gastroesophageal reflux after repair of congenital diaphragmatic hernia. J Pediatr Surg 1993;28:48

Leape LL, Holder TM, Franklin JD, et al: Respiratory arrest in infants secondary to gastroesophageal reflux. Pediatrics 1977;60:924

Maclean AD, Houghton-Allen BW: Upper esophageal web in childhood. Pediatr Radiol 1975;3:240

Marshall JB, Kretschmar JM, Diaz-Arias AA: Gastroesophageal reflux as a pathogenic factor in the development of symptomatic lower esophageal rings. Arch Intern Med 1990;150:1669

McCauley RGK, Darling DB, Leonidas JC, et al: Gastroesophageal reflux in infants and children: a useful classification and reliable physiological technique for its demonstration. AJR Am J Roentgenol 1978;130:47

McVeagh P, Howman-Giles R, Kemp A: Pulmonary aspiration studies by radionuclide milk scanning and barium swallow roentgenology. Am J Dis Child 1987;141:917

O'Hara SM: Pediatric gastrointestinal nuclear imaging. Radiol Clin North Am 1996;34:845

Peters ME, Crummy AB, Wojtowycz MM, et al: Intramural esophageal pseudodiverticulosis: a report in a child with a sixteen-year follow-up. Pediatr Radiol 1982;12:262

Piepsz A, Georges B, Perlmutter N, et al: Gastroesophageal scintiscanning in children. Pediatr Radiol 1981;11:71

Riccabona M, Maurer U, Lackner H: The role of sonography in the evaluation of gastro-oesophageal reflux—correlation to pH-metry. Eur J Pediatr 1992;151:655

Scott RB, O'Loughlin EV, Gall DG: Gastroesophageal reflux in patients with cystic fibrosis. J Pediatr 1985;106:223

Seibert JJ, Byrne WJ, Euler AR, et al: Gastroesophageal reflux—the acid test: scintigraphy or the pH probe? AJR Am J Roentgenol 1983;140:1087

Sigalet DL, Nguyen LT, Adolph V: Gastrointestinal reflux associated with large diaphragmatic hernias. J Pediatr Surg 1994;29:1262

Smith CD, Othersen HB, Gogan NJ, et al: Nissen fundoplication in children with profound neurologic disability: high risk and unmet goals. Ann Surg 1992;215:654

Stolar CJ, Berdon WE, Dillon PW, et al: Esophageal dilatation and reflux in neonates supported by ECMO after diaphragmatic hernia repair. AJR Am J Roentgenol 1988;151:135

Stolar CJ, Levy JP, Dillon PW, et al: Anatomic and functional abnormalities of the esophagus in infants surviving congenital diaphragmatic hernia. Am J Surg 1990;159:204

Thoeni RF, Moss AA: The radiographic appearance of complications following Nissen fundoplication. Radiology 1979;131:17

Tolia V, Calhoun JA, Kuhns LR, et al: Lack of correlation between extended pH monitoring and scintigraphy in the evaluation of infants with gastroesophageal reflux. J Lab Clin Med 1990;115:559

Trinh TD, Benson JE: Fluoroscopic diagnosis of complications after Nissen antireflux fundoplication in children. AJR Am J Roentgenol 1997;169:1023

Vandenplas Y, Derde MP, Peipsz A: Evaluation of reflux episodes during simultaneous esophageal pH monitoring and gastroesophageal reflux scintigraphy in children. J Pediatr Gastroenterol Nutr 1992;14:256

Weaver JW, Kaude JV, Hamlin DJ: Webs of the lower esophagus: a complication of gastroesophageal reflux? AJR Am J Roentgenol 1984;142:289

Wesley JR, Coran AG, Sarahan TM, et al: The need for evaluation of gastroesophageal reflux in brain-damaged children referred for feeding gastrostomy. J Pediatr Surg 1981;16:866

West KW, Stephens B, Rescorla FJ, et al: Postoperative intussusception: experience with 36 cases in children. Surgery 1988;104:781

Westra KW, Derkx HH, Taminiau JA: Symptomatic gastroesophageal reflux: diagnosis with ultrasound. J Pediatr Gastroenterol Nutr 1994;19:58

Westra SJ, Wolf BHM, Staalman CR: Ultrasound diagnosis of gastroesophageal reflux and hiatal hernia in infants and young children. J Clin Ultrasound 1990;18:477

Winters C Jr, Spurling TJ, Chobanian SJ, et al: Barrett's esophagus: a prevalent, occult complication of gastroesophageal reflux disease. Gastroenterology 1987;92:118

Wolfson BJ, Allen JL, Panitch HB, et al: Lipid aspiration pneumonia due to gastroesophageal reflux: a complication of nasogastric lipid feedings. Pediatr Radiol 1989;19:545

Yulish BS, Rothstein FC, Halpin TC Jr: Radiographic findings in children and young adults with Barrett's esophagus. AJR Am J Roentgenol 1987;148:353

Hiatal Hernia

Astley R, Carre IJ, Langmead-Smith R: A 20-year prospective follow-up of childhood hiatal hernia. Br J Radiol 1977;50:400

Achalasia

Ambrosino MM, Genieser NB, Banguru BS, et al: The syndrome of achalasia of the esophagus, ACTH insensitivity and alacrima. Pediatr Radiol 1986;16:328

Berquist WE, Byrne WJ, Ament ME, et al: Achalasia: diagnosis, management, and clinical courses in 16 children. Pediatrics 1983; 71:798

Hammond PD, Moore DJ, Davidson GP, et al: Tandem balloon dilatation for childhood achalasia. Pediatr Radiol 1997;27:609

Holzman MD, Sharp KW, Ladipo JK, et al: Laproscopic surgical treatment for achalasia. Am J Surg 1997;173:308

Lelli JL, Drongowski RA, Coran AG: Efficacy of transthoracic modified Heller myotomy in children with achalasia—a 21 year experience. J Pediatr Surg 1997;32:338

Starinsky R, Berlovitz J, Mores AJ, et al: Infantile achalasia. Pediatr Radiol 1984;14:113

Walton JM, Tougas G: Botulinum toxin use in pediatric esophageal achalasia: a case report. J Pediatr Surg 1997;32:916

C h a p t e r   6

MISCELLANEOUS ESOPHAGEAL ABNORMALITIES

ALAN E. SCHLESINGER and BRUCE R. PARKER

ESOPHAGEAL VARICES

Esophageal varices are secondary to portal hypertension in children and are discussed more thoroughly in Section VI, Part III. The primary modality for identifying esophageal varices now is endoscopy rather than imaging studies. However, varices may be found in the evaluation of hematemesis or coincidentally when imaging studies are performed for other reasons. Rarely, paraesophageal varices cause sufficient irregularity of the esophagus so that they can be seen as paraspinous widening on chest radiographs (Fig. 1A, B). Computed tomography (CT) and magnetic resonance imaging may incidentally identify the varices when performed for other indications (Fig. 1C, D). Angiography (Fig. 1E) is typically reserved for patients undergoing embolization procedures. Ultrasound (US), especially color Doppler US, performed for evaluation of hepatic disease may also demonstrate varices incidentally. Recently, transnasal endoluminal US with a 20-MHz transducer has been shown to be more sensitive in the detection of esophageal varices than endoscopy. Barium esophagogram is the standard imaging modality for identifying varices, which appear as serpentine filling defects in the barium column (Fig. 2). Barium paste gives better mucosal relief than liquid barium, but is not always found palatable by children.

The primary treatment modality for esophageal varices, other than treatment of the underlying portal hypertension, is endoscopic sclerotherapy. Agha described acute complications following sclerotherapy, including mucosal ulceration, luminal narrowing, sinuses, fistulas, dissection, and perforation. Chronically, one may find strictures, mural defects, dysmotility, and obstruction.

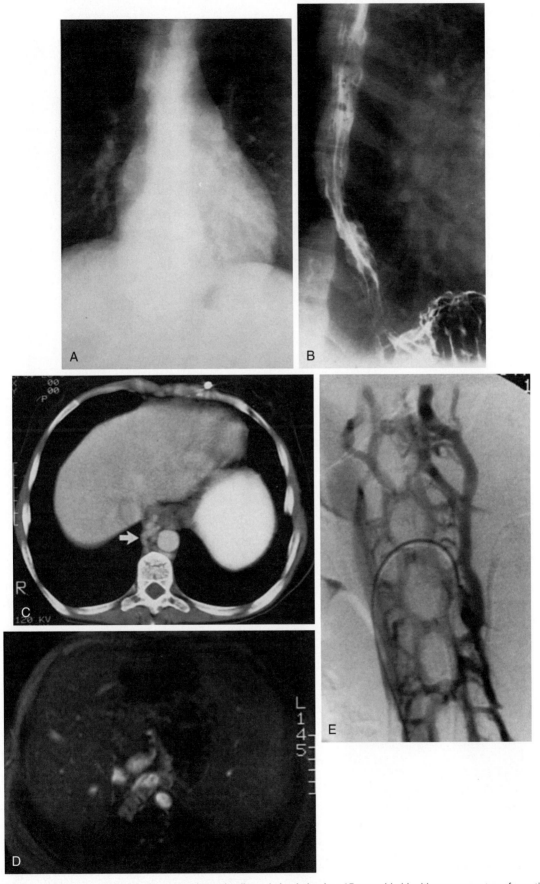

FIGURE 1. Marked esophageal and paraesophageal collateral circulation in a 15-year-old girl with cavernous transformation of the portal vein. **A,** Coned-down anteroposterior view of the chest reveals paravertebral widening at the level of the diaphragm. **B,** Esophagogram demonstrates serpentine filling defects in the distal esophagus and the gastric fundus consistent with varices. **C,** Computed tomography scan at the thoracoabdominal junction demonstrates multiple varices in the paraesophageal region *(arrow).* **D,** Magnetic resonance imaging using gradient-recalled echo sequence demonstrates right paraesophageal varices to good advantage. **E,** Angiogram using digital subtraction technique demonstrates massive bilateral paravertebral collateral venous flow.

NEOPLASMS

Esophageal tumors are extraordinarily rare in children and are usually benign. Hamartomas, leiomyomas, and hemangiomas have been reported. Leiomyomatosis, a rare neoplastic disorder causing leiomyomatous thickening of all or a portion of the esophagus, has been reported in children as well. CT demonstrated marked esophageal thickening. One of the most common pseudoneoplasms demonstrated is an inflammatory polyp secondary to chronic gastroesophageal reflux (Fig. 3). Carcinomas are even more rare and have been reported following caustic esophagitis and achalasia. Mediastinal tumors, such as lymphoma, teratoma, or neuroblastoma, may displace the esophagus, but usually do not involve it primarily.

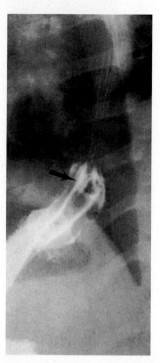

FIGURE 3. Inflammatory gastroesophageal polyp *(arrow)* presented as a filling defect on upper gastrointestinal series in a 10-year-old boy with hiatal hernia. (Courtesy of Dr. S. Kirschner, Nashville, TN.)

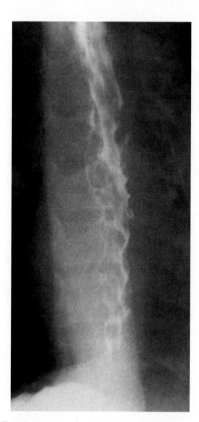

FIGURE 2. Esophagogram demonstrates multiple serpentine filling defects in the esophagus resulting from varices in a 7-year-old girl with cavernous transformation of the portal vein and secondary portal venous hypertension.

■ **Esophageal neoplasms include the following:**
1. Benign
   - Hamartomas
   - Leiomyomas
   - Hemangiomas
   - Leiomyomatosis
2. Malignant
   - Carcinoma (rare, but can be seen after caustic esophagitis or achalasia)

SUGGESTED READINGS

Esophageal Varices

Agha FP: The esophagus after endoscopic injection sclerotherapy: acute and chronic changes. Radiology 1984;153:37

Isikawa T, Saeki M, Tsukune Y, et al: Detection of paraesophageal varices by plain film. AJR Am J Roentgenol 1985;144:701

Liu, JB, Miller LS, Feld RI, et al: Gastric and esophageal varices: a 20 MHz transnasal endoluminal US. Radiology 1993;187:363

Rose JD, Roberts GM, Smith PM: The radiological appearance of the esophagus after sclerotherapy for varices. Clin Radiol 1985;36:355

Neoplasms

Guest AR, Strouse PJ, Hiew CC, et al: Progressive esophageal leiomyomatosis with respiratory compromise. Pediatr Radiol 2000; 30:247

PART VI

STOMACH AND PROXIMAL DUODENUM

ALAN E. SCHLESINGER
BRUCE R. PARKER

Chapter 1

NORMAL STOMACH AND DUODENUM

ALAN E. SCHLESINGER and BRUCE R. PARKER

NORMAL ANATOMY

The stomach normally lies below the left hemidiaphragm and extends obliquely caudad and mediad to the pyloroduodenal flexure. Embryologically, the stomach begins as a straight tube that rotates clockwise 90 degrees around its long axis. The original posterior portion of the stomach becomes the left margin. Its differential growth is greater than the opposite side, resulting in a longer, greater curvature to the left and a shorter, lesser curvature to the right. The stomach is relatively fixed at its proximal end by the esophagogastric junction and at its distal end by the fixed retroperitoneal position of the first portion of the duodenum. Additionally, the stomach is attached to neighboring organs by four major peritoneal folds: the gastrophrenic, the gastrohepatic, the gastrosplenic, and the gastrocolic ligaments.

The stomach is divided into three portions. The fundus is the most bulbous portion and is that part superior to the esophagogastric junction. The body of the stomach is the portion bounded on either side by the greater and lesser curvatures, typically becoming slightly narrower in caliber as it reaches the distal portion. The gastric antrum and pylorus are the most distal portions of the stomach, having a slightly thicker wall than the fundus or body.

The normal shape, size, and position of the stomach are variable, depending on the volume of gastric content and the position, age, and body habitus of the individual. In infancy, the stomach appears high and transverse on contrast studies in most patients (Fig. 1). The more longitudinal, J-shaped stomach is uncommonly seen in infants, but is characteristic in older children and adults (Fig. 2). Although the appearance of the fundus and body may vary, the position and appearance of the pylorus are relatively similar from patient to patient.

The fundus and the greater curvature of the body normally exhibit marginal indentations caused by the normal folds in the mucosa, the gastric rugae. The pattern is inconstant, but rugal folds can usually be seen in most normal stomachs unless they are overdistended during barium examination. The mucosal contour is best evaluated with a small amount of contrast material spread over the surface. Double-contrast studies of the stomach bring the mucosa into sharp relief, but cannot always be performed in young children. The rugae are least prominent in early infancy and become progressively more obvious in older patients (see Fig. 2).

Normal peristaltic waves can typically be seen even in neonates, although gastric motor activity increases with age. Normally, peristalsis is coordinated from the proximal to the distal stomach and is propulsive. The gastric antrum and pyloric region frequently demonstrate muscular spasm, which interrupts the normal peristaltic propulsive waves (Fig. 3). Gastric emptying time is far more variable in children than in adults, especially in infants. Although maintenance of the supine position and gaseous distention of the stomach, which typically occur in infants, may have a role in delayed gastric emptying, the effect of the delayed opening of the antrum and pylorus is probably most significant. It is not uncommon for a normal baby to have sufficient antropyloric spasm for contrast material to remain in the stomach for as long as 20 or 25 minutes before finally passing into the small intestine.

The duodenum, the most proximal portion of the small intestine, begins at the pyloroduodenal junction.

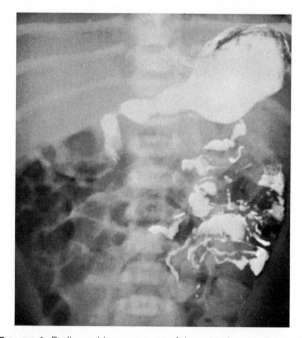

FIGURE 1. Radiographic appearance of the normal stomach in early life. The stomach in this 6-day-old infant is high, conical in shape, and transverse. Rugal markings are not prominent.

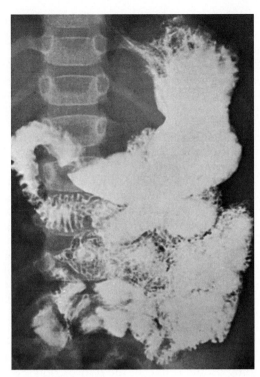

FIGURE 2. The stomach in a 4-year-old boy is J-shaped with prominent rugal folds in the fundus.

mobile. The second or descending portion extends from the neck of the gallbladder and is in intimate contact with the head of the pancreas. The common bile duct enters its midportion. The third portion is once again horizontal and courses back to the left across the spine. Anteriorly, it is covered by peritoneum and is crossed by the superior mesenteric artery and vein. The fourth portions ascends along the left side of the aorta where it turns ventrally to become the jejunum at the level of the duodenojejunal flexure. The flexure is still retroperitoneal, keeping it fixed in the normal situation, and is further held in place by the ligament of Treitz. Of importance is that the proximal portion of the duodenum receives its blood supply from the celiac axis, while the superior mesenteric artery supplies blood to the distal duodenum. Thus, while the stomach and first and second portions of the duodenum are derived from the embryonic foregut, most of the third and all of the fourth portion of the duodenum are of midgut origin and are often involved in midgut volvulus, which is discussed in Section II, Part IV.

EXAMINATION OF THE UPPER GASTROINTESTINAL TRACT

FLUOROSCOPIC CONTRAST STUDIES

Contrast studies of the upper gastrointestinal tract under fluoroscopic control (upper gastrointestinal [GI] series) continue to be the standard examination for most abnormalities of the stomach and duodenum.

The first portion of the duodenum begins at the pylorus and ends approximately at the neck of the gallbladder. It is almost completely covered by peritoneum, but is the only portion of the normal duodenum that is relatively

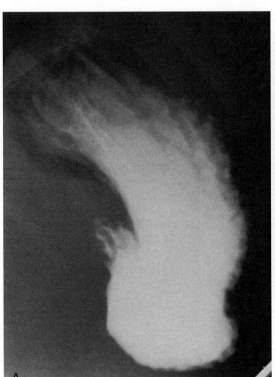

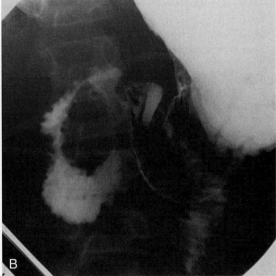

FIGURE 3. Pyloric spasm. **A,** Upper gastrointestinal tract series in a 7-year-old girl with crampy abdominal pain shows antropyloric spasm 30 minutes after barium ingestion. **B,** After parenteral administration of an anticholinergic agent, there was easy passage of barium through an anatomically normal pylorus and duodenum.

Barium is the most commonly used contrast material. Water-soluble contrast is typically used for patients in whom an intestinal perforation is suspected. Although more expensive, low-osmolar nonionic contrast material has largely replaced the older forms of water-soluble contrast media in the GI tract when perforation is suspected (especially in neonates and young infants, in whom smaller volumes of contrast are needed). However, the higher osmolar contrast agents are still used occasionally for therapeutic purposes in neonates with meconium plug syndrome or meconium ileus and in older patients with cystic fibrosis who have distal intestinal obstruction syndrome. The former is discussed more thoroughly in Section II, Part IV, and the latter in Section VI, Part VII. The low-osmolar nonionic contrast materials are sometimes used for upper GI examinations in patients with intestinal obstruction. Again, this is predominantly in newborns, especially those who are suspected of having necrotizing enterocolitis or of having feeding intolerance secondary to strictures from previous necrotizing enterocolitis. The advantages of isotonic solutions of low-osmolar nonionic contrast include lack of large fluid shifts, absence of contrast dilution, lack of injury to the bowel mucosa, low absorption from the bowel, and relatively low risk of pulmonary edema if the isotonic contrast is aspirated. In patients with subtle bowel perforation not identified by contrast extravasation at the time of the examination, perforation can be detected on delayed radiographs by renal excretion of the contrast that is absorbed by the peritoneum.

In patients who are old enough to cooperate, double-contrast examinations are useful in many instances. In these cases, a higher density barium is used, and effervescent agents are administered to produce the double contrast. Double-contrast studies are generally accepted as the upper GI imaging examination of choice in adults. However, they require longer fluoroscopy times and a larger number of films than does the standard single-contrast examination, and we do not use double-contrast examinations routinely in children. In fact, the examination in children should be tailored to the specific clinical question to be answered in order to limit the radiation exposure. Intermittent fluoroscopy should always be used instead of constant fluoroscopy, careful collimation should be used, and photo spot-film cameras or digital fluoroscopy should be used in place of standard film–screen combination spot films. If available, pulsed fluoroscopy is recommended. Infants and young children, of necessity, are studied in the recumbent position. In older children, especially when double-contrast studies are performed, the examination can be performed with a combination of recumbent and upright spot images.

Older children can be kept fasting overnight if the study is performed early in the morning. Children under 1 year of age have the potential for dehydration with this length of restriction, and we have found a 3-hour period sufficient to empty the normal stomach of foodstuffs. In infants who do have retained material in the stomach, a nasogastric tube should be placed, and most of the retained material can be withdrawn satisfactorily. If aspiration of the gastric contents through a tube is performed, the aspirate should be examined for the presence of bile or blood as a possible clue to the diagnosis of the infant's problem.

Most babies, having been kept fasting for 3 hours, will readily take barium from a bottle. The babies are generally more accepting of the bottle while they are in the supine position, even though this may introduce more air than if fed while in the prone position. The tube and nipple technique for examining swallowing is described in Section VI, Part V, Chapter 1, page 1539. Routine examination includes complete evaluation of the esophagus, the stomach, and the duodenum to the duodenojejunal junction. We routinely obtain spot images of the esophagus, stomach, duodenal bulb, and duodenal sweep (including an anteroposterior supine image demonstrating the duodenal–jejunal junction, the anatomic marker for the location of the ligament of Treitz). In addition, we obtain a lateral view of the duodenal sweep to confirm the posterior, retroperitoneal position of the duodenum. We typically obtain a supine spot image of the abdomen at the completion of the study to include the opacified proximal small bowel loops in lieu of an overhead radiograph. Obviously, specific additional views will be necessary at times depending on the results of the fluoroscopic examination. Because it is not necessary to include the pelvis in the radiographic field during upper GI examination, it is imperative that gonadal shielding be used in all children.

> ■ A lateral view of the duodenal sweep (to confirm the posterior, retroperitoneal position of the C-loop) should be obtained in addition to the frontal view of the duodenum.

ULTRASONOGRAPHY

Ultrasound (US) of the upper GI tract is becoming more widely used. Findings are discussed under specific disease entities in Section VI, Part VI, Chapters 2, page 1587 and 3, page 1593. Cohen, Haller, et al. have pointed out the technical advantages gained by filling the stomach with fluid prior to US evaluation. Their technique is particularly critical when US is used for the detection of gastroesophageal reflux and quite useful in the evaluation for pyloric stenosis and other lesions in the gastric outlet. Right posterior oblique positioning helps to displace air in the antrum with fluid to better visualize the pyloric region. US evaluation of the duodenum is most useful in neonates and is discussed in Section II, Part IV, page 104.

RADIONUCLIDE GASTRIC EMPTYING STUDIES

Radionuclide gastric emptying studies are usually performed at the time of evaluation for gastroesophageal reflux. The infant is fed a liquid meal of approximately

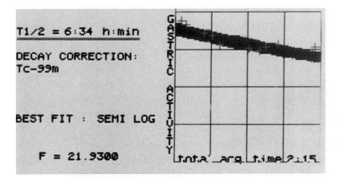

FIGURE 4. Delayed gastric emptying after administration of ^{99m}Tc sulfur colloid in formula (same patient as in Section VI, Part VI, Chapter 3, Fig. 25, page 1610). Half–gastric emptying time was 6½ hours; normal is 60 to 90 minutes. (Courtesy of Michael L. Goris, M.D., Stanford, CA.)

CROSS-SECTIONAL IMAGING

There are occasional reports of computed tomography and magnetic resonance imaging findings in benign diseases of the stomach in the pediatric population. These are often incidental to an examination being performed for other reasons. Most authors agree that the only real utility of these expensive studies for gastric lesions in children is when malignancy is being considered in the differential diagnosis or when a proven malignancy is being staged.

SUGGESTED READINGS

Cohen HL, Haller JO, Mester A, et al: Neonatal duodenum: fluid-filled US examination. Radiology 1987;164:805

Cohen MD: Choosing contrast media for the evaluation of the gastrointestinal tract of neonates and infants. Radiology 1987; 162:447

Cohen MD, Weber TR, Grosfeld JL: Bowel perforation in the newborn: diagnosis with metrizamide. Radiology 1984;150:65

Gelfand MJ, Wagner GC: Gastric emptying in infants and children: limited utility of 1-hour measurement. Radiology 1991;178:379

Miller J: Upper gastrointestinal tract evaluation with radionuclides in infants. Radiology 1991;178:326

Miller JH, Kemberling CR: Ultrasound of the pediatric gastrointestinal tract. Semin Ultrasound CT MR 1987;8:349–365

Stringer DA, Daneman A, Brunelle F, et al: Sonography of the normal and abnormal stomach (excluding hypertrophic pyloric stenosis) in children. J Ultrasound Med 1986;5:183–188

the same volume as a normal feeding. Technetium-99m sulfur colloid is typically added to the initial portion of the feeding, with the dose based on the child's age and weight. The examination time varies by institution. Gelfand and Wagner favor the increased accuracy of a 2-hour examination, while Miller evaluates the infants for 90 minutes. Miller gives the lower limit of normal gastric emptying as 45% at 60 minutes and 60% at 90 minutes (Fig. 4).

Chapter 2

CONGENITAL GASTRIC AND DUODENAL ABNORMALITIES

ALAN E. SCHLESINGER and BRUCE R. PARKER

GASTRIC DUPLICATIONS

Congenital duplications of the stomach are rare. Gastric duplications arise most typically along the greater curvature of the stomach, often in the antrum. Patients may present with vomiting, hematemesis, or melena. Large duplications may be palpable on physical examination. Small duplication cysts within the submucosa or muscularis likely develop from persistent vacuoles within the primitive foregut epithelium, whereas larger cysts likely result from anomalous separation of the endoderm and notocord. Ueda et al. reported a case of gastric duplication in association with aberrant pancreas. Vertebral anomalies are only rarely reported with gastric duplications. Tubular duplications may involve both the stomach and the esophagus. When large, gastric duplications may impinge on the gastric lumen and may be readily identified on barium study as an intramural, extraluminal mass (Fig. 1). Rarely, the duplications may communicate with the lumen of the stomach or esophagus.

The imaging diagnosis can often be made with sonography. The cyst is typically anechoic (Fig. 2). The wall of the cyst typically demonstrates an inner thin echogenic line representing the mucosa and an outer

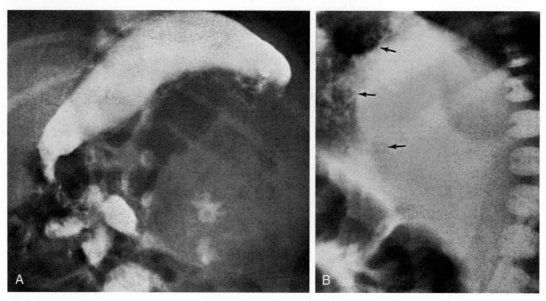

FIGURE 1. Gastric duplication. **A,** In the anteroposterior projection, a large soft tissue mass is seen deforming the greater curvature of the stomach and displacing it cephalad. **B,** On lateral examination, the stomach is seen to be displaced posteriorly by the large gastric duplication *(arrows)*.

hypoechoic muscular layer ("bowel wall signature"). Echogenic material within the cyst probably represents residua of hemorrhage, infection, or inspissated secretions. Endoscopic ultrasound has also been reported in the evaluation of gastric duplication cysts. Computed tomography (CT) and magnetic resonance imaging (MRI) can also identify these cystic masses. The cysts typically have low attenuation on CT. On MRI, these cysts usually have low signal on T_1-weighted images and high signal on T_2-weighted pulse sequences unless there is associated hemorrhage. Scintigraphy can be useful in the evaluation of gastric duplication cysts because sodium pertechnetate will accumulate in ectopic gastric mucosa. The imaging differential diagnosis is discussed in Table 1.

■ Sonographic findings with gastric duplication cyst include the following:
- Common
    1. Intramural cystic gastric mass
    2. Anechoic fluid
    3. "Bowel wall signature"
- Less common: increased echogenicity of fluid resulting from hemorrhage, infection, or proteinaceous fluid

■ Computed tomography (CT)/magnetic resonance imaging (MRI) findings with gastric duplication cyst include the following:
- Common
    1. Intramural cystic gastric mass
    2. Cyst fluid with low attenuation on CT;

    low signal on T_1-weighted and high signal on T_2-weighted MRI
- Less common
    1. Increased attenuation of fluid on CT as a result of hemorrhage, infection, or proteinaceous fluid
    2. Increased signal intensity of fluid on T_1-weighted MRI as a result of hemorrhage or elevated protein in cyst fluid

GASTRIC DIVERTICULA

True congenital gastric diverticula, in which all elements of the gastric wall appear, represent incomplete duplications and can be seen on upper gastrointestinal (GI) series when filled with barium. They are quite rare in children and are usually asymptomatic; most occur near the esophagogastric junction. Intramural diverticula are seen typically in adults and arise near the gastric antrum. Large antral diverticula can cause partial gastric outlet obstruction by compression on the antropyloric region (Fig. 3).

Table 1 ■ DIFFERENTIAL DIAGNOSIS OF GASTRIC DUPLICATION CYST

When presenting as an intramural mass:
    Intramural gastric tumor
    Inflammatory pseudotumor
    Ectopic pancreas
When communicating with gastric lumen:
    gastric diverticulum

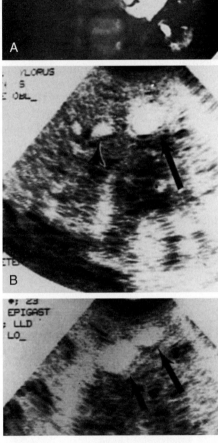

FIGURE 2. Gastric duplication. **A,** Upper gastrointestinal series in a 3-day-old boy with a history of projectile vomiting. The narrowed pyloric channel *(arrow)* in frontal and prone oblique projections suggests an extrinsic pressure defect. **B,** Transverse *(top)* and sagittal *(bottom)* ultrasound images demonstrate a fluid-filled cyst adjacent to the antrum *(arrow)* with a fluid-filled duodenal bulb *(arrowhead)* distal to it. On the sagittal sonogram, the *arrows* demonstrate the bi-lobed anechoic duplication cyst.

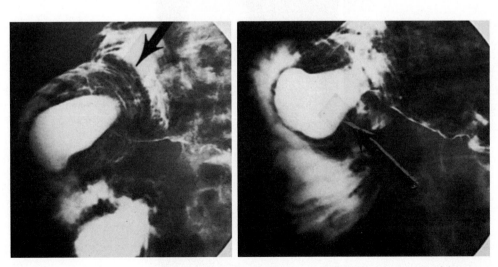

FIGURE 3. Gastric diverticulum. On upper gastrointestinal series, the coiled-spring appearance of intussusception is identified *(arrow)*. On the right, the barium-filled diverticulum is seen to be featureless, with the air-filled antrum proximal to it and the barium-filled duodenal sweep distal to it. The diverticulum originated at the gastroduodenal junction and was lined with gastric mucosa.

MICROGASTRIA

Congenital microgastria with failure of rotation of the stomach is a rare anomaly in which fetal rotation of the stomach fails to occur, and the greater and lesser curvatures do not develop. Also, there is no differentiation into fundus, body, antrum, and pyloric canal. The tiny tubular stomach remains in the midsagittal plane and is joined from above and behind at its summit by the esophagus (Fig. 4). The duodenum projects directly ventrad from the pyloric end. The gastroesophageal junction is incompetent and gastroesophageal reflux is present. The esophagus is dilated and appears to take over the storage function of the inadequate stomach. Vomiting from birth, hematemesis, weight loss, and secondary anemia are the most common presenting features. Microgastria, although reported as an isolated abnormality, is often associated with other congenital anomalies, including renal anomalies, asplenia, polysplenia, anomalous lung lobation, esophageal atresia, malrotation, duodenal atresia, hydrocephalus, anal atresia, congenital heart disease, microphthalmia, arhinencephaly, single nostril, and upper extremity limb reduction defects. The common association between microgastria and upper extremity limb reduction defects has led to the term *microgastria–limb reduction complex*. Agastria, or complete lack of gastric development, is the most extreme form of microgastria.

PYLORIC AND PREPYLORIC ATRESIAS, STENOSES, AND WEBS

Congenital pyloric and prepyloric atresias, stenoses, and webs are rare. They represent variations of the same entity and vary anywhere from an intraluminal diaphragm causing minimal obstruction to complete discontinuity between the gastric antrum and the pylorus or duodenum. The cause and pathogenesis of these lesions is not known. Although originally believed to be caused by a failure of canalization of the early fetal solid gastric epithelium (as is seen in duodenal atresia), more recently it has been suggested that the atresia, stenosis, or web may be secondary to an intrauterine vascular accident (as is the most common cause of jejunal and ileal atresia). The association of pyloric atresia and epidermolysis bullosa has been described, and the genetic mutation responsible for this combination of abnormalities has been identified. Because the obstruction is complete in patients with atresia, these patients typically present in the first hours or days after birth (see Section II, Part IV, Chapter 4, page 113).

Because most congenital obstructive lesions more distal in the proximal duodenum, such as atresia, stenosis, webs, and diaphragms, also present at birth (see Section II, Part IV, Chapter 4, page 113), clinical differentiation can be difficult. Patients with stenoses or webs of the pylorus (rather than complete atresia) may present later in life, including adulthood (as is the case with more distal duodenal stenoses or webs), because the obstruction is incomplete (Fig. 5). Some webs presenting at an older age may be related to ulcer disease rather than representing congenital defects. Radiographically, the air- and/or fluid-filled stomach is usually dilated. With atresia, there may be no air distal to the body of the stomach. With stenoses and webs, there may be varying degrees of distal air seen. In patients with incomplete obstruction, webs are more common than stenoses and are seen on upper GI series as circumferential thin filling defects in the antrum. Stenoses can cause variable obstruction to the antegrade flow of contrast.

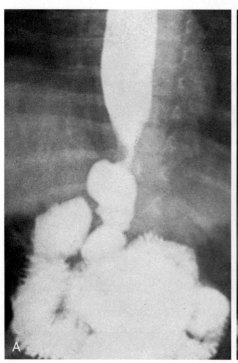
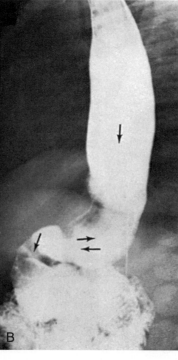

FIGURE 4. Congenital microgastria with failure of rotation of the stomach in a 6-month-old infant. Frontal **(A)** and lateral **(B)** projections demonstrate the stomach to be small and tubular in the midsagittal plane of the abdomen. The cardia is incompetent; the dilated esophagus serves as a storage organ *(top arrow)* and compensates for the inadequate stomach *(pair of lower arrows)*. The first portion of the duodenum comes directly off the pylorus and is directed ventrad *(left lower arrow)*.

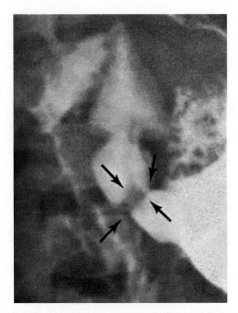

FIGURE 5. Congenital incomplete prepyloric membrane in a 2-year-old girl with nearly lifelong vomiting. The membrane *(arrows)* caused an incomplete pyloric obstruction, and in the upper gastrointestinal series produced a transverse filling defect at the prepyloric level. At surgery, a membrane with a central defect was found and removed. (Courtesy of Dr. E. Salzman, Denver, CO.)

GASTRIC VOLVULUS

Gastric volvulus is an uncommon condition of which two types have been described. As mentioned previously, the stomach is fixed by four ligaments that represent peritoneal folds. If the stomach is not fixed properly, it can rotate along an axis perpendicular to its long axis so that the pylorus comes to lie superiorly. This is known as mesenteroaxial volvulus and is associated with eventration of the left hemidiaphragm. There may be obstruc-

tion to both the gastric inlet and gastric outlet. Plain radiographs of the chest and abdomen show a large distended stomach below an elevated left hemidiaphragm (Fig. 6). The stomach may also rotate around its long axis, a condition known as organoaxial volvulus. This is most commonly seen in association with large hiatal hernias, particularly of the paraesophageal type. Of the two types of gastric volvulus, the mesenteroaxial type represents a true emergency because the twist can compromise the blood supply to the stomach. Organoaxial volvulus is much less common and may, in fact, be chronic in nature. Upper GI series is usually necessary to make the diagnosis of organoaxial volvulus. Uc et al. described a patient with both gastric volvulus and wandering spleen, entities that are both caused by anomalous intraperitoneal visceral attachments.

> - Meseneroaxial volvulus represents a true emergency as ischemia of the stomach may occur
> - Organoaxial volvulus is much less common and may be chronic

ECTOPIC PANCREAS

Ectopic pancreas (Fig. 7) is an uncommon anomaly in which pancreatic tissue is found in the antropyloric region or, less commonly, in the duodenum. Typically, ectopic pancreas is an incidental finding, but occasionally symptoms occur, including pain, GI bleeding, or obstruction. Gastroduodenal prolapse has also been reported. Typically, there is a mound of tissue seen on upper GI series projecting into the barium-filled lumen. The mass is umbilicated, and a central niche may be

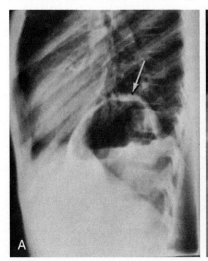
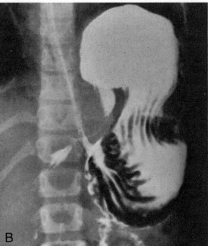
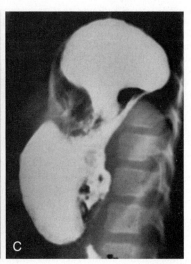

FIGURE 6. Mesenteroaxial volvulus in a 7-year-old girl with abdominal pain and distention. **A,** On lateral chest examination, eventration of the diaphragm is demonstrated *(arrow).* **B,** Two radiographs from the upper gastrointestinal series demonstrate the gastroesophageal junction to be in a relatively normal position. The gastric outlet in this instance lies superiorly and posteriorly. At surgery, the volvulus was easily reduced, and the diaphragmatic eventration repaired. (Courtesy of Dr. V. Condon, Salt Lake City, UT.)

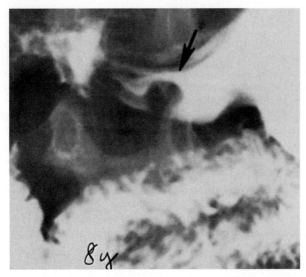

FIGURE 7. Aberrant pancreas. A rounded filling defect *(arrow)* is demonstrated along the inferior margin of the prepyloric antrum. In this case, the pathognomonic central umbilication is not identified.

seen representing an attempt at duct formation. This entity can also be identified sonographically.

SUGGESTED READINGS

Gastric Duplications

Agha, FP, Gabriele OF, Abdulla FH: Complete gastric duplication. AJR Am J Roentgenol 1981;137:406

Dittrich JR, Spottswood SE, Jolles PR: Gastric duplication cyst: scintigraphy and correlative imaging. Clin Nucl Med 1997;22:93

Egelhoff JC, Bisset GS, Strife JL: Multiple enteric duplications in an infant. Pediatr Radiol 1986;16:160–161

Hulnick DH, Balthazar EJ: Gastric duplication cyst: GI series and CT correlation. Gastrointest Radiol 1987;12:106-108

Kangarloo H, Sample WF, Hansen G, et al: Ultrasonic evaluation of abdominal gastrointestinal tract duplication in children. Radiology 1979;131:191–194

Moccia WA, Astacio JE, Kande JV: Ultrasonographic demonstration of gastric duplication in infancy. Pediatr Radiol 1981;11:52

Skandalakis JE, Gray SW, Ricketts RR: Stomach. *In* Skandalakis JE, Gray SW (eds): Embryology for Surgeons, 2nd ed. Baltimore, Williams & Wilkins, 1994:150–183

Takahara T, Torigoe T, Haga H, et al: Gastric duplication cyst: evaluation by endoscopic ultrasonography and magnetic resonance imaging. J Gastroenterol 1996;31:420

Torgerson CL, Young DW, Vaid YN, et al: Intestinal duplication: imaging with Tc-99m sodium pertechnitate. Clin Nucl Med 1996; 21:968

Ueda D, Taketazu M, Itoh S, et al: Case of gastric duplication cyst with aberrant pancreas. Pediatr Radiol 1991;21:379

Wieczorek RL, Seidman I, Ranson JH, et al: Congenital duplication of the stomach: case report and review of the English literature. Am J Gastroenterol 1984;79:597–602

Gastric Diverticula

Flacks K, Stelman HH, Matsumoto PJH: Partial gastric diverticula. Am J Roentgenol Radium Ther Nucl Med 1965;94:339–342

Microgastria

Aintablian NH, Slim MS, Antoun BW: Congenital microgastria. Pediatr Surg Int 1987;2:307

Blank E, Chisholm AJ: Congenital microgastria: a case report with a 26 year follow-up. Pediatrics 1973;51:1037–1041

Cunniff C, Williamson-Kruse L, Olney AH: Congenital microgastria and limb reduction defects. Pediatrics 1993;91:1192

Dorney SF, Middleton AW, Kozlowski K, et al: Congenital microgastria. J Pediatr Gastroenterol Nutr 1987;6:307

Gorman B, Shaw DG: Congenital microgastria. Br J Radiol 1984;57: 260–262

Hasegawa S, Kohno S, Tamura K, et al: Congenital microgastria in an infant with VACTERL association. J Pediatr Surg 1993;28:782

Hochberger O, Swoboda W: Congenital microgastria: a follow-up observation over six years. Pediatr Radiol 1974;2:207–208

Lurie IW, Magee CA, Sun CC, et al: 'Microgastria–limb reduction' complex with congenital heart disease and twinning. Clin Dysmorphol 1995;4:150

Ramos CT, Moss RL, Musemeche CA: Microgastria as an isolated anomaly. J Pediatr Surg 1996;31:445

Shackelford G, McAlister WH, Brodeur AE, et al: Congenital microgastria. Am J Roentgenol Radium Ther Nucl Med 1973;118:72–76

Pyloric and Prepyloric Atresias, Stenoses, and Webs

Bronsther B, Nadeau MR, Abrams MW: Congenital pyloric atresia: a report of three cases and review of the literature. Surgery 1971;69: 130–136

Cetinkursun S, Ozturk H, Celasun B, et al: Epidermolysis bullosa associated with pyloric, esophageal, and anal atresia: a case report. J Pediatr Surg 1995;30:1477

Cremin BJ: Congenital pyloric antral membranes in infancy. Radiology 1969;92:509–512

DeGroot WG, Postumu R, Hunger AGW: Familial pyloric atresia associated with epidermolysis bullosa. J Pediatr 1978;92:429–431

Dolan CR, Smith LT, Sybert VP: Prenatal detection of epidermolysis bullosa letalis with pyloric atresia in a fetus by abnormal ultrasound and elevated alpha-fetoprotein. Am J Med Genet 1993;47:395

Felson B, Berkman YM, Hoyumpa AM: Gastric mucosal diaphragm. Radiology 1969;92:513–517

Hasegawa T, Kubota A, Imura K, et al: Prenatal diagnosis of congenital pyloric atresia. J Clin Ultrasound 1993;21:278

Korber JS, Glasson MJ: Pyloric atresia associated with epidermolysis bullosa. J Pediatr 1977;90:600–601

Maman E, Maor E, Kachko L, et al: Epidermobullosa, pyloric atresia, aplastic cutis congenital: histopathological deliniation of an autosomal recessive disease. Am J Med Genet 1998;78:127

Mellerio JE, Pulkkinen L, McMillan JR, et al: Pyloric atresia-junctional epidermolysis bullosa syndrome: mutations in the integrin beta4 gene (ITGB4) in two unrelated patients with mild disease. Br J Dermatol 1998;139:862

Orense M, Garcia Hernandez JB, Celorio C, et al: Pyloric atresia associated with epidermolysis bullosa. Pediatr Radiol 1987;17:435

Pulkkinen L, Kim DU, Uitto J: Epidermolysis bullosa and pyloric atresia: novel mutations in the beta4 integrin gene (ITGB4). Am J Pathol 1998;152:157

Gastric Volvulus

Campbell JB, Rappaport LN, Skerket LB: Acute mesentero-axial volvulus of the stomach. Radiology 1972;103:153–156

Uc A, Kao SC, Sanders KD: Gastric volvulus and wandering spleen. Am J Gastroenterol 1998;93:1146

Ziprkowski MN, Teele RL: Gastric volvulus in childhood. Am J Gastroenterol 1979;132:921–925

Ectopic Pancreas

Allison JW, Johnson JF, Barr LL, et al: Induction of gastroduodenal prolapse by antral heterotopic pancreas. Pediatr Radiol 1995;25:50

Eklof O, Lassrich A, Stanley P, et al: Ectopic pancreas. Pediatr Radiol 1973;1:24–27

Hayes-Jordan A, Idowu O, Cohen R: Ectopic pancreas as the cause of gastric outlet obstruction in a newborn. Pediatr Radiol 1998;28:868

Kilman WJ, Berk RN: The spectrum of radiographic features of aberrant pancreatic rests involving the stomach. Radiology 1977; 123:291–296

Chapter 3

ACQUIRED GASTRIC AND DUODENAL DISORDERS

ALAN E. SCHLESINGER and BRUCE R. PARKER

HYPERTROPHIC PYLORIC STENOSIS

Hypertrophic pyloric stenosis (HPS) represents the most common cause of gastric outlet obstruction, either congenital or acquired. Although incidence figures vary from one country to another, approximately 1 in 500 liveborn children in the United States will develop pyloric stenosis. Although the age of the child at the onset of symptoms is usually 3 to 6 weeks, with a range of 1 week to 3 months, HPS has been described in the first week of life and occasionally in older children. The disease is unusual in premature infants. There is a positive family history in less than 5% of cases, but there is an increased incidence of pyloric stenosis in twin siblings of affected patients. Although the traditional history of the patient being a firstborn male in the family is not always true, there is a definite male preponderance, and firstborns do seem to be more affected than their younger siblings. In the United States, 80% to 85% of affected patients are males.

ETIOLOGY

The cause of HPS is not known. A genetic component in the etiology of this disease is well established, but the identification of a precise genetic locus has not yet been determined. The pathophysiology seems to be one of work hypertrophy of the circular muscle of the pylorus. This mucosa becomes markedly hypertrophied as if under constant stimulation (Fig. 1). Although a variety of theories as to the cause of this work hypertrophy have been put forward, none has been proven. There has been controversy regarding the association between HPS and congenital anomalies. Several studies in the surgical literature describe an increased incidence of inguinal hernia, undescended testicle, hypospadias, duplex pelvicalyceal system, hydronephrosis, and vesicoureteral reflux. However, a large retrospective review of 274 infants evaluated for HPS with ultrasound (US) by Fernbach and Morello suggested that the incidence of renal anomalies in the 126 patients with HPS was similar to that in the 148 patients without HPS.

Weiskittel et al. reported two cases of evolving HPS in which normal US scans were followed 1 to 2 weeks later by US findings diagnostic of HPS. These findings lend credence to the belief that the disease is acquired after birth and evolves over a course of days to weeks. Latchaw et al. described three older infants in whom classical pyloric stenosis developed after prolonged transpyloric jejunal feeding tube placement.

CLINICAL FINDINGS

The babies typically present with a history of vomiting that is initially mild and is often interpreted as gastroesophageal reflux with excess "spitting up." Careful history taking often reveals that the vomiting started relatively early in life, although the child may not have presented for medical attention until 6 weeks of age or older. As the relative degree of obstruction increases, in the classical case, the vomiting ultimately becomes projectile. The projectile vomiting progresses rapidly, and dehydration is common when medical attention is not sought speedily. The vomitus typically is not bile stained. Approximately 5% of the patients will be mildly jaundiced.

DIAGNOSIS

Physical examination is often diagnostic. Peristaltic waves may actually be seen on the abdominal wall progressing from the left upper quadrant across the epigastrium. The hypertrophied pyloric muscle may be palpated in the midepigastrium by an experienced pediatric surgeon or pediatrician. However, especially with the advances in US evaluation of pyloric stenosis, there has been a definite trend toward reliance on imaging rather than clinical history and physical examination. While some have bemoaned the loss of clinical skills in the evaluation of this entity and have argued that imaging increases the financial cost of the work-up of HPS, physical examination does not necessarily lead to earlier diagnosis, and may lead to false positive studies and unnecessary laparotomies, others have argued that US can lead to earlier diagnosis (prior to development of alkalosis and weight loss), has no radiation, and is relatively inexpensive.

Some have advocated the upper gastrointestinal (GI) series as the first examination in patients with symptoms

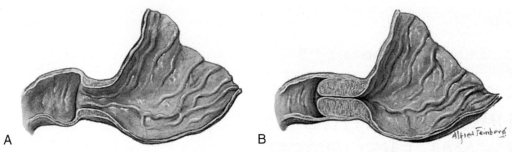

FIGURE 1. The morbid anatomic changes in hypertrophic pyloric stenosis. **A,** A normal stomach in a 4-week-old infant. Note that the pyloric muscle is slightly thicker than that of the body of the stomach. **B,** Marked thickening of the pyloric muscle is noted secondary to hypertrophy of the circular layer. This thickened muscle is elongated, projecting into the more proximal portion of the stomach. The pyloric canal is elongated and constricted. The pyloric muscle also bulges into the base of the duodenal cap.

of HPS for two reasons: an upper GI series is more cost effective as the first imaging examination compared to US (because a follow-up upper GI series is more frequently ordered after a negative US than vice versa), and, although US may be quite accurate in the diagnosis of HPS, it will not be diagnostic in infants with vomiting from other causes. Nevertheless, others have argued that an "US first" approach has other less tangible benefits, such as no radiation, better patient and parental acceptance, and lack of oral contrast. We recommend US as the first imaging study in patients with nonpalpable olives if the clinician wishes to distinguish between HPS and gastroesophageal reflux *and* will empirically treat reflux if the US is negative. If the referring clinician states that he or she will document reflux (or attempt to exclude other diagnoses) by upper GI series if the US is negative, we recommend the upper GI series as the initial sreening study rather than US to avoid increased cost in performing both studies.

Ultrasonography

US typically is performed with linear transducers with a frequency of 5 MHz or higher. The pylorus is frequently more easily seen if the stomach is filled with a dextrose–water solution or formula. With the patient in the supine or right posterior oblique position, the gallbladder is identified, and the pylorus is typically found just medial to the gallbladder. Even if air- or barium-filled bowel obscures the pylorus, it can often be visualized by using the liver as an acoustic window. Images of the pylorus should be obtained in both transverse and longitudinal projections.

An experienced examiner can frequently make the diagnosis by qualitative assessment of the thickness of the pyloric wall and length of the pyloric channel, but great interest has been focused on trying to determine accurate measurements of the pyloric muscle thickness, pyloric muscle length, and length of the pyloric channel. To perform the measurements accurately, great care much be taken to image the pylorus properly. On the transverse scans, the pylorus should look like a doughnut, with the echolucent hypertrophied muscle surrounding the echogenic gastric mucosa (Fig. 2).

Although asymmetry in the "doughnut" can sometimes be seen, careful positioning will usually show a high degree of symmetry. The echolucent ring of hypertrophied muscle may sometimes appear nonuniform on the transverse scan. Typically, the near and far fields appear more echogenic than the sides (Fig. 3). Spevak and her colleagues have shown this to be secondary to the anisotropic effect of the sound waves encountering the circular muscle fibers in a perpendicular orientation in the near and far fields and more tangentially later-

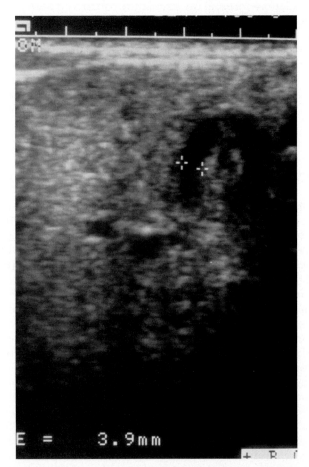

FIGURE 2. Transverse ultrasound of the pylorus demonstrates thickened muscle, measuring 3.9 mm. The characteristic findings of hypertrophic pyloric stenosis were present at surgery.

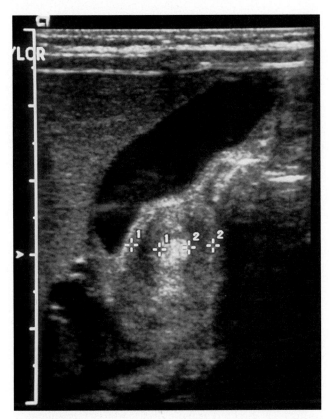

FIGURE 3. Transverse scan in a proven case of hypertrophic pyloric stenosis. Note that the echogenicity in the near field and far field is greater than that seen in the lateral aspects of the thickened pyloric muscle.

ally. On longitudinal scans, the hypertrophied muscle should be of equal thickness on both sides of the echogenic central mucosa (Fig. 4). Cohen et al. have demonstrated a US "double track" sign, which they believe is reliable.

The pyloric muscle thickness should be measured on both transverse and longitudinal scans, and these measurements should be in close agreement. The boundary between the antrum and pyloric muscle can usually be identified, with an appearance not unlike that seen on barium studies (see below). The length of the pyloric muscle can then be measured. In the same position, the length of the pyloric channel (Fig. 5), as demonstrated by the echogenic gastric mucosa, can also be measured. Keller et al. compared US measurements of the thickened pylorus with measurements at surgery, finding excellent correlation in each of 17 cases. The sonographic measurement was actually smaller than the anatomic measurement in all cases.

In the original descriptions of the technique by Teele and Smith and by Blumhagen, a measurement of pyloric wall thickness of 4 mm was judged to be the upper limit of normal. In later reports, measurements of pyloric muscle length suggested a normal upper limit of 17 mm, while the pyloric channel length was believed to be up to 13 mm in normal patients.

Subsequent to the initial reports, a number of studies have been performed suggesting that, in fact, the difference between the pyloric measurements of normal and abnormal patients was somewhat smaller than originally anticipated. Stunden et al. studied 200 consecutive infants with persistent vomiting and determine measurements for overall diameter of the pylorus, thickness of the pyloric muscle, and length of the pyloric canal. Although there was a statistically significant difference in all measurements between the normal group and the group with pyloric stenosis, there was a very small overlap between normals and abnormals based on diameter and muscle wall thickness. However, there was complete separation of the two groups based on channel length. Blumhagen et al. did a similar study on 319 infants in whom they measured the thickness of the pyloric muscle, the length of the pyloric muscle, and the length of the pyloric channel. In their study, there was significant overlap between normals and abnormals in measurement of channel length, less overlap in measurement of muscle length, and no overlap in measurement of muscle thickness. The actual values from both studies are given in Table 1.

O'Keefe et al. studied antropyloric muscle wall thickness in 145 babies with vomiting or regurgitation and also found overlap in muscle thickness measured by US in patients with and without HPS. All babies with measurements of 3 mm or more had pyloric stenosis, whereas none of the babies with measurements less than 2 mm had HPS. Of the six infants with measurements of 2.0 to 2.9 mm, two had HPS, two had pylorospasm, and one each had milk allergy and gastritis.

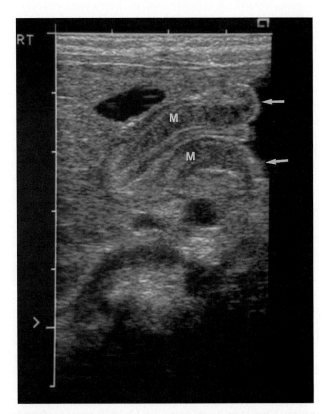

FIGURE 4. Longitudinal scan of hypertrophic pyloric stenosis demonstrates thickening of the pyloric muscle (M) characteristic of hypertrophic pyloric stenosis. The hypertrophied muscle (arrows) impresses on the fluid-filled antrum.

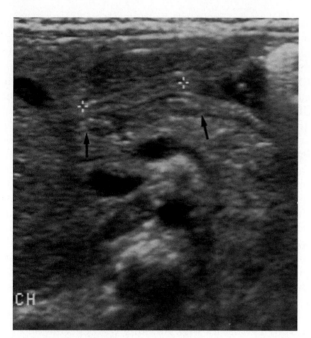

FIGURE 5. Longitudinal scan demonstrates the length of the pyloric canal as demonstrated by the cursor marks. The length of the hypertrophied pyloric muscle *(arrows)* can also be demonstrated.

Westra et al., in contrast, found that none of the three measurements was satisfactory for absolutely differentiating abnormal from normal patients and devised a formula for pyloric volume that, in their experience, was more reliable than any of the other indicators. Ozsvath et al. have shown a significant correlation between the pyloric muscle volume and palpability of the pyloric olive by pediatric surgeons in a study of 60 infants with HPS. Others have advocated a pyloric muscle index calculated using pyloric length, pyloric muscle thickeness, and pyloric diameter. Finkelstein and colleagues suggested that the volume of retained fluid in the stomach may predict the presence of pyloric stenosis. They recommend measuring gastric contents before deciding which imaging study (US or upper GI) to perform, using the volume as a predictor of the likelihood of pyloric stenosis. Like Cohen and Haller, we have not found this a useful technique.

Although the value of measurements of the pylorus varies from one study to another, most experienced sonographers have become very comfortable with the technique. In our experience, the criteria of Blumhagen et al. have proved extremely accurate. However, the age of the patient and the duration of the patient's symptoms should be considered when interpreting a case of possible HPS with borderline measurements on US, because HPS is a progressive process that starts at a few weeks of age and evolves with time. Therefore, a bordeline measurement in a very young infant (1 to 2 weeks of age) with a very short duration of symptoms may represent very early HPS even though the pyloric muscle thickness or pyloric canal length measurements do not meet the strict criteria for HPS. In such cases, the study can be repeated in 5 to 7 days if the patient's symptoms persist or progress.

US has been shown to definitely improve the ability to correctly diagnose HPS in patients with nonpalpable olives. A large study by Hernanz-Schulman et al. of 152 infants with suspected HPS and nonpalpable olives demonstrated 100% accuracy of sonography in categorizing the patients as normal, having HPS, or having pylorospasm. Van der Schouw et al. demonstrated the utility of US when used in conjunction with clinical and laboratory data in children with suspected HPS. In a study of 105 infants with possible HPS, they analyzed the utility of history, clinical signs and symptoms, and laboratory data with and without US data. Their study demonstrated that addition of US data greatly increased the ability to predict HPS in the study group.

Swischuk and his colleagues have described a number of pitfalls in the sonographic diagnosis of pyloric stenosis. The most important of these is mistaking the antrum for the pylorus, but careful examination usually helps to distinguish these two anatomic areas. Other diseases that can mimic pyloric stenosis on sonographic examination are antropyloric gastritis, with or without ulcer disease, and chronic granulomatous disease of childhood. Swischuk et al. also pointed out the need for careful examination technique, because inaccurate placement of the transducer in a plane tangential to the wall of the normal pylorus or antrum can simulate a thickened pylorus, and an overfilled stomach with a posteriorly directed antrum may lead to a false-negative diagnosis.

Contrast Upper Gastrointestinal Series

Prior to the advent of real-time US imaging, the contrast upper GI series was used for diagnosis and may still be more widely utilized than US by radiologists with limited pediatric sonographic experience. The upper GI series is also often utilized when US is normal or equivocal. Riggs and Long described eight plain radiographic findings that are suggestive of the diagnosis when present, but we have never found an instance when an

Table 1 ■ **PYLORIC MEASUREMENTS IN THE DIAGNOSIS OF HYPERTROPHIC PYLORIC STENOSIS (HPS)***		
	STUNDEN ET AL.	**BLUMHAGEN ET AL.**
Pyloric muscle thickness (mm)		
With HPS	3–5	3.5–6.0
Without HPS	1–3	1.0–3.1
Pyloric canal length (mm)		
With HPS	18–28	11–25
Without HPS	5–14	5–22
Pyloric muscle length (mm)		
With HPS	NA	14–29
Without HPS	NA	5.0–26.5
Pyloric diameter (mm)		
With HPS	9–19	NA
Without HPS	7–12	NA

*Data from Stunden et al. (1986) and Blumhagen et al. (1988).

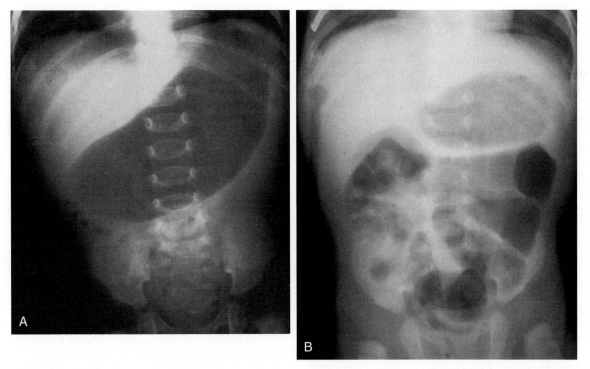

FIGURE 6. Plain radiographs in pyloric stenosis. **A,** Abdomen radiograph demonstrating marked dilatation of the stomach with little gas in the distal bowel in a patient with documented pyloric stenosis. **B,** Abdominal radiograph in a child with surgically documented pyloric stenosis, demonstrating a relatively normal-sized gastric air bubble for a crying baby and gas throughout the rest of the gastrointestinal tract, including the colon.

abnormal scout radiograph has precluded the need for US or barium study. Indeed, the plain radiographs may be quite normal even when HPS is present (Fig. 6). In rare instances, pyloric stenosis is associated with isolated gastric pneumatosis that disappears after the stomach is decompressed (Fig. 7).

In order to obtain a technically satisfactory barium study, many suggest that a nasogastric tube should be passed and the stomach emptied. When we use a tube,

we try to place the tube in the antrum with the patient in the prone oblique position so as not to require large amounts of contrast material. Barium is injected via the tube under fluoroscopic control, and spot images are obtained as needed.

Most of the infants, those with and without HPS, will show some degree of pylorospasm. Generally, barium will finally pass the antropyloric region within 1 to 10 minutes, but may be delayed as long as 20 to 25 minutes.

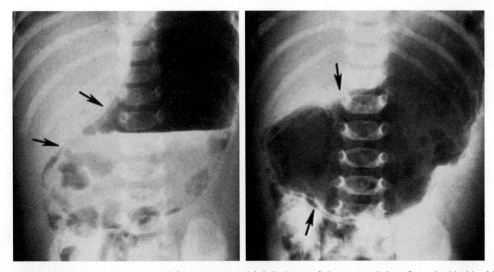

FIGURE 7. Gastric pneumatosis. Upright **(left)** and supine **(right)** views of the stomach in a 6-week-old girl with pyloric stenosis. The stomach is distended with gas and liquid. Intramural gas can be identified *(arrows)*. The pneumatosis disappeared within 24 hours after decompression with gastric intubation. (Courtesy of Dr. J. Leonidas, New Hyde Park, NY.)

Spasm may mimic HPS on both US and barium study. When spasm is severe, Currarino suggests putting the infant supine and pressing into the abdomen from left to right. With HPS, the pyloric muscle mass pushes into the air-filled antrum of the stomach, permitting a diagnosis to be made. If the barium does not pass out of the stomach because of severe HPS, the US scan will be markedly abnormal even to the less experienced sonographer.

The radiographic signs of HPS on upper GI series are remarkably constant from one patient to another (Fig. 8). The pyloric channel is narrowed (the "string sign") and almost always curved upward posteriorly. Barium may be caught between folds overlying the hypertrophied muscle, and parallel lines (the "double string sign") may be seen (Fig. 9). The enlarged muscle mass looks much like an "apple core lesion," with undercutting of the distal antrum and proximal duodenal bulb, although the latter may be seen in normal patients. The "shoulder sign" is caused by impression of the hypertrophied muscle on the air- or barium-filled atrum at the juncture of the stomach wall and hypertrophied pyloric muscle. The "pyloric tit" can be seen along the lesser curve just proximal to the impression of the pyloric mass and may be the result of a persistent peristaltic wave blocked by the mass of the hypertrophied pyloric muscle. The "beak sign" is noted as the thick muscle narrows the barium column as it enters the pyloric channel. Virtually all of the above signs can be seen transiently in infants, especially those with some degree of pylorospasm. The study should be continued sufficiently long to document the persistence of the findings in order to assure the diagnosis of pyloric stenosis. On occasion, an associated antral web or diaphragm may be identified (see Fig. 8).

- ■ Upper GI series findings in HPS include the following:
  - Gastric distension on scout view
  - Narrowed, elongated, curved pyloric channel
  - Double string sign
  - Undercutting of distal antrum and proximal duodenal bulb
  - Shoulder sign
  - "Pyloric tit" on lesser curve
  - "Beak sign"

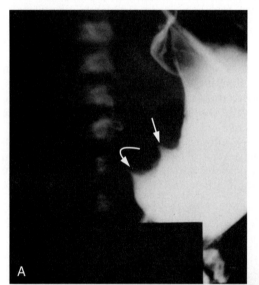

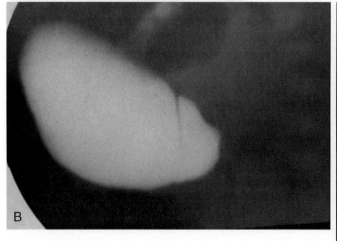

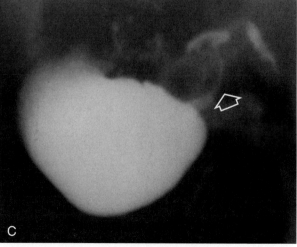

FIGURE 8. A, Typical upper gastrointestinal (GI) series in a patient with pyloric stenosis. The markedly narrowed pylorus curves upward and posteriorly to the duodenal bulb, which shows an impression of the hypertrophied muscle in the base. The hypertrophied muscle can also be seen impressing itself on the lesser curvature of the stomach, causing the "pyloric tit" *(arrow)* to appear slightly above it. The barium column narrows sharply as it enters the pylorus, causing the "beak sign" *(curved arrow)*. **B,** A portion of an upper GI series in a patient with pyloric stenosis demonstrates a linear filling defect in the barium column, suggesting an antral web. **C,** A little later in the study, the characteristic "string sign" *(open arrow)* of pyloric stenosis is seen. Both the pyloric stenosis and antral web were corrected at surgery.

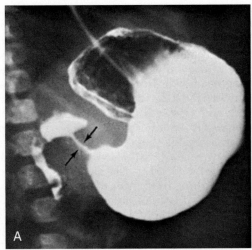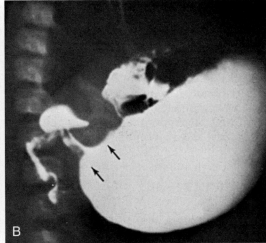

FIGURE 9. Characteristic findings of hypertrophic pyloric stenosis in a 7-week-old boy with a 4-week history of vomiting. **A,** The pyloric canal is narrowed and elongated *(arrows)*, and the base of the duodenal bulb is stretched by the pyloric mass. **B,** The pyloric canal is narrow, demonstrating a "double string sign." Indentation of the hypertrophied muscle on the lesser curvature is identified by the *double arrows.*

DIFFERENTIAL DIAGNOSIS

The most common antropyloric abnormality mimicking HPS on upper GI series is pylorospasm. Although spasm may also make the pyloric muscle appear thicker on US, this is a transient phenomenon usually distinguishable from HPS. Gastric and duodenal ulcers and gastritis (see below) can mimic the findings of HPS, especially on US. Rarer entities, such as eosinophilic gastroenteritis, have also been shown to mimic HPS on US. Focal foveolar hyperplasia, a polypoid antral mass that can extend into the pylorus, is a rare entity in children and presents with gastric outlet obstruction. Although the upper GI appearance may mimic HPS, sonography can differentiate this entity from HPS because the lobulated lesion causing the increased diameter of the pylorus is superficial to (on the lumenal side of) the normal muscle layer of the pylorus. However, there has recently been a report of coexistent HPS and focal foveolar hyperplasia.

> ■ It is important to confirm the persistence of UGI findings of HPS to avoid false positive diagnosis of HPS due to pylorospasm.

TREATMENT

Surgical pyloromyotomy is the traditional therapy for infants with HPS. However, laproscopic pyloromyotomy has been advocated recently by some pediatric surgeons. Several attempts have been made to treat HPS by peroral balloon dilatation. Hayashi et al. performed this procedure on six patients. In five patients, the muscular ring was incompletely disrupted, and pyloromyotomy was still necessary. In the sixth patient, the ring was disrupted but the mucosa was torn, requiring surgical repair.

Following surgical pyloromyotomy, both the US and the upper GI series findings may remain abnormal for several months, even in asymptomatic patients. Thus the diagnosis of incomplete surgical repair requires a history of persistent vomiting as well as a positive imaging study (Fig. 10). Jamroz et al. have suggested that the upper GI series may be more sensitive than US in detecting incomplete pyloromyotomy.

In most countries, patients are treated with pyloromyotomy, although in Sweden there has been extensive experience with successful nonsurgical therapy. A recent report by Author et al. from Japan

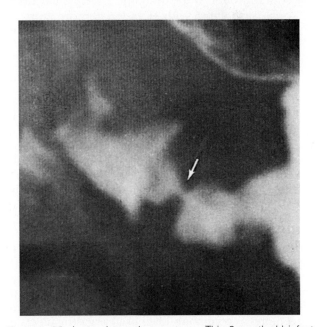

FIGURE 10. Incomplete pyloromyotomy. This 9-month-old infant had been treated surgically for pyloric stenosis 7½ months earlier. He continued to vomit and did not gain weight adequately. The distal portion of the pyloric channel *(arrow)* at the base of the duodenal bulb did not widen under lengthy fluoroscopic observation. The site of incomplete pyloromyotomy was identified and corrected with surgery.

described the US evolution of HPS in four patients with sequential US examinations during medical treatment of HPS. The authors demonstrated that the length of the canal decreased first, followed by decrease in the pyloric muscle thickness. In a second study by Nagita et al. from Japan in 23 infants with HPS that were treated medically, repeated US examinations demonstrated that symptoms resolved before pyloric muscle thickening improved. In the 21 patients who recovered without surgery, the US normalized between 4 and 12 months.

PEPTIC ULCER DISEASE

The understanding of peptic ulcer disease in children and adults has changed dramatically during the last decade with elucidation of the involvement of *Helicobacter pylori* in chronic antral gastritis and peptic ulcer disease. In fact, there is evidence that, although gastritis and peptic ulcer disease are more prevalent in adults than children, colonization with *H. pylori* likely occurs during childhood in most cases. This organism is present in the stomach of 10% of children in developed countries (but in 30% to 40% of children from lower socioeconomic groups) and in from 80% to 100% of children in developing countries. Eradication of the organism with antibiotic therapy is associated with resolution of antral gastritis and ulcers and low recurrence rate of symptoms. There is mounting evidence linking *H. pylori*–associated chronic antral gastritis and gastric adenocarcinoma and gastric lymphoma.

> ■ Although antral gastritis and peptic ulcer disease associated with *H. pylori* is more common in adults than children, colonization with *H. pylori* likely occurs in childhood in most cases.

Peptic ulcers in children occur far less frequently than in adults. Peptic ulcers can be classified as to region of involvement (gastric or duodenal) and presence or absence of a known etiology (primary or secondary). In the neonatal period, gastric ulcers (often presenting with hematemesis or with free peritoneal air resulting from gastric perforation) are more common than duodenal ulcers (see Section II, Part IV). After the neonatal period, gastric ulcers are significantly less common than duodenal ulcers in children and tend to be secondary to chronic systemic diseases (such as cystic fibrosis or Crohn's disease) or ulcerogenic drugs rather than primary. These secondary ulcers tend not to recur after standard medical therapy. Duodenal ulcers are three times as commonly diagnosed as gastric ulcers in infants and children. Although duodenal ulcers also tend to be secondary in children under 10 years of age, primary duodenal ulcers occur with greater frequency in older children. *Helicobacter pylori* gastritis is found in 90% to 100% of pediatric patients with duodenal ulcer

disease. Children with duodenal ulcer disease caused by ulcerogenic drugs or other medical causes of secondary peptic ulceration typically respond to histamine$_2$ (H$_2$) receptor antagonists alone and tend to have no recurrence, whereas patients with primary duodennal ulcers associated with *H. pylori* gastritis require combination therapy with H$_2$ receptor antagonists and antibiotics to eradicate the *H. pylori* infection and prevent recurrence. However, occasionally surgery with proximal gastric vagotomy is required. With advances in ulcer therapy with H$^+$/K$^+$-ATPase inhibitors and antibiotic therapy for *H. pylori*, surgery for bleeding and perforation resulting from ulcer disease has decreased dramatically, but surgery for obstruction related to ulcer disease has not changed significantly.

It may be difficult to determine the etiology of peptic ulcer disease because many of the diseases reported to be associated with peptic ulcers are also treated with ulcerogenic drugs that may be the immediate cause of the ulcers. Patients with cystic fibrosis may have a deficient defense mechanism because of abnormal intestinal mucus, but they are often treated with ulcerogenic drugs and are subject to intense emotional stress, and the etiology of ulcers in these patients is probably multifactorial. Patients with Zollinger-Ellison syndrome have severe abdominal pain, intractable peptic ulcers, and gastric hypersecretion. Non–beta islet cell tumors of the pancreas are implicated as the cause. Rarely seen in children, the syndrome has been described in patients as young as 7 years old.

The radiologic appearance of ulcers in children is much like that in adults (Fig. 11). Barium is the contrast material of choice unless perforation is suspected, in which case a low-osmolar nonionic contrast agent should be used. Gastric ulcers are more likely to be in the antrum than the body or the fundus of the stomach. Ulcers in both stomach and duodenum will demonstrate a barium-filled niche with radiating folds representing surrounding mucosal inflammation. In the gastric antrum, "button ulcers" may be seen (Fig. 12). Giant duodenal ulcers are even more rare in children than in adults (Fig. 13). They usually require surgical therapy.

The study of Drumm et al. confirmed in children the high false-negative rate of single-contrast barium studies for ulcer disease, when compared with endoscopy, that has been demonstrated previously in adults. Double-contrast studies of the stomach and duodenum may have a higher sensitivity but are difficult to perform in young children and usually result in a higher radiation dose at any age. Endoscopy appears to be the most sensitive diagnostic procedure.

Although US is not used routinely in evaluation for ulcer disease, Hayden et al. found 7 children of 600 being investigated for vomiting with gastric ulcers demonstrated by other means who also had US abnormalities. US abnormalities included thickening of the antropyloric mucosa, elongation of the antropyloric canal, persistent spasm, and delayed gastric emptying. Although other authors have reported US findings in gastritis and peptic ulcer disease in children, US has not been widely accepted for imaging these entities in children.

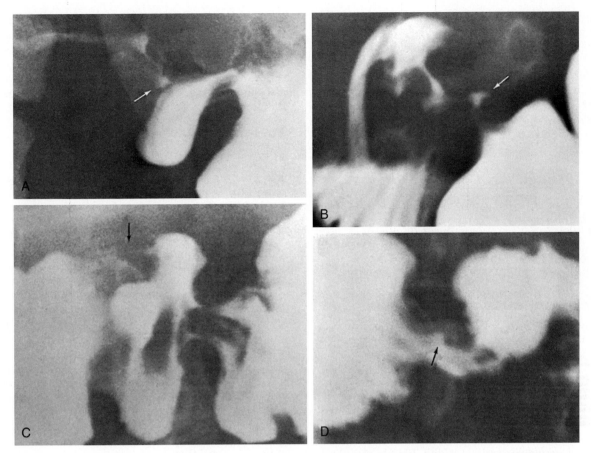

FIGURE 11. Peptic ulcers. **A,** Postbulbar ulcer *(arrow)* in a 9-year-old girl with a long history of vomiting and weight loss. **B,** Pyloric channel ulcer *(arrow)* in a 6-year-old boy. **C,** Large duodenal ulcer *(arrow)* in the bulb of a boy 9 years of age. Note the marked deformity of the duodenal bulb and the edematous folds. **D,** Small channel ulcer *(arrow)* in an 11-year-old boy with abdominal pain and melena.

GASTRITIS

Gastritis is a nonspecific term for inflammation of the mucosa of the stomach. A number of etiologies have been implicated in childhood gastritis, and the common ones are discussed here (Table 2).

CHEMICAL GASTRITIS

Chemical gastritis can be secondary to the ingestion of a variety of substances and can be of extreme severity, even leading to death. Although alkali ingestion more commonly causes esophagitis (see Section VI, Part V, Chapter 4, page 1561), about 20% of patients who ingest these substances will also develop mild to moderate degrees of antral gastritis. More common agents implicated in the direct production of gastritis are calcium chloride, zinc chloride, iron sulfate tablets, and acids (Fig. 14). Button batteries typically contain alkaline electrolytes that can cause esophageal and/or gastric irritation, but theoretical risk also exists from mercury leakage.

Following the ingestion of corrosive agents, plain radiographs, including horizontal-beam views, should be obtained to exclude free air prior to performing contrast studies. If there is a high level of suspicion of perforation, water-soluble contrast can be administered initially. If there is no evidence of perforation, double-contrast studies of the stomach are most useful if they can be performed. The most common of the corrosive agents is calcium chloride. It is likely that some free hydrochloric acid is formed in the stomach by hydrolysis of calcium chloride, and it is this acid that is the direct cause of the severe gastritis. Most commonly, by the time contrast studies are performed, there has already been severe edema, spasm, and narrowing of the distal

Table 2 ■ DIFFERENTIAL DIAGNOSIS OF GASTRITIS
Infectious
Helicobacter pylori
Opportunistic infection
Cytomegalovirus
Toxoplasmosis
Cryptosporidium
Chemical gastritis
Ménétrier's disease
Eosinophilic gastritis
Chronic granulomatous disease
Crohn's disease
Graft-versus-host disease

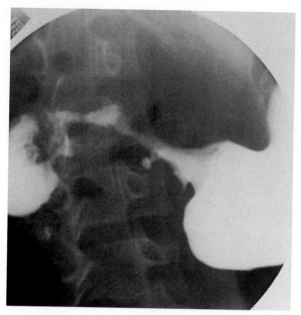

FIGURE 12. A polypoid "button" gastric ulcer in the pyloric channel with marked narrowing and fibrosis of the chronically inflamed pylorus.

stomach. Secondary calcification in the gastric wall, with cicatricial constrictions, has been found several weeks after the original ingestion. Extensive necrosis of the stomach, with almost complete obstruction, has been reported from the ingestion of zinc chloride also. Again, typically, the distal body and antrum of the stomach are primarily involved. Ingested ferrous sulfate tablets can lead to complete gastric outlet obstruction with scarring

of the antrum. Vomiting and hematemesis generally occur almost immediately after ingestion, and death has been reported. Intramural air in the stomach has been reported in cases of gastritis of various causes, although it is more common in adults than in children.

MÉNÉTRIER'S DISEASE

Markedly enlarged gastric folds, so-called giant rugal hypertrophy, can be seen with Ménétrier's disease. This is an uncommon, self-limited disease in children that likely is not the same as the adult disease. The cause in children is unknown. Hypersensitivity response, autoimmune disease, and cytomegalovirus (CMV) infection have all been implicated but not proved. Children usually present with abdominal pain or with nausea and vomiting. Because of an associated protein-losing enteropathy, peripheral edema, ascites, and pleural effusions are frequently found. Gastric hemorrhage is rare. On upper GI series, there is marked enlargement of the fundal rugae, especially along the greater curvature, with sparing of the antropyloric region (Fig. 15). US demonstrates thickened mucosa and rugal hypertrophy when the stomach is empty or partially filled, according to Gassner et al. When the stomach is completely filled with fluid, the hypertrophied rugae characteristically collapse. High-resolution sonography suggests that the gastric wall thickening may occur maximally in the submucosal layer of the stomach, and that serial sonography may be useful in following the course of the disease. Furthermore, endoscopic US has also been advocated in diagnosis of Ménétrier's disease in adults.

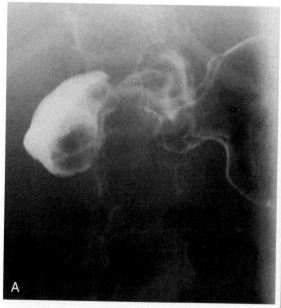
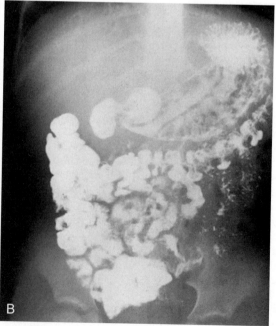

FIGURE 13. Giant duodenal ulcer confirmed at endoscopy in a 7-year-old boy with vomiting and hematemesis. **A,** Upper gastrointestinal series demonstrates a large collection of contrast in the ulcer. **B,** Persistent barium in the ulcer at 2 hours after ingestion is a useful diagnostic sign.

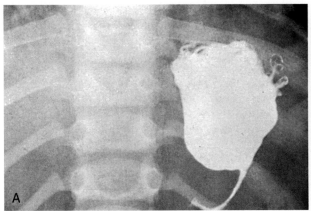
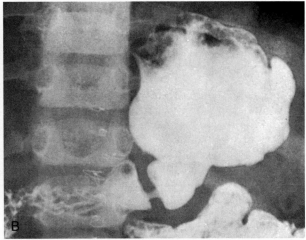

FIGURE 14. Severe necrotizing gastritis caused by zinc chloride. **A,** Eight weeks after ingestion of soldering solution, the distal third of the stomach is constricted to a lumen a few millimeters in diameter with almost complete obstruction of the pylorus. **B,** Thirteen months after surgery, function of the deformed remaining portion of the stomach is normal.

Markedly enlarged gastric rugae may also be seen in gastrointestinal lymphangiectasia (Fig. 16).

■ Ménétrier's disease in children likely is not the same as the adult disease.

INFECTIOUS GASTRITIS

Helicobacter pylori has been described in association with gastritis and peptic ulcer disease since 1982 (see above). Antral gastritis is present in virtually every patient, adult or child, from whom the organism is cultured, and gastric or duodenal ulcers have been described in many. Morrison et al. described a pattern of enlarged gastric folds in the body and antropyloric regions of the stomach in half of their patients with biopsy-proven *H. pylori* infection. Although fold thickening, when present in this disease, is mild, there have been reports of marked gastric fold thickening mimicking malignancy on both upper GI series and computed tomography (CT). These findings often reverse after medical therapy for *H. pylori*.

Infectious gastritis has been described in adults with acquired immunodeficiency syndrome (AIDS). Falcone et al. described 11 patients with AIDS who had gastric abnormalities. Five of these had infections with CMV, *Toxoplasma gondii*, or *Cryptosporidium;* the other six had Kaposi's sarcoma or lymphoma. CMV, one of the most common causes of gastritis in AIDS, typically involves the esophagus, the esophagogastric junction, and the antropyloric portion of the stomach. CMV involving the antropyloric region has been reported to cause pyloric obstruction in a child with human immunodeficiency virus (HIV). CMV gastritis often causes deep ulcerations, submucosal masses resulting from edema, or focal abscesses. Perforation can occasionally occur. *Cryptospo-*

ridium, a protozoan, can also cause antral narrowing. Thickened gastric folds can be seen in children with AIDS and *H. pylori,* but can also occur in children with AIDS as a result of cryptosporidiosis or gut-associated lymphoid tissue, a lymphoproliferative disorder. Interestingly, the prevalence of *H. pylori* in adult patients with AIDS is lower than in age-matched HIV-negative controls. Postulated explanations include antimicrobial therapy or HIV-realted host factors, such as hypochlorhydria or inadequate inflammatory response, causing impairment of successful colonization of the organism.

EOSINOPHILIC GASTRITIS

Eosinophilic gastritis has been reported, occurring either alone or, more commonly, as part of a more diffuse gastroenteritis involving particularly the small intestine. It is typically of an allergic or hypersensitivity etiology and generally responds well to steroids. The disease usually causes a strikingly nodular pattern in the gastric antrum with relative sparing of the body and fundus (Fig. 17). Two cases have been reported that sonographically mimicked HPS.

CHRONIC GRANULOMATOUS DISEASE OF CHILDHOOD

Chronic granulomatous disease of childhood is a syndrome of recurrent infection, usually bacterial or fungal, whose underlying pathophysiology is one of disordered phagocytosis. The most common GI manifestation is chronic antral gastritis (Fig. 18). US examination demonstrates an abnormally thickened antropyloric wall. This finding simulates HPS, but occurs in patients beyond infancy. Upper GI series reveals narrowing of the antropyloric lumen secondary to chronic inflammation and fibrosis. Involvement of the proximal duodenum may also occur. Rarely, surgical intervention is required.

CROHN'S DISEASE

Crohn's disease is more common in the upper gastrointestinal tract than previously thought. Lenaerts et al. reported endoscopic involvement of the esophagus, stomach, and duodenum in 69 of 230 children with Crohn's disease. In 13 of the patients, radiologic studies were negative. However, these studies were not performed using double-contrast technique, which is im-

perative to find the aphthous ulcers that characterize the early stages of the disease. These will be found radiographically most typically in the antrum, pylorus, and duodenum (Fig. 19), but can be seen in the more proximal stomach as well as the distal esophagus. This relatively high prevalence of Crohn's disease in the stomach and duodenum (with low radiographic detection rate) has been confirmed in other more recent studies. In a prospective endoscopic study in children and adolescents with Crohn's disease by Cameron, biopsies demonstrated evidence of disease in the eophagus in 16%, the gastric body in 46%, the gastric antrum in 36%, and the duodenum in 21%. In a prospective

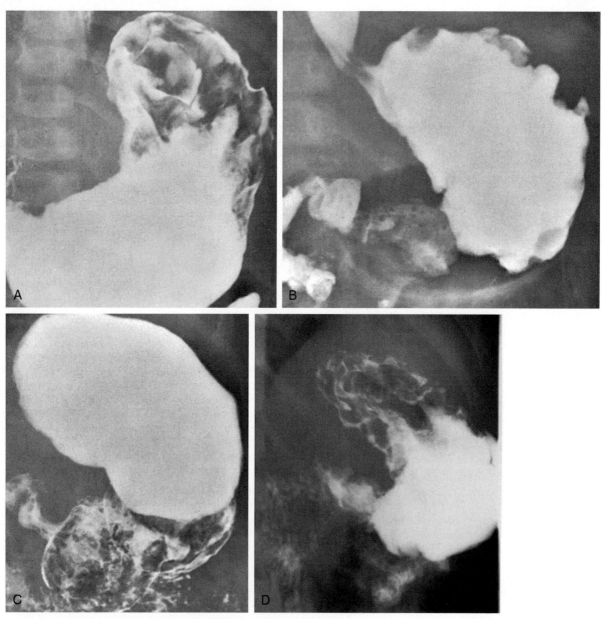

FIGURE 15. Ménétrier's disease. Prone **(A)** and supine **(B)** projections of the stomach show rugal hypertrophy in a 3½–year-old girl with periorbital edema. Hypoproteinemia was found on laboratory studies. **C,** Three months later, serum protein values were normal, as were the gastric rugae. **D,** Giant rugal hypertrophy in a 2-year-old boy with hyperproteinemia, diffuse edema, and pleural effusions. Note that the body and antrum of the stomach are normal.

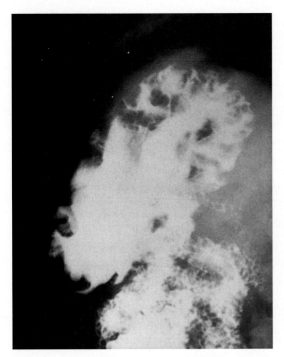

FIGURE 16. Lymphangiectasis of the stomach demonstrates giant rugal hypertrophy involving all parts of the stomach.

study of 31 children with presumed Crohn's disease by Mashako et al., clinical symptoms of upper GI tract involvement were present in 5 (16%) and radiographic findings in only 1 (3%), while endoscopic abnormalities were found in 13 (42%), and specific histologic evidence of granulomas was found on endoscopic biopsies in 12 children (39%). Finally, in a study of 41 children with Crohn's disease by Ruuska et al., upper GI endoscopy revealed esphagitis in 16, esophageal ulcer in 2, gastritis in 22, duodenal inflammation or ulcers in 18, and granulomas on biopsy in 10 children. These studies

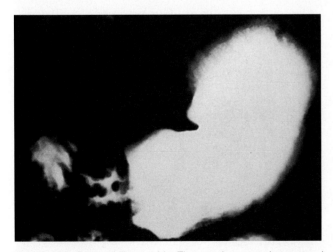

FIGURE 17. Eosinophilic gastritis. The gastric antrum is narrowed with polypoid filling defects in this adolescent girl with peripheral eosinophilia. Diagnosis was documented by biopsy. Note that the proximal portion of the stomach is entirely normal.

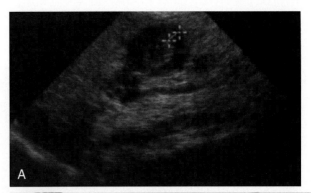

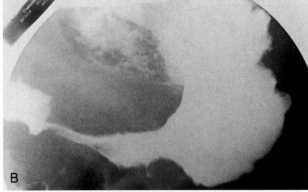

FIGURE 18. Chronic granulomatous disease of childhood in a 2-year-old boy. **A,** Ultrasound demonstrates persistently marked thickening of the antropyloric wall. **B,** Upper gastrointestinal series demonstrates a long, narrowed antrum and pylorus, which were noted to be fixed on fluoroscopic examination.

suggest that endoscopy with biopsy may be helpful to evaluate extent of involvement or to confirm the diagnosis in children with Crohn's disease.

GRAFT-VERSUS-HOST DISEASE

Graft-versus-host disease (GVHD) most typically affects the small intestine and the colon, but can affect the stomach. The findings are nonspecific, but suggestive when other clinical signs of GVHD are present. Mucosal inflammation and irregularity may be identified on upper GI series, while CT or US, as well as upper GI series, may demonstrate thickening of the gastric wall (Fig. 20). Involvement of the stomach is more common in the acute or subacute phase of GVHD than in the chronic phase. In the acute phase, this is related to edema. In the chronic phase, fibrosis is more likely the cause. Patients with GVHD may also acquire CMV gastroenteritis, with imaging findings indistinguishable from GVHD itself.

DUODENITIS

Duodenitis has been a historically contentious subject for radiologists. It is an uncommon finding in children, who are more likely to have antral gastritis than duoden-

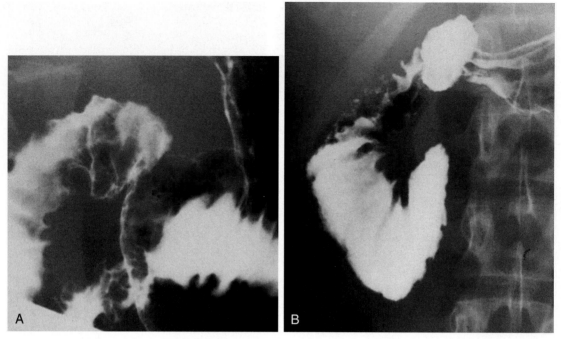

FIGURE 19. A and **B,** Crohn's disease. Marked mucosal fold hypertrophy of the duodenal bulb and postbulbar portion of the duodenum was shown at endoscopy and biopsy to be secondary to previously undetected Crohn's disease.

ditis. Large mucosal folds in the duodenal bulb are best seen on double-contrast upper GI examination. The accuracy of upper GI series in the diagnosis of duodenitis has been questioned. Levine et al., in a series of 50 adults having upper GI series and endoscopy, found the radiographs to have 50% false-positive and 50% false-negative results. However, more recently, a study by Long et al. of 75 children who underwent upper GI series and endoscopy with biopsy (15 with mild biopsy-proven duodenitis, 9 with severe biopsy-proven duodenitis, and 51 controls) revealed that upper GI series had a sensitivity of 46% and a specificity of 98% (compared to 54% and 92%, respectively, for visual inspection at upper endoscopy).

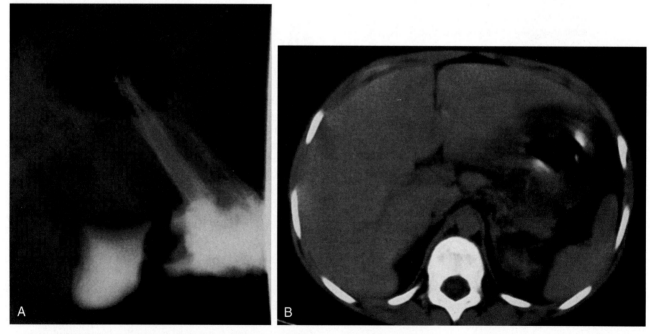

FIGURE 20. Graft-versus-host disease. **A,** Upper gastrointestinal series demonstrates the body of the stomach to be rigid, with effacement of the mucosa secondary to submucosal infiltration. **B,** Computed tomography scan demonstrates edema of the gastric wall in this 14-year-old girl with graft-versus-host disease who had bone marrow transplant for acute lymphocytic leukemia. Similar findings have been described elsewhere in the gastrointestinal tract.

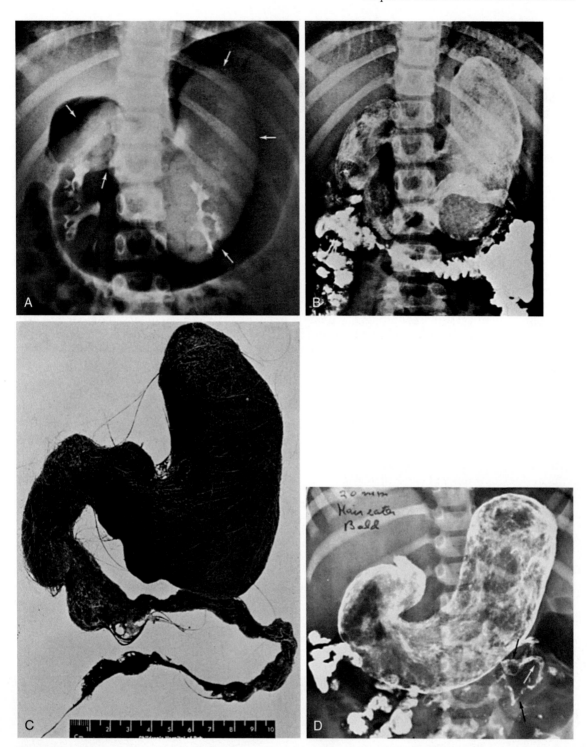

FIGURE 21. Trichobezoar in a 10-year-old girl with anemia and left upper quadrant mass. **A,** A large soft-tissue mass *(arrows)* is seen in the dilated, air-filled stomach. **B,** Barium is trapped in the trichobezoar, demonstrating the mass extending through the duodenum and into the proximal jejunum. **C,** Surgical specimen. **D,** Trichobezoar in a 20-month-old girl. The mass of hair fills the gastric lumen. The *arrows* demonstrate pieces of the trichobezoar in the duodenum and jejunum.

BEZOARS

Occasionally, ingested materials accumulate in the stomach and form nonopaque foreign bodies called bezoars. *Trichobezoars,* or hairballs, usually result from swallowing of hair plucked from the head or fibers from fur rugs, garments, or woolen clothing and blankets. Over a period of time, an intraluminal mass develops, representing matted hair and trapped food particles, taking the shape of the stomach (Fig. 21). Young girls are the most commonly affected. *Phytobezoars,* or food balls, are composed of mucilaginous masses; they develop most frequently following the ingestion of high-fiber vegetables and fruits. Swallowed shellac or tar may also form gastric foreign bodies. Alternatively, certain foods may mimic bezoars, but the findings disappear with time (Fig. 22). A similar appearance can also be seen in infants as a result of curdled milk.

Plain radiographs of patients with bezoars may show an appearance like that of the stomach shortly after the ingestion of a normal meal. Horizontal-beam plain radiographs typically demonstrate a rim of air surrounding the intragastric mass. Bezoars of all types produce filling defects in the stomach after the ingestion of barium. After the free barium has been expelled from the stomach, the barium that has adhered to the surface of the bezoar or has been absorbed by it can cast a persistent, mottled shadow of increased density. Small bezoars are frequently movable, may be of almost any shape, and are found in any position.

Newman and Girdany have demonstrated the US and CT characteristics of trichobezoars (Fig. 23). US demonstrates a broad band of increased echogenicity in the stomach with prominent acoustic shadowing. CT demonstrates an intragastric mass with entrapped air and debris. A case report of a trichobezoar in a child described a low signal mass on both T_1- and T_2-weighted magnetic resonance imaging (MRI).

TUMORS AND TUMOR-LIKE CONDITIONS

True neoplasms of the stomach are relatively uncommon in childhood (Table 3). Polyps have been described in several of the polyposis syndromes, including Peutz-Jeghers syndrome (hamartomatous polyps), Gardner's syndrome (adenomatous polyps), familial polyposis (adenomatous polyps), and juvenile polyposis (juvenile polyps). Recent studies have shown that gastrodudenal polyps may be seen in up to 83% of patients with familial polyposis syndrome, a finding that suggests that lifelong endoscopic surveillance of the upper GI tract is warranted. The potential for malignant transformation of adenomatous polyps has long been known. However, an increased risk of malignancy (both GI and extraintestinal) has recently been reported in patients with Peutz-Jeghers syndrome as well, including a case report of

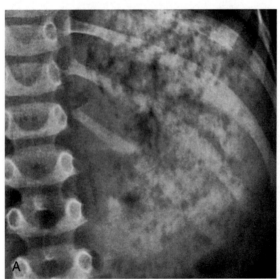
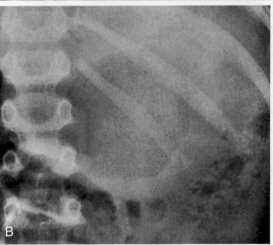
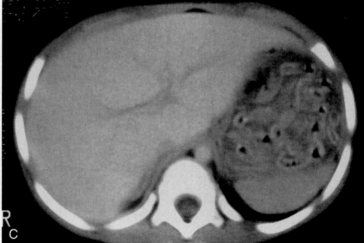

FIGURE 22. Food simulating a gastric bezoar in a 3-year-old girl. **A,** Shortly after a breakfast of four bowls of dry cereal was consumed. **B,** Twenty-four hours later, the stomach appears normal. **C,** Computed tomography section without oral or intravenous contrast in another patient demonstrates a heterogeneous "mass" containing air and curvilinear regions of higher attenuation. This patient had recently eaten macaroni and cheese, and delayed scans confirmed resolution of this pseudo-mass.

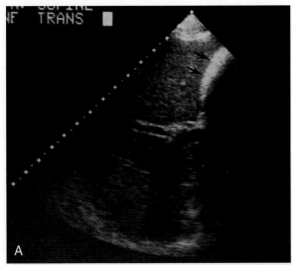

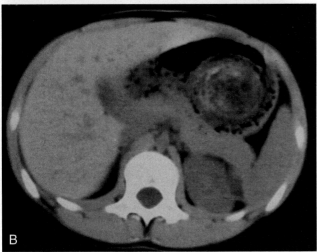

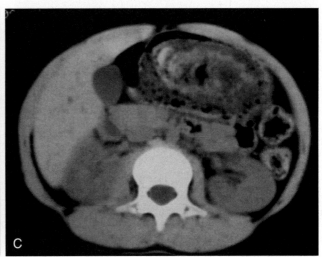

FIGURE 23. Gastric bezoar. **A,** Transverse ultrasound scan in the epigastrium demonstrates a broad band of increased echogenicity in the region of the stomach *(arrows),* with clear shadowing posteriorly. This appearance persists regardless of the angle or plane of imaging. **B** and **C,** Axial computed tomography sections through the fundus and antrum of the stomach demonstrate an intragastric mass consisting of compressed concentric rings with entrapped air, debris, and barium (from an upper gastrointestinal series 10 days previously). (From Newman B, Girdany BR: Gastric bezoars—sonographic and computed tomographic appearance. Pediatr Radiol 1990;20:526, with permission.)

gastric adenocarcinoma in a child. Gastroduodenal intussusception has been described in patients with Peutz-Jeghers syndrome and hamartomatous gastric polyps. Double-contrast studies of the stomach are most useful for evaluation of these various forms of polyps (Fig. 24).

Isolated gastric polyps (without true polyposis syn-

dromes) typically are benign hyperplastic polyps or are polyps related to pancreatic heterotopias. Hyperplastic polyps of the stomach may simulate HPS, and a patient with coexistent hyperplastic polyp and HPS has been reported. Intussuscepted hyperplastic gastric polyps may also masquerade as a duodenal duplication cyst. There have been rare reports of gastric hamartomatous polyps, including associated gastroduodenal intussusception.

Inflammatory fibroid polyps are more typically seen in the small intestine (Fig. 25), but can appear anywhere in the upper GI tract, including the stomach and duodenum. In fact, reports of these lesions in the stomach and duodenum have been appearing with increasing frequency. Their cause is unclear, and they have gone by a variety of names in the past. The histologic appearance varies slightly between areas of the GI tract, and the gastric lesions frequently contain elements histologically characterized as neurilemmomas. They are always benign, can be either polypoid or sessile, originate in the submucosa, and are best seen on double-contrast studies of the stomach or duodenum. They are also easily identified on CT.

Inflammatory pseudotumor is a benign mass of unclear etiology (either reactive or neoplastic) that has

Table 3 ■ DIFFERENTIAL DIAGNOSIS OF GASTRIC MASS

Polyp
  Hamartomatous
  Adenomatous
  Juvenile
  Hyperplastic
  Inflammatory fibroid
Inflammatory pseudotumor
Teratoma
Stromal tumors
  Leiomyoma
  Leiomyoblastoma
  Leiomyosarcoma
  Gastrointestinal stromal tumors
Carcinoma
Lymphoma

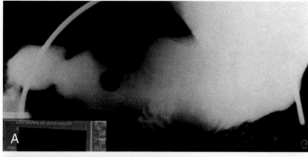

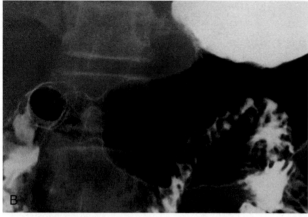

FIGURE 24. Solitary benign gastric polyp in a 14-year-old boy. Single **(A)** and double-contrast **(B)** upper gastrointestinal series demonstrate the intragastric polyp. No evidence of polyposis syndromes was found on extensive evaluation.

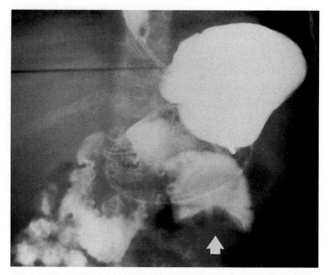

FIGURE 25. Inflammatory fibroid polyp of the jejunum presenting with symptoms of gastric outlet obstruction. (Same patient as in Section VI, Part VI, Chapter 1, Fig. 4, page 1587.)

been reported in most organ systems. It has also been called plasma cell granuloma and is characterized histologically by proliferative myofibroblasts, fibroblasts, histiocytes, plasma cells, and lymphocytes. Inflammatory pseudotumor involving the stomach has been reported in a 5-year-old child: CT revealed a partially calcified gastric mass arising from the lesser curve and infiltrating the gastrohepatic ligament; MRI demonstrated a mass that was lower in signal than the adjacent stomach on both T_1- and T_2-weighted images that enhanced after intravenous gadolinium administration.

Gastric teratomas have been described in neonates and young infants, predominantly affecting boys. They most commonly present with evidence of proximal GI obstruction or GI hemorrhage (Fig. 26). There has been one case report of a malignant gastric teratoma in a 4-month-old child; CT and US demonstrated a multilobulated mass.

Malignant lesions of the stomach are extremely rare. The most common malignancy involving the stomach in children is lymphoma, usually of the non-Hodgkin's variety. These lesions present with markedly enlarged gastric folds, usually in the body or pyloric region. CT typically shows marked thickening of the gastric wall as a result of diffusely infiltrative tumor (Fig. 27). Rarely, they may present as "bull's-eye" lesions simulating melanomatous lesions in adults (Fig. 28). Carcinomas have been described in teenagers. There is recent evidence that gastric carcinoma in children may have more aggressive clinical and pathologic features compared to that in older patients. Recently, the association of gastric carcinoma and lymphoma with *H. pylori* has been described.

Both benign and malignant stromal tumors have been

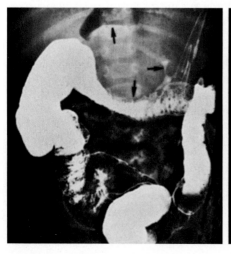
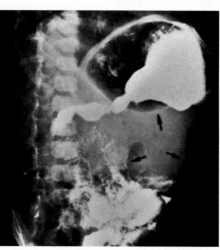

FIGURE 26. Gastric teratoma. Frontal and oblique views from a barium enema and upper gastrointestinal series demonstrate a large mass impinging on the stomach and transverse colon *(arrows)*. At surgery, the mass was found to arise directly from the stomach, and teratoma was documented histologically.

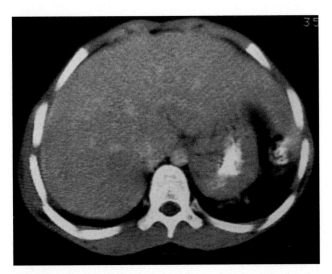

FIGURE 27. Non-Hodgkin's lymphoma of the stomach of a 14-year-old boy. The wall of the entire stomach is uniformly thickened on computed tomography scan. Findings were confirmed at laparotomy.

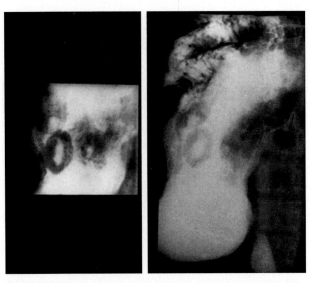

FIGURE 28. Upper gastrointestinal series in a 16-year-old boy with diffuse non-Hodgkin's lymphoma demonstrates "bull's-eye" lesions throughout the stomach that were confirmed at endoscopy and microscopy to be lymphoma.

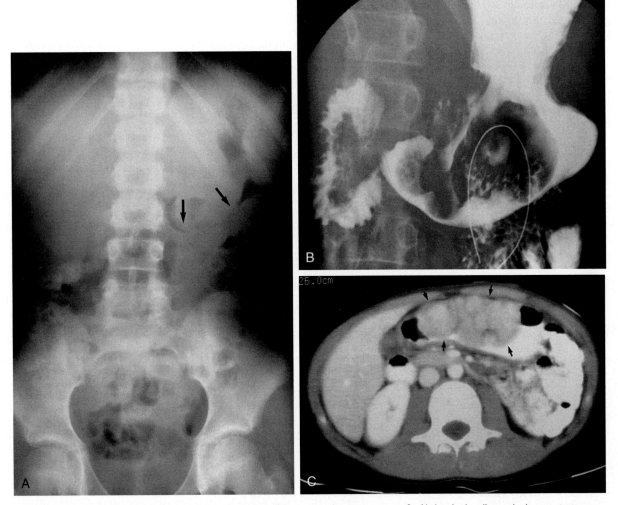

FIGURE 29. A 12-year-old girl with gastrointestinal (GI) autonomic nerve tumor. **A,** Abdominal radiograph demonstrates a soft tissue mass *(arrows)* impinging on the lesser curve of the stomach. **B,** Overhead image from an upper GI series confirms a gastric filling defect. **C,** Axial computed tomography section after oral and intravenous contrast reveals a soft tissue mass *(arrows)* with heterogeneous enhancement originating from the wall of the lesser curvature of the stomach.

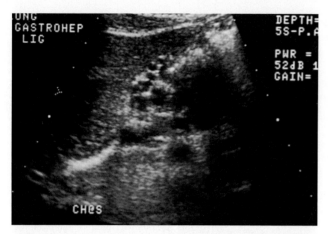

FIGURE 30. Ultrasound of the gastrohepatic ligament demonstrates multiple dilated vessels within the ligament—an appearance virtually diagnostic of varices.

described in the stomach in children, but are rare. Well-differentiated smooth muscle tumors include leiomyoma, leiomyoblastoma, and leiomyosarcoma. Because they are typically submucosal, the diagnosis can be made on upper GI series, but thickening of the submucosal region on US or CT is usually more suggestive of the correct diagnosis. CT is particularly useful to demonstrate the extragastric component of the tumor which may occur with the malignant varieties. Leiomyomas and leiomyosarcomas have been reported with increasing frequency in the GI tract (including the stomach and the duodenum) as well as in various extragastrointestinal sites in immunocompromised patients (both patients with AIDS and HIV-negative patients).

The term *gastrointestinal stromal tumor* (GIST) has been applied to less well-differentiated stromal tumors of the GI tract (as has the term *gastrointestinal stromal sarcomas* for their malignant counterpart). GIST may affect the stomach in children or adults. More recently, a broadened spectrum of the phenotypic expression of GIST has been appreciated, including smooth muscle,

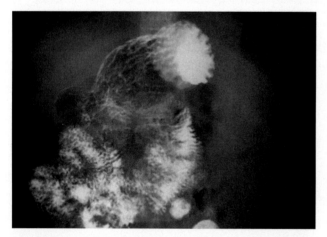

FIGURE 31. Gastric varices in an 8-year-old boy with cavernous transformation of the portal vein and massive splenomegaly. Note the serpentine filling defects throughout the fundus and lesser curvature of the stomach. Varices were confirmed by endoscopy.

peripheral nerve sheath, or neuronal differentiation. A specific subset of GIST that has received attention recently in adults and children is the gastrointestinal autonomic nerve tumor (GANT) (Fig. 29), which shows immunohistochemical reaction for markers of neurons of the autonomic enteric plexus. A report of four pediatric patients with GANT involving the stomach described imaging with plain radiographs, upper GI series, and CT. These studies revealed intramural gastric masses, of which one was multilobular and one had a large exophytic component.

Other than inflammatory polyps, primary neoplasms of the duodenum are extraordinarily rare. Both the stomach and the duodenum may be affected by tumors arising elsewhere in the abdomen that invade or displace them.

VARICES

Patients with portal hypertension may develop gastric and duodenal varices in addition to those in the esophagus. On US or CT, varices may be found in the gastrohepatic ligament (Fig. 30) and the gastric wall. On upper GI series, gastric varices are most commonly found in the fundus and along the lesser curvature, appearing as serpentine filling defects (Fig. 31). A similar appearance may less commonly be seen in the antrum of the stomach or the proximal duodenum.

SUGGESTED READINGS

Hypertrophic Pyloric Stenosis

Abbas AE, Weiss SM, Alvear DT: Infantile hypertrophic pyloric stenosis: delays in diagnosis and overutilization of imaging modalities. Am Surg 1999;65:73

Atwell JD, Levick P: Congenital hypertrophic pyloric stenosis and associated anomalies in the genitourinary tract. J Pediatr Surg 1981;16:1029

Bidair M, Kalota SJ, Kaplan GW: Infantile hypertrophic pyloric stenosis and hydronephrosis: is there an association? J Urol 1993; 150:153

Blumhagen JD: The role of ultrasonography in the evaluation of vomiting in infants. Pediatr Radiol 1986;16:267–270

Blumhagen JD, Maclin L, Krauter D, et al: Sonographic diagnosis of hypertrophic pyloric stenosis. AJR Am J Roentgenol 1988;150:1367

Breaux CS Jr, Georgeson KE, Royal SA, et al: Changing patterns in the diagnosis of hypertrophic pyloric stenosis. Pediatrics 1988;81:213

Bufo AJ, Merry C, Shah R, et al: Laparoscopic pyloromyotomy: a safer technique. Pediatr Surg Int 1998;13:240

Chen EA, Luks FI, Gilchrist BF, et al: Pyloric stenosis in the age of ultrasonography: fading skills, better patients? J Pediatr Surg 1996; 31:829

Chung E, Coffey R, Parker K, et al: Linkage analysis of infantile pyloric stenosis and markers from chromosome 9q11-q33: no evidence for a major gene in this candidate region. J Med Genet 1993;30:393

Cohen HL, Haller JO: Hypertrophic pyloric stenosis: volumetric measurement of nasogastric aspirate to determine imaging modality [Letter]. Radiology 1991;179:877

Cohen HL, Schechter S, Mastel AL, et al: Ultrasonic "double track" sign in hypertrophic pyloric stenosis. J Ultrasound Med 1987;6:136

Currarino G: The value of double contrast examination of the stomach with pressure "spots" in the diagnosis of infantile hypertrophic pyloric stenosis. Radiology 1964;83:873–878

Fernbach SK, Morello FP: Renal abnormalities in children with hypertrophic pyloric stenosis—fact or fallacy? Pediatr Radiol 1993; 23:286

Finkelstein MS, Mandell GA, Tarbell KV: Hypertrophic pyloric stenosis: volumetric measurement of nasogastric aspirate to determine the imaging modality. Radiology 1990;177:759

Foley LC, Slovis TL, Campbell JB, et al: Evaluation of the vomiting infant. Am J Dis Child 1989;143:660

Forman HP, Leonidas JC, Kronfeld CD: A rational approach to the diagnosis of hypertrophic pyloric stenosis: do the results match the claims? J Pediatr Surg 1990;25:202

Geer LL, Gaisie G, Mandell VS, et al: Evolution of pyloric stenosis in the first week of life. Pediatr Radiol 1985;15:205–206

Godbole P, Sprigg A, Dickson JA, et al: Ultrasound compared with clinical examination in infantile hypertrophic pyloric stenosis. Arch Dis Child 1996;75:335

Graham DA, Mogridge N, Abbott GD, et al: Pyloric stenosis: the Christchurch experience. N Z Med J 1993;106:57

Greason KL, Thompson WR, Downey EC, et al: Laparoscopic pyloromyotomy for hypertrophic pyloric stenosis: report of 11 cases. J Pediatr Surg 1995;30:1571

Haller JO, Cohen HL: Hypertrophic pyloric stenosis: diagnosis using US. Radiology 1986;161:335

Hayashi AH, Giocomantonio JM, Lau HYC, et al: Balloon catheter dilatation for hypertrophic pyloric stenosis. J Pediatr Surg 1990;25:1119

Hernanz-Schulman M, Sells LL, Ambrosino MM, et al: Hypertrophic pyloric stenosis in the infant without a palpable olive: accuracy of sonographic diagnosis. Radiology 1994;193:771

Holland AJ, Freeman JK, LeQuesne GW, et al: Idiopathic focal foveolar hyperplasia in infants. Pediatr Surg Int 1997;12:497

Hulka F, Campbell JR, Harrison MW, et al: Cost-effectiveness in diagnosing infantile hypertrophic pyloric stenosis. J Pediatr Surg 1997;32:1604

Hummer-Ehret BH, Rohrschneider WK, Oleszczuk-Raschke K, et al: Eosinophilic gastroenteritis mimicking hypertrophic pyloric stenosis. Pediatr Radiol 1998;28:711

Jamroz GA, Blocker SH, McAliser WH: Radiographic findings after incomplete pyloromyotomy. Gastrointest Radiol 1986;11:139–141

Katz ME, Blocker SH, McAlister WH: Focal foveolar hyperplasia presenting as an antral-pyloric mass in a young infant. Pediatr Radiol 1985;15:136

Keller H, Waldmann D, Greiner P: Comparison of preoperative sonography with intraoperative findings in congenital hypertrophic pyloric stenosis. J Pediatr Surg 1987;22:950

Konvolinka CW, Wernuth CR: Hypertrophic pyloric stenosis in older infants. Am J Dis Child 1971;122:76–79

Latchaw LA, Jacir NN, Harris BH: The development of pyloric stenosis during transpyloric feedings. J Pediatr Surg 1989;24:823

Macdessi J, Oates RK: Clinical diagnosis of pyloric stenosis: a declining art. BMJ 1993;306:553

Mandell GA: Association of antral diaphragms and hypertrophic pyloric stenosis. Am J Roentgenol Radium Ther Nucl Med 1978;131:203–206

McAlister WH, Katz ME, Perlman JM, et al: Sonography of focal foveolar hyperplasia causing gastric outlet obstruction in an infant. Pediatr Radiol 1988;18:79

Mercado-Deane MG, Burton EM, Brawley AV, et al: Prostaglandin-induced focal foveolar hyperplasia simulating pyloric stenosis in an infant with cyanotic heart disease. Pediatr Radiol 1994;24:45

Nagita A, Yamaguchi J, Amenoto K, et al: Management and ultrasonographic appearance of infantile hypertrophic pyloric stenosis with intravenous atropine sulfate. J Pediatr Gastroenterol Nutr 1996;23:172

O'Keefe FN, Stansberry SD, Swischuk LE, Hayden CK: Antropyloric muscle thickness at US in infants: what is normal? Radiology 191;178:827

Okorie NM, Dickson JA, Carver RA, et al: What happens to the pylorus after pyloromyotomy? Arch Dis Child 1988;63:1339

Ozsvath RR, Poustchi-Amin M, Leonidas JC, et al: Pyloric volume: an important factor in the surgeon's ability to palpate the pyloric "olive" in hypertrophic pyloric stenosis. Pediatr Radiol 1997;27:175

Riggs W Jr, Long L: The value of the plain film roentgenogram in pyloric stenosis. Am J Roentgenol Radium Ther Nucl Med 1971;112:77–82

Sauerbrei EE, Paloschi GGB: The ultrasonic features of hypertrophic pyloric stenosis, with emphasis on the post-operative appearance. Radiology 1983;147:503–506

Shen Z, She Y, Ding W, et al: Changes in pyloric tumor of infantile hypertrophic stenosis before and after pyloromyotomy. Pediatr Surg Int 1989;4:322

Shopfner CE, Kalmon EH, Coin CG: The diagnosis of hypertrophic pyloric stenosis. Am J Roentgenol Radium Ther Nucl Med 1964;91:796

Shuman FI, Darling DB, Fisher JH: The radiographic diagnosis of congenital hypertrophic pyloric stenosis. J Pediatr 1967;71:70–74

Spevak MR, Ahmadjian JM, Kleinman PD, et al: Sonography of hypertrophic pyloric stenosis: frequency and cause of nonuniform echogenicity of the thickened pyloric muscle. AJR Am J Roentgenol 1992;158:129

Steinicke O, Roelsgaard M: Radiographic follow-up in hypertrophic pyloric stenosis. Acta Paediatr Scand 1960;49:4–16

Stunden RJ, LeQuesne GW, Little KET: The improved ultrasound diagnosis of hypertrophic pyloric stenosis. Pediatr Radiol 1986;16:200

Swischuk LE, Hyaden CK Jr, Stansberry SD: Sonographic pitfalls in imaging of the antropyloric region in infants. Radiographics 1989;9:437

Teele RL, Smith EH: Ultrasound in the diagnosis of idiopathic hypertrophic pyloric stenosis. N Engl J Med 1997;296:1149–1150

van der Schouw YT, van der Velden MT, Hitge-Boetes C, et al: Diagnosis of hypertrophic pyloric stenosis: value of sonography when used in conjunction with clinical findings and laboratory data. AJR Am J Roentgenol 1994;163:905

Weiskittel DA, Leary DL, Blane CE: Ultrasound diagnosis of evolving pyloric stenosis. Gastrointest Radiol 1989;14:22

Westra SJ, de Groot CJ, Smits NJ, et al: Hypertrophic pyloric stenosis: use of the pyloric volume measurement in early US diagnosis. Radiology 1989;172:615

White MC, Langer JC, Don S, et al: Sensitivity and cost minimization analysis of radiology versus olive palpation for the diagnosis of hypertrophic pyloric stenosis. J Pediatr Surg 1998;33:913

Yamamoto A, Kino M, Sasaki T, et al: Ultrasonic follow-up of the healing process of medically treated hypertrophic pyloric stenosis. Pediatr Radiol 1998;28:177

Peptic Ulcer Disease

Azarow K, Kim P, Shandling B, et al: A 45-year experience with surgical tratment for peptic ulcer disease. J Pediatr Surg 1996;31:750

Blecker U: Helicobacter pylori disease in childhood. Clin Pediatr (Phila) 1996;35:175

Blecker U: Helicobacter pylori-associated gastroduodenal disease in childhood. South Med J 1997;90:570

Block WM: Chronic gastric ulcer in childhood: a critical analysis of the literature with report of a case in an eleven-year-old boy. Am J Dis Child 1963;85:566–574

Bujanover Y, Reif S, Yahav J: Helicobacter pylori and peptic ulcer disease in the pediatric patient. Pediatr Clin North Am 1996;43:213

Chan KL, Tam PK, Saing H: Long-term follow-up of childhood duodenal ulcers. J Pediatr Surg 1997;32:1609

Drumm B, Rhoads JM, Stringer DA, et al: Peptic ulcer disease in children: etiology, clinical findings and clinical course. Pediatrics 1988;82:410–414

Dunn S, Weber TR, Grosfeld JL, et al: Acute peptic ulcer in childhood. Arch Surg 1983;118:656–660

Farthing MJ: Helicobacter pylori infection: an overview. Br Med Bull 1998;54:1

Girdany BR: Peptic ulcer in childhood. Pediatrics 1953;12:56

Goggin N, Rowland M, Imrie C, et al: Effect of Helicobacter pylori eradication on the natural history of duodenal ulcer disease. Arch Dis Child 1998;79:502

Gormally SM, Kierce BM, Daly LE, et al: Gastric metaplasia and duodenal ulcer disease in children infected by Helicobacter pylori. Gut 1996;38:513

Hayden CK Jr, Swischuk LE, Rytting JE: Gastric ulcer disease in infants: US findings. Radiology 1987;164:131–134

Huang FC, Chang MH, Hsu HY, et al: Long-term follow-up of duodenal ulcer disease in children before and after eradication of Helicobacter pylori. J Pediatr Gastroenterol Nutr 1999;28:76

Jones NL, Sherman PM: Helicobacter pylori infection in children. Curr Opin Pediatr 1998;10:19

Kato S, Abukawa D, Furuyama N, et al: Helicobacter pylori reinfection rates in children after eradication therapy. J Pediatr Gastroenterol Nutr 1998;27:543

Kuipers EJ, Uyterlinde AM, Pena AS, et al: Long-term sequelae of Helicobacter pylori gastritis. Lancet 1995;345:1525

Kumar D, Spitz L: Peptic ulceration in children. Surg Gynecol Obstet 1987;159:63–66

Meining A, Behrens R, Lehn N, et al: Different expression of Helicobacter pylori gastritis in children: evidence for a specific pediatric disease? Helicobacter 1996;1:92

Purelekar SG, Lubert J: Ultrasound demonstration of giant duodenal ulcer. Gastrointest Radiol 1983;8:29–31

Rosenquist CJ: Clinical and radiographic features of giant duodenal ulcer. Clin Radiol 1969;20:324

Rowland M, Drumm B: Helicobacter pylori infection and peptic ulcer disease in children. Curr Opin Pediatr 1995;7:553

Rowland M, Drumm B: Clinical significance of Helicobacter pylori infection in children. Br Med Bull 1998;54:95

Sherman PM: Peptic ulcer disease in children: diagnosis, treatment, and the implication of Helicobacter pylori. Gastroenterol Clin North Am 1994;23:707

Stringer DA, Daneman A, Brunelle F, et al: Sonography of the normal and abnormal stomach (excluding hypertrophic pyloric stenosis) in children. J Ultrasound Med 1986;5:183

Gastritis

Baker A, Volberg F, Summer T, et al: Childhood Menetrier's disease: four new cases and discussion of the literature. Gastrointest Radiol 1986;11:131

Bar-Ziv J, Barki Y, Weizman Z, Urkin J: Transient protein-losing gastropathy (Menetrier's disease) in childhood. Pediatr Radiol 1988;18:82–84

Bass DH, Millar AJ: Mercury absorption following button battery ingestion. J Pediatr Surg 1992;27:1541

Bowen A III, Gibson MD: Chronic granulomatous disease with gastric antral narrowing. Pediatr Radiol 1980;10:119–120

Burns B, Gay BB: Menetrier's disease of the stomach in children. Am J Roentgenol Radium Ther Nucl Med 1968;103:300–306

Cameron DJ: Upper and lower gastrointestinal endoscopy in children and adolescents with Crohn's disease: a prospective study. J Gastroenterol Hepatol 1991;6:355

Chalouplea JC, Gay BB, Caplan D: Campylobacter gastritis simulating Menetrier's disease by upper gastrointestinal radiography. Pediatr Radiol 1990;20:200–201

Coad NAG, Shah KJ: Menetrier's disease in childhood associated with cytomegalovirus infection: a case report and review of the literature. Br J Radiol 1986;59:515–620

Derchi LE, Biggi GARE, Cicio GR, et al: Sonographic findings of Menetrier's disease: a case report. Gastrointest Radiol 1982;7: 323–325

Dohmen K, Harada M, Ishibashi M, et al: Ultrasonographic studies on abdominal complications in patients receiving marrow-ablative chemotherapy and bone marrow or blood stem cell transplantation. J Clin Ultrasound 1991;19:321

Drumm B, O'Brien A, Cutz E, Sherman P: *Campylobacter pylori*–associated primary gastritis in children. Pediatrics 1987;80:192–195

Edwards PD, Carrick J, Turner J, et al: Helicobacter pylori-associated gastritis is rare in AIDS: antibiotic effect or a consequence of immunodeficiency? Am J Gastroenterol 1991;86:1761

Falcone S, Murphy BJ, Weinfeld A: Gastric manifestations of AIDS: radiographic findings on upper gastrointestinal examination. Gastrointest Radiol 1991;16:95

Franken EA Jr: Caustic damage of the gastrointestinal tract: roentgen features. Am J Roentgenol Radium Ther Nucl Med 1973;118:77–85

Gassner I, Strasser K, Bart G, et al: Sonographic appearance of Menetrier's disease in a child. J Ultrasound Med 1990;9:537

Gelfand DW, Dale WJ, Ott DJ, et al: Duodenitis: endoscopic-radiologic correlation in 272 patients. Radiology 1985;157:577–581

Granot E, Matoth I, Korman SH, et al: Functional gastrointestinal obstruction in a child with chronic granulomatous disease. J Pediatr Gastroenterol Nutr 1986;5:321

Gratten-Smith D, Harrison LF, Singleton EB: Radiology of AIDS in the pediatric patient. Curr Probl Diagn Radiol 1992;21:79

Griscom NT, Kirkpatrick, JA, Girdany BR, et al: Gastric antral narrowing in chronic granulomatous disease of childhood. Pediatrics 1974;54:456–460

Haller JO, Cohen HL: Gastrointestinal manifestations of AIDS in children. AJR Am J Roentgenol 1994;162:387

Hummer-Ehret BH, Rohrschneider WK, Oleszczuk-Raschke K, et al: Eosinophilic gastroenteritis mimicking hypertrophic pyloric stenosis. Pediatr Radiol 1998;28:711

Kopen PA, McAliser WH: Upper gastrointestinal and ultrasound examinations of gastric antral involvement in chronic granulomatous disease. Pediatr Radiol 1984;14:91–93

Kost KM, Shapiro RS: Button battery ingestion: a case report and review of the literature. J Otolaryngol 1987;16:252

Lenaerts C, Roy CC, Vaillancourt M, et al: High incidence of upper gastrointestinal tract involvement in children with Crohn disease. Pediatrics 1989;83:777

Leonidas JC, Beatty EC, Wenner HA: Menetrier disease and cytomegalovirus infection in childhood. Am J Dis Child 1973;126:806–808

Manson DE, Stringer DA, Durie PR, et al: The radiologic and endoscopic investigation and etiologic classification of gastritis in children. J Can Assoc Radiol 1990;41:201

Marks MP, Lanza MV, Kahlstrom EJ, et al: Pediatric hypertrophic gastropathy. AJR Am J Roentgenol 1986;147:1031–1034

Mashako MN, Cezard JP, Navarro J, et al: Crohn's disease lesions in the upper gastrointestinal tract: correlation between clinical, radiological, endoscopic, and histologic features in adolescents and children. J Pediatr Gastroenterol 1989;8:442

McDonald GB, Shulman HM, Sullivan KM, et al: Intestinal and hepatic complications of human bone marrow transplantation. Part I. Gastroenterology 1986;90:460

Morrison S, Dahms BB, Hoffenbert E, et al: Enlarged gastric folds in association with Campylobacter pylori gastritis. Radiology 1989;171: 819–821

Narla LD, Hingsbergen EA, Jones JE: Adult diseases in children. Pediatr Radiol 1999;29:244

Ott DG, Gelfand DW, Wu WC, et al: Sensitivity of single- vs double-contrast radiology in erosive gastritis. AJR Am J Roentgenol 1982;138:263–266

Paciorek M, D'Altorio R, Gleeson G: Resolution of giant gastric folds after eradication of Heliocobacter pylori. J Clin Gastroenterol 1997;25:696

Pugh TF, Fitch SJ: Invasive gastric candidiasis. Pediatr Radiol 1986;16: 67–68

Ruuska T, Vaajalahti P, Arajarvi P, et al: Prospective evaluation of upper gastrointestinal mucosal lesions in children with ulcerative colitis and Crohn's disease. J Pediatr Gastroenterol Nutr 1994;19:181

Scharschidt BF: The natural history of hypertrophic gastropathy (Menetrier's disease): report of a case with 16-year follow-up and review of 120 cases from the literature. Am J Med 1977;63:644–652

Smith FJ, Taves DH: Gastroduodenal involvement in chronic granulomatous disease of childhood. Can Assoc Radiol J 1992;43:215

Stringer DA, Daneman A, Brunelle F, et al: Sonography of the normal and abnormal stomach (excluding hypertrophic pyloric stenosis) in children. J Ultrasound Med 1986;5:183–188

Takaya J, Kawamura Y, Kino M, et al: Menetrier's disease evaluated serially by abdominal ultrasonography. Pediatr Radiol 1997;27:178

Teele RL, Katz AJ, Goldman H, et al: Radiographic features of eosinophilic gastroenteritis (allergic gastroenteropathy) of childhood. AJR Am J Roentgeol 1979;132:575–580

Theoni RF, Goldberg HI, Ominsky S, et al: Detection of gastritis by single and double contrast radiography. Radiology 1983;148: 621–626

Tio TL: Large gastric folds evalued by endoscopic ultrasonography. Gastrointest Endosc Clin N Am 1995;5:683

Tootla F, Lucas RJ, Bernacki EG, et al: Gastroduodenal Crohn's disease. Arch Surg 1976;3:855–857

Turner CJ, Lipitz LR, Pastore RA: Antral gastritis. Radiology 1974;113: 305–312

Urban BA, Fishman EK, Hruban RH: Heliocobacter pylori gastritis mimicking gastric carcinoma at CT evaluation. Radiology 1991; 179:689

Victoria MS, Nangia BS, Jindrak K: Cytomegalovirus pyloric obstruction in a child with acquired immune deficiency syndrome. Pediatric Infect Dis 1985;4:550

Duodenitis

Levine MS, Turner D, Ekberg O, et al: Duodenitis: a reliable radiologic diagnosis? Gastrointest Radiol 1991;16:99

Long FR, Kramer SS, Markowitz RI, et al: Duodenitis in children:

correlation of radiologic findings with endoscopic and pathologic findings. Radiology 1998;206:103

Bezoars

McCracken S, Jongeward R, Silver TM, et al: Gastric trichobezoar: sonographic findings. Radiology 1986;161:123–124

Naik DR, Bolia A, Boon AW: Demonstration of a lactobezoar by ultrasound. Br J Radiol 1987;60:506–508

Newman B, Girdany BR: Gastric trichobezoars—sonographic and computed tomographic appearance. Pediatr Radiol 1990;20:526

Sinzig M, Umschaden HW, Haselbach H, et al: Gastric trichobezoar with gastric ulcer: MR findings. Pediatr Radiol 1998;28:296

Tumors and Tumor-like Conditions

Aideyan UO, Kao SC: Gastric adenocarcinoma metastatic to the testes in Peutz-Jeghers syndrome. Pediatr Radiol 1994;24:496

Bahk YW, Ahn JC, Choi HJ: Lymphoid hyperplasia of the stomach presenting as umbilicated polypoid lesions. Radiology 1971;100: 277–280

Balsam D, Segal S: Two smooth muscle tumors in the airway of an HIV-infected child. Pediatr Radiol 1992;22:552

Bethel CA, Bhattacharyya N, Hutchinson C, et al: Alimentary tract malignancies in children. J Pediatr Surg 1997;32:1008

Bourke CJ, Mackay AJ, Payton D: Malignant gastric teratoma: case report. Pediatr Surg Int 1997;12:192

Bowen B, Ros PR, McCarthy MJ, et al: Gastrointestinal teratomas: CT and US appearance with pathologic correlation. Radiology 1987; 162:431–433

Brooks GS, Frost ES, Wesselhoeft C: Prolapsed hyperplastic gastric polyp causing gastric outlet obstruction, hypergastrinemia, and hematemesis in an infant. J Pediatr Surg 1992;27:1537

Buck JL, Harned RK, Lichtenstein JE, et al: Peutz Jeghers syndrome. Radiographics 1992;12:365

Cacciaguerra S, Miano AE, Di Benedetto A, et al: Gastric carcinoma with ovarian metastases in an adolescent. Pediatr Surg Int 1998; 14:98

da Santos G, Zucoloto S: Inflammatory fibroid polyp: review of the literature. Arq Gastroenterol 1993;30:107

Defago MR, Higa AL, Campra JL, et al: Carcinoma in situ arising in a gastric hamartomatous polyp in a patient with Peutz-Jeghers syndrome. Endoscopy 1996;28:267

Denzler TC, Harned RK, Pergam CJ: Gastric polyps in familial polyposis coli. Radiology 1979;130:63–66

Desai DC, Neale KF, Talbot IC, et al: Juvenile polyposis. Br J Surg 1995;82:14

Dixon WL, Fazzari PJ: Carcinoma of the stomach in a child. JAMA 1976;235:2414–2415

Domizio P, Talbot IC, Spigelman AD, et al: Upper gastrointestinal pathology in familial adenomatous polyposis: result from a prospective study of 102 patients. J Clin Pathol 1990;43:738

Dunnick NR, Harell GS, Parker BR: Multiple "bull's-eye" lesions in gastric lymphoma. Am J Roentgenol 1976;126:965

Gengler JS, Ashcraft KW, Slattery P: Gastric teratoma: the sixth reported case in a female patient. J Pediatr Surg 1995;30:889

Goedde TA, Rodriguez-Bigas MA, Herrera L, et al: Gastroduodenal polyps in familial adenomatous polyposis. Surg Oncol 1992;1:357

Ha C, Haller JO, Rollins NK: Smooth muscle tumors in immunocompromised (HIV negative) children. Pediatr Radiol 1993;23:413

Hizawa K, Iida M, Matsumoto T, et al: Cancer in Peutz-Jeghers syndrome. Cancer 1993;72:2777

Kerr JZ, Hicks MJ, Nuchtern JG, et al: Gastrointestinal autonomic nerve tumors in the pediatric population: a report of four cases and a review of the literature. Cancer 1999;85:220

Kim S, Chung CJ, Fordham LA, et al: Coexisting hyperplastic antral polyp and hypertrophic pyloric stenosis. Pediatr Radiol 1997;27:912

Kodet R, Snajdauf J, Smelhaus V: Gastrintestinal autonomic nerve tumor: a case report with electronic microscopic and immunohisto-chemical analysis and review of the literature. Pediatr Pathol 1994;14:1005

Lauwers GY, Erlandson RA, Casper ES, et al: Gastrointestinal autonomic nerve tumors: a clinicopathological, immunohistochemical, and ultrastructural study of 12 cases. Am J Surg Pathol 1993;17:887

Lee ES, Locker J, Nalesnik M, et al: The association of Epstein-Barr virus and smooth-muscle tumors occurring after organ transplantation. N Engl J Med 1995;332:19

Lichtman S, Hayes G, Stringer DA, et al: Chronic intussusception due to antral myoepithelioma. J Pediatr Surg 1986;21:955–956

Marcello PW, Asbun HJ, Veidenheimer MC, et al: Gastroduodenal polyps in familial adenomatous polyposis. Surg Endosc 1996;10:418

McClain KL, Leach CL, Jenson HB, et al: Association of Epstein-Barr virus with leiomyosarcomas in young people with AIDS. N Engl J Med 1995;332:12

McGill TW, Downey EC, Westbrook J, et al: Gastric carcinoma in children. J Pediatr Surg 1993;28:1620

McLoughlin LC, Nord KS, Joshi VV, et al: Disseminated leiomyosar-coma in a child with acquired immune deficiency syndrome. Cancer 1991;67:2618

Megibow AJ, Balthazar EJ, Hulnick DH, et al: CT evaluation of gastrointestinal leiomyomas and leiomyosarcomas. AJR Am J Roentgenol 1985;144:727–731

Nakamura S, Yao T, Aoyagi K, et al: Helicobacter pylori and primary gastric lymphoma: a histopathologic and immunohistochemical analysis of 237 patients. Cancer 1997;79:3

Odes HS, Krawiec J, Yanai-Inbar I, et al: Benign lymphoid hyperplasia of the stomach. Pediatr Radiol 1981;10:244–246

Orlow SJ, Kamino H, Lawrence RL: Multiple subcutaneous leiomyo-sarcomas in an adolescent with AIDS. Am J Pediatr Hematol Oncol 1992;14:265

Rugge M, Busatto G, Cassaro M, et al: Patients younger than 40 years with gastric carcinoma: Helicobacter pylori genotype and associated gastritis phenotype. Cancer 1999;85:2506

Sanna CM, Loriga P, Dessi E, et al: Hyperplastic polyp of the stomach simulating hypertrophic pyloric stenosis. J Pediatr Gastroenterol Nutr 1991;13:204

Schneider K, Kickerhoff R, Bertele RM: Malignant gastric sarcoma—diagnosis by ultrasound. Pediatr Radiol 1986;16:69–70

Schroeder BA, Wells RG, Sty JR: Inflammatory fibroid polyp of the stomach in a child. Pediatr Radiol 1987;17:71

Sharon N, Kenet G, Toren A, et al: Helicobacter pylori-associated gastric lymphoma in a girl. Pediatr Hematol Oncol 1997;14:177

Shimer GR, Helwig EB: Inflammatory fibroid polyps of the intestine. Am J Clin Pathol 1984;81:708

Siegel MJ, Shackelford GD: Gastric teratomas in infants: report of 2 cases. Pediatr Radiol 1978;7:197–200

Spigelman AD, Williams CB, Talbot IC, et al: Upper gastrointestinal cancer in patients with familial autonomatous polyposis. Lancet 1989;2:783

Suster S: Gastrointestinal stromal tumors. Semin Diagn Pathol 1996; 13:297

Taratuta E, Krinsky G, Genega E, et al: Pediatric inflammatory pseudotumor of the stomach: contrast-enhanced CT and MR imaging findings. AJR Am J Roentgenol 1996;167:919

Theuer CP, Kurosaki T, Taylor TH, et al: Unique features of gastric carcinoma in the young: a population-based analysis. Cancer 1998; 83:25

Thomas JR, Mrak RE, Linuit N: Gastrointestinal autonomic nerve tumor presenting as a high-grade sarcoma: case report and review of the literature. Dig Dis Sci 1994;39:2051

Uddin N, Abernethy LJ: Gastroduodenal intussusception with a gastric antral polyp. Pediatr Radiol 1998;28:460

Wu YK, Tsai CH, Yang JC, et al: Gastroduodenal intussusception due to Peutz-Jeghers syndrome: a case report. Hepatogastroenterology 1994;41:134

Wurlitzer FP, Mares AJ, Isaacs H Jr, et al: Smooth muscle tumors of the stomach in childhood and adolescence. J Pediatr Surg 1973;8: 421–427

Part VII

SMALL INTESTINE

BRUCE R. PARKER

The small intestine is a long, convoluted, musculomembranous tube that begins at the pylorus and ends at the ileocecal valve. Its length and pattern are variable; its three major divisions are the duodenum, jejunum, and ileum. The jejunum accounts for approximately three fifths of the small bowel; the remaining two fifths is ileum. The proximal third of the small intestine commonly fills the left upper abdominal quadrant, the middle third occupies the midportion of the abdomen and the right upper quadrant, and the terminal third lies on the right side of the abdomen and pelvis. The caliber of the lumen gradually diminishes from proximal to distal, with the diameter of the terminal ileum being about one third smaller than the first portion of the jejunum. The external surface of the tube is smooth and devoid of permanent folds or creases. The internal surface is thrown into transverse and spiral folds, the plicae circulares of the submucosa, which are covered by the villous folds of mucous membrane. These folds greatly increase the secreting and absorbing surface and facilitate digestion by retarding the passage of intestinal content.

IMAGING STUDIES

Plain radiographs are often nonspecific in patients with small intestinal disease but are extremely useful in identifying adynamic ileus, intestinal obstruction, free air secondary to intestinal perforation, pathologic calcification, and masses large enough to displace normal structures. The *contrast small intestinal series* remains the mainstay of small bowel imaging. Barium is still the most frequently used contrast agent, with the more expensive water-soluble nonionic agents reserved for specific indications such as potential perforations. Although *ultrasound* (US) is limited by the intraluminal air of the intestine, it can often identify thickened bowel wall and intestinal and mesenteric masses, including abscesses and intussusceptions, and has increasing utility in a variety of disease entities as discussed throughout this chapter. Doppler studies have demonstrated value in the evaluation of inflammatory processes. *Computed tomography* (CT) has ever-increasing utility in the intestinal tract. Good opacification of the bowel lumen is critical for adequate CT evaluation of the intestine and mesentery. CT is useful in a wide variety of disorders, including, but not limited to, inflammatory bowel disease and its complications, intra-abdominal abscesses, and mass lesions. *Scintigraphy* plays a limited role in small bowel disease but may be useful in cases of abdominal pain or intestinal bleeding, especially where ectopic gastric mucosa is suspected. The value of scintigraphy in inflammatory disease of the intestinal tract is still debated. *Magnetic resonance imaging* (MRI) of intestinal disease has been little studied in children. Intestinal motion and the lack of satisfactory intestinal contrast agents severely limits the usefulness of MRI except in evaluation of mass lesions.

CONGENITAL OBSTRUCTION

Most abnormalities of the small intestine of genetic or developmental origin present in the newborn period, frequently with small bowel obstruction (Table 1). The most emergent of these conditions is midgut volvulus

Table 1 ■ DIFFERENTIAL DIAGNOSIS OF CONGENITAL SMALL BOWEL OBSTRUCTION
Midgut malrotation
Midgut volvulus
Peritoneal (Ladd's) bands
Small bowel atresia
Meconium ileus
Duplication cysts
Colonic lesions mimicking small bowel obstruction
Colonic atresia
Anorectal malformations
Aganglionosis
Meconium plug syndrome

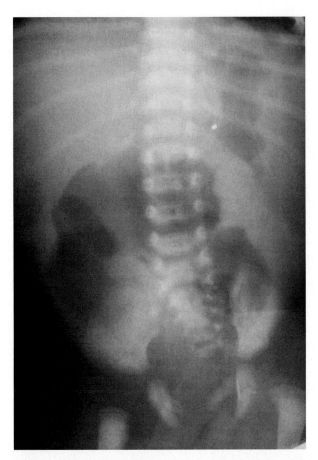

FIGURE 1. Small bowel obstruction in a newborn with midgut volvulus. Dilated loops of small bowel suggest obstruction but are nonspecific as far as etiology.

secondary to midgut malrotation. The midgut is defined as that part of the intestinal tract supplied by the superior mesenteric artery (SMA). Thus the midgut extends from near the juncture of the second and third portions of the duodenum to the level of the anatomic splenic flexure.

MIDGUT VOLVULUS/MALROTATION

The midgut is that portion of the bowel that herniates into the extraembryonic coelomic cavity in the early first trimester. The bowel rotates 90 degrees as it herniates into the yolk sac and rotates another 270 degrees as it re-enters the embryonic coelomic cavity. This process can be arrested at any point. If the bowel fails to return to the embryonic abdominal cavity, the baby is born with an omphalocele. The bowel may return but fail to undergo some or all of the normal rotation. This can result in an appearance ranging from complete midgut malrotation to normal anatomy except for a high-riding cecum in the right upper quadrant. The importance of this process is that the mesenteric attachment normally runs obliquely from a fixed point behind the SMA to a fixed point behind the cecum. If the cecum is not properly located in the right lower quadrant, the mesentery is fixed at only one point, behind the SMA,

and may twist on itself, leading to midgut volvulus. Because the mesentery contains the vessels supplying and draining the small intestine, bowel necrosis may occur in a very short interval of time.

Most patients with *midgut volvulus* present in the neonatal period, but increasing numbers of cases are being reported in older children. The presentation is usually one of bilious emesis with or without abdominal distention. Plain films typically demonstrate high-grade proximal small bowel obstruction with air–fluid levels on horizontal beam radiographs (Fig. 1). The traditional means of diagnosis has been a contrast enema to determine the position of the cecum (Fig. 2). However, patients may have midgut malrotation with other causes of obstruction, so that a contrast examination from above with a water-soluble agent is more definitive. A "corkscrew" appearance of the duodenum and proximal jejunum is usually seen because of the twisted mesentery (Fig. 3). Ultrasound may also demonstrate the abnormality with the "whirlpool sign," a swirling pattern in the affected loop of bowel (Fig. 4*B*).

> ■ Imaging findings in midgut malrotation:
> Contrast enema
> • Cecum abnormally positioned
> Upper gastrointestinal series
> • Abnormal position of duodenojejunal junction
> • "Corkscrew" appearance of duodenum and proximal jejunum if volvulus is present
> Ultrasound
> • Reversal of positions of superior mesenteric artery and vein (half or more of cases)
> • "Whirlpool" pattern in mesenteric vessels if volvulus is present

Obstruction associated with midgut malrotation may occur at almost any age from the presence of *Ladd's bands*. These are bands of peritoneum that, because of cecal malposition, cross anterior to the bowel rather than posterior to it. The third portion of the duodenum is most frequently affected (Fig. 5), but other areas of obstruction, even the colon, have been described.

Patients with *midgut malrotation* who do not develop volvulus at birth may remain asymptomatic throughout life. Midgut volvulus can present beyond infancy, but most patients with malrotation who present with intestinal obstruction later in life do so because of crossing peritoneal bands. Malrotation presenting beyond infancy may have unusual manifestations. Jackson et al. described a 16-month-old boy with malrotation and intermittent midgut volvulus who presented with failure to thrive and intestinal malabsorption. The normal alignment of the SMA and superior mesenteric vein as seen on US, MRI, and CT is sometimes inverted in patients with malrotation, with the vein being found to the left of the artery (Fig. 4*A*). This may be a helpful clue in patients with unexplained abdominal pain. However,

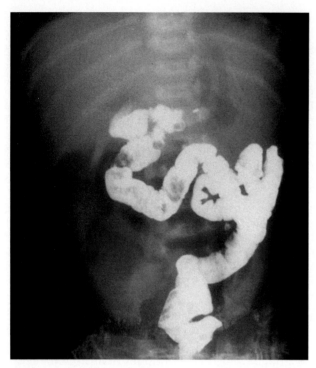

FIGURE 2. Malrotation. Contrast enema shows the cecum and ascending colon to be in the right upper quadrant in this newborn with midgut volvulus.

complete inversion of the vessels can be secondary to adjacent masses, and partial inversion of the vessels can be found in normal persons. Zerin and Di Pietro, using ultrasound to study nine patients with proven malrotation, found that six of them had inversion and three did not.

SMALL BOWEL ATRESIA

Small bowel atresias are the most common causes of small bowel obstruction at birth. They are caused by in utero vascular accidents, usually in the mid-second trimester. The devascularized bowel becomes necrotic and is resorbed, leaving an atretic area of varying length. Several forms of atresia have been described surgically, but imaging studies do not differentiate between them. The embryonic abdominal cavity is a sterile environment, but leakage of meconium may lead to inflammation of the peritoneum, a chemical peritonitis most commonly known as *meconium peritonitis.*

Plain film findings in small bowel atresia are typically dilated loops of small bowel with air–fluid levels on horizontal beam radiographs (Fig. 6). One can sometimes differentiate between jejunal and ileal atresia by the number of obstructed loops of small bowel seen, but the differentiation is not clinically important. This is true because multiple atresias may be present, and the surgeon is obliged to evaluate the entire small bowel regardless of preoperative imaging findings. If meconium peritonitis has occurred, peritoneal calcifications may be seen (Fig. 7). The most frequent finding is linear

calcification under the free edge of the liver, but any portion, or all portions, of the peritoneum may be involved. The association of meconium peritonitis with small bowel obstruction is virtually diagnostic of small bowel atresia.

Contrast enemas are typically performed to confirm the suspected diagnosis of atresia. Although not specific, the finding of *microcolon,* or unused colon, is highly suggestive of the diagnosis (Fig. 8). Because the atresia did not occur until mid-third trimester, meconium formed before the etiologic event may be noted on contrast enema even though the small bowel is completely obstructed at birth. Because the normally produced succus entericus is a major component of meconium, and continues to be produced, proximal jejunal atresia may not produce an obvious microcolon. The colon, however, is usually less distensible than in normal infants. Of note is that, even with extreme microcolon, the rectum may be of normal caliber. Reports of colonic perforation during contrast enema in patients with atresias exist, but reasonable care during the study prevents this complication. As long as water-soluble contrast material is used, and the baby is well hydrated, colonic perforation should not lead to any significant complication for the infant, who will require surgery in any event.

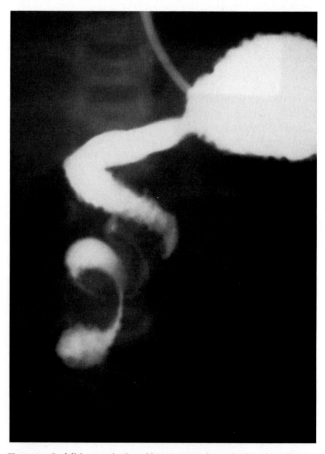

FIGURE 3. Midgut volvulus. Upper gastrointestinal series demonstrates a "corkscrew" appearance of the distal duodenum and proximal jejunum in a newborn with midgut volvulus.

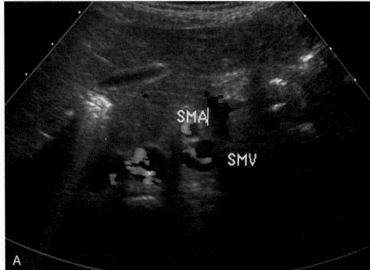

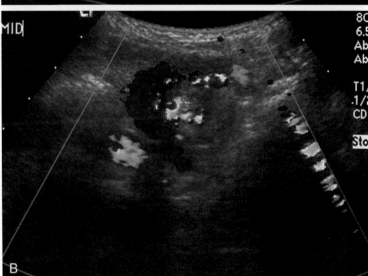

FIGURE 4. A, Malrotation. Doppler ultrasound scan shows the superior mesenteric artery to be anterior and to the right of the superior mesenteric vein. **B,** "Whirlpool sign" in midgut volvulus. Single frame from a dynamic clip demonstrates the swirling motion of the mesenteric vessels around the volvulated loop of bowel. *See Color Plate*

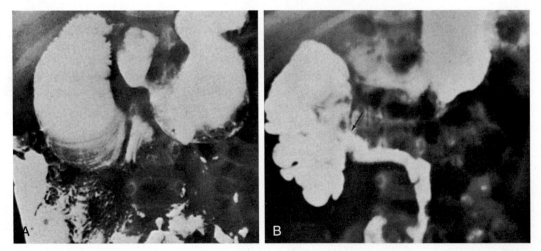

FIGURE 5. Incomplete obstruction of the third portion of the duodenum secondary to duodenal bands in a boy 5 years of age. **A,** The first and second portions of the duodenum are markedly dilated. The small intestine distal to the usual site of the ligament of Treitz lies below the duodenum and to the right. **B,** Delayed film demonstrates the terminal ileum and cecum to be on the right, although the cecum is higher than its usual position *(arrow).*

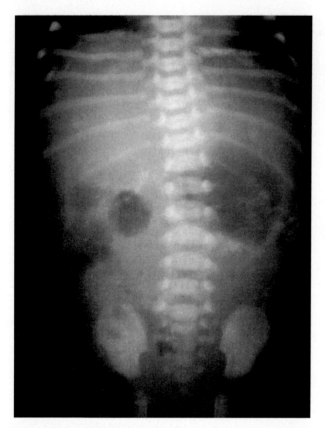

FIGURE 6. Small bowel obstruction in a newborn with ileal atresia.

MECONIUM ILEUS

The most common mimic of small bowel atresias clinically and on plain films is meconium ileus. This condition occurs in babies who in 99% of cases will be

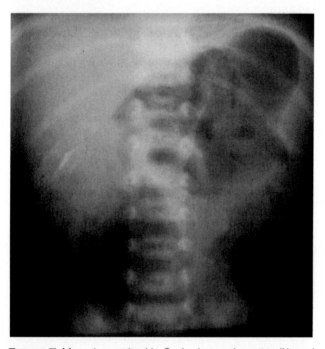

FIGURE 7. Meconium peritonitis. Supine image shows small bowel obstruction and a linear calcification under the free edge of the liver in a neonate with small bowel atresia.

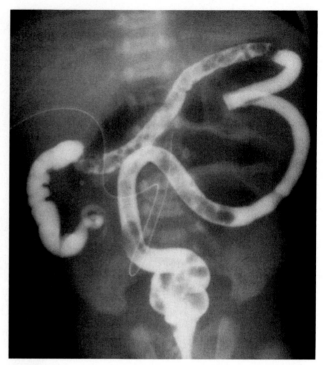

FIGURE 8. Small bowel atresia. Contrast enema demonstrates a "microcolon," or unused colon, in a newborn with ileal atresia. Note the normal rectum and the meconium pellets.

found to have *cystic fibrosis* (CF). The lack of normal pancreatic enzymes leads to thick, tenacious meconium that collects in the distal ileum and cecum, causing obstruction (Fig. 9). A differentiating feature from atresias is that theses babies may not have pronounced air–fluid levels on horizontal beam radiographs. These babies may also have microcolon on contrast enemas, but, if contrast can be refluxed into the small bowel, the correct diagnosis may be made. US can identify clumps of meconium, but, because these may also occur proximal to an atresia, the finding is not diagnostic. Therapeutic enemas for meconium ileus have largely given way to new clinical therapeutic measures.

COLONIC ABNORMALITIES

Colonic abnormalities may mimic small intestinal obstruction. These entities are discussed in Section VI, Part VIII, page 1649.

NECROTIZING ENTEROCOLITIS

Necrotizing enterocolitis is not obstructive during its acute phase, but its complications may lead to obstruction in infancy. The disease usually develops between 5 days and 2 weeks of life but has been reported in the first day of life and at several months of age. The pathophysiology is not certain but is probably a combination of mucosal ischemia and infection. Affected neonates often are premature infants who may have had positive pressure ventilation. The babies develop abdominal distention often associated with blood in the stools.

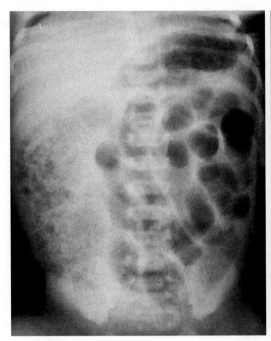 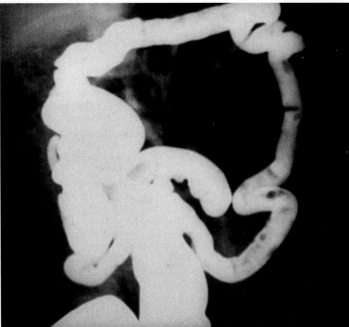

FIGURE 9. Meconium ileus. Plain radiograph demonstrates dilated loops of bowel with a large collection of bubbly meconium in the right lower quadrant. Contrast enema demonstrates a microcolon.

Initial radiographs generally show a nonspecific ileus. The diagnostic features that may develop include pneumatosis intestinalis, portal venous air, and free intraperitoneal air if perforation has occurred (Fig. 10A). Strictures may occur weeks to months after the acute episode (Fig. 10B). The colon is more commonly affected than the small bowel. The babies present with partial obstruction, often manifested as increased frank emesis, increased gastric residuals, and abdominal distention.

ACQUIRED OBSTRUCTION

Acquired intestinal obstruction in older children may be due either to intrinsic or extrinsic abnormalities affecting the small intestine. The plain film findings may help identify the level of obstruction but, in many cases, may show nonspecific changes of incomplete obstruction or adynamic ileus.

ADYNAMIC ILEUS

Although adynamic (paralytic) ileus can simulate mechanical obstruction on plain films, certain signs, if present, are useful in distinguishing the two entities. Supine radiographs of the abdomen show dilated loops of bowel in both entities. The lack of rectal gas is not a useful sign, especially in young children, because air rises out of the dependent rectum on supine films. Generalized adynamic ileus causes both small intestine and colon to dilate, whereas obstruction usually causes proximal dilatation with reduced caliber of the distal bowel. Air–fluid levels on horizontal beam films can be seen with both mechanical and adynamic ileus. In the

former, they are relatively short and are at different levels in the loop of bowel (Fig. 11), whereas in the latter, they are longer and at the same level within a loop (Fig. 12). Decubitus views are frequently more successful in demonstrating the long levels of adynamic ileus than are upright films. Unfortunately, there are a significant number of children in whom differentiation is not possible. This is especially true of children with a focal ileus affecting the small intestine but not the colon. There are other children in whom partial small intestinal obstruction mimics adynamic ileus. CT has been used in adults to identify obstruction, particularly of the closed-loop variety. Jabra and Fishman have reviewed CT findings in 20 children with small bowel obstruction and have found the procedure a helpful adjunct in diagnosis, especially in children with postsurgical adhesions.

INCARCERATED HERNIA

Incarcerated hernias are a less frequent cause of small intestinal obstruction than in the past, possibly owing to the increased performance of elective outpatient herniorrhaphy. Most incarcerated hernias are inguinal and, occasionally, umbilical. The diagnosis is made on clinical grounds, but plain films may be used to confirm the diagnosis and to rule out bowel perforation (Fig. 13).

ADHESIONS

Adhesions are a common cause of obstruction in patients who have undergone prior abdominal surgery. Adhesive bands can obstruct the small intestine even at a site distant from the original surgical site. Plain films are useful in corroborating the clinical suspicion and in rul-

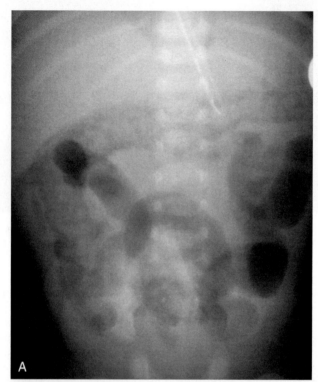

FIGURE 10. Necrotizing enterocolitis. **A,** Pneumatosis intestinalis paralleling the bowel wall. **B,** Portal venous gas.

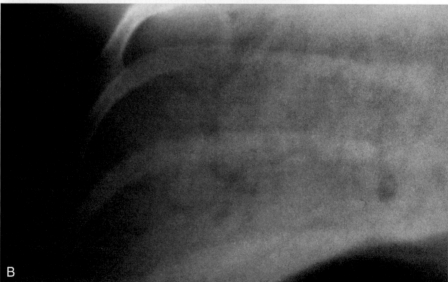

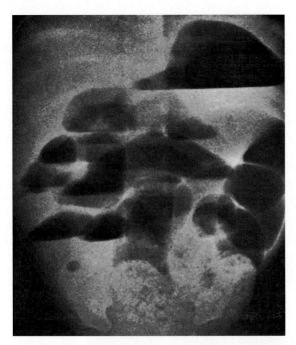

FIGURE 11. Small intestinal obstruction secondary to postoperative adhesions. Upright radiograph of the abdomen demonstrates multiple air–fluid levels at different levels throughout the abdomen.

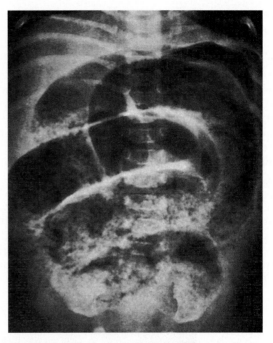

FIGURE 13. Intestinal obstruction secondary to incarcerated inguinal hernia. Supine radiograph of the abdomen demonstrates multiple dilated loops of small intestine.

ing out intestinal perforation (Fig. 14). Adhesions can also occur in children who have had peritonitis, usually from appendicitis or inflammatory bowel disease.

DUODENAL HEMATOMA

Duodenal hematomas are generally secondary to blunt abdominal trauma and are discussed in Section VI, Part VI, Chapter 3, page 1593. Occasionally, they may occur in patients with a bleeding disorder who have a diagnos-

tic or therapeutic procedure involving the duodenum: They can occur in Henoch-Schöenlein purpura and on occasion may be found as an initial finding in child abuse. We have seen one child who was severely thrombocytopenic following bone marrow transplantation for leukemia. Endoscopic biopsy of the duodenum was performed to confirm the suspected diagnosis of graft-versus-host disease (GVHD). Several days later, the patient developed jaundice. US and CT examination revealed a massive duodenal hematoma with partial obstruction of the common bile duct (Fig. 15).

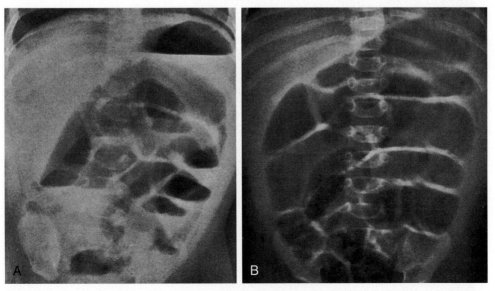

FIGURE 12. Gastroenteritis. **A,** Upright radiograph of the abdomen demonstrates multiple dilated loops of bowel with air–fluid levels approximately at the same level within each individual loop. Gas is seen within the rectosigmoid region. **B,** Supine view of the abdomen demonstrates multiple dilated loops of bowel.

SUPERIOR MESENTERIC ARTERY SYNDROME

The superior mesenteric artery syndrome is a condition in which the third portion of the duodenum is trapped between the SMA and the root of the mesentery. Originally described in young adult women, the syndrome usually occurs in asthenic persons who develop vomiting following sudden weight loss secondary to either illness or voluntary dieting. Subsequently, the syndrome was described in adolescents, but its existence as a real entity has been doubted by many. Marchant et al. reviewed their experience with 13 patients ranging in age from 4 to 18 years in whom the SMA syndrome was treated surgically in 9 children with resolution of symptoms. Plain films may show gastric dilatation, but the stomach may be decompressed by the vomiting. Barium study shows a high-grade partial obstruction of the third portion of the duodenum (Fig. 16). Fluoros-copy demonstrates to-and-fro motion of the barium in the dilated proximal portions of the duodenum. The findings are not specific and may be seen with Ladd's bands and focal ileus or functional obstruction of the proximal jejunum, as may be seen with inflammatory bowel disease. Oritz et al. described SMA syndrome in five members of a family of eight, raising the question of genetic disposition.

An acute form of SMA syndrome following scoliosis treatment has been called the *cast syndrome* because it was initially identified in children receiving full body casts for scoliosis. We have also seen the syndrome following placement of spinal rods even without a cast. Presumably, the abrupt straightening of the spine changes the angle at which the SMA branches from the aorta, causing duodenal compression. Massive gastric dilatation is the rule, and gastric perforation has been described (Fig. 17). Decompression by nasogastric tube is usually effective.

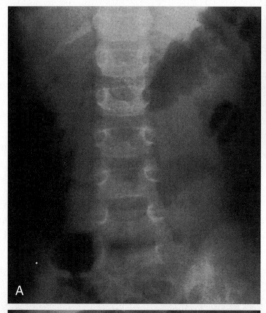
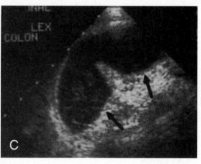
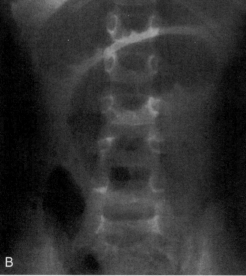

FIGURE 14. Postoperative adhesions causing intestinal obstruction. **A,** Focally dilated loops of bowel in a 4-year-old girl 3 weeks following surgery for a ruptured appendix. **B,** Coronal ultrasound scan demonstrates dilated fluid-filled loops of bowel. **C,** Plain film 2 days later shows a markedly dilated air–fluid loop of bowel *(arrows)* in the midportion of the abdomen. Adhesions were lysed at exploratory laparotomy.

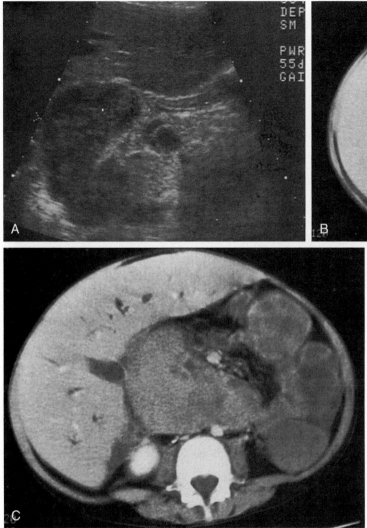

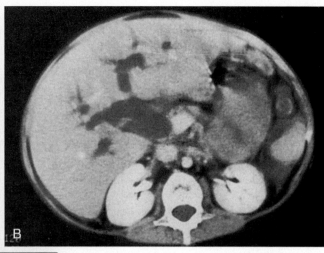

FIGURE 15. Duodenal hematoma secondary to endoscopic biopsy in a thrombocytopenic patient. **A,** Ultrasound scan demonstrates a hypoechoic lesion in the region of the pancreatic head and duodenum. **B,** Computed tomography (CT) scan section through the upper abdomen demonstrates marked dilatation of the common bile duct and intrahepatic ducts. **C,** CT scan section slightly more inferiorly demonstrates a large intramural hematoma of the duodenum. The hematoma resolved gradually over a prolonged course.

ABNORMALITIES MIMICKING OBSTRUCTION

Duodenal dilatation is a common manifestation of *intestinal pseudo-obstruction.* This entity is discussed in Section VI, Part VIII, page 1649. Another congenital abnormality that can mimic obstruction is *segmental dilatation of the small bowel.* This rare disorder is characterized by segmental dilatation, which may appear as a single dilated loop with an air–fluid level on plain film and a focally dilated loop of bowel, usually ileum, on barium study (Fig. 18). Transit time is normal, and surgery is curative.

TUMORS

Tumors of the small intestine, benign or malignant, are rare in children. Polyposis of the small bowel usually occurs in children with the polyposis syndromes, which are described in Section VI, Part VIII, page 1649. Patients usually present with blood in the stools and crampy abdominal pain secondary to recurrent enteroenteric intussusceptions. Distal ileal polyps may produce ileocolic intussusception. Barium studies reveal

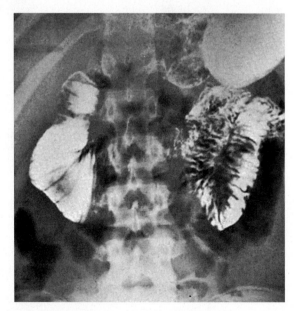

FIGURE 16. Superior mesenteric artery syndrome in a 15-year-old boy with 4 weeks of vomiting and a 32-lb weight loss. The second and third portions of the duodenum are markedly dilated secondary to a partial obstruction. The distal bowel was normal.

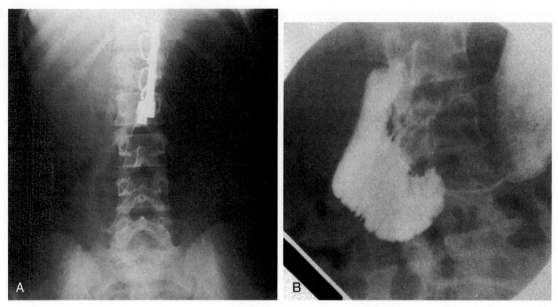

FIGURE 17. Cast syndrome. **A,** Supine radiograph of the abdomen 1 day after insertion of corrective rods for scoliosis demonstrates massive dilatation of the stomach. **B,** Spot film from an upper gastrointestinal series demonstrates characteristic obstruction of the duodenum at the level of the third portion. The symptoms resolved over the course of 1 week with nasogastric tube drainage.

polypoid filling defects. The polyps can also be identified on US and CT. In children with blue rubber bleb nevus syndrome, hemangiomas can cause polypoid defects in the stomach, colon, and small bowel. Tyrrel

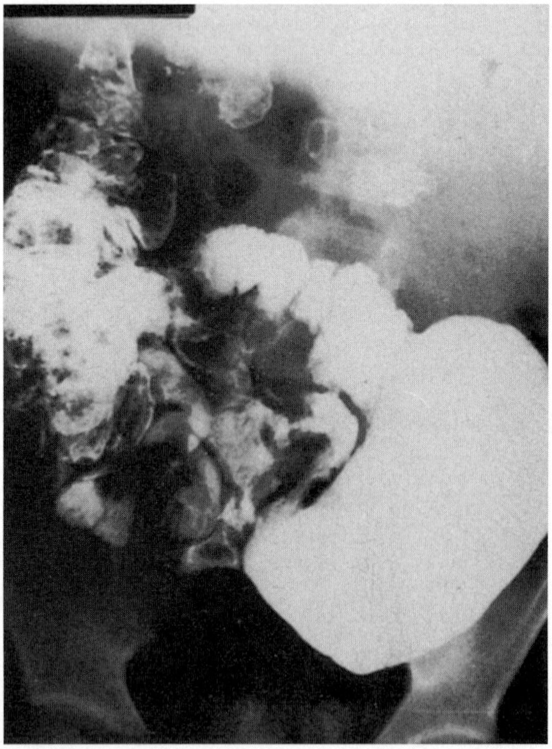

FIGURE 18. Segmental dilatation of the small bowel. Small bowel series demonstrates dilatation of a focal loop of ileum in the left lower quadrant. The patient's symptoms were relieved following removal of the abnormal portion of small intestine. (Courtesy of Dr. John Ratcliffe, Brisbane, Australia.)

et al. reported the CT diagnosis of intussusception in a young woman with the blue rubber bleb nevus syndrome. Unusual tumors in childhood include lipomas, fibromas, neurofibromas, and leiomyomas.

Malignant tumors of the small intestine in children, other than lymphoma, are exceedingly rare. The benign tumors mentioned above have their malignant counterparts. Patients with several of the polyposis syndromes can develop gastrointestinal (GI) malignancies. Malignant carcinoid has been reported in children.

BURKITT'S LYMPHOMA

Burkitt's lymphoma is a B cell lymphoma with a predilection for abdominal organs, particularly the distal ileum. It is the most common lead point in children over the age of 4 years with ileocolic intussusception (Fig. 19). Patients present with variable symptoms, including nausea, vomiting, change in bowel habits, GI bleeding, or a right lower quadrant mass. Half of all patients with the sporadic form of Burkitt's lymphoma (formerly called American Burkitt's lymphoma) have involvement of the terminal ileum, and in 25% of patients the disease is limited to this site. Mesenteric lymph nodes are usually involved. Plain film findings may be normal, show evidence of obstruction secondary to intussusception, or show a noncalcified mass. If a mass is obvious, either clinically or radiographically, US is the appropriate imaging study. Lymphoma is often hypoechoic or anechoic, so US may enable a specific diagnosis to be suggested (Fig. 20). The small-bowel lesion is usually eccentric and the lumen is frequently dilated. The involved lymph nodes may be focal or may infiltrate the mesentery and encase the mesenteric vessels. The nodal masses are also of decreased echogenicity. CT also

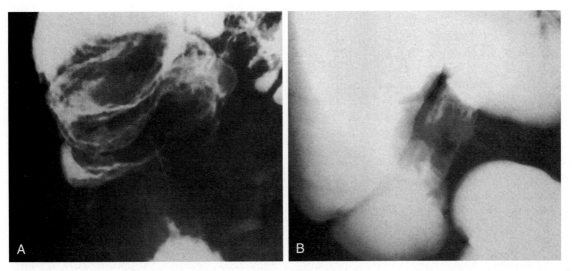

FIGURE 19. Burkitt's lymphoma presenting as intussusception. **A,** Spot film from a barium enema demonstrates and intussusceptum within the cecum. **B,** Reflux into the small intestine reveals an ileocecal mass that proved to be Burkitt's lymphoma.

shows the mesenteric masses and infiltration of bowel wall with dilatation of bowel lumen. Both US and CT may demonstrate ascites. Barium studies may show polypoid involvement of the mucosa, infiltration of the wall, dilatation and ulceration of the bowel wall, or effacement of the mucosa mimicking inflammatory bowel disease. The effect of the adjacent mesenteric masses can be seen. The tumor may also involve other abdominal sites, and careful evaluation of the retroperitoneal organs, liver, and spleen is mandatory during US and CT.

DEVELOPMENTAL CYSTS

Several different types of developmental cysts may present in infancy or later in childhood, depending largely on the size of the cyst. The most frequent location for a *duplication cyst* of the intestinal tract is the region of the terminal ileum and ileocecal valve. The next most common areas are the esophagus, stomach, and duodenum, but these cysts can be located anywhere in the GI tract. Multiple duplications have been reported. Duplication cysts, by definition, contain mucosal and muscular layers. The majority are localized, somewhat spherical, and noncommunicating. Some duplication cysts are tubular, paralleling significant lengths of bowel, and may communicate with the normal intestinal lumen. Presenting symptoms depend on the location and size of the duplication. Obstruction can occur anywhere there is a duplication cyst and is the most frequent cause of symptoms. Many are large enough to be palpable. Abdominal pain may be related to distention of the cyst or peptic disease if the cyst

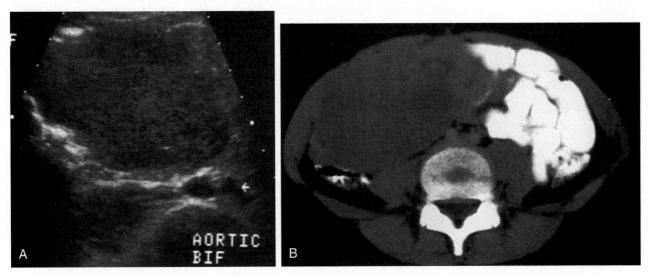

FIGURE 20. Burkitt's lymphoma in a 14-year-old boy who presented with a large abdominal mass. **A,** Ultrasound (US) scan demonstrates a hypoechoic mass anterior to the aortic bifurcation that, on multiple scans, extended both superiorly and inferiorly. **B,** Computed tomography scan demonstrates the mass extending from just in front of the psoas muscle to the anterior abdominal wall. Percutaneous needle biopsy under US control demonstrated Burkitt's lymphoma.

contains gastric mucosa. Distal ileal duplication may cause intussusception, and volvulus may occur at any site in the small intestine where a duplication is present. GI bleeding may occur from a communicating duplication containing gastric mucosa. Brown et al. reported a baby with delayed diagnosis as the cyst intermittently decompressed itself by emptying its contents into the adjacent, partially communicating bowel lumen.

Plain radiographic examination is usually unrewarding unless the duplication is large enough to cause a mass effect on adjacent structures, intestinal obstruction is present, or calcification in the wall is identified (Fig. 21A). US identifies the duplication as anechoic (Fig. 21B). Sometimes a specific sonographic diagnosis can be suggested if the echogenic mucosa surrounded by a thin hypoechoic halo representing the muscular layer is identified. Occasionally, the cysts will be multilocular. Echogenic debris may be seen, probably secondary to hemorrhage or mucosal secretions. Caspi et al. described an infected duplication cyst with mixed echogenicity that mimicked a pelvic abscess. Those duplications containing gastric mucosa may be identified by technetium-99m pertechnetate scintigraphy. CT is not indicated once US demonstrates the cystic nature of the duplication but will show low attenuation surrounded by an enhancing wall. Contrast studies of the intestinal tract may demonstrate the lumen of communicating duplications, but are more likely to demonstrate just the mass effect.

Other intraperitoneal cysts arise within the mesentery or omentum. In children with mesenteric cysts, the most common presenting symptoms are abdominal pain, abdominal distention, and vomiting. Ros et al. pointed out that the terms *mesenteric cyst* and *omental cyst* are synonymous and include a group of lesions that have differing histologic and radiologic features. They include enteric duplication cysts with their enteric lining, double muscle layer, and neural elements, as discussed above.

Lymphangiomas (Fig. 22) have only an endothelial lining, are usually multiloculated, and may contain chyle. They typically present as painless abdominal distention with a palpable mass. The cyst may be adherent to small intestine, causing partial obstruction and vomiting and requiring surgical resection of involved bowel loops. Plain films show a large mass displacing intestinal loops. Dilated loops may be seen in patients with partial obstruction. GI contrast studies show displacement of bowel with no communication. US demonstrates the multilocular nature of the mass with fine septations. Most of the mass is anechoic, but some of the loculated spaces may be hypoechoic or even echogenic, depending on the chyle or blood content. Echogenic debris is commonly seen. CT also demonstrates the septa and loculation. The attenuation values of the fluid range from near-fat to near-water, depending on the content of the fluid. The septa may enhance with intravenous contrast injection. MRI studies of patients with lymphangioma show characteristics of the cyst ranging from fluid with low-intensity signal on T_1-weighted images to fat with high-intensity signal.

Nonpancreatic pseudocysts can arise in the mesentery. They have a fibrous wall without a lining. They are frequently hemorrhagic or infected, with increased echogenicity on US and increased attenuation values on CT compared with water. *Enteric cysts* are much like duplication cysts but have an enteric lining without a muscle layer and with no ganglion cells. *Mesothelial cysts* have a mesothelial lining, are unilocular, and are anechoic on US. *Intraperitoneal teratomas* are typically cystic (Fig. 23). Identification of multitissue origin, especially when fat and calcium are seen, can lead to the

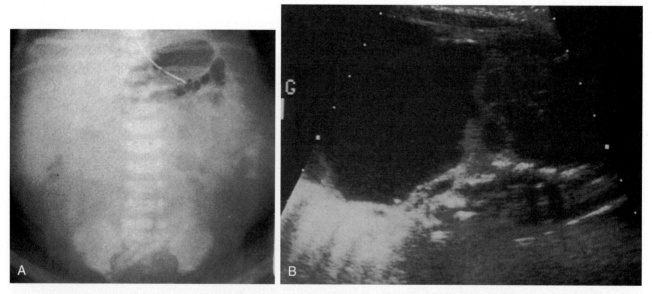

FIGURE 21. Ileal duplication cyst. **A,** Plain radiograph of the abdomen in a newborn infant demonstrates a paucity of bowel gas and marked abdominal distention. **B,** Abdominal ultrasound scan demonstrates a large, hypoechoic structure with acoustic enhancement adjacent to thickened loops of small intestine. At surgery, multiple noncommunicating ileal duplication cysts were found.

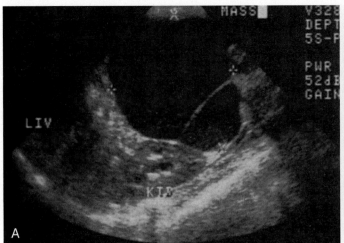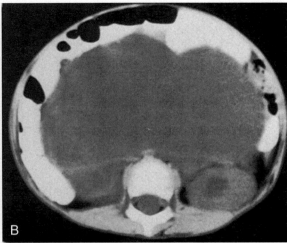

FIGURE 22. Mesenteric lymphangioma. **A,** Longitudinal ultrasound scan through the upper abdomen demonstrates a septated, hypoechoic mass abutting the liver *(LIV)* and right kidney *(KID)*. **B,** Computed tomography scan confirms the massive fluid-filled structure displacing contrast-filled loops of bowel. The right-sided septation is again seen, even in an unenhanced scan.

correct diagnosis. Because there is sufficient overlap of imaging findings among the different types of cysts, histologic examination is the only sure diagnostic study, but the characteristics of lymphangioma, a more difficult surgical problem than the other types, may lead, in some cases, to the correct preoperative diagnosis.

Omphalomesenteric remnants are the residua of the embryologic yolk stalk and present in different forms, some of which may be cystic. *Meckel's diverticulum* occurs when the enteric end of the duct fails to undergo normal involution. It may contain mucosa from any portion of the GI tract. The patients usually present with right lower quadrant pain and may have occult blood in the stools. The diverticula are difficult to image, and the diagnosis is often made at surgery (Fig. 24). A small bowel series rarely may show the diverticulum emanating from the terminal ileum. If gastric mucosa is present, a technetium scan may show the lesion, but significant numbers of false positives and false negatives decrease the reliability of the study. On rare occasions, the entire omphalomesenteric duct persists as a connection from the terminal ileum to the umbilicus. The clinical diagnosis is easily made by the presence of stool at the umbilicus. Imaging is rarely used but may show a subumbilical abscess.

INFECTIOUS DISEASES

The most common intestinal infection in children in North America and Europe is viral gastroenteritis. Parasites and bacteria as well as viruses are worldwide causative agents of acute gastroenteritis in children. The resultant severe diarrhea and vomiting with subsequent dehydration is, tragically, still a leading cause of childhood morbidity and mortality throughout the underdeveloped countries of the world.

VIRAL GASTROENTERITIS

Viral gastroenteritis in the United States is most commonly secondary to rotavirus infection. Associated upper respiratory symptoms are common and may precede the GI presentation, which usually begins with vomiting followed by severe watery diarrhea. Imaging studies are not generally indicated, but plain films are occasionally requested to rule out other causes for the patient's symptoms. The most common finding is fluid-filled loops of nondilated bowel with multiple air–fluid levels on horizontal beam radiographs. Depending on the time course and degree of motility disturbance, nonob-

FIGURE 23. Intraperitoneal teratoma. Computed tomography scan demonstrates a large intraperitoneal mass with multiple components of different attenuation values equal to those of water and of fat displacing bowel loops. A benign teratoma was removed at surgery.

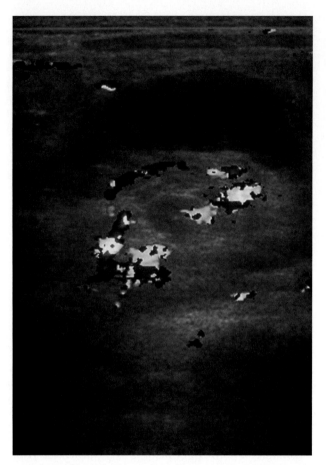

FIGURE 24. Meckel's diverticulum. Ultrasound scan demonstration of volvulus (note whirlpool sign) around a thick-walled cystic structure found to be a twisted Meckel's diverticulum at surgery. *See Color Plate*

structive dilatation of bowel loops may occur. Contrast studies are not indicated but, if performed for other reasons, will show dilution of barium from fluid retention, minimal thickening of mucosal folds, and either rapid or delayed transit time, depending on the chronicity of the disease. Disordered peristalsis is commonly seen. Capitanio and Greenberg described pneumatosis intestinalis in two infants with rotavirus enteritis.

US is not indicated for clinically obvious gastroenteritis but, if performed for other reasons, will show fluid-filled loops of bowel with vigorous peristalsis. Enlarged mesenteric lymph nodes may be found. Thickening of the bowel wall and increased Doppler signal may occur when the clinical course has been a prolonged one. Siegel and colleagues have shown the ability of US to differentiate the causes of bowel wall thickening. In their series, viral gastroenteritis was not associated with increased bowel wall vascularity.

BACTERIAL ENTEROCOLITIS

Bacterial enterocolitis is much less common than the viral form. *Shigella, Salmonella, Escherichia coli, Yersinia enterocolitica,* and *Campylobacter fetus* are the most commonly identified bacterial agents in the United States. *Vibrio cholerae* is the most common infectious bacterial

agent in Asia. The symptoms are similar to those of viral gastroenteritis, but frequently are accompanied by high fever and systemic toxicity. Typhoid fever and tuberculosis are less commonly seen than in prior years and are less common in children than in adults. The plain film findings in bacterial gastroenteritis are similar to those described above for viral disease. Contrast studies in those cases caused by the common bacteria are also nonspecific. *Yersinia,* typhoid, and tuberculosis all have a predilection for the terminal ileum (Fig. 25) and *Yersinia* may simulate Crohn's disease (Fig. 26). A cobblestone pattern may be seen. Typhoid may cause prominent lymphoid hyperplasia. Puylaert et al. diagnosed typhoid fever in a 12-year-old girl with the US findings of enlarged mesenteric lymph nodes and mural thickening of the terminal ileum and cecum accompanied by hepatic portal lymphadenopathy and splenomegaly. *Yersinia* can cause mesenteric adenitis with associated abdominal pain sometimes mimicking appendicitis. Matsumoto et al. performed US on eight children and young adults with *Yersinia* terminal ileitis. Thickening of the ileal wall was present in all eight patients and mesenteric lymphadenopathy in six. Tuberculous involvement of the terminal ileum may cause small bowel obstruction, presumably from adherent bowel loops. Ascites may be present. Pulmonary tuberculosis is probably the source of the GI infection, and chest radiographs should always be obtained in suspected cases.

PARASITIC ENTEROCOLITIS

Parasitic enterocolitis is most frequently caused by *Giardia lamblia* in the Western Hemisphere, and usually results from drinking contaminated water. In the west-

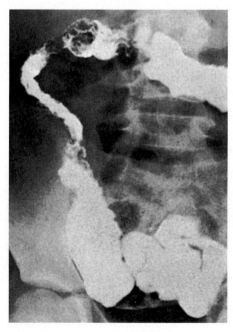

FIGURE 25. Ileocecal tuberculosis. Persistent spasm and stenosis of the terminal ileum, cecum, and ascending colon are identified on this radiograph.

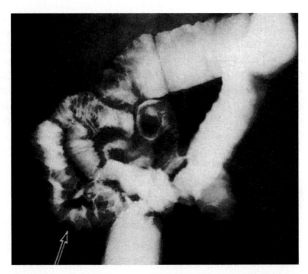

FIGURE 26. *Yersinia* enterocolitis. Barium enema demonstrates "thumbprinting" *(arrow)* in the cecum and ascending colon in a 1-year-old girl. The ileum is dilated, with thickened folds. *Yersinia enterocolitica* was cultured from mesenteric nodes removed at the time of exploratory laparotomy.

ern United States, virtually all of the natural mountain streams have become infested with *Giardia*. Although the protozoan easily infects otherwise normal people, it is an especially common etiologic agent in patients with acquired immunodeficiency syndrome (AIDS) who develop enteritis. On barium studies, giardiasis produces thickened mucosal folds in the duodenum and jejunum associated with rapid transit time and dilution of the contrast material (Fig. 27).

Helminthic enteritis can be caused by a variety of worms, of which *Ascaris lumbricoides* causes the most striking and diagnostic radiographic abnormalities. The disease results from swallowed larvae that grow into adult worms in the intestinal tract. Barium studies outline the characteristic vermiform organisms, which may appear singly or in clumps. The live worms may ingest barium, permitting visualization of their intestinal tracts. Infections with *Strongyloides stercoralis*, tapeworms, roundworms, and hookworms may all occur.

ACQUIRED IMMUNODEFICIENCY SYNDROME

AIDS is substantially less common in children than in adults, but the number of affected children is growing. Most early cases in children were secondary to transmission of the human immunodeficiency virus through contaminated blood products. Patients treated for hemophilia were at particular risk. Presently, according to Haney et al., 80% or more of affected children have acquired the virus from their mothers via transplacental passage. The presenting symptoms and signs are nonspecific and related to the affected organ systems. Enteritis is most frequently caused by the common pathogens described above, but may follow infection with opportunistic organisms such as cytomegalovirus (CMV), *Mycobacterium avium-intracellulare,* and the ubiquitous fungi, especially *Candida albicans.* Extrapulmonic *Pneumocystis carinii* infection is being reported with

increasing frequency. Candidiasis most commonly affects the esophagus, but any of the organisms can infect any part of the GI tract. Nonspecific edema of the affected intestine is the most frequently found abnormality on barium studies. Effacement of the mucosal pattern is common, especially with *Cryptosporidium* infection. Sivit, Taylor, et al. described an 8-month-old girl who developed small bowel obstruction secondary to adhesions formed by serosal plaques of CMV infection. Pneumatosis intestinalis has been reported, although the cause is unclear. US and CT demonstrate thickening of the bowel wall, with intra-abdominal and retroperitoneal lymphadenopathy being the most frequent finding. Both Kaposi's sarcoma and lymphoma have been reported in the intestine, mesentery, and pancreas of affected children, but less frequently than in adults.

INFLAMMATORY BOWEL DISEASE

CROHN'S DISEASE

Crohn's disease is also commonly known as *regional enteritis,* with the terms *segmental enteritis* and *terminal ileitis* less frequently used. The peak incidence is in young adulthood, but 25% of patients present in childhood, adolescence, or the teenage years. The disease has been reported in infants less than 1 year of age. Crohn's disease is characterized by segmental transmural granulomatous inflammation of the intestine. It may be localized to one segment or involve several segments with normal bowel between them. The terminal ileum is the most frequently involved segment, but the disease has been described everywhere in the GI

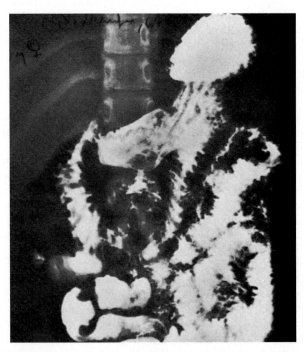

FIGURE 27. Giardiasis. Small intestinal examination in a 10-year-old girl with a history of nausea, vomiting, diarrhea, and weight loss. The mucosal folds of the duodenum and proximal jejunum are markedly thickened. Giardia was identified in the stool.

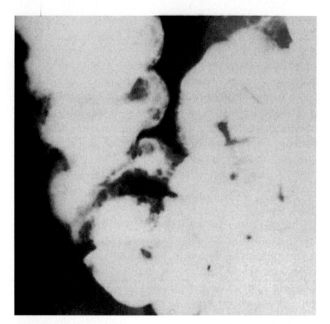

FIGURE 28. Crohn's disease. Coned-down view of the ileocecal valve demonstrates the typical "bird beak" deformity of the terminal ileum and thickening of the wall, causing separation from the ileocecal valve.

tract from the mouth to the anus. The intestinal lumen is narrowed by edematous and fibrotic thickening of the wall and by spasm. The mucosal layer is extensively destroyed, and ulcers are usually present.

Most children with Crohn's disease present with the insidious onset of GI symptoms, including diarrhea, abdominal pain, anorexia, abdominal mass, or fistula in ano. Extraintestinal manifestations of the disease may accompany or precede the GI symptoms and include failure to thrive with delayed puberty, fever, aphthous stomatitis, arthralgias, arthritis, sacroiliitis, and erythema nodosum. Digital clubbing is found in 25% to 33% of affected children. A smaller number of patients present acutely with right lower quadrant pain and fever mimicking appendicitis.

Plain film evaluation of the abdomen in patients with inflammatory bowel disease may be normal. During an acute exacerbation of the disease, plain films are more likely to show nonspecific abnormalities such as adynamic ileus and bowel wall thickening. Occasionally, a focally abnormal loop with edematous wall can be identified, strongly suggesting acute inflammation.

Barium contrast small intestinal series continues to be the most frequently utilized diagnostic imaging examination for the evaluation of the jejunoileal manifestations of Crohn's disease. The terminal ileum is the most frequently involved area (Fig. 28), but more proximal disease with sparing of the terminal ileum has been reported. The earliest change is granularity, probably reflecting mucosal edema. More prominent mural edema and increased mucosal secretion result in the thickening of mucosal folds and effacement of the mucosal pattern. More typical early findings include nodular irregularity with linear and transverse ulceration. The characteristic "rose thorn" ulcer is less

commonly seen and is not pathognomonic, as once believed. Extensive ulceration can lead to a spiculated appearance. The intersection of multiple linear and transverse ulcers leads to a cobblestone appearance (Fig. 29). This pattern has also been described as pseudopolypoid, but this is inaccurate because these pseudopolyps are really areas of mantained mucosa adjacent to denuded areas and ulcers filled with barium. Spasm of involved segments is frequently seen.

■ **Imaging findings in Crohn's Disease:**
Plain films
- Frequently normal or nonspecific
- In acute exacerbations, may see narrowed bowel loop with edema and/or thickened wall

Contrast small bowel study
- Mucosal edema
- Thickening of mucosal folds and effacement of mucosa ("moulage sign")
- Linear and transverse ulceration leading to cobblestone pattern
- Rose thorn ulcers
- Pseudopolyps
- Severe luminal narrowing and fibrosis
- Enteroenteric fistulas

Computed tomography
- Findings similar to those on small bowel series
- More sensitive to mesenteric thickening, abscess formation, and, questionably, fistulas

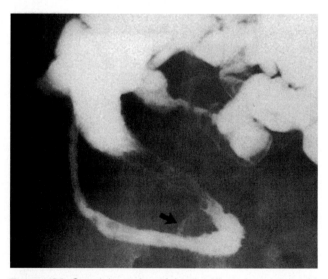

FIGURE 29. Coned-down view of the distal ileum in a patient with documented Crohn's disease demonstrates marked separation of bowel loops secondary to mesenteric thickening, a cobblestone pattern in the bowel mucosa, and multiple "rose thorn ulcers" throughout the affected loop. A walled-off fistulous tract (arrow) was identified.

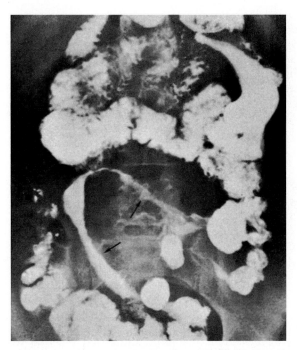

FIGURE 30. Crohn's disease in a 14-year-old girl. Small bowel series demonstrates markedly narrowed and rigid loop of jejunum. The *upper arrow* points to an extreme narrowing, the so-called string sign.

Edema, fibrosis, and spasm lead to narrowing of the intestinal lumen that may be so profound as to be labeled the "string sign" (Fig. 30). The narrowing is accompanied by persistent ulcers. The mesentery becomes inflamed, thickened, and fibrotic, causing separation and retraction of bowel loops. Enlarged mesenteric lymph nodes may cause mass effect on adjacent loops of bowel (Fig. 31). Postinflammatory polyps may be seen. These are filiform projections of submucosa covered by mucosa on all sides. They represent healing of undermined mucosal and submucosal remnants and ulcers and are almost always multiple.

The diagnostic accuracy of barium studies is quite good. Lipson et al. compared barium small bowel series with ileoscopy and biopsy results in 46 children with suspected regional enteritis of the terminal ileum. Although ileoscopy agreed with the biopsy results in all 20 positive cases, the small bowel series had a sensitivity of 90% and a specificity of 96%. The major source of misdiagnosis was pronounced lymphoid hyperpasia on the barium study, which led to diagnostic errors in two cases.

Imaging studies other than small bowel series are being used with increasing frequency in the evaluation of patients with regional enteritis, although this is more the case in adults than in children. Nuclear scintigraphy using a variety of radiopharmaceuticals can be used to identify areas of active inflammation, although with questionable success in some studies, and has been successful in differentiating primary bowel disease from adjacent abscesses. These studies are not often performed in children because of concern over the long-range effects of the isotopes used, particularly indium-111.

US is not used for primary diagnosis in Crohn's disease but is more apt to be requested for evaluation of complications such as abscesses. US can, however, demonstrate thickening of the bowel wall and separation of bowel loops. The bowel wall appears stiff as well as thickened, and no peristalsis in the affected loop can be demonstrated. A halo of submucosal edema may give a target-like appearance to the bowel wall when seen transversely, and a "double track" appearance when imaged longitudinally. Large abscesses can be identified, but small abscesses are difficult to distinguish from matted loops of inflamed bowel. Doppler US is useful in identifying areas of active inflamation, which show increased Doppler signal in and surrounding the thickened bowel wall.

CT is becoming more widely used in adults with regional enteritis, but in children is reserved for the evaluation of complications. CT readily identifies bowel wall thickening, luminal narrowing and stricture formation, and mesenteric changes such as lymphadenopathy, fibrofatty proliferation, and phlegmon formation (Fig. 32). CT can be used to identify complications when US is inconclusive.

The major intra-abdominal complications of regional enteritis are enteroenteric fistulas, sinus tracts, and abscesses (Fig. 33). CT is the most sensitive imaging study for elucidation of these complications. Barium studies can identify fistulas if the examination is carefully monitored so that premature filling of a bowel loop can be seen. Sinus tracts to the skin can be injected. We use water-soluble contrast for such injections in the event of an unanticipated intraperitoneal leak. Abscesses are among the most common complications of regional enteritis. CT will identify over 90% of abscesses and is the best modality for their guided percutaneous drainage.

Several studies have demonstrated that MRI may be complementary to CT in selected adult cases. MRI has been particularly useful in the evaluation of anorectal fistulas.

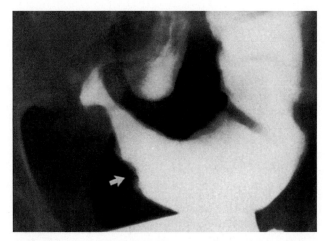

FIGURE 31. Coned-down view of the proximal ileum in a patient with Crohn's disease. Extrinsic filling defects secondary to mesenteric adenopathy are identified *(arrow)*.

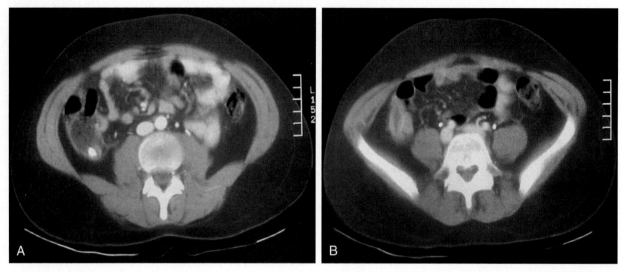

FIGURE 32. Crohn's disease. Computed tomographic sections through the lower abdomen **(A)** and pelvis **(B)** demonstrate thickening of the bowel wall and mesentery.

BEHÇET'S SYNDROME

Findings similar to those of Crohn's disease can be seen in other inflammatory diseases. Behçet's syndrome is a multiorgan process with inflammatory changes and ulceration anywhere in the GI tract. The esophagus, terminal ileum (Fig. 34), and right colon are most commonly affected. This syndrome may also have pulmonary artery aneurysms (see Section IV, Part VII, Chapter 6, page 1073).

FUNCTIONAL AND INFILTRATIVE DISEASES

There are a large number of diseases of disparate etiologies that affect the small intestine in similar, thus nonspecific, ways. Abnormalities of intestinal motility are frequently associated with abnormalities of mucosal folds identified on contrast examinations of the small bowel and with intestinal dilatation, either generalized or focal.

PROTEIN-LOSING ENTEROPATHIES

Celiac disease is the most common cause of intestinal malabsorption in childhood. The disease is also known as nontropical sprue or gluten enteropathy because the cause is gluten intolerance. Gluten is a protein present in the food grains most commonly used by humans. Most affected children present with failure to thrive, abdominal distention, and diarrhea. Diarrhea is considered one of the hallmarks of the disease but is not present in 10% of patients with celiac disease. Affected adolescents have delayed puberty, anorexia, and clinical findings related to the hypocalcemia and hypoproteinemia of malabsorption. Imaging studies are only adjunctive at best, and diagnosis relies on a combination of clinical findings and small-bowel biopsy. Plain films in patients with celiac disease may show nonspecific small-bowel dilatation. The classic findings on barium small-bowel series are dilatation, thickened mucosal folds, flocculation, and segmentation. The last two findings, however, are uncommonly seen with modern-day barium preparations. The mucosal folds may be abnormal with thinning or thickening and reversal of the mucosal patterns of jejunum and ileum. The duodenum may show mucosal erosions or thickened nodular folds. CT is not indicated for evaluation, but, if performed, may demonstrate mesenteric lymphadenopathy which resolves with the institution of a gluten-free diet.

Intestinal lymphangiectasia is a severe protein-losing enteropathy characterized by dilatation of intestinal lymphatics resulting in protein loss as lymph leaks into the lumen of the intestine. The disease can be secondary to developmental abnormalities of the intestinal lymphatics, which may be associated with abnormal lymphatics elsewhere in the body. Intestinal lymphangiectasia has been found in patients with Noonan's syndrome. Lymphangiectasia can also be secondary to diseases that cause obstruction of the intestinal lymphatics or increase in the intralymphatic pressure. Patients typically have diarrhea and hypoproteinemia. Symptoms related to malabsorption may also be present. Barium studies are nonspecific, with mild dilatation and thickened folds (Fig. 35). A substantial number of affected children may have normal barium examinations. US findings have been described but are nonspecific and related to the edema, with thickening of the walls of the intestine and gallbladder, ascites, and a thickened mesentery.

Patients with *immunodeficiency syndromes* may have a clinical and radiographic picture similar to that in patients with celiac disease. Some affected patients will have radiographic findings of lymphoid hyperplasia, especially prominent in the distal ileum. Small, relatively uniform polypoid mucosal filling defects are seen, characteristically with a central barium-filled umbilication. The latter is not seen uniformly, but its presence in a number of the polypoid defects suggests the correct nature of the lesions. Reactive lymphoid hyperplasia can also be seen in patients with gastroenteritis, both

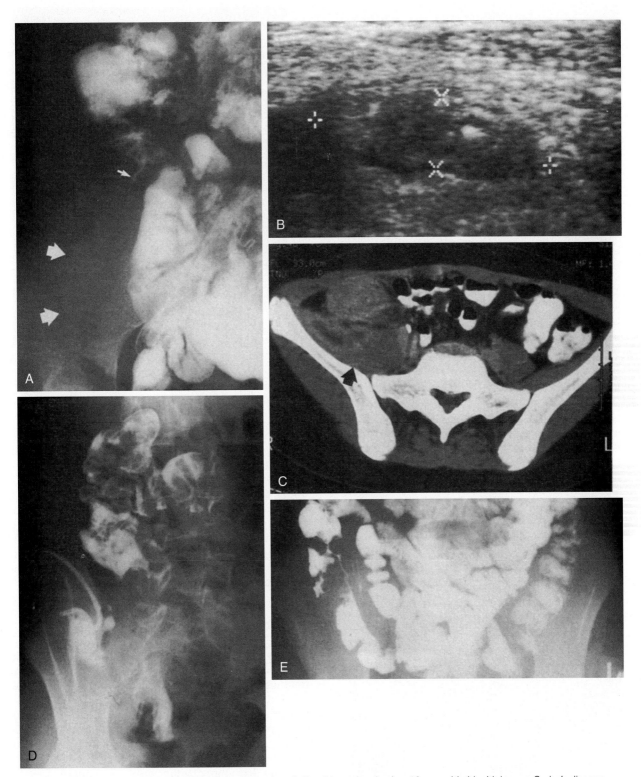

FIGURE 33. Crohn's disease with abscess formation. **A,** Small bowel series in a 13-year-old girl with known Crohn's disease who presented with fevers and right lower quadrant tenderness. A walled-off fistulous tract *(small arrow)* leads to a right lower quadrant mass *(large arrows)*, causing separation of bowel loops and extrinsic compression defect on the barium-filled small intestine. **B,** Ultrasound examination of the right lower quadrant demonstrates an area of hypoechogenicity with a bright echo within it. **C,** Computed tomography (CT) scan section through the right lower quadrant demonstrates a large abscess *(arrow)* deep to the markedly thickened and edematous cecum. Under CT guidance, a drainage tube was placed. **D,** Eight days later, injection of contrast material through the drainage tube demonstrates communication with the small bowel. **E,** Six weeks later, small bowel series demonstrates leak of contrast material from the markedly narrowed terminal ileum into a small residual mass. The patient was asymptomatic at the time of this examination.

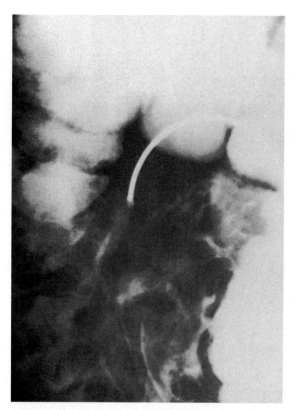

FIGURE 34. Behçet's syndrome. Coned-down pressure spot film of the terminal ileum in a patient with known Behçet's syndrome demonstrates a cobblestone pattern similar to that seen in Crohn's disease. (Courtesy of Dr. P. S. Moskowitz, Los Gatos, CA.)

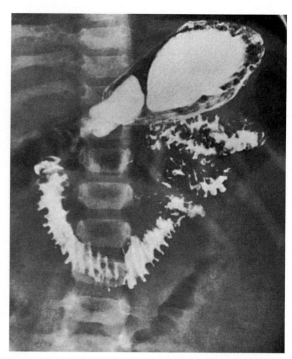

FIGURE 36. Whipple's disease in a 2½-year-old boy. Upper gastrointestinal series demonstrates marked thickening of the duodenal and jejunal folds.

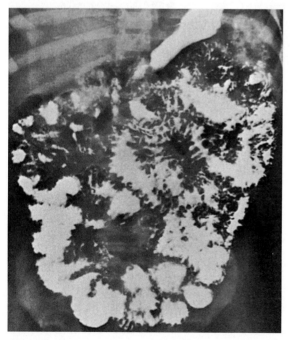

FIGURE 35. Small bowel series in a 3½-year-old girl with intestinal lymphangiectasia demonstrates mucosal folds that are markedly coarsened and thickened.

infectious and allergic, and in some otherwise normal persons. Lymphoid hyperplasia of the terminal ileum may act as a lead point for ileocolic intussusception.

Other causes of protein-losing enteropathy include allergic gastroenteropathy, Whipple's disease (Fig. 36), inflammatory bowel disease, infectious mononucleosis, and polyarteritis nodosa; Ménétrier's disease is discussed in Section VI, Part VI, Chapter 3, page 1593. The radiologic findings in the GI tract may be nonspecific or related to underlying intestinal disease such as regional enteritis.

CYSTIC FIBROSIS

CF may present in the newborn period with meconium ileus (see above). Older children show duodenal abnormalities such as dilatation, thickened folds, and filling defects that may represent abnormal collections of mucus adherent to the mucosa. Patients with CF have a surprisingly high rate of duodenal ulcer disease, which has suggested the lack of a protective mechanism in the duodenum because of the abnormal secretions. As patients live longer, the most prominent intestinal abnormality is the distal intestinal obstruction syndrome (DIOS), formerly known as meconium ileus equivalent. Patients present with colicky abdominal pain and a palpable right lower quadrant mass, representing impacted fecal material in the ileocolic region. Because mild to severe constipation is a common concomitant of CF, the term *DIOS* is reserved for those patients who also have signs and symptoms of small bowel obstruction.

Plain films show small-bowel dilatation with air–fluid levels and bubbly fecal material in the right lower

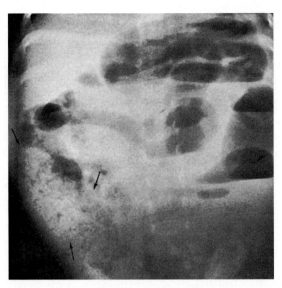

FIGURE 37. Distal intestinal obstructive syndrome in a 2-month-old infant with cystic fibrosis. Upright radiograph of the abdomen demonstrates bubbly stool in the right lower quadrant *(arrows)* with multiple air–fluid levels, suggestive of distal small intestinal obstruction.

quadrant (Figs. 37 and 38). Although most patients respond to enemas using mucolytic agents, we still occasionally perform contrast enemas under fluoroscopic control. Diatrizoate meglumine is the most widely used agent but is very expensive in the volumes needed for teenagers and adults, who are the most likely affected CF patients. We have had good success using a hypertonic solution of powdered sodium diatrizoate in warm water. For best results, reflux into the terminal ileum is necessary. Patients with CF may also have malabsorption with dilated intestinal loops showing thickened folds. Patients with *Shwachman syndrome* may have malabsorption with nonspecific findings on barium studies.

GRAFT-VERSUS-HOST DISEASE

GVHD is a reaction of donor lymphocytes against host cells. Although GVHD can be seen in patients undergoing solid organ transplantation, it is more common in patients undergoing bone marrow transplantation. Furthermore, bone marrow transplantation is more commonly performed in children than is solid organ transplantation because of its utility in hematologic and

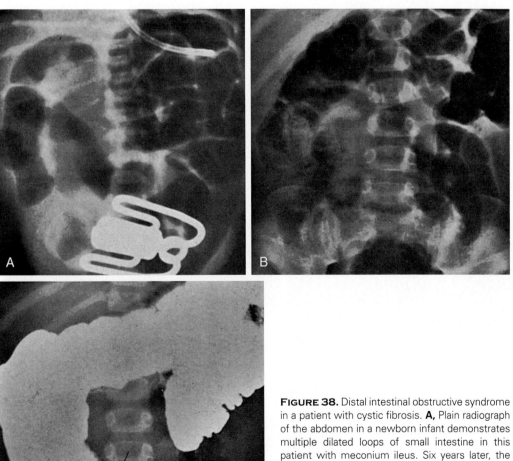

FIGURE 38. Distal intestinal obstructive syndrome in a patient with cystic fibrosis. **A,** Plain radiograph of the abdomen in a newborn infant demonstrates multiple dilated loops of small intestine in this patient with meconium ileus. Six years later, the patient presented with clinical signs of obstruction and a palpable right lower quadrant mass. **B,** Plain film of the abdomen demonstrates inspissated fecal material in the right lower quadrant and multiple dilated loops of small intestine. **C,** Barium enema demonstrates inspissated fecal material in the cecum and terminal ileum *(arrow).*

immunodeficiency states as well as in leukemia, lymphoma, and widespread malignancies such as metastatic neuroblastoma. Acute GVHD occurs within the first 3 months following transplantation. Patients with GI manifestations have severe diarrhea and crampy abdominal pain. Frequent accompaniments are skin rash, liver dysfunction, and hematologic complications. Plain films show a pattern of adynamic ileus with separation of bowel loops, thickening of the bowel wall, and air–fluid levels. Less commonly seen are pneumatosis intestinalis and ascites. On occasion, the abdomen may be completely gasless. Contrast studies are usually not necessary but will show severe edema of the bowel wall, poor coating of the mucosa, luminal narrowing, and rapid transit time. Chronic fibrosis, not unlike that seen in chronic radiation enteritis, may occur. US reveals thickening of the bowel wall, sometimes with a sonolucent ring in the submucosal layer (Fig. 39A). The bowel lumina are filled with fluid, and ascites can be identified. Concomitant findings can be seen on CT, which can also demonstrate mesenteric thickening (Fig. 39B).

HENOCH-SCHÖNLEIN PURPURA

Henoch-Schönlein purpura is an idiopathic anaphylactoid reaction characterized by a diffuse angiitis. In the small intestine, the disease manifests itself with bleeding into the bowel wall, causing submucosal filling defects and enteroenteric intussusception (Fig. 40). Findings related to the angiitis on contrast studies include segmental dilatation and stenosis, bowel wall thickening with separation of bowel loops, and coarsening and loss of the normal mucosal fold pattern. The submucosal hematomas may act as a lead point for intussusception. The characteristic skin rash is usually diagnostic, but the GI manifestations may precede its appearance.

INTUSSUSCEPTION

Intussusception is the invagination or telescoping of one portion of intestine into the contiguous distal segment (Fig. 41). The proximal segment is known as the intussusceptum, while the distal portion is the intussuscipiens. Idiopathic intussusception is the most common cause of small intestinal obstruction in the infant-toddler age group, with the peak incidence between 2 months and 3 years of life. About 50% of the affected patients present during the first year of life, with another 24% presenting during the second year. Idiopathic intussusception has been described in newborns and in adults, but its appearance outside the peak age group should always alert one to the possibility of a pathologic lead point, as discussed at the end of this section. Approximately two thirds of the patients are boys. Over 90% of intussusceptions are ileocolic, with enteroenteric and colocolic being uncommon. Some investigators believe, however, that undiagnosed ileoileal intussusception may be the lead point for ileocolic intussusception. Other authors have postulated hypertrophied Peyer's patches or reactive lymphoid hyperplasia of the terminal ileum as lead points.

The affected child usually has a history of abrupt onset of intermittent abdominal pain, sometimes following a prodromal period with symptoms of upper respiratory infection or gastroenteritis. The bouts of pain quickly come closer together, and vomiting or diarrhea may ensue. Lethargy is a frequent occurrence, often quite profound. In some cases, lethargy may be the presenting complaint in a patient with only minimal GI symptoms. Vomiting or diarrhea may lead to dehydration, which exaggerates the lethargy. Blood may appear in the stool. The mixture of stool, blood, and blood clots has been described as having a currant jelly appearance that, when present, is highly suggestive of intussuscep-

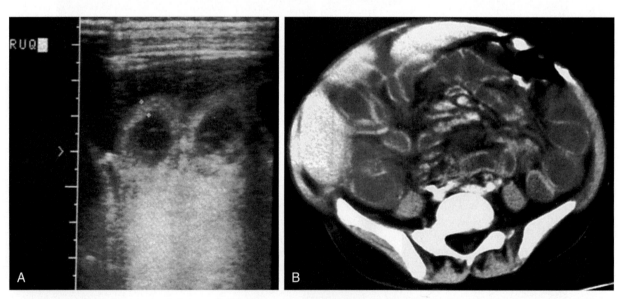

FIGURE 39. Graft-versus-host disease. **A,** Ultrasound scan of the right upper quadrant demonstrates markedly thickened bowel wall surrounded by ascitic fluid. **B,** Computed tomography scan demonstrates edematous bowel wall throughout the small intestine.

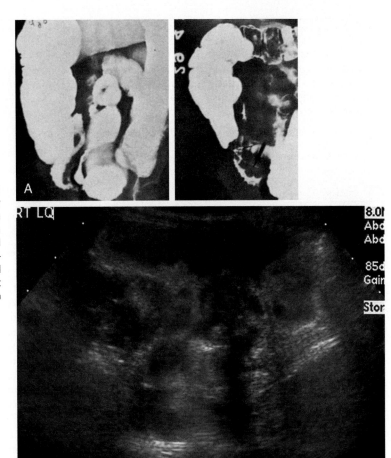

FIGURE 40. Henoch-Schönlein purpura. **A,** Barium enema performed in a 4-year-old boy with a 7-day history of vomiting, bloody diarrhea, and abdominal pain. Filling *(left)* and postevacuation *(right)* films from a barium enema demonstrate marginal filling defects in the distal ileum *(arrow)*. The diagnosis of Henoch-Schönlein purpura was made when the characteristic rash developed during hospitalization. **B,** Ultrasound scan of a different patient demonstrates polypoid projections in the ileum secondary to intramural bleeding.

tion. Patients who delay in seeking medical attention may become toxic, with fever, leukocytosis, and peritoneal signs on physical examination. Otherwise, physical examination either is unremarkable or discloses a palpable abdominal mass, most commonly located in the right upper quadrant but that may be found anywhere in the course of the colon. On rare occasions, the intussusception may be seen or palpated at the anus.

Plain abdominal radiographs are indicated regardless of how high the clinical index of suspicion is for the diagnosis of intussusception. Eklöf and Hartelius compared plain film findings in patients with proven intussusception to those with suspected intussusception who were later found not to have the disease (Table 2). The combination of diminished colonic stool and gas, especially when accompanied by a visible soft tissue mass, makes the likelihood of intussusception very high (Fig. 42). In some patients, the plain film will be normal. A horizontal beam film is useful to rule out bowel perforation and to evaluate the degree of obstruction. A

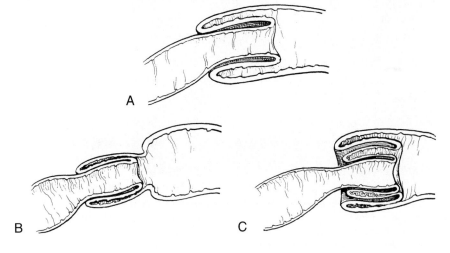

FIGURE 41. The common types of infantile intussusception, in longitudinal section. **A,** Ileocecal. **B,** Ileoileal, a type not visualized by barium enema. **C,** Ileoileocecal (double intussusception).

FINDINGS	CONFIRMED INTUSSUSCEPTION (100 PATIENTS) NO. OF CASES	SUSPECTED INTUSSUSCEPTION, NORMAL ON FOLLOW-UP (100 PATIENTS) NO. OF CASES
Sparse intestinal gas	89	45
Sparse fecal content	82	19
Discernible liver tip	66	58
Discernible mass	61	5
Small bowel in right upper quadrant	58	28
Air–fluid levels—nondilated bowel	56	75
Normal fecal content	18	81
Normal gas pattern	11	55
Air–fluid levels—dilated bowel	8	3
Ascites	0	0

Table 2 ■ PLAIN FILM ANALYSIS IN PATIENTS WITH SUSPECTED INTUSSUSCEPTION

Modified from Eklöf O, Hartelius H: Reliability of the abdominal plain film diagnosis in pediatric patients with suspected intussusception. Pediatr Radiol 1980;9:199.

cross-table lateral horizontal beam film is more likely to demonstrate the soft tissue mass than the supine film. On the cross-table lateral film, Johnson and Woisard pointed out an inappropriate craniocaudal separation of gas-filled bowel loops in the upper abdomen, representing the gasless telescoped bowel interposed between the site of initiation of the intussusception and the leading edge of the intussusception. This sign was present in 4 of 12 patients, a mass was seen in 5 patients, and no specific sign was present in 3, all of whom had documented intussusception.

US is being used with increasing frequency in patients in whom intussusception is suspected but whose clinical presentation and plain film findings are nondiagnostic. In other circumstances, when US is performed for evaluation of acute abdominal discomfort, an unsuspected intussusception may be found. US is not indicated when there is a high clinicoradiologic suspicion of intussusception. The US findings are very suggestive, if

not frankly pathognomonic. On transverse scan, a doughnut configuration may be seen. There is a central echogenic area representing the mucosa of the intussusceptum and a larger sonolucent rim representing the edematous wall of the intussusceptum. In other cases, a target sign will be seen, with concentric rings of alternating sonolucency and echogenicity. If there is fluid in the lumen of the intussusceptum, the central core may appear sonolucent, with the next layer being the echogenic mucosa (Fig. 43). Depending on the degree of edema and compression of the bowel wall, the layers of the intussuscipiens may also be seen, producing the appearance of multiple concentric rings. On longitudinal scan, the appearance of the doughnut has been likened to a kidney, with the sonolucent wall being reniform and surrounding the echogenic mucosa, which simulates the kidney's peripelvic fat. These characteristic signs will be found along the course of the intussusception, but are most easily recognized near the leading edge of the intussusceptum. Swischuk and Stansberry reported the sonographic detection of small amounts of free intraperitoneal fluid in two patients with uncomplicated intussusception. A lead point is rarely seen with US, even in patients ultimately shown to have one at contrast enema or surgery. Pracros et al. reported the sonographic findings in a series of 145 patients with intussusception, all of whom had a positive US scan. Of eight patients who had lead points, identified at surgery or by other means, only two were identified at US examination. Adamsbaum et al. described the sonographic appearance of an enterogenous cyst acting as a lead point in which the cyst was just distal to the pseudokidney. Kenney, however, described a similar appearance in a patient in whom fluid was trapped in intussuscepted mesentery.

CT is not part of the evaluation of suspected intussusception, but may demonstrate intussusception when performed for other reasons. Knowles et al. used CT to diagnose transient intussusception in two adults with regional enteritis and severe abdominal pain. Both US and CT have been successful in identifying enteroenteric intussusceptions, an increasingly described complication of abdominal surgery, especially in patients with cerebral palsy.

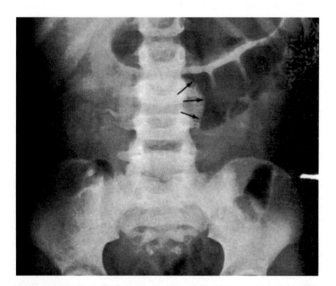

FIGURE 42. Ileocolic intussusception in a 4½-year-old patient. The leading edge of the intussusceptum is seen on this radiograph within the air column of the transverse colon (arrows). No gas can be seen in the cecum or ascending colon. The intussusception was successfully reduced with hydrostatic pressure.

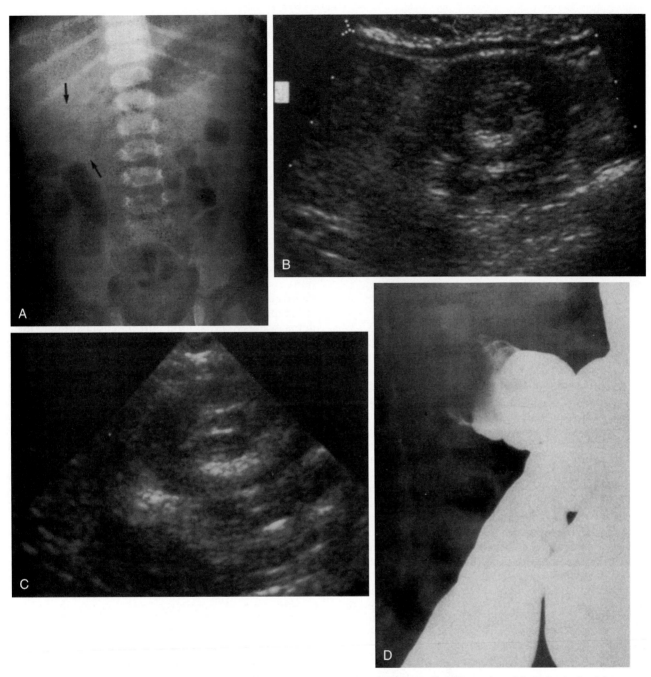

FIGURE 43. Ileocolic intussusception. **A,** Supine plain radiograph demonstrates a dilated loop of small intestine in the right midabdomen with a large soft tissue mass *(arrows)* in the right upper quadrant. **B,** Longitudinal ultrasound scan transverse to the intussusception demonstrates a target sign. The central lucency is due to fluid within the lumen, which is surrounded by an echogenic layer surrounded by another lucent layer representing edema in the wall of the intussusceptum. **C,** Longitudinal ultrasound scan of the intussusception demonstrates a pseudokidney sign with the edematous wall surrounding the echogenic mucosa. **D,** Barium enema demonstrates the characteristic "coiled spring" appearance of intussusception in the hepatic flexure.

REDUCTION TECHNIQUES

Hydrostatic reduction of ileocolic intussusception under fluoroscopic control is probably the earliest therapeutic procedure introduced into pediatric radiology. Although there are significant procedural variations among experienced radiologists, certain principles are generally accepted. Absolute contraindications to hydrostatic reduction are intestinal perforation, frank peritonitis, and hypovolemic shock (Table 3). Even patients with prolonged symptoms before diagnosis and small intestinal obstruction on plain films may have their intussusceptions reduced, but with a lower success rate and a higher rate of perforation than in uncomplicated cases. Stephenson et al. reported a higher success rate with proximal intussusceptions than with more distal ones. Fever, leukocytosis, and abdominal tenderness may be signs of early peritonitis but are nonspecific

Table 3 ■ IMAGING-GUIDED REDUCTION OF INTUSSUSCEPTION

Absolute Contraindications
  Peritonitis
  Free intraperitoneal air

Relative Contraindications
  High-fever, leukocytosis, abdominal tenderness (especially rebound tenderness)
  Small bowel obstruction
  Severe dehydration or profound lethargy

Hydrostatic Reduction
  Be sure patient is well hydrated.
  Mild sedation may help.
  Maintain pressure head no greater than 3 ft H_2O.
  Make three attempts of 3 min each.
  Be sure buttocks are well sealed.
  Reduction is incomplete unless substantial amounts of small bowel are easily filled.

Pneumatic Reduction
  Use available devices to control pressure.
  Start at 80 mm Hg; do not exceed 120 mm Hg.
  Limit attempt to 4 min.
  Even after small bowel is filled with air, evaluate cecum for residual mass.

abnormalities. An abdominal physical examination by an experienced surgeon is a useful precaution before undertaking fluoroscopically monitored reduction.

The likelihood of success seems to be enhanced if the patient is well hydrated and sedated for the procedure. Some experienced pediatric radiologists use a balloon catheter to help maintain a high pressure head, but many others are concerned about the development thereby of a closed-loop obstruction with a possibly increased hazard of perforation. A large rubber catheter with tight taping together of the buttocks usually produces a sufficient seal if reduction is possible and has a safety valve function if reduction cannot be performed. A commonly used technique is the "rule of threes." The hydrostatic pressure is kept at 3 feet and three attempts at reduction are made for 3 minutes each. Many experienced pediatric radiologists, however, will use higher pressures and perform more frequent attempts for longer periods of time. Palpation of the abdomen increases the intra-abdominal pressure in an uncontrolled fashion and should not be performed.

When the contrast column meets the head of the intussusceptum, a concave filling defect appears. This frequently presents a curvilinear spiral pattern that resembles the coil of a bedspring (Fig. 44). The appearance is produced by a steady puddling of the barium in the compressed lumen between the head and the sleeve of the invagination and is not present until the barium mixture has worked itself into the folds between the intussusceptum and the intussuscipiens. The concavity flattens, and the head of the barium column moves unevenly toward the ileocecal valve.

When contrast flows freely through the valve, reduction of the colonic portion of the intussusception is usually complete (Fig. 45). The edematous valve, which can simulate an incomplete reduction of the intussusception or lead point, may remain swollen for several days. US can confirm that the filling defect is caused by the edematous margins of the ileocecal valve. In ileo-ileocolic intussusception, the ileocolic component may be reduced completely, with persistence of the ileoileal lesions in the smal bowel.

The end point of a successful reduction is flooding of the small bowel with contrast material to prove the ileocolic intussusception has been reduced and to reduce an ileoileal intussusception that may have acted as a lead point (Fig. 46). Reported rates of successful hydrostatic reduction in uncomplicated patients are about 85%. Approximately 5% of these patients will have recurrence, half within 48 hours. A successful second reduction can frequently be accomplished. When hydrostatic reduction fails, patients are brought to surgery. A phenomenon well known to surgeons is easy manual reduction after induction of anesthesia. Collins et al. were able to reduce 21 of 31 intussusceptions by contrast enemas in the operating room after the children were anesthetized. Each patient had had a failed previous attempt at reduction in the radiology department. Koumanidou and colleagues report a significantly lower success rate for hydrostatic reduction if enlarged lymph nodes are noted at the time of US examination.

Although barium has been the traditional contrast material used for hydrostatic reduction, most pediatric centers advocate using water-soluble contrast agents because of presumed decreased hazard in the event of perforation. Schmitz-Rode et al., based on results of an experimental study, suggested that lower viscosity contrast agents such as water-soluble media, especially when

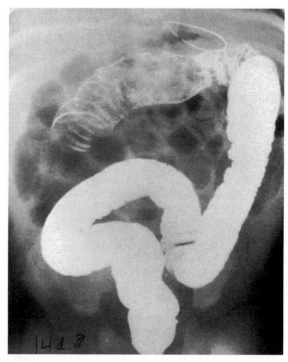

FIGURE 44. Intussusception. Barium enema demonstrates a coiled spring appearance in a 14-day-old infant. Note the lack of fecal material in the descending colon, the sigmoid colon, and the rectum.

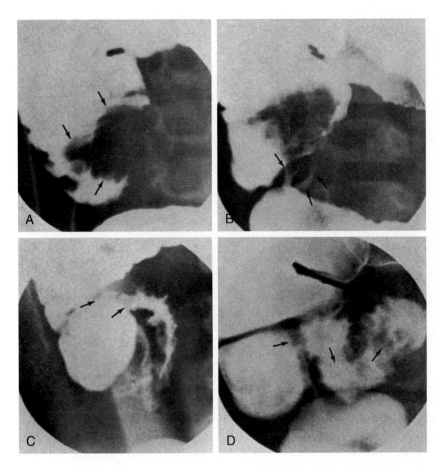

FIGURE 45. Serial radiographic changes at the ileocecal valve during hydrostatic reduction of an intussusception in an 18-month-old infant. **A,** The intussusceptum has been moved proximally from the transverse colon into the cecum, where it causes a filling defect. **B,** The appendix is beginning to fill, and the cecal filling defect is smaller. **C,** The terminal ileum is beginning to fill, and the cecal filling defect has disappeared. **D,** The terminal ileum is normally dilated, with normal mucosal relief.

used with a large-bore tube, are theoretically more successful than barium, although not as successful as air.

Pneumatic reduction of intussusception under fluoroscopic control has been practiced in China for several decades and has gained acceptance in the rest of the world. Specific devices for control of pressure are required, with most studies being performed at 80 to 120 mm Hg (Fig. 47). Success rates are higher than with hydrostatic reduction, and fluoroscopy times are lower in experienced hands. Complication rates are similar to those in hydrostatic reduction, but the complications are potentially less morbid. Advocates of pneumatic reduction point out its ease, the reduced likelihood of peritonitis in the event of perforation, and the reduced expense, at least when compared with the use of water-soluble contrast material. The pneumatic reductions are usually faster, reducing radiation exposure. As with hydrostatic reduction, the filling of large portions of small bowel is necessary for assurance of adequate reduction. Hedlund et al., however, described three patients in whom extensive reflux of air occurred without successful reduction. They point out the importance of examining the cecum for a persistent filling defect even after air refluxes into the small intestine.

Shiels, Kirks, and colleagues have studied the relative merits of air reduction and hydrostatic reduction and favor the former because of higher success rates, lower radiation dose, and decreased serious complications. Paterson and colleagues have shown equally good effect with carbon dioxide, suggesting its more rapid absorp-

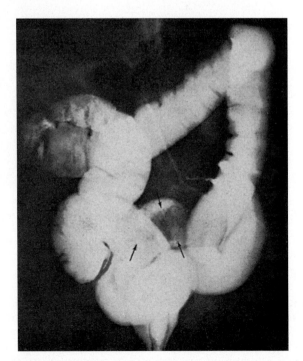

FIGURE 46. Residual ileoileal intussusception *(arrows)* in the terminal ileum following hydrostatic reduction of the colic component of an ileoileocolic intussusception, the leading edge of which was originally in the splenic flexure.

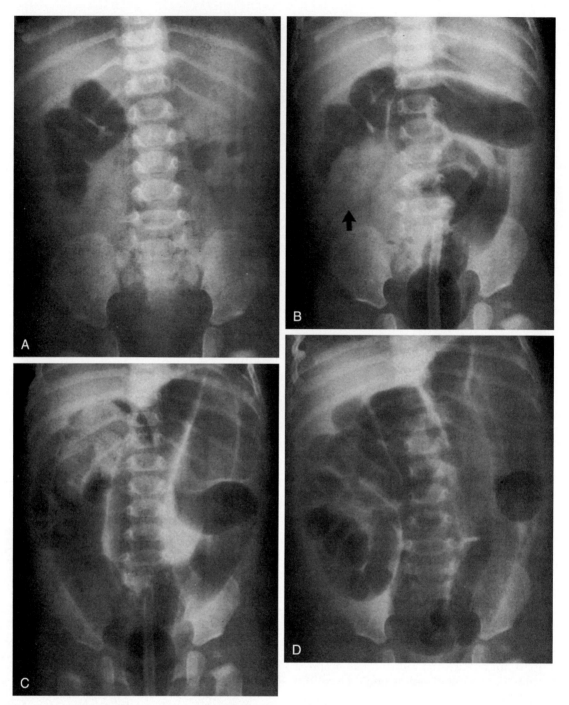

FIGURE 47. Pneumatic reduction of intussusception. **A,** Plain radiograph demonstrates a dilated loop of small intestine in the right upper quadrant. A mass was palpated in this region. **B,** Initial injection of air into the colon demonstrates a right upper quadrant mass *(arrow)*. **C,** Further distention of the colon with air reveals the mass to better advantage. At this point, the pressure was changed from 60 to 80 mm Hg. **D,** Following complete reduction of the intussusception, numerous air-filled loops of small intestine are seen, and a soft tissue mass is no longer present. (Courtesy of Dr. Liu Ai-Qin, Macao.)

tion than room air may be an advantage. Daneman, Alton, Ein and colleagues found comparable perforation rates between the two procedures. Gorenstein and colleagues reported improved rates of reduction with three attempts at air reduction compared with one attempt. Lui and colleagues suggested that 4 minutes of attempted air reduction is sufficient if reduction is possible.

The most worrisome complication of hydrostatic or pneumatic reduction is intestinal perforation, which occurs at sites of bowel necrosis, usually in the colon. Campbell's study of hydrostatic reduction reported 55 perforations in over 14,000 cases (0.4%), with one death. Stein et al. reported 7 perforations in 199 cases (2.5%) and no deaths with pneumatic reduction. If the surgeons are ready to take the patient to surgery

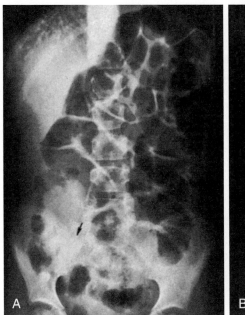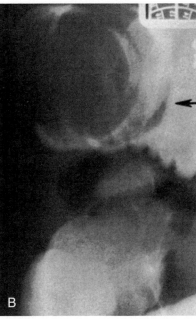

FIGURE 48. Ileocolic intussusception in an 8½-year-old child with cystic fibrosis. **A,** Plain radiograph demonstrates a soft tissue mass *(arrow)* in the right lower quadrant. Dilated small bowel loops are seen. **B,** Spot film in the transverse colon demonstrates characteristic findings of intussusception. Successful hydrostatic reduction was accomplished.

immediately, perforation with air is more bothersome to the radiologist than to the patient. Shiels, Kirks, et al. reported no perforations in 75 patients who underwent pneumatic reduction. Britton and Wilkinson suggested that the absence of free fluid, small bowel obstruction, and trapped fluid at US examination make the success of pneumoreduction highly likely. Royal reported one case of hypovolemic shock after pneumoreduction.

US has been used as the controlling imaging technique for both hydrostatic and air reduction of intussusception. These techniques have yet to be widely adopted.

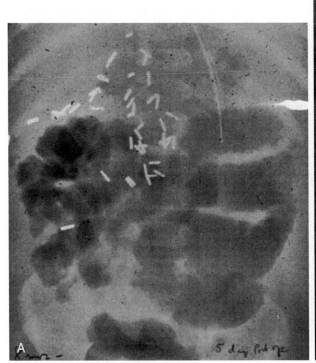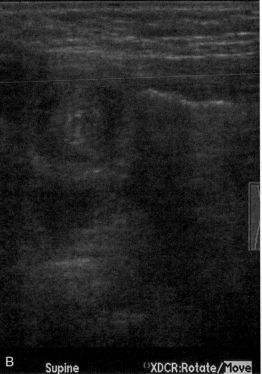

FIGURE 49. Postsurgical intussusception. **A,** Intestinal obstruction is seen on the plain radiograph of an 8-month-old patient 5 days following removal of a right-sided Wilms' tumor. Small intestinal intussusception was relieved surgically. **B,** Ultrasound scan of a different patient who developed intermittent pain after a laparotomy shows an enteroenteric intussusception in the right midabdomen. The patient underwent spontaneous reduction.

SECONDARY INTUSSUSCEPTION

Approximately 5% of intussusceptions in childhood are secondary to lead points. In the older child, adolescent, and teenager, lymphoma of the small bowel, usually Burkitt's lymphoma, is the lead point. Duplication cysts, polyps, and other congenital lesions act as lead points. Patients with CF and chronic constipation have a higher than normal incidence of intussusception (Fig. 48). Postoperative intussusception is being recognized with increasing frequency. Plain film findings are those of small intestinal obstruction (Fig. 49A). Contrast studies are usually not rewarding because the majority are enteroenteric, but US or CT may disclose the lesion (Fig. 49B). West et al. reported 36 patients with postoperative intussusceptions of which 5 were ileocolic and 31 involved only small bowel. Hydrostatic reduction was successful in two cases of ileocolic intussusception and one case of distal ileoileal intussusception.

SUGGESTED READINGS

Congenital Obstruction

Ashley LM, Allen S, Teele RL: A normal sonogram does not exclude malrotation. Pediatr Radiol 2001;31:354

Berrocal T, Lamas M, Gutierrez J, et al: Congenital anomalies of the small intestine, colon, and rectum. Radiographics 1999;5:1219

Chao HC, Kong MS, Chen JY, et al: Sonographic features related to volvulus in neonatal intestinal malrotation. J Ultrasound Med 2000;19:371

Jackson A, Bisset R, Dickson AP: Malrotation and midgut volvulus presenting as malabsorption. Clin Radiol 1989;40:536

Pracros JP, Sann L, Genin G, et al: Ultrasound diagnosis of midgut volvulus: the "whirlpool" sign. Pediatr Radiol 1992;22:18

Shatzkes D, Gordon DH, Haller JO, et al: Malrotation of the bowel: malalignment of the superior mesenteric artery-vein complex shown by CT and MR. J Comput Assist Tomogr 1990;14:93

Zerin JM, Di Pietro MA: Mesenteric vascular anatomy at CT: normal and abnormal appearances. Radiology 1991;179:739

Zerin JM, Di Pietro MA: Superior mesenteric vascular anatomy at US in patients with surgically proved malrotation of the midgut. Radiology 1992;183:693

Acquired Obstruction

Akin JR Jr: The anatomic basis of vascular compression of the duodenum. Surg Clin North Am 1974;64:1361

Jabra A, Fishman E: Small bowel obstruction in the pediatric patient: CT evaluation. Abdom Imaging 1997;22:466–470

Marchant EA, Alvear DT, Fagelman KM: True clinical entity of vascular compression of the duodenum in adolescence. Surg Gynecol Obstet 1989;168:381

Munns SW: Hyperalimentation for superior mesenteric artery (cast) syndrome following correction of spinal deformity. J Bone Joint Surg Am 1984;66:1175

Oritz C, Cleveland RH, Blickman JG, et al: Familial superior mesenteric artery syndrome. Pediatr Radiol 1990;20:588

Pentlow BD, Dent RG: Acute vascular compression of the duodenum in anorexia nervosa. Br J Surg 1981;68:665

Ratcliffe J, Tait J, Lisle D, et al: Segmental dilatation of the small bowel: report of three cases and literature review. Radiology 1989;171:827

Tumors

Alford B, Coccia P, L'Heureux P: Roentgenographic features of American Burkitt's lymphoma. Radiology 1977;124:763

Dunnick NR, Reaman GH, Head GL, et al: Radiographic manifestations of Burkitt's lymphoma in American patients. AJR Am J Roentgenol 1979;132:1

Jenkin RD, Sonley MJ, Stephens CA, et al: Primary gastrointestinal tract lymphoma in childhood. Radiology 1969;92:763

Magrath IT: Malignant non-Hodgkin's lymphomas. *In* Pizzo PA, Poplack DG (eds): Principles and Practice of Pediatric Oncology. Philadelphia, JB Lippincott, 1989:433–434

Miller JH, Hindman BW, Lam AH: Ultrasound in the evaluation of small bowel lymphoma in children. Radiology 1980;135:409

Tyrrel RT, Baumgartner BR, Montemayor KA: Blue rubber bleb nevus syndrome: CT diagnosis of intussusception. AJR Am J Roentgenol 1990;154:105

Vade A, Blane CE: Imaging of Burkitt lymphoma in pediatric patients. Pediatr Radiol 1985;15:123

Cysts

Adamsbaum C, Sellier N, Helardot P: Ileocolic intussusception with enterogenous cyst: ultrasonic diagnosis. Pediatr Radiol 1989;19:325

Barr LL, Hayden CK Jr, Stansberry SD, et al: Enteric duplication cysts in children: are their ultrasonographic wall characteristics diagnostic? Pediatr Radiol 1990;20:326

Bender TM, Ledesma-Medina J, Oh KS: Radiographic manifestations of anomalies of the gastrointestinal tract. Radiol Clin North Am 1991;29:335

Bowen B, Ros PR, McCarthy MJ, et al: Gastrointestinal teratomas: CT and US appearance with pathologic correlation. Radiology 1987;162:431

Bower RJ, Sieber WKN, Kiesewetter WB: Alimentary tract duplications in children. Ann Surg 1978;188:669

Brown D, Schlesinger A, Komppa G: Ileal duplication cyst: repeated spontaneous decompression delays diagnosis. Mil Med 1989;154:553–555

Caspi B, Schachter M, Lancet M: Infected duplication cyst of ileum masquerading as an adnexal abscess—ultrasonographic features. J Clin Ultrasound 1989;17:431

Egelhoff JC, Bisset GS III, Strife JL: Multiple enteric duplications in an infant. Pediatr Radiol 1986;16:160

Egozi E, Ricketts R: Mesenteric and omental cysts in children. Am Surg 1997;63:287–290

Geer LL, Mittelstaedt CA, Staab EV, et al: Mesenteric cyst: sonographic appearance with CT correlation. Pediatr Radiol 1984;14:102

Gilchrist AM, Sloan JM, Logan CJH, et al: Case report: gastrointestinal bleeding due to multiple ileal duplications diagnosed by scintigraphy and barium studies. Clin Radiol 1990;41:134

Haller JO, Schneider M, Kassner EG, et al: Sonographic evaluation of mesenteric and omental masses in children. AJR Am J Roentgenol 1978;130:269

Harvey PJ, Whitley NO: CT of benign cystic abdominal masses in children. AJR Am J Roentgenol 1984;142:1279

Ilstad ST, Tollerud DJ, Weiss RG, et al: Duplications of the alimentary tract. Ann Surg 1988;208:184

Lamont AC, Starinsky R, Cremin BJ: Ultrasonic diagnosis of duplication cysts in children. Br J Radiol 1984;57:463

Nicolet V, Grignon A, Filiatrault D, et al: Sonographic appearance of an abdominal cystic lymphangioma. J Ultrasound Med 1984;3:85

Rifkin MD, Kurtz AB, Pasto ME: Mesenteric chylous (lymph-containing) cyst. Gastrointest Radiol 1983;8:267

Ros PR, Olmsted WW, Moser RP Jr, et al: Mesenteric and omental cysts: histologic classification with imaging correlation. Radiology 1987;164:327

Teele RL, Henschke CT, Tapper D: The radiographic and ultrasonographic evaluation of enteric duplication cysts. Pediatr Radiol 1980;10:9

Infectious Diseases

Bohrer SP: Typhoid perforation of the ileum. Br J Radiol 1966;39:37

Bradford BF, Abdenour GE Jr, Frank JL, et al: Usual and unusual radiologic manifestations of acquired immunodeficiency syndrome (AIDS) and human immunodeficiency virus (HIV) infection in children. Radiol Clin North Am 1988;26:341

Brandon J, Glick SN, Teplick SK: Intestinal giardiasis: the importance of serial filming. AJR Am J Roentgenol 1985;144:581

Brody PA, Fertig S, Aron JM: *Campylobacter* enterocolitis: radiographic features. AJR Am J Roentgenol 1982;139:1199

Capitanio MA, Greenberg SB: Pneumatosis intestinalis in two infants with rotavirus gastroenteritis. Pediatr Radiol 1991;21:361

Eckberg O, Sjostrum B, Brahme F: Radiological findings in *Yersinia* ileitis. Radiology 1977;123:15

Haney PJ, Yale-Loehr AJ, Nussbaum AR, et al: Imaging of infants and children with AIDS. AJR Am J Roentgenol 1989;152:1033

Hodes HL: Gastroenteritis with special reference to rotavirus. Adv Pediatr 1980;27:195

Jones B, Fishman EK: CT of the gut in the immunocompromised host. Radiol Clin North Am 1989;27:763

Katz M: Parasitic infections. J Pediatr 1975;87:165

Matsumoto T, Iida M, Sakai T, et al: Yersinia teminal ileitis: sonographic findings in eight patients. AJR Am J Roentgenol 1991;156:965

Nagi B, Duggal R, Gupta R, et al: Tuberculous peritonitis in children. Pediatr Radiol 1987;17:282

Puylaert JBCM, Kristjánsdóttir S, Golterman KL, et al: Typhoid fever: diagnosis by using sonography. AJR Am J Roentgenol 1989;153:745

Siegel M, Friedland J, Hildebolt C: Bowel wall thickening in children: differentiation with US. Radiology 1997;203:631–635

Sivit CJ, Josephs SH, Taylor GA, et al: Pneumatosis intestinalis in children with AIDS. AJR Am J Roentgenol 1990;155:133

Sivit CJ, Taylor GA, Patterson K, et al: Bowel obstruction in an infant with AIDS. AJR Am J Roentgenol 1990;154:803

Inflammatory Bowel Disease

Balthazar EJ: CT of the gastrointestinal tract: principles and interpretation. AJR Am J Roentgenol 1991;156:23

Beets-Tan R, Beets G, van der Hoop A, et al: Preoperative MR imaging of anal fistulas: does it really help the surgeon? Radiology 2001;281:75–84

Berlinger L, Redmond P, Purow EK, et al: Computed tomography in Crohn's disease. Am J Gastroenterol 1982;77:533

Buck JL, Dachman AH, Sobin LH: Polypoid and pseudopolypoid manifestations of inflammatory bowel disease. Radiographics 1991;11:293

Desai RK, Tagliabue JR, Wegryn SA, et al: CT evaluation of wall thickening in the alimentary tract. Radiographics 1991;1:771

Dinker E, Dittrich M, Peters H, et al: Real-time ultrasound in Crohn's disease: characteristic features and clinical implications. Pediatr Radiol 1986;16:8

Dubois RS, Rothschild J, Silverman A, et al: The varied manifestations of Crohn's disease in children and adolescents. Am J Gastroenterol 1978;69:203

Gore RM: CT of inflammatory bowel disease. Radiol Clin North Am 1989;27:717

Hyer W, Beattie R, Walker-Smith J, et al: Computed tomography in chronic inflammatory bowel disease. Arch Dis Child 1997;76:428–431

Jabra AA, Fishman EK, Taylor GA: Crohn disease in the pediatric patient: CT evaluation. Radiology 1991;179:495

Jones B, Fishman EK, Hamilton SR, et al: Submucosal accumulation of fat in inflammatory bowel disease: CT/pathologic correlation. J Comput Assist Tomogr 1986;10:759

Kirks DR, Currarino G: Regional enteritis in children: small bowel disease with normal terminal ileum. Pediatr Radiol 1978;7:10

Lindquist BL, Jarnerot G, Wickbom G: Clinical and epidemiological aspects of Crohn's disease in children and adolescents. Scand J Gastroenterol 1984;19:502

Lipson A, Bartram CI, Williams CB, et al: Barium studies and ileoscopy compared in children with suspected Crohn's disease. Clin Radiol 1990;41:5

Park RHR, McKillop JH, Duncan A, et al: Can [111]indium autologous mixed leucocyte scanning accurately assess disease extent and activity in Crohn's disease? Gut 1988;29:821

Quillin S, Siegel M: Gastrointestinal inflammation in children: color Doppler ultrasonography. J Ultrasound Med 1994;13:751–756

Riddlesberger MM Jr: CT of complicated inflammatory bowel disease in children. Pediatr Radiol 1985;15:384

Scott WW Jr, Fishman EK, Kuhlman JE, et al: Computed tomography evaluation of the sacroiliac joints in Crohn disease: radiologic/clinical correlation. Skeletal Radiol 1990;19:207

Shirkhoda A: Diagnostic pitfalls in abdominal CT. Radiographics 1991;11:969

Siegel M, Friedland J, Hildebolt C: Bowel wall thickening in children: differentiation with US. Radiology 1997;203:631–635

Stringer DA: Imaging inflammatory bowel disease in the pediatric patient. Radiol Clin North Am 1987;25:93

Stringer DA, Cleghorn GJ, Durie PR, et al: Behçet's syndrome involving the gastrointestinal tract—a diagnostic dilemma in childhood. Pediatr Radiol 1986;16:131

Tolia V, Kuhns LR, Chang CH, et al: Comparison of indium-111 scintigraphy and colonoscopy with histologic study in children for evaluation of colonic chronic inflammatory bowel disease. J Pediatr Gastroenterol Nutr 1991;12:336

Vlymen WJ, Moskowitz PS: Roentgenographic manifestations of esophageal and intestinal involvement in Behçet's disease in children. Pediatr Radiol 1981;10:193

Yeh H-C, Rabinowitz JG: Granulomatous enterocolitis: findings by ultrasonography and computed tomography. Radiology 1983;149:253

Functional and Infiltrative Diseases

Bartram CI, Small E: The intestinal radiological changes in older people with pancreatic cyst fibrosis. Br J Radiol 1971;44:195

Berk RN, Lee FA: The late gastrointestinal manifestations of cysticic fibrosis of the pancreas. Radiology 1973;106:337

Bova JG, Friedman AC, Weser E, et al: Adaptation of the ileum in nontropical sprue: reversal of the jejunoileal fold pattern. AJR Am J Roentgenol 1985;144:299

Djurhuus MJ, Lykkegaard E, Pock-Steen OC: Gastrointestinal radiological findings in cystic fibrosis. Pediatr Radiol 1973;1:113

Dorne HL, Jequier S: Sonography of intestinal lymphangiectasia. J Ultrasound Med 1986;5:13

Fisk JD, Shulman HM, Greening RR, et al: Gastrointestinal radiographic features of human graft-vs-host disease. AJR Am J Roentgenol 1981;136:329

Glasier CM, Siegel MJ, McAlister WH, et al: Henoch-Schönlein syndrome in children: gastrointestinal manifestations. AJR Am J Roentgenol 1981;136:1081

Gorske K, Winchester P, Grossman H: Unusual protein-losing enteropathies in children. Am J Roentgenol Radium Ther Nucl Med 1969;92:739

Haworth EM, Hodson CJ, Pringle EM, et al: The value of radiological investigations of the alimentary tract in children with the celiac syndrome. Clin Radiol 1968;107:158

Herzog DB, Logan R, Looistra JB: The Noonan syndrome with intestinal lymphangiectasia. J Pediatr 1976;88:270

Jones B, Bayless TM, Fishman EK, et al: Lymphadenopathy in celiac disease: computed tomographic observations. AJR Am J Roentgenol 1984;142:1127

Jones B, Fishman EK, Kramer SS, et al: Computed tomography of gastrointestinal inflammation after bone marrow transplantation. AJR Am J Roentgenol 1986;146:691

Koletzko S, Stringer DA, Cleghorn GJ, et al: Lavage treatment of distal intestinal obstruction syndrome in children with cystic fibrosis. Pediatrics 1989;83:727

Lanning P, Simila S, Sioramo I, et al: Lymphatic abnormalities in Noonan's syndrome. Pediatr Radiol 1978;7:106

Maile CW, Frick MP, Crass JR, et al: The plain abdominal radiograph in acute gastrointestinal graft-vs-host disease. AJR Am J Roentgenol 1985;145:289

Marn CS, Gore RM, Chahremani GG: Duodenal manifestations of nontropical sprue. Gastrointest Radiol 1986;11:30

Martinez-Frontanilla LA, Silverman L, Meagher DP Jr: Intussusception in Henoch-Schönlein purpura: diagnosis with ultrasound. J Pediatr Surg 1988;23:375

Rubinstein S, Moss RB, Lewiston NJ: Constipation and meconium ileus equivalent in patients with cystic fibrosis. Pediatrics 1986;78:473

Schimmelpenninck M, Zwaan F: Radiographic features of small intestinal injury in graft-versus-host disease. Gastrointest Radiol 1982;7:29

Taussig LM, Saldino RM, di Sant'Agnese PA: Radiographic abnormalities of the duodenum and small bowel in cystic fibrosis of the pancreas (mucoviscidosis). Radiology 1973;106:369

Weizman Z, Stringer DA, Durie PR: Radiologic manifestations of malabsorption: a nonspecific finding. Pediatrics 1984;74:530

Intussusception

Adamsbaum C, Sellier N, Helardot P: Ileocolic intussusception with enterogenous cyst: ultrasonic diagnosis. Pediatr Radiol 1989;19:325

Alzen G, Funke G, Truong S: Pitfalls in the diagnosis of intussusception. J Clin Ultrasound 1989;17:481

Bisset GS III, Kirks DR: Intussusception in infants and children: diagnosis and therapy. Radiology 1988;168:141

Bramson R, Shiels W 2nd, Eskey C, et al: Intraluminal colon pressure dynamics with Valsalva maneuver during air enema study. Radiology 1997;202:825–828

Britton I, Wilkinson A: Ultrasound features of intussusception predicting outcome of air enema. Pediatr Radiol 1999;29:705–710

Campbell JB: Contrast media in intussusception. Pediatr Radiol 1989;19:293

Collins DL, Pinckney LE, Miller KE: Hydrostatic reduction of ileocolic intussusception: a second attempt in the operating room with general anesthesia. J Pediatr 1989;115:204

Daneman A, Alton D, Ein S, et al: Perforation during attempted intussusception reduction in children—a comparison of perforation with barium and air. Pediatr Radiol 1995;25:318

Daneman, A, Alton D, Logo E, et al: Patterns of recurrence of intussusception in children: a 17-year review. Pediatr Radiol 1998;28:913–919

Ein SH, Stephen CA: Intussusception: 354 cases in 10 years. J Pediatr Surg 1971;6:16

Eklöf O, Hartelius H: Reliability of the abdominal plain film diagnosis in pediatric patients with suspected intussusception. Pediatr Radiol 1980;9:199

Gorenstein A, Raucher A, Serour F, et al: Intussusception in children: reduction with repeated, delayed air enema. Radiology 1998;206:595–598

Gu L, Zhu H, Wang S, et al: Sonographic guidance of air enema for intussusception reduction in children. Pediatr Radiol 2000;30:339–342

Hedlund GL, Johnson JF, Strife JL: ileocolic intussusception: extensive reflux of air preceding pneumatic reduction. Radiology 1990;174:187

Johnson JF, Woisard KK: Ileocolic intussusception: new sign on the supine cross-table lateral radiograph. Radiology 1989;170:483

Kenney IJ: Ultrasound in intussusception: a false cystic lead point. Pediatr Radiol 1990;20:348

Knowles MC, Fishman EK, Kuhlman JE, et al: Transient intussusception in Crohn disease: CT evaluation. Radiology 1989;170:814

Koumanidou C, Vakaki M, Pitsoulakis G, et al: Sonographic detection of lymph nodes in the intussusception of infants and young children. AJR Am J Roentgenol 2002;178:445–450

Lui K, Wong H, Cheung Y, et al: Air enema for diagnosis and reduction of intussusception in children: clinical experience and fluoroscopy time correlation. J Pediatr Surg 2001;36:479–481

Paterson C, Langer J, Somers S, et al: Pneumatic reduction of intussusception using carbon dioxide. Pediatr Radiol 1994;24:296–297

Pracros JP, Tran-Minh VA, Morin De Finfe CH, et al: Acute intestinal intussusception in children. Contribution of ultrasonography (145 cases). Ann Radiol (Paris) 1987;30:525

Royal S: Hypovolemic shock after air reduction of intussusception. Pediatr Radiol 2001;31:184–186

Schmitz-Rode T, Müller-Leisse C, Alzen G, Comparative examination of various rectal tubes and contrast media for the reduction of intussusceptions. Pediatr Radiol 1991;21:341

Shiels WE II, Bisset GS III, Kirks DR: Simple device for air reduction of intussusception. Pediatr Radiol 1990;20:472

Shiels W 2nd, Kirks D, Keller G, et al: John Caffey Award: Colonic perforation by air and liquid enemas: comparison study in young pigs. AJR Am J Roentgenol 1993;160:931–935

Shiels WE II, Maves CK, Hedlund GL, et al: Air enema for diagnosis and reduction of intussusception: clinical experience and pressure correlates. Radiology 1991;181:169

Stein M, Alton DJ, Daneman A: Pneumatic reduction of intussusception: five-year experience. Radiology 1992;183:681

Stephenson CA, Seibert JJ, Strain JDO, et al: Intussusception: clinical and radiographic factors influencing reducibility. Pediatr Radiol 1989;20:57

Swischuk LE, Hayden CK, Boulden T: Intussusception: indications for ultrasonography and an explanation of the doughnut and pseudo-kidney signs. Pediatr Radiol 1985;15:388

Swischuk LE, Stansberry SD: Ultrasonographic detection of free peritoneal fluid in uncomplicated intussusception. Pediatr Radiol 1991;21:350

West KW, Stephens B, Rescorla FJ, et al: Postoperative intussusception: experience with 36 cases in children. Surgery 1988;104:781

White SJ, Blane CE: Intussusception: additional observations on the plain radiograph. AJR Am J Roentgenol 1983;139:511

PART VIII

COLON

BRUCE R. PARKER

ANATOMY AND DEVELOPMENT

The colon, or large intestine, extends from the cecum in the right lower quadrant to the anus. The cecum and ascending colon are usually fixed by peritoneal attachments, although the cecum can be on a mesentery, which makes it mobile during imaging examinations. The ascending colon extends to the hepatic flexure, which is subjacent to the underside of the liver. The transverse colon extends across the upper abdomen and is on a mesentery, allowing it substantial positional mobility. The highest visualized point in the left upper quadrant on barium enema, the radiographic splenic flexure, is actually the distal end of the transverse colon. The anatomic splenic flexure is the most proximal fixed point of the descending colon. The fixed colon descends into the left lower quadrant, where the mobile sigmoid colon on a mesentery runs between the descending colon and rectum. The colon in children, especially the sigmoid and transverse components, is often more redundant than in adults. The cecum in young children may be relatively more cephalad than it is in older children or adults.

The proximal colon, from cecum to mid- or distal transverse colon, is derived from the embryonic midgut and receives its blood supply from the superior mesenteric artery. It participates in the extracoelomic migration of the midgut described in Section VI, Part VII, page 1616. The portion of colon from the transverse colon through the rectum is derived from the hindgut and receives its blood supply from the inferior mesenteric artery. In the early embryo, it empties into the cloaca along with portions of the genitourinary tract, but is separated by a developing septum from these structures. The anal canal is formed by the joining of the distal-most portion of the hindgut to an invagination of the ectoderm of the embryonic rump.

IMAGING STUDIES

Plain radiographs are useful in the evaluation of colonic disease. The air-filled colon is usually easily distinguished from small bowel in children beyond 1 year of age. This differentiation is not always easy in infants. The supine film shows the anatomy well and is satisfactory for the evaluation of stool content, intramural air, and pathologic calcifications. A horizontal beam film is valuable when anatomic or functional obstruction or free air is a concern.

The standard examination of the colon continues to be the *contrast enema*. Barium is still the most commonly used contrast medium, with water-soluble agents being reserved for patients with potential perforations or for therapeutic interventions. Double contrast barium enemas, as described in adults, can easily be performed in children, even in infants, and are especially useful in patients with suspected mucosal lesions such as inflammatory bowel disease or in the evaluation of children with lower intestinal bleeding or who are suspected of having polyps.

Ultrasound (US) is useful in specific diseases such as appendicitis, neutropenic colitis, and tumors. It is also very useful in the search for complications of colonic disease, such as abscesses. *Computed tomography* (CT) is also useful in the evaluation of tumors, abscesses and other intra-abdominal, extracolonic manifestations of colonic disease. *Magnetic resonance imaging* (MRI) has yet to achieve a defined role in the evaluation of colonic diseases in children.

CONGENITAL AND FUNCTIONAL DISORDERS

The majority of congenital and developmental abnormalities of the colon present in the newborn period.

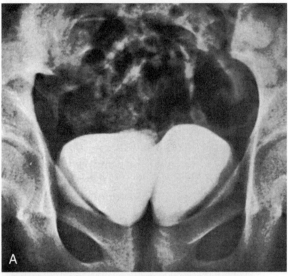
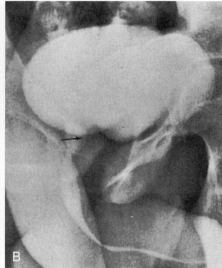
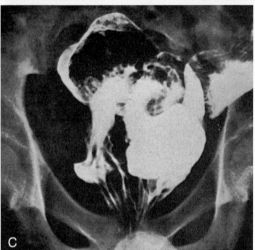

FIGURE 1. Duplication of the bladder and entire colon in a 15-year-old boy who had been treated in the newborn period for anal atresia. **A,** Frontal radiograph of the pelvis after excretory urography shows two bladders. Each upper urinary tract emptied into the bladder on its respective side. **B,** Voiding urethrogram. A single urethra *(arrow)* originated from the right side. **C,** Barium enema demonstrates two rectums. Surgical exploration revealed duplication of the colon from appendix to rectum.

CONGENITAL DISORDERS

Duplication cysts are much less frequently found in the colon than in the small bowel and are usually localized. Noncommunicating cysts may be palpable or lead to symptoms of obstruction, if large. Sonography demonstrates an anechoic mass. Contrast enemas show an extraluminal mass effect. Localized duplications occasionally communicate with the lumen and can fill with air or contrast material. A rare entity is complete duplication of the colon, which is associated with duplication of the urinary bladder (Fig. 1).

In patients with *midgut malrotation,* the cecum is usually in the midpelvis and the ascending colon is midline, running cephalad to join with a shortened distal transverse colon and left colon, which are in normal position (Fig. 2). In rare circumstances, peritoneal bands cross anterior to the transverse colon, causing partial obstruction (Fig. 3). When the left kidney is ectopic or absent, the splenic flexure may be positioned more medially and inferiorly than is the normal situation.

COLONIC OBSTRUCTION

Obstruction of the colon in the newborn infant may be either anatomic or functional (Table 1). Anatomic obstruction includes rare forms such as colon atresia and stenosis and a collection of entities grouped together as anorectal malformations. The most common functional disorder is aganglionosis, or Hirschsprung's disease. A group of poorly understood disorders (meco-

---

Table 1 ■ COLONIC OBSTRUCTION IN THE NEWBORN

Colonic atresia and stenosis
Anorectal malformations (imperforate anus, anal atresia)
Aganglionosis
Small left colon syndrome
Meconium plug syndrome
Pararectal masses
   Anterior meningocele
   Presacral teratoma
   Presacral neuroblastoma

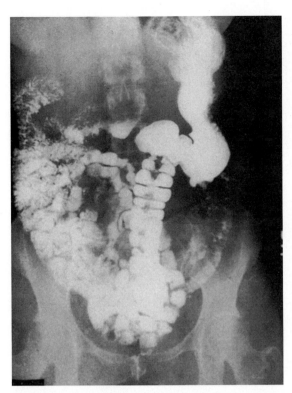

FIGURE 2. Anteroposterior view of the abdomen in a young woman with symptoms of duodenal ulcer disease shows complete malrotation of the midgut. The cecum and ascending colon are in the midline while the portions of the colon derived from the embryonic hindgut are in normal position.

nium plug and neonatal small left colon syndromes, etc.) cause transient self-limited functional obstruction. In small left colon syndrome, there is no anatomic obstruction of the colon as in anorectal atresia or colonic atresia. Extracolonic masses such as anterior sacral meningoceles, presacral teratomas, and presacral neuroblastomas may obstruct the rectum. Older children may have obstruction from aganglionosis, "functional" constipation, cystic fibrosis, intussusception, and extracolonic masses such as rhabdomyosarcoma.

Anatomic Obstruction

Colon Atresia and Stenosis

Colon atresia and stenosis are both quite rare. Plain films are not specific, but dilatation of the proximal colon, is common, although not easily recognized (Fig. 4A). Contrast enemas show a distal microcolon with an inability to opacify the proximal dilated colon (Fig. 4B). The lesion is most characteristically located in the distal transverse colon. Findings are often confusing, and a frequent error is the assumption that microcolon is secondary to the more common small bowel obstruction and inability to adequately fill the noncompliant proximal colon. Difficulty in filling the entire colon, or at least most of it, in patients with small bowel atresia or meconium ileus is uncommon. In patients with colon atresia, typically nothing proximal to the midtransverse colon is opacified.

Anorectal Malformations

The most common type of anorectal malformation is associated with ectopic termination of the primitive hindgut so that either the anus is ectopic or there is a fistula to the vagina, the posterior urethra, or, rarely, another structure. The relation of the distal rectum to the puborectalis muscle subdivides these lesions into high (supralevator) and low (infralevator) malformations, a classification with important surgical implications regarding treatment as well as predicting continence (Fig. 5).

High Malformations (Supralevator). The male patient with high anorectal malformation usually has a fistula to the posterior urethra through the prostate gland and less commonly to the bladder. With a rectourinary fistula, there may be gas and meconium in the bladder (Fig. 6).

The female patient usually has a rectovaginal fistula. There may be a separate vaginal and urethral orifice or a single urogenital sinus with bowel entering from behind and the urethra from in front. There may be gas and meconium in the vagina or uterus. There may be giant "hydrometrocolpos," easily imaged by US. Spinal and genitourinary anomalies are common (Fig. 7).

Low Malformations (Infralevator). In low anorectal malformations, the bowel passes through the levator

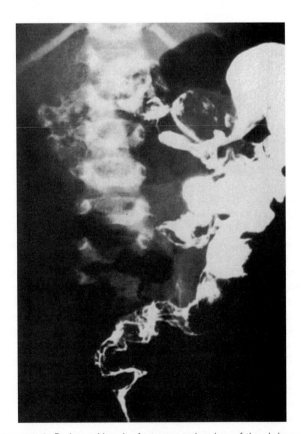

FIGURE 3. Peritoneal bands. Anteroposterior view of the abdomen following barium enema demonstrates partial obstruction of the transverse colon by peritoneal bands crossing anterior to it. The cecum is malpositioned. (Courtesy of Dr. William Schey, Chicago, IL.)

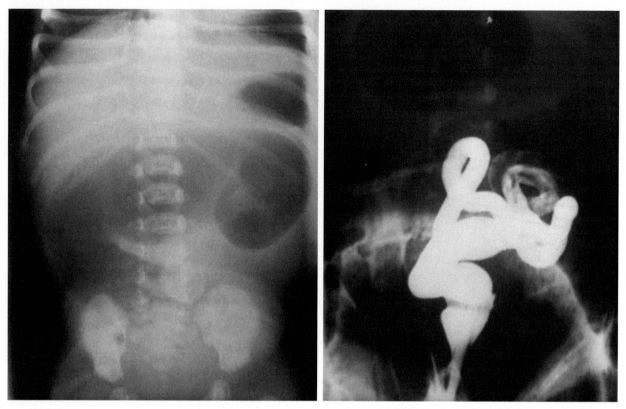

FIGURE 4. Colon atresia. **A,** Plain radiograph demonstrates bean-shaped dilated loop in mid and right abdomen. **B,** Contrast enema demonstrates distal microcolon with nonfilling of proximal colon.

sling. There may be a fistula to the lower portion of the urethra, low vagina, or perineal surface. In the male infant, there may be a thickened midline cord of tissue running from the anal dimple to the base of the scrotum, and meconium may appear at the scrotum within a day of birth. A rectoperineal fistula may simulate the anal opening but is easily recognized by a position on the perineum anterior to the normal anal rosette, which is usually present because it arises from a different embryologic anlagen.

Imaging Studies. Although the infant with a high anorectal malformation may have a fistula to the bladder, plain films usually do not show gas in the bladder, presumably because of meconium plugging. Because these infants are usually treated by colostomy, the distal limb can be injected with contrast medium to look for a fistula. Of interest, some of these patients have calcifications in the abdomen (Fig. 8) that prove to be meconium enteroliths in the lumen of the colon. Speculation has centered on stasis as well as on effect of urine on the meconium as their cause.

Distal colostomy studies (loopograms) with water-soluble agents show the bowel to "beak" as it enters through the levator sling. A rectum that terminates above the levator usually does not show this beak. In the female infant, a vaginal fistula is commonly large enough to allow decompression of gas.

Plain films in the lateral projection, with the infant inverted, were initially recommended with the rationale that gas will rise to the distal rectum and identify its distance from the anal dimple marked with a radi-opaque marker. Although many measurements and lines have been advanced (pubosacral, pubococcygeal), these are not safe guidelines. The ischial bone had lines drawn through its middle and its inferior margin; the latter were generally believed to conform to the level of the puborectalis levator sling. These lines are unreliable because the bowel moves up and down as the infant cries and strains. US and, potentially, MRI are more useful in evaluating the distance, although similarly subject to the dynamic interaction between an atretic bowel and the pelvic floor (Fig. 9).

Uroradiologic evaluation for all affected infants, not only those with high anomalies, is always warranted. Voiding cystography (for reflux) with concurrent assessment of lumbosacral deformities may be useful even with sonographically normal kidneys. Some of the genitourinary problems are structural (missing kidneys, crossed ectopia), and easily evaluated with US. Prenatal US can suggest anorectal malformations on the basis of a dilated bowel in conjunction with associated vertebral and other anomalies.

■ Recommended imaging studies in anorectal malformations:
  • Plain radiographs of abdomen, pelvis, spine
  • Skeletal radiographs as indicated by physical examination findings
  • Ultrasound of abdomen, pelvis, and spinal cord

- Magnetic resonance imaging of pelvis and spinal cord, if needed after inconclusive ultrasound
- Contrast studies through all perineal orifices

Infants with anorectal malformations, especially of the supralevator variety, should have evaluation for associated anomalies, particularly skeletal, renal, cardio-vascular, and upper gastrointestinal. Anal atresia is a component of the VACTERL complex (vertebral anomalies, anal atresia, cardiac anomalies, tracheoesophageal fistula, renal anomalies, and limb anomalies).

Small Left Colon Syndrome

The small left colon syndrome mimics aganglionosis in newborns, with a transition zone at the splenic flexure on contrast enema (Fig. 10). These children are virtually

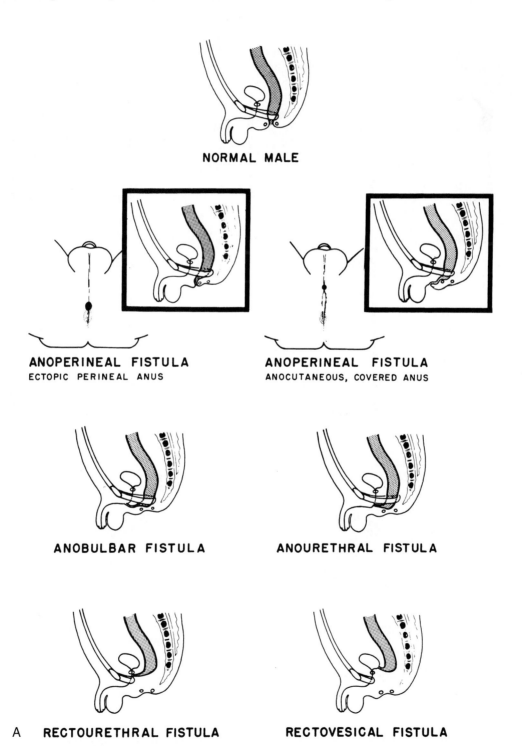

NORMAL MALE

ANOPERINEAL FISTULA
ECTOPIC PERINEAL ANUS

ANOPERINEAL FISTULA
ANOCUTANEOUS, COVERED ANUS

ANOBULBAR FISTULA

ANOURETHRAL FISTULA

A   **RECTOURETHRAL FISTULA**

RECTOVESICAL FISTULA

FIGURE 5. A, Schematic diagram of ectopic termination of the hindgut in the male.

Illustration continued on following page

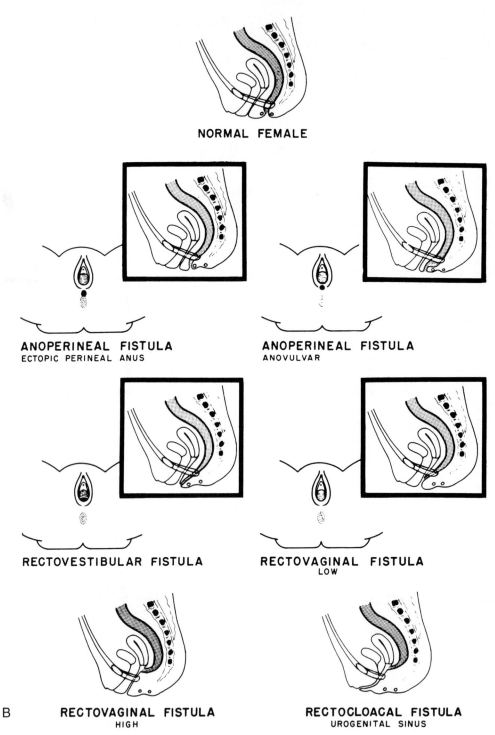

NORMAL FEMALE

ANOPERINEAL FISTULA
ECTOPIC PERINEAL ANUS

ANOPERINEAL FISTULA
ANOVULVAR

RECTOVESTIBULAR FISTULA

RECTOVAGINAL FISTULA
LOW

B   **RECTOVAGINAL FISTULA**
HIGH

RECTOCLOACAL FISTULA
UROGENITAL SINUS

FIGURE 5. *Continued.* **B,** Schematic diagram of common sites of ectopic termination of the hindgut in the female. (From Santulli TV: *In* Mustard WT et al [eds]: Pediatric Surgery, 2nd ed. St. Louis, Mosby–Year Book, 1969, with permission.)

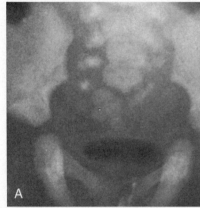

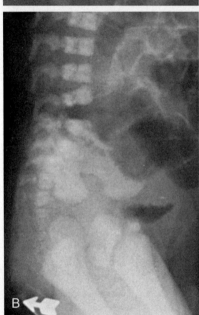

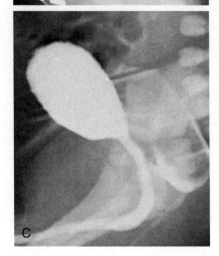

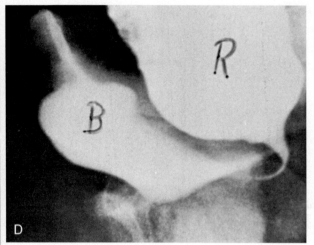

FIGURE 6. High anorectal malformation. Frontal **(A)** and lateral **(B)** projections delineate a rectoprostatic fistula and gas in the bladder of a male infant with lumbar block vertebrae (note the narrowed interspace between L4 and L5 and the abnormal sacrum). There are numerous lumbar coronal clefts; these are nine times as common in males as in females and are often seen in infants with imperforate anus. (**A** and **B** from Berdon WE, Baker DH, Santulli TV, Amoury R: The radiologic evaluation of imperforate anus. An approach correlated with current surgical concepts. Radiology 1968;90:466–471, with permission.) **C,** Voiding cystogram demonstrates a rectoprostatic fistula in another patient. Note how the rectum bulges inferiorly below the level of the fistula. This accounts for the spuriously small distance sometimes seen between rectal gas and anal marker in such patients, although the bowel is high above the puborectalis sling. **D,** Voiding cystogram identifies a rare *rectovesical* fistula in a male infant. Interposition of müllerian structures practically excludes direct fistulous connection between the rectum and urinary tract in the female.

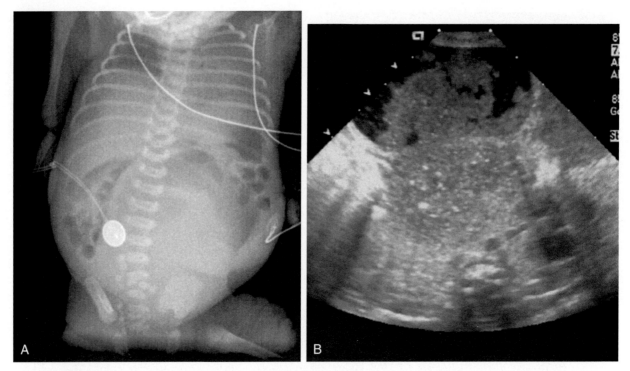

FIGURE 7. Anorectal malformation. **A,** Plain radiograph demonstrates a huge abdominal mass and sacral anomalies. **B,** Ultrasound scan demonstrates a dilated posterior rectum filled with meconium and an anterior fluid-filled mass with particulate matter and clumps of meconium secondary to a rectovaginal fistula.

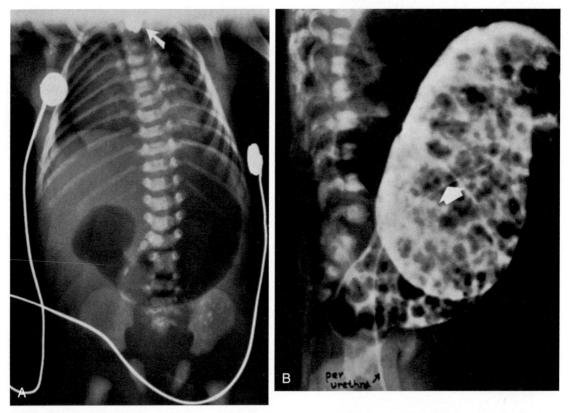

FIGURE 8. Calcified intraluminal meconium. **A,** Newborn male with multiple anomalies, including esophageal atresia, duodenal atresia, and imperforate anus. Note multiple calcifications of intraluminal meconium. There was no peritonitis at operation. **B,** Newborn male with imperforate anus. Many foci of meconium calcifications had been seen on plain films. Urethral catheterization led to easy passage of the catheter *(arrow)* into the rectum. Dense contrast makes filling defects of the intraluminal meconium seem "radiolucent." No peritonitis was noted at operation. (**B** courtesy of Dr. J. Dorst, Baltimore, MD.)

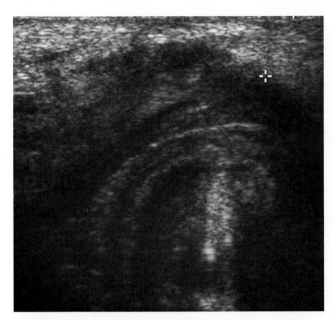

FIGURE 9. Anorectal malformation. Ultrasound scan demonstrates the distance between the anal dimple and the distal rectum in this baby with infralevator anal atresia.

always infants of diabetic mothers, which should raise the likelihood of this diagnosis instead of aganglionosis. Spontaneous resolution is invariable.

Meconium Plug Syndrome

The meconium plug syndrome is distal colonic obstruction by a vermiform plug of tenacious meconium. Rectal examination or the insertion of an enema tip frequently induces passage of the plug and relief of symptoms. Contrast enema outlines the plug, which appears in the sigmoid because it is displaced proximally by the pressure of the enema (Fig. 11). One fourth of affected patients will be found to have aganglionosis and another one fourth will have cystic fibrosis. Appropriate follow-up studies are in order if symptoms persist after passage of the plug.

Functional Obstruction

Functional disorders of the colon produce clinical and radiologic findings of constipation, obstruction, or both, without a mechanical defect being identified. They can be developmental, as with colonic aganglionosis, or acquired, as with some forms of intestinal pseudo-obstruction.

Colonic Aganglionosis (Hirschsprung's Disease)

Colonic aganglionosis, or Hirschsprung's disease, occurs in about 1 in 5000 live births. It presents in the newborn period in 80% of cases. Beyond the neonatal period, aganglionosis can present at any age, even in adults, although it is more frequently identified in younger children. The disease results from absence of

the myenteric plexus secondary to failure of migration of neural crest cells throughout the total length of the gastrointestinal (GI) tract. Because the normal migration is continuous from proximal to distal, that portion of the GI tract distal to the site of arrest is aganglionic. Skip areas are not seen (Fig. 12). So-called zonal aganglionosis has been described, but the focal lack of ganglion cells is probably secondary to a different cause and is extremely rare. The transition from innervated to aganglionic bowel is found in the anorectosigmoid region in 73% of patients, the descending colon in 14%, and the more proximal colon in 10%, according to Swenson et al. Total colonic aganglionosis occurs in 3% of patients as reported in the literature, but the incidence may be closer to 1%. Nearly all patients who present beyond infancy have short-segment disease involving only the distal colon. Because the normal myenteric plexus cells are necessary for relaxation of the colon, the pathophysiology is persistent irregular contraction of the aganglionic segment causing functional obstruction.

Males are more frequently affected than females in short-segment aganglionosis, whereas the sex incidence is equal with long-segment disease. A familial incidence has been identified in some patients with total aganglionosis and long-segment involvement. The disease is associated with trisomy 21 in about 3% of cases and with a variety of other congenital abnormalities in sporadic instances.

Newborns and infants with aganglionosis most commonly present with abdominal distention, with or without bilious emesis. Plain films typically suggest distal colonic obstruction but can be confused with partial small bowel obstruction when the transition point from normal to aganglionic bowel is in the proximal colon (Fig. 13).

Patients beyond infancy present with a history of constipation usually dating to the first weeks of life, although the onset of symptoms is sometimes delayed. Fecal soiling is very rare, and its presence is suggestive of functional constipation rather than aganglionosis. The classic presentation of the wan, lethargic patient with protuberant abdomen, but otherwise wasted-appearing and with failure to thrive, is very uncommon other than in areas of the world that are medically underserved. Definitive diagnosis is made by distal colonic biopsy, but radiographic evaluation is useful in differentiating aganglionosis from other causes of megacolon and for evaluating the length of the involved colon segment.

Plain film examination reveals extensive amounts of stool throughout a dilated colon. Depending on the level of transition, a small distal colon empty of stool may be identified (Fig. 14). Dilated, air-filled loops of small intestine may be seen, but the signs of intestinal obstruction frequently present in newborns are uncommon in older children.

Either barium or water-soluble contrast agents can be utilized to evaluate a child for aganglionosis. Water-soluble media are now more commonly used because, whatever the reason for the constipation, patients are likely to retain barium for extended periods of time. Water-soluble agents may even be therapeutic if the

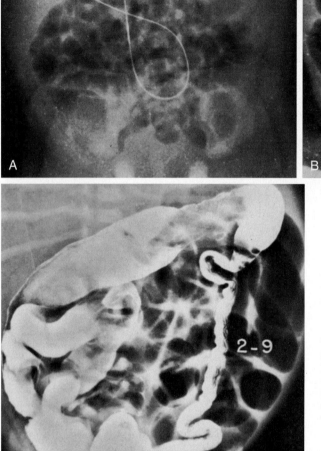
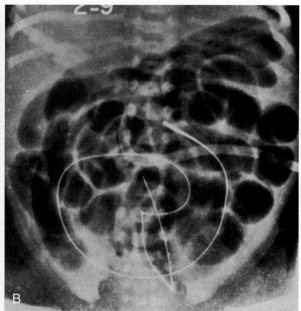

FIGURE 10. Small left colon syndrome. **A,** Normal plain radiograph on day 2 of infant of diabetic mother. Infant had passed large amounts of meconium (umbilical vein catheter in place). There was mild respiratory distress with pneumomediastinum after cesarean section. **B,** Patient on day 3; distention has developed (umbilical arterial catheter now in place). **C,** Contrast enema shows transition at splenic flexure typical of small left colon syndrome. The case is of interest because of normal films the previous day and a history of large amounts of meconium already having been evacuated. We believe "obstruction" in such patients is due to peristaltic problems, not "meconium plug."

patient has functional constipation. Historically, patients do not receive a bowel preparation before contrast enema because the presence of stool in the dilated portion of the bowel makes the identification of a transition zone easier. The older the patient, however, the less likely cleansing enemas are to cause confusion. Digital rectal examination preceding contrast enema does not interfere with making the diagnosis. A large-bore straight rubber catheter cut to have only a single end-hole is inserted no more than 1 cm into the anal canal and taped in place. The buttocks of young children can be taped tightly. Initial filling takes place with the patient recumbent, left side down, and spot films of the rectum in lateral projection are obtained, following which the patient is turned supine and anteroposterior films are obtained. The examination is terminated if the characteristic findings of aganglionosis are present. If not, the examination is continued until a transition zone is identified or until the colon is filled.

The most frequently identified sign of aganglionosis on contrast enema is the presence of a transition zone between a normal or variably narrowed, stool-free aganglionic distal segment and a dilated, stool-filled proximal segment (Figs. 15 and 16). The transition zone cannot always be identified, but it is more reliably present in older children than in neonates. Although the radiographic transition zone does not correspond exactly to the histologic transition zone, it is close enough to be a guide to the surgeon. The final decision as to the true level of transition is made in the operating room with serial biopsies and frozen sections until normal ganglion cells are found.

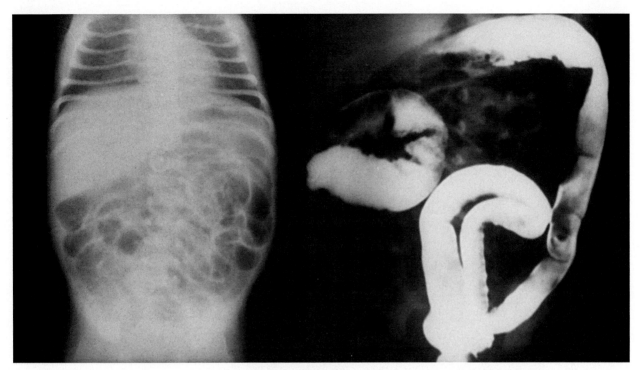

FIGURE 11. Meconium plug syndrome. Contrast enema demonstrates a vermiform filling defect in a baby with a distended abdomen. The symptoms resolved after the meconium plug was evacuated.

In general, the normal rectum is more capacious than the sigmoid colon. This relationship may be reversed with anorectal aganglionosis and has led to the derivation of a "rectosigmoid index." There are so many factors that affect colonic caliber in this disease, however, that a quantitative assessment of the rectosigmoid relationship may be misleading.

Because the aganglionic segment has disordered motor function, irregular contraction waves will be seen in about 20% of patients. These can be either smooth (Fig. 17) or spiky (Fig. 18) and are a very reliable diagnostic indicator when present. When the diagnosis cannot be made at the time of the enema, delayed films occasionally may be helpful if barium was the contrast

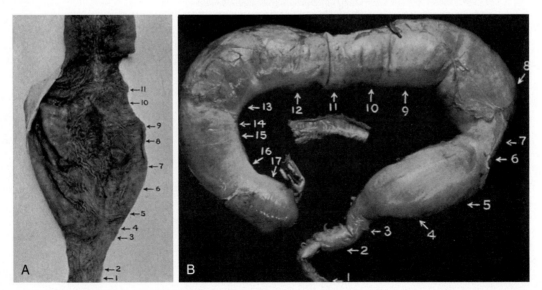

FIGURE 12. Absence of the myenteric plexus in the rectum and terminal segment of the sigmoid colon in congenital megacolon. **A,** Photograph of an enlarged colon that shows the small rectum distal to the dilated sigmoid. In blocks of tissue taken from sites marked by *arrows,* there were no ganglion cells in levels 1 through 7, a few at level 8, and normal numbers at levels 9 through 11. **B,** Photograph of an entire megacolon that shows the small rectum. There were no ganglion cells at levels 1 through 4, scanty ganglion cells at levels 5 through 7, and normal numbers at levels 8 through 17. (From Whitehouse FR, Kernohan JW: Myenteric plexus in congenital megacolon. Arch Intern Med 1948;82:75, with permission.)

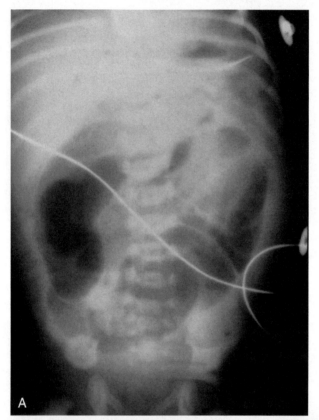

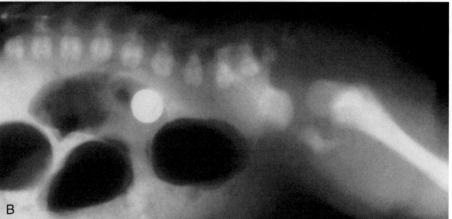

FIGURE 13. Aganglionosis. **A,** Supine and **B,** prone lateral abdominal radiographs demonstrate dilated bowel loops with air–fluid levels suggesting distal intestinal obstruction.

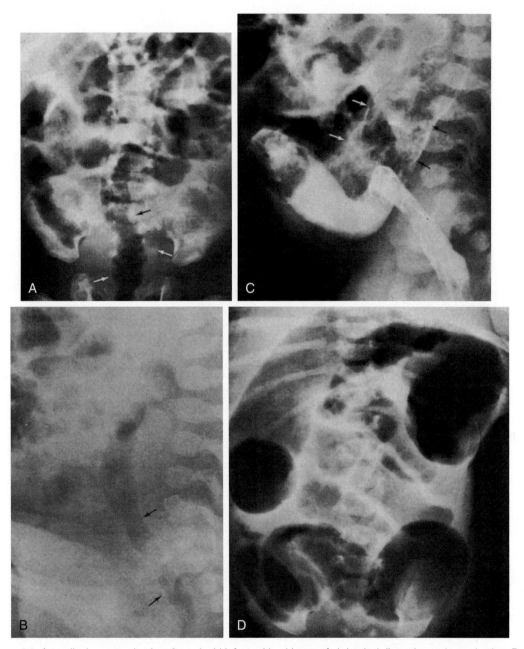

FIGURE 14. Aganglionic megacolon in a 6-week-old infant with a history of abdominal distention and constipation. Frontal **(A)** and lateral **(B)** radiographs of the abdomen demonstrate the small caliber of the air-filled rectum *(arrows)*. **C,** Lateral view of a barium enema demonstrates a transition zone between the narrowed rectosigmoid colon and the dilated descending colon. **D,** Frontal radiograph 3 days after the barium enema demonstrates the abdomen to be distended with markedly dilated loops of colon. Some dilatation of small bowel is also seen. The baby required emergency transverse colostomy for necrotizing enterocolitis of Hirschsprung's disease.

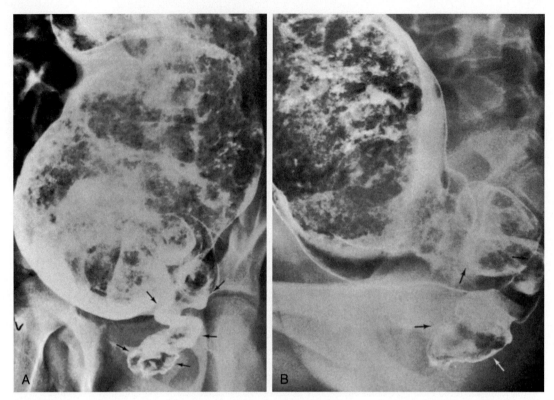

FIGURE 15. Megacolon secondary to aganglionosis of the rectum and distal sigmoid colon. Oblique **(A)** and lateral **(B)** projections of barium enema demonstrate an abrupt transition from the narrow caliber of the rectosigmoid to the large caliber of the more proximal sigmoid colon. This 14-year-old girl had been obstipated since birth.

agent used. By 24 hours after an enema that completely filled the colon, the barium should have moved to the left side of the colon, and, by 48 hours, it should be gone except for minor rectal residual. Retention at 48 hours is suspect for aganglionosis but certainly not diagnostic. A pattern of mixed stool and barium on delayed films a useful sign, but it is seen uncommonly. Most pediatric radiologists now forego the delayed films because patients with a high suspicion of disease will probably undergo the safe procedure of suction biopsy.

■ Signs of Hirschsprung's disease after barium enema:
  • Transition zone (usually rectosigmoid), often subtle during the first week of life
  • Abnormal, irregular contractions of aganglionic segment (rare)
  • Thickening and nodularity of colonic mucosa proximal to transition zone (rare)
  • Delayed evacuation of barium
  • Mixed barium–stool pattern of delayed radiographs
  • Distended bowel loops on plain film fill almost immediately after contrast enema (confirming that they mostly represent colon)

The major complication of colonic aganglionosis is *Hirschsprung-associated enterocolitis* (Fig. 19). This is a potentially fatal entity seen most frequently in the first month of life. Affected patients are gravely ill with fever, abdominal distention, diarrhea, and sepsis. Contrast enemas are generally contraindicated if Hirschsprung-associated enterocolitis is suspected, but water-soluble contrast enemas may be used if the diagnosis is in doubt. Plain films show intestinal distention usually associated with air–fluid levels. US demonstrates thickened bowel wall and ascites. The diagnosis is usually clinically obvious, and, generally, the only imaging examination requested is plain films to look for evidence of intestinal perforation. In rare instances, older children who have had surgical therapy for aganglionosis develop acute distention that usually responds to conservative treatment. The distention may be secondary to a very short segment of aganglionic bowel that is left in place to permit the anus to remain in its normal anatomic position. Coran and Teitelbaum have reviewed the clinical aspects of recent advances in the management of aganglionosis.

Miscellaneous Functional Disorders

Neuronal intestinal dysplasia is a much rarer form of myenteric plexus abnormality in which most children present with constipation, although rectal bleeding has been described. Clinically, colonic involvement may mimic aganglionosis, but histologic examination reveals

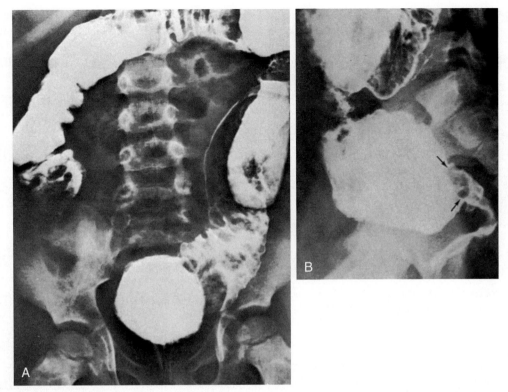

FIGURE 16. Aganglionosis of the rectum in a 5-year-old boy. Frontal **(A)** and lateral **(B)** projections of a barium enema demonstrate the transition zone between the small caliber of the rectum and the large sigmoid *(arrows, **B**)*.

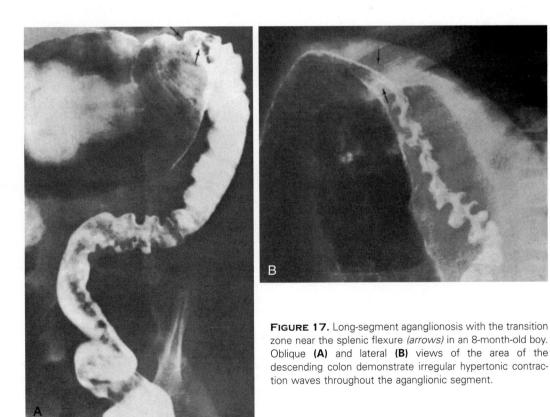

FIGURE 17. Long-segment aganglionosis with the transition zone near the splenic flexure *(arrows)* in an 8-month-old boy. Oblique **(A)** and lateral **(B)** views of the area of the descending colon demonstrate irregular hypertonic contraction waves throughout the aganglionic segment.

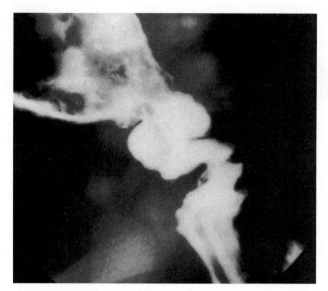

FIGURE 18. Rectal aganglionosis. Lateral view of a barium enema demonstrates spiky irregular contractions of the aganglionic segment of the rectum.

hyperplastic submucosal and myenteric plexuses, giant neurons, and ganglia within the lamina propria. The abnormal neuromuscular activity leads to intestinal pseudo-obstruction. Barium enema demonstrates a flaccid megacolon. Small bowel series shows poor motor activity of the involved portions of the intestine, with focal areas of dilatation and delayed passage of barium. Neuronal dysplasia has been found in the proximal intestine of patients with colonic aganglionosis and can be associated with neurofibromatosis and multiple endocrine neoplasia (MEN) syndrome type IIB. MEN syndrome type IIA can also mimic the presentation of colonic aganglionosis, but rectal biopsy shows giant ganglia.

Intestinal pseudo-obstruction has been associated with non-neurogenic causes, including scleroderma, amyloidosis, and endocrinopathies, especially hypothyroidism (Fig. 20); drugs; and electrolyte disturbances. These entities affect the intestinal smooth muscle, leading to disordered motility. An idiopathic form of myopathic intestinal pseudo-obstruction is being described with increasing frequency. These children present with periodic vomiting, abdominal distention, constipation, urinary retention, and weight loss. Plain films demonstrate dilated loops of bowel with air–fluid levels suggestive of obstruction but that really represent severe adynamic ileus (Fig. 21). Barium studies are nonspecific, showing poor motor activity in affected parts of the bowel. Megacolon is typically found with contrast enema. Associated myogenic abnormalities of the urinary tract may be found.

Pyschogenic constipation is a pejorative term used for children who develop severe constipation without gross or microscopic pathologic abnormalities. In many instances, no definite emotional disturbance is recognized, and a better, although ambiguous, term is *functional constipation*. Patients typically stool normally

during the first year or two of life, but the disease has been reported in infants. The affected children suffer severe constipation, which may lead to anal fissures and painful defecation. Encopresis is very common in this disease as opposed to colonic aganglionosis, in which it virtually never occurs. Plain films demonstrate a capacious rectum filled with scybalous

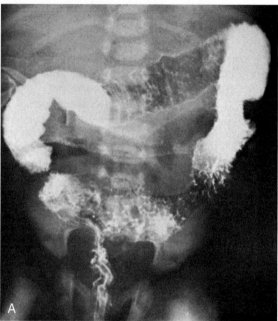

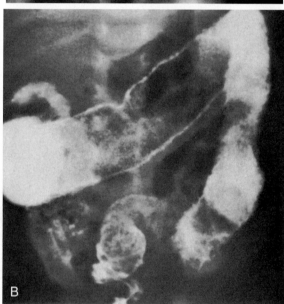

FIGURE 19. Enterocolitis. **A,** Lethal enterocolitis in aganglionosis in a boy 12 days of age whose diagnosis was missed in the immediate newborn period. Barium enema (given elsewhere during a period of fever, foul diarrhea, and shock) demonstrates dilated bowel to the low sigmoid with edematous mucosa of this ganglionic bowel that had severe enterocolitic involvement. The film accompanied the patient, who was dead on arrival at the hospital. **B,** Enterocolitis in a 3-week-old boy with aganglionic megacolon. Contrast enema demonstrates a granular appearance to the mucosa, with small ulcerations.

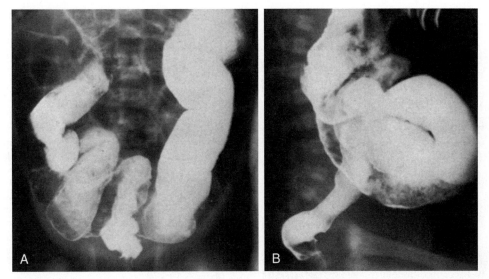

FIGURE 20. Frontal **(A)** and lateral **(B)** views of the abdomen following barium enema in a patient with congenital hypothyroidism. Obstipation was present before the other signs of hypothyroidism became manifest. An apparent transition from small-caliber rectum to dilated sigmoid mimics aganglionosis. (Courtesy of Dr. F. A. Lee, Pasadena, CA.)

material. Stool may back up all the way to the cecum, and secondary small bowel dilatation may be seen. Contrast studies are usually not necessary but, if performed, will show a colon dilated to the anus and filled with fecal material (Fig. 22). Anal aganglionosis may give a similar appearance.

NEOPLASMS

Colonic neoplasms are rare in children. The majority are benign juvenile polyps. The hereditary polyposis syndromes (Table 2) are less common, and primary

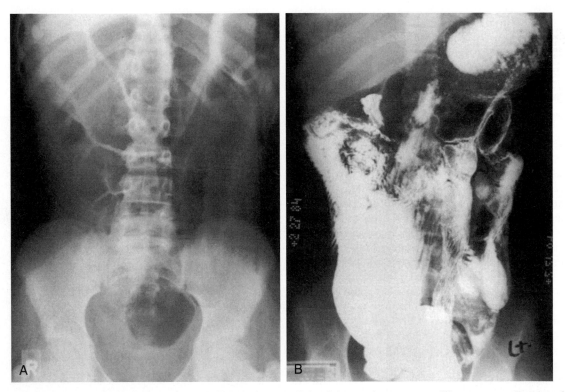

FIGURE 21. Intestinal pseudo-obstruction. **A,** Plain radiograph of the abdomen demonstrates diffuse gaseous dilatation of the small bowel. **B,** Small intestinal series reveals diffuse dilatation of the bowel with no focal obstructive lesion identified. At surgery, no mechanical obstruction was identified. Ganglion cells were present in the myenteric plexus but were abnormal.

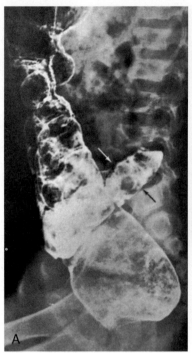 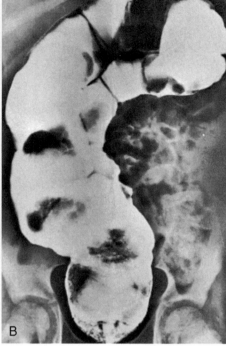

FIGURE 22. Functional (psychogenic) megacolon. **A,** Lateral projection following barium enema demonstrates markedly enlarged rectum that is filled with stool. The normal rectal shelf is well seen. **B,** Frontal projection during barium enema demonstrates scybalous material throughout the distal colon down to and including the low rectum. A rectal biopsy demonstrated normal ganglion cells.

malignancies of great rarity. The double contrast enema is the examination of choice in children who present with rectal bleeding or who are suspected, for any reason, of having a benign or malignant colonic neoplasm. Scattered reports have suggested that US may be helpful in determining the depth of wall involvement in colorectal carcinomas. These cancers are so rare in children that they can reasonably be evaluated, as are those in adults when they occur.

JUVENILE POLYPS AND POLYPOSIS SYNDROMES

Juvenile polyps have been considered either postinflammatory in nature or hamartomatous. They may be single or multiple, sessile or pedunculated, and are benign with no reported tendency to become malignant (Fig. 23). The majority are diagnosed in children under age 10 years who present with painless rectal bleeding. Juvenile polyps primarily occur in the rectosigmoid region and are less frequently found in the transverse, ascending, and cecal portions of the colon, in that order. They are typically under 2 cm in diameter and may be as small as 2 to 3 mm. *Juvenile polyposis coli* is an uncommon syndrome consisting of multiple juvenile polyps found in children who have a family history of colorectal malignancy. Associated abnormalities include midgut malrotation, amyotonia congenita, hypertelorism, and hydrocephalus. Juvenile polyps are found in the *Cronkhite-Canada syndrome*, which does not occur in children.

Adenomatous polyps are found in several of the inherited polyposis syndromes (Table 2) and have significant malignant potential. *Familial polyposis* is an autosomal dominant disorder characterized by numerous tiny adenomatous polyps scattered throughout the colon. The majority of patients have a family history of colonic polyps or cancers. Others may develop their disease as a result of a new genetic mutation. All immediate family members, even if asymptomatic, should be studied for polyposis. The malignant potential approaches 100%, and total colectomy is usually performed. Rectal bleeding, diarrhea, and crampy abdominal pain are the common presenting symptoms. Double contrast barium enema demonstrates a myriad of tiny polyps that have been likened to a shag carpet (Fig. 24).

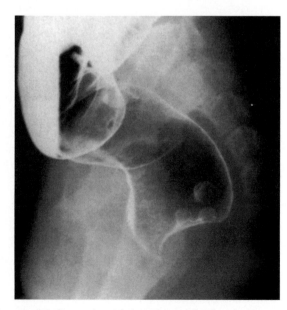

FIGURE 23. Prone view of the rectum following double contrast barium enema demonstrates multiple sessile and pedunculated juvenile polyps, all of which measured less than 2 cm in diameter. No polyps were identified in the remainder of the colon.

Table 2 ■ INHERITED GASTROINTESTINAL POLYPOSIS SYNDROMES

SYNDROME	GASTROINTESTINAL LESIONS	PATHOLOGIC NATURE OF POLYPS	EXTRAINTESTINAL LESIONS	PREDISPOSITION TO CANCER	INHERITANCE
Familial adenomatous colonic polyposis	Polyposis limited to colon and rectum	Adenomatous	None	Marked (colonic adenocarcinoma develops in most untreated patients)	Autosomal dominant
Peutz-Jeghers syndrome	Generalized polyposis, but polyps of small intestine are consistent	Hamartomatous	Melanin spots of lips, buccal mucosa, and digits	About 2%–3% risk of GI cancer, often involving duodenal region	Autosomal dominant
Gardner syndrome	Polyps of colon and rectum (rarely small intestine)	Adenomatous	Osseous and soft-tissue tumors, usually multiple (globoid osteomas of the mandible with overlying fibromas are characteristic); also seen are osteomas of the calvaria with overlying fibromas, epidermoid cysts, lipomas, and especially after an operation, desmoid tumors and wound fibromatosis	Marked, as in familial adenomatous colonic polyposis but with additional risk of carcinoma of pancreaticoduodenal region	Autosomal dominant
Generalized juvenile polyposis	Usually colon and rectum but may involve small intestine and stomach	Hamartomatous	None	Probable, but magnitude of risk uncertain	Autosomal dominant
Turcot syndrome	Colonic polyps	Adenomatous	Tumors of brain	In brain (not reported in GI tract)	Autosomal recessive

From Erbe RW: Inherited gastrointestinal-polyposis syndromes. N Engl J Med 1976;294:1101, with permission.

The appearance is reminiscent of lymphoid hyperplasia (Fig. 25), but the polyps are of variable size, do not have central umbilication, and affect the whole colon. Lymphoid hyperplasia shows filling defects of uniform size, many of which have central umbilication, and is predominantly found in the left colon with progressively diminished involvement in the more proximal portions of the colon (see below).

Gardner's syndrome is an autosomal dominant disorder in which adenomatous polyps of the colon are associated with multiple osseous and soft tissue tumors, the more common of which are cranial and facial osteomas. The potential for cancers of the colon and of the pancreas is high. *Turcot's syndrome* is an autosomal recessive disease that presents more commonly in adults than in children. Although adenomatous polyps are found in the colon, they usually do not become malignant. Malignant brain tumors do develop, however. The polyps in *Peutz-Jeghers syndrome* are more likely to be found in the proximal portions of the GI tract than in the colon (Fig. 26). These polyps are hamartomatous and the malignant potential is low. If colonic polyps are present, however, they may be adenomatous with malignant potential. The characteristic clinical appearance is melanosis of the lips, buccal mucosa, and digits.

MALIGNANT LESIONS

Colorectal carcinoma is quite rare in children. It is usually found in teenage boys but has been reported even in infancy and in patients of both sexes. Although there is an increased incidence of carcinoma in patients with polyposis syndromes, these cancers usually do not appear until adulthood. Mucinous adenocarcinoma is the most common histologic variety in children. There is some evidence that environmental factors or diet may be involved in childhood colonic cancers. Chromosomal abnormalities have been discovered in patients with predisposing polyposis syndromes and with the sporadic variety of colon cancer. The most common symptoms are pain, change in bowel habits, weight loss and anorexia, anemia, rectal bleeding, and an abdominal mass. Plain films may be normal, show irregularity in the bowel gas pattern, or demonstrate partial obstruction. The mucinous tumors may have punctate calcification in the primary area (Fig. 27*A*) and in metastatic deposits. Air-contrast barium enema demonstrates findings like those described in adults. Because diagnosis is often delayed as a result of a low index of suspicion on the part of physicians, the tumors tend to be larger at presentation than is frequently true in adults (Figs. 27*B* and 28). Cures have not been reported other than following complete surgical resection. Initial metastases are to liver, lymph nodes, and other intra-abdominal sites. Generalized carcinomatosis may occur.

The colon is a less frequent primary site for the development of *lymphoma* than is the small intestine. The US characteristics are similar, with a large hypoechoic mass usually extending well beyond the bowel itself (Fig. 29). CT characteristics are similar to those discussed in Section VI, Part VII, page 1616.

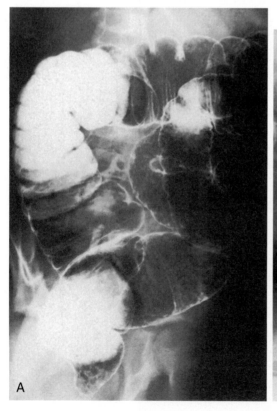
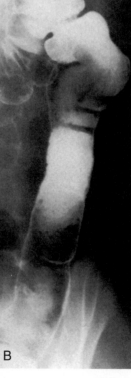

FIGURE 24. Familial adenomatous polyposis. **A,** Double contrast barium enema in an 11-year-old boy whose father had had a total colectomy for familial polyposis. Numerous mucosal filling defects of varying sizes are seen throughout the entire colon. None of the lesions appear umbilicated. The patient underwent total colectomy at the age of 15. **B,** Coned-down view of the descending colon during air-contrast barium enema in the patient's sister, age 9 years. Multiple filling defects seen in face are similar to those seen in lymphoid hyperplasia (compare with Fig. 25). Note the marginal filling defects, however, which suggest the presence of polyps. Colonoscopy confirmed the diagnosis of familial adenomatous polyposis.

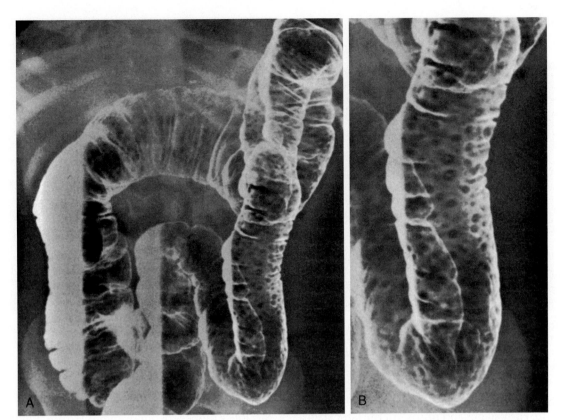

FIGURE 25. Lymphoid hyperplasia demonstrating multiple umbilicated polypoid filling defects throughout the colon, although more prominently seen in the left colon than the right. Right lateral decubitus view **(A)** and close-up of the sigmoid and descending portions of the colon **(B)** demonstrate the filling defects to be of relatively uniform size, with many of them having a central umbilication. (Courtesy of Dr. Marie Capitano, Philadelphia, PA.)

BENIGN LYMPHOID HYPERPLASIA

Benign lymphoid hyperplasia is not a neoplasm but may be mistaken for polyposis (see Fig. 25). The filling defects seen on air-contrast barium enema represent patches of lymphoid tissue in the mucosa and submucosa with an increased size and number of lymph follicles. They are uniform, frequently umbilicated, and found predominantly in the left side of the colon. They are typically 2 to 3 mm in diameter. Larger hyperplastic lymphoid patches may be seen in patients with inflammatory bowel disease and hypogammaglobulinemia. Rectal bleeding has been described with benign lymphoid hyperplasia, but the association is probably fortuitous.

INFLAMMATORY AND INFECTIOUS DISEASES (Table 3)

NONSPECIFIC CHRONIC ULCERATIVE COLITIS

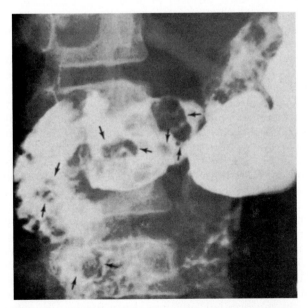

FIGURE 26. Multiple polyposis of the duodenum *(arrows)* in a 12-year-old boy who also had polyps in the stomach, small intestine, and colon. Examination of his mouth demonstrated the typical melanin patches of Peutz-Jeghers syndrome.

Nonspecific chronic ulcerative colitis is an idiopathic inflammatory disease of the colon affecting older children and young adults. An infantile form has been described that is devastating and often fatal (Fig. 30). The disease is characterized by mucosal inflammation,

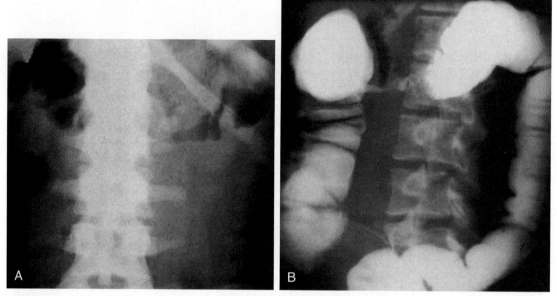

FIGURE 27. Carcinoma of the colon in a 16-year-old boy. **A,** Plain radiograph of the abdomen demonstrates focal narrowing in the midportion of the transverse colon with associated stippled calcifications. **B,** Oblique view during barium enema demonstrates a circumferential mass in the same area. Histologic examination confirmed the diagnosis of mucinous adenocarcinoma of the colon.

edema, and ulceration. It is accompanied by submucosal edema in the early stages and fibrosis in the later stages. Transmural disease is uncommon. The disease may be localized in the distal colon or spread to involve the entire colon and the terminal ileum. Fatal outcomes are less common recently than in years past but still occur. Colonic carcinoma is a frequent complication, especially in patients who present with total colonic involvement or who respond poorly to therapy. Although the cancers do not arise in childhood, prophylactic total colectomy is often offered to patients in the high-risk group.

Bloody diarrhea may appear explosively in as many as one third of affected patients, but the majority present with progressive chronic diarrhea. Many children present with non-GI symptoms, of which severe growth retardation is the most common and clinically striking. Arthritis may precede the colon symptoms. Typically, it is monarticular or pauciarticular, affecting large joints. Seronegative spondyloarthropathy is seen in some affected males. Skin rashes, uveitis, digital clubbing,

stomal ulcers, and hepatic dysfunction may occur in variable numbers of children but less frequently than in adults.

Plain films are most frequently nonspecific but may show evidence of mucosal edema (Fig. 31A). Occasional patients present with toxic megacolon in which marked dilatation of the large bowel, primarily the transverse colon, is seen. These patients should not undergo contrast enemas because of the high risk of perforation.

Double contrast barium enema is the imaging procedure of choice. Stringer et al. have demonstrated its efficacy in children, in whom it is almost comparable to endoscopy for diagnosis. The disease always affects the rectum, with contiguous proximal involvement. Skip areas do not occur, although different parts of the colon may not be equally affected. The earliest change seen with air-contrast enema is a fine granularity of the colonic mucosa. This may be accompanied by haustral thickening secondary to edema of the submucosa. The mucosa becomes progressively more irregular as the disease progresses, and ulcers can be seen (Fig. 31B). In the early stages, they may be small enough to be confused with normal innominate grooves (Fig. 32), but the associated mucosal irregularity and edema should lead to the correct interpretation. The ulcers may become large, so-called collar button ulcers. Pseudopolyposis may occur when islands of residual mucosa are surrounded by areas of denuded mucosa (Figs. 31C and 33). The colonic wall becomes stiff, shortened, and tubular—the "lead pipe" colon—secondary to fibrosis of the submucosa (Fig. 34). With total colonic involvement, the terminal ileum may also be involved, so-called backwash ileitis (Fig. 35). Late-stage disease produces presacral thickening, and retroperitoneal fibrosis is a rare complication (Fig. 36).

Table 3 ■ INFLAMMATORY BOWEL DISEASE OF THE COLON
Gastroenteritis—transient
Other infectious colitides
Ulcerative colitis
Crohn's disease
Pseudomembranous colitis
Hemolytic uremic syndrome
Behçet's syndrome
Radiation colitis
Neutropenic colitis

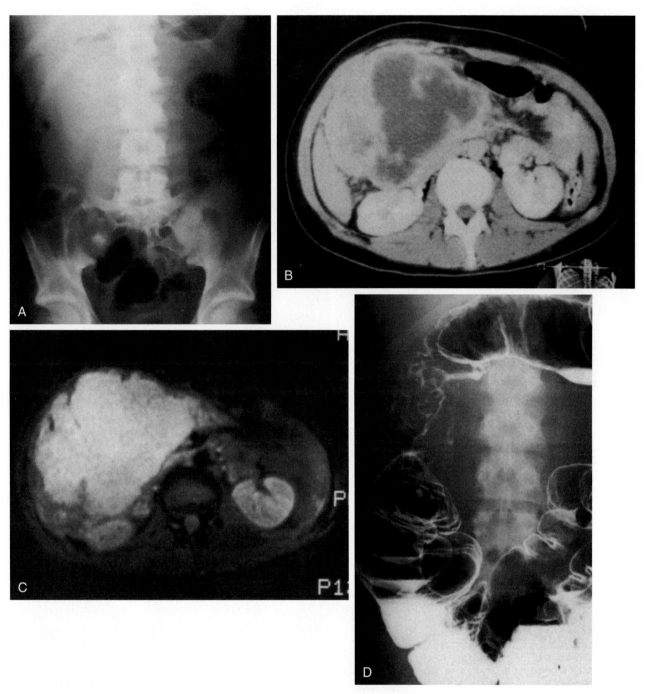

FIGURE 28. Carcinoma of the colon. **A,** Plain radiograph of the abdomen performed following the palpation of an abdominal mass in a 14-year-old boy demonstrates a large mass in the right upper quadrant, displacing normal intra-abdominal structures. **B,** Because a presumptive diagnosis of Burkitt's lymphoma was made, a computed tomography scan was performed that shows the right-sided mass to have central areas of nonenhancement that were initially thought to be areas of necrosis within a lymphomatous tumor. **C,** T$_2$-weighted spin-echo magnetic resonance image of the right upper quadrant demonstrates the marked irregularity of the mass and the high signal intensity suggestive of malignant tumor. **D,** Following a needle biopsy, which revealed signet cells, a barium enema was performed, which demonstrates a large infiltrating carcinoma of the right side of the colon. Histologic examination confirmed the diagnosis of mucinous adenocarcinoma of the colon.

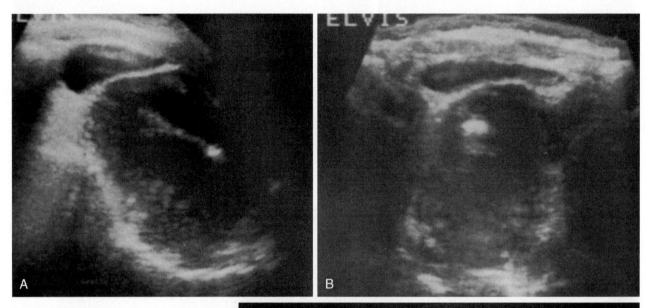

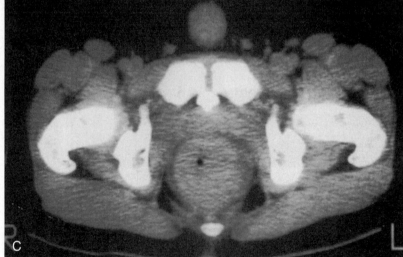

FIGURE 29. Perirectal lymphoma in a 14-year-old boy. Longitudinal **(A)** and transverse **(B)** ultrasound scans of the pelvis demonstrate a large hypoechoic mass completely surrounding the rectum. The bright shadow echoes within the mass is residual rectal gas. Displacement of the bladder is noted. **C,** Computed tomography scan section through the pelvis demonstrates the markedly narrowed rectal lumen surrounded by the mass of lymphomatous tissue. Histologic examination revealed lymphocytic lymphoma.

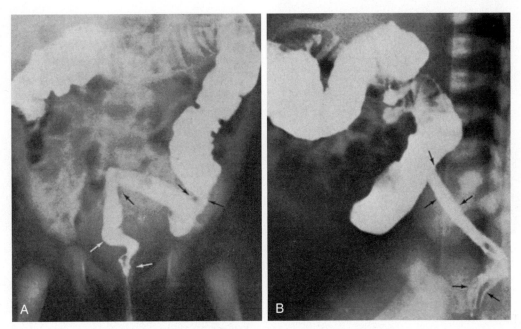

FIGURE 30. Infantile ulcerative colitis in a 3-week-old girl with rectal bleeding. Frontal **(A)** and lateral **(B)** projections during barium enema demonstrate tubular narrowing of the rectum and sigmoid colon *(arrows)* with an abrupt transition zone. The findings were suggestive of aganglionosis, but biopsy revealed ulcerative colitis.

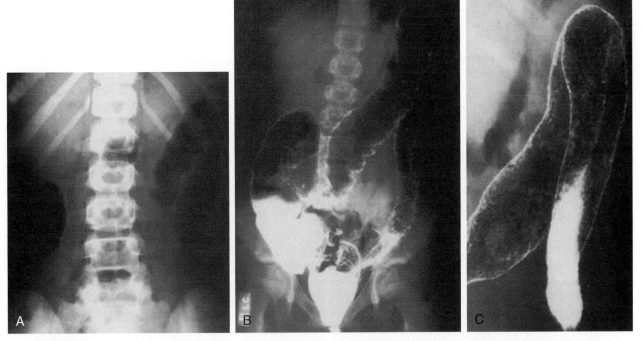

FIGURE 31. Ulcerative colitis in a 14-year-old girl. **A,** Plain radiograph demonstrates "thumbprinting" of the distal transverse colon, suggesting mucosal and submucosal edema. **B,** Double contrast enema demonstrates granularity and irregularity of the colonic mucosa. Small ulcerations are seen throughout the transverse colon and the descending colon. The entire colon was involved. **C,** Coned-down view of the splenic flexure demonstrates multiple areas of pseudopolyps.

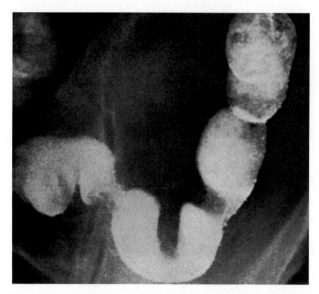

FIGURE 32. Innominate grooves. Coned-down view of the distal descending and proximal sigmoid colon demonstrates regular, small spiculations that should not be confused with the ulceration of inflammatory bowel disease. The innominate grooves are less commonly seen in children than in adults.

- ■ Imaging findings in ulcerative colitis:
Plain films
  - Bowel wall edema and luminal narrowing
Double contrast enemas
  - Mucosal granularity and edema
  - Ulceration
  - Haustral thickening
  - Pseudopolyposis
  - Colonic wall stiff, shortened, tubular
  - "Backwash" ileitis
Computed tomography
  - Complications such as abscesses

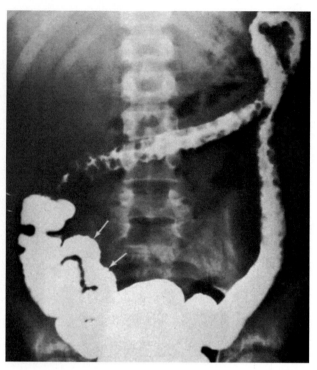

FIGURE 33. Ulcerative colitis with pseudopolyposis and "backwash ileitis" in a 15-year-old boy. There are multiple round marginal filling defects in the transverse and descending portions of the colon, reflecting retained islands of normal mucosa between areas of denuded mucosa. The terminal ileum is rigid and lacks a normal mucosal pattern.

CT is used less frequently in patients with ulcerative colitis than in patients with Crohn's disease and is infrequently requested in children, who are more likely subjected to colonoscopy. Durno and colleagues reported the inability of abdominal MRI to distinguish between types of inflammatory bowel disease in children in general, although the accuracy in ulcerative colitis was good in a very small patient sample.

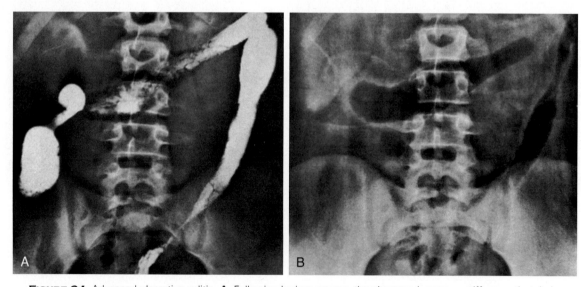

FIGURE 34. Advanced ulcerative colitis. **A,** Following barium enema, the shortened, narrow, stiff, smooth, tubular appearance is evident. **B,** The air-filled colon on plain radiograph demonstrates strikingly similar findings.

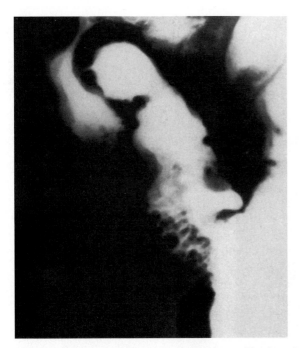

FIGURE 35. Backwash ileitis in a teenage boy with ulcerative colitis. Although the terminal ileum is distensible, it is irregular, with marginal filling defects and mucosal inflammation. The cecum is markedly fibrotic and contracted.

CROHN'S DISEASE

Crohn's disease is discussed in Section VI, Part VII, page 1616. The disease can affect the colon as well as the small intestine. An important differentiating feature from ulcerative colitis is the frequent sparing of the rectum and the presence of skip areas with involved portions of colon separated from one another by uninvolved portions. Ulceration and edema are noted on air-contrast barium enemas. The ulcers are initially small and superficial (aphthous) but eventually develop the characteristic "rose thorn" configuration. A cobblestone pattern like that in the small intestine may be seen (Fig. 37A, B). As in the small intestine, fistulas, sinus tracts, and abscesses can develop (Fig. 37C). Crohn's disease is more likely to lead to colonic strictures than is ulcerative colitis. CT is very useful in evaluation of the complications of the disease (Fig. 38), as noted in Section VI, Part VII, page 1611, but clinicians still favor colonoscopy for evaluation of the colonic manifestations of Crohn's disease.

PSEUDOMEMBRANOUS COLITIS

Pseudomembranous colitis is characterized by fever, diarrhea, and colonic mucositis. The condition most commonly follows antibiotic therapy, often in debilitated or postoperative patients (Fig. 39). The toxin produced by *Clostridium difficile* is the most important cause of antibiotic-associated pseudomembranous coli-

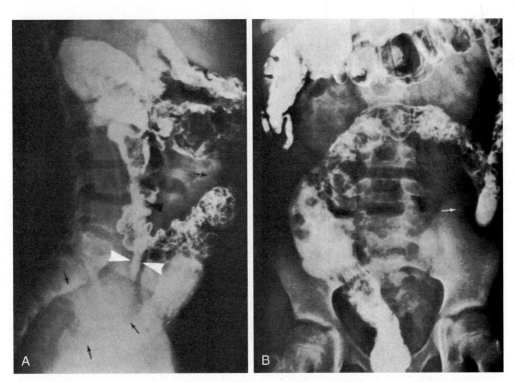

FIGURE 36. Ulcerative colitis with pseudopolyposis and retroperitoneal fibrosis. **A,** Lateral view following excretory urography and barium enema demonstrates marked thickening of the presacral soft tissues *(arrows)*. The anterior margin of the sacrum is sclerotic. The ureters are dilated *(arrowheads)*. **B,** Frontal projection demonstrates the rectum and sigmoid to be fixed by the retroperitoneal fibrosis *(arrow)*, the presence of which was confirmed at surgery.

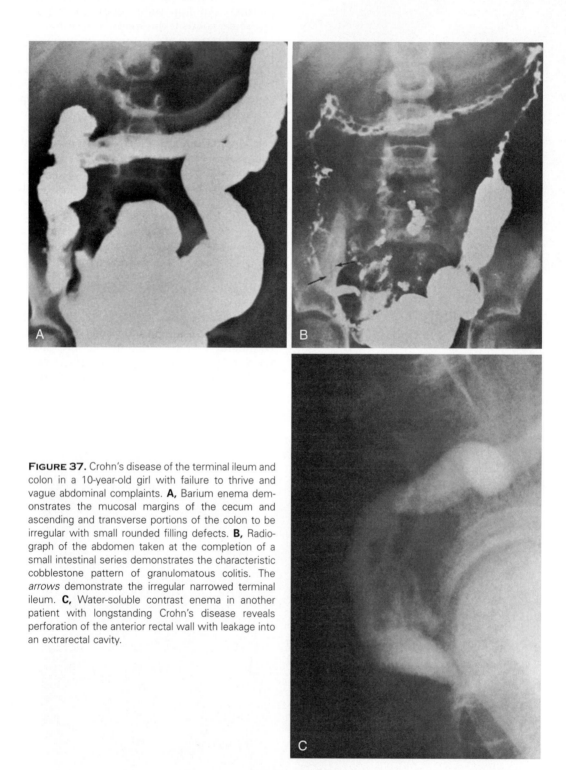

FIGURE 37. Crohn's disease of the terminal ileum and colon in a 10-year-old girl with failure to thrive and vague abdominal complaints. **A,** Barium enema demonstrates the mucosal margins of the cecum and ascending and transverse portions of the colon to be irregular with small rounded filling defects. **B,** Radiograph of the abdomen taken at the completion of a small intestinal series demonstrates the characteristic cobblestone pattern of granulomatous colitis. The *arrows* demonstrate the irregular narrowed terminal ileum. **C,** Water-soluble contrast enema in another patient with longstanding Crohn's disease reveals perforation of the anterior rectal wall with leakage into an extrarectal cavity.

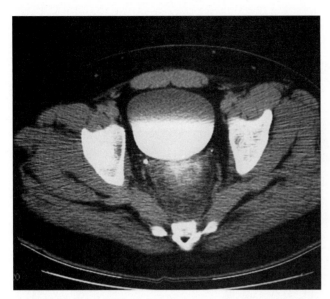

FIGURE 38. Crohn's disease. Computed tomography of the pelvis in a 14-year-old boy with known Crohn's disease and new onset of fever and diarrhea. The rectum and distal sigmoid have narrowed lumina and thickened walls. No abscess was identified.

tis, but it may also be responsible for enterocolitis in infants and children who have not received antibiotics. The radiographic findings are similar to those of the other colitides, and the diagnosis is a clinical one. Some authors have suggested a specific CT pattern in adults, but studies in children have not borne out these findings. Blickman and colleagues found that circumferential colonic wall thickening was the only consistent feature on CT in children.

HEMOLYTIC UREMIC SYNDROME

The hemolytic uremic syndrome (HUS) usually has a GI prodrome preceding clinical evidence of renal involvement. Evidence implicates a bacterial toxin. Colitis is common, and barium enema is frequently requested before the correct diagnosis has been made. The findings are nonspecific, but "thumbprinting" is a frequent manifestation (Fig. 40). Toxic megacolon has been reported in HUS, as has a case of HUS with colonic perforation (Fig. 41).

BEHÇET'S SYNDROME

Behçet syndrome can affect virtually any part of the GI tract. Severe ulceration in the colon can occur, although the radiographic findings are not specific (Fig. 42).

RADIATION COLITIS

Patients with radiation colitis do not usually undergo imaging examinations during the acute phase, when diarrhea is the prominent clinical feature. Eventually, fibrosis may occur, leading to the affected portions of

the colon being stiff with fibrotic walls and loss of the normal mucosal pattern (Fig. 43). The normally mobile portions of the colon are fixed.

NEUTROPENIC COLITIS

Neutropenic colitis is a specific entity in patients with hematopoietic disorders. In children, acute lymphocytic leukemia is the most common underlying disease, with acute myelogenous leukemia also being associated with colitis. Although the colitis may be due to bacterial overgrowth in immunocompromised patients, leukemic children are almost invariably in relapse rather than remission. The prognosis is grave, with most affected leukemic children dying. The disease most often affects the cecum, hence the other commonly used name, *typhlitis.* Abdominal pain, diarrhea, and distended abdomen are the most common presenting symptoms.

The patients are often too ill to come to the radiology department, and portable radiography and US are the most commonly performed studies. The radiographs show focal ileus in the right lower quadrant. Often a sentinel loop of dilated terminal ileum may be seen. We have had two patients who developed pneumatosis coli as a preterminal event (Fig. 44). US demonstrates a markedly thickened cecal wall that may be either hyperechoic or hypoechoic. Intraluminal fluid may be identified (Fig. 45). US can also identify associated

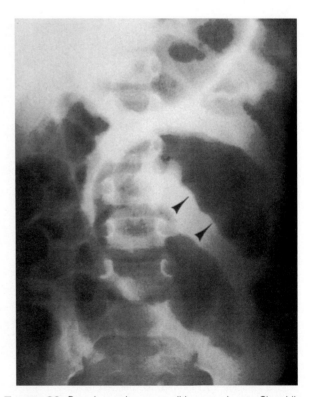

FIGURE 39. Pseudomembranous colitis secondary to Clostridium toxin. Anteroposterior view of the abdomen in a 7-year-old boy who received 1 week of antibiotic therapy for otitis media demonstrates dilatation of a loop of sigmoid colon with typical thumbprinting *(arrowheads).*

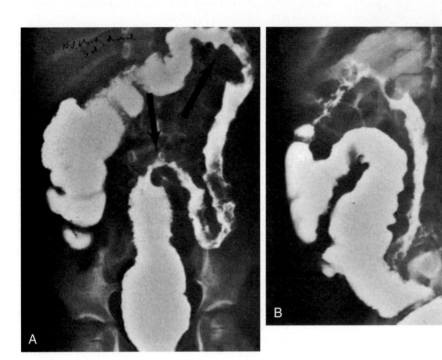

FIGURE 40. Hemolytic–uremic syndrome. Frontal **(A)** and lateral **(B)** radiographs following barium enema demonstrate irregular, narrow, spiculated areas from the distal transverse colon to the distal sigmoid colon *(arrows)*. The clinical and radiographic gastrointestinal abnormalities preceded the abnormalities of the kidneys and blood.

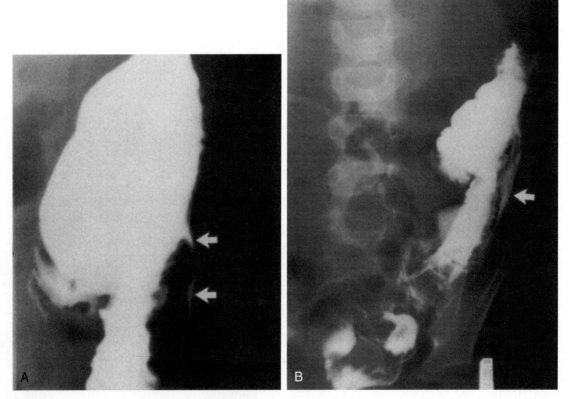

FIGURE 41. Hemolytic uremic syndrome. **A,** Coned-down view of the hepatic flexure during barium enema demonstrates a fistulous tract *(arrows)*. **B,** Delayed radiograph demonstrates extravasated contrast material *(arrow)* tracking along the lateral paracolic gutter. (From Liebhaber MI, Parker BR, Morton JA, et al: Abdominal mass and colonic perforation in a case of the hemolytic-uremic syndrome. Am J Dis Child 1977;131:1168, with permission.)

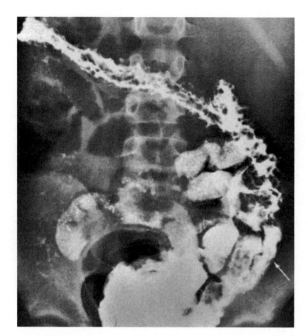

FIGURE 42. Behçet's syndrome. Barium enema demonstrates a cobblestone pattern in the colon with coarse ulceration. The patient also had ulcerative esophagitis. (Courtesy of Dr. W. Berdon, New York, NY.)

ascites. If the cecum has perforated, an abscess may be seen.

INFECTIOUS COLITIS

The infectious colitides are usually caused by the same agents discussed in Section VI, Part VII, page 1616, in the section on Infectious Diseases. Imaging studies are rarely needed and usually show a nonspecific colitis when performed.

FIBROSING COLONOPATHY

Fibrosing colonopathy was first described in 1994 in patients with cystic fibrosis receiving lipase replacement therapy. The most common contrast enema findings are colonic strictures, loss of haustra, and colonic shortening. MRI has been reported to be of value in these patients, but contrast enema is still recommended as the primary imaging modality. As the doses of pancreatic enzymes are adjusted, this disease may disappear.

APPENDICITIS

The vermiform appendix serves no significant physiologic function in humans, but inflammation of this atavistic organ is the most common reason for abdominal surgery in children. Early diagnosis is important because morbidity increases after the appendix perforates. Death from appendicitis, even in the most complicated cases, is much rarer in children than in adults but

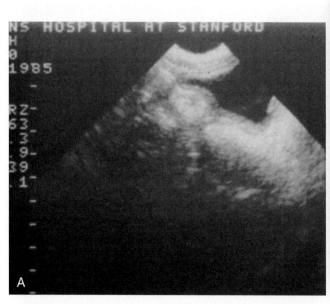

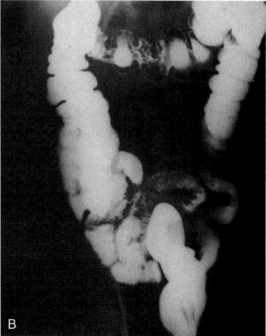

FIGURE 43. Radiation colitis. **A,** Pelvic ultrasound scan in an 8-year-old boy who had received radiation therapy for a pelvic tumor 3 years prior to the study. The echogenic area adjacent to the bladder is fixed bowel with no peristalsis. **B,** Barium enema demonstrates narrowing, rigidity, and loss of haustration in the distal descending and sigmoid portions of the colon.

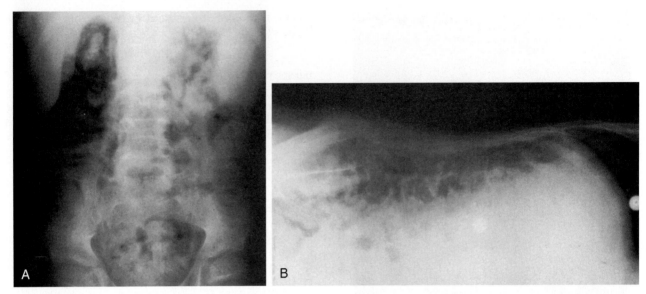

FIGURE 44. Neutropenic colitis. Anteroposterior **(A)** and decubitus **(B)** views of the abdomen of a 9-year-old boy with leukemia and chemotherapy-induced neutropenia demonstrate air diffusely throughout the colonic wall. These films were obtained 10 days following an episode of acute neutropenic colitis.

certainly occurs. However, because the history and physical findings in children with suspected appendicitis are often atypical, patients without appendicitis are often sent to surgery. According to Kottmeier, 11% to 32% of children undergoing appendectomy have a normal appendix. Therefore, imaging examinations can play a useful adjunctive role when the clinical findings are ambiguous.

According to Shandling and Fallis, the actual incidence of appendicitis in children is unknown, but the annual rate of appendectomy in the United States is about 4 in 1000 children under age 14 years. Appendicitis occurs most frequently in children over 2 years of age, but can occur in infancy and even in the neonate. The disease occurs secondary to obstruction of the appendix. Transmural inflammation occurs rapidly. Young children are particularly susceptible to perforation because delayed diagnosis is more frequent than in older children and adults. Perforation can lead to generalized peritonitis, but a local abscess adjacent to the appendix is more likely because the perforation is usually contained by the omentum. Pain, vomiting, and anorexia are common symptoms, but younger children often do not localize the pain to the right lower quadrant. Abdominal tenderness, fever, and leukocytosis are common accompaniments. Surgery is performed

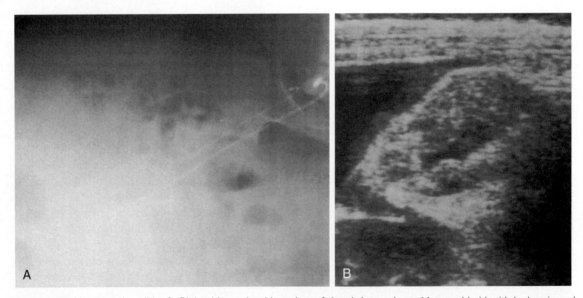

FIGURE 45. Neutropenic colitis. **A,** Right-side-up decubitus view of the abdomen in an 11-year-old girl with leukemia and severe abdominal pain demonstrates a mottled appearance in the right lower quadrant. **B,** Ultrasound scan of the right lower quadrant demonstrates the cecal wall to be markedly thickened. Fluid is seen within the cecal lumen, and ascites is present.

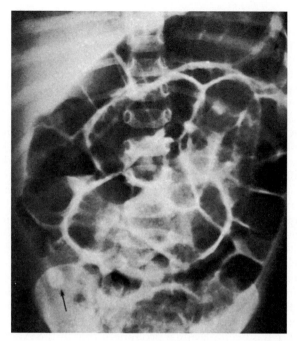

FIGURE 46. Acute appendicitis with abscess formation. Anteroposterior view of the abdomen demonstrates marked distention of the small intestine and colon with a right lower quadrant appendicolith *(arrow)* in a 14-month-old boy with peritonitis and periappendiceal abscess.

without imaging studies when the diagnosis is clinically obvious.

IMAGING FINDINGS

Patients with appendicitis and an atypical clinical presentation often undergo plain film radiography. Pain usually leads to abdominal splinting with subsequent scoliosis of the lumbar spine, concave toward the side of pain. Dilated loops of bowel are seen, sometimes focally in the right lower quadrant but more often throughout the abdomen when perforation has occurred (Fig. 46). When an abscess has formed, a mass effect on the air-filled cecum may be seen. On horizontal beam films, a right lower quadrant air–fluid level that has no discernible mucosal pattern is presumptive evidence of an abscess (Fig. 47). Abscesses most commonly have a mottled appearance on supine films, but a featureless air collection may be seen as well. The radiographic appearance of distal small intestinal obstruction may be found in patients with appendiceal abscesses.

Appendicoliths are calcific concretions in the appendix that are considered compelling evidence of appendicitis in symptomatic patients. Many surgeons will operate on these children without further imaging studies. According to Shimkin, they occur in up to 50% of children with appendicitis. They may be round or oval and uniformly calcified or, more frequently, lamellated. Appendicoliths are multiple 30% of the time (Fig. 48).

Before the introduction of sonographic evaluation of appendicitis, barium enemas were requested in patients in whom the diagnosis was not clinically evident. Non-filling of the appendix was considered a positive sign for appendicitis, but this finding is also present in 5% to 10% of normal persons. Cecal spasm is seen, and a mass effect on the cecum may be present if an abscess has formed. All of these signs are nonspecific and can be found in other conditions. Barium enemas are rarely performed any longer in patients suspected of having appendicitis.

■ Imaging findings in appendicitis:
Plain films
- Ileus, often localized to right lower quadrant
- Spinal splinting
- Appendicolith
- Apparent obstruction, most commonly found in younger children
- Abscess with mass effect and/or atypical air collection

Ultrasound
- Appendiceal diameter >6 mm
- Noncompressible
- Appendicolith with acoustic shadowing
- Periappendiceal fluid

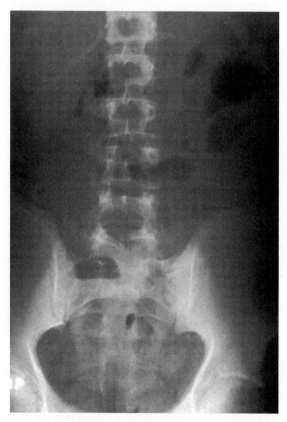

FIGURE 47. Upright view of the abdomen in a 15-year-old boy with signs and symptoms of appendicitis. A featureless air–fluid level is noted in the right lower quadrant. Computed tomography (CT) scan confirmed the presence of the abscess, which was drained under CT control.

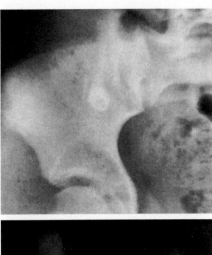

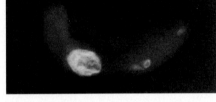

FIGURE 48. Calcified appendicoliths are seen in a coned-down anteroposterior view of the right lower quadrant and in the resected appendix of a 10-year-old girl with acute appendicitis.

- • Perforation may decompress the appendix
- • Abscess

Computed tomography
- • Dilated appendix
- • Appendicolith
- • Abscess

The role of US in the evaluation of possible appendicitis was described by Puylaert in 1986. Numerous studies demonstrating its efficacy in adults have appeared, as well as several series in children. A 5.0- or 7.5-MHz linear array transducer is used, depending on the size of the patient and the depth of the appendix from the skin. Transverse and longitudinal scans are performed over the point of maximal tenderness. Graded compression displaces other loops of bowel, permits higher resolution imaging, and differentiates compressible normal bowel from the inflamed noncompressible appendix. If the appendix is not identified, a complete scan of the lower abdomen and pelvis should be performed because of the variability of appendiceal position (Fig. 49). The normal sonographic anatomy of the right lower quadrant was well described by Abu-Yousef and Franken.

The inflamed appendix almost always measures more than 6 mm in diameter in children as well as adults and is noncompressible (Fig. 50). A "target sign" has been described with respect to the order of hypoechoic and hyperechoic layers, depending on the acuity of the process. In most instances of obstructive appendicitis, as typically found in children, the center of the target is hypoechoic because of fluid or pus in the lumen of the appendix (Fig. 51A). This is surrounded by a circle of echogenic mucosa that is, in turn, surrounded by a hypoechoic edematous appendiceal wall. When the appendix is not markedly inflamed and the lumen is collapsed, multiple concentric rings corresponding to the layers of the appendiceal wall may be identified. Longitudinal images will be comparable in nature but ovoid rather than circular (Fig. 51B). Appendicoliths will be seen more commonly than on plain films since not all of them calcify (Fig. 52). Perforation and abscess formation can be identified at sonography by the presence of periappendiceal fluid, intraperitoneal fluid, and a mass of mixed echogenicity (Fig. 53). Perforation without abscess may lead to a false-negative examination because the decompressed appendix may be difficult to find. The presence of unexplained fluid, however, should alert the examiner to the possibility, and further studies such as CT or scintigraphy should be undertaken.

CT has been playing a prominent role in the evaluation of appendicitis for a decade, but has recently become more widely used in children. The technique varies between institutions, but helical CT has been shown to be superior to standard CT in this patient population (Fig. 54). Not enough information is yet available to determine whether or not multidetector CT will offer further advantages. Some centers do only unenhanced scans, some use intravenous contrast only, and some use oral contrast, rectal contrast, or both. The majority of articles have shown greater sensitivity and specificity for CT as compared to US. CT is considered the better imaging study in the hands of radiologists and technologists who have limited experience with US in children. Conversely, in experienced hands, the accuracy of US approaches that of CT. As radiologists have become more aware of the potential long-term hazards of radiation from CT in children, increasing emphasis is being placed on dose reduction. Pena and colleagues have emphasized a protocol wherein US is the first imaging study utilized in clinically equivocal cases. If the US is negative or equivocal, CT is then performed. This protocol has increased the overall accuracy rate of clinical/imaging diagnosis and significantly reduced the false-positive rate of preoperative diagnosis. CT has also played a major role as the imaging modality of choice for abscess drainage by interventional radiologists (Fig. 55).

Scintigraphic studies may also be useful in the diagnosis of appendicitis, although they are not widely used. Navarro and Weber used indium-111–labeled white blood cells and found them particularly useful when perforation had led to a false-negative US scan. Menneman et al. used technetium-99m–labeled white blood cells in the evaluation of acute appendicitis in children. They found the scan useful to rule out appendicitis in that they had no false negatives. However, 24% of their cases had abnormal but nondiagnostic studies.

Text continued on page 1687

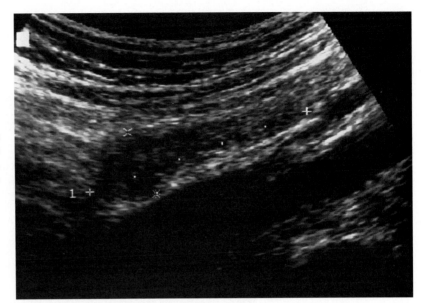

FIGURE 49. Appendicitis. Ultrasound scan of the right lower quadrant shows a noncompressible tubular structure measuring more than 6 mm. Nonperforated appendicitis was found at surgery.

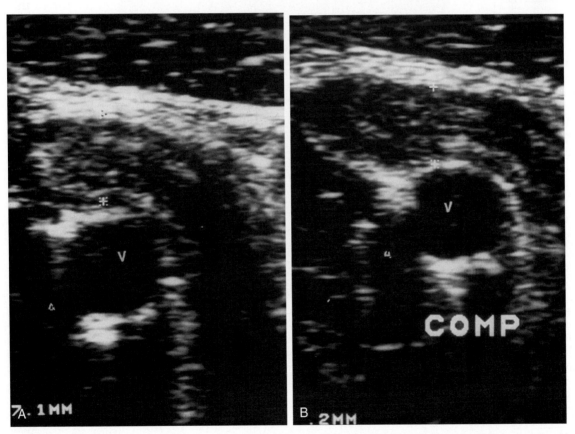

FIGURE 50. Appendicitis. Compression ultrasound scan demonstrates little change in the caliber of a dilated appendix with and without compression. The patient was exquisitely tender under the transducer.

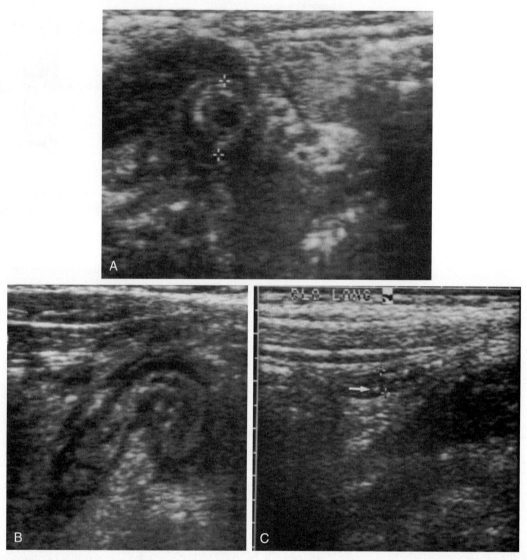

FIGURE 51. Ultrasound examination of patients with appendicitis. **A,** Transverse ultrasound scan of the appendix demonstrates the characteristic "target sign." In this case, the innermost portion is sonolucent, compatible with fluid or pus. **B,** Longitudinal view of another patient demonstrates the alternating hyperechoic and hypoechoic layers with an outermost hypoechoic layer, suggesting periappendiceal fluid. **C,** Longitudinal ultrasound scan of the right lower quadrant demonstrates a dilated, noncompressible appendix. The bright echo within the appendix represents an appendicolith with acoustic shadowing *(arrow).*

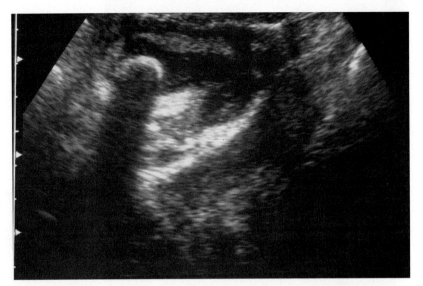

FIGURE 52. Appendicolith. Ultrasound scan of the right lower quadrant shows a calcification with acoustic shadowing in a dilated appendix.

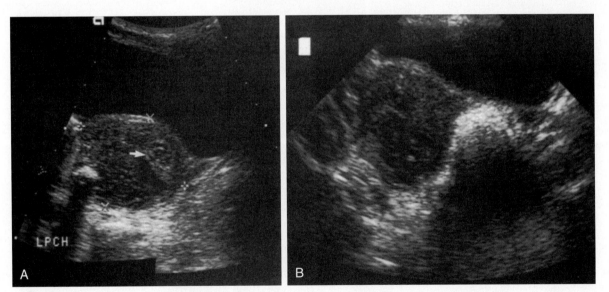

FIGURE 53. Periappendiceal abscesses. **A,** Transverse ultrasound scan of the pelvis demonstrates a large mass of mixed echogenicity behind the bladder. Within the mass is the appendix *(arrow),* showing a typical "target sign." **B,** Longitudinal ultrasound scan in another patient demonstrates a mass of mixed echogenicity behind the bladder. In this case, the appendix itself was not seen because of decompression secondary to perforation.

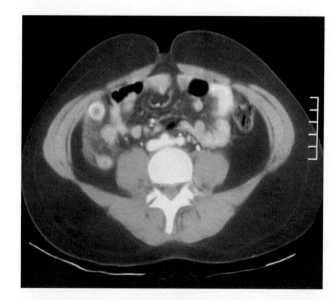

FIGURE 54. Appendicitis. Computed tomography demonstrates a dilated appendix with no evidence of abscess formation.

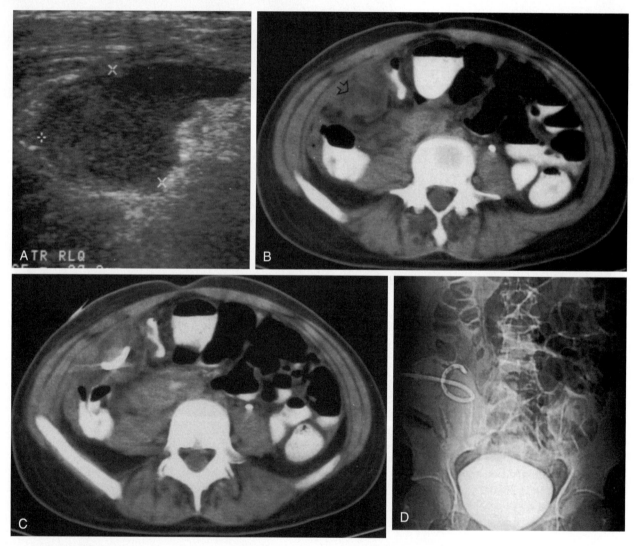

FIGURE 55. Percutaneous drainage of an appendiceal abscess. **A,** Transverse ultrasound scan through the right lower quadrant demonstrates a large mass of mixed echogenicity. The appendix itself was not identified. **B,** Computed tomography (CT) scan demonstrates a mass in the right lower quadrant *(arrow)* of mixed attenuation characteristic of an abscess. **C,** A percutaneous drainage catheter was placed under CT control. The tip of the catheter can be seen within the center of the abscess cavity. **D,** CT scanogram following placement of the catheter demonstrates its course and positioning in the right lower quadrant.

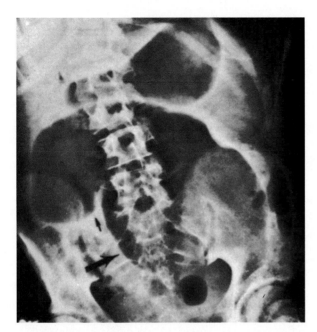

FIGURE 56. Cecal volvulus. Anteroposterior view of the abdomen in a 20-year-old man with abdominal distention and vomiting demonstrates a markedly distended cecum in the lower portion of the abdomen *(arrows).* Note the typical "coffee bean" configuration. (Courtesy of Dr. Donald Darling, Boston, MA.)

Although most abscesses will be adjacent to the appendix, distant spread can occur. Diffuse peritonitis is less common in children over age 2 than in infants. Slovis et al. described three patients with hepatic abscesses and two patients with portal pylephlebitis following complicated appendicitis. Zerin described an intrathoracic appendiceal abscess in a 10-year-old girl with a previously undetected Bochdalek's hernia.

MISCELLANEOUS DISORDERS

VOLVULUS OF THE COLON

Volvulus of the colon is quite rare in children. *Cecal volvulus* may occur in children with a malpositioned cecum secondary to partial midgut malrotation. Plain films show the dilated cecum displaced to the midabdomen (Fig. 56), and the diagnosis can be confirmed by contrast enema. *Sigmoid volvulus* is equally rare in children and may be related to a congenital defect in the sigmoid mesentery. The sigmoid can rotate 180 degrees, causing ischemia, infarction, perforation, and peritonitis. Plain films demonstrate a dilated loop of bowel extending from the left lower quadrant to the right upper quadrant (Fig. 57). Contrast enema will demonstrate the spiral torsion and may actually cause the sigmoid to untwist. Reinarz et al. described splenic flexure volvulus as a complication of intestinal pseudo-obstruction in infancy.

PNEUMATOSIS COLI

Pneumatosis coli is itself a benign disorder but is often a sign of grave underlying disease. It is most commonly seen in adults with chronic partial obstruction. In children, it has been seen in patients with cystic fibrosis, leukemia, collagen-vascular disorders, acquired immunodeficiency syndrome, and neutropenic colitis (see Fig. 44) and following organ transplantation (Fig. 58), presumably secondary to drug therapy. It is a rare complication of steroid therapy. Patients may have asymptomatic pneumatosis coli for months. Pneumoperitoneum rarely, if ever, occurs. Pneumatosis coli may be seen in newborns with necrotizing enterocolitis, in whom it is a more ominous finding (see Section VI, Part VII, page 1616).

FIGURE 57. Sigmoid volvulus in a 10-year-old boy with acute crampy abdominal pain. **A,** Anteroposterior view of the abdomen demonstrates a markedly dilated loop of colon extending from the left lower quadrant to the right upper quadrant. **B,** Lateral view of barium enema demonstrates a spiral twist at the level of the sigmoid torsion *(arrow).* (Courtesy of Dr. Eugene Blank, Portland, OR.)

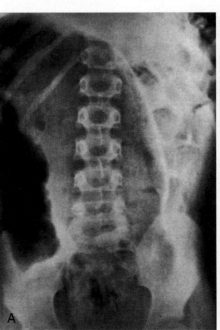
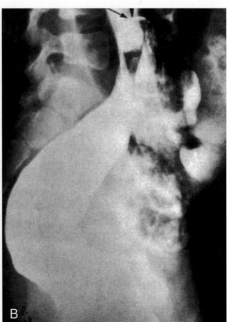

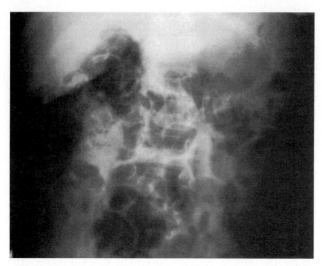

FIGURE 58. Pneumatosis coli in a 4-year-old boy 5 months after cardiac transplantation. Note the air in the wall of the transverse colon outlining the mucosa, which appears as a thin white line.

SUGGESTED READINGS

Congenital and Functional Disorders

Colonic Obstruction

Aslam A, Grier D, Duncan A, et al: The role of magnetic resonance imaging in the preoperative assessment of anorectal anomalies. Pediatr Surg Int 1998;14:71

Berrocal T, Lamas M, Guiterrez J, et al: congenital anomalies of the small intestine, colon, and rectum. Radiographics 1999;19:1219

deSouza N, Gilderdale D, MacIver D, et al: High-resolution MR imaging of the anal sphincter in children: a pilot study using endoanal receiver coils. AJR Am J Roentgenol 1997;169:201

Kangarloo H, Sample WF, Hansen G, et al: Ultrasonic evaluation of abdominal gastrointestinal tract duplication in children. Radiology 1979;131:191

Kluth D, Lambrecht W: Current concepts in the embryology of anorectal malformations. Emin Pediatr Surg 1997;6:180

Kottra JJ, Dodds WJ: Duplication of the large bowel. Am J Roentgenol Radium Ther Nucl Med 1971;113:310

McHugh K: The role of radiology in children with anorectal anomalies; with particular emphasis on MRI. Eur J Radiol 1998;26:194

McHugh K, Dudley N, Tam P: Pre-operative MRI of anorectal anomallies in the newborn period. Pediatr Radiol 1995;25(Suppl 1):33

Moss R: The failed anoplasty: successful outcome after reoperative anoplasty and sigmoid resection. J Pediatr Surg 1998;33:1145

Nievelstein R, Vos A, Valk J: MR imaging of anorectal malformations and associated anomalies. Eur Radiol 1998;8:573

Taccone A, Martucciello G, Dodero P, et al: New Concepts in preoperative imaging of anorectal malformation. New concepts in imaging of ARM. Pediatr Radiol 1992;22:196

Warf B, Scott R, Barnes P, et al: Tethered spinal cord in patients with anorectal and urogenital malformations. Pediatr Neurosurg 1993;19:25

Sonada N, Matsuzaki S, Ono A, et al: Duplication of the caecum in a neonate simulating intussusception. Pediatr Radiol 1985;15:427

Yucesan S, Zorludemir V, Olcay I: Complete duplication of the colon. J Pediatr Surg 1986;21:962

Colonic Aganglionosis (Hirschsprung's Disease)

Coran A, Teitelbaum D: Recent advances in the management of Hirschsprung's disease. Am J Surg 2000;180:382

Cremin BJ: The early diagnosis of Hirschsprung's disease. Pediatr Radiol 1974;2:23

Fotter R: Imaging of constipation in infants and children. Eur Radiol 1998;8:248

Haney PJ, Hill JL, Chen-Chik JS: Zonal colonic aganglionosis. Pediatr Radiol 1982;12:258

Johnson JF, Cronk RL: The pseudotransition zone in long segment Hirschsprung's disease. Pediatr Radiol 1980;10:87

Kilcoyne RF, Taybi HT: Conditions associated with congenital megacolon. Am J Roentgenol Radium Ther Nucl Med 1970;108:615

Krishnamurthy S, Schuffler MD: Pathology of neuromuscular disorders of the small intestine and colon. Gastroenterology 1987;93:610

Pochaczevsky R, Leonidas JC: The "rectosigmoid index": a measurement for the early diagnosis of Hirschsprung's disease. Am J Roentgenol Radium Ther Nucl Med 1975;123:770

Rosenfield NS, Ablow RC, Markowitz RI, et al: Hirschsprung disease: accuracy of the barium enema examination. Radiology 1984;150:393

Schey WL, White H: Hirschsprung's disease: problems in the roentgen interpretation. Am J Roentgenol Radium Ther Nucl Med 1971;112:105

Schiller M, Levy P, Shawa RA, et al: Familial Hirschsprung's disease—report of 22 affected siblings in four families. J Pediatr Surg 1990;25:322

Siegel MJ, Shackelford GD, McAlister WH: The rectosigmoid index. Radiology 1981;139:497

Swenson O, Sherman JO, Fisher JH: Diagnosis of congenital megacolon: an analysis of 501 patients. J Pediatr Surg 1973;8:587

Whitehouse FR, Kernohan JW: Myenteric plexus in congenital megacolon. Arch Intern Med 1948;82:75

Yunis E, Sieber WK, Akers DR: Does zonal aganglionosis really exist? Pediatr Pathol 1983;1:33

Other Functional Disorders

Case Records of the Massachusetts General Hospital: Intestinal neuronal dysplasia associated with long-segment Hirschsprung's disease. N Engl J Med 1991;325:1865

Glassman M, Spivak W, Mininberg D, et al: Chronic idiopathic intestinal pseudo-obstruction: a commonly misdiagnosed disease in infants and children. Pediatrics 1989;83:603

Khan AH, Desjardins JG, Youssef S, et al: Gastrointestinal manifestations of Sipple syndrome in children. J Pediatr Surg 1987;22:719

Puri P, Lake B, Nixon HH, et al: Neuronal colonic dysplasia: an unusual association of Hirschsprung's disease. J Pediatr Surg 1977;12:681

Schärli AF, Meier-Ruge W: Localized and disseminated forms of neuronal intestinal dysplasia mimicking Hirschsprung's disease. J Pediatr Surg 1981;16:164

Schuffler MD: Chronic intestinal pseudo-obstruction syndromes. Med Clin North Am 1981;65:1331–1357

Staple TW, McAlister WH, Anderson MS: Plexiform neurofi bromatosis of the colon simulating Hirschsprung's disease. Am J Roentgenol Radium Ther Nucl Med 1964;91:840

Neoplasms

Bartram CI, Thornton A: Colonic polyp patterns in familial polyposis. AJR Am J Roentgenol 1984;142:305

Berk RN: Polypoid lesions of the colon. Postgrad Radiol 1981;1:29

Bryne WJ, Jimenez JF, Euler AR, et al: Lymphoid polyps (focal lymphoid hyperplasia) of the colon in children. Pediatrics 1982;69:598

Capitanio MA, Kirkpatrick JA: Lymphoid hyperplasia of the colon in children: roentgen observations. Radiology 1970;94:323

Cremin BJ, Louw JH: Polyps in the large bowel in children. Clin Radiol 1970;21:195

Dodds WJ: Clinical and roentgen features of the intestinal polyposis syndromes. Gastrointest Radiol 1976;1:127

Erbe RW: Inherited gastrointestinal-polyposis syndromes. N Engl J Med 1976;295:1101

Franken EA, Bixler D, Fitzgerald JF, et al: Juvenile polyposis of the colon. Ann Radiol (Paris) 1975;18:499

Howell J, Pringle K, Kirschner B, et al: Peutz-Jeghers polyps causing colocolic intussusception in infancy. J Pediatr Surg 1981;16:82

Lamego CM, Torloni H: Colorectal adenocarcinoma in childhood and adolescence: report of 11 cases and review of the literature. Pediatr Radiol 1989;19:504

Laufer I, deSa D: Lymphoid follicular pattern: a normal feature of the pediatric colon. AJR Am J Roentgenol 1978;130:51

Lewis CT, Riley WE, Georgeson K, et al: Carcinoma of the colon and rectum in patients less than 20 years of age. South Med J 1990;83:383

Pratt CB, George SL: Epidemic colon cancer in children and

adolescents. *In* Correa P, Haenszel W (eds): Epidemiology of Cancer of the Digestive Tract. Boston, Martinus Nijhoff, 1982:127–145

Radin DR, Fortgang KC, Zee CS, et al: Turcot syndrome: a case with spinal cord and colonic neoplasms. AJR Am J Roentgenol 1984;142:475

Rao BN, Pratt CB, Flaming ID, et al: Colon carcinoma in children and adolescents. Cancer 1985;55:1322

Schatello CR, Pickren WJ, Grace JT Jr: Generalized juvenile gastrointestinal polyposis: a hereditary syndrome. Gastroenterology 1970; 58:699

Inflammatory and Infectious Diseases

Abramson SJ, Berdon WE, Baker DH: Childhood typhlitis: its increasing association with acute myelogenous leukemia. Radiology 1983; 146:61

Archibald RB, Nelson JA: Necrotizing enterocolitis in acute leukemia: radiographic findings. Gastrointest Radiol 1978;3:63

Atkinson GO Jr, Gay BB, Ball TI Jr, et al: *Yersinia enterocolitica* colitis in infants: radiographic changes. Pediatr Radiol 1983;146:113

Balachandran S, Hayden CK Jr, Swischuk LE: Filiform polyposis in a child with Crohn disease. Pediatr Radiol 1984;14:171

Bartlett JG: Antimicrobial agents implicated in *Clostridium difficile* toxin–associated diarrhea or colitis. Johns Hopkins Med J 1981; 149:6

Blickman J, Boland G, Cleveland R, et al: Pseudomembranous colitis: CT findings in children. Pediatr Radiol 1995;25(Suppl 1):157

Bolandi L, Ferrentino M, Trevisani F, et al: Sonographic appearance of pseudomembranous colitis. J Ultrasound Med 1985;4:489

Brunner D, Feifarek C, McNeely D, et al: CT of pseudomembranous colitis. Gastrointest Radiol 1984;9:73

Cammerer RC, Anderson DL, Boyce HW Jr, Burdick GE: Clinical spectrum of pseudomembranous colitis. JAMA 1976;235:2502

Chamovitz BN, Hartstein AI, Alexander SR, et al: *Campylobacter jejuni*–associated hemolytic-uremic syndrome in a mother and daughter. Pediatrics 1983;71:253

Crisci K, Greenberg S, Wolfson B, et al: Contrast enema findings of fibrosing colonopathy. Pediatr Radiol 1997;27:315

Davidson M, Bloom AA, Kugler MK: Chronic ulcerative colitis of childhood: an evaluative review. J Pediatr 1965;67:471

Devroede GJ, Taylor WF, Sauer WG, et al: Cancer risk and life expectancy of children with ulcerative colitis. N Engl J Med 1971;285:17

Diner WC, Barnard HJ: Toxic megacolon: Semin Rotentgenol 1973; 8:433

Durno C, Sherman P, Williams T, et al: Magnetic resonance imaging to distinguish to type and severity of pediatric inflammatory bowel diseases. J Pediatr Gastroenterol Nutr 2000;30:170

Eklöf O, Gierup J: The retrorectal soft tissue space in children: normal variations and appearances in graulomatous colitis. Am J Roentgenol Radium Ther Nucl Med 1970;108:624

Frick MP, Maile CW, Crass JR, et al: Computed tomography of neutropenic colitis. AJR Am J Roentgenol 1984;143:763

Goldstein SJ, Crooks DJM: Colitis in Behçet's syndrome: two new cases. Radiology 1978;128:321

Gore RM, Marn CS, Kirby DF, et al: CT findings in ulcerative, granulomatous and indeterminate colitis. AJR Am J Roentgenol 1984;143:279

Grand RJ, Homer DR: Approaches to inflammatory bowel disease in childhood and adolescence. Pediatr Clin North Am 1975;22:835

Hamilton JR, Bruce GA, Abdourhaman M, et al: Inflammatory bowel disease in children and adolescents. Adv Pediatr 1979;26:311

Hunter TB, Bjelland JC: Gastrointestinal complications of leukemia and its treatment. AJR Am J Roentgenol 1984;142:513

Hymans JS, Berman MM, Helgason H: Nonantibiotic-associated enterocolitis caused by *Clostridium difficile* in an infant. J Pediatr 1981;99:750

Joffe N: Diffuse mucosal granularity in double-contrast studies of Crohn's disease of the colon. Clin Radiol 1981;32:85

Karjoo M, McCarthy B: Toxic megacolon of ulcerative colitis in infancy. Pediatrics 1976;57:962

Karmali MA, Steele BT, Petric M, et al: Sporadic cases of haemolytic-uraemic syndrome associated with faecal cytotoxin and cytotoxin-producing *Escherichia coli* in stools. Lancet 1983;1:619

Kawanami T, Bowen A, Girdany BR: Enterocolitis: prodrome of the hemolytic-uremic syndrome. Radiology 1984;151:91

Kelvin FM, Oddson TA, Rice RP, et al: Double contrast barium enema in Crohn disease and ulcerative colitis. AJR Am J Roentgenol 1978;131:207

Kirks DR: The radiology of enteritis due to hemolytic-uremic syndrome. Pediatr Radiol 1982;12:179

Liebhaber MI, Parker BR, Morton JA, et al: Abdominal mass and colonic perforation in a case of the hemolytic-uremic syndrome. Am J Dis Child 1977;131:1168

Loughran CR, Tappin JA, Whitehouse GH: The plain abdominal radiograph in pseudomembranous colitis due to *Clostridium difficule*. Clin Radiol 1982;33:277

McNamara MJ, Chalmers AG, Morgan M, et al: Typhlitis in acute childhood leukemia: radiological features. Clin Radiol 1986;37:83

Stringer DA, Cleghorn GJ, Daneman A, et al: Behçet's syndrome involving the gastrointestinal tract: a diagnostic dilemma in childhood. Pediatr Radiol 1986;16:131

Stringer DA, Sherman PM, Jakowenko N: Correlation of double-contrast high-density barium enema, colonoscopy, and histology in children with special attention to disparitis. Pediatr Radiol 1986; 16:298

Tochen ML, Campbell JR: Colitis in children with the hemolytic-uremic syndrome. J Pediatr Surg 1977;12:213

Vlymen WJ, Moskowitz PS: Roentgenolgraphic manifestations of esophageal and intestinal involvement in Behçet's disease in children. Pediatr Radiol 1981;10:193

Wagner ML, Rosenberg HS, Fernbach JJ, et al: Typhlitis: a complication of leukemia in childhood. Am J Roentgenol Radium Ther Nucl Med 1971;109:341

Winthrop JD, Balfe DM, Shackelford GD, et al: Ulcerative and granulomatous colitis in children. Radiology 1985;154:657

Zerin J, Kuhn-Fulton J, White S, et al: Colonic strictures in children with cystic fibrosis. Radiology 1995;194:223

Appendicitis

Abu-Yousef MM, Franken EA Jr: An overview of graded compression sonography in the diagnosis of acute appendicitis. Semin US CT MR 1989;10:352

Borushok KF, Jeffrey RB Jr, Laing FC, et al: Sonographic diagnosis of perforation in patients with acute appendicitis. AJR Am J Roentgenol 1990;154:275

Dilley A, Wesson D, Munden M, et al: The impact of ultrasound examinations on the management of children with suspected appendicitis: a 3-year analysis. J Pediatr Surg 2001;36:303

Fedyshin P, Kelvin FM, Rice RP: Nonspecificity of barium enema findings in acute appendicitis. AJR Am J Roentgenol 1984;143:99

Garcia CJ, Rosenfeld NS: The barium enema in the diagnosis of acute appendicitis. Semin US CT MR 1989;10:314

Jeffrey RB Jr, Laing FC, Townsend RR: Acute appendicitis: sonographic criteria based on 250 cases. Radiology 1988;167:327

Johnson JF, Coughlin WF: Plain film diagnosis of appendiceal perforation in children. Semin US CT MR 1989;10:306

Kao SCS, Smith WL, Abu-Yousef MM, et al: Acute appendicitis in children: sonographic findings. AJR Am J Roentgenol 1989;153:375

Kottmeier PK: Appendicitis. *In* Welch KJ, Randolph JG, Ravitch MM, et al (eds): Pediatric Surgery. St Louis, Mosby–Year Book, 1986: 989–994

Lowe L, Penney M, Stein S, et al: Unenhanced limited CT of the abdomen in the diagnosis of appendicitis in children: comparison with sonography. AJR Am J Roentgenol 2001;176:31

Lowe L, Perez R Jr, Stein S, et al: Appendicitis and alternate diagnosis in children: findings on unenhanced limited helical CT. Pediatr Radiol 2001;31:569

Menneman PL, Marcus CS, Inkelis SH, et al: Evaluation of children with possible appendicitis using technetium 99m leukocyte scan. Pediatrics 1990;85:838

Navarro DA, Weber PM: Indium-111 imaging in appendicitis. Semin US CT MR 1989;10:321

Nunez D Jr, Yrizarry JM, Casillas VJ, et al: Percutaneous management of appendiceal abscesses. Semin US CT MR 1989;10:348

Pena B, Taylor G, Fishman S, et al: Costs and effectiveness of ultrasonography and limited computed tomography for diagnosis appendicitis in children. Pediatrics 2000;106:672

Puylaert JB: Acute appendicitis: US evaluation using graded compression. Radiology 1986;158:355

Rice RP, Thompson WM, Fedyshin PJ, et al: The barium enema in appendicitis: spectrum of appearances and pitfalls. Radiographics 1984;4:393

Shandling B, Fallis JC: Acute appendicitis. *In* Behrman RE, Vaughn VC III (eds): Nelson Textbook of Pediatrics. Philadelphia, WB Saunders, 1987:810–813

Shimkin PM: Radiology of acute appendicitis. AJR Am J Roentgenol 1978;130:1001

Sivit C, Applegate K, Stallion A, et al: Imaging evaluation of suspected appendicitis in a pediatric population: effectiveness of sonography versus CT. AJR Am J Roentgenol 2000;175:977

Sivit C, Dudgeon D, Applegate K, et al: Evaluation of suspected appendicitis in children and young adults: helical CT. Radiology 2000;216:430

Sivit C, Newman K, Chandra R: Visualization of enlarged mesenteric lymph nodes at US examination: clinical significance. Pediatr Radiol 1993;23:471–475

Slovis TL, Haller JO, Cohen HL, et al: Complicated appendiceal inflammatory disease in children: pylephlebitis and liver abscess. Radiology 1989;171:823

Van Sonnenberg E, Wittich GR, Gasola G, et al: Periappendiceal abscesses: percutaneous drainage. Radiology 1987;163:23

Vignault F, Filiatrault D, Brandt ML, et al: Acute appendicitis in children: evaluation with US. Radiology 1990;176:501

Wantanabe M, Ishii E, Hirowatari Y, et al: Evaluation of abdominal lymphadenopathy in children by ultrasonography. Pediatr Radiol 1997;27:860–864

Zerin JM: Intrathoracic appendicitis in a ten-year-old girl. Invest Radiol 1990;25:1162

Miscellaneous Disorders

Andersen JF, Eklöf O, Thomasson B: Large bowel volvulus in children. Pediatr Radiol 1981;11:129

Berger RB, Hillmeier AC, Stahl RS, et al: Volvulus of the ascending colon: an unusual complication of nonrotation of the midgut. Pediatr Radiol 1982;12:298

Campbell JR, Blank E: Sigmoid volvulus in children. Pediatrics 1974;53:702

Hernanz-Schulman M, Kirkpatrick J Jr, Schwachman H, et al: Pneumatosis intestinalis in cystic fibrosis. Radiology 1986;160:497

Kirks DR, Swischuk LE, Merten DF, et al: Cecal volvulus in children, AJR Am J Roentgenol 1981;136:419

Knight PJ, Morse TS: Splenic flexure volvulus. J Pediatr Surg 1981;16:744

Reinarz S, Smith WL, Franken EA, et al: Splenic flexure volvulus: a complication of pseudoobstruction in infancy. AJR Am J Roentgenol 1985;145:1303

Sivit CJ, Josephs SH, Taylor GA, et al: Pneumatosis intestinalis in children with AIDS. AJR Am J Roentgenol 1990;155:133

Wood RE, Herman CJ, Johnson KW, et al: Pneumatosis coli in cystic fibrosis. Am J Dis Child 1985;129:246

Yeager AM, Kanof ME, Kramer SS, et al: Pneumatosis intestinalis in children after allogeneic bone marrow transplantation. Pediatr Radiol 1987;17:18

PART IX

ABDOMINAL TRAUMA

CARLOS J. SIVIT

Abdominal trauma in children most commonly occurs following blunt force injury. Over 80% of injuries in childhood are the result of blunt trauma. Abdominal injury is second in frequency to head injury in children. The most common reported mechanism is motor vehicle crashes, followed by auto–pedestrian injuries. Other common injuries relate to falls from a height and bicycle injuries. In young children, injuries may result from intentional trauma.

Computed tomography (CT) is the imaging method of choice in the evaluation of abdominal and pelvic injury after blunt trauma in hemodynamically stable children. Evaluation with CT allows for accurate detection and quantification of injury to solid and hollow viscera. CT also identifies and quantifies intraperitoneal and extraperitoneal fluid and blood and can detect active bleeding. Additionally, CT demonstrates associated bony injury to ribs, spine, and pelvis. The role of CT in the evaluation of injured children includes establishing the presence or absence of visceral and bony injury, detecting active bleeding and estimating associated blood loss, identifying injury requiring close monitoring and operative intervention, and excluding an intra-abdominal or pelvic source of blood loss. The increase in CT screening of injured children over the past two decades, along with improvements in supportive care, has played a large role in the nonoperative management of most solid viscus injuries. The rapid evaluation of injured children with CT has resulted in improved triage and has contributed to reduced morbidity and mortality in these patients.

INDICATIONS

Indications for imaging following blunt trauma include physical examination or laboratory findings suggestive of abdominal injury. These include hematuria, abdominal bruising or ecchymosis, abdominal distention, abdominal pain, absence of bowel sounds, vomiting, decreased hematocrit, and blood per rectum or naso-pharyngeal tube aspirate. Children should be hemodynamically stable prior to CT. An unstable patient needs to be stabilized or to proceed directly to surgery for evaluation. If they require rapid imaging, hemodynamically unstable children can be examined at the bedside with sonography.

The most common indication for CT in children is hematuria. Several points to be noted regarding hematuria and abdominal injury include (1) the majority of children with hematuria do not have urinary tract injury, (2) non–urinary tract injury is observed more frequently than urinary tract injury in children with hematuria, and (3) asymptomatic hematuria is a low-risk indicator for abdominal injury.

Clinical variables that have been associated with a high risk of injury include gross hematuria, abdominal tenderness, lap belt ecchymoses, and a low trauma score. Lap belt ecchymoses represent an important high-risk marker for injury. These linear ecchymoses across the lower abdomen or flank are seen in belted passengers involved in motor vehicle crashes. The ecchymoses show the pattern of the lap belt. They are associated with a complex of injury to the lumbar spine, bowel, and bladder accounting for the majority of injuries to belted motor vehicle passengers.

Two clinical findings that are frequently used as indications for CT but have a low diagnostic yield in predicting injury are asymptomatic hematuria and neurologic impairment in the absence of abdominal signs and symptoms. Abdominal injuries in both of these groups have been shown to be uncommon and minor in significance.

TECHNIQUE

A precise protocol is critical to minimize the length of the examination and maximize the information obtained. Children should be placed on the table supine with their hands above their heads because the hands will produce beam-hardening artifacts that will degrade the image. Monitoring devices and metallic leads should be moved from the scanning plane because they will yield streak artifacts. Gastric distention should be relieved because artifacts may arise from air–fluid interfaces. Sedation is rarely required prior to CT. However, excessive patient motion will result in image degradation. Therefore, in select instances, a short-acting sedative may be necessary to obtain diagnostic images.

The use of intravenous (IV) contrast by rapid bolus injection is essential to maximize opacification of solid viscera and ensure adequate injury detection. We administer 2 ml/kg with a maximum amount of 120 ml. IV contrast is necessary because solid viscus laceration or hematoma may be relatively isodense to unenhanced or poorly enhanced solid viscera. Additionally, the use of IV contrast allows for the detection of active hemorrhage. Scanning of the pelvis should be delayed by several minutes after IV contrast injection to optimize bladder distention by IV contrast.

There is a great deal of controversy regarding the use of oral contrast following blunt trauma. Potential advantages to the use of oral contrast include (1) enhanced detection of small intramural or mesenteric hematomas, (2) improved delineation of the pancreas from surrounding bowel, and (3) detection of oral contrast extravasation as a sign of bowel rupture. Potential disadvantages include (1) time constraints and decreased bowel motility in injured children, which limits the ability to opacify much beyond the proximal small bowel; (2) creation of artifacts from air–contrast interfaces in the stomach; and (3) the possibility of vomiting with resultant aspiration. If oral contrast is utilized, dilute (2%) water-soluble contrast material should be administered 20 to 30 minutes prior to scanning.

CT FINDINGS IN ABDOMINAL TRAUMA

HEPATIC INJURY

The liver is the most frequently injured viscus following blunt trauma. Most injury occurs in the posterior segment of the right lobe. The effects of blunt force are maximized in this location because the posterior right lobe is fixed by the coronary ligaments, which limits its movement while the rest of the liver is free to move. This results in shearing forces centered in the posterior segment of the right lobe. A laceration appears as a nonenhancing region of varying configuration (Fig. 1). It may be linear or branching. Lacerations may be associated with either an intraparenchymal or a subcapsular hematoma.

The liver is surrounded by a thin capsule that in turn is covered by peritoneal reflection of thin connective tissue. The presence of hemoperitoneum associated with hepatic injury principally relates to whether the liver capsule remains intact at the site of injury. In several large series, hepatic injury was associated with hemoperitoneum in approximately two thirds of cases. Associated hemoperitoneum may be seen throughout

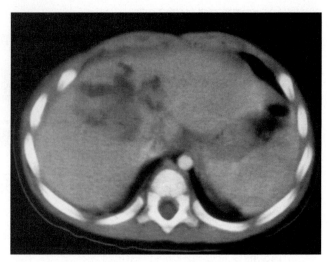

FIGURE 1. Hepatic laceration. Contrast-enhanced computed tomography scan through the upper abdomen demonstrates a complex hepatic laceration.

the greater peritoneal cavity. Often the largest fluid pockets are located in the pelvis.

Hepatic injury may not be associated with intraperitoneal hemorrhage if the injury does not extend to the surface of the liver, if the hepatic capsule is not disrupted, or if there is extension to the liver surface in the bare area of the liver, which is devoid of peritoneal reflection (Fig. 2). The bare area is the site of insertion of the coronary ligaments. Injury extending to the bare area may lead to associated retroperitoneal hemorrhage, with blood often surrounding the right adrenal gland or extending into the anterior pararenal space.

Circumferential zones of periportal low-attenuation may be seen in the liver following trauma (Fig. 3). The presence of these low attenuation zones does not indicate hepatic injury. They are likely due to intravascular third-space fluid losses following fluid resuscitation. The fluid extends to the periportal lymphatics,

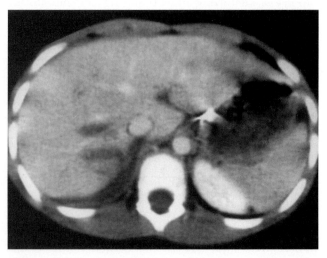

FIGURE 2. Hepatic laceration through the bare area. Contrast-enhanced computed tomography scan through the upper abdomen demonstrates a laceration extending into the bare area of the liver.

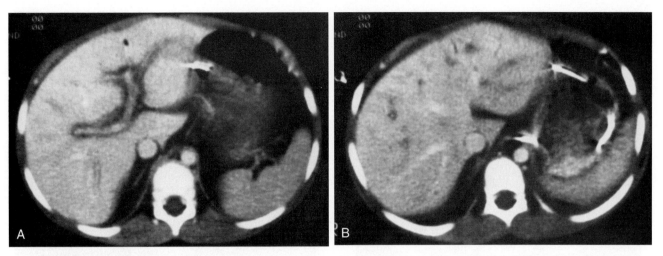

FIGURE 3. Periportal low-attenuation zones. Contrast-enhanced computed tomography scan through the liver demonstrates circumferential periportal low-attenuation zones surrounding the right and left main portal veins **(A)** and surrounding peripheral portal venules **(B)**.

which are located within the portal triad. Thus the periportal zones of low attenuation result from distention of these lymphatics.

There have been a number of grading scales proposed to quantify the severity of hepatic injury. The scales emphasize the anatomic extent of the injury, including capsular integrity, extent of subcapsular collection, extent of parenchymal disruption, and state of the vascular pedicle. In children, these scales are not predictive of need for operative management because the vast majority of hepatic injury can be successfully managed nonoperatively regardless of severity.

SPLENIC INJURY

Splenic injury is also common after blunt trauma. It is frequently associated with other organ injuries. Splenic lacerations have a variable appearance ranging from linear to a branching pattern. Because the spleen is much smaller than the liver, complex injury results in shattering or fragmentation of the organ (Fig. 4). Associated intraparenchymal or subcapsular hematoma may be present (Fig. 5). As with hepatic injury, associated intraperitoneal hemorrhage is not always present, and retroperitoneal hemorrhage may be present. If the splenic capsule remains intact, there is no associated hemoperitoneum. The absence of associated hemoperitoneum is seen in approximately 25% of splenic injuries. Blood can track into the retroperitoneum after splenic injury. This typically occurs with injury extending to the splenic hilum. In these instances, blood extends along the splenorenal ligament into the anterior pararenal space surrounding the pancreas (Fig. 6).

As with hepatic injury, various injury grading scales have been reported for quantifying injury to the spleen. As is true for hepatic injury, these scales are not measures of required treatment, because nonoperative

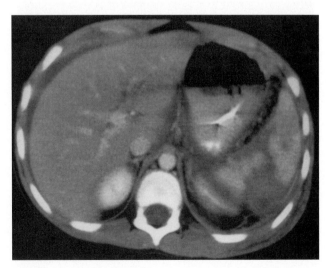

FIGURE 4. Shattered spleen. Contrast-enhanced computed tomography scan through the upper abdomen shows a shattered spleen.

FIGURE 5. Splenic laceration with associated intraparenchymal hematoma. Contrast-enhanced computed tomography scan through the upper abdomen demonstrates a splenic laceration with associated intraparenchymal hematoma posteriorly.

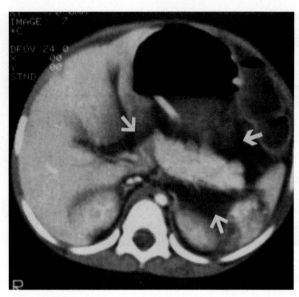

FIGURE 6. Splenic injury with retroperitoneal extension of hemorrhage. Contrast-enhanced computed tomography scan through the upper abdomen shows a splenic laceration associated with blood in the anterior pararenal space *(arrows)* surrounding the pancreas.

management is successful in the majority of splenic injuries.

Pitfalls that may result in false-positive diagnosis of splenic injury include heterogeneous splenic enhancement early during the bolus, and splenic lobulations and clefts that mimic a laceration. The heterogeneous splenic enhancement is due to differences in enhancement between red and white pulp in the spleen. This artifact can be avoided by instituting a delay of at least 70 seconds prior to scanning after the administration of IV contrast. Splenic clefts and lobulations typically have smooth contours and thus can be differentiated from lacerations, which typically have irregular contours.

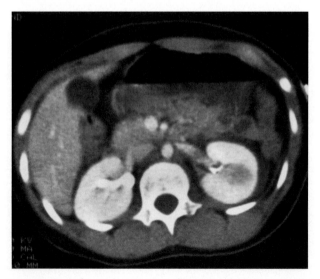

FIGURE 7. Left renal contusion. Contrast-enhanced computed tomography scan through the midabdomen shows a rounded focus of low attenuation in the midpole of the left kidney indicative of contusion.

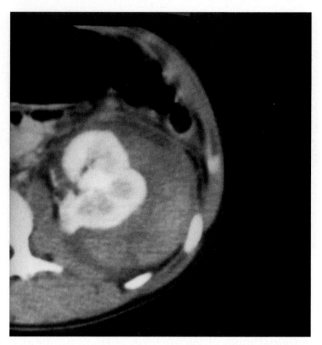

FIGURE 8. Subcapsular renal hematoma. Contrast-enhanced computed tomography through the midabdomen demonstrates a large left-sided subcapsular hematoma compressing the left renal parenchyma.

RENAL INJURY

The kidney is the third most frequently injured abdominal viscera in children. Renal parenchymal injury typically results from direct impact, whereas vascular and collecting system injury usually results from deceleration. The most common renal injury is the parenchymal contusion, which is manifested on CT by a focal or diffuse region of delayed contrast enhancement (Fig. 7). The contusion represents an organ bruise characterized by microscopic areas of hemorrhage and surrounding edema. The involved kidney may also appear larger on CT as a result of the associated edema.

Renal injury may be complicated by perirenal hematoma, which may be subcapsular or perinephric. These two types of hematoma can be differentiated on the basis of CT features: a subcapsular hematoma is limited in its extension by the renal capsule and will therefore exert greater mass effect on renal parenchyma (Fig. 8), whereas a perinephric hematoma is distributed throughout the perirenal space and typically demonstrates less mass effect on renal parenchyma.

Renal collecting system injury results in urinary extravasation of IV contrast medium (Fig. 9). Delayed scanning with CT may be useful in detecting such extravasation. Urine leakage typically remains encapsulated in the perirenal space and is referred to as a urinoma. Occasionally, hemorrhage or urinary extravasation may extend into the pelvis, owing to direct communication between the perirenal space in the abdomen and the prevesical extraperitoneal space in the pelvis in some patients.

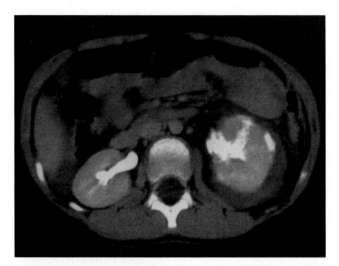

FIGURE 9. Renal collecting system injury. Contrast-enhanced computed tomography scan through the midabdomen shows a left renal laceration with extravasation of intravenous contrast into the perirenal space. Also note low-attenuation perinephric fluid.

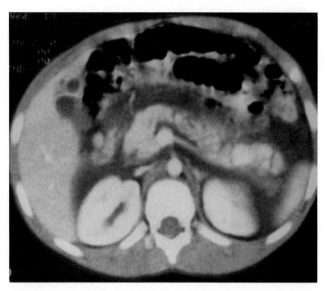

FIGURE 11. Pancreatic injury with associated peripancreatic fluid. Contrast-enhanced computed tomography scan through the upper abdomen shows fluid in the anterior pararenal space surrounding the pancreas. Also note fluid dissecting between the splenic vein and pancreas.

PANCREATIC INJURY

Pancreatic injury is relatively uncommon in children. Injury typically results from direct compression of the gland against the vertebral column. The most common mechanism is from a bicycle handlebar injury. Direct signs of injury may be difficult to identify owing to the small size of the gland, the paucity of surrounding fat, and the minimal separation of fracture fragments (Fig. 10). Pancreatic injury can be complicated by pancreatitis and by peripancreatic fluid collections, which may evolve into pancreatic pseudocysts. Trauma is the leading cause of pancreatitis in children.

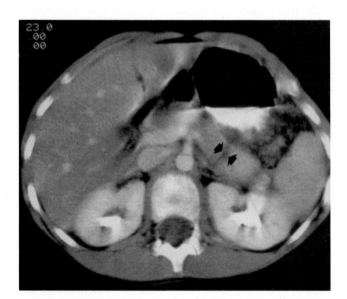

FIGURE 10. Pancreatic injury. Contrast-enhanced computed tomography scan through the upper abdomen demonstrates a laceration through the junction of the body and tail of the pancreas (arrows).

The best indicator of pancreatic injury at CT is unexplained peripancreatic fluid (fluid in the anterior pararenal space or lesser sac) (Fig. 11). This finding may be seen more often than the actual laceration. Fluid in the anterior pararenal space may also dissect between the pancreas and splenic vein.

Pancreatic injury is only one cause of fluid in the anterior pararenal space. Other causes include third-space intravascular fluid loss, blood extending from injury to the spleen or bare area of the liver, blood or bowel contents from a duodenal injury, and blood or urine dissecting from a renal injury after disruption of the renal fascia. Additional CT signs of pancreatic injury include diffuse gland enlargement, stranding of peripancreatic fat, and thickening of the anterior renal fascia.

A false-positive diagnosis of pancreatic injury may result from the partial volume effect caused by the gland's small size and undulating nature. This pitfall may be avoided by obtaining repeat sections through the pancreas utilizing thinner collimation.

PERITONEAL FLUID AND HEMORRHAGE

The attenuation values of blood in the peritoneal cavity vary widely dependent on whether it is unclotted blood (hemoperitoneum), clotted blood, or active hemorrhage. Many factors affect the measured attenuation values for peritoneal fluid on CT, including measurement technique, fluid location within the field, artifacts, and delayed fluid enhancement following IV contrast administration. Unclotted hemoperitoneum has attenuation values that range from 20 to 60 H.U. Approximately one third of fluid pockets will demontrate attenuation values of less than 30 H.U. Low-attenuation fluid (<60 H.U.) in the acutely injured child may also

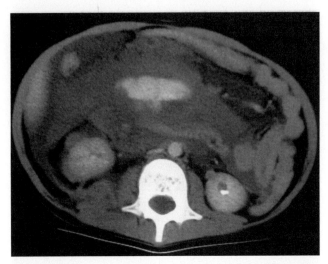

FIGURE 12. Active hemorrhage. Contrast-enhanced computed tomography scan through the midabdomen shows a focal high-attenuation collection representing intravenous contrast extravasation from a mesenteric arterial tear.

represent bile, urine, bowel contents, third-space fluid losses or pre-existing ascites.

Clotted blood has higher attenuation values (60 to 90 H.U.) than free-flowing blood because of the greater density and hemoglobin content. Because clotted blood is typically seen adjacent to the site of injury, the presence of focal, higher attenuation clotted blood has been described as the "sentinel clot" sign and is a marker for the principal site of hemorrhage. This may occasionally be useful in localizing the site of injury.

Children are typically excluded from CT if ongoing bleeding is clinically evident. Occasionally, CT may demonstrate active hemorrhage in children who appear hemodynamically stable. The amount of hemoperitoneum noted on CT is not a measure of ongoing hemorrhage. Rather, it reflects the cumulative amount of bleeding occurring between the time of injury and the time that CT was obtained. The only sign of active hemorrhage on CT is focal or high-attenuation areas (>90 H.U.) (Fig. 12). CT is useful in these cases not only in identifying the active bleeding but in localizing the site of hemorrhage. This finding may occasionally be observed only on delayed scanning.

The absence of peritoneal fluid or blood does not exclude the presence of hepatic or splenic injury. Over one third of hepatic injuries and one fourth of splenic injuries in children have no associated peritoneal fluid. The relatively high prevalence of hepatic and splenic injury without associated peritoneal fluid has significant implications for imaging strategies for evaluating injured children. Sonography is highly sensitive in the detection of peritoneal fluid. However, the sensitivity of sonography in the detection of solid viscus injury has not been as good, with over one third of injuries missed in some studies. Thus, if one relies on identifying peritoneal fluid as a marker for hepatic and splenic injury, one will miss a significant number of injuries.

BOWEL INJURY

Bowel injury is uncommon after blunt trauma in children. Injury can result in intramural hematoma or bowel rupture. Associated mesenteric injury is often present. Most injuries are noted in children who have been involved in motor vehicle crashes and who display lap belt ecchymoses. The clinical diagnosis of bowel injury may be challenging. Clinical signs and symptoms may be absent, minimal, or delayed. Increased morbidity and mortality are associated with delayed diagnosis.

Intramural hematoma results from hemorrhage into the bowel wall, typically through a partial-thickness tear. The most common location is the duodenum. The injury can usually be managed nonoperatively. Large hematomas can result in a proximal small bowel obstruction. The CT appearance is that of focal bowel wall thickening. Large hematomas may appear dumbell shaped (Fig. 13). No extraluminal air or contrast material should be present.

Bowel rupture most commonly occurs in the mid to distal small intestine. The most common site is the jejunum. Extraluminal air is noted on CT in only approximately one third of cases. Review of the examination at a wide window setting is helpful in the detection of small amounts of extraluminal air (Fig. 14). The prevalence of extravasation of oral contrast material is even lower, ranging from 0% to 12% in published series. The most frequent CT findings associated with bowel rupture are "unexplained" peritoneal fluid (moderate to large amounts of fluid in the absence of solid viscus injury or bony pelvic fracture) (Fig. 15). Approximately one half of children with moderate to large amounts of peritoneal fluid as the only finding on CT following blunt trauma have a bowel injury. Additional CT findings seen with bowel rupture include abnormally intense bowel wall enhancement (Fig. 16), focal bowel wall discontinuity, bowel dilatation, bowel wall thickening, and streaky infiltration of mesenteric

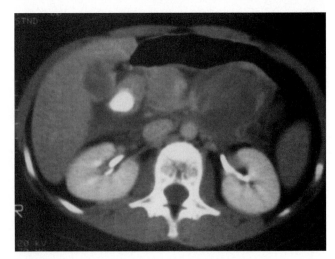

FIGURE 13. Duodenal hematoma. Contrast-enhanced computed tomography scan through the upper abdomen demonstrates a rounded duodenal hematoma to the left of midline.

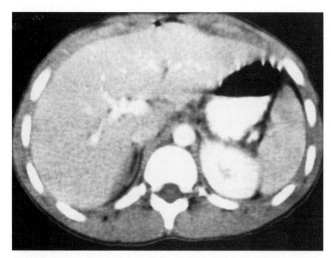

FIGURE 14. Bowel rupture with associated extraluminal air. Contrast-enhanced computed tomography scan through the upper abdomen shows a small collection of extraluminal air anterior to the left lobe of the liver.

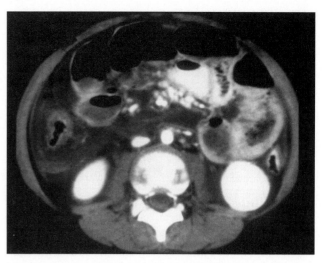

FIGURE 16. Bowel rupture with abnormally intense bowel wall enhancement and bowel wall thickening. Contrast-enhanced computed tomography scan through the midabdomen demonstrates focally thick-walled bowel loops anterior to the left kidney. Note the associated intense bowel wall enhancement. At surgery, jejunal rupture was noted.

fat. The latter finding may result from either associated mesenteric injury or chemical irritation of the mesentery from spilled intestinal contents.

BLADDER INJURY

Bladder injury is also uncommon in children. Bladder rupture can be intraperitoneal or extraperitoneal. Combined injuries may occur. Extraperitoneal bladder rupture occurs more frequently than intraperitoneal rupture in children. Approximately two thirds of posttraumatic bladder ruptures are extraperitoneal in location. Intraperitoneal rupture typically results from

shearing of the distended bladder by a lap belt, whereas extraperitoneal rupture often results from laceration by a bony spicule from a pelvic fracture.

The use of delayed scanning on CT before imaging the pelvis is essential in order to maximize bladder distention so as to demonstrate extravasation of IV contrast material in children with bladder rupture (Fig. 17). The Foley catheter should be clamped prior to IV contrast administration. CT cystography may also be performed in children with suspected bladder rupture. During this procedure, dilute iodinated contrast is instilled into the bladder in a retrograde fashion, followed by clamping of the Foley catheter. Images are then obtained through the pelvis over several minutes.

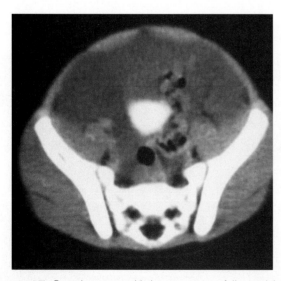

FIGURE 15. Bowel rupture with large amount of "unexplained" peritoneal fluid. Contrast-enhanced computed tomography (CT) scan through the upper pelvis shows a large amount of peritoneal fluid. The patient did not have any other abnormalities noted on CT. At surgery, a jejunal rupture was noted.

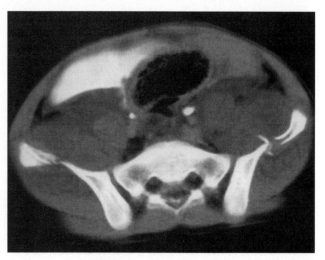

FIGURE 17. Intraperitoneal bladder rupture. Contrast-enhanced computed tomography scan through the upper pelvis shows high-attenuation fluid in the right lateral pelvic recess secondary to intraperitoneal bladder rupture.

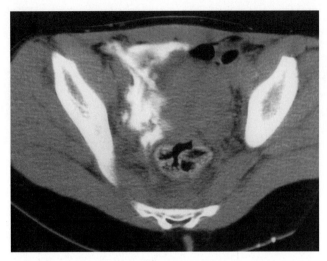

FIGURE 18. Extraperitoneal bladder rupture. Contrast-enhanced computed tomography scan through the pelvis shows high-attenuation fluid adjacent to the pelvic side walls and low-attenuation fluid posterior to the rectum. These fluid collections are extraperitoneal in location, consistent with extraperitoneal bladder rupture.

The location of extravasated IV contrast material on CT is useful in differentiating intraperitoneal from extraperitoneal bladder rupture. This distinction is important because an extraperitoneal bladder rupture is typically managed nonsurgically, whereas an intraperitoneal rupture requires immediate surgical repair. Intraperitoneal fluid in the pelvis will be located in the lateral perivesical spaces superior to the bladder and anterior to the rectosigmoid colon. Extraperitoneal pelvic fluid will be localized in the perivesical space that surrounds the bladder superiorly and anteriorly to the umbilicus and posteriorly behind the rectum. Thus, if pelvic fluid is noted lateral to the bladder or behind the rectum, it is extraperitoneal in location (Fig. 18). Fluid superior and anterior to the bladder may be intraperitoneal or extraperitoneal. If fluid superior to the bladder is extraperitoneal, it will extend superiorly and anteriorly to the level of the umbilicus. If fluid superior to the bladder is intraperitoneal, it will be in a more lateral location (see Fig. 17) and typically be contiguous with fluid in the lateral pericolic spaces.

HYPOPERFUSION COMPLEX

A characteristic complex of findings on CT associated with hypovolemic shock in severely injured children has been characterized as the "hypoperfusion complex." The majority of these children have had arterial hypotension on admission. The hypotension may be transiently corrected, and it may be believed that the child is hemodynamically stable enough to undergo CT, but the child may subsequently develop rapid hemodynamic decompensation.

CT findings in all children with the hypoperfusion complex include diffuse intestinal dilatation with fluid; abnormally intense contrast enhancement of bowel wall, mesentery, kidneys, aorta, and inferior vena cava; and diminished caliber of the aorta and inferior vena cava (Fig. 19). Variable findings include periportal low-attenuation zones; intense adrenal, pancreatic, and mesenteric enhancement; decreased pancreatic and splenic enhancement; peritoneal and retroperitoneal fluid; and bowel wall thickening.

The hypoperfusion complex is a marker for a tenuous hemodynamic state and a high-risk indicator for a poor outcome. The mortality rate in children with this constellation of findings at CT is over 80%.

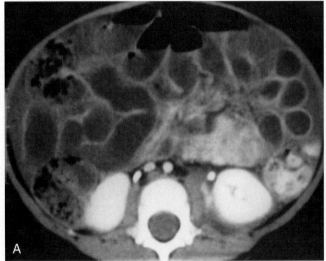
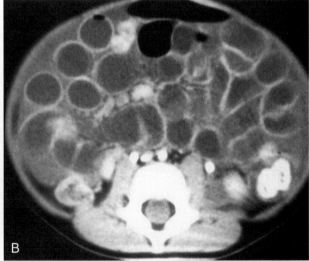

FIGURE 19. Hypoperfusion complex. Contrast-enhanced computed tomography scans through the upper **(A)** and mid **(B)** abdomen demonstrate diffuse intestinal dilatation with fluid, intense contrast enhancement of bowel wall, and diminished caliber of the great vessels indicative of systemic hypoperfusion.

SONOGRAPHY IN THE ASSESSMENT OF ABDOMINAL TRAUMA

Interest has been growing over the past decade in the use of sonography for the assessment of abdominal injury in children and adults. Initial studies utilizing sonography focused primarily on identifying hemoperitoneum. More recent studies have also attempted to evaluate the accuracy of sonography for the diagnosis of solid viscus injury. It is clear that sonography has important limitations in the evaluation of the abdomen in injured children. First, it does not provide any diagnostic information regarding injury to the bony pelvis or lumbar spine. Additionally, sonography cannot be used in the diagnosis of hollow viscus injury. Finally, sonography has been shown to miss approximately one fourth to one third of solid viscus injuries. An important issue that should not be overlooked when evaluating the impact of CT as the primary screening modality for children following abdominal trauma relates to the value of a normal examination. A normal CT examination may prevent unnecessary surgical exploration owing to its ability to provide a comprehensive evaluation of the abdomen and pelvis. It would be difficult to provide such a comprehensive assessment with sonography. As a result, CT remains the primary imaging modality for assessing pediatric abdominal injury. Nevertheless sonography has a useful role in the hemodynamically unstable patient because it can be performed at the bedside prior to taking the patient to the operating room. In this role, it serves as a fast, noninvasive replacement of diagnostic peritoneal lavage.

SUGGESTED READINGS

Basile KE, Sivit CJ, O'Riordan MA, et al: Acute hemoperitoneum in children: prevalence of low-attenuation fluid. Pediatr Radiol 2000; 30:168

Bensard DB, Beaver BL, Besner GE, et al: Small bowel injury in children after blunt abdominal trauma: is diagnostic delay important? J Trauma 1996;41:476

Benya EC, Bulas DI, Eichelberger MR, et al: Splenic injury from blunt abdominal trauma in children: follow-up evaluation with CT. Radiology 1995;195:685

Bond SJ, Eichelberger MR, Gotschall CS, et al: Nonoperative management of blunt hepatic and splenic injury in children. Ann Surg 1996;223:286

Brick SH, Taylor GA, Potter BM, et al: Hepatic and splenic injury in children: role of CT in the decision for laparotomy. Radiology 1987;165:643

Coley BD, Mutabagani KH, Martin LC, et al: Focused abdominal sonography for trauma (FAST) in children with blunt abdominal trauma. J Trauma 2000;48:902

Cooper C, Silverman PM, Davros WJ, et al: Delayed contrast enhancement of ascitic fluid on CT: frequency and significance. AJR Am J Roentgenol 1993;161:787

Federle MP, Yagan N, Peitzman AB, et al: Abdominal trauma: use of oral contrast material for CT is safe. Radiology 1997;205:91

Hara H, Babyn PS, Bourgeois D: Significance of bowel wall enhancement on CT following blunt abdominal trauma in childhood. J Comput Assist Tomogr 1989;13:430

Hollingsworth CL, Bisset GS: CT evaluation of pediatric abdominal trauma: pitfalls and quandaries. Emerg Radiol 2001;8:67

Hulka F, Mullins RJ, Leonardo V, et al: Significance of peritoneal fluid as an isolated finding on abdominal computed tomographic scans in pediatric trauma patients. J Trauma 1998;44:1069

Jamieson DH, Babyn PS, Pearl R: Imaging gastrointestinal perforation in pediatric blunt abdominal trauma. Pediatr Radiol 1996;26:188

Levine CD, Patel US, Silverman PM, et al: Low attenuation of acute traumatic hemoperitoneum on CT scans. AJR Am J Roentgenol 1996;166:1089

Lin-Dunham JE, Narra J, Benya EC, et al: Aspiration after administration of oral contrast material in children undergoing abdominal CT for trauma. AJR Am J Roentgenol 1997;169:1015

Luks F, Lemire A, St-Vil D, et al: Blunt abdominal trauma in children: the practical value of sonography. J Trauma 1993;34:607

McGahan JP, Richards JR: Blunt abdominal trauma: the role of emergent sonography and a review of the literature. AJR Am J Roentgenol 1999;172:897

Miller K, Kou D, Sivit CJ, et al: Pediatric hepatic trauma: does clinical course support intensive care unit stay? J Pediatr Surg 1998;33:1459

Morgan DE, Nallamala LK, Kenny PJ, et al: CT cystography: radiographic and clinical predictors of bladder rupture. AJR Am J Roentgenol 2000;174:89

Neisch AS, Taylor GA, Lund DP, et al: Effect of CT information on the diagnosis and management of acute abdominal injury in children. Radiology 1998;206:327

Orwig D, Federle MP: Localized clotted blood as evidence of visceral trauma on CT: the sentinel clot sign. AJR Am J Roentgenol 1989;153:747

Patrick LE, Ball TI, Atkinson GO, et al: Pediatric blunt abdominal trauma: periportal tracking at CT. Radiology 1992;183:689

Patten RM, Spear RP, Vincent LM, et al: Traumatic laceration of the liver limited to the bare area: CT findings in 25 patients. AJR Am J Roentgenol 1993;160:1019

Ruess L, Sivit CJ, Eichelberger MR, et al: Blunt hepatic and splenic trauma in children: correlation of a CT injury severity scale with clinical outcome. Pediatr Radiol 1995;25:321

Ruess L, Sivit CJ, Eichelberger MR, et al: Blunt abdominal trauma in children: impact of CT on operative and nonoperative management. AJR Am J Roentgenol 1997;169:1011

Shankar KR, Lloyd DA, Kitteringham L, et al: Oral contrast with computed tomography in the evaluation of abdominal trauma in children. Br J Surg 1999;86:1073

Sievers EM, Murray JM, Chen D, et al: Abdominal computed tomography scan in pediatric blunt abdominal trauma. Am Surg 1999;65:968

Sivit CJ, Cutting JP, Eichelberger MR: CT diagnosis and localization of rupture of the bladder in children with blunt abdominal trauma: significance of contrast material in the pelvis. AJR Am J Roentgenol 1995;164:1243

Sivit CJ, Eichelberger MR: CT diagnosis of pancreatic injury in children: significance of fluid separating the splenic vein and pancreas. AJR Am J Roentgenol 1995;165:921

Sivit CJ, Eichelberger MR, Taylor GA: CT in children with rupture of the bowel caused by blunt trauma: diagnostic efficacy and comparison with hypoperfusion complex. AJR Am J Roentgenol 1994;163:1195

Sivit CJ, Eichelberger MR, Taylor GA, et al: Blunt pancreatic trauma in children: CT diagnosis. AJR Am J Roentgenol 1992;158:1097

Sivit CJ, Frazier AA, Eichelberger MR: Prevalence and distribution of hemorrhage associated with splenic injury in children. Radiology 1995;197:298

Sivit CJ, Kaufman RA: Commentary: Sonography in the evaluation of children following blunt trauma? Is it to be or not to be? Pediatr Radiol 1995;25:326

Sivit CJ, Peclet MH, Taylor GA: Life-threatening intraperitoneal bleeding: demonstration with CT. Radiology 1989;171:430

Sivit CJ, Taylor GA, Bulas DI, et al: Blunt trauma in children: significance of peritoneal fluid. Radiology 1991;178:185

Sivit CJ, Taylor GA, Bulas DI, et al: Post-traumatic shock in children: CT findings associated with hemodynamic instability. Radiology 1992;182:723

Sivit CJ, Taylor GA, Eichelberger MR, et al: Significance of periportal low-attenuation zones following blunt trauma in children. Pediatr Radiol 1993;23:388

Sivit CJ, Taylor GA, Newman KD, et al: Safety-belt injuries in children with lap-belt ecchymosis: CT findings in 61 patients. AJR Am J Roentgenol 1991;157:111

Stalker HP, Kaufman RA, Towbin R: Patterns of liver injury in childhood: CT analysis. AJR Am J Roentgenol 1986;147:1199

Strouse PJ, Bradley JC, Marshall KW, et al: CT of bowel and mesenteric trauma in children. Radiographics 1999;19:1237

Taylor GA, Eggli KD: Lap-belt injuries of the lumbar spine in children. AJR Am J Roentgenol 1988;150:1355

Taylor GA, Eichelberger MR: Abdominal CT in children with neurologic impairment following blunt trauma. Ann Surg 1989;210:229

Taylor GA, Eichelberger MR, O'Donnell R: Indications for computed tomography in children with blunt abdominal trauma. Ann Surg 1991;213:212

Taylor GA, Eichelberger MR, Potter BM: Hematuria: a marker of abdominal injury in children after blunt trauma. Ann Surg 1988; 208:688

Taylor GA, Fallat ME, Eichelberger MR: Hypovolemic shock in children: abdominal CT manifestations. Radiology 1987;164:479

Taylor GA, Guion CJ, Potter BM, et al: CT of blunt abdominal trauma in children. AJR Am J Roentgenol 1989;153:155

Taylor GA, Kaufman RA, Sivit CJ: Active hemorrhage in children after thoracoabdominal trauma: clinical and CT features. AJR Am J Roentgenol 1994;162:401

Taylor GA, O'Donnell BA, Sivit CJ, et al: Abdominal injury score: a clinical score for the assignment of risk in children after blunt trauma. Radiology 1994;190:689

Taylor GA, Sivit CJ: Posttraumatic peritoneal fluid: is it a reliable indicator of intraabdominal injury in children? J Pediatr Surg 1995;30:1644

SECTION VII

Urinary Tract and Retroperitoneum

JACK O. HALLER

SANDRA K. FERNBACH

KATE A. FEINSTEIN

ALAN DANEMAN

JAMES S. DONALDSON

DOUGLAS F. EGGLI

JOHN R. STY

PART I

OVERVIEW

JACK O. HALLER
DOUGLAS F. EGGLI
JAMES S. DONALDSON

DIAGNOSTIC PROCEDURES, EXCLUDING NUCLEAR MEDICINE

JACK O. HALLER*

CONTRAST MEDIA FOR RADIOGRAPHIC PROCEDURES

Contrast media are pharmaceuticals that alter tissue characteristics to enhance information obtained on diagnostic images. Contrast media available for intravenous (IV) use in radiography (Table 1) are categorized as high-osmolality contrast media (HOCM) and low-osmolality contrast media (LOCM). Considerations in choice are the concentration of iodine achieved within plasma and urine, economic factors, and safety factors.

After IV injection of contrast material, a peak level in the plasma occurs within the first minute. This peak is followed by a rapid decline in the plasma level resulting from renal excretion, dilution of the material from mixing within the vascular space, and rapid diffusion of the molecules into extravascular and extracellular compartments.

The quality of visualization on an excretory urogram or computed tomography (CT) scan is related to the initial level of contrast material present within plasma and available for glomerular filtration and excretion by the kidney. Visibility by urography is related to concentration of contrast material in the urine and the urine volume. Distention of collecting structures further enhances the duality of a diagnostic urogram.

HIGH-OSMOLALITY CONTRAST MEDIA

A monomer ionic contrast medium in solution has two dissolved ions per molecule, a cation and a large organic iodine-containing anion. As salts of diatrizoate, iothalamate, or iodamide, these media have sodium, meglumine, or a combination as the cation. These compounds are listed in Table 1 and grouped according to iodine content.

The first eight products of group 1 are designed primarily for cystography, urethrography, vaginography, retrograde pyelography, antegrade pyelography, and ureterostomy studies. The latter agents of this group may also be used thus, but are more often used for IV

infusion urography or infusion CT enhancement, inferior vena cavogram, renal venography, and arterial injection digital subtraction angiography. The compounds of group 2 are used for IV urography, venography, and bolus IV enhancement of CT scans, abdominal and selective angiography, IV digital subtraction arteriography, or any of the above-mentioned urologic procedures if properly diluted. The agents of group 3 are used primarily for aortography and selective arteriography. They could be used for excretory urography or other vascular procedures, but their high viscosity makes injection through a small needle difficult.

Dosage of contrast material is based on grams of iodine administered in relation to body mass. It is appropriate to use a dosage of approximately 300 mg of iodine per kilogram. This represents approximately 1.0 ml/kg in the most commonly used forms of diatrizoate or iothalamate. The total dose for excretory urography is usually 2.0 ml/kg in children or 3.0 ml/kg in the newborn (Fig. 1).

Speed of injection is important for the resultant plasma concentration of contrast material. After rapid injection, there is an increase in serum osmolality within 3 minutes, a decrease in serum sodium concentration, and an increase in heart rate. The osmotic effect is particularly significant in young infants. A mean increase of 3% in serum osmolality is observed in adults. Excretion occurs rapidly by renal glomerular filtration. Contrast medium is concentrated in the proximal tubules by water and sodium resorption occurring at this level. Because of a high osmotic load, these contrast media also produce diuresis, opposing tubular resorption. The iodine-bearing anion is osmotically active and nonreabsorbable, leading to a diuresis of salt and water. There is less diuretic effect from sodium salts than from the meglumine salts. Additional water resorption occurs in the distal tubules and collecting ducts. The major influence on water resorption at this level is produced by antidiuretic hormone.

Contrast excretion begins immediately on initial circulation through the kidney and peaks at 10 to 20 minutes. At least 50% of injected contrast material is excreted within 2 to 3 hours of injection and 100% is cleared within 24 hours. In patients with renal failure, contrast material remains in the circulation for much longer and may eventually be excreted vicariously from

---

*This chapter is based on the work of Dr. Beverly P. Wood and Dr. Guido Currarino from the prior edition of this book.

Table 1 ■ CONTRAST AGENTS

HIGH-OSMOLALITY IONIC MEDIA (HOCM)					
Contrast Agents (Manufacturer*)	Anion Chemical Structure	Salt (% Concentration)	Iodine Content (mg/ml)	Osmolality (mOsm/kg H_2O)	Viscosity (cps, 37°C)
Group 1: Low-iodine concentration					
Cystografin Dilute (S)	Diatrizoate	Meglumine (18)	85	—	—
Cystografin (S)	Diatrizoate	Meglumine (30)	141	—	—
Reno-M-30 (S)	Diatrizoate	Meglumine (30)	141	—	—
Hypaque Cysto (W)	Diatrizoate	Meglumine (30)	141	—	—
Urovist Cysto (B)	Diatrizoate	Meglumine (30)	141	—	—
Urovist Cysto Ped (B)	Diatrizoate	Meglumine (30)	141	—	—
Cysto Conray II 17.2% (M)	Iothalamate	Meglumine (17.2)	81	—	—
Cysto Conray (M)	Iothalamate	Meglumine (43)	202	—	—
Hypaque (Sodium) 25% (W)	Diatrizoate	Sodium (25)	150	695	1.17
Hypaque (Meglumine) 30% (W)	Diatrizoate	Meglumine (30)	141	633	1.43
Reno-M-DIP (S)	Diatrizoate	Meglumine (30)	141	643	1.4
Urovist Meglumine DIU/CT (B)	Diatrizoate	Meglumine (30)	141	640	1.4
Conray-30 (M)	Iothalamate	Meglumine (30)	141	750	1.5
Conray-43 (M)	Iothalamate	Meglumine (43)	202	100	2.0
Renovue-DIP (S)	Iodamide	Meglumine (24)	111	500	1.8
Group 2: Medium-iodine concentration					
Hypaque (Sodium) 50 (W)	Diatrizoate	Sodium (50)	300	1515	2.43
MD-50 (M)	Diatrizoate	Sodium (50)	300	1546	2.4
Urovist Sodium-300 (B)	Diatrizoate	Meglumine (60)	300	1550	2.4
Hypaque (Meglumine) 60% (W)	Diatrizoate	Meglumine (60)	282	1415	4.1
Reno-M-60 (S)	Diatrizoate	Meglumine (60)	282	1500	4.2
Angiovist-282 (B)	Diatrizoate	Meglumine (60)	282	1400	4.08
Angiovist-292 (B)	Diatrizoate	Meglumine (60); sodium (8)	292	1500	3.93
Renografin 60 (S)	Diatrizoate	Meglumine (52); sodium (8)	292.5	1511	4.0
MD-6 (M)	Diatrizoate	Meglumine (52); sodium (8)	292.5	1539	4.5
Renovist II (S)	Diatrizoate	Meglumine (28.5); sodium (29.1)	309	1616	3.4
Conray 325 (M)	Iothalamate	Sodium (54.3)	325	1700	3.0
Conray 60 (M)	Iothalamate	Meglumine (60)	282	1500	4.0
Renovue-65 (S)	Iodamide	Meglumine (65)	300	1590	6.4
Group 3: High-iodine concentration					
Diatrizoate Meglumine 76% (S)	Diatrizoate	Meglumine (76)	358	1761	9.2
Hypaque-76 (W)	Diatrizoate	Meglumine (66); sodium (0)	370	2016	8.32
Renografin-76 (S)	Diatrizoate	Meglumine (66); sodium (10)	370	1689	8.4
MD-76 (M)	Diatrizoate	Meglumine (66); sodium (10)	370	2140	9.1
Renovist (S)	Diatrizoate	Meglumine (34.3); sodium (35)	370.5	1720	5.5
Hypaque-M 75 (W)	Diatrizoate	Meglumine (50); sodium (25)	385	2108	7.99
Angiovist-370 (B)	Diatrizoate	Meglumine (66); sodium (10)	370	2100	8.4
Conray-400 (M)	Iothalamate	Sodium (66.8)	400	2100	4.5
Angio-Conray (M)	Iothalamate	Sodium (80)	480	2500	9.0
Vascoray (M)	Iothalamate	Meglumine (52); sodium (26)	400	2150	9.0
Hexabrix (M)	Ioxaglate	Meglumine (39.3); sodium (16.9)	320	600	7.5
Omnipaque-180 (W)	Iohexol	Nonionic (38.8)	180	408	2.0
Omnipaque-240 (W)	Iohexol	Nonionic (51.8)	240	504	3.4
Omnipaque-300 (W)	Iohexol	Nonionic (64.7)	300	672	6.3

*B = Berlex Laboratories, Inc. (Cedar Knolls, NJ); M = Mallinkrodt, Inc. (St. Louis, MO); S = E.R. Squibb & Sons, Inc. (New Brunswick, NJ); W = Winthrop Laboratories (New York, NY).

Table continued on following page

Table 1 ■ CONTRAST AGENTS CONTINUED

LOW-OSMOLALITY MEDIA (LOCM)					
Contrast Agents (Manufacturer*)	Anion Chemical Structure	Salt (% Concentration)	Iodine Content (mg/ml)	Osmolality (mOsm/kg H$_2$O)	Viscosity (cps, 37°C)
Omnipaque-350 (W)	Iohexol	Nonionic (75.5)	350	844	10.4
Isovue-128 (S)	Iopamidol	Nonionic (26)	128	290	1.4
Isovue-300 (S)	Iopamidol	Nonionic (61)	300	616	4.7
Isovue-370 (S)	Iopamidol	Nonionic (76)	370	796	9.4
Optiray-160 (M)	Ioversol	Nonionic (34)	160	355	1.9
Optiray-240 (M)	Ioversol	Nonionic (51)	240	502	3.0
Optiray-320 (M)	Ioversol	Nonionic (68)	320	702	5.8

mucosal surfaces, including the small bowel and gall-bladder.

Factors affecting the chemotoxicity of contrast material include concentration, site of injection, speed of injection, specific chemical action, and osmolality. The physiologic effects related to osmolality include hypervolemia, cellular diuresis, urinary diuresis, altered vascular and glomerular endothelial permeability, vessel

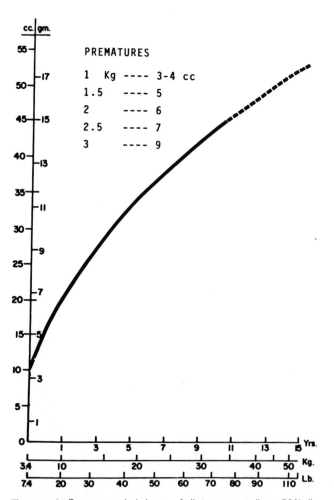

FIGURE 1. Recommended doses of diatrozoate sodium, 50% (in cubic centimeters and corresponding grams of iodine), for excretory urography according to age and weight of the patient. Similar high doses also apply to other urographic agents. Doses for premature infants are as shown.

dilatation with decreased resistance and blood pressure, increased blood flow, pain, and sinus bradycardia and conduction delays.

LOW-OSMOLALITY CONTRAST AGENTS

These contrast agents were introduced to the United States and Canada in 1985, but have been in use for a longer period in Europe. Agents include iohexol (Omnipaque), iopamidol (Isovue), iopromide, and ioversol (Optiray), which are triiodinated contrast agents—nonionic, monomeric compounds with hydrophilic side chains. Ioxaglate (Hexabrix) is a monoacid dimer containing six iodine atoms per molecule, and is an ionic dimeric salt.

LOCM have an iodine content ranging from 128 to 320 mg/ml and an osmolality range from 290 to 702 mOsm/kg. Normal serum osmolality is 285 mOsm/kg. Agents with low iodine content are most suitable for intra-arterial digital subtraction arteriography. Those with iodine content of 240 to 300 mg/ml are used for excretory urography, venography, venous injection digital subtraction arteriography, and bolus IV enhancement for CT scans. The media with high iodine content, 320 to 370 mg/ml, are used for aortography and selective arteriography.

LOCM have little or no effect on serum osmolality, serum sodium, vasodilation, hemodilation, red blood cell morphology, or vascular permeability. There is little or no effect on the blood–brain barrier, fewer electrocardiographic changes, and fewer alterations in myocardial contractility, cardiac output, and left ventricular, pulmonary artery, and aortic pressures. There is less endothelial damage, and lower release or activation of vasoactive substances, including complement activation, histamine release, and acetylcholinesterase inhibition. Diminished effect on coagulation pathways has been demonstrated. These effects are attributed to the lower osmolality and the reduced chemotactic effect of the molecules. Of importance is reduction in the nephrotoxic effect noted with HOCM, including proteinuria, altered renal blood flow, and urinary enzyme excretion. There is a notable improvement in the patient's experience, with less or no pain, heat, nausea, vomiting, or anxiety. Improved patient comfort has resulted in improved image quality.

Evidence has indicated definite advantages to adoption of LOCM; however, they are more costly, averaging from 10 to 20 times the price of HOCM. Current criteria for the use of LOCM advised by the American College of Radiology for use of LOCM are as follows:

1. Patients with a history of a previous adverse reaction to contrast material, with the exception of a sensation of heat, flushing, or a single episode of nausea or vomiting
2. Patients with a history of asthma or allergy
3. Patients with known cardiac dysfunction, including recent or potentially imminent cardiac decompensation, severe arrhythmias, unstable angina pectoris, recent myocardial infarction, and pulmonary hypertension
4. Patients with generalized severe debilitation
5. Any other circumstances where, after due consideration, the radiologist believes there is a specific indication for the use of LOCM

In infants and children, considerations include very small size, prematurity, significant cardiac disease, congestive failure, dehydration, severe asthma or allergies, previous reaction to contrast material, renal insufficiency, and sickle cell anemia. A major consideration is degradation of the resulting examination resulting from pain, heat, or vomiting.

ADVERSE REACTIONS

Contrast reactions represent the most common complications of intravascular contrast administration and are observed in 2% to 10% of patients receiving HOCM. Most reactions are minor and do not require treatment. Reactions that require treatment but are not life threatening occur in a small but significant number of patents. Life-threatening reactions such as laryngeal and facial edema, cardiac arrhythmias, severe bronchospasm, pulmonary edema, and cardiovascular collapse are detected in 1 in 3000 to 1 in 14,000 patients undergoing contrast studies. Most patients with potentially fatal reactions are successfully resuscitated. Contrast reactions are classified as idiosyncratic and nonidiosyncratic. Idiosyncratic reactions are "allergic-type" reactions and include hives, itching, facial and laryngeal edema, bronchospasm, and circulatory collapse. Nonidiosyncratic reactions result from direct toxic effects of contrast material and contrast hyperosmolality and include nausea, vomiting, cardiac arrhythmias, pulmonary edema, and cardiovascular collapse. The existence of a known allergy doubles the frequency of a contrast reaction and quadruples the rate of severe reactions. Recurrent reactions have been reported in from 15% to 60% of patients with a history of previous contrast reaction, and nearly 20% of such patients developed identical severe reactions. There is a higher frequency of reactions when the total iodine dose exceeds 20 g.

Although there is significantly greater contrast binding by serum globulin in patients who experience contrast reactions, it has been suggested that most reactions are not the result of immunoglobulin E–antigen interactions. Contrast reactions are considered to be "anaphylactoid" or allergy-like rather than "anaphylactic." Contrast material may induce histamine release from basophils and mast cells and may affect both the complement and coagulation systems.

Several disease processes may be aggravated by the administration of intravascular contrast material. Hypertensive crisis, related to catecholamine release, may result in patients with pheochromocytoma. Contrast-induced sickle cell crisis can occur in patients with sickle cell anemia. Patients with hyperthyroidism may develop thyroid storm. Contrast nephropathy may occur following intravascular contrast administration. The patient at risk for developing contrast nephropathy has existing azotemia, diabetes mellitus, severe congestive failure, multiple contrast studies, or renal tubules filled with uric acid precipitates (as in those undergoing rapid tumor lysis). It is inadvisable to administer contrast media for CT in patients clinically at risk for azotemia.

A study by Katayama et al. of 337,647 cases in Japan indicates that nonionic contrast media reduce significantly the incidence of all reactions and specifically the incidence of severe and potentially life-threatening adverse reactions. The incidence of adverse reactions was 3.13% among patients given LOCM compared to 12.66% among those given HOCM. Severe reactions occurred in 0.04% of LOCM patients compared with 0.22% of HOCM patients. The choice of contrast medium itself was found to be a major risk factor for adverse reactions. Low-risk patients given HOCM experienced a higher incidence of severe adverse reactions than high-risk patients given LOCM. In children under 1 year of age, the incidence of all adverse reactions is 0.7% with HOCM and 0.4% with LOCM. The risk of death is very low with either HOCM or LOCM. Severe nonfatal reactions with HOCM are rare, but approximately 80% can be avoided by using LOCM.

Nevertheless, it is important to be aware that both mild and severe adverse reactions may occur with any IV contrast material. Immediate treatment of contrast reactions includes the use of antihistamine drugs, epinephrine administered subcutaneously, intravascular volume expansion, and oxygen. Pretreatment with a two-dose corticosteroid regimen given 12 and 2 hours before HOCM administration has been shown to lower the reaction rate in high-risk patients to that observed in a large group of patients receiving LOCM without pretreatment. This regimen does not protect completely against reactions to contrast material, and patients at high risk should receive LOCM.

CONTRAST AGENTS FOR MAGNETIC RESONANCE IMAGING

Contrast agents for magnetic resonance imaging (MRI) improve the diagnostic information on magnetic resonance (MR) images by either decreasing proton relaxation times or altering proton density. MR contrast agents with large magnetic moments are found in the proximity of tissue protons and stimulate relaxation of nuclei, decreasing T_1 and T_2 relaxation times. MRI contrast media are used to improve the inherent contrast differences between magnetically similar tissues, to directly evaluate organ function, to estimate perfusion of an organ, to delineate the gastrointestinal tract, or to localize high concentrations of antigenic determinants. Paramagnetic substances are ions, atoms, or molecules that align with an external magnetic field, then return to their random orientation when the field is removed. Strongly paramagnetic substances, such as the Gd^{3+} in gadopentetate dimeglumine (with seven unpaired electrons), produce proton relaxation enhancement, resulting in a significant reduction in T_1 and T_2 times for neighboring protons and a resultant increase in MR signal intensity. Superparamagnetism is a property of iron oxide particles and preferentially reduces the T_2 relaxation time by induction of local field inhomogeneity. There is little effect on T_1 relaxation. Binding of metal ions to multidentate chelates by electrostatic forces effectively reduces their toxicity, prevents intracellular deposition, facilitates rapid and complete renal excretion, and controls biodistribution. The paramagnetic substances considered for use as contrast agents include transition series metals (Fe^{3+} or Mn^{2+}, with up to five unpaired electrons), lanthanide metals (Gd^{3+}, up to seven unpaired electrons), or nitroxide spin labels (pyrroxiamide, one or more unpaired electrons). Gadolinium–diethylenetriaminepentaacetic acid (Gd-DTPA) dimeglumine was approved in 1988 for clinical use. The characteristics of Gd-DTPA dimeglumine are as follows:

- T_1 relaxivity: 4.5 to 5.1 mmol/sec
- Water solubility: high
- Clinical dose: 0.1 mmol/kg
- Half-life: 90 minutes
- Distribution: extracellular fluid space–glomerular filtration
- Osmolality: 1900 mOsm/kg

Gd-DTPA is excreted by glomerular filtration, with 90% excreted within 24 hours. Rapid renal clearance and low toxicity are important features of this contrast material. The high osmolality is of little importance because of the small volume administered.

Other compounds are being developed for enhancement of the extracellular fluid space and detection of defects in the blood–brain barrier. Contrast agents with other distributions desired are those that alter relaxation time of the liver by reticuloendothelial cell uptake or hepatobiliary excretion, oral gastrointestinal tract enhancement, or those for blood volume and perfusion indicators. The porphyrins or paramagnetically labeled specific antibodies may be developed as tumor-specific contrast agents.

EXCRETORY UROGRAPHY

This radiographic examination utilizes the physiology excretion of iodine-labeled contrast media injected IV for visualization of the renal cortex, medulla, and collecting system. Anatomic detail of the renal parenchyma and collecting system and general information concerning renal function are obtained. The study requires good excretion of iodinated contrast material, and appropriate filming to document the nephrographic phase and excretion of contrast material into the pelvocaliceal collecting system. Injection of iodinated contrast media is also utilized to evaluate these renal structures by CT scanning. Excretory urography has previously been the imaging method of choice for the kidney and collecting system; it has been supplanted by ultrasound (US), radionuclide studies, and CT.

Following bolus IV injection of contrast media, the material is excreted by glomerular filtration into the proximal renal tubules, where water is resorbed. The nephrographic phase of the urogram is best seen in the first minute after injection and is directly related to the amount of contrast present in the urine (measured in milligrams per milliliter) and the volume of urine (milliliters per minute). The nephrographic phase provides an estimate of renal function as well as information on renal size and parenchymal contour. A poorly visible nephrogram may indicate a technical problem in achieving optimal plasma concentration of contrast material or some degree of renal failure or diminished renal function. A dense and prolonged nephrogram indicates obstruction of the renal collecting system or renal tubules, hypotension, hypovolemia, or acute tubular necrosis. There is diminished tubular flow and increased water resorption with resultant higher tubular concentration of iodine. Microscopically, there are interstitial edema and dilated tubules filled with cellular debris. The dense nephrogram may remain for a prolonged period, often 24 hours or longer, with little or no opacification of the collecting system.

Opacification of urine in the pelvocaliceal collecting system reflects the plasma concentration of contrast material (in milligrams per milliliter) and is enhanced by dehydration and diminished by dilution during diuresis and high tubular flow. Diminished glomerular filtration also results in reduced opacification.

Promptness and density of the nephrogram and opacification of the collecting structures provides a general estimate of quality of renal function, but it is not a sensitive indicator of function. The usual reduced glomerular filtration in the neonate results in a very poor nephrogram. Renal scintigraphy may compensate for this limitation (see Section VII, Part I, Chapter 2, page 1722).

PROCEDURAL FEATURES

Bowel preparation is unnecessary in infants and children, except for the very constipated patient, in whom 24 to 48 hours of liquids and oral stool softener may be helpful. Use of tomography avoids the necessity of bowel preparation. Deliberate dehydration should be avoided. A light meal or clear fluids several hours before the study followed by withholding of feeding for 2 to 4 hours is helpful in decreasing the stomach content and lessens the possibility of aspiration if vomiting occurs. The filming sequence is initiated with a frontal radiograph of the abdomen to identify any calcifications or masses. Following this preliminary radiograph, IV access is established and contrast material is injected in a steady bolus at a moderate rate. If there is any indication of extravasation, such as swelling or pain, injection must be halted. Extravasated contrast material can produce pain, edema, and necrosis of subcutaneous tissues and skin. Such reactions are less severe with LOCM than with HOCM. Extravasation may be treated by use of warm, wet soaks to hasten resorption of the contrast material. Dosage of either contrast material is between 2 and 3 ml/kg to obtain adequate iodine concentration in the tubules and collecting systems. There is a diuretic effect with HOCM; visualization with LOCM, which does not produce diuresis, is equivalent. The injected dose volume is calculated by weight or surface area of the patient.

The filming sequence is tailored to the individual examination. An initial frontal radiograph within 1 to 2 minutes of injection, collimated over the region of the kidneys, is used for visualization of the nephrographic phase of the study. Assessment of this radiograph is used to determine subsequent filming, which may include tomography or oblique views of the kidneys. On routine

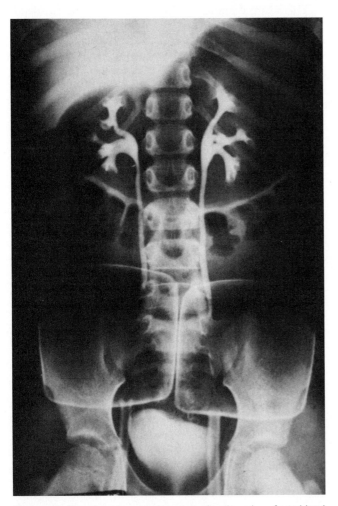

FIGURE 2. Excretory urogram demonstrating the value of combined ureteral compression and carbonated beverage in an older child.

examination, a radiograph at approximately 8 minutes allows visualization of the kidneys and their collecting systems, including the bladder. This is collimated over the entire abdomen with the patient prone or supine. In the prone position, the higher specific gravity of the contrast material allows better visualization of the renal pelves and ureters. Oblique views may provide visualization of the more anterior and posterior aspects of the kidneys and the lower ureters and trigonal region of the bladder. Some radiologists use carbonated beverages to provide better visualization of the kidneys through the window of the distended stomach (Fig. 2).

In many circumstances an abbreviated examination is adequate, postoperative patients may require only an abdominal film to examine the kidney, ureters, and bladder 8 minutes after contrast injection.

ULTRASOUND EXAMINATION OF THE UROGENITAL TRACT

Ultrasonography is the most widely used general examination of the urinary system in infants and children. The widespread use of obstetric US has resulted in early detection of many urinary tract abnormalities that would otherwise have become manifest only later. Early identification and treatment of such abnormalities prevents many of the more severe sequelae, such as obstructive nephropathy.

Ultrasound is an inexpensive and easily accessible technique for screening, identification, and characterization of urinary abnormalities and for follow-up examination postoperatively or following other appropriate treatment. Common indications for US of the urinary tract include

1. Possible fetal anomalies (in utero screening)
2. Palpable abdominal mass
3. Renal enlargement
4. Unexplained infection, fever, pyuria, failure to thrive
5. Urinary tract infection, in either girls or boys
6. Hematuria
7. Abnormal pattern of urination
8. The presence of anomalies that may be associated with urinary anomalies—limb, vertebral, cardiac, anal
9. Physical characteristics that are associated with renal neoplasia—hemihypertrophy, visceromegaly, sporadic aniridia
10. Hypertension
11. Serologic findings of diminished renal function or impending renal failure
12. Positive family history of urinary abnormalities

The small physical habitus of infants and children, the absence of abdominal fat, and the lack of ionizing radiation make US an ideal method of examination of the kidneys and bladder. Variable transducer power (3.5, 5.0, or 7.5 MHz), variation in focal length, and variation in design of transducers (sector scanners, phased array, linear array) allow for a variety of tailored approaches. Real-time US scanning is the most practical method of examination. Children are scanned in the supine, decubitus, or prone position. The liver provides an excellent acoustic window for the upper pole of the right kidney and the spleen may be useful as an acoustic window for the left kidney. On occasion, bowel gas may obscure part of the kidney, but a posterolateral approach can be used to improve visualization.

It is advisable to initiate the urogenital US examination in young children with an examination of the bladder. The full bladder of an infant usually empties when the transducer is placed in the suprapubic region. Kidneys are ideally visualized in the longitudinal, or coronal, and transverse planes. Examination of other retroperitoneal and pelvic structures, including the uterus and ovaries and the adrenal glands, may be performed at the same time that the urinary tract is evaluated. Signs or symptoms referable to the urinary tract may also originate from adjacent structures.

ULTRASOUND CHARACTERISTICS OF THE UROGENITAL SYSTEM

The kidneys are ovoid solid organs with fine, medium-level echoes arising from the cortex, a well-delineated corticomedullary junction with brightly echoic arcuate arteries, and pyramid-shaped, relatively large medullary rays that are hypoechoic, owing to the large fluid volume within the tubules. Cortical echogenicity in the neonate and young infant is higher than in older children. By comparison, the medullary pyramids are more hypoechoic in this age group (Fig. 3). The cortical echogenicity is comparable to the liver and spleen in the

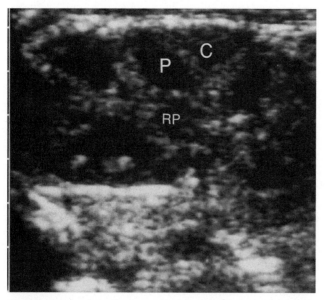

FIGURE 3. Ultrasonographic appearance of a normal kidney in a 4-week-old infant in the longitudinal plane shows large, hypoechoic renal pyramids, normal cortex, and a small amount of fluid in the renal pelvis. *C,* cortex; *P,* pyramids; *RP,* renal pelvis.

neonate and young infant, but diminishes progressively as the child grows older. The renal pyramids are proportionately larger in comparison with the cortex in the newborn. With increasing maturity they lose their hypoechogenicity. The transition from the infant renal echo pattern to that of the child occurs between 6 and 9 months (Fig. 4). The central, highly echoic sinus results from vascular structures interfacing with fat around the renal pelvis. The newborn infant has little renal sinus fat and a very small hilum. With maturity, the highly echoic hilar structures develop and are similar to those of an adult by the time the child reaches his or her teens. With diuresis or dilatation of the pelvoinfundibular portion of the collecting system, separation of the hyperechoic renal sinus echo is noted and is termed sinus *splitting.*

US examination of the kidneys provides detailed anatomic information concerning the neonatal kidney at a time when visualization by excretory urography is poor owing to low glomerular filtration, poor concentration of IV-administered contrast material, and overlying bowel gas. Furthermore, administration of large volumes of contrast material in a neonate sensitive to changes in vascular volume is ill advised. HOCM have potentially harmful effects on vascular volume and serum osmolality. Although US provides excellent anatomic detail, it does not provide functional data.

The adrenal glands of the neonate are one third the size of the kidneys and are visualized by longitudinal US examination as inverted Y- or V-shaped structures, and by transverse scan as oval structures superior and slightly medial to the upper pole of each kidney. The adrenal cortex is hyperechoic and the central medulla is hypoechoic (Fig. 5). Adrenal size decreases by 50% in the first 3 weeks of life. Vascular structures—the aorta, inferior vena cava, and renal veins and arteries—are identified using color flow Doppler examination to identify the vessels, and duplex and color flow to provide information about vascular flow and resistance.

The bladder is examined early in the study because spontaneous micturition resulting from stimulation from the transducer often occurs. If the bladder is empty early in the study, it may fill by the end, particularly in a patient receiving IV fluids. The wall of the bladder is thick but smooth in a partially filled or unfilled bladder. The wall is smooth and thin in a filled bladder. Neither the urethra nor the ureters are visualized if normal. Propulsion of urine from the distal ureter into the bladder results in a turbulent jet of fluid that may be observed during IV urography, cystography, or US. In the last, the ureteral jet is seen as a hyperechoic stream of bubbles. Color Doppler US depicts ureteral jets more frequently and with greater reliability than real-time US alone. Absence of a jet or an abnormal angle of flow may signify reflux.

The uterus and ovaries are visualized using the fluid-filled bladder as a "window" (Fig. 6). These are easily identified in the first month because of maternal hormonal stimulation but thereafter become smaller and more difficult to visualize until menarche. The premenarcheal uterus and ovaries are small, but, with the onset of menses, the uterus becomes larger with

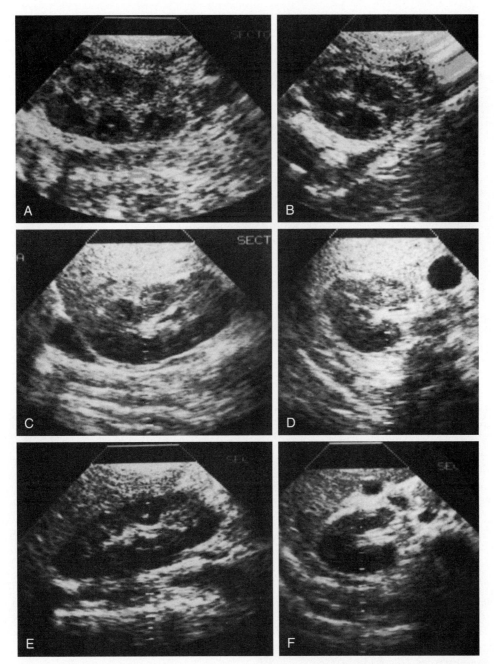

FIGURE 4. Normal US pattern of the right kidney in three children. Longitudinal sections are on the *left* and transverse sections are on the *right*. **A** and **B,** 3-month-old infant. **C** and **D,** 3½-year-old child. **E** and **F,** 8-year-old child. The central echogenic oval area is produced by hilar structures. The renal parenchyma is much less echogenic than the adjacent liver. Note the large and hypoechogenic pyramids of infancy in **A** and **B.**

clearly identified characteristics, including a central endometrial hyperechoic strip surrounded by a hypoechoic zone. The ovaries in the young child are high in the abdomen, usually measuring somewhat less than 1 cm in length, but they may be identified within the pelvis after 8 years. Normal ovaries contain numerous small cysts several millimeters in diameter.

The testis can be visualized within the scrotum or in the inguinal canal. High-frequency transducers provide excellent resolution. The testis is ovoid with the comma-shaped epididymis and appendix identified

superiorly. A homogeneous medium-echo pattern is present throughout the testis and a slightly hyperechoic central hilum is identified. Fine septations are occasionally seen. Color Doppler identification of arterial and venous flow is helpful in evaluation of possible testicular torsion, to be differentiated from epididymitis or orchitis.

High-resolution real-time US examination of the retroperitoneum is accurate in identifying abnormalities of the kidneys, the perirenal space, or the renal collecting system.

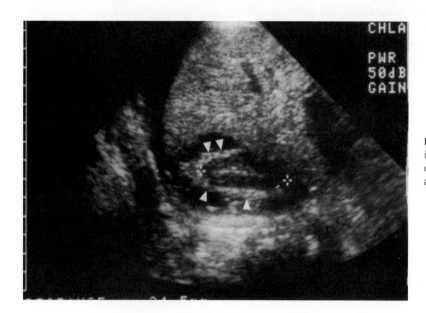

FIGURE 5. Transverse plane sonogram of the normal infant adrenal gland (surrounded by a small amount of fluid) shows the hyperechoic cortex *(arrowheads)* and hypoechoic medulla (marked with *cursors*).

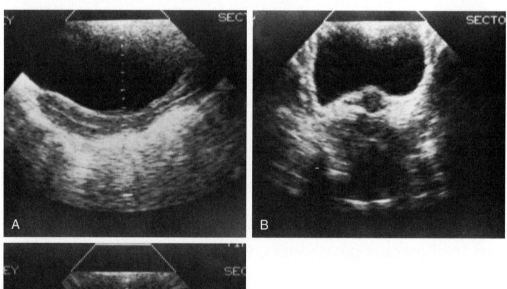

FIGURE 6. Pelvic US scan through the bladder in a 6½-year old girl. **A,** Longitudinal section showing the uterus with its echogenic central canal. **B** and **C,** Transverse sections at different levels show the bladder as square-shaped. The uterus indents the posterior wall of the bladder centrally. The iliac and psoas muscles are seen along the lateral wall of the bladder and should not be mistaken for ovaries.

DOPPLER ULTRASOUND

Doppler US, particularly color Doppler imaging, has the potential to replace invasive vascular procedures. Blood flow parameters currently being measured with Doppler US include peak velocity, mean velocity, volume flow rate, flow impedance, and pulsatility. It is possible to estimate the velocity of a moving object emitting or reflecting sound waves by the measured Doppler shift. The great advantage of pulsed Doppler lies in quantification of precise flow characteristics derived from time and velocity spectra. Doppler US is valuable for the detection of flow, to confirm arterial perfusion of organ transplants, or to exclude venous thrombosis. Doppler US identifies the direction of flow. Spectral analysis is helpful in recognizing and quantifying vascular disease by comparison of peak velocities and quantification of impedance from time–velocity waveforms. Change in impedance may be pathologic, as in the renal artery or peripheral arteries of a transplanted kidney, in which it heralds vascular rejection. Doppler US is also used for tissue characterization, because tumors may have specific flow patterns that allow evaluation of their vascular morphology. Quantification of flow evaluates hypertension in the kidneys, duplex Doppler US is used for detection of stenosis or occlusion of the renal artery, renal vein thrombosis, and postoperative evaluation of renal transplants.

Duplex Doppler provides a display of the relative blood flow velocity. In arterial Doppler, the waveform has a systolic and a diastolic component. The large arteries exhibit high pulsatility with a prominent systolic wave and a reverse (negative) wave in diastole. The pulsatility of the renal artery and its branches is lower with progressive dampening of flow as the caliber of the renal artery branch is decreased to the level of the arcuate arteries. Initial diastolic velocity is one half the peak systole, with progressive dampening of flow but persistence of flow in late diastole. Venous flow does not exhibit such a waveform but is represented by a continuous audible hum and uniform, rhythmic wave produced by pulsations of adjacent structures.

Testicular torsion and ischemia may be differentiated from epididymitis, tumor, orchitis, or appendix torsion using color Doppler sonography. This technique is accurate in older children and adolescents and is also successfully used in infants and young children. It may also be utilized in characterization of abdominal tumors, arteriovenous malformations or hemangiomas, and abnormalities of large vessels.

FETAL ULTRASOUND OF UROGENITAL ABNORMALITIES

Prenatal US examination of the fetus is now performed with greater frequency, particularly in cases of suspected fetal abnormalities. More than one third of the anomalies detected in the fetus are urogenital. Urinary anomalies are discovered incidentally during routine screening or in cases of oligohydramnios, abnormal serum α-fetoprotein, abnormal fetal growth pattern, or family history of renal disease. Suspicion of urinary tract abnormalities identifies the infant requiring a more complete investigation and possible treatment soon after birth. On occasion, early delivery or prenatal therapeutic intervention is warranted.

Fetal kidneys and bladder are visualized by US between 15 and 20 weeks of gestation. The pelvocaliceal systems and ureters are not seen unless dilated. The adrenal gland is visualized early in the third trimester of pregnancy. It is noteworthy that moderate dilatation of the calices and pelvis is identified in utero early in the third trimester. This represents normal fetal diuresis at this time and is not an abnormal finding. Postnatal confirmation of normal collecting systems may be accomplished in these patients. Obstructed collecting systems, renal cystic dysplasias, and oligohydramnios syndrome with hypoplastic lungs (Potter's sequence) are identified by US examination early in the third trimester.

Significant dilatation of the pelvocaliceal system postnatally may not be apparent in the first 24 to 48 hours of life because of low glomerular filtration and relative dehydration of the neonate. Studies after this time will identify collecting system dilatation that was previously obscure in babies with collecting system obstruction, prune-belly syndrome, or vesicoureteral reflux.

In the second half of gestation, fetal urine plays a major role in the formation of amniotic fluid. Oligohydramnios in the second trimester commonly reflects bilateral severe renal malformations, or severe urinary tract obstruction. These infants present with Potter facies, hypoplastic lungs and thorax, abnormalities of the limbs, and severe bilateral renal dysplasia. The kidneys may be difficult to visualize, although large fluid-filled bladder and ureters are seen. Bilateral multicystic kidney or severe cystic renal dysplasia is identified in utero, appearing much as it does postnatally. Posterior urethral valves or prune-belly syndrome is suggested by dilated ureters. Unfortunately, by the time in utero diagnosis is possible, significant damage has occurred to the parenchymal development of the kidneys, and intervention does not significantly improve the outcome.

VOIDING CYSTOURETHROGRAPHY AND OTHER UROLOGIC PROCEDURES

VOIDING CYSTOURETHROGRAPHY

Antegrade voiding cystourethrography is the examination of choice for evaluation of the bladder, for identification of vesicoureteral reflux, and for study of the anatomy of the male urethra. A well-lubricated small catheter is advanced through the urethra into the bladder, and the bladder is filled by gravity pressure (fluid at a height of approximately 2.5 to 3.0 ft) using the contrast agents designated in group 1 in Table 1, or any other dilute sterile contrast media with an iodine concentration of 80 to 100 mg/ml. Sufficient contrast is introduced into the bladder to produce the urge to void in older children, often visible fluoroscopically by relaxation of the internal sphincter just prior to voiding. Average bladder volumes vary from 10 to 15 ml in the newborn infant to 300 ml in older children.

Radiographs in the study include the static cystogram followed by voiding films. The voiding films are obtained to include the trigonal region of the bladder and the urethra during voiding with the patient in a steep oblique position. Most examiners prefer the patient voiding against the placed catheter. Voiding films are useful for evaluation of the bladder and the urethra (particularly the male urethra) and also for the diagnosis of vesicoureteral reflux, which may occur only during voiding. Following voiding, a film of the kidneys identifies reflux that occurred during the examination. (Many institutions use double voiding and even triple voiding, which increase the percentage of refluxing ureters detected. As a consequence, radiation and time increase as well.) For evaluation of specific lesions within the bulbous or penile urethra, leaving the catheter in place near the urethral ampulla causes partial obstruction and distention of the ampullary region of the urethra proximally for more detailed evaluation. A postvoiding film of the bladder to evaluate bladder residual is not helpful because residual may reflect the artificial situation of the cystogram, rather than inability to empty the bladder. Residual obtained on initial catheterization if the patient has previously voided is more significant. False residual urine occurs in patients with reflux who refill an empty bladder from their ureters.

In patients with neurogenic bladder and meningomyelocele, voiding is usually impossible, and evaluation to detect reflux is the most important part of the study. In these instances, the bladder is filled, with a single or several films obtained over the kidneys and ureters to evaluate reflux. The bladder is then emptied through the catheter.

Because cystourethrography includes radiation to the region of the gonads, videotape recording, digital image storage, or the use of 105-mm film is preferable to overhead filming or fluoroscopic spot films. Fluoroscopic examination by a physician is preferable in young or uncooperative patients.

RETROGRADE URETHROGRAPHY

Retrograde urethrograms are rarely obtained in children. A small catheter is introduced into the anterior urethra to or slightly past the level of the ampulla with the meatus obliterated. With the patient in a steep oblique position, a small amount of contrast material is rapidly injected through a syringe for evaluation of the urethra to the level of the external sphincter. Spasm of the external sphincter prevents filling of the posterior urethra. This examination is most frequently utilized to evaluate possible urethral rupture following straddle injury or pelvic trauma. Another technique uses a Foley catheter with the balloon distended and taped to the perineum with the tip extending into the vagina.

VAGINOGRAPHY

A vaginogram is utilized to evaluate vaginal size, a common urogenital orifice, the presence of a cervix, or a vaginal mass. The technique is used in cases of ambiguous genitalia or common urogenital sinus. A small catheter is introduced into the vagina and taped. If possible, another catheter is introduced anteriorly into the urethra and bladder, particularly when evaluating a common urogenital sinus. Contrast is injected under fluoroscopic control with the patient in a steep oblique or lateral view. Lateral and oblique views are valuable to establish the interrelationships of the urogenital structures.

GENITOGRAPHY

Genitography is a procedure most useful for children with suspected intersex or whose sexual differentiation by external genitalia is indeterminate. Most of these children are masculinized females. Karyotyping is used to determine the sexual chromosomal component, and genitography is used to detail the anatomy of the urethra, vagina, and possible presence of a uterus. Genitography is carried out by catheterization of the urethra and urinary bladder. Following this, a second catheter may be placed just dorsally and may enter a vagina that communicates with the proximal urethra. Some examiners also prefer to place a catheter within the rectum, possibly with a small amount of contrast material within the rectum. A standard cystourethrogram is performed for evaluation of the bladder and urethra. During this procedure there may be reflux of contrast material into the vagina that enters a masculinized urethra. If this does not occur, use of a second posterior catheter is helpful. Injection by hand into the urethra with the tip of the catheter placed in the posterior urethra will also often delineate a vagina and its associated cervix. These studies are best performed with the patient in the true lateral position.

US or MRI may be used to establish the presence of a uterus and gonads and the anatomy of the phalus.

RETROGRADE PYELOGRAPHY

Uncommonly performed, this procedure is usually done as an adjunct to cystoscopy, with the urologist placing retrograde catheters within the ureter. The examination is used most frequently in children with a blind-ending ureter, either duplex or single. Following placement of the ureteral catheters by the urologist, sterile contrast medium is injected carefully and multiple oblique views are obtained to identify the anatomic relationships.

VESICOSTOMY STUDY

In patients with a simple vesicostomy, a small Foley catheter is inserted into the bladder through the stoma;

the balloon is inflated and used to occlude the vesicostomy site. A cystogram is then performed, filling the bladder by gravity introduction of contrast material.

NEPHROSTOMY AND URETEROSTOMY STUDIES

These examinations are performed by gravity introduction or low-pressure manual injection of iodinated contrast material into the indwelling catheter, or through a small catheter inserted into the stoma with the tip advanced to the desired location. Both procedures are performed with fluoroscopic guidance.

COMPUTED TOMOGRAPHY

Computed tomography, a cross-sectional imaging technique, produces high-resolution images of the body. Its sensitivity is related to fine differentiation of tissue attenuation. Computer analysis of attenuation and location and reconstruction produces the consequent images. High-quality CT can be performed in patients of all ages, although relative immobility is required. Reassurance, explanation of the procedure, the presence of a parent, sedation, and immobilization all contribute to the production of a successful diagnostic study. Electron beam or multidetector helical CT scanners obviate the need for sedation in most patients. A nasogastric tube within the stomach or other radiopaque materials within the abdomen degrade the image. If a nasogastric tube is used for administration of oral contrast material, or if one is already present, it should be repositioned within the esophagus during abdominal imaging. Neither overlying bones nor gas within the gastrointestinal tract degrade the CT image. Because of the small amount of intraperitoneal fat in children, IV contrast material is essential for visualization of vessels and organs. Fluid-filled or collapsed loops of bowel mimic the attenuation of solid structures, masses, cysts, or lymph nodes; thus opacification of the gastrointestinal tract with very dilute contrast agents is recommended under most circumstances (Fig. 7). Rectal administration of dilute contrast is helpful in evaluation of the pelvis. For evaluation of calcification, a precontrast limited scan is obtained followed by IV administration of contrast material. IV contrast enhancement is required for visualization of renal lesions and the vessels of the abdomen. An IV bolus of contrast material is administered by hand injection, although a power injector should be considered for use in older teenagers.

Scanning is started after at least half the volume of contrast material is administered. Careful visual monitoring of the IV line is important during injection to be sure that extravasation is not occurring. Slow, steady administration of contrast material over 60 to 180 seconds is advised. Under some circumstances, delayed scanning is used to evaluate appearance and excretion of contrast material within or surrounding renal lesions. This is useful for evaluating areas of inflammation. With ultrafast scanning, the entire dose of contrast material is administered prior to the scan. Dynamic contrast-enhanced scanning visualizes the inferior vena cava and the aorta. It also shows progression of contrast through the cortex, medulla, and collecting system of the kidney (Fig. 8); thus, contrast-enhanced CT (CECT) not only is useful for anatomic evaluation of structures but also provides physiologic information concerning renal function and vascularity of lesions.

NORMAL ANATOMY

On an unenhanced scan, the kidney is of slightly lower or the same attenuation as liver and spleen without differentiation of the cortex and medulla. The renal pelvis is situated medially and slightly anteriorly and contains urine of low water attenuation. Following bolus IV injection of contrast material and rapid scanning, there is initially an even opacification of the renal cortex followed by symmetric opacification of the medulla, followed by a diffuse nephrogram. This pattern proceeds to opacification of the pelvocaliceal system and ureters, then the bladder. The renal artery and vein are visualized with bolus injection, as are the aorta and inferior vena cava.

The adrenal glands are located just cephalad and slightly medial to the upper poles of the kidneys and anterior to the diaphragmatic crura. They are linear or have the appearance of an inverted V or Y (Fig. 9). The psoas muscle is ovoid, of low attenuation, and smallest at the level of the renal pelvis, becoming progressively larger as it travels caudad. The aorta and inferior vena cava are oval and located immediately anterior, to the left and right, respectively, of the vertebrae. Retroperitoneal lymph nodes are small, normally less than 1 cm in diameter.

Evaluation of pelvic structures requires contrast material within the large and small bowel and the bladder. Pelvic lymph nodes, when enlarged, can be distinguished from contrast-filled bowel loops. The uterus is immediately retrovesical in older girls; the ovaries may be seen in older girls, but are not usually identified in girls under 8 to 10 years of age.

CLINICAL USES

CT has multiple uses for evaluation of intraabdominal disease in children. In patients with suspected congenital anomalies, CT identifies the presence, location, and possible abnormalities of kidneys. CT is useful in the evaluation of patients with a kidney that has diminished or absent function. CT is used to evaluate the kidneys and other organs of children with abdominal trauma. Patients with significant trauma present with hematuria, hypotension, rigid abdomen, or abdominal bruising or discoloration. The kidney is frequently involved in children with trauma to the liver, spleen, pancreas, or duodenum. CT examination for abdominal trauma should be performed with IV contrast material. Use of gastrointestinal contrast is optional.

CECT is utilized in the evaluation of intrarenal or

perirenal abscess, lobar nephronia, focal bacterial nephritis, and xanthogranulomatous pyelonephritis. The area involved does not show enhancement initially, although in some instances there is delayed enhancement of the involved regions. In suspected infection or trauma, the demonstration of intraperitoneal or retroperitoneal fluid by CT is helpful.

CT examination is excellent in the evaluation of abdominal masses. CT identifies location, organ of origin, involvement of neighboring structures, vascular supply, vascular involvement, and the presence of intraperitoneal or retroperitoneal fluid. Evaluating differing tissue characteristics by attenuation on CT successfully identifies fat, gas, calcium, water, or soft tissue density. CT identifies gas in an abscess; fat present in teratomas or fatty tumors; and masses of water density that are found in abscesses, pseudocysts, or lymphoceles. Old hematomas may present as water density. Masses of soft tissue density are solid neoplasms, inflammatory masses, or recent hematoma. IV contrast enhancement of mass

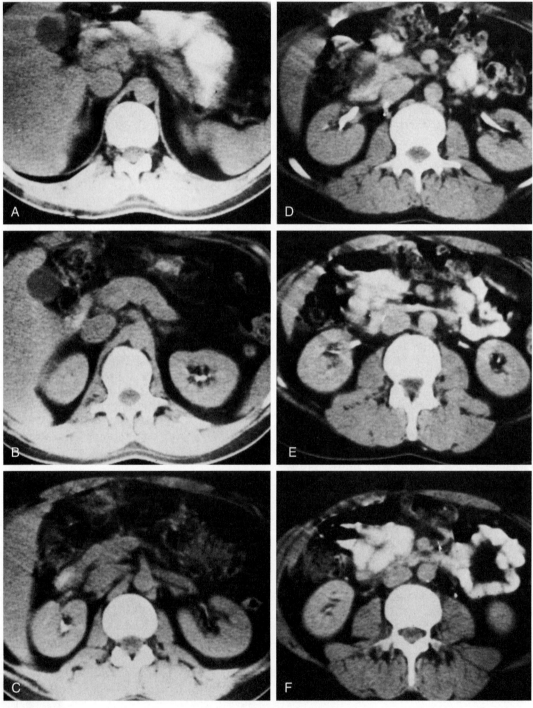

FIGURE 7. Six CT sections of the adrenal and renal areas obtained after IV injection of contrast material and opacification of the gastrointestinal tract by very diluted contrast agent. The abundant retroperitoneal fat in this patient permits excellent visualization of the kidneys and other retroperitoneal structures.

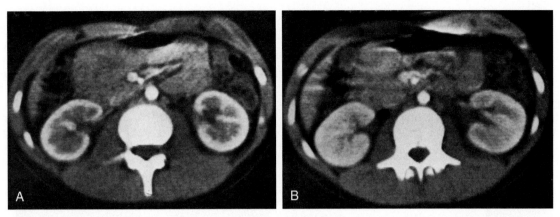

FIGURE 8. Dynamic CT scans of the kidneys after a bolus injection of contrast agent. A dense opacification of the cortex **(A)** is followed a few seconds later by early opacification of the medulla **(B)**.

lesions identifies vascularity and areas of necrosis or cysts, and differentiates normal renal parenchyma from renal tumor or hemangioma. Frequently, low-attenuation areas of necrosis, hemorrhage, or cysts are present in solid neoplasms. Calcification is best demonstrated on unenhanced CT, which is a useful preliminary in the evaluation of a mass. CECT is essential for recognition of small tumors and in evaluation of tumor extension.

After identifying a renal or extrarenal abdominal mass, the retroperitoneal space is inspected for direct tumor invasion, vascular invasion or encasement, lymph node involvement, and vertebral or spinal canal extension. The large vessels may be displaced, compressed, or encased, or may contain a tumor thrombus that presents as a low-attenuation defect within the lumen of the vessel outlined by contrast material. Pulmonary parenchymal metastases, often not visible by chest radiograph, are identified by lung CT scan at the initial work-up of the abdominal mass. Liver metastases and lymph node metastases are also evaluated.

Simple renal cyst, abscess, or old hematoma appears on an unenhanced scan as a water-density mass (Fig. 10) Following IV contrast injection, the cyst or hematoma will maintain its original attenuation, but septations within the cyst and a rim of tissue forming the wall will show enhancement. Hydronephrosis appears as a rim of functional renal parenchyma surrounding the water-density collecting system. Aside from abscess, focal infection such as xanthogranulomatous pyelonephritis or lobar nephronia (focal bacterial nephritis) demonstrates enhancement with a low-attenuation center surrounded by enhancing renal parenchyma. Examination of the ureters and bladder is always included in the evaluation of the urinary tract.

MAGNETIC RESONANCE IMAGING

MRI is a sectional diagnostic technique that depends on proton density, T_1 and T_2 relaxation, flow phenomena, magnetic susceptibility, and diffusion. Image quality is determined by homogeneity of the magnetic field and gradient strength, magnetic field strength, and utilization of surface or specifically designed coils to increase signal-to-noise ratio. Advantages include good spatial resolution, excellent contrast resolution, multiplanar imaging, and the lack of ionizing radiation. Vascular

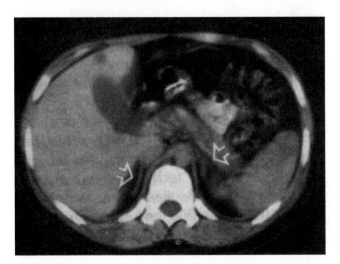

FIGURE 9. CT appearance of the adrenal glands *(arrows)* in a 4-year-old boy. The right gland is shown as a short thin line, the left as an inverted V.

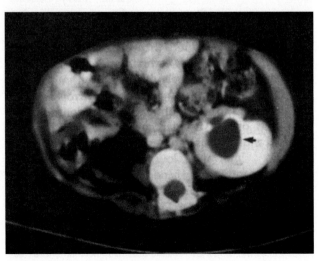

FIGURE 10. CT with IV contrast shows a simple renal cyst *(arrow)* of water density in a solitary kidney.

contrast materials used include Gd-DTPA, a paramagnetic agent that undergoes glomerular filtration, and larger molecular-weight agents. Lipid suppression techniques are helpful in the abdomen, particularly after contrast enhancement, by removing the contribution of high signal from fat. Degradation resulting from metallic foreign material and patient motion may considerably affect the image. Use of surface coils, the ability to reduce motion artifact, and the development of appropriate contrast materials and faster scanning times have resulted in improved imaging. Patient sedation is required in very young or agitated patients in order to obtain sufficient immobility during the scan.

The standard planes in which imaging is performed using MR are the axial, coronal, and sagittal planes. Bony structures are easily evaluated with a low signal cortex and high signal central marrow only in older children. Blood within vessels is identified as a flow void or by vascular contrast techniques. Abdominal musculature shows a long T_1 and short T_2 relaxation time, with low signal intensity on T_1-weighted sequences. Urine and other water-density structures show a long T_1 and T_2 relaxation time, low signal intensity on T_1-weighted and higher signal intensity on T_2-weighted scans. Fat shows a short T_1 relaxation time, with high signal on both T_1- and T_2-weighted sequences. The kidney is easily visualized with intermediate signal on T_1-weighted sequences. The renal cortex has an intermediate signal close to that of the spleen, while the medullary pyramids show a lower intensity signal on T_1-weighted images. On T_2-weighted scans, the renal signal is high uniformly. The renal collecting system and artery and vein are visualized as water and flow voids, respectively. The adrenal glands are seen superior and slightly medial to the kidney.

MRI is utilized for pelvic structures, including the uterus and ovaries in girls and the testes in boys (Fig. 11). The bladder wall is imaged against the low water signal of urine. The uterus shows an intermediate signal on

both T_1- and T_2-weighted images. MRI is particularly well suited for evaluation of pelvic structures because of good soft tissue contrast, excellent regional anatomic visualization, multiplanar capabilities, and absence of respiratory degradation. No patient preparation is required. Furthermore, there are no known biologic effects associated with this technique.

Unfortunately MRI is not always a readily available modality. Cost is higher than other imaging modalities, and patient cooperation or sedation is necessary. Newer techniques that address some problems are the fast scan techniques (e.g., rapid acquisition relaxation enhancement [RARE] and half-Fourier acquisition single-shot turbo spin-echo [HASTE]), including gradient-echo and fast spin-echo techniques and three-dimensional acquisition for improved sequencing of studies and more useful data acquision.

CLINICAL USES

MRI is of value in evaluating intrarenal or pararenal masses, assessing tissue character, determining effects on surrounding structures, and evaluating neurovascular invasion. Contrast material is not required in differentiating an intrarenal mass from normal renal tissue, although the use of gadolinium compounds is promising.

Renal hemorrhage and renal or perirenal abscess are well identified by MR, using the known signal characteristics of these materials—high signal intensity on T_1- and T_2-weighted imaging in the case of an abscess, and variable signal intensity from a hematoma depending on its age.

The adrenal gland is better evaluated by CT owing to its suprarenal location and horizontal orientation; in the case of neuroblastoma, however, MRI is useful to evaluate the relationship of the tumor to the diaphragm, the liver, the vena cava and aorta, and the spinal canal and spinal cord, and to visualize bone marrow metastases.

MR study of renal tumors identifies the unicentric or multicentric intrarenal origin of the mass(es); its relationship to neighboring tissues; and tumor invasion of the renal vein, inferior vena cava, or pelvis. The uniform, intermediate signal intensity characteristics, on T_1-weighted imaging, of a Wilms' tumor are interspersed with foci of hemorrhage, necrosis, and cyst formation. These regions, on T_1-weighted images, are usually of increased signal intensity. MRI is an accurate indicator of para-aortic lymphadenopathy, and liver metastases can be identified with short repetition time and echo time sequences or T_2-weighted sequences.

Neuroblastoma shows an inhomogeneous long T_1 and T_2 relaxation time. Retroperitoneal spread of the tumor, encasement or invasion of the inferior vena cava and aorta, or displacement of these vessels is identified. MRI is particularly helpful for evaluating contiguous spread of the tumor, metastases to the liver, and, most important, transforaminal, intraspinal extradural extension of neuroblastoma with displacement of the spinal cord. The axial and coronal planes are utilized in this

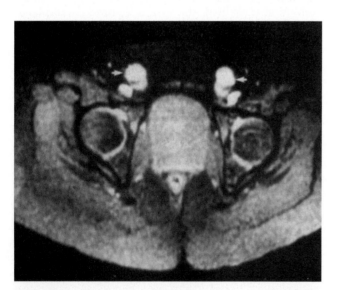

FIGURE 11. Pelvic MRI of a boy with undescended testes, using fat-suppression technique, shows normal pelvic structures and testes *(arrows)*.

evaluation. A coronal or sagittal T_1-weighted image of the spine also can indicate bone marrow replacement by low-signal metastatic disease.

MRI is useful in evaluation of retroperitoneal neoplasms and pelvic neoplasms of ovarian, bladder, prostate, uterine, vaginal, or muscular origin. Primitive neuroectodermal tumors, tumors of mesenchymal origin, germ cell tumors, teratomas, and rhabdomyosarcomas and variants are well evaluated in multiplanar MRI. A true T_1-weighted sequence for the anatomic evaluation and a true T_2-weighted sequence should be obtained in any work-up.

Hematoma within a tumor, following solid organ trauma, or in the psoas muscle is well visualized. Acute hemorrhage produces low signal intensity on T_1-weighted imaging; subacute hemorrhage shows short T_1 and T_2 relaxation times with high signal on T_1- and T_2-weighted sequences; and old hemorrhage shows low signal on T_1-weighed imaging, representing methemoglobin and hemosiderin.

Transplanted kidney evaluation in the case of acute or chronic rejection shows generalized enlargement of the kidney and loss of the corticomedullary differentiation on T_1-weighted sequences. Hydronephrosis, hematoma, lymphocele, abscess, or perirenal fluid may be identified.

Use of surface coils results in improved resolution with improved signal-to-noise ratio, but limitation in the field of view. However, evaluation of the adrenal gland, kidneys, retroperitoneum, bladder, or gonads is effectively performed.

There are constantly new uses of MRI such as static-dynamic MR urography for the various causes of urinary tract dilatation. This technique allows for evaluation of the functional aspects as well as morphologic aspects of pediatric renal disease.

VASCULAR STUDIES

Diagnostic vascular procedures performed in children include inferior vena cava cavography, abdominal aortography, selective renal arteriography, digital subtraction angiography, and other studies such as renal venography and selective venous renin studies. These studies have been largely supplanted by CT angiography and MR angiography and venography.

INFERIOR VENA CAVOGRAPHY

Contrast evaluation of the inferior vena cava may be used in infants and children with suspected spontaneous thrombosis or tumor thrombus of the renal vein or inferior vena cava. Constriction or occlusion of the inferior vena cava has been evaluated by cavography in patients with tumors, but this procedure is largely obviated by real-time US, CT, and MR. In children, a transfemoral percutaneous approach to the inferior vena cava is utilized.

ABDOMINAL AORTOGRAPHY

Abdominal aortography is utilized in evaluation of renovascular hypertension, possible arteriovenous malformation, trauma, and occasionally complex retroperitoneal tumors. In the early weeks of life, an umbilical artery line may be used for injection of small volumes of contrast material. After this time, a percutaneous transfemoral artery approach is utilized.

SELECTIVE RENAL ARTERIOGRAPHY

This technique is utilized for evaluation of renal artery stenosis at its origin, renal artery hypoplasia, or multiple renal artery stenoses. It is the technique used for visual evaluation of the renal artery of a transplanted kidney. The percutaneous transfemoral approach is used.

DIGITAL SUBTRACTION ANGIOGRAPHY

Digital subtraction angiography is utilized with an arterial catheter, a central venous catheter, or a peripheral venous injection. A scout film, used as a digital mask, is followed by rapid-sequence filming with a rapid bolus injection. This technique is helpful in diagnosis of renal or other abdominal arterial abnormalities.

SUGGESTED READINGS

Contrast Media for Radiographic Procedures

Baltaxe HA, Mooring P, Kugler J, et al: Comparative hemodynamic effect of metrizamide and Renografin 76 in infants with congenital heart disease. AJR Am J Roentgenol 1983;140:1097–1101

Bettman MA: Ionic versus nonionic contrast agents for intravenous use: are all the answers in? Radiology 1990;175:616–618

Bettman MA, Geller SC, McCleenan B, et al: Current use of low-osmolality contrast agents: results of a survey. AJR Am J Roentgenol 1989;153:1079–1083

Brismar J, Jacobsson BF, Jorulf H: Miscellaneous adverse effects of low-versus high-osmolality contrast media: a study revised. Radiology 1991;179:19–23

Caro JJ, Trindade E, McGregor M: The risks of death and of severe nonfatal reactions with high- vs low-osmolality contrast media: a meta-analysis. AJR Am J Roentgenol 1991;156:825–832

Current criteria for the use of water soluble contrast agents for intravenous injections. ACR Bull 1990; Oct:7–8

Debatin JF, Cohan RH, Leder RA, et al: Selective use of low-osmolar contrast media. Invest Radiol 1991;26:17–21

DiSessa TG, Zednikova M, Hiraishi S, et al: The cardiovascular effects of metrizamide in infants. Radiology 1983;148:687–691

Elam EA, Door RT, Lagel KE, et al: Cutaneous ulceration due to contrast extravasation: experimental assessment of injury and potential antidotes. Invest Radiol 1991;26:13–16

Evens RG: Low-osmolality contrast media: good news or bad? Radiology 1988;169:277–278

Fareed J, Walenga JM, Saravia GE, et al: Thrombogenic potential of nonionic contrast media. Radiology 1990;174:321–325

Fischer HW: Catalog of intravascular contrast media. Radiology 1986;159:561–563

Gerstman BB: Epidemiologic critique of the report on adverse reactions to ionic and nonionic media by the Japanese Committee on the Safety of Contrast Media. Radiology 1991;178:787–790

Harvey L, Caldicott WJH, Kuruc A: The effect of contrast media on immature renal function. Radiology 1983;148:429–432

Katayama H, Yamaguchi K, Kozuka T, et al: Adverse reactions to ionic and nonionic contrast media: a report from the Japanese Committee on the Safety of Contrast Media. Radiology 1990;175:621–625

Kaufmann HJ (ed): Contrast Media in Pediatric Radiology. Berlin, Schering AG, 1987

Magill HL, Clarke EA, Fitch SJ, et al: Excretory urography with johexol: evaluation in children. Radiology 1986;161:625–630

McClennan BL: Ionic and nonionic iodinated contrast media: evolution and strategies for use. AJR Am J Roentgenol 1990;155:225–233

Miller DL, Chang R, Wells WT, et al: Intravascular contrast media: effect of dose on renal function. Radiology 1988;167:607–611

Mishkin MK, Edeiken J: The current efficacious use of water soluble contrast agents for intravascular injections. Progress report of the Committee on Drugs and Contrast Media. ACR Bull 1988; Nov:9–10

Newhouse JH, Murphy RX Jr: Tissue distribution of soluble contrast: effect of dose variation and changes with time. AJR Am J Roentgenol 1981;136:463–467

Newman B, Caldicott WJH, Michelow P: Contrast media and renal function in the immature kidney. Invest Radiol 1987;22:608–612

Palmer FJ: The R.A.C.R. Survey of Intravenous Contrast Media Reactions final report. Australas Radiol 1988;32:426–428

Reuter SR: The use of conventional vs lower-osmolar contrast agents: a legal analysis. AJR Am J Roentgenol 1988;151:529–531

Saini S, Modic MT, Hamm B, et al: Advances in contrast-enhanced MR imaging. AJR Am J Roentgenol 1991;156:235–254

Steinberg EP, Anderson GF, Powe NR, et al: Use of LOCM in a price sensitive environment. AJR Am J Roentgenol 1988;151:271–274

Wolf GL, Arenson RL, Cross AP: A prospective trial of ionic vs nonionic contrast agents in routine clinical practice. AJR Am J Roentgenol 1989;152:939–944

Adverse Reactions

Bagg MNJ, Horwitz TA, Bester L: Comparison of patient responses to high- and low-osmolality contrast agents injected intravenously. AJR Am J Roentgenol 1986;147:185–187

Bettmann MA, Holzer JF, Trombly ST: Risk management issues related to the use of contrast agents. Radiology 1990;175:629–631

Brasch RC: Allergic reactions to contrast media: accumulated evidence. AJR Am J Roentgenol 1980;134:797–801

Cohan RH, Dunnick NR, Bashore TM: Treatment of reactions to radiographic contrast material. AJR Am J Roentgenol 1988;151:253–270

Katayama H, Yamaguchi K, Kozuka T, et al: Adverse reactions to ionic and nonionic contrast media: a report from the Japanese Committee on the Safety of Contrast Media. Radiology 1990;175:621–628

Lasser EC: Pretreatment with corticosteroids to prevent reactions to IV contrast material: overview and implications. AJR Am J Roentgenol 1988; 150:257–259

Lasser EC, Berry CC, Talner LB: Pretreatment with corticosteroids to alleviate reactions to IV contrast material. N Engl J Med 1987;317:845–849

Moore RD, Steinberg EP, Powe NR, et al: Frequency and determinants of adverse reactions induced by high osmolality contrast media. Radiology 1989;170:727–732

Rasuli P, McLeish WA, Hammond DI: Anticoagulant effects of contrast materials: in vitro study of iohexol, ioxaglate, and diatrizoate. AJR Am J Roentgenol 1989;152:309–311

Excretory Urography

Diament M, Kangarloo H: Dosage schedule for pediatric urography based on body surface area. AJR Am J Roentgenol 1983;140:815–816

Egeblad M, Gottlieb E: Radiation dose measurements in intravenous pyelography. Ann Radiol (Paris) 1975;18:21–24

Seppanen U, Torniainen P, Kivinitly K: Radiation gonad doses received by children in intravenous urography and micturition cysto-urethrography. Pediatr Radiol 1979;8:169–172

Ultrasound Examination of the Urogenital Tract

Avni EF, Brion LE: Ultrasound of the neonate urinary tract. Urol Radiol 1983;5:177–183

Berland LL, Koslin DB, Routh WD, et al: Renal artery stenosis: prospective evaluation of diagnosis with color duplex US compared with angiography: Work in progress. Radiology 1990;174:421–423

Burks DD, Markey BJ, Burkhard TK, et al: Suspected testicular torsion

and ischemia: evaluation of color Doppler sonography. Radiology 1990;175:815–821

Desberg AL, Paushter DM, Lammert GK, et al: Renal artery stenosis: evaluation with color Doppler flow imaging. Radiology 1990;177:749–753

Grant EG, Tessler FN, Perrelia RR: Clinical Doppler imaging. AJR Am J Roentgenol 1989;152:707–717

Haller JO, Berdon WE, Friedman AP: Increased renal cortical echogenicity: a normal finding in neonates and infants. Radiology 1982;142:173–174

Hricak H, Slovis TL, Callen CW, et al: Neonatal kidneys: sonographic-anatomic correlation. Radiology 1983;147:699–702

Keller MS: Renal Doppler sonography in infants and children. Radiology 1989;172:603–604

Jequier S, Paltiel H, Lafortune M: Ureterovesical jets in infants and children: duplex and color Doppler US studies. Radiology 1990;175:349–353

Kraus RA, Gaisie G, Young LW: Increased renal parenchymal echogenicity: causes in pediatric patients. Radiographics 1990;10:1009–1018

Lewis BD, James EM, Charboneau JW, et al: Current applications of color Doppler imaging in the abdomen and extremities. Radiographics 1989;9:599

Makland NF, Wright C, Rosenthal SJ: Gray-scale ultrasonic appearances of renal transplant rejection. Radiology 1979;131:711–717

Marshall JL, Johnson ND, De Campo MP: Vesicoureteric reflux in children: prediction with color Doppler imaging: Work in progress. Radiology 1990;175:355–358

McInnis AW, Felman AH, Kaude JV, et al: Renal US in the neonatal period. Pediatr Radiol 1981;12:15–20

Merritt CRB: Doppler color flow imaging. J Clin Ultrasound 1987;15:591

Mitchell DG: Color Doppler imaging: principles, limitations, and artifacts. Radiology 1990;177:1–10

Nelson TR, Pretorius DH: The Doppler signal: where does it come from and what does it mean? AJR Am J Roentgenol 1988;151:439–447

Oppenheimer DA, Carroll BA, Yousem S: Sonography of the normal neonatal adrenal gland. Radiology 1983;146:157–160

Platt JF, Ellis JH, Rubin JM, et al: Intrarenal arterial Doppler sonography in patients with nonobstructive disease: correlation of resistive index with biopsy findings. AJR Am J Roentgenol 1990;154:1223–1227

Scoutt LM, Zawin ML, Taylor KWJ: Doppler US: Part II. Clinical applications. Radiology 1990;174:309–319

Taylor KJW, Holland S: Doppler US: Part I. Basic principles, instrumentation, and pitfalls. Radiology 1990;174:297–307

Computed Tomography

Berger PE, Kuhn PJ, Brusehaber J: Techniques for computed tomography in infants and children. Radiol Clin North Am 1981;19:399–408

Dachner JN, Boillot B, Eurin D, et al: Rational use of CT in acute pyelonephritis: findings and relationships with reflux. Pediatr Radiol 1993;23:281–285

Dalla-Palma L, Pozzi-Mucelli F, Pozzi-Mucelli RS: Delayed CT findings in acute renal infection. Clin Radiol 1995;50:364–370

Doppman JL, Cornblath M, Dwyer AJ, et al: Computed tomography of the liver and kidneys in glycogen storage disease. J Comput Assist Tomogr 1982;6:67–71

Fernbach SK, Feinstein KA, Donaldson JS, Baum ES: Nephroblastomatosis: comparison of CT with US and urography. Radiology 1988;166:153–156

Fishman EK, Hartman DS, Goldman SM, Siegelman SS: The CT appearance of Wilms' tumor. J Comput Assist Tomogr 1983;7:659–665

Fultz PJ, Hampton WR, Totterman MS: Computed tomography of pyonephrosis. Abdom Imaging 1993;18:82–87

Heneghan JP, Dalrymple NC, Verga M, et al: Soft-tissue rim sign in the diagnosis of ureteral calculi with use of unenhanced helical CT. Radiology 1997;202:709–711

Herman TE, Shackelford GD, McAlister WH: Pseudotumoral sarcoid granulomatous nephritis in a child: case presentation with sonographic and CT findings. Pediatr Radiol 1997;27:752–754

Kirks DR: Computed tomography of pediatric urinary tract disease. Urol Radiol 1983;5:199–208

Kirks DR: Practical techniques for pediatric computed tomography. Pediatr Radiol 1983;13:148–155

Kuhn JP, Berger PE: Computed tomography in the evaluation of blunt trauma in children. Radiol Clin North Am 1981;19:495–501

Kuhn JP, Berger PE: Computed tomography of the kidney in infancy and childhood. Radiol Clin North Am 1981;19:445–461

Nguyen MM, Das S: Pediatric renal trauma. Urology 2002;59:762–66; discussion 766–767

Perez-Brayfield MR, Gatti JM, Smith EA, et al: Blunt traumatic hematuria in children: is a simplified algorithm justified? J Urol 2002;167:2543–2546; discussion 2546–2547

Quillin SP, Brink JA, Heiken JP, et al: Helical (spiral) CT angiography for identification of crossing vessels at the ureteropelvic junction. AJR Am J Roentgenol 1996;166:1125–1130

Rohrschneider WK, Weirich A, Rieden K, et al: US, CT, and MR imaging characteristics of nephroblastomatosis. Pediatr Radiol 1998;28:435–443

Siegel MJ: Protocols for helical CT in pediatrics. In Silverman PM (ed): Helical (Spiral) Computed Tomography: A Practical Approach to Clinical Protocols. New York, Lippincott–Raven, 1998:179–224

Siegel MJ, Balfe DM, McClennan BL, et al: Clinical utility of CT in pediatric retroperitoneal disease: 5 years experience. AJR Am J Roentgenol 1982;138:1011–1017

Siegel MJ, Glasier CM, Sagel SS: CT of pelvic disorders in children. AJR Am J Roentgenol 1981;137:1139–1143

Siegel MJ, Luker GD: Pediatric applications of helical (spiral) CT. Radiol Clin North Am 1995;33:997–1022

Smith RC, Rosenfield AT, Choe KA, et al: Acute flank pain: comparison of non-contrast-enhanced CT and intravenous urography. Radiology 1995;194:789–794

Strouse PJ, Bates DG, Bloom DA, Goodsitt MM: Non-contrast thin-section helical CT of urinary tract calculi in children. Pediatr Radiol 2002;32:326–332

Szolar DH, Kammerhuber F, Altziebler S, et al: Multiphasic helical CT of the kidney: increased conspicuity for detection and characterization of small (< 3-cm) renal masses. Radiology 1997;202:211–217

Tublin ME, Tessler FN, McCauley TR, Kesack CD: Effect of hydration status on renal medulla attenuation on unenhanced CT scans. AJR Am J Roentgenol 1997;168:257–259

Magnetic Resonance

Aerts P, Van Hoe L, Bosmans H, et al: Breath-hold MR urography using the HASTE technique. AJR Am J Roentgenol 1996;166:543–545

Baker ME, Blinder R, Spritzer CE, et al: MR evaluation of adrenal masses at 1.5 T. AJR Am J Roentgenol 1989;153:307–312

Bennett HF, Debiao L: MR imaging of renal function. Magn Reson Imaging Clin 1997;5:107–126

Borthne A, Nordshus T, Reiseter T, et al: MR urography: the future gold standard in paediatric urogenital imaging? Pediatr Radiol 1999;29:694–701

Borthne A, Pierre-Jerome C, Nordshus T, Reiseter T: MR urography in children: current status and future development. Eur Radiol 2000;10:503–511

Choyke PL: MR imaging of the kidneys and retroperitoneum. In Categorical Course Syllabus on MRI. Oakbrook, IL, Radiological Society of North America, 1990:165–173

Choyke PL, Frank JA, Girton ME, et al: Dynamic Gd-DTPA-enhanced MR imaging of the kidney: experimental results. Radiology 1989;170:713–720

Cohen MD: The visualization of major blood vessels by magnetic resonance in children with malignant tumors. Radiographics 1985;5:441

Dunnick NR: Adrenal imaging: current status. AJR Am J Roentgenol 1990;154:927–936

Ellenberg SS, Lee JKT, Brown JJ, et al: Renal masses: evaluation with gradient-echo Gd-DTPA–enhanced dynamic MR imaging. Radiology 1990;176:333–338

Fichtner J, Spielman D, Herfkens R, et al: Ultrafast contrast enhanced magnetic resonance imaging of congenital hydronephrosis in a rat model. J Urol 1994;152:682–687

Fukuda Y, Watanabe H, Tomita T, et al: Evaluation of glomerular function in individual kidneys using dynamic magnetic resonance imaging. Pediatr Radiol 1996;26:324–328

Hattery R, King BF: Technique and application of MR urography. Radiology 1995;194:25–27

Heiken JP, Lee JKT: MR imaging of the pelvis. Radiology 1988;166:11–16

Henning J, Friedburg H: Clinical applications and methodological developments of the RARE technique. Magn Reson Imaging 1988;6:391–395

Hussain S, O'Malley M, Jara H, et al: MR urography. Magn Reson Imaging Clin N Am 1997;5:95–106

Kier R, McCarthy S: MR characterization of adrenal masses: field strength and pulse sequence considerations. Radiology 1989;171:671–674

Kikinis R, Schulthess GK, Jäger P, et al: Normal and hydronephrotic kidney: evaluation of renal function with contrast-enhanced MR imaging. Radiology 1987;165:837–842

Kneeland JB, Hyde JS: High-resolution MR imaging with local coils. Radiology 1989;171:1–7

Knesplova L, Krestin GP: Magnetic resonance in the assessment of renal function. Eur Radiol 1998;8:201–211

Krestin GP: Magnetic resonance imaging of the kidneys: current status. Magn Reson Q 1994;10:2–21

Laissy JP, Faraggi M, Lebtahi R, et al: Functional evaluation of normal and ischemic kidney by means of gadolinium-DOTA enhanced turbo flash MR imaging: a preliminary comparison with 99mTc-MAG3 dynamic scintigraphy. Magn Reson Imaging 1994;12:413–419

Lenz GW, Haacke EM, Masaryk TJ, et al: In-plane vascular imaging: pulse sequence design and strategy. Radiology 1988;166:875–882

Nolte-Ernsting CC, Bucker A, Adam GB, et al: Gadolinium-enhanced excretory MR urography after low-dose diuretic injection: comparison with conventional excretory urography. Radiology 1998;209:147–157

O'Malley ME, Soto JA, Yucel EK, Hussain S: MR urography: evaluation of a three-dimensional fast spin-echo technique in patients with hydronephrosis. AJR Am J Roentgenol 1997;168:387–392

Pettigrew RI, Avruch L, Dannels W, et al: Fast-field-echo MR imaging with Gd-DTPA: physiologic evaluation of the kidney and liver. Radiology 1986;160:561–563

Podolak MJ, Hedlund LW, Evans AJ, et al: Evaluation of flow through simulated vascular stenoses with gradient echo magnetic resonance imaging. Invest Radiol 1989;24:184–189

Regan F, Bohlman ME, Khazan R, et al: MR-urography using HASTE imaging in the assessment of ureteric obstruction. AJR Am J Roentgenol 1996;167:1115–1120

Reuther G, Kiefer B, Wandl E: Visualization of urinary tract dilatation: value of single-shot MR urography. Eur Radiol 1997;7:1276–1281

Rohrschneider WK, Becker K, Hoffend J, et al: Combined static-dynamic MR urography for the simultaneous evaluation of morphology and function in urinary tract obstruction. II. Findings in experimentally induced ureteric stenosis. Pediatr Radiol 2000;30:523–532

Rohrschneider WK, Hoffend J, Becker K, et al: Combined static-dynamic MR urography for the simultaneous evaluation of morphology and function in urinary tract obstruction. I. Evaluation of the normal status in an animal model. Pediatr Radiol 2000;30:511–522

Rothpearl A, Frager D, Subramanian A, et al: MR urography: technique and application. Radiology 1995;194:125–130

Rothschild PA, Crooks LE, Margulis AR: Direction of MR imagining. Invest Radiol 1990;25:275–281.

Roy C, Saussine C, Jahn C, et al: Evaluation of RARE-MR urography in the assessment of ureterohydronephrosis. J Comput Assist Tomogr 1994;18:601–608

Semelka RC, Hricak H, Tomei E, et al: Obstructive nephropathy: evaluation with dynamic Gd-DTPA–enhanced MR imaging. Radiology 1990;175:797–803

Sigmund G, Stoever B, Zimmerhackl LB, et al: RARE-MR-urography in the diagnosis of upper urinary tract abnormalities in children. Pediatr Radiol 1991;1991:416–420

Staatz G, Nolte-Ernsting CC, Adam GB, et al: Feasibility and utility of respiratory-gated, gadolinium-enhanced T1-weighted magnetic resonance urography in children. Invest Radiol 2000;35:504–512

Tang Y, Yamashita Y, Namimoto T, et al: The value of MR urography that uses HASTE sequences to reveal urinary tract disorders. AJR Am J Roentgenol 1996;167:1497–1502

Verswijvel GA, Oyen RH, Van Poppel HP, et al: Magnetic resonance imaging in the assessment of urologic disease: an all-in-one approach. Eur Radiol 2000;10:1614–1619

Vascular Studies

Anglade MC, Derhy S, Delvalle A, et al: Abdominal venous thrombosis: applications of gradient-echo magnetic resonance imaging. Diagn Intervent Radiol 1989;1:61–67

Stanley P, Miller JH (eds): Pediatric Angiography. Baltimore, Williams & Wilkins, 1982

Wagner ML, Singleton EB, Egan ME: Digital subtraction angiography in children. AJR Am J Roentgenol 1983;140:127–133

Choice of Imaging Procedures

Cramer BM, Schlegel EA, Thureroff JW: MR imaging in the differential diagnosis of scrotal and testicular disease. Radiographics 1991;11:9–21

DeVun DA, Merritt CRB: Ultrasonography of testicular masses. Appl Radiol 1991;Jan:26–29

Gatsonis C, McNeil BJ: Collaborative evaluations of diagnostic tests: experience of the Radiology Diagnostic Oncology Group. Radiology 1990;175:571–575

C h a p t e r   2

NUCLEAR IMAGING OF THE KIDNEYS AND URINARY TRACT

DOUGLAS F. EGGLI

Imaging of the kidneys and urinary tract is an important part of pediatric nuclear medicine. Scintigraphic techniques compliment the anatomic imaging modalities by evaluating normal physiology and the pathophysiology of disease states. Together, the demonstration of alterations in anatomy, coupled with alterations in physiology, provides a more complete diagnostic picture of problems in the pediatric genitourinary (GU) tract. Scintigraphic studies can quantitatively measure numerous physiologic parameters. Studies include dynamic renal imaging, with or without pharmacologic interventions, renal cortical imaging, isotope cystography, and quantitative measurements of glomerular filtration rate (GFR) and effective renal plasma flow (ERPF). Physiologic processes that can be evaluated include renal flow, renal function (both tubular and glomerular), absolute and differential renal function, drainage of the collecting systems, and bladder function, including bladder volumes. Disease processes that can be evaluated include vesicoureteral reflux (VUR), pyelonephritis, renal ectopia, obstructive uropathy, hypertension, and complications of renal transplantation. Radiopharmaceuticals include tubular transport and glomerular filtration agents. Both types are typically labeled with technetium-99m.

A more detailed discussion of the diseases affecting the kidneys and urinary tract in children is included elsewhere in this text. This chapter is primarily focused on the discussion of nuclear medicine approaches to the evaluation of the pediatric GU tract.

Nuclear medicine GU procedures are minimally invasive, requiring no more than bladder catheterization and venous access. Intravenous hydration accompanies most pharmacologic challenge tests. Most GU tract procedures require no patient preparation. Sedation should rarely be required. Radiation exposure to the GU tract is similar to radiographic and computed tomography (CT) procedures. Radiation exposures to gonads, bone marrow, and whole body are typically less than 10% of the target organ exposures.

Renal function is evaluated both qualitatively and quantitatively. Qualitative evaluation includes visual evaluation of blood flow to the kidneys, extraction and concentration of the radiopharmaceutical by the cortex, and excretion. The radiopharmaceutical should appear in the kidneys within one flow frame of when the aorta appears and then peak rapidly. The cortex should rapidly extract and concentrate the tracer, peaking by 3 to 4 minutes. The cortex should clear half of its activity by 6 to 8 minutes. Excreted activity should be seen in the renal pelvis by about 6 minutes after injection, and activity should appear in the bladder by 10 to 12 minutes. Dynamic images are acquired digitally every 15 to 30 seconds using a computer. Time–activity curves permit quantitative measurements of renal function. Differential function is measured and time–activity curves representing renal function are generated from regions of interest drawn around the kidneys and drainage system. Normal differential function is symmetric around 50% with a margin of ± 5%. On dynamic studies with tubular transport agents, activity within the cortex should peak within 3 to 4 minutes, and the clearance half-time (peak to half-peak) should be 6 to 8 minutes.

Testicular scintigraphy was once a significant component of pediatric nuclear medicine. Although it still has a high level of diagnostic accuracy in the evaluation of the acutely painful scrotum, it has largely been replaced by color and power Doppler ultrasound. Sonography is rapid and accurate and avoids the use of ionizing radiation.

RADIOPHARMACEUTICALS

Four radiopharmaceuticals are in common use in renal and GU tract studies. They are technetium-99m MAG$_3$ (mercaptoacetyltriglycine), technetium-99m DTPA (diethylenetriaminepentaacetic acid), technetium-99m DMSA (dimercaptosuccinic acid), and technetium-99m sulfur colloid. MAG$_3$ is the agent of choice for most dynamic renal imaging. DMSA is used for renal cortical imaging. Sulfur colloid is used for isotope cystography. Radiopharmaceutical dosages are usually calculated on a microcurie (μCi) per kilogram of body surface area basis, with minimum and maximum doses for each study type.

Technetium-99m MAG$_3$ is a tubular transport agent functionally similar to *para*-aminohippurate and its imaging analog *ortho*-iodohippurate (OIH), labeled with iodine-131 or iodine-123. MAG$_3$ is extracted from renal plasma blood flow and actively transported into the proximal tubular cell and again actively transported against a gradient into the tubular lumen. MAG$_3$ is highly protein bound so that it remains in the vascular space and does not distribute into extracellular water. Unlike OIH, it does not distribute into red blood cells, so its total volume of distribution is smaller than OIH. As a result its calculated quantitative plasma clearance is about half of that of OIH. Renal transit parameters, however, are virtually identical. The rapid transit and clearance parameters of MAG$_3$ make it the preferred radiopharmaceutical for dynamic renal imaging. Clearance half-time is in the 6 to 8 minute range. Quantitative ERPF measurements can be obtained as part of a MAG$_3$ study.

Technetium-99m DTPA is a glomerular filtration agent. It can be used for dynamic renal imaging as well as quantitative GFR measurements. Quantitative GFR measurements can be made using either a camera-based technique as part of an imaging study or by measuring plasma clearance from blood samples. Approximately 20% to 25% of the DTPA in the renal blood flow is cleared in each pass through the kidney, resulting in a clearance half-time of about 25 to 30 minutes. Technetium-99m MAG$_3$ is more than 90% cleared in a single pass through the kidney. Therefore, its clearance half-time is much shorter than that of DTPA. In a standard 30-minute dynamic renal scan, kidney function is evaluated through in excess of three clearance half-times for MAG$_3$ compared to a single clearance half-time for DTPA. DTPA is less protein bound than MAG$_3$. Protein binding is variable and depends on the commercial preparation. There is enough protein binding of DTPA that quantitative GFR measurements must be corrected for it. Alternatively, iodine-125–labeled iothalamate can be used for quantitative GFR measurements.

Technetium-99m DMSA is a tubular transport agent. It is actively transported into the proximal tubular epithelial cell by the organic acid active transport mechanism. Because DMSA contains a sulfhydryl group in its structure, it binds to other sulfhydryl groups in the cytosol of the tubular cell and is not excreted. This permits static imaging of the renal cortex in multiple projections. Fifty percent of the injected DMSA dose is retained in the renal cortex 2 hours after injection. Typically, no activity is visualized in the renal pelvis at that time. DMSA is not accumulated in the medullary portions of the kidney.

Technetium-99m sulfur colloid is an inert, radiolabeled, nonabsorbable colloidal particle of about 0.1 μ in size. It is used as a passive label and is employed whenever systemic absorption of the radiotracer needs to be avoided. It is used to radiolabel the saline that is infused into the bladder for isotope cystography. For the same reason, it is used as the label for most gastrointestinal tract transit studies. When sulfur colloid is administered systemically, it is rapidly trapped by the reticuloendothelial system of the liver, spleen, and bone marrow.

Finally, although not in common use and not readily commercially available, glucoheptonate (GH) should be mentioned. Technetium-99m GH is partially filtered and partially excreted by tubular secretion, with approximately 7% to 10% of the injected dose remaining in the renal cortex 2 hours after injection. This permits information about dynamic renal function and cortical architecture to be obtained with a single radiopharmaceutical. However, the functional parameter of cortical clearance cannot be evaluated because of the cortical retention, and retention of concentrated radiopharmaceutical in a dilated renal pelvis may make cortical activity difficult to image. Because of these limitations, GH is not routinely used in clinical practice and, as a result, currently has limited availability in the United States.

ISOTOPE CYSTOGRAPHY

Isotope cystography is performed to diagnose VUR. Similar to contrast cystography, the bladder is filled in a retrograde fashion to maximum distention with saline and radiopharmaceutical. At peak filling, oblique straining images can be obtained in children old enough to cooperate. An upright voiding sequence followed by a postvoid image typically completes the study. The radiopharmaceutical of choice for isotope cystography is technetium-99m sulfur colloid. It is a nonabsorbable colloidal particle. The usual dose is in the 0.5- to 1.0-mCi (18- to 37-MBq) range. Technetium-99m DTPA and technetium-99m pertechnetate can also be used for isotope cystography, but it is possible that either of these two radiopharmaceuticals could be absorbed across an inflamed bladder mucosa and be subsequently excreted by the kidneys, simulating VUR when none exists. Quantitative measurements of DTPA absorption across the bladder mucosa are used to follow adult patients with chronic cystitis. Radiation exposure to the bladder wall from radiolabeled sulfur colloid is in the 20- to 30- mrem range, not dissimilar to the radiation exposure to the bladder from low-dose intermittent pulsed fluoroscopy. The radiation dosage to the bone marrow and gonads with isotope scintigraphy, however, is in the 1- to 3-mrem range, more than 10-fold lower than pulsed fluoroscopy.

Compared to contrast cystography, the scintigraphic study has low anatomic resolution. When anatomic detail is required, a contrast cystogram must be performed. This includes patients who have suspected structural abnormality of the GU tract and the first study on all males, to exclude posterior urethral valves. Anatomic detail is insufficient to evaluate calyceal morphology with isotope cystography; however, using ureteral and renal pelvic configuration, isotope cystography employs the same 5-grade international reflux grading system as contrast cystography (Fig. 1). The advantages of isotope cystography include the low radiation exposure to bone marrow and gonads and the ability to image continuously, which increases the sensitivity for the detection of grade II and III reflux 2 to 2½ times over contrast cystography. The ability to quantita-

tively measure bladder volumes and reflux rates and volumes is an additional benefit.

Patients with reflux do not reflux every time the bladder is filled. Studies of cyclic bladder filling show that filling the bladder multiple times increases the detection of VUR. The incremental value of cyclic filling, however, falls off significantly after the second bladder filling. Data from cyclic bladder filling studies show that a standard single-fill cystogram probably misses up to 27% of grade I reflux, 38% of grade II reflux, and 12% of grade III reflux.

Isotope cystography should be used for all follow-up studies in patients with documented VUR, and for the screening of asymptomatic siblings of patients with reflux, and can be used for the initial cystogram in female patients over 1 year of age who present with an uncomplicated urinary tract infection.

It is important that siblings of patients with documented VUR be screened for reflux. Studies show that about 45% of asymptomatic siblings of patients with documented VUR also have reflux. Reflux in the asymptomatic siblings is grade II or higher in 70% (Fig. 2). It is particularly important to screen younger siblings. Grade III or higher reflux was seen in 50% of siblings under the age of 1 year. Screening for renal scarring may also be appropriate because 23% of the refluxing asymptomatic siblings were found to have

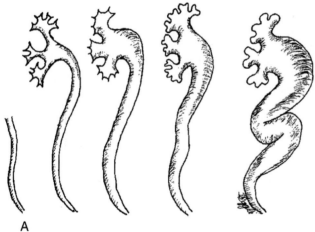

A

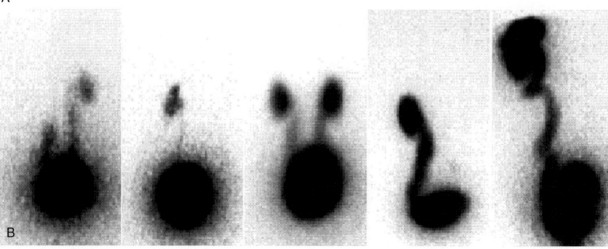

B

FIGURE 1. A, Conceptual diagram of the 5-grade grading system for vesicoureteral reflux, grades I through V, from left to right. B, Scintigraphic grading of VUR demonstrated in a series of images from five different patients. The images are obtained posteriorly. The first image demonstrates grade I reflux on the left and grade III on the right. The second image demonstrates grade II reflux on the left. Note that the ureter is not dilated. The third image demonstrates bilateral grade III reflux with ureteral dilatation and mild dilatation of the renal pelvis. The fourth image demonstrates grade IV reflux with both tortuosity and dilatation of the ureter and dilatation of the renal pelvis. The last image demonstrates grade V reflux with a corkscrew ureter and massively dilated renal pelvis. (A from and B adapted from Eggli DF, Tulchinsky M: Scintigraphic evaluation of pediatric urinary tract infection. Semin Nucl Med 1993;23:199–218, with permission.)

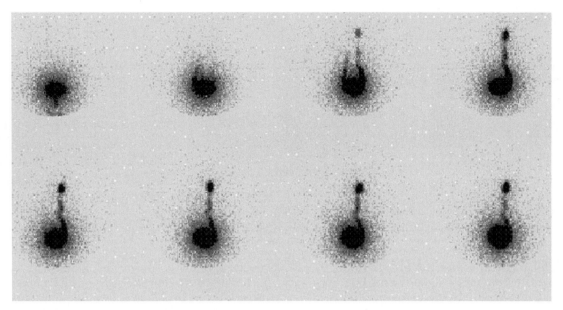

FIGURE 2. Bilateral VUR in a sibling screening exam. Grade I reflux is seen on the left and grade IV on the right. Note the tortuous right ureter.

renal scarring, presumptive evidence of silent pyelonephritis.

RENAL CORTICAL SCINTIGRAPHY

Renal cortical scintigraphy is typically performed with DMSA. The most common clinical indications include the evaluation of pyelonephritis and renal scarring, the calculation of differential function, and the evaluation of renal ectopia and dysplasia. Differential function calculation is independent of size, morphology, and, when a geometric mean methodology is employed, differences in renal depth.

Animal research has shown that the sensitivity and specificity of renal cortical imaging with DMSA approach 95%. Imaging must be done at a minimum with a pinhole collimator. Parallel-hole collimation lacks sufficient anatomic detail for reliable diagnosis. Electronic magnification cannot substitute for the true increase in resolution that can be achieved with pinhole collimation. Sensitivity can be further increased by performing single-photon emission computed tomography (SPECT) with a multiheaded gamma camera. This, however, is accomplished at the cost of specificity. Although sensitivity with multiheaded SPECT increases to between 97% and 100%, specificity decreases toward 90% or slightly higher. SPECT cortical tomography requires a higher DMSA dose to be administered than is required for planar imaging, and younger children may require sedation. When SPECT is performed, the camera should have two or more heads. Single-head SPECT acquisition is worse than pinhole imaging. Contrast-enhanced CT and magnetic resonance imaging have been shown to have sensitivity and specificity similar to renal cortical imaging with pinhole collimation. Both studies are more expensive, and CT provides significantly higher bone marrow exposure. Ultrasound, even when power Doppler is employed, is less sensitive than any of the studies mentioned above. Ultrasound has been shown to detect only 40% to 50% of the abnormalities seen with DMSA imaging. Inclusion of color or power Doppler improves this only minimally. Intravenous urography misses 75% of DMSA abnormalities.

The usual dose of technetium-99m DMSA for renal cortical imaging is 50 µCi (2 MBq) per kilogram, with a minimum dose of 350 to 500 µCi (13 to 18.5 MBq) and a maximum dose of 3 mCi (111 MBq). Radiation exposure to the radiation-sensitive organs (bone marrow and gonads) is very low with DMSA. Bone marrow receives 0.022 rads/mCi. Ovaries, testes, and the whole body receive even less. The highest radiation dose is to the kidney cortex, where DMSA actively accumulates. The cortical dose is approximately 0.9 rads/mCi. Total kidney exposure is about two thirds of the cortical exposure. Most children being evaluated for urinary tract infection receive a DMSA dose in the 0.5- to 1.0-mCi range (18.5 to 37 MBq).

DMSA is extracted by and accumulates in the proximal convoluted tubule. It does not accumulate in the loop of Henle, the renal medulla, or the collecting systems. This results in the appearance of a rim of cortical activity surrounding photon-deficient central collecting systems (Fig. 3). DMSA will provide a more reliable estimate of differential function than either MAG3 or DTPA if one of the kidneys has delayed function. In children, static images with pinhole collimation are obtained in multiple projections 1½ to 2 hours after injection. The usual projections are posterior, both posterior obliques, and both laterals. Anterior views with obliques are obtained in patients with renal ectopia and significant scoliosis, where one kidney can be expected to be more anteriorly located. Geometric

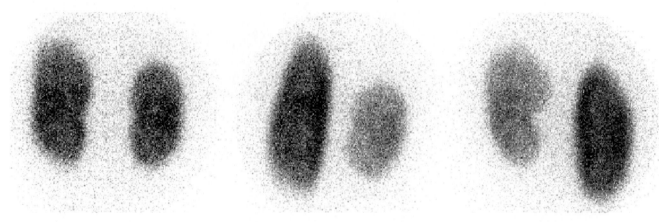

FIGURE 3. Normal DMSA renal study. Images are posterior, left posterior oblique, and right posterior oblique.

mean calculations of differential function, which correct for depth discrepancies, should be made if there is a significant left-to-right renal depth discrepancy.

Renal cortical scintigraphy can be used to evaluate both pyelonephritis and renal scarring. Both are seen as areas of diminished radiotracer accumulation. In acute pyelonephritis, decreased radiotracer accumulation results from the combination of interstitial edema and swelling, which produce secondary ischemia and decreased delivery of the radiotracer, and from paralysis of the cellular active transport mechanism by toxic superoxides that result from white blood cell lysis (Fig. 4). In scarring, loss of functioning tubules results in reduced tracer accumulation. Renal configuration aids in the separation of acute and chronic abnormality. Volume loss is the hallmark of scarring, whereas acute pyelonephritis demonstrates preservation of renal volume and contours. In very small cortical defects, it may be difficult to determine whether a defect visualized is acute pyelonephritis or scar without a follow-up study.

Healing of the defect created by acute pyelonephritis is age dependent. In children under 1 year of age, it may take 3 months or longer for tubular function to recover in an area of adequately treated and resolved pyelonephritis, whereas the kidneys of older children and teenagers return to normal in as little as 2 weeks. The likelihood of scarring after an acute infection is also age related. Younger children are more likely to scar than older children. Scarring following an acute episode of pyelonephritis is unusual in teenagers.

DIURESIS RENOGRAPHY

Diuresis renography is usually performed to evaluate hydronephrosis detected by ultrasound. It is a quantitative pharmacologic challenge test, which measures the response of the kidney to hydration and a diuretic challenge. If a hydronephrotic collecting system washes out promptly following a fluid and diuretic challenge, it is not obstructed. A detailed protocol has been described in a consensus report developed by the Pediatric Nuclear Medicine Council of the Society of Nuclear Medicine and the Society of Fetal Urology. The hallmark of the protocol is standardization of the acquisition parameters so that washout results can be reliably and reproducibly measured. The theory is that maximal hydration (15 ml/kg 5% dextrose in 0.45-normal saline [D_5 $_{0.45}$NS] given intravenously) and diuresis (1 mg/kg

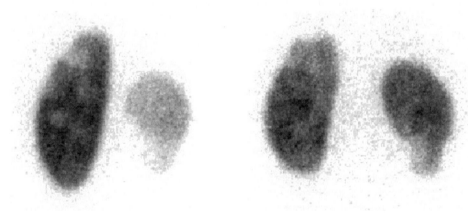

FIGURE 4. Acute pyelonephritis with old scarring. Left posterior oblique (LPO) and right posterior oblique pinhole views from a DMSA renal scan. The LPO view shows two areas of decreased DMSA accumulation with preservation of contours, one in the upper pole laterally and one in the midkidney. On the right side, the lower pole is shriveled, indicating volume loss and scar.

furosemide given intravenously) are required to evaluate the possibility of obstructive uropathy. Because a filling bladder physiologically obstructs the ureterovesical junction, continuous bladder drainage with a bladder catheter is essential. A bladder catheter also permits ongoing evaluation of the patient's response to diuresis and correction of any fluid imbalance. It also reduces the bone marrow and gonadal radiation dose. Technetium-99m MAG3 is the radiopharmaceutical of choice for diuresis renography. Because of its rapid cortical clearance, very little activity is likely to be retained in the cortex at the time of diuretic administration. Retained cortical activity could artificially prolong the washout half-time calculation.

The dose of MAG3 for diuretic renography is 50 to 100 µCi (1.85 to 3.7 MBq) per kilogram, with a minimum dose of 1 mCi (37 MBq) and a maximum dose of 5 mCi (185 MBq). For DTPA, the dose is 100 to 200 µCi (3.7 to 7.4 MBq) per kilogram, with a minimum dose of 2 mCi (74 MBq) and a maximum dose of 10 mCi (370 MBq). The study is a quantitative pharmacologic challenge test and requires intravenous access and bladder catheterization. The study has two phases. The first phase, prior to diuretic administration, evaluates renal function—flow, extraction, and excretion. The second phase, following diuretic administration, evaluates drainage. By closely monitoring urine output, the response to diuresis can be better evaluated.

Interpretation of results includes visual analysis of the images, inspection of the time–activity curves, and quantitative parameters. With standardization of the acquisition parameters, those patients who are clearly not obstructed and those who clearly are obstructed are easy to differentiate. In the absence of obstruction, following diuretic administration, the radioactivity in the renal pelvis visually washes out rapidly and the postdiuretic washout curve falls rapidly to baseline. When obstruction is present, activity visually persists in the renal pelvis and the washout curve either plateaus or continues to rise.

Quantitative analysis of washout is most valuable when there is some but incomplete washout. Calculation of a washout half-time will place most of the visually indeterminate patients into either the obstructed or nonobstructed categories, leaving a significantly smaller number of indeterminate results. Diuresis renography correlates well with the more invasive Whitaker pressure–perfusion test. Following diuretic administration, washout half-times can be measured either from the point of furosemide injection or from the point where the time–activity curve begins to drop. If the patient has been adequately intravenously hydrated, the two points should converge. An initial plateau on the time–activity curve before washout begins usually implies inadequate prehydration. A washout half-time of 10 minutes or less indicates no significant obstruction (Fig. 5). A washout half-time of 20 minutes or longer indicates a urodynamically significant obstruction (Fig. 6). Half-times between 10 and 20 minutes are indeterminate and require further follow-up.

After surgical correction of obstruction, the washout half-time may not return to the normal range for several months. The more dilated the system is prior to surgery, the more slowly it improves. However, function in these patients should remain stable.

Flow rate–dependent partial obstruction (beer drinker's kidney) presents a distinctive pattern on diuresis renography. After diuretic challenge, the washout curve initially falls promptly and then either plateaus or begins to rise again. This produces a biphasic washout curve. These patients have a partially obstructing lesion. Urine output rises incrementally following diuretic administration and peaks at about 15 minutes. Initially, these partially obstructing lesions can accommodate the increasing urine flow rate, and the washout curve falls. Once the urine flow rate exceeds the capacity of the partial obstruction, the curve either flattens or begins to rise, indicating that the drainage system has become functionally obstructed at a higher urine flow rate.

Several patient factors can confound the interpretation of diuretic renography studies. They include the degree of renal maturity, volume capacity of the dilated system, the degree of impairment of renal function, and the degree of obstruction. The goal of diuresis renography is to achieve maximal hydration and maximal diuresis in order to offset these confounding factors. These factors, however, must be considered when the study is interpreted.

Neonatal and infant kidneys are functionally immature and do not achieve an adult level of function until between 1 and 2 years of age. Under 6 months of age, urine production is low, and the urine produced is poorly concentrated. GFR is about half that at 1 year of age, and the immature kidney is less responsive to diuretic stimulation. Renal function under 1 month of age is halved again. Diuresis renography should be avoided if possible in the first month of life. Diuretic doses can be increased in patients with immature renal function. This will result in a more appropriate diuretic response.

Not all collecting systems are equally dilated. The more dilated the collecting system is, the more urine flow is required to achieve adequate washout. This is most problematic when massive dilation is coupled with immature or impaired renal function. Inadequate washout as a result of too little urine flow compared to the capacity of the collecting system may result in the appearance of obstruction when none exists.

Impaired renal function, like immaturity of renal function, leads to less urine volume produced. Studies have shown, however, that kidneys with GFRs as low as 10 ml/min per kidney can still achieve a significant diuretic response when the diuretic dose is adequate. The dose of diuretic administered can be scaled based on the creatinine level to achieve adequate diuresis in most patients.

Finally, most obstructions are partial. The result of the study predicts which partial obstructions are significant and are likely to result in the loss of renal function over time. The loss of function is secondary to back-pressure or infection upstream from the obstructing lesion. The more significant the partial obstruction, the greater the back-pressure, and the longer the washout half-time.

The most difficult cases combine multiple confounding factors. Although diuresis renography typically pro-

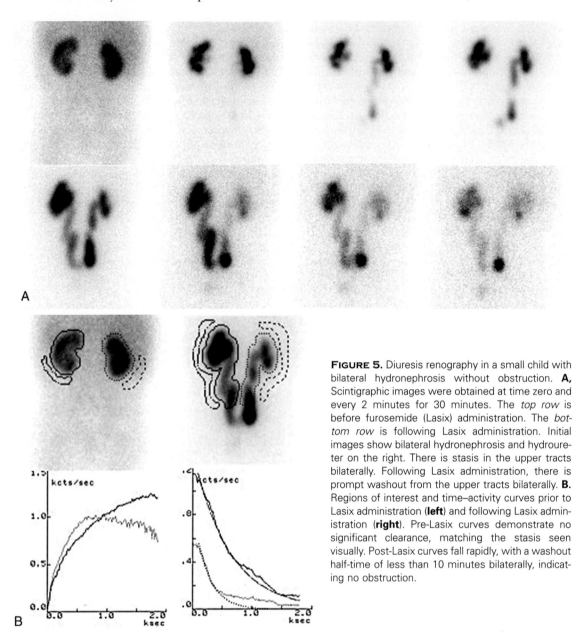

FIGURE 5. Diuresis renography in a small child with bilateral hydronephrosis without obstruction. **A,** Scintigraphic images were obtained at time zero and every 2 minutes for 30 minutes. The *top row* is before furosemide (Lasix) administration. The *bottom row* is following Lasix administration. Initial images show bilateral hydronephrosis and hydroureter on the right. There is stasis in the upper tracts bilaterally. Following Lasix administration, there is prompt washout from the upper tracts bilaterally. **B.** Regions of interest and time–activity curves prior to Lasix administration (**left**) and following Lasix administration (**right**). Pre-Lasix curves demonstrate no significant clearance, matching the stasis seen visually. Post-Lasix curves fall rapidly, with a washout half-time of less than 10 minutes bilaterally, indicating no obstruction.

duces highly reliable and reproducible results, these cases must be interpreted with caution.

ANGIOTENSIN-CONVERTING ENZYME INHIBITION SCINTIGRAPHY

Angiotensin-converting enzyme (ACE) inhibition scintigraphy is performed to evaluate patients suspected of having hypertension of a renovascular origin. It can also be used to evaluate the hemodynamic significance of a known renal artery stenosis. Anatomy and physiology do not always follow hand-in-hand in renal artery stenosis. Animal models suggest that the degree of renal artery stenosis has to be in excess of 90% to trigger the renin–angiotensin axis. ACE inhibition scintigraphy can

be used to determine whether or not a renal artery stenosis is likely to be the cause of a patient's hypertension. This is conceptually similar to coronary artery disease, myocardial perfusion imaging, and the diagnosis of ischemic heart disease. Not all renal artery stenoses produce hypertension. A renal artery stenosis produces renovascular hypertension only when the stenosis is severe enough to result in activation of the renin-angiotensin axis.

The renin-angiotensin axis is responsible for maintaining perfusion pressure to the kidneys and, indirectly, the whole body. When a decrease in perfusion pressure is detected at the juxtaglomerular complex, renin is released. Through a series of reactions, the renin is converted initially into angiotensinogen, then into angiotensin I, and subsequently by the action of ACE to angiotensin II, which is an extremely potent vasoconstrictor. Peripheral vasoconstriction then restores perfusion pressure to the kidneys. A hemodynamically significant renal artery stenosis will reduce the perfusion pressure to the affected kidney enough to activate the renin–angiotensin axis.

ACE inhibition scintigraphy can be performed either with oral captopril (0.7 mg/kg with a maximum dose of 50 mg) or intravenous enalaprilat (0.04 mg/kg IV). Intravenous enalaprilat is preferred over oral captopril. When IV enalaprilat is used, the imaging study can start 15 minutes after enalaprilat administration. Variable absorption of oral captopril limits its utility. When captopril is used, a delay of 1 hour or longer is required. A negative study with oral captopril is of uncertain significance and may represent a false-negative result because of inadequate absorption.

Mild hydration is part of the preparation for ACE inhibition scintigraphy. We hydrate intravenously with 5 ml/kg D_5 $_{0.45}$NS. Adequate prehydration prevents a hypotensive response to enalaprilat. It also prevents a false-positive result, which can occur when intravascular volume depletion systemically activates the renin-angiotensin axis. Activity in the renal pelvis interferes with the evaluation of cortical transit. A small dose of furosemide (lasix), approximately 0.25 mg/kg, can be used with the study to keep the renal pelvis washed out. If Lasix is used, a bladder catheter will also probably be required.

Renal function in most hypertensive children is normal, permitting a challenge study to be performed first. Either DTPA or MAG3 can be used for ACE inhibition scintigraphy. When DTPA is used, differential

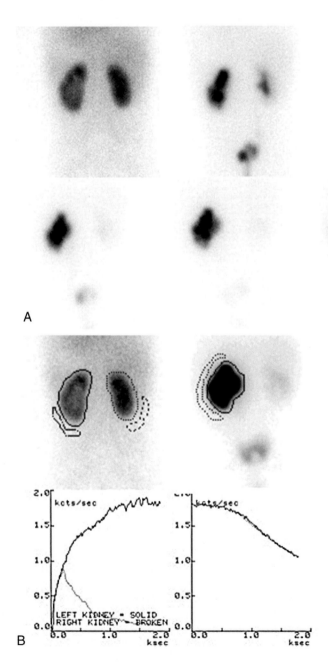

FIGURE 6. A, Hydronephrosis with obstruction. **A,** Scintigraphic images were obtained at time zero and every 2 minutes for 30 minutes. The *top row* is before furosemide (Lasix) administration. The *bottom row* is following Lasix administration. The initial nephrogram image on the left shows a prominent central photon deficiency with splaying of the cortex and enlargement of the left kidney. Over 30 minutes, the left renal pelvis fills but does not drain. The right kidney functions and drains normally. After Lasix administration, visually there is no washout. **B,** Regions of interest and time–activity curves prior to Lasix administration (**left**) and following Lasix administration (**right**). The pre-Lasix curve of the left kidney demonstrated progressive accumulation of tracer. The right kidney curve is normal. After Lasix administration, there is visually indeterminate washout from the left kidney, but the washout half-time is 30 minutes, in the obstructed range.

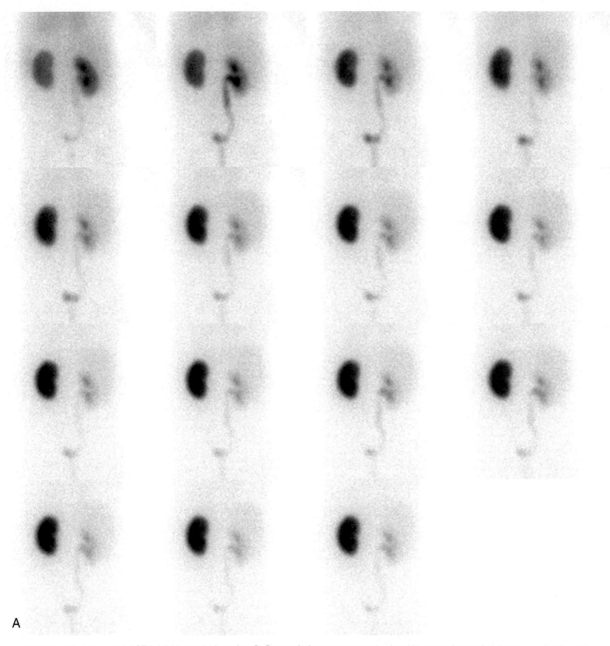

A

FIGURE 7. Abnormal ACE inhibition scintigraphy. **A,** Dynamic images were obtained in posterior projection every 2 minutes for 30 minutes. Fifteen minutes after challenge with 0.04 mg/kg intravenous enalaprilat, images demonstrate a pattern of cortical retention on the left, while the right side functions normally.   *Illustration continued on opposite page*

function is reduced on the affected side. On a MAG_3 study, cortical transit is prolonged and differential function is at most minimally affected. The kidney develops a pattern of cortical retention of radiopharmaceutical similar to the pattern seen in acute tubular necrosis (Fig. 7). Technetium-99m MAG_3 is more sensitive for detecting a hemodynamically significant renal artery stenosis than DTPA and is the preferred radiopharmaceutical. The combination of oral captopril and DTPA increases the likelihood of a false-negative result. If renal artery stenosis is responsible for the patient's hypertension, then scintigraphy following challenge with an ACE inhibitor should be abnormal. If the

challenge study is normal, a renovascular origin of the patient's hypertension is unlikely. If the challenge study is abnormal, a baseline study without the ACE inhibitor must be performed. If the baseline study is normal, a renovascular origin is likely.

RENAL TRANSPLANT EVALUATION

Doppler and power Doppler ultrasound along with biopsy are the primary methods of evaluating transplanted kidneys. However, scintigraphy can be used to demonstrate a number of complications of transplant

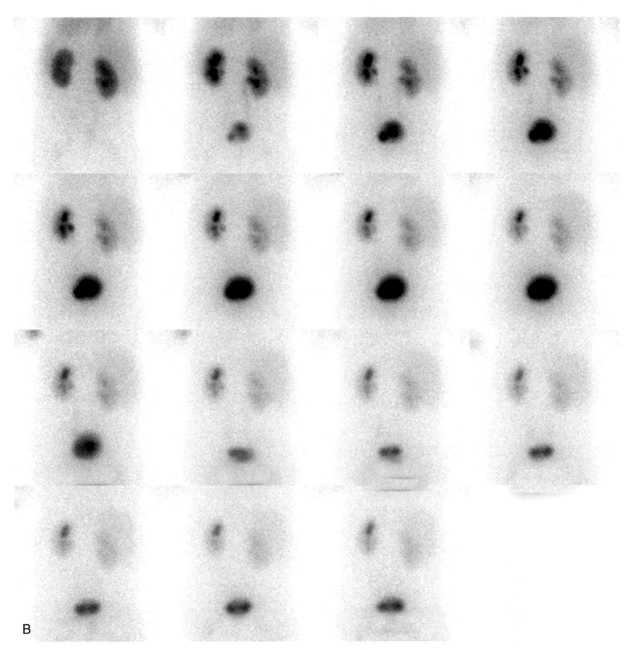

B

FIGURE 7. *Continued.* **B,** A subsequent baseline study without ACE challenge shows normal function on the left. This confirms a hemodynamically significant renal artery stenosis on the left.

surgery. Vascular compromise, including either renal artery or renal vein thrombosis, is readily evaluated using dynamic renal imaging. The usual clinical setting is a post-transplant patient with little or no urine output. Absence of vascular flow is a surgical emergency. If flow is present, a pattern of progressive parenchymal accumulation without excretion into the urine suggests acute tubular necrosis. Fluid collections around the kidney, such as hematoma, urinoma, or lymphocele, may be demonstrated. Scintigraphy may show extravasation of radiopharmaceutical into the fluid collection and confirm the diagnosis of a urinoma. Both hematomas and lymphoceles are photon-deficient collections, but are readily separated temporally. Hematomas occur early after transplantation and lymphoceles occur weeks to months later.

Chapter 3

SCINTIGRAPHIC ADRENAL IMAGING

DOUGLAS F. EGGLI

Adrenal scintigraphy is largely limited to evaluation of tumors of the adrenal medulla. Like much of nuclear medicine, anatomic detail is limited, but scintigraphic studies may be both sensitive and specific for pathophysiologic processes, both benign and malignant.

Radiopharmaceuticals specific for tumors of neuroendocrine origin are in common clinical use. They are methyl-iodobenzylguanidine (MIBG) labeled with iodine-131 or iodine-123 and octreotide labeled with indium-111. MIBG is a norepinephrine analog that is taken up by the amine reuptake and scavenging system in tissues of neutral origin. MIBG labeled with iodine-131 is commercially available, whereas MIBG labeled with iodine-123 is only available in those institutions capable of iodinating the MIBG molecule. Octreotide is composed of the eight N-terminal peptides of the somatostatin molecule and binds to the cellular somatostatin receptors, which are overexpressed by a number of tumors, including those of neuroendocrine origin.

Neuroblastoma is the most commonly scintigraphically imaged neuroendocrine tumor in children. The evaluation of neuroblastoma usually includes both MIBG imaging and bone imaging with a technetium-99m–labeled organophosphate compound, either ethylene diphosphonate or methylene diphosphonate. MIBG detects soft tissue disease that, except for the primary tumor itself, is not seen on bone scans. However, it may be difficult to determine on MIBG scans whether abnormal activity is in bone or bone marrow. Bone-scanning agents are reported to demonstrate more bone metastases than MIBG. Although bone-scanning agents are taken up in the primary tumor in approximately two thirds of cases, as previously noted, they are not taken up in soft tissue metastases. MIBG labeled with iodine-123 provides higher quality images in a shorter period of time than MIBG labeled with iodine-131, but is not generally available, so that most MIBG scans are done with iodine-131. MIBG positivity is not specific for malignancy. Benign neural tumors such as ganglioneuromas may demonstrate MIBG accumulation.

Bone metastases may occur anywhere in either the axial or appendicular skeleton, making screening of the whole body with bone scanning a useful tool. The lesions are often subtle and are frequently mixed "hot and cold." In long bones, they tend to occur in the metaphyses, adjacent to metabolically active growth

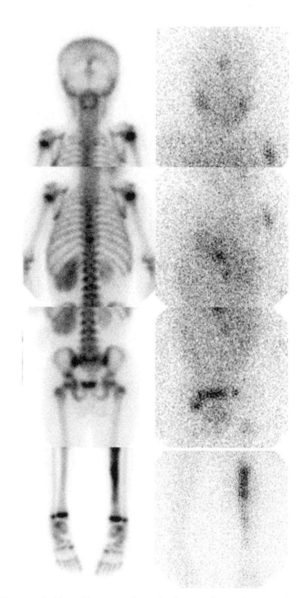

FIGURE 1. Neuroblastoma. Posterior images from a bone scan and MIBG scan obtained within days of each other on the same patient. Both studies show metastatic lesions in the posterior skull, midthoracic spine, posterior pelvis, and left tibia. A right proximal humeral metastasis seen on MIBG is not well seen on bone scan in this projection, but was seen on other views. The bone scan provides better anatomic localization of the MIBG-positive lesions. Normal MIBG accumulation is seen in the salivary glands and faintly in the heart and liver.

centers, so careful patient positioning and reliable resolution of the growth plates is required (Fig. 1).

Positron emission tomography (PET) with fluorine-18 fluorodeoxyglucose has utility as a nonspecific tumor imaging agent. Its role relative to more tumor-specific radiopharmaceuticals in neuroendocrine tumors is still evolving. PET imaging, once predominantly a research technique, is now widely available clinically and is approaching price competitiveness with MIBG. Like other nuclear medicine techniques, PET images often lack anatomic detail. The clinical value of PET images can be enhanced by registration and fusion with anatomic images from computed tomography or magnetic resonance imaging.

Octreotide labeled with indium-111 is not commonly used to image neuroblastoma. As neuroblastomas dedifferentiate toward anaplastic, they shed their somatostatin receptor, resulting in a false-negative scan. Octreotide, however, is an ideal radiopharmaceutical for imaging pheochromocytoma, which may rarely occur in childhood. The sensitivity of octreotide for pheochromocytoma is in excess of 90% and is greater than that of MIBG. MIBG, though, is more specific.

Chapter 4

INTERVENTIONAL PROCEDURES IN THE URINARY SYSTEM

JAMES S. DONALDSON

Interventional radiology plays a significant role in the management of children with genitourinary diseases. It is beyond the scope of this text to discuss many technical details; the goal is to provide the readers with enough information that they know some of the capabilities of an interventional service. Familiarity with the spectrum of procedures will help the diagnostic radiologist know when to recommend consultation and involvement by the interventional radiology service.

PERCUTANEOUS NEPHROSTOMY

Drainage of an obstructed kidney by placement of a nephrostomy is the most commonly performed interventional procedure in children (Fig. 1). Common indications include ureteropelvic junction obstruction in a child with solitary kidney or with impaired renal function and obstruction in a child with a failed pyeloplasty. Less common indications include fungal ball obstruction in an infant, obstruction resulting from a pelvic tumor or abscess, and renal calculi and inability to stent cystoscopically. A Whitaker test is occasionally needed to differentiate a dilated nonobstructed system from obstruction. The Whitaker test is performed by puncturing and infusing the collecting system at a constant rate while pressure measurements are obtained.

The nephrostomy in the infant is a more challenging procedure than in older children because of the small anatomy and the elasticity of the retroperitoneal tissues. Care must be taken in the infant to avoid decompression of the collecting system during guidewire exchanges.

The percutaneous nephrostomy results in a temporary urinary diversion until the cause of obstruction can be corrected. Securing devices such as the Cope loop within the collecting system and meticulous care of the external part of the catheter will prevent children from inadvertently pulling their catheters out.

URETERAL STENTING

Ureteral stents can be placed retrograde via a cystoscope under control of a urologist, or they may be placed in an antegrade fashion through a nephrostomy tract by interventional radiologists (Fig. 2). A retrograde approach is generally the first approach taken and is less invasive, but is sometimes not possible. Indications for ureteral stent placement include ureterovesical junction obstruction following reimplantation for reflux, ureteropelvic obstruction resulting from failed pyeloplasty, ureteral obsruction following renal transplantation, traumatic ureteral transection, ureteral calculus, ureteral obstruction caused by pelvic tumor, or primary ureteral stenosis.

Antegrade percutaneous access into the collecting system allows instrumentation of the ureter and usually

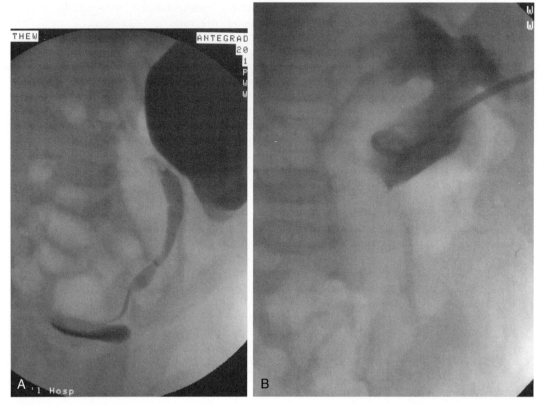

FIGURE 1. Nephrostomy for ureteropelvic junction obstruction. **A,** Antegrade nephrostomy in this 1-week-old child demonstrates stenosis at the ureteropelvic junction. **B,** A percutaneous nephrostomy was performed to assess amount of renal function in this kidney prior to pyeloplasty surgery.

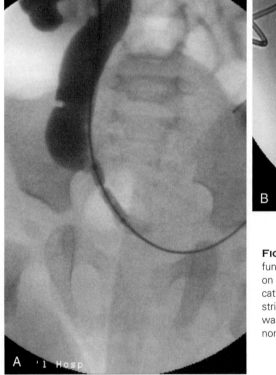

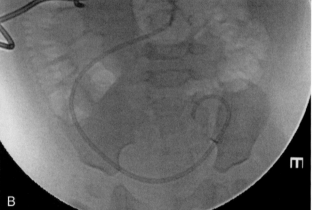

FIGURE 2. Ureterovesical obstruction on the side of the functioning kidney in a patient with a multicystic dysplastic kidney on the opposite side. Severe tortuosity of the ureter made catheterization of the distal ureter, balloon dilatation of the stricture (**A**) and double-J stent placement (**B**) difficult. The stent was removed after 6 weeks, leaving a widely patent and nonrefluxing ureter.

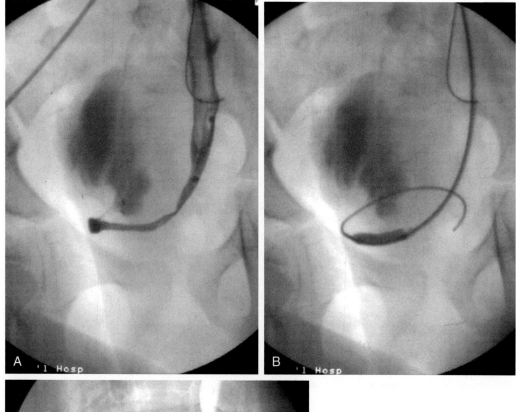

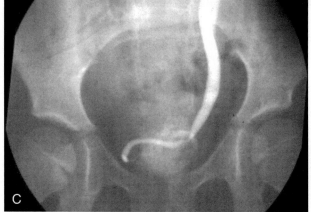

FIGURE 3. Ureterovesical obstruction following ureteral reimplantation for vesicoureteral reflux in a 5-year-old girl who developed obstruction of the distal ureter. **A,** Antegrade nephrostogram reveals tight stenosis of the surgically altered distal ureter. **B,** The stenosis was successfully passed and balloon dilatation was performed. **C,** Following dilatation, the ureter drained well despite the radiographic appearance, and a stent was not placed.

passage of small guidewires into the bladder. A stricture can be dilated if necessary, permitting passage of the stent. If a ureteral stricture cannot be crossed during initial access and instrumentation, the collecting system should be decompressed with a nephrostomy tube for several days. Another attempt should be made to cross the stricture before considering it a failure of percutaneous management.

Stent placement may provide the definitive treatment in the setting of a postoperative stricture or ureteral transection or rupure. A nephrostomy tube is generally left overnight, and a challenge of capping the nephrostomy tube is usually performed prior to removal of the nephrostomy tube. The internal stent allows diversion of urine without the need for external catheters. Successful dilatation can be performed without stent placement; however, stent placement is recommended in most situations (Fig. 3).

PERCUTANEOUS NEPHROLITHOTOMY

Large stones and staghorn calculus are the most common indication for the need for percutaneous stone extraction. Percutaneous endoscopic stone removal is generally preferred over an open flank surgical procedure because it is less invasive. Success rates for percutaneous techniques and open surgery are similar.

The procedure is usually staged into two procedures.

During the first procedure, a nephrostomy is placed preferably into the calyx containing the stones for removal. During the next procedure, usually performed the following day, the nephrostomy tract is dilated up to 30 French (except in infants and small children, in whom a smaller sheath will be introduced) and a sheath is placed. Through the sheath, the endoscope is introduced and the stones are extracted. These procedures are usually done in conjunction with a urologist, who performs the endoscopic portion of the exam.

TRAUMA TO THE GENITOURINARY TRACT

Many patients with renal injuries resulting from blunt trauma can be managed nonoperatively by interventional radiology. Patients with severe renal injuries defined by computed tomography scan and clinical evidence of ongoing bleeding should be evaluated with arteriography, and selective embolization of arterial bleeding should be performed. Renal vein injuries require immediate surgery. Complications following renal biopsies include fistulas to the collecting system and to the venous system (arteriovenous fistulas). Arteriography is indicated in these situations, with superselective embolization of the site of bleeding (Fig. 4).

Renal fracture with disruption of the renal collecting system and formation of a urinoma can sometimes be managed nonoperatively. Percutaneous drainage of the urinoma and diversion of urine by placement of a percutaneous nephrostomy and/or ureteral stent allows diversion of urine from the disrupted collecting system.

RENOVASCULAR DISORDERS

The results of percutaneous transluminal renal artery angioplasty (PTRA) in children are not as encouraging as those in adults with fibromuscular disease, but certainly there are indications for use of this procedure (Fig. 5). The location and length of the lesion are important predictors of success, as in adult series. Short, nonostial stenoses respond most favorably, with reported technical and clinical success rates of 80% to 100%. Long lesions and those involving the ostium are much less likely to respond. Initial success of PTRA in children with Takayasu's arteritis has been reported, but long-term patency is not known. The middle aortic syndrome and Williams syndrome may be indistinguishable angiographically; neither responds well to PTRA.

Intrarenal segmental stenoses may not be accessible for PTRA, and segmental embolization with infarction of the ischemic portion of renal parenchyma may be therapeutic in managing some children with hypertension (Fig. 6).

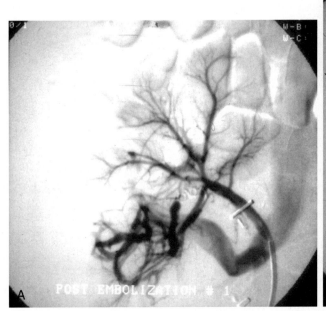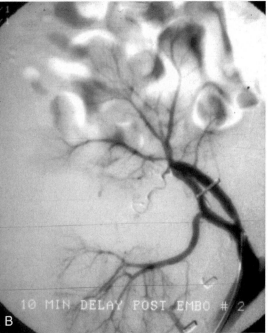

FIGURE 4. Embolization of arteriovenous fistula postbiopsy. Two days following a percutaneous biopsy of this patient's transplant kidney, the child continued to have gross hematuria. **A,** Angiogram revealed a large arteriovenous fistula. **B,** Selective coil embolization of the segmental artery resulted in occlusion of the fistula and infarction of only a small portion of renal parenchyma.

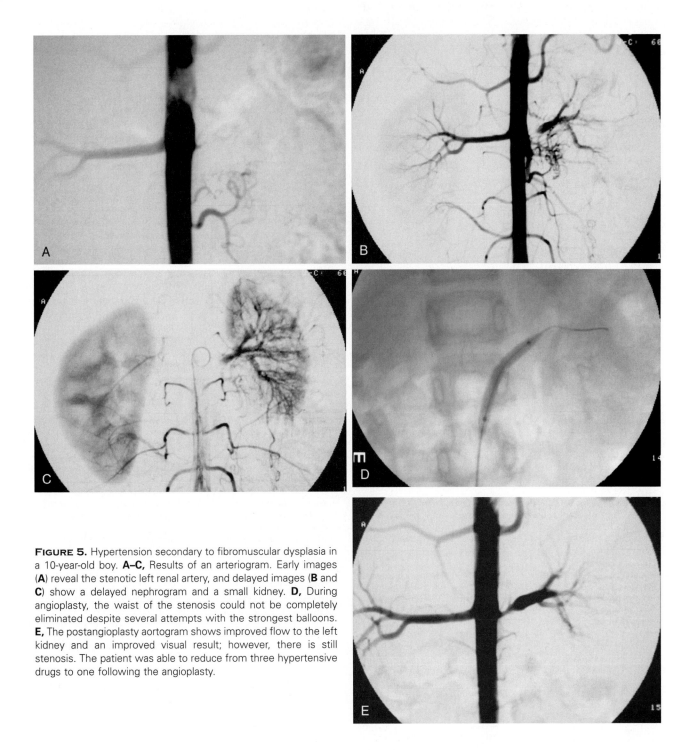

FIGURE 5. Hypertension secondary to fibromuscular dysplasia in a 10-year-old boy. **A–C,** Results of an arteriogram. Early images (**A**) reveal the stenotic left renal artery, and delayed images (**B** and **C**) show a delayed nephrogram and a small kidney. **D,** During angioplasty, the waist of the stenosis could not be completely eliminated despite several attempts with the strongest balloons. **E,** The postangioplasty aortogram shows improved flow to the left kidney and an improved visual result; however, there is still stenosis. The patient was able to reduce from three hypertensive drugs to one following the angioplasty.

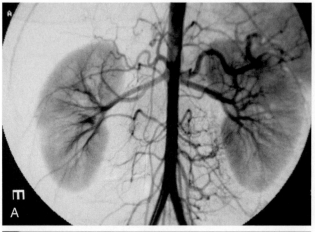

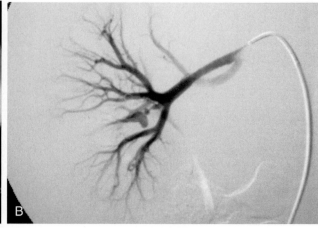

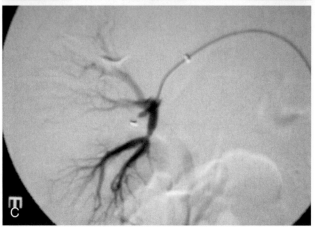

FIGURE 6. Segmental stenosis and embolization in a 14-year-old boy taking three hypertensive drugs. **A,** The patient underwent an aortogram which at first review appears normal. **B,** A selective renal arteriogram, however, reveals a tight lower pole segmental stenosis with distal aneurysm typical of fibromuscular dysplasia. This lesion could not be dilated with balloon angioplasty. **C,** The renal segment was embolized with a combination of liquid agents (ethanol), particles (polyvinyl alcohol), and microcoils. The patient improved following embolization, reducing to one hypertensive drug, but was unable to completely eliminate medical therapy.

SUGGESTED READINGS

Bryant K, Maxfield C, Rabalais G: Renal candidiasis in neonates with candiduria. Pediatr Infect Dis J 2000;18:959–963

Guzzetta PC, Potter BM, Ruley EJ, et al: Renovascular hypertension in children: current concepts in evaluation and treatment. J Pediatr Surg 1989;24:1236

Haas CA, Reigle MD, Selzmann AA, et al: Use of ureteral stents in the management of major renal trauma extravasation: is there a role? J Endourol 1998;12:545–549

Hagiwara A, Sakaki S, Goto H, et al: The role of interventional radiology in the management of blunt injury: a practical protocol. J Trauma 2001;51:526–531

Holden S, McPhee M, Grabstald H: The rationale of urinary diversion in cancer patients. J Urol 1979;121:1

Holloway WR, Weinstein SH: Percutaneous decompression: treatment for respiratory distress secondary to multicystic dysplastic kidney. J Urol 1990;144:113–115

Jackman SV, Hedican SP, Peters CA, Docimo SG: Percutaneous nephrolithotomy in infants and preschool children: experience with a new technique. Urology 1998;52:697–701

Koral K, Saker M, Morello F, et al: Percutaneous nephrostomy in infants: improved success with two step technique. *In* Scientific Astracts from the Society of Cardiovascular and Interventional Radiology meeting, 2000, p 269

Mansi MK, Alkhudair WK: Conservative management with percutaneous intervention of major blunt renal injuries. Am J Emerg Med 1997;15:633–637

Martin LG, Rees CR, O'Bryant T: Percutaneous angioplasty of renal arteries. *In* Strandness DE, Van Breda A (eds): Vascular Diseases: Surgical and Interventional Therapy. New York, Churchill Livingstone, 1994;721–741

Millward S: Percutaneous nephrostomy: a practical approach. J Vasc Interv Radiol 2000;11:955–964

Riedy MJ, Lebowitz RL: Percutaneous studies of the upper urinary tract in children with special emphasis on infants. Radiology 1986;160:231–235

Sclafani SJ, Becker JA: Interventional radiology in the treatment of retroperitoneal trauma. Urol Radiol 1985;7:219–230

Staples DP, Ginsberg NJ, Johnson ML: Percutaneous nephrostomy: a series and review of the literature. AJR Am J Roentgenol 1978;130:75

Towbin RB, Ball WS: Pediatric interventional radiology. Radiol Clin North Am 1988;26:419–440

PART II

NORMAL FINDINGS AND ANATOMIC VARIANTS

SANDRA K. FERNBACH
KATE A. FEINSTEIN

KIDNEY

INTERNAL ANATOMY

A coronal section of the kidney reveals that it is composed of two distinct regions: the outer cortex and the inner medulla (Fig. 1). Within the cortex are the nephrons. The medulla is composed of 8 to 18 pyramids that terminate in the renal papillae at the level of the calices. Two or more pyramids may drain into the same papilla (confluent papilla). Two or more papillae may drain into a single calix (compound calix). Compound calices are typically located in the poles of the kidney and produce the unusual lucency sometimes seen on ultrasound (US) in these regions. Renal cortex can extend centrally between the pyramids (column of Bertin) and may simulate a renal tumor on excretory urography, unless the calix that is beneath it is well seen (Fig. 2). US or nuclear scans using cortical agents can easily identify this variant, which occurs more often at the junction of the middle and upper group of calices or between the two central renal echo complexes of a duplex kidney.

In newborns and infants, the kidneys have a larger medullary and a smaller cortical volume than in later life. On US, the neonatal renal cortex is moderately hyperechoic, close to the echogenicity of the adjacent liver and spleen. The pyramids are relatively hypoechoic (Fig. 3). This pattern can suggest hydronephrosis, especially on prenatal US studies. After a few years of age, the echogenicity of each is close to that of adult kidneys, making the corticomedullary differentiation much less distinct on US. However, the corticomedullary differentiation remains well appreciated on contrast-enhanced computed tomography (CECT) and magnetic resonance imaging (MRI) (Fig. 4). Corticomedullary differentiation is rarely seen on excretory urography.

RENAL ARTERIES AND VEINS

The kidney is usually supplied by a single artery arising from the aorta. After the renal artery enters the renal hilum, behind and slightly above the renal vein, it divides into anterior and posterior branches that, in turn, generally divide into superior and inferior branches (Fig. 5). Variations exist at all levels. About 20% to 30% of kidneys have a second or accessory renal artery that also arises from the aorta. The renal artery (or arteries) arise more distally from the aorta than normal in kidneys with ectopia (pelvic kidney and crossed renal ectopy) or fusion (horseshoe kidney).

The renal vein lies anterior and slightly inferior to the renal artery (see Fig. 5). The left renal vein is longer than the right, coursing anterior to the aorta, and it receives the ipsilateral suprarenal and gonadal veins before entering the inferior vena cava. The main renal artery and vein can be well shown with Doppler US, CECT, and gadolinium-enhanced MRI. Smaller intrarenal vessels can be demonstrated with all three techniques, but CECT and MRI allow processing of the data after their acquisition (postprocessing), in particular, maximum intensity projection reconstructions that enhance detection of accessory vessels.

Prominent vessels may produce nonobstructive impressions on the renal pelvis or caliceal system. Less frequently, a vessel may cause true obstruction of an infundibulum (Fig. 6) or even the renal pelvis. On US, echolucency of hilar vessels can simulate mild hydronephrosis; the use of color Doppler US clearly differentiates vascular structures from a dilated renal pelvis.

MEASUREMENTS

The wide range of normal findings makes sequential measurements of greater value than a single measure-

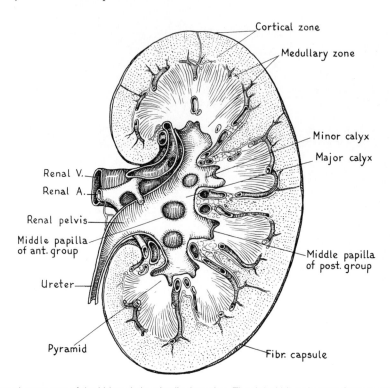

FIGURE 1. Macroscopic anatomy of the kidney in longitudinal section. The right kidney is seen from the back; the renal artery is posterior to the renal vein. (Redrawn from Kelly HA, Burnam CF: Diseases of the Kidneys, Ureters and Bladder, 2nd ed. New York, Appleton, 1922.)

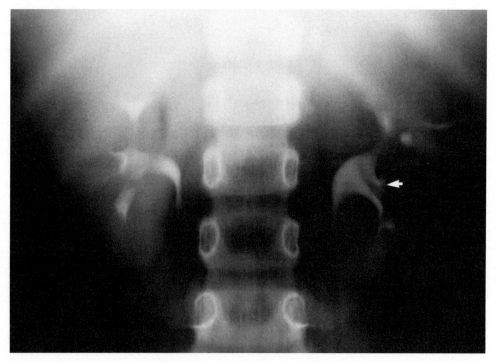

FIGURE 2. A column of Bertin has produced spreading of the calices of the left kidney, simulating a renal mass. The centrally located single calix *(white arrow)* is draining this ectopic tissue. Note also the oblique vascular impression on the lower pole infundibulum (major calix).

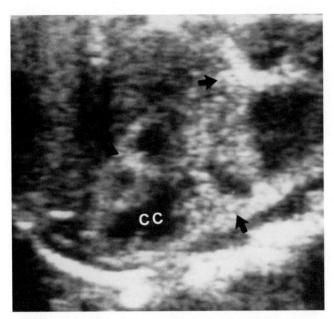

FIGURE 3. Supine sagittal renal ultrasound demonstrates the sharp corticomedullary differentiation common in infancy and early childhood. The large hypoechoic triangular renal pyramids in the upper pole can be attributed to a compound caliceal system *(CC)*. The echogenic tissue peripheral to the pyramids is the cortex *(arrows)*.

ment. For example, a kidney studied during an acute infection may be swollen, making prior renal scarring impossible to detect initially. Measurements of the kidney can be made with all imaging modalities, but standards for renal size have been developed for urography and US only (Fig. 7). Kidney length is the most commonly measured parameter. Determinations of renal width, cortical thickness, and parenchymal area may also be made and can be used to evaluate renal growth.

At urography, these measurements should be made only on films obtained with the child in the supine projection. The length of the kidney has been correlated to age (see Fig. 7*A*), body height, and weight, and with the height of the first three or four lumbar vertebral bodies. At urography, the renal length is equal to the height of about five vertebral bodies (including intervening disk spaces) in newborns, 4½ vertebral bodies in infants and children up to 1½ years, and 4 vertebral bodies in older children. The left kidney may be slightly longer than the right; in adults, the difference may reach 15 mm. Kidneys with duplicated ureters are also longer than normal kidneys.

The width of the kidney is approximately 50% of renal length and is relatively thicker in neonates than in older children. Cortical thickness is measured as that part of the renal parenchyma that lies outside a line drawn through the tips of the renal calices on frontal films of an

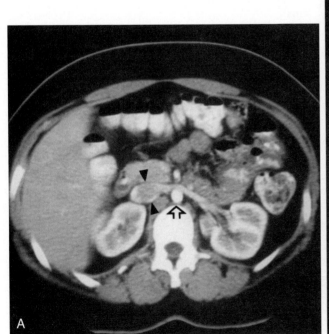

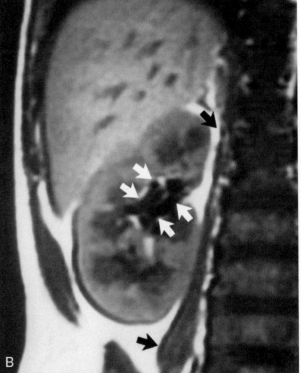

FIGURE 4. Corticomedullary differentation. **A,** On axial contrast-enhanced computed tomography, the cortex is enhancing during the early phase of the bolus infusion of contrast material. The medullary tissue beneath remains unopacified. The aorta *(open arrow)* is intensely opacified. Laminar flow of unopacified blood is responsible for the uneven appearance of the contrast in the inferior vena cava *(arrowheads)*. **B,** On coronal magnetic resonance imaging, the different signals of the cortex and the medulla allow them to be easily differentiated, even without contrast material. The tubular structures at the hilum *(white arrows)* are the signal voids of the hilar vessels. Note also how the psoas muscle *(black arrows)* is thin at the upper portion of the kidney and broader distally.

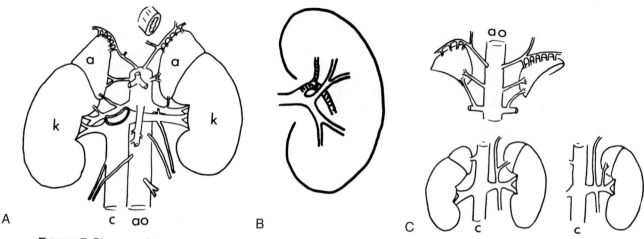

FIGURE 5. Diagrams of the arterial supply and venous return of kidneys and adrenal glands. **A,** The renal artery courses to the kidney behind and slightly higher than the renal vein. The left renal vein is longer than the right and courses in front of the aorta and behind the superior mesenteric artery. *a* = adrenal gland; *ao* = aorta; *c* = vena cava; *k* = kidney. **B,** Common branching of the renal artery into a posterior and an anterior major branch. The posterior branch *(hatched vessels)* usually describes a downward loop. **C,** Vascular supply of the adrenal gland. The arteries originate from the aorta *(ao)* and renal arteries *(top)*. The right adrenal vein drains into the vena cava *(c)*, whereas the left vein drains into the left renal vein via the phrenic vein *(bottom left)* or directly *(bottom right)*.

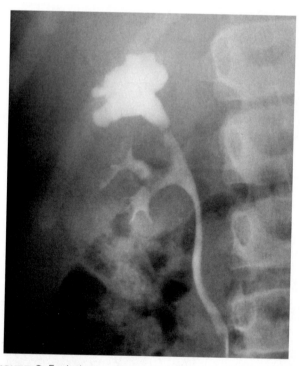

FIGURE 6. Extrinsic vascular compression on upper pole infundibulum. During excretory urography, the upper pole infundibulum and compound caliceal system are dilated above the linear defect produced by a crossing vessel. The other calices have a normal caliber. When this appearance is associated with persistent right upper quadrant pain (and nuclear scintigraphy documents obstruction), the process is referred to as Fraley's syndrome and may require surgery.

excretory urogram (Fig. 8). This line is roughly parallel to the outer border of the kidney. The upper pole is normally slightly thicker than the lower pole, and the renal cortex is slightly thinner in the center of the kidney. The polar thickness is essentially the same on the two sides. Extra cortical tissue may be noted about the renal hilum and may impinge from above or below on the renal pelvis (suprahilar or infrahilar bulge; hilar lips).

Renal length is now more frequently measured with US than excretory urography. Measurements of renal length should be made with the child supine; such values will tend to be slightly higher than those obtained with the child in the prone position. US standards for kidney length relative to age, height, weight, and body surface have also been developed. Specific US standards have been developed for preterm infants and myelodysplastic children. Normal US values for renal length are shown in Figure 7*B* and 7*C.* The values obtained by US are generally lower than those derived from urographic films, with the difference being a bit less than 1 cm in the first 5 years of life and a bit more than 1 cm after that. Kidney volume may also be estimated by US according to the formula

$$\text{Volume} = \text{length} \times \text{width} \times \text{anteroposterior diameter} \times 0.523$$

using the maximal measurement for each parameter. The length is measured on coronal scans, the width and anteroposterior (AP) diameter on transverse images. Intraobserver variation in the measurements, although generally not clinically significant, is magnified when calculating the renal volume and may, in children over 2 years, result in kidney volumes that deviate by 2 to 3 years' normal renal growth. If differential is symmetric

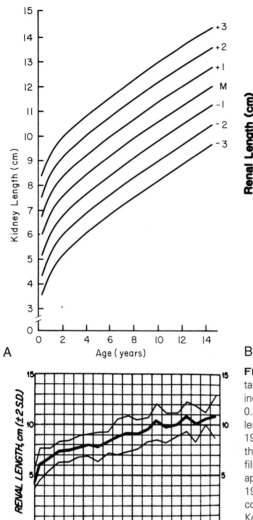

A

B   **Age**

FIGURE 7. Kidney length in centimeters. **A,** Measurements obtained from supine urographic films and correlated with age, including values for 3 SD above and below the mean *(M)*. The SD is 0.75 cm. (Modified from Currarino G, Williams B, Dana K: Kidney length correlated with age: normal values in children. Radiology 1984;150:703.) **B,** Sonographic measurements correlated with age; the values are slightly lower than those obtained from urographic films. (From Han BK, Babcock DS: Sonographic measurements and appearance of normal kidneys in children. AJR Am J Roentgenol 1985;145:611, with permission.) **C,** Ultrasound measurements correlated with age, including ±2 SD. (From Rosenbaum DM, Korngold E, Teele RL: Sonographic assessment of renal length in normal children. AJR Am J Roentgenol 1984;142:467, with permission.)

C

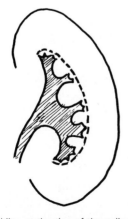

FIGURE 8. Dashed line at the tips of the calices parallels the edge of the kidney. The corticomedullary junction and arcuate arteries are located approximately at the junction of the middle and outer thirds of the intervening renal parenchyma.

(i.e., 50/50) differences in length and volume estimate may not be clinically significant.

COMPENSATORY HYPERTROPHY

Contrary to reports in the early literature, compensatory hypertrophy can begin in utero. Children with one multicystic dysplastic kidney may be born with a contralateral kidney that is significantly larger than the norm. Lack of expected compensatory hypertrophy may indicate that the functioning kidney may be compromised by a second process, such as vesicoureteral reflux. Compensatory hypertrophy is more rapid in infants than in older children and adults. It has also been described in a kidney contralateral to a severely obstructed but functioning kidney.

Following unilateral nephrectomy, the remaining normal kidney displays accelerated growth over a 2-year period. This solitary kidney will reach a length that is several standard deviations above the mean.

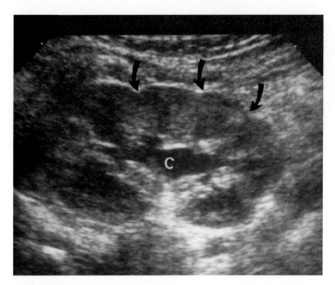

FIGURE 9. Residual fetal lobulations are responsible for scalloped border of the kidney *(arrows)* on this sagittal sonogram. The central renal echo complex *(C)* is separated. The corticomedullary differentiation is not as pronounced as in Figure 3.

SHAPE

The primitive fetal kidney comprises multiple renal lobules that fuse to form the kidney. The junction of these lobules sometimes persists and can be seen as a scalloping of the cortical border (Fig. 9). These fetal lobulations become increasingly effaced throughout childhood but are noted in about 10% of adults. Fetal lobulations can be differentiated from cortical scarring by their position: Fetal lobulations indent between the calices, but scarring occurs directly peripheral to a calix. The junctional parenchymal defect observed with renal US (Fig. 10) is similarly derived from a variation in the fusion of the fetal renunculi or lobules. It appears as a thick, triangular, echogenic notch in the anterosuperior or posteroinferior aspect of the kidney (more often on the right) and mimics a cortical scar. The junctional

parenchymal defect may be connected to the renal hilum by an echogenic line called the interrenicular septum (Fig. 10).

In infants, the kidney is more rounded and relatively broader than in adults. The poles are folded into a relatively narrow renal sinus. The left kidney is apt to be triangular in shape, with a distinct bulge along its lateral aspect, the so-called dromedary kidney.

POSITION AND MOBILITY

The left kidney is higher than the right in at least two thirds of people. In 5% to 10%, the left kidney is lower, and, in the remainder, the kidneys are at the same height. On supine films, the center of the renal pelvis of the left kidney is opposite the lower half of L1, whereas that of the right kidney is usually at the level of the superior half of L2.

The distance between the spine and the medial aspect of the upper caliceal system should be the same on each side. Medial deviation of the upper calices suggests focal parenchymal scarring. Downward or lateral displacement suggests adrenal mass, left upper pole mass, or obstruction of a left upper pole ureter. During urography, on rarely needed lateral films, the anterior surface of the kidney projects over the anterior surface of the spine. This same relationship is clearly demonstrated on axial computed tomography (CT) scans and MRI.

The cephalocaudal position of the kidney is determined by its relation to the underlying psoas muscle. The upper pole is medial and dorsal to the lower because the psoas muscle broadens as it passes inferiorly. Reversed obliquity (lower pole more medial) and increased obliquity (lower pole more lateral) are occasional normal variants. Reversed obliquity can also be seen in horseshoe kidney and in myelodysplastic children with lumbar kyphosis and psoas muscle atrophy, the so-called pseudohorseshoe kidney. Unusual orientations or positions of the kidney may warrant additional

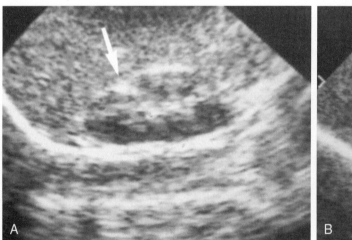
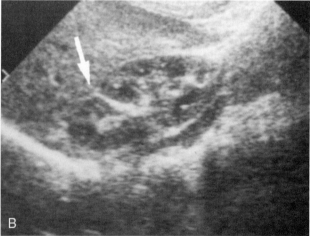

FIGURE 10. Longitudinal ultrasound of the right kidney in two infants showing a junctional parenchymal defect **(A)** and a renicular septum **(B)** *(arrows)*. Both are normal findings, probably related to a demarcation of embryonic reniculi.

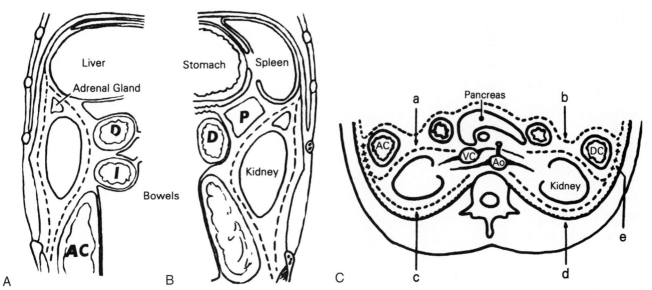

FIGURE 11. Sagittal sections of the abdomen at the level of the right kidney **(A)** and left kidney **(B)**. The liver, right adrenal gland, stomach, spleen, and left kidney are labeled, for orientation. The relationship of the right kidney to the duodenum *(D)*, ileum *(I)*, and ascending colon *(AC)* is demonstrated in **A**. In **B**, the pancreas *(P)* and duodenum *(D)* are also labeled. **C**, An axial (transverse) section of the abdomen at the level of the kidneys outlines the following spaces: the *anterior perirenal space* between the kidney and the anterior renal fascia *(broken line a)*; the *anterior pararenal space* between the anterior perirenal space *(broken line a)* and the posterior peritoneal layer *(broken line b)*; the *posterior perirenal space* between the kidney and the posterior renal fascia *(broken line c)*; and the *posterior pararenal space* between the posterior renal fascia *(broken line c)* and the transversalis fascia *(broken line d)*. The lateroconal fascia *(e)* is also shown. For orientation, the pancreas and kidney are labeled, as are the aorta *(Ao)*, the inferior vena cava *(Vc)*, and the ascending *(AC)* and descending *(DC)* colon.

imaging to exclude the presence of a flank mass or ureteral duplication with an obstructed pole.

The kidneys move slightly caudally with each inspiration and also move caudally about one vertebral body when the patient moves from the supine to the prone position. The mobility of the left kidney is greater than that of the right. In the prone position, both kidneys no longer rest on the psoas muscle. They acquire a more vertical axis and also rotate anteriorly on their long axis, causing them to appear broader.

ANATOMIC RELATIONSHIPS

Knowledge of the relationship of the kidney to adjacent structures and organs is essential for evaluating the location and spread of renal and pararenal neoplasms, infections, and fluid collections. A large portion of the posterior surface of the left kidney is in contact with the diaphragm above, along the posterior costophrenic sulcus. The renal capsule, anterior and posterior renal fascia, posterior layer of the peritoneal membrane (parietal peritoneum), and transversalis fascia respectively delimit the following potential spaces in the region of the kidneys: subcapsular, perirenal, and anterior and posterior pararenal. The relationships between these potential spaces, adjacent structures, and the route of spread of disease are shown in Figure 11. Intraperitoneally, in front of the right kidney and the proximal descending duodenum, is a posterior extension of the infrahepatic recess termed *Morison's pouch*, an important

space for fluid collections. It is bordered superiorly by the right transverse colon and posteriorly by the right kidney and adrenal gland. This pouch is continuous medially with the lesser omental sac through the foramen of Winslow.

PELVOCALICEAL SYSTEM AND URETER

The renal pelvis varies in size from a small and poorly defined sac to a large, box-like structure. The pelvis may lie entirely within (intrarenal) or almost entirely beyond (extrarenal) the renal sinus. A redundant and partially extrarenal pelvis may be flattened along its medial aspect by the psoas muscle and thus appear square instead of funnel shaped. In newborns and small infants, the pelvis is often relatively small and intrarenal and usually points medially instead of downward.

The configuration of the pelvocaliceal system is quite variable, even from side to side. In most kidneys, the pelvis branches into two major infundibula (or major calices). The inferior infundibulum is commonly broad and short and is connected with a larger number of calices than the upper infundibulum. In some, the major calices are poorly defined and the lesser calices appear to originate from the renal pelvis. Also normal are the elongated, spider-like calices that are often associated with a small or bifid renal pelvis.

Each kidney has about 8 to 13 minor calices. These have a cup-shaped appearance that is due to protrusion

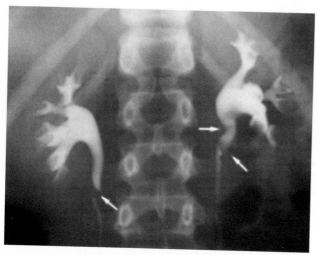

FIGURE 12. Excretory urogram in a 14-year-old girl showing several defects on the ureteropelvic junction and proximal ureter *(arrows)*, presumably caused by aberrant renal arteries.

of the renal papilla into the calix. Two or more papillae may enter one calix (compound calix). Most calices are directed laterally and either slightly anteriorly or posteriorly. Calices that are directed medially are seen in malrotated kidneys.

The number of calices demonstrated on an excretory urogram may change from study to study in the same child. The actual calices that opacify may also vary; different calices may be visualized on sequential studies.

The transition between the renal pelvis and the ureter, or ureteropelvic junction (UPJ), may be sharply or poorly defined. Both extrinsic filling defects and local narrowing are commonly observed at the UPJ without resultant hydronephrosis. An inferior polar artery may produce a small extrinsic defect or notch in the ureter near the UPJ (Fig. 12). A sharp kink without obstruction is occasionally seen in the proximal portion of the ureter as a transient or constant finding. Folds in the upper ureter (Fig. 13), mild elongation and tortuosity of the ureter, and mild widening of the midureter are all seen in infant urograms. They are believed to be a persistence of fetal characteristics and disappear in early childhood.

An atypical course of the ureter medial or lateral to the psoas muscle may simulate a paravertebral mass or retroperitoneal fibrosis, a process that is rare in childhood. In athletic children, psoas muscle hypertrophy may produce anterolateral displacement of the kidney and ureter. When the proximal right ureter deviates medially, looping over the L4 pedicle, retrocaval ureter should be suspected. In childhood, the ureters are mobile and can be displaced medially or laterally by dilated bowel loops.

Just above the pelvic brim, one or both ureters often show an oblique defect as a result of adjacent iliac vessels (Fig. 14). This may be accompanied by a mild degree of hydroureteronephrosis above; the dilatation diminishes in the prone and oblique projections because the extrinsic pressure is relieved. Oblique views, rarely needed, usually confirm that the defect is on the posterior aspect of the ureter.

On most urograms, only segments of the ureter are seen on any single film. When the ureter is visible throughout its course, one should search for a distal obstruction of either congenital (primary megaureter, simple ureterocele) or acquired etiology. When both ureters are visualized throughout, other causes should be sought: vesicoureteric reflux, atony of infection, even diabetes insipidus. A distended bladder will impede drainage from the ureters and produce hydroureteronephrosis; in this setting, a postvoid abdominal film demonstrates normal-caliber ureters.

The ureter enters the bladder along the lateral angle of the trigone. Within the bladder wall, it courses first through the bladder musculature in a slightly oblique direction downward and medially. It then continues submucosally for a much longer segment to end in the corner of the trigone. This anatomic arrangement allows the intramural portion of the ureter to act as a one-way valve during emptying and filling of the bladder and is a major factor in the prevention of vesicoureteral reflux.

BLADDER

The bladder is divided into the dome (vertex), body, and base (fundus). The posterior aspect of the bladder base is formed by the trigone, a triangular space limited by the two ureteral orifices superolaterally and by the

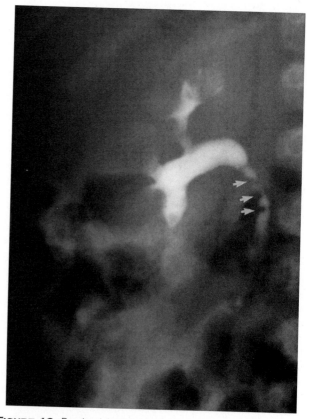

FIGURE 13. Retained fetal folds are responsible for the multiple nonobstructive filling defects *(arrows)* in the proximal portion of the ureter. In most children, these disappear over time.

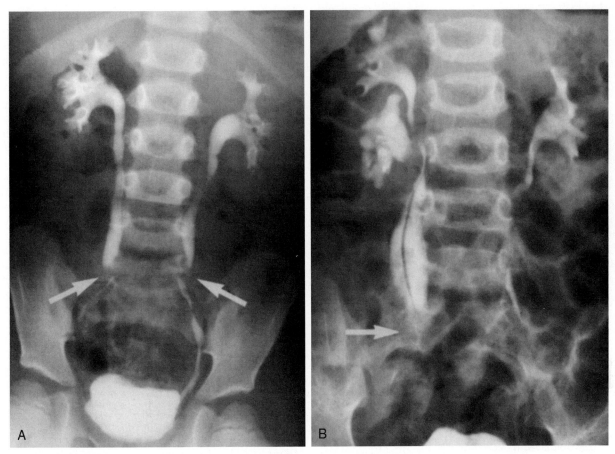

FIGURE 14. A, Extrinsic defects of the ureter caused by the underlying iliac vessels that are sometimes associated with mild, transient dilatation proximally *(arrows).* This dilatation usually disappears with the patient in the oblique position, prone, or upright. **B,** Incomplete ureteral duplication on the right with two ureters joining at the level of the sacral promontory and iliac vessels. Mild dilatation of both ureters above this level may be caused by iliac vessels, as in **A,** or by ureteroureteral reflux.

internal urethral meatus inferiorly in the midline. When the bladder is incompletely filled, a ridge between the two ureteral orifices (the trigonal or interureteric ridge) may produce a transverse linear defect visible on both frontal and oblique views during cystography. Occasionally oblique films may also demonstrate a prominent band of the detrusor muscle as a sharp defect along the anterior wall of the bladder, just above the bladder neck.

The bladder normally has a smooth contour. During voiding, it may develop fine serrations and contour irregularities, especially along the posterior wall, as a result of detrusor muscle contractions (Fig. 15). These should not be mistaken for diverticula or neurogenic changes.

In infants and young children, the incompletely filled bladder may transiently herniate a portion of its infero-lateral wall into a dilated internal inguinal ring (Fig. 16). This phenomenon can be seen on voiding cystoure-thrography (VCUG) or excretory urography. There may be an associated ipsilateral inguinal hernia. These "bladder ears" disappear when the bladder is distended. Bladder ears are uncommon in older children and adults.

The bladder is easily compressed and deformed by bowel loops, particularly if they are distended with gas or

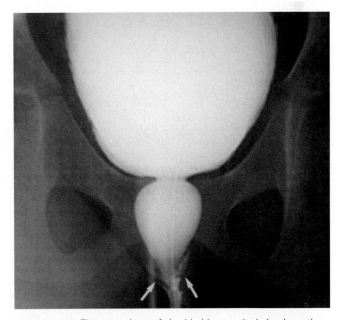

FIGURE 15. Fine serrations of the bladder, particularly along the detrusor muscle, are a normal finding during voiding and may simulate tiny cellules. They are due to contractions of the detrusor muscle. The "spinning top" urethra is normal. A small amount of contrast has refluxed into the vagina *(arrows).*

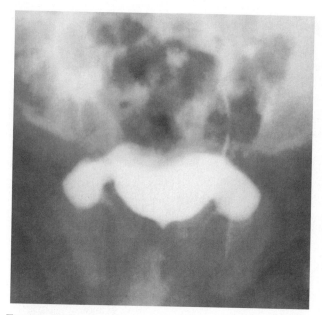

FIGURE 16. Transitory hernias of the bladder ("bladder ears") in a normal infant.

fecal material. In postpubertal girls, the uterus may produce an indentation on the dome of the bladder centrally or slightly to one side. Gas in the rectum projecting through the contrast-filled bladder may simulate a ureterocele (Fig. 17).

In newborns and very young infants, the entire bladder is normally higher than in later life. The floor of the bladder is slightly above the level of the symphysis pubis in newborns and is at or slightly below this level in older children.

The normal bladder capacity increases with age from 30 to 50 ml in newborns to about 100 ml at 1 year, 200 ml at 5 years, and 300 to 400 ml from age 10 to adult life.

A commonly used formula to estimate bladder capacity in ounces up to 11 years is the patient's age in years plus 2 ounces. However, other authors estimate bladder capacity differently, stressing that a linear model does not work well, especially after toilet training has occurred.

During excretory urography or CECT, a jet of opacified urine from one or both ureters may be seen extending toward the opposite wall of the bladder (Fig. 18). A jet of urine can also be demonstrated as a stream of echogenic bubbles entering the urine-filled bladder along the posterior bladder wall with both standard and color Doppler US. Visualization of a jet is a good indication that the ureter is not obstructed but does not correlate well with the presence or absence of vesicoureteral reflux.

The bladder normally contracts concentrically throughout the entire phase of micturition but, in some patients, may be transiently divided into two functional units: the base and the rest of the bladder. The degree and force of contraction in each of these segments may appear independent of the other. Neonates and infants are known to have intermittent urination or incomplete bladder emptying as a normal phenomenon.

When the child is prone during an excretory urogram, the contrast material collects in the anterosuperior portion of the bladder and the nonopacified urine is at the posteroinferior aspect (trigone) of the bladder. A frontal film done in this position projects normal ureteral orifices beneath the bladder contrast, causing them to look as if they have an abnormally low insertion.

BLADDER NECK

The term *bladder neck* refers to the poorly delineated junction between the bladder and the urethra at the

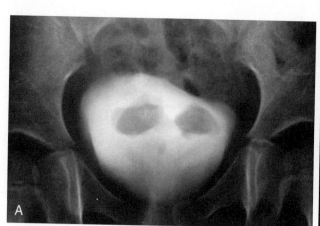
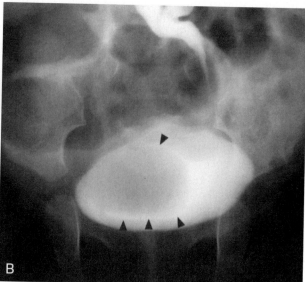

FIGURE 17. False and true ureterocele. **A,** Bowel gas projecting over the contrast-filled bladder simulates bilateral ureteroceles on this film from a voiding cystourethrogram. **B,** The true ectopic ureterocele is intravesical and has an acute angle with the bladder wall. Note how pooled contrast has created a halo about it *(arrowheads)*. On this film from an excretory urogram, the calices from a left pelvic kidney project over the lumbosacral junction.

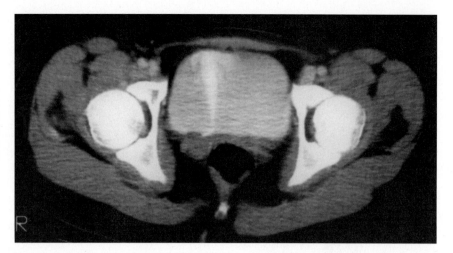

FIGURE 18. Contrast-enhanced computed tomography demonstration of jet effect. Contrast propelled from the right ureter streams across the urine-filled bladder as a bolus. As the bolus hits the front wall of the bladder, it is sprayed medially and laterally.

level of the internal urethral sphincter. The appearance of the bladder neck on VCUG is quite variable, especially in girls. In most normal children, the area is funnel shaped and has a smooth outline. In some girls, both the bladder neck and proximal urethra are markedly dilated during voiding. This is a normal variant and does not indicate obstruction or a neurogenic bladder.

At the beginning of voiding, the bladder floor descends and becomes funnel shaped and is in continuity with the proximal urethra. In some children with myelomeningocele, and occasionally also in otherwise normal children, the bladder base and pelvic floor descend to a marked degree during voiding. When the bladder is empty, the bladder base ascends to its normal resting position and again becomes relatively flattened.

URETHRA

FEMALE URETHRA

Pathology of the female urethra is rare in children. It is the absence of urethral pathology and the infrequency of bladder anomalies that make screening nuclear cystography a reasonable choice in young girls being evaluated for urinary tract infections. The female urethra is short, straight, and without any significant radiographic landmarks. It has both an internal sphincter at the bladder neck and an external sphincter just above the pelvic floor (Fig. 19*A*). During voiding it becomes cylindrical or conical and may be slightly directed anteriorly.

Variations in the urethral appearance are normal. For example, during voiding, the proximal portion of the urethra may dilate ("spinning top urethra"), simulating the exceedingly rare distal urethral obstruction (see Fig. 15). However, in children with incontinence, this finding may be pathologic, an indication of detrusor–sphincter dyssynergia. In some normal girls, the urethra may be dilated or narrowed focally or throughout its length. Longitudinal folds may extend the length of the urethra when it is not completely distended.

The urethra can be seen well on AP films centered over this region (see Fig. 15). Such positioning also removes the gonads from the direct beam, a technique

used to decrease gonadal exposure during VCUG. Lateral films of the pelvis and urethra produce a high gonadal exposure and should be avoided unless a specific anatomic problem such as urogenital sinus or prolapsing ureterocele is suspected or present. Although reflux into the vagina may decrease the clarity with which the urethra is seen, this rarely produces a clinical problem and is a frequent finding when girls void while supine.

MALE URETHRA

The male urethra is divided into a posterior and an anterior segment (Figs. 19 and 20). The posterior or prostatic urethra extends from the bladder neck to, and including, the short segment of urethra related to the urogenital diaphragm (membranous portion). Its proximal half or two thirds is surrounded by the prostate and the lower third by the external urethral sphincter. An impression along the dorsal midportion of the prostatic

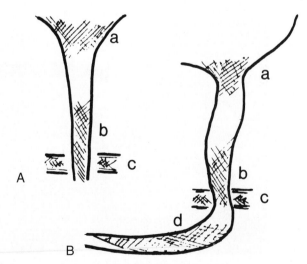

FIGURE 19. Diagram of the musculature of the bladder neck and urethra in the female **(A)** and in the male **(B)** shows the internal urethral sphincter at the bladder neck *(a)*, the external urethral sphincter *(b)*, the musculature of the urogenital diaphragm and pelvic floor *(c)*, and the bulbocavernosus muscle *(d)*.

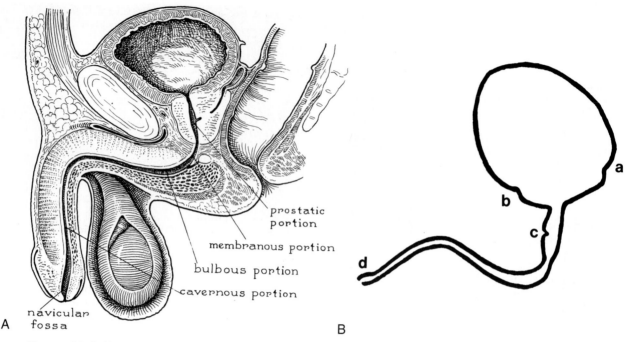

FIGURE 20. A, Normal male urethra, showing variations in caliber of the different segments. **B,** Diagram of the bladder and urethra in the male. The indentation on the posterior surface of the bladder is caused by the trigonal ridge *(a)*, and the indentation on the anterior contour of the bladder is caused by a prominent band of the detrusor *(b)*. The indentation in the midportion of the prostatic urethra anteriorly is called the incisura *(c)*. The fossa navicularis at the distal end of the urethra is also shown *(d)*.

urethra is the verumontanum (Fig. 21*A*). This can be seen on VCUG as an oval extrinsic defect about 5 mm long.

The *incisura* is a fold or ridge along the anterior aspect of the proximal prostatic urethra. The *superior urethral crest* is an uncommonly visualized Y-shaped fold extending from the bladder neck to the verumontanum. The *inferior urethral crest,* also in the posterior urethra, is a longitudinal fold that takes origin from the lower aspect of the verumontanum and extends down the posterior wall of the verumontanum (Fig. 21*A*). Distally, its bifurcation into an inverted Y may produce thin filling defects in the urethra (plicae colliculae or fins) that are variably visualized. They may simulate posterior urethral

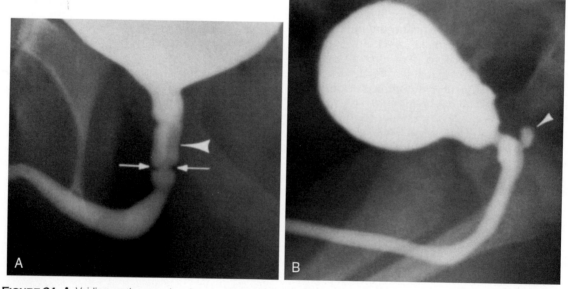

FIGURE 21. A, Voiding urethrogram in a 9-year-old boy showing some normal anatomic variants in the posterior urethra: the verumontanum and the inferior urethral crest and fins *(arrowhead)*. A thin mucosal fold encircles the urethra at the level of the fins without obstruction *(arrows)*. **B,** Normal voiding urethrogram in male infant showing opacification of an enlarged utricle *(arrowhead)*.

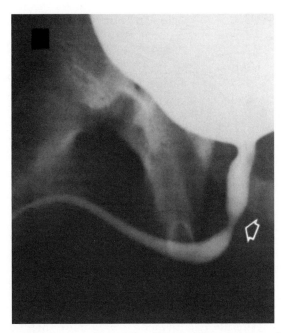

FIGURE 22. Cystourethrogram in a 12-year-old boy demonstrating a normal urethra. The slight narrowing of the urethra at the junction between the posterior and the anterior urethra corresponds to the urogenital diaphragm *(arrow).*

valves but are not associated with any secondary changes of urethral obstruction.

The prostatic utricle is a urethral diverticulum of variable size, inconstantly seen dorsally at the apex of the verumontanum (Fig. 21 *B*). The utricle, a remnant of the müllerian system, is more frequently seen and is larger in children with penoscrotal hypospadias, which carries an increased incidence of intersex anomalies, and in children with prune-belly (triad, Eagle-Barrett) syndrome.

Just below and on each side of the utricle are the openings from the ejaculatory ducts, rarely seen during standard contrast studies. Uncommonly demonstrated are the numerous ducts draining the prostate gland, arrayed in rows longitudinally along the posterior urethra. Contrast refluxes into them most frequently in the presence of obstruction or dysfunctional voiding but can be noted during a normal examination.

On VCUG, the urogenital diaphragm (Figs. 19 *B* and 22) produces a smooth, nonobstructive area of circumferential narrowing at the transition between the posterior and anterior urethra. This short segment of the posterior urethra is referred to as the membranous urethra and is the site of the external sphincter. On retrograde studies, the sphincter acts as an obstruction, allowing contrast to pass through to, but not distend, the prostatic urethra.

The anterior urethra (cavernous urethra, spongy urethra) is divided into a proximal and a distal segment. The proximal segment, the bulbar urethra, extends from just beyond the membranous urethra to the suspensory ligament, at the level of the symphysis pubis. It lies on the bulbocavernosus muscle, which sends fibers around its dorsal surface. Along the dorsolateral aspect of the anterior urethra are the paired corpora cavernosa, which arise from and attach to the rami of the pubic arch, one on each side of the midline. Beneath these is the corpus spongiousum, through which the anterior urethra courses.

On the floor of the bulbar urethra are the two openings of the Cowper's gland ducts. The paired parasagittal glands are located proximally, at the level of the urogenital diaphragm. Obstruction of a duct results in secretions building up within it. The distended duct produces an obtuse, extrinsic filling defect along the ventral surface of the urethra. Visualization of the ducts is unusual and is more likely to follow resolution of obstruction, with contrast refluxing into a previously dilated segment of the duct.

The distal segment of the anterior urethra, the pendulous or penile urethra, extends from the suspensory ligament to the urethral meatus. Rarely, an indentation along the ventral aspect of the urethra is noted at the level of the suspensory ligament, perhaps caused by fibers of the ligament itself. When a boy voids in the upright position, narrowing at this level may also be due to the extrinsic pressure of the urinal, the so-called urinal artifact.

The penile urethra has a uniform caliber except at the level of the glans penis. The slight dilatation there, the fossa navicularis, is a site where a small balloon may be lodged to perform a retrograde urethrogram (Figs. 20 *B* and 23). A focal dilatation along the dorsal aspect of the fossa navicularis is called a dorsal diverticulum or the lacuna magna; it may present with hematuria or dysuria. During voiding, contrast may pool beneath the glans penis and the prepuce (Fig. 24).

Incomplete relaxation, spasm, or contractions of the external urethral sphincter may produce transient narrowing of the distal half of the posterior urethra and simulate stenosis. Similar processes in the bulbocavernosus muscle may produce narrowing of the bulbar urethra seen on retrograde urethrograms.

Further details on the anatomy and physiology of micturition are described in Section VII, Part V.

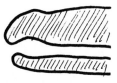

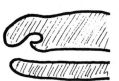

FIGURE 23. Diagram of the distal segment of the male urethra. **Top,** A localized widening of the urethra at the level of the glans penis is a normal finding corresponding to the fossa navicularis. **Bottom,** In abnormal situations there is a deep outpouching or diverticulum in the dorsal part of the fossa navicularis called the lacuna magna.

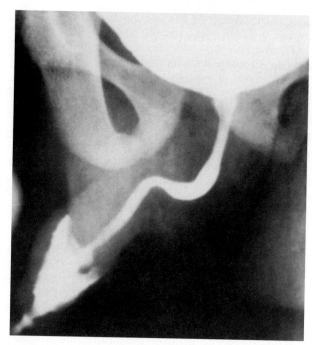

FIGURE 24. Voiding urethrogram in a 5-year-old uncircumcised boy with phimosis. Note the collection of contrast material enclosed by the prepuce.

GENITAL TRACT

FEMALE GENITAL TRACT

The main anatomic features of the female genital tract are diagrammed in Figures 25 and 26. During the last 2 months of gestation, maternal estrogen crosses the placenta and produces hypertrophy of the fetal female

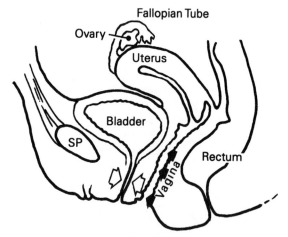

FIGURE 25. Female genitourinary tract. On this sagittal section, the bladder is seen directly behind the symphysis pubis (SP). The urethra (between open arrows) passes inferiorly from it. Behind the urethra is the vagina, with its corrugated walls (black arrows). The walls of the uterus (labeled) surround the endometrial cavity. The ovary and fallopian tube, shown here, would not appear in a midline section such as this because they are located several centimeters from the midline. The rectum is the most dorsal tubular structure.

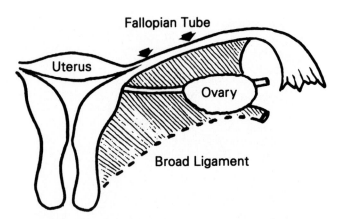

FIGURE 26. Female reproductive tract. This coronal section clearly demonstrates the relationship between the midline uterus and endometrial cavity (EC) and the parasagittal ovary, fallopian tube (arrows), and broad ligament (hatched area).

genital structures. Prenatal US can detect the swollen vagina, uterine enlargement (cervix more than body), and ovarian cysts, some as large as 10 cm. Such cysts regress in the neonatal period, as do the uterine and vaginal changes.

The neonatal vaginal epithelium is markedly hypertrophied and contains an increased number of cellular layers and an increased amount of intracellular glycogen. The prominent mucosa can, to the naked eye, simulate a neoplasm. Vaginal and cervical secretions are increased and may take the form of a creamy or bloody discharge.

At birth, the vagina is 40 to 45 mm in length. As the estrogen effect regresses, the vagina decreases in length and becomes straight and smooth walled. Its length is again 40 to 45 mm at 2 to 3 years of age and increases to 5 to 6 cm at 7 years, to 8 cm at 10 years, and to 11 cm at age 11 years.

At birth, the uterus measures 2.3 to 4.6 cm (mean 3.4 cm) in length and 0.8 to 2.2 cm (mean 1.3 cm) in width. At this age, the cervix is normally wider than the body of the uterus. In the first few weeks after birth, the uterus decreases in size to a length of 2 to 3 cm and a width of 0.5 to 1.0 cm. In this same period, it acquires an infantile configuration, with the width of the cervix being less than or the same as the width of the uterus.

A gradual increase in the size of the uterus starts at 7 to 8 years of age, with a more dramatic growth spurt at puberty. Both uterine size and ovarian volume increase as the patient matures; the changes can be correlated with the Tanner stage of development. The uterine length is 3.5 to 4.0 cm at 9 years, and 5.5 cm at 13 years. The postpubertal uterus measures 5 to 8 cm in length and 1.6 to 3.0 cm in width and achieves an adult configuration, with the width of the uterine body being greater than the width of the cervix. US demonstrates an echogenic endometrium in almost all girls, from the neonatal period forward (Fig. 27).

The ovaries are frequently seen in the neonatal period because of the maternal estrogen effect. They become progressively smaller in the first 2 years of life. After this, until age 5 years, they are inconstantly visualized with

US; in this period, the ovary measures 0.5 to 1.5 cm in length and 0.3 to 0.5 cm in width. After age 5 years, although the ovaries are not much bigger, one or both ovaries are seen in 80% to 90% of children. An ovary is considered to be enlarged when it measures more than 2.2×1.1 cm during the first 5 years or more than 2.7×1.4 cm from 6 years to puberty. The ovary grows dramatically at puberty, reaching 5.0 cm in length and 1.5 to 3.0 cm in width. Its shape also changes from a prolate ellipse to ovoid. US can be used to determine ovarian volume using the formula

$$\text{Volume} = 0.525 \times \text{length} \times \text{width} \times \text{thickness}$$

with volume being roughly half the product of the length, width, and thickness. Girls who were small for gestational age at birth (intrauterine growth retardation) have a smaller than normal uterus and ovaries. Additionally, they may, as adults, have fertility problems because they also have a decreased number of primordial follicles.

Normal ovaries will frequently contain small follicular cysts, even in prepubertal girls. The cysts may measure up to a few centimeters but are usually only a few millimeters (Fig. 28). The small amounts of free fluid frequently seen in the pelvis in female children may be related to rupture of these cysts.

MALE GENITAL TRACT

The main anatomic features of the male genital tract are illustrated in Figures 20, 29, and 30. There are two testes, one in each scrotal sac. The usual contents of the scrotal sac are the spermatic cord, the testis (and appendix testis), and the epididymis (and appendix epididymis). The anatomy of the epididymis is as drawn in Figure 30, but variations are reported and may be visible with US. On longitudinal testicular sonograms, the head of the epididymis is usually demonstrated as a triangular

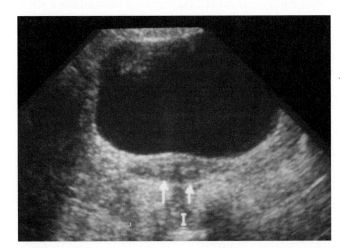

FIGURE 27. On transverse bladder sonogram, the uterus in this neonate is seen as a diamond-shaped retrovesical structure with two separate endometrial stripes (arrows)—a uterus didelphys.

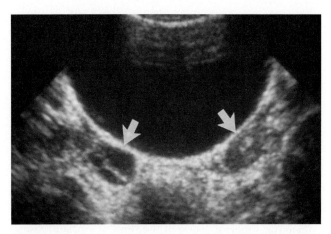

FIGURE 28. On transverse bladder sonogram, the well-distended bladder allows great visualization of both ovaries (arrows). The right ovary contains multiple small cysts that make it appear slightly less echogenic.

structure located along the superior pole of the testis. It has a homogeneous echogenicity similar to that of the testis.

Asymmetry of the scrotal sac at birth should suggest herniation of bowel contents into the scrotum, perinatal torsion of the testicle, or hydrocele (free fluid) on the too-large side. An abnormally small scrotal sac may be due to nondescent of the testes or prenatal torsion and infarction of the testis.

The testes derive their blood supply from the testicular or internal spermatic arteries that arise from the anterolateral aspect of the abdominal aorta, below the renal arteries but above the inferior mesenteric artery. Each artery descends over the psoas muscle and courses through the inguinal canal within the spermatic cord. The epididymis receives its blood supply from branches of the inferior vesical artery. The draining veins of each testis join the vein of the ipsilateral epididymis to form the pampiniform plexus. This ascends in the spermatic cord, enters the inguinal canal through two or three venous channels, and terminates in the testicular vein. The right testicular vein drains into the inferior vena cava just below the renal vein; as a rare variant it may drain directly into the right renal vein. The left testicular vein drains into the left renal vein. This difference in drainage accounts for the fact that most varicoceles are left sided.

The testicular length is about 15 mm at birth, 20 mm at 4 to 10 years, 30 mm at 12 to 13 years, and about 40 mm thereafter. US measurement of testicular volume is reliable and easily performed and may be used to evaluate questions of both normal (bilateral) development or possible unilateral damage after hernia or varicocele repair.

On US, the testis is a homogeneous, moderately echogenic structure. A linear, intensely echogenic structure noted along the posterior aspect of the testis on longitudinal scans is the mediastinum testis, a focal infolding of the tunica albuginea, the membrane that covers the testis. A focal area of slightly less echogenic tissue can be observed along the testicular hilum; this is the rete testis. Intratesticular vessels, well shown with color and power Doppler, may produce hypoechoic bands on standard US.

ADRENAL GLANDS

The right adrenal gland is a triangular structure located on the superior pole of the right kidney behind and to the right of the inferior vena cava. The left adrenal gland has a semilunar shape and is located along the antero-medial surface of the superior pole of the left kidney, lateral to the aorta, and may extend above the kidney in only 50% of children. Both adrenals are contained within the superior recess of the renal (Gerota's) fascia, to which they are firmly adherent.

Each adrenal gland receives blood from three separate arteries: a superior adrenal artery that originates from the inferior phrenic artery, a middle adrenal artery that comes directly from the aorta at the level of the celiac axis, and an inferior adrenal artery that arises

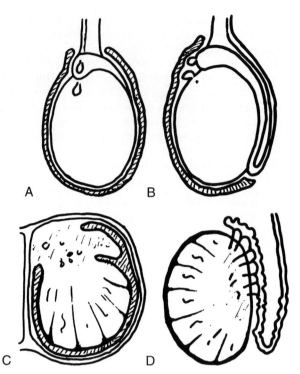

FIGURE 30. Diagram of a normal left testis. Frontal **(A)** and lateral **(B)** views show the epididymis and the proximal part of the spermatic cord. The appendix epididymis (above) and the appendix testis (below) are also shown. The sac of the tunica vaginalis *(hatched area)* is shown in coronal **(A)** and sagittal **(B)** section. **C,** Axial section showing attachment of the testis to the posterior wall of the scrotum, and the relationship of the vaginal sac to the testis and epididymis *(hatched area)*. **D,** Sagittal section without the tunica vaginalis showing the relationship of the epididymis to the testis.

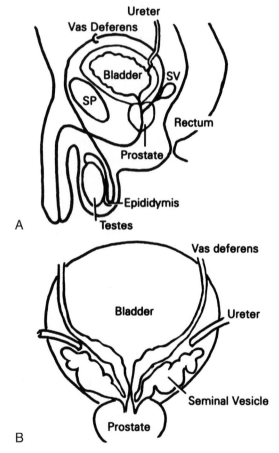

FIGURE 29. Male reproductive anatomy. **A,** This sagittal section demonstrates the relationship of the bladder to the prostate, seminal vesicles *(SV)*, and vas deferens. The urethra is shown to arise from the bladder base, to course through lobes of the horseshoe-shaped prostate gland, and to pass anteriorly through the penis. The path of the vas deferens from testicle to prostatic urethra is also shown. **B,** This coronal retrovesical diagram shows the relationship between the ureter and the vas deferens and seminal vesicle.

from the main renal artery. The gland drains through a single vein. On the right, the vein enters directly into the inferior vena cava at the T11 to T12 level; on the left, the adrenal vein drains either directly into the renal vein or indirectly via the inferior phrenic vein (see Fig. 5C).

The adrenal gland is composed of a cortex and a medulla. The cortex is from mesoderm and the medulla has neural crest origin. During fetal life and for a short period postnatally, a transient fetal cortex is present between the true or permanent cortex and medulla. The fetal cortex is initially quite large, but it decreases in late pregnancy and even more rapidly in the first few weeks of life. The position and relatively large size of the adrenal glands may make them vulnerable to birth trauma. Adrenal gland hemorrhage can also occur in response to other perinatal stresses. Adrenal hemorrhage can simulate other neonatal masses such as neuroblastoma and rare cortical tumors. Sequential US studies or MRI (to detect hemosiderin within the hemorrhage) may be useful. Involution of the hemorrhage may produce fine calcifications that may remain throughout life and may be dense enough to be seen on abdominal radiographs.

Normal adrenal glands are not visualized on plain films or with excretory urography but may be seen with US, CT, or MRI. Because of their large size in the neonate, they are almost always demonstrated on US

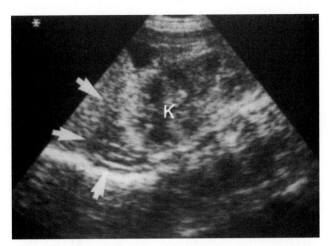

FIGURE 31. Longitudinal ultrasound (US) scan of the right adrenal gland *(arrows)* in a newborn. The adrenal glands in the newborn period are relatively large and are easier to recognize by US than in later life. *K* = kidney.

performed in this period (Fig. 31). Later, they may be hard to see with US. The left adrenal gland is more difficult to visualize than the right. In the neonate, the adrenal medulla and adjacent vascular fetal cortex are hyperechoic and the cortex is prominent and hypoechoic, probably as a result of the residual fetal cortical tissue. After the first year of life, when the fetal cortex has involuted, the adrenal gland becomes hypoechoic throughout, without the clear differentiation between the cortex and medulla. The gland also changes shape, becoming more triangular, with three distinct vertical ridges or limbs directed anteromedially, laterally, and posteriorly. These ridges can be seen on transverse US images but are more frequently and better demonstrated on CT. On axial superior CT or MRI sections, the adrenal gland appears as a thin, linear structure, but on lower sections it has an inverted Y or V shape.

SUGGESTED READINGS

Kidney

Renal Anatomy

Auh YH, Rubinstein WA, Markisz JA, et al: Extraperitoneal paravesical spaces: CT delineation with US correlation. Radiology 1986;159:319

Auh YH, Rubinstein WA, Markisz JA, et al: Intraperitoneal paravesical spaces: CT delineation with US correlation. Radiology 1986;159:311

Currarino G, Williams B, Dana K: Kidney length correlated with age: normal values in children. Radiology 1984;150:703

Dodds WJ, Darweesh RM, Lawson TL, et al: The retroperitoneal spaces revisited. AJR Am J Roentgenol 1986;147:1155

Erwin BC, Carroll BA, Muller H: A sonographic assessment of neonatal renal parameters. J Ultrasound Med 1985;4:217

Fernbach SK, Davis TM: The abnormal renal axis in children with spina bifida and gibbus deformity—the pseudohorseshoe kidney. J Urol 1986;136:1258

Gross GW, Boal DK: Sonographic assessment of normal renal size in children with myelodysplasia. J Urol 1988;140:784

Haller JO, Berdon WE, Friedman AP: Increased renal cortical echogenicity: a normal finding in neonates and infants. Radiology 1982;142:173

Han BK, Babcock DS: Sonographic measurements and appearance of normal kidneys in children. AJR Am J Roentgenol 1985;145:611

Hoffer FA, Hanabergh AM, Teele RL: The interrenicular junction: a

mimic of renal scarring on normal pediatric sonograms. AJR Am J Roentgenol 1985;145:1075

Kenney IJ, Wild SR: Renal parenchymal junctional line in children: ultrasonic frequency and appearance. Br J Radiol 1987;60:865

Lafortune M, Constantin A, Breton G, et al: Sonography of hypertrophied column of Bertin. AJR Am J Roentgenol 1986;146:53

McClennan BL, Lee JKT, Peterson RR: Anatomy of the perirenal area. Radiology 1986;158:555

Rosenbaum DM, Korngold E, Teele R: Sonographic assessment of renal length in normal children. AJR Am J Roentgenol 1984;142:467

Schlesinger AE, Hedlund GL, Pierson WP, et al: Normal standards for kidney length in premature infants: determination with US. Work in progress. Radiology 1987;164:127

Schlesinger AE, Hernandez RJ, Zerin JM, et al: Interobserver and intraobserver variations in sonographic renal length measurements in children. AJR Am J Roentgenol 1991;156:1029

Vade A, Lau P, Smick J, et al: Sonographic renal parameters as related to age. Pediatr Radiol 1987;17:212

Zerin JM, Meyer RD: Sonographic assessment of renal length in the first year of life: the problem of "spurious nephromegaly." Pediatr Radiol 2000;30:52

Compensatory Hypertrophy

Heymans C, Breysem L, Proesmans W: Multicystic kidney dysplasia: a prospective study on the natural history of the affected and contralateral kidney. Eur J Pediatr 1998;157:673

Hill LM, Nowak A, Hartle R, et al: Fetal compensatory hypertrophy with a unilateral functioning kidney. Ultrasound Obstet Gynecol 2000;15:191

Rottenberg GT, De Bruyn R, Gordon I: Sonographic standards for a single functioning kidney in children. AJR Am J Roentgenol 1996;167:1255

Pelvocaliceal System and Ureter

Jequier S, Paltiel H, Lafortune M: Ureterovesical jets in infants and children: duplex and color Doppler US studies. Radiology 1990; 175:349

Kaufman RA, Dunbar JS, Gole DE: Normal dilatation of the proximal ureters in children. AJR Am J Roentgenol 1981;137:945

Bladder and Urethra

Berger RM, Maizels M, Morgan GC, et al: Bladder capacity (ounces) equals age (years) plus 2 predicts normal bladder capacity and aids in diagnosis of abnormal voiding patterns. J Urol 1983;129:347

Bis KG, Slovis TL: Accuracy of ultrasonic bladder volume measurements in children. Pediatr Radiol 1990;20:457

Blane CE, Zerin JM, Bloom DA: Bladder diverticula in children. Radiology 1994;190:695

Fairhurst JJ, Rubin CM, Hyde I, et al: Bladder capacity in infants. J Pediatr Surg 1991;26:55

Fernbach SK, Feinstein KA: Abnormalities of the bladder in children: imaging findings. AJR Am J Roentgenol 1994;162:1143

Fernbach SK, Feinstein KA, Schmidt MB: Pediatric voiding cystourethrography: a pictorial guide. Radiographics 2000;20:155

Holmdahl G, Hanson E, Hanson M, et al: Four-hour voiding observation in healthy infants. J Urol 1996;156:1809

Kaefer M, Zurakowski D, Bauer SB, et al: Estimating normal bladder capacity in children. J Urol 1997;158:2261

Saxton HM, Borzykowski M, Mundy AR, et al: Spinning-top urethra: not a normal variant. Radiology 1988;168:147

Zerin JM, Chen E, Ritchey ML, et al: Bladder capacity as measured at voiding cystourethrography in children: relationship to toilet training and frequency of micturition. Radiology 1993;87:803

Genital Tract

Cassorla FG, Golden SM, Johnsonbaugh RE, et al: Testicular volume during early infancy. J Pediatr 1981;99:742

Cohen HL, Eisenberg P, Mandel F, et al: Ovarian cysts are common in premenarchal girls: a sonographic study of 101 children 2–12 years old. AJR Am J Roentgenol 1992;159:89

Cohen HL, Haller JO: Pediatric and adolescent genital abnormalities. Clin Diagn Ultrasound 1989;24:187

Cohen HL, Shapiro MA, Mandel FS, et al: Normal ovaries in neonates and infants: a sonographic study of 77 patients 1 day to 25 months old. AJR Am J Roentgenol 1993;160:583

Cohen HL, Tice HM, Mandel FS: Ovarian volume measured by US: bigger than we think. Radiology 1990;177:189

Daniel WA Jr, Feinstein RA, Howard-Peebles P, et al: Testicular volume in adolescents. J Pediatr 1982;101:1010

de Bruin JP, Dorland M, Bruinse HW, et al: Fetal growth retardation as a cause of impaired ovarian development. Early Hum Dev 1998; 51:39

Griffin IJ, Cole TJ, Duncan KA, et al: Pelvic ultrasound measurements in normal girls. Acta Paediatr 1995;84:536

Haber HP, Mayer EI: Ultrasound evaluation of uterine and ovarian size from birth to puberty. Pediatr Radiol 1994;24:11

Holm K, Mosfeldt Laursen E, Brocks V, et al: Pubertal maturation of the internal genitalia: an ultrasound evaluation of 166 healthy girls. Ultrasound Obstet Gynecol 1995;6:175

Ibanez L, Potau N, Enriquez G, et al: Reduced uterine and ovarian size in adolescent girls born small for gestational age. Pediatr Res 2000;47:575

Ivarsson SA, Nillson KO, Persson PH: Ultrasonography of pelvic organs in prepubertal and postpubertal girls. Arch Dis Child 1983;58:352

Munn CS, Kiser LC, Wetzner SM, et al: Ovary volume in young and premenopausal adults: US determination. Work in progress. Radiology 1986;159:731

Nussbaum AR, Sanders RC, Jones MD: Neonatal uterine volume morphology as seen on real-time US. Radiology 1986;160:641

Orsini LF, Salardi S, Pilu G, et al: Pelvic organs in premenarcheal girls: real-time ultrasonography. Radiology 1984;153:113

Rigsby CK, Siegel MJ: CT appearance of pediatric ovaries and uterus. J Comput Assist Tomogr 1994;18:72

Schmahmann S, Haller JO: Neonatal ovarian cysts: pathogenesis, diagnosis, and management. Pediatr Radiol 1997;27:101

Thomas RD, Dewbury KC: Ultrasound appearances of the rete testis. Clin Radiol 1993;47:121

Turek PJ, Ewalt DH, Snyder HM, et al: Normal epididymal anatomy in boys. J Urol 1994;151:726

Adrenal Glands

Kangarloo H, Diament MJ, Gold RH, et al: Sonography of the adrenal glands in neonates and children: changes in appearance with age. J Clin Ultrasound 1986;14:43

Mitty HA: Embryology, anatomy, and anomalies of the adrenal gland. Semin Roentgenol 1988;23:271

Oppenheimer DA, Carroll BA, Yousem S: Sonography of the normal neonatal adrenal gland. Radiology 1983;146:157

Rosenberg ER, Bowie JD, Andreotti RF, et al: Sonographic evaluation of the fetal adrenal glands. AJR Am J Roentgenol 1982;139:1145

Scott E, Thomas A, McGarrigle HH, et al: Serial adrenal ultrasonography in normal neonates. J Ultrasound Med 1990;9:279

PART III

KIDNEY

SANDRA K. FERNBACH
KATE A. FEINSTEIN
JOHN R. STY

Chapter 1

CONGENITAL RENAL ANOMALIES

SANDRA K. FERNBACH

ANOMALIES OF ROTATION

The metanephros has its origin in the fetal pelvis and, in this site, has its renal pelvis oriented anteriorly. As the kidney ascends to its normal position, the renal pelvis and hilum normally rotate 90 degrees medially (Fig. 1). Kidneys that are located inferior to a normal position (i.e., those that fail to ascend completely) generally maintain some degree of the earlier anterior orientation of the renal pelvis; they are described as incompletely rotated. Such malrotation can also be observed, but is much less frequent, in normally positioned kidneys. The renal pelvis of normally positioned kidneys may also be overrotated and be oriented posteriorly or, even more rarely, be rotated into a lateral position.

Kidneys that are in a normal position also have, as a rule, a normal renal axis. A line drawn from the upper caliceal system to the lower parallels the psoas muscle, with the upper pole medial to the lower. The intimate

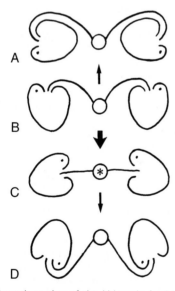

FIGURE 1. Normal rotation of the kidney in fetal life and various types of renal malrotation. **A,** Reversed rotation, which is rare. **B,** Primitive fetal position of the kidney with the hilum pointing forward. A persistent fetal position is referred to as an absent or incomplete rotation; this is the most common form of renal malrotation. **C,** Normal postnatal position with the hilum pointing medially and slightly forward. **D,** Overrotation, which is rare. All these anomalies of rotation may be unilateral or bilateral.

relationship of the kidney to the psoas muscle also results in the superior and medial portion being more dorsal than the inferior and lateral portion of the kidney, which rests on the bulkier aspect of the psoas. Anomalies of ascent and fusion anomalies produce abnormalities of the renal axis and of the normal relationship of the kidney to the psoas muscle.

RENAL ECTOPIA AND ANOMALIES OF FUSION

Most forms of renal ectopia and renal fusion anomalies are associated with anomalies of other organ systems. Spinal anomalies (such as segmentation anomalies, partial/complete sacral agenesis, and most dysraphic processes), cardiac anomalies, and limb anomalies are associated with renal ectopia, agenesis, and fusions. When other specific anomalies of the gastrointestinal tract (esophageal atresia, imperforate anus) are present, the affected child is said to have the VACTERL association, a linkage of *v*ertebral, *a*norectal, *c*ardiac, *t*racheo-*e*sophageal, *r*enal, and *l*imb anomalies. The limb anomalies, originally described as affecting the radial aspect of the forearm and hand, have been extended to other lesions of the upper extremity and hand as well as the lower extremities. Anomalies of the urethra have also been described in boys with the VACTERL association.

When magnetic resonance imaging (MRI) is used to evaluate spinal anomalies, previously unappreciated renal anomalies may be detected (Figs. 2 and 3). Some renal anomalies described below have specific associations, each detailed in its section.

IPSILATERAL RENAL ECTOPIA (SIMPLE UNCROSSED RENAL ECTOPIA)

Pelvic Kidney (Inferior Ectopia)

The normal ascent to the renal fossa may be incomplete and the kidney may remain in the pelvis or be located anywhere between the bony pelvis and the renal fossa. In early gestation, the kidney takes its blood supply from the middle sacral artery. As the kidney ascends, the blood supply changes; the lower vessels atrophy as vessels with a more cephalad origin develop. In turn, "renal" arteries develop from the iliac artery and then,

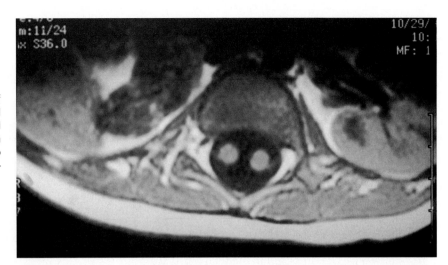

FIGURE 2. Magnetic resonance imaging of unilateral (right) renal agenesis. Vertebral anomalies prompted this study. The axial image shows a normal left kidney and a bowel loop in the right renal fossa. Note also the split spinal cord, indicating diastemato-myelia. (Courtesy of Joan A. Zawin, MD.)

sequentially, higher sites on the aorta. A kidney that is in a lower than normal position will usually retain its earlier blood supply and, as described above, will have some degree of abnormal rotation of the renal pelvis (Figs. 4 and 5).

■ Anomalies of ascent are associated with variations in rotation of the pelivicaliceal system and persistence of a more primitive vascular supply.

Because the embryology of the adrenal gland is independent of the kidney, it will be in its expected position whenever the kidney is absent or does not reach the renal fossa. However, the adrenal gland may develop an elongated or elliptical shape rather than its normal triangular or y configuration. Differentiation of the adrenal cortex from the medullary tissue remains clear (Fig. 6). The elongated gland is easily recognized as such; the elliptical adrenal may, with its echogenic medulla simulating the central echo complex, be mistaken for a hypoplastic kidney in the renal fossa.

The pelvic kidney is an extremely low-lying kidney that has, for many years, been considered to be a poorly functioning, dysmorphic structure, and in many instances it is. Statistically, it will suffer vesicoureteral reflux more often than a normal kidney and may, in about 10% of children, be the only kidney. In some children, both kidneys are in the pelvis and may be fused into a single unit, the so-called cake kidney. Anomalies of rotation and blood supply are to be expected. The adrenal gland is usually in a normal position, but will have an abnormal conformation.

In some children, anomalies of other organ systems prompt the sonogram that detects the pelvic kidney; in others, it may be discovered prenatally. Many are not detected until adult life. For example, a maternal pelvic kidney can interfere with normal engagement of the fetal head and, therefore, precipitate a cesarean section.

On ultrasound (US), the pelvic kidney may have a normal appearance (Fig. 7), but it frequently does not

(Figs. 7 and 8). The pelvocaliceal system may be predominantly extrarenal, resulting in images in which the kidney lacks the usual echogenic central renal echo complex. Corticomedullary differentiation may be indistinct. Hydronephrosis may be present without obstruction as a result of the extrarenal location of the pelvocaliceal, system but ureteropelvic junction obstruc-

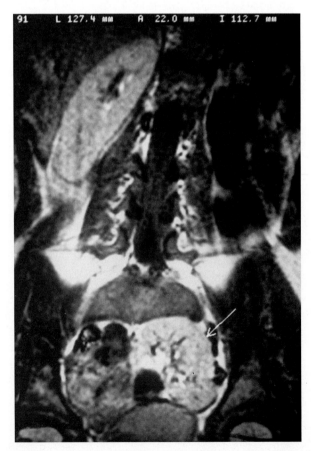

FIGURE 3. Magnetic resonance imaging (MRI) of pelvic kidney. A diagnosis of scoliosis and plain films showing vertebral anomalies preceded this MRI study. The coronal scan demonstrates a normally positioned and normal-appearing right kidney and an unsuspected left pelvic kidney *(arrow)*. (Courtesy of Joan A. Zawin, MD.)

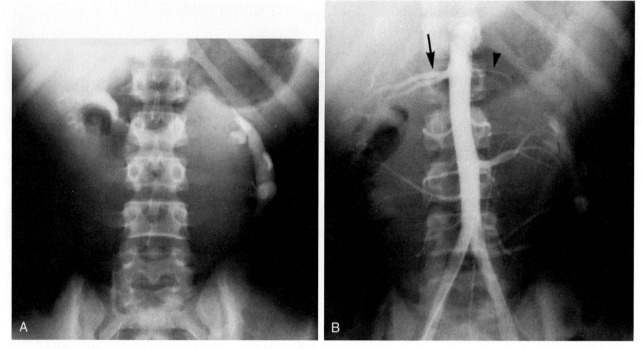

FIGURE 4. Failure of the kidney to ascend to normal position as seen on excretory urography and angiography. **A,** The abnormal orientation of the left renal pelvis and calices is typical of a kidney with inferior ectopia. The right kidney is in a normal position and is normally rotated. **B,** The right kidney has a normal origin of its artery *(arrow)*. The left kidney has its blood supply arising two vertebral levels below the usual origin of the left renal artery. The small, normally positioned vessel *(arrowhead)* is supplying the normally positioned adrenal gland.

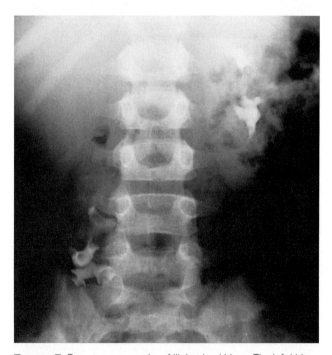

FIGURE 5. Excretory urography of iliolumbar kidney. The left kidney is in a normal position and the right partially overlies the right iliac bone. Note the abnormal rotation of the right renal pelvis.

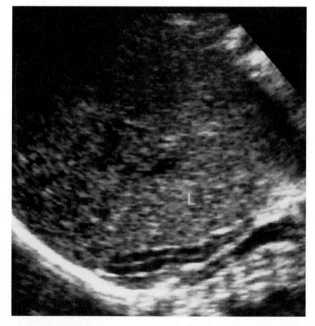

FIGURE 6. Abnormal ultrasound appearance of the adrenal gland with renal ectopia or agenesis. The adrenal gland, just beneath the liver *(L),* is elongated. The lucent tissue at the periphery is the cortex. The bright central stripe in the adrenal medulla is the medulla.

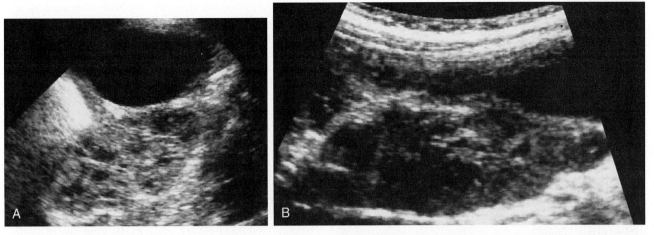

FIGURE 7. Renal ultrasound of normal and abnormal (pelvic) kidney. **A,** The normal kidney is adjacent to the urine-filled bladder. Normally lucent medullary tissue is easily distinguished from the cortex. **B,** In the abnormal pelvic kidney, the upper and lower poles are shrunken and the corticomedullary differentiation is indistinct.

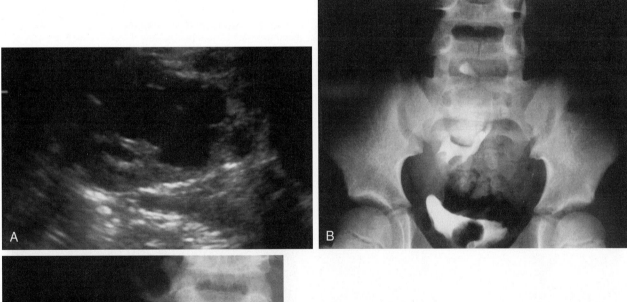

FIGURE 8. Pelvic kidney with focal abnormality of caliceal system. **A,** Longitudinal ultrasound (US) demonstrates that the kidney is just above the bladder. A central fluid collection does not have the appearance of a hydronephrotic renal pelvis and could represent a simple cyst. The parenchyma of the upper and lower pole has a normal appearance. **B,** On excretory urography, the kidney is seen to overlie the sacrum. The upper and lower caliceal systems are widely separated. **C,** A retrograde injection of the ureter was performed and proved that the fluid collection seen on US is in a distended caliceal system draining the midportion of the kidney.

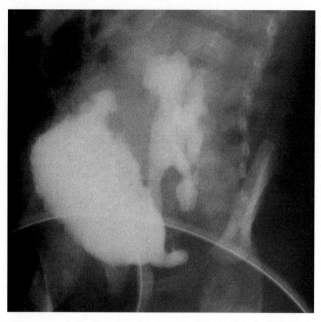

FIGURE 9. Reflux into a pelvic kidney. The bladder is moderately trabeculated, in this child a sign of a neurogenic bladder associated with a spinal cord anomaly. Reflux fills and distends the ureter and pelvocaliceal system, indicating grade V reflux.

tion is common in the pelvic kidney because of the abnormal orientation of the ureter to the renal pelvis, an insertion that impedes drainage. Because of the high incidence of vesicoureteral reflux in the pelvic or contralateral kidney (up to 70%), radionuclide or radiographic cystography is recommended (Fig. 9). Renal cortical scintigraphy using DMSA can be employed to both locate and define morphology of ectopic kidneys. Nuclear scintigraphy is useful to distinguish obstructive from nonobstructive hydronephrosis when urinary tract surgery is contemplated because the child has vesicoureteral reflux or repeated urinary tract infections. Excretory urography usually provides limited evaluation of the pelvic kidney because the kidney may function poorly or, even when functioning well, may be hard to see because of the overlying shadows of the sacrum and gastrointestinal tract.

Thoracic Kidney (Superior Ectopia)

The kidney may continue its ascent through the retroperitoneum and enter the thorax (Fig. 10). Superior ectopia may occur as an isolated lesion but is more often part of a larger intrathoracic herniation of subdiaphragmatic structures through the foramen of Bochdalek. Because congenital diaphragmatic hernia occurs about

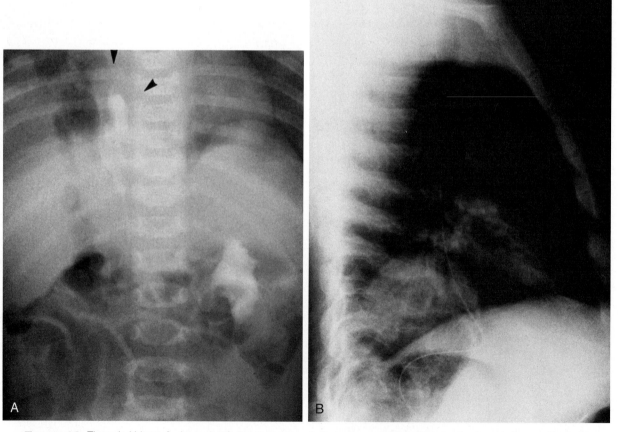

FIGURE 10. Thoracic kidney. **A,** An oval soft tissue mass projects in the posterior sulcus on the lateral chest radiograph. **B,** Anteroposterior film from excretory urography. The left kidney has a normal appearance; the right kidney projects above the medial aspect of the right diaphragm. Also projecting above the diaphragm are several bowel loops, indicating that the kidney displacement occurred as a result of a hernia.

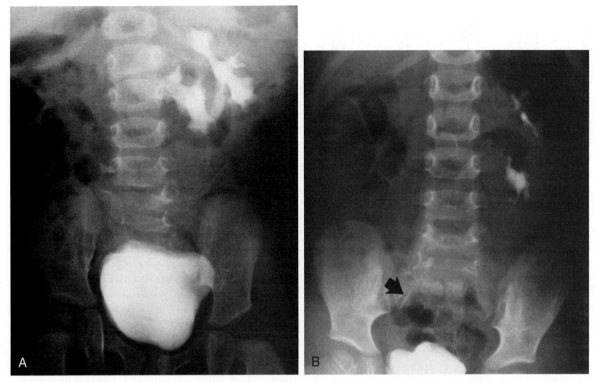

FIGURE 11. Excretory urography of crossed renal ectopia. **A,** Segmentation anomalies of the sacrum, subtle in this child, are one of the skeletal anomalies associated with crossed renal ectopia. The dysplasia of the left hip (shallow acetabular roof and delayed ossification of femoral head) is due to neurologic problems related to the sacral anomaly. **B,** As seen in a different child, the lower kidney is usually ectopic, and its ureter *(arrow)* crosses the midline to insert into the bladder in a normal position.

seven times more frequently on the left than the right, superior renal ectopia is also more frequently left sided. The thoracic kidney tends to function well and usually has its blood supply from a normally positioned renal artery, although it may also have an accessory artery arising from the thoracic aorta. The adrenal gland is usually in its normal location in the retroperitoneum.

On chest radiographs, the thoracic kidney, located in the posterior mediastinum, may be mistaken for the usual neurogenic tumors that develop in this region: neuroblastoma, ganglioneuroblastoma, or ganglioneuroma (Fig. 10). If the adjacent spine has an abnormal appearance, intrathoracic meningocele or neurenteric cyst would be included in the differential diagnosis. Renal cortical scintigraphy, US or computed tomography (CT) can define the mass as being renal and may detect other herniated tissue or organs not appreciated with plain radiographs. Excretory urography can demonstrate the kidney, and MRI can also define it, but these are not commonly used for diagnosis (Fig. 10).

CROSSED RENAL ECTOPIA

This term is used when the bulk of both kidneys is on one side of the spine; a portion of the lower kidney, the one that has usually moved from its normal position, may extend over the spine (Fig. 11). It is seen in 1 in 3000 to 1 in 8000 children, with boys more often affected than girls. Usually, the ureter from the lower kidney usually crosses the midline to insert into the bladder in its normal position, contralateral to the ureter from the upper kidney. Departure from this pattern is rare, but does occur (Fig. 12). There is also variation in the alignment of the two kidneys. Although the majority are oriented in a completely superior–inferior or vertical axis, the lower kidney may be obliquely related to the superior kidney (Fig. 11). The absolute position of the upper kidney can also be ectopically low, with the position of the crossed kidney varied.

Approximately 90% of these kidneys will be fused and encompassed by a common renal fascia; hence the term *crossed fused renal ectopia* is frequently used. With standard imaging, it is impossible to differentiate those that are fused from the few that are in close apposition. However, in most clinical settings this information is not relevant. As expected in any type of inferior ectopia, the renal arterial vascularity may be anomalous and the renal pelvis, especially of the lower kidney, may be malrotated. Because each kidney is drained by its own ureter, multicystic dysplasia can develop in one of the kidneys. The occasional case report of unilateral crossed ectopy may be due to involution of an affected upper kidney.

Imaging demonstrates an empty renal fossa on one side (with abnormal adrenal configuration) and an apparently enlarged kidney on the other side. The demonstration of two separate renal pelves and a larger

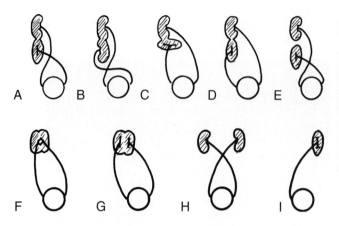

FIGURE 12. Diagram of various types of renal crossed ectopia. **A,** Unilateral fused kidney (inferior renal ectopia), the most common form. **B,** Sigmoid or S-shaped kidney. **C,** L-shaped kidney. **D,** Unilateral fused kidney (superior renal ectopia). **E,** Crossed ectopia without fusion. **F,** Unilateral disk kidney. **G,** Unilateral lump kidney. **H,** Bilateral crossed ectopia. **I,** Crossed ectopia of a solitary kidney (solitary crossed renal ectopia).

than normal amount of renal parenchyma may raise the possibility of a duplex kidney. Excretory urography or CT will show the separate ureters, each entering its appropriate trigone. Careful coronal or sagittal US and renal cortical scintigraphy may allow visualization of a small indentation, a niche, between the two kidneys even when fusion has occurred (Fig. 13). If one kidney has multicystic dysplasia, it will show typical US changes while the adjacent kidney will appear normal. It is important to exclude vesicoureteral reflux, known to occur with increased incidence into the lower kidney, by performing radionuclide cystography or voiding cysto-urethrography.

HORSESHOE KIDNEY

This common anomaly, noted in 1 in 500 to 1 in 1000 autopsies, takes its name from the U shape produced by the fusion of the lower poles of the kidneys (Fig. 14). The bridging tissue, known as the *isthmus,* is commonly composed of functioning parenchyma or, less commonly, fibrous tissue. Not every horseshoe kidney is symmetrically related to the spine; some are a bit more to the left or right, almost a transition to crossed renal ectopia (Fig. 15). In virtually all, the fusion occurs

inferiorly; superior fusion has been reported but is rarely seen.

There is an increased incidence of ureteral duplication, ureteropelvic junction obstruction, and vesicoureteral reflux in horseshoe kidneys (Figs. 16 and 17). The ureteropelvic junction obstruction develops from the mechanical obstruction of the ureters passing over the tissue of the isthmus. However, as with pelvic kidneys, dilatation of the pelvocaliceal system should not always be interpreted as obstruction because an extrarenal pelvis, also a common finding, can simulate obstruction. Multicystic dysplasia has been described in one segment of a horseshoe kidney; involution of the involved segment can produce a changing radiographic appearance of the functioning segments.

The segment of kidney that is over the spine is prone to injury from direct trauma. Wilms' tumor also occurs more frequently in horseshoe kidneys than in normal kidneys. In adults, stone formation and transitional cell cancer is more common in horseshoe than normal kidneys.

The fusion produces an abnormal renal axis; the lower pole of each kidney is more medial than the upper. The isthmus is intimately related to the inferior mesenteric artery. The kidneys are also abnormally low in the retroperitoneum. For this reason, the vascular

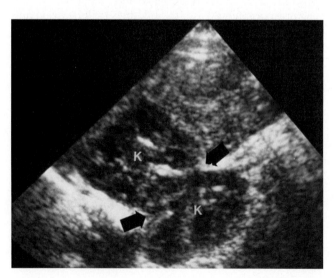

FIGURE 13. Renal ultrasound of crossed renal ectopia. There is a well-defined indentation or niche *(arrows)* at the junction between the two kidneys *(K).*

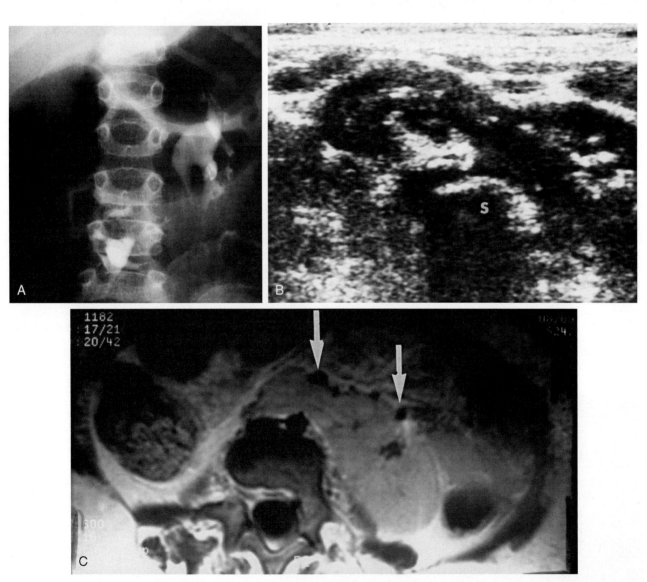

FIGURE 14. Horseshoe kidney showing fusion of the inferior poles, spreading apart of the superior poles, and failure of rotation. The renal pelves enter the kidneys on their anterior aspect. (Redrawn from Kelly HA, Burnam CF: Diseases of the Kidneys, Ureters and Bladder, 2nd ed. New York, Appleton, 1922.)

FIGURE 15. Transition between crossed renal ectopia and asymmetric horseshoe kidney. **A,** The axis of the left kidney is abnormal, with the lower pole directly below the upper. The right kidney overlies the spine. **B,** The confluence of the kidneys is anterior to the spine *(S)*, and the kidneys are asymmetrically related to the spine. **C,** The fused kidneys are anterior to and to the left of the spine. Note the the multiple signal voids of the renal vessels along the anterior aspect of the kidney *(arrows).* (Courtesy of Joan A. Zawin, MD.)

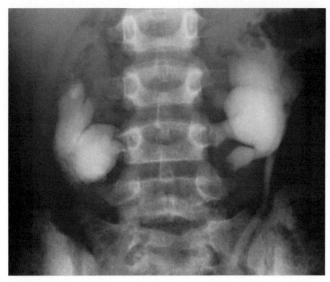

FIGURE 16. Excretory urography of horseshoe kidney with bilateral ureteropelvic junction obstruction. The abnormal renal axes, with the lower poles medial to the upper poles, is typical in horseshoe kidney. The moderate dilatation of each renal pelvis suggests obstruction, which was proven with subsequent scintigraphy.

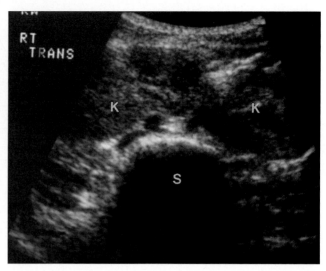

FIGURE 18. Renal ultrasound of horseshoe kidney. On this transverse image, the two kidneys (K) are connected in the midline, in front of the spine (S).

supply of the horseshoe kidney is variable. Multiple renal arteries may arise directly from the aorta or from a single vessel that itself arises from the aorta. Unless surgery is contemplated, the anatomy of the vascular supply need not be defined.

Although horseshoe kidney can be an incidental finding, it occurs in association with trisomy 18, imperforate anus (more often with high than low imperforate anus), cardiac anomalies, and Turner's syndrome, which itself has an increased incidence of aortic coarctation. Horseshoe kidney also occurs more frequently in infants of diabetic mothers and, in this setting, may be a form fruste of the caudal regression syndrome, also more common in these infants.

Prenatal and postnatal US may demonstrate the upper portion of each kidney in a low but otherwise normal paraspinal location and the low position of the "lower pole" of the kidneys. Postnatal US, usually done because of associated anomalies or an abnormal prenatal US, may demonstrate the isthmus anterior to the spine, especially when mild compression is used to displace interposed bowel loops (Fig. 18). The abnormal renal axis can be appreciated while scanning; the unusual orientation of the transducer when trying to obtain a sagittal view of the kidney should suggest the diagnosis. Occasionally the horseshoe kidney will be an incidental finding on MRI done because of obvious or suspected vertebral abnormality. Contrast studies are rarely performed for diagnosis but display the abnormal renal axis well (Figs. 16 and 17). An abnormal renal axis should suggest a horseshoe kidney, but in children with spinal dysraphism the abnormal axis may be due to a secondary kyphosis of the spine and underdevelopment of the psoas muscles. This is the pseudohorseshoe kidney (Fig. 19). Rarely, the anatomy of the asymmetric horseshoe kidney may be difficult to demonstrate, and

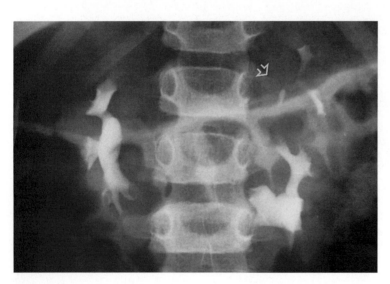

FIGURE 17. Excretory urography of horseshoe kidney with ureteral duplication. The abnormal axis of the kidneys, pointing toward the isthmus of parenchyma anterior to the spine, is a classic sign of horseshoe kidney. The left kidney is composed of two moieties, with the upper one (arrow) having a more delicate appearance than the lower.

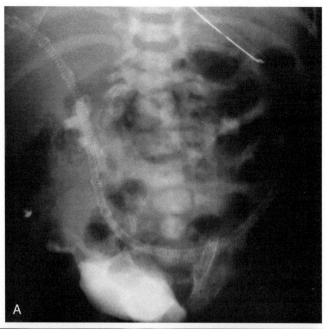

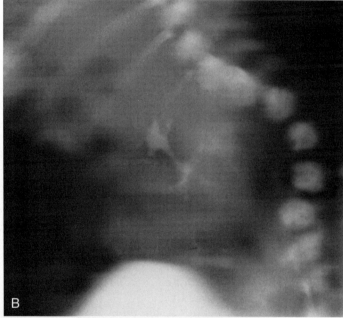

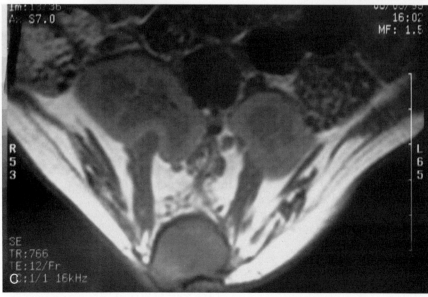

FIGURE 19. Pseudohorseshoe kidney. **A** and **B,** The abnormal renal axis on an anteroposterior film from an excretory urogram is related to the spinal kyphosis. The orientation of the kidney is also abnormal on the lateral view, with the upper pole anterior to the lower. **C,** Axial magnetic resonance imaging section through the lower abdomen in a second child with sacral agenesis demonstrates how the atretic psoas musculature poorly supports the kidneys and contributes to the midline position of the nonfused kidneys. With other imaging techniques, the separation between them might not be apparent. (Courtesy of Joan A. Zawin, MD.)

differentiation from an abdominal mass may require additional imaging.

RENAL AGENESIS

BILATERAL RENAL AGENESIS

This lethal anomaly occurs in about 1 in 4000 live births. Males are affected about three times as often as females. Although the incidence is usually sporadic, renal agenesis in some families appears to be an inherited trait and may be transmitted in association with lesser degrees of renal dysplasia. Bilateral renal agenesis may be an isolated finding or associated with other anomalies, especially those of the hindgut. Prenatal diagnosis is possible because the lack of urine production results in profound oligohydramnios. Also, the kidneys, usually seen by US in the 15th week of pregnancy, are not seen in a normal or anomalous position. Careful US examination detects the absence of bladder filling and emptying, a phenomenon seen at regular intervals on prenatal studies.

■ Oligohydramnios can result from a number of processes that result in a diminished production of urine.

If diagnosis is not made until birth, the child will manifest Potter's sequence: pulmonary hypoplasia; abnormal facial features (micrognathia, deep folds beneath the eyes, flattening of the ears); and deformities of the limbs (tightly apposed fingers, dislocated hips, club feet). The pulmonary hypoplasia may present as respiratory distress or pneumothorax and pneumomediastinum. Bedside US may be used to exclude another, possibly treatable, cause of Potter's sequence, especially if the clinical stigmata are mild.

The absence of the kidney in the renal fossa results in an unusual configuration of the adrenal gland, as described above in the section Pelvic Kidney (Inferior Ectopia). Because renal ectopia is also associated with this appearance of the adrenal gland, the entire abdomen and pelvis should be evaluated before making the diagnosis of renal agenesis. It may be difficult to exclude a pelvic kidney in an infant whose empty bladder precludes full examination of the pelvic contents or one with imperforate anus with a large amount of stool or air in the pelvis. For this reason, additional imaging is occasionally warranted. Nuclear renal cortical scintigraphy can detect an obscured or dysplastic kidney or confirm the complete absence of functioning renal parenchyma. Cystography, once advocated as a way to demonstrate the unusually small bladder, is rarely necessary because of these other studies.

UNILATERAL RENAL AGENESIS

Present in about 1 in 1000 to 1 in 1500 live births, unilateral renal agenesis is sometimes detected prenatally, or when postnatal US is done because of anomalies in the skeletal, gastrointestinal, or cardiovascular systems (Fig. 20). It is frequently seen in association with anomalies of the cervical spine (Klippel-Feil syndrome) and the lumbosacral spine, with or without rectal and anal anomalies. The ipsilateral adrenal gland is usually present owing to its separate embryology, but it may be absent in about 8% of patients.

Unilateral renal agenesis may be silent until puberty when, especially in females, the associated genital tract anomalies become clinically apparent. Associated anomalies of the genital tract are multiple (Table 1). In males, many are silent; occasionally a seminal vesicle cyst can simulate a ureterocele. In females, the anomalies may present with absence of menses, increasing abdominal or pelvic mass, or pelvic pain. The association of unilateral renal agenesis with genital tract problems in females, especially absence or hypoplasia of the vagina, is given the name Mayer-Rokitansky-Küster-Hauser syndrome (Fig. 21).

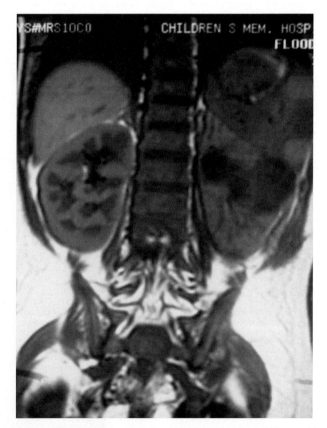

FIGURE 20. Magnetic resonance imaging of solitary kidney with aberrant bowel simulating multicystic dysplastic kidney. The coronal image demonstrates a normal right kidney. The mesentery and bowel loops in the left renal fossa could be mistaken for a multicystic dysplastic kidney. (Courtesy of Joan A. Zawin, MD.)

Table 1 ■ GENITAL ANOMALIES ASSOCIATED WITH UNILATERAL RENAL AGENESIS

Female
Absence/hypoplasia of the vagina
Absence of the uterus
Failure of fusion of midline structures (müllerian derivatives)
   Bicornuate uterus, duplicated uterus
   Obstructed hemivagina and hemiuterus → hydrocolpos,
     hematocolpos, hematosalpinx
Gartner's duct cyst—can present per vagina
Ipsilateral absence of the uterine horn and fallopian tube
   (unicornuate uterus)

Male
Ipsilateral anomalies
   Absence of the epididymis
   Absence of the seminal vesicle
   Absence of the vas deferens
   Absence/hypoplasia of the testis
   Seminal vesicle cyst

■ Unilateral renal agenesis is associated with genital anomalies in both girls and boys. The genital anomalies may be clinically silent and difficult to detect until puberty.

Some kidneys absent at birth may have been present in utero. Kidneys with multicystic dysplasia have been reported to involute so completely that the renal vasculature is no longer detectable, even at surgery. The dual pathway to unilateral renal agenesis may explain why some children have associated anomalies (true agenesis, a severe intrauterine insult) and other do not (involution of multicystic dysplastic kidney, a more limited process). The dual pathway may also explain why about 80% of children with unilateral renal agenesis lack the ipsilateral ureter and hemitrigone of the bladder (true agenesis) and why 20% have a normally developed bladder and a distal ureter of varying length (involution of multicystic dysplastic kidney). The fact that cystic dysplasia of the testis has been seen in association with two lesions of the genitourinary tract, multicystic dysplastic kidney and unilateral renal agenesis, may be another indication that the two processes may be linked.

The plain film finding of an abnormally positioned splenic or hepatic flexure (bowel falling toward the empty fossa) is inconstant and dependent on the amount of gas in the colon and the position of the child when the film is obtained. During a contrast enema, the direction of contrast flow is reversed in the region of the splenic flexure. Neither conventional radiographs nor contrast enema are used for diagnosis of unilateral renal agenesis. Instead, methods that directly image the renal fossa and remainder of the abdomen are employed.

US of the renal fossa demonstrates absence of the kidney and the abnormally configured adrenal gland. Whenever the renal fossa is empty, renal ectopia should be excluded before the diagnosis of unilateral renal agenesis is made. The contralateral kidney should be measured because, even in the very young, compensatory hypertrophy can be appreciated. Although uterine and vaginal anomalies are common associations, US in early childhood, before these structures reach adult size, may be inconclusive. In some settings, other imaging studies (nuclear studies, CT) may be necessary to differentiate a very small and poorly functioning kidney from an absent one. CT and MRI have been used to evaluate the associated genital anomalies (Fig. 21).

Because of the increased incidence of vesicoureteral reflux into a solitary kidney and the need to protect its parenchyma, a study to exclude reflux is recommended early in the child's life.

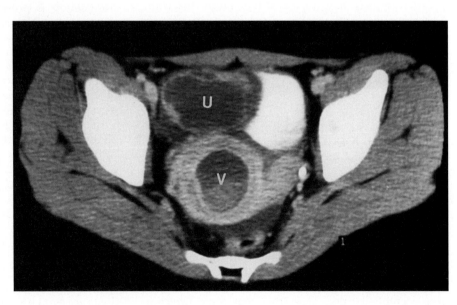

FIGURE 21. Computed tomography of Mayer-Rokistansky-Küster-Hauser syndrome: female genital anomalies associated with ipsilateral renal agenesis. The obstructed hemivagina (V) is filled with menstrual debris, as is the hemiuterus (U) above. On higher sections, the dilated fluid-filled fallopian tube could be identified. The nonobstructed system projects to the left of the dilated vagina.

CONGENITAL RENAL HYPOPLASIA

OLIGOMEGANEPHRONIA (OLIGOMEGANEPHRONIC RENAL HYPOPLASIA)

The uniformly small kidney detected in childhood may indeed be a congenitally small kidney, an anomaly derived from an embryologic misadventure. However, such a kidney is rarely detected on prenatal US. It may develop when, after pre- or postnatal renal vein thrombosis, the kidney shrinks and yet retains its normal morphology and some function.

At times, bilaterally small kidneys are noted in a child with anomalies of the central nervous system, usually microcephaly associated with some degree of mental retardation. Specific abnormalities of chromosome 4, a deletion or ring, have been noted in many of these patients. Pathologically, the small kidneys have fewer than normal nephrons but the nephrons are, as the name *oligomeganephronia* implies, much larger than normal. Oligomeganephronia has also been diagnosed in children with a small solitary kidney or a kidney with a single papilla, again giving weight to the theory that either an embryologic insult affected the quantity of the metanephric blastema or the metanephric blastema, originally normal, did not grow and differentiate normally.

HYPOPLASIA AND DYSPLASIA WITH ECTOPIC URETERAL INSERTION

Another form of hypoplastic kidney is associated with ectopic insertion of the ureter. The abnormal origin of the ureter from the wolffian duct produces an abnormal relationship between the ureter and the metanephric blastema. The ureter does not reach the greatest concentration of blastema, and the kidney thus induced is both hypo- and dysplastic. This process is much more frequent in girls than boys, and the ectopic insertion, most commonly in the vagina, is associated with primary incontinence. The small, poorly functioning kidney may be impossible to detect with excretory urography or US (Fig. 22). Nuclear scintigraphy and contrast-enhanced CT (CECT) are both useful when this diagnosis is being considered.

ASK-UPMARK KIDNEY (SEGMENTAL RENAL HYPOPLASIA)

When first described, segmental renal hypoplasia was thought to be a congenital process. However, analysis of the pattern of scarring and the pathologic changes have reversed the original hypothesis and it is now believed to be an acquired phenomenon. More common in females, the scarring is often detected during an evaluation for hypertension. Specific pathologic changes have been described and include thinning of the parenchyma over a clubbed calix, suggesting that renal infection

(pyelonephritis) with secondary scarring may be the cause of the change.

CONGENITAL RENAL DYSPLASIA

MULTICYSTIC DYSPLASTIC KIDNEY

This form of cystic renal disease is often confused with the autosomal forms of renal cystic disease. It usually occurs sporadically, but, in some families, appears to have autosomal linkage. Also, in contrast to the autosomal forms of renal cystic disease, the renal dysplasia is due to or associated with ureteral atresia, distal ureteral obstruction (simple ureterocele), or ectopic ureteral insertion. The affected kidney has no or negligible renal function. This condition is most often diagnosed prenatally or in the neonatal period (see Section II, Part V, Chapter 4, page 113). However, if not discovered in the neonate, then it may be detected in the older child.

■ Multicystic dysplastic kidney is a nonheritable disorder and is associated with obstruction of urinary drainage on the affected side; both autosomal recessive and autosomal dominant polycystic kidney disease are inherited and are not associated with obstruction of the renal pelvis or ureter.

The cysts, of varying size, may be several centimeters and easily seen, usually in a random array within the renal tissue (Fig. 23*A*). No normal parenchyma is discerned. The occasional hydronephrotic variant of multicystic dysplastic kidney may be difficult to differentiate from the much more common true hydronephrosis because it has a centrally located cyst that simulates a dilated renal pelvis. Nuclear imaging can be useful to evaluate the hydronephrotic variant, lest a treatable obstruction is present, as well as the potentially obstructed contralateral kidney; there is virtually no function in the kidney with multicystic dysplasia (Fig. 24). In a few children, the multicystic dysplastic kidney consists of only a few large cysts (Fig. 23*B*). Because the one functioning kidney has vesicoureteric reflux about 25% of the time, nuclear cystography or voiding cystourethrography is recommended.

At one time the multicystic dysplastic kidney was always removed. This practice is no longer universal.

CYSTIC RENAL DISEASE

AUTOSOMAL RECESSIVE POLYCYSTIC KIDNEY DISEASE

This rare disorder affects both kidneys and liver with ectasia and fibrosis. In the kidneys, the ectasia primarily involves the collecting tubules; in the liver, the biliary ducts are similarly affected. Liver fibrosis, not present at

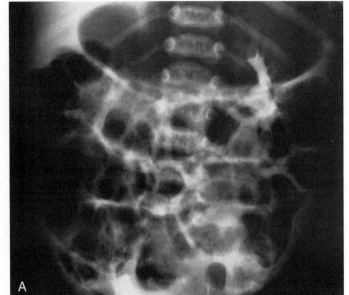

FIGURE 22. Renal hypoplasia and dysplasia with ectopic ureteral insertion. **A,** On excretory urography, the left kidney concentrates and excretes contrast. The right kidney is not visible. **B,** The ureteral orifice, located in the vagina, was injected for retrograde ureterography. The ectopic right ureter is thin and morphologically bizarre. The caliceal system above is also abnormal in appearance.

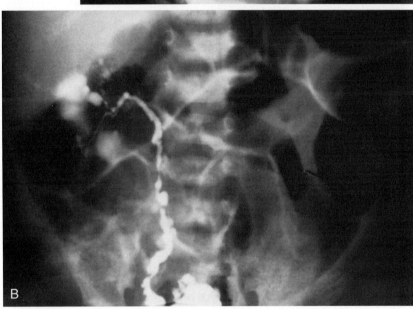

birth, also develops. The degree of fibrosis and ectasia is not parallel in the same organ, and the degrees of involvement of the liver and kidney tend to be inversely proportional to each other. A small segment of children with autosomal recessive polycystic kidney disease (ARPKD) will also have Caroli's disease, or cystic dilatation of the intrahepatic biliary ducts. (For information on the severe form of ARPKD, see Section II, Part V, Chapter 5, page 223.)

As in the neonate, the kidneys tend to be large, extending up to 10 cm. The dilated collecting tubules create intense echogenicity within the medulla (Fig. 25). Because the cortex is spared, it may appear relatively hypoechoic, creating an echolucent rim at the periphery of the kidney; this is an inconstant finding. Occasionally, the increased medullary echogenicity will define the triangular pyramids and simulate the nephrocalcinosis of renal tubular acidosis. A clearly visible "cyst" may be a true cyst or a trapped calix. High-frequency US

probes may allow direct visualization of the dilated tubules arranged in a fan-like configuration reminiscent of the spoke-wheel pattern noted on excretory urography or CECT as a result of contrast pooling in the tubules (Fig. 26). Imaging other than US is seldom necessary. The appearance of affected kidneys with magnetic resonance (MR)–urography has been reported; the dilated tubules were identified as hyperintense, linear, radial patterns in the medulla, extending to the cortex. MR-urography also showed a few small cortical cysts in about half of the few children studied.

Not all children with ARPKD present and die in infancy. Those with initially adequate (even if not normal) renal function may not have their disease detected until later in the first decade. These children may have their renal abnormality found when US studies are being done for nonrelated purposes and may have little clinical renal or liver disease attributable to the ARPKD at that time. Some present in the second

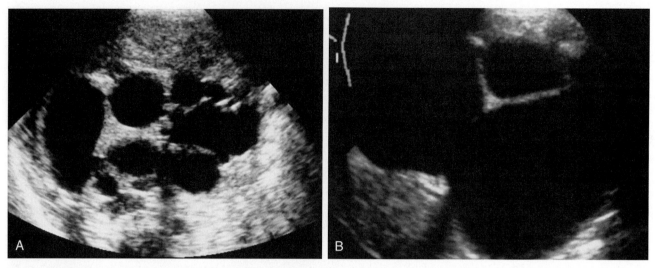

FIGURE 23. Renal ultrasound of multicystic dysplastic kidney. **A,** The coronal scan demonstrates multiple noncommunicating cysts of varied size. No normal renal architecture can be identified. **B,** This multicystic dysplastic kidney is composed of a few very large cysts. At times this appearance can mimic a hydronephrotic kidney.

decade with renal failure and require dialysis or renal transplantation. Late complications include systemic hypertension and those derived from the hepatic fibrosis: portal hypertension with subsequent hypersplenism and gastroesophageal varices.

AUTOSOMAL DOMINANT POLYCYSTIC KIDNEY DISEASE

The pathophysiology of this very common form of polycystic kidney disease (PKD) affects multiple organs: kidneys, liver, and pancreas. Ovarian cysts have been described as being part of the pathologic process but, according to recent references, may not be so. Both the renal and liver cysts become larger and more numerous with increasing age; patients usually present with renal failure or hypertension in their fourth or fifth decade. An association with cysts of the seminal vesicles has been consistently noted. Affected adults have an increased incidence of uric acid stones. There are two forms of the disease inherited as an autosomal dominant trait; the one with a milder phenotype (PKD2) presents later and has less morbidity than the more severe form (PKD1).

Spontaneous mutations are frequently responsible for the disease; thus, screening parents and siblings of affected children, although routine, may not yield additional cases. Screening can be done with US in adults, in whom one would expect the disease to be more advanced. Screening very young children with US may be inconclusive because detectable cysts may not be present in the first or second decade. CT can demonstrate millimeter-size cysts but is not generally used to screen young family members. Affected kidneys will be large, will contain multiple cysts, and will still retain a normal renal shape. The kidneys may be asymmetrically involved, and disease within a single kidney can show segmental variation.

Symptoms of autosomal dominant PKD (ADPKD) (renal failure, hypertension) rarely develop in childhood. The cysts that affect other organs are also usually absent or asymptomatic in childhood. However, occasionally a child may present with a unilaterally enlarged kidney and hematuria. In this setting, US or CT is performed because of the presumption of neoplasm; this may show conglomerate cysts, often appearing as a multicystic mass, and the numerous other cysts that may be only a millimeter or two in size scattered through the cortex of both kidneys. If there has been bleeding into one of the cysts, producing rapid enlargement of the cyst, the child may present with flank pain. The affected cyst may have an atypical appearance on US or CT,

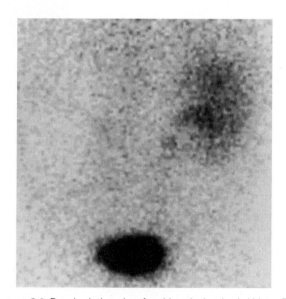

FIGURE 24. Renal scintigraphy of multicystic dysplastic kidney. The isotope defines the single functioning kidney. No isotope is present in the contralateral multicystic dysplastic kidney.

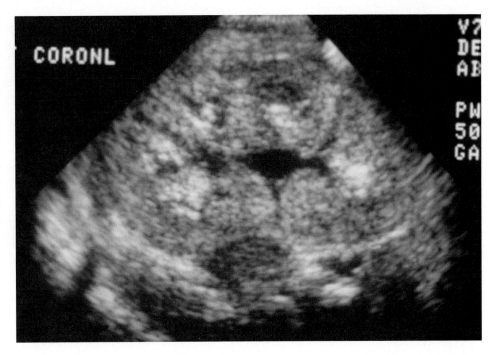

FIGURE 25. Renal ultrasound of autosomal recessive polycystic kidney disease. The dilated tubules in the medulla have produced numerous interfaces and, hence, the increased echogenicity of the medulla. The normal cortex, frequently seen as a lucent rim, cannot be identified in this patient.

making the differential diagnosis more difficult and raising the possibility of cystic nephroma unless additional geographically distant cysts are identified. Sometimes a totally asymptomatic child has ADPKD detected when urinary tract evaluation is being performed for unrelated symptoms (Fig. 27).

About 15% of patients with ADPKD have an aneurysm of the circle of Willis. Because the consequences of aneurysm rupture are so profound, screening with magnetic resonance angiography for aneurysms is recommended in patients with ADPKD. This is usually not performed in childhood because aneurysm rupture is rare in this period and because additional studies indicate that the incidence of aneurysms increases with age.

SIMPLE RENAL CYSTS

Although renal cysts are commonly seen as a consequence of aging and may be present in as much as 50% of the population over the age of 50, they are uncommon in the pediatric population. When kidneys were primarily evaluated with excretory urography, renal

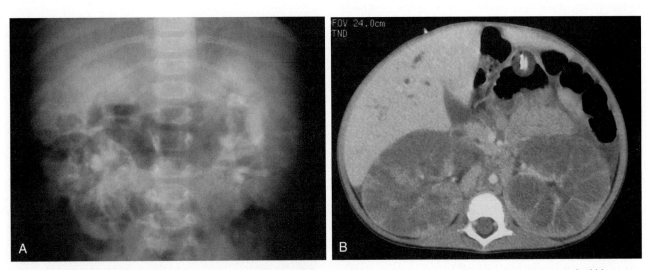

FIGURE 26. Autosomal recessive polycystic kidney disease (ARPKD). **A,** On excretory urography, contrast trapped within the dilated collecting tubules creates a streaky or spoke-wheel appearance to the renal parenchyma. **B,** Noncontrast computed tomography scan demonstrates that the pathologic process is medullary. The dilated tubules have produced a linear pattern that can be clearly seen in a few regions. Cortical thinning, present along the anterior aspect of each kidney, is not a typical finding because ARPKD usually spares the cortex.

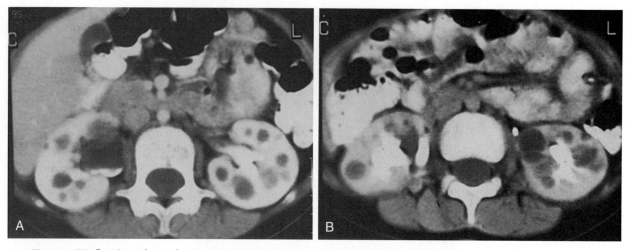

FIGURE 27. Dominant form of polycystic kidney disease (positive family history) in a 10-year-old girl. Contrast-enhanced computed tomography at two levels shows multiple cysts throughout both kidneys.

cysts were rarely diagnosed in children. In that era, detection of a presumed cystic lesion raised the specter of cystic Wilms' tumor and was believed to warrant additional evaluation, including angiography. With wider use of US, simple renal cysts have become a recognized entity in the pediatric population. Renal cysts have even been observed with prenatal US. The etiology of these cysts is unknown, and most will resolve, but detection of a fetal renal cyst warrants additional or sequential studies to exclude cyst-associated syndromes or multicystic dysplastic kidney. Although most simple cysts are idiopathic, they are a recognized acquired finding in children with acquired immunodeficiency syndrome (AIDS).

If the cyst meets the criteria deemed to indicate a simple cyst, no further imaging is necessary. The US criteria for a simple cyst are the same in children as in adults: a thin, almost imperceptible wall; no internal echogenicity; spherical shape; and good through-transmission (Fig. 28). When the above criteria cannot be met, CT is recommended to exclude cystic Wilms' tumor or cystic nephroma (multilocular renal cyst). Again, to be confident of the diagnosis of simple cyst, the same CT criteria used in adults with presumed simple cysts must be met: a density less than 15 H.U. on non-CECT, imperceptible wall, and no internal architecture. When more than one cyst is observed with US, CT may be necessary to exclude ADPKD. If the cyst is detected during an evaluation for urinary tract infections and these continue, it may be necessary to perform a contrast study. A caliceal diverticulum can simulate a simple cyst on US, and stasis within it can result in infection and, over time, stone formation. A caliceal diverticulum will fill with contrast on delayed films during excretory urography or CECT. Multiple cysts may not be cysts at all but enlarged calices in patients with infundibulopelvic stenosis (Fig. 29).

Most simple cysts are asymptomatic and managed with benign neglect. Intervention is warranted if the cyst is large and positioned such that it may contribute to pathologic fracture of the kidney, or if the cyst is causing obstruction of the collecting system.

ACQUIRED RENAL CYSTS

As mentioned above, children with AIDS may develop renal cysts. Cysts also develop, as in adults, in children with renal failure who receive both hemo- and peritoneal dialysis. The number of cysts increases as the years on dialysis increase. With US, the involved kidneys are generally smaller and more echogenic than normal; the cysts are scattered throughout the parenchyma and have a typical appearance of simple cysts (Fig. 30).

MISCELLANEOUS CYSTIC DISEASES

Glomerulocystic Disease

This rare condition can be inherited as an autosomal dominant disease and is sometimes present in children

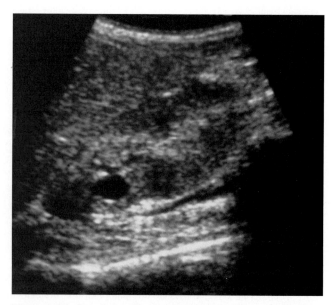

FIGURE 28. Renal ultrasound of simple cyst. The small fluid collection in the right upper pole shows the changes of a simple cyst: thin wall, no internal septations, and good through-transmission.

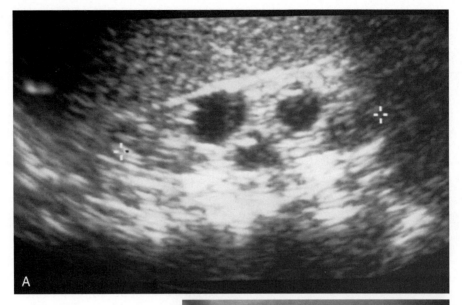

FIGURE 29. Infundibulopelvic stenosis simulating autosomal dominant polycystic kidney disease. **A,** A sagittal image from renal ultrasound demonstrates multiple "cysts" scattered throughout the kidney in this child with the VACTERL association. **B,** At cystography, contrast refluxes into the abnormal pelvocaliceal system. Contrast refluxing from the bladder demonstrates that the ureter has a greater caliber than the renal pelvis, infundibula, and calices. The most peripheral portion of each calix is rounded. The rounded calices produced the cystic spaces seen with ultrasound.

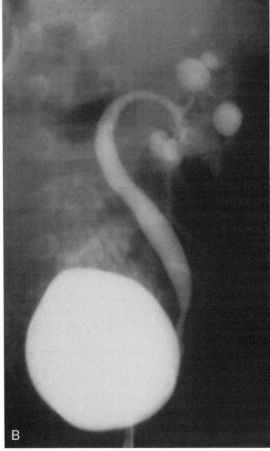

with a family history of ADPKD. The kidneys are usually of normal size but have also been described as enlarged and, when studied with US, have increased echogenicity regardless of size. Those patients who present with glomerulocystic disease and small kidneys are believed to have a recognized but even rarer variant that has a sporadic inheritance. Glomerulocystic disease also is identified in some children with malformation syndromes but may not be present in all children with the

syndrome. Such syndromes are discussed later in this chapter. The pathology is reproducible: cystic dilatation of Bowman's capsule and the proximal convoluted tubules.

The size of the kidney is not helpful in making the radiologic diagnosis because, as said above, although most affected kidneys are normal sized, glomerulocystic disease is also seen in small and large kidneys. The echogenicity is not only increased but may have a

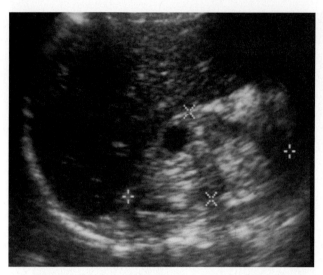

FIGURE 30. Renal ultrasound of acquired cysts in a child on dialysis. The sagittal sonogram illustrates the increased echogenicity of the kidney, which is small for the child's age. A single cyst is present.

specific pattern. Tiny cysts, smaller than those typical for ADPKD, have been described in the cortex. In contrast to ARPKD, the medulla has a normal US appearance.

Infantile Microcystic Renal Disease

This is a rare disease, inherited as an autosomal recessive disorder, that presents in early life with nephrotic syndrome of the Finnish type. The kidneys are of normal size and have dilatation of the proximal convoluted tubules. Initially thought to have no radiologic changes, infantile microcystic renal disease does have US abnormalities: small cortical cysts and increased echogenicity of the kidney with loss of the corticomedullary junction.

Juvenile Nephronophthisis and Medullary Cystic Disease

These diseases are frequently linked because of the similarities in pathology. The kidney is studded with small (< 1 cm) cysts that increase in size and number over time; these develop from dilated tubules. Glomerulosclerosis is also present in both. The clinical symptoms, polydipsia and polyuria and later renal failure, are noted in the first decade in those with juvenile nephronophthisis and in the third decade or beyond in medullary cystic disease.

Medullary Sponge Kidney (Cacchi-Ricci Disease)

Medullary sponge kidney is a disease more frequently diagnosed in adults than children and is generally considered a noninherited disorder. Most often it is an incidental finding, but it may be associated with stone formation, hematuria, and urinary tract infection. It has also been described in children with the Beckwith-Wiedemann syndrome. The radiologic changes are due to the focal dilatation of the collecting tubules. The number of renal pyramids involved is variable.

Plain abdominal radiographs may demonstrate, especially in older patients, multiple tiny calculi in the medulla. When intravenous contrast is given, streaky linear densities (pooled contrast) develop in the affected papillae. The normal papillary blush noted in children receiving a bolus injection of contrast can simulate the pathologic process; close observation reveals that the tubules are opacified but not dilated. Sonography can demonstrate the calcifications in the tubules before they are visible on abdominal radiographs and may also visualize the dilated tubules.

Malformation Syndromes with Renal Cysts

Renal cysts are reported in many syndromes; in some they are a constant and defining feature, but in others they may be present in only a percentage of those children with the syndrome. Some syndromes in which the presence of cysts is an integral part of the definition of the syndrome include Zellweger syndrome (cerebrohepatorenal syndrome) and Meckel's syndrome. Cystic renal disease is also reported in but not limited to Alagille, Bardet-Biedl, Cumming, orofaciodigital types I, II, and VI, and Joubert's (especially those with retinal dystrophy) syndromes. Over 80 syndromes have some form of cystic renal disease associated with them.

The most commonly recognized syndrome with renal cysts is tuberous sclerosis, an autosomal dominantly inherited phakomatosis. Like other phakomatoses, it is associated with pathology of many organ systems. Skin lesions are multiple: angiofibromas (previously incorrectly called adenoma sebaceum) on the face, a depigmented area ("ash leaf") on the trunk, and a pigmented area of thickened skin in the sacral region (shagreen patch). Rhabdomyomas develop in many organs, including the heart. Characteristic brain anomalies include subependymal hamartomas, anomalies of the corpus callosum, and occasional development of a subependymal giant cell astrocytoma. Clinically, the child may have seizures and mental retardation. Two different processes may develop in the kidney. One, the angiomyolipoma, is a benign neoplasm infrequently seen in childhood that may grow throughout life. In childhood, a second process, the development of multiple simple cortical cysts, is more frequently observed and may be present in as many as one third of children with tuberous sclerosis. The radiologic appearance of the affected kidneys is not unlike that of ADPKD. Interestingly, the loci of the major genes for tuberous sclerosis and ADPKD are close to each other on chromosome 16.

Children with Beckwith-Wiedemann syndrome, another syndrome with renal cysts, are usually identified at birth because of the association of macroglossia, macrosomia, visceromegaly, and omphalocele. The increased incidence of nephrogenic rests and Wilms' tumor in these children is well recognized and has resulted in surveillance radiologic studies of the kidneys. Review of these has indicated that many other renal malformations are present in this population. Medullary renal cysts may be noted in 13% to 19%. Other processes (nephrocalcinosis, nephrolithiasis, hydronephrosis) have also been described in children with Beckwith-Wiedemann syndrome.

ANOMALIES OF THE PELVOCALICEAL SYSTEM

CALICEAL DIVERTICULUM

This focal outpouching of the caliceal system, usually in the upper pole, is believed to be developmental in origin, being present in both pediatric and adult studies with about the same frequency of about 4.5 per 1000 excretory urograms. Although it is often an incidental finding, stasis in the caliceal diverticulum can be associated with both urinary tract infection and stone formation within the diverticulum.

The caliceal diverticulum may be seen with US, appearing as a rounded fluid collection, simulating a solitary renal cyst (Figs. 31*A* and 32*A*). The size may vary from a few millimeters to several centimeters and may increase over time. On excretory urography and CT, the caliceal diverticulum does not fill during the early parenchymal phase, again looking like a renal cyst (Fig. 31*B*). However, delayed films demonstrate its thin connection to the adjacent fornix of a minor calix when contrast fills the diverticulum (Figs. 31*C* and 32*B*).

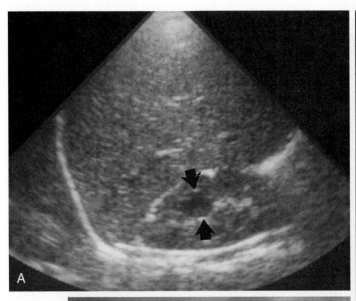

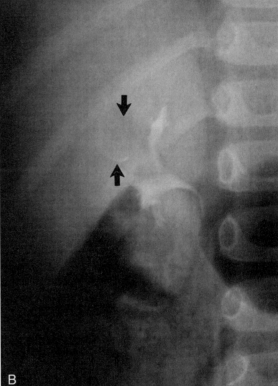

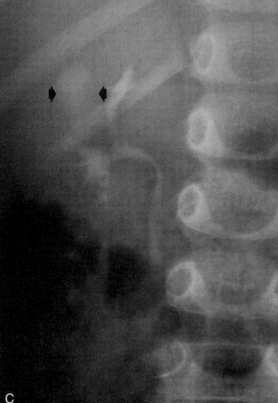

FIGURE 31. Caliceal diverticulum. **A,** Sagittal renal ultrasound reveals that the medulla contains a cystic structure a few millimeters in diameter *(arrows)*. **B,** Early film from excretory urogram. As the parenchyma opacifies, a nonenhancing region is noted adjacent to the calices *(arrows)*. A tiny amount of contrast has entered the diverticulum, creating a semilunar density along its inferior aspect. **C,** On a late film from excretory urogram, contrast is seen in the caliceal system and has now filled and opacified the diverticulum *(arrows)*.

When the caliceal diverticulum is the cause of a clinical problem, it must be ablated, usually surgically. In adults, both lithotripsy of stones within the diverticulum and percutaneous ablation of the cavity have decreased the invasiveness of the treatment; these techniques have not yet been widely applied to children.

INFUNDIBULOPELVIC STENOSIS

This anomaly is considered to be very rare but may be underreported. The kidney has a very specific appearance on contrast studies. The renal pelvis and infundibula are narrowed but not entirely obliterated; the calices become rounded (Fig. 29). Despite the cyst-like appearance of the calices on contrast studies, renal sonography may be normal or demonstrate the caliceal changes. The function of the kidney may be normal but may also be severely compromised.

CONGENITAL MEGACALICES (MEGACALICOSIS)

This rare anomaly is associated with abnormal development of the renal medulla that causes all of the calices to be filled maximally. The ensuing stasis may produce

infection and stones (Fig. 33A). Surgery is rarely indicated, except for removal of stones if these are serving as a nidus of secondary infection. The process can be focal, unilateral, or bilateral. Boys are more commonly affected than girls. Occasionally, megacalices are associated with primary megaureter.

The classically described changes are multiple: nephromegaly, thinning of the parenchyma at the expense of the renal medulla, visualization of a large number of calices, calices that are polygonal and fit close together like a mosaic, shortening of the infundibula, and mild dilatation of the renal pelvis despite the absence of ureteropelvic junction obstruction (Fig. 33B). Twenty or more calices may be seen in each kidney. Most changes can be demonstrated with US, excretory urography, CT, or MRI. Nuclear diuresis renography may be useful to exclude mild, intermittent but significant obstruction as a cause of the dilated pelvocaliceal system.

URETEROPELVIC JUNCTION OBSTRUCTION

Ureteropelvic junction obstruction occurs in about 3 in 1000 live births more often in boys than girls. It occurs more often on the left than the right, is bilateral in 10% to 20% of cases, and is seen in association with inferior

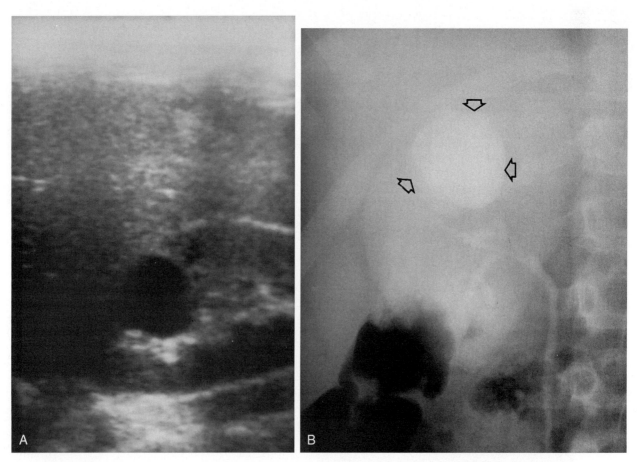

FIGURE 32. Caliceal diverticulum. **A,** Sagittal renal ultrasound demonstrates a rounded fluid collection along the anterior aspect of the right kidney. **B,** On a late film from excretory urogram, contrast is seen filling a slightly larger caliceal diverticulum *(arrows)* than in Figure 31.

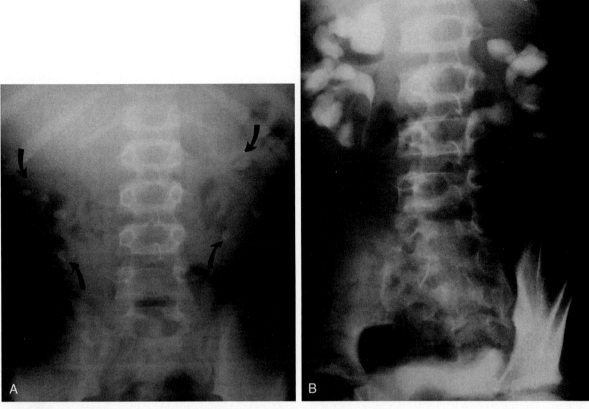

FIGURE 33. Congenital megacalices. **A,** Multiple calculi are present in each kidney on the abdominal radiograph. *Arrows* are on the upper and lower calculi in each kidney. **B,** After contrast injection, contrast fills the many polygonal-shaped calices. Note the relative nephromegaly despite the thinning of the tissue over the calices. The renal pelvis is not dilated.

ectopia and lower pole duplication, both incomplete and complete (Fig. 34). Older children who first present with ureteropelvic junction obstruction are, like adults, likely to have extrinsic compression from crossing vessels as the etiology.

Children with gross ureteropelvic junction obstruction present with abdominal mass. In fact, the most frequent cause of neonatal abdominal mass is ureteropelvic junction obstruction. Plain abdominal radiographs will show soft tissue fullness and bulging of the ipsilateral flank. If excretory urography is performed, the obstructed kidney will have delayed opacification and delayed excretion of contrast material. Contrast pools in the obstructed tubules adjacent to the dilated calices, producing *caliceal crescents* (Fig. 35*A*). Delayed films are necessary to visualize the renal pelvis (Fig. 35*B*); prone films are most useful because they move contrast from the calices to the anteriorly located renal pelvis. Prone positioning will also promote filling of the ureter, allowing differentiation of a ureteropelvic junction obstruction from a ureterovesical junction obstruction. Preoperative retrograde ureterography, once the norm, is not usually performed now because newer imaging techniques make the diagnosis much more secure (Fig. 36). Diuretic renography is commonly performed to evaluate possible UPJ obstruction. Both renal function and drainage are demonstrated. MR-

urography may come to be an important tool in the diagnosis of ureteropelvic junction obstruction but is yet in the trial stages (Fig. 37).

■ Ureteropelvic junction obstruction is the most common cause of an abdominal mass in a neonate.

Postoperative evaluation has changed over the years. Excretory urography has been used to document, grossly, the function of the kidney. Visualization of the size and configuration of the pelvocaliceal system allows comparison to preoperative contrast studies. However, postoperative evaluation of the pelvocaliceal system and overlying parenchymal thickness can be made with US without the need for injection of contrast or ionizing radiation if a preoperative examination is available for comparison. A good test of differential renal function is the nuclear renogram. This, too, can be compared with the preoperative studies. Interestingly, some authors report a definite improvement in function in the majority of their patients, whereas other describe only a stabilization of the renal function.

Text continued on page 1784

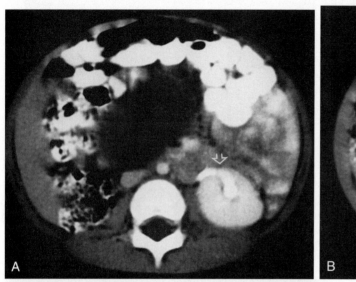

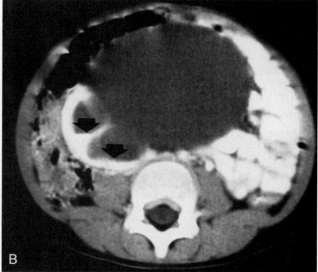

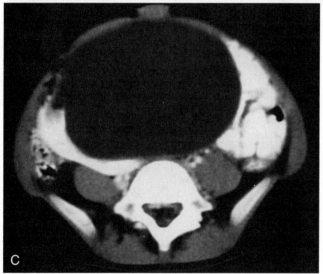

FIGURE 34. Ureteropelvic junction obstruction in kidney with inferior ectopia. **A,** Computed tomography scan at the level of the inferior liver edge demonstrates that the left kidney is underrotated, with its renal pelvis directed anteriorly *(arrow).* A large fluid collection anterior to the spine is an unopacified portion of the right renal pelvis. **B,** A few centimeters below **A,** the renal parenchyma of the right kidney is seen. The dilated calices have contrast layering dependently *(arrows)* but contain a large amount of unopacified urine, as does the enormous renal pelvis, which, as above, is anterior and to the left of the spine. **C,** The dilated renal pelvis is seen to extend to the level of the iliac crests and continues to extend across the midline.

Illustration continued on opposite page

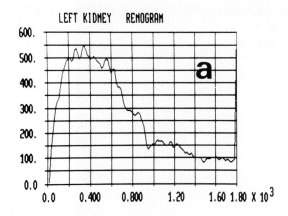

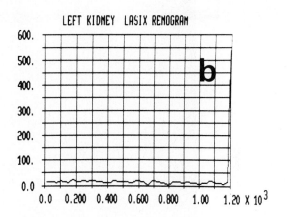

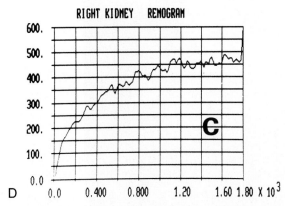

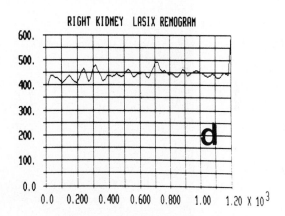

FIGURE 34. *Continued.* **D,** Diuretic renogram of the left kidney is normal *(a)*. The left kidney rapidly excretes the remaining isotope *(b)* after the child is given Lasix (furosemide). The obstructed right kidney takes the isotope in more slowly and does not concentrate it as well *(c)*. It responds poorly to the diuretic, with much isotope remaining in the kidney *(d)*.

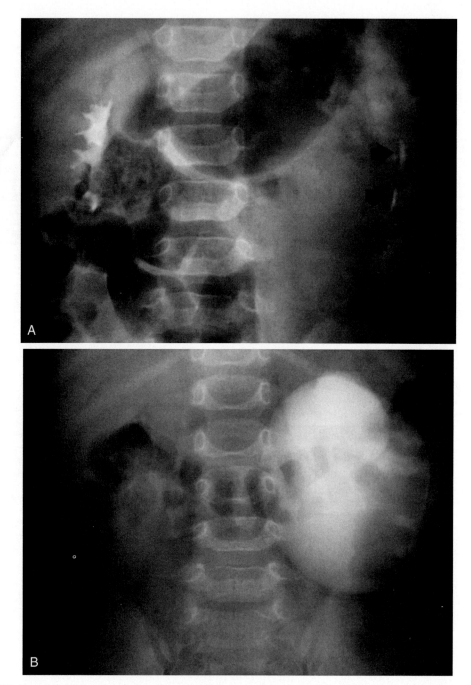

FIGURE 35. Ureteropelvic junction obstruction with caliceal crescents. **A,** On this 10-minute excretory urography film, the right kidney appears normal, with contrast in a normal pelvocaliceal system. On the left, a few crescentic collections are present at a great distance from the spine *(arrows)*. **B,** On the 1-hour prone film, the dilated left renal pelvis is seen to extend from the spine to the lateral abdominal wall. It is obscuring the calices.

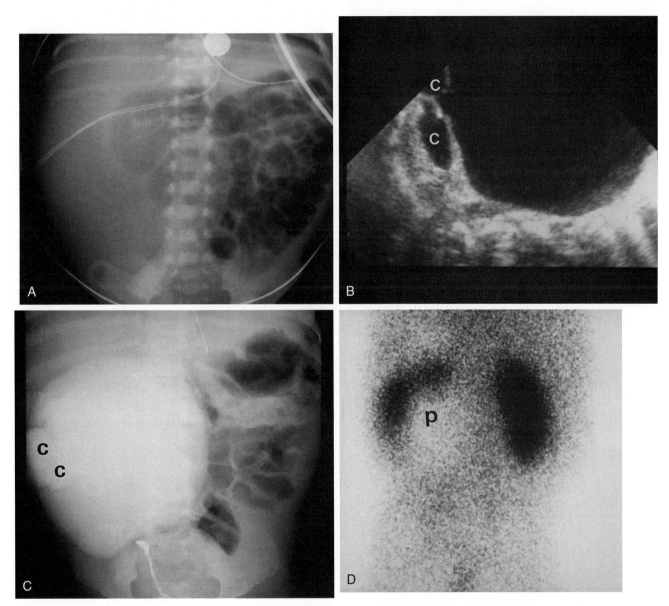

FIGURE 36. Right ureteropelvic junction obstruction. **A,** In this neonate (note umbilical clamp), bowel loops are displaced from right to left by a soft tissue mass. **B,** Transverse renal sonogram showed that the soft tissue mass was a markedly dilated renal pelvis associated with dilated calices *(C)*. **C,** A retrograde injection confirms that the obstruction is at the level of the renal pelvis. Again the renal pelvis is shown to be much more dilated than the calices *(C)*. **D,** Renal scintigraphy with ⁹⁹ᵐTc mercaptotriglycylglycine demonstrates a normal left kidney. On the right, the thinned renal parenchyma is displaced superiorly and laterally by the dilated renal pelvis, seen as the photopenic region *(P)*.

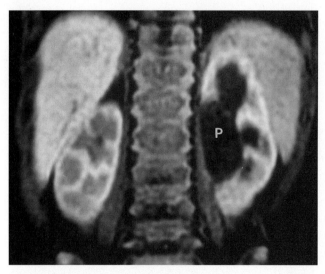

FIGURE 37. Ureteropelvic junction obstruction. Coronal magnetic resonance imaging section obtained after injection of gadolinium demonstrates a normal right kidney with a well-defined corticomedullary junction. On the left, the corticomedullary junction is poorly seen. The pelvis *(p)* and the caliceal system are dilated.

SUGGESTED READINGS

Renal Ectopia and Anomalies of Fusion

Renal Ectopia

Barnewolt CE, Lebowitz RL: Absence of a renal sinus complex in the ectopic kidney of a child: a normal finding. Pediatr Radiol 1996;26:318

Dretler SP, Olsson C, Pfister RC: The anatomic, radiologic, and clinical characteristics of the pelvic kidney: an analysis of 86 cases. J Urol 1971;105:623

Fernbach SK: Urethral abnormalities in male neonates with VATER association. AJR Am J Roentgenol 1991;156:137

Fernbach SK, Glass RB: The expanded spectrum of limb anomalies in the VATER association. Pediatr Radiol 1988;18:215

Hertz M, Rubenstein ZJ, Shahin N, et al: Crossed renal ectopia: clinical and radiological findings in 22 cases. Clin Radiol 1977;289:339

Hoffman CK, Filly RA, Callen PW: The "lying down" adrenal sign: a sonographic indicator of renal agenesis or ectopia in fetuses and neonates. J Ultrasound Med 1992;11:533

Jimenez-Hefferman A, Rebollo AC, Garcia-Martin M, et al: Tc-99m DMSA and Tc-99m MAG3 findings in crossed renal ectopia. Clin Nucl Med 1998;239:255

Kenney PJ, Robbins GL, Ellis DA, et al: Adrenal glands in patients with congenital renal anomalies: CT appearance. Radiology 1985; 155:181

N'Guessen G, Stephens FD, Pick J: Congenital superior ectopic (thoracic) kidney. Urology 1984;24:219

Nussbaum AR, Hartman DS, Whitley N, et al: Multicystic dysplasia and crossed renal ectopia. AJR Am J Roentgenol 1987;149:407

Horseshoe Kidney

Cook WA, Stephens FD: Fused kidneys: morphologic study and theory of embryogenesis. Birth Defects Orig Artic Series 1977;13:327

Fernbach SK, Davis TM: The abnormal renal axis in children with spina bifida and gibbus deformity—the pseudohorseshoe kidney. J Urol 1986;136:1258

Lippe B, Geffner ME, Dietrich RB, et al: Renal malformations in patients with Turner syndrome: imaging in 141 patients. Pediatrics 1988;82:852

Mandell GA, Maloney K, Sherman NH, et al: The renal axes in spina bifida: issues of confusion and fusion. Abdom Imaging 1996;21:541

Mesrobian HJ, Kelalis PP, Hrabovsky E, et al: Wilms' tumor in horseshoe kidneys: a report from the National Wilms' Tumor Study. J Urol 1985;133:1002

Pitts WR Jr, Muecke EC: Horseshoe kidneys: a 40-year experience. J Urol 1975;113:743

Strauss S, Dushnitsky T, Peer A, et al: Sonographic features of horseshoe kidney: a review of 34 patients. J Ultrasound Med 2000;19:27

Unilateral and Bilateral Renal Agenesis

Cascio S, Paran S, Puri P: Associated urological anomalies in children with unilateral renal agenesis. J Urol 1999;162(3 Pt 2):1081

Daneman A, Alton DJ: Radiographic manifestations of renal anomalies. Radiol Clin North Am 1991;29:351

Fedele L, Bianchi S, Agnoli B, et al: Urinary tract anomalies associated with unicornuate uterus. J Urol 1996;155:847

Li YW, Sheih CP, Chen WJ: Unilateral occlusion of duplicated uterus with ipsilateral renal anomaly in young girls: a study with MRI. Pediatr Radiol 1995;25(Suppl 1):S54

McGahan JP, Myracle MR: Adrenal hypertrophy: possible pitfall in the sonographic diagnosis of renal agenesis. J Ultrasound Med 1986; 5:265

O'Neill MJ, Yoder IC, Connolly SA, et al: Imaging evaluation and classification of developmental anomalies of the female reproductive system with an emphasis on MR imaging. AJR Am J Roentgenol 1999;173:407

Palmer LS, Andros GJ, Maizels M, et al: Management considerations for treating vesicoureteral reflux in children with solitary kidneys. Urology 1997;49:604

Roodhoft AM, Birnholz JC, Holmes LB: Familial nature of congenital absence and severe dysgenesis of both kidneys. N Engl J Med 1984;310:1341

Schlegel PN, Shin D, Goldstein M: Urogenital anomalies in men with congenital absence of the vas deferens. J Urol 1996;155:1644

Song JT, Ritchey ML, Zerin JM, et al: Incidence of vesicoureteral reflux in children with unilateral renal agenesis. J Urol 1995;153:1249

Tanaka YO, Kurosaki Y, Kobayashi T, et al: Uterus didelphys associated with obstructed hemivagina and ipsilateral renal agenesis: MR findings in seven cases. Abdom Imaging 1998;23:437

Tarry WF, Duckett JW, Stephens FD: The Mayer-Rokitansky syndrome: pathogenesis, classification, and management. J Urol 1986;136:648

Valenzano M, Paoletti R, Rossi A, et al: Sirenomelia: pathological features, antenatal ultrasonographic clues, and a review of current embryogenic theories. Hum Reprod Update 1999;5(11):82

van den Ouden D, Blom JH, Bangma C, et al: Diagnosis and management of seminal vesicle cysts associated with ipsilateral renal agenesis: a pooled analysis of 52 cases. Eur Urol 1998;33:433

Wojcik LJ, Hansen K, Diamond DA, et al: Cystic dysplasia of the rete testis: a benign congenital lesion associated with ipsilateral urological anomalies. J Urol 1997;158:600

Multicystic Dysplastic Kidney

al-Khaldi N, Watson AR, Zuccollo J, et al: Outcome of antenatally detected cystic dysplastic kidney disease. Arch Dis Child 1994;70:520

Avni EF, Thoua Y, Lalmand B, et al: Multicystic dysplastic kidney: natural history from in utero diagnosis and postnatal followup. J Urol 1987;138:1420

Blane CE, Ritchey ML, DiPietro MA, et al: Single system ectopic ureters and ureteroceles associated with dysplastic kidney. Pediatr Radiol 1992;22:217

Gordon AC, Thomas DF, Arthur RJ, et al: Multicystic dysplastic kidney: is nephrectomy still appropriate? J Urol 1998;140(5 Pt 2):1231

Hashimoto BE, Filly RA, Callen PW: Multicystic dysplastic kidney in utero: changing appearance on US. Radiology 1986;159:107

Heymans C, Breysem L, Proesman W: Multicystic kidney dysplasia: a prospective study on the natural history of the affected and the contralateral kidney. Eur J Pediatr 1998;157:673

Jeon A, Cramer BC, Walsh E, et al: A spectrum of segmental multicystic renal dysplasia. Pediatr Radiol 1999;29:309

John U, Rudnik-Schoneborn S, Zerres K, et al: Kidney growth and renal function in unilateral multicystic dysplastic kidney. Pediatr Nephol 1998;12:567

Kazmazyn B, Zerin JM: Lower urinary tract abnormalities in children with multicystic dysplastic kidney. Radiology 1997;203:223

Kessler OJ, Ziv N, Livne PM, et al: Involution rate of multicystic renal dysplasia. Pediatrics 1998;102:E73

Kleiner B, Filly RA, Mack L, et al: Multicystic dysplastic kidney: observations of contralateral disease in the fetal population. Radiology 1986;161:27

Lazebnik N, Bellinger MF, Ferguson JE 2nd, et al: Insights into the pathogenesis and natural history of fetuses with multicystic dysplastic kidney disease. Prenat Diagn 1999;19:418

Perez LM, Naidu SI, Joseph DB: Outcome and cost analysis of operative versus nonoperative management of neonatal multicystic dysplastic kidneys. J Urol 1998;160(3 Pt 2):1207

Rottenberg GT, De Bruyn R, Gordon I: Sonographic standards for a single functioning kidney in children. AJR Am J Roentgenol 1996;167:1255

Rottenberg GT, De Bruyn R, Gordon I: The natural history of the multicystic dysplastic kidney in children. Br J Radiol 1997;70:347

Rudnik-Schoneborn S, John U, Deget F, et al: Clinical features of unilateral multicystic renal dysplasia in children. Eur J Pediatr 1998;157:666

Selzman AA, Elder JS: Contralateral vesicoureteral reflux in children with a multicystic kidney. J Urol 1995;153:1252

Simoneaux SF, Atkinson GO, Ball TI: Cystic dysplasia of the testis associated with multicystic dysplastic kidney. Pediatr Radiol 1995; 25:379

Snodgrass WT: Hypertension associated with multicystic dysplastic kidney in children. J Urol 2000;164:472

Strife JL, Souza AS, Kirks DR, et al: Multicystic dysplastic kidney in children: US follow-up. Radiology 1993;186:785

Vinocur L, Slovis TL, Perlmutter AD, et al: Follow-up studies of multicystic dysplastic kidneys. Radiology 1988;167:311

Webb NJ, Lewis MA, Bruce J, et al: Unilateral multicystic dysplastic kidney: the case for nephrectomy. Arch Dis Child 1997;76:31

White R, Greenfield SP, Wan J, et al: Renal growth characteristics in children born with multicystic dysplastic kidneys. Urology 1998; 52:874

Zerin JM, Baker DR, Casale JA: Single-system ureteroceles in infants and children: imaging features. Pediatr Radiol 2000;30:139

Zerin JM, Leiser J: The impact of vesicoureteral reflux on contralateral renal length in infants with multicystic dysplastic kidney. Pediatr Radiol 1998;28:683

Cystic Renal Disease

Autosomal Recessive Polycystic Kidney Disease

Blickman JG, Bramson RT, Herrin JT: Autosomal recessive polycystic kidney disease: long term sonographic findings in patients surviving the neonatal period. AJR Am J Roentgenol 1995;164:1247

Jung G, Benz-Bohm G, Kugel H, et al: MR cholangiography in children with autosomal recessive polycystic kidney disease. Pediatr Radiol 1999;29:463

Kern S, Zimmerhackl LB, Hildebrandt F, et al: RARE-MR-urography— a new diagnostic method in autosomal recessive polycystic kidney disease. Acta Radiol 1999;40:543

Lonergan GJ, Rice RR, Suarez ES: Autosomal recessive polycystic kidney disease: radiologic-pathologic correlation. Radiographics 2000;20:837

Roy S, Dillon MJ, Trompeter RS, et al: Autosomal recessive polycystic kidney disease: long term outcome of neonatal survivors. Pediatr Nephrol 1997;11:302

Wisser J, Hebisch G, Froster U, et al: Prenatal sonographic diagnosis of autosomal recessive polycystic kidney disease (ARPKD) during the early second trimester. Prenat Diagn 1995;15:868

Zerres K, Mucher G, Becker J, et al: Prenatal diagnosis of autosomal recessive polycystic kidney disease (ARPKD): molecular genetics, clinical experience and fetal morphology. Am J Med Genet 1998; 76:137

Zerres K, Rudnik-Schoneborn S, Deget F, et al: Autosomal recessive polycystic kidney disease in 115 children: clinical presentation, course and influence of gender. Acta Pediatr 1996;85:437

Autosomal Dominant Polycystic Kidney Disease

Butler WE, Barker FG 2nd, Crowell RM: Patients with polycystic kidney disease would benefit from routine magnetic resonance angiographic screening for intracerebral aneurysms: a decision analysis. Neurosurgery 1996;38:506

Danaci M, Akpolat T, Bastemir M, et al: The prevalence of seminal vesicle cysts in autosomal dominant polycystic kidney disease. Nephrol Dial Transplant 1998;13:2825

Hateboer N, van Dijk MA, Bogdanova N, et al: Comparison of phenotypes of polycystic kidney disease types 1 and 2. European PKD1-PKD2 Study Group. Lancet 1999;353:103

Jain M, LeQuesne GW, Bourne AJ, et al: High-resolution ultrasonography in the differential diagnosis of cystic diseases of the kidney in infancy and childhood: preliminary experience. J Ultrasound Med 1997;16:235

MacDermot KD, Saggar-Malik AK, Economides DL, et al: Prenatal diagnosis of autosomal dominant polycystic kidney disease (PKD1) presenting in utero and prognosis for very early onset disease. J Med Genet 1998;35:13

Nakajima F, Shibahara N, Arai M, et al: Intracranial aneurysms and autosomal dominant polycystic kidney disease: followup study by magnetic resonance angiography. J Urol 2000;164:331

Stamm ER, Townsend RR, Johnson AM, et al: Frequency of ovarian cysts in patients with autosomal dominant polycystic kidney disease. Am J Kidney Dis 1999;34:120

Simple and Acquired Renal Cysts

Acquired cystic kidney disease in children undergoing continuous ambulatory peritoneal dialysis. Kyushu Pediatric Nephrology Group. Am J Kidney Dis 1999;34:242

Blazer S, Zimmer EZ, Blumenfeld Z, et al: Natural history of fetal simple renal cysts detected in early pregnancy. J Urol 1999;162 (3 Pt 1):812

Leichter HE, Dietrich R, Salusky IB, et al: Acquired cystic renal disease in children undergoing long-term dialysis. Pediatr Nephrol 1988;2:8

Zinn HL, Rosberger ST, Haller JO, et al: Simple renal cysts in children with AIDS. Pediatr Radiol 1997;27:827

Glomerulocystic Disease, Nephronophthisis, Medullary Cystic Disease, and Medullary Sponge Kidney

Ala-Mello S, Jaaskelainen J, Koskimies O: Familial juvenile nephronophthisis: an ultrasonographic follow-up of seven patients. Acta Radiol 1998;39:84

Bernstein J: Glomerulocystic kidney disease—nosologic considerations. Pediatr Nephrol 1993;7:464

Blowey DL, Querfeld U, Geary D, et al: Ultrasound findings in juvenile nephronophthisis. Pediatr Nephrol 1996;10:22

Chuang YF, Tsai TC: Sonographic findings in familial juvenile nephronophthisis-medullary cystic disease complex. J Clin Ultrasound 1998;26:203

Dedeoglu IO, Fisher JE, Springate JE, et al: Spectrum of glomerulocystic kidneys: a case report and review of the literature. Pediatr Pathol Lab Med 1996;16:941

Fitch SJ, Stapleton FB: Ultrasonographic features of glomerulocystic disease in infancy: similarity to infantile polycystic kidney disease. Pediatr Radiol 1986;16:400

Jain M, LeQuesne GW, Bourne AJ, et al: High-resolution ultrasonography in the differential diagnosis of cystic diseases of the kidney in infancy and childhood: preliminary experience. J Ultrasound Med 1997;16:235

Patriquin HB, O'Regan S: Medullary sponge kidney in childhood. AJR Am J Roentgenol 1985;145:315

Sharp CK, Bergman SM, Stockwin JM, et al: Dominantly transmitted glomerulocystic kidney disease: a distinct genetic entity. J Am Soc Nephrol 1997;8:77

Malformation Syndromes with Renal Cysts

Boltshauser E, Forster I, Deonna T, et al: Joubert syndrome: are the kidneys involved? Neuropediatrics 1995;26:320

Borer JG, Kefer M, Barnewolt CE, et al: Renal findings on followup of patients with Beckwith Wiedemann syndrome. J Urol 1999;161:235

Chance PF, Cavalier L, Satran D, et al: Clinical nosologic and genetic aspects of Joubert and related syndromes. J Child Neurol 1999; 14:660

Choyke PL, Siegel MJ, Craft AW, et al: Screening for Wilms tumor in children with Beckwith-Wiedemann syndrome or idiopathic hemihypertrophy. Med Pediatr Oncol 1999;32:196

Choyke PL, Siegel MJ, Oz O, et al: Nonmalignant renal disease in pediatric patients with Beckwith-Wiedemann syndrome. AJR Am J Roentgenol 1998;17:733

Cook JA, Oliver K, Mueller RF, et al: A cross sectional study of renal involvement in tuberous sclerosis. J Med Genet 1996;33:480

Dibbern KM, Graham JM, Lachman RS, et al: Cumming syndrome: report of two additional cases. Pediatr Radiol 1998;28:798

Dippell J, Varlam DE: Early sonographic aspects of kidney morphology in Bardet-Biedl syndrome. Pediatr Nephrol 1998;12:559

Ewalt DH, Sheffield E, Sparagana SP, et al: Renal lesion growth in children with tuberous sclerosis complex. J Urol 1998;160:141

Fitzpatrick DR: Zellweger syndrome and associated phenotypes. J Med Genet 1996;33:863

Gershoni-Baruch R, Nachieli T, Leibo R, et al: Cystic kidney dysplasia and polydactyly in 3 sibs with Bardet-Beidl syndrome. Am J Med Genet 1992;44:269

Haug K, Khan S, Fuchs S, et al: OFD II, OFD VI, and Joubert syndrome manifestations in 2 sibs. Am J Med Genet 2000;91:135

Martin SR, Garel L, Alvarez F: Alagille's syndrome associated with cystic renal disease. Arch Dis Child 1996;74:232

North KN, Hoppel CL, De Girolami U, et al: Lethal neonatal deficiency of carnitine palmitoyltransferase II associated with dysgenesis of the brain and kidneys. J Pediatr 1995;127:414

O'Dea D, Parfrey PS, Harnett JD, et al: The importance of renal impairment in the natural history of Bardet-Biedl syndrome. Am J Kidney Dis 1996;27:776

Odent S, Le Marec B, Toutain A, et al: Central nervous system malformations and early end-stage renal disease in oro-facio-digital syndrome type I: a review. Am J Med Genet 1998;75:389

O'Hagan AR, Ellsworth R, Secic M, et al: Renal manifestations of tuberous sclerosis complex. Clin Pediatr 1996;35:483

Puechel SM, Oyer CE: Cerebrohepatorenal (Zellweger) syndrome: clinical, neuropathological, and biochemical findings. Childs Nerv Syst 1995;11:639

Sampson JR, Maheshwar MM, Aspinwall R, et al: Renal cystic disease in tuberous sclerosis: the role of the polycystic kidney disease 1 gene. Am J Hum Genet 1997;61:843

Sepulveda W, Sebire NJ, Souka A, et al: Diagnosis of the Meckel-Gruber syndrome at eleven to fourteen weeks' gestation. Am J Obstet Gynecol 1997;176:316

Silverstein DM, Zacharowicz L, Edelman M, et al: Joubert syndrome associated with multicystic kidney disease and hepatic fibrosis. Pediatr Nephrol 1997;11:746

Whitfield J, Hurst D, Bennett MJ, et al: Fetal polycystic kidney disease associated with glutaric aciduria type II: an inborn error of metabolism. Am J Perinatol 1996;13:131

Wright C, Healicon R, English C, et al: Meckel syndrome: what are the minimum diagnostic criteria? J Med Genet 1994;31:482

Anomalies of the Pelvocaliceal System

Caliceal Diverticulum

Monga M, Smith R, Ferral H, et al: Percutaneous ablation of caliceal diverticulum: long-term follow up. J Urol 2000;163:28

Patriquin H, Lafortune M, Filiatrault D: Urinary milk of calcium in children and adults: use of gravity-dependent sonography. AJR Am J Roentgenol 1985;144:407

Timmons JW, Malek RS, Hattery RR, et al: Caliceal diverticulum. J Urol 1975;114:6

Congenital Megacalices (Megacalicosis)

Garcia CJ, Taylor KJ, Weiss RM: Congenital megacalyces: ultrasound appearance. J Ultrasound Med 1987;6:163

O'Reilly PH: Relationship between intermittent hydronephrosis and megacalicosis. Br J Urol 1989;64:125

Sethi R, Yang DC, Mittal P, et al: Congenital megacalyces: studies with different imaging modalities. Clin Nucl Med 1997;22:653

Vargas B, Lebowitz RL: The coexistence of congenital megacalyces and primary megaureter. AJR Am J Roentgenol 1986;147:313

Ureteropelvic Junction Obstruction

Anderson N, Clautice-Engle T, Allan R, et al: Detection of obstructive uropathy in the fetus: predictive value of sonographic measure-ments of renal pelvic diameter at various gestational ages. AJR Am J Roentgenol 1995;164:719

Conway JJ, Maizels M: The "well tempered" diuretic renogram: a standard method to examine the asymptomatic neonate with hydronephrosis or hydroureteronephrosis. A report from combined meetings of the Society for Fetal Urology and members of the Pediatric Nuclear Medicine Council–the Society of Nuclear Medicine. J Nucl Med 1992;33:2047

Coret A, Morag B, Katz M, et al: The impact of fetal screening on indications for cystourethrography in infants. Pediatr Radiol 1994;24:516

Docimo SG, Silver RI: Renal ultrasonography in newborns with prenatally detected hydronephrosis: why wait? J Urol 1997;156:1387

Dremsek PA, Gindl K, Voitl P, et al: Renal pyelectasis in fetuses and neonates: diagnostic value of renal pelvis diaimeter in pre and postnatal sonographic screening AJR Am J Roentgenol 1997;168:1017

Fernbach SK, Maizels M, Conway JJ: Ultrasound grading of hydronephrosis: introduction to the system used by the Society for Fetal Urology. Pediatr Radiol 1993;23:478

Fernbach SK, Zawin JK, Lebowitz RL: Complete duplication of the ureter with ureteropelvic junction obstruction of the lower pole of the kidney: imaging findings. AJR Am J Roentgenol 1995;164:701

Frauscher F: Value of contrast-enhanced color Doppler imaging for detection of crossing vessels in patients with ureteropelvic junction obstruction. Radiology 2000;217:916

Herndon CD, McKenna PH, Kolon TF, et al: A multicenter outomes analysis of patients with neonatal reflux presenting with prenatal hydronephrosis. J Urol 1999;162(3 Pt 2):1203

Houben CH, Wischermann A, Bomer G, et al: Outcome analysis of pyeloplasty in infants. Pediatr Surg Int 2000;16:189

Joseph DB, Bauer SB, Colodny AH, et al: Lower pole ureteropelvic junction obstruction and incomplete renal duplication. J Urol 1989;141:896

Lim GY, Jang HS, Lee EJ, et al: Utility of the resistance index ratio in differentiating obstructive from nonobstructive hydronephrosis in children. J Clin Ultrasound 1999;27:187

McAleer IM, Kaplan GW: Renal function before and after pyeloplasty: does it improve? J Urol 1999;162(3 Pt 2):1041

McCarthy CS, Sarkar SD, Izquierdo G, et al: Pitfalls and limitations of diuretic renography. Abdom Imaging 1994;19:78

McGrath MA, Estroff J, Lebowitz RL: The coexistence of obstruction at the ureteropelvic and ureterovesical junctions. AJR Am J Roentgenol 1987;149:403

Mitsumori A, Yasui K, Akaki S, et al: Evaluation of crossing vessels in patients with ureteropelvic junction obstruction by means of helical CT. Radiographics 2000;20:1383

Ross JH, Kay R, Knipper NS, et al: The absence of crossing vessels in association with ureteropelvic junction obstruction detected by prenatal sonography. J Urol 1998;160(3 Pt 1):973

Rouviere O, Lyonnet D, Berger P, et al: Ureteropelvic junction obstruction: use of helical CT for preoperative assessment—comparison with intrarterial angiography. Radiology 1999;213:668

Rushton HG, Salem Y, Belman AB, et al: Pediatric pyeloplasty: is routine retrograde pyelography necessary? J Urol 1994;152(2 Pt 2):604

Stocks A, Richards D, Frentzen B, et al: Correlation of prenatal renal pelvic anteroposterior diameter with outcome in infancy. J Urol 1996;155:1050

Takla NV, Hamilton BD, Cartwright PC, et al: Apparent unilateral ureteropelvic junction obstruction in the newborn: expectation for resolution. J Urol 1998;160(6 Pt 1):2175

Yerkes EB, Adams MC, Pope JC 4th, et al: Does every patient with prenatal hydronephrosis need voiding cystourethrography? J Urol 1999;162(3 Pt 2):1218

Zerin JM: Hydronephrosis in the neonate and young infant: current concepts. Semin Ultrasound CT MR 1994;15:306

Chapter 2

RENAL NEOPLASMS

KATE A. FEINSTEIN

NEPHROBLASTOMATOSIS COMPLEX

Nephrogenesis is completed by the 36th gestational week. A focus of fetal metanephric blastema or embryonal renal tissue that persists into infancy is called a nephrogenic rest. Multiple foci or diffuse nephrogenic rests are termed *nephroblastomatosis*. Nephroblastomatosis is identified in about 1% of neonatal autopsies, but these areas are usually no longer found after 4 months of age. Genetic abnormalities and syndromes may be associated with nephroblastomatosis; however, the majority of patients with nephroblastomatosis do not have these abnormalities. Malignant transformation of the fetal metanephric blastema may occur, with development of Wilms' tumor (nephroblastoma), or nephroblastomatosis may resolve spontaneously.

Nephrogenic rests can occur anywhere in the kidney depending on when nephrogenesis is interrupted. These may be located in the renal lobe (intralobar) or in the cortex enveloping the renal lobe (perilobar). The two types of nephrogenic rests have different appearances, malignant potential, and associated genetic abnormalities.

Intralobar nephrogenic rests are less common than perilobar nephrogenic rests. The intralobar nephrogenic rests are more likely to degenerate into Wilms' tumor. These tend to be few, located randomly in the renal lobe. Intralobar nephrogenic rests are seen in patients with sporadic aniridia, Drash syndrome (male pseudophermaphrodism and nephritis), and WAGR syndrome (Wilms' tumor, aniridia, genital anomalies, and mental retardation). Patients with sporadic aniridia have a 30% to 40% risk of developing Wilms' tumor, the greatest likelihood of all of the genetic and syndromic abnormalities associated with nephroblastomatosis.

Perilobar nephrogenic rests are multiple, located at the corticomedullary junction or in the cortex. Also called diffuse perilobar nephrogenic rests or diffuse perilobar nephroblastomatosis, these are found in hemihypertrophy and in Beckwith-Wiedemann (macroglossia, macrosomia, and omphalocele), Perlman (fetal gigantism and multiple congenital anomalies), and trisomy 18 syndromes. Patients with hemihypertrophy and Beckwith-Wiedemann syndrome have about a 5% risk of developing Wilms' tumor.

Microscopic nephrogenic rests cannot be identified radiologically. Diffuse perilobar nephroblastomatosis and multifocal nephroblastomatosis can be evaluated with ultrasonography, computed tomography (CT), and magnetic resonance imaging (MRI). In diffuse perilobar nephroblastomatosis, the affected kidney may be enlarged. On sonography, corticomedullary differentiation is absent. The regions of nephroblastomatosis may be hypo- or isoechoic with respect to normal renal cortex (Fig. 1). Multifocal nephroblastomatosis is more difficult to identify on sonography.

CT is more sensitive than sonography for the evaluation of nephroblastomatosis. On CT, the areas of nephroblastomatosis are well defined because they enhance less than normal renal cortex (Fig. 2). Bulky masses of nephroblastomatosis may distort the pyelocaliceal system. Involvement may be symmetric or asymmetric (Fig. 3). In diffuse perilobar nephroblastomatosis, a thick rind of lower attenuation tissue encases normally enhancing but architecturally distorted parenchyma. In multifocal nephroblastomatosis, multiple round masses of low attenuation are present. Flat or plaque-like areas of involvement may be difficult to identify on CT.

On MRI, nephroblastomatosis appears hypointense relative to normal renal parenchyma after contrast administration on T_1-weighted sequences and iso- or hyperintense on T_2-weighted sequences. On T_1-weighted sequences without contrast administration, the areas of nephroblastomatosis cannot be distinguished from normal renal parenchyma. The signal intensity of nephroblastomatosis is homogeneous.

Children with genetic abnormalities or syndromes associated with nephroblastomatosis should be monitored to detect Wilms' tumor development because the prognosis for Wilms' tumor is best with small lesions. Children with hemihypertrophy or Beckwith-Wiedemann syndrome are at additional risk for developing other embryonal tumors such as hepatoblastoma and adrenal cell carcinoma. No large studies have been performed to establish the optimal screening interval for Wilms' tumor surveillance; however, large tumors with metastases developing in a 6-month time period are reported. A baseline CT of nephroblastomatosis-related genetic abnormalities or syndromes at 6 months of age or at diagnosis, if the patient is older than 6 months, followed by ultrasonographic examinations every 3 to 4 months until the child is 7 years of age, is recommended based on results from the National Wilms' Tumor Studies. An area of nephroblastomatosis that grows larger and rounder is suspicious for malignant degeneration.

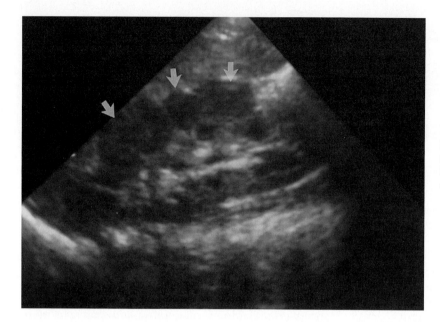

FIGURE 1. Diffuse perilobar nephroblastomatosis. Sagittal sonogram shows an enlarged right kidney with lobulated contour and hypoechoic cortical masses *(arrows)*.

WILMS' TUMOR

Wilms' tumor is the most common abdominal malignancy of childhood. It occurs predominantly in the toddler, but has been described in teenage children and adults. The most common renal tumor in the neonatal period is congenital mesoblastic nephroma; however, there have been reports of Wilms' tumor in neonates as well as in fetuses. As discussed in the Nephroblastomatosis Complex section, certain syndromes and genetic abnormalities predispose to Wilms' tumor development (Fig. 4). Bilateral Wilms' tumors almost exclusively occur in patients with nephroblastomatosis. Most

Wilms' tumors arise from the renal parenchyma; however, extrarenal Wilms' tumors may develop rarely in the abdomen or distant sites.

In the National Wilms' Tumor Study Group 5 (NWTS 5), the tumor stage is determined operatively. The grade is established on pathologic examination. The classical triphasic Wilms' tumor contains blastemal, stromal, and epithelial elements. Tumors with favorable histology do not contain any anaplastic changes. The prognosis for tumors with favorable histology is excellent, even for the higher stages. In Europe, the staging system is based completely on the radiologic findings. Tumors are classified on their imaging appearances, and chemotherapy is given before definitive surgery is performed. Tumors with extension into the inferior vena cava or invasion through the renal capsule are

FIGURE 2. Diffuse perilobar nephroblastomatosis with symmetric involvement. On the contrast-enhanced computed tomography scan, the kidneys are enlarged and multiple round, peripheral masses of low attenuation are present. Architectural distortion at this level is pronounced; in the medial portion of the right kidney, only a peripheral area of normally enhancing kidney *(arrowheads)* is present.

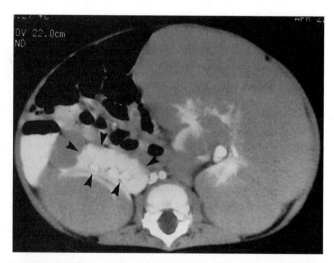

FIGURE 3. Diffuse perilobar nephroblastomatosis with asymmetric involvement. On the contrast-enhanced computed tomography (CT) scan, the left kidney is much larger than the right. The architecture of the kidneys is distorted. A portion *(arrowheads)* of normally enhancing right kidney consists of parenchyma and calices.

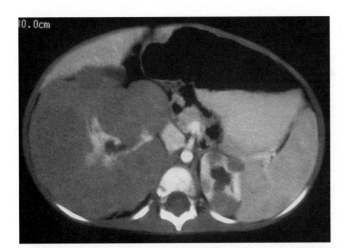

FIGURE 4. Diffuse perilobar nephroblastomatosis and right Wilms' tumor. Contrast-enhanced computed tomography (CT) scan shows round, peripheral masses enhancing less than normal renal parenchyma in the upper pole of the left kidney. The right kidney has a thick rind of lobulated, hypoattenuating tissue. Biopsy showed Wilms' tumor on the right and a nephrectomy was performed. On CT, no discreet mass was identified on the right.

easier to resect after tumor shrinkage from chemotherapy.

Radiologic evaluation of Wilms' tumor is focused on identifying the site(s) of involvement, extension, and metastases in order to assist in surgical planning. The preoperative imaging protocol in NWTS 5 includes abdominal and pelvic sonography, abdominal and pelvic CT, chest CT, and conventional chest radiography. Ultimately, the data will be analyzed to determine what modalities are most beneficial.

On sonography, Wilms' tumor is an intrarenal mass of heterogeneous echogenicity. Some Wilms' tumors may contain cystic components, either portions of ob-

structed and entrapped pyelocaliceal systems or hemorrhagic and necrotic tumor. Extension into the inferior vena cava and right atrium are characteristic routes of tumor growth and can be well visualized with sonography, CT, and MRI (Fig. 5). The tumor typically forms a pseudocapsule but may invade the renal capsule, seed the peritoneal space, or grow directly into the mesentery and omentum. Hepatic metastases are also possible. The contralateral kidney may contain a smaller Wilms' tumor or nephroblastomatosis. Synchronous or metachronous bilateral Wilms' tumor may occur in up to 10% of patients.

On CT, Wilms' tumor is generally spherical and intrarenal. It may contain small amounts of fat or fine calcification (Figs. 6 and 7); the metanephric blastema cell is a pleuripotential embryonal cell. Dystrophic calcifications occur as well. Calcifications are seen in about 9% of Wilms' tumors. The tumor enhances less than renal parenchyma. In patients who have been screened ultrasonographically because of genetic or syndromic conditions, the tumor is usually less than 4 cm in diameter. Children who are evaluated because of physical examination abnormalities generally have tumors larger than 10 cm in diameter. CT and conventional radiographs of the chest are used to identify pulmonary metastases. On MRI, Wilms' tumor is isointense with respect to normal renal parenchyma in T_1-weighted sequences and hyperintense with respect to normal renal parenchyma on T_2-weighted sequences. After contrast administration, Wilms' tumor is hypointense relative to normal renal parenchyma. The signal intensity is inhomogeneous.

For patients enrolled in NWTS 5, surgery begins with a complete abdominal exploration before attention is given to the kidneys. The unaffected kidney is initially visualized and palpated to evaluate it for masses or areas of superficial nephroblastomatosis before the en bloc resection of the affected kidney. Analysis of the radio-

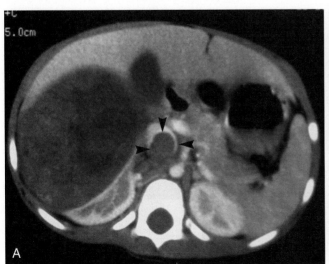
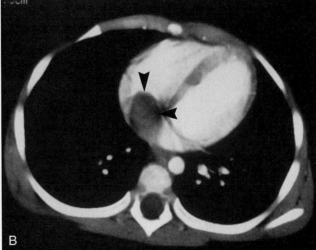

FIGURE 5. Wilms' tumor extending into the inferior vena cava and right atrium. **A,** Contrast-enhanced computed tomography (CT) scan reveals a large, round, heterogeneous mass in the right kidney that enhances less than normal renal parenchyma. Contrast material opacifies the lateral and anterior margins of the inferior vena cava containing hypoattenuating tumor (arrowheads). **B,** The tumor (arrowheads) extends into the right atrium.

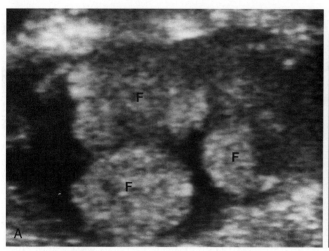
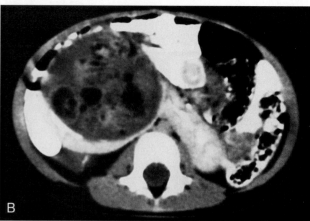

FIGURE 6. Wilms' tumor containing fat in a horseshoe kidney. **A,** Axial sonogram of part of the Wilms' tumor demonstrates hyperechoic fat-containing lobules *(F)*. **B,** Contrast-enhanced computed tomography (CT) shows the areas of fat in the mass. The isthmus of renal parenchyma extends across the midline.

logic data in NWTS 5 may change this approach. Excisional biopsy of lung nodules is done to ensure that the stage of the tumor is correctly assigned. Patients with bilateral disease have a staging surgery as well. The results of the surgical stage and the histologic examination determine therapy. In patients with bilateral disease, treatment is according to the tumor histology and the higher stage side, with a later nephron-sparing surgery.

CLEAR CELL SARCOMA OF THE KIDNEY

Clear cell sarcoma of the kidney was considered a sarcomatous subtype of Wilms' tumor before 1978, when it was reclassified as a separate entity from Wilms'

tumor. Formerly, it was called bone metastasizing renal tumor of childhood. It occurs in an age group similar to that of Wilms' tumor, and its imaging features are not distinct from Wilms' tumor (Fig. 8). Clear cell sarcoma has a predilection for bone metastases, usually occurring after diagnosis of the primary site. A pathologic diagnosis of clear cell sarcoma necessitates an evaluation of the skeletal system. The NWTS 5 recommends both bone scintigraphy and a conventional radiographic skeletal survey. The prognosis is poor because of the aggressive behavior of the tumor.

RHABDOID TUMOR OF THE KIDNEY

Rhabdoid tumor of the kidney was considered a sarcomatous variant of Wilms' tumor before 1978, when it

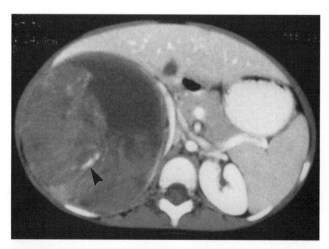

FIGURE 7. Wilms' tumor containing calcification. Contrast-enhanced computed tomography (CT) reveals fluid-attenuating material anteromedially, most likely hemorrhage, in the large heterogeneous mass. Linear calcification is present posteriorly *(arrowhead)*.

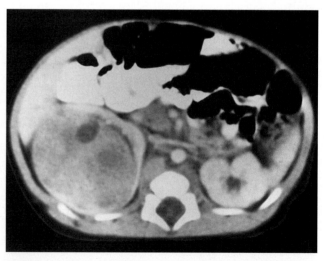

FIGURE 8. Clear cell sarcoma of the kidney. Contrast-enhanced computed tomography (CT) shows a large, round heterogeneous right kidney mass. The mass was identified on antenatal sonography, and the CT was performed on the second day of life.

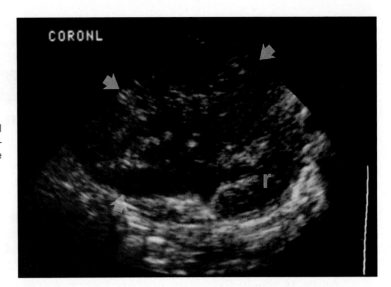

FIGURE 9. Congenital mesoblastic nephroma. On coronal sonography, the large, round mass *(arrows)* is predominantly solid, with foci of hyperechogenicity. A portion of the normal kidney *(r)* is present inferomedially.

was reclassified as a separate entity from Wilms' tumor. As with clear cell sarcoma of the kidney, it has imaging features similar to those of Wilms' tumor, but it occurs in a slightly younger age group. Rhabdoid tumor of the kidney has a distinct metastatic pattern: It is frequently associated with primary or metastatic central nervous system lesions. After tissue diagnosis, MRI of the brain is recommended. Rhabdoid tumor has the worst prognosis of all of the childhood renal tumors.

MESOBLASTIC NEPHROMA

Formerly, mesoblastic nephroma was thought to be an infantile type of Wilms' tumor; however the patients with this diagnosis all had excellent outcomes. The tumor is composed of spindle cells and does not have the typical histology of Wilms' tumor. Although most common in the neonatal period, it has been reported in adults, older children, and fetuses. On sonography, mesoblastic nephroma is predominantly solid and may contain cystic components (Fig. 9). The mass may distort and displace the pyelocaliceal system. On CT, congenital mesoblastic nephroma may be homogeneous or heterogeneous. Enhancement patterns are variable. The tumor although benign has been known to metastasize.

MULTILOCULAR CYSTIC RENAL TUMOR

Multilocular cystic renal tumor occurs predominantly in boys during infancy and toddler stages and in women in their seventh and eighth decades. When the cystic mass has blastemal elements within its septa, it is called cystic partially differentiated nephroblastoma. Multilocular cystic tumors with septa containing completely differentiated tissue are called cystic nephroma. Partially differentiated cystic nephroblastoma is found in the child more commonly than cystic nephroma. Cystic neph-

roma is identified in women. This benign tumor may recur locally if incompletely excised.

Partially differentiated cystic nephroblastoma and cystic nephroma cannot be distinguished based on imaging features. The multilocular cystic renal tumor may involve the entire kidney or a small portion. Sonography is more sensitive than CT for septa identification (Fig. 10). The septa may appear thin or thick. The pyelocaliceal system may be distorted and displaced. On CT, the septa enhance but the locules do not (Fig. 11).

RENAL CELL CARCINOMA

Renal cell carcinoma is rare in childhood. It has been reported as a secondary malignant neoplasm after chemotherapy or radiation therapy. Calcification and ossification occur more commonly in children than in adults. In the second decade of life, a solid renal mass is equally likely to be a renal cell carcinoma or a Wilms' tumor. In the first decade of life, a solid renal mass is much more likely to be a Wilms' tumor.

Well-defined intrarenal lesions have been described on sonography and CT (Fig. 12). In some case reports, the tumor has been of increased attenuation relative to renal parenchyma. About 25% of renal cell carcinomas contain calcifications. Renal cell carcinoma enhances less than normal renal parenchyma.

MEDULLARY CARCINOMA OF THE KIDNEY

Medullary carcinoma of the kidney was described as a distinct entity in 1995. It has been identified almost exclusively in patients of African descent with sickle cell trait or hemoglobin SC disease. The tumor develops in the renal medulla, infiltrates the cortex, and encases the renal pelvis, causing caliectasis while reniform shape is maintained (Fig. 13). Medullary carcinoma metastasizes rapidly to regional lymph nodes and lung.

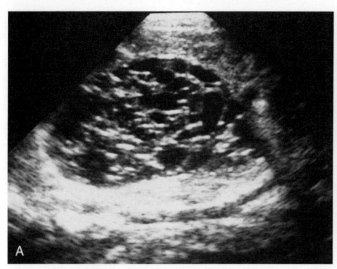

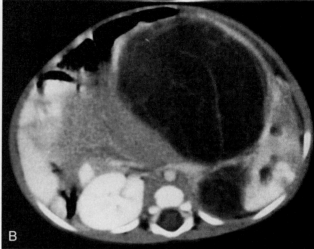

FIGURE 10. Partially differentiated cystic nephroblastoma. **A,** Sagittal sonogram of the left kidney reveals a cystic mass containing many septa and locules of varying sizes. **B,** Contrast-enhanced computed tomography (CT) reveals the hypoattenuating mass with very delicate-appearing septa.

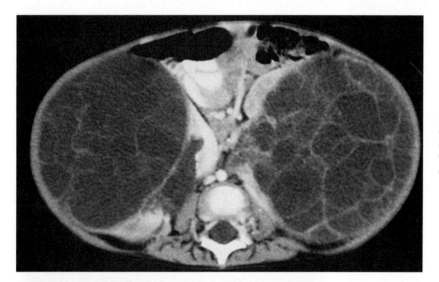

FIGURE 11. Bilateral partially differentiated cystic nephroblastoma. Contrast-enhanced computed tomography (CT) shows the septa, with similar attenuation to renal parenchyma, coursing through low-density masses.

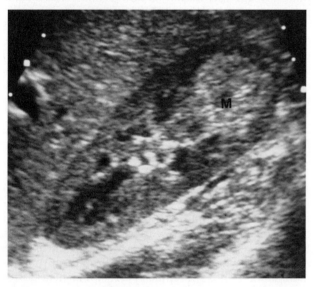

FIGURE 12. Renal cell carcinoma. Sagittal sonogram of the right kidney shows a round, hyperechoic mass *(M)* in the lower pole.

RENAL ANGIOMYOLIPOMA

Angiomyolipomas and cysts are the hamartomatous renal lesions seen in children with tuberous sclerosis. The majority of children with tuberous sclerosis have angiomyolipomas by 10 years of age. Angiomyolipomas occur in at least 50% of patients with tuberous sclerosis and may be the only manifestation of the disease.

Angiomyolipomas contain a variable amount of fat and can be mistaken for Wilms' tumor or renal cell carcinoma if the history of tuberous sclerosis is not elicited. Bilateral lesions are seen in tuberous sclerosis (Fig. 14). The vascular supply for angiomyolipoma is characteristic and consists of tortuous, dilated vessels with aneurysm formation.

On sonography, angiomyolipoma is hyperechoic. Lesions larger than 4 cm may be selectively embolized or surgically removed to prevent life-threatening hemorrhage. Ultrasonographic screening to monitor angi-

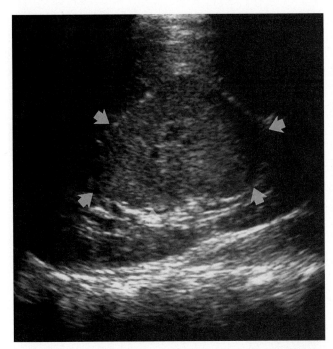

FIGURE 13. Medullary carcinoma of the kidney. Sagittal sonogram of the right kidney shows a mass *(arrows)* isoechoic to parenchyma effacing and abutting the pelvis.

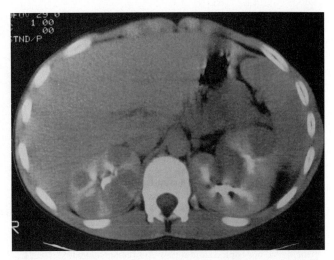

FIGURE 15. Non-Hodgkin's lymphoma of the kidneys. Contrast-enhanced computed tomography (CT) demonstrates multiple, round hypoattenuating cortical masses.

omyolipoma size is recommended every 2 to 3 years before puberty and then annually after puberty.

RENAL LYMPHOMA

Lymphoma of the kidney is due to hematogenous spread or extension from retroperitoneal sites; the kidney does not normally contain lymphoid tissue, making primary renal lymphoma rare. Non-Hodgkin's lymphoma involving the kidneys is more common than Hodgkin's lymphoma; however, it occurs seldom.

CT is better than sonography for demonstrating renal lesions. On CT, there may be multiple round masses that enhance less than normal renal parenchyma (Fig. 15). On sonography, the mass(es) may be occult. The kidney may be normal in appearance. Nephromegaly may be the only finding. Hypo-, iso-, and hyperechoic subcortical masses have been described (Fig. 16).

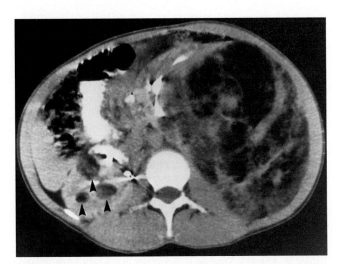

FIGURE 14. Angiomyolipomas of the kidneys. Contrast-enhanced computed tomography (CT) depicts a large angiomyolipoma in the left kidney and three smaller ones *(arrowheads)* in the right kidney.

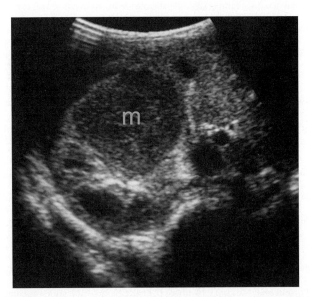

FIGURE 16. Non-Hodgkin's lymphoma of the kidney. Axial sonogram of the right kidney shows a hypoechoic mass *(m)* replacing the anteromedial portion of the kidney.

SUGGESTED READINGS

Nephroblastomatosis Complex

Beckwith JB: Questions and answers: Wilms' tumor screening. AJR Am J Roentgenol 1995;164:1294

Borer JG, Kaefer M, Barnewolt CE, et al: Renal findings on radiological follow-up of patients with Beckwith-Wiedemann syndrome. J Urol 1999;161:235

Choyke PL, Siegel MJ, Craft AW, et al: Screening for Wilms' tumor in children with Beckwith-Wiedemann syndrome or idiopathic hemihypertrophy. Med Pediatr Oncol 1999;32:196

Gallant JM, Barnewolt CE, Taylor GA, et al: Radiologic-pathologic conference of Children's Hospital Boston: bilateral asymptomatic renal enlargement. Pediatr Radiol 1997;27:614

Gylys-Morin V, Hoffer FA, Kozakewich H, et al: Wilms' tumor and nephroblastomatosis: imaging characteristics at gadolinium-enhanced MR imaging. Radiology 1993;188:517

Hoyme HE, Seaver LH, Jones KL, et al: Isolated hemihyperplasia (hemihypertrophy): report of a prospective multicenter study of the incidence of neoplasia and review. Am J Med Genet 1998;79:274

Lonergan GJ, Martinez-Leon MI, Agrons GA, et al: Nephrogenic rests, nephroblastomatosis, and associated lesions of the kidney. Radiographics 1998;18:947

Rohrschneider WK, Weirich A, Rieden K, et al: US, CT, and MR imaging characteristics of nephroblastomatosis. Pediatr Radiol 1998;28:435

White KS, Kirks DB, Bove KE: Imaging of nephroblastomatosis: an overview. Radiology 1992;182:1

Wilms' Tumor

Andrews MA, Amparo EG: Wilms' tumor in a patient with Beckwith-Wiedemann syndrome: onset detected with 3-month serial sonography. AJR Am J Roentgenol 1992;159:835

Applegate KE, Ghei M, Perez-Atayde AR: Prenatal detection of a Wilms' tumor. Pediatr Radiol 1999;29:64

Ballock RT, Wiesner GL, Myers MT, et al: Hemihypertrophy: concepts and controversies. J Bone Joint Surg Am 1997;79:1731

Carrico CWT, Cohen MD, Zerin JM, et al: Wilms' tumor imaging: patient costs and protocol compliance. Radiology 1997;204:627

Cohen MD: Commentary: imaging and staging of Wilms' tumors: problems and controversies. Pediatr Radiol 1996;26:307

De Kraker J, Delemarre JF, Lilien MR, et al: Misstaging in nephroblastoma: causes and consequences. A report of the Sixth Nephroblastoma Trial and Study of the International Society of Paediatric Oncology. Eur J Pediatr Surg 1999;9:153

Fernbach SK, Feinstein KA: Renal tumors in children. Semin Roentgenol 1995;30:200

Geller E, Smergel EM, Lowry PA: Renal neoplasms of childhood. Radiol Clin North Am 1997;35:1391

Godzinski J, Tournade MF, de Kraker J, et al: The role of preoperative chemotherapy in the treatment of nephroblastoma: the SIOP experience. Societe Internationale d'Oncologie Pediatrique. Semin Urol Oncol 1999;17:28

Goske MJ, Mitchell C, Reslan WA: Imaging of patients with Wilms' tumor. Semin Urol Oncol 1999;17:11.

Graf N, Tournade MF, de Kraker J: The role of preoperative chemotherapy in the management of Wilms' tumor. The SIOP studies. International Society of Pediatric Oncology. Urol Clin North Am 2000;27:443

Kullendorff C-M, Wiebe T: Wilms' tumour in infancy. Acta Paediatr 1998;87:747

Lowe LH, Isuani BH, Heller RM, et al: Pediatric renal masses: Wilms' tumor and beyond. Radiographics 2000;20:1585

Meisel JA, Guthrie KA, Breslow NE, et al: Significance and management of computed tomography detected pulmonary nodules: a report from the National Wilms' Tumor Study Group. Int J Radiat Oncol Biol Physics 1999;44:579

Neville HL, Ritchey ML: Wilms' tumor: overview of National Wilms' Tumor Study Group results. Urol Clin North Am 2000;27:435

Porteus MH, Narkool P, Neuberg D, et al: Characteristics and outcome of children with Beckwith-Wiedemann syndrome and Wilms' tumor: a report from the National Wilms' Tumor Study Group. J Clin Oncol 2000;18:2026

Scott DJ, Wallace WHB, Hendry GMA: With advances in medical imaging can the radiologist reliably diagnose Wilms' tumours? Clin Radiol 1999;54:3217

Slasky BS, Bar-Ziv J, Freeman AI, et al: CT appearance of involvement of the peritoneum, mesentery and omentum in Wilms' tumor. Pediatr Radiol 1997;27:14

Suzuki K, Miyake H, Tashiro M, et al: Extrarenal Wilms' tumor. Pediatr Radiol 1993;23:149

Wootton-Gorges SL, Albano EA, Riggs JM, et al: Chest radiography versus chest CT in the evaluation for pulmonary metastases in patients with Wilms' tumor: a retrospective review. Pediatr Radiol 2000;30:533

Clear Cell Sarcoma of the Kidney

Argani P, Perlman EJ, Breslow NE, et al: Clear cell sarcoma of the kidney: a review of 351 cases from the National Wilms' Tumor Study Group Pathology Center. Am J Surg Pathol 2000;24:4

Glass RBJ, Davidson AJ, Fernbach SK: Clear cell sarcoma of the kidney: CT, sonographic, and pathological correlation. Radiology 1991;180:715

Khalil RM, Aubel S: Clear cell sarcoma of the kidney: a case report. Pediatr Radiol 1993;23:407

Rhabdoid Tumor of the Kidney

Agrons GA, Kingsman KD, Wagner BJ, et al: Rhabdoid tumor of the kidney in children: a comparative study of 21 cases. AJR Am J Roentgenol 1997;168:447

Chung CJ, Lorenzo R, Rayder S, et al: Rhabdoid tumors of the kidney in children: CT findings. AJR Am J Roentgenol 1995;164:697

Mesoblastic Nephroma

Goldberg J, Liu P, Smith C: Congenital mesoblastic nephroma presenting with hemoperitoneum and shock. Pediatr Radiol 1994;24:54

Hartman DS, Lim Lesar MS, Madewell JE, et al: Mesoblastic nephroma: radiologic-pathologic correlation of 20 cases. AJR Am J Roentgenol 1981;136:69

Schlesinger AE, Rosenfield NS, Castle VP, et al: Congenital mesoblastic nephroma metastatic to the brain: a report of two cases. Pediatr Radiol 1995;25:S73

Willert JR, Feuser J, Beckwith JB: Congenital mesoblastic nephroma: a rare cause of perinatal anemia. J Pediatr 1999;134:248

Wootton SL, Rowen SJ, Griscom NT: Congenital mesoblastic nephroma. Radiographics 1991;11:719

Multilocular Cystic Renal Disease

Agrons GA, Wagner BJ, Davidson AJ, et al: Multilocular cystic renal tumor in children: radiologic-pathologic correlation. Radiographics 1995;15:653

Hartman DS, Davis CJ, Sanders RC, et al: The multiloculated renal mass: considerations and differential features. Radiographics 1987;7:29

Madewell JE, Goldman SM, Davis CJ, et al: Multilocular cystic nephroma: a radiographic-pathologic correlation of 58 patients. Radiology 1983;146:309

Renal Cell Carcinoma

Allison JW, James CA, Figarola MS: Pediatric case of the day: renal cell carcinoma in a child with tuberous sclerosis. Radiographics 1999;19:1388

Donnelly LF, Rencken IO, Shardell K, et al: Renal cell carcinoma after therapy for neuroblastoma. AJR Am J Roentgenol 1996;167:915

Fenton DS, Taub JW, Amundson GM, et al: Renal cell carcinoma occurring in a child 2 years after chemotherapy for neuroblastoma. AJR Am J Roentgenol 1993;161:165

Kabala JE, Shield J, Duncan A: Renal cell carcinoma in childhood. Pediatr Radiol 1992;22:203

Pursner M, Petchprapa C, Haller JO, et al: Renal carcinoma: bilateral breast metastases in a child. Pediatr Radiol 1997;27:242

Sostre G, Johnson JF, Cho M: Ossifying renal cell carcinoma. Pediatr Radiol 1998;28:458

Medullary Carcinoma of the Kidney

Davidson AJ, Choyke PL, Hartman DS, et al: Renal medullary carcinoma associated with sickle cell trait: radiologic findings. Radiology 1995;195:83

Davis CJ, Mostofi FK, Sesterhenn IA: Renal medullary carcinoma: the seventh sickle cell nephropathy. Am J Surg Pathol 1995;19:1

Kalyanpur A, Schwartz DS, Fields JM, et al: Renal medulla carcinoma in a white adolescent. AJR Am J Roentgenol 1997;169:1037

Pickhardt PJ: Renal medullary carcinoma: an aggressive neoplasm in patients with sickle cell trait. Abdom Imaging 1998;23:531

Renal Angiomyolipoma

Carter TC, Angtuaco TL, Shah HR: Ultrasound case of the day: large, bilateral angiomyolipomas of the kidneys with tuberous sclerosis. Radiographics 1999;19:555

Ewalt DH, Sheffield E, Sparagana SP, et al: Renal lesion growth in children with tuberous sclerosis complex. J Urol 1998;160:141

Lemaitre L, Claudon M, Dubrulle F, et al: Imaging of angiomyolipomas. Semin Ultrasound CT MR 1997;18:100

Tchaprassian Z, Mognato G, Paradias G, et al: Renal angiomyolipoma in children: diagnostic difficulty in 3 patients. J Urol 1998;159:1654

Renal Lymphoma

Fernbach SK, Glass RBJ: Uroradiographic manifestations of Burkitt's lymphoma in children. J Urol 1986;135:986

Hartman DS, Davis CJ, Goldman SM, et al: Renal lymphoma: radiologic-pathologic correlation of 21 cases. Radiology 1982;144:759

Weinberger E, Rosenbaum DM, Pendergrass TW: Renal involvement in children with lymphoma: comparison of CT with sonography. AJR Am J Roentgenol 1990;155:347

C h a p t e r   3

UROLITHIASIS, NEPHROCALCINOSIS, AND TRAUMA TO THE URINARY TRACT

JOHN R. STY

UROLITHIASIS

INCIDENCE AND ETIOLOGY

The incidence of urolithiasis varies according to geographic areas. The incidence of urolithiasis in children in the United States is 1 in 1000, with 7000 hospital admissions per year, slightly lower than the incidence in Europe and considerably lower than that in Asia. In children, the risk is greatest in southern California and in the southeastern states, which is actually also considered the "stone belt" in the United States in adults.

The etiology also varies somewhat according to geographic regions. Bladder stones have been noted to be endemic in developing countries such as those in Southeast Asia, which include Thailand, Indonesia, and India. The high prevalence of these stones is attributed to the predominately cereal-based and low-protein diet. In contrast, in developed countries in Europe and North America, upper tract or kidney stones predominate. It is also been demonstrated that, as industrialization progresses in a geographic area, there tends to be a shift from lower tract to upper tract stones. In the United Kingdom and certain European countries, approximately 30% to 90% of patients have infection stones, whereas in the United States and Scandinavia, metabolic disorders are the most common cause of kidney stones.

In contrast to the marked male predominance of urolithiasis in adults, there is equal to slightly higher male prominence in children. In several studies of children with urolithiasis, 6% to 10% are blacks and 72% to 90% are whites. Recurrence rates reported range from 6% to 50%, with mean interval to recurrence of 3 to 5 years.

MECHANISMS OF STONE FORMATION AND COMPOSITION OF STONES

Urinary tract stone formation is a complex process involving three main factors: (1) the concentration of the precipitating substances and their urine solubilities, (2) promoters, and (3) inhibitors of crystallization and aggregation.

The process by which the formation of urinary stones occurs is thought to be nucleation. The concentration of stone-forming ions in the urine is critical in stone production. When the concentration of these ions are excessively high, there is a tendency for their activity product, the product of these free ion concentrations, to increase also. When this product exceeds its urine solubility, there exists a state of supersaturation, and this is the actual driving mechanism for stone formation. It is explained by the tendency of urine to form stone crystals, as a result of ionic activity of calcium and calcium oxalate. A crystal or foreign body initiates formation in urine that is supersaturated with crystalizing salts. The concentration of the stone-forming ions in the urine and the urinary pH are major factors related to stone formation. Other conditions affect this process that determine whether this state of supersaturation will further progress into what is termed a *metastable state*. For instance, urine pH influences the solubility of certain ions. Increasing the urine pH increases the solubility of uric acid, but a high pH decreases calcium phosphate solubility. The pH also affects the availability of inhibitors of crystal formation, thereby influencing the state of saturation of certain stone-forming ions.

Crystallization inhibitors include magnesium, pyrophosphate, and citrate, which inhibit spontaneous nucleation and growth of calcium crystals. Inhibitors of crystallization act by binding certain lithogenic ions, thereby decreasing their concentration in the urine. The complexes formed by this process are more soluble. Therefore, the pre-ion activity and the saturation for the specific crystal are reduced. Citrate and pyrophosphate, the most commonly known inhibitors, act by binding to calcium. Magnesium and sodium bind oxalate. Any pyrocalcinin inhibits calcium oxalate crystallization by adsorbing to crystal surfaces. Other inhibitors include glycosaminoglycans, uropontin, and Tamm-Horsfall mucoprotein.

Developmental anomalies of the urinary tract promote urinary stasis and associated infection and predispose a child to stone formation. Physical damage to the urothelium from infection or the presence of a foreign body to serve as a nidus for bacterial colonization also potentate stone formation. The stone matrix theory invokes an organic matrix of urinary protein and serum providing a framework for deposition of crystals.

Calcification of the urinary tract can occur in the form of nephrocalcinosis, focal dystrophic calcification, or urolithiasis. Crystals in the kidney or urinary drainage system are identified in a wide range of renal, urologic, endocrine, and metabolic abnormalities. A distinction is drawn between urolithiasis (stones in the urinary tract) and nephrocalcinosis (increase in calcium content of the kidney). Many different types of stones may be identified in the urinary tract in children.

Urinary stones are of the following types: calcium, magnesium ammonium phosphate (struvite calculi), citric acid, cystine, and xanthine. Calcium-containing stones are the most common of all stones; infection-related stones (struvite and carbonate–apatite) account for 10% to 25%. Calcium stones and struvite are moderately to markedly radiopaque. Uric acid stones are unusual and account for less than 5% of urinary stones. They are radiolucent in pure form but relatively radiopaque when mixed calcium salts or struvite. Cystine stones are uncommon and are moderately radiopaque because of their physical density and higher

effective atomic number compared with adjacent fluid and tissue. These may occur in mixed form with calcium oxalate or calcium phosphate. Xanthine stones that occur in pure form are radiolucent (Table 1).

The etiology of renal stones in children is (1) infection; (2) developmental anomalies of the urinary tract; (3) immobilization or steroid therapy; (4) metabolic disorders, such as hypercalcemia and hypercalciuria, hyperoxaluria, uricosuria, cystinuria, and xanthinuria; and (5) idiopathic.

Stones Caused by Urinary Stasis, Foreign Body, and Chronic Urinary Tract Infection

Stasis of urine resulting from urinary obstruction or neurogenic bladder promotes calculus formation, often as a result of chronic infection, urothelial damage with defective distal tubular acidification, and persistently alkaline urine. Urinary tract anomalies in association with other risk factors predispose patients to urolithiasis by promoting stasis of urine and heterogeneous nucleation. Infection leads to injury of the uroepithelial lining. Resultant bacterial and inflammatory cellular debris acts as a nidus for stone formation, and growth at lower solute concentrations in effect hastens the process of crystallization. This is what has been referred to as heterogeneous nucleation.

Infection stones compromise approximately 25% of the total number of urolithiasis cases in North American children, compared to 50% in European children. Two thirds of the patients with infection stones are less than 5 years of age. This type of stone also has predominately renal location noted in 70%.

Thirty percent of the patients have an anatomic lesion that probably contributes to stone formation. These include ureteropelvic junction obstruction, neurogenic bladder, and obstructed megaureter. Vesicoureteral reflux is noted in 10% of patients. Urinary diversions are also considered risk factors. Other risk factors for infection stone formation include ileal loops, large loop residuals, and hyperchloremic acidosis or ureteral dilatation.

These calculi are predominately struvite, although mixed stones (carbonate–apatite) have been noted.

Table 1 ■ RADIOLUCENCY OF URINARY STONES

MINERAL COMPOSITION	OPACITY
Calcium stones	
Calcium oxalate (mono or dehydrate)—small dense stippled	+++
Calcium oxalate and apatite	+++
Calcium phosphate—laminated	+++
Calcium hydrogen phosphate	+++
Magnesium ammonium phosphate—staghorn calculus	++
Struvite + calcium phosphate	++
Cystine	+
Uric acid	−
Xanthine	−
Matrix	−

Stones other than these that develop with infection are said to be infection-associated stones and are not classified as infection stones per se. Urease-splitting bacteria, especially *Escherichia coli, Pseudomonas aeruginosa, Proteus mirabilis, Kliebsiella,* and *Proteus vulgaris,* are responsible for forming these stones. The mechanism by which stones are formed involves the release of ammonia when the urease from the bacteria acts on urea in the urine. This increases urine pH and urine ammonium, which substantially binds with phosphate and magnesium ions, forming struvite stones. These stones increase in size, filling the pelvicaliceal system and forming a staghorn configuration, which often requires some form of surgical removal. Bacteria may be interspersed within the structure of the stone, making antibiotic penetration difficult, and thus making infection recurrent or persistent. For this reason, it is essential not only to treat aggressively with appropriate antibiotics but also to ensure complete removal of all stone fragments. The recurrence rate following initial management is over 10%, and, in those cases associated with anatomic abnormalities, the median interval to recurrence following initial surgery is approximately 1 year.

Idiopathic Hypercalciuria

Hypercalciuria is the most common metabolic etiology attributed to urolithiasis in both children and adults. There are several causes of hypercalciuria, the most common of which is idiopathic hypercalciuria (IH). IH is caused by a combination of absorptive and renal hypercalciuria excretion. It is more common in white children, and it affects both sexes but with a male predominance. Family history is positive for urolithiasis in 50% of children with IH, and an autosomal dominant pattern has been suggested.

The most common clinical feature of hypercalciuria is gross or microscopic hematuria, which may occur with or without urolithiasis. Flank pain is a frequent symptom, as well as dysuria, frequency, and enuresis. Within 5 years of the onset of hematuria, without therapy, the risk for urolithiasis is estimated to be approximately 20%.

Other clinical conditions that may cause increased urine calcium excretion (secondary hypercalciuria) include chronic diuretic use, sarcoidosis, primary hyperparathyroidism, distal renal tubular acidosis (RTA), and prolonged immobilization. Chronic diuretic use, especially of furosemide can cause nephrocalcinosis and nephrolithiasis. This is particularly evident in premature infants with chronic lung disease or patients with congestive heart failure who are on prolonged therapy. Sarcoidosis, a chronic granulomatous disorder the cause of which is unknown, may be associated with hypercalciemia and stone formation. This is attributed in some part to renal damage by the granulomata but mainly to the hypercalciemia and hypercalciuria. Primary hyperparathyroidism is characterized by increased serum parathyroid hormone concentrations and increased calcitriol production, causing increased intestinal absorption, tubular reabsorption, and bone resorption of calcium. These cause markedly increased serum and urine calcium concentrations. In hyperparathyroid stone formers, surgical removal of the parathyroid is necessary.

Distal RTA is a disorder caused by a defect in the production and maintenance of the hydrogen ion gradient in the distal tubule. It is characterized by normal anion gap acidosis with hyperchloremia. The risk for stone formation is attributed to (1) increased urine pH promoting precipitation of calcium phosphate stones, (2) increased calcium excretion, and (3) low urine citrate. The low urine citrate is attributed to a defect in renal citrate metabolism, acidosis, low glomerular filtration rate, and hypokalemia. The hypercalciuria is due to the metabolic acidosis. When a chronic acidosis exists, the homeostatic body buffers retain hydrogen ions in the bone. Consequently, calcium salts are dissolved from the bone and tubular calcium reabsorption decreases, causing increased urine calcium excretion.

Immobilization as short as several weeks also may result in hypercalciuria. This is attributed to increased calcium mobilization from bone leading to increased calcium excretion. Other disorders causing calcium urolithiasis include vitamin D excess, especially if accompanied by large doses of oral calcium; malignancies with metastatic bone disease; juvenile rheumatoid arthritis; and idiopathic hypercalciemia of infancy.

Hyperoxaluria

Oxalate is one of the end products of normal metabolism. Its main route of excretion is via the kidneys. The majority of urine oxalate is derived from endogenous metabolism, with ascorbate and glyoxylic acid as the main precursors. Only approximately 10% of urine oxalate is derived from diet. Hyperoxaluria accounts for 2% of children with calcium urolithiasis. Specific clinical disorders may result in malabsorption, promoting increased oxalate absorption, and these disorders comprise what is know as enteric hyperoxaluria. The absorption of oxalate is increased by decreased intraluminal calcium and free fatty acids as well as by increase permeability of the gastrointestinal mucosa to oxalate caused by inflammatory small bowel disease, ileal resection, pancreatic disorders, and fat malabsorption. There are two main categories of this condition, both of which cause marked increase in oxalate biosynthesis from glyoxylate that accumulates behind the metabolic block. One type is associated with the deficiency of hepatic peroxismal alanine:glyoxylate aminotransferase, and the second category is due to deficiency of glyoxylate reductase.

Uric Acid Lithiasis

Uric acid stones account for 5% of stones in childhood. Their formation occurs with low urine pH as well as low urine volume. Uric stones may also occur with increase in urine ammonium concentration secondary to urinary tract infection, dehydration, or starvation. Uric acid is the end product of purine metabolism, which is handled by the kidney and partly by the gastrointestinal tract.

Hyperuricosuria is the greatest predisposing factor, and this can occur with a high-purine diet, intake of drugs (salicylates, probenecid, etc.), obesity, and alcohol intake. Hereditary diseases causing hyperuricemia, such as Lesch-Nyhan syndrome, where there is a deficiency of hypoxanthine guanine phosphoribosyltransferase and superactivity of phosphoribosylpyrophosphate synthetase, also cause marked hyperuricemia, uricosuria, and uric acid stones.

The more common reason for hyperuricemia and hyperuricosuria is increased purine biosynthesis, as in lymphoproliferative or myeloproliferative disorders. Uric acid urolithiasis is estimated to occur in as many as 40% of these patients. During the active stage of tumor reduction following chemotherapy or radiation therapy, precipitation of uric acid crystals within the collecting tubules may produce intrarenal urinary obstruction, oliguria, and anuria. Uric acid stones may also occur in polycythemia.

Cystinuria

Cystinuria is a genetic disorder with autosomal recessive transmission. It is characterized by abnormalities in the renal and intestinal transport mechanisms of cystine, ornithine, lysine, and arginine. There is an increase in urine excretion of these dibasic amino acids, with normal or decreased plasma levels. This defect is of no clinical consequence per se except that, once the solubility limit is exceeded, cystine stone formation occurs. Cystinuria occurs account for 5% of urolithiasis in children in the United States and approximately 1% of all patients with urolithiasis. It can occur anytime from infancy to adulthood, although the mean age of occurrence is in the second to third decade of life. Other clinical disorders associated with cystinuria are hemophilia, retinitis pigmentosa, Down syndrome, muscular dystrophy, and hereditary pancreatitis, as well as mental illness and retardation.

Xanthinuria

Xanthinuria is an autosomal recessive disorder of purine metabolism with inability to convert hypoxanthine and xanthine to uric acid. Serum and urinary uric acid levels are low, and urinary excretion of xanthine and hypoxanthine results. Xanthine urolithiasis occurs in about 25% to 30% of affected patients, most of whom are asymptomatic. The stones are radiolucent.

Idiopathic Stones

Idiopathic stones, without predisposing factors, represent 30% to 40% of urinary tract stones found in childhood. Calcium phosphate or calcium oxalate is the usual composition. Idiopathic calcium stones may have a nucleus of urate, indicating that the primary disease is uric acid lithiasis rather than primary calcium stone disease.

LOCATION OF STONES

Approximately half of urinary stones are located only in the kidney, a third only in the ureter, 15% in the kidney and ureter, and the remainder in the bladder. Multiple stones may occupy several locations.

Kidney Calculi

The pelvocaliceal system is the most common site of stone location, and stones within the renal pelvis or calices are either single or multiple. They range in size from sand-like to large conglomerate masses. When the stone produces a cast of the pelvocaliceal system, it is termed a *staghorn calculus*. The staghorn calculus is usually a struvite stone, but occasionally results from uric acid, cystine, or calcium oxalate. These patients usually have pre-existing hydronephrosis with upper urinary tract dilatation and stasis. The ureteropelvic junction obstruction results from stones and chronic infection with resulting cortical loss and interstitial renal fibrosis. Calculi may form in congenital caliceal diverticula, congenitally obstructed calices, and the dilated tubules of medullary sponge kidney. Congenital genitourinary anomalies are present in over one third of patients and in virtually all cases related to infection.

Ureteral Calculi

These calculi presumably originate in the pelvocaliceal system or, rarely, proximal to an obstruction of a ureter. Ureteral stones in a ureter that is otherwise normal are usually located in the distal several centimeters of the ureter. Such stones cause variable obstruction of the ureter. Sonography will detect dilatation of the obstructed ureter and pelvis proximal to the ureteral stone, and an echogenic stone with shadowing may be seen, even in the absence of calcification identified radiographically. Initially the obstructed ureter shows hyperperistalsis, but with prolonged obstruction the ureter becomes atonic. Intravenous urography, in the event of acute high-grade obstruction, shows a dense, prolonged nephrogram with marked delay in excretion of contrast material into the pelvocaliceal system. Passage of the stone from the ureter into the bladder will produce edema at the ureterovesical junction and residual dilatation of the ureter.

Bladder Stones

Stones within the bladder may originate from the upper urinary tract or from within the bladder, most commonly as a result of chronic bladder infection, neurogenic bladder, hypotonic bladder, or an intravesical foreign body. These stones are single or multiple and frequently laminated. They may reach a very large size. Stones also form in a bladder diverticulum, Kock pouch, or urachal remnant.

Urethral Calculi

Urethral calculi are rare and occur only in males. They may originate in the more proximal urinary tract; form locally, secondary to prolonged obstruction; or form within a urethral diverticulum or prostatic utricle. Stasis and infection are important in their formation.

CLINICAL PRESENTATION AND DIAGNOSIS

The most common clinical manifestation of urolithiasis is pain, occurring in 50% to 75% of children. The pain varies from nonspecific to vague, dull, or sharp abdominal or flank pain that may be either localized or radiating. The classical renal colic experienced in adults, described as intermittent, excruciating, and usually radiating through the groin, is quite rare in children.

Other features include hematuria, occurring in 50% to 90% of children. Symptoms such as urgency, dysuria, frequency, and fever as well as pyuria with or without bacteriuria or documented urinary tract infection are noted in approximately 40% of patients. The younger the patient, the more likely that urinary tract infection symptoms as well as incidental findings on imaging will lead to the diagnosis of renal stones; in older children, pain is the most frequent initial symptom. Obstructive symptoms such as urinary retention may also occur, especially in bladder or urethral stones. At times other symptoms are seen, such as nausea and vomiting as well as failure to thrive, which is especially evident in patients with concomitant metabolic acidosis or RTA.

The initial medical management is directed at relieving pain, which may require narcotics; treatment of the concurrent infection; and promoting passage of the stone, if possible, by adequate hydration with two times maintenance requirements to increase urine output. Stones measuring less than 6 mm frequently pass spontaneously. Subsequent measures are taken to prevent further stone formation by maintaining adequate fluid intake with the goal of at least the calculated maintenance requirements. This is the mainstay of therapy in all types of urolithiasis. With low urine volume, the concentration of all stone-forming ions increases, predisposing to stone formation.

The evaluation of urolithiasis in terms of calculus detection and evaluation of the morphology and function of the kidneys continues to change with the advances in imaging technology. The most significant advance is the use of helical or spiral computed tomography (CT) for the accurate delineation of renal and ureteral calculi in the acute setting. This frequently provides an accurate, rapid, and cost-effective method of patient evaluation. The alternative approach is to use a standard radiograph of the abdomen to detect the ureter or ureteral calculi. Non–contrast-enhanced helical or spiral CT scanning has its greatest impact in patients with negative abdominal radiographs or in those with suspected urinary calculi and in whom renal but not ureteral calculi are seen (Fig. 1). Combined

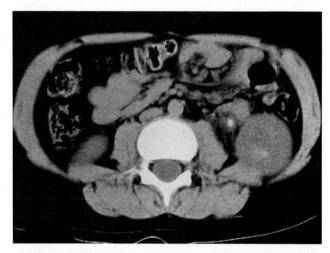

FIGURE 1. Noncontrast computed tomography scan of the mid-abdomen shows an enlarged left kidney with soft calcification in the renal pelvis and a thickened ureter with an impacted small calcium oxalate stone.

abdominal radiography and sonography may be used for calculus detection and the demonstration of obstruction. Sonography, however, is an operator-dependent technique requiring expertise, experience, and adequate imaging equipment for satisfactory results.

NEPHROCALCINOSIS

Nephrocalcinosis is uncommon in children. In nephrocalcinosis, calcium accumulates in the tubules, tubular epithelium, or interstitial tissue. The term *nephrocalcinosis* implies multifocal or diffuse renal calcifications. Bilateral renal involvement, when present, distinguishes nephrocalcinosis from focal dystrophic calcification resulting from local causes; the latter is more likely to be both irregular and unilateral. Focal dystrophic calcification can be caused by neoplasm, inflammation, or trauma.

The pattern of nephrocalcinosis can be peripheral, central, or mixed. This indicates predominant involvement of cortical or medullary tissue or both, respectively. Calcification in conditions such as oxalosis frequently involves both the medullary and cortical portions of the kidney, causing a mixed pattern. Peripheral calcifications may be observed in vascular disorders; this usually gives a tram-track type of appearance. Diseases such as RTA and hypercalciuria result in medullary calcification. Cortical necrosis and chronic glomerulonephritis are most often associated with cortical calcifications. Usually nephrocalcinosis is confined to the medullary regions of the kidney; more rarely, calcifications are noted only within the renal cortex.

MEDULLARY NEPHROCALCINOSIS

Medullary nephrocalcinosis represents over 90% of nephrocalcinosis seen in childhood. This abnormality is characterized by triangular patterns of fine, or occasionally coarse, calcification that correspond to the medullary pyramids. Metabolic conditions associated with hypercalcemia are the most frequent cause of medullary renal calcification in children (Table 2). RTA is the most commonly associated syndrome. Nephrocalcinosis as well as urolithiasis in these patients are usually the result of the combination of hypercalciuria, alkaline urine, and decreased citrate elimination. Nephrocalcinosis occurs in type I RTA, in which there is a defect in hydrogen ion metabolism. Type I RTA is a persistent disease and is found predominantly in girls older than 2 years and in adults of both sexes. In three quarters of the patients with the persistent type I form of RTA, there is nephrocalcinosis or urolithiasis.

Type I RTA is characterized by a constellation of biochemical disorders that include hyperchloremic acidosis in excessive urinary loss of sodium, potassium, calcium, and phosphate. Early in the disease, it is difficult to detect calcification unless sonography or CT is used (Figs. 2 and 3). Sonography is relatively sensitive for the detection of medullary calcification, particularly in children; this is demonstrated at regions of increased echogenicity in the medullary portions of the kidneys. Sonographically detectable medullary calcification may occur in low-birth-weight infants who have been treated with long-term furosemide therapy.

Calcium in the renal parenchyma must reach a critical density before radiographic detection is possible. Consequently, in the early minimal calcification stage,

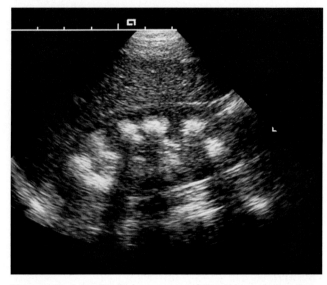

FIGURE 2. A longitudinal sonogram of the kidney shows dense hyperechoic pyramids with shadowing secondary to medullary calcinosis.

radiographs of the kidney are normal. Prompt treatment may arrest the irreversible pathologic process and prevent progressive renal damage; therefore, early detection is crucial. Sonography appears to offer a greater sensitivity than radiography for detection of renal calcification. Standard radiography may show normal-size or occasional large kidneys with medullary sponge disease. Likewise, grouped rounded/linear calcifications or small, poorly defined or large, course granular calcifications can be identified in the pyramids. Sonography demonstrates absence of the normal hypoechoic papillary structures. This is the earliest sign. Also seen with this abnormality are hyperechoic rims at the corticomedullary junction plus around the tip and sides of the pyramids. A solitary focus of hyperechogenicity at

Table 2 ■ CAUSES OF MEDULLARY NEPHROCALCINOSIS

Hypercalciuria
Endocrine
  Hyperparathyroidism
  Cushing syndrome
  Diabetes insipidus
  Hyperthyroidism
Alimentary
  Milk alkali syndrome
  Hypervitaminosis D
Skeletal
  Metastases
  Immobilization
Renal
  Renal tubular acidosis
  Medullary sponge kidney
Drugs
  Furosemide
  Steroids
Miscellaneous
  Idopathic hypercalciuria
  Idiopathic hypercalcemia

Hyperoxaluria
Primary
Secondary

Hyperuricosuria

Urinary stasis

Dystrophic calcification
Renal papillary necrosis

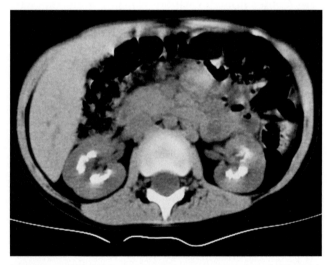

FIGURE 3. A noncontrast computed tomography of the midabdomen shows calcifications in the renal pyramids with normal-size kidneys secondary to medullary calcinosis.

the tip of the pyramids near the fornix may also represent medullary calcinosis. Although late in the disease there is increased echogenicity of the pyramids with or without shadowing, a shadow will not occur with small or minimal calcification.

Calcification along the sides or at the apices of the pyramids have been noted in normal adult cadaveric kidneys. Identical deposits in adult cadaveric kidney slices have been demonstrated with high-resolution radiography. The concentration of calcium is high in the peritubular fluid spaces, and that calcium is normally removed from this region by lymphatic mechanisms. If the amount of calcium exceeds the capacity of the lymphatic clearance, microscopic calcium aggregates accumulate in the renal medulla. These microscopic calcifications may coalesce to form a plaque and may migrate toward the calyceal epithelium, eventually perforating the calyx to form a nidus for urolithiasis. This process is known as the Anderson-Carr-Randall progression of calculus formation.

Studies have evaluated renal calcium deposits in children and suggested a sonographic demonstration of the Anderson-Carr-Randall progression theory. Patriquin et al. found that, in patients with diseases that predisposed them to nephrocalcinosis, sonography showed hyperechoic pyramids in 50% of children. Of these, seven had CT examinations and two had abdominal radiographs that proved the abnormality to be due to calcium. It is most likely that the hyperechoic false negatives on sonography in the others were due to calcium deposits not yet apparent with other imaging techniques. The pattern of calcium deposition seen in this group of patients appears to follow the Anderson-Carr-Randall progression postulate. The areas of extensive medullary hyperechogenicity correlated with the location of calcium plaques seen in cadaver kidney slices.

CORTICAL NEPHROCALCINOSIS

The calcifications in this entity are restricted to the renal cortical area. A rare infantile form of primary hyperoxaluria is the best-known etiology of cortical calcification, presenting as homogeneously dense renal cortex on ultrasound or CT. The kidneys are initially enlarged but do not show shadowing from the markedly hyperechoic cortex.

Bilateral renal cortical necrosis secondary to hypotension and cortical ischemia in the neonate results in bilateral cortical calcification, which appears several weeks after the onset of acute renal failure. The calcifications are diffuse, punctate, or tram-track. Streaks of calcification may be present in the columns of Bertin. Branching calcifications correspond to vascular structures following renal vein thrombosis. Diffuse cortical calcification is also described in transplant rejection. Bilateral chronic pyelonephritis and chronic glomerulonephritis have rarely been associated with cortical calcification. Inhomogeneous cortical and med-

ullary calcifications have been reported with acquired immunodeficiency syndrome and associated with mycobacterium avium-intracellulare infections.

TRAUMA TO THE GENITOURINARY TRACT

Accidental injuries are a significant source of morbidity and a major cause of death in childhood. Genitourinary injury accounts for 2% of such injuries. In children sustaining multiple injuries, urinary tract trauma is second in frequency only to central nervous system trauma. In childhood, renal trauma is most commonly due to vehicular or pedestrian accidents, falls, and contact sports.

Approximately 1 in 1000 pediatric hospital admissions is the result of trauma that includes renal injury. Renal injury is more common during the second decade of life than the first. The kidney seems to be more prone to injury in children than adults. This is attributed to the following specific anatomic factors:

1. The kidneys are proportionately larger in size in children than adults.
2. There is less perirenal fat, and the muscles of the flank and abdomen are less well developed.
3. Gerota's facia is underdeveloped and incomplete until the age of 10 years.
4. The lower ribs are more elastic.
5. The kidneys are in closer approximation to other organs, and the paravertebral musculature is underdeveloped.
6. The kidneys have a more delicate structure, including persistence of fetal lobulation.

In spite of the increased vulnerability of children to renal injury, recovery is usually more rapid and complete than in adults, and there is a lower incidence of significant pre-existing disease.

Most childhood renal injuries are caused by blunt trauma. Approximately 10% of children who exhibit manifestations of renal injury after trauma have pre-existing renal abnormalities. Ectopic kidneys and hydronephrotic kidneys are more susceptible to injury with minimal trauma. No treatment is required in many of these cases, but others require surgical correction of the underlying pathology. On rare occasions, a traumatized kidney may contain a tumor; in this age group, it is most often a Wilms' tumor.

Blunt injuries to the kidney are most commonly associated with rapid deceleration. During deceleration, the kidney, which is mobile within Gerota's fascia, may be thrust against the ribs laterally or the vertebral column medially. Likewise, a fractured rib may be displaced medially to lacerate the kidney. During rapid deceleration, the renal vessels are stretched. Because the media and adventitia are more elastic than the intima, a tear may occur in the intima of the renal vessels, resulting in a subintimal dissection, luminal obstruction, and renal artery thrombosis. Similar mechanisms may lead to arterial spasm without intimal tear; this causes decreased renal perfusion and places the kidney at risk for vascular occlusion. Primary lacerations of the vessels, most often the renal vein, can also occur. This is more common on the left side because the left renal vein is longer.

Penetrating renal injuries are much less common in children than in adults. Iatrogenic renal injury is also a common source of penetrating trauma. This occurs during various biopsy procedures, antegrade urography, and percutaneous nephrostomy.

CLASSIFICATION OF RENAL INJURIES

There are several proposed classifications of renal injuries. The primary subgroups are minor and major renal injury, and the role of the radiologist is to define the extent of the renal injury as a guide to treatment, possible surgery, and predictable complications. Minor injuries include:

1. Parenchymal contusions without a tear in the capsule
2. Superficial cortical lacerations without extension to the collecting system and with intact capsule
3. Laceration at the fornices, with small parenchymal lacerations that communicate with the collecting system

Major injuries include the following:

1. Deep parenchymal laceration with extension from the capsular surface to the collecting system. Capsule may be intact or disrupted. Significant subcapsular hemorrhage is present.
2. Shattered kidney. The kidney is disrupted into multiple fragments with extension into the collecting system and the capsular surface. The capsule may be intact or disrupted. Significant perirenal hematoma is present.
3. Vascular pedicle injury with subintimal flap, vascular avulsion, spasm, or vascular thrombosis
4. Ureteropelvic junction avulsion and laceration

The diagnosis of renal injury is made from a history of trauma, flank pain, tenderness, and hematuria. The signs and symptoms may be subtle to profound (shock). Hematuria is almost always present, unless the renal artery is completely occluded, in which case hematuria may be absent.

Helical CT is the imaging modality of choice for evaluating the kidneys in blunt trauma. Unsuspected injuries of other organs are detected in approximately 10% of all children with signs of renal trauma. Sonography is less frequently used in evaluating renal trauma. Studies evaluating the use of sonography in trauma have been increasingly reported in radiology and clinical emergency medicine literature. Generally these studies can be grouped into two types: those that describe (1) the use of sonography to rapidly detect intraperitoneal fluid and a hemodynamically unstable patient to

confirm the presence of hemoperitoneum and (2) the use of sonography to detect intraperitoneal fluid and/or organ injury in a hemodynamically stable patient. However, in approximately 20% to 30% of children with solid organ injuries, no peritoneal fluid can be identified. Similar findings are noted in adult trauma. This statistic suggests that a trauma sonographic examination to assess for free intraperitoneal fluid alone would miss a significant number of abdominal injuries. Therefore, abdominal ultrasound must include organ assessment in addition to fluid identification to fully evaluate intra-abdominal injury.

The purpose of imaging in renal injury is to access accurately the extent of insult. Renal injury can be categorized on the basis of CT findings. CT demonstrates traumatic abnormalities better than any other noninvasive examination. Extravasation of contrast-opacificied urine is sometimes identified on CT, especially if delayed images are obtained.

The most common renal injury is a localized contusion. Renal contusion occurs in more than one half of traumatic insults. The capsule, collecting system, and renal vessels remain unaffected by the insult, but the parenchyma itself is injured. Hemorrhage and parenchymal edema are confined by the intact capsule. Renal blood flow is reduced in proportion to the magnitude of the contusion and the degree of compression of the intrarenal vessels. Reduced renal blood flow can result in a transient decrease in urine output. The most frequent clinical findings, however, are microscopic or gross hematuria and flank pain. An intrarenal hematoma appears on CT as a focal region that lacks enhancement after contrast administration (compared to the decreased or delayed enhancement of the contusion). CT of the contused kidney shows one or more regions of decreased function, which are imaged as areas of poor or delayed enhancement on the nephrogram phase. Intrarenal hematomas are usually poorly marginated. A traumatic renal infarction also fails to enhance and is distinguished from a hematoma by its sharply marginated, wedge-shaped appearance. This abnormality results from the occlusion of one or more intrarenal or polar arterial branches.

Subcapsular hematoma is imaged as fluid in the periphery of the kidney separated from Gerota's fascia by fat. This fluid is usually lenticular in shape and indents the adjacent renal parenchyma. Unenhanced CT images obtained within several hours of injury show that subcapsular hematoma has a slightly higher attenuation than the kidney. Subsequently scans show diminished attenuation as the hematoma liquefies.

When the renal capsule is lacerated, a perirenal hematoma results. Even though the hematoma may be sizable and can result in a clinically detectable flank mass, the hemorrhage remains confined and exsanguination is rare. With this injury, CT shows poor function, a nonenhancing intrarenal mass, and perirenal fluid. It also shows that the fluid is confined by Gerota's fascia. A perirenal hematoma may be an isolated injury, but more frequently it is associated with subcapsular hematoma. In addition to perirenal accumulations, the fluid may extend along the course of the ureter, in the interfascial space or interconal fascia, into an anterior pararenal space, and into the psoas compartment. Rupture into the peritoneal cavity is uncommon. Hypertension may result because of the Goldblatt phenomenon.

Severe renal injury is diagnosed when there is a complete renal laceration, renal fracture, or pulped kidney. The term *complete renal laceration* had been used to define a parenchymal injury that extends into a collecting system and results in urine extravasation. Communication between the collecting system and a perirenal hematoma with this injury can result in urinary obstruction by an intraluminal clot. *Renal fracture* describes a transection of the kidney into two segments. Renal fractures tend to occur along the interlobar divisions; therefore, there is often preservation of the blood supply. A shattered kidney indicates multiple fractures.

Injuries to the vascular pedicle are extremely uncommon in children. Nonpenetrating vascular injuries are produced by obstruction of the pedicle as a result of the lateral renal displacement. Different types of arterial injury may result. If the vessels are completely severed, a large hematoma results. Extravasation is very uncommon. Renal perfusion ceases at the time of injury, and total renal ischemia follows. More commonly, the intima of the renal artery is torn, but the outer muscular layer remains intact. Blood flow at first is decreased; thrombosis develops lateral to the sight of the intimal tear and renal perfusion ceases. Because this process takes a variable amount of time, it is usually impossible to determine the length of time the kidney has been without adequate blood supply. A helical CT should be performed immediately. CT in cases of renal artery damage show lack of contrast enhancement of the kidney, extravasation, and a large retroperitoneal hematoma, and provide information concerning the anatomy of the renal artery and vein.

URETERAL INJURY

Injury to the ureter is uncommon in childhood. The right ureter is more vulnerable to injury than the left, and the mechanism of injury is believed to be compression of the renal pelvis and the upper ureter against the lower portion of the rib cage or the upper lumbar transverse processes. This injury may occur because of the mobility of the spine in the pediatric patient. The diagnosis of this injury may be delayed, and less than half the patients are diagnosed initially. This injury is readily identified with excretory urography or CT. Obliteration of the psoas muscle outline and a focal mass may be seen. There is extravasation of contrast into the perihilar, peripelvic space. Hematuria is not a reliable sign, although it is present in 60% of the patients with this injury. The site of injury is the ureteropelvic junction or the proximal 4 cm of the ureter. Management is surgical. Complications including strictures and fistulas may result if this injury is overlooked; the ureter may also be entrapped by delayed retroperitoneal fibrosis.

BLADDER INJURY

Bladder injuries result most often from blunt trauma and less often from penetrating injuries. The urinary bladder in the child occupies a more abdominal location than in the adult; it is therefore more vulnerable to rupture with blunt abdominal trauma. Pelvic fractures are frequently associated. With severe injuries, rupture may occur. Bladder rupture can occur in an extraperitoneal or intraperitoneal location (or, rarely, both). Extraperitoneal rupture is the most common variety of bladder injury, accounting for more than 80% of the injuries to the urinary bladder. The injury involves the inferior portion of the bladder near the bladder neck. Intraperitoneal rupture can result in a situation of urine reabsorption, which can produce azotemia and severe acidosis. Because there is a broad area of urinary bladder in infants that is covered by peritoneum, any injury to the urinary bladder in an infant is more likely to result in intraperitoneal extravasation than it would in the older child or adult. Signs and symptoms of bladder trauma include hematuria, abdominal pain, painful urination, and urinary retention.

Radiographs are the initial imaging study performed in the evaluation of abdominal or pelvic trauma. The presence of pelvic fracture raises the possibility of bladder or uretheral injury. CT with intravenous contrast material more accurately demonstrates the soft tissue and the osseous abnormalities in the pelvis. The CT findings in bladder injury include localized contrast extravasation, free intraperitoneal contrast extravasation, and paravesicular low-attenuation fluid that shows evidence of contrast accumulating on delayed images. Filling defects in the bladder as a result of clot may also be identified. In cases of bladder rupture, increased soft tissue density is sometimes visible and the pelvis is marked by extravasation of blood and urine.

Extraperitoneal rupture is usually associated with fracture of the superior ramus of the pubis, and is managed conservatively or with drainage and repair. Girls are usually managed by transurethral catheter and boys by suprapubic drainage. Intraperitoneal rupture and laceration may become apparent only when the bladder is distended or during an attempted void and is seen in a steep oblique or lateral projection on cystourethrography. The bladder is usually not deformed. The extravasated contrast may outline loops of bowel or accumulate in the pericolic recesses.

URETHERAL INJURY

Injuries to the urethra result from straddle injuries, pelvic fractures, and occasionally mechanical manipulations such as cystoscopy, uretheral surgery, or catherization. The areas of the male urethra that are particularly vulnerable to injury are the lower portion of the posterior urethra at the urogenital diaphragm, at which point the urethra is firmly fixed to the surrounding structures, and the bulbous urethra, which is vulnerable in straddle injury. The classical injury to the proximal urethra involves shearing the prostatic urethra at the superior leaf of the urogenital diaphragm. This is slightly less common in children because the pelvis is more flexible. In boys, lower abdominal trauma may result in partial or complete vesicourethral avulsion. In girls, much less frequently, a similar injury may result in rupture of the vesicourethrovaginal septum. Urethral tears may be complete or partial. In avulsion of the urethra or complete rupture, the ends of the urethra may remain in good apposition or they may be widely separated. The extravasation of blood and surrounding hematoma into the prostate and about the base of the bladder results in a palpable mass on rectal examination. Laceration of the urogenital diaphragm or tear of the urethra may cause extension of hematoma and urine extravasation into the perineal region. The classical signs of urethral injury include inability to void, urethral pain, and hematuria.

Injury to the bulbous urethra from external trauma is usually the result of a straddle injury and may be associated with fractures. Complete tears are infrequent, but there is usually dorsal urethral rupture (Fig. 4). Urinary retention, hematuria, perineal swelling, and ecchymosis are often present. In the case of a contusion or minor laceration, the lesion may not be detected but will later result in a stricture.

Radiographic diagnosis is established with retrograde urography carried out with a catheter placed in the region of the fossa navicularis or slightly further in the urethra, minimal inflation of the balloon, and hand injection of the contrast. Catheterization of the posterior urethra and bladder should be initially avoided because further trauma can result. Following insertion of a suprapubic catheter, a voiding cystourethrogram may be obtained to evaluate the position and alignment of the uretheral segments and degree of laceration. In the case of avulsion of the posterior urethra, the base of the bladder is elevated and flattened. Incomplete tears of the urethra result in compression of the bladder from the lateral aspects. The compression is often asymmetric. If a catheter is already in place, a urethrogram may be performed by placing a second small catheter beside the indwelling catheter.

The management of urethral trauma differs depending on the site of injury. With prostatomembranous uretheral injury, immediate surgery is performed. This may consist of uretheral realignment or a limited exploration with placement of a suprapubic catheter with delayed repair. The majority of pediatric urologists employ the latter approach. However, immediate urethral approximation is performed for complex posterior urethral injuries associated with rectal perforation, massive pelvic hematomas with superior displaced bladders, and associated injuries of the bladder neck. The incidence of stricture formation with immediate repair versus delayed repair is approximately 70% as compared with 100%. Impotence may occur in approximately 40% after immediate repair and 15% with delayed repair. Incontinence occurs in 20% of patients with immediate repair and 5% with delayed repair. Eventual urethral strictures are repaired by immobilization of the urethra, excision of the stricture, and end-to-end anastomosis using a perineal approach.

Distal uretheral injuries in children are most often associated with iatrogenic etiologies. Urethral strictures may develop following posterior urethral valve ablation.

Urethral injuries in girls are rare but do result from blunt abdominal trauma in vehicular accidents associated with pelvic fractures. Injury will also involve the vagina, and urethrovaginal fistulas may result. Management involves initial suprapubic drainage and delayed

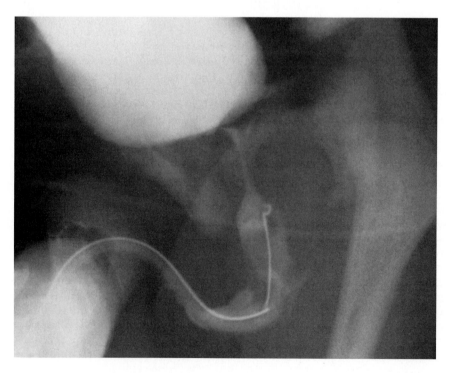

FIGURE 4. A retrograde urethrogram shows blood within the urethra and a tear in the dorsal urethra. This was in an infant who sustained physical abuse.

urethroplasty. These injuries are not well demonstrated with radiologic examination, but a retrograde urethrogram may be performed using syringe injection.

Scrotal Injury

Minor degrees of scrotal trauma are common in boys; however, severe injuries to the testes are rare. Testicular injuries in childhood are most commonly the result of a severe direct blow to the scrotum or a straddle injury; penetrating injuries are distinctly rare. Damage to the testicle occurs when it is forcibly compressed against the pubic bone. Because of the small size and mobility of the testes in a prepubertal child, testicular injuries are exceedingly rare in this age group. A significant injury from a relatively minor trauma suggests a testicular lesion. The right testis is slightly more prone to injury than the left. Physical examination of the scrotum is difficult because of hematocele or hematoma.

A spectrum of injuries can occur as a result of scrotal trauma. Traumatic epididymitis, a noninfectious inflammation of the epididymis, frequently follows a blow to the scrotum. This usually presents several days after the insult. A typical history in this circumstance includes a recent blow to the scrotum causing temporary acute pain; however, after a pain-free interval, the scrotal pain redevelops over several days. The typical abnormalities noted on physical examination may include scrotal erythema and edema and a tender, indurated epididymis. Urinalysis is normal. Doppler sonography is the imaging modality of choice. It will rule out more severe testicular injury and demonstrate the epididymal hyperemia typical of epididymitis. The usual treatment is conservative and is similar to that of nontraumatic epididymitis.

Scrotal trauma also can result in an intratesticular hematoma or a rent of the tunica albuginea, which often can be seen with high-resolution gray-scale images. When the physical findings and sonography demonstrate the tunica albuginea to be intact, surgical intervention is not required. However, if there is any question of testicular laceration, immediate scrotal exploration with hematoma drainage and repair of the laceration is performed.

Blood within the tunica vaginalis, known as hematocele, can be a sign of significant testicular injury. Hematocele can be suspected on physical examination when there is contusion and ecchymosis of the scrotal wall. Sonography identifies the hematocele as a fluid-filled structure contained within the tunica vaginalis with greater echogenicity than the usual hydrocele fluid. In this circumstance, as long as there is no testicular rupture, surgery is not indicated. Again, often scrotal exploration is performed because a large hematocele resolves more rapidly with drainage.

Finally, trauma can induce testicular torsion. The findings on physical examination in this circumstance are identical to those in nontraumatic testicular torsion. Doppler sonography can exclude torsion by identifying arterial blood flow within the testes.

In conclusion, trauma of the scrotum can potentially result in multiple broad-ranging injuries. Most patients with testicular injury should be evaluated with static as well as Doppler sonography to aid the differential diagnosis. Sonography is extremely useful to analyze blood flow, and distinguish testicular from extratesticular pathology. When the imaging study is equivocal, or if the clinical findings alone suggest a testicular injury, emergency scrotal exploration is needed. Patients who do not require surgery can be managed with symptomatic treatment and repeat sonographic imaging.

SUGGESTED READINGS

Urolithiasis

Alon US: Nephrocalcinosis. Curr Opin Pediatr 1997;9:160–165

Alon US, Scagliotti D, Garola RE: Nephrocalcinosis and nephrolithiasis in infants with congestive heart failure treated with furosemide. J Pediatr 1994;125:149–151

Begun FP, Foley WD, Peterson A, et al: Patient evaluation: laboratory and imaging studies. Urol Clin North Am 1997;24:97–116

Bushinsky DA: Nephrolithiasis. J Am Soc Nephrol 1998;9:917–924

Cochat P: Primary hyperoxaluria type 1 [clinical conference]. Kidney Int 1999;55:2533–2547

Dick PT, Shuckett BM, Tang B, et al: Observer reliability in grading nephrocalcinosis on ultrasound examinations in children. Pediatr Radiol 1999;29:68–72

Downing GJ, Egelhoff JC, Daily DK, et al: Furosemide-related renal calcifications in the premature infant: a longitudinal ultrasonographic study. Pediatr Radiol 1991;21:563–565

Goodyer P, Saadi I, Ong P, et al: Cystinuria subtype and the risk of nephrolithiasis [see comments]. Kidney Int 1998;54:56–61

Greenbaum LA: Renal colic as the presenting sign of Cushing syndrome: a case report. Clin Pediatr 1998;37:263–264

Gu LL, Daneman A, Binet A, Koch SW: Nephrocalcinosis and nephrolithiasis due to subcutaneous fat necrosis with hypercalcemia in two full-term asphyxiated neonates: sonographic findings. Pediatr Radiol 1995;25:142–144

Hubert J, Blum A, Cormier L, et al: Three-dimensional CT-scan reconstruction of renal calculi: a new tool for mapping-out staghorn calculi and follow-up of radiolucent stones. Eur Urol 1997;31:297–301

Jantarasami T, Larew M, Kao SC, et al: Ultrasound demonstration of nephrocalcinosis in William's syndrome. J Clin Ultrasound 1989;17:533–534

Karlowicz MG, Adelman RD: What are the possible causes of neonatal nephrocalcinosis? Semin Nephrol 1998;18:364–367

Kimme-Smith C, Perrella RR, Kaveggia LP, et al: Detection of renal stones with real-time sonography: effect of transducers and scanning parameters. AJR Am J Roentgenol 1991;157:975–980

Kraus SJ, Lebowitz RL, Royal SA: Renal calculi in children: imaging features that lead to diagnoses: a pictorial essay. Pediatr Radiol 1999;29:624–630

Langlois V, Bernard C, Scheinman SJ, et al: Clinical features of X-linked nephrolithiasis in childhood. Pediatr Nephrol 1998;12:625–629

Liberman SN, Halpern EJ, Sullivan K, et al: Spiral computed tomography for staghorn calculi. Urology 1997;50:519–524

Nimkin K, Lebowitz RL, Share JC, et al: Urolithiasis in a children's hospital: 1985–1990. Urol Radiol 1992;14:139–143

Pak CY: Kidney stones. Lancet 1998;351:1797–1801

Parekh RS, Smoyer WE, Bunchman TE: Diagnosis and management of primary hyperoxaluria type 1 in infancy [see comments]. Pediatr Transplant 1997;1:48–54

Polinsky MS, Kaiser BA, Baluarte HJ, et al: Renal stones and hypercalciuria. Adv Pediatr 1993;40:353–384

Rosen CL, Brown DF, Sagarin MJ, et al: Ultrasonography by emergency physicians in patients with suspected ureteral colic. J Emerg Med 1998;16:865–870

Rosenfeld DL, Preston MP, Salvaggi-Fadden K: Serial renal sonographic evaluation of patients with Lesch-Nyhan syndrome. Pediatr Radiol 1994;24:509–512

Sakhaee K: Pathogenesis and medical management of cystinuria. Semin Nephrol 1996;16:435–447

Santos-Victoriano M, Brouhard BH, Cunningham RJ 3rd: Renal stone disease in children. Clin Pediatr 1998;37:583–599

Scheinman SJ: Nephrolithiasis. Semin Nephrol 1999;19:381–388

Schurman SJ, Norden AG, Scheinman SJ: X-linked recessive nephrolithiasis: presentation and diagnosis in children [see comments]. J Pediatr 1998;132:859–862

Watts RW, Deltas CC: Primary hyperoxaluria. Contrib Nephrol 1997;122:143–159

Wickham JE: Treatment of urinary tract stones. BMJ 1993;307:1414–1417

Nephrocalcinosis

Alon US: Nephrocalcinosis. Curr Opin Pediatr 1997;9:160–165

Dick PT, Shuckett BM, Tang B, et al: Observer reliability in grading nephrocalcinosis on ultrasound examinations in children. Pediatr Radiol 1999;29:68–72

Downing GJ, Egelhoff JC, Daily DK, et al: Furosemide-related renal calcifications in the premature infant: a longitudinal ultrasonographic study. Pediatr Radiol 1991;21:563–565

Francois M, Tosivint I, Mercadal L, et al: MR imaging features of acute bilateral renal cortical necrosis. Am J Kidney Dis 2000;35:745–748

Gu LL, Daneman A, Binet A, Kooh SW: Nephrocalcinosis and nephrolithiasis due to subcutaneous fat necrosis with hypercalcemia in two full-term asphyxiated neonates: sonographic findings. Pediatr Radiol 1995;25:142–144

Karlowicz MG, Adelman RD: What are the possible causes of neonatal nephrocalcinosis? Semin Nephrol 1998;18:364–367

Patriquin H, Robitaille P: Renal calcium deposition in children: sonographic demonstration of the Anderson-Carr progression. AJR 1986;146:1253–1256

Wickham JE: Treatment of urinary tract stones. BMJ 1993;307:1414–1417

Trauma to the Genitourinary Tract

Abdalati H, Bulas DI, Sivit CJ, et al: Blunt renal trauma in children: healing of renal injuries and recommendations for imaging follow-up. Pediatr Radiol 1994;24:573–576

Abou-Jaoude WA, Sugarman JM, Fallat ME, Casale AJ: Indicators of genitourinary tract injury or anomaly in cases of pediatric blunt trauma. J Pediatr Surg 1996;31:86–90

Batislam E, Ates Y, Germiyanoglu C, et al: Role of title classification in predicting urethral injuries in pediatric pelvic fractures. J Trauma 1997;42:285–287

Benya EC: Imaging pediatric blunt abdominal trauma: computed tomography versus ultrasonography. Pediatr Radiol 1998;28:71–78

Bode PJ, Edwards MJ, Kruit MC, van Vugt AB: Sonography in a clinical algorithm for early evaluation of 1671 patients with blunt abdominal trauma. AJR Am J Roentgenol 1999;172:905–911

Brown SL, Elder JS, Spirnak P: Are pediatric patients more susceptible to major renal injury from blunt trauma? A comparative study. J Urol 1998;160:138–140

Carpio F, Morey AF: Radiographic staging of renal injuries. World J Urol 1999;17:66–70

Chung SE, Frusch DP, Fordham LA: Sonographic appearance of extratesticular fluid and fluid-containing scrotal masses in infants and children: clues to diagnosis. AJR Am J Roentgenol 1999;173:741–745

Daudia A, Hassan TB, Ramsay D: Trauma to a horseshoe kidney. J Accid Emerg Med 1999;16:455–456

Dewbury K: Scrotal ultrasound. Br J Hosp Med 1997;57:10–14

Dewire DM, Begun FP, Lawson RK, et al: Color Doppler ultrasonography in the evaluation of the acute scrotum. J Urol 1992;147:89–91

Elshihabi I, Elshihabi S, Arar M: An overview of renal trauma. Curr Opin Pediatr 1998;10:162–166

Goldman SM, Sandler CM: Upper urinary tract trauma—current concepts. World J Urol 1998;6:62–68

Grasso SN, Keller MC: Diagnostic imaging in pediatric trauma. Curr Opin Pediatr 1998;10:299–302

Herbener TE: Ultrasound in assessment of the acute scrotum. J Clin Ultrasound 1996;24:405–421

Kass EJ, Lundak B: The acute scrotum. Pediatr Clin North Am 1997;44:1251–1266

Kratzik CH, Hain A, Kuber W, et al: Has ultrasound influenced the therapy concept of blunt scrotal trauma? J Urol 1989;142:1243–1246

Learch TJ, Hansch LP, Ralls PW: Sonography in patients with gunshot wounds of the scrotum: imaging findings and their value. AJR Am J Roentgenol 1995;165:879–883

Levy JB, Baskin LS, Ewalt DH, et al: Nonoperative management of blunt pediatric major renal trauma. Pediatr Urol 1993;42:418–424

Lewis CA, Mitchell MJ: The use of real-time ultrasound in the management of scrotal trauma. Br J Radiol 1991;65:792–795

Marcos HB, Noone TC, Semelka RC: MRI evaluation of acute renal trauma. J Magn Reson Imaging 1995;8:989–990

Martinez-Piñeiro L Jr, Cerezo E, Cozar JM, et al: Value of testicular ultrasound in the evaluation of blunt scrotal trauma without haematocele. Br J Urol 1992;69:286–290

Mayor B, Gudinchet E, Wicky S, et al: Imaging evaluation of blunt renal trauma in children: diagnostic accuracy of intravenous pyelography and ultrasonography. Pediatr Radiol 1995;25:214–218

McAleer IM, Kaplan GW, Scherz HC, et al: Genitourinary trauma in the pediatric patient. Pediatr Urol 1993;42:563–568

McGahan JP, Richards JR: Blunt abdominal trauma: the role of emergent sonography and a review of the literature. AJR Am J Roentgenol 1999;172:897–903

McGahan JP, Richards JR, Jones CD, Gerscovich EO: Use of ultrasonography in the patient with acute renal trauma. J Ultrasound Med 1999;18:207–213

Morey AF, Bruce JE, McAninch JW: Efficacy of radiographic imaging in pediatric blunt renal trauma. J Urol 1996;156:2014–2018

Mulhall JP, Gabram SG, Jacobs LM: Emergency management of blunt testicular trauma. Acad Emerg Med 1995;2:639–643

Skoog SJ: Benign and malignant pediatric scrotal masses. Pediatr Clin North Am 1997;44:1229–1250

Stein JP, Kaji DM, Eastman J, et al: Blunt renal trauma in the pediatric population: indications for radiographic evaluation. Pediatr Radiol 1994;44:406–410

Taylor GA: Assessing the impact of imaging information on clinical management and decision making in pediatric blunt trauma. Pediatr Radiol 1998,28:63–65

Wessels H, McAninch JW: Testicular trauma. Images Clin Urol 1992;750

Chapter   4

SPECIAL INFECTIONS

SANDRA K. FERNBACH

ACUTE BACTERIAL PYELONEPHRITIS (ACUTE PYELONEPHRITIS, RENAL OR PERIRENAL ABSCESS)

The terminology of acute kidney infections underwent scrutiny and revision in the early 1990s. A seminal article described how our understanding of the pathophysiology of infection, clearly demonstrated by ultrasound (US) and computed tomography (CT), required that the previous system of categorizing renal infection be changed. Focal processes (previously termed *lobar nephronia, renal phlegmon, or cellulitis*) were shown to occur frequently in a nonlobar distribution. The term *acute bacterial pyelonephritis* was used to encompass all aspects of acute bacterial inflammation, focal and diffuse, and was extended to include severe or complicated infections, including renal abscess.

Children with urinary tract infections (UTIs) present a unique challenge to the clinician and radiologist. The usual signs, symptoms, and laboratory tests that allow distinction between kidney infections and lower UTIs are less reliable in children than in adults. Because the treatment of upper UTIs is so different from that of lower UTIs, it is crucial to make this differentiation as quickly and precisely as possible. This role is given to radiology. Imaging is important to determine if a kidney infection is present, how much of the kidney is involved, and whether antibiotic treatment alone will suffice. Two additional questions are put to the radiologist: When do we image a child with UTI? What modality(ies) do we use?

The techniques, indications, value, and problems with both voiding cystourethrography and nuclear cystography are addressed in Section II, Part V, Chapter 2, page 22. Some form of cystography is usually performed after an acute UTI even though as many as two thirds of these studies will be normal and children with known pyelonephritis or renal scarring may not have reflux. Cystography can be done either subacutely (during the hospitalization) or after a short period (about a month) during which the child receives prophylactic antibiotics. Sonicated material placed into the bladder via catheter can be used in combination with US to diagnose reflux but remains in limited clinical use.

When a child is not responding appropriately to antibiotics, renal US is done to exclude the rare parenchymal abscess that needs drainage. Renal US is more frequently performed, especially in the acute period, to detect structural anomalies that might hinder successful treatment of the infection or that might predispose the child to subsequent infections. However, many obstructive lesions of the urinary tract are detected by prenatal US, long before the children present with infection. Thus, some authors, but not the American Academy of Pediatrics, have suggested that renal US can be eliminated in children with acute UTI.

Pyelonephritis can be demonstrated with many imaging modalities. Despite the number of sonographic changes produced by pyelonephritis, gray-scale US is a modality not particularly sensitive to pyelonephritis, and the infected kidney frequently appears normal. Specific non-Doppler US signs of acute pyelonephritis are renal swelling, loss of definition of the corticomedullary junction, thickening of the walls of the upper urinary tract, renal sinus hyperechogenicity, and focal area(s) of abnormal echogenicity. During an acute infection, the parenchyma may develop small anechoic regions that are not true abscesses; response of these to conservative treatment can be monitored with serial US studies.

Renal abscess is a rare complication and is more often seen in children who are immunocompromised or have diabetes mellitus or sickle cell disease. On US, a true abscess appears as a rounded hypoechoic region with good through-transmission (Fig. 1). The abscess wall becomes thicker as the process progresses. Contrast-enhanced CT (CECT) demonstrates a renal abscess as a rounded region that fails to enhance when contrast is given; this appearance differentiates it from the wedge-shaped, poorly enhancing regions of pyelonephritis (Fig. 2). A thick wall around the abscess is an inconstant finding. Concern about the radiation dose given by CT studies in the pediatric population may limit its use to the subset of children in whom renal abscess is suspected. An enlarging abscess can be drained under US or CT guidance.

Acute infection produces wedge-shaped areas with decreased perfusion on Doppler US. These can be demonstrated with color Doppler US but are better shown with power Doppler. Power Doppler US not as sensitive to pyelonephritis as renal scintigraphy performed well with DMSA but may detect only about 80% of the lesions seen with CECT.

Renal cortical scintigraphy, CECT, and magnetic resonance imaging (MRI) are all used to detect focal areas of pyelonephritis (Figs. 2 and 3). Pyelonephritis-induced areas of ischemia and tubular dysfunction

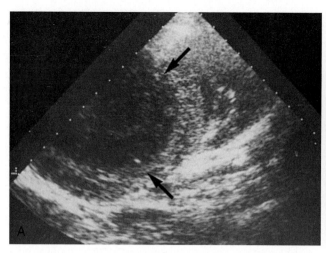 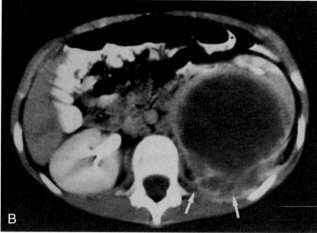

FIGURE 1. Longitudinal ultrasound scan **(A)** of a renal abscess demonstrates a large hypoechoic mass with good through-transmission. A few scattered echoes within the center of the mass suggest that the contents are a thickened fluid or that there are poorly seen septations. The wall of the mass is thickened and more echogenic than the central portion of the mass. **B,** Postcontrast CT. (Courtesy of Dr. A'Delbert Bowen, Pittsburgh, PA.)

become evident after the intravenous injection of isotope, iodinated contrast material, or gadolinium, respectively. In each instance, the injected material does not enter the abnormal parenchyma as much as the normal. CECT changes of acute pyelonephritis (Fig. 2) are focal or diffuse swelling, loss of the definition of the corticomedullary junction, and wedge-shaped, poorly enhancing regions (broadening from center to periphery). Gadolinium-enhanced MRI, using inversion–recovery sequences, demonstrates infected parenchyma as bright regions. Detection of abnormal regions is equally successful with MRI than with renal cortical scintigraphy and eliminates the radiation of CT studies. Furthermore, MRI has a high interobserver agreement for lesions, eliminating another potential pitfall with renal cortical scintigraphy. However, the limited accessibility and high cost of MRI has restricted its clinical use for this purpose.

Renal cortical scintigraphy can be performed by tagging technetium-99m with either dimercaptosuccinic acid (DMSA) or, less frequently, glucoheptonate (GHA). The sensitivity of renal scintigraphy is enhanced

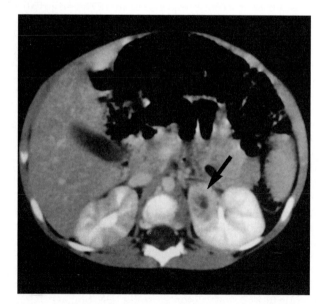

FIGURE 2. Multiple findings of pyelonephritis are evident on this contrast-enhanced computed tomography scan of acute pyelonephritis. Swelling of the left kidney causes it to appear diffusely larger than the right. Along the anteromedial aspect of the left kidney is an abscess; it is seen as a region with very low Hounsfield units values surrounded by a poorly enhancing region *(arrow)*. On the right, multiple poorly enhancing, wedge-shaped regions extend from the renal pelvis to the periphery, another sign of acute pyelonephritis.

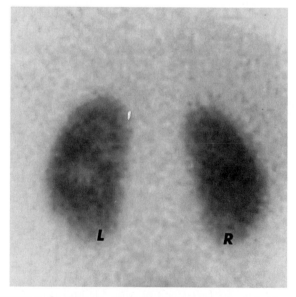

FIGURE 3. On this technetium-99m glucoheptonate study of acute pyelonephritis, obtained from behind, the right kidney appears normal. The infected left kidney diffusely has less isotope than the right and also has some focal areas with even less isotope, an indication of tubulointerstitial edema and diminished blood flow.

when pinhole collimation or single-photon emission CT (SPECT) imaging is added. Unfortunately, a first ^{99m}Tc-DMSA or -GHA study cannot tell active disease from scarred regions because both produce photopenic areas; similarly, an area of nonsuppurative acute pyelonephritis can not be differentiated from an abscess (Fig. 3). Photopenic regions may not regain a normal appearance for up to 5 months, even in the absence of scarring. Gallium-67 SPECT imaging is both sensitive and specific for pyelonephritis and can readily differentiate scars from active infection, but this technique is unlikely to proliferate because of the relatively large radiation dose, especially to growth plates, with this isotope. (Experts in nuclear medicine disagree with this paragraph.)

Excretory urography is rarely performed for diagnosis of UTI. In most instances, the study is normal even when renal infection is present, and, when abnormal, poorly displays the extent of the infection. Multiple described excretory urography findings of renal infection include focal or diffuse renal enlargement, poor uptake and poor excretion of contrast material, and narrowing of the pelvicaliceal system as a result of parenchymal edema.

XANTHOGRANULOMATOUS PYELONEPHRITIS

Xanthogranulomatous pyelonephritis (XPN) is a chronic pyelonephritis that is rare in childhood, being more classically described in females in their fifth through seventh decades. However, it can occur in childhood, even affecting infants. The process, virtually always unilateral, more often involves the entire kidney but may affect only a segment. Contralateral renal hypertrophy is identified in about half of the patients. The infection, usually caused by *Proteus mirabilis* and, less commmonly, *Escherichia coli* or *Staphylococcus aureus*, results in necrotic loss of renal parenchyma. In about 80% of cases, the process dissects into the perirenal space and produces focal adhesions. Further extension of the infection is responsible for some of the less common presentations, including fistulous tracts to skin, psoas muscle, colon, and bronchi. The infected region is composed of areas of multiple abscesses. Grossly, the areas of chronic infection have a nodular yellow appearance. Microscopically, fibrogranulomatous tissue and nodules of lipid-filled macrophages (foam or xanthoma cells) are noted in addition to the areas of necrotic parenchyma. Inflammatory cells are also present.

Both the diffuse and segmental forms have been reported in association with anatomic renal anomalies such as ureteropelvic junction obstruction (more often diffuse) or an obstucted infundibulum or upper moiety in a duplex system (segmental). An association with vesicoureteric reflux has also been noted. A staghorn calculus may be the cause of or secondary to an obstruction at the renal pelvis; smaller renal calculi may also be present.

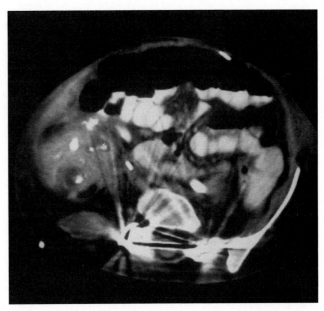

FIGURE 4. Contrast-enhanced computed tomography of xanthogranulomatous pyelonephritis. Metal-induced artifacts are produced by the spinal fixation hardware in this child with spina bifida. The right kidney contains multiple stones. Two stones are surrounded by low-density regions of abscess or tissue necrosis. The process has extended into the perirenal tissues, which are edematous and poorly defined, and into the soft tissues beneath the right abdominal wall, which are thickened.

The focal and diffuse forms can both be tumefactive and simulate other renal masses; in childhood, Wilms' tumor may be suggested. The child may have flank pain or a palpable renal mass. Although few children have hematuria, most have anemia at presentation. Weight loss or failure to thrive may occur. Most affected children will have pyuria. Typical symptoms and signs of acute UTI may be absent. Some children will have a history of repeated UTIs with a poor response to antibiotic therapy.

The radiologic findings of XPN are multiple. Plain abdominal radiographs may show a flank mass with calculi. The kidney is initially enlarged but may decrease in size with longer infections. Excretory urography, no longer a primary modality used in this setting, would show focal or diffuse renal enlargement and focal or diffuse nonfunction or diminished function. More often US is performed as the first study in children with UTI, hematuria, or flank mass. In the diffuse form, US has been reported to show a massively enlarged but reniform kidney; the parenchyma may have increased echogenicity. As the process progresses, the kidney is replaced by necrotic tissue and may appear filled with fluid and debris; the appearance may overlap with that of pyonephrosis. Occasionally, echogenic calculi are demonstrated within the calices, but it may be difficult to appreciate a large calculus in the renal pelvis. In the focal form, the abnormal segment is adjacent to normal-appearing parenchyma. Extension of the process into the perirenal space or adjacent structures may be shown with US but is easier to see with CECT (Fig. 4). CECT also demonstrates the intrarenal calcifications, the necrotic tissue, the nodules of granulation tissue, and lack of function (Fig. 4). MRI findings, reported in a few adult patients, indicate that MRI clearly depicts extrarenal extension but has not proven diagnostically more accurate than CECT.

Increased recognition of the process in children and increased familiarity of the imaging findings have decreased the need for previously used aggressive diagnostic procedures such as retrograde pyelography and renal angiography. Occasionally, if the diagnosis is in doubt, fine-needle aspiration can be used to differentiate the process from a true renal tumor. When the entire kidney is involved, nephrectomy is performed. Focal disease may be treated with resection of the affected parenchyma or nephrostomy (for drainage) with systemic antibiotics.

PYONEPHROSIS

This term applies to the presence of infected material (pus) in the pelvicaliceal system, most often associated with an obstruction. In children, the obstruction is frequently congenital, at the ureteropelvic junction. Prompt diagnosis and treatment (drainage) preserves renal function. Delayed diagnosis may result in severe or chronic renal parenchymal infection and has been implicated in the development of XPN. The organisms most frequently cultured when pyonephrosis is drained are *E. coli* and *Proteus,* also the most common organisms cultured in children with XPN.

The affected child presents with the usual signs and symptoms of UTI. The urine culture will be positive. Hematuria frequently accompanies the infection.

The diagnosis cannot be made with plain films or excretory urography. However, plain films may show a calculus in the renal pelvis, contributing to or caused by the obstruction. The inability of the kidney to concentrate contrast produces either poor or nonvisualization on excretory urography, a nonspecific finding. US is useful to diagnose pyonephrosis when the fluid within the dilated pelvicaliceal system contains gravity-dependent echogenic debris, the pus and particulate matter (crystals) that develop above an obstruction (Fig. 5). However, in some children the fluid may have few internal echoes and be impossible to differentiate from that with uncomplicated hydronephrosis. The renal parenchyma must be carefully assessed to exclude an abscess.

CT can demonstrate the hydronephrotic pelvicaliceal system with gravity-dependent debris below the urine, as seen on US. Calculi may be better appreciated. CT may be used to evaluate the parenchyma, especially to exclude the presence of abscesses. Parenchymal loss may be better seen than with US.

Immediate treatment consists of drainage of the obstructed system, usually under US or CT guidance, and organism-specific antibiotics. If calculi are present, they need to be removed either surgically or with extracorporeal shock wave lithotripsy. To prevent recurrence, the site and cause of the obstruction need to be determined and corrected.

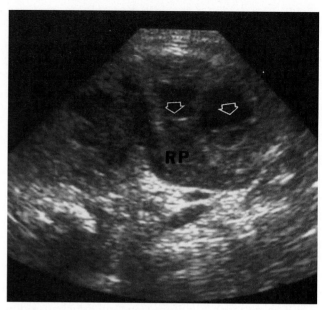

FIGURE 5. Ultrasound scan of pyonephrosis. The pelvicaliceal system is dilated, and debris fills the renal pelvis *(RP).* Debris is also layered beneath the urine in the lower pole calices *(arrows)* and is mixed with the urine in the upper pole calices.

FUNGAL INFECTIONS

Fungal infections rarely occur in a normal host. In pediatrics, the population most frequently affected with urinary tract fungal infections are premature neonates. Children immunocompromised by a malignancy or its treatment, by human immunodeficiency virus (HIV)–induced disease, or on corticosteroids or other immunosuppressive medications may also develop fungal infections. Other predisposing circumstances include open wounds (burns, surgery) and central vascular catheters.

The most common fungal disease involving the urinary tract is *candidiasis,* most often caused by *Candida albicans. Candida* is responsible for about 80% of renal fungal infections. Early reports indicated that about 10% of extremely premature infants had a candidal infection during their initial hospitalization, but a recent large prospective multicenter study by Saiman et al. documented that the risk for candidemia is lower, about 1.2%. In many infants, thrush or other colonization of the gastrointestinal tract precedes the candidemia, presumably the source of renal candidiasis (hematogenous spread). Significant other risk factors for candidemia include a gestational age less than 32 weeks, a 5-minute Apgar score less than 5, shock, disseminated intravascular coagulopathy, prior use of intralipid and parenteral nutrition, and treatment with histamine$_2$ blockers.

Premature neonates are an unusual subpopulation of those who present with UTI. Boys are more frequently involved than girls, with the ratio being as much as 10:1 in those with extremely low birth weight (<1000 g). In this population, the most commonly cultured organism is *Klebsiella*, but *C. albicans* accounts for about 15% of UTIs.

Candida species are the most frequently detected fungal infections in the neonatal nursery. *Candida* infections can manifest as a septic process, or focally infect the brain, the globe, or the urinary tract. The bladder may become infected via the urethra if the perineal skin is colonized. Hematogenous seeding of the kidney produces parenchymal disease that may later pass into the pelvicaliceal system and, from there, the bladder. Neonates with urinary tract involvement may develop hypertension, oliguria, or anuria, changes that could mistakenly attributed to a vascular clot induced by an umbilical artery catheter. Diagnosis of renal candidiasis is made when urine, obtained in a sterile manner, contains *Candida;* when urine and an otherwise sterile body fluid contain *Candida;* or when urine contains *Candida* and changes of candidiasis are demonstrated with renal US.

Because of their fragile state, these neonates are usually studied with bedside US. In the parenchymal phase, the kidneys may be enlarged or have small fluid collections thought to represent abscesses. Increased cortical echogenicity is a described finding in those infants with parenchymal fungal infection but may be difficult to differentiate from the increased cortical echogenicity typical of premature neonates. Fungus balls (mycetomas, fungal bezoars) within the pelvicaliceal system appear as echogenic, nonshadowing structures (Fig. 6) and may cause upper urinary tract obstruction. The initial US is likely to show the mycetoma in those patients with candiduria, but, in a few infants, serial studies are needed before a mycetoma is identified. With treatment, the fungus balls may slowly resolve or calcify. US is likely to show parenchymal disease or fungus balls in about 40% of neonates with

candiduria. Infections limited to the bladder may produce bladder wall thickening or gravity-dependent debris within the bladder lumen.

Doppler US is a complementary part of the examination. It can document normal blood flow, excluding a vascular cause of the oliguria or anuria.

In older children, the presentation is that of a typical UTI: fever, chills, dysuria, and flank pain. Most affected children will have one or more of the risk factors described above.

Medical treatment has proven successful in almost all cases of renal involvement, almost eliminating the need for nephrectomy. Systemic antifungal medication may be augmented by local drainage/installation of antifungal medication. *Candida* infection of the central nervous system has more dire consequences, being associated with long-term psychomotor changes.

The second most common fungal infection that involves the urinary tract, *Aspergillosis*, develops secondary to disease elsewhere, usually in the lungs. The affected population is slightly different than those who develop renal candidiasis, with few premature neonates. Instead, the other immunosupressive processes that are associated with renal candidiasis (see above) underlie the aspergillosis infection of the urinary tract. Diagnosis is usually made with US. A focal renal abscess has the appearance of a mass. A fungus ball may develop in the renal pelvis or bladder. In adults, rare instances of associated ureteral disease have been reported and may result in hydronephrosis.

Blastomycosis is a rare fungal infection that can involve the urinary tract but more commonly involves (in decreasing frequency) the lungs, the skin, the bones, and the central nervous system. Pulmonary disease is seen in over 80% of patients and is the source from which other sites become infected (hematogenous spread). *Cryptococcosis* usually involves the central nervous system (meninges and parenchyma) in immunocompromised patients. A few reports describe renal changes, including papillary necrosis and abscess formation, but there are no reports of imaging in an affected pediatric population.

TUBERCULOSIS OF THE URINARY TRACT

Although genitourinary tract tuberculosis is a major cause or infertility in third world nations, involvement of the genital tract is rarely encountered in the pediatric population, especially in North America, where UTI is seen instead. A rise in the number of tuberculosis cases has been documented to parallel the spread of HIV-related illness.

Primary pulmonary tuberculosis may spread hematogenously to many organs. Although the kidney is the most commonly seeded site, accounting for as much as 30% of extrapulmonary disease, urinary tract tuberculosis remains an uncommon and perhaps underdiagnosed clinical problem in childhood. The lower urinary

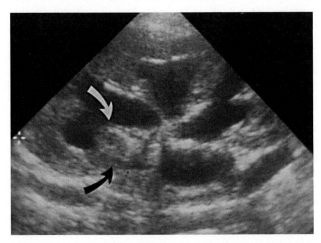

FIGURE 6. Ultrasound of left kidney in a premature infant with urinary candidiasis showing hydronephrosis and a small fungus ball in the right upper collecting system *(arrows)*. (Courtesy of Dr. Beverly Wood, Los Angeles, CA.)

tract is infected by antegrade seeding (submucosal, lymphatic) from the infected upper tract. Urinary tract disease may become apparent years after the initial infection as a result of reactivation of the original deposits of the bacterium; the lungs, mediastinum, and pleura have frequently healed without scarring by the time the renal disease is detected. Usual urinary tract symptoms at presentation are frequency and dysuria. Abdominal and flank pain more commonly occur in affected children than adults. Sterile pyuria is noted in about 25% of cases and may be accompanied by microscopic hematuria or urine with an acid pH. Diagnosis is made by urine culture and specific staining of the urine for *Mycobacterium tuberculosis,* augmented by skin testing and, when applicable, biopsy of affected structures.

The bacterium is deposited in at the corticomedullary junction, where tubercles form, enlarge, coalesce, and spread the infection to both the cortex and the medulla. Early treatment may prevent irreversible changes of parenchymal loss and fibrosis. The radiographic appearance of the affected kidney is dependent on the stage of the disease at the time of detection. There may be no change acutely. Although the hematogenous process infects both kidneys, radiologically unilateral disease is the rule. Parenchymal necrosis is associated with loss of renal parenchyma and, later, dystrophic calcification. Calcifications can be in the form of small, poorly seen nodules or the markedly calcified kidney that has undergone autonephrectomy. Focal disease with secondary stricture formation in the pelvicaliceal system may result in dilatation of the calix or calices above.

Plain films may demonstrate calcifications. Excretory urography shows changes that parallel the pathologic process. Acutely, edema or large tubercles can compress and distort the caliceal system. Later, poor or delayed renal function may be noted. As tubercles coalesce and cavitation develops, contrast may pool in the parenchyma. The classical moth-eaten appearance of a calix is due to focal edema and usually precedes adjacent papillary necrosis. Strictures of a calix, infundibulum, or the renal pelvis form late and cause obstruction with focal dilatation or hydronephrosis.

Ureteral changes rarely occur without visible renal disease. The ureteral disease also changes with time, from an acute inflammatory process of the mucosa producing irregularity on contrast studies to later granuloma formation associated with ureteral nodularity or notching. The normal undulant course of the ureter may be lost as the ureter becomes narrowed and straightened or beaded. Lower ureteral strictures may form with consequent hydroureteronephrosis.

The involvement of the bladder similarly progresses from the mucosa to bladder wall. The initial mucosal irregularity is followed by bladder wall thickening. Eventual fibrosis and contraction of the bladder produces voiding abnormalities as well as a small-volume bladder on imaging. Bladder wall calcification can develop but is rare in childhood. Vesicoureteral reflux is a frequent result of any form of bladder tuberculosis.

On CT, the infection may be difficult to differentiate from other infections that produce parenchymal thinning, necrosis, and calcification, such as XPN and pyonephrosis.

Multiple-drug antituberculous medication is routinely given when genitourinary tuberculosis is diagnosed. Surgery is needed to treat strictures of the upper and lower urinary tract but should not be performed hastily, because some apparent strictures are areas of edema that will regress during treatment and because all developing strictures may not be clinically apparent for several months. Bladder augmentation may be needed.

SCHISTOSOMIASIS (BILHARZIASIS)

Humans are an intermediate host in any infection with the *Schistosoma* species. Of the three schistosoma species that affect humans (*japonicum, mansoni, haematobium*) only *S. haematobium* produces changes in the urinary tract.

Also referred to a bilharziasis, primary infection with *S. haematobium* is rare in North America and Europe but is common in parts of Africa and the Middle East. However, increased immigration from and travel to and from these regions has extended the infected population beyond the endemic regions. In all studies, boys and men outnumber female patients. Most of the literature reports pediatric and adult patients together.

The cercaria stage of the parasite lives in fresh water, enters the bodies of bathers, and there goes through its life cycle. Acutely, there may be a flu-like illness associated with some lymphadenopathy, sun sensitivity, and eosinophilia (Katayama syndrome).

The fluke migrates and establishes itself in the venules of the bladder wall, just beneath the mucosa. At this site, it produces large quantities of ova that break out of the venules and pass into the surrounding tissues (both bladder and adjacent ureter) or into the bladder lumen directly or via the ureter. This process is associated with hematuria, which can be gross or microscopic. Protein and eosinophils may be detected in the urine. Urine samples can be tested for ova (because of the diurnal rhythm of the parasite, the best sampling time is midday), but only about 45% of those with infection proven by other techniques, including serology, will have ova in their urine. Later clinical and radiographic changes are due to the ova and the host response to them.

As many as 50% of those patients proven to have schistosomiasis will be asymptomatic. About 50% will show changes on US, the technique most frequently used to assess the urinary tract in endemic regions. Not surprisingly, the bladder is more likely to demonstrate changes on imaging than is the upper tract. Acutely, little change may be appreciated with US. The subacute inflammatory response manifests as bladder wall thickening (most common in children under 10 years) and mucosal irregularity, which can progress to polyp/ pseudopolyp formation (most common in children ages 10 to 14 years). Fewer acute changes are seen in adults, but bladder wall fibrosis may develop later in the course of the disease. Calcification of the bladder wall occurs when large amounts of ova are deposited in it and is seen almost exclusively in adults.

US can also be used to evaluate the response of the bladder to treatment. Severe bladder changes regress more quickly and more dramatically than minor ones. Recurrence of the early bladder changes, sometimes referred to as resurgence, is more common in those whose initial studies demonstrated more pronounced disease and in those who continue to have exposure to the parasite.

The lower ureter, especially the segment close to the bladder, shows pathologic changes that parallel those noted in the bladder. Dilatation of the pelvicaliceal system may follow. Such changes are more frequently seen in those 10 to 19 years of age. When antiparisitic medications are given, these abnormalities regress, but less often and less completely than abnormalities in the bladder.

Excretory urography is uncommonly performed in affected children, partially because of the medical circumstances in the endemic regions, and partially because it does not demonstrate the changes as well. However, as on US, lower tract changes are more obvious. The ureters have diminished numbers of peristaltic waves and may appear dilated as a result of distal ureteral edema. Later, distal ureteral strictures develop, especially in the intravesical portion. Ureteral changes may ascend and take the form of multiple stenoses or granulomas. Bilateral disease is the rule, although the changes are usually not symmetric. Secondary dilatation of the upper tract may occur.

Genital pathology can develop but is rarely encountered in a pediatric population. Reproductive problems (infertility/ectopic pregnancy) follow schistosome-induced adnexal inflammation. Prostatic fibrosis has been described in adult males.

SUGGESTED READINGS

Acute Pyelonephritis

Alon US, Ganapathy S: Should renal ultrasonography be done routinely in children with first urinary tract infection? Clin Pediatr (Phila) 1999;38:21

American Academy of Pediatrics, Committee on Quality Improvement, Subcommittee on Urinary Tract Infection: Practice Parameter: the diagnosis, treatment, and evaluation of the initial urinary tract infection in febrile infants and young children. Pediatrics 1999;103(4 Pt 1):843

Chan YL, Chan KW, Yeung CK, et al: Potential utility of MRI in the evaluation of children at risk of renal scarring. Pediatr Radiol 1999;29:856

Dacher JN, Pfister C, Monroc M, et al: Power Doppler sonographic pattern of acute pyelonephritis in children: comparison with CT. AJR Am J Roentgenol 1996;166:1451

Darge K, Troeger J, Duetting T, et al: Reflux in young patients: comparison of voiding US of the bladder and retrovesical space with echo enhancement versus voiding cystourethrography for diagnosis. Radiology 1999;210:201

Dascher JN, Avni F, Francois A, et al: Renal sinus hyperechogenicity in acute pyelonephritis: description and pathological correlation. Pediatr Radiol 1999;29:179

Ditchfield MR, Nadel H: The DMSA scan in paediatric urinary tract infection. Australas Radiol 1998;42:318

Jequier S, Jequier JC, Hanquinet S: Acute childhood pyelonephritis:

predictive value of positive sonographic findings in regard to later parenchymal scarring. Acad Radiol 1998;5:344

Laguna R, Silva F, Orduna E, et al: Technetium-99m MAG3 in early identification of pyelonephritis in children. J Nucl Med 1998;39:1254

Lonergan GJ, Pennington DJ, Morrison JC, et al: Childhood pyelonephritis: comparison of gadolinium-enhanced MR imaging and renal cortical scintigraphy for diagnosis. Radiology 1998;207:377

Paterson A, Frush DP, Donnelly LF: Helical CT of the body: are settings adjusted for pediatric patients? AJR Am J Roentgenol 2001;176:297

Piepsz A, Blaufox MD, Gordon I, et al: Consensus on renal cortical scintigraphy in children with urinary tract infection. Semin Nucl Med 1999;29:160

Poutschi-Amin M, Leonidas JC, Palestro C, et al: Magnetic resonance imaging in acute pyelonephritis. Pediatr Nephrol 1998;12:579

Rossleigh MA, Farnsworth RH, Leighton DM, et al: Technetium-99m dimercaptosuccinic acid scintigraphy studies of renal cortical scarring and renal length. J Nucl Med 1998;39:1280

Sorantin E, Fotter R, Aigner R, et al: The sonographically thickened wall of the upper urinary tract system: correlation with other imaging methods. Pediatr Radiol 1997;27:667

Stokland E, Hellstrom M, Jacobsson B, et al: Evaluation of DMSA scintigraphy and urography in assessing acute and permanent renal damage in children. Acta Radiol 1998;39:447

Talner LB, Davidson AJ, Lebowitz RL, et al: Acute pyelonephritis: can we agree on terminology? Radiology 1994;192:297

Yen TC, Tzen KY, Chen WP, et al: The value of Ga-67 renal SPECT in diagnosing and monitoring complete and incomplete treatment in children with acute pyelonephritis. Clin Nucl Med 1999;24:669

Xanthogranulomatous Pyelonephritis and Pyonephrosis

Cousins C, Somers J, Broderick N, et al: Xanthogranulomatous pyelonephritis in childhood: ultrasound and CT diagnosis. Pediatr Radiol 1994;24:210

Hammadeh MY, Nicholls G, Calder CJ, et al: Xanthogranulomatous pyelonephritis in childhood: pre-operative diagnosis is possible. Br J Urol 1994;73:83

Levy M, Baumal R, Eddy AA: Xanthogranulomatous pyelonephritis in children: etiology, pathogenesis, clinical and radiologic features and management. Clin Pediatr 1994;33:360

Matthews GJ, McLorie GA, Churchill BA, et al: Xanthogranulomatous pyelonephritis in pediatric patients. J Urol 1995;153:1958

Perez LM, Netto JM, Induhara R, et al: Xanthogranulomatous pyelonephritis in an infant with an obstructed upper pole renal moiety. Urology 1999;54:744

Quinn FM, Dick AC, Corbally MT, et al: Xanthogranulomatous pyelonephritis in childhood. Arch Dis Child 1999;81:483

Schneider K, Helmig FJ, Eife R, et al: Pyonephrosis in childhood—is ultrasound sufficient for diagnosis? Pediatr Radiol 1989;19:302

Takamizawa S, Yamataka A, Kaneko K, et al: Xanthogranulomatous pyelonephritis in childhood: a rare but important clinical entity. J Pediatr Surg 2000;35:1554

Fungal Infections

Benjamin DK Jr, Fisher RG, McKinney RE Jr, et al: Candidal mycetoma in the neonatal kidney. Pediatrics 1999;104(5 Pt 1):1126

Bryant K, Maxfield C, Rabalais G: Renal candidiasis in neonates with candiduria. Pediatr Infect Dis J 1999;18:959

Eliakim A, Dolfin T, Korzets Z, et al: Urinary tract infection in premature infants: the role of imaging studies and prophylactic therapy. J Perinatol 1997;17:305

Hitchcock RJ, Pallett A, Hall MA, et al: Urinary tract candidiasis in neonates and infants. Br J Urol 1995;76:252

Khoory BJ, Vino L, Dall'Agnola A, et al: Candida infections in newborns: a review. J Chemother 1999;11:367

Saiman L, Ludlington E, Pfaller M, et al: Risk factors for candidemia in neonatal intensive care unit patients. The National Epidemiology of Mycosis Survey study group. Pediatr Infect Dis J 2000;19:319

Wise GJ, Talluri GS, Marella VK: Fungal infections of the genitourinary system: manifestations, diagnosis, and treatment. Urol Clin North Am 1999;26:701

Tuberculosis of the Urinary Tract

Chattopadhyay A, Bhatnagar V, Agarwala S, et al: Genitourinary tuberculosis in pediatric surgical practice. J Pediatr Surg 1997;32:1283

Engin G, Acuna B, Acuna G, et al: Imaging of extrapulmonary tuberculosis. Radiographics 2000;20:471

Ferrie BG, Rundle JS: Genitourinary tuberculosis in patients under twenty-five years of age. Urology 1985;25:576

Harisinghani MG, McLoud T, Shepard JO, et al: Tuberculosis from head to toe. Radiographics 2000;20:449

Weinberg AC, Boyd SD: Short-course chemotherapy and role of surgery in adults and pediatric genitourinary tuberculosis. Urology 1988;31:95

Schistosomiasis

Hatz CF: The use of ultrasound in schistosomiasis. Adv Parasitol 2001;48:225

Palmer PE: Schistosomiasis. Semin Roentgenol 1998;33:6

Richter J: Evolution of schistosomiasis-induced pathology after therapy and interruption of exposure to schistosomes: a review of ultrasonographic studies. Acta Trop 2000;77:111

Wagatsuma Y, Aryeetey ME, Sack DA, et al: Resolution and resurgence of Schistosoma haematobium-induced pathology after community-based chemotherapy in Ghana, as detected by ultrasound. J Infect Dis 1999;179:1515

Whitty CJ, Mabey DC, Armstrong M, et al: Presentation and outcome of 1107 cases of schistosomiasis from Africa diagnosed in a non-endemic country. Trans R Soc Trop Med Hyg 2000;94:531

Chapter 5

RENOVASCULAR DISORDERS

JOHN R. STY

RENAL FAILURE

ACUTE RENAL FAILURE

Renal failure represents a sudden decrease in and eventual cessation of renal function as a result of a pathophysiologic event and is characterized by oliguria or anuria, electrolyte imbalance, acidosis, and progressive increase in serum creatinine and urea levels. Clinical conditions that may produce acute renal failure (ARF) include hypotension, shock, renal ischemia, rhabdomyolysis, drug toxicity, nephrotoxicity, sepsis, asphyxia, autoimmune disease, urinary tract obstruction, and primary renal disease. Acute renal failure in the child population is almost 20% of the adult incidence. Among children, however, age-related incidence is highest in the neonate/infant population and is comparable to the incidence in adults. Intensive care is needed in about 40% of these children. For all ages, hemolytic–uremic syndrome is the most common etiology (40%). Surgery for congenital heart disease, trauma, and major congenital gastrointestinal disease accounts for 65% of cases during the neonatal period. The overall mortality is approximately 20%. Primary renal disease accounts for less than 10% of cases and frequently is the etiology for the majority of patients who require chronic renal replacement therapy.

ARF is frequently an event secondary to other organ failure, and the majority of the mortality arises from severe congenital disease.

Prerenal Acute Renal Failure

Seen most commonly in the neonate and infant, prerenal ARF results from hypoperfusion of an otherwise normal kidney and may be the end result of hemorrhage, dehydration, shock, hypoxemia, or congestive heart failure. The infant kidney is vulnerable to hypoperfusion because renal blood flow is proportionately lower in neonates and infants, and glomerular filtration is low, especially in infants with respiratory abnormalities. Traumatic delivery, prenatal hypoxia, placental hemorrhage, renal vein thrombosis, or administration of large doses of hypertonic contrast material may precipitate ARF.

The normal full-term infant produces between 15 and 50 ml of urine per 24 hours during the first 48 hours of life and 50 to 100 ml/kg/day during the next month. The term oliguria indicates urine output of less than 1 ml/hour. Renal failure is defined as anuria or oliguria when the blood urea nitrogen level is greater than 20 mg/dl and the serum creatinine level is greater than 1 mg/dl.

Information from radionuclide studies, when combined with sonography, is useful in differentiating prerenal, renal, and postrenal causes of ARF. By evaluating renal perfusion, function, and excretion, prerenal conditions, such as renal artery thrombosis or stenosis, can be distinguished from renal causes such as acute tubular necrosis (ATN) and from postrenal causes such as obstruction or extravasation of urine. Functional evaluation requires a measurement of effective renal plasma flow (ERPF) with ^{131}I-orthoiodohippurate (^{131}I-OIH), a measurement of glomerular filtration rate (GFR) with ^{99m}Tc-diethylenetriaminepentaacetic acid (^{99m}Tc-DTPA) and determination of the filtration fraction (or ratio of GFR to ERPF).

Prerenal ARF has a delayed ^{131}I-OIH uptake peak and a decreased ERPF and infiltration fraction. ATN is characterized by delayed ^{131}I-OIH uptake, but filtration fraction in this condition most often tends to be high. The uptake of the radiopharmaceutical in the later phase of the study is related to prognosis, although the time taken for the eventual return to normal function cannot be predicted.

Neonates with anuria or oliguria from prerenal or renal pathology may show an abnormal renal parenchymal appearance on sonography. The most common pattern is usually diffusely increased cortical echogenicity. Evaluation of the renal arteries may provide additional information. Any increase in intra-arterial pressure results in decreased flow. The diastolic flow occurs at the lowest pressure during the cardiac cycle, so it will decrease or be absent before systolic Doppler flow curves are affected appreciably. The etiologies of increased intra-arterial resistance to flow can be classified as intravascular, perivascular, and perirenal. Any decrease in the size of the lumen of small intrarenal arteries or arterioles leads to increased resistance to flow. However, compression of small vessels by intrarenal edema, such as occurs in renal vein thrombosis, may result in an identical arterial Doppler pattern. Also, obstruction of the urinary tract leads to similar Doppler findings.

Intrinsic Acute Renal Failure

This category of renal failure is associated with an insult to the renal parenchyma. The conditions that are responsible for prerenal ARF may result in intrinsic ARF if the ischemic event is severe and prolonged. Renal cortical and renal medullary necrosis, hemolytic–uremic syndrome, acute immune-related nephropathies, rhabdomyolysis, and Tamm-Horsfall proteinuria result in intrinsic ARF. ATN, renal cortical necrosis, or renal medullary necrosis reflects the etiology, length, and severity of the ischemia. ATN from hypoperfusion, hypoxia, shock, and disseminated intravascular coagulation contributes to the development of ARF. Renal artery or renal vein thrombosis frequently produces ARF in the neonate.

Renal Cortical Necrosis

In renal cortical necrosis, the cortex of both kidneys is affected in a similar manner with a similar distribution. Renal sonography characteristically shows the pattern of increased cortical echogenicity and accentuation of the corticomedullary junction. The renal pyramids usually are not affected and remain hypoechoic. Sonography is useful evaluating parenchymal renal disease because it will estimate renal size and assess the changes in renal parenchyma. Frequently early in the course of the disease, sonography is normal except for slight neph-romegaly. Eventually, abnormal increased echogenicity is visible, usually being prominent in the glomerular and subcortical region. This increased echogenicity is frequently the result of fine calcification and collagen deposition. Depending on the severity and duration of the process, sonography can be used to detect the parenchymal changes that occur in acute cortical necrosis and to follow the renal findings sequentially.

Renal Medullary Necrosis

In renal medullary necrosis (papillary necrosis) the ischemic event occurs predominantly in the interstitium of the renal pyramids. There is ischemic necrobiosis of the medulla (loops of Henle and vasa recta) secondary to interstitial edema or intrinsic vascular obstruction. The etiologies include pyelonephritis, obstruction, sickle cell disease, nephrotoxic chemicals, and renal vein thrombosis. It occasionally follows or is associated with dehydration, hemophilia, severe infantile diarrhea, and high-dose intravenous contrast.

Historically, this abnormality was divided into central medullary and papillary categories. It is now appreciated, however, that these actually represent variations of the same pathophysiologic process. These terms are sometimes used to indicate the areas of greatest involvement in individual cases. Current terminology includes three forms of papillary necrosis. Necrosis "in situ" occurs when the necrotic papilla detaches but remains unextruded within its bed. In the medullary form, partial sloughing of the papilla results in a single irregular cavity located concentrically or eccentrically in the papilla, with the long axis paralleling the long axis of the papilla and communicating with the calyx. The papillary form occurs when the entire papilla is sloughed. The process can be localized or diffuse. Bilateral distribution results from systemic etiologies. The unilateral disease can be seen in obstruction, renal vein thrombosis, and acute bacterial nephritis.

The imaging findings are variable. The kidneys may be large or small, as seen in analgesic nephropathy. In the acute stage there may be bilateral renal enlargement. The margins of the kidney are usually reniform and smooth. When contrast is used to evaluate the urinary tract, there is frequently diminished density in the nephrogram phase. The fornices widen as a result of necrotic shrinkage, and the calyces may be club shaped when the papilla detaches. On occasion there will be displacement to the collecting system from an enlarged septal cortex that is edematous. Intraluminal filling defects occur when there are contained sloughed papillae. On occasion, calcifications can be seen in the papillae and may be ring-like if attached to the papillae. Sonography shows highly echogenic papillae. In the medullary form of necrosis, the process is limited to the center of the papilla, whereas, in the papillary type, the entire papilla becomes necrotic. The papillary form usually shows symmetric involvement. Late stages seen on excretory urography or sonography reflect this type of pattern. In the medullary form, there is sinus formation and intrapapillary cavitation. Small rings indicate the segment of necrotic tissue contained in the central cavities. In the papillary form of necrosis, the urogram or sonogram is unremarkable until the necrotic papillae separate and a sonolucent ring is demonstrated around the sloughed papillae. When the process is complete, club-like calices remain. With severe combined necrosis (cortical and medullary), the affected kidney becomes smaller secondary to diffuse or focal scarring. Similar imaging findings are seen with reflux nephropathy.

Hemolytic–Uremic Syndrome

Hemolytic–uremic syndrome is characterized by the rapid onset of microangiopathies, thrombocytopenia, hemolytic anemia, and renal failure of varying degrees. The pathology is a microangiopathy that includes endothelium swelling and thrombus formation. The kidney is the main target of involvement, although the intestines, lung, and brain may be affected. The syndrome is initiated by a viral respiratory or gastrointestinal infection. In most cases of hemolytic–uremic syndrome, the following symptoms occur in otherwise healthy infants: fever, vomiting, bloody diarrhea, and abdominal discomfort. The child, usually around 3 years of age, may become critically ill with signs and symptoms that include pallor, irritability, seizures, heart failure, hypertension, gastrointestinal bleeding, and oliguria. A few have only minimal renal manifestations, indicated by a transient decrease in the volume of urine output. ARF that lasts for 1 to 4 weeks is followed by slow improvement. In most cases recovery is complete, but some children have permanent neurologic or renal damage. In approximately 20% of cases, there is a progressive deterioration of renal function that may lead to chronic uremia.

During the acute phase of hemolytic–uremic syndrome, radiographs of the abdomen may show renal enlargement. Frequently the colon is distended with air. "Thumbprinting" may be identifiable in the colon wall. In most patients, renal size returns to normal as the disease resolves, but, in those who sustain a more severe injury, there is eventually shrinking of the kidney, and calcification may develop in regions of the cortex.

Sonography is useful in hemolytic–uremic syndrome for estimating renal size and assessing the changes in the renal parenchyma. Early in the disease, sonography is normal or shows minimal nephromegaly. Eventually, abnormal increased echogenicity is visible, usually being most prominent in the glomerular and subcortical regions. The degree of cortical echogenicity correlates with the severity of the illness.

The renal arterial narrowing that occurs in hemolytic–uremic syndrome causes resistance to blood flow that can be demonstrated on Doppler examination. With severe disease, intrarenal arterial flow may not be detectable, or systolic Doppler signals are identified and diastolic Doppler shifts are absent or reversed. With clinical improvement, early diastolic flow reappears and Doppler signal is absent at the end of dyastole. With complete regression of arterial obstruction, the Doppler signal pattern returns to normal. Doppler studies in these children may be utilized to help determine the severity of the illness and predict the course of recovery.

Tamm-Horsfall Proteinuria

Tamm-Horsfall protein, a normal protein found in the luminal side of the distal tubule, has been identified in the interstitial tissue of kidneys in patients with vesicoureteral reflux and reflux nephropathy. It has also been identified as a causative agent in tubular obstruction in patients with proteinuria secondary to asphyxia, sepsis, administration of hypertonic agents, or other etiologies of ARF. This protein probably elicits a cellular immune response by the lymphocytes of individuals with renal damage, and it is thought to be a humoral response to a foreign antigen within the kidney. In neonates, Tamm-Horsfall proteinuria occurs, which may result in anuria and oliguria. On sonography, Tamm-Horsfall proteinuria is characterized by normal-appearing renal cortex and hyperechoic medulla (Fig. 1). With resolution, the medullary pyramids become hypoechoic.

There have been rare cases of transient neonatal nephromegaly that simulates recessive polycystic kidney disease. In some cases, urography performed early in life in infants with bilateral renal enlargement reveals findings characteristic or thought to be characteristic of recessive polycystic kidney disease, but repeat urography later in life reveals normal architecture and renal size. The cause of the nephromegaly is thought to be transient intratubular obstruction of unknown etiology. This may be due to the interaction between urographic contrast media and Tamm-Horsfall protein. Consequently, these children should be studied sequentially, and parents and siblings should be studied with sonography.

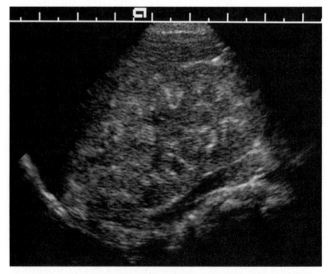

FIGURE 1. Longitudinal renal sonogram in a neonate. The image shows normal, slightly increased echogenicity in the renal cortex and a hyperechoic medulla with Tamm-Horsfall proteinuria.

Nephropathy of Sickle Cell Anemia

Nephropathy of sickle cell anemia involves the entire renal parenchyma. Microscopy reveals cortical changes of dilatation and engorgement of capillary tufts, glomerulosclerosis, increased mesangial matrix, and iron deposition in the glomerular epithelium and glomerular basement membrane. Glomerular, cortical, and medullary capillaries show engorgement and contain sickled erythrocytes. Renal function and structural alterations have been described in sickle cell disease. These include a defective ability to concentrate the urine and a defect in hydrogen ion production that leads to deterioration of the metabolic homeostatic mechanisms. An abnormally high GFR, ERPF, and tubular excretion of *para*-iminohippuric acid have been identified. These abnormally high values are found in children and tend to decrease until about the age of 40. A low creatinine clearance rate can occur in children with sickle cell disease; this is probably associated with glomerular abnormalities. Histologically, glomerular sclerosis may progress to complete obliteration of the glomerular tufts.

In sickle cell disease, the red blood cells tend to develop their abnormal sickle shape in the renal medulla because of the local high osmolality and low oxygen tension in this region. The sickled cells cause sludging in the vessels of the medulla, leading to occlusion and necrosis. Blunting of the calyces and cortical hypertrophy, with or without papillary necrosis, result in the characteristic imaging finding of the infundibular collecting system that is sometimes termed *sickle cell calyectasis.*

Nephromegaly, usually bilateral, is common in sickle cell disease. Enlarged kidneys with bizarre-looking collecting system may suggest this disorder. Small kidneys are the end result of infarction and fibrosis. A perirenal hematoma can occur as a complication of renal infarction. However, most of the findings related to the urinary system are found in children who have had the disease well established years prior.

Sonographic examination of the kidney shows diffuse enlargement, hyperechogenicity, and loss of well-defined cortical medullary tissue. Magnetic resonance imaging (MRI) indicates changes peculiar to sickle cell disease and is characterized by decreased cortical signal relative to medulla on T_1-weighted and T_2-weighted images. These changes reflect abnormality of iron deposition in the renal cortex.

Henoch-Schönlein Purpura

Henoch-Schönlein purpura is a cause of nephritis in children between the ages of 3 and 10. It is usually preceded by upper respiratory infection 1 to 3 weeks before the onset of the syndrome. Clinical manifestations are found in the skin, joints, gastrointestinal tract, and kidneys. The pattern and degree of renal involvement vary widely, with reported incidences ranging from 20% to 90%. The urinary system abnormality and Henoch-Schönlein purpura are sometimes transient and may go undetected unless examination of the urinary sediment is performed. Twenty percent to 30% of patients have hematuria, and 30% to 70% have proteinuria. The clinical features of renal involvement are similar to those of acute poststreptococcal glomerulonephritis. In Henoch-Schönlein purpura, the whole clinical spectrum of glomerulonephritis may occur. If the proteinuria is profound, it may lead to nephrotic syndrome and is accompanied by renal insufficiency. Clinical signs of renal involvement may follow or coincide with the appearance of the purpura, but they rarely antedate it. The incidence of renal involvement is higher in patients with recurrent attacks of purpura and in patients with abdominal manifestations. Henoch-Schönlein purpura is usually a self-limited disease, but in some cases it can be complicated by hypertension and chronic renal failure.

The imaging findings in Henoch-Schönlein purpura are similar to those of acute glomerulonephritis. Sonographic findings include normal or bilaterally enlarged kidneys with diffuse increase in echogenicity of the renal cortex. The cortical echogenicity may be greater than that of the adjacent liver, and the medullary pyramids appear prominent in contrast to the hyperechoic cortex. The echogenicity of the renal cortex decreases with the regression of the acute disease, the urographic findings in Henoch-Schönlein purpura likewise are similar to those characteristic findings found in acute glomerulonephritis. In a few patients, intramural hematomas may be seen in the bladder wall as well as the ureter. Testicular involvement is described in 2% to 3% of patients. Painful scrotal hematomas occasionally mimic testicular torsion. An uncommon complication is the development of unilateral hydronephrosis and ureteral beading that may be due to ureteral fibrosis.

Systemic Lupus Erythematosus

Systemic lupus erythematosus involves the kidneys in 50% to 75% of patients. The prognosis is poor in children with renal involvement, with only 50% surviving 5 years following the diagnosis. Sonography demonstrates kidneys that are normal or slightly increased in size. The renal cortex is echogenic, and there is accentuation of the corticomedullary junction. At times within the cortex are multiple, variable-sized and -shaped areas of decreased echogenicity. Abnormal creatinine clearance correlates with the degree of abnormality identified in the renal cortex. Renal size correlates directly with the degree of renal impairment. The smaller the kidneys, the more abnormal the echo pattern.

Rhabdomyolysis

Rhabdomyolysis will occur after severe muscle injury or secondary to toxic drug reactions. If extensive systemic disruption of muscles results and there is a release of sarcoplasm into the systemic circulation, an elevation of levels of myoglobin and creatine phosphokinase occurs. ARF develops from inspissated myoglobin plugs in the renal tubules and the loops of Henle, decreased glomerular filtration secondary to toxic effect of myoglobin, and direct nephrotoxicity. If patients are imaged with bone-seeking radiopharmaceuticals, the kidneys are enlarged and show intense uptake. The sonographic examination usually shows normal to slightly enlarged kidneys with markedly increase echoes throughout.

Acute Cortical Necrosis

Acute cortical necrosis is a very uncommon disorder with patchy or entire necrosis of the renal cortex. Also involved are the proximal convoluted tubules secondary to the distention of the glomerular capillaries with dehemoglobulinized red blood cells, and medulla with 1 to 2 mm of peripheral cortical sparing. This disorder occurs in patients with severe dehydration, fever and infection, hemolytic–uremic syndrome, transfusion reactions, heart failure, burns, snakebites, and hyperacute renal transplant rejection. The imaging findings depend on the stage and severity of the disease. Early there are diffusely enlarged smooth kidneys. Sonography will show a hyperechoic cortex, and the radionuclide studies will demonstrate paired renal perfusion. If contrast is used, there is absent or a faint nephrogram phase. Late in the disease, usually after 1 month, the kidneys become small. Tramline or punctate calcification along the margins of viable and necrotic tissue occur. Sonography at this stage will show a hyperechoic cortex with acoustic shadowing.

Leukemia

Kidney involvement with leukemia may present at the time of diagnosis or may appear during relapse. The most common manifestation is asymptotic renal enlargement. Leukemic infiltration is usually diffuse, resulting in bilateral nephromegaly, but focal masses occasionally are encountered. With severe infiltration, there may be significant functional compromise. Impaired renal function interferes with the elimination of chemotheraputic agents and metabolic products, resulting in systemic toxicity. Nephromegaly is not synomous with leukemia infiltration because it can result in these children from uric acid nephropathy, renal vein thrombosis (which is associated with a high white blood cell count), renal infection, and obstructed uropathy (secondary to uric acid stones) or lymphopathy.

The sonographic findings of leukemic involvement of the kidneys include degrees of renal enlargement, loss of corticomedullary demarcation, distortion of the renal pelvocalyceal system, and hypoechoic masses. One or more hypoechoic lesions may result from leukemic lesions. Renal parenchymal changes can occasionally antedate a clinical relapse.

Sonography is useful in evaluating renal complications of leukemia and its therapy. Uric acid nephropathy may be present at the time of diagnosis and may progress with therapy as a result of cell lysis. The sonographic findings include nephromegaly, a thickened and echogenic cortex, and loss of normal corticomedullary demarcation. Chronic changes associated with uric acid

nephropathy include renal cortical thinning and increased renal sinus echoes (resulting from deposition of fat).

On computed tomography (CT), leukemic involvement of the kidneys presents as unilateral or bilateral nephromegaly, focal masses, and pelvocaliceal distortion or dilatation. Pelvocaliceal dilatation may result from obstruction by retroperitoneal adenopathy. Renal leukemic masses are usually slightly hypodense or isodensed in normal parenchyma on unenhanced images, and may demonstrate uniform enhancement approximately equal to that of the surrounding parenchyma after contrast medium is administered.

Hematuria is uncommon in children with leukemia. It is usually the result of thrombocytopenia and clotting abnormalities. There is no indication for imaging of leukemic children with hematuria, although excretory urography, sonography, or CT may be performed to detect focal renal disease or urinary tract obstruction. Hematuria can occur secondary to hemorrhagic cystitis, which is most commonly seen with cyclophosphamide therapy.

Investigation with any of the imaging techniques shows a thickened bladder wall and, frequently, intraluminal clots. The bladder wall of leukemic patients may be thickened as a result of hemorrhagic cystitis, leukemic infiltration, or infection. These abnormalities are readily identified on sonography.

Postrenal Acute Renal Failure

Postrenal ARF results from obstruction to the flow of urine from the collecting system. Prenatal urinary tract obstruction produces renal failure in the newborn. This is frequently associated with bilateral hydronephrosis caused by obstruction at the level of the bladder or bladder outlet. A neurogenic bladder can result in a thickened and/or dilated bladder and bilateral dilatation of the collecting systems and ureters. The bladder and bladder outlet may be obstructed by congenital anomalies such as posterior urethral valves or polyps, or it may be obstructed by a pelvic mass such as a tumor distorting the bladder base. Congenital anomalies of the spine should be sought with radiographs and spinal cord sonography in neonates, if not clinically apparent. Posterior urethral valves may be diagnosed by sonography with demonstration of a dilated posterior urethra. Voiding cystourethrograms should be performed for optimal visualization of the posterior urethral valve. A pelvic mass such as a sacrococcygeal teratoma or hydrometrocolpos may produce extrinsic obstruction of the bladder outlet. These entities can readily be diagnosed with sonography or standard radiographs.

Megacystic microcolon–malrotation–intestinal hypoperistalsis syndrome occurs in girls who are born with a grossly distended abdomen. The onset of symptomatology is the neonatal period. Clinical manifestations include abdominal distention, decreased or absent bowel movements, bilious vomiting, absent or decreased bowel sounds, thin abdominal muscles, bilateral flank masses, and a large midline abdominal mass (bladder). Radiologic manifestations include microcolon, malrotation, intestinal hypoperistalsis, dilated small bowel, megacystis, hydronephrosis, hydroureter, and absence of anatomic bladder outlet obstruction. Vesicoureteral reflux is frequently present.

In older children, postrenal ARF can result from trauma to the pelvis or ureters, extrinsic tumors obstructing the bladder or ureters, calculi, or blood clots. ARF will also be superimposed on previously unrecognized mild chronic uropathy.

CHRONIC RENAL FAILURE

The diagnosis of chronic renal failure is rarely suspected on clinical grounds alone until the GFR has fallen below 20 to 25 ml/min/1.73 m². Up to this level the remaining functioning nephrons are capable of regulating body chemistry through adaptive alterations in tubular function, either intrinsic or secondary to events such as development of hyperparathyroidism.

Chronic renal failure may be congenital or acquired; it also may be primary or secondary to a systemic condition. In cases of congenital maldevelopment of the urinary tract, end-stage renal disease usually develops within 10 to 15 years of the time of diagnosis. Because of the protracted course, children are much more susceptible to deleterious effects of chronic renal failure on nutritional status and growth. In contradistinction, acquired lesion such as glomerulonephritis rarely occur during infancy and early childhood. Progression to end-stage renal disease, however, is frequently more accelerated in this population. Even so, these patients do have an excellent chance to grow and develop.

Because of the slow evolution of chronic renal disease in most children, the manifestations that are identified are frequently nonspecific. Chronic renal failure may be detected in the course of evaluation of a child for failure to thrive, urinary tract infection, hypertension, abdominal masses, or urinary abnormalities such as hematuria or proteinuria. Cardiomegaly, uremic myocarditis and pericarditis, congestive heart failure, pleural effusion and pulmonary edema, peripheral edema, and systemic hypertension are common systemic manifestations of chronic renal failure. Peptic ulcers, ulcerated necrotic lesions of large and small bowel, uremic colitis, pancreatitis, malabsorption syndrome, and ascites are gastrointestinal manifestations. Esophageal varices occur in older patients with renal tubular ectasia and hepatic fibrosis.

Renal osteodystrophy is a frequent complication of chronic renal insufficiency, with a common feature of generalized increase in bone density. The vertebral body shows sclerosis of the upper and lower thirds (rugger-jersey vertebrae) in some severely affected and untreated patients; the skeleton is markedly demineralized. Cortical erosion resulting from secondary hyperparathyroidism is common and is best demonstrated along the radial side of the middle phalanges of the second and third fingers and in the medial aspect of the proximal metaphyses of the humerus, femur, and tibia. Bone reabsorption is also observed in the lateral and medial ends of the clavicle. Loss of the lamina dura

around the teeth and a "peppered" demineralization of the calvarium are attributed to the hyperparathyroidism. Metaphyseal changes, also in part the result of hyperparathyroidism, may be indistinguishable from typical rickets, and the growing ends of long bones are irregularly mineralized and markedly disorganized. Metaphyseal fractures, slipping of weight-bearing epiphyses, genu valgum, bowing of long bones, sharp angulation of long bones at the metaphyses, and deformation of the thorax and pelvis are present with longstanding disease. Brown tumors rarely occur in childhood. Also related to renal osteodystrophy are arterial and periarticular soft tissue calcifications, which may be small, linear, or the size of a tumor.

Imaging studies of the kidneys are required in patients with chronic renal failure. Sonography is the most useful because it can determine the size and configuration of the kidney independent of the renal function. Reduced renal size often indicates an irreversible loss or maldevelopment of renal parenchyma. A dilated collecting system will direct the evaluation toward obstructive uropathy or severe reflux. Renal cystic disease will be apparent.

Radionuclide imaging has helped in the assessment of the relative amount of renal tissue in each kidney, detection of urinary tract obstruction, and quantification of GFR. Excretory urography is rarely useful because the low GFR will not allow adequate visualization of the urinary tract. Voiding cystourethrography is required if there is a history of prior urinary tract infections or an abnormal voiding pattern or if abnormalities of the urinary tract are detected on sonography. The voiding cystourethrogram will assess for bladder outlet obstruction and bladder morphology and will detect vesicoureteral reflux.

HEMODIALYSIS

Management of ARF consists of supportive care until the kidney recovers from the acute insult. Acute dialysis or arteriovenous hemofiltration is utilized, especially if the patient has increased intravascular volume with pulmonary edema, hypertension hyperkalemia, or asymptomatic uremia.

Solute transport is obtained by hemofiltration or hemodialysis. Hemofiltration reproduces the glomerular filtration function of the kidney. With hemodialysis, solute transport occurs by diffusion with elimination of uremic substances according to their molecular weight. In hemofiltration, waste products are removed by convective transport, which is independent of their molecular weight but depends on the molecular weight of solute and the rate of flow of the filtrate.

The patient's arterial blood is brought in contact with a dialysis solution across a series of semipermeable membranes within the dialyzer and is returned as dialyzed blood to the patient's venous system. An arteriovenous fistula is created to allow ready access to the patient's arterial and venous circulation. The most common complication resulting in fistula failure is a stenosis in the vein proximal to the fistula. A venous obstruction is demonstrated by venous injection of contract material. Venous injection with an inflated pressure cuff near the axilla may opacify the fistula and part of the artery. Injection by puncture of the graft may be used in patients with a bridging graft between the artery and vein. Catheterization of the brachial artery may be required to visualize completely the arterial side of the fistula. Aneurysms at the site of anastomosis or in the graft, excessive arterial–venous shunting, and arterial insufficiency distal to the fistula are other types of complications. Another method of vascular access is used occasionally for temporary hemodialysis. This is a catheter system in the right atrium with a double lumen introduced through a subclavian or jugular vein. Its complications include improper position of the catheter, kinks, and thrombosis at the catheter tip. Advantages of this route are potential use of the catheter to maintain the patient's nutrition with amino acids and calories.

Patients on long-term periodic hemodialysis may develop small or large cortical renal cysts. Single or multiple neoplasms, usually adenomas or carcinomas, may develop in association with the cysts.

RENAL TRANSPLANTATION

Terminal renal failure is estimated to occur in 2 patients per 1 million population per year. Slightly less than one half of children with end-stage renal disease are expected to have normal functional outcome following appropriate therapy. Available therapy for the uremic child is chronic dialysis or live or cadaveric renal transplantation. Renal transplantation is the preferred method of treatment for children who have end-stage renal disease. Primary renal disease that has resulted in end-stage renal failure is an important consideration because the pathologic process that affected the native kidneys can reoccur in the allograft (Table 1). Focal glomerulosclerosis is the most common specific glomerular disease that causes end-stage renal disease in childhood. It is also the most common glomerular

Table 1 ■ RENAL FAILURE RECURRENCE AND GRAFT LOSS

DISEASE*	RECURRENCE RATE (%)	SEVERITY	GRAFT FAILURE (%)
FSGS	25–30	High	50
MPGN type I	70	Mild	25
MPGN type II	100	Low	10
SLE	5–50	Low	5
HSP	50–75	Mild	10
HUS	10–20	Moderate	5

*FSGS = focal segmental glomerulosclerosis; HSP = Henoch-Schölein purpura; HUS = hemolytic–uremic syndrome; MPGN = mebranoproliferative glomerulonephritis; SLE = systemic lupus erythematosus.

disease that has the potential for recurrence in the allograft.

Two metabolic diseases that can cause end-stage renal disease in children are cystinosis and oxalosis. Cystine crystals are identifiable in the allografts of transplant recipients who have cystinosis; they apparently have little effect on allograft function. There is a poor outcome of renal transplantation in patients with oxalosis. These patients have a high incidence of recurrence of oxalite deposition in the transplanted kidney.

In preparation for renal transplantation, it is necessary to minimize the risk of rejection. Mechanisms of rejection are based on T-cell–mediated (cellular) and B-cell–mediated (humoral) immune mechanisms, and genetically related cell surface antigens represented in the human leukocyte antigen (HLA) system. The HLA system is the major antigen matching technique in evaluation of donor sources. Presensitization of the recipient may have occurred from previous organ transplants or blood transfusions. It has been observed, however, that there is enhanced graft survival in patients receiving more than 10 blood transfusions, and a program of donor-specific transfusions is sometimes undertaken to decrease the risk of presensitization. In preparation for a pediatric renal transplant, renal biopsy is mandatory to establish the histologic changes of the underlying renal disease and to exclude the risk of occurrence of the original disease in the transplanted kidney. Nephrectomy is not routine. It is indicated in patients with hydronephrosis in whom post-transplant urinary tract infections may still occur or in those with severe hypertension or massive proteinuria. It is important that the bladder and urethra be adequate for effective urine collection and voiding to completion. If the urinary tract has previously been diverted, reversal of the diversion is required. It is important to avoid surgical reconstruction in an immunocompromised patient and to minimize the potential for urinary tract infection or sepsis.

In the technique of transplantation commonly used, the aorta or iliac artery is the site of arterial anastomosis, with the renal vein entering the inferior vena cava or common iliac artery. The transplanted kidney is placed in the retroperitoneum in older children, and in children under 20 kg the kidney is located intraperitoneally. The ureter is reimplanted via transvesical or intravesical antirefluxing technique.

The surgical aspects of graft preservation in renal transplant patients have dramatically improved. The problems of immunosuppression and diminishing the incidence of vascular and urologic complications remain.

Immediate complications from transplant related to physiologic alterations may result from the implantation of the donor kidney. Because an adult kidney will sequester a volume of between 250 and 300 ml of blood, a substantial percentage of the blood volume and cardiac output of a small child will enter the kidney. Thus hypotension, renal ischemia, and vascular thrombosis can occur. The transplanted kidney may excrete a large volume of fluid, approaching the blood volume of a young infant on an hourly basis. This requires careful maintenance of an expanded blood volume and good cardiac output while maintaining normal glucose and electrolyte balance and avoiding hypertension. Factors influencing graft survival include severity and type of underlying disease; the high incidence of urologic abnormalities, which must be corrected in children; donor–recipient organ size discrepancy with necessary alteration in recipient graft site; small recipient vessel size; and need for larger, more proximal recipient vessels, including the aorta, vena cava, and iliac arteries. Recipient survival is improved in children over the age of 5 because of the decreased incidence of vascular thrombosis when compared to the younger age group.

The introduction of cyclosporine therapy has markedly improved allograft survival but has also introduced cyclosporine nephrotoxicity into the differential diagnosis of graft dysfunction. Cyclosporine nephrotoxicity does not primarily affect tubular cells: rather, it has a vasoconstrictive effect that decreases ERPF and perfusion indices of the kidney. It has become clear that certain complications of renal transplantation occur at specific times after transplantation.

Renal allografts show better survival in children with urologic disease and normal bladder function compared with those in whom urinary transport is impaired and higher bladder pressures are maintained. It is postulated that the diuresis and reduced concentrating ability of the renal allograft diminish the effectiveness of the transplant ureter. Inefficient ureteral urine transport leads to diminished renal blood flow and diminished glomerular filtration and eventual ischemia, necrosis, and graft loss, particularly when combined with the effects of rejection. Survival is better in children with primary reflux or pyelonephritis compared with children with posterior urethral valves or other severe, longstanding obstructive uropathies.

Vascular Complications of Pediatric Renal Transplantation

Vascular complications of transplantation include thrombosis, renal vascular hypertension related to anastomotic or postanastomotic renal artery narrowing, and peripheral thromboembolic disease. Other causes of malfunction of a renal allograft after surgery include dehydration, ATN, hyperacute or accelerated rejection, cyclosporine toxicity, and infection. Sonography is the screening examination of choice in evaluating anatomic abnormalities. The hemodynamic information obtained with Doppler is useful. The Doppler examination is a reliable indicator of the patency of newly anastomosed vessels and of flow in the intrarenal arteries and veins as well as into the postbiopsy arteriovenous fistula. The renal artery and its anastomosis to the iliac artery are usually seen well with real-time and Doppler sonography; the detection of renal artery stenosis in a graft is much easier than in a native kidney. The renal artery is followed from the hilum to the iliac anastomosis. The Doppler pattern changes from a pan-diastolic flow in the renal artery to the typically high-resistance pattern

with reversed early diastolic flow in the iliac artery distal to the graft. Narrowing is identified by a zone of high-frequency Doppler shift. The flow pattern beyond the stenosis and within the kidney may be normal or may show a parvus-tardus pulse.

Complications of Pediatric Renal Transplantation

Surgical complications usually present early after transplantation. Urologic complications of transplant may be as high as 30% in pediatric patients. Urinary fistulas at the site of bladder reimplantation can lead to urine leaks and urinoma formation. Wound infection and wound abscesses occur early in the postoperative period. Injury during surgery to the lympathics of the recipient can cause lymphocele formation. This frequently appears in the second or third month after transplantation. Hematomas are identified in the immediate postoperative period. The lesions, if of sufficient size, can put pressure on the graft, its collecting system, or the urinary bladder, which results in obstruction. Intrinsic obstruction can be caused by ureteral stenosis, blood clots, or early calculi formation. Renal artery stenosis at the anastomotic site is a late complication.

Other Complications

Transplantation and immunosuppression therapy have been associated with increased incidence of malignancy. Lymphomas are the most common tumors seen in pediatric allograft recipients. Primary Epstein-Barr virus (EBV) infection has been linked to the development of post-transplant lymphoproliferative syndrome (LPS) by initiating B-cell proliferation. Children are particularly at risk for LPS because a primary infection is more common at young ages. The treatment of EBV-associated LPS is disappointing, but decrease in immunosuppression or removal of the graft with cessation of immunosuppression has been suggested to be effective, especially in the initial stages of the B-cell proliferation. The use of interferon-alfa and acylovir has been recommended with variable results. Multidrug regimens and sequential immunosuppression have been reported as risk factors for development of malignancy with pediatric transplant.

Avascular necrosis has been reported to occur in 10% to 20% of pediatric allograft recipients. The most commonly involved bones are the femoral head or femoral condyles, but multiple bone involvement is not unusual. Pain is the initial clinical manifestation. The exact etiology is unclear, but corticosteroid therapy and secondary hyperparathyroidism have been postulated in the pathogenesis.

Immunosuppressive treatment used for the prevention of rejection renders transplant patients susceptible to infection. Infections of the urinary tract and surgical wounds with *Staphylococcus aureus* and *Escherichia coli* are common during the first few weeks post-transplant; after this period, opportunistic infections increase. The most common viral infections are caused by cytomegalovirus, herpesvirus, and varicella-zoster. Cytomegalic infection results in significant morbidity and mortality in immunocompromised children.

Graft Rejection

Long-term living related donor graft survival rates generally are higher than those for cadaveric donor grafts. Long-term survival rates are better in pediatric patients than in adult patients. Increased pretransplant risk factors in the adult patients and complications directly attributable to the process of aging are the possible explanations for this difference. Graft loss after 10 years continues to be a problem despite low mortality rates. The major detriments to graft survival are episodes of rejection, death of the patient with a functioning graft, and progressive renal failure from chronic rejection or intrinsic disease. Decline in graft function is suggested to be the result of both indolent immunologic attack and the same nonimmune mechanisms that damaged the native kidneys. Systemic hypertension, glomerular hyperfiltration, and hypercholesterolemia may cause glomerular sclerosis and interstitial fibrosis, resulting in progressive loss of renal function. The effects of protein intake on glomerular perfusion and optimal protein intake to improve long-term functions of pediatric recipients remain to be determined.

Graft rejection is the recipient's response to an allograft and is related to antigenic stimulation of cytotoxic T lymphocytes to develop interleukin-2 receptors and promote interleukin-1 release from macrophages. Rejection is classified as hyperacute, accelerated acute, acute, and chronic. Hyperacute rejection may be seen within hours of transplantation and is the result of antibodies against the graft tissue that are already present in the host prior to the transplantation. Hyperacute rejections are rare with modern assays for presensitization. Accelerated acute rejection occurs in the initial week of transplantation in poorly matched living donor grafts. It can also be caused by presensitization. It is characterized by fever, pain, hypertension, and oliguria. Acute rejection occurs within the first year, usually within several months of the transplant, and presents with pain, fever, and oliguria. Acute rejection occurs because T or B cells must be stimulated, and rejection response needs a week or more to occur.

There are other causes of graft dysfunction in the first days or week after transplantation. These include ATN, obstructive uropathy, perirenal fluid collection, cyclosporine toxicity, acute renal vein thrombosis, and renal infection. The clinical spectrum of findings in all are similar: decrease in urine output, elevated serum creatinine, pain, fever, and leukocytosis.

Doppler sonography is extremely sensitive in evaluating the increasing intrarenal impedance that is associated with acute vascular rejection. If serial measurements can be obtained by performing a baseline study after operation, then the patient's resistive index (RI)

Table 2 ■ RESISTIVE INDICES (TRANSPLANT RECIPIENTS)			
	EARLY RI	LATE RI	RENAL SIZE
Normal	↑	Baseline (2 wk)	↑ slightly
Acute tubular necrosis	↑	Baseline (2 wk)	↑ slightly
Acute rejection	↓	↑ >5 days	↑
Cyclosporine toxicity	No change	No change	No change

can be compared to his or her own baseline rather than population norms. A single measurement of intrarenal impedance is disappointing in distinguishing ATN and cyclosporine toxicity from acute rejection. To evaluate the alterations in intrarenal arterial resistance commonly found in the transplant kidney, an anatomic study as well as pulsed Doppler is needed. In normal postoperative patients and ATN patients, RIs become elevated immediately after surgery and return to baseline after 2 weeks (Table 2). Renal volume increases slightly. With cyclosporine toxicity, there is frequently no change in RI or renal volume. With acute rejection, the RI shows an initial slight decrease and then there is a rapid and progressive rise after 5 days. Renal volume increases during this time. When acute vascular rejection is effectively treated with cyclosporine, which prevents proliferation of T cells, or with polyclonal or modified monoclonal antibodies, the T cells do not attack the graft antigen; the resulting decrease in intrarenal resistance is dramatic, and is well identified with Doppler sonography.

Chronic rejection is insidious and asymptomatic, and results in loss of graft function months to years after transplantation. It seems to be the result of multiple episodes of unsuccessfully treated acute rejection. It is characterized histologically by an arteritis and tubular atrophy. The glomeruli are smaller than normal and may become hyalinized. With chronic rejection, there is vascular intimal proliferation in the interlobar and arcuate arteries. This decreases the diameter of small vessels, will increase acoustic impedance, and will cause lower or absent diastolic flow.

Morphologically, renal changes can be seen in the allograft with rejection. There is wall thickening of the renal collecting system. However, moderate thickening may be seen in urinary tract infection, reflux, or obstruction. Enlarged and sonolucent pyramids, areas of decreased parenchymal echogenicity, alteration in sharpness of the corticomedullary junction, and an increase in corticomedullary ratio are all indicators of rejection. Sonography is considered the most valuable diagnostic aid in evaluating postoperative renal transplant failure. Sonography is used for the initial investigation of a failing graft. Diagnosis is usually established with a renal biopsy.

RENAL VEIN THROMBOSIS AND RENAL ARTERY THROMBOEMBOLISM

RENAL VEIN THROMBOSIS

Renal vein thrombosis, either unilateral or, less commonly, bilateral, produces a flank mass in the neonate. This disorder, although uncommon, is the most common renal vascular abnormality in the neonate, and is discussed in Section II, Part V, Chapter 6, page 231. A good prognosis is indicated if renal scintigraphy demonstrates mild renal compromise. Usually within a few weeks of the onset of renal vein thrombosis, the affected kidney shows a decrease in size. In most circumstances, however, there is a return of function. In a small number of cases, a radiographically identifiable reticular pattern of calcification develops in the intrarenal veins. These calcifications are particularly well demonstrated on CT. The finding is virtually pathognomonic of previous renal vein thrombosis (Fig. 2).

RENAL ARTERY THROMBOEMBOLISM

This disorder is discussed in Section II, Part V, Chapter 6, page 231.

SYSTEMIC ARTERIAL HYPERTENSION

Hypertension is present in approximately 2% to 4% of all children, and severe hypertension occurs in at least 10% of these. The underlying causes of significant hypertension in the pediatric population differ considerably from those of adults. Although the prevalence of hypertension in children is lower than in adults, second-ary, or clinically identifiable, etiologies of hypertension account for a much higher proportion of hypertension, approximately 90% in children less than 10 years of age. In children, most secondary hypertension is due to renal parenchymal disease, whereas endocrine and renal vascular disorders account for a greater percentage of secondary hypertension in adults. Approximately 60% to 80% of hypertension in children less than 10 years of age has an identifiable associated renal lesion. Essential hypertension accounts for 10% of the hypertension seen in this age group, versus over 90% in adults. The incidence of essential hypertension in the young appears to increase with age. In general, the higher the blood pressure and the younger the child, the more likely a secondary cause underlies the hypertension. Although management of essential hypertension is important, in children the primary efforts of physicians should be directed toward uncovering any secondary, potentially correctable, etiology (Table 3).

Although hypertension is uncommon in newborns, certain infants have an increased risk. They include premature infants hospitalized in neonatal intensive care units, infants with a history of umbilical catheriza-tion, and infants with bronchopulmonary dysplasia. The most frequent causes of neonatal hypertension include renal artery thrombosis, renal artery stenosis, congenital renal malformations, coarctation of the aorta, and bronchopulmonary dysplasia. From infancy to 6 years of age, renal parenchymal disease, renal artery stenosis, and coarctation are the most common etiologies. From 6 to 10 years of age, renal parenchymal disease and renal artery stenosis remain as major causes of elevated diastolic pressures. Primary or essential hypertension begins to be seen during this time, usually causing milder elevations in blood pressure.

There is debate concerning the appropriate use of diagnostic imaging in hypertensive children. Imaging studies are indicated, however, for all hypertensive children with a history of neuroectodermal disorder or

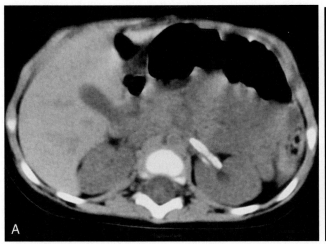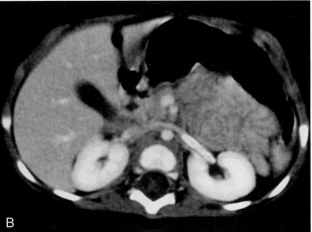

FIGURE 2. A, Nonenhanced computed tomography (CT) scan of the upper abdomen in an infant with linear calcification in the renal vein. **B,** Enhanced CT scan of the upper abdomen showing patency of the renal vein and normal renal function. This finding is secondary to renal vein thrombosis in the neonatal period.

Table 3 ■ HYPERTENSIVE CONDITIONS

Primary Hypertension
(cause not known)
Obesity, positive family
history

Cardiovascular
Coarctation
Renal artery stenosis
Williams syndrome
Neurofibromatosis
Systemic arteritis
Takayasu's arteritis
Henoch-Schönlein purpura

Renal
Structural abnormalities
Obstruction
Reflux
Glomerulonephritis (acute
and chronic)
Chronic renal failure
Diabetic nephropathy
Renal trauma

Endocrine
Hyperthyroidism
Congenital adrenal
hyperplasia
Primary aldosteronism
Hyperparathyroidism

Neurologic
Increased intracranial
hypertension
Guillain-Barré syndrome
Familial dysautonomia

Oncologic
Neuroblastoma
Pheochromocytoma
Adrenal adenocarcinoma

Drug Ingestion
Cocaine
Corticosteroids
Oral contraceptives
Sympathomimetics
Phencyclidine

multiple endocrine neoplasias. Imaging also should be performed when laboratory studies suggest the presence of pheochromocytoma or renovascular disease. The severity of the hypertension and the age of the child also bear on the need for diagnostic imaging. Adolescents with mild labile hypertension and no laboratory abnormalities are most likely to have essential hypertension; this group does not require diagnostic imaging studies.

Sonography can be used for the initial evaluation of children with hypertension. A normal examination does not exclude renal etiology; however, identification of renal abnormalities on sonography narrows the differential diagnosis and aids in the selection of additional testing. When sonography demonstrates a specific renal abnormality, such as a renal cystic disease or hydronephrosis, additional anatomic imaging studies should be performed, such as voiding cystourethrography. If sonography demonstrates unilateral or bilateral renal hypoplasia, the findings should be correlated with those of clinical examination and laboratory studies to determine whether this is due to renovascular disease or parenchymal disease. Sonography sometimes demonstrates specific abnormalities of the aorta and renal arteries, such as thrombosis or narrowing. Most intraabdominal mass lesions are detected on sonography. CT is an accurate (better than 95%) technique for detection of adrenal tumors. Pheochromocytoma also is imaged satisfactorily by CT in both adrenal and extra-adrenal sites. The later category includes tumors arising along the course of the ureters, in the organ of Zuckerkandl, or in the bladder wall.

RENAL PARENCHYMAL ABNORMALITIES

In children, the most common etiology of hypertension is renal disease. Renal pathology responsible for hypertension can be grouped into disorders that predomi-

nately involve the parenchyma and those that involve major renal arteries (i.e., medical renal disease and renal vascular disease). The kidneys maintain blood pressure levels by two primary mechanisms and multiple secondary mechanisms. The primary mechanisms are those in which some function of the kidney itself responds directly to changes in arterial blood pressure and in turn causes a feedback phenomenon on the vascular system to return the blood pressure to its previous level. The renin–angiotensin system, one of the primary mechanisms, releases angiotensin in response to falling blood pressure; the multiple effects of angiotensin then cause the pressure to return to normal. Another primary mechanism is the renal blood volume pressure control mechanism. The secondary renal mechanism for blood pressure control include the effects of multiple extrinsic factors acting on the two primary kidney pressure control mechanisms to alter their control characteristics. For example, aldosterone affects the kidney by causing water and salt retention and is an important secondary renal pressure control mechanism. Also, antidiuretic hormone mildly affects renal pressure control. The nervous system, acting primarily through the sympathetic nervous system, may have long-term effects on kidney function that could alter pressure control capability.

Acute glomerulonephritis is the most common cause of acute hypertension in all pediatric age groups, accounting for approximately 70% of cases of renal vascular hypertension. It is an acute inflammatory process of presumed immunologic origin affecting the kidneys, in which the lesions are located predominantly in the glomerulus. It may follow infection with a number of bacteria or viruses, or it may be part of a systemic disease. The organisms that most frequently cause this condition are Group A β-hemolytic streptococci. Certain specific serial types (1, 4, 12, 17, 18, and 49) are most often associated with acute glomerulonephritis. In this disease, there is increase in blood pressure that decreases again to normal within a few weeks. The normal blood pressure level does not correlate with the pathologic findings in the kidney. Nevertheless, the more severe the nephritis, which is indicated by hematuria, oliguria, and uremia, the more significant the hypertension. Cardiac failure and hypertensive encephalopathy occasionally complicate the disease. The mechanism of hypertension in acute glomerulonephritis is not fully understood but is probably the result of generalized vasospasm. Whether all of this occurs through neurogenic or hormonal influences is unknown. Slowing of the pulse, however, such as occurs with nephrotoxic hypertension (without heart failure), also occurs in experimental animals whose blood pressure is elevated by angiotensin or norepinephrine.

Chronic glomerulonephritis is uncommon in childhood. Renal biopsy establishes the diagnosis. It has been noted that nephritis associated with Henoch-Schönlein purpura commonly leads to a type of chronic glomerulonephritis. Familial nephritis is also a chronic form of glomerulonephritis. If renal failure is associated with chronic glomerulonephritis, hypertension is frequent. In other cases in which the disease is mild and does not seriously affect renal function or the general health of the patient, hypertension is unusual.

Nephritis is associated with collagen–vascular abnormalities. For example, nephritis can occur in patients with systemic lupus erythematosus, dermatomyositis, scleroderma, and polyarteritis nodosa. Hypertension caused by renal involvement may precede the other manifestations of these disorders; therefore, the etiology of unexplained hypertension in childhood must be investigated, and renal pathology should be considered as a possible etiology. Other chronic diseases that destroy renal tissue by inflammation or scarring can also be associated with elevated blood pressure; examples include reflux nephropathy, radiation nephritis, necrosis of glomeruli with fibrinoid necrosis of renal vessels and end-stage cystinosis, and chemical nephrotoxicity. Reflux nephropathy is one of the more common etiologies of hypertension in childhood.

Chronic pyelonephritis, with or without obstructive uropathy, can be associated with hypertension. There is disagreement concerning the frequency with which chronic pyelonephritis is the basis of persistent hypertension. It is also unclear why hypertension should be present in some patients and absent in others. Hypertension is more likely to occur in those patients who have endarteritis. In adults with hypertension, 10% are found to have histologic evidence of chronic pyelonephritis on renal biopsy. These considerations indicate that there are probably many factors involved in hypertension with chronic pyelonephritis.

Imaging studies in patients with suspected hypertension secondary to renal parenchymal disease includes a sonographic examination for evaluation of the kidneys and collecting system. Sonography is able to evaluate renal volume, the presence or absence of scars, and corticomedullary anatomy. Reflux can be excluded by radiographic or radionuclide cystography, and dimercaptosuccinic acid (DMSA) renal scans will identify scarring. In suspected renal vascular disease, Doppler sonography and arteriography, particularly using digital subtraction techniques and measurement of peripheral and renal plasma renins, are extremely sensitive indicators of renal vascular pathology.

RENOVASCULAR HYPERTENSION

Renal artery narrowing occurs in all age groups and is a well-documented cause of hypertension. Obstruction to renal blood flow may be due to

1. Structural renal artery anomalies (multiple renal arteries of variable caliber, hypoplasia, or aneurysms)
2. Localized muscular and fibrous thickening of the renal artery (generation of elastic tissue with active fibrosis and fibrinoid degeneration)
3. Thrombosis
4. Trauma
5. Distortion and compression associated with a renal mass, such as a Wilms' tumor, cyst, or intrarenal hemorrhage

6. Extrarenal compression in the renal artery
7. Disorders that cause vascular disease within the kidneys

Approximately 5% to 10% of children and adolescents who are referred to centers for evaluation of severe hypertension are subsequently found to have clinically significant renal vascular lesions. Many children who are eventually found to have renovascular hypertension are not symptomatic at initial presentation, and, when symptoms are present, they are frequently nonspecific. Younger children often present with increased irritability, behavioral changes, or failure to thrive, whereas in older children, lethargy and headaches are frequent complaints. Asymptomatic left ventricular hypertrophy, congestive heart failure, or neurologic complications, including encephalopathy, Bell's palsy, seizures, and cerebral hemorrhage, occasionally occur in all ages. Children may have midaortic syndrome, occasionally manifested by claudication, but abdominal angina is rare.

Fibrous dysplasia comprises a group of conditions that are by far the more common causes of renal artery stenosis in children (Table 4). These lesions are considered congenital dysplasias and cause maldevelopment of the fibrous muscular and elastic tissues of the renal arteries. They are subcategorized according to the layer of the arterial wall that is involved. The classification is important because each type of fibrous dysplasia has a distinct histologic and angiographic feature and occurs in a different clinical setting.

Primary intimal fibroplasia is an etiology of renovascular hypertension seen more frequently in children than in adults. This lesion is characterized by circumferential accumulation of collagen inside the internal elastic lamina. Angiographically this causes a smooth, fairly focal stenosis, usually involving the midportion of the renal artery or its branches. Although this disease most often is localized in the renal arteries, it may occur also as a generalized disorder with involvement of the

Table 4 ■ ETIOLOGY OF RENOVASCULAR HYPERTENSION	
Fibrous and fibromuscular dysplasia	Vascular malformations
Inflammatory disease	Arteriovenous malformation (renal)
Takayasu's arteritis	Renal artery aneurysm
Kawasaki disease	Thromboembolism
Irradiation	Renal transplant artery stenosis
Moyamoya disease	Rejection
Inherited conditions	Adhesions
Williams syndrome	Anastomic stenosis (end-to-end)
Neurofibromatosis	Turbulent flow (end-to-side)
Syndromes	Other causes
Klippel-Trénaunay-Weber syndrome	Congenital rubella
Feuerstein-Mims syndrome	Compression by masses
Rett syndrome	Congenital fibrous bands
Degos-Kohlmeier disease	Post-traumatic
Marfan syndrome	Retroperitoneal fibrosis
Atherosclerosis	
Hyperlipidemias	

vessels of the aortic arch, upper and lower extremities, and mesenteric vessels.

Perimedial or subadventitial fibrodysplasia is another of the fibrous dysplasias that is encountered in childhood. This causes a very tight stenotic lesion that pathologically consists of dense collagen in the renal artery of variable length and thickness. The collagen is deposited in the outer border of the media. Angiographically, this causes a beaded arterial appearance as well as diffuse narrowing of the renal arteries. Frequently, evidence of collateral circulation is seen at the time of the angiogram (Fig. 3). This disease occurs almost exclusively in girls older than 10 years of age. It occurs only in renal arteries or branches and is more common on the right. Approximately 15% of cases are bilateral.

Fibromuscular hyperplasia is an extremely rare disease that may occur in childhood. This is the only renal arterial obstructive lesion in which there is true hyperplasia of the smooth muscle cells. The renal artery shows concentric thickening of its wall resulting from proliferating smooth muscle and fibrous tissue. Angiographically, this lesion presents as a smooth stenosis of the renal artery or its branches and may be indistinguishable from intimal fibroplasia.

Medial fibroplasia is the most common cause of nonarteriosclerotic renovascular disease in adults. This disease is encountered rarely in childhood. Pathologically, the internal elastic membrane is focally and variably thinned. In the alternating thickened areas, much of the medial musculature is replaced by collagen. Angiographically, medial fibrodysplasia demonstrates a string-of-beads appearance typically involving the distal two thirds of the main renal artery and its branches. Any of the areas of aneurysmal dilatation frequently are seen. The areas of dilatation are greater in caliber than the normal renal artery, and collateral circulation is absent. These features are important in differentiating medial fibroplasia from perimedial fibroplasia.

Stenotic arterial lesions are seen in childhood with neurofibromatosis 1 (NF1). Vascular pathology occurs in the kidneys, heart, and gastrointestinal tract. It consists of fibrosis and thickening of the intima, proliferation of neural tissue in the arterial wall, perivascular nodular proliferations, and occasionally aneurysmal dilatation. In the kidney, arterial stenosis usually occurs at the origin or in the proximal third of the main renal artery. Angiographically, it is difficult to distinguish from intimal fibroplasia. Renal artery involvement can produce hypertension. Hypertension in children with NF1 also can occur with pheochromocytoma.

There are various other rare causes of hypertension in childhood. Takayasu's arteritis is sometimes associated with renal stenosis. The main renal arteries are occasionally involved in polyarteritis nodosa. Fibrotic renal artery narrowing can occur following radiation therapy. The middle aortic syndrome is a pathologic disorder characterized by nonspecific stenosing arteritis that affects the aorta and the major branches, including the renal arteries. It is thought to be a form of Takayasu's disease, and an autoimmune mechanism has been postulated. This disease can extensively involve the subdiaphragmatic aorta or, in some cases, may spare the aorta and primarily involve the renal or splanchnic vessels. The inflammatory process generally does not involve the iliac vessels.

Many tests have been devised to aid in the diagnosis of children with suspected renovascular hypertension. However, for more than 30 years, arteriography has been the standard examination. New technologies have been used to supplement the information gained from arteriography, thereby aiding in the selection of the best option for treatment. Still, direct intra-arterial digital

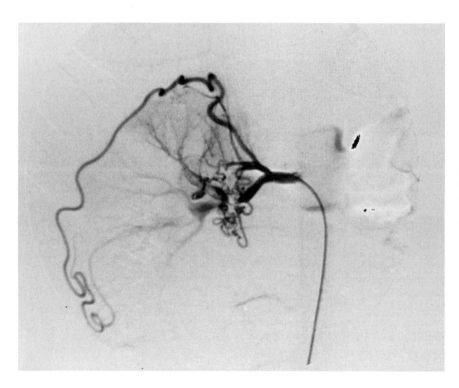

FIGURE 3. Selective right renal angiogram shows multiple stenotic renal arteries as well as intrarenal and capsular collateral circulation in a hypertensive 10-year-old female with fibrodysplasia.

subtraction angiography has allowed identification of arterial lesions using lower volumes of dilute contrast.

Direct sampling of blood for measurement of renin from the renal veins, branches of the renal veins, and infra- and suprarenal inferior vena cava has proved to be a useful diagnostic tool. In patients with significant unilateral renal artery stenosis, increased plasma renin activity (PRA) is anticipated from the underperfused kidney, with suppression of PRA on the contralateral side. This difference may also be pronounced in patients who have bilateral renal artery stenosis with unequal degrees of stenosis, although this has not been consistently observed. Lateralization is usually not apparent in children with significant aortic involvement or bilateral renal artery stenosis, which appear equal by angiography. However, lateralization in patients with bilateral disease may be misleading because of the formation of collateral vessels. Technically, if possible, sampling from segmental renal veins may be useful to confirm more distal arterial defects or to guide the decision making prior to therapeutic intervention. Routine measurement of renal vein PRA with every angiographic procedure is not often practiced, and it is suggested that measurement of renal vein activity be done only if it will affect subsequent treatment.

Noninvasive or less invasive diagnostic procedures have been used to study children with suspected renovascular hypertension. Renal sonography with duplex Doppler scanning and radionuclide scintigraphy have been used as adjunct diagnostic tools, but the sensitivity and specificity of these methods, when compared to arteriography, has not permitted substitution for angiography. Duplex sonography combines anatomic (direct visualization of renal vessels) and functional (color Doppler evaluation of renal blood flow) measurements in one noninvasive examination. Sonography is probably best at detecting lesions of the main renal arteries, including arteriovenous malformations and renal artery aneurysms. This technique is useful in children with midaortic syndrome or renal artery stenosis resulting from NF1. Furthermore, Doppler studies occasionally suggest bilateral renal artery stenosis in children with acute renal parenchymal disease, including acute glomerulonephritis, renal hemorrhage, and leukemic infiltration.

Radionuclide scintigraphy is widely used as an ancillary diagnostic tool. Among the radiopharmaceuticals available for renal scintigraphy, ^{99m}Tc-DTPA, ^{123}I-OIH, and ^{99m}Tc-mercaptotriglycylglycine (MAG-3) are preferred. ^{99m}Tc-DTPA and ^{123}I-OIH allow the estimation of differential renal blood flow and GFR. Several studies in children have employed ^{99m}Tc-DMSA, which, in contrast to DTPA, is incorporated in the proximal tubular cells and is a sensitive indicator of renal parenchymal disease. The sensitivity of pre- versus postcaptopril-enhanced DMSA scanning compared with the angiography is approximately 75% in children with hypertension. Comparison of pre- and postcaptopril scanning significantly increases specificity of the tests. Unfortunately, captopril-enhanced DMSA scanning produces both false-positive and false-negative results in children. Symmetric bilateral renal artery stenosis and very poor renal function may yield false-negative examinations. An additional problem with renal scintigraphy is that it does not allow detail study of the renovascular anatomy. That is why the International Committee on the Use of Radionuclides recommends the use of MAG$_3$.

Reduction of elimination of hypertension, prevention of hypertension-induced morbidity, and preservation or renal function are all therapeutic objectives. Various treatment options permit individualization of therapy, although technical expertise and physician preference are usually evident in the regimen. Well performed ace inhibition scintigraphy determines whether or not a renal artery stenosis is actually producing hypertension.

COARCTATION OF THE AORTA

Coarctation of the aorta can be discreet or involve a sizable segment. It occurs at the junction of the aortic arch and the descending aorta. A fibrous ridge usually extends into the aorta that narrows its orifice. A sharp indentation is present on the lateral aortic wall at the site of aortic narrowing. The most common site of coarctation is opposite the ductus arteriosus. More than half the patients with coarctation of the aorta have a bicuspid aortic valve. In older infants and children, isolated coarctation of the aorta leads to left ventricular hypertrophy and the development of collateral blood flow. Among patients who have developed large collateral vessels, systolic and continuous murmurs may be heard over the thorax.

Radiographic patterns of coarctation differ between the symptomatic infant and the asymptomatic infant or child. In a symptomatic infant, there is generalized cardiomegaly; the pulmonary vascularity is increased if a ventricular septal defect is present. Left ventricular pressure and volume overload cause pulmonary venous hypertension as well as pulmonary edema. Coarctation syndrome is the most frequent cause of pulmonary venous hypertension in the second to third weeks of life. In the asymptomatic infant or child with coarctation of the aorta, heart size is usually normal on radiographs, but there is a prominent left cardiac contour reflecting left ventricular hypertrophy. Poststenotic dilatation of the descending aorta immediately distal to the coarctation causes a figure-of-3 configuration. The proximal portion of the "3" is formed by the distal aortic arch and the dilated left proximal subclavian artery. The distal part is formed by the poststenotic dilatation of the aorta beyond the area of coarctation, which forms the center of the "3." Notching of the inferior margins of the posterior segments of ribs three through eight is often found in older children with coarctation. The superior aspect of the notch is frequently sclerotic. Notching of the ribs is due to collateral blood flow through dilated intercostal arteries.

Echocardiography in infants with coarctation of the aorta is most useful in determining associated anomalies, including aortic and mitral valves and the presence or absence of a ventricular septal defect. Discrete narrowing of the site of juxtaductal coarctation as well narrowing of the aortic isthmus may also be demonstrated on echocardiography. Doppler evaluation, including color Doppler sonography, is extremely useful in identifying coarctation in infants. In infants, a juxtaductal coarctation of the aorta is suggested on angiography when injection with contrast material into the aortic root fills a patent ductus arteriosus, and if the pulmonary artery and the descending aorta are simultaneously visualized. A preductal coarctation is suggested if the descending aorta fills from the pulmonary artery via a patent ductus arteriosus. Left ventriculography is needed to document the presence and location of a ventricular septal defect. Aortography will also show the extensive collateral arterial system involving the intercostal, internal mammary, and other thoracic arteries above the level of the coarctation in the older child. A bicuspid aortic valve is frequently demonstrated.

In older infants and children with coarctation of the aorta, MRI is the modality of choice for complete diagnostic evaluation. In the parasagittal oblique projection, the entire aortic arch may be displayed in a single series acquisition. Both juxtaductal and diffuse isthmus hypoplasia of the aortic arch are demonstrable on MRI. It is important to identify the location, length, and severity of the aortic narrowing and the presence or absence of collateral vessels. Segmented gradient-echo techniques may be utilized to demonstrate the alterations in flow dynamics in the aorta adjacent to the lesion. It is also important to assess the aortic valve because of the increased incidence of bicuspid aortic valve in patients with coarctation. The subclavian artery must be delineated because this vessel is frequently used in repair of coarctation.

RENAL ARTERY ANEURYSMS AND RENAL ARTERIOVENOUS FISTULAS

These lesions are rare in childhood. Renal artery aneurysms may occur as primary lesions, secondary to sepsis, or in association with renal artery stenosis, often in NF1. Aneurysms of the renal artery are described in Kawasaki disease. Aneurysms may be singled or multiple. Most aneurysms are saccular, and clot or calcification within the aneurysm occasionally occurs (Fig. 4). Hematuria or flank pain may be a sign of an aneurysm. Real-time Doppler sonography or MRI is sensitive in identifying these lesions.

Arteriovenous fistulas may be congenital or acquired, secondary to penetrating trauma or blunt trauma to the kidney, renal biopsy, or renal surgery. Arteriovenous fistulas are also seen in primary renal neoplasms. Calcification or clot may occur. Hematuria is common, and a bruit may be heard on physical exam. A large arteriovenous fistula may result in congestive heart failure. Turbulent flow, a large feeding vessel, and a large draining vein are identified by Doppler sonography or angiography.

ENDOCRINE CAUSES OF HYPERTENSION

Hypertension in childhood can be due to an endocrine dysfunction. The most common form in childhood is iatrogenic, resulting from the exogenous administration of adrenocortical steroids or related synthetic derivatives. Unlike the situation with mineralocorticosteroids, hypertension produced by glucocorticosteroids is not affected by the amount of dietary sodium or

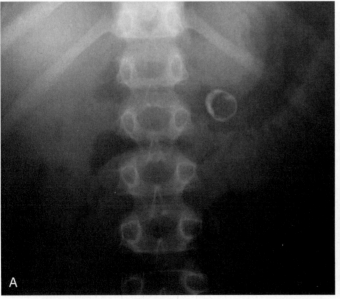
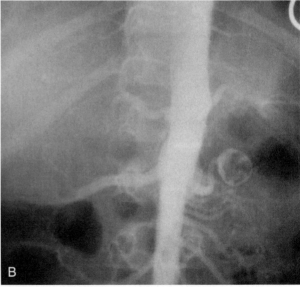

FIGURE 4. A, Standard radiograph of the upper abdomen shows an eccentric calcified ring immediately to the left of the second lumbar vertebra. **B,** Arteriogram shows that the left renal artery enters this calcified aneurysm and partially fills with contrast.

the severity of extracellular alkalosis. These children do not usually require diagnostic studies because the etiology is apparent.

Abnormalities of the adrenal gland associated with hypertension include pheochromocytoma, Cushing's syndrome, adrenal adenoma, adrenocortical carcinoma, adrenogenital syndrome, and primary aldosteronism. Hypertension is also associated with neuroblastoma.

Pheochromocytoma is a tumor that arises from neural crest derivatives. These cells occur in sites that include the adrenal glands, the thoracic and abdominal sympathetic chains, the organ of Zuckerkandl, the bladder wall, and the periureteral region. About 10% of pheochromocytomas are diagnosed in children. Approximately 70% of pheochromocytomas in children arise in the adrenal gland, and they are most often unilateral. Thirty percent of the cases are extrarenal, occurring as either single or multiple tumors.

Three distinct forms of pheochromocytoma have been identified: primary sporadic, malignant metastatic, and familial forms. The primary sporadic benign pheochromocytoma accounts for 85% of cases and most often occurs as an isolated adrenal lesion. Metastatic malignant pheochromocytoma accounts for about 5% to 10% of pediatric cases. Malignant pheochromocytoma cannot be identified reliably by simple pathologic examination of the primary lesion and requires demonstration of metastases. A lesion is clearly a metastatic lesion if, pathologically, pheochromocytoma can be demonstrated in tissue that normally does not contain chromaffin cells, such as liver, lung, lymph node, or bone. These are frequent sites of metastatic locations.

About 10% of pheochromocytomas in children are associated with a familial condition. These children often have multiple pheochromocytomas. Cases that occur as an isolated familial occurrence usually demonstrate an autosomal dominant pattern of inheritance. Other cases occur in association with one of several syndromes, including neuroectodermal disorders (NF1, von Hippel-Lindau disease, and tuberous sclerosis) and multiple endocrine neoplasia types IIA, IIB, and III.

Multiple endocrine neoplasia type IIA (Sipple's syndrome) consists of the association of pheochromocytoma that is often bilateral with medullary carcinoma of the thyroid and tumors of the parathyroid glands. Cases with this constellation of findings and mucosal neuromas are designated type IIB. The submucosal neuromas are found in the lips, tongue, eyelids, and gastrointestinal tract. Adrenal-medullary hyperplasia as a precursor of pheochromocytoma is nearly universal in the type II syndromes. Because of these findings, patients with type II syndrome should undergo bilateral adrenalectomy.

Although pheochromocytoma is an uncommon cause of hypertension in children, this lesion is included in the differential diagnosis. Hypertension associated with pheochromocytoma can be persistent or paroxysmal, with the former being more common in childhood. These tumors secrete various proportions of epinephrine and norepinephrine, which frequently cause high blood levels of vasoactive hormones. Norepinephrine may represent as much as 90% of the total released catecholamines. It has been observed that both epinephrine and norepinephrine are elaborated by tumors that are located in the adrenal glands, but norepinephrine is the only substance that is secreted by pheochromocytomas located in an extra-adrenal location. Norepinephrine tends to produce sustained hypertension; this occurs in approximately 90% of pediatric cases of pheochromocytoma.

Although approximately 80% of children with pheochromocytoma are hypertensive, this tumor accounts for only 5% of all pediatric cases of hypertension. This is usually sustained hypertension, but paroxysmal hypertensive crisis occur. These children sometimes exhibit other manifestations of sympathetic overstimulation, including flushing, diaphoresis (55%), tachycardia and palpations (30%), and dizziness (30%). Other symptoms include fever, headache, tremor, and blurred vision.

Adrenal etiology of hypertension is suspected on the basis of clinical symptomatology and laboratory results. Standard radiographs of the abdomen occasionally show calcification with the adrenal lesions, but this is not specific. Sonography is helpful for the evaluation of this region as well of the retroperitoneum. Abdominal CT with oral and IV contrast or MRI is also a sensitive imaging procedure for evaluation of the adrenal glands. The diagnostic evaluation should begin with a physical examination and laboratory evaluation (serum blood urea nitrogen and creatinine and urinalysis). In children with symptoms suggesting a pheochromocytoma, urine should be screened for catecholamines, vanillylmandelic acid, and metanephrines. Urinary metanephrines are elevated in 95% of patients; urinary vanillylmandelic acid is elevated in approximately 90%.

Most often pheochromocytomas are moderate size at presentation. Internal areas of low attenuation secondary to hemorrhage are not uncommon on CT. More than 10% will have dystrophic calcifications. Pheochromocytomas may be exophytic and locally invasive. This suggests malignancy. Without contrast media, pheochromocytomas usually appear relatively homogeneous on CT, with attenuation values approximately those of renal parenchyma. Intense enhancement occurs in most cases; a mild appearance or a peripheral rim around a nonenhancing center is another finding. The larger the lesion, the more hemorrhage or necrosis is seen. Demonstration of hepatic metastasis or lymph node enlargement underscores the malignant nature in some patients.

Sipple's syndrome is suggested when CT shows nephrolithiasis associated with an adrenal mass that has characteristics of a pheochromocytoma. Patients with von Hippel-Lindau disease and at-risk family members have an increased risk for the development of pheochromocytoma and renal cell carcinoma.

In patients with clinical findings that suggest pheochromocytoma and in whom abdominal CT is normal, CT of the chest and neck should be performed. Indium-111 labeled pentatreotide (octreotide) scintigraphy is a useful supplementary study. This radiopharmaceutical, a somatostatin analog is accumulated in

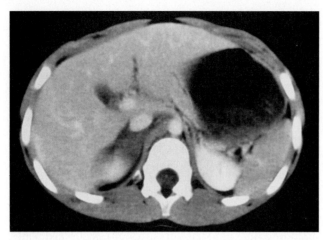

FIGURE 5. Contrast-enhanced upper abdominal computed tomography examination shows a minimally enhancing 1.5-cm adrenal cortical adenoma. The lesion is small and noninvasive.

neurosecretory tumors such as pheochromocytoma and neuroblastoma. Most pheochromocytomas of sufficient size cause scintigraphically demonstrable uptake of octreotide. Radioiodine labeled metaiodobenzylguanidine (MIBG) can also be used to image pheochromocytoma, but is less sensitive than In-111 octreotide, is more expensive, requires imaging over more days, and gives the patient a higher radiation exposure.

Cushing's syndrome may occur secondary to adrenocortical hyperplasia or an adrenocortical tumor: adenoma (Fig. 5) or adenocarcinoma (Fig. 6). There is increased cortical production of glucocorticoids, particularly cortisol, with resultant increased renin production. Congenital adrenal hyperplasia *(adrenogenital syndrome)* is associated with hypertension secondary to increased release of glucocorticoids. *Conn's syndrome* is hyperaldosteronism secondary to adrenal adenoma or adrenal

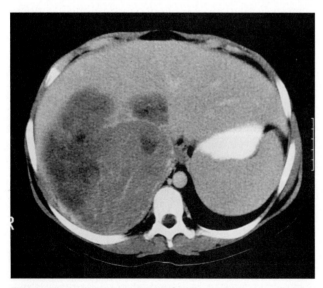

FIGURE 6. Upper abdominal contrast-enhanced computed tomography examination of the abdomen shows an enhancing large adrenal mass with metastatic liver disease. This is an adrenal carcinoma.

carcinoma and is distinctly uncommon in childhood. The increased production of aldosterone results in increased resorption of water from the distal renal tubule, increased vascular volume, resultant depression of the juxaglomerular apparatus, and subsequent decreased levels of circulating renin. The diagnosis is made by high urinary excretion of aldosterone and decreased blood renin levels.

SUGGESTED READINGS

Renal Failure

Alwaidh MH, Cooke RW, Judd BA: Renal blood flow velocity in acute renal failure following cardiopulmonary bypass surgery. Acta Paediatr 1998;87:644-649

Choyke PL, Grant EG, Hoffer FA, et al: Cortical echogenicity in the hemolytic uremic syndrome: clinical correlation. J Ultrasound Med 1988;7:439–442

Cramer BC, Jequier S, de Chadarevian JP: Factors associated with renal parenchymal echogenicity in the newborn. J Ultrasound Med 1986;5:633–638

Dittrich S, Dahnert I, Vogel M, et al: Peritoneal dialysis after infant open heart surgery: observations in 27 patients. Ann Thorac Surg 1999;68:160–163

Filiatrault D, Perreault G: Transient acute tubular disease in a newborn and a young infant: sonographic findings. J Ultrasound Med 1985;4:257–258

Flynn JT: Causes, management approaches, and outcome of acute renal failure in children. Curr Opin Pediatr 1998;10:184–189

Habib R: Nephrotic syndrome in the 1st year of life. Pediatr Nephrol 1993;7:347–353

Jeong YK, Kim IO, Kim WS, et al: Hemolytic uremic syndrome: MR findings of CNS complications. Pediatr Radiol 1994;24:585–586

Kaplan BS, Meyers KE, Schulman SL: The pathogenesis and treatment of hemolytic uremic syndrome. J Am Soc Nephrol 1998;9:1126–1133

Kelsch RC, Sedman AB: Nephrotic syndrome. Pediatr Rev 1993;14:30–38

Kozlowski K, Brown RW: Renal medullary necrosis in infants and children. Pediatr Radiol 1978;7:85–89

Lande IM, Glazer GM, Sarnaik S, et al: Sickle-cell nephropathy: MR imaging. Radiology 1986;158:379–383

Luciano R, Gallini F, Romagnoli C, et al: Doppler evaluation of renal blood flow velocity as a predictive index of acute renal failure in perinatal asphyxia. Eur J Pediatr 1998;157:656–660

Maxvold NJ, Smoyer WE, Gardner JJ, et al: Management of acute renal failure in the pediatric patient: hemofiltration versus hemodialysis. Am J Kidney Dis 1997;30:S84–S88

McLaughlin MG, Swayne LC, Rubenstein JB, et al: Transient acute tubular dysfunction in the newborn: CT findings. Pediatr Radiol 1990;20:363–364

Mendley SR, Langman CB: Acute renal failure in the pediatric patient. Adv Ren Replace Ther 1997;4:93–101

Moghal NE, Brocklebank JT, Meadow SR: A review of acute renal failure in children: incidence, etiology and outcome. Clin Nephrol 1998;49:91–95

Ogura H, Takaoka M, Kishi M, et al: Reversible MR findings of hemolytic uremic syndrome with mild encephalopathy. AJNR Am J Neuroradiol 1998;19:1144–1145

Patriquin HB, O'Regan S, Robitaille P, et al: Hemolytic-uremic syndrome: intrarenal arterial Doppler patterns as a useful guide to therapy. Radiology 1989;172:625–628

Platt JF, Rubin JM, Ellis JH: Lupus nephritis: predictive value of conventional and Doppler US and comparison with serologic and biopsy parameters. Radiology 1997;203:82–86

Polito C, Papale MR, La Manna A: Long-term prognosis of acute renal failure in the full-term neonate. Clin Pediatr 1998;37:381–385

Salusky IB, Goodman WG: Renal osteodystrophy in dialyzed children. Miner Electrolyte Metab 1991;17:273–280

Siegel NJ, Van Why SK, Devarajan P, et al: Pathogenesis of acute renal failure. *In* Barrat TM, Avner ED, Harmon WE (eds): Pediatric

Nephrology. Baltimore, Lippincott Williams & Wilkins, 1999:1109–1118

Vergesslich KA, Sommer G, Wittich GR, et al: Acute renal failure in children: an ultrasonographic-clinical study. Eur J Radiol 1987;7:263–265

Walker JT, Keller MS, Katz SM: Computed tomographic and sonographic findings in acute ethylene glycol poisoning. J Ultrasound Med 1983;2:429–431

Wong SN, Lo RN, Yu EC: Renal blood flow pattern by noninvasive Doppler ultrasound in normal children and acute renal failure patients. J Ultrasound Med 1989;8:135–141

Dialysis

Bay WH, Henry ML, Lazarus JM, et al: Predicting hemodialysis access failure with color flow Doppler ultrasound. Am J Nephrol 1998;18:296–304

Litherland J, Lupton EW, Ackrill PA, et al: Computed tomographic peritoneography: CT manifestations in the investigation of leaks and abnormal collections in patients on CAPD. Nephrol Dial Transplant 1994;9:1449–1452

Robbin ML, Oser RF, Allon M, et al: Hemodialysis accesses graft stenosis: US detection. Radiology 1998;208:655–661

Stafford-Johnson DB, Wilson TE, Francis IR, et al: CT appearance of sclerosing peritonitis in patients on chronic ambulatory peritoneal dialysis. J Comput Assist Tomogr 1998;22:295–299

Renal Transplantation

Babcock DS, Slovis TL, Han BK, et al: Renal transplants in children: long-term follow-up using sonography. Radiology 1985;156:165–167

Bay WH, Henry ML, Lazarus JM, et al: Predicting hemodialysis access failure with color flow Doppler ultrasound. Am J Nephrol 1998;18:296–304

Bereket G, Fine RN: Pediatric renal transplantation. Pediatr Clin North Am 1995;42:1603–1628

Gottlieb RH, Voci SL, Cholewinski SP, et al: Sonography: a useful tool to detect the mechanical causes of renal transplant dysfunction. J Clin Ultrasound 1999;27:325–333

Hildell J, Aspelin P, Nyman U, et al: Ultrasonography in complications of renal transplantation. Acta Radiol Diagn 1984;25:299–304

Hoyer PF, Schmid R, Wunsch L, et al: Color Doppler energy—a new technique to study tissue perfusion in renal transplants. Pediatr Nephrol 1999;13:559–563

Litherland J, Lupton EW, Ackrill PA, et al: Computed tomographic peritoneography: CT manifestations in the investigation of leaks and abnormal collections in patients on CAPD. Nephrol Dial Transplant 1994;9:1449–1452

Matas AJ, Chavers BM, Nevins TE, et al: Recipient evaluation, preparation, and care in pediatric transplantation: the University of Minnesota protocols. Kidney Int Suppl 1996;53:S99–S102

Mutze S, Turk I, Schonberger B, et al: Colour-coded duplex sonography in the diagnostic assessment of vascular complications after kidney transplantation in children. Pediatr Radiol 1997;27:898–902

Oliver JH 3rd: Clinical indications, recipient evaluation, surgical considerations, and the role of CT and MR in renal transplantation. Radiol Clin North Am 1995;33:435–446

Platt JF, Ellis JH, Korobkin M, et al: Helical CT evaluation of potential kidney donors: findings in 154 subjects. AJR Am J Roentgenol 1997;169:1325–1330

Robbin ML, Oser RF, Allon M, et al: Hemodialysis access graft stenosis: US detection. Radiology 1998;208:655–661

Salgado O, Garcia R, Rincon O, et al: Acute tubular necrosis in renal transplantation evaluated by color duplex sonography. Transplant Proc 1996;28:3337–3339

Snider JF, Hunter DW, Moradian GP, et al: Transplant renal artery stenosis: evaluation with duplex sonography. Radiology 1989;172:1027–1030

Stafford-Johnson DB, Wilson TE, Francis IR, et al: CT appearance of sclerosing peritonitis in patients on chronic ambulatory peritoneal dialysis. J Comput Assist Tomogr 1998;22:295–299

Stringer DA, O'Halpin D, Daneman A, et al: Duplex Doppler sonography for renal artery stenosis in the post-transplant pediatric patient. Pediatr Radiol 1989;19:187–192

Surratt JT, Siegel MJ, Middleton WD: Sonography of complications in pediatric renal allografts. Radiographics 1990;10:687–699

Toki K, Takahara S, Kokado Y, et al: Comparison of CT angiography with MR angiography in the living renal donor. Transplant Proc 1998;30:2998–3000

Townsend RR, Tomlanovich SJ, Goldstein RB, et al: Combined Doppler and morphologic sonographic evaluation of renal transplant rejection. J Ultrasound Med 1990;9:199–206

Vergesslich KA, Khoss AE, Balzar E, et al: Acute renal transplant rejection in children: assessment by duplex Doppler sonography. Pediatr Radiol 1988;18:474–478

Renal Vein Thrombosis and Renal Artery Thromboembolism

Adelman RD, Karlowicz MG: What is the appropriate workup and treatment for an infant with an umbilical artery catheter-related thrombosis? Semin Nephrol 1998;18:362–364

Ahluwalia JS, Kelsall AW, Diederich S, et al: Successful treatment of aortic thrombosis after umbilical catheterization with tissue plasminogen activator. Acta Paediatr 1994;83:1215–1217

Alexander AA, Merton DA, Mitchell DG, et al: Rapid diagnosis of neonatal renal vein thrombosis using color Doppler imaging. J Clin Ultrasound 1993;21:468–471

Cremin BJ, Davey H, Oleszczuk-Raszke K: Neonatal renal venous thrombosis: sequential ultrasonic appearances. Clin Radiol 1991;44:52–55

Ford KT, Teplick SK, Clark RE: Renal artery embolism causing neonatal hypertension: a complication of umbilical artery catheterization. Radiology 1974;113:169–170

Hibbert J, Howlett DC, Greenwood KL, et al: The ultrasound appearances of neonatal renal vein thrombosis. Br J Radiol 1997;70:1191–1194

Kavaler E, Hensle TW: Renal artery thrombosis in the newborn infant. Urology 1997;50:282–284

Keidan I, Lotan D, Gazit G, et al: Early neonatal renal venous thrombosis: long–term outcome. Acta Paediatr 1994;83:1225–1227

Laplante S, Patriquin HB, Robitaille P, et al: Renal vein thrombosis in children: evidence of early flow recovery with Doppler US. Radiology 1993;189:37–42

Lin GJ, Yang PH, Wang ML: Neonatal renal venous thrombosis—a case report describing serial sonographic changes. Pediatr Nephrol 1994;8:589–591

Loges RJ, Tulchinsky M, Boal DK, et al: Tc-99m MAG3 renography in renal vein thrombosis secondary to Finnish-type congenital nephrotic syndrome. Clin Nucl Med 1994;19:888–891

Nuss R, Hays T, Manco-Johnson M: Efficacy and safety of heparin anticoagulation for neonatal renal vein thrombosis. Am J Pediatr Hematol Oncol 1994;16:127–131

Orazi C, Fariello G, Malena S, et al: Renal vein thrombosis and adrenal hemorrhage in the newborn: ultrasound evaluation of 4 cases. J Clin Ultrasound 1993;21:163–169

Ricci MA, Lloyd DA: Renal venous thrombosis in infants and children. Arch Surg 1990;125:1195–1199

Seibert JJ, Lindley SG, Corbitt SS, et al: Clot formation in the renal artery in the neonate demonstrated by ultrasound. J Clin Ultrasound 1986;14:470–473

Wright NB, Blanch G, Walkinshaw S, et al: Antenatal and neonatal renal vein thrombosis: new ultrasonic features with high frequency transducers. Pediatr Radiol 1996;26:686–689

Systemic Arterial Hypertension

Bartosh SM, Aronson AJ: Childhood hypertension: an update on etiology, diagnosis, and treatment. Pediatr Clin North Am 1999;46:235–252

Berenson GS: The control of hypertension in African-American children: the Bogalusa Heart Study. J Nat Med Assoc 1995;87:614–617

Chandar JJ, Sfakianakis GN, Zilleruelo GE, et al: ACE inhibition scintigraphy in the management of hypertension in children. Pediatr Nephrol 1999;13:493–500

Daniels SR: Consultation with the specialist. The diagnosis of hypertension in children: an update. Pediatr Rev 1997;18:131–135

Decsi T, Soltesz G, Harangi F, et al: Severe hypertension in a ten-year-old boy secondary to an aldosterone-producing tumor identified by adrenal sonography. Acta Paediatr Hung 1986;27: 233–238

Dillon MJ: The diagnosis of renovascular disease. Pediatr Nephrol 1997;11:366–372

Falkner B, Sadowski RH: Hypertension in children and adolescents. Am J Hypertens 1995;8:106s–110s

Feld LG, Springate JE, Waz WR: Special topics in pediatric hypertension. Semin Nephrol 1998;18:295–303

Goonasekera CD, Dillon MJ: Reflux nephropathy and hypertension. J Hum Hypertens 1998;12:497–504

Harshfield GA, Hanevold CD: Ambulatory blood pressure monitoring in the evaluation of pediatric disorders. Pediatr Ann 1998;27: 491–494

Hohn AR: Diagnosis and management of hypertension in childhood. Pediatr Ann 1997;26:105–110

Ishijima H, Ishizaka H, Sakurai M, et al: Partial renal embolization for pediatric renovascular hypertension secondary to fibromuscular dysplasia. Cardiovasc Intervent Radiol 1997;20:383–386

Jones BV, Egelhoff JC, Patterson RJ: Hypertensive encephalopathy in children. AJNR Am J Neuroradiol 1997;18:101–106

Mittal BR, Kumar P, Arora P, et al: Role of captopril renography in the diagnosis of renovascular hypertension. Am J Kidney Dis 1996;28: 209–213

Muller-Berghaus J, Homoki J, Michalk DV, et al: Diagnosis and treatment of a child with the syndrome of apparent mineralocorticoid excess type 1. Acta Paediatr 1996;85:111–113

National High Blood Pressure Education Program Working Group on Hypertension Control in Children and Adolescents: Update on the 1987 Task Force Report on High Blood Pressure in Children and Adolescents: a working group report from the National High Blood Pressure Education Program. Pediatrics 1996;98:649–658

Ng CS, de Bruyn R, Gordon I: The investigation of renovascular hypertension in children: the accuracy of radio-isotopes in detecting renovascular disease. Nucl Med Commun 1997;18:1017–1028

O'Neill JA Jr: Long-term outcome with surgical treatment of renovascular hypertension. J Pediatr Surg 1998;33:106–111

Sadowski RH, Falkner B: Hypertension in pediatric patients. Am J Kidney Dis 1996;27:305–315

Schwartz RB, Bravo SM, Klufas RA, et al: Cyclosporine nuerotoxicity and its relationship to hypertensive encephalopathy: CT and MR findings in 16 cases. AJR Am J Roentgenol 1995;165:627–631

Sharma S, Thatai D, Saxena A, et al: Renovascular hypertension resulting from nonspecific aortoarteritis in children: midterm results of percutaneous transluminal renal angioplasty and predictors of restenosis. AJR Am J Roentgenol 1996;166:157–162

Sinaiko AR: Hypertension in children. N Engl J Med 1996;335:1968–1973

Sinaiko A, Michael A: Reflux nephropathy and hypertension: more whys and wherefores. Lancet 1996;347:633–634

Taylor AT Jr, Fletcher JW, Nally JV Jr, et al: Procedure guideline for diagnosis of renovascular hypertension. Society of Nuclear Medicine. J Nucl Med 1998;39:1297–1302

Tyagi S, Kaul UA, Satsangi DK, et al: Percutaneous transluminal angioplasty for renovascular hypertension in children: initial and long-term results. Pediatrics 1997;99:44–49

Wells TG, Belsha CW: Pediatric renovascular hypertension. Curr Opin Pediatr 1996;8:128–134

Yiu VW, Dluhy RP, Lifton RP, et al: Low peripheral plasma renin activity as a critical marker in pediatric hypertension. Pediatr Nephrol 1997;11:343–346

PART IV

URETER

JACK O. HALLER

Chapter 1

OBSTRUCTIVE LESIONS OF THE BODY OF THE URETER

JACK O. HALLER

OBSTRUCTIONS BETWEEN THE URETEROPELVIC AND URETEROVESICAL JUNCTIONS

Most ureteral obstructions occur at the ureteropelvic (UPJ) or ureterovesical (UVJ) junction. Obstructive lesions between these two points are very uncommon and include retrocaval ureter, retroiliac ureter, ureteral obstruction caused by other vessels, ureteral valves, acquired ureteral strictures, ureteral neoplasms, and extrinsic lesions affecting the ureter.

RETROCAVAL URETER

Retrocaval or circumcaval ureter (Fig. 1A) is an uncommon anomaly in which the right ureter, in its course to the bladder, passes behind the inferior vena cava, emerges between the cava and the aorta, and then curves around and in front of the cava to return to its normal position in the pelvis. This anomaly results from abnormal persistence of the subcardinal vein in the definitive inferior vena cava. Two types are described (Table 1). In the first type (low loop), the ureter descends from the renal pelvis and crosses behind the inferior vena cava near its bifurcation. It then curves medially and upward, forming a reversed J appearance (Fig. 1B). Ureteral obstruction at this level is common. In the second type (high loop), the renal pelvis and upper ureter lie nearly horizontally so that the retrocaval element of the ureter is at the level of the renal pelvis. A variable degree of ureteral obstruction at this level may be present but is less often seen than in the first type. In both types, dilatation of the upper tract above the lesion is caused in part by compression of the ureter by the vena cava, but a kink of the ureter at this level, local adhesions, an intrinsic ureteral stricture, or an adynamic ureteral segment may be the principal cause of the obstruction.

Retrocaval ureter is more common in males than in females and usually manifests in adult life, perhaps because the hydronephrosis is slow to develop. Often the lesion is asymptomatic and is discovered as an incidental finding. The diagnosis is made on the excretory urogram and is confirmed by retrograde ureterography and an inferior vena cavogram. The lesion may also be demonstrated by contrast-enhanced computed tomography (CECT) or magnetic resonance imaging (MRI). This condition is often associated with Turner's syndrome.

RETROILIAC URETER

Retroiliac ureter is rare. The affected ureter courses behind one or both iliac vessels rather than in front of them (see Fig. 1A). The proximal ureter and the pelvocaliceal system are variously dilated. In the lateral or steep oblique projection, the anterior defect of the ureter at the level of the iliac vessels may be recognized. The anomaly may be corrected surgically by excision of the involved ureteral segment and reanastomosis. The lesion should be differentiated from the defect in the posterior aspect of the ureter normally caused by the iliac vessels. This is sometimes associated with slight dilatation of the proximal ureter; with the patient upright or prone, these ureters drain without residual dilatation.

URETERAL OBSTRUCTION CAUSED BY OTHER VESSELS

Ureteral obstructions caused by other vessels are also rare. The vessel most often involved is an ovarian artery, the hypogastric artery, or one of its branches (Fig. 2A). Usually the obstruction is in the lower third of the ureter, and in many instances an intrinsic ureteral stricture coexists. Vascular impressions are occasionally seen and may be normal (Fig. 2B).

URETERAL VALVES

Only a few cases of ureteral valves have been reported. These valves are said to consist of a cusp-like fold or an iris diaphragm composed of ureteral mucosal and smooth muscle fibers (Fig. 2C). They are commonly found in the lower third of the ureter, but have been reported in the middle or upper third of the ureter as well.

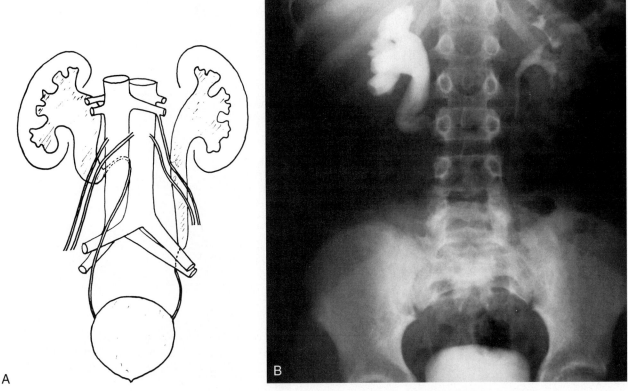

FIGURE 1. **A,** Anatomy of a retrocaval ureter on the right and a retroiliac ureter on the left. **B,** Retrocaval ureter. Excretory urogram shows right hydronephrosis. The dilated right ureter hooks retrocavally in front of the right L3 pedicle.

URETERAL STRIATIONS

These longitudinal mucosal folds may be seen in normal ureters but are often a sign of inflammatory disease, reflux, or previous obstruction. They must be distinguished from submucosal hemorrhage and collateral circulation from compensated renal vein thrombosis.

ACQUIRED STRICTURES

Acquired strictures of the body of the ureter are uncommon. They may be due to a local surgical procedure, instrumentation, or ureteral stones or periureteral infection; may be a complication of Henoch-Schönlein purpura, periarteritis nodosa, tuberculosis, or granulomatous disease of childhood; may be the result of submucosal hemorrhage in patients on anticoagulant medication; or may follow local radiation.

PRIMARY NEOPLASMS

Primary neoplasms of the renal pelvis and ureters are very rare in children. Involvement of the pelvocaliceal system by Wilms' tumor, and Wilms' tumor implants in the ureter, may occur. Instances of benign and usually pedunculated fibrous polyps in the upper third of the ureter (Fig. 3), occasionally bilateral, have been reported. They may cause hematuria or obstruction (rare) and have no malignant potential. They are more common in adults.

EXTRINSIC LESIONS

Extrinsic lesions causing ureteral displacement or obstruction include many of the primary or secondary retroperitoneal processes described in Section VII, Part VIII, page 1909. Extra-adrenal paraspinal neuroblastoma and ganglioneuromas are the most common primary retroperitoneal neoplasms that may affect the ureter extrinsically (Fig. 4). Other primary neoplasms of the area include teratoma, rhabdomyosarcoma, lipomatous tumors, and lymphangiomas. The ureters are commonly displaced by enlarged retroperitoneal lymph nodes from lymphoma, leukemia, Wilms' tumor, neuro-

Table 1 ■ RETROCAVAL URETER
Low Loop
Behind inferior vena cava at bifurcation
"Reverse J" appearance
Dysfunction common
High Loop
Behind inferior vena cava at ureteropelvic junction
Obstruction uncommon
Kinks/adhesions
Intrinsic stricture
Both Types
Males > females
Presents in adulthood

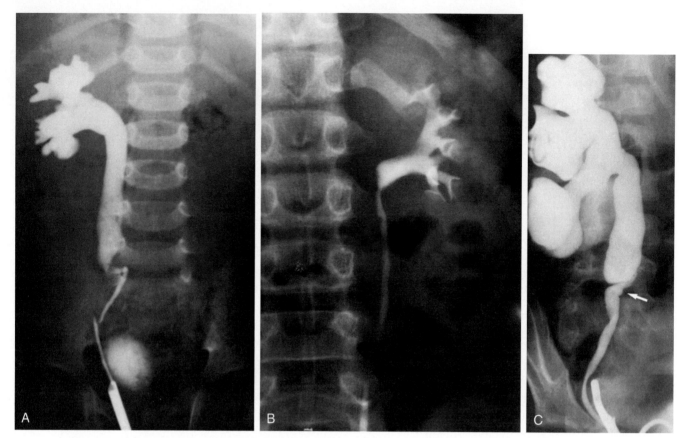

FIGURE 2. A, Right retrograde ureteropyelogram in a 2½–year-old child with partial obstruction of the ureter at the level of the iliac vessels, secondary to an overlying hypogastric artery. **B,** Vascular impressions along left ureter. **C,** Right retrograde pyelogram in a 3½–year-old child with a congenital midureteral obstruction caused by a valve-like mucosal fold *(arrow)*.

blastoma, and gonadal neoplasms. Of the acquired non-neoplastic retroperitoneal processes, the best known are appendiceal abscess and retroperitoneal hematoma or fibrosis. In the differential diagnosis, certain anatomic variants should be kept in mind, particularly congenital malpositions of the kidney, normal meandering of the ureter over the psoas muscle, displacement of the ureter by asymmetric enlargement of the psoas muscle, and displacement of the ureters by distended bowel, especially a large colon in patients with severe constipation. Ultrasound (US) or CECT scans may be helpful when the diagnosis is in doubt.

DISTAL URETERAL OBSTRUCTIONS

Obstructions of the distal end of the ureter are relatively common. They are characterized by dilatation of the ureter (megaloureter) and by failure of the ureter to empty normally on postvoiding films of an excretory urogram or on delayed films of a retrograde pyelogram. The obstruction may be further documented by a diuretic renogram and, in difficult cases, by pressure–flow studies. Two types of distal ureteral obstruction are described: (1) megaureter resulting from an organic lesion, and (2) primary megaureter, which is mostly

functional in origin. Obstruction of the distal end of a refluxing ureter in the presence of vesicoureteral reflux may also occur.

MEGAURETER FROM ORGANIC CAUSES

Instances have been reported of atresia of the distal end of the ureter with marked ureteral dilatation presenting as an abdominal mass. Primary organic obstructions in the distal end of the ureter or at the UVJ caused by congenital narrowing or fibrosis of the area also exist, but their incidence is not known (Fig. 5). Extravesical ectopic ureters without ureterocele occurring in a duplicated or unduplicated upper tract are often partially obstructed at their distal end. Ureters associated with an intravesical or an ectopic ureterocele are obstructed in varying degrees at their termination. UVJ obstruction may also be observed in cases of posterior urethral valves or neurogenic bladder caused by markedly thickened, stiff, and poorly functioning bladder musculature. An acquired distal ureteral obstruction may also be caused by a calculus, blood clot, or fungus ball; may be a complication of a surgical procedure (usually ureteral reimplantation); or may result from severe local infection or from compression by an extrinsic mass (Table 2; Fig. 6).

PRIMARY MEGAURETER

This type of megaureter (Fig. 7), also called primary obstructive megaureter, functional megaureter, ureteral achalasia, and aperistaltic, adynamic, or atonic distal ureter, is an uncommon nonhereditary lesion, probably congenital, caused by an adynamic distal segment about 0.5 to 4 cm in length that prevents normal, caudal propagation of ureteral peristalsis. The disorder is seen in patients of any age, is apparently more common in males than in females, and is frequently bilateral, especially in children less than 1 year of age. Three fourths of cases are unilateral, with the left ureter being involved more than the right. The affected ureter is variously dilated, but tapers down rather abruptly to a curved, short distal segment that in the roentgenogram appears normal in caliber or slightly narrowed. The dilatation is often limited to, or is most marked in, the lower half of the ureter. Diffuse dilatation with involvement of the pelvocaliceal system also occurs, but even in these cases the dilatation is more severe in the lower ureter.

The ureter is usually straight or only mildly tortuous, in contrast to megaureters resulting from reflux, lower urinary tract obstruction, or prune-belly syndrome, in which the ureters tend to be elongated and tortuous (Table 3). The renal parenchyma is usually of normal

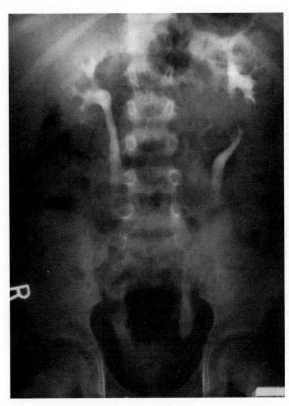

FIGURE 4. Lateral deviation of ureter caused by neuroblastoma, with primary megaureter. A 10-minute film from an excretory urogram demonstrates lateral deviation of the left kidney and proximal ureter by a mass. The child also has bilateral primary megaureter, for which he was being studied.

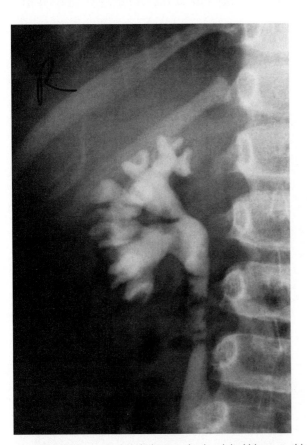

FIGURE 3. Mild hydronephrosis is seen in the right kidney on this excretory urogram. Filling defects in the ureter were resected and found to be polyps.

thickness, but in more severe cases it is variously atrophic. The distal segment of the ureter appears grossly normal, with normal ganglion cells without evidence of organic narrowing on probing with ureteral catheters, but histologically, it shows hypoplasia and atrophy of muscle fibers and an increase in collagen tissue. The remaining muscle fibers are predominantly circular, and in severe cases there is little or no muscle tissue present. The proximal dilated segment of the ureter shows muscular hypertrophy. The ureteral orifices are cystoscopically normal.

The symptoms include recurrent urinary tract infection, abdominal pain, and hematuria. Ureteral stone formation has been reported. Not uncommonly, the lesion is discovered as an incidental finding in asymptomatic patients. The findings on excretory urography and by US reflect the pathologic changes in the ureter and kidney. The short, nondilated distal segment of the ureter can be seen on postvoiding films. The voiding cystogram shows no organic or functional abnormalities of the bladder or urethra. Vesical reflux is not a feature of the disorder but does occur in some children. As seen fluoroscopically, the opacified ureter shows normal or hyperactive peristalsis with waves starting in the proximal ureter and increasing in amplitude, and fading distally into the dilated portion of the ureter. Antiperistaltic waves may be observed. Retrograde ureterogra-

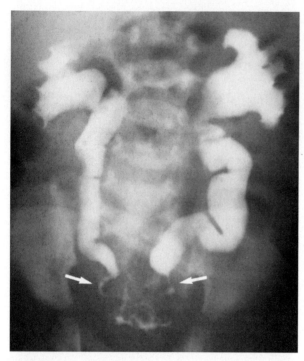

FIGURE 5. Postvoiding film of a cystourethrogram in a newborn infant showing bilateral reflux and bilateral ureterovesical junction obstruction caused by stenosis of the distal ureteral segments *(arrows).*

Table 2 ■ CAUSES OF URETERAL OBSTRUCTION

Retrocaval ureter	Acquired strictures
Retroiliac ureter	Polyps
Other vessels	Extrinsic lesions (masses)
Valves	Primary megaureter
Clot	Calculus, fungus ball

phy shows the changes more clearly than excretory urography.

Renal agenesis and other contralateral abnormalities have been described. Ipsilaterally, megacalicosis may occur.

URETEROVESICAL JUNCTION OBSTRUCTION AND REFLUX

The coexistence of vesicoureteral reflux and obstruction of the distal end of the refluxing ureter is not uncommon. The reflux may be primary and caused by a congenital anomaly of the UVJ, or it may be secondary to a lower urinary tract obstruction, neurogenic bladder, or other functional voiding disorders. Extravesiculation of the intramural portion of the ureter has been suggested as a possible cause of obstruction in some cases. This segment of the ureter is composed of only

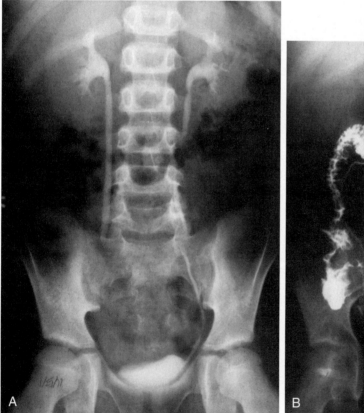

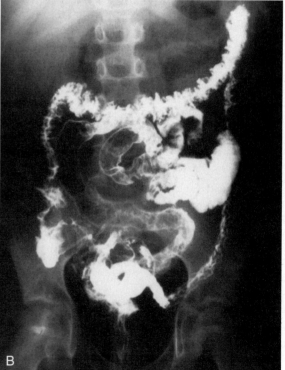

FIGURE 6. Effect of Crohn's disease on the right ureter. **A,** A 10-minute film from an excretory urogram shows that the right ureter is mildly dilated, straight, and visible only to the pelvic rim. **B,** Late film from a small bowel follow-through shows extensive Crohn's disease, especially in the right lower quadrant.

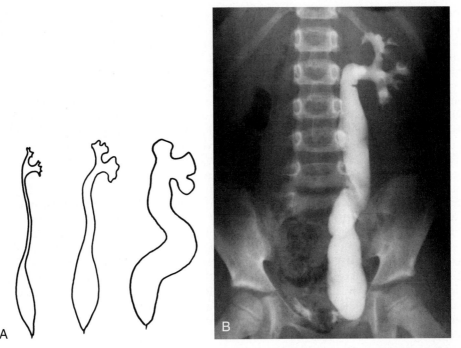

FIGURE 7. A, Appearance of the pelvocaliceal system and ureter in three examples of primary megaureter of different severity. **B,** Post–voiding cystourethrogram in a 6½–year-old girl showing left-sided ureteral reflux and ureterovesical junction obstruction with changes suggesting primary megaureter. The ureteral dilatation is diffuse but most pronounced in the lower segment. The renal pelvis and calices are very little affected.

circular muscle fibers, which would prevent normal progress of ureteral peristalsis and cause a functional obstruction. Reflux may also be observed in some patients with primary megaureter (see Table 3).

URETERAL DUPLICATION

Duplication of the renal pelvix and ureter (Fig. 8) is one of the most common anomalies of the urinary tracts. It may be partial or complete. Incomplete duplication ranges from bifid pelvis to two ureters joining anywhere along their course and continuing inferiorly as a single structure. In completely duplicated systems, the two ureters are separate throughout their entire course. The ureter draining the upper pole of the kidney normally inserts in the bladder more caudally and more medially than the lower pole ureter (Weigert-Meyer rule), and has a longer submucosal tunnel than the lower pole ureter. Embryologically, the more cranial of the two ureteric buds from the mesonephric duct separates from the latter duct later, and is thus carried caudiomedially, yet the more cranial ureteral portion of the

metanephros unites with the more cranial ureteric bud. This renders the inferior and medially inserting ureter the drain for the upper pole. In all types of duplication, the affected kidney is often longer than the opposite organ, and the lower pelvocaliceal system is usually larger and has more calices and a better defined pelvis than the proximal one. Ureteral duplication may be bilateral, but unilateral is six times more common.

Ureteral duplication is of no clinical importance unless it is complicated by another congenital lesion or an acquired process. *Ureteral ectopia* with or without ureterocele is one of the principal anomalies associated with ureteral duplication. *Congenital UPJ obstruction* is

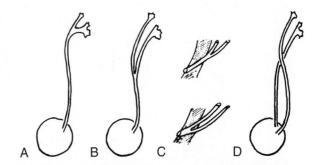

FIGURE 8. Various forms of ureteral duplication. **A,** Bifid pelvis. **B,** Partial duplication, with the two ureters joining in the mid-lumbar area (Y ureter). **C,** Incomplete duplication, with the two ureters joining very near the bladder or within the bladder wall (V ureter). **D,** Complete duplication, with the two ureters draining into the bladder separately; the ureter draining the upper part of the kidney normally ends slightly below and medial to the lower pole ureter (Weigert-Meyer law).

Table 3 ■ TYPES OF MEGAURETER
Primary
Congenital ureterovesical junction obstruction
Prune-belly syndrome
Refluxing megaureter
Megaureter caused by stone
Bladder outlet obstruction

occasionally seen in patients with complete ureteral duplication and affects preferentially the larger, inferior renal pelvis. *Vesicoureteral reflux* and *urinary tract infections* are not uncommon and occur more frequently in completely duplicated systems (both ureters draining into the bladder) than in unduplicated ureters. In completely duplex systems, the reflux may involve both ureters but more often is limited to the lower pole ureter. Reflux limited to the upper pole ureter is rare. Ureteroureteral reflux may occur in double ureters joining in the lumbar area (Y ureters), when urine flowing from one limb of the Y ascends into the other limb rather than passing down the common stem.

When renal function is adequate, duplication of the pelvocaliceal system and ureter is visible on the excretory urogram, but it is sometimes difficult by this method to determine whether the duplication is partial or complete; retrograde studies are more helpful for this purpose. The diagnosis of a duplicated upper tract by US may be difficult or impossible unless a prominent segment of renal cortex (column of Bertin) is present between these two pelvocaliceal systems (Fig. 9). It may be clearly established by CECT by demonstration of two separate pelvocaliceal systems and two ureters (two proximal ureters and a single distal ureter in the case of incomplete duplication). A section through the intermediate area of the kidney may result in a "faceless" kidney without major renal vessels or other pelvic structures.

When the superior component of a duplicated system is not visualized on the excretory urogram, as is fre-quently the case in patients with ureteral ectopia with or without ureterocele, the diagnosis is established or is suspected from the appearance of the opacified lower collecting system (Fig. 10A). In such cases the visualized calices are fewer than usual and the proximal calices may be short and broad. The distance between the upper-most medial calix and the spine is increased compared with the opposite side. The longitudinal axis of the kidney tends to be perpendicular or is reversed, and the visualized calices and pelvis are displaced laterally and downward by the dilated nonvisualized pelvocaliceal system ("drooping lily" appearance). The opacified ipsilateral ureter frequently is displaced laterally by a dilated, nonvisualized upper pole ureter (Fig. 10B). US is a very important diagnostic tool in further defining the anatomy. The dilated upper pole pelvis, thin renal parenchyma, and dilated unopacified ureter are easily identified by this method (Fig. 10C–E). When the nonvisualized system is not dilated, the urographic findings may be very subtle, and, in some cases, the urogram and US are entirely normal. CECT may be diagnostic in these cases.

VARIANTS OF URETERAL DUPLICATION

ACCESSORY URETER/URETERAL STUMP

Possibly related to ureteral duplication, an accessory ureter is a tubular structure originating from the distal

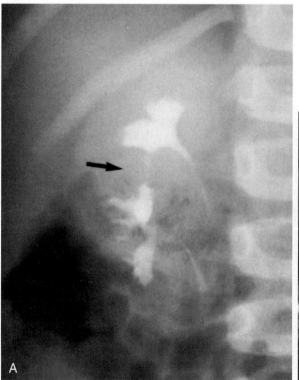
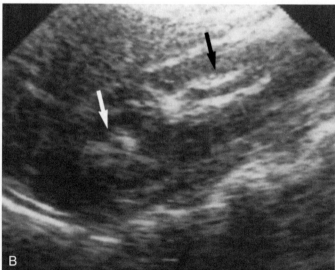

FIGURE 9. A, Excretory urogram in an 11-month-old infant with upper tract duplication on the right. Abundant cortical tissue separates the two pelvocaliceal complexes *(arrow).* **B,** Renal ultrasound on the same patient demonstrates two pelvocaliceal complexes *(arrows).*

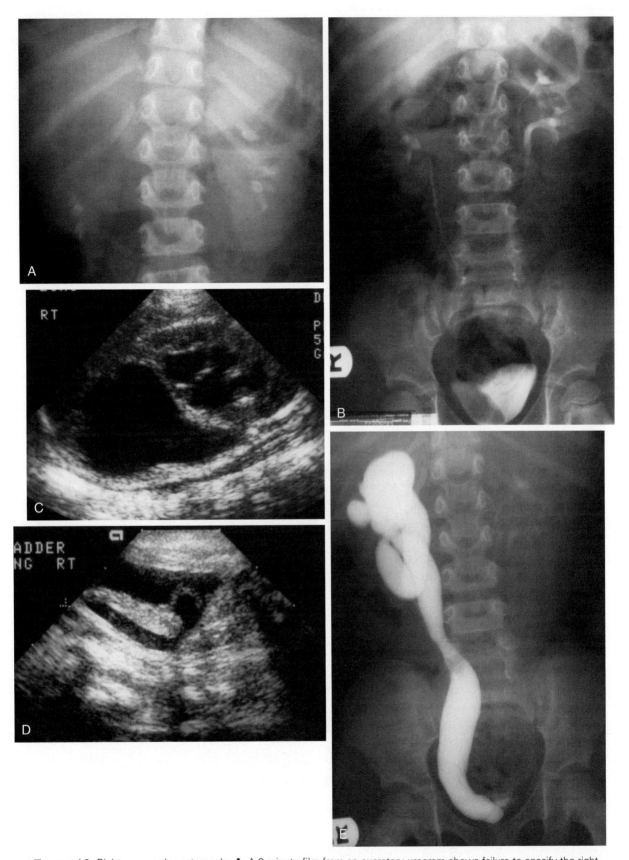

FIGURE 10. Right upper pole ureterocele. **A,** A 3-minute film from an excretory urogram shows failure to opacify the right upper pole (negative pyelogram) and a "drooping lily" right lower pole. **B,** A 15-minute film shows bilateral duplicated systems with obstruction of the right upper pole and a filling defect along the right half of the bladder representing the ureterocele. **C,** Longitudinal ultrasound of the right kidney shows marked hydronephrosis of the upper pole of the kidney. The lower pole shows mild dilatation of the collecting system as well. **D,** Longitudinal scan of the pelvis shows the right ureter dilated and ending in a ureterocele that extends into the bladder. **E,** Voiding cystourethrogram demonstrates reflux into the ureterocele and right upper pole as well as mild reflux into the left kidney.

segment of a ureter and extending cephalad along the normal ureter to end blindly proximally without connection to the pelvocaliceal system or renal parenchyma. The ureteral stump varies from a few centimeters to a narrow patent cord that extends almost to the kidney. The anomaly is demonstrated by excretory urography and is further delineated by retrograde ureterography (Fig. 11).

URETERAL TRIPLICATION

Ureteral triplication (Fig. 12) is a rare anomaly in which three ureters arise from the kidney, one from the upper pole, the second from the midzone of the kidney, and the third from the lower pole. The three ureters may drain separately in the bladder or one may end ectopically in the urethra; the parenchyma drained by the ectopic ureter is usually small and poorly functioning. In a second type, two of the three ureters may join in the lumbar area to form a single Y-shaped ureter that drains usually in the bladder, together with a normal upper pole ureter. In a third type, the three ureters join in the lumbar area to form a common distal ureter that drains in the bladder. More than half the cases of ureteral triplication defy

the Weigert-Meyer rule. Four ureters emanating from a single kidney have been described.

SUPERNUMERARY KIDNEY

Supernumerary kidney is another rare anomaly in which there is an accessory third kidney that is not attached or is very loosely attached to the normal ipsilateral kidney. In the first type, the accessory and the adjacent normal kidneys are drained by a common Y-shaped ureter. In the second type, the accessory kidney has a separate ureter that drains usually in the bladder, and sometimes in the urethra or vagina.

URETERAL ECTOPIA

An ectopic ureter is one that drains in an abnormal location (outside the posterolateral angle of the trigone) either within the bladder or extravesically. Extravesical ureteral ectopia is more common and clinically more important than the intravesical type. It is also more common in girls than in boys, with some anatomic and functional differences between the two sexes (Table 4). It is more common in ureteral duplication anomalies (68% to 80%).

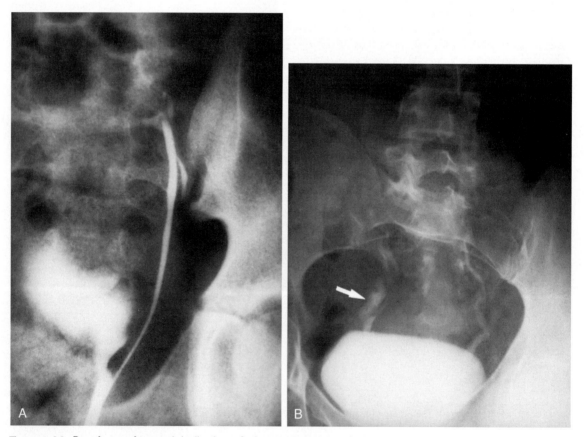

FIGURE 11. Rare forms of ureteral duplications. **A,** An accessory ureter is demonstrated on this retrograde ureterogram ascending blindly on the left pelvic brim. **B,** A voiding cystourethrogram demonstrates reflux into the normal left and right ureters and a blind-ending ureteral stump on the right *(arrow).*

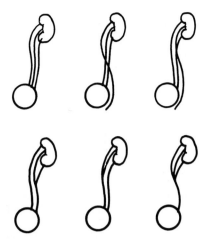

FIGURE 12. Types of ureteral triplication. **Top,** Complete triplication: all three ureters enter the bladder separately or one may end ectopically outside the bladder, sometimes in association with a ureterocele. **Bottom,** Incomplete triplication: two ureters or all three ureters join in the lumbar area and drain in the bladder by two orifices or only one orifice.

INTRAVESICAL URETERAL ECTOPIA

Two types of intravesical ureteral ectopia are recognized: lateral and caudal. In lateral ectopia, the more common of the two, one or both ureters (the lower pole ureter in a duplicated system) drain in the bladder more laterally and craniad than normal. The intramural submucosal tunnel of the affected ureter tends to be short or otherwise defective, leading to reflux in many cases. In the second type, one or both ureters (the lower pole ureter in a duplicated system) drain caudad and medial to the usual site along a line extending from the normal lateral corner of the trigone to the bladder neck. These ureters are probably less prone to reflux than the lateral type.

EXTRAVESICAL URETERAL ECTOPIA IN GIRLS

This form of ureteral ectopia (Fig. 13) is associated with a duplicated system in at least 85% of the cases, and affects the upper pole ureter in practically all cases.

Partial or complete duplication of the opposite system is common, and sometimes the anomaly is bilateral. The ectopic ureter may end in the urethra or in the vestibule, or less commonly in the vagina. A common presenting complaint is continuous leakage of urine in the context of an otherwise normal voiding pattern. Leakage of urine is observed even if the anomalous ureter ends in the proximal urethra, owing to relative weakness of the external urethral sphincter in girls. The renal parenchyma drained by the ectopic ureter is often dysplastic. The ectopic-ending ureter is frequently dilated and tortuous but may be normal in size, and sometimes it ends superiorly in a minute collecting system and a diminutive upper pole. The ipsilateral, lower pole ureter may be normal in size or dilated and is frequently the site of reflux. Reflux and upper tract dilatation may also be observed on the opposite side. The function of the renal segment drained by an ectopic ureter is usually decreased and may be absent. The corresponding pelvocaliceal system and ureter may be visualized only on delayed films of an excretory urogram. A nonfunctioning second system is suspected when the visualized pelvocaliceal system is displaced downward and laterally and by the other indirect signs of duplication described above.

When the aberrant ureter empties in the urethra, reflux into the ectopic ureter is occasionally demonstrated in the voiding study. A vaginogram may show reflux in the affected ureter if this terminates in the vagina (Figs. 14 and 15). US is a valuable adjunct to excretory urography and may be diagnostic when the anomalous ureter is dilated. The course of this ureter may be followed down to and beyond the bladder. A vaginal ectopic ureter may be shown by US to be connected with a urine-filled vagina. A diethylenetriaminepentaacetic acid (DTPA) or more commonly MAG$_3$ renal scan may show essentially the same findings as the excretory urogram, and a dimercaptosuccinic acid (DMSA) scintigram may be useful in evaluation of the renal parenchyma. Renal function may be detected on the renal scan that is not apparent on the urogram. CECT or MRI may reveal a second ureter that is not demonstrated by other methods.

Single (unduplicated) ureteral ectopia in girls is uncommon and usually unilateral. The corresponding kidney is frequently small and dysplastic and may be

Table 4 ■ EXTRAVESICAL URETERAL ECTOPIA		
	GIRLS	**BOYS**
Duplicated System	More common	Less common
	Inserts into urethra, vestibule, vagina	Inserts into prostatic urethra, bladder neck, genital ducts
	Urethral-ending ureter refluxes	Same
	Ectopic ureter normal	Same
	Drains atropic nubbin	Same
	Lower pole refluxes	Same
	Chief complaint: continuous urine leakage	Chief complaint: infection
Single System	Uncommon	Uncommon
	Associated with small, often ectopic kidney	Associated with dysplastic kidney
	May insert in urethra, vestibule, vagina	May insert in seminal vessicle
	Gartner's duct cyst	Ejaculatory duct wolffian tissue posterior to bladder

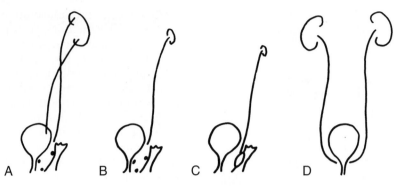

FIGURE 13. Various types of ureteral ectopia in females. **A,** In this variant, the most common of the group, the ectopic ureter drains into the urethra, in the perineum near the ureteral meatus, or in the vagina low or near the vault. On the affected side, there is a ureteral duplication and the affected ureter is the one draining the upper pole of the kidney, which is frequently small and dysplastic. **B** and **C,** Same type of ureteral ectopia as in **A,** but without ureteral duplication. Occasionally, the ectopic ureter drains into a Gartner's duct cyst in the wall of the vagina **(C)** and, in such cases, the corresponding kidney may be absent. **D,** Bilateral single ureteral ectopia (no ureteral duplication), in which the two ureters terminate at the bladder neck or in the proximal urethra. This uncommon anomaly occurs almost exclusively in females and is usually associated with a wide bladder neck, a defective internal sphincter and sometimes a malformed urethra, and urinary incontinence.

ectopic. Sometimes the ectopic ureter is connected with a minute dysplastic kidney (renal aplasia), or ends blindly superiorly without renal tissue (renal agenesis). The anomalous ureter may terminate in the urethra, vestibule, or vagina. Occasionally, a single ectopic ureter ends in a blind cystic structure in the lateral wall of the vagina (Gartner's duct cyst) (Fig. 16); in these cases the ipsilateral kidney is usually nonfunctioning and may be absent. Sometimes a Gartner's duct cyst is found in the wall of the vagina without a demonstrable ureter or kidney on that side.

Bilateral unduplicated ureteral ectopia (no ureter entering the bladder; see Fig. 13*D*) is a rare anomaly

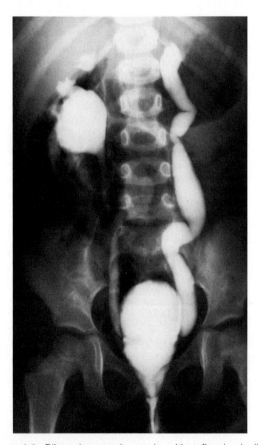

FIGURE 14. Bilateral ureteral ectopia with reflux in duplicated systems. Voiding cystourethrogram shows grade II–III reflux into both upper and lower pole collecting systems on the right and grade V reflux into an atrophic left upper pole "nubbin." The ureter from the left upper pole ended in the vagina.

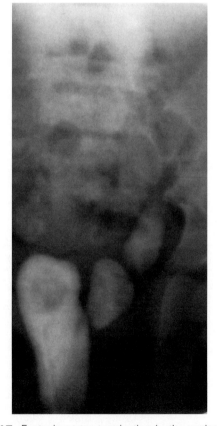

FIGURE 15. Ecotopic ureter terminating in the vagina. Contrast injected into the vagina is seen filling the left ureter.

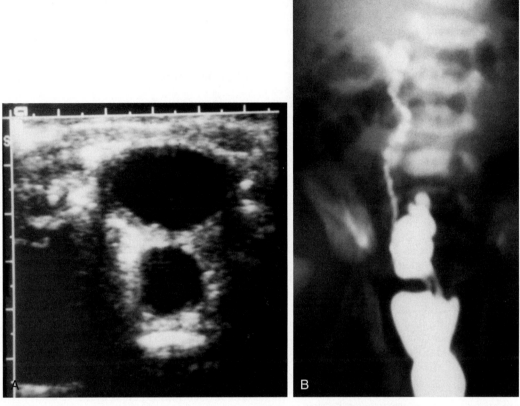

FIGURE 16. Ectopic ureter ending in Gartner's duct cyst. **A,** Transverse ultrasound scan of the pelvis shows a cystic structure posterior to the bladder. **B,** Voiding cystourethrogram shows filling of the bladder through the Gartner's cyst and through the ureter to the upper pole.

affecting females almost exclusively. The two ureters terminate at the bladder neck or in the proximal urethra. This form of ureteral ectopia is usually accompanied by defective formation of the trigone and base of the bladder, a wide bladder neck, a deformed internal sphincter, and in some cases a short and broad urethra. Incontinence is the rule even after reimplantation of both ureters.

EXTRAVESICAL URETERAL ECTOPIA IN BOYS

Extravesical ureteral ectopia also occurs in males but much less commonly than in females. As described in the female, the anomaly commonly involves the upper pole ureter in a duplex system, but also may occur in a single, unduplicated ureter. The anomalous ureter may insert in the prostatic urethra, sometimes near the bladder neck and much less often in the genital ducts (Fig. 17). Ureteral ectopia to the posterior urethra (usually ending slightly above or at the level of the verumontanum, sometimes in the utricle) is seen most often in duplicated systems and almost always affects the upper pole ureter (Figs. 18 and 19). The renal parenchyma drained by the ectopic ureter is commonly small and dysplastic and often nonfunctioning. The opposite

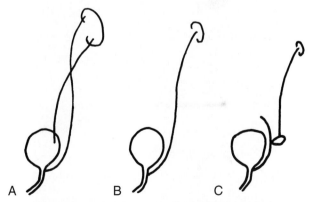

FIGURE 17. Ureteral ectopia in males. **A,** In most cases, the ectopic ureter ends in the posterior urethra. As in the female, the upper tract on the side of the lesion is often duplicated and the ectopic ureter is regularly the one draining the upper part of the kidney, which frequently is dysplastic. **B,** Ectopic ureter connected to the posterior urethra without ureteral duplication. **C,** Ectopic ureter connected to a seminal vesicle, vas deferens, or ejaculatory duct. Ureteral ectopia to the male genital tract frequently is not associated with ureteral duplication, and the corresponding kidney is generally small and dysplastic or absent.

upper tract may be duplicated. Urinary tract infection is the most common clinical manifestation. Urinary incontinence is not a problem in boys because the ectopic ureter drains above the strongly developed external urethral sphincter. The urographic and sonographic features are similar to those described in girls.

In ureteral ectopia to the genital tract in males, the affected ureter is almost always single (unduplicated) and ends in a markedly dilated seminal vesical, the vas deferens, the ejaculatory duct, or a mass of ill-defined, tortuous tubular structures located behind the trigone of the bladder. Some of these structures probably represent a persistent and markedly dilated and distorted embryonic common distal duct for the wolffian (spermatic) duct and primitive ureter. The ipsilateral kidney is usually very small and severely dysplastic or absent, and the affected ureter may be atretic. Cryptorchidism or testicular hypoplasia on the side of the lesion is common. Pain on voiding and straining to void are common clinical manifestations. Epididymo-orchitis is a common complication. A mass may be felt between the rectum and the bladder on rectal examination. The excretory urogram almost invariably reveals no renal function on the affected side, and commonly shows an extrinsic mass deforming the base of the bladder posterolaterally. The voiding cystogram often shows an extrinsic deformity of the posterior wall of the bladder and may reveal reflux of contrast material in the ipsilateral ejaculatory duct. The cystic nature of the mass may be demonstrated by US. The lesion may also be demonstrated by computed tomography or MRI, and the status of the upper tracts may be studied by a renal scintigram.

URETEROCELE

Ureterocele is a globular expansion of the terminal segment of the ureter projecting into the lumen of the bladder. The anomaly is relatively common and is of two types: (1) intravesical ureterocele, which is located entirely within the bladder; and (2) ectopic ureterocele, which is usually large and extends to the bladder neck area and proximal urethra. Both forms may be associated with a duplicated or an unduplicated system.

INTRAVESICAL URETEROCELE

This form of ureterocele, also called stenotic, orthotopic, simple, or adult-type ureterocele, is much more common in adults than in children, suggesting that it may be acquired in many cases. In children, it is more frequently associated with significant hydrouteronephrosis. It is produced by a herniation of the very distal end of the ureter into the bladder, where it presents as a rounded cystic mass usually less than 1 cm in diameter, but occasionally much larger. The ureterocele is located at the lateral angle of the trigone, and is entirely within the bladder. The ureteral orifice is on the surface of the ureterocele and is variously stenotic, a feature that may be responsible in part for the anomaly. Embryologically, it may be due to persistence of Chwalla's membrane. The lesion is often bilateral and, although it is commonly seen in single (unduplicated) ureters, it may also involve the upper and sometimes the lower pole ureter of a duplicated system. Intravesical ureterocele is often discovered as an incidental asymptomatic finding, but, when large, it may be associated with a more severe degree of ureteral obstruction and may obstruct the bladder outlet. Stone formation within the ureterocele has been reported. Reflux into the ureter may occur.

The urographic findings are characteristic. The affected ureter is variously dilated but seldom more than 1 cm in diameter. The dilatation involves predominantly the lower half of the ureter, but the entire ureter, pelvocaliceal system, and renal parenchyma may also be affected in more severely obstructed cases. In the early films of an excretory urogram, the lesion generally presents as a round, radiolucent defect at the trigone. As contrast material collects within the bladder and in the ureterocele, it outlines a rounded or cystic mass surrounded by a radiolucent halo representing the nonopacified wall of the ureterocele. This is the well-known "cobra head" or "spring onion" formation characteristic of the lesion (Fig. 20). A radiolucent filling defect is usually the only finding on retrograde cystography. Some intravesical ureteroceles may be large and extend to the bladder area, simulating an ectopic ureterocele, but even in such cases the contrast material

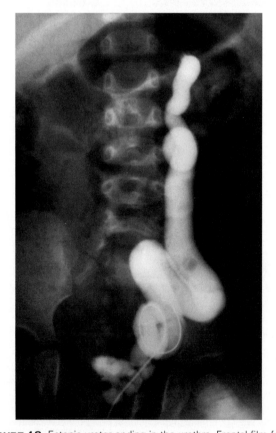

FIGURE 18. Ectopic ureter ending in the urethra. Frontal film from a voiding cystourethrogram shows that the catheter has exited the posterior urethra and entered the left ureter. Contrast is seen extending cephalad to an atrophic upper pole.

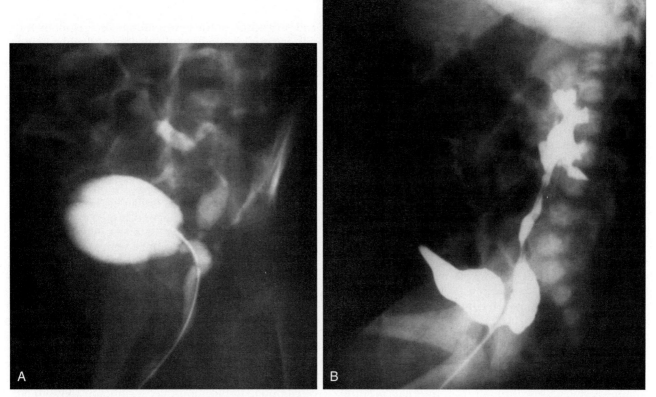

FIGURE 19. Ectopic ureter ending in the posterior urethra. **A,** Voiding cystourethrography in this patient demonstrates reflux into ureter emanating off the posterior urethra. **B,** In another patient, a catheter is seen traversing the urethra and exiting the posterior urethra into the ureter and ureteropelvic junction.

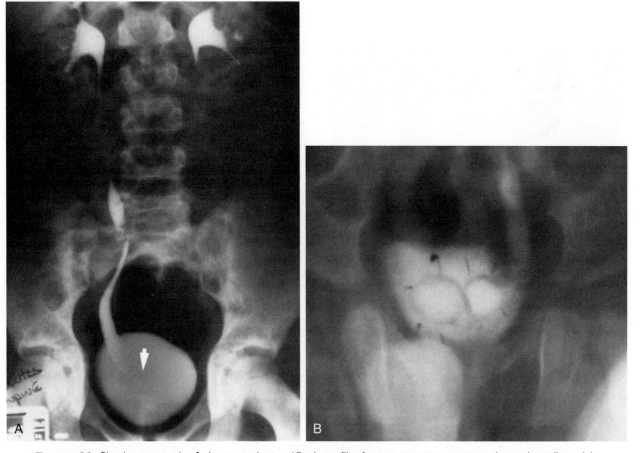

FIGURE 20. Simple ureterocele. **A,** In one patient, a 15-minute film from an excretory urogram shows the solitary right ureter ending in the typical "cobra head" appearance of a ureterocele. **B,** Coned-down view of the bladder in this second patient demonstrates two "cobra heads" *(black marks),* one from each simple ureter.

usually outlines the lower part of the mass. A large ureterocele may be shown by US as a cystic mass protruding into the lumen of the bladder. A dilated ureter connecting with the ureterocele may also be demonstrated by this method.

ECTOPIC URETEROCELE

Ectopic or infantile ureterocele (Figs. 21 through 24) is one of the most important urologic disorders in children and is the most common cause of bladder outlet obstruction in girls (Table 5). It is more common than the intravesical type, and is five to seven times more frequent in females than males. It is unilateral in 90% of the cases and bilateral in 10%. Its anatomy differs from that of an intravesical ureterocele in several respects. Ectopic ureteroceles most often occur in a duplicated system and almost always are connected with the upper pole ureter. An ectopic ureterocele of a similar configuration also occurs in unduplicated ureter, more commonly in boys than in girls. In both types, the ureter connected with the ureterocele enters the bladder wall at the normal site, descends toward the bladder neck submucosally, passes through the internal urethral sphincter, and terminates ectopically in the proximal urethra. In contrast to simple ureterocele, in which the "cyst" is formed by herniation of the distal end of the ureter, the ectopic ureterocele represents a dilatation and protrusion of the entire submucosal segment of the ureter into the lumen of the bladder and at the bladder neck.

The ectopic ureterocele has a broad base and tends to be larger than the simple intravesical type, and characteristically is located more inferiorly in the bladder and extends to the bladder neck area and proximal urethra. Its orifice is almost always in the posterior urethra and may be stenotic, but more often it is patent, and the ureterocele is obstructed by the sphincteric action of the bladder neck. In many cases no ureteral orifice can be found at endoscopy or at surgery. In rare instances, the ureterocele has a patulous orifice in the bladder, even though the dilated submucosal ureter extends downward through the bladder neck to end blindly in the urethra. This anatomic arrangement is termed *cecoureterocele*. A typical ureterocele with an acquired perforation resulting from infection or previous bladder instrumentation may acquire a similar configuration.

The ureterocele may obstruct the bladder neck or the opposite ureteral orifice (see Fig. 21), and, in patients with ureteral duplication, it may deform the musculature of the adjacent ureter so that reflux into the lower pole ureter occurs (40% to 50% of cases). Reflux may also occur on the opposite side (15%), where a partial or complete duplication tract is common (35% to 50% of cases). Reflux into the ureter connected with the ureterocele is very unusual. Occasionally, the ureterocele herniates into the urethra, causing urethral obstruction, or may evert, appearing as a diverticulum

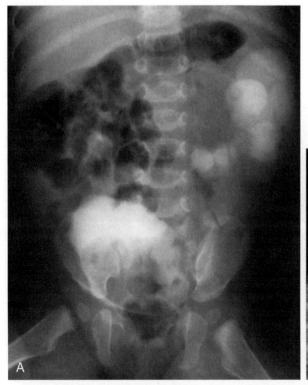
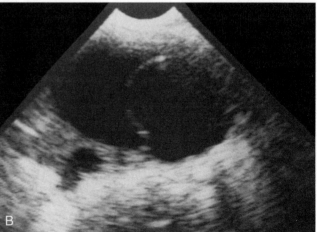

FIGURE 21. Left upper pole ureterocele. **A,** A large ureterocele is seen on this excretory urogram occupying the left lower half of the bladder (filling defect), partially obstructing the left lower pole and completely obstructing the right kidney. **B,** Longitudinal ultrasound of the bladder shows the ureterocele distally and a bit of dilated ureter proximally.

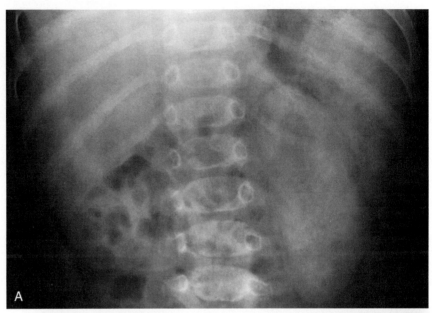

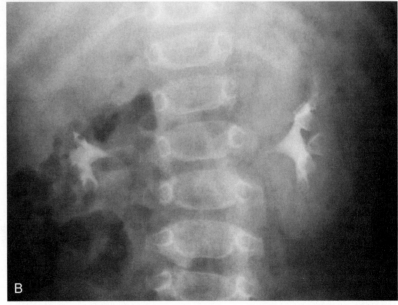

FIGURE 22. Bilateral upper pole obstruction. **A,** A 1-minute film from an excretory urogram shows radiolucent areas in the upper poles as a result of delayed opacification. **B,** A 15-minute film shows the bilateral "drooping lilies."

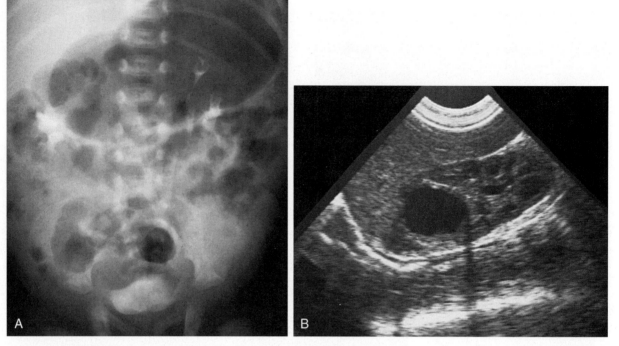

FIGURE 23. Right upper pole ureterocele. **A,** A 10-minute film from an excretory urogram shows a normal-appearing duplicated left collecting system. On the right, the lower pole is opacified but not the upper pole. **B,** Longitudinal scan of the right upper quadrant show an echo-free area in the upper half of the right kidney representing the obstructed upper pole.

(Fig. 25); in females, it may present as a fleshy mass at the external urethral meatus resembling a prolapsed urethra.

The ureter connected with the ureterocele is often dilated and tortuous. Its proximal segment and the corresponding pelvocaliceal system may also be very large but sometimes are only mildly dilated. Sometimes the entire ureter is of normal size and ends in a point at the level of the kidney. The adjacent ureter and the opposite ureter(s) are commonly dilated. In the majority of cases, the proximal moiety of the kidney on the affected side (the entire kidney in an unduplicated ureter) is hypoplastic and dysplastic and may be further reduced in size by pressure atrophy and infection.

Table 5 ■ ECTOPIC URETEROCELE
Most common cause of bladder outlet obstruction in girls
90% present under 3 yr of age, one fourth present as newborns
Clinical manifestations
Urinary tract infection
Failure to thrive
Urinary retention
Flank pain
5–7 times more frequent in males
Simple ectopic ureterocele more common in boys
Most often in duplicated systems
Connected to upper pole moiety
Enters at normal orifice, migrates to ectopic location
Bigger, more inferiorly located than simple ureterocele
May occlude other side
May cause contralateral reflux
May cause urethral obstruction
May present as an intralabial mass

More than 90% of the cases are discovered in children under 3 years of age, and in more than one fourth of the cases the diagnosis is made in the newborn period and is often suspected on the basis of a prenatal US. Urinary tract infection is the most common presenting clinical manifestation. Failure to thrive, difficulty in voiding, urinary retention, flank pain, and sometimes chronic renal failure are prominent manifestations of the anomaly in older infants and in children. Dribbling of urine is not a feature of the disorder.

The excretory urogram shows no function of the renal parenchyma drained by the ureterocele-bearing ureter in 90% of the cases and poor function in 10%. The affected ureter is very seldom visualized. In the usual type of ureterocele associated with a duplex system, the visualized pelvocaliceal system is displaced downward and laterally, and the ureter is frequently displaced laterally by the dilated, nonvisualized upper tract. The excretory urogram in patients with ectopic ureterocele in a single unduplicated ureter usually shows no function on the side of the lesion.

In most cases, the ureterocele is clearly shown by the excreted contrast material accumulated in the bladder as a rounded and usually eccentrically placed filling defect (Table 6). Occasionally, the defect is lobulated. A double ureterocele, one on each side of the midline, is seen in bilateral cases. The outline of the ureterocele is usually clearly defined by the contrast material except for the lower margin of the mass, which is confluent with the base of the bladder and bladder neck. This is in contrast to simple or intravesical ureteroceles, which are usually completely outlined. On the voiding cystourethrogram, the negative defect of the ureterocele is commonly obscured by the concentrated contrast mate-

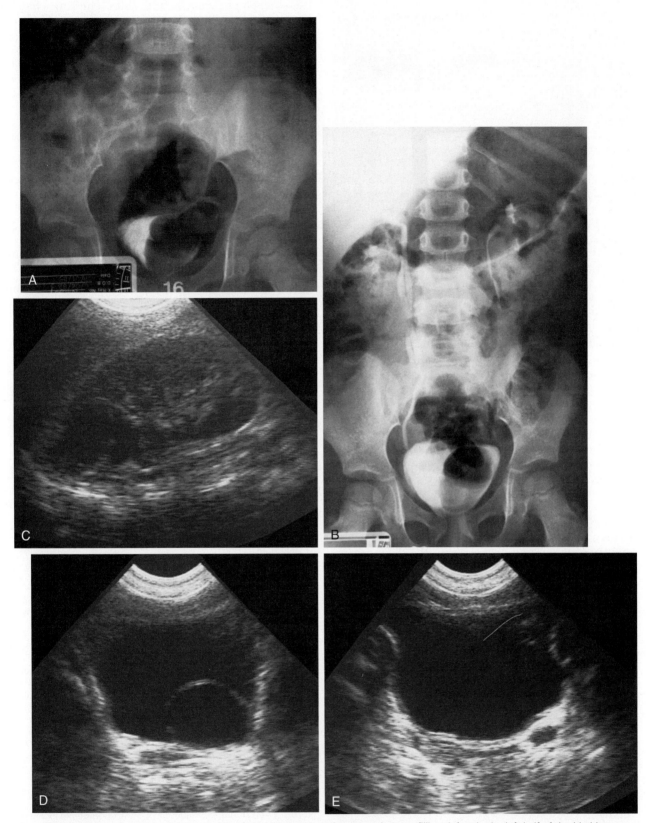

FIGURE 24. Left upper pole ureterocele. **A,** Voiding cystourethrogram shows a filling defect in the left half of the bladder. **B,** A 10-minute film from an excretory urethrogram shows a double system on the right but only a single, normal-appearing collecting system and ureter on the left. A filling defect is seen in the bladder. **C,** Ultrasound of the left kidney shows an echo-free (hydronephrotic) left upper pole. **D,** Transverse scan of the bladder demonstrates the left upper pole ureterocele appearing as a cystic mass in the bladder. **E,** Transverse scan more cephalad shows the dilated left upper pole ureter.

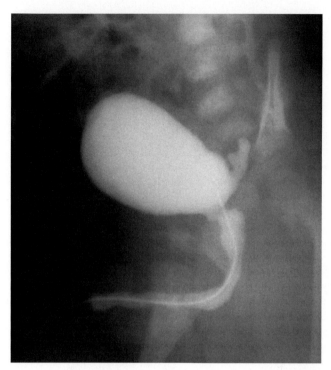

FIGURE 25. A diverticulum-like structure is seen on this film from a voiding cystourethrogram. Subsequent films confirmed an everting ureterocele.

rial but may be seen well during early filling of the bladder. If the bladder is overdistended, by contrast material or during voiding, the cystic mass may be decompressed and flattened against the bladder wall and may even evert, simulating a paraureteral diverticulum. The voiding cystogram may show prolapse of the ureterocele into the urethra.

US is a valuable adjunct to cystourethrography and excretory urogram and may establish the diagnosis in many cases. The main findings include the demonstration of an intravesical cystic lesion of variable size attached to the posterolateral wall of the bladder (cyst within cyst), associated with a cystic structure in the upper pole of the kidney and two dilated ureters on the side of the ureterocele. US is also valuable in the evaluation of the rest of the upper tracts and size of

the renal parenchyma on both sides. The same changes shown by excretory urography may be detected by renal scintigraphy, including decreased function at the superior pole of the kidney and often a photon-deficient area in the bladder corresponding to the ureterocele. The nuclear renogram may show function in the kidney or part of the kidney connected with the ureterocele that is not visualized by excretory urography.

SUGGESTED READINGS

Avni FE, Nicaise N, Hall M, et al: The role of MR imaging for the assessment of complicated duplex kidneys in children: preliminary report. Pediatr Radiol 2001;31:215

Amis ES, Cronan JJ, Pfister RC: Lower moiety hydronephrosis in duplicated kidneys. Urology 1985;26:82

Berdon WE: Contemporary imaging approach to pediatric urologic problems. Radiol Clin North Am 1991;29:605

Bisset GS, Strife JL: The duplex collecting system in girls with urinary tract infection: prevalence and significance. AJR Am J Roentgenol 1987;148:497

Blair D, Rigsby C, Rosenfield AT: The nubbin sign on computed tomography and sonography. Urol Radiol 1987;9:149

Bloom RA, Crooks EK, Wise HA: Complete ureteral triplication with ectopia. Urology 1984;25:176

Braverman RM, Lebowitz RL: Occult ectopic ureter in girls with urinary incontinence: diagnosis using CT. AJR Am J Roentgenol 1991;156:365

Caldamone AA: Duplication anomalies of the upper tract in infants and children. Urol Clin North Am 1991;12:75

Churchill BM, Abara EO, McLorie GA: Ureteral duplication, ectopy and ureteroceles. Pediatr Clin North Am 1987;34:1273

Cremin BJ: A review of ultrasonic appearances of posterior urethral valves and ureteroceles. Pediatr Radiol 1986;16:357

Currarino G: Single vaginal ectopic ureter and Gartner's duct cyst with ipsilateral renal hypoplasia (or agenesis). J Urol 1982;128:988

Docimo SG, Lebowitz RL, Retik AB, et al: Congenital midureteral obstruction. Urol Radiol 1989;11:156

Gosalbez R Jr, Gosalbez R, Piro C, et al: Ureteral triplication and ureterocele: report of 3 cases and review of the literature. J Urol 1991;145:105

Gylys-Morin VM, Minevich E, Tackett LD, et al: Magnetic resonance imaging of the dysplastic renal moiety and ectopic ureter. J Urol 2000;164:2034

Hawas N, Noah M, Pattel PJ: Blind-ending ureter: clinical significance? An analysis of 13 cases with review of the literature. Eur Urol 1987;13:39

Herman TE, McAlister OH: Radiographic manifestations of congenital anomalies of the lower urinary tract. Radiol Clin North Am 1991;29:365

Horgan JG, Rosenfield NS, Weiss RM, Rosenfield AT: Is renal ultrasound a reliable indicator of a nonobstructed duplication anomaly? Pediatr Radiol 1984;14:388

Hulnick DH, Bosniak MA: Faceless kidney: CT sign of renal duplicity. J Comput Assist Tomogr 1986;10:771

Jednak R, Kryger JV, Barthold JS, Gonzales R: A simplified technique of upper pole heminephrectomy for duplex kidney. J Urol 2000;164:1326

Kass EJ, Fink-Bennett D: Contemporary techniques for the radioisotopic evaluation of the dilated urinary tract. Urol Clin North Am 1990;17:273

Keating MA, Retik AB: Management of dilated obstructed ureter. Urol Clin North Am 1990;17:291

King BF, Hattery RR, Lieber MM, et al: Congenital cystic disease of the seminal vesicle. Radiology 1991;178:207

Korogi Y, Takahashi M, Fujimura N, et al: Computed tomography demonstration of renal dysplasia with a vaginal ectopic ureter. J Comput Tomogr 1986;10:273

Lautin EM, Haramati N, Frager D, et al: CT diagnosis of circumcaval ureter. AJR Am J Roentgenol 1988;150:591

MacDonald GR: The ectopic ureter in men. J Urol 1986;135:1269

Matsumoto J: Acquired lesions involving the ureter in childhood. Semin Roentgenol 1986;21:166

Table 6 ■ IMAGING FINDINGS IN ECTOPIC URETEROCELE
Poor or nonfunction in upper pole
"Drooping lily" appearance
Filling defect in bladder
Often double filling defect
Filling defect on early filling of bladder
May evert, simulating diverticulum
May show urethral mass
Ultrasound
"Cyst" in bladder
Obstructed "cystic" upper pole
Nuclear medicine studies
Decreased function in upper pole
Photon-deficient area in bladder

N'Guessan G, Stephens FD: Supernumerary kidney. J Urol 1983; 130:649

Nussbaum AR, Dorst JP, Jeffs RD, et al: Ectopic ureter and ureterocele: their varied radiographic manifestations. Radiology 1986;159:227

Parker MD, Clark RL: Urothelial striations revisited. Radiology 1996;198:89

Peters CA, Mandell J, Lebowitz RL, et al: Congenital obstructed megaureters in early infancy: diagnosis and treatment. J Urol 1989;142:641

Pfister RC, Hendren WH: Primary megaureter in children and adults: clinical and pathophysiologic features of 150 ureters. Urology 1978;12:160

Reinberg Y, Alaibadi H, Johnson P, Gonzalez R: Congenital ureteral valves in children: case report and review of the literature. J Pediatr Surg 1987;22:379

Reitelman C, Perlmutter AD: Management of obstructing ectopic ureterocele. Urol Clin North Am 1990;17:318

Sen S, Ahmed S: Single system ureteroceles in childhood. Aust N Z J Surg 1988;58:903

Share JC, Lebowitz RL: Ectopic ureterocele without ureteral and calyceal dilatation (ureterocele disproportion): findings on urography and sonography. AJR Am J Roentgenol 1989;152:567

Tilley EA, Dow CJ: Cranial blind-ending branch of a bifid ureter: report of 3 cases. Br J Urol 1988;62:127

Wasserman NF: Inflammatory disease of the ureter. Radiol Clin North Am 1996;34:1131

Zaontz MR, Kass EJ: Ectopic ureter opening into seminal vesicle cyst associated with ipsilateral renal agenesis. Urology 1987;24:523

Zerin JM: Uroradiologic emergencies in infants and children. In Kirks DR (ed): Emergency Pediatric Radiology: A Problem Oriented Approach. Reston, VA, American Roentgen Ray Society 1995: 181–188

Chapter 2

VESICOURETERAL REFLUX

JACK O. HALLER

Vesicoureteral reflux (VUR) refers to the retrograde passage of urine from the bladder into the ureter and often to the calices. It is a common and important childhood problem that is generally regarded as abnormal at all ages (Table 1). It is a risk factor for the development of pyelonephritis. VUR causes neither urinary tract infections nor renal damage.

NORMAL URETEROVESICAL JUNCTION

The anatomic relationship of the distal ureter to the bladder wall is important in preventing reflux (Fig. 1A). Normally the distal ureter courses through the bladder musculature at an oblique angle, and then continues submucosally to end in the lateral corner of the trigone. The submucosal ureteral tunnel contains only longitudinal fibers, in contrast to the extravesical ureter, which contains both longitudinal and circular fibers. Some longitudinal fibers continue to the opposite ureteral orifice along the trigonal ridge, while others fan out to the trigone or are in continuity with the musculature of the proximal urethra. The ureterovesical junction (UVJ) acts as a passive flap valve. Continence is assured by apposition of the roof and floor of the submucosal tunnel when intravesical pressure increases, and is enhanced by the action of the intrinsic local musculature. Size of the ureteral orifice; proper obliquity, length, diameter, and flexibility of the tunnel; and adequate support of the tunnel by the bladder musculature are also important in preventing reflux. Normally the submucosal ureter measures 0.5 cm in the newborn, 1.0 cm at 12 years, and 2.0 cm in adults, with a tunnel-to-length ratio in children of 5:1. A ratio of at least 3:1 is necessary for UVJ competence. In patients with reflux, the ratio may be as low as 1.5:1. In general, the larger the ureteral orifice and the shorter the submucosal tunnel, the more severe the reflux.

CAUSES OF REFLUX

The most common cause of reflux is a developmental anomaly of the UVJ in which the ureteral orifice is too large, and the submucosal ureter has a deficiency in longitudinal muscle fibers or is too short and/or too wide, or both too short and too wide (Table 2). This type of reflux, often referred to as *primary reflux,* is seen more frequently in girls than in boys, with some predilection for girls with fair skin and blonde or red hair. It is rarely seen in African-Americans. Numerous familial cases have been reported, including siblings, twins, and members of consecutive generations. A much less common type of reflux is that caused by an abnormally formed bladder wall with an inadequate detrusor musculature and diminished support of the submucosal tunnel. Prune-belly syndrome, a large smooth-walled bladder from other causes, and primary paraureteral or Hutch diverticula are examples.

Table 1 ■ REFLUX FACTS

- African-Americans have lower incidence.
- Hispanics have questionable lower incidence.
- There is a family history to reflux: parent–child or sibling–sibling.
- Children with reflux have twice the incidence of pyelonephritis.
- 50% of children with postinfectious nephropathy do not have reflux.
- Cyclic voiding studies increase reflux detection.
- Filling the bladder to capacity increases reflux detection.
- The prevalence of VUR in children without UTI is almost equal to that in children with UTI.
- Bladder infections do not cause VUR.
- UTI is independent of the presence of reflux.
- Sterile VUR in the absence of increased voiding pressures or bladder dysfunction does not produce renal scars or other damage.
- New scars usually do not develop after puberty.
- Despite the initial severity or persistence of VUR, renal growth rates will remain unaffected.
- VUR and asymptomatic bacturia does not result in scars.
- In the treatment of VUR, there is no difference between continuous antibiotic prophylaxis or just treating episodes of UTI vis-à-vis renal scar development.
- Most patients with VUR do not demonstrate defects at DMSA scintigraphy, and those children with defects often do not have VUR.
- Symptomatic and asymptomatic VUR have the same natural history and resolution.
- Bladder urodynamics are related to the presence and resolution of VUR.
- UTI per se does not result in end-stage kidney disease.
- Breakthrough infections, changes in renal function or growth, and new or progressive scarring are seen with equal frequency in both medical and surgical treatment of reflux.
- Sterile VUR in the absence of increased voiding pressures or bladder dysfunction does not produce renal damage.

DMSA = dimercaptosuccinic acid; UTI = urinary tract infection; VUR = vesicoureteral reflux.

A *secondary type* of reflux is seen in patients with bladder outlet obstruction (e.g., posterior urethral valves) or with neurogenic bladder disease. It is in part caused by thinning and weakening of the UVJ musculature precipitated by chronically increased intravesical pressure; however, the fact that reflux in these disorders may be absent and is frequently unilateral suggests the possibility of an associated congenital weakness of the UVJ. Many girls who have reflux have signs of bladder instability both clinically and in urodynamic studies, but the relation between these findings and reflux is not well defined. In some cases reflux and urinary tract infections may improve or resolve when bladder instability is treated. Although lesser degrees of urinary tract obstruction per se do not seem to cause reflux in patients with a completely normal UVJ, they may precipitate reflux (with spreading of infection to the upper tracts and kidneys) in people with valves of borderline competence, as the result of local edema and cellular infiltration, causing further weakening of the UVJ. Recent bladder surgery, indwelling catheters, foreign bodies, bladder calculi, and other local irritants may also cause reflux in a marginally competent UVJ.

On rare occasions, reflux is *iatrogenic* following surgery on the UVJ, particularly in unsuccessful ureteral reimplantations or following unroofing of a ureterocele.

REFLUX AND URETERAL DUPLICATION

Vesicoureteral reflux may be more common in people (mostly girls) with complete ureteral duplication than in those with single, unduplicated ureters. The reflux may affect both ureters but is more often limited to the ureter draining the lower pole. The corresponding renal parenchyma (lower renal pole) is especially prone to secondary atrophic changes. This variant of primary reflux is probably caused by a defectively formed UVJ accompanying a lateral ureteral ectopia (see Section VII, Part IV, Chapter 1, page 1834). Reflux limited to the upper pole ureter in people with complete ureteral duplication is quite rare.

GRADING OF REFLUX

The severity of reflux is commonly judged according to the degree of dilatation of the upper tracts on the voiding cystourethrogram. International criteria for grading reflux are shown in Figure 1*B* and are described in the legend. Although simple and easy to use, this and other similar classifications reflect only the appearance of the upper tracts and do not take into consideration other important factors such as the age and sex of the patient, the presence of intrarenal reflux or urinary tract obstruction, the severity of the changes on the excretory urogram, renal function, cystoscopic findings, and the presence or absence of associated disorders (e.g., ureteral duplication, ureteral ectopia, ureterocele, bladder diverticula, prune-belly syndrome, urethral obstruction, or neurogenic bladder).

NATURAL HISTORY OF REFLUX

Reflux has a tendency to improve and to disappear spontaneously during the first decade of life, often during the preschool years. This tendency is attributed to a maturation process of the UVJ with age, with an increase in the length of the intramural ureter and strengthening of its musculature. Mild reflux (grades I and II) with normal-sized ureters and ureteral orifices has a favorable prognosis and disappears with time in more than 80% of the cases, whereas more severe forms of reflux with dilated ureters have a lower incidence of spontaneous recovery (grade III, about 50%; grade IV, 30%; grade V, rarely). Reflux associated with a large ureteral orifice and short submucosal tunnel at cystoscopy is not likely to subside. Reflux occurring in an ectopically ending ureter or associated with a large paraureteral diverticulum also tends to persist, especially if the ureter ends in the diverticulum. Reflux occurring in patients with lower urinary tract obstruction may disappear following correction of the lesion

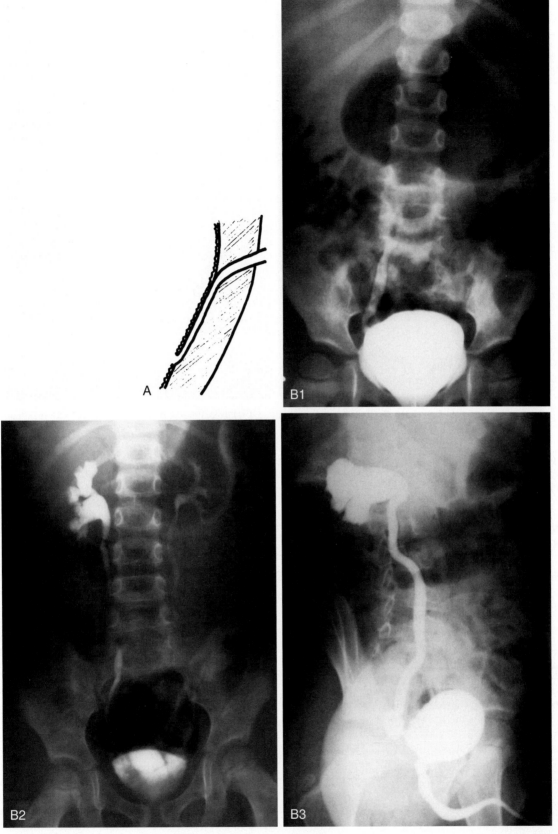

FIGURE 1. A, Course of the distal segment of the ureter within the bladder wall. The ureter at first traverses the bladder musculature almost perpendicularly and then descends submucosally for a much longer segment (submucosal tunnel). **B,** Grades of reflux. *1,* grade 1 reflux into right ureter; *2,* grade 2 reflux on the left where the calyces are preserved and grade 3 reflux on the right where they are blunted; *3,* grade 4 reflux into the lower pole collecting system on the right with intrarenal reflux.

Illustration continued on following page

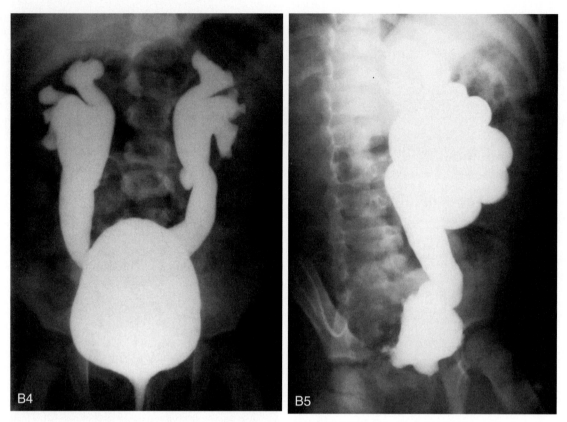

FIGURE 1. *Continued.* **B,** Grades of reflux. *4,* grade 4 reflux bilaterally; *5,* grade 5 reflux on left.

but is considered permanent if it is still present 1 year postoperatively. Reflux occurring in neurogenic bladder disease also tends to persist.

EFFECTS OF REFLUX ON THE KIDNEY

CHANGES IN THE UPPER URINARY TRACTS

The appearance of refluxing ureters and pelvocaliceal systems on *cystourethrograms* is quite variable, ranging

Table 2 ■ CAUSES OF REFLUX

Primary
Developmental
　Anomalous development at the ureterovesical junction
　Prune-belly syndrome
　Diverticula

Secondary
Bladder outlet obstruction
　Posterior urethral valves
　Neurogenic bladder
　Bladder dyssynergia
　Postoperative bladder
　Indwelling catheter
　Foreign body
　Bladder calculi
　Iatrogenic
　Ureterocele surgery

from normal-sized upper tracts to extreme upper tract dilatation and marked ureteral tortuosity (Figs. 2 through 5). These changes may reflect only an increased volume and decreased motility of the ureters, but in some cases a developmental defect of the ureter related either to in utero reflux or to an inadequate development of the ureteral musculature is suspected (e.g., prune-belly syndrome). In some patients, reflux is accompanied by marked ballooning of the pelvocaliceal system without evidence of ureteropelvic junction (UPJ) obstruction (Fig. 6). The phenomenon is transient, the renal pelvis empties promptly, and the excretory urogram shows no discrepancy between the size of the pelvis and that of the ureter. The finding reflects an increased elasticity of unknown cause in the upper collecting systems.

A similar distention of the pelvocaliceal system during cystourethrography may also be seen in association with an organic UPJ obstruction, evidenced by delayed emptying of the collecting system at cystourethrography, excretory urography, or diuretic renal scan. The obstruction may be related to local scarring from infection or kinks in the ureter or to overlying aberrant vessels or fibrous bands that have become significant with time. Occasionally, a primary congenital UPJ obstruction and primary reflux coexist as associated anomalies.

Some patients with reflux develop an obstruction at the UVJ over time. Despite this obstruction, reflux usually continues. On direct inspection and catheterization at cystoscopy, the ureteral orifice and distal ureter are not stenotic, suggesting a functional rather than an

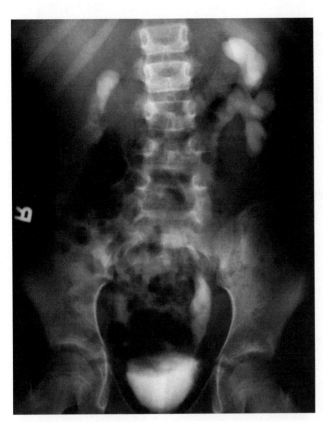

FIGURE 2. Reflux nephropathy. A 10-minute film from an excretory urogram shows a small, atrophic, but functioning right kidney. The parenchyma is markedly thinned. The left kidney shows dilated collecting as well.

organic basis for the obstruction. Reflux may also occur in association with primary megaureter.

As seen in *excretory urograms*, the ureters and pelvocaliceal systems of patients with reflux are often normal even if they appear dilated in the cystourethrogram. Minor urographic changes observed in patients with reflux include mild dilatation of the lower ureter, fullness of the entire ureter, and visualization of the entire ureter in more than one film. Longitudinal striations of the pelvis and proximal ureter on the side of the reflux are not uncommon (Fig. 7A). They probably represent mucosal wrinkles that occur when a dilated pelvis and proximal ureter are seen in a partially collapsed state. In more severe cases, the refluxing upper tracts are grossly dilated, with clubbing of the calices (Fig. 7B) and elongated and tortuous ureters. Ureteral peristalsis is generally poor, especially in the presence of urinary infection. Kinks in the proximal ureter or distal segment of the ureter are common.

INTRARENAL REFLUX

In patients with reflux to the calices, one may observe a transient pyelotubular and interstitial reflux of contrast material extending outward in a wedge-shaped pattern from one or more papillae to the renal cortical surface (Fig. 8). Intrarenal reflux is generally seen in children under 4 years of age and occurs most often in infants. It

is seen in less than 10% of patients with VUR in these age ranges and most often when VUR is severe or when it occurs at high intravesical pressure. Intrarenal reflux is often limited to the upper pole of the kidney, an area where compound papillae (i.e., more than one papilla per calix) are most numerous, but may occur also in the lower pole or other areas of the kidneys, or may be generalized. It is believed that the morphology of the opening of the collecting ducts of Bellini on the renal papilla is partly responsible for intrarenal reflux. The opening of these ducts on compound, flat-topped papillae are round and therefore less resistant to retrograde flow than the slit-like openings of the ducts of simple or conical papillae. It is possible that, in high-pressure VUR, all the papillae are affected by intrarenal reflux. The fact that intrarenal reflux does not occur in all infants and that it is rarely seen after age 4 years suggests an additional local defect that improves with age. Intrarenal reflux is an important finding because of its close relation to renal scarring (see below).

REFLUX AND URINARY TRACT INFECTIONS

Urinary tract infections are a common pediatric problem, affecting especially infants and children of preschool years, with a tendency to recur and to damage the kidney. Urinary tract infections, like reflux, decrease with age and are uncommon in older children and adolescents. In infancy, they occur with an equal frequency in both sexes and are often present as part of generalized sepsis, and may be associated with vomiting, anorexia, and failure to thrive. After 3 to 6 months of age, urinary tract infections occur predominantly in

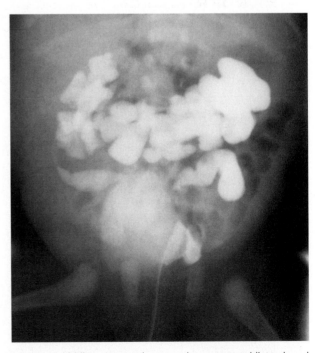

FIGURE 3. Voiding cystourethrogram demonstrates bilateral grade V reflux in a horseshoe kidney.

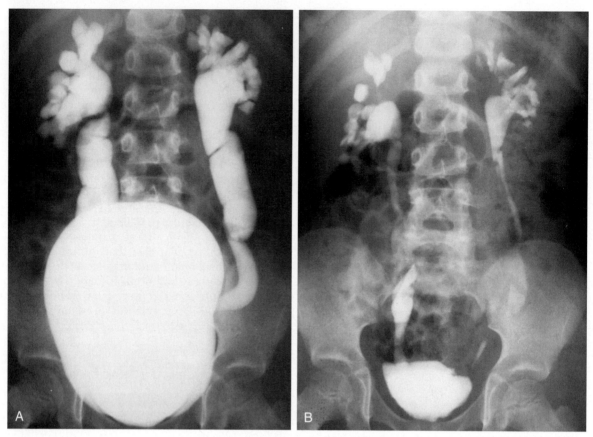

FIGURE 4. Voiding cystogram **(A)** and postvoiding film **(B)** in a 5-year-old girl with recurrent urinary tract infections. The cystourethrogram shows a large, smooth-walled bladder with severe (grade V) reflux bilaterally. The postvoiding film shows only mild to moderate pelvocaliectasis and very mild ureterectasis. Renal parenchymal loss is present bilaterally.

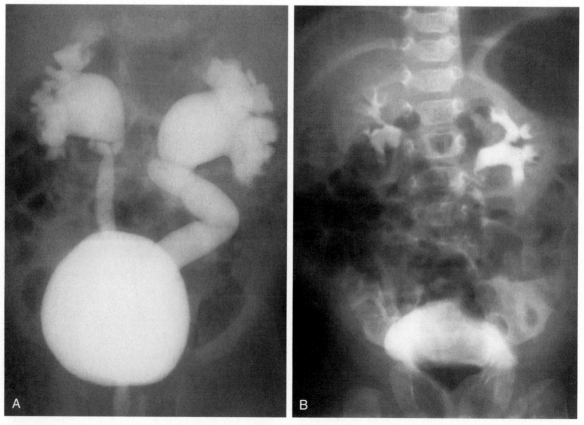

FIGURE 5. Voiding cystourethrogram (VCUG) **(A)** and excretory urogram **(B)** in a 3½–year-old girl with recurrent urinary tract infections. The VCUG shows severe (grade IV–V) reflux bilaterally and the excretory urogram is normal.

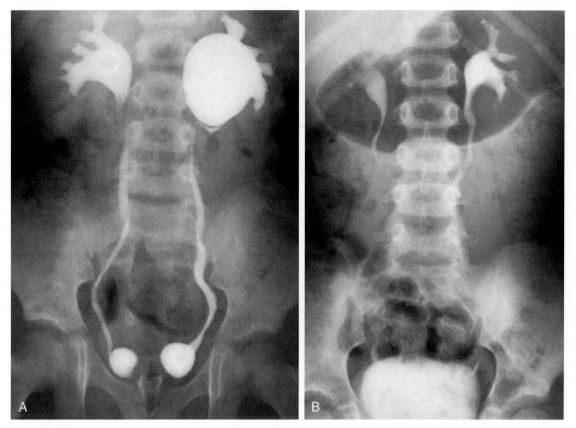

FIGURE 6. Post–voiding cystourethrogram film **(A)** and excretory urogram **(B)** in a 5½–year-old girl with recurrent urinary tract infections. The postvoiding film shows bilateral reflux with ballooning of the left renal pelvis and bilateral paraureteral (Hutch) bladder diverticula. The excretory urogram is entirely normal.

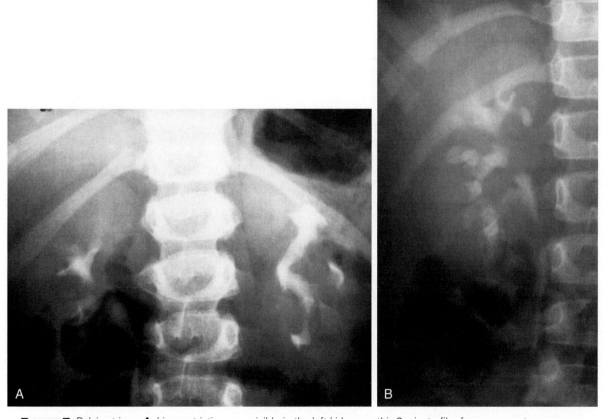

FIGURE 7. Pelvic stripes. **A,** Linear striations are visible in the left kidney on this 3-minute film from an excretory urogram. **B,** Reflux and papillary necrosis is noted in the upper pole calyces as demonstrated on this voiding cystourethrogram.

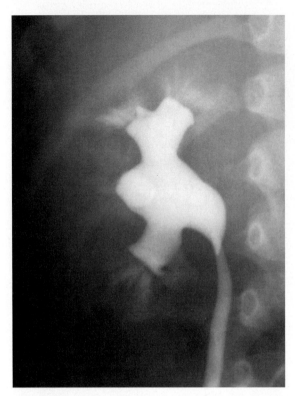

FIGURE 8. Right-sided ureteral reflux and diffuse intrarenal reflux in a 2-year-old girl.

girls (Table 3). Symptoms referable to the lower urinary tract are common in some children, whereas in others the clinical features are those of pyelonephritis with flank pain, chills, and fever. The distinction between cystitis and pyelonephritis may be difficult by clinical and laboratory methods. Renal changes of acute pyelonephritis may be clearly shown in a dimercaptosuccinic acid (DMSA) renal scan. The diagnosis of urinary tract infection depends on laboratory confirmation of significant bacterial counts in cultures of properly collected urine specimens. The infecting organisms are most often gram-negative bacteria of fecal flora, especially *Escherichia coli*.

In girls, the infection originates in the perineum and ascends to the bladder via the short urethra. The port of entry of infection in males is more difficult to explain. Stasis of urine in the bladder as a result of an obstruction or a functional abnormality of the bladder may foster

Table 3 ■ URINARY TRACT INFECTION
Decreases with age
Incidence
M = F in infants
F > M at 3–6 mo
Increases with
Stasis (dysfunctional voiding)
Indwelling catheter
Calculi
Local irritants

growth of bacteria that would otherwise be eliminated by complete emptying of the bladder. The resistance of the bladder mucosa to infection may also be altered by intravesical catheters, calculi, or local irritants. Other factors, less well understood, may predispose to or aggravate urinary infections, some related to an increased bacterial virulence, others to a decrease in host resistance. One of the factors enhancing bacterial activity is the ability of certain bacteria, particularly certain strains of *E. coli* (B-fimbriated *E. coli*) to adhere to the urothelium. This property enhances bacterial colonization and invasiveness, in part by increasing the resistance to the normal clearing of bacteria from the urinary draining system by unobstructed urine flow and bladder emptying. Propagation of infection from the bladder to the upper tracts and to the kidneys occurs mainly by way of reflux, which can be demonstrated in many patients with recurrent urinary tract infection (70% of patients age less than 1 year, 25% at 1 year, 10% at 12 years, and 5% in adults). Reflux seems to compensate for virulence in some organisms (*E. coli* in patients with pyelonephritis); with reflux, the bacteria does not require special virulence.

The view that reflux is an important factor in the origin of renal infection is supported by the frequent cessation of renal infections following a successful reimplantation of the refluxing ureters. The procedure, however, does not seem to prevent the recurrence of cystitis (in girls). As already indicated, bladder infection may precipitate reflux by weakening a marginally competent UVJ with propagation of infection to the kidney. The decreased incidence of renal infections with age is probably in large part related to a decreased incidence of reflux secondary to normal maturation of the UVJ.

RENAL SCARRING

Renal scarring is a common and potentially serious problem in patients with reflux and urinary tract infections (pyelonephritis). The lesion, often referred to also as *reflux nephropathy* or chronic atrophic pyelonephritis, is characterized by one or more areas of renal cortical atrophy that is almost always associated with blunting or distortion of the underlying calix or group of calices, retraction of the papillae, and reduction of the medullary zone. Histologically, the affected kidneys show areas of cortical loss with tubular destruction and atrophy, and interstitial fibrosis. Obliteration of glomeruli, arteriolar changes, and minor signs of interstitial inflammation may also be observed.

The scarring characteristically has a focal or segmental pattern with a predisposition for the upper pole (38%), and less frequently for the lower pole. Multiple areas of scarring may also be seen in other parts of the kidney, and in some cases the process affects the whole kidney diffusely. The areas of scarring result in one or more clefts or depressions of various size in the outline of the kidney. They are sharply demarcated from the adjacent normal renal parenchyma and are usually wedge shaped, with the apex at a calix or group of calices. The unaffected renal parenchyma may be

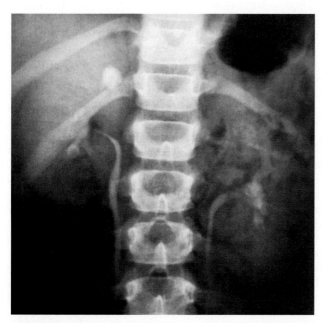

FIGURE 9. A 5-minute film from an excretory urogram shows the right upper pole calyx close to the spine because the parenchyma between the upper pole calyx and the spine has been destroyed by reflux. This phenomenon is referred to as medial deviation of the upper pole calyx.

hypertrophied, sometimes simulating a renal mass (pseudotumor). When the process is diffuse and severe, it results in global renal atrophy. When the process is bilateral, it is usually asymmetric. The calices of the affected area of the kidney are close to the surface of the kidney and closer together than normal. When the renal poles are affected, the distance between the most medial polar calices and the spine is decreased (Fig. 9). The parenchymal changes are seen best in the early phase of the excretory urogram, especially in tomographic sections, and may be clearly visible in contrast-enhanced computed tomography. They are frequently detected by ultrasound (US) as areas of depression in the outline of the kidney. Nuclear scintigraphy, using a cortical agent such as DMSA, is especially sensitive in detecting renal cortical scars.

Renal scarring, like urinary tract infections, is much more common in girls than in boys and is uncommon in African-Americans. In early life, it is regularly associated with reflux and is seen in about one third of patients who have both urinary tract infection and reflux. Reflux (and infections) may be absent in older children and adolescents with renal scarring, probably because reflux tends to disappear with age. These clinical observations have suggested that renal scarring is a consequence of reflux associated with bacteriuria. Scarring may be seen in refluxers and nonrefluxers—reflux is not necessary to develop scars. The observation that scars are located preferentially in the renal poles, where compound papillae and intrarenal reflux predominate, has suggested the theory that intrarenal reflux may play an important role in the development of renal scars. Although sterile intrarenal reflux does not seem to cause parenchymal scarring, except perhaps in some

severe cases, there is evidence both clinically and from animal experiments that renal scars probably result from the intrarenal reflux of infected urine. VUR is of paramount importance in the transport of bacteria from the bladder to the upper tract.

Renal scarring has been interpreted as an event that occurs in the first few months of life, perhaps following the first episode of infantile pyelonephritis, and that usually remains stable thereafter. It has also been suggested that all the areas of the kidneys that are susceptible to intrarenal reflux (i.e., all the refluxing or compound papillae) are affected simultaneously ("big bang theory"), while all the unaffected areas of the kidney are drained by a single conical papilla and are therefore more resistant to intrarenal reflux. According to this theory, infants with urinary tract infection and reflux are at greater risk of developing renal scars than older children with reflux and urinary infections.

It may take a few weeks to several months for the scars to become apparent on conventional studies after the precipitating bout of infected intrarenal reflux. The process is generally already well established when the child is first examined and usually does not progress. Some apparently new renal scars that are seen in follow-up urograms may represent the end stage of an old insult to the kidney, which was not previously apparent. Also, what appears to be a progression of a previously demonstrated scar in follow-up urograms may only reflect continuing growth and hypertrophy of adjacent normal renal tissue contrasting with a fixed atrophic area.

HYPERTENSION AND END-STAGE RENAL DISEASE

Systemic arterial hypertension is a relatively common complication of reflux nephropathy, occurring probably in 10% to 20% of children with unilateral or bilateral renal scarring, with an increased risk after 15 years of age. Hypertension may develop 10 or more years after ureteral reimplantation for reflux, as well as in patients in whom reflux has subsided spontaneously; in fact, most older children and young adults with hypertension and scarred kidneys fail to show reflux when the hypertension is first noted. The hypertension seen in these patients is probably vascular in origin. The plasma renin is elevated, but an elevated renin may also be found in patients with reflux nephropathy who do not have hypertension.

Reflux nephropathy is also associated with some frequency with decreased renal function of varying severity, and is a relatively common cause of end-stage renal disease (ESRD) requiring chronic dialysis and renal transplantation. It probably occurs in 10% to 20% of all cases of ESRD, but how many children with scarred kidneys eventually develop this complication is difficult to establish owing to the varying degree of severity and extent of the scarring. Reflux may not be demonstrated at the time of diagnosis because of previous ureteral reimplantation or because of spontaneous resolution of the reflux. As with hypertension, ESRD resulting from reflux nephropathy is seen most commonly in older children, adolescents, and young adults, with an increased risk in patients with hypertension. The ESRD of these patients is probably the result of a decrease in the number of nephrons plus an acquired glomerulosclerosis caused by an increased workload (hyperperfusion) of the unaffected glomeruli.

OTHER EFFECTS OF REFLUX ON THE KIDNEY

Clinical observations of patients with longstanding VUR suggest that sterile reflux is usually well tolerated, except perhaps when it is severe or occurs at high intravesical pressure so that some degree of renal atrophy may result from the "water-hammer effect" of the reflux on the kidney (hydrostatic damage).

Males with primary VUR (reflux not associated with lower urinary tract obstruction or neurogenic bladder) are not as prone to develop urinary tract infection as are females, and can tolerate reflux without complications for many years.

Reflux in patients with urinary tract infection may cause a decreased growth rate of the affected kidney followed by resumption of the normal growth rate when the infection is fully under control. During an episode of acute pyelonephritis, the affected kidney may be enlarged up to 50% of its original size, a possibility that should be kept in mind when interpreting serial measurements of kidney size in refluxing patients.

TREATMENT

Eradication of infection and prevention of recurrences are the main therapeutic objectives in children with reflux, with emphasis on infants and small children who are at particularly high risk of developing renal scars. These objectives may be attained by long-term suppressive medication with antibiotics until the patient is 4 to 5 years of age or until reflux ceases. Medical treatment is often sufficient in patients with grades I and II reflux. An antireflux procedure is necessary in many patients with grades III and IV reflux, and is usually indicated in grade V reflux. The success rate of ureteral reimplantation is high (up to 95%) in patients with grade I and II reflux but decreases as the size of the infected ureter increases (a 60% success rate in grade V has been reported). A nonsurgical, closed antireflux procedure, recently introduced and commonly used with satisfactory results in many types of reflux, consists of an endoscopic, intravesical injection of a small amount of Teflon paste in the bladder behind the submucosal ureteral tunnel (Fig. 10). The injected Teflon paste elevates and narrows the ureteral tunnel, and causes a localized protrusion of the bladder wall at the lateral angle of the trigone containing the ureteral orifice (newer materials to be injected are being tested in clinical trials constantly). This defect is seen by US as an echogenic focus with a distal shadowing. Urinary tract infections may still occur following a successful antireflux procedure, but they are mostly limited to the bladder. The main objective of an antireflux procedure is to prevent propagation of infection from the bladder to the upper tract and kidney.

IMAGING STUDIES

The major objective in the evaluation of children with urinary tract infections is to diagnose or exclude reflux, existing renal scarring, and structural or functional abnormalities of the urinary tract that may predispose to reflux and infection, particularly anomalies that may require prompt surgical treatment. The diagnostic modalities available to study these patients include conventional and nuclear cystourethrography for the evaluation of reflux, conventional cystourethrography for the study of the lower urinary tract, and excretory urography, US, and diethylenetriaminepentaacetic acid renal scan for the evaluation of the upper tract (Table 4). The DMSA scan is used when a more detailed study of the renal parenchyma is indicated. The choice of methods depends in large part on individual preference and on the experience of the examiner; the age, sex, and race of the patient; whether an initial or a follow-up examination is being done; and the cost of and time required to perform the procedure.

It is generally agreed that an investigation is indicated in all patients after the first documented urinary tract infection, particularly infants and young children in whom early detection of reflux and treatment of infection are critical for the prevention of renal scarring. A conventional cystourethrogram followed by excretory urography is the traditional procedure in such cases. A more common current practice is to start the investigation with a conventional cystourethrogram carried out when the infection is under control with antibiotics. If the cystourethrogram is normal or shows only grade I to II reflux, it is followed by US of the upper tracts. If the cystourethrogram shows a higher grade of reflux or is otherwise abnormal, it is followed by an excretory urogram. In the newborn period, the renal nuclear scan is often more informative than the urogram. Another method that has been recommended is to start the investigation with a conventional cystourethrogram in males and a nuclear cystogram in females, followed in both sexes by US of the upper tracts if reflux is not present, or by a DMSA renal scan if there is reflux. In hospitalized patients with severe urinary tract infection, US may be the initial study even at the height of the infection; when the infection is cleared, or earlier if necessary, a conventional cystourethrogram is carried out and is followed by an excretory urogram or a nuclear renal scan if there is reflux, or by US of the upper tract if reflux is not evident. In the investigation of asymptomatic patients who may have reflux (e.g., siblings of patients with the disorder), a nuclear cystogram may be sufficient as the initial study, followed by other procedures when necessary. In teenage girls with urinary tract infection, no previous history of urinary tract disease,

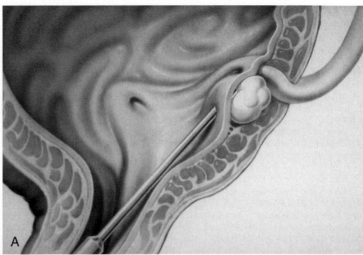

FIGURE 10. Subureteric Teflon injection. **A,** Diagrammatic representation of Teflon injection under entrance of ureter into bladder. **B,** Longitudinal sonogram of the right ureterovesical junction (UVJ) shows a dilated ureter entering the bladder. At the UVJ, there is echogenic material with posterior shadowing. **C,** Transverse ultrasound scan shows echogenic foci and shadowing at both UVJs at the trigone.

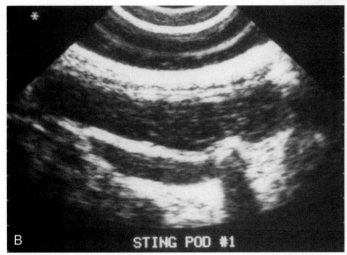

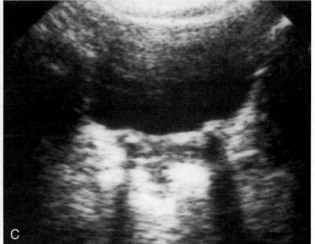

and only clinical signs of cystitis, US of the upper tracts may be the only procedure necessary. In follow-up examinations and in postreimplantation studies, a nuclear cystogram may replace the voiding cystogram for evaluation of reflux and US may be used to monitor the upper tracts.

Table 4 ■ USE OF IMAGING STUDIES

Voiding cystourethrogram
  Defines anatomy (urethra in males)
  Accurate grading of reflux
Nuclear studies
  Decreased ability to see urethra in males
  Decreased gonadal dose
  Continuous imaging
  Don't need to see urethra in girls
  Grading of reflux is mild, moderate, severe
  Can be used as initial study in girls
  Good for screening familial reflux

SUGGESTED READINGS

Alon U, Berant M, Pery M: Intravenous pyelography in children with urinary tract infection and vesicoureteral reflux. Pediatrics 1989; 83:332

Andriole VT: Urinary tract infections: recent developments. J Infect Dis 1987;156:865

Arant BS: Medical management of mild and moderate vesicoureteral reflux: follow-up studies of infants and young children—a preliminary report of the Southwest Pediatric Nephrology Group. J Urol 1992;148:1683–1687

Arnold AJ, Brownless SM, Carty HM, Rickwood AM: Detection of renal scarring by DMSA scanning: an experimental study. J Pediatr Surg 1990;25:391

Assael BM, Guez S, Marra G, et al: Congenital reflux nephropathy: a follow-up of 108 cases diagnosed perinatally. Br J Urol 1998;82: 252–257

Ben-Ami T, Gayer G, Hertz M, et al: Natural history of reflux in the lower pole of duplicated collecting systems: a controlled study. Pediatr Radiol 1989;19:308

Ben-Ami T, Rozin M, Hertz M: Imaging of children with urinary tract infection: a tailored approach. Clin Radiol 1989;40:64

Ben-Ami T, Sinai L, Hertz M, Boichis H: Vesicoureteral reflux in boys: review of 196 cases. Radiology 1989;173:681

Bisset GS III, Strife JL: Duplex collecting system in girls with urinary tract infection: prevalence and significance. AJR Am J Roentgenol 1987;148:497

Blake NS, O'Connell E: Endoscopic connection of vesico-ureteric reflux by subureteric Teflon injection: follow-up ultrasound and voiding cystography. Br J Radiol 1989;62:443

Connolly LP, Treves ST, Zurakowski D, Bauer SB: Natural history of vesicoureteral reflux in siblings. J Urol 1996;156:1805–1807

Decter RM, Roth DR, Gonzales ET Jr: Vesicoureteral reflux in boys. J Urol 1988;140:1089

Diard F, Nicolau A, Bernard S: Intra-renal reflux: new cause of medullary hyperechogenicity? Pediatr Radiol 1987;17:154

Dillon MJ, Goonasekera CDA: Reflux nephropathy. J Am Soc Nephrol 1998;9:2377–2383

Ditchfield MR, De Campo JF, Cook DJ, et al: Vesicoureteral reflux: an accurate predictor of acute pyelonephritis in childhood urinary tract infection? Radiology 1994;190:413–415

Farkas A, Moriel EZ, Lupa S: Endoscopic correction of vesicoureteral reflux: our experience with 115 ureters. J Urol 1990;144:534

Farnsworth RH, Rossleigh MA, Leighton DM, et al: The detection of reflux nephropathy in infants by [99m]technetium dimercaptosuccinic acid studies. J Urol 1991;145:542

Fernback SK, Feinstein KA: Abnormalities of the bladder in children: imaging findings. AJR Am J Roentgenol 1994;162:1143–1150

Garin EH, Campos A, Homsy Y: Primary vesicoureteral reflux: review of current concepts. Pediatr Nephrol 1998;12:249–256

Gedroye WMW, Chaudhuri R, Saxton HM: Normal and near-normal calyceal pattern in reflux nephropathy. Clin Radiol 1988;39:615

Ginalski J-M, Michaud A, Genton N: Renal growth retardation in children: sign suggestive of vesicoureteral reflux. AJR Am J Roentgenol 1985;145:617

Goldraich NP, Goldraich IJ: Follow-up of conservatively treated children with high and low grade vesicoureteral reflux: a prospective study. J Urol 1992;148:1688–1692

Goldraich NP, Ramos OL, Goldraich IH: Urography versus DMSA scan in children with vesicoureteric reflux. Pediatr Nephrol 1989;3:1

Gross GW, Lebowitz RL: Infection does not cause reflux. AJR Am J Roentgenol 1981;137:929–932

Hanson S, Jodal U, Noren L, Bjure J: Untreated bacteriuria in asymptomatic girls with renal scarring. Pediatrics 1998;84:964–968

Hellström M, Jacobsson B, Marild S, Jodal U: Voiding cystourethrography as a predictor of reflux nephropathy in children with urinary-tract infections. AJR Am J Roentgenol 1989;152:801

Hollowell JG, Altman HG, Snyder HM 3rd, Duckett JW: Coexisting ureteropelvic junction obstruction and vesicoureteral reflux: diagnosis and therapeutic implications. J Urol 1989;142:490

International Reflux Study Committee: Medical versus surgical treatment of primary vesicoureteral reflux: a prospective international reflux study in children. J Urol 1981;125:277–283

Jequier S, Forbest PA, Nogrady MB: The value of ultrasonography as a screening procedure in a first documented urinary tract infection in children. J Ultrasound Med 1985;4:393

Jequier S, Jequier JC: Reliability of voiding cystourethrography to detect reflux. AJR Am J Roentgenol 1989;153:807–810

Kenda R, Kenig T, Sile M, Zupancic Z: Renal ultrasound and excretory urography in infants, and young children with urinary tract infection. Pediatr Radiol 1989;19:299

Kenny PJ: Imaging of chronic renal infections. AJR Am J Roentgenol 1990;155:485

Lebowitz RL: The detection and characterization of vesicoureteral reflux in the child. J Urol 1992;148:1640–1642

Lebowitz RL, Mandell J: Urinary tract infection in children: putting radiology in its place. Radiology 1987;165:1

Lebowitz RL, Olbing H, Parkkulainen KV, et al: International system of radiographic grading of vesicoureteric reflux. Pediatr Radiol 1985;15:105

Leighton DM, Mayne V: Obstruction in the refluxing urinary tract: a common phenomenon. Clin Radiol 1989;40:271

Lenaghan D, Whitaker JG, Jensen F, Stephens FD: The natural history of reflux and long-term effects of reflux on the kidney. J Urol 1976;115:728–730

Lerner GR, Fleischmann LE, Perlmutter AD: Reflux nephropathy. Pediatr Clin North Am 1987;34:747

Mason WG Jr: Urinary tract infections in children: renal ultrasound evaluation. Radiology 1989;153:109

McLorie GA, Alaibadi H, Churchill BM, et al: [99m]Technetium-dimercapto-succinic acid renal scanning and excretory urography in diagnosis of focal renal scans in children. J Urol 1989;142:790

McLorie GA, McKenna PH, Jumper BM, et al: High grade vesicoureteral reflux: analysis of observational therapy. J Urol 1990;144:537

Nancarrow PA, Lebowitz RL: Primary vesicoureteral reflux in blacks with posterior urethral valves: does it occur? Pediatr Radiol 1988;19:31

Reid BS, Bender TM: Radiographic evaluation of children with urinary tract infections. Radiol Clin North Am 1988;26:393

Roberts JA: Pathogenesis of nonobstructive urinary tract infections in children. J Urol 1990;144:475

Sargent MA: What is the normal prevalence of vesicoureteral reflux? Pediatr Radiol 2000;30:723

Seruca H: Vesicoureteral reflux and voiding dysfunction: a prospective study. J Urol 1989;142:494

Shanon A, Feldman W: Methodologic limitations in the literature on vesicoureteral reflux: a critical review. J Pediatr 1990;117:171

Shapiro E, Slovis TL, Perlmutter AD, Kuhns LR: Optimal use of [99m]technetium-glucoheptonate scintigraphy in the detection of pyelonephritic scarring in children: a preliminary report. J Urol 1988;140:1175

Shimada K, Matsui T, Ogino T, et al: Renal growth and progression of reflux nephropathy in children with vesicoureteral reflux. J Urol 1988;140:1097

Skoog SJ, Belman AB: Primary vesicoureteral reflux in the black child. Pediatrics 1991;87:538

Sillen U: Vesicoureteral reflux in infants. Pediatr Nephrol 1999;13:355–361

Smellie JM: Urinary tract infection, vesicoureteric reflux, and renal scarring. Semin Urol 1986;4:82

Smellie JM, Prescod NP, Shaw PJ, et al: Childhood reflux and urinary infection: a follow-up of 10–41 years in 226 adults. Pediatr Nephrol 1998;12:727–736

Smellie JM, Shaw PJ, Prescod NP, Bantock HM: [99m]Tc dimercaptosuccinic acid (DMSA) scan in patients with established radiological renal scarring. Arch Dis Child 1988;63:1315

Strife JL, Bisset GS 3rd, Kirks DR, et al: Nuclear cystography and renal sonography: findings in girls with urinary tract infection. AJR Am J Roentgenol 1989;153:115

Sty JR, Wells RG, Starshak RJ, Schroeder BA: Imaging in acute renal infection. AJR Am J Roentgenol 1987;148:471

Tamminen-Mobius T, Brunier E, Ebel KD, et al: Cessation of vesicoureteral reflux for five years in infants and children allocated to medical treatment. J Urol 1992;148:1662–1666

Verber IG, Strudley MR, Meller ST: [99m]Tc dimercaptosuccinic acid (DMSA) scan as the first investigation of urinary tract infection. Arch Dis Child 1988;63:1320

White RHR: Vesicoureteric reflux and renal scarring. Arch Dis Child 1989;64:407

P A R T   V

BLADDER

JACK O. HALLER

URACHAL ANOMALIES

In early fetal life, the bladder extends to the umbilicus, where it is in continuity with the allantois. As the fetus grows, the cephalad part of the bladder narrows to form a channel, the urachus, that obliterates into a fibrous cord during the fourth to fifth month of gestation. Failure of the urachus to regress may result in one of four disorders: patent urachus, urachal sinus, urachal diverticulum, and urachal cyst (Fig. 1). In patent urachus, the urachus develops normally but fails to obliterate, resulting in a vesicoumbilical fistula (Fig. 2). In urachal sinus, the urachus is closed at the level of the bladder but remains patent at the umbilicus. In urachal or vesicourachal diverticulum, the urachus is obliterated at the level of the umbilicus but communicates with the bladder (Fig. 3). In urachal cyst, the urachus is obliterated at both ends but remains patent in its midportion; there may be multiple small urachal cysts as a result of segmental obliteration of the urachus.

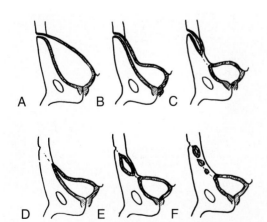

FIGURE 1. Development of the urachus and types of urachal anomalies. **A,** Appearance of the bladder in early fetal life, before development of the urachus. **B,** Patent urachus (vesicoumbilical fistula). **C,** Urachal sinus. **D,** Urachal (vesicourachal) diverticulum. **E** and **F,** Urachal cyst(s).

All these abnormal structures are related to the anterior abdominal wall, mainly on the inner surface, extraperitoneally, and usually in the midline. They frequently occur as isolated lesions. Small urachal remnants were found by sonography in a series of 60 of 100 consecutive infants and children. However, they may be seen in association with other anomalies. A patent urachus is not uncommon in patients with severe congenital lower urinary tract obstructions, but is unusual in posterior urethral valves. A vesicourachal diverticulum is a frequent finding in prune-belly syndrome. A patent urachus also may be seen in this syndrome. Urachal sinuses and cysts are likely to become infected, and malignant neoplasms developing in urachal remnants have been reported in adults and in a few children.

- Urachal anomalies are
  - Remnants of allantois
  - Associated with urethral obstruction
  - Not associated with posterior urethral valves
  - Associated with prune-belly syndrome
  - Associated with urachal (adeno-) carcinoma in adults

Leakage of urine at the umbilicus suggests the presence of patent urachus; the diagnosis is confirmed by catheterization of the bladder through the umbilicus or by voiding cystourethrography (VCUG) with films in the lateral projection. The diagnosis of urachal sinus can be made only by catheterization and opacification of the umbilical fistula, demonstrating a downward course of the tract toward the bladder. Urachal or vesicourachal diverticula are best demonstrated on a cystogram in the lateral projection. The diagnosis of urachal cyst is more difficult (Figs. 4 and 5). The cystogram may show only an extrinsic compression defect on the dome of the bladder in the midline or slightly to one side. Ultrasound (US), computed tomog-

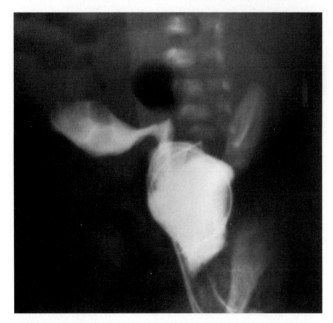

FIGURE 2. Oblique film from a voiding cystourethrogram shows a fistulous tract leading from the dome of the bladder toward the umbilicus, consistent with a patent urachus.

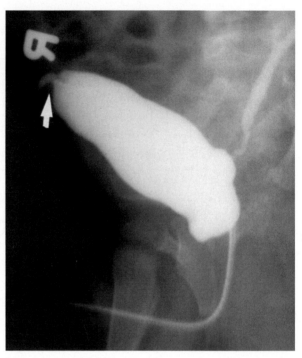

FIGURE 3. A voiding cystourethrogram in a child with prune belly syndrome demonstrates a small urachal diverticulum from the dome of the bladder *(arrow)*.

raphy (CT), or magnetic resonance imaging (MRI) may show the lesion more effectively. Percutaneous catheter drainage of an infected urachal cyst under US guidance may be carried out prior to excision.

BLADDER DIVERTICULA

Most bladder diverticula are localized outpouchings of the bladder mucosa between fibers of the detrusor muscles (pseudodiverticula), resulting from a congenital or acquired defect in the bladder wall. The neck of the diverticulum varies greatly from a few millimeters in

diameter to very large. Small diverticula, less than 2 cm in diameter, are sometimes called saccules. Bladder diverticula may be primary (idiopathic), secondary, or iatrogenic (postoperative) (Table 1).

Primary or idiopathic diverticula are the most common, are seen more often in males than in females, and may be single or multiple. They occur anywhere in the bladder, but most frequently in the trigonal area. A common type of bladder diverticulum, referred to as

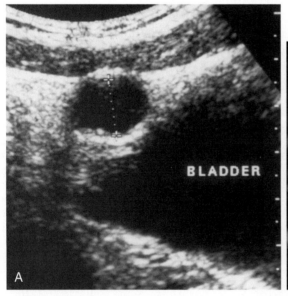

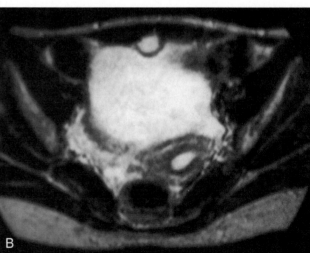

FIGURE 4. Urachal cyst. **A,** Longitudinal ultrasound scan of the midline pelvis shows an echo-free mass at the dome of the bladder. **B,** T$_2$-weighted magnetic resonance imaging confirms the cystic nature of the mass under the umbilicus, typical of a urachal cyst.

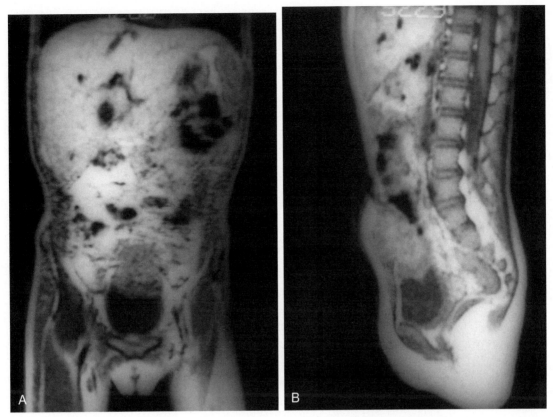

FIGURE 5. T$_1$-weighted coronal **(A)** and sagittal **(B)** magnetic resonance imaging sections show low-signal debris in a supravesical mass attached to the umbilicus. An infected urachal cyst was subsequently removed at surgery.

paraureteral diverticulum, or Hutch diverticulum after the author who first described it, is located laterally and cephalad to the ureteral orifice (Fig. 6). The ureter enters the bladder near the base of the diverticulum, but, if the diverticulum is large, it may engulf the ureteral meatus and the ureter may empty into the diverticulum. Associated vesicoureteral reflux is present in about half of the cases and may be expected to occur when the ureter terminates in the diverticulum. A large diverticulum originating from the trigonal area of the bladder may expand posteriorly and caudally and may cause bladder outlet obstruction.

Bladder diverticula of the primary type, often multiple, may be seen in several syndromes, including cutis laxa, Ehlers-Danlos syndrome, fetal alcohol syndrome,

Menkes' syndrome, and Williams syndrome. Secondary diverticula are seen mostly in patients with posterior urethral valves or other severe lower urinary tract obstructions and in patients with neurogenic bladder disease. They are the result of chronically increased intravesical pressure with hypertrophy of bladder musculature. They may occur anywhere in the bladder but are most common in the paraureteral area. Iatrogenic diverticula are seen most often in the anterior wall of the bladder at the site of a previous vesicostomy or suprapubic drainage catheter, and at the ureterovesical junction (UVJ) following ureteral reimplantation.

Bladder diverticula may become visible only during voiding when contractions of the bladder force urine into the diverticulum (Fig. 7). Diverticula with a narrow neck empty much slower than those with a large neck and are best seen when the bladder is empty. Those located in the anterior or posterior wall of the bladder may be visible only in lateral or steep oblique views. The size of the diverticulum and the width of its neck are best judged on films obtained with the x-ray beam angled tangentially to the area. Bladder diverticula may also be demonstrated and evaluated by US.

MEGACYSTIS

Megacystis is a descriptive term for a large, smooth-walled bladder. The finding may be a normal variant or a congenital anomaly of little clinical significance. A large,

Table 1 ■ TYPES AND CAUSES OF BLADDER DIVERTICULA

Primary (congenital, idiopathic)
Multiple syndromes: cutis laxa, Ehlers-Danlos, fetal alcohol, Menkes', Williams

Secondary
Posterior urethral valves
Urethral obstruction
Neurogenic bladder

Iatrogenic
Vesicostomy site
Suprapubic drainage site
Urethral reimplantation site

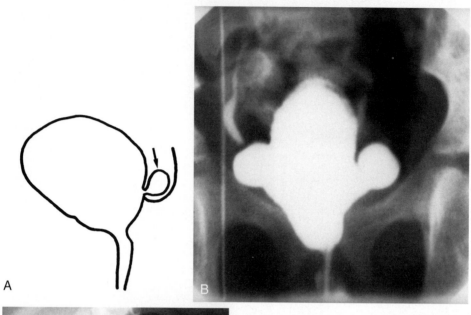

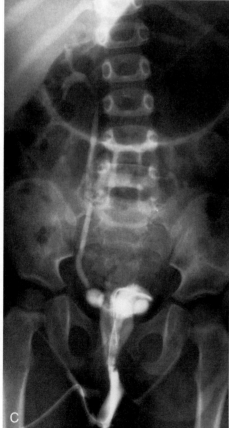

FIGURE 6. A, Diagram of a paraureteral bladder diverticulum (Hutch diverticulum) located immediately above the ureterovesicle junction *(arrow)*. When the diverticulum is very large, the ureter may end in the diverticulum. Hutch diverticula are frequently associated with ureteral reflux on the same side. **B** and **C,** Two cases of bilateral Hutch diverticulae are demonstrated on pre- **(B)** and postvoiding **(C)** films. Contrast is also noted in the vagina, as is grade III reflux on the right.

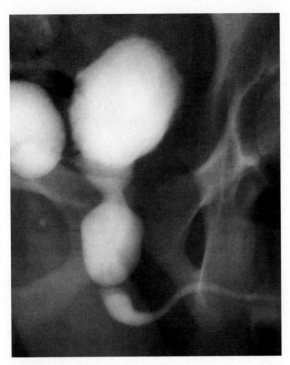

FIGURE 7. A large bladder diverticulum is noted on the right during the voiding phase of this voiding cystourethrogram.

smooth-walled bladder may also be seen in patients who produce an excessive amount of urine chronically (e.g., patients with diabetes insipidus). The ureters in these patients may be dilated as well. A large, smooth-walled bladder may also be seen in true neurogenic disease, but this is quite uncommon in children; in most cases, true neurogenic disease in children is associated with a hypertonic, trabeculated bladder. A large, smooth-walled bladder is a common finding in prune-belly syndrome.

CYSTITIS

Acute hemorrhagic cystitis, cyclophosphamide (Cytoxan) cystitis, and nonspecific nodular or localized tumor-like or bullous cystitis are the most important forms of pediatric cystitis of radiologic interest seen in the United States (Table 2).

Acute hemorrhagic cystitis (Fig. 8) is one of the most

Table 2 ■ CYSTITIS

Forms of Cystitis
Hemorraghic
Cyclophosphamide
Tumoral
Eosinophilic

Imaging Findings
Thick-walled, irregular bladder
Localized bladder wall thickening } All enhance on CT & MRI
Tumoral mass

CT = computed tomography; MRI = magnetic resonance imaging.

---

common causes of gross hematuria in children. Dysuria and frequent urination of relatively sudden onset are other common symptoms. The disorder may occur throughout childhood but most often in children 5 to 7 years of age. It is a self-limited disease that generally subsides in a few days to 2 or 3 weeks without sequelae. Adenovirus and *Escherichia coli* have been cultured in more than one third of the cases. On the excretory urogram or cystogram, the bladder may be rounded, spastic, and small, and may show contour irregularities, thickening of the mucosal folds, or a cobblestone pattern. These findings may be diffuse or limited to the base of the bladder or bladder trigone. Mild ureterectasis may be present, and reflux is sometimes demonstrated.

Cyclophosphamide cystitis is a sterile inflammatory reaction of the bladder mucosa occurring in patients with leukemia or other neoplasia who are receiving this drug. Cyclophosphamide is converted by the liver to the active metabolite acrolein, which is excreted in the urine and affects the bladder mucosa by direct contact. Gross hematuria is the main clinical manifestation. An acute and a chronic form of cyclophosphamide cystitis are described. The acute form usually develops a few days or weeks after initiation of treatment, occasionally after the first dose. Cystoscopy shows diffuse mucosal edema, inflammation, submucosal hemorrhages, and occasionally areas of necrosis, and the cystogram often reveals a small spastic bladder with nodular mucosal irregularities, especially at the level of the bladder trigone. Blood clots may be observed within the bladder, and vesicoureteral reflux may be demonstrated. The process generally clears following withdrawal of the drug, increased hydration, and a period of bladder drainage. The chronic form is a much more serious problem, usually developing 2 to 3 months after initiation of therapy, sometimes only after its completion. It is commonly manifested by continuous or intermittent painless hematuria. The bladder becomes contracted and fibrotic, with diffuse mucosal telangiectases. The cystogram shows a markedly contracted bladder with elevation and deformity of the bladder base and occasionally UVJ obstruction or reflux.

Tumoral cystitis is an uncommon inflammatory process of the bladder, usually presenting with clinical symptoms of acute or subacute cystitis, and characterized by a nodular inflammatory mass (or masses) of the bladder, often mimicking a bladder neoplasm (Fig. 9). The process has a predilection for the base of the bladder and bladder trigone and may cause ureteral obstruction. The gross appearance and the histologic features are quite variable, with changes classified descriptively as bullous cystitis, cystitis cystica, proliferative cystitis, cystitis follicularis, cystitis granularis, and eosinophilic cystitis. The cause of this disorder or group of disorders is not clear. In some instances, the changes may be the sequelae of bacterial or viral infection. Allergy and hypersensitivity reaction have been implicated in eosinophilic cystitis. Cystoscopy and biopsy may be necessary for diagnosis.

Eosinophilic cystisis is an inflammatory process that presents with dysuria, hematuria, proteinuria, fre-

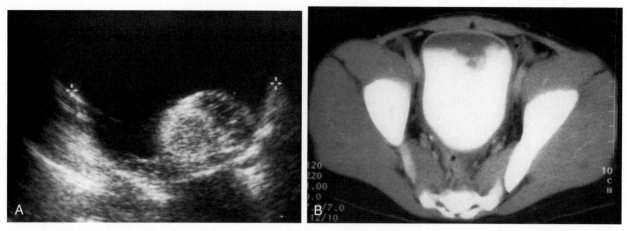

FIGURE 8. Hemorrhagic cystitis. **A,** Transverse sonogram of the bladder shows an echogenic mass consistent with a blood clot. **B,** Computed tomography of the bladder with a delayed scan shows bladder wall enhancement consistent with inflammation; also evident are filling defects representing blood clots.

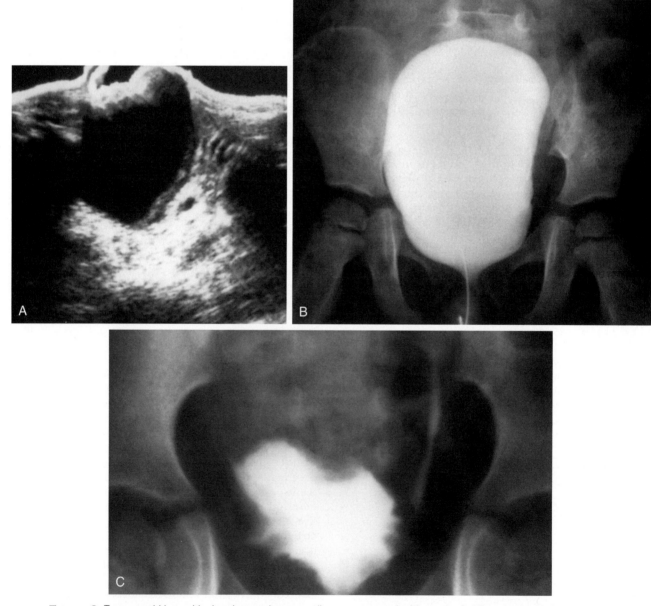

FIGURE 9. Two-year-old boy with chronic granulomatous disease presented with pyuria. **A,** Ultrasound examination of the bladder show focal bladder wall thickening at the left posterior wall with a small echo-free area representing an abscess. **B,** Voiding cystourethrogram shows straightening and mass effect on lateral aspect of bladder. **C,** Bullous cystitis with multiple filling defects along the bladder wall is seen on this excretory urogram. Clinical information suggested infection, which cleared after antibiotic therapy.

quency, and pain. The cause is unclear. Some have associated it with injury, drugs, infections, food reactions, and other allergens. It may present as a mass anterior to the rectum simulating a rhabdomyosarcoma. It may also appear as localized bladder wall thickening. Suspected by eosinophils in the urine and/or peripheral blood, the diagnosis is confirmed by biopsy. It is treated with steroids, and the bladder returns to normal in 2 to 3 weeks.

NEOPLASMS OF THE BLADDER

Neoplasms of the bladder, urethra, and prostate in children are uncommon. Hematuria and urinary retention are the most frequent clinical manifestations. An abdominal mass may be palpated in some cases. The Intergroup Rhabdomyosarcoma Study staging system for neoplasms of the bladder is given in Table 3.

Rhabdomyosarcoma is, in both sexes, the most common and the most important neoplasm of the lower urinary tract and accounts for about 10% of all rhabdomyosarcomas seen in children. Histologically, the tumor may be embryonal, alveolar, or polymorphic. The embryonal type is by far the most common, and in about one fourth of the cases it has a lobulated, polypoid appearance resembling a bunch of grapes, hence the name *sarcoma botryoides* often used for this variant. The tumor is discovered most often during the first 2 or 3 years of life, occasionally at birth. In more than half of the cases, the neoplasm arises from the prostate. Symptoms usually include hematuria, frequency, urinary retention, and obstruction (i.e., hydronephrosis). In the rest of the cases, it originates in the bladder frequently from the area of the trigone and occasionally from the dome (Fig. 10). The tumor is locally invasive and frequently extends toward the bladder outlet, causing urethral obstruction. In females, rhabdomyosarcoma may also arise from the vagina and uterine cervix and invade the same areas of the bladder. When local extension is present, it may not be possible to determine the site of origin.

The neoplasm also tends to spread to regional and retroperitoneal lymph nodes. Lymph node involvement or distant tumor spread is found at initial diagnosis in 10% to 20% of patients. Distant metastases, particularly to the lungs, bones, and liver, also occur but usually only late in the disease. MRI and CT are used to assess these metastases. Lymph node enlargement is seen, as well as local extension from the bladder, prostate, and vagina into regional lymph nodes and muscle. T_1-weighted MRI is used for fat invasion and lymph node spread, while T_2-weighted images document soft tissue invasion (fat suppression technique). CT is less time consuming and less expensive that MRI, and is superior for imaging lung metastases. CT and MRI are comparable for detecting liver metasteses.

An overall survival rate of more than 70% is observed following surgical removal of at least part of the tumor, chemotherapy, and radiation. The prognosis is generally worse when the tumor occurs in the first year of life. When the neoplasm originates in the bladder, the excretory urogram and cystourethrogram show a large and often lobulated filling defect in the posteroinferior aspect of the bladder. When it originates in the prostate, the cystogram usually shows an upward displacement of the bladder floor or a smooth, lobulated mass at the base of the bladder (Fig. 11), and the urethrogram may reveal elongation and displacement of the posterior urethra, and sometimes a lobulated filling defect in the posterior urethra. The bladder may be enlarged and the ureters may be obstructed. US, CT, and MRI are used to evaluate the extent of the tumor and to detect local and retroperitoneal lymph node involvement.

Other primary malignant neoplasms of the lower urinary tracts are very rare. Instances have been reported of epithelial bladder tumors, usually of the papillary type and of low malignancy, as well as instances of leiomyosarcoma and primary lymphoma of the bladder and malignant neoplasms of the urachus. The bladder may also be involved secondarily by leukemia and lymphoma.

Among the benign neoplasms, hemangioma of the bladder is probably the most common. It presents as a discrete solitary mass of variable size, usually projecting from the dome of the bladder. Hematuria is the most common clinical finding. Hemangioma of the skin may be observed in 20% to 30% of the cases. Neurofibromas of the bladder may occur as part of systemic neurofibromatosis or as an isolated lesion (Fig. 12). Other reported benign neoplasms of the bladder include fibromas, fibromatous polyps, blood clots (Fig. 13), inverted papilloma, and nephrogenic adenoma of the bladder. Isolated instances of benign neurofibroma and leiomyoma of the prostate have been reported. Posterior urethral polyps are described in the next section.

DYSFUNCTIONAL VOIDING DISORDERS OF UNKNOWN CAUSE AND CLASSIC NEUROGENIC BLADDER

NORMAL ANATOMY AND FUNCTION

The muscles related to bladder continence and micturition are the detrusor muscle of the bladder, the musculature of the bladder neck and proximal urethra (internal urethral sphincter), and the external urethral

---

Table 3 ■ INTERGROUP RHABDOMYOSARCOMA STUDY STAGING SYSTEM FOR NEOPLASMS OF THE BLADDER

I. Localized tumor, completely resected
II. A. Localized tumor, grossly resected with microscopic residual
   B. Tumor with regional disease or lymph node involvement, completely resected
   C. Tumor with regional disease or involved lymph nodes, grossly resected with microscopic residual
III. A. Gross residual tumor after biopsy only
   B. Distant metastases present at diagnosis.

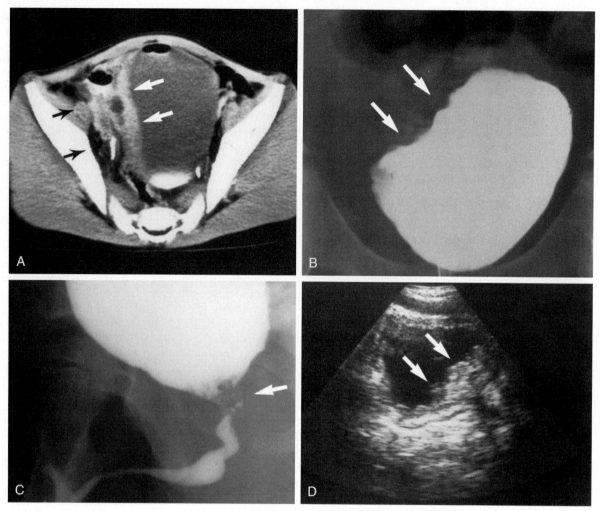

FIGURE 10. A and **B,** Rhabomyosarcoma originating from the right side of the bladder superiorly in a 9-year-old boy with hematuria. Cystogram in the frontal projection is shown in **A** and computed tomography scan section through the lesion is shown in **B** (*arrows* point to the lesion). **C** and **D,** Rhabomyosarcoma originating from the base of the bladder and bladder neck area in a 4-year-old boy with hematuria. Voiding cystogram in the right posterior oblique projection is shown in **C** (*arrow* points to the lesion), and a sagittal midline ultrasound section outlining the lesion is shown in **D** (*arrows).*

sphincter (Fig. 14). The urethra is also affected indirectly, at the level of the urogenital diaphragm, by the striated voluntary muscles of the pelvic floor; a contraction of these muscles results in elevation of the pelvic floor, compressing the urethra.

The muscles of micturition are under the control of the autonomic nervous system (parasympathetic with center at S2 to S4, and sympathetic with center at T10 to L2) and of the voluntary somatic nerves (via the pudendal nerves with center at S2 to S4). The various nerves and muscles involved in bladder control and normal bladder filling and emptying are closely interrelated. Parasympathetic stimulation results in increased tone of the detrusor and, as a secondary phenomenon, in relaxation of the bladder neck. Sympathetic stimulation results in a contraction of the bladder neck and a decrease in the tone of the detrusor. A voluntary contraction of the external sphincter and perineal muscles narrows the urethra and, indirectly, causes an increase in the tone of the bladder neck and relaxation of the detrusor.

The activity of the sacral (parasympathetic) micturition center (S2 to S4) is modulated by impulses from a pontine micturition center that is under the (voluntary) control of cortical areas of the brain. During bladder filling at a physiologic filling rate in normal people, intravesical pressure remains relatively low until a certain point of detrusor stretch is reached, when reflex activity causes increased tone of the detrusor and an urge to void. If the conditions for micturition are not favorable (or during voluntary interruption of micturition), bladder emptying can be prevented, up to a certain bladder volume and pressure, by voluntary cortical inhibition of the sacral micturition center, which depresses the tone of the detrusor, and by voluntary impulses from the motor cortex to the sacral nuclei of the pudendal nerves, which cause a contraction of the external sphincter and, secondarily, an increased tone of the internal sphincter and a relaxation of the detrusor.

The act of micturition is a complex function requiring several years to develop, from a single spinal cord reflex

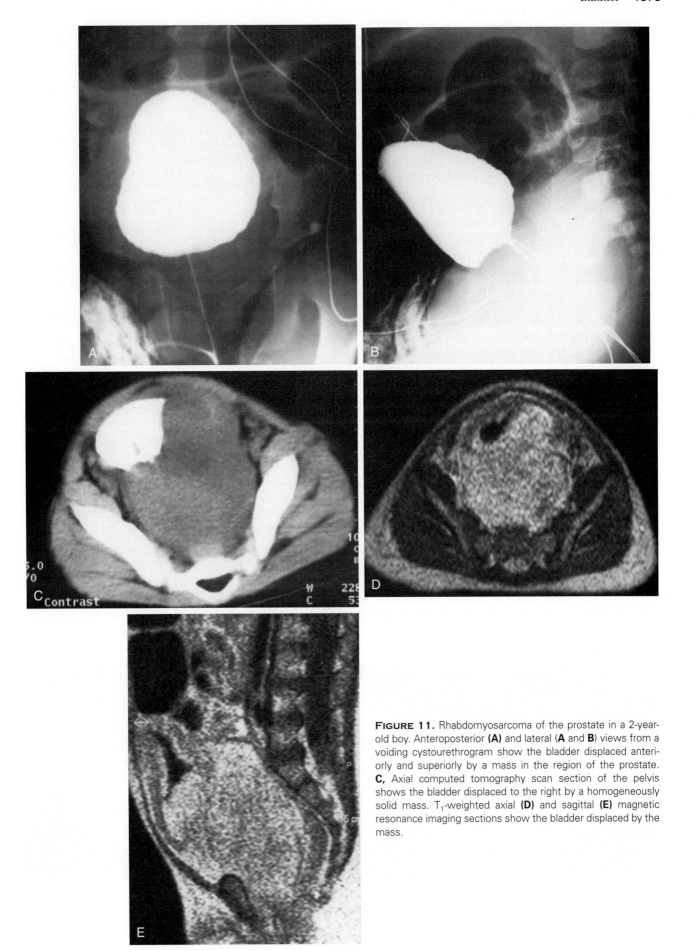

FIGURE 11. Rhabdomyosarcoma of the prostate in a 2-year-old boy. Anteroposterior **(A)** and lateral **(A** and **B)** views from a voiding cystourethrogram show the bladder displaced anteriorly and superiorly by a mass in the region of the prostate. **C,** Axial computed tomography scan section of the pelvis shows the bladder displaced to the right by a homogeneously solid mass. T_1-weighted axial **(D)** and sagittal **(E)** magnetic resonance imaging sections show the bladder displaced by the mass.

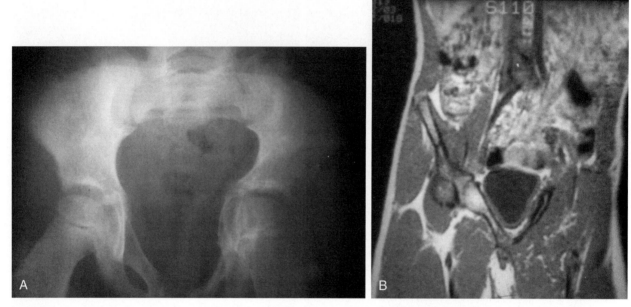

FIGURE 12. Effect of neurofibromatosis on the bladder. **A,** Plain film of the pelvis shows distortion of the left pelvic wall and medial displacement of the left obturator fat line. **B,** T_1-weighted coronal magnetic resonance imaging section shows a mass extending from the pelvic inlet down through the obturator foramen and down the leg.

action in infancy (infantile bladder) to complete bladder control, both conscious and subconscious, which is attained in the vast majority of children during the fourth year. The remaining children acquire full bladder control in subsequent years, with only 2% to 3% still showing some nocturnal enuresis or daytime frequency at puberty.

DYSFUNCTIONAL VOIDING DISORDERS

Under this heading are included some functional disorders of the bladder and urethral musculature manifested in some patients by a delay in maturation of bladder control, in others by a hyperreflexia of the

detrusor muscle with normal external sphincter activity, and in still others by a lack of coordination of the detrusor and the external sphincter. The so-called lazy bladder syndrome of infrequent voiders is also included in this group. The causes of these disorders are not certain. There are no demonstrable neurogenic organic lesions, the spine is normal roentgenographically, and there is no abnormality of the spinal cord demonstrable by MRI or other methods.

Enuresis

A child who wets at age 5 years or older is considered a "bedwetter" by the American Psychiatric Association. Clearly, children should have bladder control and be out

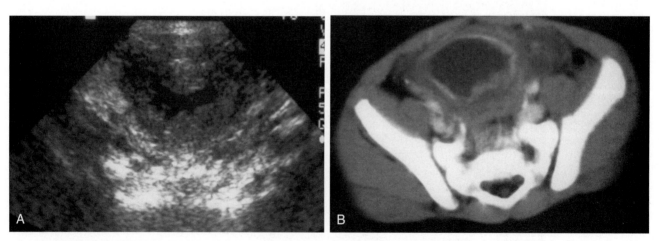

FIGURE 13. Bladder hematoma. **A,** Transverse sonogram of the bladder reveals a thick, irregular wall. **B,** Computed tomography scan section of the pelvis shows bladder wall enhancement and low-attenuation areas in the bladder wall as well as larger blood collections at the left lateral bladder wall.

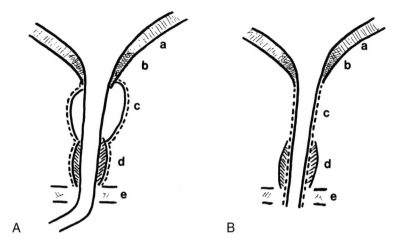

FIGURE 14. Diagram of the muscles of micturition in the male **(A)** and in the female **(B).** These muscle include *a*, detrusor of the bladder (smooth muscle fibers, autonomic innervation); *b*, bladder neck musculature (smooth muscle fibers, autonomic innervation); *c*, fibers of the detrusor of the bladder extending to the capsule of the prostate and external urethral sphincter in the male, and to the entire urethra underneath the external sphincter muscle in the female; *d*, external urethral sphincter (striated muscles, somatic innervation) muscles of the pelvic floor (striated muscles, somatic innervation); and *e*, muscles of the pelvic floor (striated muscles, somatic innervation).

of diapers by the time they attend school. Some of the common accepted facts about children with enuresis are presented in Table 4.

Urodynamic studies are often normal and are usually reserved for treatment nonresponders. Rarely, one will find a duplicated system in which the upper pole ureter empties below the urethral sphincter or at some other site (vagina, perineum, or uterus) that results in constant wetness. This is most common in girls (see Section VII, Part IV, Chapter 1, Fig. 14, page 1844). Nocturnal enuresis occurs in both sexes and may respond to anticholinergics, whereas daytime frequency is more common in boys and apparently does not respond to anticholinergics.

Unstable Bladder in Children

This relatively common disorder, also called detrusor instability and idiopathic detrusor hyperreflexia, is characterized by uninhibited (involuntary) detrusor contractions and normal external sphincter activity. It is seen usually in children between 3 and 14 years (median 6 to 8 years) and is more common in girls than in boys. The clinical manifestations include frequent daytime voiding and urge to void that may result in episodes of incontinence. Nocturnal enuresis is common. The patients may react to detrusor contractions by increasing the external sphincter and perineal muscular activity and frequently assume characteristic postures or develop special maneuvers to prevent urine loss. Vesicoureteral reflux and urinary tract infections are not

uncommon, and chronic constipation and soiling may be present. The patient can void on command, and the act of voiding is usually well coordinated.

Increased thickness of the bladder wall is demonstrated by US. On VCUG, the bladder is commonly smaller than normal and hypertonic, and may be smooth in outline or slightly trabeculated. Vesicoureteral reflux may be observed. The urethra may show transient narrowing at the level of the external sphincter with proximal urethral dilatation ("spinning top" urethra in females). The patient can void with a sustained flow without residual urine in the bladder at the end of voiding. Signs and symptoms of transient detrusor contractions may be noted during the examination, including urge to void at lower bladder volumes, intermittent slowing or cessation or even reversal of the flow of contrast material in the tubing, and intermittent widening of the bladder neck and proximal urethra during bladder filling. The upper urinary tracts are usually normal. Bladder instability is a generally benign disorder that tends to resolve spontaneously with age.

Detrusor–External Sphincteric Dyssynergia

This relatively uncommon type of voiding dysfunction, also called non-neurogenic neurogenic bladder, syndrome of vesicoureteral incoordination, and Hinman syndrome, is the most severe of the group. It is characterized by an incoordination, or dyscoordination, in the activity of the detrusor muscle and that of the external sphincter. The two muscles tend to contract at the same time, preventing efficient emptying of the bladder and leading to a chronically increased intravesical pressure and obstructive changes in the bladder and upper urinary tracts similar to those seen in classical neurogenic bladder (see below).

The condition occurs with equal frequency in boys and girls and is commonly encountered between ages 2 and 13 years. Recurrent urinary infections, nighttime wetting, and daytime urgency and frequency are common manifestations. Dribbling between voidings, possibly an overflow phenomenon, may be observed. Voluntary initiation of voiding may be difficult, requiring much straining. The distended and firm bladder is

---

Table 4 ■ COMMON OBSERVATIONS OF CHILDHOOD ENURESIS

- Daytime control precedes nightime control.
- 15%–20% of 5-year-old children wet the bed.
  - 15% of these become spontaneously continent each year.
  - 1% have enuresis over age 15 years.
  - Diurnal (day and night) wetters = 20%.
- Primary and secondary eneuretics are equal in evaluation, treatment, and response to therapy.
- Positive family history is frequent.
- Cystic fibrosis and sickle cell patients have higher incidence of nocturnal eneuresis.

sometimes present on physical examination. Episodes of urinary retention may also be observed. An occasional patient presents with clinical signs of chronic uremia. Many children with this disorder also have bowel dysfunction manifested by chronic constipation and soiling. A wide range of behavioral or psychological disturbances is common and may contribute to the severity of the symptoms and affect the response to therapy.

US shows an increased thickness of the bladder wall, and, on VCUG, the scout film may show a large amount of feces in the colon. The bladder is commonly enlarged, hypertonic, and variously trabeculated, and may point upward and to the right as in classic neurogenic bladder. Unilateral or bilateral reflux is also common, occurring in about 50% of the patients. The refluxing upper tracts are frequently dilated. The bladder neck and urethra appear normal, but the area of the external sphincter may show a constant or intermittent narrowing (spasm) of the urethra at that level with dilatation proximally. In girls, the urethra may assume a "spinning top" configuration (Fig. 15). Large postvoiding residue in the bladder is very common.

The excretory urogram may show unilateral or bilateral upper tract dilatation that is sometimes severe. Atrophy of the renal parenchyma may be present, and renal function may be decreased. The more severe urographic changes are seen in patients with reflux and

urinary tract infections. In some cases, the urinary tract changes are already developed at the time of the first examination. Voiding cystograms obtained in early life may show that the bladder was originally smooth, indicating that the trabeculation is an acquired and progressive phenomenon.

The uncoordinated activity of the detrusor and external sphincter muscles tends to improve in late childhood or early adolescence, but, in the meantime, the secondary changes in the upper tracts may have progressed to chronic uremia. Current treatment consists of biofeedback training and an intensive and prolonged bladder retraining program, including frequent and "relaxed" voiding with complete emptying of the bladder and other forms of behavior modification.

Megacystic or Lazy Bladder Syndrome of Infrequent Voiders

This disorder, characterized by a dilated hypotonic and hyporeflexic bladder, is seen predominantly in girls and usually becomes manifest between 2 and 6 years of age with recurrent urinary tract infections, infrequent voiding, passage of small amounts of urine, and sometimes overflow or stress incontinence. The child may delay voiding for long periods of time and usually voids only once or twice a day. Constipation and soiling are common. The excretory urogram is usually normal. The cystourethrogram demonstrates a large, smooth-walled bladder with a decreased sensation of fullness. Initiation of voiding may be difficult and require much straining and coaxing. Urine flow may be interrupted. The bladder neck and urethra appear normal during voiding, and postvoiding bladder residue is common. Reflux is not present or is very mild. Urodynamic studies show a hypotonic large-capacity bladder with elevation of intravesical pressure during filling occurring well beyond the level when urge to void is normally expected. The detrusor contractions are small, ineffective, unsustained, or absent, with normal activity of the external sphincter in the electromyelogram (EMG). Environmental or psychological factors and urinary retention from habitual neglect may play a role in the etiology of the condition. These lazy bladders should be distinguished from the large, smooth, and thin-walled bladders seen in some patients with severe reflux (see Section VII, Part IV, Chapter 2, page 1853), which are probably caused by a myogenic failure resulting from the constant passage of urine from the bladder to the ureters and back to the bladder.

CLASSIC NEUROGENIC BLADDER

Causes

In contrast to adult patients, in whom neurogenic bladder is most often due to an acquired, usually traumatic spinal cord lesion, the vast majority of children affected with this disorder have a myelomeningocele or a related myelodysplastic anomaly (occult spinal dysraphism, sacral agenesis).

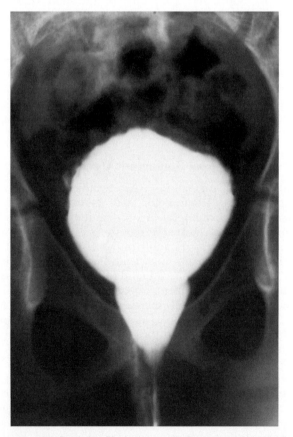

FIGURE 15. Posterior ("spinning top") female urethra. Voiding cystourethrogram demonstrates a dilated posterior urethra (spinning top) in this girl with bladder dysynergia.

Myelomeningocele

Myelomeningocele resulting from faulty closure of the neural canal is the most common cause of neurogenic bladder in children. It can occur at any level of the spine (cervical–thoracic, 2% to 5%; lumbar, 26%; lumbosacral, 47%; sacral, 20%). This disorder occurs in 1 to 2 in 1000 live births, and the clinical types include

1. Complete rachischisis—absence of the vertebral arches in the lumbar region, an underdeveloped cord, and no covering on the nerve elements
2. Myelomeningocele—a soft tissue sac covered by a transparent membrane extruding from the back and exposure of neural elements and cerebrospinal fluid
3. Meningocele—a soft tissue sac covered by atrophic skin that covers the bony defect of the spine

Antenatal diagnosis is made by means of ultrasound (see Section II, Part VII, Chapter 1, Fig. 1, page 266). α-Fetoprotein screening has allowed early detection of the lesion and, when desired, termination of the pregnancy. The roentgenograms of the affected area show widening of the neural canal, defective posterior neural arches, absence of the posterior spinous processes, and widened interpedicular distance involving several segments, with elongated and flattened or defective pedicles.

Occult Spinal Dysraphism

Occult spinal dysraphism (occult myelodysplasia) is a group of congenital anomalies of the spinal cord in which the overlying skin is intact, although cutaneous stigmata of the disorder may be present, such as local hair overgrowth, hyperpigmentation, hemangioma, a skin dimple, or an ill-defined soft-tissue mass caused by a lipoma. These anomalies include tethered cord, diastematomyelia, intraspinal lipoma, dermoid cyst, and hamartoma. Roentgenograms of the spine may show osseous changes similar to those seen in myelomeningocele, and sometimes scoliosis, vertebral fusion, segmentation defects, or broad vertebral bodies. In simple tethered cord, the abnormalities may be subtle, and in some cases the spine appears entirely normal. In the evaluation of the vertebral column in children with suspected occult spinal dysraphism, one should keep in mind that small midline defects in the posterior arch of one or two vertebrae, often at the lumbosacral junction without widening of the neural canal or thinning of the pedicles, are very common. They are secondary to incomplete fusion of the neural canal and are considered to be normal variants. Clinical manifestations of occult spinal dysraphism may be delayed several years.

Sacral Agenesis

Sacral agenesis is often partial, involving one or more distal sacral segments and the coccyx. If the entire sacrum or most of the sacrum is deficient, the iliac bones are close together and may be fused in the midline, the distal segments of the lumbar spine are commonly defective or missing, and occasionally the entire lumbosacral spine is absent. Maternal diabetes is common in patients with complete or almost complete sacral agenesis (15% to 20% of the cases). Lesser degrees of sacral agenesis, hypoplasia of one side of the sacrum with sacral scoliosis, segmentation defects, and other sacral anomalies may also be associated with neurologic abnormalities, including neurogenic bladder, and may occur as isolated lesions or in association with congenital anorectal anomalies.

Trauma

Trauma to the spinal cord, nerve roots, or pelvic nerves, often from external sources, is the most common cause of acquired neurogenic bladder. Trauma may occur at any level. Spinal roentgenograms may show vertebral fractures or dislocations. A special form of spinal cord injury, often at the level of C7 to T1, may complicate a difficult, usually breech, delivery. The vertebral column in these patients may appear normal radiographically. Paraplegia following relatively minor trauma may occur in patients with hemophilia (intraspinal hematoma) or achondroplasia (narrow spinal canal). Neurogenic bladder may also be caused by injury to the nerve supply of the bladder during surgical correction of congenital anorectal anomalies or Hirschsprung's disease, excision of a pelvic tumor, or extensive pelvic dissection for other reasons.

Other Causes

Primary or secondary intraspinal neoplasms, paravertebral neoplasms extending into the neural canal, vertebral neoplasms or osteomyelitis, epidural abscesses, and transverse myelitis are other recognized causes of neurogenic bladder at all ages.

Functional Changes

Based on the level of the causative lesion and the functional aspects of voiding, several types of neurogenic bladder have been observed in experimental animals and sometimes in pure forms also in humans. The best-known types include

1. Uninhibited hyperreflexic bladder resulting from an acquired disease of the cerebral cortex
2. Uninhibited hyperreflexic bladder resulting from a congenital or acquired lesion of the spinal cord above the sacral centers, resulting in an interruption of the inhibitory impulses from higher centers and a purely reflex bladder
3. Autonomic bladder resulting from a lesion affecting the sacral center or the neural pathways connecting the sacral center with the bladder, causing separation of the bladder from the spine and loss of the sacral micturition reflex

Although well-defined clinical and radiographic features have been attributed to these and other postulated forms of neurogenic bladder, these classifications are often impractical because the primary lesion may be incomplete or is not sharply limited, and because motor and sensory nerve fibers may be involved to a different degree. Also, the clinical and radiographic features may be greatly modified by the duration of the disease and previous urinary tract infections. In addition, the vast majority of cases of neurogenic bladder in pediatrics fall in the large, heterogeneous group of hyperreflexic bladders caused by sacral and suprasacral lesions and are frequently complicated by detrussor–external sphincter dyssynergia.

Clinical Manifestations

The principal clinical manifestation in most children with a neurogenic bladder is a dysfunction of the detrusor, usually associated with a dysfunction of the external sphincter. In mild or early cases, there may be only night and day wetting and urinary urgency and frequency. In severe advanced cases, there is total loss of bladder sensation and urinary control, with constant dribbling of urine, urine retention, and overflowing incontinence. The urethral resistance is usually increased, and it may not be possible to empty the bladder by manual compression. Between these two extremes are all grades of severity and combinations of symptoms. Urinary tract infections with episodes of sepsis and pyelonephritis are common complications, and in some patients there is a deterioration of renal function that may lead to chronic uremia. Urinary calculi are not uncommon.

Radiographic Investigations

The excretory urogram provides information on the status of the spine and upper tracts. Early in the disease, the urogram can be entirely normal. Dilatation of the upper tracts may not be observed until after repair of the myelomeningocele (Fig. 16). In advanced cases, one or both kidneys may show decreased function and loss of parenchyma. One or both upper urinary tracts may be dilated, even in the absence of reflux. UVJ obstruction attributed to a thickened, heavily trabeculated bladder may be observed. Often, in the resting state, the bladder neck area has a funnel-like configuration, with contrast material in the bladder extending downward into the proximal urethra. US of the kidneys and upper urinary tracts may be a useful alternative to the excretory urogram in the initial evaluation and in follow-up studies. The diethylenetriaminepentaacetic acid renogram is also of special value in the evaluation of renal function and upper tract dilatation, and the dimercaptosuccinic acid scan may be used to detect cortical loss or pyelonephritis.

The cystourethrogram is used to evaluate the anatomy of the bladder neck and the urethra and to demonstrate reflux. As a functional study, it complements the urodynamic investigation and contributes information regarding the amount of urine at the time of catheterization, bladder capacity, sensation of bladder fullness, behavior of the detrusor muscle and urethral sphincter during bladder filling and voiding, ability to stop and start micturition voluntarily, the voiding pattern, effect of Credé's maneuver on bladder emptying, and amount of residual urine in postvoiding films. When a VCUG recorded on videotape is combined with a synchronous multichannel urodynamic study, continuously recording flow rates, intravesical and rectal pressures, and the EMG findings (synchronous, cine, or pressure–flow cystometrography, or videocystourodynamic study), it may be possible to compare and correlate more precisely the various phases of filling and emptying and the behavior of the bladder, bladder neck, and external sphincter with a corresponding display of the urodynamic changes at each level.

Early in the course of the disease and in mild cases, the VCUG may show no abnormalities or only minor changes. In more advanced cases, residual urine at the time of catheterization is common. Full distention of the bladder or retrograde filling is often impossible. The bladder is usually hypertonic and may be round, smooth, or trabeculated (Fig. 17). Paraureteral diverticula may be demonstrated. The bladder may become elongated, pointing upward and often to the right. Whether hypertonic or relatively smooth, the bladder may be small, of normal size, or large, depending on the status of the urethral resistance and previous or current infections. A purely atonic, large, and smooth-walled bladder of the type seen in adults with isolated sensory nerve root disease is uncommon in children. In patients with gross incontinence, voiding may occur during filling of the bladder. Once the bladder is filled, voiding may be initiated spontaneously or may be obtained only with Credé's maneuver. Sometimes voiding continues in an uncontrolled fashion with a good and sustained stream or intermittently. The patient may or may not be able to stop and start micturition voluntarily.

On voiding films, the bladder neck and proximal urethra are frequently dilated. At the level of the external sphincter, the urethra is usually narrowed intermittently or constantly as a result of external sphincter hyperactivity, sometimes from local denervation, muscle atrophy, and fibrosis. The urethra above the narrow sphincter area is dilated, sometimes resembling posterior urethral valves in males. Reflux of contrast material into the prostatic ducts may be observed (see Fig. 17B). The bulbocavernosus muscle may be spastic, causing a constant or intermittent narrowing of the bulbar urethra. Normal function of the pelvic floor musculature observed in some cases is characterized by an exaggerated relaxation of these muscles with a marked descent of the pelvic floor during urination and an incomplete ascent at the end of micturition. Vesicoureteral reflux is frequent and is often associated with variable ureterectasis. The reflux is often bilateral but may be limited to one side for a long period of time. Residual urine in the bladder at the end of the procedure is a common finding.

Evaluation of the Artificial Urinary Sphincter

Artificial urinary sphincters are designed to alleviate urinary incontinence in patients with low urethral resistance, normal or near-normal detrusor function

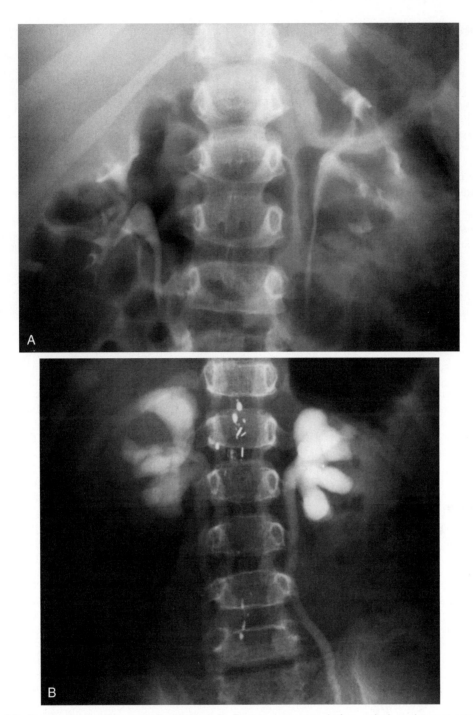

FIGURE 16. Renal effects of neurogenic bladder. **A,** Excretory urogram before spinal cord tumor was removed demonstrated normal renal parenchymal thickness and normal collecting systems. **B,** Two years after spinal surgery, the excretory urogram now shows loss of renal parenchyma and blunting of all the calyces. Surgical clips and Pantopaque are noted in the spinal canal.

and bladder compliance, and absence of significant bladder diverticula or vesicoureteral reflux. Reflux, when present, can be corrected prior to the implantation of the sphincter.

The artificial sphincter most commonly used at this time is the AMS 800 (American Medical Systems). The device, shown diagrammatically in Figure 18, is composed of a pump or bulb with a control assembly, a regulator pressure balloon or reservoir, an inflatable

cuff, and connecting tubes. The pump with the attached control assembly is implanted in the scrotum above the testis or in one of the labia majora, the balloon reservoir is placed beneath the fascia of the anterior abdominal wall near the bladder, and the inflatable cuff is implanted around the bladder neck. An isotonic solution of iodinated contrast material is used as hydrostatic fluid to fill the system. The cuff may be deflated manually by squeezing the pump. With this maneuver, the content of

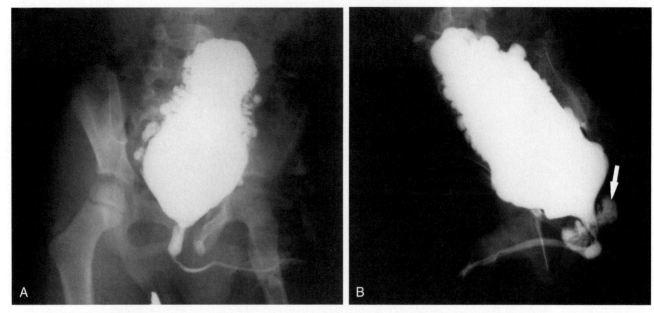

FIGURE 17. A and **B,** Voiding cystourethrograms of two children with neurogenic bladder both demonstrate multiple cellules and bladder trabeculation. The child in **B** also had reflux into the prostatic bed *(arrow)*.

the pump is forced into the reservoir through a one-way valve in the control assembly; the pump refills promptly by withdrawing fluid from the cuff through another one-way valve in the control assembly, thus deflating the cuff and allowing emptying of the bladder; a resistor in the control assembly causes a slow refilling of the cuff from the reservoir.

A functional failure of the device is manifested most commonly by recurrence of urinary incontinence, sometimes by urinary retention (and overflow incontinence), and is caused most often by loss of fluid from the

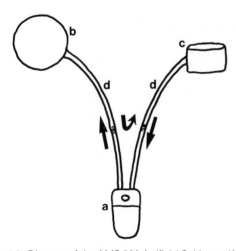

FIGURE 18. Diagram of the AMS 800 Artificial Sphincter (American Medical System). The device is composed of a combined pump and control assembly with an off/on button *(a)*, a regulator pressure balloon or balloon reservoir *(b)*, an inflatable cuff *(c)*, and tubes connecting the reservoir and cuff to the pump-control assembly *(d)*. *Arrows* indicate the possible direction of flow of the hydraulic fluid within the system, controlled by two one-way valves and a resistor circuit in the control assembly.

system. Although the site of leakage (most often the cuff) cannot be recognized in abdominal roentgenograms, it may be possible to determine in most cases from abdominal films that loss of fluid from the system has occurred. It is important that the films be exposed with the same technical factors used in the baseline films obtained routinely immediately after implantation. The site of leakage can be determined at the time of surgery. When the fluid loss is complete, the entire system is empty and invisible roentgenographically; in less severe cases, the system is partially collapsed with a decrease in the thickness of the cuff sleeve and a decrease in diameter or loss of the spherical shape of the balloon reservoir. A significant fluid loss from the device may only be associated with a difference of a few millimeters in balloon diameter compared to the baseline study.

Urinary retention, frequently associated with overflowing incontinence, is most often the result of failure of the bulb to deflate, and is usually due to kinks in the tubing that may be apparent only on lateral or oblique views or fluoroscopically. Migration of the deflated pump into the inguinal canal with failure to palpate the pump is an uncommon cause of sphincteric failure with urinary retention. Erosion of the bladder neck and proximal urethra by the cuff is an infrequent but serious complication resulting in bladder neck obstruction, urinary retention, detrusor hyperreflexia, and sometimes incontinence. Hematuria, dysuria, and pain when the pump is activated are common manifestations. Local erosion caused by the cuff may result in contour irregularities of the area and local extravasation of contrast material demonstrable by cystourethrography, retrograde urethrography, and cystourethroscopy.

Other causes of malfunction of the device not recognizable on plain abdominal films include a decreased bladder compliance, worsening of the existing abnormalities such as vesicoureteral reflux or bladder diverticula, and development of inhibited bladder contractions or hypertonicity leading to increased intravesical pressure relative to the pressure within the cuff. Some of these complications can be demonstrated by cystourethrography or other urographic procedures. In some cases, the underlying abnormality can be diagnosed only by urodynamic studies.

SUGGESTED READINGS

Amis ES, Blaivas JG: The role of the radiologist in evaluation voiding dysfunction. Radiology 1990;175:317

Avni EF, Matos C, Diard F, Schulman CC: Midline omphalovesical anomalies in children: contributions of ultrasound imaging. Urol Radiol 1988;10:189

Batista J, Bauer S, Shefner J, et al: Urodynamic findings in children with spinal cord ischemia. J Urol 1995;154:1183

Bauer S: Neuropathology of the lower urinary tract. In Kelalis PP, King LR, Belman AB (eds): Clinical Pediatric Urology, 3rd ed. Philadelphia, WB Saunders, 1992:399

Bauer SB: Neurogenic bladder dysfunction. Pediatr Clin North Am 1987;34:1121

Boemers T, van Gool J, de Jong T, et al: Urodynamic evaluation of children with caudal regression syndrome (caudal dysplasia sequence). J Urol 1994;151:1041

Burbige KA, Lebowitz RL, Colodny AH, et al: The megacystis-megaureter syndrome. J Urol 1984;131:1133

Cacciarelli AA, Kass EJ, Yang SS: Urachal remnants: demonstration in children. Radiology 1990;174:473

Connor J, Betrus G, Fleming P, et al: Early cystometrograms can predict the response to intravesical instillation of oxybutinin chloride in myelomeningocele patients. J Urol 1994;151:1045

Erickson D, Bartholomew T, Marlin A: Sonographic evaluation and conservative management of newborns with myelomeningocele and hydronephrosis. J Urol 1989;142:592

Fernandes E, Vermier R, Gonzalez R: The unstable bladder in children. J Pediatr 1991;118:831

Flood HD, Ritchey ML, Bloom DA, et al: Outcome of reflux in children with myelodysplasia managed by bladder pressure monitoring. J Urol 1994;152:1574

Fotter R, Kopp W, Klein E, et al: Unstable bladder in children: functional evaluation by modified cystourethrography. Radiology 1986;161:811

Henly DR, Farrow GM, Zincke H: Urachal cancer: the role of conservative surgery. Urology 1993;42:635

Herman TE, McAllister WH: Radiographic manifestations of the lower urinary tract. Radiol Clin North Am 1991;29:365

Hernanz-Schulman M, Lebowitz FL: The elusiveness and importance of bladder diverticula in children. Pediatr Radiol 1985;15:399

Hill LM, Kislak S, Belfar HL: Sonographic diagnosis of urachal cysts in utero. J Clin Ultrasound 1990;18:434

Jodal U, Koskimies I, Hanson E, et al: Infection pattern in children with vesicoureteral reflux randomly allocated to operation or long-term antibacterial prophylaxis. J Urol 1992;148:1650–1652

Khowry AE, Churchill BM: The artificial urinary sphincter. Pediatr Clin North Am 1987;34:1175–1207

Kindo A: Cystourethrogram characteristics of bladder instability in children. Urology 1990;35:242

Klein FA: Unusual bladder tumors in children. In Broecker BH, Klein FA (eds): Pediatric Tumors of the Genitourinary Tract. New York, Alan R. Liss, 1998:177

Klimberg I: The development of voiding control. Am Urol Assoc Update Series 1988;7:161

Koff SA: Evaluation and management of voiding disorders in children. Urol Clin North Am 1988;15:769

Kumar A, Aggarwal S: Case report: the sonographic appearance of cyclophosphamide-induced acute haemorrhagic cystitis. Clin Radiol 1990;41:289

Leicher-Duber A, Schumacher R: Urachal remnants in asymptomatic children: sonographic morphology. Pediatr Radiol 1991;21:200

Levine LA, Richie JP: Urologic complications of cyclophosphamide. J Urol 1989;141:1063

Levine PM, Gonzales ET Jr: Congenital bladder diverticula causing ureteral obstruction. Urology 1985;25:273

Maurer HM, Ragab A: Rhabdomyosarcoma. In Fern Brett DJ, Vietti TJ (eds): Clinical Pediatric Oncology, 4th ed. St. Louis, Mosby–Year Book, 1991:491–515

Mundy AR: Detrusor instability. Br J Urol 1988;62:393

Noe HN: The role of dysfunctional voiding in failure or complication of ureteral reimplantation for primary reflux. J Urol 1985;134:1172

Ozbek SS, Pourbagher MA, Pourbagher A: Urachal remnants in asymptomatic children: gray scale and color Doppler. J Clin Ultrasound 2001;29:218

Peterson NE, Silverman A, Campbell JB: Eosinophilic cystitis and coexistent eosinophilic gastroenteritis in an infant. Pediatr Radiol 1989;19:484

Poggiani C, Teani M, Auriemma A, et al: Sonographic detection of rhabdomyosarcoma of the urinary bladder. Eur J Ultrasound 2001;13:35

Rafal RV, Markicz JA: Urachal carcinoma: the role of magnetic resonance imaging. Urol Radiol 1991;12:184

Rose SC, Hansen ME, Webster GD, et al: Artificial urinary sphincters: plain radiography of malfunction and complications. Radiology 1988;168:403

Rozenberg H, Abdelkader T, Hussein AA: Laparascopic excision of voluminous bladder diverticulum. Prog Urol 1994;4:91

Saxton HM, Borzyskowski M, Mundy AR, Vivian GC: Spinning top urethra: not a normal variant. Radiology 1988;168:147

Schulman SL, Quyinn CK, Plachter N, Kodman-Jones C: Comprehensive management of dysfunctional voiding. Pediatrics 1999;103:E31

Sidi AA, Peng W, Gonzalez R: Vesicoureteral reflux in children with myelodysplasia: natural history and results of treatment. J Urol 1986;136:329

Siegel MJ: Pelvic tumors in childhood. Radiol Clin North Am 1997;75:1455

Spindel MR, Bauer SB, Dyro FM, et al: The changing neurologic lesion in myelodysplasia. JAMA 1987;258:1630

Steinhard G: Prostatic suppuration and destruction in patients with myelodysplasia: a newly recognized entity. J Urol 1988;140:1002

Taylor GA, Lebowitz RL: Artificial urinary sphincters in children: radiographic evaluation. Radiology 1985;155:91

Verhagen PC, Nikkels PG, de Jong T: Eosinophilic cystitis. Arch Dis Child 2001;84:344

Wan J, Greenfield S: Enuresis and common voiding abnormalities. Pediatr Clin North Am 1997;44:117

Wein AJ: Lower urinary tract function and pharmacologic management of lower urinary tract dysfunction. Urol Clin North Am 1987;14:273

Wein AJ, English WS, Whitmore KE: Office urodynamics. Urol Clin North Am 1988;15:609

PART VI

URETHRA

JACK O. HALLER

POSTERIOR URETHRAL VALVES*

Posterior urethral valves (PUV) that are not diagnosed antenatally and are not apparent clinically in the newborn period may present in the first months or years of life with urinary tract infections, sepsis, voiding disorders, hematuria, vomiting, failure to thrive, urinary retention, and palpable kidneys. In some of these patients, there may be a history of respiratory distress in the newborn period that gradually subsided. There are still other patients with PUVs that have caused little or no change in the urinary tract and who may present during childhood or later life with only functional voiding disorders or urinary tract infections. The diagnosis can be made on the basis of imaging findings (Table 1).

Following transurethral resection or fulguration of the obstructing valvular structures, the cystourethrogram commonly shows a prompt decrease in the dilatation of the posterior urethra, but in about one fourth of the patients the dilatation persists despite a widely patent, unobstructed urethra, possibly as the result of prostatic gland hypoplasia. Residual valve tissue with obstruction is not uncommon, and stricture formation at the site of the previous urethral valves, or in the membranous urethra as a complication of surgery, may occur. Urethroscopy is usually more reliable than the urethrogram in the diagnosis of these lesions. Persistent reflux may require ureteral reimplantation.

The upper tract dilatation generally improves following surgery and sometimes disappears. A persisting dilatation may be due to a residual or acquired urethral obstruction, continuing vesicoureteral reflux, or poor ureteral peristalsis. Ureteral obstruction at the ureterovesical junction (UVJ) resulting simply from muscular hypertrophy of the bladder is uncommon. A more common cause of upper tract dilatation and apparent UVJ obstruction is the so-called valve–bladder syndrome, in which the upper tract dilatation without reflux is due to a stiff, noncompliant bladder, best seen when the bladder is full. Persistent bladder dysfunction (detrusor instability without urethral sphincter dysfunction) and urinary incontinence may also be seen postoperatively. Patients with residual upper tract dilatation or recurrent urinary tract infections and deterioration of renal function are investigated by voiding cystourethrography (VCUG) for evidence of reflux or urethral stricture, and to determine the size and shape of the bladder and, to some extent, the function of the bladder during voiding. Urodynamic studies may be indicated if a functional disorder of the bladder is suspected. The upper tracts are evaluated by ultrasound (US) and by excretory urography if renal function permits. Diuretic diethylenetriaminepentaacetic acid renal scintigraphy and sometimes a Whitaker test may be necessary to differentiate a functional from an obstructive ureterectasis. The renal parenchyma is best followed by dimercaptosuccinic acid scans.

Refinements in surgical approach and in pre- and postoperative management of patients with PUV have

---

Table 1 ■ IMAGING FINDINGS WITH POSTERIOR URETHRAL VALVES

Ultrasound
Renal cysts
Bilateral (unilateral) hydronephrosis
Thick-walled bladder
Actual valves may be demonstrated

Voiding Cystourethrogram
Dilated posterior urethra
Actual valves may be demonstrated
Reflux into prostatic and/or ejaculatory ducts
Thick bladder neck
Trabeculated bladder
Reflux (50% of cases)

---

*For a discussion of posterior urethral valves in the antenatal and perinatal periods, see Section II, Part V, Chapter 4, page 204.

resulted in a significant improvement in the initial results. However, the long-term results continue to be disappointing. A large percentage of patients with PUV show progressive deterioration of renal function to chronic renal insufficiency with growth failure, systemic arterial hypertension, renal osteodystrophy and other complications of chronic renal failure, and in many cases end-stage renal disease requiring dialysis and renal transplantation. End-stage renal disease may be reached within a few months to 15 or more years after the diagnosis of PUV.

POSTERIOR URETHRAL POLYPS

This uncommon lesion of the male posterior urethra, also called congenital polyp of the verumontanum, consists of an elongated, freely movable polypoid mass on a long stalk originating from the region of the verumontanum (Table 2; Fig. 1). It is a benign hamartomatous lesion composed of a fibroconnective tissue core containing smooth muscle elements, blood vessels, nests of glandular cells, and sometimes neural tissue. It is covered by a transitional cell epithelium, sometimes with metaplastic changes of the glandular type. The lesion is usually diagnosed in children between 3 and 6 years of age, but has been reported in infants and adults. The symptoms are those of intermittent urethral obstruction with straining on voiding, abnormal voiding pattern, and urinary retention. Hematuria and urinary tract infections may also be observed. On the excretory urogram before voiding, the tip of the polyp is frequently located at the level of the bladder neck, causing a small rounded filling defect at that level. In the voiding phase of a cystourethrogram, the polyp moves downward into the distal posterior urethra and occasionally into the bulbar urethra. Sometimes the polyp becomes impacted in the posterior urethra, obstructing urine flow. At the end of voiding, the polyp is displaced backward to the level of the bladder outlet by the contraction of the external urethral sphincter. Bladder trabeculations, vesicoureteral reflux, and upper tract dilatation may be present.

Table 2 ■ POSTERIOR URETHRAL POLYPS

Originates at verumontanum
Usually found at 3–6 years of age
Hamartoma with muscle, neural, and vascular tissue
Stalk is present
Signs/symptoms
    Intermittent urethral obstruction
    Urinary retention
    Hematuria
    Infections
    Bladder tics
Imaging findings
    Filling defect at bladder neck–midurethra
    Vesicoureteral reflux
    Dilatation of upper tracts

PROSTATIC UTRICLE AND MÜLLERIAN DUCT CYSTS

The *prostatic utricle* is a small, epithelium-lined diverticulum of the prostatic urethra. It is located in the verumontanum between the two openings of the ejaculatory ducts and extends backward and slightly upward for a very short distance within the medial lobe of the prostate. It is a normal anatomic variant representing the remnant of the fused caudal ends of the müllerian ducts, and thus is the homolog of the female vagina and uterine cervix. The utricle is occasionally seen on the routine VCUG as a tiny diverticulum of a few millimeters in length. In some apparently normal males, the utricle may be much larger, measuring up to 1 cm or more in length, sometimes reaching the base of the bladder or even a higher level (Fig. 2). Prostatic utricles, often quite large, are seen with some frequency in male hypospadias, especially in the more severe types. They are not uncommon in prune-belly syndrome, and may be seen in patients with imperforate anus and rectoposterior urethral fistula, and in patients with Down syndrome. Occasionally prostatic utricle is bifid, reflecting the bifid nature of its precursors, namely the paired müllerian ducts. Urine may be stored in a large utricle, resulting in infection and voiding frequency.

> ■ Prostatic utricle
> • Occurs in prostatic urethra
> • Located between ejaculatory ducts
> • Müllerian remnant
> • Seen with prune-belly syndrome, Down syndrome, imperforate anus

A *müllerian duct cyst*, or cyst of the prostatic utricle, is a cystic dilatation of an obstructed utricle occurring in patients with otherwise normal lower urinary tract and external genitalia. The obstruction has been attributed to congenital valves or mucosal folds, local infection, or desquamation of the epithelium. Müllerian cysts are rare and are most often discovered in adults. They vary greatly in size from a few centimeters in diameter to a large pelvic mass displacing the bladder upward and forward and sometimes obstructing the urethra. Stone formation within these cysts has been reported. Sometimes these cysts are found to communicate with the urethra by a minute tract. In some cases, it has been possible to opacify a müllerian cyst following insertion of a small catheter into the utricle at urethroscopy. The cystic nature and location of the pelvic mass is readily determined by US, computed tomography, or magnetic resonance imaging.

> ■ Müllerian duct cyst
> • Obstructive utricle
> • Rare
> • Presents as pelvic mass

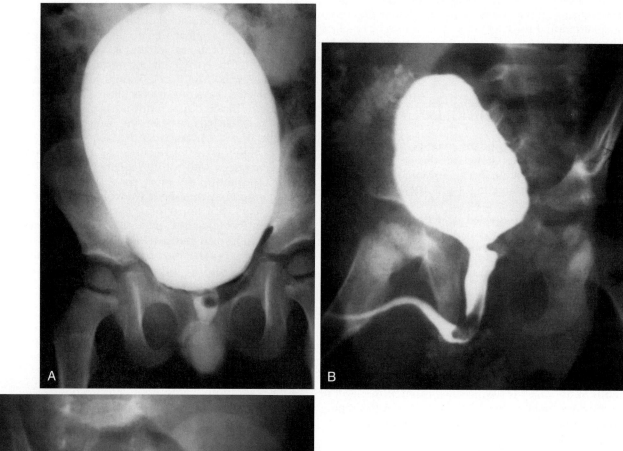

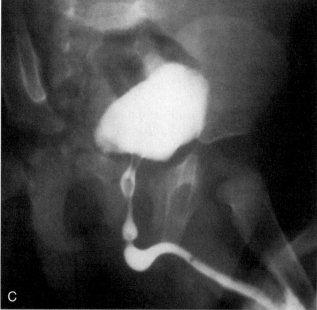

FIGURE 1. Urethral polyps. In case one, frontal **(A)** and oblique **(B)** views during a voiding cystourethrogram show a filling defect representing a polyp on a stalk that flipped back and forth from posterior to anterior urethra. **C,** Case two shows a polyp on a stalk. The polyp is seen in the posterior urethra while the stalk extends to the bladder neck.

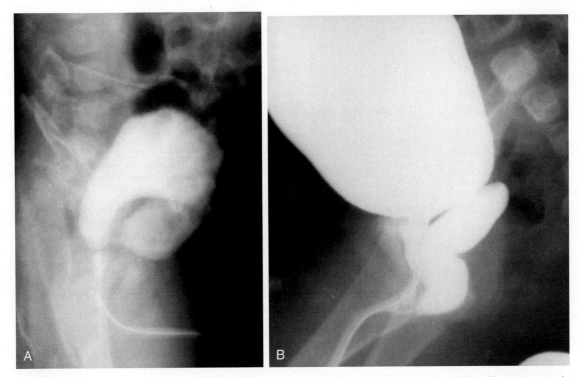

FIGURE 2. Utricle. **A,** In case one, voiding cystourethrography reveals small and large diverticulum-like structures that emanate in both cases off the posterior urethra. **B,** In case two, the catheter actually enters the utricle.

ABNORMALITIES OF COWPER'S GLANDS

The bulbourethral or Cowper's glands are two pea-sized bodies located behind the distal end of the posterior urethra between the two layers of the urogenital diaphragm (Fig. 3). They are the homolog of the Bartholin's glands of the female. Their ducts are directed forward through the bulb of the corpus spongiosum to end in the ventral aspect of the bulbar urethra. The ducts of these glands, and sometimes also the glands themselves, may be opacified during VCUG,

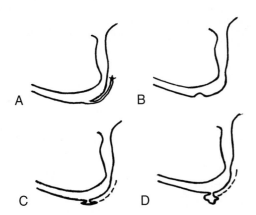

FIGURE 3. Various configurations of cowperian ducts and Cowper's glands that may be observed on urethrography. **A,** Filling of the duct up to the gland. **B,** Opening of the cowperian duct is obliterated, causing a small mass on the floor of the bulbar urethra. **C** and **D,** Diverticular cavities originate in the floor of the bulbar urethra; the proximal portion of the duct usually is not opacified in these cases.

probably owing to an anomaly of their orifice (Fig. 4). This finding, as a rule, is of no clinical significance. On occasion, these dilated ducts form a globular cavity on the ventral surface of the bulbar urethra, suggesting a diverticulum. It is suspected that many diverticula of the bulbar urethra reported in the earlier literature were in fact dilated cowperian ducts. Possibly related to these ducts is the finding of a small rounded defect or mound in the floor of the bulbar urethra, occasionally seen on routine voiding urethrograms. At urethroscopy, these lesions appear cystic, and, on unroofing, they are found to be filled with clear fluid, or sometimes blood-tinged fluid. They are believed to represent obstructed cowperian ducts. Instances have been reported of very large congenital retention cysts of these ducts causing urethral obstruction.

MEGALOURETHRA, ANTERIOR URETHRAL DIVERTICULA, AND ANTERIOR URETHRAL VALVE

These uncommon anomalies of the male urethra are considered together because of common features and transitional forms suggesting a spectrum of related deformities. Their causes and modes of development are uncertain.

Fusiform megalourethra, the rarest of the group, is characterized by a diffuse ectasia of the penile urethra secondary to an absence or partial deficiency of the corpus spongiosum and corpora cavernosa without distal obstruction. The penis is large, misshapen, and flabby, with a redundant and wrinkled skin. Erections

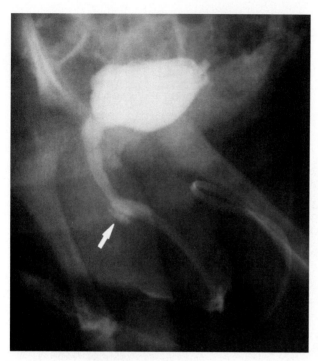

FIGURE 4. Voiding cystourethrography shows filling of Cowper's gland inferior to the urethra at the penoscrotal junction *(arrow)*.

are not possible owing to the defective corpora cavernosa. During voiding, the urethra and penis become markedly distended. The patient voids with a poor urinary stream. On the voiding or retrograde urethrogram, the penile urethra is markedly dilated and fusiform, tapering both distally and proximally into a relatively normal urethra. The proximal urethra may be dilated. Sometimes the anomaly affects a small portion of the urethra, as shown in Figure 5. The anomaly may occur as an isolated lesion but is seen more commonly in patients with prune-belly syndrome. The clinical symptoms and prognosis vary with the severity of the associated anomalies.

■ Megalourethra occurs in two types:
  • Fusiform—no corpora cavernosa or spongiosa
  • Scaphoid—no corpora spongiosa

Scaphoid megalourethra is much more common than the fusiform type. It consists of a localized saccular dilatation of the penile urethra apparently caused by a localized absence or underdevelopment of the corpus spongiosum. The corpora cavernosa are intact. The penis is normal in size or somewhat enlarged and appears shorter dorsally than ventrally, causing a mild dorsal chordee. Ventrally, the penis is soft and baggy with a redundant skin. During voiding, the affected part of the urethra balloons markedly, causing a large, smooth bulge in the ventral surface of the penis. The patient voids with a poor stream. During voiding or during an erection, the penis and pendulous urethra assume a scaphoid configuration. The dilated segment

of the urethra blends gradually with a normal urethra distally and proximally. The proximal urethra may be slightly dilated. Associated anomalies in the rest of the urinary tract are much less common than in fusiform megalourethra. Scaphoid megalourethra may also occur in association with prune-belly syndrome, partial or complete.

Anterior urethral diverticulum is a saccular outpouching of the ventral aspect of the anterior urethra into the corpus spongiosum, usually near the penoscrotal junction. A circumferential thinning and local fibrosis of the corpus spongiosum may be present. The corpora cavernosa are intact. The communication of the urethra with the diverticulum is usually wide and centrally placed. The diverticulum has a well-defined, valve-like anterior lip, and a less well-defined posterior lip. During voiding, urine distends the diverticulum and displaces the anterior lip of the diverticulum forward and against the dorsal wall of the urethra, obstructing the flow of urine. A tense bulge on the ventral aspect of the penis at the level of the diverticulum is observed during voiding.

The diagnosis is made by VCUG. The urethra proximal to the diverticulum is dilated, with a sharp demarcation with the unobstructed distal urethra. The lateral edges of the roof of the diverticulum may be seen on the lateral projection as two thin horizontal lines. The posterior lip is usually not well delineated. The lesion is not well shown on a retrograde urethrogram. Bladder trabeculations, bladder diverticula, and vesicoureteral reflux may be present. The upper tracts may be dilated, and there may be loss of renal parenchyma. The symptoms depend on the degree of obstruction. They include poor urinary stream, a penile mass during voiding, urinary tract infections, and in rare cases stone formation within the diverticulum.

An *anterior urethral valve* is a semilunar fold very much like the anterior lip of a urethral diverticulum. It originates in the floor of the urethra near the penoscrotal junction. It is directed backward, and is anchored laterally in such a way as to be raised up against the dorsal aspect of the urethra during voiding, obstructing the flow of urine (Figs. 6 and 7). It differs from a urethral diverticulum in that it lacks a posterior lip, and usually causes a lesser degree of localized swelling of the ventral aspect of the penis during micturition. No abnormalities of the corpus spongiosum or corpora cavernosa are present. It is possible that an anterior urethral valve originates from an anterior urethral diverticulum with loss of the posterior lip. The clinical manifestations and complications on radiographic appearance are the same as those described for anterior urethral diverticula but are often milder. The differential diagnosis from urethral diverticulum may be possible only at endoscopy or at the time of surgery.

■ Anterior urethral valve
  • Fold in floor of urethra
  • At penoscrotal junction
  • No corpora deficiency

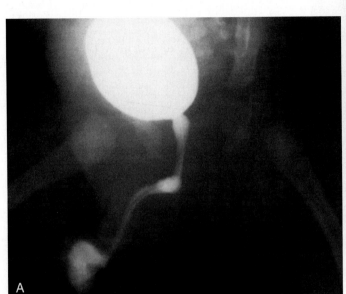

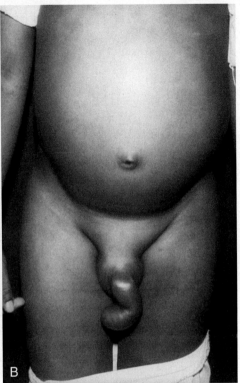

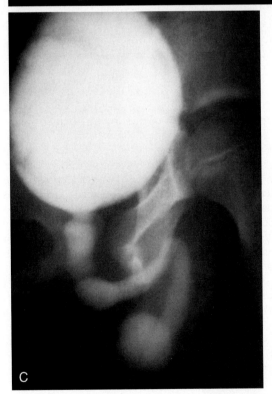

FIGURE 5. Megalourethra. **A,** In one patient, a voiding cystourethrogram shows dilatation of the anterior penile urethra. **B,** Postvoid photo of the same child. **C,** A second boy with dilatation of the anterior urethra resulting from partial absence of the corpora spongiosa.

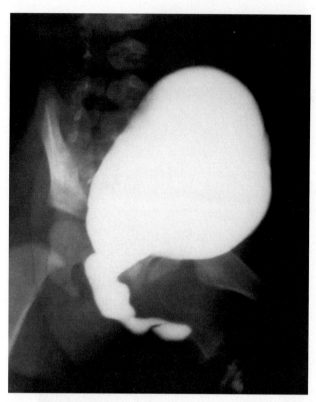

FIGURE 6. Anterior urethral valve. Both voiding cystourethrogram films show a filling defect emanating from the floor of the anterior urethra causing proximal obstruction.

URETHRAL DUPLICATIONS AND ACCESSORY URETHRAL CHANNELS

These developmental anomalies are characterized by the presence of an accessory urethra, complete or partial, occurring in the setting of a single bladder and a single penis (Figs. 8 and 9). According to the location of the accessory urethral opening on the dorsal or ventral aspect of the penis, urethral duplications are divided into epispadic (the most common type) and hypospadic types, respectively.

In the *epispadic type,* the accessory urethra originates from the bladder, bladder neck area, or proximal urethra, or rarely from a minute cavity (probably a rudimentary bladder) located behind the pubic symphysis and in front of the normal bladder. The accessory dorsal urethra courses through the dorsal aspect of the penis to end in an epispadic position anywhere between the glans and the root of the penis. Sometimes the epispadic, accessory urethra ends blindly proximally (incomplete urethral duplication). The normal urethra ends at the tip of the penis (in rare cases the normal urethra ends in a hypospadic location).

In the *hypospadic type,* the accessory ventral urethra often originates from the bladder and ends in a hypospadic position, while the normal urethra ends at the tip of the penis (in rare cases both urethras are in a hypospadic location). In other cases, the accessory urethra originates from the penile part of the normal urethra and ends in a hypospadic location, or there is a hypospadic accessory urethra ending blindly proximally (incomplete form). In a rare but important variant of urethral duplication of the hypospadic type, referred to as Y duplication, H-type (ano-) urethral fistula, urethroanal fistula, or urethroperineal fistula, a normally

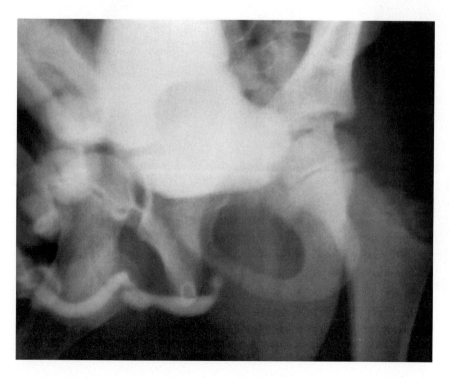

FIGURE 7. Another case of filling defect in the urethra representing an anterior urethral valve.

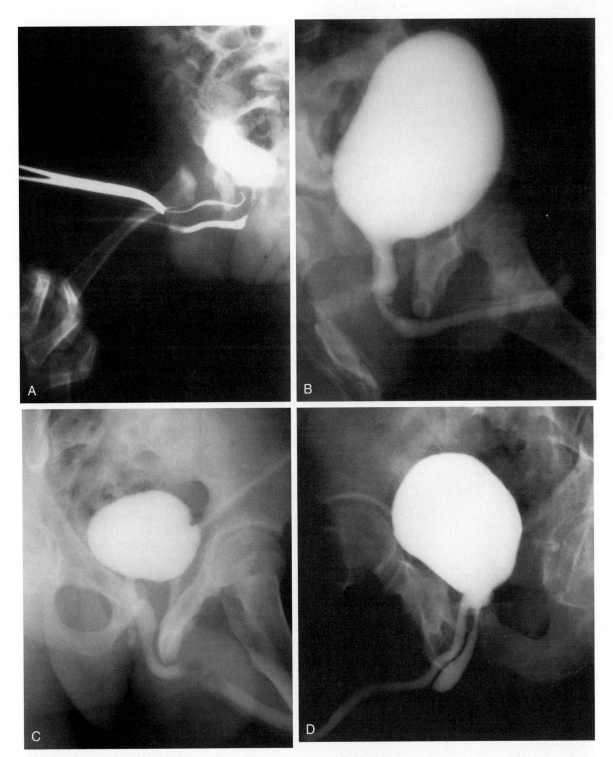

FIGURE 8. Double urethra. Two dorsal (**A** and **B**) and two ventral (**C** and **D**) accessory urethras are seen on these voiding cystourethrograms. None was completely patent from bladder to external penis.

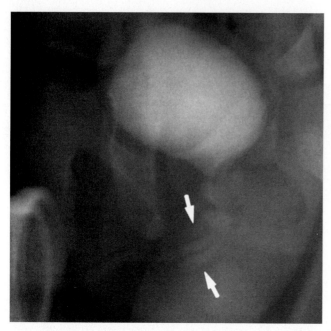

FIGURE 9. Three urethras are seen on this voiding film from a voiding cystourethrogram. There are dorsal and ventral accessory urethras *(arrows).*

placed but usually stenotic urethra (hypoplastic anterior urethra from the bulb to a point 1 to 2 cm from the external meatus) is associated with an accessory urethral channel that originates from the midprostatic urethra

and terminates in the anal canal or in the perineum near the anus (Fig. 10).

- ■ Urethral duplication
  - • May be complete or incomplete
  - • Occur in sagittal plane
  - • Epispadic (dorsal) type usually abortive
  - • Hypospadic (ventral) type is more functional
  - • Other types forked
  - • Perineal a rare variant

Accessory urethras may be asymptomatic or may cause double urinary stream, urinary incontinence, urinary tract infections, and urinary retention. The diagnosis is made by VCUG or catheterization and opacification of both urethras.

URETHRAL STRICTURES

Urethral strictures are almost entirely limited to males. They are relatively uncommon but constitute an important and often serious problem that may be difficult to treat. In most cases, the stricture is iatrogenic or is secondary to external trauma or infection (Fig. 11). Sometimes the cause of the stricture is unknown.

Iatrogenic strictures account for about two thirds of

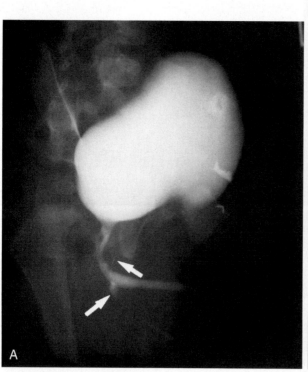
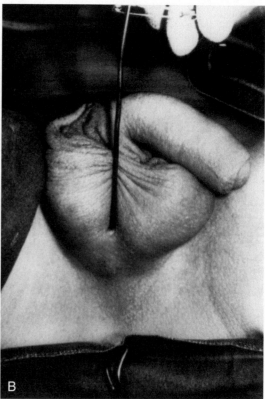

FIGURE 10. Perineal double urethra. **A,** Voiding film from a voiding cystourethrogram shows a normal urethra and an accessory urethra proceeding inferiorly to the perineum *(arrows).* **B,** A probe is seen in the perineal urethra.

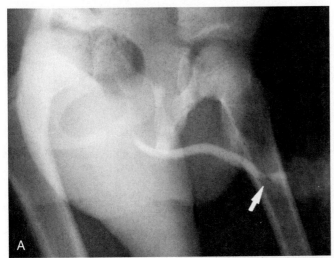

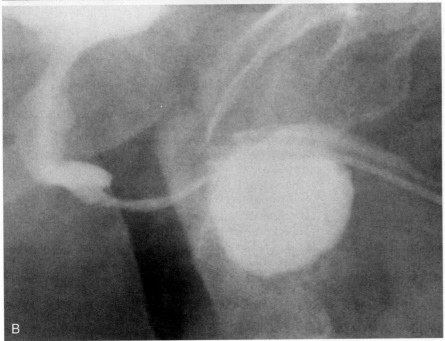

FIGURE 11. A, A stricture *(arrow)* is seen in the distal urethra in this 8-year-old boy whose father abused him by twisting his penis when he did not behave. **B,** A large urethral abscess cavity is seen filling with contrast on this voiding cystourethrogram. A hypospadius repair had become infected.

the cases. Urethral strictures following urethral instrumentation are located predominantly near the penoscrotal junction, an area that is particularly vulnerable to internal trauma. Pelvic fractures, penetrating injuries, direct blows to the perineum, and straddle injuries are the most common forms of external trauma. The membranous urethra is the area most often injured owing to its fixation by the urogenital diaphragm. Strictures from straddle injuries are usually located in the bulbar urethra. Urethral infections are uncommon causes of urethral strictures in children as opposed to young adults, in whom urethral strictures are often due to *Neisseria gonorrhoeae* infection. The strictures caused by *Neisseria* predominate in the bulbar urethra and are usually multiple. Urethral strictures of unknown cause in symptomatic boys are not rare. They are located most often in the bulbar urethra (Fig. 12) and are usually very short and diaphragm-like. They may be the result of unrecognized external trauma or urethritis, or may develop as a sequela of cowperian duct infection or rupture of one of the cowperian duct cysts mentioned above. The possibility of a congenital stricture is suggested in some cases, particularly when there is a family history of a similar lesion (Fig. 13).

■ Urethral strictures can be iatrogenic (two thirds), traumatic, or secondary to infection (gonococcal).

The clinical manifestations of urethral strictures include poor urinary stream, straining to void, urinary retention, painful urination, hematuria, urinary infections, and recurrent epididymitis. The diagnosis is readily established by VCUG when the bladder can be catheterized. Compression of the distal penis during

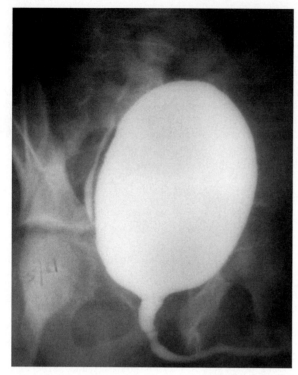

FIGURE 12. Urethral fold. Proximal to the urogenital diaphragm, a radiolucent line is seen in the posterior urethra on this voiding film of a voiding cystourethrogram.

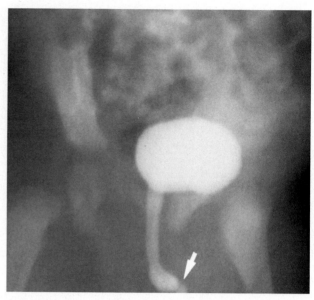

FIGURE 13. Congenital urethral membrane. A linear filling defect is seen in the distal urethra in this newborn *(arrow)*. The child presented with a poor urinary stream.

voiding (choke urethrogram), or a retrograde urethrogram, results in distention of the normal urethra and a better delineation of the true extent of the stricture. A voiding urethrogram using the contrast material accumulated in the bladder at the end of an excretory urogram may be the only radiographic procedure available to study the urethra when catheterization of the bladder or a retrograde urethrogram is not possible. The urethra proximal to the stricture may be dilated. Bladder trabeculation, vesicoureteral reflux, and upper tract dilatation may coexist. In the interpretation of the urethrogram, it is important to keep in mind that normal areas of narrowing at the level of the urogenital diaphragm, or narrowing caused by spasm of the bulbocavernosus or external sphincter muscles, may simulate a stricture.

MEATAL STENOSIS IN BOYS AND DISTAL URETHRAL STENOSIS IN GIRLS

Meatal stenosis in males is seen most frequently in patients with hypospadias and as an acquired process in circumcised boys. Except for severe cases, meatal steno-

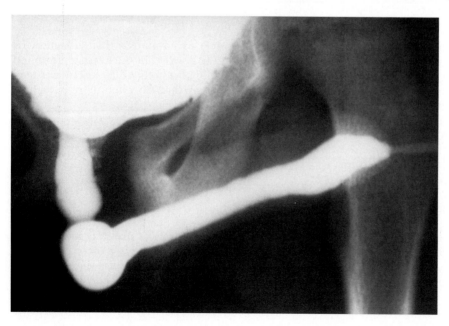

FIGURE 14. Meatal stenosis. Voiding film from a voiding cystourethrogram shows a dilated urethra to the meatus, where the stream suddenly becomes markedly attenuated.

sis is not believed to be as important as was once suggested. On the voiding cystogram, the urethra is generally dilated throughout, in contrast with the thin urinary stream outside the penis (Fig. 14). Narrowing of the distal female urethra as a result of spasm of the external sphincter with proximal urethral dilatation is common on routine VCUGs in young girls, and some consider it to be a normal variant, but it can also be observed in some girls with unstable bladders (bladder dysynergia) (see Section VII, Part V, Fig. 15, page 1876).

SUGGESTED READINGS

Appel RA, Kaplan GW, Brock WA, Streit D: Megalourethra. J Urol 1986;135:747

Baker AR, Neoptolemos JP, Wood KF: Congenital anterior urethral diverticulum: a rare cause of lower urinary tract obstruction in childhood. J Urol 1985;34:751

Beurton D, Magnier M, Cukier J: Bladder tumors in children. Prog Clin Biol Res 1984;162B:289

Brock WA, Kaplan GW: Lesions of Cowper's glands in children. J Urol 1979;122:121

Brown WC, Dillon PW, Hensle TW: Congenital urethral-perineal fistula: diagnosis and new surgical management. Urology 1990; 36:157

Bruce R, Alton D: Duplication of urethra with communication to the rectum. Pediatr Radiol 1986;16:79

Bueschen AJ, Royal SA: Urethral meatal stenosis in a girl causing severe hyponephrosis. J Urol 1986;136:1302

Caro P, Rosenberg H, Snyder HM: Congenital urethral polyp. AJR Am J Roentgenol 1986;147:1041

Colodny AH, Lebowitz RL: Lesions of the Cowper's ducts and glands in infants and children. Urology 1978;11:321

Currarino G: Large prostatic utricles and related structures, urogenital sinus and other forms of urethrovaginal confluence. J Urol 1986;136:1270

Currarino G, Fugua F: Cowper's glands in the urethrogram. Am J Roentgenol Radium Ther Nucl Med 1972;116:838

Currarino G, Stephens FD: An uncommon type of bulbar urethral stricture, sometimes familial, of unknown cause: congenital versus acquired. J Urol 1981;126:658

Devine CJ Jr, Gonzalez-Serva L, Strecker JF Jr, et al: Utricular configuration in hypospadias and intersex. J Urol 1980;123:407

Duckett JW: Hypospadias. In Gillenwater JY, Grayhack JT, Howard SS, et al (eds): Adult and Pediatric Urology. St. Louis, Mosby–Year Book, 1987;1880

Fernbach SK, Maizels M: Posterior urethral valves causing urinary retention in an infant with duplication of the urethra. J Urol 1984;132:353

Forster RS, Garrett RA: Congenital urethral polyps. J Urol 1986; 136:670

Glassberg KI: Current issues regarding posterior urethral valves. Urol Clin North Am 1985;12:175

Gordon I, Ransley PG, Hubbard CS: ^{99m}Tc DTPA scintigraphy compared with intravenous urography in followup of posterior urethral valves. Br J Urol 1987;60:447

Hernanz-Schulman M, Lebowitz RL: The elusiveness and importance of bladder diverticula in children. Pediatr Radiol 1985;15:399

Higashi TS, Takizawa K, Suzuki S, et al: Mullerian duct cyst: ultrasonographic and computed tomographic spectrum. Urol Radiol 1990; 12:39

Ikoma F, Shima H, Yabumoto H: Classification of enlarged prostatic utricle in patients with hypospadias. Br J Urol 1985;57:334

Karnak I, Senocak ME, Buyukpamukcu N, Hicsonmez A: Rare congenital anomalies of the anterior urethra. Pediatr Surg Int 1997;12:407

Khuri FJ, Hardy BE, Churchill BM: Urologic abnormalities associated with hypospadias. Urol Clin North Am 1981;8:565

Kolte SP, Joharapurkar SR: Anterior urthral valves, a rare cause of obstruction. Indian J Pediatr 2001;68:83

Levitt SB, Reda EF: Hypospadias. Pediatr Ann 1988;17:48

Lima SVC, Pereira CS: Giant diverticulum of the anterior urethra. Br J Urol 1984;56:335

Lindner A, Jonas P, Hertz M, Many M: Scaphoid megalourethra: a report of 2 cases. Br J Urol 1980;52:143

Linsenmeyer TA, Friedland GW: Duplicated urethra communicating with the seminal vesicle. Urol Radiol 1988;10:210

Maddeen NP, Turnock RR, Rickwood AMK: Congenital polyps of the posterior urethra in neonates. J Pediatr Surg 1986;21:193

Maizels M, Stephens FD, King LR, Firlit CF: Cowper's syringocele: a classification of dilatations of Cowper's gland duct based upon clinical characteristics of eight boys. J Urol 1983;129:111

Mortensen PHG, Johnson HW, Coleman GU: Megalourethra. J Urol 1985;134:358

Moskowitz PS, Newton NA, Lebowitz RL: Retention cysts of the Cowper's duct. Radiology 1976;120:377

Musselman P, Kay R: The spectrum of urinary tract fibroepithelial polyps in children. J Urol 1986;136:476

Netto NR, Lemos GC, Claro JF, Hering FL: Congenital diverticulum of male urethra. Urology 1984;24:239

Ortolano V, Nasrallah FP: Urethral duplication. J Urol 1986;136:909

Parkhouse HF, Barratt TM, Dillon MJ, et al: Long-term outcome of boys with posterior urethral valves. Br J Urol 1988;62:59

Podesta ML, Medel R, Castera R, Ruarte AC: Urethral duplication in children: surgical treatment and results. J Urol 1998;160:1830

Prasad N, Vivekandhan KG, Ilangovan G, Prabakaran S: Duplication of the urethra. Pediatr Surg Int 1999;15:419

Psihramis KE, Colodny AH, Lebowitz RL, et al: Complete patent duplication of the urethra. J Urol 1986;136:63

Rittenberg MH, Hulbert WC, Snyder HM 3rd, Duckett JW: Protective factors in posterior urethral valves. J Urol 1988;140:993

Salle JL, Sibai H, Rosenstein D, et al: Urethral duplication in the male: review of 16 cases. J Urol 2000;163:1936

Shrom SH, Cromie WJ, Duckett JW Jr: Megalourethra. Urology 1981;17:152

Tank ES: Anterior urethral valves resulting from congenital urethral diverticula. Urology 1987;30:467

Tejani A, Butt K, Glassberg K, et al: Predictors of eventual end stage renal disease in children with posterior urethral valves. J Urol 1986;136:857

Thurnher S, Hricak H, Tanagho EA: Mullerian duct cyst: diagnosis with MR images. Radiology 1988;168:25

PART VII

ADRENAL GLAND

ALAN DANEMAN

This chapter outlines the imaging and the pathology of the adrenals encountered in pediatrics. For a more specific discussion of neonatal adrenal conditions, the reader is referred to Section II, Part V, Chapter 10, page 239.

IMAGING

The adrenal glands can be visualized on antenatal sonography as early as the second trimester (Fig. 1A). During the neonatal period, the glands are relatively large because of the presence of the fetal cortex, and both adrenals can thus be very well visualized on sonography (Fig. 1B) (see also Section II, Part V, Chapter 10, Fig. 1, page 240). Once the fetal cortex has involuted, the glands are more difficult to visualize in detail on sonography; therefore, computed tomography (CT) and magnetic resonance imaging (MRI) play a more important role in imaging the adrenal glands in the older infant and child.

On both CT and MRI, both adrenal glands (Fig. 2) are usually easily visualized at all ages and are found anteromedial to the upper pole of the ipsilateral kidney. The left adrenal lies lateral to the left diaphragmatic crus and aorta, posterior to the stomach and tail of the pancreas, and medial to the spleen. The right adrenal lies lateral to the right diaphragmatic crus, medial to the right lobe of the liver, and posterior to the inferior vena cava. In the older infant and child, the adrenal glands are usually thinner than the adjacent diaphragmatic crura on axial CT and magnetic resonance (MR) images.

Plain abdominal radiographs, excretory urography, and angiography were used extensively in the past in patients with known or suspected adrenal disease. However, these modalities cannot show subtle changes in the adrenal gland or extent of disease as well as modern cross-sectional imaging modalities and are therefore seldom used today.

More recently, positron emission tomography (PET) scanning has been used for evaluation for recurrent or metastatic adrenal neoplasms, mainly neuroblastoma but also adrenocortical carcinoma. Initial reports have shown that this modality is sensitive in detecting disease, sometimes more accurately than CT or MRI. The radiation exposure from PET scanning is comparable to that from other radiologic techniques and nuclear medicine. Because of these initial promising results, this technique may become a standard approach to evaluation when the modality is more widely available. PET may localize disease, and CT or MRI depict the anatomy, better.

ADRENAL MASSES

Adrenal masses may be due to neoplasms, hemorrhage, abscess, and cysts. For special consideration of masses in the neonatal period, the reader is referred to Section II, Part V, Chapter 10, page 239.

NEOPLASMS

Neoplasms of the adrenal gland may arise from the medulla or the cortex. Those neoplasms from the medulla are of neural crest origin and may occur not only in the medulla but also in the sympathetic nerve chains. These neoplasms include neuroblastoma, ganglioneuroma, and pheochromocytoma. Those lesions arising from the cortex include adrenocortical carcinoma and adenoma. Rarely other neoplasms occur, including smooth muscle tumors in children with acquired immunodeficiency syndrome (AIDS).

Medullary Neoplasms

Neuroblastoma

Neuroblastoma is the most common extracranial solid neoplasm and accounts for almost 10% of all neoplasms seen in pediatrics (see also Section II, Part V, Chapter 10, page 239). These tumors may arise not only

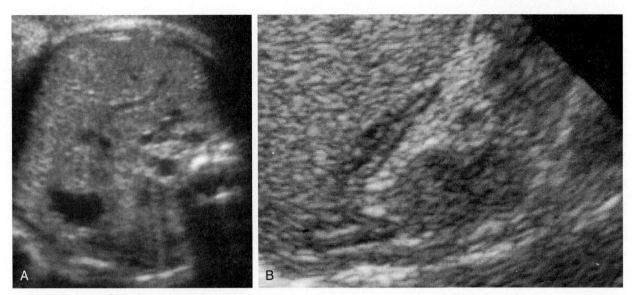

FIGURE 1. Antenatal and postnatal sonograms of normal right adrenal. **A,** On the antenatal sonogram, the right adrenal has a V shape in transverse view of the upper abdomen of the fetus. **B,** In the neonate, the longitudinal scan reveals the right adrenal has a reversed Z shape. (See also Section II, Part V, Chapter 10, Fig. 1, page 240.)

in the adrenal glands but also anywhere along the sympathetic nerve chains from the neck down into the pelvis. Neuroblastoma arises in the abdomen in three quarters of the children with this lesion, and, of these, one half to two thirds of lesions occur in the adrenal gland. The remainder occur elsewhere from sympathetic nerve tissue. Among abdominal neoplasms, neuroblastoma is the second most common after Wilms' tumor.

Neuroblastoma and ganglioneuroma belong to a group of related neoplasms arising from neural crest tissue that are distinguished by their degree of cell maturation and cellular differentiation. Neuroblastoma accounts for the vast majority of these lesions and has the most primitive and malignant cells. It is composed of small round cells that may be characteristically arranged in rosettes. Ganglioneuroma, on the other hand, represents the most differentiated end of the spectrum and is benign. Lesions with mixed histology are termed *ganglioneuroblastomas* and represent an intermediate mixed group.

Most children with neuroblastoma present between 1 and 5 years of age, with a median age of almost 2 years. However, the lesion may present in the neonatal period, and it has also been detected in the fetus by antenatal sonography. Less commonly, it may be present in older children and teenagers. Both sexes are affected equally.

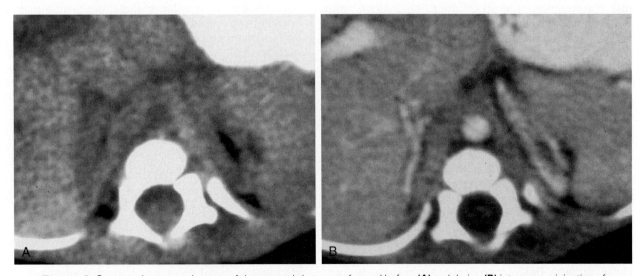

FIGURE 2. Computed tomography scan of the upper abdomen performed before **(A)** and during **(B)** intravenous injection of contrast in a full-term neonate with normal adrenal glands. The right adrenal can be seen lying behind the inferior vena cava, lateral to the right crus of the diaphragm and medial to the right lobe of the liver. The left adrenal lies behind the stomach, lateral to the left diaphragmatic crus and medial to the spleen. In the scan performed during intravenous injection of contrast, the adrenals enhance dramatically, probably as a result of the large sinusoids in the fetal cortex, which persists in the neonate.

Neuroblastoma has been found in association with neurofibromatosis type 1 and aganglionosis of the colon.

Most neuroblastomas present as a palpable mass. This may be an incidental finding in an otherwise apparently healthy child, or it may be brought to attention in children with otherwise relatively minor abdominal trauma. However, children may also present with symptoms and signs related to local tumor invasion, metastatic disease, or the effects of production of hormones such as catecholamines and vasoactive intestinal polypeptides (VIP). Local invasion may be into the kidneys, or there may be encasement and narrowing of the renal vessels (which may cause hypertension) and ureters (causing hydronephrosis). Invasion through the intervertebral foramina into the extradural intraspinal space, which occurs less commonly than with neuroblastomas in the chest, may cause cord and nerve compression that may lead to paraparesis and paraplegia or bladder and bowel dysfunction. Metastatic disease may be present in over 50% of patients at presentation. The most common sites include local and distant lymph nodes (e.g., cervical nodes), bone, bone marrow, liver, and skin. The pattern of metastatic disease is age related (see Section II, Part V, Chapter 10, page 239). Symptoms and signs therefore include skeletal pain, and metastatic lesions to the metaphyses of the long bones may give a clinical picture simulating an arthritis. Metastases to the orbits may cause proptosis and periorbital ecchymoses. The raised levels of catecholamines may lead to hypertension, and VIP may cause diarrhea. An interesting phenomenon is presentation with the signs of opsomyoclonus with nystagmus and ataxia, which occurs as a result of nonmetastatic distant effects on the cerebellum.

There have been several classification systems for staging neuroblastoma. The international neuroblastoma staging system is shown in Table 1. According to this classification, the distribution of patients with neuroblastoma at presentation is as follows: stage 1, 20%; stage 2, 10%; stage 3, 15%; stage 4, 50%; and stage 4S, 4%. The diagnosis of neuroblastoma can be made by tissue biopsy, but a combination of a positive bone marrow aspirate and an increase of urinary catecholamine metabolites (vanillylmandelic acid and homovanillic acid) is also sufficient evidence to confirm the diagnosis. The urinary level of catecholamine metabolites is increased in almost 90% of neuroblastoma.

The treatment of patients with neuroblastoma depends on several factors, including the stage of the disease at the time of presentation and the response to initial therapy. Surgery, chemotherapy, and radiation therapy all have a role to play. Primary surgical resection is the modality of choice for more localized tumors and chemotherapy for those that are unresectable. Radiation is used for localized disease that does not respond to chemotherapy. Delayed surgical resection may be performed for initially unresectable lesions once they have decreased sufficiently in size.

The prognosis of neuroblastoma depends on the age of the patient, the stage of disease at presentation, and the site of tumor. A favorable prognosis is seen mainly in

Table 1 ■ INTERNATIONAL NEUROBLASTOMA STAGING SYSTEM	
Stage 1	Localized tumor confined to the area of origin; complete gross excision, with or without microscopic residual
Stage 2A	Unilateral tumor with incomplete gross excision; ipsilateral and contralateral lymph nodes negative microscopically
Stage 2B	Unilateral tumor with complete or incomplete gross excision with positive ipsilateral regional lymph node identifiable contralateral lymph nodes negative microscopically
Stage 3	Tumor infiltrating across the midline with or without regional lymph node involvement; or unilateral tumor with contralateral regional lymph node involvement; or midline tumor with bilateral regional lymph node involvement
Stage 4	Dissemination of tumor to distant lymph nodes, bone marrow, liver, and/or other organs (except as defined in stage 4S)
Stage 4S	Localized primary tumor as defined for stage 1 or 2 with dissemination limited to liver, skin, and/or bone.

those patients presenting under 1 year of age, in those with lower stages of disease, and with lesions that arise in extra-abdominal sites. Those patients with localized disease may have an 80% 2-year survival, compared to 5% for those with bone metastases. There are several biologic markers that may also affect prognosis. A poor prognosis is seen particularly with N-*myc* oncogene amplification (more than 10 copies) but is also seen with allelic loss of chromosome 1p and with diploid (decreased DNA) karyotype. In contrast, a favorable prognosis is seen with an unamplified N-*myc* oncogene, a well-differentiated stroma, absence of abnormalities of chromosome 1, and triploid karyotypes.

Adrenal neuroblastomas and those arising from the adjacent retroperitoneal area are usually easily identified with sonography, CT, or MRI because the size of the mass is usually considerable at the time of presentation (Figs. 3 through 5). Very small masses are uncommon, and in these cases CT and MRI may play a more important role than sonography (Fig. 6). These cross-sectional imaging modalities have obviated the necessity for plain radiographs and urography in these children. On sonography, the masses usually have a variety of echogenic appearances. Areas of hyperechogenicity may represent calcification, and these areas do not always have acoustic shadowing (Fig. 3). Anechoic areas resulting from cystic, hemorrhagic, or necrotic changes may be present but are seen less commonly than in Wilms' tumors. Mainly cystic lesions may be present, particularly in neonates (see Section II, Part V, Chapter 10, Fig. 13, page 249). On CT, the lesions have an attenuation equal to or less than that of muscle, and calcification may be present in 85% of cases. The calcification may be coarse, globular, finely stippled, or curvilinear (see Figs. 4, 7, and 15). After intravenous contrast injection, the lesions enhance very heterogeneously, reflecting areas of vascularity more clearly in

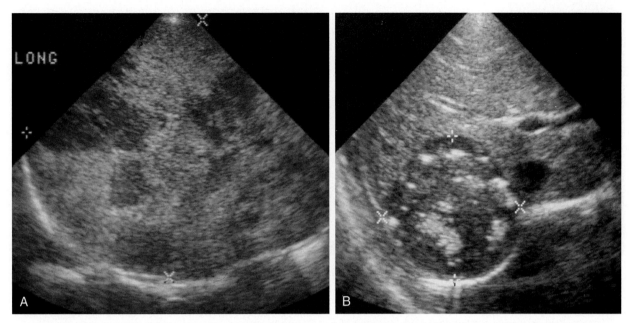

FIGURE 3. Longitudinal **(A)** and transverse **(B)** sonograms of the right upper quadrant in two children with adrenal neuroblastoma. **A,** The neuroblastoma has a heterogeneous echogenicity with hyperechoic and hypoechoic areas. **B,** Very small globular hyperechoic areas represent calcification without acoustic shadowing.

contrast to areas of necrosis, hemorrhage, and cystic change. On MRI, the lesions have a low signal on T_1- and high signal on T_2-weighted images.

With all modalities, it is essential to assess extent of tumor within the abdomen as clearly as possible. In this regard, sonography tends to underestimate the full extent, and for this reason CT and MRI are required for evaluation after initial sonography. Local spread may be to lymph nodes (Fig. 7) and direct invasion into the kidneys or liver (Fig. 8). The ureters may be obstructed. There may be direct or lymph node spread behind the crura into the thorax. The transverse scans of CT may overestimate invasion into adjacent solid viscera such as

the kidney and liver, and the longitudinal sagittal and coronal scans of sonography or MRI are more helpful in this regard. Sagittal and coronal reconstruction of axial CT images with the newer generation of CT scanners should be used if renal or hepatic invasion is in question.

Independent of which modality is used, the full extent of spread in the abdomen is best assessed when one defines the anatomy of the major vessels of the abdomen clearly (Figs. 7 through 9). Whatever cross-sectional technique is used, the technique should be optimized to define the vessels to best advantage: use of color or power Doppler sonography, use of a power injector for intravenous contrast administration for CT, or use of

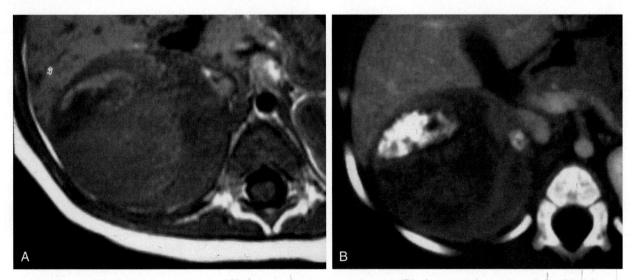

FIGURE 4. Magnetic resonance image **(A)** and computed tomography scan **(B)** of upper abdomen in patient with right adrenal neuroblastoma. The mass is well defined, with a large area of calcification anterolaterally. The mass displaces the inferior vena cava slightly forward. The spinal canal is uninvolved.

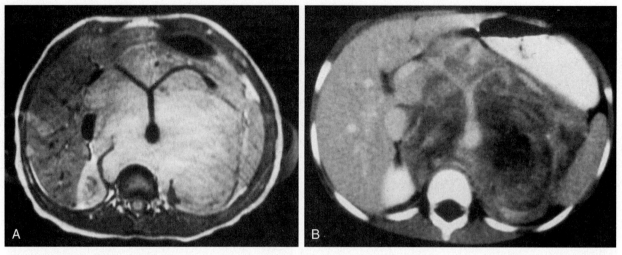

FIGURE 5. T$_1$-weighted magnetic resonance image **(A)** and computed tomography scan **(B)** of the upper abdomen in patient with upper abdominal retroperitoneal neuroblastoma. In both scans, the large mass is noted crossing the midline and there is displacement of the aorta forward, with encasement of the aorta, celiac axis, and proximal portions of the splenic and hepatic arteries. The inferior vena cava is displaced anteriorly and to the right. Display of the vasculature in this manner, independent of whichever modality is used, is essential for accurate evaluation of extent of disease preoperatively and during follow-up.

MR arteriography and MR venography together with gadolinium if necessary. Neuroblastomas may push major vessels aside but even more characteristically encase the vessels (Figs. 5 and 8). Defining the position of the vessels well and determining the relationship of the tumor tissue to the vessels enables one to define extent of tumor accurately and determine operability. Furthermore, compression or encasement of the renal vessels may lead to renal atrophy as a result of ischemia or infarction. Neuroblastoma rarely invades into major veins, which occurs more frequently with Wilms' tumor. However, rarely neuroblastoma may even extend up the inferior vena cava into the heart (Fig. 10).

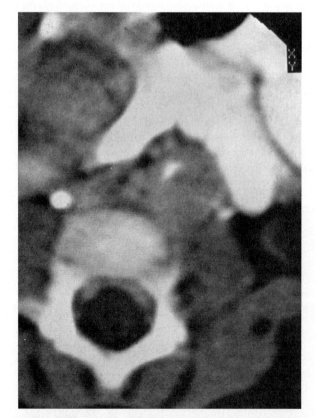

FIGURE 6. Computed tomography scan of abdomen in patient with retroperitoneal neuroblastoma who had presented with opsomyoclonus. There is a small retroperitoneal mass that is well defined and has a small area of calcification anteromedially. The left ureter is displaced laterally, and the contrast-filled bowel loops are displaced forward. Neuroblastoma masses of this size are less common than the larger lesions.

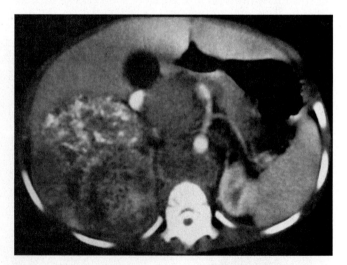

FIGURE 7. Computed tomography scan of upper abdomen during intravenous contrast injection shows a large right adrenal mass with punctate and globular calcification, mainly anteriorly. Lobular masses in the retroperitoneum extending anteriorly represent lymph node metastases. The inferior vena cava and aorta are displaced anteriorly and the celiac axis is displaced toward the left.

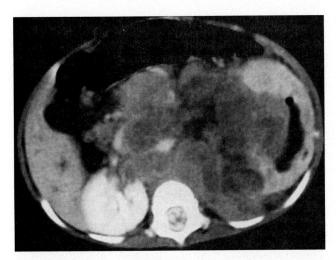

FIGURE 8. Computed tomography scan of upper abdomen shows large retroperitoneal neuroblastoma with a very irregular lobulated border that has invaded and displaced the left kidney inferolaterally, causing hydronephrosis. There is encasement and displacement of the aorta, right renal artery, and inferior vena cava.

Intraspinal extension occurs less commonly with abdominal neuroblastomas than with those arising in the chest, and even less commonly with those arising in the adrenal gland than those from the retroperitoneum. However, significant intraspinal extension may be present without the presence of overt clinical symptoms or signs. Therefore, it is essential to evaluate the intraspinal contents in all children with neuroblastoma in order to determine the presence or absence of extradural spread because this may affect therapy. MRI defines intraspinal spread exceptionally well without the need for intrathecal contrast (Fig. 11). The tumor is easily seen if it involves the intervertebral foramina or extra-

dural space. Intraspinal involvement may be limited to one vertebral level, or the tumor may grow as a sheet of tissue or in a more nodular or mass-like manner more extensively along several levels. Furthermore, involvement may include sites at a distance from the primary intra-abdominal lesion (Fig. 12).

In the past CT was used after intrathecal injection of contrast (e.g., metrizamide) to evaluate the intraspinal contents in these children (Figs. 12 and 13). However, the newer generation CT scanners can depict the detail of the spinal canal very well without the need for intrathecal contrast injection (Figs. 14 and 15). In scans done after intravenous contrast injection, the spinal cord, surrounding thecal sac, and adjacent soft tissue structures are easily identified, making visualization of any intraspinal tumor simple. In infants, sonography may also be able to detect intraspinal extension before there is complete ossification of the posterior elements of the vertebrae.

Other features that may be present in the abdomen in patients with neuroblastoma include metastases to the liver. This may be in the form of single or multiple nodules or masses, or it may be infiltrative, particularly in neonates. Rarely, peritoneal seeding with nodules and ascites may be present. Metastases to bone are best identified with radionuclide bone scans or ^{131}I-metaiodobenzylguanidine (MIBG) scans. MRI has the advantage over other cross-sectional imaging because it can also be used to assess the bone marrow when evaluating patients with neuroblastoma of the abdomen or other sites.

Imaging plays an important role in patient evaluation after surgery or chemotherapy. Regular follow-up is required after surgery to assess the tumor bed for local recurrence, and this is best achieved with CT. Similarly, follow-up is essential in nonoperable tumors to assess

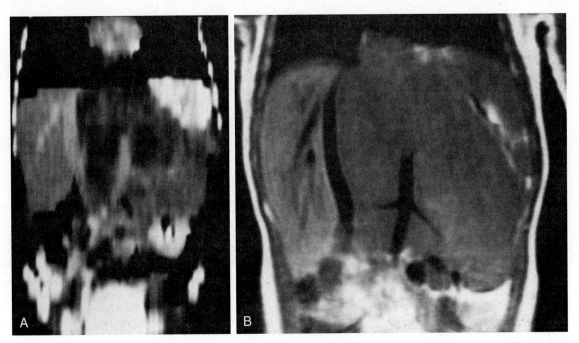

FIGURE 9. Coronal reconstruction of computed tomography scan **(A)** and coronal magnetic resonance image **(B)** show large retroperitoneal neuroblastoma encasing the aorta and the renal arteries and displacing the inferior vena cava to right.

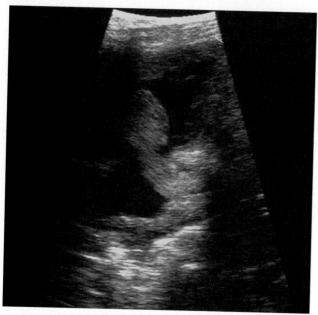

FIGURE 10. Longitudinal sonogram of lower thorax reveals an echogenic tumor thrombus of abdominal neuroblastoma that has extended up the inferior vena cava into the right atrium and forward into the right ventricle. (Courtesy of Dr. Michel Panuel, Marseilles, France.)

response to chemotherapy and to determine the most appropriate time for delayed surgery. If the lesion responds to chemotherapy, there is usually a regression in size of the mass, which shrinks to a very small amount of soft tissue that often becomes more calcified (Fig. 16).

However, biopsy is sometimes necessary to determine whether residual tissue is fibrosis or viable tumor. Renal atrophy may also occur following treatment and may be the result of surgical trauma, chemotherapy, or radiation.

Ganglioneuroma

Ganglioneuromas represent the mature form of neural crest neoplasms and are benign, in contrast to their more malignant relative, the neuroblastoma. They are composed of mature ganglion cells and nerve fibers and are usually well encapsulated. This type of neural crest tumor is far less frequent than neuroblastoma, and may be seen to develop from maturation of a previous known malignant neuroblastoma or may be found de novo.

Most ganglioneuromas occur in the posterior mediastinum. Only one third occur in the abdomen, and most are paravertebral and are seldom in the adrenal gland. They have been documented in association with neurofibromatosis. These tumors usually occur in older children, who are often asymptomatic. They may therefore be found incidentally on abdominal sonography or chest radiographs performed for some other reason. Occasionally they may cause symptoms resulting from growth into the intervertebral foramina causing cord compression. Rarely do they present with myoclonic encephalopathy, diarrhea, or hypertension. Urinary catecholamine levels are usually normal.

The imaging appearances of ganglioneuromas are similar to those of neuroblastoma, and the abdominal

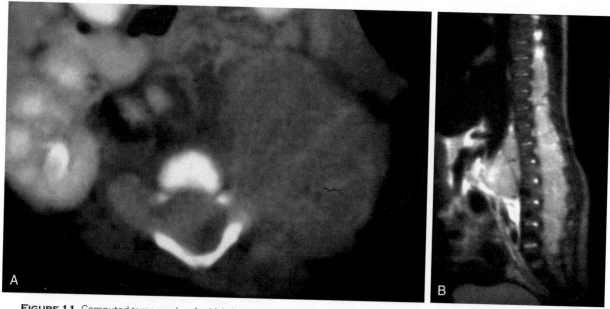

FIGURE 11. Computed tomography of midabdomen **(A)** and sagittal magnetic resonance imaging of spine **(B)** in patient with retroperitoneal neuroblastoma that has invaded the spinal canal, causing expansion of the canal. **A,** The large left retroperitoneal mass is easily seen and is noted filling the spinal canal, which is enlarged. The mass extends through a right intervertebral foramen into the region of the right psoas muscle. **B,** The retroperitoneal tumor can be seen in front of the vertebral bodies, and there is a marked amount of tumor involving several levels of the thoracolumbar spine, causing expansion of the spine particularly in the lumbar region.

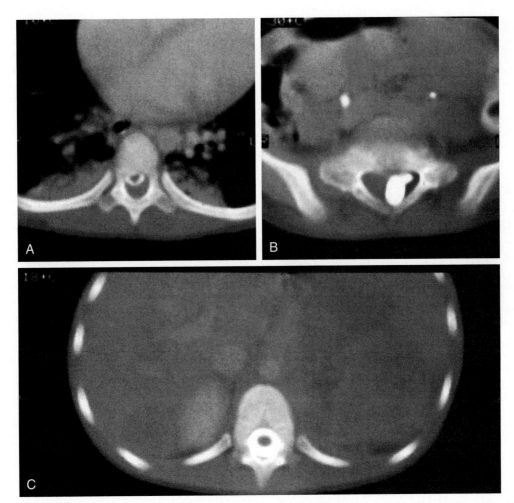

FIGURE 12. Computed tomography scans through chest **(A)**, upper pelvis **(B)**, and upper abdomen **(C)** in patient with large left adrenal neuroblastoma. This study has been performed after injection of intrathecal metrizamide to outline the thecal sac. The large tumor mass is noted in the left adrenal in the upper abdomen. Displacement of the thecal sac is noted in the lower chest and in the pelvis due to spinal canal involvement. This involvement is at sites which are distant from the primary.

lesions may even encase the aorta and inferior vena cava and their branches. The definitive diagnosis therefore depends on histologic examination of tumor tissue. In some of the patients with abdominal ganglioneuromas, surgical removal may be difficult, particularly if the mass is large, adjacent to vital structures, encasing vessels, or extending into the intervertebral foramina. Clinicians may prefer to manage these patients non-operatively, particularly if they are asymptomatic. In such cases, regular clinical and imaging follow-up is mandatory. There are 10 patients documented in the literature with abdominal ganglioneuromas that developed malignant peripheral nerve sheath tumors in the mass many years later. Seven of these had had previous abdominal radiation as part of the therapy for a neuroblastoma that then matured into a benign gan-glioneuroma, but three did not. CT or MRI is essential as part of the follow-up protocol. Changes in the appear-ance of the mass or an increase in size should alert one to the possibility of malignant degeneration and should be followed by biopsy. Follow-up of ganglioneuromas

managed nonoperatively should probably be for the rest of the patient's life, but it is uncertain how often imaging should be done.

Pheochromocytoma

Pheochromocytoma is an uncommon neoplasm in children. Five percent of all pheochromocytomas occur in children, accounting for well under 1% of all neoplasms seen in large pediatric centers. It is a potentially curable secretory tumor arising from chro-maffin cells in the adrenal gland or in extra-adrenal sites. In children, 70% of pheochromocytomas occur in the adrenal gland and 24% have bilateral adrenal involvement. Thirty percent of patients have extra-adrenal lesions, and most of these occur in the upper abdomen. Other less common extra-adrenal sites in-clude the sympathetic chain anywhere from the base of the skull down into the pelvis; more rarely, they may occur in the urinary bladder, spermatic cord, and vagina. Multiple lesions are present in 30% to 70% of

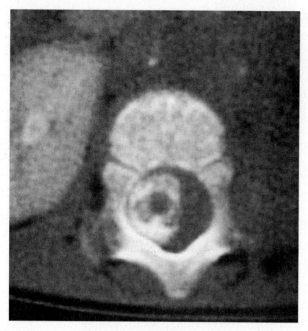

FIGURE 13. Computed tomography scan showing spine after intrathecal injection of metrizamide. The thecal sac is compressed on the left due to extradural intraspinal extension from the left-sided neuroblastoma, which has caused some erosion of the vertebral body and pedicle.

children, and this is seen mainly in those with a family history of pheochromocytoma. Malignancy is present in 10% of lesions in adults but is much less frequent in children. The diagnosis of malignancy is often made on the basis of metastases rather than histology.

Pheochromocytoma usually presents in older children but has been reported in infants. It is frequently familial and is inherited as an autosomal dominant trait. Familial pheochromocytoma has been described in the multiple endocrine neoplasia syndrome type II in association with medullary thyroid carcinoma and parathyroid hyperplasia. Pheochromocytoma may also be seen in association with neurofibromatosis, other neurocutaneous syndromes, and hemihypertrophy.

Clinical presentation is usually related to the secretion of catecholamines, predominantly epinephrine and norepinephrine. Patients may present with hypertension, sweating, headaches, visual blurring, papilledema, flushing, tachycardia, diarrhea, hypertensive encephalopathy, and weight loss. Chronic diarrhea may be due to production of VIP. Rarely, the patient may present with symptoms resulting from metastatic spread or from the local effects of the tumor. Although tumors may range in size from 1 to 10 cm in diameter at presentation, they are usually between 2 and 5 cm. They are well encapsulated and highly vascular and may contain some necrosis and hemorrhage.

Accurate and noninvasive localization of these tumors, which may be multiple, is an important prerequisite for successful surgical management. Furthermore, preoperative delineation of any local invasion or metastatic disease is important because the malignant potential of these lesions is difficult to assess on histologic grounds. Evaluation of a child suspected of having a pheochromocytoma requires careful imaging not only of the adrenal area but also of other possible extraadrenal sites because these lesions are often multiple. Although sonography may easily depict lesions in and adjacent to the adrenal glands, it is less sensitive than CT and MRI for lesions in the mid- and lower abdomen, particularly in older children.

On sonography, the lesions may be homogeneously

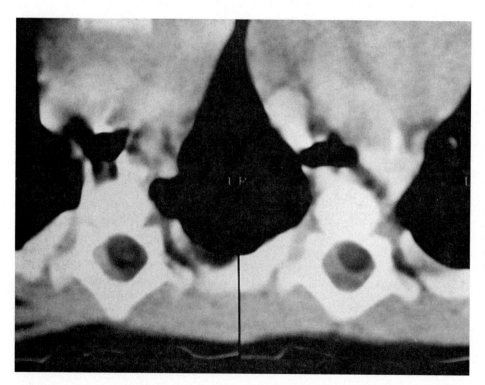

FIGURE 14. Computed tomography scan sections of the chest in patient with upper abdominal neuroblastoma shows extension of tumor sheet into the spinal canal posteriorly and on the right, displacing the thecal sac anteriorly and to the left. This tumor sheet can be seen after intravenous injection of contrast and does not necessarily require intrathecal injection of contrast.

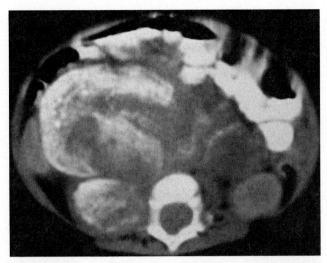

FIGURE 15. Computed tomography scan of full-term neonate with huge retroperitoneal right-sided neuroblastoma that is seen crossing the midline and is a lobulated mass that shows heavy calcification. The bowel filled with contrast is displaced anteriorly and toward the left. Note that the spinal canal is enlarged and deformed as a result of a large amount of tumor mass filling the spinal canal.

echoic but may also be heterogeneous, with areas of decreased echogenicity caused by hemorrhage and necrosis and areas of increased echogenicity that may represent hemorrhage and, less commonly, calcification (Fig. 17). On CT, the lesions have a soft tissue attenuation, and enhancement may be diffuse, mottled, or rim-like. Hypertensive crises can be provoked by contrast material, which elevate the plasma catecholamines. They are more often caused by angiography than intravenous injection for CT. Angiography is seldom required today for localization of these lesions and has been replaced by CT, MRI and ^{131}I-MIBG scans. On MRI, pheochromocytomas have a low signal on T_1- and high signal on T_2-weighted images, with a pattern of intense enhancement and slow washout after administration of gadolinium diethylenetriaminepentaacetic acid. The radionuclide ^{131}I-MIBG is also accurate in localizing these lesions but does not show the anatomy as well as CT or MRI. Evaluation of the chest is also important, even though pheochromocytomas less commonly occur in this region. Chest CT is particularly important in those patients suspected of having malignant lesions.

Surgical removal of all known lesions is usually curative. However, clinical follow-up is essential, together with urinary catecholamine determinations to detect possible recurrence or development of other new lesions.

CORTICAL NEOPLASMS

Adrenocortical neoplasms are uncommon in children. Most occur in children over the age of 3, but they can occur rarely in neonates. Girls are three times more commonly affected than boys. Carcinomas are three times more common than adenomas. The vast majority

are functioning, and the most common endocrine abnormality is overproduction of androgens. Girls present with virilization and boys with pseudoprecocious puberty. Often there is a mixed endocrine dysfunction with the effects of overproduction of glucocorticoids and mineralocorticoids also present. This is in contrast to adrenal hyperplasia, where there are usually only the effects of overproduction of single hormone types. Less commonly, patients with adrenocortical neoplasms may present with only Cushing's syndrome, feminization, or hyperaldosteronism. It is uncommon for these lesions to be nonfunctioning in children; when this occurs, the masses may be found incidentally. It is impossible from the endocrine status of the child to predict whether the lesions are carcinomas or adenomas. Only a small number of these lesions present with a palpable mass, and these are usually carcinomas. Presentation with metastatic disease is rare.

At presentation, the masses are usually small but are usually over 1.5 cm, and it is extremely rare in children to see adrenocortical neoplasms present as smaller adrenal nodules. However, on occasion the masses may be huge, and, although these are usually carcinomas, they may still represent adenomas. Even the smaller lesions are easily documented with sonography, CT, or MRI (Fig. 18). Sonography is usually the initial modality used to evaluate the adrenals, but CT and MRI are particularly important to evaluate the very large lesions and local invasion and spread.

On all three modalities, the smaller lesions tend to have a fairly homogeneous appearance, and areas of hemorrhage, necrosis, and calcification are usually seen more commonly in the larger lesions, which are usually carcinomas (Figs. 19 through 21). In these larger lesions, there is often a central scar evident with radiating linear bands that represent areas of necrosis

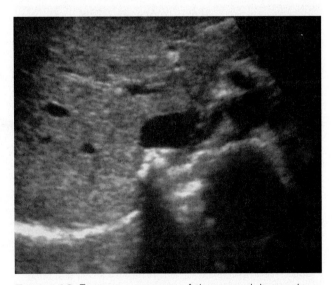

FIGURE 16. Transverse sonogram of the upper abdomen shows hyperechoic foci caused by globules of calcification with posterior acoustic shadowing lying behind the inferior vena cava. This scan was done following chemotherapy in a patient with right adrenal neuroblastoma and shows the residual calcification after reduction in size of the mass.

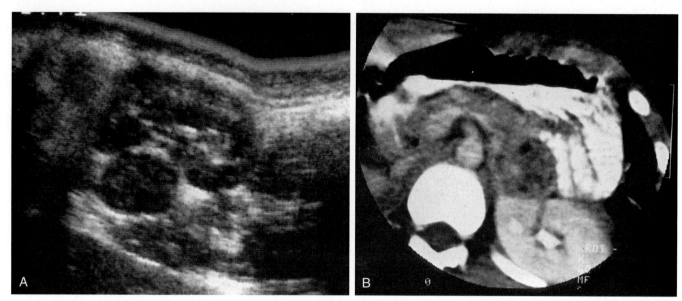

FIGURE 17. A, Longitudinal prone sonogram in an 8-year-old girl shows left adrenal pheochromocytoma anterior to the left kidney. The mass is well defined and slightly heterogeneous in echogenicity, with no calcification. **B,** Computed tomography scan of a 17-year-old girl with left adrenal neuroblastoma anterior to the left kidney. The mass is well defined and heterogeneous in attenuation. At age 11, a right adrenal pheochromocytoma had been removed.

and calcification (Fig. 21). This is a characteristic appearance seen in some of the larger lesions and may help to differentiate these neoplasms from other masses in the suprarenal area. It is not always possible to predict accurately which masses are malignant unless there is local spread and invasion or metastatic disease (Fig. 20). Initially, the lesions displace surrounding viscera, but large carcinomas may invade the kidney or grow into the inferior vena cava.

Metastatic disease from these lesions most commonly occurs to the lungs, liver, and bone, but other unusual sites have been reported. Complete resection of the primary tumor is essential for survival. Chemotherapy has had a major effect on improved outcome in recent years. Larger and infiltrating tumors and those with metastatic disease do more poorly. Adenomas clearly have a good prognosis if they are removed completely, but clinical and imaging follow-up are essential because

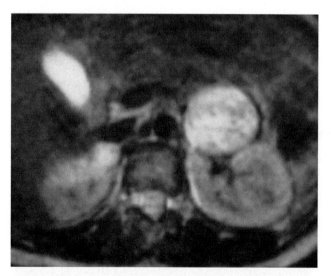

FIGURE 18. T$_2$-weighted magnetic resonance image of the upper abdomen in a 12-year-old boy with bilateral adrenal neuroblastoma. The lesions have high signal intensity on T$_2$ weighting. The right adrenal lesion lies between the upper pole of the right kidney and the inferior vena cava and the large left adrenal lesion lies in front of the kidney and to the left of the aorta. Both lesions are well defined.

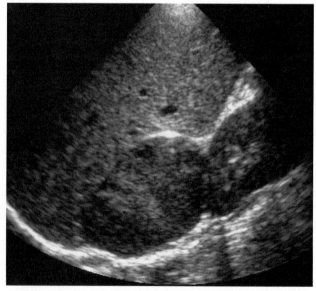

FIGURE 19. Longitudinal sonogram in a 14-year-old girl shows an incidental finding of a right adrenal adenoma that was nonfunctioning. The adenoma is well defined between the liver and the right kidney. It has a slightly heterogeneous echogenicity.

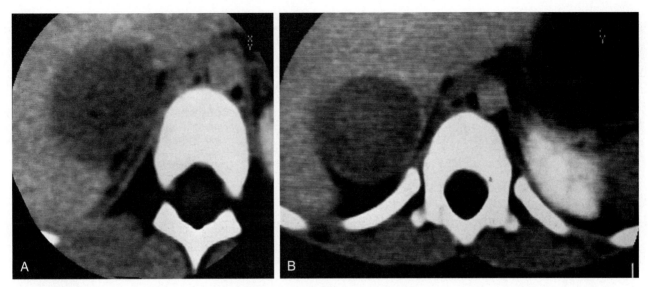

FIGURE 20. Computed tomography scans of the upper abdomen in a 3-year-old girl with right adrenocortical adenoma **(A)** and a 5-year-old girl with right adrenocortical carcinoma **(B).** Both lesions have low attenuation with no calcification. They are well defined, and, in the adenoma, a part of the normal adrenal is noted posterior to the mass. With small adrenocortical lesions, it is difficult to differentiate adenoma from carcinoma, as in these two cases.

the histologic differences between adenoma and carcinoma are not clear in all cases.

Other Adrenal Neoplasms

Smooth muscle tumors have been described recently in the adrenal glands of children with AIDS. These tumors have been more frequently described in the small and large bowel in children with AIDS but have also occasionally been reported at other sites. These lesions are leiomyomas and may arise in the walls of adrenal vascular structures. They are usually unilateral but may be bilateral. Their presence appears to be linked to the Epstein-Barr virus.

OTHER MASSES

Other adrenal mass lesions are uncommon in children beyond the neonatal period. These include hemorrhage, cysts and infection.

Adrenal hemorrhage occurs most commonly in the neonatal period. However, it may occur in older children following blunt abdominal trauma, and usually

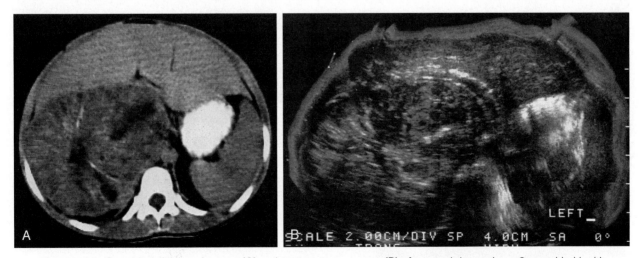

FIGURE 21. Computed tomography scan **(A)** and transverse sonogram **(B)** of upper abdomen in an 8-year-old girl with precocious puberty. The scans show a large right adrenal mass with very heterogeneous echogenicity and attenuation. There is a radial pattern of calcification noted in the mass, together with adjacent areas of decreased attenuation caused by some necrosis, which is more characteristic of adrenocortical carcinomas. The mass is relatively well defined.

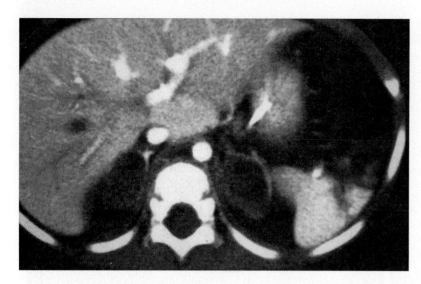

FIGURE 22. Computed tomography scan of upper abdomen in a patient with blunt abdominal trauma shows laceration to the anterior aspect of the spleen and bilateral adrenal hemorrhages resulting from the trauma.

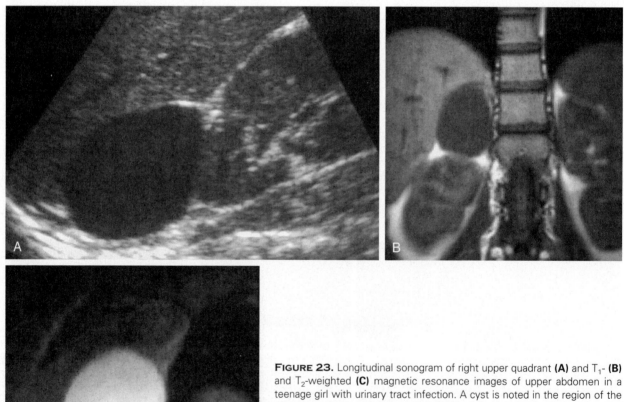

FIGURE 23. Longitudinal sonogram of right upper quadrant **(A)** and T_1- **(B)** and T_2-weighted **(C)** magnetic resonance images of upper abdomen in a teenage girl with urinary tract infection. A cyst is noted in the region of the right adrenal. The cyst is well defined with a smooth wall and no solid components on either ultrasound or magnetic resonance imaging.

traumatic lesions are also present in other viscera as well (Fig. 22). Even if both adrenal glands are involved, there are no signs of adrenal insufficiency. Adrenal hemorrhage may also occur in bleeding diatheses, with vasculitis, or as a complication of meningococcemia or adrenal angiography.

Large *adrenal cysts* may be found in older children. These are usually endothelial lined and may be found incidentally (Fig. 23). If cross-sectional imaging reveals that they have a thin, smooth wall without any evidence of solid components, and there is no evidence of endocrine dysfunction, hypertension, infection, or metastatic disease, they can be managed conservatively because adrenal neoplasms seldom have large cystic components and never present as thin, smooth-walled cystic structures without solid components in these older children.

ADRENAL HYPERPLASIA

Adrenal hyperplasia usually presents in the neonatal period (see Section II, Part V, Chapter 10, page 239). However, adrenocortical hyperplasia may also be seen in older children, in which case it can be primary or secondary. Primary hyperplasia usually results in Cushing's syndrome and much less commonly in primary aldosteronism. Secondary hyperplasia may be present in patients who produce excessive endogenous adrenocorticotropic hormone (ACTH), such as those with Cushing's disease or ectopic ACTH production, or in patients receiving ACTH administration, such as in infantile spasms.

In older children, the adrenal glands are not easily visible on sonography. If the glands are easily visible on

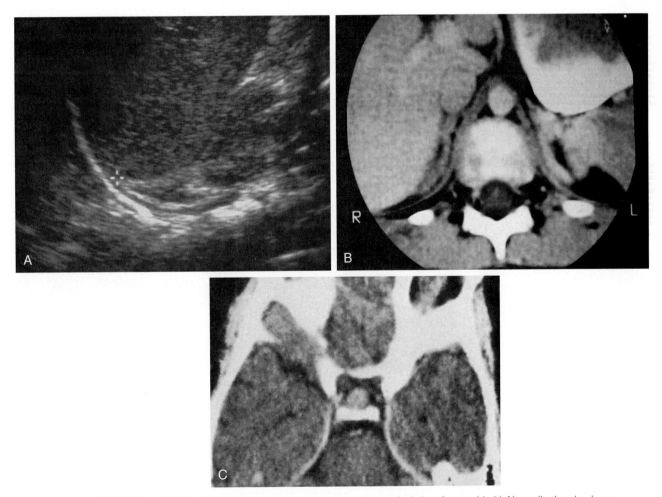

FIGURE 24. A, Enlarged right adrenal gland resulting from adrenal hyperplasia in a 3-year-old girl. Normally the glands are not as easily seen on sonography at this age. **B** and **C,** Computed tomography (CT) scan sections of a 12-year-old girl with Cushing's syndrome. **B,** CT section of upper abdomen reveals markedly enlarged, thickened adrenal glands. The glands are symmetrically involved with no evidence of small nodules. **C,** In the CT section of the head, a pituitary adenoma is noted, which is the cause of the adrenal hyperplasia in this teenager.

sonography, one should consider the diagnosis of adrenal hyperplasia (Fig. 24A). CT and MRI play a more important role in imaging the adrenals in this age group of children suspected of having adrenal hyperfunction. The adrenal glands may appear bilaterally, symmetrically, and evenly enlarged (Fig. 24B). If the adrenal limbs are thicker than the adjacent crura, adrenal hyperplasia should be considered. Enhancement of the glands on CT may be increased relative to that seen in normal glands. Occasionally the adrenal enlargement may not be even, and one may see one or more smaller nodular areas in one or both adrenal glands. However, it is important to note that finding normal-sized glands does not rule out adrenal hyperplasia. Those children with adrenal hyperplasia and without a known source of ACTH should have MRI of the brain and pituitary to exclude pathology in this region as a source of adrenal stimulation (Fig. 24C).

SUGGESTED READINGS

Krebs TL, Wagner BJ: MR imaging of the adrenal gland. Radiographics 1998;18:1425–1440

Paterson A: Adrenal pathology in childhood, a spectrum of disease. Eur Radiol 2002;12:2491–2508

Shady KL, Brown JJ: MR imaging of the adrenal glands. Magn Reson Imaging Clin N Am 1995;3:73–85

PART VIII

RETROPERITONEAL MASSES

JACK O. HALLER

The retroperitoneum is a potential space that extends along the posteriormost aspect of the abdominal cavity from the level of the diaphragms to the pelvic brim. It meets the abdominal parietal peritoneum anteriorly (see Section VII, Part II, Fig. 11, page 1745). The anterior and posterior renal fasciae fuse laterally to form the lateroconal fascia. Masses located within the retroperitoneal space or pelvis often involve structures of the urogenital tract. These masses originate from the urogenital tract itself or in proximity to it. Masses that originate within the urogenital tract are discussed in Section II, Part V, Chapter 5, page 223; Section VII, Part II, page 1739 and Part III, Chapter 2, page 1787; and Section VIII, Parts I, page 1917 and II, page 1939. Those located outside the urinary tract arise from structures normally present within this space, including the adrenal glands, kidneys, lymph nodes, lymphatic channels, sympathetic ganglia or other neural tissue, and iliopsoas muscle.

PERIRENAL FLUID COLLECTIONS

Subcapsular fluid collections around the kidney are due to renal lacerations with consequent perirenal hematoma, perirenal abscess, or urinoma from an obstructed draining system. A *subcapsular hematoma* is a collection of blood beneath the renal capsule, which remained intact following renal laceration from abdominal trauma. Most subcapsular hematomas are located along the posterolateral aspect of the kidney. The kidney parenchyma may appear flattened by the hematoma. Occasionally, persistent compression of the renal parenchyma or structures in the renal pedicle with associated fibrosis result in systemic hypertension (see Systemic Arterial Hypertension in Section VII, Part III, Chapter 5, page 1814).

A *perirenal hematoma* is a collection of blood in the perirenal space. In this case there is a laceration or rupture of the renal parenchyma and also the renal capsule, often from penetrating trauma. The perirenal space is a potential space formed from the posterior and anterior renal fascia of Gerota. This space contains the adrenal gland, kidney, renal pelvis, and upper ureter. It extends inferiorly as a cone-shaped potential space to the iliac fossa. Perirenal hematomas are located posterior and inferior to the kidney and extend downward to the pelvis. Although often larger, they produce less renal compression than subcapsular hematomas.

A *subcapsular abscess* results from contiguous spread of inflammation into the subcapsular space from an associated renal parenchymal abscess. Such an abscess may represent extravasation of infected urine from an obstructed renal collecting system. Perirenal abscesses are extracapsular and are posterolateral and inferior in location and extend inferiorly. A *urinoma* results from a spontaneous rupture of a caliceal fornix secondary to acute or chronic obstruction of the renal collecting system or from trauma. It is a rare complication of surgery, although it may be the result of postoperative obstruction. Perirenal urinoma present in utero or at birth results from fetal urinary obstruction, usually secondary to obstructing posterior urethral valves.

The presence of perirenal fluid collections and their extent are easily demonstrated by real-time ultrasound (US) examination. Computed tomography (CT) with intravenous contrast material is also helpful in identification of these abnormalities. Both methods demonstrate the nature and extent of the underlying renal parenchymal or collecting system abnormality. Chronic extravasation of urine may result in formation of a fibrotic pseudocapsule with a perinephric cyst. Such cysts may surround the kidney or be located near the pelvis and proximal ureter.

OTHER PRIMARY RETROPERITONEAL TUMORS

Primary tumors of the adrenal cortex and medulla and renal tumors have been discussed in Section VII, Part III, Chapter 2, page 1787 and Part VII, page 1894. The retroperitoneum is also the site of origin of neoplasms of neuroectodermal origin outside the adrenal medulla,

Table 1 ■ PRIMARY RETROPERITONEAL TUMORS

Neuroectodermal Tumors Outside of Adrenal Medulla
Extra-adrenal neuroblastoma
Ganglioneuroblastoma
Ganglioneuroma
Primitive peripheral neuroectodermal tumor
Neurofibroma/sarcoma/schwannoma

Tumors of Fatty Origin
Lipoma
Lipoblastoma
Lipoblastomatosis
Liposarcoma (rare)

lipomatous tumors, rhabdomyosarcoma, undifferentiated sarcoma, tumors of germ cell ectodermal origin, mesenchymomas, lymphoma, and lymphangioma. Neuroectodermal neoplasms arising in the retroperitoneum outside of the adrenal medulla may originate from tissue of the sympathetic (autonomic) nervous system, including extra-adrenal neuroblastoma, ganglioneuroblastoma, and ganglioneuroma, or may result from neuroectoderm, as in the case of a primitive peripheral neuroectodermal tumor (Table 1). Extra-adrenal pheochromocytoma also arises in the retroperitoneum. The site of origin of all of these tumors is in the paravertebral gutter, with resultant anterior and lateral displacement of other retroperitoneal structures, including the kidneys, ureters, and inferior vena cava. Uncommon neuroectodermal tumors are paraganglioma, neurofibroma, neurofibrosarcoma, neurilemmoma, and schwannoma. Although occasionally isolated tumors, they are seen often as multiple tumors in patients with neurofibromatosis.

Tumors of fatty origin are often quite large at the time of diagnosis and are usually benign. These include lipoma, lipoblastoma, and liposarcoma-like lipoblastomatosis (see Table 1). Lipoma is a clearly delineated tumor; lipoblastoma is extensive and locally invasive, and is difficult or impossible to remove completely. Histologically, lipoblastoma shows adult liposarcoma-like cells. Its appearance on imaging studies may be similar to lipoma, but some cases examined by CT have shown areas of relatively increased attenuation, which on pathologic examination have been shown to be regions of myxoid material. Liposarcoma is extremely rare in children, but is locally invasive and also metastatic to distant sites. A lipoma is identified easily on abdominal radiographs by its radiolucent appearance, with clear delineation of adjacent soft tissue structures such as the kidneys, liver margin, and psoas muscle. Abdominal US examination reveals a large, ill-defined mass with homogeneous hyperechogenicity. A characteristic very-low-attenuation mass on CT scan, often with poor delineation of its margins and diffuse displacement of surrounding structures, is characteristic. Magnetic resonance imaging MRI also demonstrates a homogeneous mass as high signal on T_1- and T_2-weighted scan sequences. The boundaries of the mass are clearly delineated because of the marked contrast in signal intensity with surrounding structures.

RHABDOMYOSARCOMA AND UNDIFFERENTIATED SARCOMAS

Rhabdomyosarcoma (RMS) accounts for 5% to 8% of childhood cancer and presents in a wide variety of histologic types and patterns of spread of tumor. The

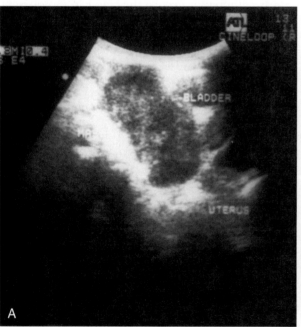 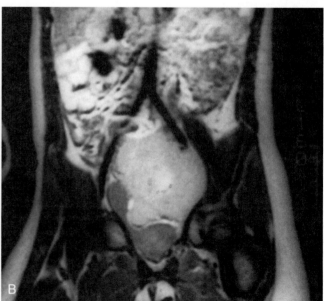

FIGURE 1. Rhabdomyosarcoma. **A,** Longitudinal sonogram of the pelvis demonstrates a large echogenic mass posterior and cephalad to the bladder. **B,** Coronal T_2-weighted magnetic resonance imaging section shows the mass indenting the bladder superiorly and encasing the left iliac artery.

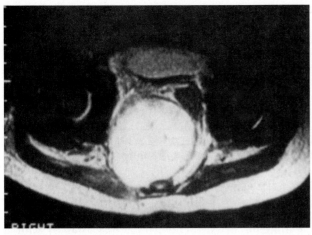

FIGURE 2. Midline, deeply located presacral rhabdomyosarcoma in a 1-year-old child. Well-defined, spherical, high-signal-intensity tumor is identified on T_2-weighted magnetic resonance imaging section.

Table 2 ■ IRS-TNM STAGING SYSTEM

Staging based on clinical, radiographic, and laboratory examination (plus histologic biopsy):
A: Localized tumor with favorable histology and clinically negative nodes
B: Locally extensive tumor with favorable histology and clinically negative nodes
C: Any size tumor with clinically involved regional nodes and/or unfavorable histology
D: Distant metastasis
   Tumor
      T-1: Confined to anatomic site of origin
         (a) <5 cm in size
         (b) ≥5 cm in size
      T-2: Extension or fixation to surrounding tissues
         (a) <5 cm in size
         (b) ≥5 cm in size
   Regional lymph nodes
      N-0: regional nodes not clinically involved
      N-1: regional nodes clinically involved by tumor
      N-X: clinical status of regional nodes unknown
   Metastases
      M-0: no distant metastasis
      M-1: metastases present

tumors infiltrate locally invade lymphatics and blood vessels, and frequently present with distant hematogenous metastases to the lungs, bone marrow, and bone. The histologic appearance of RMS seen in young children is characterized as embryonal, alveolar, or mixed RMS. The sarcomas of the genitourinary tract arise in the bladder and prostate and present with a polypoid appearance, hematuria, urinary obstruction, and a characteristic mucosanguineous mass of tissue termed *sarcoma botryoides,* in children less than 4 years of age. Prostatic RMS presents as a large pelvic mass surrounding and obstructing the urethra or producing constipation. It has two age peaks: 2 to 6 and 14 to 18 years of age.

On imaging studies, bladder RMS reveals bladder wall thickening, and/or a soft tissue mass at the bladder base (Fig. 1). If the mass is in the prostate, it will elevate the bladder and elongate the urethra. MRI is the modality of choice for staging and treatment planning. MRI reveals a mass of muscle intensity and greater than

muscle intensity on T_1-weighted images (less than fat). On T_2-weighted images, the intensity increases. It enhances with gadolinium-diethylenetriaminepentaacetic acid. Distant metastases are best evaluated with CT.

Retroperitoneal pelvic tumors may be quite large at the time of diagnosis, with wide infiltration. This is because they are often not well encapsulated. Their deep location within the body results in late identification of the mass and late presentation with obstruction of the bowel or bladder or sacral nerve root involvement (Fig. 2). Retroperitoneal lymph nodes, bone marrow metastases, and distant hematogenous metastases to the lungs are common at presentation (Fig. 3). Common sites of metastases are lungs, lymph nodes, bone, bone marrow, liver, and brain. Ten percent to 20% of patients have metastases at time of initial diagnosis. The newest staging system is a combination of the Intergroup Rhabdomyosarcoma Study (IRS) system and the tumor, nodes, metastasis (TNM) system (Table 2). Treatment of genitourinary RMS is chemotherapy followed by surgical excision of residual disease after 4 to 5 months. Radiation is added if the tumor is relatively chemotherapy resistant. Follow-up is best achieved by CT.

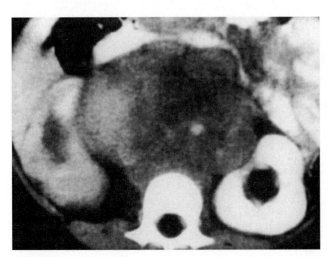

FIGURE 3. Retroperitoneal metastatic node mass from a testicular rhabdomyosarcoma in a 7-year-old boy. Both renal pelves are obstructed by the node mass.

GERM CELL TUMORS

Germ cell tumors are benign or malignant tumors derived from the primordial germinal epithelial layer cells in extragonadal or gonadal sites. These tumors account for 3% of malignant tumors of children and adolescents. Two thirds of these tumors are extragonadal in origin. Forty-one percent of germ cell tumors occur in the sacrococcygeal region, and most are benign. Thoracic germ cell tumors are located in the anterior superior mediastinum. Abdominal germ cell tumors are usually located in the retroperitoneal space, though occasional involvement of the stomach, omentum, and liver is described.

Germ cell tumors include germinoma, embryonal carcinoma, endodermal sinus tumor, choriocarcinoma, polyembryoma, gonadoblastoma, and teratoma. A teratoma (Fig. 4) arises from pluripotent cells and is composed of a variety of tissues foreign to the organ of its anatomic site of origin. The component tissues are poorly organized and in various stages of maturation, and the lesion may be solid, multicystic, or a single large cyst. Neonatal teratomas occur 80% of the time in the sacrococcygeal region. Other sites include the jaw, nasopharynx, intracranial cavity, retroperitoneum, mediastinum, and gonads.

α-Fetoprotein is produced in immature germ cell tumors of children. Germ cell tumors with trophoblastic elements (choriocarcinomas) produce β-human chorionic gonadotropin.

OTHER SARCOMAS

Other sarcomas occasionally seen in children and adolescents include fibrosarcoma, neurofibrosarcoma, malignant fibrous histioytoma, hemangiopericytoma, leiomyosarcoma, and liposarcoma.

HODGKIN'S DISEASE AND NON-HODGKIN'S LYMPHOMA

Malignant lymphomas are neoplasms of the cells of the immune system. Because these cells circulate through the body, all lymphomas are generalized disease from the time of origin. The lymphomas present with a mediastinal mass 50% to 70% of the time, and the vast majority of patients with lymphoma present with the

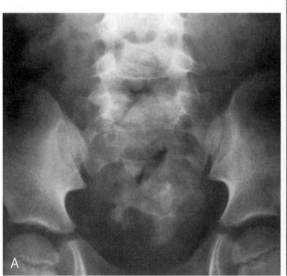

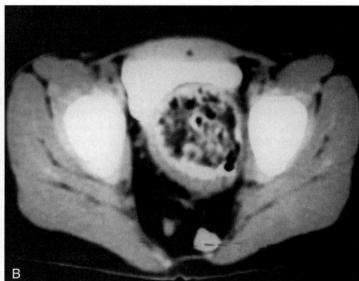

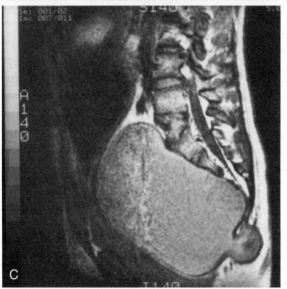

FIGURE 4. Retroperitoneal teratoma (ASP syndrome). **A,** Plain film of the sacrum shows a "scimitar" anomaly of the lower sacral segments. **B,** Computed tomography scan demonstrates calcium and asymmetric fat posterior to the bladder. **C,** Sagittal T_1-weighted magnetic resonance imaging section of the pelvis in another patient shows a presacral mass that proved at surgery to be a benign teratoma.

Table 3 ■ STAGING OF HODGKIN'S DISEASE

STAGE	DEFINITION
I	Involvement of a single lymph node region or single organ
II	Involvement of two or more lymph node regions on the same side of the diaphragm or involvement of one lymph node region and an organ site on the same side of the diaphragm
III	Involvement of lymph node regions on both sides of the diaphragm, often with spleen involvement or involvement of an extralymphatic organ or site
IV	Diffuse, disseminated involvement of one or more extralymphatic organs or tissues, either with or without lymph node involvement

tumor above the diaphragm in the supraclavicular regions, axillae, or mediastinum. Abdominal involvement is most likely to involve only the liver and spleen; however, those lymphomas with small noncleaved cells frequently present with abdominal tumors, most frequently in or around the gastrointestinal tract.

Burkitt's lymphoma presents with abdominal tumor in all except a very small number of cases. Clinical manifestations are abdominal pain or swelling, sometimes with a symptom complex characterized by intussusception, nausea and vomiting, gastrointestinal bleeding, and intestinal perforation. Palpation of a right iliac fossa mass is quite common, and lymphadenopathy in these patients is inguinal or iliac in distribution. Abdominal sites of involvement, retroperitoneal adenopathy, and involvement of the jaw are common for Burkitt's lymphoma. Initial presentation with retroperitoneal masses is uncommon and more likely to be associated with the lymphomas related to pharmacologic immunosuppression.

Hodgkin's disease generally spreads from one adjacent nodal area to another until late in the disease. The currently used staging classification for Hodgkin's disease is shown in Table 3.

RETROPERITONEAL LYMPHANGIOMA AND HYGROMA

A retroperitoneal lymphangioma is a benign tumor of congenital lymphatic origin. On US examination, it is most commonly a multilocular cystic mass containing clear or slightly turbid fluid. Occasionally, the mass is unilocular. Debris levels may be seen within the cystic spaces. The mass is commonly large. The histologic classification of these masses is simple, cavernous, or cystic lymphangioma. A cystic lymphangioma, or hygroma, consists of multiple dilated, poorly developed lymphatic channels. Although it may present early as a palpable abdominal mass, the soft nature of this lesion may render it difficult to identify on physical examination. The mass may compress adjacent structures, particularly displacing and obstructing the ureters. The

cystic spaces are lined with endothelium and contain multiple thin septa and chylous fluid.

A lymphangioma is easily identified by US examination, which shows multiple, apparently noncommunicating, fluid-containing cystic regions separated by thin septa. CT examination also reveals the cystic nature, although the septa are not easily visible. Rarely, hemorrhage or infection may complicate a lymphangioma.

IDIOPATHIC RETROPERITONEAL FIBROSIS

Rarely seen in children, this abnormality is characterized by dense fibroblastic sheets of tissue, often with an inflammatory component. The ureters, aorta, and inferior vena cava are involved by this tissue. This abnormality results as a complication of treatment with methysergide in adults. Clinical symptoms include flank pain, urinary tract obstruction, and lower extremity edema. Occasionally systemic hypertension secondary to renal artery involvement is noted. The diagnosis may be suspected by evaluation of the course of the ureters and retroperitoneum by CT and by identification of ureteral obstruction and high-signal streaks of fibroblastic tissue by T_2-weighted coronal MRI. US examination shows homogeneous soft tissue masses involving the retroperitoneum.

RETROPERITONEAL HEMATOMA OR ABSCESS

Hematoma of the retroperitoneum is most commonly the result of severe blunt abdominal trauma or a surgical procedure. Spontaneous retroperitoneal hematoma, usually affecting the psoas muscle, is seen in patients with hemophilia and other bleeding diatheses (Fig. 5). Patients receiving anticoagulant therapy may also pre-

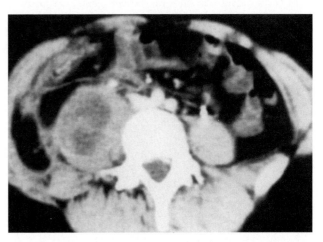

FIGURE 5. Psoas muscle hematoma in a teenage boy with known hemophilia and 6 days of back pain. Contrast-enhanced computed tomography shows psoas mass with low-attenuation center.

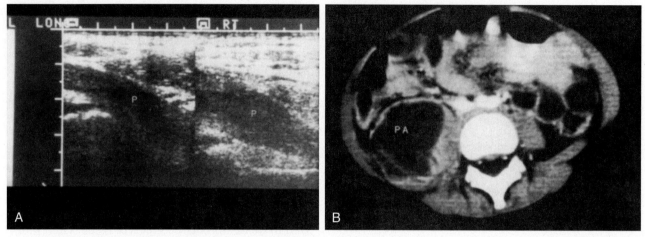

FIGURE 6. Psoas abscess in a 16-month-old child limping on the right leg. **A,** Hip ultrasound shows edema of the psoas tendon *(P).* **B,** Computed tomography shows a large, liquefied psoas muscle abscess *(PA).* Organism was β-hemolytic streptococcus group B.

sent with this abnormality. On US examination, the psoas muscle is enlarged with initially hyperechoic regions seen in the area of hemorrhage. As the blood cells break down, the area of hemorrhage becomes hypoechoic. CT examination reveals an enlarged psoas muscle with high attenuation or isoattenuation initially, later seen as a low-attenuation region. MRI accurately identifies and documents the age of the hemorrhage.

Retroperitoneal abscess is usually of hematogenous origin and the result of distant infection such as osteomyelitis with resultant septicemia. Tuberculosis is a common cause of psoas abscess and may be associated with paraspinal abscess and extradural, intraspinal abscess extension. Osteomyelitis secondary to tuberculosis or another organism involving adjacent vertebrae is common. Psoas abscesses are also seen as a result of appendicitis or inflammatory bowel disease. Gram-negative bacteria are the etiologic factors. Retroperitoneal abscess may be demonstrated by gallium scan, US examination, or CT examination (Fig. 6). US reveals a sonolucent region within the psoas muscle with associated fluid along the margins of the psoas. CT shows a low-attenuation lesion within the psoas muscle with rim enhancement after injection of intravenous contrast material. US is useful as a guide for diagnostic and therapeutic drainage of these abscesses.

SUGGESTED READINGS

Bloom DA, Schofield D, Hoffer FA: Radiologic-pathologic conference of Children's Hospital Boston: a palpable pelvic mass in an adolescent girl. Pediatr Radiol 1997;27:888

Ecklund K, Taylor GA, Schofield DH: Radiologic-pathologic conference of Children's Hospital Boston: abdominal mass in a prepubertal girl. Pediatr Radiol 1997;27:832

Groff DB: Pelvic neoplasms in children. J Surg Oncol 2001;77:65

Hussain HK, Kingston JE, Domizio P, et al: Imaging-guided core biopsy for the diagnosis of malignant tumors in pediatric patients. AJR Am J Roentgenol 2001;176:43

Iinuma Y, Iwafuchi M, Uchiyama M, et al: A case of Currarino triad with familial sacral bony deformities. Pediatr Surg Int 2000;16:134

Kim EE, Valenzuela RF, Kumar AJ, et al: Imaging and clinical spectrum of rhabdomyosarcoma in children. Clin Imaging 2000;Sept 24:257

Kirks DR, Merten DF, Filston HC, Oakes WJ: The Currarino triad: complex of anorectal malformation, sacral bony abnormality, and presacral mass. Pediatr Radiol 1984;14:220

McHugh K, Pritchard J: Problems in the imaging of three common paediatric solid tumours. Eur J Radiol 2001;37:72

Ng WT, Ng TK, Cheng PW: Sacrococcygeal teratoma and anorectal malformation. Aust N Z J Surg 1997;67:218

Parker BR: Leukemia and lymphoma in childhood. Radiol Clin North Am 1997;35:1495

Ruymann FB, Grovas AC: Progress in the diagnosis and treatment of rhabdomyosarcoma and related soft tissue sarcomas. Cancer Invest 2000;18:223

Siegel MJ: Pelvic tumors in childhood. Radiol Clin North Am 1997;35:1455

SECTION VIII

REPRODUCTIVE ORGANS

JACK O. HALLER

HARRIS L. COHEN

PART I

ABNORMALITIES OF THE MALE GENITAL TRACT

HARRIS L. COHEN

JACK O. HALLER

NORMAL SCROTAL ANATOMY

The normal infant testicle is 1.0 cm long. In early childhood, the testicle is largest by 2 to 3 months of age, with a volume of 2 cm³. This somewhat more prominent size is probably related to the androgen surge of the first months of life that subsequent declines. By 6 months of age, the average pediatric testicle is somewhat smaller than it is at 2 months of age. Testicular volume increases slowly until pubescence, when a greater degree of enlargement usually occurs with a rise in gonadotrophins. In a 1966 study of 300 healthy Swiss boys and 300 healthy Swiss men, Prader found a 2- to 5-cm³ testicular volume at age 12, a 5- to 10-cm³ volume at the beginning of testicular growth at age 13, and a 15- to 25-cm³ volume after a rapid growth spurt at about 15 years of age. These measurements are obviously related to the ages of puberty in a given population. Testicular growth ceased at about 18 years of age. At that time the average testicular volume was 15 to 25 cm³.

The development of secondary sexual characteristics in males is a good indicator of testosterone production by the testicle's Leydig cells. Testicular size is a good indicator of tubular function and spermatogenesis. In the adolescent, the left testis is marginally smaller than the right. The mature postpubescent testicle measures 2.5 × 3.0 × 4.0 cm. The normal testes should be ovoid and symmetric on physical examination as well as all imaging examinations.

IMAGING MODALITIES

Ultrasound (US), including Doppler in all its forms (i.e., duplex, color, and power Doppler), is the main diagnostic imaging tool for evaluating the scrotum. Computed tomography (CT) may be used for the analysis of intrapelvic or intra-abdominal extension of intrascrotal masses but is predominantly used to denote spread, particularly metastatic, of testicular or other intrascrotal tumors. Magnetic resonance imaging (MRI) has been used in the search for undescended testes that remains in an intra-abdominal position. MRI, like CT, can be used to analyze metastatic spread of testicular tumor. Its uses in intra-abdominal, intrapelvic, and intrascrotal imaging are currently evolving.

Scrotal US has developed into a highly accurate imaging modality for determining the presence of testes within the scrotum, evaluating echogenicity patterns of the testes to identify normal versus abnormal testes, and evaluating the testicular adnexa, particularly each epididymis. US is highly accurate in determining whether an intrascrotal abnormality is testicular or extratesticular and whether it is cystic or solid.

SCROTAL ULTRASOUND TECHNIQUE

Scrotal US is performed using a high-frequency transducer. As with other body areas, the choice of an US transducer seeks a compromise between the better near-field resolution obtained with a high-frequency (e.g., 7.5- or 10-MHz) transducer and the better penetration afforded by lower frequency transducers (e.g., 3.5 MHz). The superficial position of testes in the normally thin-walled scrotum allows excellent imaging with a transducer of 7.5 MHz or higher. Some authors limit their examinations to linear array transducers only. Others, including ourselves, include views obtained with a sector or vector transducer so that both testes can be examined, in full, side by side. This allows better analysis of differences in echogenicity, an important point in analyzing patients for testicular torsion, particularly when the torsion is subacute. At times, a lower frequency transducer may be necessary to analyze the scrotum and its contents when it is enlarged by, for example, a large amount of hydrocele (Fig. 1) or its wall is thickened by edema or trauma. This is more often a problem in adult

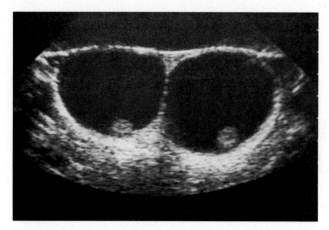

FIGURE 1. On transverse plane ultrasound, two normal testes are seen as small echogenic structures within a very enlarged scrotum of a young child with large hydroceles. Typically, high-frequency transducers (e.g., 7.5 MHz) are used for improved near-field resolution of superficial structures such as the testes. In cases, such as this one, with large hydroceles, a lower frequency transducer (e.g., 3.5 MHz) may be needed to better penetrate the longer distance between the anterior and posterior scrotal walls and actually image the testes.

imaging, but the technique can be helpful for evaluation of the postpubertal adolescent.

More often, in children, the technical difficulties for US imaging relate to the small size of the scrotum and its contents. Examiner persistence will often prove rewarding. Some examiners cup the scrotum with one hand while holding the transducer in the other. A small palpated lesion may be more easily positioned for US evaluation by having the sonologist or the older or more cooperative patient hold the area of concern between two fingers while the examiner places the transducer directly on it.

Longitudinal (Fig. 2), transverse (Fig. 3), and coronal US views are taken of each hemiscrotum. Transverse views, particularly with a convex array transducer (Fig. 3), allow the best side-by-side comparison of both testicles and their adnexae, especially when checking for differences in size and echogenicity. Occasionally, one may accomplish the same with a linear array transducer with a footprint that encompasses the entire scrotum. Coronal views using the near-field testicle as an ultrasonic window may help in evaluating the contralateral testicle. However, because of differences in depth

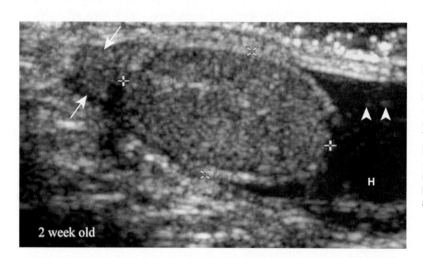

FIGURE 2. Hydrocele with some contained meconium in the normal testis of a 2-week-old boy as seen on ultrasound in the longitudinal plane. *Crosses* mark off the right testicle. The triangular structure *(arrows)* superior to it is the epididymis. The relatively echoless area inferior to it is part of a hydrocele *(H)*. This hydrocele has some debris *(arrowheads)* within it consistent with some meconium. The walls of the scrotum are seen surrounding the testicle and can best be individually identified anterior and posterior to the hydrocele.

FIGURE 3. Two normal testes of a teenager are seen as homogeneously echogenic on ultrasound in the transverse plane. This image was obtained using a convex linear array probe that allowed imaging of most of both testes. These transducers can show both testes in their entirety in most cases and are therefore an improvement over linear array transducers (limited by the size of their footpad) for side-by-side comparisons of testes.

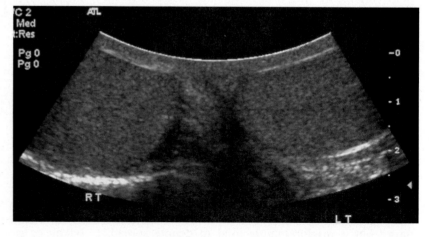

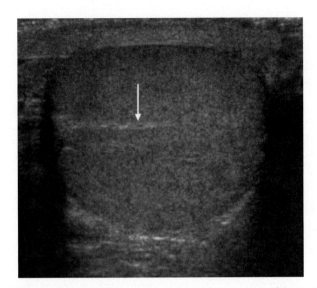

FIGURE 4. On transverse plane ultrasound, an *arrow* points to a linear echogenicity within a normal testicle that is the mediastinum testis.

of beam penetration for each testicle, coronal views are not optimal for echogenicity comparisons between testicles.

The adolescent scrotum is examined in a manner similar to that used with the adult scrotum. A folded towel is used as a bridge to lift the scrotum off the thighs. Holding the ends of the towel, the patient can control positioning, thus alleviating some of the discomfort of inadvertent motion during the examination of the painful scrotum. The bridge helps cup the scrotum, decreasing the size of the area to be examined. Furthermore, both testicles can be seen better for side-by-side comparison when they are placed closer to each other.

IMAGING FINDINGS ON SCROTAL ULTRASOUND

On US examination, the testes should be homogeneously echogenic. A highly echogenic linear density (seen posteriorly and superiorly) represents the mediastinum testis (Fig. 4), the inward extension of the testicle's tightly adherent covering, the tunica albuginea (Fig. 5). The mediastinum tends not to be well seen until postpubescence. Fibrous septa extending from the mediastinum testes, which are not typically seen on US examination, divide the testes into greater than 250 lobules. The spermatic cord, draining veins, lymphatics, nerves, vas deferens, and a single testicular artery run within the mediastinum testis.

The head of the epididymis (Fig. 6) sits atop the superior pole of each testicle. The head is continuous with the epididymal body and tail, which travel inferiorly along the posterolateral margin of the testicle. The epididymal head is about three to four times the diameter of the epididymal body and tail. It is more readily imaged as a structure separate from the testes as compared to the epididymal body or tail. The echoge-

nicity of the epididymis is normally homogeneous and equal to or slightly greater or lesser than that of the testes.

The scrotal wall should be between 3 and 6 mm thick. Beneath the scrotal wall are the two layers of the tunica vaginalis (see Fig. 5), the outer (parietal) and the inner (visceral) layers that are the residua of the processus vaginalis (peritoneum that descended with the testicle from the abdomen). The visceral layer covers the testicle on its anterior border and is attached to the tunica albuginea. Between the tunica's two layers is a potential space that may contain as much as 1 to 2 ml of fluid in normal patients. It is here that the fluid of hematocele or hydrocele may accumulate.

Three small, persistent, vestigial remnants of the mesonephric and müllerian duct systems may occasionally be seen when a normal testicle is surrounded by significant fluid (hydrocele). These are the appendix testis (Fig. 7) (a remnant of the müllerian duct), attached to the testicle's upper pole (and the most common one to potentially torse); the appendix epididymis (a remnant of the mesonephron), attached to the head of the epididymis; and the vas aberrans (a remnant of the mesonephron), attached to the epididymis at the junction of its body and tail. These remnants may become diseased. Torsion of any of them can result in scrotal pain, swelling, local erythema, and clinical complaints similar to those of testicular torsion. The torsed mass may be imaged, but it may be difficult to distinguish which of the three remnants is the torsed one.

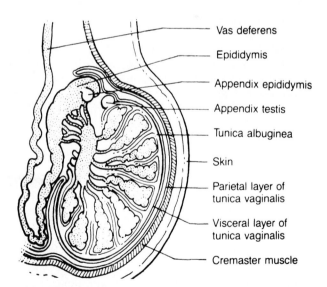

FIGURE 5. Schematic drawing of scrotum and its contents as seen in the longitudinal plane through a single testicle. Note the tunica albuginea surrounding the lobules of the testes. The tunica albuginea, in turn, is surrounded by the visceral layer of the tunica vaginalis and the more superficial parietal layer of the tunica vaginalis. (From Cohen HL, Sivit C [eds]: Fetal and Pediatric Ultrasound: A Casebook Approach. New York, McGraw-Hill, 2001. Reproduced with permission of McGraw-Hill Companies.)

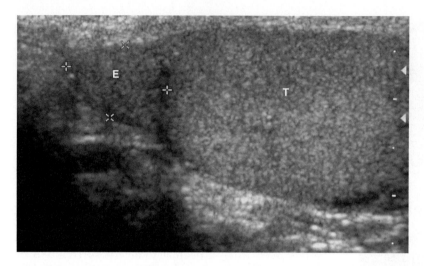

FIGURE 6. *Crosses* mark off the head of the epididymis *(E)*, which sits atop the superior testicle *(T)*, in this longitudinal plane ultrasound. The normal epididymal body and tail, which travel along the side of the testicle, are more difficult to separate from normal testicle.

CONGENITAL ABNORMALITIES OF THE TESTES

MONORCHIDISM AND ANORCHIDISM

Monorchidism, the presence of a single testicle, is seen in 1 of every 5000 males. It is four times more common than anorchidism. US, MRI, CT, or laparoscopy may be used to prove that there is no undescended testicle(s) (cryptorchidism) simulating mon- or anorchidism. When a blind-ending spermatic vessel is found at surgery, it suggests anorchidism, probably on the basis of an intrauterine vascular insult. No further ipsilateral exploration for an undescended testicle is necessary.

CRYPTORCHIDISM

By 32 weeks' gestational age, the testes have descended into the scrotum via the inguinal canal in 93% of all male fetuses. By 6 weeks of age, only 4% of term infants have a nonpalpable testicle. Of these, 20% have true cryptorchidism (undescended testes). Cryptorchidism occurs bilaterally in 10% to 33% of cases. It is more common on the right (70%). It may be familial. Beyond the age of 1 year, the prevalence of true cryptorchidism in the male population remains unchanged at 0.7% to 1%.

Most cases of nonpalpable testicles are related to testicular agenesis or dysgenesis. The disruption of testicular descent, in cases of cryptorchidism, usually occurs within or just above the external inguinal ring. Occasionally the testicle may be intra-abdominal. In rare cases, an undescended testicle may be in a femoral location. The undescended testicle that remains within the abdomen has known malignant potential. It is at 10 to 40 times greater risk for developing a future malignancy than either of a pair of normally descended testes. Seminoma is the most common tumor that develops. Other germ cell–type tumors, such as embryonal carcinoma or teratocarcinoma, may occur. The risk of malignancy in the contralateral, normally descended testicle is also increased as compared with the risk in a

testicle of someone with two normally descended gonads. Patients with bilateral nondescent in which one testicle developed a neoplasm stand a 25% chance that a neoplasm will occur in the remaining testicle.

Men with unilateral cryptorchidism are less fertile than men after unilateral orchiectomy. The cause is thought to be due to immobilizing antibodies that develop to the patient's sperm. This was noted in one third of a group of 33 infertile men with cryptorchidism.

The occurrence of an inguinal hernia (Fig. 8) ipsilateral to an undescended testicle is common. Ten percent to 20% of affected patients have an associated genitourinary abnormality, such as vesicoureteral reflux, hydronephrosis, horseshoe kidney, renal ectopia, or renal agenesis. Rare and unusual cases of testicular absence in association with ipsilateral absence of the spermatic duct and the kidney point to a developmental abnormality of the entire urogenital ridge.

The cause of cryptorchidism is not clear; it may be

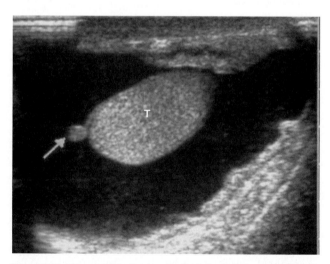

FIGURE 7. Ultrasound in the longitudinal plane through testicle. An *arrow* points to a small circular structure extending off the testicle *(T)* that is a normal appendix testis. It was readily seen on this image because of the presence of a large hydrocele. It would otherwise probably not be imaged.

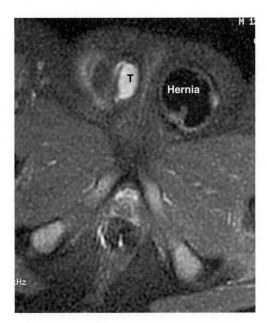

FIGURE 8. Inguinal hernia on T$_2$-weighted magnetic resonance imaging study with fat suppression in the axial plane. A child with a history of cryptorchidism and growth hormone therapy that allowed the right testicle to descend is noted to have a normal-appearing testicle *(T)* within the scrotum, seen as a homogeneously intense area, medial to a right inguinal hernia. On the left side of the scrotum, a testicle was neither palpated nor imaged. Bowel from a left inguinal hernia is noted. (Courtesy of Dr. David Bluemke.)

hormonal in nature or mechanical (lack of proper fixation of the testis or an abnormal gubernaculum), or a combination of the two. Cryptorchidism is the rule in cases of male pseudohermaphroditism, gonadal dysgenesis, and true hermaphroditism. It occurs with some frequency in males with hypospadias.

IMAGING EVALUATION

US is commonly the initial procedure for localization of a testis not palpable within the scrotum. US is excellent for denoting a testis or nubbin of testis in the high scrotum or inguinal area (Fig. 9A). It can usually, but not always, differentiate between testicle and node when imaging a mass in the inguinal area. Lymph nodes (Fig. 9B) (which are not an uncommon finding in the inguinal region of children) often have echogenic fat in their central hilar areas and a relatively specific blood flow pattern into the central hilum and extending out to the remainder of the node.

MRI is generally more effective than CT for intra-abdominal testes because of its ability to provide multi-planar images and the fact that it may also give more information about the texture of the testis. Normal testes have homogeneous high signal on T$_2$-weighted images (Fig. 8). Finding normal testes on MRI is aided by fat suppression techniques.

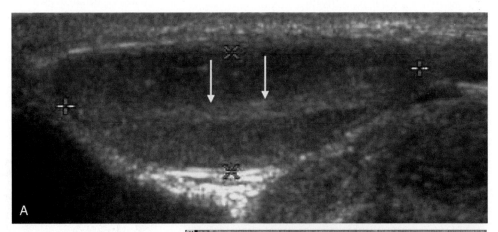

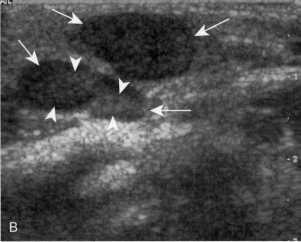

FIGURE 9. Analysis of groin for undescended testes. **A,** Inguinal testis on ultrasound in the transverse plane to groin and longitudinal plane through testis. *Crosses* mark off the borders of a normal undescended testicle found in the right groin of a child. *White arrows* point to the testicle's mediastinum. Color Doppler denoted normal flow to the testicle, which appeared homogeneous and normal. Its superficial position required a high-frequency transducer (10 MHz). Often in the past, but less so these days, a stand-off pad would be needed for sufficient distance between transducer head and testicle to allow better images. **B,** Lymph nodes in groin on ultrasound in the transverse plane to groin. Two oval structures *(arrows)* are noted in the right groin of a child with undescended testes. The presence of two similar structures goes against the possibility that either is a testicle. The fact that each is somewhat lobular rather than smooth goes against either being a typical normal testicle. The contained brighter echogenicity *(arrowheads)* within the inner at least three fourths of the more inferior mass is typical of the fat noted in benign nodes and not a testicle.

SURGICAL TREATMENT

Surgical treatment for undescended testes consists of orchiopexy, whenever possible. It is carried out, especially in cases of intra-abdominal testes, because of the great risk for developing testicular neoplasia. The orchiopexy should be performed in early childhood. In light of the occasional occurrence of spontaneous descent during the first year of life, surgical correction early in the second year of life is advised. Although orchiopexy may not reduce the risk for malignant degeneration, the exteriorized testicle is more easily followed both clinically and by US. The undescended testes are usually small and hypoplastic, although usually of equal echogenicity compared to the normal testicle.

Early orchiopexy also hopefully aids the fertility potential of affected patients. Undescended testes are said to be normal histologically until the second year of life, when progressive tubular changes may develop. Somewhat problematic for this concept is the fact that these histologic findings may be noted in the contralateral descended testicle as well. A review by Giwercman et al. of the US and Doppler findings of 75 maldescended testes studied 2 to 11 years after orchiopexy showed 53% of the testes to be abnormal by either position, volume, structure, or perfusion. Of interest is the fact that 19 cases had surgery within the first 2 years of life, but 49 of the testes had operative intervention at a later time. There was no correlation of abnormal US findings and the time of surgical intervention.

POLYORCHIDISM

Polyorchidism is a rare condition that is most often discovered at puberty because of a scrotal mass. Usually the mass consists only of a small accessory testicle in addition to two normal testes or two unequal testes, both smaller than the contralateral normal one, each with an individual epididymis and a shared vas deferens allowing spermatogenesis from each.

HYDROCELE

A hydrocele (see Fig. 7) is the most common scrotal mass in a child. Figure 10 is a schematic drawing of several types of hydrocele. The most common type after the first year of life is the scrotal hydrocele. Hydroceles represent fluid accumulated within the layers of the tunica vaginalis, which, although predominantly anterior to each testicle, appears to surround the testicle except for the area of the epididymal head. The proximal portion of the processus vaginalis typically closes before 18 months of age. This prevents abdominal contents from entering the scrotum and the tunica vaginalis. Residual fluid from testicular descent is responsible for noncommunicating hydroceles reported in at least 15% of male fetuses beyond 28 weeks of life. Such physiologic hydroceles occur in at least 16 of every 1000 newborns and tend to resolve spontaneously by fluid resorption by 6 to 9 months of age. The processus vaginalis is closed in 50% to 75% of individuals by the

time they are born and in most of the remainder of children by the end of the first year of life. If the processus fails to close, there will be communication between the peritoneal cavity and the scrotum. A communicating hydrocele can develop in such patients. Enlarging hydroceles may be due to an intrascrotal cause such as neoplasm, infection, or torsion. Increasing hydrocele without an intrascrotal cause suggest a patent processus vaginalis and the presence of an associated inguinal hernia. At times, a hernia, denoted by the presence of bowel within the scrotum, can be diagnosed by US, particularly if the bowel is surrounded by fluid (Fig. 11). However, air-filled bowel may obscure US analysis of the scrotum.

It is well known that the patent processus of fetal life allows the possible descent of meconium into the scrotum in cases of meconium peritonitis. This meconium can calcify within the scrotum as it can within the abdomen. US may image the calcified meconium as one or several small echogenic masses within the scrotum but not within the testicle. Obviously, pus, air, urine, or cerebrospinal fluid (in patients with ventriculoperitoneal shunts) or even blood from blunt trauma to, for example, the spleen, may also enter the scrotum from the peritoneal cavity as long as the processus vaginalis remain patent.

In most cases in the child or adolescent, a hydrocele is idiopathic. Acquired hydroceles occur mostly in patients with a normally closed funicular process following scrotal trauma or as a complication of epididymitis or orchitis, testicular torsion, or intrascrotal neoplasms (reactive hydrocele).

A hydrocele may vary in size according to the amount of contained fluid. There may be small amounts of fluid, not detectable clinically, to moderate to larger amounts contained within the scrotum. Scrotal US shows the cystic nature of the hydrocele as it appears to surround the normal homogeneously echogenic testes. Septations

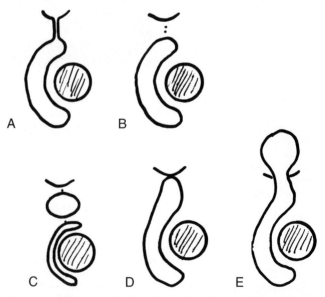

FIGURE 10. Diagram of various types of hydrocele. **A,** Congenital or intermittent hydrocele. **B,** Scrotal hydrocele. **C,** Hydrocele of the cord. **D,** Inguinoscrotal hydrocele. **E,** Abdominoscrotal hydrocele.

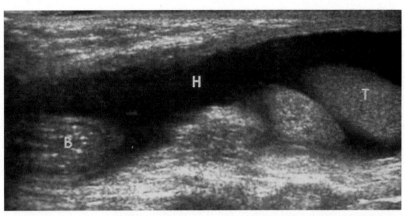

FIGURE 11. Bowel herniated into scrotum as seen on ultrasound in the longitudinal plane. This teenager had an enlarged scrotum as a result of a contained hydrocele *(H)*. Within the hydrocele were several loops of bowel, with the largest denoted by the letter *B*. The testicle *(T)* is seen inferiorly within the enlarged scrotum.

and debris may be present in a hydrocele, particularly if the hydrocele is infected or hemorrhagic. Echogenic debris (Fig. 12) is often seen in the fluid of many chronic hydroceles. The exact etiology for this is unknown. Cholesterol crystals have been shown to be the cause of this in some adults with chronic hydrocele. Calcifications may occasionally develop within the scrotum of patients with chronic hydroceles and chronic inflammation, purportedly from shed cells and disturbed hydrocele resorption. Nuclear medicine scintigraphy with technetium pertechnetate, once a popular imaging method, shows a hydrocele as a photon-deficient area that may mimic the lack of flow to a testicle in cases of testicular torsion, a space-occupying mass such as bowel in a patient with an intrascrotal hernia, or intrascrotal hematoma in a patient after trauma. The evolution of scrotal imaging away from nuclear medicine examinations and toward US examination has helped avoid this potential diagnostic confusion.

Less common types of hydroceles (see Fig. 10) of congenital origin include hydrocele of the cord, inguinoscrotal hydrocele, and abdominoscrotal hydrocele. In hydrocele of the cord, or funicular hydrocele, the processus vaginalis is obliterated in its proximal and distal end, and the hydrocele is contained in the patent funicular space between these two points. In inguinoscrotal hydrocele, the processus vaginalis is obliterated only at the internal inguinal ring, and the hydrocele extends cephalad from the scrotum into the inguinal canal. In abdominoscrotal hydrocele (Fig. 13), there also is closure of the funicular process at the internal inguinal ring; the hydrocele is very large and forms a dumbbell-shaped cystic mass that protrudes into the retroperitoneal space of the anterior abdominal wall above the inguinal area. The inguinal mass can be made to vary in size depending on the pressure placed on either the inguinal or the scrotal end of the abdominoscrotal hydrocele. The abdominoscrotal hydrocele presents as an inguinal or intra-abdominal mass and must be considered when evaluating lower abdominal masses occurring in the first year of life. They are discovered at abdominal palpation in children with scrotal hydroceles or by noting that a hydrocele evaluated by US extends above the scrotum and into the inguinal region and/or abdomen. They are treated by total excision of the mass through an extensive inguinal incision.

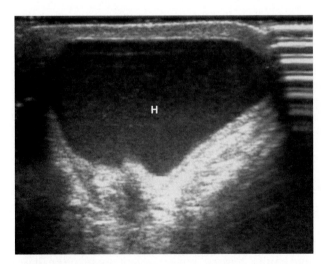

FIGURE 12. Echogenic fluid in chronic hydrocele as seen on ultrasound in the transverse plane. Debris fills the fluid of a large right hydrocele *(H)* in an older teenager. This image does not include the normal testicle, which was seen in another portion of the affected hemiscrotum. In an infant, the contained debris may be related to meconium. In an older patient such as this one, it is most often due to contained cholesterol crystals, often found in the fluid of chronic hydroceles. Proteinaceous, hemorrhagic, or infectious material may also be considered as less likely possibilities.

HEMATOCELES

Hematoceles (Fig. 14) are complex extratesticular fluid collections containing hemorrhagic material separating the layers of the tunica vaginalis. Acutely, after fibrin deposition, hemorrhage is echogenic on US examination. With time the contained hemorrhage become less echogenic and the fluid may become more typical of hydrocele. Such hematoceles may contain low-level echoes similar to chronic hydroceles or septations seen more often in cases of infected hydroceles.

Hematoceles may develop from scrotal trauma but may also accumulate from distal trauma (e.g., bleeding from an injured spleen) if there is a patent processus vaginalis. In cases of scrotal trauma, unless there is an associated break in the testicle's tunica albuginea or testicular blood flow is compromised, the presence of a hematoceles and even a testicular fracture is not a definitive indication for surgery.

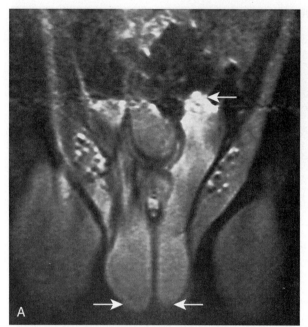

FIGURE 13. Abdominoscrotal hydrocele. **A,** A tubular white structure *(arrows)* is seen extending from each side of the scrotum superiorly into the abdominal cavity on a T_1-weighted magnetic resonance imaging section in the coronal plane. The superior extent of the structure on the right is not well seen on this image. This child had bilateral abdominoscrotal hydroceles. He presented with an enlarged scrotum and palpable inguinal area masses whose size changed with scrotal compression. (From Cohen HL, Sivit C [eds]: Fetal and Pediatric Ultrasound: A Casebook Approach. New York, McGraw-Hill, 2001. Reproduced with permission of McGraw-Hill Companies.) **B,** On ultrasound in the longitudinal plane, a right-sided tubular, fluid-filled structure extended from the scrotum *(S)* to above the inguinal area *(arrow)* in another child with an abdominoscrotal hydrocele. *See Color Plate*

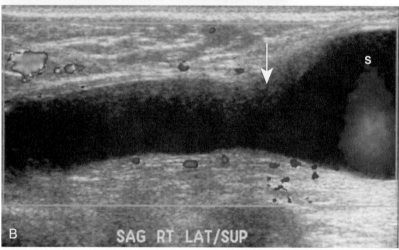

Various US findings may be seen in patients who have had scrotal trauma. In one study by Anderson et al. of 19 blunt traumas, the authors noted four hematoceles, two epididymal hematomas, two cases of post-traumatic epididymitis, two cases of post-traumatic hydrocele, and seven cases of testiclar rupture.

Testicular rupture (Fig. 15) is thought to be uncommon, occurring mostly in athletes or in vehicular or industrial accidents. It is usually caused by a nonpenetrating crush injury in which the testis is trapped between the pubic ramus and the crushing object. A tear develops in the tunical albuginea, with subsequent hemorrhage and extravasation of seminiferous tubules and other testicular contents into the potential space of the tunica vaginalis. On US there is often bizarre heterogeneous echogenicity to the testicular parenchyma, often caused by infarction and hemorrhage; irregularity of the normally smooth testicular border; and, on occasion, nonvisualization of any normal testicular parenchyma. The testes may be displaced into the inguinal canal. A reactive hydrocele or hematocele

(because of concomitant bleeding) may occur. Discrete fracture lines are unusual. Testicular tumors may predispose a testis to rupture. One must be wary of the possibility that a bizarre heterogeneous echogenicity in a traumatized scrotum may actually be a hematoma that has displaced a normal testicle (Fig. 16), often superiorly.

SCROTAL WALL THICKENING

Not all scrotal enlargement is due to contained fluid. In older adults, massive scrotal enlargement often has a component of scrotal wall thickening. This is less common in children. Certainly in either age group, the scrotal wall may be thickened by contained infection or hemorrhage. Occasionally, a child with nephrotic syndrome may present with an enlarged scrotum made up predominantly of an edematous and therefore thickened scrotal wall (Fig. 17).

TESTICULAR TORSION

Testicular torsion is a relatively common clinical problem that, if left uncorrected, leads to the serious consequences of ischemic necrosis of the testicle and loss of testicular function. Torsion may occur at any age but is seen most often in adolescent boys between 11 and 18 years of age, perhaps because of the increase in testicular growth and weight during this time. Torsion may also be seen with some frequency in the newborn period, often as result of a torsion that occurred antenatally (see Section II, Part V, Chapter 11, page 252).

CLINICAL FINDINGS

Testicular torsion represents 20% of cases of acute scrotal pathology in the postpubertal male. The normal testicle is strongly attached to the epididymis, which in turn is applied to the posterior scrotal wall. If these attachments fail to develop properly, the testis, suspended within the tunica vaginalis, may rotate and the spermatic cord undergo torsion (the clapper-in-a-bell phenomenon), with compromise of blood flow to the testis and epididymis. After 2 hours, the cells of spermatogenesis are damaged. They are said to be destroyed by 6 hours. Detorsion is necessary for testicular viability. Surgery within 24 hours leads to 60% to 70% testicular salvage, but after 24 hours salvage is only 20%. Because this condition is considered a bilateral phenomenon, preventive orchiopexy is often performed on the contralateral nontorsed testicle. Hadziselimovic found pre-existing contralateral testicular abnormality in 58% of

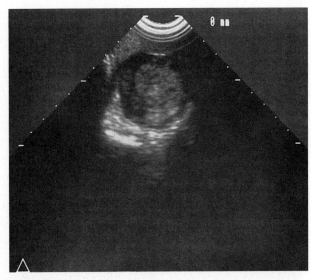

FIGURE 15. On transverse plane ultrasound, a small amount of hydrocele surrounds an irregularly shaped and heterogeneously echogenic mass that is a fractured testis. The fracture occurred from a direct blow with a hammer.

38 boys with acute torsion who underwent contralateral testicular biopsy at the time of surgery. This finding gives credence to the concept that torsion is a bilateral phenomenon and supports the current clinical approach of saving viable twisted testes and removing the nonviable testes.

The patient with acute torsion is, classically, a pubertal male who develops sudden acute scrotal pain. The pain may waken him or develop suddenly during the daytime waking hours. The pain may radiate to the groin or abdomen. Nausea or vomiting occur occasionally. Dysuria is not present, and urinalysis results are negative. Patients may occasionally have fever. Leukocytosis may be present. In some cases there is a history of previous episodes of scrotal pain and tenderness, suggesting previous episodes of torsion with spontaneous detorsion. A history of recent trauma to the testis or strenuous physical exercise is occasionally elicited. An important finding on physical examination that helps make the diagnosis is noting a change in testicular axis from the testis' normal vertical (north to south) positioning in the scrotum to a horizontal one. Within hours of torsion, the patient develops a reddened scrotum, with or without enlargement. The differential diagnostic possibilities include acute idiopathic scrotal edema, hemorrhage into a testicular tumor, and torsion of an intrascrotal hernial sac. Epididymitis, epididymo-orchitis, and torsion of appendages of the testicle or epididymis may also simulate testicular torsion.

IMAGING FINDINGS

US is the key initial imaging tool and often the only diagnostic tool necessary to make the diagnosis and suggest surgical exploration. The typical image of a testicle that has undergone acute torsion is one of a normal-sized to enlarged testicle of normal to decreased

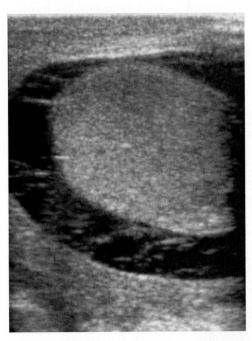

FIGURE 14. On longitudinal plane ultrasound, fluid with contained echogenic material surrounds the normal testicle of a 14-year-old who was kicked in the scrotum several days before. This was hemorrhagic material consistent with a hematocele.

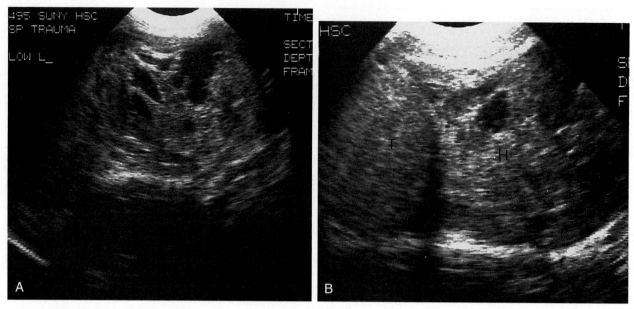

FIGURE 16. Scrotal hematoma simulating testicular fracture. **A,** On ultrasound in the transverse plane, this solid mass with irregular borders and heterogeneous echogenicity was thought to be a testicular fracture in the lower half of the scrotum by a covering house officer. Irregular borders suggesting a tunica albuginea fracture would have required surgical intervention. **B,** An orthogonal view in the longitudinal plane of the hemiscrotum in **A** shows the mass of concern to be not the testicle, but rather a hematoma *(H)*. A normal testicle *(T)* was imaged in a more superior portion of the scrotum (to the reader's left), where it had been pushed by the hematoma. The ultrasound examination was performed 6 days after trauma to the patient's scrotum.

echogenicity. Enlargement and hypoechogenicity are thought to be due to venous congestion. The echogenicity pattern is usually homogeneous. Comparing the echogenicity of the affected testicle with that of the contralateral normal testicle (Fig. 18A) can be of great help. This is best seen on transverse images. Many high-frequency linear array transducers with small footpads are able to show only the medial portions of each testicle for side-by-side comparison. Additional imaging with a high-frequency curved array transducer will allow more complete imaging of both testes in the transverse plane, if they have not been completely imaged with the linear array transducer.

Epididymal enlargement may be an early finding in some cases of torsion. At least 10% of cases of torsion have associated reactive hydroceles. A torsion for which US examination is not performed for more than 48 hours after symptomatology, and the diagnosis of which is therefore delayed (the pejorative term *missed torsion* is often incorrect) (Fig. 18B), may show hetero-

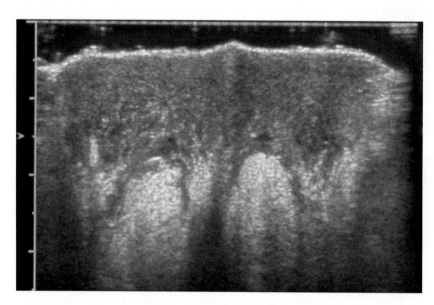

FIGURE 17. A 5-year-old with an enlarged scrotum was noted on ultrasound in the transverse plane to have normal testes deep to the thick, soft tissues of the scrotum. This thickening was due to scrotal wall edema in this patient with nephrotic syndrome that had not been diagnosed prior to the ultrasound exam.

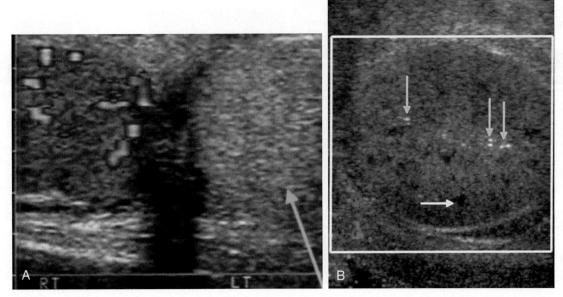

FIGURE 18. Testicular torsion. **A,** Acute left testicular torsion on color Doppler ultrasound in the transverse plane. The right testicle is more echopenic than the left testicle. Often the acutely torsed testicle is more echopenic than the normal one. However, in this case color flow is seen only in the right testicle. The left testicle, despite having the more normal echogenicity pattern, has no color flow and is, therefore, torsed. Note that the high-frequency linear array transducer image used does not allow imaging and comparison cutoff of the lateral aspects of each testicle. **B,** Delayed diagnosis of testicular torsion on color Doppler ultrasound in the longitudinal plane. An enlarged testicle with heterogeneous echogenicity and no contained color flow is seen in this teenager whose testicle had, by history, torsed 4 days prior to his seeking medical care. Echoless areas (*horizontal arrow* points to one) are consistent with destroyed areas of testicular parenchyma. A few bright echoes *(vertical arrows)* were consistent with areas of hemorrhage. *See Color Plate*

geneous or increased echogenicity because of contained hemorrhage/hemorrhagic necrosis.

The key element in the US diagnosis of testicular torsion is Doppler. Doppler allows rapid evaluation of testicular blood flow. Earlier conventional duplex Doppler could listen for absent or decreased arterial flow in the spermatic cord, but intratesticular flow was, at times, difficult to evaluate by this method owing to the smallness of the intratesticular vessels and the necessity to image an individual vessel before insonating it. Lesser sensitivity of Doppler at that time made nuclear medicine pertechnetate studies the gold standard for analysis of patients with possible testicular torsion. Color Doppler US provided a more sensitive tool that was easier to use and that has improved over subsequent years. It allowed a triplex display of gray-scale real-time images of the testes with simultaneous display of vascular flow as a color signal that could be insonated for its spectral pattern.

Color Doppler of a testicle without torsion (Fig. 19) shows readily evident vascular color flow within the testicle. Insonation of the vessels proves them to be arterial or venous. Classically, color Doppler of testicular torsion shows no arterial signals from the testis or the spermatic cord. Normal flow was noted in cases with 0 degrees of experimental torsion. Of concern to imagers and clinicians is the fact that no abnormality of color flow was detected in two rabbits with 180 degrees of testicular rotation. Of six rabbits with 360 degrees of

rotation, four testes showed reduced or absent flow with color Doppler at 24 hours after the injury, but only one of these rabbits had an abnormal nuclear medicine examination. From this work, it was concluded that color Doppler was better than nuclear medicine scintigraphy for evaluating cases of torsion of less than 540 degrees. The sonologist, however, is warned to be wary not only of a lack of flow but of reductions in flow when comparing a testis of concern to the opposite normal testis.

Color Doppler US is also a convenient and reliable procedure for evaluation patients with known or suspected testicular torsion following manual or spontaneous detorsion to determine if the therapy has been successful and normal vascular flow can be detected.

Power Doppler is a more sensitive form of triplex Doppler that can pick up even more subtle (10 to 15 dB) vascular signal and show it as a bright color US image. It has helped make nondiagnostic US studies much rarer. The fact that power Doppler, unlike color Doppler, does not provide information on flow direction is irrelevant in the analysis of flow in the testicle.

State-of-the-art color or power Doppler methods have made US the gold standard for the imaging and preoperative diagnosis of testicular torsion. Identification by Doppler of arterial (and venous) flow in the center of a testicle goes against the diagnosis of torsion. Flow may be normal in a torsed testicle that spontaneously detorsed. Color flow comparison to the contralat-

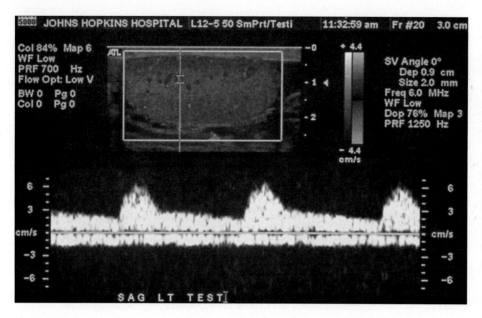

FIGURE 19. Normal color Doppler flow in a testicle. The upper half of the image shows the gray-scale image of a normal testicle. Color within the testicle fills vessels with moving blood flow. Insonation of a point in the upper third of the testicle provides a spectral pattern (lower half of the image) that shows classical arterial signal with its systolic and diastolic components above the baseline and relatively unchanging and continuous venous signal below it. Arterial color Doppler flow signal obtained in the center of a testicle proves there is no torsion. *See Color Plate*

eral testis is helpful and necessary, particularly when torsion may be less than complete (less than 540 degrees in rabbits), in which case the diagnosis may be suggested not by a lack of flow but by an asymmetry of blood flow.

Testicular torsion can occur in undescended testes as well. If the affected testis is in the inguinal canal, pain, swelling, redness, and tenderness in the groin may be observed. Torsion of an intra-abdominal testis in postnatal life may present with abdominal pain and other findings suggesting acute appendicitis.

TESTICULAR TORSION IN THE FETUS AND NEWBORN

The torsion that occurs or is first diagnosed in the newborn period usually presents as a painless, firm scrotal mass often associated with bluish-red discoloration of the scrotum. It may present as scrotal enlargement that may simulate hydrocele. The affected testis is generally nonviable. If the torsion occurred in intrauterine life, one is imaging the neonatal equivalent of a temporally older (delayed diagnosis) torsion.

Antenatal torsion may be diagnosed on fetal US examination. It must be considered if the fetal testicle or testicles are heterogeneous in echogenicity or of asymmetric size (Fig. 20). Diagnosis in the newborn is also made by noting similar imaging findings. Imaging homogeneous testes that are symmetric in size and of normal echogenicity and denoting central arterial flow goes against torsion. The antenatal US analysis may be limited by fetal lie, fetal positioning in that lie, and maternal size. Neonatal US analysis may be difficult because the small scrotum is difficult to image. The presence of hydrocele seen in many newborns actually aids diagnosis by allowing easier imaging of the testicle.

TORSION OF TESTICULAR AND EPIDIDYMAL APPENDAGES—SIMULATORS OF TESTICULAR TORSION

Testicular (and epididymal) appendages may torse. This condition occurs most typically in the 6- to 12-year-old group and represents 5% of cases of acute scrotal pathology in the child and young adolescent. Early in the course of testicular appendix torsion, patients may have localized pain, a pea-sized mass in the area of the upper pole of the testis suggesting the diagnosis, and, at times, a pinpoint discoloration ("blue dot" sign) seen through the overlying scrotal skin. However, within hours the clinical picture may become indistinguishable from that of classical testicular torsion, albeit in a somewhat younger age group. In such cases, US will show normal testicular echogenicity and normal testicular vascular flow. Normal testicular/epididymal appendages are not seen unless there is significant hydrocele surrounding a testicle (see Fig. 7). They are usually small and circular or comma shaped. Often, US, can image the enlarged torsed appendage as a small circular mass (Fig. 21) of variable echogenicity (sometimes with increased echogenicity, sometimes echopenic with increased echogenicity peripherally) near the testicle or epididymis of the affected side. This mass represents the twisted and edematous appendage. Some authors have noted associated epididymal swelling. Although the ability to denote vascular flow to these enlarged appendices via color Doppler is not consistent or, therefore, helpful, color Doppler certainly allows rapid identification of color flow in the testicle, so as to negate the possibility of testicular torsion.

EPIDIDYMITIS

Epididymitis is the most common cause of an acute painful scrotum in the postpubescent male. The cause is usually bacterial, although in pediatric and adolescent patients, epididymitis may be viral (e.g., mumps). Although common in adolescents who are active sexually, it is important to distinguish between scrotal swelling and testicular pain resulting from epididymitis, requiring antibiotics for treatment, and that resulting from testicular torsion, usually requiring urgent surgical exploration. In the adolescent (under 20 years of age), the ratio of epididymitis to torsion cases has been reported as 3:2. After age 20, that ratio is 9:1. These ratios may become somewhat different as sexually transmitted disease becomes more epidemic in the adolescent population. Epididymitis may be seen at an earlier age than adolescence and even, occasionally, in newborns, most usually on a nonsexual basis.

Although the pain of epididymitis usually develops more gradually than in classical cases of testicular torsion (i.e., over a 1- to 2-day period), the clinical picture may simulate torsion. Unlike patients with torsion, patients with epididymitis are often febrile, and at least half complain of dysuria. There is often scrotal edema, testicular tenderness, and a reactive hydrocele. An enlarged epididymis may be palpated. Pyuria is common, and nausea, vomiting, and leukocytosis may be present.

The infection usually responds to antibiotics. The infecting agents include *Staphylococcus, Streptococcus aureus, Escherichia coli, Klebsiella, Pseudomonas*, and in adolescents also *Neisseria gonorrhoeae* and *Chlamydia trachomatis*. Often no organism can be demonstrated. The infection usually reaches the epididymis through the spermatic ducts. Occasionally, infection is via a hematogenous or lymphatic route. Causative factors include urinary tract infections, urethral instrumentation and indwelling catheters, distal urethral obstruction, and reflux of urine from the urethra into the seminal ducts as a result of a congenitally patulous orifice, an ectopic ureter draining into the vas deferens, and an ectopic vas draining into the bladder or ureter. Epididymitis has also been reported in patients with a rectourethral fistula, in patients following scrotal trauma, and in association with meningitis, sepsis, Kawasaki disease, and Henoch-Schönlein purpura.

Complications of epididymitis include direct spread of the infection to the testis (i.e., epididymo-orchitis),

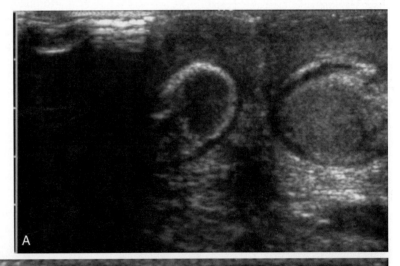

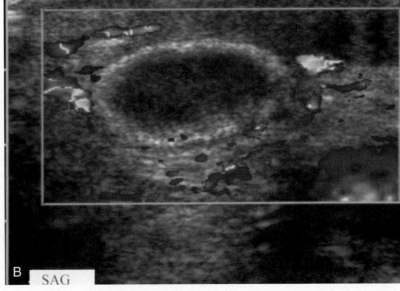

FIGURE 20. Antenatal testicular torsion. **A,** Two testes with torsion of different ages seen on ultrasound in the transverse plane. Two testes of a newborn with scrotal swelling are seen deep to a more superficial thickened scrotal wall. The right testicle is echopenic with a somewhat echogenic periphery, suggesting an old torsion. The grayer left testicle does not appear particularly abnormal on this image, although its periphery is more echogenic than the remainder of its parenchyma. Color Doppler showed no flow in either testicle. Both testes were proven to be torsed at postnatal surgery. The left testicle's torsion probably occurred later in fetal life. There are tiny hydroceles bilaterally. The small scrotum of this newborn allowed it to be seen completely by the high-frequency (14 MHz) linear array probe despite its small footpad. **B,** Torsed right testis as seen on ultrasound in the longitudinal plane. No color flow is seen within the echopenic parenchyma or the surrounding echogenic periphery of this neonate's testicle, torsed during fetal life. *See Color Plate*

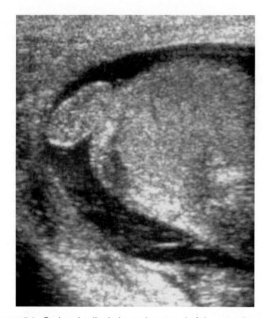

FIGURE 21. On longitudinal plane ultrasound of the superior portion of the scrotum, a prominent oval structure is seen superior to the testicle of a child who presented with sudden testicular pain. The oval structure is of equal echogenicity to the testicle. However it is larger than a normal testicular appendix. It is a torsed testicular appendage. Color flow of the testicle was normal, proving there was no testicular torsion. There is some debris in a small surrounding hydrocele.

which can be seen in as many as 20% of cases. Less usually, an abscess may develop within the scrotum or testes and require drainage. In unusual cases, acute epididymitis may impede testicular blood flow, resulting in focal or diffuse infarction of the testis or epididymis even in the absence of torsion.

Epididymitis evaluated by gray-scale US shows enlargement of the epididymis (Fig. 22A) and commonly a reactive hydrocele. The usual area of involvement is the head of the epididymis, just superior to the testicle. It can also occur in other areas such as the epididymal body or tail. The echogenicity of the enlarged epididymis may be normal, slightly decreased, or slightly increased. In chronic cases, the epididymis is typically hyperechoic. The affected area of epididymis, although enlarged, usually maintains its normal shape. The diagnosis is supported by color Doppler US showing increased flow to the affected epididymis (Fig. 22B).

In most cases of epididymitis, the adjacent testis is usually normal in appearance. With spreading of the infection to the testicle, the homogeneous echogenicity pattern of the testicle is lost. Most often, an echopenic area of involvement is seen within the testicle directly adjacent to the area of involved epididymis, suggesting the diagnosis of epididymo-orchitis (Fig. 23). Although possibly caused by lymphatic or blood-borne organisms, this hypoechoic area is usually caused by direct spread from the epididymis. Color Doppler usually shows

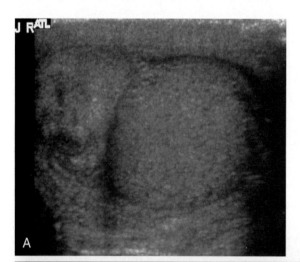

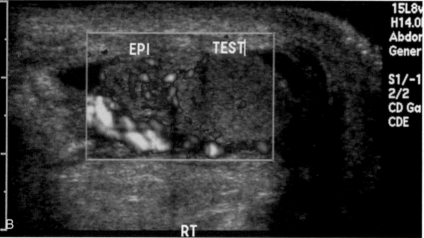

FIGURE 22. A, Ultrasound of the left testicle in the longitudinal plane. The epididymis of this teenager is very large compared to the normal testicle. The patient had epididymitis. **B,** Color Doppler ultrasound of the right testicle, longitudinal plane. Flow to the prominent epididymis of this 10-year-old with epididymitis is greater than that to the testicle. *See Color Plate*

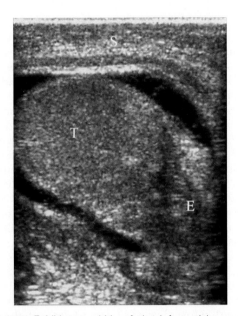

FIGURE 23. Epididymo-orchitis of the left testicle as seen on ultrasound in the longitudinal plane. The scrotum is somewhat thickened, and there is a hydrocele. An enlarged and echopenic portion of the epididymis *(E)* is seen inferiorly and is difficult to separate from the testicle *(T)*. The testicle is echopenic where it is in contact with the inflamed epididymis. The findings are consistent with extension of the infection into the testicle as orchitis.

increased flow to the involved portion of adjacent testicle as well as the epididymis.

Testicular ischemia may play a role in the development of the associated orchitis, because the inflamed and edematous epididymis compresses terminal branches of the spermatic vessels (making this ischemic peripheral area more susceptible to bacterial invasion). The testicular mass of focal orchitis may simulate tumor on US examinations, but the clinical presentation, its association with an enlarged epididymis, and its resolution within weeks with appropriate antibiotic therapy and "tincture of time" helps confirm the infectious etiology and epididymo-orchitis diagnosis.

Testicular scintigraphy with ^{99m}Tc pertechnetate is not often used today. In cases of epididymitis, it can show increased blood flow with increased uptake of the nuclide in the scrotum both during perfusion and in the tissue phase. In the younger patient when epididymitis may be secondary to a congenital anomaly, a voiding cystourethrogram may be performed. Abnormalities such as reflux of contrast into a vas deferens may be imaged.

SCROTAL COMPLICATIONS OF HENOCH-SCHÖNLEIN PURPURA

Henoch-Schönlein purpura is a generalized vasculitis of unknown cause characterized clinically by a purpuric rash, abdominal pain, joint manifestations, and often hematuria. Severe vasculitis of the testis may result in scrotal swelling and tenderness. Sometimes the process is complicated by testicular torsion. Not uncommonly, the scrotum alone is involved by severe purpura and

swelling, simulating an intrascrotal problem. Imaging may be indicated to exclude testicular torsion. A standoff pad or some of the newer higher frequency linear array probes (e.g., 10 MHz), or a combination of the two, can help image the superficial scrotal wall.

TESTICULAR MASSES

Asymptomatic testicular enlargement may be idiopathic or be caused by such conditions as juvenile hypothyroidism with precocious puberty, X-linked megalotestis syndrome, congenital adrenal hyperplasia, and metastatic tumor. Patients with unilateral cryptorchidism may develop compensatory enlargement of the intrascrotal testes. Testicular US is the primary imaging modality used to rule out neoplasm. The finding of homogeneous normal testicular echogenicity makes a tumor an unlikely possibility, although follow-up examination may aid in assuring the absence of an isoechoic lesion.

TESTICULAR AND PARATESTICULAR NEOPLASMS

PRIMARY TESTICULAR NEOPLASMS

Testicular neoplasms are usually a problem of young adults, representing the most common solid tumors of 20- to 35-year-old men. They are uncommon in infants and children, representing 1% to 1.5% of all childhood malignancies. When they do occur in children, they tend to occur in the very young, with a peak incidence of 2 years of age and 60% of the cases occurring in those less than 2 years of age. Such tumors usually present as a painless, nontender, and firm scrotal mass often of weeks' to months' duration. Scrotal pain and tenderness may occur if torsion of the affected testis supervenes. The increased weight of the testicle with a tumor may be responsible for the torsion. Testicular tumors are occasionally bilateral. Signs of precocious puberty or gynecomastia may be present in some cases.

General Imaging Information

The predominant imaging tool for the analysis of the scrotum and its contents is diagnostic US. This is true as well for the evaluation for and of intratesticular tumors. Abdominal US, CT, or MRI is often performed for detection of pelvic or retroperitoneal lymph node enlargement as well as in the search for solid organ metastases. Chest radiographs and CT are used to search for pulmonary metastases. Laboratory serum analysis for testicular tumor markers such as serum α_1-fetoprotein and human chorionic gonadotropin (HCG) can help suggest the primary diagnosis, but are more often used to identify recurrences and analyze effectiveness of therapy.

Scrotal US shows most testicular neoplasms to be hypoechoic (Fig. 24). The image is nonspecific and may be simulated by infarcts, granulomas, and focal orchitis. Contained anechoic areas within such tumors either represent cystic components or more often are evidence of focal necrosis as the tumor outstrips its blood supply. Acute hemorrhage would appear echogenic; older hemorrhage evolves from echogenic to echoless areas as fibrin is deposited and then dissolves. Testicular teratomas are usually less homogeneous than other testicular neoplasms in that, just as in other areas of the body, they show cystic areas, echogenic fat-containing areas, and echogenic foci with posterior shadowing corresponding to intratumoral calcifications or dental structures. Reactive hydroceles are seen in association with testicular tumors in at least 15% to 20% of cases.

CLASSIFICATION OF PRIMARY NEOPLASMS

Primary testicular tumors are classified according to their tissue of origin:

1. Germ cell tumors (yolk sac carcinoma, teratoma, teratocarcinoma, choriocarcinoma, seminoma) occurring as pure histologic patterns or in various combinations (mixed germ cell tumors)
2. Gonadal stromal tumors (Sertoli–granulosa cell, Leydig cell, or granulosa cell tumors)
3. Germ cell plus stromal cell tumors (gonadoblastoma)
4. Tumors of supporting tissues (fibroma, leiomyoma, hemangioma)

Germ Cell Tumors

The majority (65% to 75%) of childhood testicular tumors are germinal cell in type. This is in contrast to the case among adults, in whom almost all (95%) testicular tumors are germinal cell in type. Among adults, these

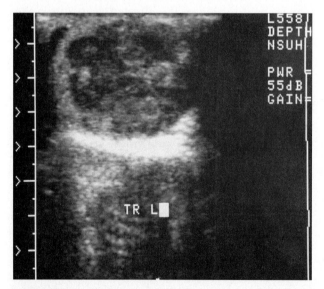

FIGURE 24. On ultrasound in the transverse plane, a predominantly echopenic mass takes up almost the entirety of this patient's left testicle. There is some residual normal tissue at the periphery seen predominantly to the reader's left. This was a seminoma, which is not a typical testicular tumor of childhood.

are typically choriocarcinoma, seminoma, teratocarcinoma, and embryonal carcinoma, which are rare in children.

Yolk sac tumor (also known as yolk sac carcinoma, orchioblastoma, endodermal sinus tumor, or embryonal carcinoma of infancy) is by far the most common germ cell tumor (80% to 90%) in children and therefore the most common testicular neoplasm in children. Three fourths of yolk cell tumors are diagnosed by 24 months of age. They may be aggressive and invade the tunica, distorting the testicular contour. Frequent hemorrhage, particularly after clot dissolution, causes echo-free areas within this typically echopenic, somewhat well-circumscribed mass. An elevated serum α-fetoprotein level is a tumor marker in approximately 90% of affected patients.

Testicular teratoma represents 10% to 15% of childhood germinal cell tumors, usually developing in children between 3 months and 5 years of age. The mean age of diagnosis is 18 months, with 65% of cases diagnosed before 2 years of age. Once thought universally benign, at least one third will show metastases within 5 years of diagnosis. As noted, they appear on US as complex masses with cystic and solid components (Fig. 25A). They are made up of elements derived from all three germ cell layers and may contain cartilage, bony spicules, and epidermal elements such as keratin, fibrous tissue, smooth muscle, and adipose tissue. Many of these tumors contain glial tissue. Contained calcifications and bony or dental structures are often visible on plain film (Fig. 25B). Bony and dental elements are noted as echogenic with posterior shadowing on US, while the adipose component appears echogenic but without shadowing. Prepubertal teratomas are said to almost always follow a benign course even if they contain islands of malignant germ cells (15%). Postpubertal teratomas, in contrast, are frequently malignant or are potentially malignant owing to their propensity to develop components of other germ cell tumors, resulting in teratocarcinomas. The serum HCG level in these cases is usually elevated.

It is known that an undifferentiated testicular teratoma may undergo conversion ("retroconversion") to a mature differentiated teratoma following chemotherapy. One report showed conversion of liver metastases in such a patient to benign fatty and cystic liver masses after chemotherapy.

Some pathologists support the separate categorization of dermoid cyst of the testis from teratoma because the dermoid cyst does not have a propensity to develop malignancy (see Epidermoid Cyst below).

Choriocarcinoma and *seminoma* are extremely rare testicular tumors in children but may occur as histologic components of mixed germ cell tumors.

Gonadal Stromal Tumors

Non–germinal cell types represent only 25% to 30% of pediatric testicular tumors. *Leydig cell* tumors and *Sertoli–granulosa cell* tumors are very uncommon but represent the most common gonadal stromal tumors of childhood. They are almost always benign adenomas. Almost

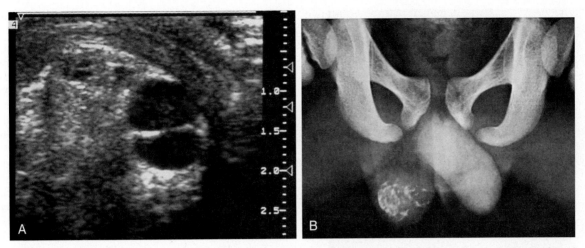

FIGURE 25. Testicular teratoma. **A,** On transverse plane ultrasound, a testicular mass with cystic, debris-filled, and echogenic areas proved to be a teratoma of this child's testicle. (Courtesy of Dr. Leslie E. Grissom.) **B,** On plain film, calcification within the scrotum of this child proved to be from a teratoma of the right testis with calcific components.

half (45%) are Leydig cell tumors, which have a peak incidence at 4 years of age and are the most common testicular malignancy in African-American children. Usually diagnosed between the ages of 2 and 9 years, Leydig cell tumors are painless but may be associated with hormone production. Patients may develop premature virilization (Fig. 26) if androgen is produced or gynecomastia if estrogen is produced. Sertoli cell tumors represent 20% of the non–germinal cell tumors. Half are diagnosed in the first year of life. Gynecomastia caused by estrogen production may occur. Tumors containing a mixture of non–germinal cell histologic patterns may occur.

Germ Cell Plus Stromal Cell Tumors

Gonadoblastomas are composed of germ cells and gonadal stromal cell elements. They are very uncommon and most often seen in older children and adolescents. Punctate dystrophic calcifications within the tumor are common and may be detected roentgen-ographically. Gonadoblastomas are frequently bilateral and generally benign. One tenth of cases, however, are associated with or develop germ cell tumors, including embryonal carcinoma, yolk sac tumor, and choriocarcinoma. Pure germ cells tumors and mixed germ cell tumors, particularly containing seminoma and gonadoblastoma, occur with some frequency in mostly adult patients born with certain disorders of sex differentiation, particularly in patients born with a Y chromosome, dysgenetic gonads, and ambiguous external genitalia.

Epidermoid Cyst

The epidermoid cyst (Fig. 27) is a benign tumor of germ cell origin that is uncommon, representing less than 1% of all testis tumors. It is most commonly found in the second to fourth decades of life. It typically consists of a simple squamous cell–lined echopenic area located within the testicular parenchyma usually just below the tunica albuginea. The wall is made up of fibrous tissue, and its lumen contains cheesy keratinized material or

FIGURE 26. This African-American child presented with precocious puberty (i.e., early virilization). On ultrasound in the longitudinal plane, multiple calcifications (bright echogenicities) are scattered in the testicular parenchyma. There is shadowing beyond one or two of the calcifications. The tumor was proven histopathologically to be a Leydig cell tumor, the most common testicular malignancy of African-American children and a common cause of early virilization. (Courtesy of Dr. Tom Smith.)

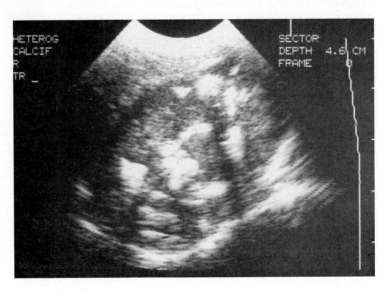

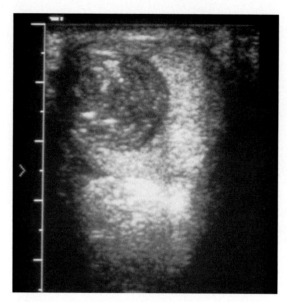

FIGURE 27. On transverse plane ultrasound, an echopenic mass with some echogenic (onion skin) layering is seen with the testicle in this young adult. This proved to be an epidermoid tumor. (Courtesy of Dr. Sheila Sheth.)

amorphous debris. These tumors do not contain elements such as sebaceous material or hair that would suggest the testicular teratoma and therefore the possibility of premalignancy. However, often one cannot definitively differentiate the US image of this mass from that of a teratoma, and histologic analysis is necessary before making a definitive diagnosis and resultant therapeutic decisions.

Patients usually present with a painless 0.5- to 4-cm nodule often picked up incidentally on routine physical examination. Occasionally, patients may present with diffuse testicular enlargement. US examination shows an echopenic mass with an echogenic wall. The "cyst" contents prevent the description as a classical cystic on US. Occasionally the wall may calcify.

Testicular Tumors Originating from Testicular Supporting Tissues

Testicular tumors originating from testicular supporting tissues are rare and mostly benign. They include leiomyoma, fibroma, hemangioma, and lymphangioma. Isolated and rare cases of leiomyosarcoma and fibrosarcoma can occur in childhood. Their US images are similar to such connective tissue tumors elsewhere in the body. They appear solid. Many originate from the cells of the tunica albuginea.

SECONDARY TESTICULAR NEOPLASMS

Testicular metastases are rare in children, representing far less than 1% of testicular tumors. Leukemia and lymphoma are the most common causes. Enlarged testes caused by leukemic or lymphomatous infiltration are

uncommon but may be the primary manifestation of these diseases.

Acute lymphocytic (lymphoblastic) leukemia (ALL) is the most common secondary testicular neoplasm in children. The lesion is often bilateral. The affected testis may be normal in size or enlarged. At least 8% of ALL patients have testicular involvement at some point during the course of their disease. There is an incidence among autopsy specimens of 92%. These enlarged testicles have focal (Fig. 28) or diffuse areas of decreased echogenicity. Areas of hemorrhage appear echogenic, and lymphatic obstruction may lead to hydrocele. Color Doppler imaging often shows significant increases in flow, often in an asymmetric pattern related to the position of the infiltrating masses within the testicle.

Testicular involvement may be present when leukemia is first diagnosed, and occasionally testicular enlargement resulting from leukemic cell infiltration is the presenting manifestation of leukemia. It is a key diagnostic consideration when analyzing patients with intrascrotal symptomatology who have undergone treatment for leukemia and are in remission. With more aggressive treatment to prevent the central nervous system of leukemics from becoming a sanctuary site for leukemic cells, the testes are now the main potential sanctuary site in boys and therefore a key area to evaluate for recurrence of leukemia. Unilateral or bilateral testicular enlargement seen in the first 2 years after bone marrow remission can be a first sign of relapse. This may be followed by bone marrow relapse and widespread metastatic disease because chemother-

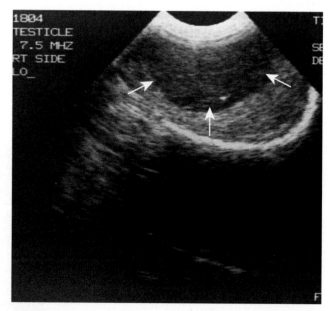

FIGURE 28. An echopenic mass *(arrows)* is seen on ultrasound in the longitudinal plane in the right testicle of this teenager with leukemia who was thought to be in remission. The testicle was enlarged. The echopenic area proved to be due to leukemic involvement of the testicle. (From Cohen HL, Sivit C [eds]: Fetal and Pediatric Ultrasound: A Casebook Approach. New York, McGraw-Hill, 2001. Reproduced with permission of McGraw-Hill Companies.)

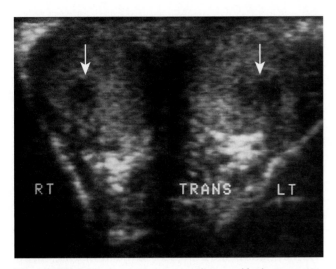

FIGURE 29. Adrenal rests as seen on ultrasound in the transverse plane. Single echopenic masses *(arrows)* are seen in both the right and left testicles of this boy with congenital adrenal hyperplasia. (Courtesy of Dr. Carlos Sivit, Cleveland, OH.)

apy is less effective in dealing with leukemic cells in the testis as compared to other organs.

ADRENAL RESTS

Adrenal rests are simulators of intratesticular tumors. At times aberrant cells from the adrenal cortex may travel with gonadal tissue and be incorporated into the testis during fetal life. With high levels of adrenocorticotropic hormone and associated cortical cell stimulation, these rests may enlarge and appear mass-like (Fig. 29). This stimulation occurs in patients with congenital adrenal hyperplasia, whether early in life as infants or later as adolescents or young adults. It can also occur in patients with Cushing's syndrome. Patients present with testicular mass or enlargement. On US, one usually sees several echopenic masses, usually in both testes. They can be echogenic. A typical color Doppler pattern has been

described in which multiple peripheral vessels radiate in a spoke-like fashion from the centers of individual rest masses. Similar rests may be found in the epididymis or spermatic cord.

TESTICULAR MICROLITHIASIS AND ITS ASSOCIATION WITH TESTICULAR TUMORS

Testicular microlithiasis is an uncommon condition characterized by calcifications within the lumina of seminiferous tubules. It is denoted on US by individual tiny, bright echogenicities (Fig. 30) within the testicular parenchyma. Some reserve the diagnosis for cases in which more than five microliths are noted on a single US image. It is usually an incidental finding. However there is an association between the presence of testicular microlithiasis and the presence or development of testicular neoplasm, particularly germ cell neoplasia. Although usually seen in young adults, the finding may be made in adolescents.

According to two major studies of prevalence of testicular microlithiasis and tumor risk by Cast et al. and Skyrme et al., there is a 0.68% to 1.1% prevalence and a 13 to 21.6 times greater risk for the presence of a testicular neoplasm. Among the 54 tumors noted by these studies, there were 28 seminomas, 14 teratomas, 8 mixed germ cell tumors, 2 Leydig cell tumors and 2 non-Hodgkin's lymphomas. Because of the association of microlithiasis and tumors, patients with testicular microlithiasis alone are followed closely both clinically and by US for possible tumor development over time.

INTRASCROTAL EXTRATESTICULAR MASSES

PARATESTICULAR RHABDOMYOSARCOMA

Primary extratesticular neoplasms are rare; 70% are benign spermatic cord tumors, and paratesticular neu-

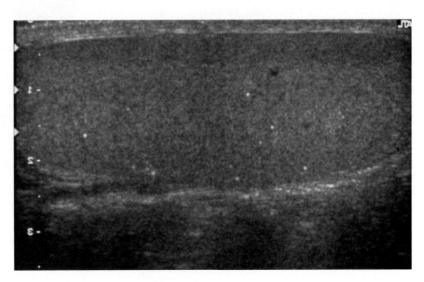

FIGURE 30. Testicular microlithiasis as seen on ultrasound in the longitudinal plane. Several tiny, bright echoes are noted within the otherwise normal right testicle of this teenager. This was an incidental finding in both his testes. There is, however, an association between testicular microlithiasis and the coexistence or future development of a testicular neoplasm.

roblastomas have been reported. Rhabdomyosarcoma is the most common malignant paratesticular mass in the child, representing 10% of intrascrotal tumors of childhood. It originates from the supporting stroma of the spermatic cord, testicular appendages, and paratesticular tunics, and is often located superior to the testis. It often presents as a painless mass in the scrotum of a young boy. There are two incidence peaks for intrascrotal rhabdomyosarcoma, one at 2 to 4 years of age and the other between 15 and 17 years. Rhabdomyosarcomas grow rapidly and are frequently large at presentation. They spread early to regional and retroperitoneal lymph nodes. Venous invasion and distant metastases, especially to the lungs, are not uncommon. There are three types of rhabdomyosarcomas: (1) the anaplastic type, (2) a type composed of round cells of uniform size, and (3) a mixed type. The mixed type is the most common (80%) and has a more favorable prognosis. Prognosis is related to the extent of the tumor at diagnosis. On US examination, the mass is predominantly echogenic with focal anechoic areas caused by necrosis. As with all extratesticular masses, if the testes are invaded, differentiating the lesion from a mass of testicular origin may be difficult.

VARICOCELES

A common mass found within the scrotum of adults or teenagers are varicoceles, which are dilated veins of the pampiniform plexus. They are thought to usually develop because of incompetence of the internal spermatic vein. Varicoceles are graded according to their size. Approximately 65% are grade I, which are defined as small varicoceles palpated with difficulty, and usually appearing as only mild thickening of the cord on physical exam. One fourth (24%) are grade II, defined as moderate in size, easily discovered on physical examination, and consisting of a mass of veins up to 2 cm in diameter. Ten percent of cases are grade III, with the varicocele made up of individual veins greater than 2 cm in diameter. The scrotum of such affected individuals is said to look like a "bag of worms."

When unilateral, 99% of varicoceles are left sided. Theoretically this is a result of increased pressure on the left renal vein with concomitant increased pressure and retrograde flow into its branch (the left spermatic vein) caused either by compression between the aorta and the superior mesenteric artery (the "nutcracker" phenomenon) or by incompetent or absent valves in the internal spermatic vein. Varicoceles most often develop on the left side of the body where the spermatic vein enters the renal vein at a right angle. This anatomy seems to be linked to a far greater chance for venous incompetence compared to the right side, where the right spermatic vein enters the inferior vena cava directly at an oblique angle. The occurrence of bilateral varicoceles is common. Because of the aforementioned facts regarding normal anatomy that seem to protect the right side, finding a solitary right-sided varicocele is extremely

uncommon. If noted, the examiner must rule out intra-abdominal neoplasm or other mass as a cause. Varicoceles are painless and may disappear on supine examination. Therefore, physical examination with the patient in standing position and, if necessary, bearing down, may be required to make the diagnosis.

The major imaging method for varicocele analysis is US. On US examination, varicoceles are tortuous, tubular, echo-free structures (Fig. 31A) that may be situated superior, lateral, and/or posterior to the testicle. Doppler examination (especially color Doppler) can confirm the vascular nature of these structures. More often the diagnosis is confirmed by having the patient perform a Valsalva maneuver, sometimes standing but even in supine position, and noting via color Doppler that the tubular vessels, which may not show evident intraluminal flow prior to the maneuver, will fill with color (Fig. 31B). Flow can be proven as venous by spectral Doppler analysis. Having the patient strain or perform a Valsalva maneuver may show the spectral pattern change (Fig. 31C) from no or little flow to a significant increase in spectral flow the equivalent of the change seen with strain and color Doppler flow.

The diagnosis of varicoceles is of great significance because of their association with infertility in the adult male (39% of infertile men have varicoceles) and their possible gonadotoxic effect on the testes over time. Surgical ligation of the varicocele is therapeutically recommended in cases when there is ipsilateral testicular volume loss of 2 ml or greater. Histologic analysis of such testicles have shown various degrees of tubal hypoplasia, decreased spermatogenesis, focal fibrosis, or arrest of germ cell maturation. Kass et al. operated on 20 grade II to III patients with left varicocele and testicular volume loss and showed that 16 had increases in left testicular volume on follow-up after ligation of the varicoceles.

There are rare instances of intratesticular varicoceles that appear on US and Doppler, as if the testicular parenchyma has been replaced by cystic areas with venous flow patterns.

OTHER EXTRATESTICULAR MASSES

Cystic masses in the epididymis are known as *spermatoceles* when they are large and as *epididymal cysts* when small. They represent a confluence of dilated efferent ductules of the testis filled with seminal plasma. Most are of idiopathic origin. They can occur in patients with chronic epididymitis and have been reported in patients whose mothers were exposed to diethylstilbestrol. On US examination, a spermatocele typically appears as solitary echo-free mass (Fig. 32) that, on occasion, may appear septated.

Epididymal sperm cell granulomas may simulate neoplasm. This typically hypoechoic solid mass with echogenicity caused by contained fibrous connective tissue is the result of an inflammatory response to the extravasation of spermatozoa. Epididymal sperm cell granulomas may present as a painless intra- or extratesticular mass.

FIGURE 31. A and **B,** Varicocele as seen on ultrasound in the transverse plane. **A,** Tubular echoless structures were noted lateral to a teenager's left kidney. One is noted to be 2.7 mm wide. **B,** This image was obtained using color Doppler and straining by the patient. Color fills several of the tubular structures. A venous spectral pattern was obtained to prove them to be varicoceles. The normal kidney is seen to the reader's left. **C,** On triplex Doppler, the top half of the image shows tubular structures in the scrotum of another teen. They appear to be those of a varicocele. The lower half of the image shows the spectral pattern over time. *Arrows* point out when the patient strained. The strain resulted in significant venous-type flow increase, proving the structures to be due to a varicocele. *See Color Plate*

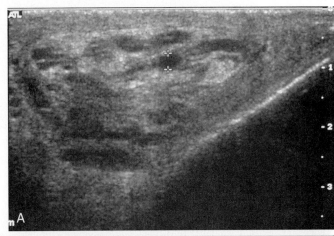

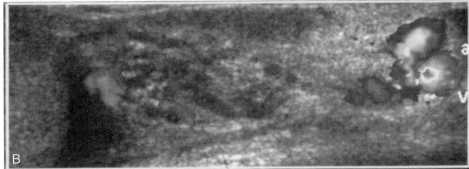

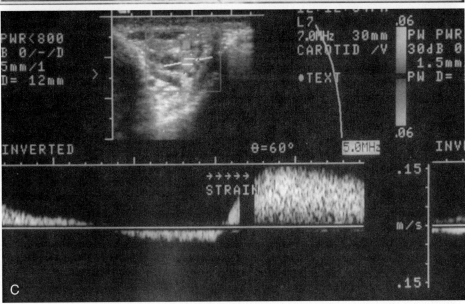

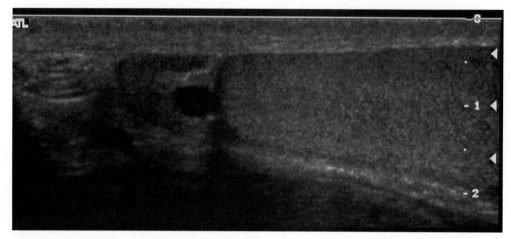

FIGURE 32. A small cystic area is seen in this teenager's epididymis on ultrasound in the longitudinal plane proved to be a spermatocele.

SUGGESTED READINGS

Anderson K, McAninch J, Jeffrey RB, Laing F: Ultrasonography for the diagnosis and staging of blunt scrotal trauma. J Urol 1983;130:933

Avila N, Premkumar A, Shawker T, et al: Testicular adrenal rest tissue in congenital adrenal hyperplasia: findings at gray-scale and color Doppler US. Radiology 1996;198:99

Benson CB, Doubilet PM, Richie JP: Sonography of the male genital tract. AJR Am J Roentgenol 1989;153:705

Brown SM, Casillas V, Montalvo B, Aldores-Saavedra J: Intrauterine spermatic cord torsion in the newborn with sonographic and pathologic correlation. Radiology 1990;177:755

Burks DD, Markey B, Burkhard T, et al: Suspected testicular torsion and ischemia: evaluation with color Doppler sonography. Radiology 1990;175:815

Cast J, Nelson W, Early A, et al: Testicular microlithiasis: prevalence and tumor risk in a population referred for scrotal sonography. AJR Am J Roentgenol 2000;175:1703

Cohen HL, Haller J: Scrotal ultrasound in the pediatric and adolescent patient. Radiol Rep 1990;2:276

Cohen HL, Shapiro M, Haller J, Glassberg K: Sonography of intrascrotal hematomas simulating testicular rupture in adolescents. Pediatr Radiol 1992a;2:296

Cohen HL, Shapiro M, Haller J, Glassberg K: Torsion of the testicular appendage. J Ultrasound Med 1992b;11:81

Cohen HL, Sivit C (eds): Fetal and Pediatric Ultrasound: A Casebook Approach. New York, McGraw-Hill, 2001

Connor S, Guest P: Conversion of multiple solid testicular teratoma metastases to fatty and cystic liver masses following chemotherapy: CT evidence of "maturation." Br J Radiol 1999;72:1114

Dambro T, Stewart R, Carroll B. The scrotum. In Rumack C, Wilson S, Charboneau J (eds): Diagnostic Ultrasound. St. Louis, Mosby, 1998:791

Ganem J: Testicular microlithiasis. Curr Opin Urol 2000;10:99

Giwercman A, Grindsted J, Hansen B, et al: Testicular cancer risk in boys with maldescended testis: a cohort study. J Urol 1987;138:1214

Gross B, Cohen HL, Schlessel J: Perinatal diagnosis of bilateral testicular torsions: beware of torsions simulating hydroceles. J Ultrasound Med 1993;12:479

Hadziselimovic F: Treatment of cryptorchidism with GnRH. Urol Clin North Am 1982;9:413

Horstman W, Middleton W, Melson G, Siegel B: Color Doppler US of the scrotum. Radiographics 1991;6:941

Jensen MC, Lee K, Halls J, Ralls P: Color Doppler sonography in testicular torsion. J Clin Ultrasound 1990;18:446

Kass E, Chandra R, Belman A: Testicular histology in the adolescent with a varicocele. Pediatrics 1987;79;996

Koff WJ, Scaletscky R: Malformations of the epididymis in undescended testes. J Urol 1990;143:340

Kurtz A, Middleton W: Ultrasound: The Requisites. St. Louis, Mosby, 1996:446

Lerner RM, Mevorach RA, Hulbert WC, Rabinowitz R: Color Doppler US in the evaluation of acute scrotal disease. Radiology 1990;176:355

McAlister WH, Sisler CL: Scrotal sonography in infants and children. Curr Probl Diagn Radiol 1990;19:207

Middleton WD, Siegel B, Melson G, et al: Acute scrotal disorders: prospective comparison of color Doppler US and testicular scintigraphy. Radiology 1990;177:177

Moore CCM: The role of routine radiographic screening of boys with hypospadias: a prospective study. J Pediatr Surg 1990;25:339

Musmanno ML, White JM: Scrotal ultrasonography as adjunct to testis biopsy in leukemia. Urology 1990;35:239

Ozcan H, Aytac S, Yagci C, et al: Color Doppler ultrasonographic findings in intratesticular varicocele. J Clin Ultrasound 1997;25:325

Ralls PW, Jensen M, Lee K, et al: Color Doppler sonography in acute epididymitis and orchitis. J Clin Ultrasound 1990;18:383

Ralls PW, Larsen D, Johnson M, Lee K: Color Doppler sonography of the scrotum. Semin Ultrasound CT MR 1991;12:109

Riebel T, Herrmann C, Wit J, Sellin S: Ultrasonographic late results after surgically treated crytorchidism. Pediatr Radiol 2000;30:151

Siegel M (ed): Male genital tract. In Pediatric Sonography, 2nd ed. New York, Raven Press, 1995:479

Skyrme R, Fenn N, Jones A, Bowsher W: Testicular microlithiasis in a UK population: its incidence, association and follow-up. BJU Int 2000;86:482

Trambert MA, Mattrey R, Levine D, Berthoty D: Subacute scrotal pain: Evaluation of torsion versus epididymitis with MR imaging. Radiology 1990;175:53

Troughton AH, Waring J, Longstaff A, Goddard P: Role of magnetic resonance imaging in the investigation of undescended testes. Clin Radiol 1990;41:178

Ulbright T, Srigley J: Dermoid cyst of the testis: a study of five postpubertal cases, including a pilomatrixoma-like variant, with evidence supporting its separate classification from mature testicular teratoma. Am J Surg Pathol 2001;25:788

Vanzulli A, DelMaschio A, Paesano P, et al: Testicular masses in association with adrenogenital syndrome: US findings. Radiology 1992;183:425

Zerin JM, DiPietro MA: Testicular infarction in a newborn: ultrasound findings. Pediatr Radiol 1990;20:329

ABNORMALITIES OF THE FEMALE GENITAL TRACT

HARRIS L. COHEN
JACK O. HALLER

IMAGING TECHNIQUES

GENERAL OVERVIEW

The key technique in the analysis of the pediatric gynecologic tract, its diseases, and the simulators of those diseases is ultrasound (US). It provides quick analysis of the uterus, ovaries, and cul-de-sac. Real-time examinations allow for rapid shifting of transducer position and the subsequent assessment of other organs (e.g., kidney for renal stones) or organ systems (e.g., the gastrointestinal tract to rule out nonperforated appendicitis), when necessary, to complete the analysis of an apparent gynecologic complaint that may have a nongynecologic cause. US performs these assessments without the use of radiation, an important issue, particularly in the young.

Computed tomography (CT) allows excellent analysis of the global contents of the pelvis in an axial plane. It is most helpful in cases in which the US examination is inconclusive, usually because of bowel gas interference. When additional information is needed, CT is particularly useful regarding localization of a pelvic mass and the assessment of its resectability. Despite this ability, once a mass is very large, the analysis of its borders and organ of origin may be limited or impossible. CT is extremely sensitive in denoting density differences among imaged structures and can note the presence of subtle areas of calcium or fat within pelvic masses. It is of major help in the analysis of the bony pelvis. Use of the technique has been limited in children because of the need to sedate (now less necessary because of quicker spiral and volume CT scanning) as well as the child's paucity of intrapelvic and intra-abdominal fat, which obscures identification of visceral borders. CT is far less helpful than US for the analysis of the normal and anomalous gynecologic tract because it does not image the ovaries (particularly normal ones) well, uses radiation, and provides initial imaging in only one plane. US surpasses CT in the ability to analyze small cysts and cystic structures, including ovarian follicles/cysts.

Magnetic resonance imaging (MRI) provides multiplanar analysis without radiation and with superior tissue resolution. These examinations have poorer spatial resolution than CT and difficulty in imaging calcium. Although MRI is making progress in providing improved analysis of uterine and other müllerian duct anomalies, it still remains a secondary exam because of its cost and the need to sedate the uncooperative patient since study times are longer than those of US or CT.

CT and MRI provide a more global view of the pelvis and abdomen than does US and are preferred for the analysis of tumor extent and metastases. They are particularly helpful and better than US in the assessment of the mesentery and peritoneum.

The aforementioned cross-sectional imaging modalities, as well as plain film, nuclear medicine, genitourinary and gastrointestinal contrast examinations, and angiography, are the imager's tools in the evaluation of the pediatric pelvis. Each has its limitations and drawbacks. The drawbacks of radiation exposure, less than optimal control of the patient's environment, and the need to sedate are of particular relevance in the pediatric patient (although they become less so with increasing patient age), and are the reason that US remains the screening examination of choice in these assessments.

DIAGNOSTIC ULTRASOUND—TECHNIQUE AND TECHNICAL FACTORS

US examinations of the pelvis are hindered by air-containing bowel. Fluid in the bladder from patient drinking or from placement via a Foley catheter lifts loops of small bowel superiorly and out of the pelvis. The fluid-filled bladder is an excellent US window for analysis of the gynecologic structures posterior and posterolateral to it. Little if any of the ultrasound beam is lost to scatter. Traditionally, neonates were examined with 7.5 MHz transducers, children with 5- or 7.5-MHz transducers, and adolescents with 5- or 3.5-MHz transducers. Newer multifrequency transducers have expanded the sonographer's choices. These transducers have a range of megahertz capability, allowing the examiner to penetrate to deeper structures requiring lower settings (e.g., 3.5 MHz) and then, with a flick of a switch, changing the same transducer's setting to, for example, 7 MHz for improved superficial scanning. Transducer choices are always a compromise between the better near-field resolution of high-frequency transducers and the better penetration of low-frequency transducers.

There have been tremendous technical improvements in US over the last decade. Sonographic resolution has improved markedly with advances in transducer technology. Improved high-resolution transducers are available. There is electronic control of transducer "focal points." Linear- and convex linear (curvilinear)–design transducers allow improved near-field analysis compared to older sector transducers while, in the case of convex linear probes, still allowing imaging of deeper structures that are longer than the transducer footprint.

Cineloop features, which have been around for more than a decade, allow the retention and review of a number of images seen prior to that of a frozen image and allow faster examination times in even the most uncooperative of children.

Doppler US and color Doppler imaging (CDI) allow rapid identification of both normal and abnormal vessels. They allow identification of the possible vascular nature of cystic masses and enable the sonologist to obtain physiologic data in addition to the usual morphologic image. Power Doppler imaging is a somewhat more sensitive imager of vascular flow compared to classical CDI, although at the cost of information on flow direction.

Transvaginal (TV) transducers have been a boon in the diagnosis of ectopic pregnancy, pelvic inflammatory disease (PID), and other intrauterine and adnexal assessments. The TV or endovaginal transducer is typically 5 to 6.5 MHz, allowing improved resolution of structures within its field of view (i.e., the uterus and the ovaries) when present in the lower pelvis. It can be placed endovaginally in sexually active teenagers, after being placed in a condom or other probe cover containing some couplant gel. Transducer gel is also used on the outside of the probe and cover for proper imaging, because air between transducer and examined part may hinder proper imaging. A full bladder is not necessary for TV imaging. However, because of the limitation of the far-field view with the higher megahertz TV transducer, many radiologists will examine a patient with routine transvesicle (through a filled bladder) technique to assess the pelvis globally, have the patient void, and then perform a transvaginal exam for additional information that may be needed. Some physicians will begin a study with the TV probe and then wait for the patient's bladder to fill or fill the bladder with a Foley catheter if an answer is not obtained or transvesicle (transabdominal; TA) images are needed. In the virginal patient, one can obtain some of the benefits of TV scanning by transperineal (translabial) scanning. The covered TV or other probe is placed at the introitus. Images in longitudinal and transverse planes are typically obtained. This method has been successfully used for the assessment of vaginal stenosis and vaginal obstruction.

Some recent work with three-dimensional ultrasound software, which has proven helpful in fetal anatomy analysis, has shown usefulness with regard to uterine anatomy, particularly for müllerian duct anomalies.

THE PEDIATRIC AND ADOLESCENT GYNECOLOGIC TRACT—WHAT IS NORMAL?

THE NORMAL OVARY

The normal ovary is an ovoid structure located in the mesovarium of the broad ligament. The two ovaries are generally located posterior or lateral (Fig. 1) to the uterus, medial and anterior to their ipsilateral iliac vessels, and adjacent to the ipsilateral obturator internus muscle. They can often be found alongside the uterus when it is examined in the axial plane and while the transducer is angled in a superoinferior direction. One can occasionally follow the fallopian tube from the cornu of the uterus laterally to find them. Contained follicles help one avoid confusing the ovary with nearby collapsed small bowel. Ovaries may be located anywhere along their embryologic course from the inferior border of the kidney to the broad ligament. The true absence of an ovary is rare. The discovery at surgery of an absent

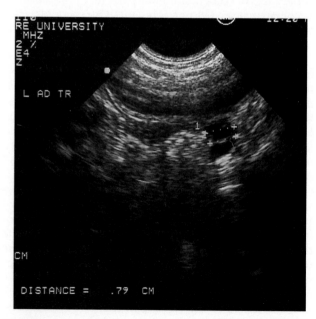

FIGURE 1. Normal left ovary as seen on ultrasound in the transverse plane. Two cysts, marked off by graticles (*crosses*), are seen lateral to the prepubertal uterus of a 6-year-old. Bladder fluid is filled in by near-field artifact.

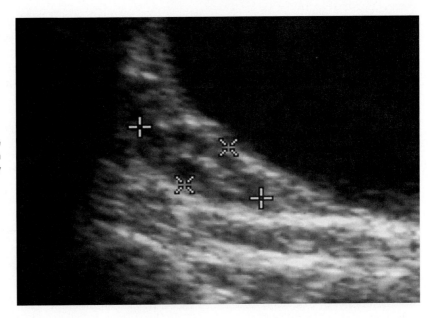

FIGURE 2. Graticles are seen measuring the length and depth of a normal left ovary on ultrasound in the longitudinal plane. A few echoless follicles are seen within the ovary.

ovary and ipsilateral fallopian tube suggests antenatal torsion with secondary necrosis. Ovaries may be involved in indirect inguinal hernias, 15% of which occur in females. Herniated ovaries can extend as low as the labia, the female equivalent of the scrotum.

Despite what has been stated in older articles, the ovaries of pediatric patients are regularly imaged by US. Cohen et al. were able to image in three dimensions 64% of the ovaries of 77 patients between newborn and 2 years of age and 78% of the ovaries of 101 premenarchal children between 2 and 12 years of age.

Adnexal volume is determined by US using the formula for a modified prolate ellipse: $\pi/6$ (or 0.523) $\times$ L $\times$ W $\times$ D, a formula often simplified as W $\times$ L $\times$ D divided by 2. Length (L) and depth (D) are usually measured on a longitudinal (parasagittal) image (Fig. 2) and width (W) on a transverse view.

Concepts of normal ovarian volumes and echogenicity have changed significantly over the last decade for adults as well as children. For example, the oft-repeated but incorrect "$3 \times 2 \times 1$ cm" (3 cm^3 volume) ovarian measurements ascribed to normal adults and older adolescents underestimate the 6 to 9.8 cm^3 mean volumes for menstruating females noted in more recent studies.

What are considered correct ovarian measurements in neonates and children have also changed in recent years aided by larger numbers of patients studied as well as better US equipment. Whereas at one time imaging ovaries in the neonatal group was considered uncommon, it is now considered the norm. Whereas once a measurement of 1 cm^3 was considered the high end of normal for children, this too has changed. In the first 3 months of life, when gonadotropin levels are highest in children (as a consequence of the decrease in neonatal estrogen and progesterone levels caused by separation from the placenta) ovarian volumes average 1.06 cm^3 but have a range of normal as high as 3.6 cm^3. The high end of the range of normal is 2.7 cm^3 for 4- to 12-month-olds and 1.7 cm^3 for 13- to 24-month-olds.

Salardi et al. and Orsini et al. noted mean volumes ranging between 0.75 and 4.18 cm^3 for 101 premenarchal girls. However, they suggested that the normal pediatric ovary was homogeneous in echogenicity (i.e., without follicles/cysts). Using older equipment, they stated that the typical ovary in a child of 6 or younger had no imaged follicles and that cysts and particularly macrocysts (defined by them as >9 mm in largest diameter) were uncommon before 11 years of age. Cohen et al.'s more recent work showed follicles/cysts in the majority of children of all ages. Cysts were noted in 80% of the imaged ovaries of a group of healthy newborns to 2-year-olds (Fig. 3), 72% of a 2- to 6-year-old group, and 68% of a 7- to 10-year-old group. Macrocysts were occasionally seen in all age groups. These more recent US findings are consistent with Rokitansky's 1861 report in the pathology literature that noted the presence of cystic follicles in the ovaries of fetuses, neonates, and children. The ovary is not a quiescent organ in childhood, but rather a dynamic organ undergoing constant internal change.

The fact that ovarian cysts are common findings in children has helped in other aspects of US diagnosis. Imaging follicle/cysts in a labial or inguinal mass in a girl with ambiguous genitalia or herniated ovary suggests that the mass is an ovary. Finding follicles in otherwise normal-appearing ovaries of a child with precocious puberty should not concern the sonologist or endocrinologist. The common finding of cysts, however, does not allow differentiation between the healthy child and the child with isosexual precocious puberty.

THE NORMAL UTERUS

Uterine shape and size change during pediatric life. In the first months of life, the high circulating gonadotropin levels that develop with the decline of maternal estrogen and progesterone after separation of the

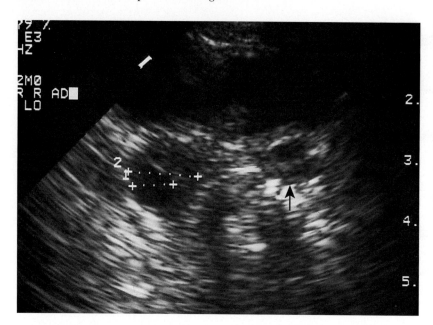

FIGURE 3. Normal ovary seen in a neonate on ultrasound in the transverse plane. Graticles mark off the width of an ovary *(2)* and a contained follicle *(1)*. Follicles/cystic areas are very common in infants such as this 2-month-old. The left adnexum *(arrow)* can also be seen with contained follicles.

neonate from the placenta influence uterine shape and size. The uterus of the newborn has a mean length of 3.5 cm, which decreases to 2.6 to 3 cm by the fourth month of life as the gonadotropin levels decrease. It is not uncommon to find on the US examination of the newborn's uterus either a hypoechoic halo around an imaged echogenic endometrial cavity stripe (Fig. 4), seen in 29% of the patients of Nussbaum's study, or endometrial cavity fluid (23%), both of which are findings far more typical of an adolescent or adult uterus under the cyclical hormonal influences of postmenarchal life.

The typical newborn's uterus is shaped like a spade (see Fig. 4), with the anteroposterior (AP) diameter of the cervix as much as twice that of its fundus. The newborn's cervix is also longer than the fundus. Nussbaum et al. noted the uterus of infant girls to be spade shaped in 58% of cases and tube shaped (AP diameter of cervix equal to AP diameter of fundus) in

32% of cases. One tenth of their cases showed the classical adult uterine shape of a pear, with the fundus wider than the cervix. Our own work shows almost all newborn uteruses to be spade shaped. After the first year of life, the typical uterus is tube shaped (Fig. 5) and remains that way for at least several years.

Identification of the uterus is important information for several clinical diagnostic work-ups, most notably evaluations of children with ambiguous genitalia. The easiest time to image the child's uterus is in the first few months of life.

Uterine length increases gradually between 3 and 8 years of age. The mean perimenarchal measurement is 4.3 cm. Salardi et al. believe that changes in uterine length and change into the adult pear shape are not solely a matter of increasing estradiol levels, but also a function of two other independent variables: age and size of the girl. There is a moderate ($r = .69$) correlation between uterine length and weight in childhood.

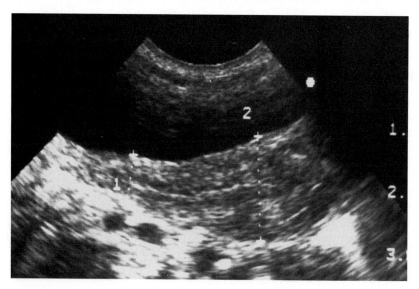

FIGURE 4. A normal neonatal uterus, which is spade shaped, is seen posterior to the echoless bladder on longitudinal plane ultrasound. Graticles marked by the number *1* show a relatively narrow uterine fundus. Graticles marked by the number *2* show the far wider cervical region of the newborn's uterus. Note the central echogenic line, which is the endometrial cavity echogenicity. (From Cohen HL: The female pelvis. *In* Siebert J [ed]: Syllabus: Current Concepts: A Categorical Course in Pediatric Radiology. Chicago, RSNA Publications, 1994:65–72, with permission.)

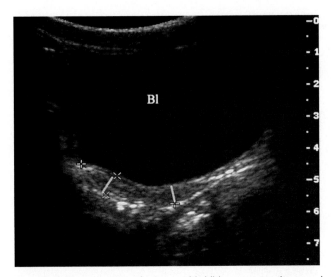

FIGURE 5. Normal uterus of a 6-year-old child as seen on ultrasound in the longitudinal plane. Lines mark off the widths of the cervical area and fundal area, which are similar.

After puberty, the typical pear-shaped (Fig. 6) uterus measures 5- to 8 cm in length. It is said to descend deeper in the pelvis and no longer maintains the typical neutral position of premenarchal life but, rather, may be anteverted or retroverted.

MRI and its multiplanar capability can help in the analysis of the uterus, particularly if a müllerian duct anomaly is suspected. MRI can help identify the tissue composition of an intrauterine septum, thereby allowing differentiation between a bicornuate uterus (Fig. 7), whose septum contains myometrium, and a septate uterus, whose septum does not contain myometrium.

EMBRYOLOGY OF THE (MALE AND) FEMALE GENITAL SYSTEM

Differentiation of the primitive gonad into a testis begins at 7 weeks of fetal life in the presence of the H-Y antigen found on the Y chromosome. If there is no

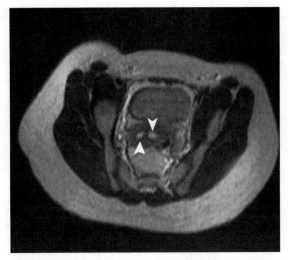

FIGURE 7. Bicornuate uterus on T_1-weighted magnetic resonance imaging in the axial plane. In the middle of the pelvis is a gray structure containing two bright echoes representing the two endometrial cavities *(arrowheads)* seen at this level. The intensity of the tissue between the cavities is the same as that of the surrounding uterus, making it consistent with uterine tissue. (From Cohen HL, Bober S, Bow S: Imaging the pediatric pelvis: the normal and abnormal genital tract and simulators of its diseases. Urol Radiol 1992;14:273–283, with permission.)

Y chromosome, ovarian differentiation begins at 17 weeks' gestation in the presence of two X chromosomes.

Development of the urinary system and genital system are closely associated. Urogenital ridges develop from the intermediate mesoderm and are situated on each side of the primitive aorta. They gives rise to parts of the genital and urinary systems.

The association of uterine and renal abnormalities is quite common, and, when there is a gynecologic anomaly, one should evaluate the renal bed to rule out ectopia or agenesis (Fig. 8). Both sexes develop two different pairs of genital ducts. Components of the wolffian (mesonephric) duct system develop into the epididymis, vas deferens, and seminal vesicles under the influence of testosterone. By 6 weeks, a müllerian (parameso-

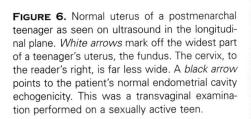

FIGURE 6. Normal uterus of a postmenarchal teenager as seen on ultrasound in the longitudinal plane. *White arrows* mark off the widest part of a teenager's uterus, the fundus. The cervix, to the reader's right, is far less wide. A *black arrow* points to the patient's normal endometrial cavity echogenicity. This was a transvaginal examination performed on a sexually active teen.

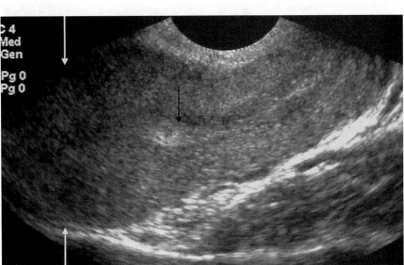

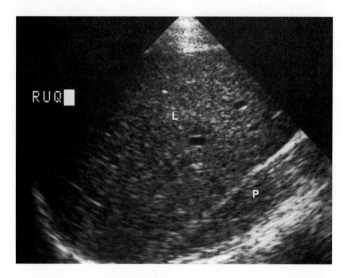

FIGURE 8. Ultrasound of the right upper quadrant in the longitudinal plane shows the liver *(L)* and right psoas muscle *(P)*. No kidney is seen between them, suggesting renal agenesis or ectopia. Nuclear medicine examination proved that there was no right renal ectopia. On the basis of right renal agenesis, the gynecologic tract was assessed in this teenager. The patient had an associated müllerian duct system abnormality—a bicornuate uterus.

nephric) duct has developed lateral to each ipsilateral wolffian (mesonephric) duct. In the female, the müllerian duct system (MDS) develops into the fallopian tubes, uterus, and upper two thirds of the vagina, and the wolffian system degenerates. External genital development proceeds along female lines except in the presence of androgens.

By 11 weeks, a Y-shaped uterovaginal primordium has developed into the two fallopian tubes and, with fusion of a large portion of the MDS of both sides, a single uterus and a single upper two thirds of the vagina. This occurs "passively" (i.e., with or without the presence of ovaries), as long as there are no testes or high levels of androgens present. The testes produce testosterone, a masculinizing hormone, and müllerian inhibiting factor, which suppresses the further development of the paramesonephric ducts.

In females, nonfusion or variably incomplete fusion of the MDS can lead to a wide spectrum of anomalies (Fig. 9). Complete nonfusion results in a didelphys uterus, in which there are two vaginas, two cervices, and two uterine bodies. Various anomalies are associated

with incomplete müllerian duct fusion. Partial fusions of only the caudal ends of the MDS result in a bicornuate uterus, in which there is variable nonfusion of the cranial portion of the uterus resulting in paired and variably separated uterine horns at the fundus that communicate with a correctly fused and, therefore, single uterine body, cervix, and vagina. The bicornuate uterus results in a wider than normal uterus that may be diagnosed on physical examination (usually when a patient is pregnant) by an anterior uterine depression or by US when two endometrial cavity echogenicities (Fig. 10) are imaged. This is usually most readily imaged during the luteal phase of the menstrual cycle or during pregnancy.

Where the MDS joins the urogenital sinus, the lower one third of the vagina develops by elongation of the primitive vaginal plate into a core of tissue that canalizes by week 20. Until late fetal life, the lumen of the vagina is separated from the vestibule of the vagina by a hymenal membrane. The hymen usually ruptures in the perinatal period, remaining as a thin fold of mucous membrane around the vaginal entry.

Male genital system development is "active," requiring the presence of testes and their production of müllerian inhibiting factor, which causes MDS involution. Dihydrotestoterone, acting locally, allows the wolffian duct system to develop into the epididymis, vas deferens, and seminal vesicles. The enzyme 5α-reductase converts testosterone intracellularly, within the target tissues, into the powerful dihydrotestosterone.

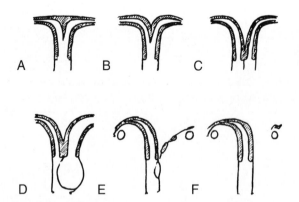

FIGURE 9. Fusion defects of the müllerian ducts (septate vagina with normal uterus not included). **A,** Uterus subseptus (uterus septus if septum extends to cervix). **B,** Uterus bicornis unicollis. **C,** Uterus duplex bicornis bicollis, and uterus didelphys with septate vagina. **D,** Uterus didelphys with congenital occlusion of one hemivagina. **E** and **F,** Rudimentary hemiuterus and unicornuate uterus.

CLINICAL PROBLEMS IN THE PELVIS OF THE FEMALE CHILD AND ADOLESCENT

UTERINE MASSES CAUSED BY VAGINAL AND/OR VAGINAL–UTERINE OBSTRUCTION

Uterine masses are uncommon in childhood. The predominant pelvic mass found in neonates and infants is a distended vagina (colpos) or uterus (metro) filled

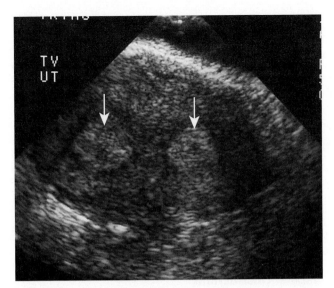

FIGURE 10. Two endometrial cavity echogenicities are seen in the uterus of a teenager on ultrasound in the transverse plane. Their presence suggests a bicornuate uterus, which was confirmed. The findings are similar to those on MRI in Figure 7. The patient was in the second half of her menstrual cycle, an easier time to see the two endometrial cavity echogenicities *(arrows)*, which tend to be wider and more echogenic closer to the time of menses.

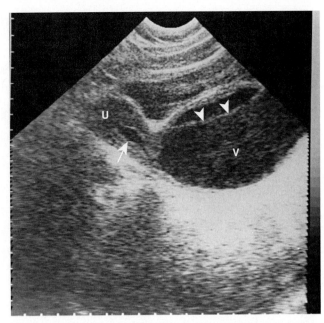

FIGURE 12. This patient presented with pelvic pain and no history of menarche. On ultrasound in the longitudinal plane, the vagina *(V)* is dilated. It contains debris with a fluid–debris level *(arrowheads)* seen in its superior portion. The uterus *(U)* has a smaller amount of contained fluid *(arrow)*. The uterus can be distinguished from the vagina by its thick muscular wall. Dilatation of the uterus and vagina with contained debris is consistent with hematometrocolpos, which this patient had because of menses and an imperforate hymen. (From Cohen H, Haller J: Pediatric and adolescent genital abnormalities. Clin Diagn Ultrasound 1988;24:187–216, with permission.)

with secretions (muco), fluid (hydro), or blood (hemato). For example, hematometrocolpos is defined as hemorrhagic material filling a distended vagina and uterus. US images are similar in appearance whether the affected individual is a neonate or a menarchal teenager. On US, the distended vagina appears as a tubular mass that is usually midline (Fig. 11), often with contained echogenicities either from accumulated cervical mucus secretions or possible hemorrhage from sloughing of a hormonally stimulated endometrial lining. The uterus can be identified separately from the vagina because the muscular uterine wall surrounding the

debris- or heme-filled endometrial cavity is thick while the vaginal wall is thin (Fig. 12).

An obstructed uterus discovered in neonatal life is usually suggested clinically by either seeing an interlabial mass or palpating a uterine mass. Pelvic US is used to confirm these findings. The mass develops in the neonate because of the influence of the high gonadotropin levels on a normal endometrial lining. If the uterus, cervix, and vagina are present and not obstructed, the neonate will soon pass cellular debris, mucoid material, or blood, the equivalent of withdrawal bleeding. If the uterus is obstructed, hydrometra, mucometra, or hematometra will develop. If the uterus and cervix are patent but the vagina is present and obstructed, hydro-, muco-, or hematometrocolpos may develop. The obstructed material may, at times, also be noted in dilated fallopian tubes. At times, the amount accumulated will only fill the vagina. If this obstructive phenomenon is not discovered in neonatal life, the endometrial effluvia will be resorbed and the obstruction will not be discovered until postmenarchal life.

Patients with neonatal hydro/hematometrocolpos can be divided into two groups: those with and those without associated cloacal (single perineal opening for bladder, vagina, and rectum) or urogenital sinus (single perineal opening for bladder and vagina) malformations.

Only a few patients with a congenital vaginal obstruction present at birth with hydrocolpos. Most patients are asymptomatic at birth and during childhood but present

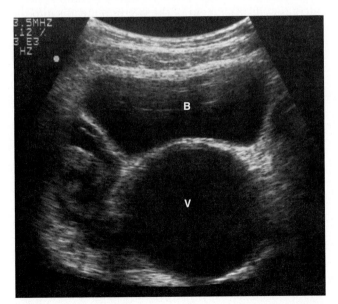

FIGURE 11. On transverse plane ultrasound, a large midline circular cystic structure is seen behind the bladder *(B)*. It was a fluid-filled, dilated vagina *(V)* (hydrocolpos) in a teen with an imperforate hymen.

in the postpubertal years because of failure of menstruation despite normal development of secondary sex characteristics. Clinical presentations include amenorrhea and cyclic crampy abdominal pains or a pelvic mass resulting from accumulation of menstrual blood in the proximal vagina (uterus and tubes). The degree of vaginal and uterine dilatation is related to the degree of obstruction (usually complete) and the time lapse between true menarche and the diagnosis. Patients with an imperforate hymen may present with a bulging, bluish cystic mass protruding from the introitus. In others, only a cystic pelvic mass is diagnosed clinically, by US, or by MRI. A vaginogram may show a shallow, blind-ending vagina in such patients.

Unlike the rarity of the diagnosis of hydro/hematometrocolpos in neonatal life, it is more common among teenagers, occurring in 1 in every 1000 to 2000 adolescent females. It is said that such masses may become large enough to result in reported cases of lymphatic or venous flow obstruction or cause hydronephrosis from mass effect on the bladder and ureters. Occasional patients will complain of a relatively recent history of difficulty with micturition.

Complete or partial vaginal and/or uterine obstructions may occur in association with various MDS anomalies. These may include vaginal agenesis associated with uterine cervix atresia, isolated atresia of the uterine cervix, and cases of absence of the vagina in the presence of an entirely normal uterus. As stated, hematocolpos or hematometrocolpos usually suggests an imperforate hymen or transverse vaginal septum. Hematometra alone, however, suggests a more unusual abnormality such as cervical dysgenesis or a partial obstruction of the uterus (e.g., only one horn of a bicornuate system).

Syndrome of Vaginal Agenesis with Rudimentary Uterus (Mayer-Rokitansky-Küster-Hauser Syndrome)

A patient with a dysgenetic MDS may have an absent or rudimentary vagina or uterus as in the Mayer-Rokitansky-Küster-Hauser syndrome. Such patients have normal karyotypes and normal secondary sex development but have associated renal (33% to 50%) and skeletal (12%) anomalies.

Vaginal agenesis, the failure of vaginal development in otherwise normal females, occurs 1 in 4000 to 5000 female births. It is the most frequent cause of primary amenorrhea (no menses by age 16) after classical Turner's syndrome with its infantile uterus. The proximal two thirds of the vagina and sometimes the entire vagina is absent. The uterus is usually rudimentary and is often bicornuate (rudimentary uterus duplex). At times, one of the two uterine anlagen will contain some functioning endometrium. Fallopian tubes are usually normal but may be hypoplastic or absent. Ovaries are almost always present and are usually anatomically and functionally normal. The external genitalia are also normal except for an absent introitus in some cases.

Vaginal agenesis may, on occasion, be familial. There is frequent association with congenital anomalies (more

so than in cases of vaginal obstruction) of other body systems, typically malformations of the upper urinary tract, including solitary kidney, renal fusion, unilateral renal ectopia, and especially pelvic kidney. Anomalies of the renal pelves and ureters as well as the occurrence of vesicoureteral reflux have been reported in these patients. Skeletal abnormalities (12%) are often vertebral, including the Klippel-Feil anomaly, but may also encompass rib anomalies, congenital hip dislocation, pectus deformity, and syndactyly. Cardiac malformations and deafness resulting from middle ear defects occur. An association of absent vagina with middle ear conductive deafness and Klippel-Feil anomaly has been described. Another entity consisting of müllerian duct aplasia, renal aplasia, and cervicothoracic somite dysplasia (MURCS) has also been described.

Vaginal Obstructions

Transverse Vaginal Septum

In transverse vaginal septum, the vagina is obliterated by fibrous connective tissue with vascular and muscular elements lined by squamous epithelium. The area of obliteration may be a thin membrane, but more commonly it involves a segment of the vagina (segmental vaginal atresia). Vaginal septa are most common in the midportion of the vagina but may affect the proximal third of the vagina near the cervix, and occasionally the distal vagina near the hymen.

An association of transverse vaginal septum or segmental atresia of the vagina with postaxial polydactyly has been described as a separate entity occurring as an autosomal recessive trait (McKusick-Kauffman syndrome). Other commonly occurring anomalies in this syndrome are those of the gastrointestinal tract, including imperforate anus and Hirschsprung's disease. Other reported anomalies include those of the eyes; the cardiovascular system; the limbs; the urinary tract, especially dilated upper systems; and the genital system, including displacement of the urethral meatus into the distal vaginal wall (female hypospadias) and duplication of the vagina and uterus. Female members of affected families may show only polydactyly and/or congenital heart disease. Male relatives may be affected by polydactyly and/or hypospadias.

Imperforate Hymen

An imperforate hymen is the simplest and most easily correctable cause of vaginal obstruction. In such cases, the vagina is obliterated by a thin membrane, the hymen, which forms at the junction of the caudal end of the müllerian ducts and the cranial end of the urogenital sinus. The imperforate hymen is not considered a müllerian anomaly because it originates from the urogenital sinus. A transperineal US approach (placing a transducer on the perineum) may more readily denote vaginal obstruction by an imperforate hymen (Fig. 13). Patients with imperforate hymen or vaginal membrane have normal external genitalia, ovaries, fallopian tubes, and uterus.

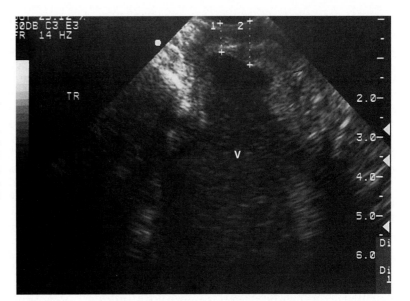

FIGURE 13. Imperforate hymen as seen on ultrasound in the transverse plane. Graticles measure a somewhat asymmetric soft tissue mass that is obstructing the vagina in this 13-year-old who presented with abdominal pain and fever. The distended vagina (V) deep to the superficial hymen has contained debris from hemorrhagic material. The uterus is too deep to be seen on this transperineal image obtained with a high-frequency transducer.

Imaging Vaginal Obstructions

US is the key diagnostic tool in neonatal life. Scattered internal echoes representing cellular and mucous debris and fluid–debris levels may be observed in the dilated obstructed vagina (see Fig. 12). US can denote the linear echogenicity of the nonobstructed coapted vagina. Pelvic MRI in the sagittal or coronal plane can show the dilated vagina (Fig. 14) as well. Although vaginal obstruction may also be noted by CT, that modality is limited to the axial plane. If a diagnosis is still not certain, a contrast vaginogram can be helpful. In cases in which an obstructed vaginal lesion exists at a high level, a vaginogram may demonstrate a short, blind-ending vagina. Placement of contrast into the vagina can help denote obstruction or narrowing on fluoroscopy. An obstructed vagina may be filled on voiding cystourethrography if there is an associated urethrovaginal communication. A congenital fistula between the urethra and vaginal proximal to a vaginal obstruction may be present.

Differential Diagnostic Considerations for a Bulging Mass at the Introitus

Although a bulging cystic mass at the introitus associated with a cystic pelvic mass detectable by US in a newborn or at puberty in an amenorrheic girl is characteristic of neonatal hydrocolpos or pubertal hematocolpos caused by an imperforate hymen, there is a differential diagnosis. The main other possibilities are complex MDS anomalies with obstructions of only a portion of the uterus (e.g., one horn) or a portion of a vagina in cases of duplication and distal obstruction of one hemivagina.

Vaginal Obstructions—Treatment Points

The vaginal obstruction in patients with congenital hydrocolpos is corrected in the newborn period. In patients presenting with hematometrocolpos at puberty, the obstruction should be corrected as promptly as

possible. This is done, in part, to avoid endometriosis as a result of distal obstruction and repeated (reverse) spillage of menstrual blood into the peritoneal cavity through the fallopian tubes. Chronic hematosalpinx can also lead to chronic epithelial changes in the fallopian

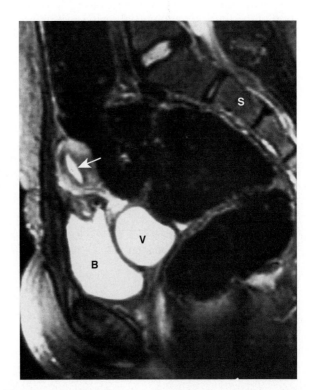

FIGURE 14. Hydrocolpos on T_1-weighted magnetic resonance imaging in the sagittal plane. A dilated, fluid-filled vagina (V) is seen posterior to the bladder (B). Fluid (seen as white on this study) filling the bladder, vagina, and endometrial cavity (arrow) all appears of similar intensity. S = sacrum. (From Cohen HL: Evaluation of the adolescent and young adult with amenorrhea: role of US. In Bluth E, Arger P, Hertzberg B, Middleton W [eds]: Syllabus: A Special Course in Ultrasound: Clinical Questions, Practical Answers. Oak Brook, IL, RSNA Publications, 1996:171–184, with permission.)

tubes, placing fertility at risk and increasing the possibility of ectopic pregnancy. Hysterectomy is indicated in patients with vaginal agenesis with rudimentary uterus and a functional endometrium, and in patients with cervical atresia occurring as an isolated lesion or in association with vaginal agenesis. A detailed evaluation of the uterus, uterine cervix, and vagina by TA and transperineal US and/or by pelvic MRI is indicated prior to any surgery (Figs. 15 and 16). At times, however, the true anatomy of the lesion will only be discovered at surgical exploration.

Müllerian Duct System Anomalies and Unilateral Hydro/hematometrocolpos

The MDS has to undergo a series of meticulous and significant changes in order to develop from a bifid system into a single uterus, a single cervix, a single vagina (upper two thirds), and two fallopian tubes. Many potential errors may occur in this embryologic process. MDS anomalies are said to be very common, occurring in at least 0.1% to 0.5% of females, with some reports indicating as high an incidence as 12%. An incomplete fusion of the distal segment of the two müllerian ducts can result in various degrees of bifidity of the uterus or vagina, or both (see Fig. 9). Abnormalities may range (in order of increasing complexity) from a septate uterus (with merely a septum separating a variable portion of the uterine endometrial cavity) to a bicornuate uterus to the more complex anomalies. Most simple abnormalities may never be discovered unless there is a problem with fertility or the ability to carry a baby to term, and then are discovered in a subsequent work-up. As an example, the bicornuate uterus is usually not discovered until later pregnancy, when the growth of

the uterus allows the clinician to feel the typical anterior depression in the upper uterus from variable separation of the upper uterus into two horns. It is the more abnormal cases, such as uterus didelphys with unilateral vaginal obstruction and unicornuate uterus (syndrome), that have been referred to as potential simulators of simple hydrocolpos.

A didelphys uterus refers to the presence of two hemiuteri, each connected with a separate fallopian tube and with a separate cervix, and often associated with a sagittal vaginal septum. This septum originates at the junction of the two cervices and ends caudally at or near the hymen. In some instances of duplex uterus with a vaginal septum, the caudal end of one hemivagina, more often the one on the left, is congenitally obstructed (uterus didelphys with septate vagina and unilateral vaginal obstruction) (Fig. 17). No hymenal tissue is found on the obstructed side. Renal agenesis, or severe renal dysplasia (and ectopic ureter), is almost always noted on the side of the vaginal obstruction. The disorder may be familial. It may present at birth with a pelvic mass caused by an accumulation of vaginal and cervical secretions within the obstructed hemivagina and hemiuterus. The ipsilateral fallopian tube may also be enlarged. More commonly, as with simpler hymenal membrane obstruction, the patient may present at puberty with cyclic abdominal pain and/or a pelvic mass or on physical examination with a cystic mass protruding from her introitus. A vaginogram may show lateral displacement of the normal patent hemivagina toward the contralateral side.

Unicornuate uterus, or rudimentary uterine horn syndrome, is at the extreme end of the spectrum of müllerian duct anomalies. One of the two müllerian ducts fails to develop or is resorbed, resulting in an

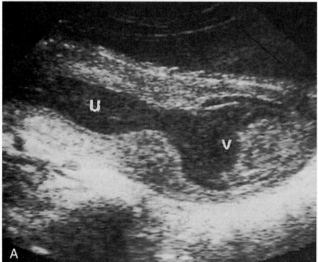
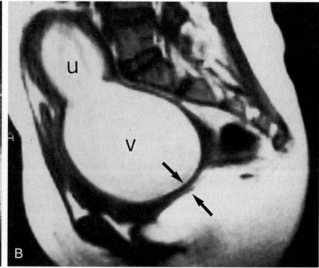

FIGURE 15. Hematometrocolpos from imperforate hymen. **A,** Ultrasound of the pelvis in the longitudinal plane shows a large midline cystic structure consistent with a distended vagina *(V)* and uterus *(U)*. The lower part of the vagina contains echogenic material. The patient is a 13-year-old girl investigated because of crampy abdominal pain and a pelvic mass. The external genitalia appeared normal on inspection. **B,** On T$_2$-weighted magnetic resonance imaging (MRI) of the pelvis in the midline sagittal plane, an enlarged vagina *(V)* and uterus *(U)* filled with material consistent with old blood are seen. The obstruction is in the distal vagina and measures probably 0.5 cm in thickness *(arrows)*. The MRI exam was obtained for presurgical planning. At surgery, this obstruction was found to be a very low vaginal septum or a very thick imperforate hymen.

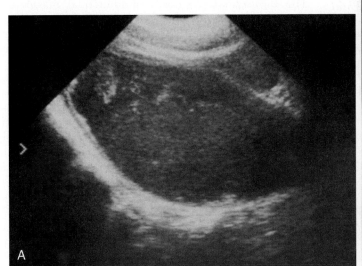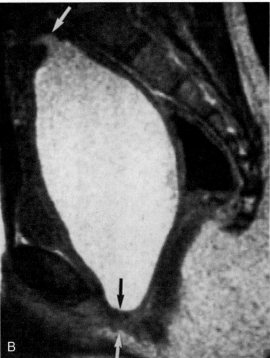

FIGURE 16. Hematocolpos from vaginal atresia in a 12-year-old girl investigated because of crampy abdominal pain and a pelvic mass. **A,** On ultrasound of the pelvis in the longitudinal plane, a large midline cystic structure containing debris consistent with hematocolpos is seen. **B,** On T_2-weighted magnetic resonance imaging (MRI) of the pelvis in the midsagittal plane, a markedly distended vagina filled with material consistent with old blood is seen. The uterus *(upper arrow)* is not enlarged. The occlusion is in the distal segment of the vagina and measures more than 0.5 cm in thickness *(lower arrows)*. The MRI was obtained for presurgical planning. At surgery, the obstruction was found to be a thick vaginal septum or a short zone of vaginal atresia.

absent or rudimentary ipsilateral tube, hemiuterus, and hemivagina. Affected patients therefore have two ovaries and only one tube, uterus, and vagina. The kidney on the side of the missing or malformed hemiuterus is almost always absent. If a rudimentary hemiuterus contains functioning endometrium, the patient may develop an accumulation of blood within this structure at the time of puberty. If the hemiuterus does not communicate with the rest of the uterus, it may appear as a cystic mass or a debris-filled one.

A minor and relatively common form of müllerian fusion defect is the simple septate vagina, in which the vagina is divided in two lateral compartments by a midline sagittal septum, without any associated uterine anomalies.

CLOACAL MALFORMATION

Cloacal malformation is an uncommon anomaly in which the rectum, vagina, and urethra end in a common terminal channel as the only outlet for the gastrointestinal, genital, and urinary systems. The anomaly represents a persistence of the primitive fetal cloaca with failure of the urogenital and the urorectal septa to develop and separate the three structures. The presence of cloacal malformation should be suspected in a newborn girl with imperforate anus and a single perineal opening (see Section II, Part V, Chapter 11, page 252).

INTERLABIAL MASSES IN YOUNG GIRLS

Several abnormalities may present as interlabial masses in female infants and young girls. They may be related to problems originating at the level of the urethral meatus or problems originating at the level of the vaginal introitus.

Interlabial Masses Associated with the Urethral Orifice

Prolapse of an ectopic ureterocele may protrude from the urethral orifice as a small cystic mass. The prolapse may be noted only during voiding. Prolapse of urethral mucosa may be noted as a small, reddened, doughnut-like mass with its central opening being the urethral meatus itself. This abnormality is most often seen in African-Americans. Cystic dilatation of an obstructed paraurethral (Skene's) gland may present as an interlabial mass located on either side of the urethral meatus, which is itself displaced in the opposite direction by the mass.

Interlabial Masses Associated with the Vaginal Introitus

Newborns with prolapse of a vaginal cyst may present with an interlabial mass arising from the vagina. These cysts arise from rests of the wolffian or müllerian duct systems or may represent epithelial inclusions originating from elements of the urogenital sinus. As previously discussed, patients with an imperforate hymen may present at birth with hydrocolpos, but more often present at puberty or beyond because of hematocolpos with a smooth cystic mass extending from the vaginal introitus. Patients with a didelphys uterus with a septate vagina may present with a similar mass because of congenital obstruction of one of the hemivaginas (Fig. 17A). Cystic dilatation of an obstructed greater vestibular or Bartholin's gland may result in a mass that may be found posterolaterally on either side of the vaginal introitus. The vaginal opening may be displaced to the opposite side by the mass. An important differential possibility that should be diagnosed quickly is the prolapse of a sarcoma botryoides or rhabdomyosarcoma of the vagina. Such a tumor is often seen as a lobulated and grape-like mass protruding from the vaginal introitus.

Differential Diagnosis

The differential diagnoses of interlabial masses are usually made on visual inspection based on the location and external appearance of the mass. Diagnosis is more difficult when the mass is very large, filling the entire vulvar area. Catheterization of the urethra and a cystogram and catheterization of the vagina and a vaginogram, as well as an US scan of the bladder and upper genitourinary tract, may be necessary to further define the lesion. CT, MRI, or excretory urography may help if continued anatomic questions remain. At times, only surgery is conclusive.

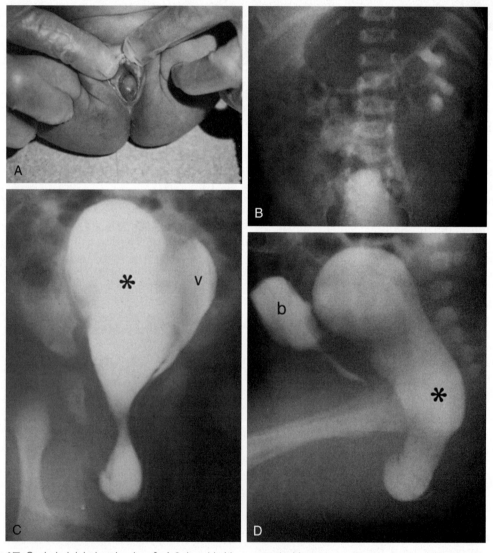

FIGURE 17. Occluded right hemivagina. **A,** A 2-day-old girl presented with a gray cystic mass at the vaginal introitus. **B,** On excretory urogram, no renal function is noted on the right (probably absent kidney). In a cystogram (not shown), the bladder was displaced forward by the mass. The patent left hemivagina could be catheterized and was found to be markedly displaced to the left. On frontal **(C)** and lateral **(D)** vaginograms, contrast material introduced through a needle inserted in the cystic mass at the introitus opacifies a markedly distended right hemivagina and uterus (unilateral hydrometrocolpos). Contrast material from previous studies is still present in the patent vagina *(V),* uterus (∗), and bladder *(b).*

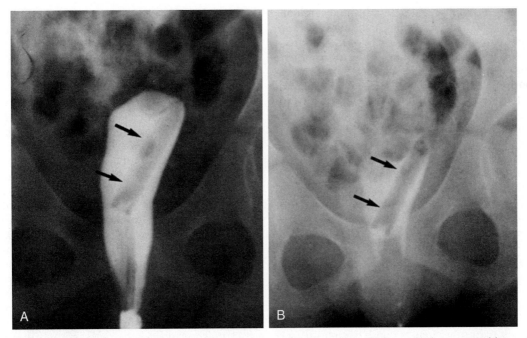

FIGURE 18. A vaginal foreign body that was not apparent on plain films of the abdomen is demonstrated by contrast vaginography *(arrows)* in the vagina of a 3½–year-old girl. **A,** Vaginogram obtained during vaginal filling. (From Jaramillo D, Lebowitz RL, Hendren WH: The cloacal malformation: radiologic findings and imaging recommendations. Radiology 1990;177:441–448.) **B,** Vaginogram obtained after removal of the catheter.

VAGINAL FOREIGN BODIES

All kinds of foreign bodies have been found in the vagina in children. Foreign bodies in the vagina of long standing may cause local inflammation, a foul-smelling discharge, and sometimes a bloody discharge. Foreign bodies are the most common cause of nonphysiologic vaginal bleeding in the prepubertal child. The most common foreign body is toilet paper. The diagnosis of a vaginal foreign body may be markedly delayed. Some foreign bodies are opaque and are easily recognized in frontal and lateral roentgenograms, but a vaginogram may be indicated for confirmation of a radiopaque foreign body or discovery of a radiolucent one (Fig. 18). US, usually performed with downward angulation through a fluid-filled bladder, can show the normal coapted vaginal mucosa as an echogenic line without shadowing (Fig. 19). Foreign bodies in the vagina will create a change to that image. Attempts at distal vaginal analysis by US may be better made by a transperineal US approach. Obviously direct inspection, when possible, whether using a Kelly cystoscope or other available tool, may make a definitive diagnosis of a vaginal foreign body. General anesthesia may be required for direct inspection of the vagina and for removal of the foreign body.

PELVIC INFLAMMATORY DISEASE

The sexually active teenager is at particularly high risk for sexually transmitted diseases. Increases in sexual activity among adolescents in the last decades has resulted in a markedly increased incidence of sexually transmitted diseases, particularly among girls.

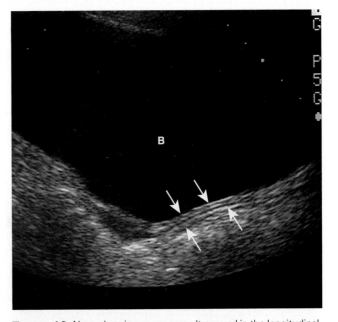

FIGURE 19. Normal vagina as seen on ultrasound in the longitudinal midline plane. The normal coapted vaginal walls *(arrows)* of this child appear as a long linear area with echogenic lines representing the outer walls and the coapted inner wall. If the vagina were obstructed, the walls would be separated and filled with material, whether echoless fluid, echogenic debris, or soft tissue mass. The vagina is seen distal (inferior) to the uterus and its most inferior portion, the cervix, as well as posterior to the fluid-filled bladder *(B)*. (From Cohen HL: Evaluation of the adolescent and young adult with amenorrhea: role of US. *In* Bluth E, Arger P, Hertzberg B, Middleton W [eds]: Syllabus: A Special Course in Ultrasound: Clinical Questions, Practical Answers. Oak Brook, IL, RSNA Publications, 1996:171–184, with permission.)

Pelvic inflammatory disease (PID) is the most serious complication of sexually transmitted diseases. PID includes a spectrum of abnormality that ranges from isolated endometritis to extension of infection into the tubes (salpingitis) and ovaries, potentially resulting in a tubo-ovarian abscess (TOA), and even extension into the peritoneum as disseminated peritonitis. Involvement of the fallopian tubes (and ovaries), often bilaterally, can lead to decreased fertility and increased chances for a future ectopic pregnancy. As far back as 1985, Weckstein reported the annual incidence of PID among 15- to 19-year-olds as 2%. The risk of PID for a sexually active 15-year-old girl was 1 in 8 as compared to the far lesser 1 in 80 for a 24-year-old woman. This risk of PID is particularly high in adolescents because of the high incidence of multiple sexual partners and the prevalence of chlamydia and gonorrhea in this age group. *Neisseria gonorrhoeae* and *Chlamydia trachomatis* are the most common etiologic agents. The infection ascends from the vagina into the "higher" portions of the gynecologic tract, the uterus and then the fallopian tubes and the ovaries.

Infected fallopian tubes may become edematous and bulky. Spread of purulent exudate from tubal openings to adjacent pelvic surfaces may result in dense adhesions and distortion of local structures. If the fimbriated ends of the fallopian tubes (salpinges) become adherent to the ovaries, the tubes may obstruct and distend with fluid, resulting in a hydrosalpinx, or with pus, resulting in a pyosalpinx (Fig. 20). Although diagnosis would be easier if echoless fluid in an obstructed vagina represented accumulated clear and noninfected fluid, echogenic fluid represented contained pus, and fluid of variable echogenicity represented accumulated secretions, this is not always true. Echoless fluid may be infected and echogenic fluid may be noninfected but made up of proteinaceous fluid or fluid with accumulated cellular debris. The infection may extend to the ovaries, resulting in a TOA (Fig. 21) with further adhesions or distortions of pelvic structures and an increase in the pelvic mass. Rupture of a TOA is an uncommon but serious complication of the disease. Following adequate antibiotic therapy, acute PID may resolve, but residual chronic changes are not uncommon, including adhesions and hydrosalpinx. It also may be difficult to know whether the finding of prominent size and/or adherence of ovaries to the uterus is of acute or chronic cause without correlation with clinical and historical information. Previous bouts of PID predispose to recurrent episodes of the same process. The long-term sequelae of PID are infertility, ectopic pregnancy, and chronic pelvic pain.

A high index of suspicion is important for the diagnosis of acute PID, particularly because symptoms and findings are often variable and nonspecific. Patients may present with lower abdominal/pelvic pain. Most patients have cervical motion tenderness, fever and leukocytosis. Many will have a vaginal discharge. Occasionally, patients may complain of right upper quadrant pain and tenderness thought to be due to perihepatitis (Fitz-Hugh–Curtis syndrome). This uncommon abnormality is rarely diagnosed by imaging. Seeing septations within fluid surrounding liver parenchyma may suggest it. A pelvic mass may be detected on physical examination. Adnexal tenderness, generally bilateral, and cervical motion tenderness, a hallmark for the clinical diagnosis, may be elicited on bimanual examination.

Laboratory findings may include a high erythrocyte sedimentation rate as well as the aforementioned leukocytosis, which has a left shift. Purulent discharge may be observed exiting from the cervix. Cultures of endocervical secretions may yield *N. gonorrhoeae* and *C. trachomatis.*

Ultrasound Findings in Pelvic Inflammatory Disease

Pelvic US is an important tool in the analysis of teenagers with clinical complaints that may suggest PID or one of its simulators. The sonographic findings vary with the extent of the disease. In early PID, or salpingitis, there may be no US findings, and the diagnosis will be

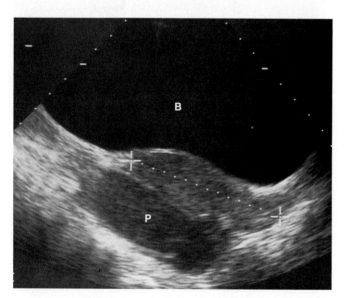

FIGURE 20. Pyosalpinx as seen on ultrasound in the longitudinal midline plane. Graticles mark off the uterus, which is posterior to the bladder. Posterior to the uterus is a tubular structure *(P)* that is fluid filled, allowing good through-transmission of sound. It contains debris, and was determined to be a pyosalpinx. *B* = bladder.

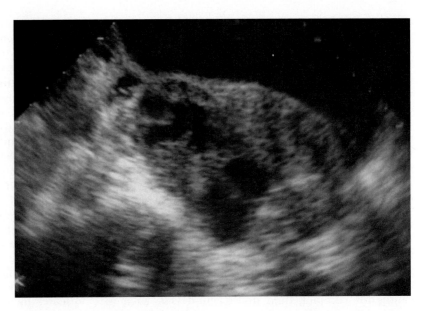

FIGURE 21. Tubo-ovarian abscess (TOA) as seen on transverse oblique plane ultrasound of the right adnexal region. To the right of the uterus and posterior to the bladder is a large, heterogeneous oval structure with contained echoless circular and tubular structures that were not typical of normal follicles or cysts on transverse or longitudinal images. This was a TOA in a teenager with a history of pelvic inflammatory disease. At times a dilated fallopian tube arising from a TOA accounts for part of the contained cystic structure, whether echoless or containing echoes. This is most likely when the structure appears tubular in at least one of the imaged planes.

based solely on clinical and laboratory evaluation. A helpful US finding in somewhat more advanced cases (i.e., there is salpingo-oophoritis) is prominent ovaries (most often bilateral) that may be adherent to the uterus. We consider an ovary of greater than 20-cm³ volume as enlarged (despite the fact that some normal patients may fit into that group) for the postmenarchal female. We use a volume of 15 to 20 cm³ as a gray zone for adnexal enlargement. We monitor patients with greater than 15-cm³ ovaries at the very least by a 6-week follow-up examination. One must be careful to remember that the presence of physiologic cysts may falsely elevate the ovarian volume. The imaging of prominent ovaries adherent to the uterus is indicative of salpingo-oophoritis. We have labeled this image, the "koala bear" sign (Fig. 22) because the ovaries resemble the ears of a koala, with the koala's face represented by the uterus. A prominent endometrial cavity echo that may be physiologic, particularly in the second half of the menstrual cycle, or increased and related to infection, represents the koala bear's nose. Adherence of the ovaries does not indicate acuity of the infection (unless old US studies are available and are normal) because it can be seen as a consequence of any previous infection in the pelvis, usually PID. These patients usually do well on antibiotic therapy.

More advanced cases of acute or, more often, chronic PID may demonstrate evidence of hydro- or pyosalpinx or TOA. Although it would be convenient if echoless dilated tubes were hydrosalpinges and echo-filled fluid within dilated tubes were suggestive of pyosalpinx, this is *not* always true. The affected tubal walls may be thickened and linear echoes may protrude from them into the tubal lumen.

A key finding suggestive of a significant bout of PID is the TOA (Fig. 22), which is said to be seen in 14% to 38% of patients hospitalized for PID. TOAs show up on US as partial or complete replacement of the normal ovarian tissue by a heterogeneous mass or an echopenic area with contained debris. When they represent only part of the imaged ovary, they may be hard to differentiate from

physiologic cysts with hemorrhage. Complete replacement of ovarian tissue allows a readier diagnosis. Cystic components of a TOA, the usual cause of its heterogeneous image, may represent the dilated fallopian tube. An orthogonal projection may help prove the presence

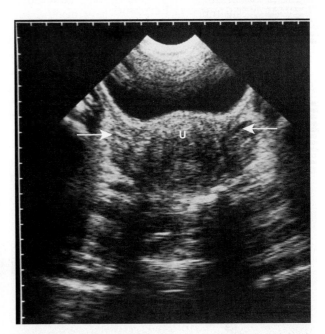

FIGURE 22. Salpingo-oophoritis as seen on ultrasound in the transverse plane. Prominent adnexa *(arrows)* hug the uterus *(U)*, suggesting they are adherent to the uterus. This is particularly well seen on the left. A triangular echogenic area within the uterus was consistent with a prominent endometrial echo, which may be happenstance in the second half of the cycle or may be related to endometrial cavity echo prominence seen in some patients with pelvic inflammatory disease (PID). We have likened this image to a koala bear's head and have called it the "koala bear" sign. Adnexal adherence does not denote acute infection in that it can be seen in patients with infection of any duration. It can be simulated by normal uterus and ovaries in a patient with significant retroflexion. Classically, the ovary of PID will be at least somewhat enlarged in acute infection.

of a true tubular structure extending beyond the confines of the ovary. The contents (debris filled) of the echopenic areas of a TOA can often be better seen by TV examination. TOAs are important to diagnose because they are usually treated aggressively with intravenous antibiotic regimens and, if necessary, percutaneous drainage or surgery.

A hemorrhagic cyst or an endometrioma—both also appearing as complex debris-filled cysts—may simulate the ultrasound image of the TOA. The images of these entities may all look alike.

The US finding of echoless fluid in the cul-de-sac can be seen in patients with PID but also in normal patients, usually because of physiologic rupture of a cyst. It is a nonspecific finding. Echogenic fluid in the cul-de-sac is of greater concern because of the possibility that the fluid is therefore proteinaceous, infected, or hemorrhagic. Hemorrhagic cul-de-sac fluid is of particular concern when considering ectopic pregnancy. Other causes for complex fluid in the cul-de-sac, such as perforated appendicitis, should be considered. Be aware that patients with ventriculoperitoneal shunts and patients undergoing peritoneal dialysis will often have cul-de-sac fluid and more significant amounts of free intraperitoneal fluid.

Normal Pregnancy/Ectopic Pregnancy

Pregnancy is a relatively common cause of pelvic mass and/or pelvic pain in postpubertal girls. It is the most common physiologic cause of secondary amenorrhea in girls over 9 years of age. It therefore must be considered in any girl after menarche, particularly (but not exclusively) if she claims a sexual history. Most pregnancies in

adolescents are not intended and occur within 1 to 2 years of becoming sexually active. Such adolescents often deny the possibility of pregnancy and ascribe complications of pregnancy to other physical causes. The examining physician should be aware of the possibility of a normal or abnormal pregnancy even with a noncontributory history. Pregnancy can be confirmed or ruled out by the appropriate laboratory tests. US can prove the presence of an intrauterine pregnancy by imaging a gestational sac within the uterus (Fig. 23), and a viable pregnancy by denoting a gestational sac with a contained embryo with normal cardiac motion.

Ectopic pregnancy is a pregnancy in a location other than the uterus. It is the cause of 6% to 11% of all maternal deaths and is the leading cause of first-trimester maternal mortality. The incidence of ectopic pregnancy in teen-age girls has increased in recent years coincident with an increase of sexually transmitted diseases in this group. The incidence is particularly increased in individuals with a prior history of PID. Antibiotic therapy for PID has been thought responsible for maintaining fertility in those patients who would otherwise have developed obstructed fallopian tubes, preventing pregnancy, but instead have patent tubes but with abnormal cilia that can limit the speed and transit of a fertilized egg to an implantation site in the uterus. Most (95% to 97%) of ectopic pregnancies occur at the ampullary end of the fallopian tube or the more proximal isthmus. When the pregnancy grows beyond the ability of the fallopian tube to contain it (8 to 12 weeks' gestational age), the tube may rupture and an abdominal crisis, usually presenting with severe hypotension or shock and possibly leading to death, may occur. Two percent to 5% of cases are cornual ectopic pregnancies, occurring at the cornua of the uterus, with

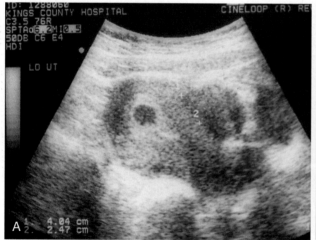 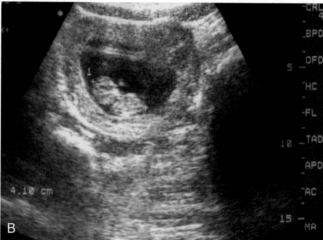

FIGURE 23. Normal intrauterine pregnancy as seen on ultrasound. **A,** Early pregnancy viewed in the midline longitudinal plane. A small, circular echoless area consistent with a gestational sac is seen within the uterus of this teenager with a several-week history of secondary amenorrhea. Immediate surrounding echogenicity is consistent with trophoblastic tissue. The gestational sac is completely surrounded by the uterus, denoting an intrauterine pregnancy and excluding it as being an ectopic pregnancy, including a cornual ectopic pregnancy, which may be surrounded only partially by uterine muscle. **B,** Older first-trimester pregnancy viewed in the longitudinal oblique plane. A fetal pole is seen in the gestational sac, which is completely surrounded by uterine muscle. Fetal heart motion was noted. This proved it to be a viable intrauterine pregnancy. This fetus was 10 weeks by measurement of crown–rump length. Modern equipment aided by endovaginal transducers will usually denote fetal heart motion and a yolk sac by 4 to 5 weeks' gestational age.

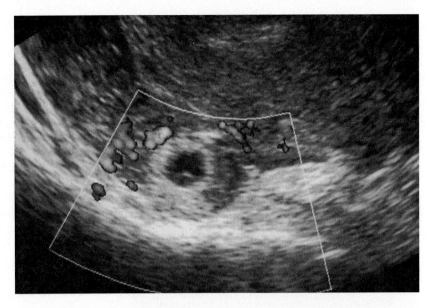

FIGURE 24. Ectopic pregnancy as seen on color Doppler ultrasound in the longitudinal oblique plane. A color Doppler box surrounds a fluid-filled circular structure with an echogenic periphery made up of trophoblastic tissue. It contains a small circular echogenic structure that proved to be a yolk sac of an early pregnancy. The fact that the circular structure is not surrounded by uterine tissue suggests that it is an ectopic gestational sac. The uterus of this teenager is superficial to the gestational sac. Of note is the fact that color Doppler flow about the ectopic gestational sac is only limited in amount. It was once hoped that reports of significant color flow around ectopic pregnancies would help make the diagnosis easier. In reality, flow is variable and equivalent flow can be seen around a physiologic corpora lutea cyst.

the embryo able to grow larger and for a longer time because of the greater expandability of the cornua because of its contained myometrium. Rare sites of ectopic pregnancy include the ovary (0.5% to 1%) and the cervix (0.1%).

The diagnosis of ectopic pregnancy is easy when a viable extrauterine gestational sac (Fig. 24) is seen with its contained embryo and heartbeat. Any time there is an ectopic pregnancy, no matter what its US image, a pseudogestational sac (i.e., some associated fluid within the endometrial cavity) may falsely simulate an intrauterine gestational sac. A normal pregnancy is never within the endometrial cavity but, rather, implanted within one of the walls deep to the endometrial cavity. A common image of concern for ectopic pregnancy is the finding of a complex or solid adnexal mass that is separate from the ipsilateral ovary. Ectopic pregnancies often have associated cul-de-sac fluid collections. When these collections are particularly large in amount and echogenic from contained hemorrhage, one must consider an ectopic pregnancy if there is a positive pregnancy test and no intrauterine pregnancy, even if an extrauterine pregnancy or mass cannot be discovered.

OVARIAN TORSION

Ovarian torsion is an uncommon but important cause of abdominal pain in the first three decades of life. It is caused by partial or complete rotation of the ovary on its pedicle, compromising first lymphatic, then venous, and finally arterial flow. Torsion of the ovary possibly leading (if not detorted) to hemorrhagic ovarian infarction is most often seen in peripubertal or older girls. It may occur in patients of all ages, including newborns, and has been shown to occur also in utero. It is said that if an ovary and its ipsilateral fallopian tube are not found at surgery, the cause is not agenesis of the ovary but antenatal torsion of the ovary and fallopian tube (tubo-ovarian torsion). Ovarian torsion usually occurs in anatomically normal ovaries (perhaps having had a recent size or weight increase with, e.g., puberty or a large physiologic cyst). Many cases, however, occur in ovaries with an associated ovarian or paraovarian mass or neoplasm. Bilateral, asynchronous ovarian torsion cases have been reported. Historically, the diagnosis of ovarian torsion has been made at surgery. More recently, US has proven a helpful tool for the diagnosis. A prompt diagnosis is important because surgical detorsion can help avoid irreversible damage to the ovary.

Clinically, affected pediatric patients may have symptoms that simulate gastroenteritis, appendicitis, intussusception, or any other acute abdominal condition affecting the child or adolescent. The classical ovarian torsion pain is sudden and acute. A subacute course of several days, however, can occur. Patients may report being awakened from sleep by their pain. Associated complaints of nausea, vomiting, or constipation may occur and mislead the clinician. Fever is rare. This fact can help differentiate right-sided torsion from classical cases of appendicitis. In contrast to appendicitis, the pain is sharp and localized immediately. At least half of patients with ovarian torsion claim prior bouts of such pain. This suggests previous bouts of torsion and detorsion. A tender pelvic mass may be felt on rectal examination. Fever and leukocytosis with a left shift are frequent laboratory findings.

Diagnostic US is the most important first imaging tool for the analysis of ovarian torsion. Ovaries involved in torsion have a variable appearance related to the degree of internal hemorrhage, stromal edema, and infarction that has occurred by the time they are imaged. The ovaries may appear cystic, cystic with septations, cystic with a debris layer, or complex with mixed solid and cystic components, as well as solid. Each of these images may suggest its own list of differential diagnostic considerations. One relatively specific US image was reported by Graif and Itzchak, who noted in 7 of 11 cases of ovarian torsion a unilaterally enlarged solid ovary with multiple peripheral (i.e., cortical zone) follicles (Fig. 25). Similar images of a large ovary with peripheral follicles can be seen with CT or MRI. The acute torsed ovary is *much* larger than a normal ovary. Ovarian volumes of 150 to 400 cm^3 are often measured. None of

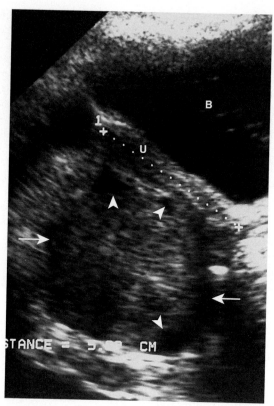

FIGURE 25. Ovarian torsion as seen on ultrasound in the longitudinal midline plane. Graticles mark off a tubular uterus that is posterior to the bladder *(B)* and anterior to a large solid mass *(arrows)* with a few peripheral cysts *(arrowheads)*. The cysts were better seen on other views. This is a relatively classical image of early torsion. Infarction or acute hemorrhage would make the internal contents of the torsed ovary more heterogeneous. (From Cohen HL, Safriel YI: Ovarian torsion. *In* Cohen HL, Sivit C [eds]: Fetal and Pediatric Ultrasound: A Casebook Approach. New York, McGraw-Hill, 2001:516, with permission.)

our cases have been less than 75 cm³ in volume. Graif et al. noted volumes of the torsed ovaries in their study to be at least 34 times larger among prepubertal and 15 times larger among postpubertal unaffected ovaries. Cul-de-sac fluid may be noted in these patients.

Reviews of CDI used in the analysis of cases of ovarian torsion are confusing with regard to its reliability. This is, in part, because Doppler signal may be difficult to obtain even in normal ovaries, particularly using transvesicle technique. In addition, there are well-documented cases of surgically proven torsed ovaries that CDI evaluation showed having peripheral and even central arterial flow. Other groups have reported success with color Doppler, particularly for determining viable versus infarcted torsed ovaries. Fleischer et al. noted that an assurance of viability can only be made by imaging central *venous* flow in a torsed ovary. Lee et al. reported an 87% diagnostic accuracy for determining viability by verifying blood flow changes at the twisted vascular pedicle itself. Their patients with no blood flow at the twisted pedicle had necrotic ovaries.

Detorsions and, if necessary, removal of a mass (e.g., cystectomy) causing torsion will hopefully save the

gonad and preserve its function. The time from clinical complaint to diagnosis and therapy plays a large role in preserving ovarian function. US analysis, with or without Doppler, is certainly time efficient.

Several case reports of adults, children, and even infants have discussed finding a detached and often freely movable and usually calcified ovary in the pelvis at some distance from the normal ovarian site. The lesion is believed to be the result of a prior episode of prenatal or postnatal torsion. Such a detached ovary may parasitize the blood supply from a bowel loop, liver, or other abdominal structure, resulting in a partially calcified cystic mass with a long vascular pedicle that may be located anywhere in the abdomen.

OVARIAN MASSES

Ovarian Cysts In Children And Adolescents

The normal pediatric ovary and its adnexa are not felt on physical examination. Non-neoplastic cysts of follicular origin (i.e., functional ovarian cysts) are the most common cause of enlargement. Follicles are seen routinely throughout childhood and are part of normal ovaries. It is a noninvoluted follicle that may become an enlarged cyst.

The increased use of US and improvements in its technology have made possible the detection of small follicles in normal ovaries occurring as normal functional variants. This has also resulted in a more frequent diagnosis of ovarian cysts in children and in a better understanding of their natural history. Where normal ovaries of children less than 10 were once considered homogeneous in echogenicity, indicating an absence of follicles, work by Cohen et al. has confirmed Rokitansky's work written in 1861 that noted the common occurrence of follicles in the pathology specimens of the fetus, child, and adult. We usually image the ovaries of girls from birth to 12 years of age.

Beyond puberty the adolescent ovary is similar to that of the adult, developing several follicles early in the menstrual cycle until a dominant follicle develops, rupturing at midcycle while the others atrophy and resorb. Occasionally one or more of these follicles fails to resorb and, instead, enlarges as a functional cyst or as a retention cyst. These cysts can reach a large size, but usually enlarge to no more than 3 cm. The majority of functional ovarian cysts are treated conservatively (i.e., watched clinically and sonographically) and resolve spontaneously. Rarely, there is a complication, the most common being ovarian torsion, which occurs, as already noted, more often in ovaries with large cysts or masses. Functional cysts may rupture and result in free cul-de-sac fluid that is usually echoless but may be echogenic. Occasionally a ruptured cyst may result in more significant amounts of peritoneal fluid. A 6-week follow-up allows analysis of the possible ovarian cyst in the other half of a different menstrual cycle so as to denote resolution or change and thereby help prove it to be a physiologic cyst and, if gone, to disprove the far less likely diagnosis of a cystic neoplasm. The classical cyst on

US exam is echoless with a sharp back wall and excellent through-transmission.

Occasionally, a cystic mass is seen near the bladder of a female fetus. This is usually due to an enlarged ovarian cyst, perhaps developing because of increased sensitivity to maternal hormone stimulation. Less likely possibilities include a duplicated portion of bowel or a diverticulum of the bladder. These possibilities may be considered and analyzed for during follow-up pelvic US evaluation of the newborn (see Section II, Part V, Chapter 11, page 252).

Hemorrhagic Ovarian Cysts

Hemorrhagic ovarian cysts (HOCs) represent a complication that occurs to physiologic/functional ovarian cysts. Functional ovarian cysts result from failure of a normal maturing follicle to involute. The follicle/cyst continues to enlarge, usually because of a temporary or persistent hormonal imbalance. Functional cysts may develop internal hemorrhage. This occurs when theca interna vessels rupture into the cyst cavity. Such HOCs can arise from ovarian follicles at any stage in their maturation, even as they undergo atresia. HOCs may develop in the corpus luteum, which develops from the dominant or graafian follicle, after ovulation.

The typical clinical presentation of a HOC is either that of sudden, severe, transient lower abdominal pain of 1 to 3 hours' duration or that of lower abdominal pain and a palpable mass. The pain is thought to result from sudden distention of the ovarian cyst by the hemorrhage. The finding can be incidental. Among 70 adolescent and adult patients with HOC studied by Baltarowich et al., only 4% were asymptomatic. Slightly more than one fourth (26%) of the patients in that series had prior, concurrent, or subsequent simple or hemorrhagic cysts. Because some individuals have a greater tendency to produce functional cysts, some may also have a greater tendency to develop hemorrhagic cysts when in a particular hormonal milieu. In the majority of cases, the clot hemolyzes and is gradually resorbed.

Hemorrhagic cysts are not an uncommon reason for a teenager to present with lower abdominal or pelvic pain and possible appendicitis. Once the patient diagnosed as having a HOC, resolution of pain and confirmation of a stable hematocrit allow conservative management and the use of "tincture of time" to follow the cyst by US to resolution. Such resolution includes the disappearance of the cyst altogether or a change in the cyst's echogenic hemorrhagic contents as a result of clot lysis.

Ultrasonographic Findings

The US diagnosis of any complicated cyst becomes more difficult when the classic US characteristics (echoless, sharp posterior wall, and strong posterior acoustic enhancement) are lost. The majority of HOCs are heterogeneous in echogenicity. In one study of 15 HOCs Baltarowich et al. reported 93% to have hypoechoic or hyperechoic areas separated by thin or thick linear

echoes or to be hypoechoic with contained lamellar-thin echoes (Fig. 26) to thick echoes in various orientations. However, HOCs may also be essentially echoless or echoless with a contained round echogenicity of variable size consistent with clot or retracting clot. They may contain fluid–debris levels. When clot fills the HOC cavity, it can be confused with a solid mass. Decreases in posterior enhancement (through-transmission) can cause confusion at times with solid masses, including neoplasm.

HOCs tend to be clearly separable from the uterus. Their size ranges widely, with Baltarowich et al. noting a size range of 2.5 to 14 cm in longest length. Most HOCs are between 2 and 3 cm. A changing US appearance over time can help make the diagnosis of HOC. Image change is expected because hemorrhage changes its US appearance with time. The initial bright echogenicity of acute hemorrhage, caused by fibrin deposition, becomes less echogenic and eventually fluid-like as the fibrin dissolves and the clot lyses. Technically, a TV examination using a higher frequency transducer (e.g., 6.5 MHz) can help improve evaluation of the contents of any complex cystic mass lying in the low pelvis and close to the transducer.

Differential Diagnosis

Hemorrhagic cysts may look very similar to TOAs or endometriomas. The associated clinical stories vary significantly. Patients with TOAs have a history or a clinical picture of PID. Patients with endometriomas have a history of very painful periods and perhaps already diagnosed endometriosis. Beyond these two imaging simulators, the differential diagnosis of the HOC would include other complex ovarian masses. One may consider a benign cystic teratoma (if it does not have a significant solid component), an ectopic preg-

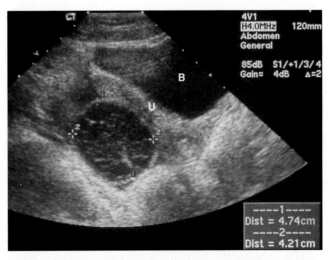

FIGURE 26. Hemorrhagic cyst as seen on longitudinal plane ultrasound. An echopenic mass, marked off by graticles and containing criss-crossing linear echogenicities, is seen in the adnexal area of a 12-year-old with acute abdominal pain. Tubo-ovarian abscess and endometrioma may look similar but present with different clinical scenarios. *B* = bladder; *U* = uterus.

nancy (but it would have to be chronic or complicated so as not to look like a gestational sac with a contained fetal pole), a torsed ovary (torsed ovaries are usually very large, with volumes >75 cm^3), or an appendiceal abscess (but an ipsilateral adnexa could be imaged in such a case).

Ovarian Cysts and Hypothyroidism

Bilateral ovarian cysts have been observed in older girls with longstanding, untreated hypothyroidism, possibly on the basis of a secondary hypothalamic–pituitary hyperfunction. Precocious puberty and galactorrhea may be present. Rapid regression of the cysts has been demonstrated following the initiation of therapy for hypothyroidism. Ovarian cysts have also been recognized prenatally in infants who postnatally were shown to have hypothyroidism.

Polycystic Ovary Syndrome

Polycystic ovary syndrome (PCOS; also known as Stein-Leventhal syndrome) is a hyperandrogenic state with resultant peripheral conversion of larger than normal amounts of estrogen. The chronic hyperestrogenic hyperandrogenic stimulation leads to chronic anovulation and is responsible for the classical bilaterally enlarged ovaries, which may be asymmetric but usually contain multiple small follicles/cysts. PCOS is the most common pathologic cause of amenorrhea, usually secondary, in the adolescent and young adult. Patients often, but far from always, suffer from the classical triad of obesity (31%), hirsutism (62%), and menstrual abnormalities (80%), including amenorrhea, irregular menses, and prolonged uterine bleeding. Laboratory diagnosis is made by noting increased luteinzing hormone: folicle-stimulating hormone ratios and elevated androstenedione levels. The syndrome is usually first noted at or shortly beyond puberty.

Imaging Findings

There are some confusing data in the literature on the diagnosis of PCOS by imaging. Part of the problem is that there is an overlap between normal US findings and the US findings reported in patients with PCOS. This is true whether patients are examined with TA or TV US probes. One must be aware of the fact that TV US will show increased numbers of ovarian follicles/cysts in both normal and PCOS patients compared to TA examinations. PCOS patients have high numbers of subcapsular follicles in their ovaries. These follicles are hyperstimulated but do not reach maturity. A dominant follicle does not develop. Typically, there are at least five cysts of 5 to 8 mm in diameter noted on TA evaluation of each ovary (Fig. 27). Follicles of classical cases should not be greater than 10 mm in diameter. Larger follicles or the presence of a single large (dominant) cyst goes against the diagnosis of PCOS. PCOS ovaries are larger and more echogenic than normal. Takahashi et al. noted mean ovarian volumes of 10.3 cm^3 in 47 affected patients, a volume significantly greater than the mean

for their control group. Among their PCOS patients, 94% had either an ovarian volume greater than 6.2 cm^3 or more than 10 follicles of 2 to 8 mm in diameter. Six percent of their patients had normal ovarian volumes and normal numbers of follicles. As we know, however, many normal adolescent have ovarian volumes greater than 6.2 cm^3. As previously noted, our US laboratory uses 15 to less than 20 cm^3 as a gray zone for ovarian enlargement and a figure of 20 cm^3 or greater as evidence of definitive enlargement of the ovary in adults and older adolescents.

A helpful indicator of PCOS is increased ovarian echogenicity (Fig. 28). This is thought to be due to pathologically proven ovarian stromal hypertrophy. Increased ovarian stroma is considered evidence of hyperandrogenism. Battaglia et al. found some PCOS ovaries to have lower ovarian arterial resistance. High androstenedione levels are linked to high uterine artery resistance. Pinkas et al. did not see differences in the resistances between PCOS patients and controls.

Other Clinical Considerations in Cases of Possible Polycystic Ovary Syndrome

The symptoms of obesity, menstrual irregularity, and hirsutism, individually or in combination, can be observed in normal patients as well as in those with other abnormalities. There are patients with familial hirsutism. Many young teenagers take a while for their cycles to become regular. Many individuals are obese. If signs of virilization are found, a work-up to rule out a virilizing adrenal or ovarian tumor is required. Certainly if a unilateral ovarian mass, usually solid, is imaged, an endocrinologically active ovarian tumor must be considered. Androgen excess may also occur in cases of idiopathic hirsutism, late-onset forms of congenital adrenal hyperplasia, exaggerated adrenarche, Cushing's disease, hyperprolactinemia, and acromegaly. Most hyperandrogenic adolescents are found to have PCOS.

Other Causes of Polycystic Ovaries

Not all polycystic ovaries are due to hyperandrogenism. Unopposed estrogen stimulation from any source can result in polycystic ovaries. Genetic deficiencies of the enzymes 21-hydroxylase, 3-β-hydroxysteroid dehydrogenase, or 11-β-hydroxylase have all been associated with polycystic ovary development.

NEOPLASMS OF THE GYNECOLOGIC TRACT IN CHILDREN AND ADOLESCENTS

NEOPLASMS OF THE VAGINA AND UTERUS

Tumors of the vagina and uterus are rare in childhood. They are usually malignant. They often present with a bloody vaginal discharge and may protrude from the introitus and be noted by inspection. Such tumors can be further imaged by vaginography. Pelvic US performed using a fluid-filled bladder or a transperineal

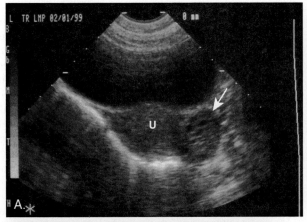

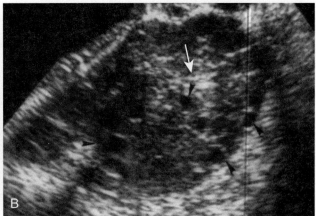

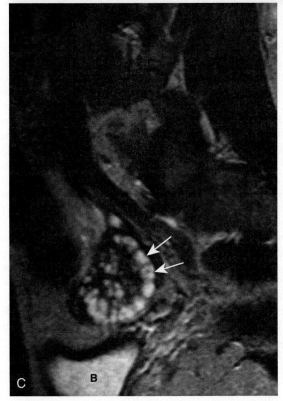

FIGURE 27. Polycystic ovarian disease. **A,** In the transverse plane, an enlarged left ovary *(arrow)* containing multiple small follicles is seen adjacent to the uterus *(U).* A similar right ovary was seen in another plane. There is some bright echogenicity within the ovary, which can be seen in polycystic ovaries. This was an older teen who was heavy and had secondary amenorrhea. She was proven to have polycystic ovary syndrome (PCOS). **B,** *Arrowheads* point to three of many small follicles seen within the ovary of a teen with PCOS using endovaginal ultrasound technique in the longitudinal oblique plane. One must be wary of the fact that endovaginal technique, using higher frequency transducers, will show more follicles in both normal and PCOS patients. In PCOS, only immature follicles, typically 5 to 8 mm at their largest, are seen. Some bright echogenicity *(arrow),* not seen in normal ovaries, is noted in the superior third of this imaged ovary. (From Cohen HL, Ruggiero-Delliturri M: Polycystic ovary syndrome. *In* Cohen HL, Sivit C [eds]: Fetal and Pediatric Ultrasound: A Casebook Approach. New York, McGraw-Hill, 2001:496, with permission.). **C,** On T_2-weighted magnetic resonance imaging in the longitudinal plane through the right abdomen. Multiple cortical cysts are seen, particularly at the periphery, of a teen proven to have PCOS. The ovary is seen superior to the bladder (B), and its follicles/cysts *(arrows)* have similar intensity (seen as white using this technique). (Courtesy of Mark Flyer, MD.)

approach with the transducer placed on the labia can help define the extent of the lesion and dismiss the possibility of simulation by a hemato/hydrocolpos from an obstructed vagina. Better definition of the origin, extent, and internal characteristics of the tumor can be obtained by CT, but particularly by multiplanar MRI. The most common neoplasms of the vagina and uterus in children are embryonal rhabdomyosarcoma, endodermal sinus tumor, and clear cell adenocarcinoma.

Embryonal rhabdomyosarcoma is the most common genital neoplasm in children of both sexes. It is generally seen before the age of 3 years but rarely at birth. It is rare in older patients. Urogenital sinus remnants are thought to be the origin of some rhabdomyosarcomas (sarcoma botryoides) usually originating from the anterior vagina near the cervix. They may occasionally arise from the cervix. Whatever the area of origin, the mass may protrude from the vaginal introitus, often with a polypoid or cluster-of-grapes appearance (botryoid variant). These rhabdomyosarcomas are aggressive tumors that spread rapidly by direct invasion of the vaginal wall and pelvic structures. The tumor may extend to the uterus, bladder, or ureters. On occasion, it may extend to the rectum. Metastases to regional lymph nodes, the lungs, and other organs may occur. Local recurrence is common.

Endodermal sinus tumor of the vagina, also known as yolk sac carcinoma or adenocarcinoma of the infant vagina, is seen usually in infants between 8 and 15 months, and rarely after the second year. It often originates in the posterior wall of the vagina (Fig. 28) and may have a polypoid appearance very similar to that of sarcoma botryoides. The tumor spreads to pelvic soft tissues, para-aortic nodes, liver, and lungs.

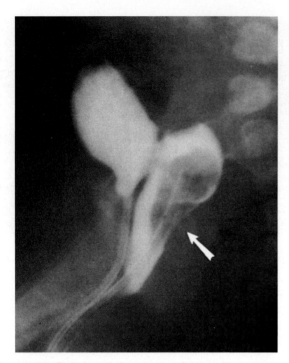

FIGURE 28. Endodermal sinus tumor of the vagina as seen on a vaginogram in the midline longitudinal plane. A mass is noted within the contrast-filled vagina of a 6-month-old girl, originating from the vagina's posterior wall. The contrast-filled bladder seen anterior to the vagina was filled by a separate injection.

Clear cell (or mesonephric) *adenocarcinoma* usually originates from the vagina and uncommonly from the cervix. It is usually seen after menarche. In the last few decades, about two thirds of patients with this tumor had a history of maternal exposure to diethylstilbestrol or related substances during the first 3 months of pregnancy. These tumors can become quite large, filling the entire vagina by the time of diagnosis. Tumor spread is via the lymphatics and to pelvic nodes. Local recurrence is common. Pulmonary metastases can occur.

OVARIAN NEOPLASMS

General Information

Ovarian neoplasms are uncommon in children. Despite this fact, they may be seen among all the age groups of pediatric life, from newborn to adolescence.

Ovarian neoplasms are commonly divided into groups based on the apparent origin of their cellular components: germ cell tumors, sex cord stromal tumors, and surface epithelial tumors. Unlike adults, in whom epithelial cell tumors are the most common ovarian tumor type, in children, germ cell tumors are the most common type. Sixty percent of all pediatric ovarian neoplasms are of germ cell origin. Of the germ cell tumors, 70% are teratomas, 25% are dysgerminomas, and 5% are endodermal sinus or yolk sac tumors. Only one fifth of pediatric ovarian tumors are epithelial cell in origin, including cystadenoma (80%) and cystadenocarcinoma (10%). The final 10% of pediatric ovarian tumors are sex cord tumors or tumors of stromal/

mesenchymal origin. Fifteen percent of those are arrhenoblastomas and 75% are granulosa–theca cell tumors. Granulosa–theca cell tumors are the most common ovarian cause of isosexual precocious puberty in children.

Greater than half of childhood ovarian tumors are diagnosed in girls between 10 and 14 years of age. The majority are teratomas, usually picked up incidentally on plain film or US examination. Ovarian tumors have variable presentations; some present with abdominal pain and some because of a mass felt on physical examination. Ovarian neoplasms are usually unilateral, but bilateral involvement may occur, particularly in the case of teratomas.

Overall, one third of all ovarian neoplasms are malignant. This percentage decreases with increasing age. A greater percentage, as many as half, of hormonally active tumors, often granulosa cell tumors, are malignant. Of the malignant lesions, 85% are germ cell tumors (dysgerminomas, immature teratomas, endodermal sinus tumor, embryonal cell carcinoma, and choriocarcinoma); 10% are stromal (Sertoli–Leydig cell, granulosa–theca cell, and undifferentiated neoplasms); and 5% are epithelial cell tumors (serous and mucinous adenocarcinoma). Malignant neoplasms tend to break through the ovary's capsule and invade adjacent organs. Metastases are most often to the peritoneum, opposite ovary, pelvic and retroperitoneal lymph nodes, omentum, liver, and abdominal organs. Involvement of peritoneal and pleural linings may lead to ascites or pleural effusions.

Underlining the fact that neoplasms are not the most common cause of noncystic ovarian masses in children and adolescents are the results of Wu and Siegel's review of 70 such masses in girls ranging in age from neonate to late adolescence. They found 16 complex masses; 7 were hemorrhagic cysts (3 predominantly cystic and 4 predominantly solid in appearance), 5 TOAs, 5 teratomas, and only 1 a malignant dysgerminoma. Of their solid-appearing adnexal masses, two were torsed ovaries, three were echo-filled hemorrhagic cysts, and only three were neoplasms (two teratomas and one dysgerminoma).

Imaging

Abdominal plain films may show a soft tissue density suggesting an abdominal or pelvic mass. Occasionally fat from a teratoma can be seen as a circular or oval radiolucency. This can readily be confirmed by denoting homogeneous echogenicity without shadowing on US or a low-density area with negative Hounsfield units (e.g., – 100 H.U.) on CT. Intrinsic tumor calcifications, often seen in teratomas, may be noted as radiodensity on plain film (see Fig. 34 below), echogenicity with posterior shadowing on US, or high-density areas (e.g., +100 or greater H.U.) on CT examination. Extrinsic compression of the bladder and bowel by ovarian masses has been reported to occasionally cause bowel obstruction or urinary complaints that have been demonstrated in the past by contrast studies of the urinary or intestinal tract. CT has replaced the intravenous urogram and barium study in many of these work-ups. Pelvic US is the initial procedure of choice to investigate patients with a possible ovarian tumor suspected clinically or radiologically. It may provide information as to the location and origin of the mass and readily differentiates a cystic from a mixed or solid lesion. Once a mass is large, its analysis by US or any other method for point of origin becomes difficult. CT or MRI studies may provide further information and may help elucidate US findings. CT is used particularly for a more global view of tumoral and metastatic involvement. CT and/or MRI are more valuable for staging tumors than is US. Table 1 shows a commonly used method for staging such tumors.

Malignant tumors in postpubertal girls are usually large in size, often 15 cm or greater by the time they are discovered. On US imaging, they are predominantly solid with contained areas of necrosis. Whereas coarse calcifications are typical of the malignant teratoma, stippled calcifications can be seen in the dysgerminoma. Endodermal sinus tumors typically have both echogenic and hypoechoic components. They grow rapidly, and patients often present because of abdominal pain, occasionally resulting from torsion or rupture of the tumor. When imaging predominantly cystic masses, the presence of contained papillary projections or evidence of capsular invasion is suggestive of malignancy. This is the case with the serous cystadenocarcinoma, a common adult malignant neoplasm that is uncommon in adolescents and rarely noted before puberty. Malignant ovarian tumors may metastasize by direct extension to adjacent structures or by hematogenous or lymphangitic spread to more distant locations. Findings beyond the ovary (i.e., significant ascites, pelvic fixation, or distant metastases) can underline concern that a given ovarian mass is malignant and probably metastatic. Again, CT and MRI will allow a more global analysis of a mass and its relationship to surrounding tissues and can help denote this. Within the abdomen, these modalities are particularly helpful in diagnosing omental involvement ("caking") and peritoneal implants (Fig. 29) and lymphadenopathy. Common sites for distal parenchymal metastases are the liver and lung.

Ovarian Tumors of Germ Cell Origin

Germ cell tumors represent the majority of pediatric ovarian neoplasms. They include mature and immature

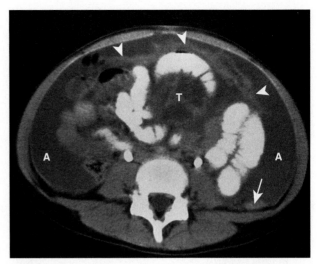

FIGURE 29. Omental "caking" and peritoneal implants in an endodermal sinus tumor as seen on computed tomography of the low abdomen in the axial plane. *Arrowheads* point to malignant omental spread ("caking") in this 13-year-old with malignant endodermal sinus tumor of the ovary. There is moderate ascites *(A)*. An *arrow* points to a posterior left-sided peritoneal metastasis. *T* = the most superior portion of the ovarian tumor. (From Cohen HL, Bober S, Bow S: Imaging the pediatric pelvis: the normal and abnormal genital tract and simulators of its diseases. Urol Radiol 1992;14:273–283, with permission.)

teratomas, dysgerminoma, endodermal sinus tumor, embryonal carcinoma, choriocarcinoma, and gonadoblastoma. About 20% of these tumors contain islands of different germ cell neoplasms and are therefore known as mixed germ cell tumors. Endodermal sinus tumor, embryonal carcinoma, and some immature teratomas are associated with elevated serum α-fetoprotein levels, a finding that may be of value in the initial diagnosis, but more so in the detection of residual tumor or recurrences on follow-up examinations. Germ cell tumors are generally unilateral, but bilateral involvement by the same or a different germ cell neoplasm may occur.

Ovarian Teratomas

Mature ovarian teratomas (or dermoid cysts) are the most common ovarian neoplasm in pediatric patients. They are less common in children and therefore more typically found in the adolescent. Although teratomas and dermoid cysts are talked about almost interchangeably, dermoids by definition contain two cell layers—mesoderm and ectoderm—whereas teratomas are made up of elements from all three germ cell layers, including the endoderm. Almost all dermoids and teratomas are benign. Malignancy is found in 2% to 10% of cases or less.

Teratomas are usually asymptomatic, and this may be why the exact numbers in older females who have not needed an US exam of the pelvis may be underestimated. One third of cases are thought to present with symptomatology. Of teratomas diagnosed in children because of symptoms, the usual history is that of a 6- to

Table 1 ■ STAGING FOR OVARIAN NEOPLASMS	
STAGE	**CHARACTERISTICS**
I	Tumor limited to one or both ovaries (with subgroups)
II	Tumor involving one or both ovaries with extension to uterus, tubes, or other pelvic areas
III	Tumor involving one or both ovaries with widespread intraperitoneal involvement
IV	Tumor involving one or both ovaries with distant metastases outside the peritoneal cavity

Adapted from Eman S, Goldstein D (eds): Pediatric and Adolescent Gynecology, 3rd ed. Boston, Little Brown, 1990:149.

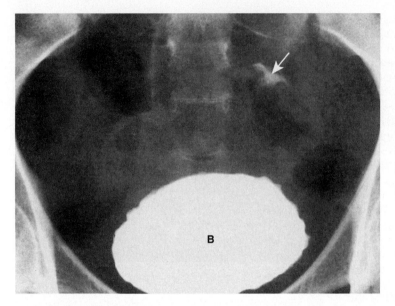

FIGURE 30. Ovarian teratoma as seen on plain film of the pelvis in the anteroposterior projection. A triangular calcification *(arrow)* is seen in the right side of the pelvis. It proved to be within a right ovarian teratoma. The finding was made incidentally during an intravenous pyelogram. *B* = bladder.

11-year-old with an abdominal mass (65% to 70% of cases) or pain secondary to torsion of or hemorrhage within the cyst. Teratomas are most often discovered by chance during pelvic US exams performed on adolescents for amenorrhea, bladder infection, PID, or pregnancy work-ups. They may occasionally be diagnosed by the incidental discovery of calcifications (particularly teeth or bone) in the adnexal area on plain film examination (Fig. 30). One fourth of ovarian teratomas are bilateral. The tumors may vary in size from those contained solely within the ovary itself to those that extend 5 to 10 cm beyond the ovary.

The US appearance of teratomas is highly variable because the varied contents of such masses. The classical US appearance shows a prominent cystic component and at least one contained mural nodule (dermoid plug, Rokitansky projection) (Fig. 31) that is often echogenic as a result of either contained fat, hair, sebum, or calcium (e.g., teeth or bone). The contained teeth and bone and perhaps other components may cause poste-

rior shadowing of the US beam. The shadowing may obscure deeper portions of the mass. This phenomenon has been called the "tip of the iceberg" sign. The anechoic component of teratomas is made up of serous fluid or sebum, which is in a fluid state when at body temperature. Fat–fluid levels and hair–fluid levels may be seen as part of the cystic component of the mass. Echogenic fat may float on top of the cystic component, or echogenic particulate matter may be the dependent component of a fluid–debris level.

Two thirds of teratomas are sonographically complex cysts with anechoic, hypoechoic, and echogenic components. One third of cases are claimed to be either purely echoless (perhaps because the solid component is at the mass's periphery and not imaged) or purely echogenic. We have seen many purely echogenic ovarian teratomas but none, yet, that was purely cystic. Occasionally, the cystic component of a teratoma may be so large or so positioned that it may simulate the bladder, or extend beyond the pelvis and have its size underestimated or its

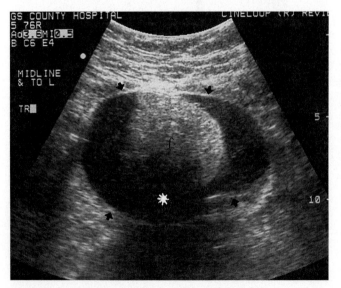

FIGURE 31. Left ovarian teratoma picked up incidentally in a teenager undergoing a pelvic ultrasound of the left pelvis in the transverse plane. A large mass *(arrows)* with a highly echogenic component *(f)* is seen. There is shadowing *(*)* distal to the central portion that represents a dermoid plug. The echogenicity is predominantly due to fat. Some calcification, which is not evident in this plane, was responsible for the shadowing. The periphery of the mass is fluid with contained debris. Some teratomas are more solid, some are more cystic. (From Ruggierro M, Awobuluyi M, Cohen H, Zinn D: Imaging the pediatric pelvis: role of ultrasound. Radiologist 1997;4:155–170, with permission.)

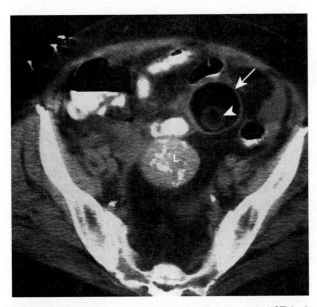

FIGURE 32. Ovarian teratoma on computed tomography (CT) in the axial plane. A circular low–Hounsfield-unit mass *(arrow)* is seen in the anterior left pelvis. The CT technique used makes its predominant component appear to be of the same low density as the air seen within nearby bowel or the fat seen in the posterior pelvis anterior to the sacrum. Its actual Hounsfield measurements were consistent with fat. It contains a mural nodule *(arrowhead)* that has no contained calcification. Incidentally noted is a midpelvic mass *(L)* with calcifications that was a calcified leiomyoma. (From Cohen HL, Safriel YI: Benign cystic teratomas of the ovaries. *In* Cohen HL, Sivit C [eds]: Fetal and Pediatric Ultrasound: A Casebook Approach. New York, McGraw-Hill, 2001:516, with permission.)

contained echogenic components missed. Septations or fluid–fluid levels within the cyst may be seen. These findings may also be demonstrated by abdominal CT (Fig. 32) or MRI. CT may show calcifications that are not seen by other methods. MRI is particularly valuable in demonstrating the fatty components of the mass. Signal characteristics on MRI reflect the composition of a teratoma. Calcium, bone, and hair have low signal intensity on both T_1- and T_2-weighted images. Fat has a high signal on T_1-weighted studies. Fluid has a high signal on T_2-weighted studies.

In a large Turkish study of 943 women with 1095 adnexal masses, including 147 pathologically proven dermoids, Ekici et al. found US to be 94% sensitive, 98% accurate, and 99% specific for differentiating mature and benign teratomas from other adnexal masses. The findings used for the diagnosis were an echogenic mass with or without acoustic enhancement, a dermoid plug, layered lines, a fat–fluid level, isolated bright echoes with acoustic shadowing within a complex mass, linear echogenicities (hair) in low-viscosity fluid, contained teeth or bone fragments, or an intraovarian echogenic mass (Fig. 33) with or without shadowing or enhancement (evidence of an intraovarian dermoid cyst).

Classical benign teratomas do not look like malignant teratomas. In analyzing ovarian masses for malignancy, noting a purely cystic ovarian mass or a mixed mass with well-differentiated epithelial elements such as hair, sebum, or teeth suggests that it is benign. A lack of

ascites helps assure this. Immature, partially differentiated malignant teratomas are uncommon and are generally solid. Well-differentiated teratomas with foci of embryonal carcinoma, endodermal sinus tumor, or other malignant germ cell neoplasms are included in this subgroup. Some immature teratomas are hormonally active and can cause precocious puberty. Immature teratomas are almost universally unilateral, but a mature teratoma may be seen in the contralateral ovary in 5% to 10% of cases.

Ovarian Dysgerminoma

Dysgerminoma is the second most common ovarian neoplasm in children and adolescents after mature teratoma. It is the most common malignant ovarian tumor of pediatric life, but is considered a low-grade malignancy. It is said to be the histologic counterpart to the testicular seminoma of boys. Imaging or inspection shows it to be solid, smooth in shape, and well encapsulated. These tumors are often large when first diagnosed. One fifth of cases have bilateral involvement. Dysgerminoma may arise in dysgenetic gonads but much less commonly than gonadoblastoma. Pure dysgerminomas are nonfunctioning tumors, but function may be observed in germinomas that contain islands of cells of other germ cell tumors. These tumors can spread locally and to retroperitoneal nodes. These tumors are very radiosensitive, and prognosis with treatment

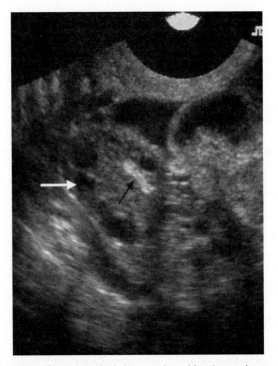

FIGURE 33. On endovaginal ultrasound, a *white arrow* points to this teenager's right ovary. A *black arrow* points to an echogenic area consistent with the fat of a small intraovarian teratoma. This was discovered after noting a large left ovarian teratoma on a transvesicle examination of the pelvis. At least one fourth of cases of teratoma are bilateral. Teratomas that do not extend beyond the borders of the ovary are not treated surgically, but followed.

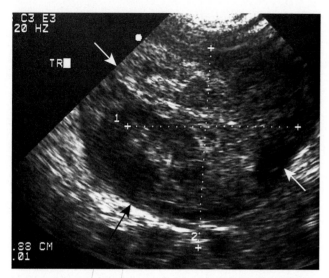

FIGURE 34. A large solid mass *(arrows)* extending beyond the measurement calipers is noted on ultrasound in the transverse plane in this 13-year-old who presented with a distended abdomen. This is an endodermal sinus tumor of the ovary. Computed tomography scan section of this patient that showed significant metastatic disease is presented in Figure 30.

is generally good, with an overall survival of more that 90%.

Endodermal Sinus Tumor

Endodermal sinus tumor (yolk sac tumor, yolk sac carcinoma, Teilum tumor) is an uncommon malignant neoplasm that can occur at any age. It is often bulky at the time of diagnosis. Its US image (Fig. 34) is predominantly solid but may contain cystic spaces within the tumor. In most cases serum α_1-fetoprotein levels are increased. Some endodermal sinus tumors secrete human chorionic gonadotropin (HCG), causing incomplete precocious puberty by stimulating estrogen production by the ovary. This can cause menstrual irregularities in postpubertal girls. The tumor is very radiosensitive, but there is a high incidence of recurrences. There is a high survival rate among treated patients.

Choriocarcinoma

Choriocarcinoma of the ovary is very uncommon, but is sometimes seen as a component of mixed germ cell tumors. It may secrete HCG.

Gonadoblastoma

Gonadoblastomas are composed of both germ cells plus sex cord–stromal cells. They usually are seen in postpubertal patients. They are considered potentially malignant because about 10% give rise to dysgerminomas and other malignant germ cell tumors. These tumors may have punctate calcifications that may be seen on plain film.

Germ Cell Neoplasms

Germ cell neoplasms, or mixed germ cell neoplasms containing seminoma, dysgerminoma, or gonadoblastoma, may be seen in some patients with intersex disorders and a Y chromosome.

Ovarian Tumors of (Surface) Epithelial Origin

Surface epithelial tumors in children are similar to those in adults and consist predominantly of the cystadenoma and cystadenocarcinoma. Cystadenomas are very uncommon before puberty and are usually unilateral. They vary in size from 3 to 30 cm. Of the two types of cystadenomas, serous cystadenomas contain clear watery fluid and the less common mucinous cystadenomas contain mucin, a jelly-like material. Most of these tumors are multiseptated cystic masses (Fig. 35) when imaged by US. Cystadenomas are benign neoplasms, but a serous papillary form is reported to be prone to rupture, with spillage of tumor material into the peritoneal cavity causing a serous papillomatosis.

Cystadenocarcinomas are much less common than their benign counterparts. They may appear similar to cystadenomas. The presence of irregular margins, thick septations, and papillary projections suggests malignancy. Ascites, omental or peritoneal implants, lymphadenopathy and hepatic metastases suggest malignant spread.

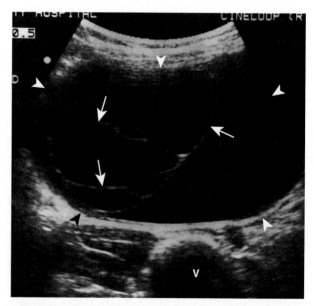

FIGURE 35. Ovarian cystadenoma in a teenager as seen on ultrasound in the transverse plane. A large cystic mass *(arrowheads)* with several intersecting septations *(arrows)* seen within its right half proved to be a cystadenoma. These are much more common tumors of the adult ovary than of the child's ovary. *V* = vertebral body. (From Ruggierro M, Awobuluyi M, Cohen H, Zinn D: Imaging the pediatric pelvis: role of ultrasound. Radiologist 1997;4:155–170, with permission.)

Ovarian Tumors of Sex Cord or Mesenchymal Origin

Sex cord (gonadal stromal) tumors are uncommon. They include granulosa–theca cell tumors (75%) and arrhenoblastoma (15%).

Granulosa–Theca Cell Tumors

Granulosa–theca cell tumors are generally large at the time of diagnosis. They are predominantly solid, but mixed solid and cystic patterns or a predominantly cystic type are also seen. Three fourths of juvenile granulosa cell tumors produce estrogen, which causes isosexual precocious puberty. Postpubertal girls with these tumors may develop abnormal menses. As already noted, greater than 50% of hormonally active childhood ovarian tumors are malignant. Nonfunctioning granulosa cell tumors are often discovered incidentally because a lower abdominal mass noted on physical examination or an ovarian mass noted by US. The vast majority of nonfunctioning granulosa cell tumors are benign, with recurrences and metastases a rarity.

Arrhenoblastomas

Arrhenoblastomas (Leydig cell tumors) are usually large and unilateral. They may be solid or cystic. They are usually well differentiated and benign, but a poorly differentiated form also occurs. Most arrhenoblastomas produce androgenic substances, causing virilization in prepubertal girls and signs of virilization, hirsutism, and oligomenorrhea or amenorrhea after puberty.

Ovarian Involvement in Leukemia

Ovarian involvement in cases of acute leukemia is a common microscopic finding, noted incidentally in 35% to 50% of autopsies performed on girls dying of acute lymphoblastic leukemia (ALL). By contrast, leukemia infiltrating the ovary, occurring as the primary site of leukemia relapse after completion of chemotherapy, is rarely identified during life. This is probably because more intensive chemotherapy has been used in recent protocols to avoid this problem. Ovarian relapse in ALL is about 50 times less common than testicular relapse. It should be considered, however, if there is asymmetric (solid) enlargement of the adnexa in such a patient. Leukemic infiltration of the ovary may present with abdominal pain and a lower abdominal mass resulting from ovarian enlargement. Involvement is usually bilateral. Patients may develop hydronephrosis.

US examination of ovaries with leukemic infiltration reveals them to be solid and usually more hypoechoic than normal because of the ready penetration by US of areas containing homogeneous arrays of infiltrated small cells. The response to chemotherapy, radiotherapy, and surgical resection of ovarian leukemic infiltration is generally poor.

Other Ovarian Tumors

Rare solid ovarian fibromas have been reported in pre- and postpubertal females. They have been associated with ascites and/or pleural effusion in Meig's syndrome. These typically benign ovarian tumors range in US appearance from anechoic to solid to calcified. If they are bilateral and calcified, one should consider basal cell nevus syndrome and its associated multiple basal cell carcinomas, as well as mandibular cysts and rib anomalies.

Differential Diagnosis of Ovarian Neoplasms

Neoplasms that may simulate solid and complex gynecologic adnexal masses include sacral and pelvic girdle tumors, retroperitoneal or pelvic soft tissue sarcomas (particularly rhabdomyosarcoma), neuroblastomas, and bowel tumors. Non-neoplastic simulators of adnexal masses include adenopathy, gynecologic (tubo-ovarian) and gastrointestinal (appendicitis, inflammatory bowel disease) inflammatory masses, endometriomas, and uterine (müllerian duct) anomalies.

SUGGESTED READINGS

Atiomo W, Pearson S, Shaw S, et al: Ultrasound criteria in the diagnosis of polycystic ovary syndrome (PCOS). Ultrasound Med Biol 2000; 26:977

Baltarowich OH, Kurtz A, Pasto M, et al: The spectrum of sonographic findings in hemorrhagic ovarian cysts. AJR Am J Roentgenol 1987; 148:901

Battaglia C, Artini P, Genazzani A, et al: Color Doppler analysis in oligo- and amenorrheic women with polycystic ovary syndrome. Gynecol Endocrinol 1997;11:105

Boechat M: Magnetic resonance imaging of abdominal and pelvic masses in children. Top Magn Reson Imaging 1990;3:25

Bulas D, Ahlstrom P, Sivit C, et al: Pelvic inflammatory disease in the adolescent: comparison of transabdominal and transvaginal sonographic evaluation. Radiology 1992;183:435

Caloia D, Morris H, Rahmani M: Congenital transverse vaginal septum: vaginal hydrosonographic diagnosis. J Ultrasound Med 1998;17:261

Carrington B, Hricak H, Nuruddin R, et al: Mullerian duct anomalies: MR imaging evaluation. Radiology 1990;176:715

Cohen HL: Evaluation of the adolescent and young adult with amenorrhea: role of US. In Bluth E, Arger P, Hertzberg B, Middleton W (eds): Syllabus: A Special Course in Ultrasound: Clinical Questions, Practical Answers. Oak Brook, IL, RSNA Publications, 1996:171

Cohen HL: The female pelvis. In Siebert J (ed): Current Concepts: A Categorical Course in Pediatric Radiology. Chicago, RSNA Publications, 1994:65

Cohen HL, Bober S, Bow S: Imaging the pediatric pelvis: the normal and abnormal genital tract and simulators of its diseases. Urol Radiol 1992;14:273

Cohen HL, Eisenberg P, Mandel F, Haller J: Ovarian cysts are common in premenarchal girls: a sonographic study of 101 children 2–12 years of age. AJR Am J Roentgenol 1992;159:89

Cohen HL, Shapiro MA, Mandel FS, Shapiro ML: Normal ovaries in neonates and infants: a sonographic study of 77 patients 1 day to 24 months old. AJR Am J Roentgenol 1993;160:583

Cohen HL, Sivit CJ (eds): Fetal and Pediatric Ultrasound: A Casebook Approach. New York, McGraw-Hill, 2001

Cohen HL, Smith W, Kushner D, et al: Imaging evaluation of acute right lower quadrant and pelvic pain in adolescent girls (ACR Appropriateness Criteria). Radiology 2000;215S:833–840

Cohen H, Tice H, Mandel F: Ovarian volumes measured by US: bigger than we think. Radiology 1990;177:189

Connor S, Guest P: Conversion of multiple solid testicular teratoma metastases to fatty and cystic liver masses following chemotherapy: CT evidence of "maturation." Br J Radiol 1999;72:1114

Cornel E, deGrier R, van Die C, Feitz W: Testicular simple cyst and teratoma: asynchronous bilateral occurrence within the first year of life. Urology 1999;54:366

Currarino G, Wood B, Majd M: Abnormalities of the genital tract. *In* Silverman F, Kuhn J (eds): Caffey's Pediatric X-Ray Diagnosis, 9th ed. St. Louis, Mosby–Year Book, 1993:1375

Davis AJ, Fein NR: Subsequent asynchronous torsion of normal adnexa in children. J Pediatr Surg 1990;25:687

Eberenz W, Rosenberg H, Moshang T, et al: True hermaphroditism: sonographic identification of ovotestes. Radiology 1991;179:429

Eisenberg P, Cohen H, Mandel F, et al: US analysis of premenarchal gynecological structures. J Ultrasound Med 1991;10:S30

Ekici E, Soysal M, Kara S, et al: The efficiency of ultrasonography in the diagnosis of dermoid cysts. Zentralbl Gynakol 1996;118:136

Emans S, Goldstein D (eds): Delayed puberty and menstrual irregularities. *In* Pediatric & Adolescent Gynecology, 3rd ed. Boston, Little Brown, 1990:149

Emans S, Goldstein D (eds): The physiology of puberty. *In* Pediatric & Adolescent Gynecology, 3rd ed. Boston, Little Brown, 1990:95

Fedele L, Dorta M, Brioschi D, et al: Magnetic resonance imaging in Mayer-Rokinstansky-Kuster-Hauser syndrome. Obstet Gynecol 1990;76:593

Fleischer AC, Brader KR: Sonographic depiction of ovarian vascularity and flow: current improvements and future applications. J Ultrasound Med 2001;20:241–250

Garel L, Filiatrault D, Brandt M, et al: Antenatal diagnosis of ovarian cysts: natural history and therapeutic implications. Pediatr Radiol 1991;21:182

Graif M, Itzchak Y: Sonographic evaluation of ovarian torsion in childhood and adolescence. AJR Am J Roentgenol 1988;150:647

Herter L, Magalnaes J, Spritzer P: Association of ovarian volume and serum LH levels in adolescent patients with menstrual disorders and/or hirsutism. Braz J Med Biol Res 1993;26:1041

Hugosson C, Jorulf H, Bakri Y: MRI in distal vaginal atresia. Pediatr Radiol 1991;21:281

Jamarillo D, Lebowitz RL, Hendren WH: The cloacal malformation: radiologic findings and imaging recommendations. Radiology 1990;177:441

Kurtz AB, Middleton WD: Ultrasound: The Requisites. St. Louis, Mosby–Year Book, 1996:202

Larsen W, Felmar E, Wallace M, Frieder R: Sertoli-Leydig cell tumor of the ovary: a rare cause of amenorrhea. Obstet Gynecol 1992;79:831

Lee E, Kwon H, Joo H, et al: Diagnosis of ovarian torsion with color Doppler sonography: depiction of twisted vascular pedicle. J Ultrasound Med 1998;17:83

Levitin A, Haller K, Cohen HL, et al: Endodermal sinus tumor of the ovary: imaging evaluation. AJR Am J Roentgenol 1996;167:791

Nussbaum A, Sanders R, Jones M: Neonatal uterine morphology as seen on real-time US. Radiology 1986;160:641

Nussbaum Blask AR, Sanders RC, Gearhart JP: Obstructed ureterovaginal anomalies: demonstration with sonography. Part 1. Neonates and infants. Radiology 1991;179:79

Orsini L, Salardi S, Pilu G, et al: Pelvic organs in premenarchal girls: real-time ultrasonography. Radiology 1984;153:113

Pais RC, Kim T, Zwiren G, Ragab A: Ovarian tumors in relapsing acute lymphoblastic leukemia: a review of 23 cases. J Pediatr Surg 1991;26:70

Pinkas H, Mashiach R, Rabinerson D, et al: Doppler parameters of uterine and ovarian stromal blood flow in women with polycystic ovary syndrome and normally ovulating women undergoing controlled ovarian stimulation. Ultrasound Obstet Gynecol 1998;12:197

Quillin S, Siegel M: Color Doppler ultrasound of children with acute lower abdominal pain. Radiographics 1993;13:293

Reed M, Griscom N: Hydrometrocolpos in infancy. Am J Roentgenol Radium Ther Nucl Med 1973;118:1

Reid R: Amenorrhea. *In* Copeland L (ed): Textbook of Gynecology. Philadelphia, WB Saunders, 1993:367

Reinhold C, Hricak H, Forstner R, et al: Primary amenorrhea: evaluation with MR imaging. Radiology 1997;203:383

Rosenblatt M, Rosenblatt R, Kutcher R, et al: Utero-vaginal hypoplasia: sonographic, embryologic and clinical considerations. Pediatr Radiol 1991;21:536

Rosenfield R: Hyperandrogenism in peripubertal girls. Pediatr Clin North Am 1990;37:1333

Ruggierro M, Awobuluyi M, Cohen H, Zinn D: Imaging the pediatric pelvis: role of ultrasound. Radiologist 1997;4:155

Salardi S, Orsini, L, Cacciari E, et al: Pelvic ultrasonography in premenarchal girls: relation to puberty and sex hormone concentrations. Arch Dis Child 1985;60:120

Scanlan KA, Pozniak M, Fagerholm M, Shapiro S: Value of transperineal sonography in the assessment of vaginal atresia. AJR Am J Roentgenol 1990;154:545

Shah R, Woolley M, Costin G: Testicular feminization syndrome: the androgen insensitivity syndrome. J Pediatr Surg 1992;27:757

Sherer D, Shah Y, Eggers P, Woods J: Prenatal sonographic diagnosis and subsequent management of fetal adnexal torsion. J Ultrasound Med 1990;9:161

Siegel MJ: Pediatric gynecologic sonography. Radiology 1991;179:593

Sisler CL, Siegel MJ: Ovarian teratomas: a comparison of the sonographic appearance in prepubertal and postpubertal girls. AJR Am J Roentgenol 1990;154:139

Steele GS, Clancy T, Datta M, et al: Angiosarcoma arising in a testicular teratoma. J Urol 2000;163:1872

Surratt J, Siegel M: Imaging of pediatric ovarian masses. Radiographics 1991;11:533

Takahashi K, Okada M, Ozaki T, et al: Transvaginal ultrasonographic morphology in polycystic ovarian syndrome. Gynecol Obstet Invest 1995;39:201

Ulbright T, Srigley J: Dermoid cyst of the testis: a study of five postpubertal cases, including a pilomatrixoma-like variant, with evidence supporting its separate classification from mature testicular teratoma. Am J Surg Pathol 2001;25:788

Weckstein L: Current perspective on ectopic pregnancy. Obstet Gynecol Surg 1985;40:259

Westrom L: Incidence, prevalence and trends of acute pelvic inflammatory disease and its consequences in industrialized countries. Am J Obstet Gynecol 1980;138:880

Woodward P, Sohaey R, Wagner B: Congenital uterine malformations. Curr Probl Diagn Radiol 1995;24:177

Wu A, Siegel MJ: Sonography of pelvic masses in children: diagnostic predictability. AJR Am J Roentgenol 1987;148:1199

PART III

ANOMALIES OF SEX DIFFERENTIATION*

HARRIS L. COHEN
JACK O. HALLER

There are various conditions that result in abnormalities or confusion with regard to a patient's sex differentiation. The etiologies of these conditions are varied. In some cases, excessive androgen stimulation of the female fetus in early gestation may lead to anatomic findings that can confuse sexual identification by phenotype. The same is true in males when there is either deficient synthesis or metabolism of testosterone or deficient end-organ sensitivity to normal testosterone. Other abnormalities that lead to abnormal sex differentiation are due to abnormalities of the sex chromosomes or gonads themselves. The external genitalia of such patients range from either deformed or ambiguous to normal. Problems of sex differentiation may be noted in patients whose genitalia are consistent with their genetic (chromosomal) and gonadal (ovary or testis) sex or in patients with inconsistency between their external genitalia and their genetic or gonadal sex (e.g., a female phenotype in a patient who has a 46,XY chromosome makeup). The following pages discuss some of these issues and the clinical conditions in which they are found.

SOME EMBRYOLOGIC POINTS REGARDING SEX DIFFERENTIATION—GONAD DIFFERENTIATION

A person's genetic sex is determined at the time of fertilization. The development of a male genital system occurs as an "active" process requiring the presence of testes and their production of müllerian inhibiting factor (MIF), which, in turn, causes müllerian duct system involution. Dihydrotestoterone (DHT), acting locally, allows the wolffian duct system to develop into the epididymis, vas deferens, and seminal vesicles. The enzyme 5α-reductase converts testosterone intracellularly, within the target tissues, into the powerful androgen DHT. Differentiation of the primitive gonad into a testis begins at 7 weeks of fetal life in the presence of H-Y antigens. H-Y antigens are found in the cell membranes of normal XY males. A locus on the Y chromosome is responsible for either H-Y antigen production or expression. If there is no Y chromosome or there is abnormal H-Y antigen expression, the gonad will passively differentiate into an ovary by perhaps as early as 12 weeks' to perhaps as late as 17 weeks' gestation when in the presence of *two* X chromosomes. Absence of two X chromosomes may lead to abnormal or streak ovaries. The ovaries, however, are said to have no apparent role in sex differentiation of the female genital tract.

SEX DIFFERENTIATION DISORDERS WITHOUT AMBIGUITY OF EXTERNAL GENITALIA

PHENOTYPIC FEMALES

The best-known sex differentiation disorders that occur without ambiguity of external genitalia in phenotypic females are the classic XO Turner's syndrome, the chromatin-positive variant of Turner's syndrome, and XX and XY gonadal dysgenesis.

Turner's Syndrome (XO Gonadal Dysgenesis)

Turner's syndrome is the most common gonadal dysgenesis associated with an abnormal karyotype in girls. It is relatively common and nonfamilial. It is characterized by an abnormal sex chromosome, gonadal dysgenesis, and a number of somatic anomalies. At least half of

*This chapter is based in significant part on Currarino G, Wood B, Majd M: Abnormalities of the genital tract. *In* Silverman F, Kuhn J (eds): Caffey's Pediatric X-Ray Diagnosis, 9th ed. St Louis, Mosby–Year Book, 1993.

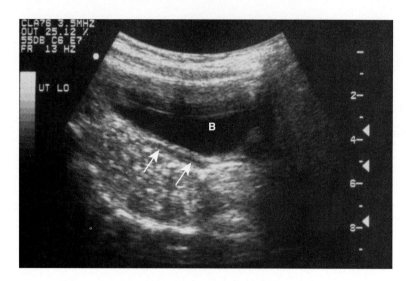

FIGURE 1. On ultrasound of the pelvis in the longitudinal midline plane, a small tubular uterus *(arrows)* is seen in this 16-year-old with primary amenorrhea. She was a 45,XO Turner's syndrome patient. Her ovaries could not be definitively identified. *B* = bladder.

affected patients have classical Turner's syndrome with an isochromatous 45,XO karyotype pattern. The second X chromosome is absent. In the case of classical Turner's syndrome, the presence of only a single X chromosome is the probable cause for the presence of streak ovaries (streaks or ridges of connective tissue in the mesosalpinges parallel to the fallopian tubes), rather than normal ovaries. Some functional ovarian elements are present in a few cases. Fallopian tubes, a uterus, and a vagina are present, and no wolffian duct derivatives are found.

Patients with classical Turner's syndrome have several somatic findings, some more common than others. Affected patients are short in stature (usually no greater than 58 inches), with a distinctive facies that includes low-set ears, a low hairline, and a high, arched palate. They classically have a short, broad, and webbed neck; widely spaced nipples; and a shield chest. Skeletal abnormalities, which are common, include cubitus valgus, short fourth and/or fifth metacarpals, and osteoporosis of hands, feet, elbows, and upper femora. Bone age is normal to slightly retarded during childhood. Steroid deficiency is considered the cause of typically retarded postpubertal bone age. Lymphedema of the extremities, particularly the hands and feet, as well as pleural effusions and ascites seen at birth may be linked to the cystic hygromas of the neck area noted in fetal life, of which the webbed neck is thought to be a residuum. Other variably seen findings include large aortic roots, coarctation of the aorta (particularly in those patients with webbed necks), and multiple pigmented nevi. One fourth of Turner's syndrome patients have renal anomalies, usually horseshoe kidneys but also including malrotation, duplication anomalies, and ureteropelvic junction obstruction. Systemic arterial hypertension is not uncommon and is thought to be of renovascular origin. However, a proven causative vascular lesion has not been imaged. Turner's syndrome patients have an increased incidence of autoimmune disorders, particularly Hashimoto's thyroiditis.

Patients with classical Turner's syndrome have a history of delayed onset of puberty, infantile internal and external genitalia, and primary amenorrhea. Young adolescents have sparse axillary and pubic hair and bilateral streak gonads. Ultrasound (US) evaluation typically shows a prepubertal uterus (Fig. 1). The prepubertal uterus, as well as the vagina, of such patients is normally formed and will respond to exogenous hormone stimulation. The dysgenetic or streak gonads are difficult to image. According to some sources, the gonads contain a normal amount of oocytes in early fetal/neonatal life, but accelerated oocyte loss leads to their depletion within the first years of life. When the adnexa are measured, they are typically less than 1 cm^3 in volume. In older adolescence, around 15 to 16 years, many Turner's syndrome patients will have pubic and axillary hair but no breast development or vaginal mucosal estrogenization.

Mosaic Turner's Syndrome

As many as one fourth of 45,XO Turner's syndrome patients have a so-called chromatin-positive pattern. Their karyotype is a mosaic consisting most often of a mixture of 45,XO and 46,XX chromosomes. Less often, there are other mosaic patterns without a Y cell line (e.g., XO/XXX or XO/XX/XXX), or 46,XX with an abnormal X chromosome. In such cases, the gonads may consist of a streak ovary on one side and a hypoplastic or normal ovary on the other side, bilateral hypoplastic ovaries, or essentially normal ovaries. External and internal genitalia are entirely female, without wolffian duct remnants. These patients usually do not have the somatic abnormalities typically attributed to classical Turner's syndrome, but many will still be short.

It is the Turner's syndrome patients with mosaic patterns, who have only partial ovarian failure, who may therefore develop secondary sex characteristics at puberty (said to occur in about 50%) and who, in some cases, may menstruate regularly. Instances of pregnancy have been reported. Although, as just noted, some (typically mosaic) Turner's syndrome patients can have estrogen production, such production requires the clinician to rule out the possibility of estrogen production from an associated theca–lutein cyst or a germ cell tumor. US is an excellent tool for this analysis.

Amenorrhea Caused by Hypergonadotropic Hypogonadism

Amenorrhea is a key indication for US of the adolescent pelvis. Primary amenorrhea is defined as a lack of menses by age 16. There are many causes of primary amenorrhea. Many of these causes may also be linked to causes of delayed or retarded sexual development as well as causes of secondary amenorrhea, defined as the cessation of menses at any point in time after menarche and before menopause.

There are other causes of hypergonadotropic hypogonadism that can lead to amenorrhea. Such patients may have secondary ovarian failure as a result of radiation (usually 800 rads or greater to the pelvis) or chemotherapy (at least transient amenorrhea occurs in 50% of women who undergo chemotherapy), or on an autoimmune basis (autoimmune oophoritis). Premature menopause, as a complication of chemotherapy or radiotherapy, is usually seen in those patients who are treated when 25 years of age or older and is unusual in adolescents. Adolescents with secondary causes of hypogonadotropic hypogonadism may have varying degrees of pubertal development.

Turner's syndrome is the primary example of the hypergonadotropic hypogonadism group of patients with primary amenorrhea. Such adolescents, who have high levels of follicle-stimulating hormone and luteinizing hormone by serum assays and yet do not have menses, are amenorrheic because of ovarian failure in which their gonadal tissues fail to respond to endogenous gonadotropins. In the pure form of the diseases that make up this group, secondary sex characteristics fail to develop and menses does not occur.

In the case of Turner's syndrome, the hypergonadotropic hypogonadism is due to a karyotype abnormality usually discovered early in life, particularly when present in its classical form. Other karyotype abnormalities placed under a broad heading of gonadal dysgenesis, including 46,XY and familial 46,XX gonadal dysgenesis, are also associated with failure of affected patients to develop secondary sexual characteristics or menses as a result of hypergonadotropic hypogonadism.

46,XY Gonadal Dysgenesis

There are patients with 46,XY gonadal dysgenesis who are phenotypically female, with streak gonads and infantile internal and external female genitalia, but who are neither typically short nor have the somatic findings of those with Turner's syndrome. These patients are usually first diagnosed as abnormal in adolescence. As with other forms of gonadal dysgenesis, such patients may not have an absent sex chromosome, but rather have abnormality of the sex chromosome that *is* present. One tenth of patients with XY gonadal dysgenesis have a deletion of the small arm of the Y chromosome linked to a testis-determining factor (and perhaps to MIF). Mosaicism may lead to the development of ovaries. If a Y chromosome is a component of the karyotype of a patient with gonadal dysgenesis and ovaries, the patient has an increased risk of developing a gonadoblastoma within a dysgenetic ovary. Imaging asymmetrically sized adnexa, especially if the larger adnexum is a solid mass, suggests the possibility of gonadoblastoma. Seminomas also occur in these patients. Inheritance of this condition is thought to be X-linked recessive or sex-limited autosomal dominant.

Familial 46,XX Gonadal Dysgenesis

Familial XX gonadal dysgenesis may be sporadic or inherited as an autosomal recessive trait. In some familial cases there is associated sensorineural deafness. The karyotype is 46,XX, and the gonads consist of bilateral streaks in some cases, while in others there may be hypoplastic ovaries or a hypoplastic ovary on one side and a streak gonad on the other. The internal and external genitalia are entirely female, without wolffian duct derivatives. Incomplete puberty may be observed in patients with residual ovarian tissue. Sexual infantilism and primary amenorrhea are typical findings in those patients with bilateral streak gonads.

PHENOTYPIC MALES

Klinefelter's Syndrome (47,XXY Seminiferous Tubular Dysgenesis)

Seminiferous tubular dysgenesis (Klinefelter's syndrome) is the most common human sex chromosome aberration. The typical 47,XXY karyotype is found in phenotypic males with primary hypogonadism. It is nonfamilial, occurring in 1 in every 750 to 1000 males. Variants have been described with less common chromosomal abnormalities, including XX/XXY or XY/XXY mosaicism, as well as XXXY, XXXXY, XXYY, or XXXYY sex chromosomal karyotypes. The external genitalia, especially the testes, are small. The testes are usually less than 3 cm in length and firm. Cryptorchidism and hypospadias are common. Progressive fibrosis of the seminiferous tubules occurs, especially after puberty, leading to azoospermia and sterility in most patients. Patients are often long legged. They are often mentally retarded or have psychological problems. The diagnosis is usually not made until after puberty. Gynecomastia develops in almost half of the older patients, and affected patients, particularly those with the more classical 47,XXY karyotype, are at an increased risk for breast cancer. Testicular and extragonadal germ cell neoplasms have been uncommonly reported.

A variant form (49,XXXXY) of Klinefelter's syndrome has somatic findings including radioulnar synostosis, coxa valga, abnormal facies, short neck, retarded bone age, hypertonia, small external genitalia, and severe mental retardation. These findings may allow diagnosis earlier than puberty.

Persistent Müllerian Duct Syndrome

Persistent müllerian duct syndrome (also known as uterine hernia syndrome and hernia uteri inguinalis) is a rare type of sexual differentiation abnormality of males caused by deficiency of MIF, the testicular hormone that causes the normal regression of the müllerian duct system in the male fetus. The patients usually have a normal 46,XY karyotype and are phenotypically male, but they have a small uterus and fallopian tubes and a small vagina connected to the posterior urethra at the level of the verumontanum. Unilateral or bilateral cryptorchidism is common. If the undescended testis is underdeveloped, the ipsilateral vas may be absent. Unilateral or bilateral inguinal hernias are common. A uterus (uteri hernia syndrome), fallopian tubes, or sometimes a testis may be found in the hernia. Uncommonly, gonadal neoplasia may occur. The disorder, typically sporadic, has been reported in siblings. The voiding or retrograde urethrogram is usually normal. In these patients, direct catheterization and injection of the utricle (noted on US as a cystic area in the region of the prostate, extending from the seminal colliculus and said to be the male analog of the uterus and vagina and residua of the fused posterior ends of the müllerian ductal system) with contrast material at urethroscopy may demonstrate a uterus and/or fallopian tubes.

DISORDERS OF SEX DIFFERENTIATION WITH AMBIGUOUS EXTERNAL GENITALIA

The four main groups with ambiguous external genitalia and problems of sex differentiation are female intersex (pseudohermaphroditism), male intersex, mixed gonadal dysgenesis, and true hermaphrodites.

PSEUDOHERMAPHRODITISM (INTERSEX)

Pseudohermaphroditism or intersex problems are abnormalities in which there is nonaccord of chromosomal, gonadal, and genital sex. Unlike true hermaphroditism, which is rare and in which the nonaccord is based on the presence of two types of gonads or elements of both type of gonads in, for example, an ovotestis, pseudohermaphroditism has nonaccord but only one gender's gonads are present. By definition male intersex patients have testes and female intersex patients have ovaries or ovarian tissue.

Female Intersex

Female intersex is usually diagnosed in neonatal life in chromosomally normal females (46,XX) with masculinized external genitalia. The cause, in cases of congenital

adrenal hyperplasia or adrenogenital syndrome, is usually increased fetal adrenal androgen production. Other cases may be due to maternal causes such as androgen ingestion in early pregnancy or, rarely, a masculinizing ovarian tumor in the mother. Excess androgen exposure leading to female intersex is thought to usually occur in the first trimester. Affected patients have normal ovaries, uterus, and fallopian tubes. They have no testicular tissue or internal wolffian ducts derivatives. In most cases the external genitalia are ambiguous (Fig. 2), with a prominent phallus or partially fused labial scrotal folds. There is a variously sized vagina connected with the posterior urethra and forming a urogenital sinus (UGS), which commonly empties at the base of the phallus (Fig. 3). There is a spectrum of possible external genital findings ranging from mild virilization manifested by mild clitoral hypertrophy to rare patients with an advanced degree of virilization and a normal-appearing but empty "scrotum," a large phallus resembling a penis, and a penile (phallic) urethra usually associated with apparent hypospadias. No gonads can be palpated in the labioscrotal folds or in the inguinal canal of such patients because they are within the pelvis. US can assess enlarged adrenal glands as well as normal uterine development in patients suspected of having this problem. Voiding cystourethrography often shows a male-type elongated urethra (Fig. 4). These patients are potentially fertile with satisfactory genital reconstruction and correct sex assignment.

Congenital Adrenal Hyperplasia

Congenital adrenal hyperplasia (see Fig. 4) is by far the most common cause of abnormal sex differentiation in females, occurring in 1 in 15,000 live births worldwide (see Section II, Part V, Chapter 10, page 239). It is due to

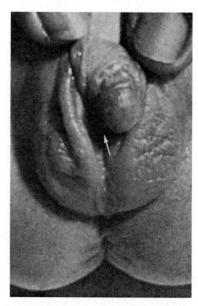

FIGURE 2. Ambiguous external genitalia in a 1-month-old infant. A phallus and scrotum are present, but no gonads are palpable. A single perineal opening was found at the base of the phallus (arrow).

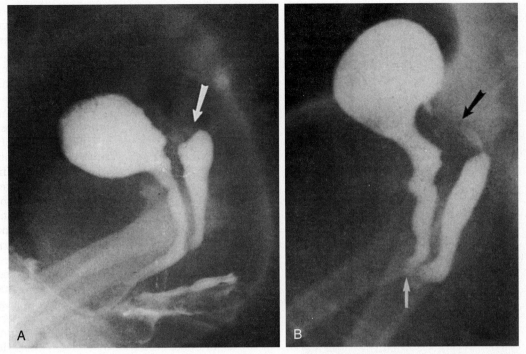

FIGURE 3. Two cases of adrenogenital syndrome showing different degrees of masculinization of the lower urogenital tract as seen on lateral views from voiding cystourethrograms (VCUGs). **A,** Urogenital sinus, the most common appearance of the lower urogenital tract in adrenogenital syndrome, in one infant. A well-developed vagina with a well-defined impression of the uterine cervix on the vaginal vault *(arrow)* joins the distal end of the urethra to form a long common sinus tract (urogenital sinus) that ends in the perineum at the base of a prominent phallus. Barium paste was applied on the perineum to show the distance between the vagina and perineum. **B,** The VCUG of a second infant with adrenogenital syndrome shows a well-developed vagina with opacification of the uterine canal *(upper arrow)* that joins the urethra very near the perineum to form an ultrashort urogenital sinus *(lower arrow)*. An enlarged clitoris, posterior fusion of the labia, and a single perineal opening were the only external signs of the disorder, which caused only mild virilization. There are patients at the opposite end of the spectrum who appear more severely masculinized, with a phallic urethra.

an inherited deficiency of enzymes involved in adrenocortical hormone biosynthesis.

Male Intersex

Male intersex patients are true males with a normal 46,XY male karyotype, present H-Y antigens, normal or mildly defective (and usually undescended) testes, but incomplete masculinization or frank ambiguity of their external genitalia. Cases of pure male intersex (pseudohermaphroditism) are usually not diagnosed until after puberty. These patients are thought to be female and may present with the clinical concern of primary amenorrhea. Other cases of male intersex have either incomplete testosterone production or early destruction or dysgenesis of the testes and do not produce testosterone. Decreased testosterone production and a lack of MIF production results in a karyotypically normal male with a female phenotype (except for partial masculinization of the external genitalia), and incomplete inhibition of the development of müllerian elements such as the uterus, vagina, and fallopian tubes (Fig. 5). Such patients usually have no secondary sexual development at puberty and may have an infantile uterus on US. If production of MIF by the testes is not affected, no internal müllerian system structures (uterus and fallopian tubes) will develop. The underly-

ing defect in these cases is an abnormality of metabolism of testosterone by the fetal testes. The biochemical defect may be decreased androgen synthesis, decreased DHT production as a result of deficiency of 5α-reductase, or a defect in the androgen receptors. In many cases the exact etiology remains unknown.

There are a variety of rarer forms of male intersex caused by deficiency of various enzymes necessary to produce testosterone. Manifestations are variable. Deficiency of enzymes affecting the synthesis of both corticosteroids and testosterone (e.g., 20,22-desmolase, 3β-hydroxysteroid dehydrogenase) or affecting only the synthesis of testosterone by the testis (17β-ketosteroid reductase) may produce infants with an entirely female phenotype with a blind-ending vaginal pouch emptying in the perineum, who may be partially masculinized with varying degrees of genital ambiguity similar to that seen in congenital adrenal hyperplasia. The testes are undescended. Defects involving the synthesis of both testosterone and corticosteroids are considered variants of congenital adrenal hyperplasia and are complicated by severe salt wasting or hypertension. At puberty, patients with decreased testosterone synthesis by the testes often show some virilization and may develop gynecomastia. Gonadal neoplasia has not been reported in these cases.

Another form of male intersex, caused by a deficiency

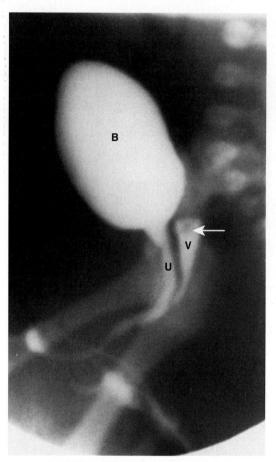

FIGURE 4. Congenital adrenal hyperplasia patient's voiding cysto-urethrogram in the lateral view (the image is not in classical position). The bladder *(B)* with an elongated male-type urethra *(U)* is noted. Posterior to it is a vagina *(V)* with a subtle impression *(arrow)* of a cervix superiorly. The patient was a 46,XX neonate from an area in Puerto Rico where congenital adrenal hyperplasia is common. (From Cohen H, Haller J: Pediatric and adolescent genital abnormalities. Clin Diagn Ultrasound 1988;24:187–216, with permission. Copyright Elsevier Science [USA].)

in 5α-reductase (Fig. 5*B*), the enzyme that converts testosterone to DHT (the locally active androgenic substance responsible for masculinization of the male's external genitalia), results in pseudovaginal perineal hypospadias. Production of testosterone and MIF is not affected. The testes are well developed and normal histologically. They may be located intra-abdominally, in the inguinal canals, or in the scrotal folds. The external genitalia are poorly masculinized, with a phallus of intermediate size resembling a clitoris more than a penis. The urethra opens at the base of the phallus (perineoscrotal hypospadias), and the vagina is a blind-ending structure of variable size emptying onto the perineum behind the urethral opening (pseudovagina), or occasionally in the urethra (UGS) (Fig. 5). There are no internal müllerian derivatives (uterus and tubes), and the epididymis, vas deferens, seminal vesicles, and ejaculatory ducts are present and empty into the vagina. There is an underdeveloped prostate. At puberty there is variable, sometimes remarkable, masculinization of the patient, with descent of the testes, increased phallus size, development of

normal axillary and pubic hair, deepening of the voice, and increased muscle mass. Spermatogenesis has been reported. Gynecomastia does not develop. Gonadal neoplasms may occur but are uncommon.

Testicular Feminization Syndrome (Androgen Receptor Defect)

Testicular feminization syndrome (Fig. 6) is a form of intersex in which 46,XY patients have well-formed testes (usually undescended within the abdomen or inguinal region) that produce androgens and MIF. The patients, however, do not have an end-organ response to the androgens. Müllerian system development is inhibited, and patients do not develop a uterus, fallopian tubes, or upper two thirds of the vagina. They do develop secondary female sexual characteristics via circulating estrogens (produced by the testes and adrenal gland). Because there is no turnoff mechanism for testosterone, there are, at times, higher than normal amounts of testosterone converted to estrogen. Patients with the complete form of the abnormality appear as phenotypically normal females, although they may have inguinal or labial masses resulting from the undescended testes (Fig. 6*B*). They have normal breast development, but pubic and axillary hair are scant. They do not suffer from acne. They may or may not have a short, blind-ending vagina behind the urethral opening. They often first present with amenorrhea. Ultrasound examination will show no uterus (Fig. 6*A*) and no ovaries. This inherited end-organ unresponsiveness to the action of endogenous or exogenous androgen (androgen resistance) is caused by a defect in a specific cytoplasmic receptor protein (cytosol receptor) that normally binds DHT to the plasma membrane and transports it to the nuclear chromatin.

The complete form of testicular feminization syndrome is seen in 1 in every 20,000 to 60,000 apparent females. It is inherited as an X-linked recessive trait, affecting 50% of the males in the same family. Affected females are carriers. After puberty, many such patients undergo gonadectomy, because any cryptorchid patient would be at risk for developing a gonadal neoplasm. These patients are treated with substitutional estrogen therapy.

Incomplete Forms of Testicular Feminization Syndrome

There is an incomplete form (10% to 20% of cases) of testicular feminization that can present earlier in life with ambiguous genitalia. Affected patients may have a predominantly female phenotype (incomplete testicular feminization), or a predominantly male phenotype (Reifenstein's syndrome). These patients have an incomplete androgen receptor defect. Those with a predominantly female phenotype have the same anatomic abnormalities as in complete testicular feminization except for the presence of mild virilization of the external genitalia in some cases (clitoromegaly and partial labial fusion), and the presence of wolffian duct derivatives that empty into the vagina (Fig. 5*A*). A

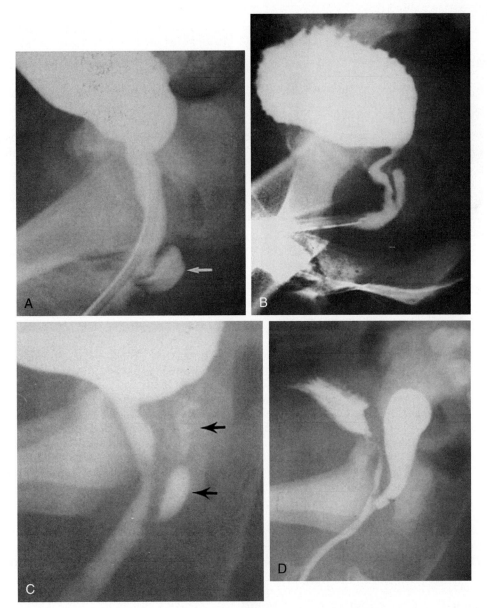

FIGURE 5. Four cases of male pseudohermaphroditism. **A,** Male pseudohermaphrodite with incomplete testicular feminization syndrome. The patient had a predominantly female phenotype. Voiding cystourethrogram (VCUG) shows a mildly elongated urethra and retrograde opacification of a short, blind-ending vaginal pouch in the perineum behind the urethra (*arrow*). Seminal ducts may end in a vaginal pouch such as this. A similar configuration can be seen in patients with complete testicular feminization syndrome and in patients with 5α-reductase deficiency. **B,** Male pseudohermaphrodite with 5α-reductase deficiency. The patient is a 3½–year-old child with ambiguous external genitalia. A retrograde urethrogram shows a urogenital sinus and a small vagina without a cervical imprint. A more common pattern in 5α-reductase deficiency is that shown in **A. C,** A male infant with severe hypospadias (perineal and scrotoperineal), bilateral cryptorchidism, small penis, and unfused scrotal folds has a VCUG that shows a utricle or blind vaginal pouch that is very short and extending off the distal aspect of the posterior urethra. *Arrows* show spermatic ducts emptying into the utricle. The male urethra is somewhat short. **D,** Male pseudohermaphrodite with severe hypospadius. Retrograde urethrogram shows a somewhat longer utricle connected with the distal end of the posterior urethra. The male urethra is somewhat short.

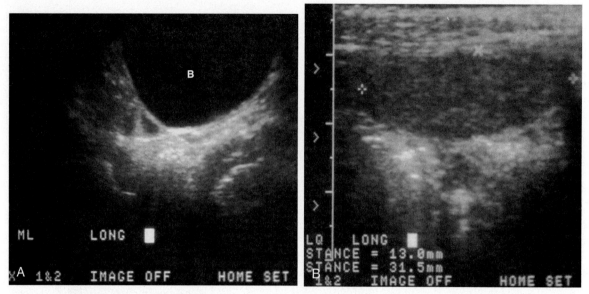

FIGURE 6. Testicular feminization syndrome. **A,** A phenotypically normal 16-year-old presented with primary amenorrhea. A pelvic ultrasound in the longitudinal plane showed no uterus posterior to the bladder. Ovaries were also not seen. Karyotyping proved the patient to be 46,XY. The patient was proven to have testicular feminization syndrome. *B* = bladder. **B,** On examination for primary amenorrhea, the patient was noted to have bilateral inguinal masses. An oval structure without contained cysts was found in the patient's left inguinal region on longitudinal plane ultrasound. The ultrasound image is that of a normal but undescended left testicle, marked off by measurement markers, which it proved to be. (**A** and **B** courtesy of Joseph Yee, M.D.)

varying degree of virilization or feminization is observed at puberty, but menses does not occur. Those patients with Reifenstein's syndrome have more advanced degree of virilization. The degree of masculinization may vary greatly even in the same family. In the most severely affected (poorly virilized) patients, there is a small phallus, and an incomplete fusion of the labial scrotal folds, or a bifid scrotum. The urethra empties at the base of the phallus, and there may be a separate vaginal pouch ending in the perineum behind the urethra (pseudovagina). More commonly, however, the patient is less severely affected (more virilized) and has a better developed penis and scrotum.

Hypospadias is the rule, ranging from perineoscrotal to penile. A large prostatic utricle (Fig. 7) or a blind vaginal pouch connected to the posterior urethra may be present. The testes tend to be smaller than normal and are often undescended. The prostate is absent. Wolffian duct derivatives are usually present but may be incompletely developed and may empty in the utricle or

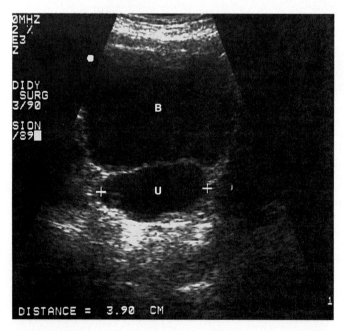

FIGURE 7. Utricle as seen on ultrasound of the pelvis in the transverse plane. A cystic mass *(U)* is noted posterior to the bladder *(B)* of a boy with significant hypospadius and incomplete testicular feminization syndrome. (From Cohen HL, Bober S, Bow S: Imaging the pediatric pelvis: the normal and abnormal genital tract and simulators of its diseases. Urol Radiol 1992;14:273–283, with permission.)

vaginal pouch. There is no uterus or fallopian tubes. The habitus is generally masculine, and most patients are reared as males. At puberty, there is some development of axillary and pubic hair but no chest or facial hair or voice changes. Postpubertal gynecomastia, azoospermia, and infertility are typical. In both types of incomplete testicular feminization, gonadal neoplasms have been reported uncommonly.

GONADAL DYSGENESIS

Mixed Gonadal Dysgenesis (Dysgenetic Male Pseudohermaphroditism)

Mixed or asymmetric gonadal dysgenesis (also known as XO/XY gonadal dysgenesis) is a relatively common form of abnormal sexual differentiation, usually occurring sporadically. Affected patient karyotypes are most often a mosaic of 45,XO and 46,XX. At times, XO/XYY or other mosaicisms are seen. These patients often have a streak gonad similar to that seen in Turner's syndrome on one side, and a usually dysgenetic (but occasionally normal) testis on the other. A fallopian tube is often present on the side of the streak gonad, and a vas deferens may be present on the side of the testis. The testis is usually intra-abdominal but can be partially or completely descended. The external genitalia cover a wide spectrum of appearances from that of an almost normal female to that of an essentially normal male with hypospadius. Most patients have ambiguous external genitalia (as seen in other intersex situations), with a phallus/clitoris of variable size, unfused labioscrotal folds, and a variously sized vagina connected with the urethra (UGS) and commonly emptying at the base of the phallus (Fig. 8). A uterus, said to be present in all cases, is usually small or rudimentary. Most patients are raised as females, but at puberty some virilization may take place (usually without gynecomastia).

Mixed gonadal (gonadal streak on one side and testicular tissue on the other) dysgenesis patients, as already noted, are at a high risk for developing gonadal neoplasia. The risk increases with increasing patient age. Gonadectomy is recommended at the time of diagnosis. Although commonly seen in XO/XY mosaicism, cases may also occur in 46,XY males with a structurally abnormal Y chromosome or in patients with the 46,XY variant of gonadal dysgenesis.

Familial 46,XY Gonadal Dysgenesis

This condition is inherited as an X-linked (or male-limited) autosomal dominant trait, but sporadic cases can occur. The disorder may be associated with camptomelic dwarfism. The karyotype is 46,XY. The gonads are variable and may be bilateral streaks, bilateral dysgenetic testes, or a streak on one side and a dysgenetic testis on the other (mixed gonadal dysgenesis). Cases with different gonadal anatomy may be observed in the same family.

Patients with bilateral streak gonads have a female

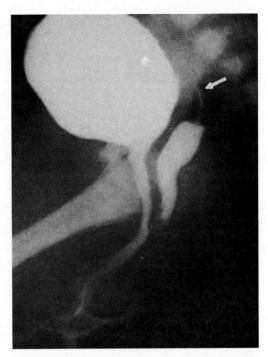

FIGURE 8. Mixed gonadal dysgenesis. A voiding cystourethrogram (lateral view) shows a urogenital sinus with a well-developed vagina in an 11-day-old with ambiguous external genitalia. There is a cervical imprint, and contrast material opacifies the uterine canal *(arrow)*.

phenotype with normal fallopian tubes, uterus, and vagina, usually clitoromegaly, and absence of wolffian duct derivatives. Sexual infantilism and amenorrhea are expected at puberty. Somatic features similar to those of Turner's syndrome may be observed. Patients with bilateral dysgenetic testes or with a mixed form of gonadal dysgenesis typically have ambiguous or incompletely masculinized external genitalia. Müllerian and wolffian duct derivatives are present but may be hypoplastic or rudimentary. At puberty, various degrees of virilization usually take place. Patients with this form of gonadal dysgenesis have the same high risk of developing gonadal tumors as those with XO/XY gonadal dysgenesis.

Drash Syndrome—Gonadal Dysgenesis, Nephropathy, and Wilms' Tumor

Drash syndrome is an uncommon form of gonadal dysgenesis and male intersex. Patients most often have a 46,XY karyotype, bilateral gonadal dysgenesis with a variable histologic pattern, ambiguous external genitalia, and intra-abdominal testes. They have chronic glomerulonephritis with histologic features similar to those of congenital nephrosis. They develop end-stage renal disease in early life. Greater than half of these patients develop a Wilms' tumor at a young age. Purportedly this occurs only in those patients with Drash syndrome who have a female phenotype. Twenty percent to 30% of patients with Drash syndrome develop gonadal neoplasia.

46,XY Gonadal Agenesis (Vanishing Testes Syndrome)

Patients with this condition are male with a 46,XY karyotype. No gonads are present, and there is an absent or incomplete male sex differentiation as a result of testicular resorption of unknown cause in early fetal life. The external genitalia are ambiguous, and there is usually complete absence of both müllerian and wolffian duct derivatives. Occasional cases may have partial development of both systems. This vanishing testes syndrome is differentiated from cases of bilateral anorchia (congenital absence of the testes), which are presumably due to resorption of the testes after the first trimester (i.e., beyond 13 to 14 weeks' gestational age). Those patients have normal male sex development and no residual müllerian structures. However, some families have individuals with 46,XY gonadal agenesis as well as individuals with bilateral anorchia, suggesting some link between the two conditions.

TRUE HERMAPHRODITISM

True hermaphroditism is a rare condition. It is a sporadic disorder in which the affected patient has both testicular and ovarian tissue in the same or contralateral gonads. More than half such patients have a 46,XX karyotype. Mosaic karyotype patterns with at least one line with a Y chromosome do exist, including XO/XY, XX/XXY, or XX/XY chimerism (30%). Fifteen percent of patients are 46,XY. All true hermaphrodites are H-Y antigen positive regardless of karyotype. In 45,XX patients, undetected Y chromosomal material is probably present and transferred to another chromosome. Half of the cases have a testis (or an ovary) on one side and an ovotestis on the other, 30% have a testis on one side and an ovary on the other, and 20% of the time there are bilateral ovotestes. The testes or ovotestes may be intra-abdominal, in the inguinal region, in the scrotal area, or in the labia majora. The ovaries of hermaphrodites are almost always intra-abdominal. The testis or the testicular portion of an ovotestis is usually dysgenetic, and spermatogenesis after puberty is rare. Ovulation occurs more commonly. Internal gonadal ducts are usually consistent with the ipsilateral gonad (i.e., a vas on the side of a testis and a fallopian tube on the side of an ovary). In the case of ovotestes, the associated internal gonadal duct is usually a fallopian tube. A uterus is found in almost all cases but is most often hypoplastic and may be bicornuate.

There is a wide spectrum of external genitalia ranging from normal male to ambiguous to female. Cryptorchidism is common. Inguinal hernias are common and, as with normal patients, can contain a gonad with its internal gonadal duct or even a uterus. About 75% of hermaphrodites are brought up as males. At puberty, there is usually some virilization as well as gynecomastia. Fertility and childbearing have been described in some 46,XX patients. Gonadal neoplasms are uncommon.

GONADAL NEOPLASIA OF PATIENTS WITH DISORDERS OF SEX DIFFERENTIATION

As discussed, the gonads in several intersex disorders (with or without ambiguous genitalia) are at an increased risk for developing neoplasms. Neoplasms are almost always germ cell in type, including seminoma or dysgerminoma and gonadoblastoma. Less commonly, patients may develop a gonadal teratoma, teratocarcinoma, yolk sac tumor, embryonal carcinoma of the adult type, or choriocarcinoma. These neoplasms are rare in patients who do not have a Y chromosome as part of their karyotype. The risk is apparently related to the H-Y antigen. One must be aware that, because the gonad may be in an unusual location (i.e., inguinal area, labia, abdomen), that is also where the neoplasm may be discovered. This is especially true for intra-abdominal gonads. The fact that, in some intersex disorders, the incidence of gonadal neoplasia is higher than in males with simple cryptorchidism suggests that there is an additional causative factor of unknown etiology.

Patients with the highest risk of developing gonadal neoplasia are those with XO/XY mixed gonadal dysgenesis and those with 46,XY gonadal dysgenesis. The incidence of a gonadal tumor in both these conditions increases from 3% to 4% by age 10 years to 10% to 20% within the second decade of life and to 70% or more in older patients. Gonadal neoplasms are less frequent (but still more common than in simple cryptorchidism) in patients with complete testicular feminization syndrome. One fifth of those patients develop a gonadal tumor after 25 years of age but have little risk of such a tumor in childhood.

Gonadal neoplasms also occur in Klinefelter's syndrome, persistent müllerian duct syndrome, incomplete testicular feminization, 5α-reductase deficiency, and true hermaphroditism, but with a risk equal to or lower than that in simple cryptorchidism.

DIAGNOSTIC EVALUATION OF PATIENTS WITH AMBIGUOUS GENITALIA

The discovery of anomalous or ambiguous genitalia in a newborn has been described as an emergency from a social perspective and hence, to many, from a clinical perspective as well. Of the seven components of sexual identity described by Hanson (chromosomes, gonads, external genital anatomy, internal genital anatomy, hormones, rearing, and psychosexual orientation), rearing has been considered key and perhaps the most important factor. Paramount in the decision on how to rear a child is the identification of the uterus, vagina, or UGS by US, contrast fistulogram, or vaginogram. These findings can then be correlated and sexual identification aided by current laboratory methods used in the treating institution. Methods used have included sex chromatin studies (buccal smear), hormone assays, analysis of blood electrolytes and metabolites, fluorescent studies for Y chromosome, culture of genital skin fibroblasts for androgen receptor binding, tests for androgen responsiveness, and of course karyotyping. Sometimes the definitive anatomic diagnosis is made only at laparoscopy or laparotomy and on the basis of gonadal biopsy. The main role of US, and a most helpful early imaging finding, is identification of the uterus, a relatively easy task in the newborn female.

Important diagnostic clues as to sexual identity and causes of gender identification confusion may be obtained from clinical history, particularly the history of maternal exposure to androgens or progestins during the first trimester of pregnancy, or the history of similar findings in other members of the newborn's family. The appearance of the external genitalia is seldom diagnostic of a specific intersex disorder, but palpable gonads in the inguinal canal, labioscrotal folds, or scrotum can exclude female pseudohermaphroditism in most cases. There are females with inguinal hernias who may have an ovary, perhaps with the fallopian tube, in the inguinal region or the labia.

A detailed radiographic study of the lower genitourinary tract (genitography) is important for diagnosis and as a guide in surgical reconstructive procedures. Patients usually have a UGS, a common terminal channel for the anterior urethra and posterior vaginal pouch. This sinus usually empties at the base of the phallus. A UGS anomaly should be suspected whenever there is a single perineal opening and any degree of ambiguity of the external genitalia. A voiding cystourethrogram (VCUG), particularly on lateral view, may outline the entire anatomy needed for evaluation. If the urethral catheter can be advanced only to the vagina, an injection with the catheter in that position may opacify the vagina, the UGS, and often the proximal urethra. If there is still confusion about the anatomy during the VCUG exam, a retrograde injection of contrast material may be attempted through a catheter

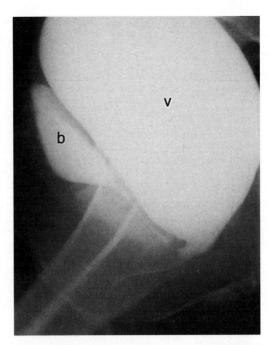

FIGURE 10. Hydrocolpos in adrenogenital syndrome. A large obstructed vagina is demonstrated in a retrograde vaginogram (lateral view) with the catheter in the vagina. The urogenital sinus of a 14-year-old girl with known adrenogenital syndrome and urogenital sinus who presented with abdominal pain and a pelvic mass. *v* = vagina, *b* = bladder.

whose tip is placed just inside the "urethral" meatus. At times, a firmer catheter (with a curved tip) manipulated under fluoroscopic control into the urethra and bladder or into the vagina may improve contrast study of the area. At times, it may be impossible to opacify all the components of the UGS anomaly at the same time. An effort should be made on the VCUG/vaginogram to determine if a uterine cervix is present. Often, if a uterus (especially if normal) is present, there is a mass impression of the cervix on the contrast filled vagina (see Fig. 4). A cervical imprint, however, may not be apparent if the vagina is not sufficiently distended or if the uterus is hypoplastic.

In some patients evaluated by VCUG/contrast vaginogram, the UGS is quite short and joined by the vagina very close to the perineal surface (Fig. 9). In other patients it is a much longer channel, joined by the vagina at a much higher level, occasionally near the bladder neck. A very high insertion of the vagina in the UGS may pose a problem at the time of vaginal reconstruction because of the danger of injuring the external urethral sphincter. In patients evaluated for abnormalities of sex differentiation/ambiguous genitalia, the vagina may vary in size from a small cavity to an organ of normal size for the patient's age. Occasionally its distal end is stenosed or is completely obliterated, resulting in hydrocolpos at birth or hematocolpos at puberty (Fig. 10).

The length of the UGS and the level of insertion of the vagina into the UGS are good indicators of the degree of virilization that has taken place, but the findings are nonspecific regarding the true sex of the patient or

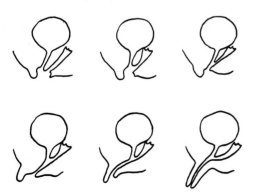

FIGURE 9. Different types of urogenital sinus are arranged in order of increasing masculinization, from an almost normal female pattern to a penile urethra. The urogenital sinus is of variable length, and the vagina may enter the urogenital sinus at various levels.

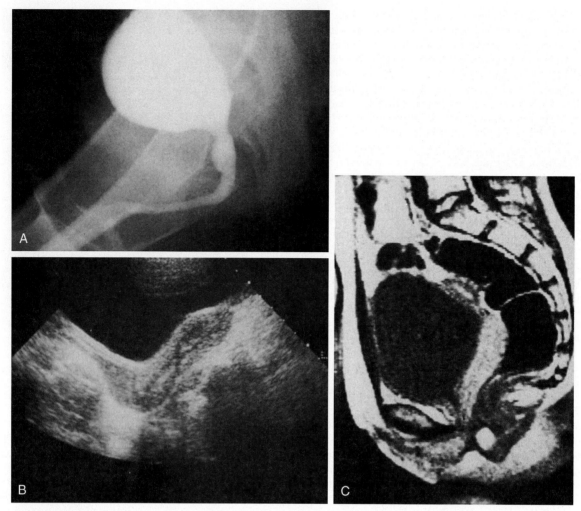

FIGURE 11. Anatomic evaluation of a 13-year-old with known adrenogenital syndrome being evaluated prior to surgical vaginoplasty. **A,** On a voiding cystourethrogram (lateral view), a phallic urethra is noted. A vagina is not seen. **B,** On ultrasound (lateral view), there is a normal adult uterus. The proximal two thirds of the vagina are noted and appear normal. **C,** On T_1-weighted magnetic resonance imaging (lateral view), the vagina is well seen throughout its course posterior to the low- to medium-intensity bladder and anterior to the low-intensity bowel. A small uterus is seen anterosuperior to it.

the type of underlying disorder. For this purpose, the presence or absence of a cervical imprint on the vaginogram is more important. A uterine cervix is present in all female intersex patients. It is a common finding among many patients with mixed gonadal dysgenesis or true hermaphroditism as well. All these groups may have a hypoplastic or rudimentary uterus that may not be noted radiographically. Cervical imprints are not seen in male pseudohermaphroditism or male hypospadias.

Pelvic US is valuable in evaluating infants with ambiguous genitalia. We find US the best tool for identification of uterine tissue. Obviously hypoplastic uterine tissue may be difficult to denote using any imaging modality. The proximal vagina may also be demonstrated, particularly if it contains urine, but the urethra and UGS cannot be studied by this method. US does not replace genitography but is of particular value when genitography is unsuccessful. Instillation of fluid in the rectum may be helpful in separating stool from a retrovesical mass. Ovaries are often seen. Fallopian tubes, unless obstructed, are more difficult to image. Some enlargement of the adrenal glands may be seen in congenital adrenal hyperplasia, but normal-sized adrenals do not rule out this diagnosis. In addition, the adrenal glands of newborns are usually prominent. US is an excellent tool for the identification of the adrenal gland in the newborn as well as the older child. Pelvic magnetic resonance imaging may also be of value (Fig. 11) in situations with complex anatomy.

SUGGESTED READINGS

Boechat MI, Westra SJ, Lippe B: Normal US appearance of ovaries and uterus in four patients with Turner's syndrome and 45,X karyotype. Pediatr Radiol 1996;26:37

Cohen HL: Evaluation of the adolescent and young adult with amenorrhea: role of US. *In* Bluth E, Arger P, Hertzberg B, Middleton W (eds): Syllabus: A Special Course in Ultrasound: Clinical Questions, Practical Answers. Oak Brook, IL, RSNA Publications, 1996:171

Cohen HL, Bober S, Bow S: Imaging the pediatric pelvis: the normal and abnormal genital tract and simulators of its diseases. Urol Radiol 1992;14:273

Cohen HL, Haller JO: Pediatric and adolescent genital abnormalities. Clin Diag Ultrasound 1988;24:187

Conte F, Grumbach MM: Pathogenesis, classification, and treatment of anomalies of sex. *In* DeGroot LJ (ed): Endocrinology. Philadelphia, WB Saunders, 1989:1810

Coran AG, Polley TZ Jr: Surgical management of ambiguous genitalia in the infant and child. J Pediatr Surg 1991;26:812

Currarino G, Wood B, Majd M: Abnormalities of the genital tract. *In* Silverman F, Kuhn J (eds): Caffey's Pediatric X-Ray Diagnosis, 9th ed. St. Louis, Mosby-Year Book, 1993;1375

Fernandes E, Fernandes E, Hollabaugh S, et al: Persistent mullerian duct syndrome. Urology 1990;36:516

Ganong W (ed): The gonads: development and function of the reproductive system. *In* Review of Medical Physiology, 17th ed. Norwalk, CT, Appleton & Lange, 1995:399

Hall JG, Gilchrist DM: Turner syndrome and its variants. Pediatr Clin North Am 1990;37:1421

Marcantonio SM, Fechner PY, Migeon CJ, et al: Embryonic testicular regression sequence: a part of the clinical spectrum of 46,XY gonadal dysgenesis. Am J Med Genet 1994;49:1

Sivit CJ, Hung W, Taylor G, et al: Sonography in neonatal congenital adrenal hyperplasia. AJR Am J Roentgenol 1991;156:141

Speiser P: Prenatal treatment of congenital adrenal hyperplasia. J Urol 1999;162:534

Zinn HL, Cohen HL: Amenorrhea in the adolescent or young adult. *In* Bluth E, Arger P, Benson C, et al (eds): Ultrasound: A Practical Approach to Clinical Problems. New York, Thieme, 2000:475

PART IV

ABNORMALITIES OF PUBERTY AND AMENORRHEA

HARRIS L. COHEN

JACK O. HALLER

Indications for the evaluation of the adolescent pelvis (often with ultrasound [US] as the first and sometimes only imaging examination) are most often complaints of abdominal pain, pelvic pain, or mass. Much of the differential diagnosis for these complaints has been reviewed in Section VIII, Parts I, II, and III. Other key clinical complaints resulting in pelvic US and other imaging evaluations, particularly in females, relate to abnormalities of development of the secondary sexual characteristics of puberty. These changes may be seen earlier than normal, as in precocious puberty, or may be delayed (delayed puberty) or fail to develop (hypogonadism, sexual infantilism) in adolescents. The other key reason for adolescent gynecologic evaluations is amenorrhea (lack of menses), whether primary or secondary. Much of what causes pubertal delay may also cause primary or secondary amenorrhea.

PUBERTY

Puberty among girls is the stage of development in between childhood and adulthood when activation of the hypothalamic–pituitary–ovarian–uterine (H-P-O-U) axis results in maturation of the gonads, resulting in an increased production of sex hormones, development of secondary sex characteristics, a growth spurt, and development of reproductive capability. The earliest signs of puberty among girls are breast development (usually occurring between 8 and 13 years) and pubic hair growth (8 to 14 years). This is followed by a growth spurt (9.5 to 14.5 years), axillary hair development, and menarche (10 to 16 years). Puberty is usually completed within about 4 years.

Puberty among males begins between 9 and 14 years of age and is completed in 3.5 to 4 years. It begins with testicular enlargement (usually occurring between 9 and 13.5 years), followed by the appearance of pubic hair (10 to 15 years), enlargement of the penis (11 to 12.5 years), and development of axillary and facial hair as well as a growth spurt (10.5 to 16 years).

PHYSIOLOGIC CHANGES AT PUBERTY AND THE NORMAL OVULATORY MENSTRUAL CYCLE

All the components necessary for menstruation can be found in the normal female at the time of birth. This is evidenced by the occasional neonatal withdrawal bleeding that may result from decreasing estrogen and progesterone levels after separation from the placenta. Ordinarily, until the age of at least 8 years, however, an unknown "central restraining mechanism" prevents the pulsatile release of gonadotropin-releasing hormone (GnRH) from the arcuate nucleus of the hypothalamus. Pulsatile release of GnRH appears necessary for ovulation and corpus luteum development. Evidence of this central control (rather than a negative feedback mechanism from ovarian hormone production) can be shown by the inhibition of GnRH production even in patients with Turner's syndrome who have no apparent functioning gonadal tissue. In early puberty, the pulsatile GnRH release is maximal only at night, but, with time, the typical adult pattern of continuous pulsatile GnRH secretion develops.

With the earliest activation of GnRH, most individuals undergo ovarian folliculogenesis without ovulation. Unopposed estrogen production leads to progressive uterine growth and endometrial proliferation. There is breast budding, physiologic leukorrhea, and accelerated linear growth of the girl. Axillary and pubic hair development are the result of ovarian and adrenal gland androgen production. The H-P-O-U axis continues to mature. Over an approximately 2-year span, cycles with subnormal progesterone production and shortened intermenstrual intervals are replaced by normal corpus luteum function and fertile cycles.

The typical ovulatory cycle has a 24- to 35-day intermenstrual interval and usually a premenstrual molimina. Longer intervals are often associated with anovulation, although the eventual menses is often associated with some corpus luteum activity. Improved nutrition and living conditions are thought to be responsible for the gradual fall in mean menarchal age over the last century. In North America, it is currently 12.4 years with a range of 9 to 17 years. Menarche usually occurs 2 to 5 years after breast bud development.

PREMATURE THELARCHE AND PREMATURE ADRENARCHE

Premature thelarche and adrenarche are relatively common, self-limited variants of normal pubertal development in girls. Premature thelarche refers to premature breast development without other signs of precocious sex maturation in girls less than 8 years of age. It usually is seen between 1 and 4 years of age. A third of cases resolve spontaneously. At puberty, breast development is normal. Premature adrenarche refers to the appearance of pubic and axillary hair without other signs of precocious sexual maturity. In both premature thelarche and premature adrenarche, bone age and patient height are normal to only slightly increased. The cause of premature thelarche or adrenarche is not certain. The levels of circulating sex hormones are usually normal. Increased end-organ sensitivity to normal levels of estrogen or androgen have been suggested as a possible cause.

In boys, premature appearance of pubic and axillary hair without other signs or only minor signs of precocious puberty is a relatively common variant of normal development that may be due to an increase in circulating androgens from premature maturation of the adrenal glands of unknown cause. There is no penile enlargement, presumably because the levels of circulating androgens are not sufficiently elevated. The bone age and growth rate are slightly increased. The rest of pubertal development occurs at a normal age.

PRECOCIOUS PUBERTY

Precocious puberty refers to the appearance of external signs of adolescence (secondary sex characteristics) before 8 years of age in girls, and before 9 years in boys. Precocious puberty and its clinical problems are more common in girls than in boys. In girls, precocious breast development (thelarche), axillary or pubic hair development (adrenarche), or menses (menarche) may occur.

Precocious puberty is divided into two main types: (1) complete, central, gonadotropin-dependent, or *true* precocious puberty; and (2) incomplete, peripheral, gonadotropin-independent, *pseudo*precocious puberty, or precocious pseudopuberty. Whereas the complete form is characteristically isosexual, with development of secondary sex characteristics that are appropriate for the patient's gender, the incomplete form may be either isosexual or heterosexual. Incomplete heterosexual precocious puberty is manifested by signs of virilization in girls, and by gynecomastia or other signs of feminization in boys.

COMPLETE OR CENTRAL ISOSEXUAL PRECOCIOUS PUBERTY

This form of precocious puberty results from premature activation of the hypothalamic–pituitary–gonadal complex, with increased production of gonadotropic and sex hormones and an early onset of ovulation or spermatogenesis. Complete precocious puberty may be idiopathic or secondary to organic central nervous system (CNS) lesions.

The cause of precocious puberty in girls is idiopathic in at least 80% of cases. Early menarche results from an idiopathic increase in the activity of the hypothalamic–pituitary–gonadal axis. About 20% of affected girls have a hypothalamic or pituitary lesion. These can be defined by computed tomography (CT) or magnetic resonance imaging (MRI). Pelvic US helps denote the presence of a normal uterus and ovaries or denote abnormalities of these organs. Less than 10% of cases of true precocious puberty in boys have an idiopathic cause. A familial tendency to early pubertal development of the idiopathic type is observed in some cases (constitutional or genetic precocious puberty).

Possible causes of precocious puberty in either sex include intracranial tumors or cysts, hydrocephalus, sequelae of intracranial inflammatory processes or trauma, and other intracranial lesions that may activate the hypothalamus by pressure or invasion. Of the CNS neoplasms that may cause true precocious puberty, hamartoma of the tuber cinereum (Fig. 1), or hypothalamic hamartoma, is the most common. This usually small CNS tumor is more common in boys than girls, is generally benign and nonprogressive, and usually cannot be surgically corrected. The tumor may be pedunculated and may appears as an excrescence on the tuber cinereum below the mammillary body. It secretes GnRH. The onset of puberty in patients with this lesion is usually at a younger age (2 years) than in patients with idiopathic precocious puberty. Use of MRI has increased the frequency of this diagnosis over the last 15 years.

Other CNS neoplasms that may cause true precocious puberty in either sex are usually located in or near the hypothalamus and include hypothalamic or optic gliomas with or without neurofibromatosis, astrocytoma, ependymoma, dysgerminoma, and prolactinoma. Suprasellar dysgerminoma (ectopic pinealoma) in boys may also cause incomplete precocious puberty through a secretion of human chorionic gonadotropin (HCG) by the tumor.

True precocious puberty may be observed in some children with longstanding untreated hypothyroidism. It is often accompanied by galactorrhea. Affected patients show little, if any, development of secondary sexual characteristics, especially pubic hair. These patients have arrested linear growth, and bone age is not advanced. All of these changes regress with treat-

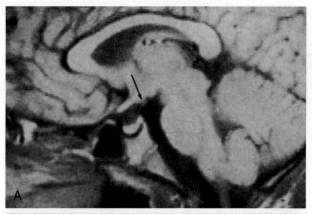

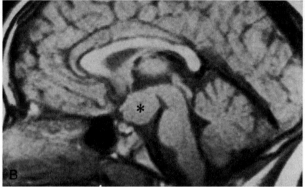

FIGURE 1. Precocious puberty caused by brain abnormality—hamartoma of the tuber cinereum. On T$_1$-weighted magnetic resonance imaging through the midline of the brain, an *arrow* (**A**) points to a small hamartoma in the brain of an 8-year-old and an *asterisk* (**B**) is seen over an unusually large hamartoma in a 7-year-old, both with a longstanding history of precocious puberty.

ment of the hypothyroidism. The increased production of gonadotropic hormones and prolactin seen in these patients may be due to a hormonal overlap in the pituitary response to thyroid deficiency.

Premature maturation of the hypothalamic–pituitary complex, increased gonadotropin secretion, and true precocious puberty may also occur after chronic exposure to endogenous or exogenous androgens and sometimes also estrogens. This is especially true when the source of the sex hormone is removed (e.g., after ending therapy for congenital adrenal hyperplasia [CAH], or after surgical removal of an androgen-secreting neoplasm or an estrogen-secreting ovarian tumor or cyst).

INCOMPLETE (PSEUDOSEXUAL) PRECOCIOUS PUBERTY IN GIRLS

Pseudosexual (or incomplete) precocious puberty in girls usually presents before 5 years of age. Excess circulating estrogens or related substances develop independently of the hypothalamus and pituitary gland. These estrogens are produced by the ovaries or adrenal glands. They may be from an exogenous source, such as food, parenteral or oral medications, creams, lotions, or other substances.

Gonadotropin levels are not high, but rather low. Gonads remain immature. The most common ovarian source are autonomous estrogen-secreting follicular (granulosa–thecal) cysts (Fig. 2). The cyst (or cysts) may rupture or regress spontaneously, resulting in a decreased estrogen level and vaginal withdrawal bleeding. They may redevelop and symptoms may recur. Other causes are tumors such as the relatively common estrogen-producing ovarian neoplasms, particularly granulosa cell (or granulosa–theca cell) tumors (Fig. 3), and rare estrogen-secreting adrenal neoplasms (adenomas or carcinomas).

McCune-Albright syndrome consists of polyostotic fibrous dysplasia, cutaneous café au lait spots and precocious puberty. The syndrome is predominantly found in females. Vaginal bleeding is often the first sign of precocious puberty, which is usually pseudoprecocious in type. Autonomously functioning ovarian cysts are seen in some cases. In others, no anatomic cause is noted. McCune-Albright syndrome occasionally presents with complete or true precocious puberty. It has been suggested that the initially partial or incomplete precocious puberty in these patients becomes complete (gonadotropin dependent) as the result of an early maturation of the hypothalamic–pituitary–gonadal complex caused by a longstanding exposure to estrogen.

Virilizing Disorders (Heterosexual Precocious Puberty)

Testosterone, as already noted, is the most potent of the circulating androgens. It is produced in normal females by the adrenal (25%), by the ovary (25%), and by peripheral conversion of Δ^4-androstenedione (50%), with only 1% typically free and biologically active. A form of pseudosexual precocity may occur in girls when either androgen levels are excessive or end organs become excessively sensitive to normal amounts of circulating androgens. In either case, this may lead to heterosexual pseudoprecocious puberty as the girls undergo virilization, developing secondary sexual characteristics of males. Clinical findings include increases in body and facial hair (hirsutism), acne, deepening of the voice, clitoromegaly, increased muscle mass, and temporal balding. Menstrual abnormalities are common among affected adolescents. Postpubertal virilized girls may become defeminized, with decreases in breast size and the development of vaginal atrophy.

Congenital Adrenal Hyperplasia

CAH is the most common form of hyperandrogenism. The increased production of androgenic substance is due in most cases to a deficiency of 21-hydroxylase, and far less commonly to deficiencies in 11β-hydroxylase or 3β-hydroxysteroid dehydrogenase (see Section II, Part V, Chapter 10, page 239).

Other Causes of Virilization in Girls

Adrenal adenomas or adrenal carcinomas may produce increased androgens and virilization. Signs of Cushing's

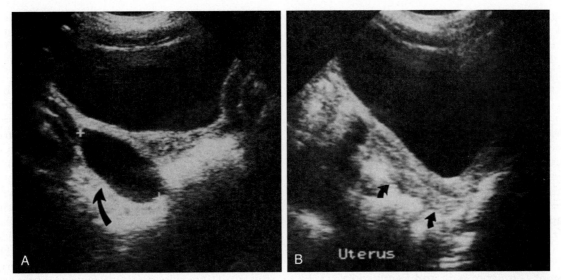

FIGURE 2. Precocious puberty due to autonomous estrogen-secreting ovarian cyst. **A,** On ultrasound in the right parasagittal plane, the right adnexum *(arrow)* of a 3-year-old with precocious puberty consists of a large cyst. The left adnexa was normal. This cyst was proven to autonomously secrete estrogen. **B,** On ultrasound in the midline longitudinal plane, the child's uterus *(arrows)* is longer than normal for her age. It is not the tubular shape typical of childhood but, rather, appears almost pear shaped, with an evident echogenic central endometrial cavity suggesting estrogenization.

syndrome may be seen in such patients as a result of associated secretion of glucocorticoid hormones by the tumor.

Some ovarian neoplasms may secrete androgens and cause virilization, including the Sertoli–Leydig cell tumors (once known as an androblastoma or arrhenoblastoma), the thecoma (luteoma), a virilizing dysgerminoma containing theca cells, or a gonadoblastoma (occurring mostly in dysgenetic gonads). Exogenous exposure to androgens or androgen-like substances may cause virilization at all ages. Again, some girls with rare anomalies of sex differentiation, such as 46,XY gonadal dysgenesis, may develop virilization at puberty, despite being phenotypically normal females at birth.

Idiopathic hirsutism and polycystic ovarian disease are also considered among the virilizing disorders of females. An increase in body and facial hair (hirsutism, hypertrichosis) occurring as the sole or predominant abnormality is a relatively common problem in otherwise normal pubertal and postpubertal girls. It may be precipitated by any of the causes of virilization. It may be seen in families or as a result of polycystic ovary syndrome (PCOS). The cause is usually idiopathic and believed to be a result of an altered response of the end organ (hair follicle) to normal levels of circulating androgens. In PCOS (see Section VIII, Part II, Fig. 28, page 1960), both ovaries are larger and more echogenic than normal. They contain many small follicular cysts. The hirsutism seen in these cases may result from an increased androgen production by the ovarian cysts.

INCOMPLETE ISOSEXUAL (PSEUDOPRECOCIOUS) PUBERTY IN BOYS

Isosexual pseudoprecocity of sexual development in boys is due to an increase in circulating androgen or androgen-like substances either because of their production by adrenal glands or testes or by their addition to the bloodstream from an exogenous source. CAH is the most common cause for excessive androgen production by the adrenal gland of either sex. Affected males are born with normal external genitalia, but, if the CAH is untreated, they soon develop signs of sexual precocity. Isosexual pseudoprecocious puberty in males, sometimes associated with signs of glucocorticoids excess, can also occur because of androgen-secreting neoplasms of the adrenal cortex (adenocarcinoma, benign adenoma). A rare cause of isosexual precocity in boys is an androgen-secreting Leydig cell tumor of the testis (benign or malignant). Several extrapituitary HCG-

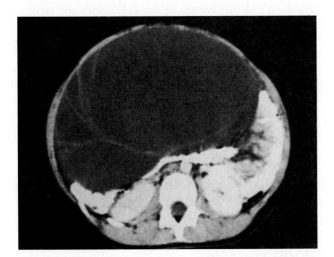

FIGURE 3. Axial computed tomography at the level of the kidneys shows a large, cystic, septated mass occupying most of the abdomen in a 10-year-old girl. The mass proved to be a juvenile granulosa cell tumor that produced estrogen and caused precocious puberty.

secreting tumors can also result in an incomplete form of isosexual precocious puberty by stimulating testosterone production by the Leydig cells of the testis (see Section VIII, Part I, Fig. 26, page 1933). These tumors include some hepatomas, hepatoblastomas, and some teratomas or chorioepitheliomas of the mediastinum and retroperitoneum. A suprasellar germinoma or ectopic pinealoma may secrete HCG and cause pseudoprecocious puberty in males through the same mechanism. A familial form of gonadotropin-independent precocious puberty in boys is caused by premature maturation and sometimes hyperplasia of the Leydig cells of the testis, with production of testosterone. Exposure to exogenous androgens or the administration of HCG for undescended testes may be further causes of incomplete virilization in males.

Adolescent Gynecomastia and Feminizing Disorders in Boys

Mild breast development may occur transiently in adolescent boys between 13 and 15 years of age. The gynecomastia, although sometimes pronounced, is seldom severe enough to require surgical correction. It is usually bilateral, is of no definitive cause, and may be familial. Usually, no source of excessive androgen is found. The gynecomastia generally regresses in 2 or 3 years, but, in a few cases, may persist into adult life. It is usually idiopathic. Pathologic causes of gynecomastia in boys, sometimes associated with other signs of feminization, may be due to exposure to exogenous estrogens, as well as the presence of an estrogen-secreting neoplasm of the testis or adrenal cortex, or a prolactin-secreting neoplasm of the pituitary gland. Gynecomastia may also be noted in Klinefelter's syndrome, congenital bilateral anorchia, acquired testicular failure, and in other conditions with some biochemical defect in testosterone production or androgen end-organ receptor.

CLINICAL AND LABORATORY EVALUATION OF PRECOCIOUS PUBERTY

A detailed medical history and physical examination can help make the correct diagnosis. A history of previous exposure to estrogen or androgenic substances should be questioned. Physical examination should denote the type and degree of pubertal development as well as the size, shape, and firmness of the testes. In complete precocious puberty, both testes are enlarged, in partial sexual precocity they are often of normal size. Unilateral testicular enlargement suggests a testicular neoplasm. The abdomen should be evaluated for a flank or pelvic mass. A detailed neurologic evaluation should be obtained, including funduscopic examination. The presence of café au lait spots should suggest the diagnosis of fibrous dysplasia or neurofibromatosis. The latter may be associated with intracranial neoplasms, mostly gliomas, in or around the hypothalamus, which may lead to increased pituitary function and precocious puberty. Laboratory studies may include luteinizing hormone (LH), follicle-stimulating hormone, and estra-diol levels; gonadotropin response to GnRH; thyroid studies; and vaginal smear in girls as well as plasma and urinary testosterone levels.

IMAGING WORK-UP OF PRECOCIOUS PUBERTY

An anteroposterior film of the left hand, including carpal bones and distal forearm, is used for bone age determination. Bone age is commonly advanced in patients with true precocious puberty and in patients with androgenic stimulation, but may be normal or only slightly increased in patients with premature thelarche or adrenarche. Normal bone ages are followed at 6-month intervals. The skeletal length is often increased early, in association with increased bone age. However, if the precocious puberty is not treated, premature fusion of the epiphyses may develop and result in a decrease in the patient's potential height.

Imaging studies (from plain film to cross-sectional imaging) may be used to denote a possible causative intra-abdominal mass.

Abdominal US, with emphasis on the adrenal area and the ovaries, has become, together with bone age determination, the primary radiologic study in the initial evaluation of patients with precocious puberty. In girls with true precocious puberty, pelvic US may show some bilateral enlargement of the ovaries and prominence of the uterus. In rare cases, a large estrogen-secreting ovarian cyst has resulted in stimulation of the hypothalamic–pituitary complex, causing true precocious puberty as described above. Small and multiple ovarian cysts/follicles may be seen in girls with true precocious puberty because of high gonadotropin levels, but may also be seen in those with isosexual pseudoprecosity. These cystic ovaries may look and be similar to those seen normally throughout childhood. Pseudoprecocity caused by the autonomous estrogen secretion of an ovarian cyst or tumor will be denoted by asymmetry of the ovaries of the child, with the autonomous mass being denoted by a larger ovary (Fig. 2A) on US exam. The finding in prepubertal girls of an increased uterine size and a well-defined central endometrial echo indicates an increase in circulating estrogen from any cause. A skeletal survey is indicated when fibrous dysplasia is suspected.

Patients with isosexual precocious puberty that is suspected to be of the complete or central type should have MRI of the brain with special attention to the tuber cinereum. Skull films are usually of limited diagnostic value but may show intracranial calcifications, enlargement of the sella turcica, signs of increased intracranial pressure, or skull changes of fibrous dysplasia.

DELAYED OR ABSENT PUBERTAL DEVELOPMENT

Puberty is considered to be delayed and should be investigated in girls when secondary sex characteristics fail to appear by 13 years of age, considered 2 standard deviations beyond the norm. Causes of pubertal delay in girls are also causes for primary amenorrhea. Evaluations for pubertal delays in boys are suggested when pubic and axillary hair or other external secondary characteristics, particularly enlargement of the testes and penis, fail to appear by age 14. Delayed puberty or failure of puberty to develop may be idiopathic (constitutional) or due to chronic systemic disorders, disorders of the hypothalamic–pituitary complex causing decreased gonadotropin secretion (secondary or hypogonadotropic hypogonadism), or primary disorders of the gonads with a secondary elevation of gonadotropic hormone secretion (primary or hypergonadotropic hypogonadism).

IDIOPATHIC (CONSTITUTIONAL) PUBERTAL DELAY

In some otherwise normal children, the onset of puberty is delayed for up to several years. When puberty eventually starts, it usually continues to completely normal secondary sexual development. These occurrences underline the fact that there may be constitutional or genetic causes for delay in the maturation of the hypothalamic–pituitary complex. Often, such children may have delay in bone age and height development. The ability to differentiate between constitutional pubertal delays in otherwise normal children and true disorders of the hypothalamic-pituitary axis may not be simple and make take years of clinical and laboratory observation.

DELAYED PUBERTY IN CHRONIC SYSTEMIC DISORDERS

Delayed puberty may occur on a physiologic basis in patients with chronic disease such as inflammatory bowel disease (Fig. 4) or long-term disorders of cardiac, pulmonary, renal, or other body systems. Patients with other long-term debilitating processes as well as anorexia nervosa may have delays in pubertal development. Such delays may also be noted in children or adolescents who undergo prolonged and vigorous physical exertion, such as long-distance running. All these possibilities must be considered in evaluation patients with amenorrhea as well. Puberty may develop or proceed normally in some of these patients following improvement or removal of the precipitating cause.

A work-up for pubertal delay may be held up for a year, if the patient has a known debilitating illness or is involved in competitive or endurance sports, such as ballet or track. As an aside, any *halt* in pubertal development is a cause for concern and endocrinologic work-up.

HYPOGONADISM CAUSED BY HYPOTHALAMIC–PITUITARY DISORDERS (HYPOGONADOTROPIC HYPOGONADISM)

Several disorders of the hypothalamic–pituitary complex result in decreased gonadotropin production and,

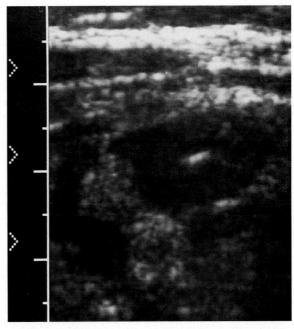

FIGURE 4. Inflammatory bowel disease as a cause of delayed puberty or primary amenorrhea. On ultrasound in the transverse plane through the right lower quadrant, an abnormally thick bowel wall is noted about a central echogenic linear area representing air in the lumen of a portion of a teenager's small bowel. The area did not compress well. The ultrasound is consistent with the proven diagnosis of Crohn's disease. This teenager presented for a work-up for amenorrhea/delayed puberty. Ultrasound showed an infantile uterus. After noting the abnormal small bowel, the history of chronic disease (i.e., long-term Crohn's disease) was elicited.

secondarily, a decrease in gonadal sex steroids. Impaired or absent gonadal function causes an absence of pubertal development. In girls, the uterus remains infantile, menses does not occur, and breast budding and other secondary sexual characteristics do not develop. In boys, the penis and scrotum are infantile and the testes remain immature and smaller than expected for the age. Pubic and axillary hair are scanty or absent, the voice remains high pitched, and there is often increased fat deposition, particularly at the hips, pelvis, abdomen, and breast. Delayed closure of the epiphyses with elongation of the limbs is observed unless there is an associated growth hormone deficiency.

Causative abnormalities include intracranial abnormalities such as craniopharyngioma, hypothalamic and optic gliomas, dysgerminoma, and other tumors of the pituitary gland and hypothalamus or adjacent areas. Other manifestations of pituitary insufficiency, such as diabetes insipidus and short stature, may be present. Hypogonadotropic or secondary hypogonadism may also be seen in histiocytosis X and certain congenital midline defects of the face, the base of the skull, and the CNS, such as septo-optic dysplasia or holoprosencephaly, which may be associated with developmental anomalies of the hypothalamus and pituitary gland resulting in hypogonadism.

Functional causes of hypogonadism include idiopathic hypopituitarism characterized by short stature resulting from growth hormone deficiency and sometimes other findings associated with deficiencies of other pituitary hormones. Cases of isolated gonadotropic deficiency, sporadic or familial, may occur in association with anosmia or hyposmia and other abnormalities that characterize Kallmann's syndrome. Isolated LH deficiency in males, sometimes familial, results in failure of pubertal development, usually associated with preservation of spermatogenesis and with gynecomastia (fertile eunuch syndrome). Hypogonadism, probably also related to abnormalities of hypothalamic function, can be observed in such syndromes as Prader-Willi and Laurence-Moon-Biedl.

HYPOGONADISM CAUSED BY GONADAL LESIONS (HYPERGONADOTROPIC HYPOGONADISM)

As previously stated, certain congenital or acquired lesions of the gonads may result in hypogonadism and failure of pubertal development. Gonadal sex steroids are decreased and, because of this, there is an increased secretion of gonadotropins by the pituitary, hence the term *hypergonadotropic* hypogonadism. Just as in hypogonadotropic hypogonadism, there is absent pubertal development in girls or boys. The key gonadal lesions in girls include Turner's syndrome, XX gonadal dysgenesis, XY gonadal dysgenesis, and a gonadal dysgenesis with galactosemia and immune oophoritis (often associated with Hashimoto's thyroiditis, hypoparathyroidism, adrenal insufficiency, pernicious anemia, chronic active hepatitis, and candidiasis). Hypergonadotropic hypogonadism can also occur among patients with normal karyotypes who develop secondary ovarian failure either by infarction, as with cases of bilateral ovarian torsion, or because of surgical removal of both ovaries, or because of radiation therapy (usually of 8 Gy [800 rads] or greater) to the pelvis or chemotherapy or autoimmune oophoritis.

Gonadal lesions in boys leading to hypogonadism include congenital bilateral anorchia with otherwise normal external genitalia caused by resorption of the testes after the 13th week of gestation (vanishing testes and functional prepubertal castrate syndromes), and acquired testicular atrophy resulting from bilateral testicular torsion, surgical injury during bilateral orchiopexy, radiation, or other causes. Absence of puberty is also observed in some genetic males born with an entirely female phenotype, including those with XY gonadal dysgenesis, and some forms of male pseudohermaphroditism with impaired biosynthesis of active sex steroids as a result of an inherited enzymatic deficiency.

DIAGNOSTIC AND HISTORICAL CONSIDERATIONS

Important information may be obtained from the patient's family history, past medical history, associated medical disorders, and physical examination. On physical examination, special emphasis should be placed on pubertal staging (Tanner classification), assessment of general growth and maturation, and detection of signs

and symptoms of CNS disease, and of systemic diseases or syndromes that may be chronic and or debilitating and therefore associated with abnormal pubertal development. Visual fields testing, gynecologic evaluation, and chromosomal analysis should be carried out as indicated. The hormonal studies include measurements of plasma androgens and estrogens, blood and urine gonadotropins, gonadotropic response to GnRH stimulation, and testosterone response to HCG stimulation. Measurements of circulating prolactin and growth hormone, as well as thyroid function tests, may be undertaken in special cases. The radiologic procedures include bone age determination, head CT or MRI, pelvic US to evaluate the size of the ovaries and uterus, and other studies as indicated.

ANALYSIS OF PATIENTS WITH AMENORRHEA

Causes of pubertal delay in girls may be similar to causes of primary or secondary amenorrhea. Primary amenorrhea is defined as a lack of menses by age 16. Secondary amenorrhea is defined as a cessation of menses at any point in time after menarche and before menopause.

Primary amenorrhea has many causes involving several systems (Table 1). It may be seen in adolescents with normal pubertal development as well as those with delayed sexual development, delayed menarche with some pubertal development, and delayed menarche

---

Table 1 ■ ETIOLOGIES OF PRIMARY AMENORRHEA

Hypothalamus
  Systemic illness
  Chronic disease
  Familial
  Stress
  Competitive athletics
  Eating disorders
  Obesity
  Drugs
Pituitary
  Idiopathic hypopituitarism
  Tumor
  Hemochromatosis
Thyroid gland
  Hypothyroidism
  Hyperthyroidism
Adrenal glands
  Congenital adrenocortical hyperplasia
  Adrenal tumor
Ovaries
  Gonadal dysgenesis
  Ovarian failure
  Polycystic ovary syndrome
  Ovarian tumor
Cervix: agenesis
Vagina
  Agenesis
  Transverse septum
Hymen: imperforate

Adapted from Emans S, Goldstein D (eds): Delayed puberty and menstrual irregularities. In Pediatric and Adolescent Gynecology, 3rd ed. Boston, Little Brown, 1990:149.

plus virilization. We have already reviewed many of its causes. They include hypogonadotropic hypogonadism, hypergonadotropic hypogonadism, pseudohermaphroditism, female adolescents with virilization, PCOS, eugonadism estrogenization with genital obstruction (e.g., hematometra/hematometrocolpos), and uterine aplasia or hypoplasia. Secondary amenorrhea is often due physiologically to pregnancy and pathologically to PCOS.

SUGGESTED READINGS

Battaglia C, Artini P, D'Ambrogio G, et al: The role of color Doppler imaging in the diagnosis of polycystic ovary syndrome. Am J Obstet Gynecol 1995;172:108

Cohen HL, Bober S, Bow S: Imaging the pediatric pelvis: the normal and abnormal genital system and simulators of its diseases. Urol Radiol 1992;14:273

Cohen HL, Eisenberg P, Mandel F, Haller J: Ovarian cysts are common in premenarchal girls: a sonographic study of 101 children 2–12 years old. AJR Am J Roentgenol 1992;159:89

Cohen HL, Shapiro MA, Mandel FS, Shapiro ML: Normal ovaries in neonates and infants: a sonographic study of 77 patients 1 day to 24 months old. AJR Am J Roentgenol 1993;160:583

Cohen HL: Evaluation of the adolescent and young adult with amenorrhea: role of US. In Bluth E, Arger P, Hertzberg B, Middleton W (eds): Syllabus: A special course in Ultrasound: Clinical Questions, Practical Answers. Oak Brook, IL, RSNA Publications 1996;171

Currarino G, Wood B, Majd M: Abnormalities of the genital tract. In Silverman F, Kuhn J (eds): Caffey's Pediatric X-Ray Diagnosis, 9th ed. St. Louis, Mosby-Year Book, 1993:1375

Daya S: Habitual abortion. In Copeland L (ed): Textbook of Gynecology. Philadelphia, WB Saunders, 1993:204

Emans S, Goldstein D (eds): Delayed puberty and menstrual irregularities. In Pediatric and Adolescent Gynecology, 3rd ed. Boston, Little Brown, 1990a:149

Emans S, Goldstein D (eds): The physiology of puberty. In Pediatric and Adolescent Gynecology, 3rd ed. Boston, Little Brown, 1990b:95

Falsetti L, Pasinetti E, Mazzani M, Gastaldi A: Weight loss and menstrual cycle: clinical and endocrinological evaluation. Gynecol Endocrinol 1992;6:49

Ganong W (ed): The gonads: development and function of the reproductive system. In Review of Medical Physiology, 17th ed. Norwalk, CT, Appleton & Lange, 1995:399

Herter L, Magalnaes J, Spritzer P: Association of ovarian volume and serum LH levels in adolescent patients with menstrual disorders and/or hirsutism. Braz J Med Biol Res 1993;26:1041

Larsen W, Felmar E, Wallace M, Frieder R: Sertoli-Leydig cell tumor of the ovary: a rare cause of amenorrhea. Obstet Gynecol 1992;79:831

Lee PA: Neuroendocrinology of puberty. Semin Reprod Endocrinol 1988;6:13

Lee PA: Physiology of puberty. In Principles and Practice of Endocrinology and Metabolism. Philadelphia, JB Lippincott, 1990:740

Lee PA, O'Dea L: Primary and secondary testicular insufficiency. Pediatr Clin North Am 1990;37:1359

Mahoney CP: Adolescent gynecomastia: differential diagnosis and management. Pediatr Clin North Am 1990;37:1389

Polk D: Abnormalities of sexual differentiation. In Taeush H, Ballard R, Avery M (eds): Schaeffer & Avery's Diseases of the Newborn, 6th ed. Philadelphia, WB Saunders, 1991:946

Reid R: Amenorrhea. In Copeland L (ed): Textbook of Gynecology. Philadelphia, WB Saunders, 1993:367

Rosenfeld RL: Clinical Review 6: Diagnosis and management of delayed puberty. J Clin Endocrinol Metab 1990a;70:559

Rosenfield RL: Hyperandrogenism in peripubertal girls. Pediatr Clin North Am 1990b;37:1333

Schwartz ID, Root AW: Puberty in girls: early, incomplete or precocious? Contemp Pediatr 1990;7:147

Shah R, Woolley M, Costin G: Testicular feminization syndrome: the androgen insensitivity syndrome. J Pediatr Surg 1992;27:757

Starceski PJ: Hypothalamic hamartomas and sexual precocity. Am J Dis Child 1990;144:225

Takahashi K, Okada M, Ozaki T, et al: Transvaginal ultrasonographic morphology in polycystic ovarian syndrome. Gynecol Obstet Invest 1995;39:201

Tarani L, Lampariello S, Raguso G, et al: Pregnancy in patients with Turner's syndrome: six new cases and review of literature. Gynecol Endocrinol 1998;12:83

Wheeler MD, Styne DM: Diagnosis and management of precocious puberty. Pediatr Clin North Am 1990;37:1255

SECTION IX

MUSCULOSKELETAL SYSTEM

BARRY D. FLETCHER

KATHLEEN H. EMERY

THEODORE E. KEATS

TAL LAOR

RALPH S. LACHMAN

WILLIAM H. McALISTER

THOMAS E. HERMAN

KEITH A. KRONEMER

SAMBASIVA R. KOTTAMASU

H. THEODORE HARCKE

GERALD A. MANDELL

BRADLEY A. MAXFIELD

DANIELLE K. B. BOAL

E. MICHEL AZOUZ

PAUL S. BABYN

MARILYN D. RANSON

PART I

OVERVIEW

BARRY D. FLETCHER

The practice of pediatric radiology demands specialized knowledge of normal growth, development, and morphology in order to recognize and understand the numerous injuries, disease entities, syndromes, and malformations that are peculiar to infancy, childhood, and adolescence. In the past, much of this knowledge has been acquired by observations of plain radiographs. Indeed, readers of previous editions of this book will remember the superb descriptions of musculoskeletal disorders based on Dr. Caffey's original observations and later expanded on by Dr. Frederic N. Silverman. However, the intervening years since the earlier editions have seen remarkable technological advances in our specialty. Now, the growing use of other imaging modalities such as ultrasound, computed tomography (CT), magnetic resonance imaging (MRI), and nuclear scintigraphy (Table 1) has added significantly to the knowledge base. The richness of anatomic and pathologic detail that these additional imaging options have provided now warrants a substantial change in the editorial approach to the broad subject of musculoskeletal abnormalities. This section, therefore, comprises the combined specialized expertise of more than a dozen authors. Our goal is to provide the reader with the most up-to-date information about the various pathologic entities and current thinking about the use of the various imaging modalities used in the study of musculoskeletal disorders.

RADIOGRAPHY

Plain film radiography remains the primary method of detecting and analyzing skeletal abnormalities. In many cases, plain films may be the only medium needed to portray a disorder, whether it is a skeletal dysplasia, metabolic abnormality, or fracture. The spatial resolution provided by analog and the newer digital radiographs is superior to all other modalities. With radiography, radiation to the patient is minimal and the cost is low. The study and characterization of musculoskeletal dysplasias and dysostoses is based almost entirely on radiographic observations.

The skeletal survey is a commonly requested screening examination for patients with suspected genetic disorders or nonaccidental trauma. However, skeletal surveys have largely been replaced by technetium-99m methylene diphosphonate (MDP) nuclear scintigraphy for detecting metastatic disease. Even when more detailed investigation is required using other imaging modalities, radiographs are frequently used to follow the clinical course and response to treatment of such entities as arthritis, infections, metabolic disorders, and growth disorders.

Radiographs are less relevant to the study of soft tissues because of their narrow contrast range, but plain films can improve the diagnostic specificity of soft tissue lesions by depicting calcifications, fat, gas, or foreign material within the lesion or showing the extent of secondary involvement of adjacent bone.

ULTRASONOGRAPHY

The role of diagnostic ultrasound in the management of patients with musculoskeletal disorders is somewhat limited by its narrow field of view and the physical constraints of sonic transmission through bone. Nevertheless, ultrasound is inexpensive, accessible, and versatile and does not require ionizing radiation, thus making it one of the most valuable tools in the pediatric imaging armamentarium. Ultrasound is an ideal method of investigating focal soft tissue lesions and joint abnormalities. Even juxtaskeletal lesions such as periosteal abscesses can be detected with ultrasound.

Vascular neoplasms and malformations are frequent causes of soft tissue masses in children. Color Doppler ultrasonography is an ideal method of assessing flow rates of the vascular component of these lesions. For example, fast flow suggests a diagnosis of hemangioma, arteriovenous malformation, or fistula, whereas a compressible slow-flow lesion indicates the presence of a

Table 1 ■ FREQUENT APPLICATIONS OF IMAGING MODALITIES FOR THE EVALUATION OF PEDIATRIC MUSCULOSKELETAL DISORDERS

	IMAGING MODALITY*				
	XR	**US**	**CT**	**MRI**	**NM†**
Congenital disorders	+			+	
Metabolic disorders	+				
Infection	+	+	+	+	Tc, Ga
Trauma	+		+	+	Tc
Arthropathy	+	+	+	+	Ga
Soft tissue		+		+	Ga
Bone tumors	+		+	+	Tc, Ga, MIBG

*XR = radiography; US = ultrasound; CT = computed tomography; MRI = magnetic resonance imaging; NM = nuclear imaging; + indicates frequent applications.
†Tc = technetium-99m MDP; Ga = gallium-67; MIBG = iodine-131 or iodine-123 *meta*-iodobenzylguanidine (for neuroblastoma bone metastases).

venous malformation. A growing cystic lesion lacking flow is highly suggestive of a lymphatic malformation. In the presence of characteristic clinical and sonographic findings of vascular malformations, the need for further more complex or invasive procedures may be avoided.

Occasionally, the ultrasonographic appearance of a lesion will be sufficiently specific to permit an accurate diagnosis of a benign lesion such as hematoma or lipoblastoma. Conversely, disordered, complex echoes from within a mass may point to the possibility of soft tissue sarcoma—a rare diagnosis in children—and the need for further imaging and clinical investigation.

The ability of ultrasonography to depict radiolucent structures, especially cartilage, makes it an ideal modality for investigation of the highly cartilaginous immature skeleton. For example, the ability to image the morphology and location of the unossified proximal femoral epiphysis in infants has prompted major advances in the diagnosis and management of developmental dysplasia of the hip. Ultrasound may even be used to detect cartilaginous epiphyseal fractures that are invisible on radiographs. Furthermore, ultrasound is highly sensitive to the presence of excess intra-articular fluid. Therefore, ultrasound has become the primary method of diagnosing septic arthritis and, in patients with juvenile rheumatoid arthritis, of detecting joint effusion and differentiating it from synovial hypertrophy.

COMPUTED TOMOGRAPHY

CT images achieve greater contrast resolution than plain radiographs and are therefore more sensitive than radiographs to variations in bone and soft tissue density. In spite of the potential risk of adverse reactions, intravenous (IV) contrast is usually administered to further improve soft tissue contrast based on relative differences in tissue vascularization. However, CT is a major source of radiation in the pediatric population and should be restricted to use in clinical situations with clearly defined imaging goals. Radiation dose can be minimized by reducing milliamperage to levels well below those of standard protocols used for imaging adults.

CT is used primarily to assess bony structures and is a very sensitive method of detecting cortical disruption, periosteal reaction, and other osseous changes associated with infection, trauma, and neoplasia. Some tumors (e.g., osteoid osteoma) may be more readily detected by CT than other modalities. CT is superior to MRI for detecting bony sequestra associated with osteomyelitis. Although not as sensitive to differences in soft tissue contrast as magnetic resonance (MR) images, quite subtle increases in the normally hypodense marrow of older children can be seen on CT images. CT is also more sensitive than radiographs to the presence of abnormal calcifications, fat, and air within soft tissues.

CT scanning has been generally limited to the axial plane. However, this orientation and the tomographic nature of CT images complements longitudinal radiographic projections of bones, facilitating the assessment of osseous abnormalities in anatomically complex regions such as the pelvis. Furthermore, current scanners are capable of rapid production of slices as thin as 0.75 mm, which can be reconstructed in any desired plane. These multiplanar reconstructions are useful to detect and analyze subtle fractures of long bones and to show their relationship to articular structures. Data generated by narrowly collimated CT imaging can also be displayed in a three-dimensional format useful for planning surgical reconstruction procedures. The newest scanners incorporate multiple rows of detectors and are capable of true volumetric imaging. CT angiography is an additional procedure that can be performed with fast multidetector scanners and is expected to compete with MR angiography in the investigation of vascular abnormalities and for planning surgical procedures that involve major blood vessels.

MAGNETIC RESONANCE IMAGING

MRI has had a major impact on musculoskeletal imaging owing to its ability to produce high-contrast images of structures that are invisible or are poorly visualized by x-ray–based modalities. This feature is especially important in children because the immature skeleton contains a high proportion of radiolucent cartilage. With the use of high-field imagers, specialized pulse sequences, and dedicated surface coils, multiplanar images with excellent spatial and contrast resolution can be obtained. Lack of ionizing radiation and the relative safety of gadolinium-based contrast agents have enhanced the utility of this modality in the investigation of pediatric musculoskeletal disorders. In many cases, the relatively high cost of MRI is mitigated by its clinical usefulness and the potential avoidance of other costly or more invasive diagnostic procedures.

MR contrast is basically dependent on the T_1 and T_2 relaxation rates of biologic tissues and the imaging sequence employed (Table 2). In general, combinations of conventional spin-echo, fast spin-echo, and gradient-echo sequences are employed to achieve the clinical goals of each examination. Short inversion-time inversion-recovery (STIR) pulse sequences are frequently used to image musculoskeletal neoplasms. These sequences incorporate an inversion time precisely timed to null lipid signals and to maximize contrast from well-hydrated tissues, such as neoplasms, by adding signal derived from the effects of both T_1 and T_2 relaxation. Gadolinium-based paramagnetic contrast agents can also be used to increase signal intensity of tissues on T_1-weighted images. Radiofrequency pulses that selectively saturate the lipid resonance peak are frequently added to fast spin-echo sequences to suppress fat signals. This method of fat suppression is also frequently used with gadolinium-enhanced T_1-weighted sequences to achieve contrast between enhanced and otherwise similarly intense fatty tissues. Although IV contrast administration adds time, expense, and slight risk to the MR examination, its use is justified in a number of musculoskeletal imaging applications.

An important feature of MRI in this clinical setting is a lack of signal from bone and other dense tissues, including ligaments and tendons. This characteristic absence of signal provides negative contrast in comparison to muscle, which is of intermediate intensity, and yellow marrow, which is hyperintense on T_1-weighted images. In contrast, abnormal accumulations of fluid within joints and bursae are hyperintense on T_2-weighted images, as are fluid-containing lesions such as abscesses and cysts. The use of gadolinium with T_1-weighted imaging sequences can help differentiate joint effusions, which show only very slow enhancement, from rapidly enhancing vascularized tissues such as hypertrophied synovium or juxta-articular tumors. Gradient-echo sequences produce images more rapidly than spin-echo imaging, but they are dependent on T_2* relaxation. As a result, they are susceptible to artifacts caused by local variations in the magnetic field, which can be quite pronounced in the presence of bone. However, gradient-echo sequences are very useful for displaying cartilage, which appears intense on these images.

Bone bruises, indicated by alterations in marrow signal, frequently point to the presence of subtle or even radiographically undetectable microfractures. In addition, MRI is sensitive to injuries and malformations involving the physis and epiphysis. This feature permits the early detection of post-traumatic bony bridges that, when they cross the physis, can lead to deformities as growth ensues. MRI is also useful to follow the course of inflammatory conditions such as juvenile rheumatoid arthritis and hemarthroses associated with blood coagulation disorders. A major benefit of MRI is its ability to detect internal articular derangements such as meniscal and cruciate ligament tears. Indeed, percutaneous arthrography is now a nearly obsolete procedure.

Before the advent of MRI, detection and diagnosis of soft tissue lesions by radiologic means was limited. MRI may provide a specific diagnosis of lesions that contain fat and vascular elements. However, the signal characteristics of most soft tissue tumors are nonspecific because they are isointense to muscle on T_1-weighted images and hyperintense on T_2-weighted images. Furthermore, most soft tissue masses enhance on gadolinium-contrasted T_1-weighted images. Although not diagnostic, these characteristics permit precise evaluation of tumor size, configuration, and location. MRI is also valuable for assessing generalized diseases such as myofibromatosis and muscular dystrophy.

The advantage of MRI over radiography and CT for bone tumors lies mainly in its ability to display adjacent soft tissue and joint involvement in a variety of planes. The ability to obtain longitudinally oriented

Table 2 ■ RELATIVE MRI SIGNAL INTENSITIES OF NORMAL AND PATHOLOGIC TISSUES

	IMAGING SEQUENCE*				
	T_1W	T_2W	STIR	T_2* GRE	GdT_1W, FS
Muscle	2	2	2	2	2
Bone	1	1	1	1	1
Fat	3	2	0	2	0
Marrow					
Yellow	3	2	0	1–2	0
Red	2	2	2	2	2
Tendons, ligaments	1	1	1	1	1
Cartilage	2	2–3	3	3	2
Joint effusion	1	3	3	3	1
Pathologic tissues	2	3	3	3	3

T_1W = T_1-weighted spin-echo; T_2W = T_2-weighted spin-echo or fast spin-echo; STIR = short inversion-time (tau) inversion-recovery; T_2 GRE = T_2*-weighted gradient-recalled echo; GdT_1W = gadolinium-enhanced T_1-weighted; FS = fat saturation.
Scoring: 1 to 3 = least to most intense signal; 0 = nulled fat signal.

images greatly facilitates the evaluation of the extent of medullary involvement. Several MR angiographic techniques (time-of-flight, phase contrast, and gadolinium-enhanced T_1-weighted sequences) are available to map the relationship of major blood vessels to tumors to help plan surgery and determine resectability. Dynamic contrast-enhanced MRI, which is sensitive to differences in the rate of gadolinium uptake of malignant and non-neoplastic tissues, is an emerging method of depicting tumor necrosis and evaluating response of malignant tumors to preoperative chemotherapy.

MRI is the only modality that permits direct visualization of normal bone marrow. As red, hematopoietic marrow converts to yellow, fatty marrow during childhood, the marrow signal changes from hypointense to hyperintense on T_1-weighted images. This process, which begins during infancy, is most prominent in the extremities. It progresses from the distal to the more proximal portions of the appendicular skeleton and finally to the axial skeleton. On T_1-weighted images, marrow abnormalities caused by primary bone tumors, metastases, and hematologic malignancies exhibit considerably lower signal intensity than fat-containing marrow and are consequently readily visible. Thus MRI is a useful procedure to localize marrow disease prior to biopsy. In the appropriate clinical setting, a focal abnormality of marrow signal is an early indicator of osteomyelitis. Reconversion of yellow to red marrow, which can occur under a variety of physiologic and pathologic conditions, can also be observed, and subtle changes in marrow composition can be detected on images made with sequences that are highly sensitive to changes in the relative amount of fat and water.

NUCLEAR IMAGING

Skeletal scintigraphy using technetium-labeled phosphates was introduced more than three decades ago. Today, the "bone scan" is the most frequently performed pediatric nuclear imaging study. The universal acceptance of this study is based on its high sensitivity relative to skeletal radiography and the ability to perform the test easily with an acceptable radiation dose. The radiopharmaceutical most commonly used today is technetium-99m MDP. Images obtained after injection of this compound reflect a combination of pathophysiologic functions (blood flow and bone turn-over) but are nonspecific and do not provide exceptional anatomic detail. The resulting images should therefore be interpreted in the context of the patient's clinical presentation and the relevant radiologic findings. Indeed, a reasonable dictum holds that bone scans of pediatric patients should be viewed along with the appropriate bone radiographs to avoid common pitfalls in interpretation caused by the normally nonuniform distribution of radiotracer in the growing skeleton. The most problematic anatomic areas to image and interpret accurately are the growth centers. Before closure of the physes, these rapidly growing areas display especially high uptake that may overwhelm the activity associated with an adjacent pathologic lesion. The addition of single-photon emission CT helps localize such lesions because it improves the spatial resolution of activity in contiguous and overlapping structures.

Indications for skeletal scintigraphy are many and include investigation of bone pain, diagnosis of early and chronic osteomyelitis, avascular necrosis, and occult trauma, including nonaccidental trauma and stress fractures. Bone scans may reveal benign bone tumors such as osteoid osteomas that may be radiographically invisible and are useful in estimating the extent of primary tumors and evaluating osseus involvement by adjacent soft tissue neoplasms. MRI may be competitive with bone scans in some circumstances, such as early diagnosis of osteomyelitis and avascular necrosis. Nevertheless, whole-body skeletal scintigraphy is mandated for the detection of metastatic deposits and plays an important role in many oncology treatment protocols. In patients with neuroblastoma, *meta*-iodobenzylguanidine (MIBG) tagged with ^{123}I or ^{131}I is used in an effort to increase specificity and sensitivity in the diagnosis of metastatic disease.

In other clinical settings, anatomic imaging modalities are complementary to nuclear studies and are frequently requested for further evaluation of a lesion located on a scintigram. The detection or confirmation of osteomyelitis is one of the most common indications for skeletal scintigraphy. In such cases, a three-phase scintigram is recommended. This study is composed of serial "angiographic" images followed by blood pool or tissue-phase images of the suspected site obtained soon after injection of the radiopharmaceutical, followed by skeletal equilibrium images made several hours later. Three-phase scans are also recommended in patients with suspected osteoid osteoma because the blood pool images may demonstrate a small focus of intense activity, increasing diagnostic specificity for this lesion.

Gallium-67 citrate, commonly used for tagging lymphoreticular malignancies, is also bound by inflammatory leukocytes, making ^{67}Ga imaging a useful adjunct to ^{99m}Tc-MDP scintigraphy in the diagnosis of osteomyelitis, especially in the small percentage of cases in which a three-phase bone scan reveals no abnormality. [67]Ga is also taken up by both benign and malignant bone and soft tissue tumors. Gallium scintigraphy is less blood flow dependent and is more specific than ^{99m}Tc-MDP imaging. However, it is usually assigned a secondary role to ^{99m}Tc-MDP scintigraphy because of its inferior spatial resolution and the fact that imaging must be performed periodically for up to 48 to 72 hours postinjection to rule out osteomyelitis with confidence. In the absence of abnormality detected by bone or gallium scans, scintigraphy using ^{111}In-labeled leukocytes is a further strategy for the detection of musculoskeletal infections.

The problem of differentiating infarction from osteomyelitis in patients with sickle cell anemia has been addressed with some success by the use of dual, sequential bone, and bone marrow scans, the latter employing ^{99m}Tc-sulfur colloid. Abnormally low bone marrow uptake of sulfur colloid in the presence of increased osseous activity demonstrated on the bone scan is indicative of infarction, whereas normal marrow uptake is highly suggestive of infection. Similarly, an incongruently high uptake of ^{67}Ga relative to ^{99m}Tc-sulfur colloid also suggests a diagnosis of infection rather than infarction. The relative effectiveness of MRI and bone marrow scintigraphy in the diagnosis of focal and diffuse bone marrow disorders is the subject of ongoing clinical investigations.

Positron emission tomography (PET) imaging is becoming increasingly available for clinical use. PET imaging with 2-[^{18}F]fluoro-2-deoxyglucose (FDG) offers improved spatial resolution and greater sensitivity for detection of aggressive bone neoplasms. Some studies suggest that FDG-PET will be particularly effective in detecting metastatic bone lesions as compared to ^{99m}Tc-MDP scintigrams. PET may also prove to be a more effective method of determining response of malignant bone tumors to therapy.

CONCLUSION

Radiologists must be prepared to advise their clinical colleagues on the appropriate selection and application of imaging among the large number of modalities and techniques currently available for the detection and diagnosis of musculoskeletal disorders. The following chapters provide a fundamental understanding of the musculoskeletal disease processes commonly occurring in pediatric patients as well as guidance regarding the use of specific imaging modalities.

PART II

DISORDERS OF THE SOFT TISSUES

KATHLEEN H. EMERY
BARRY D. FLETCHER

■ Chapter 1

THE SOFT TISSUES

KATHLEEN H. EMERY

OVERVIEW

Alterations in the soft tissues are a frequent complaint for which pediatric patients seek medical attention. Soft tissues cover all areas of the body but are largely ignored in many radiology texts, even though they are present on virtually all imaging studies. Although the skin is the largest single organ, it is most efficiently evaluated by direct visual inspection. Suspected pathology in the deeper soft tissues, including the subcutaneous fat, muscles, fascia, blood and lymphatic vessels, nerves, and lymph nodes, that are not amenable to direct visual inspection may require imaging evaluation. At times it is the visual inspection of the skin itself that will provide important clues to underlying pathology in the deeper soft tissues. For example, the bluish discoloration over a hemangioma may trigger the need for imaging to define the lesion and its extent.

A variety of modalities are at our disposal for soft tissue evaluation. Conventional radiography is widely available, easily performed, and economical and does not require sedation. Radiographs have a relatively narrow density latitude, which limits their utility. Most soft tissues, with the exception of fat, are the same density on conventional radiographs. However, radiographs may provide important information about amount of soft tissue (too much or too little), presence or absence of abnormal radiopaque or radiolucent structures (such as calcification or air), and integrity of underlying skeletal structures. The greatest utility of radiographs for soft tissue evaluation in children is for suspected foreign body search and in helping screen the soft tissue prior to more advanced imaging.

Computed tomography (CT) provides a broader density latitude than radiography, with cross-sectional capability allowing for more precise localization of pathology. However, soft tissue contrast remains limited (particularly without intravenous contrast) and relative radiation dose high, restricting the value of CT in soft tissue evaluation.

Sonography brings unique capabilities to soft tissue evaluation. Primarily, the absence of ionizing radiation, lack of need for sedation to obtain a diagnostic study, and wide availability of high-resolution transducers to visualize superficial structures (7, 10, and even 15 MHz) make it very attractive in the pediatric population. Determining cystic or solid contents and evaluating vascularity with Doppler are distinctive pieces of information sonography can provide about soft tissue lesions. Soft tissue contrast is somewhat limited, as is field of view, making the role of sonography more restricted.

Magnetic resonance imaging (MRI) provides the most exquisite soft tissue contrast available with the added benefit of no ionizing radiation and a wide range of flexibility for field-of-view coverage as determined by the variety of coils at one's disposal. Even though magnetic resonance (MR) images may be degraded by ferromagnetic structures in the field or interest, and small foreign bodies that emit no signal may be difficult to recognize, this modality has revolutionized the radiologist's ability to diagnose soft tissue abnormalities. A normal MRI exam may help confidently exclude pathology. The cost of MRI remains high, and reliance on sedation is common in the vast majority of patients under age 8. Distracting techniques such as audio and videotapes with compatible headphones and viewing goggles may reduce the need for sedation in the 4- to 8-year-old age group. Nonetheless, MRI has proven to be a most powerful tool for evaluating focal and diffuse soft tissue pathology.

A wide variety of pathologic conditions may involve the soft tissues. Many of these, including congenital malformations and infectious and neoplastic conditions, are addressed in subsequent parts of this section. This chapter focuses on soft tissue foreign body evalua-

Table 1 ■ DIFFERENTIAL DIAGNOSIS OF SOFT TISSUE CALCIFICATION

Trauma
Myositis ossificans
Hematoma
Subcutaneous fat necrosis

Inflammation
Dermatomyositis
Scleroderma
Lupus
Ehlers-Danlos syndrome
Acne vulgaris (treated with tetracyclines)
Parasitic infection (i.e., *Taenia solium* [pork tapeworm])

Neoplasm
Pilomatrixoma
Epidermal cyst
Lipoma
Synovial sarcoma

Congenital
Fibrodysplasia ossificans progressiva
Venous malformation (phleboliths)
Albright's hereditary osteodystrophy

Metabolic
Tumoral calcinosis
Chronic renal failure
Milk-alkali syndrome
Vitamin D intoxication
Parathyroid neoplasms

Miscellaneous
Injection sites
Multiple heel sticks
Immobilization
Electroencephalogram electrodes (scalp)

tion; conditions that may cause abnormal focal or diffuse soft tissue radiodensity, calcification, or ossification (Table 1); and conditions resulting in abnormal soft tissue excess or deficiency (i.e., neuromuscular disorders).

CUTANEOUS CALCIFICATION/ OSSIFICATION

Calcification or ossification normally occurs in the teeth and bones but might arise in the skin in a variety of pathologic conditions. These may be focal or diffuse and symptomatic or asymptomatic.

CALCINOSIS CUTIS

Precipitation or deposition of hydroxyapatite crystals of calcium phosphate within cutaneous tissues is a pathologic condition known under the general term *calcinosis cutis*. Most forms of this disorder fall into one of three categories—dystrophic, metastatic, or idiopathic types—depending on the underlying disease process.

Dystrophic calcinosis cutis occurs in previously damaged tissue without an associated metabolic disturbance of the calcium:phosphorus ratio. Localized forms occur in inflammatory and traumatic lesions, including acne, ulcers, and foreign body granulomas, and following heel sticks for blood drawing in neonates. Neoplastic conditions, including epidermal cysts, lipoma, and pilomatrixoma (a benign tumor of hair matrix cell origin), are known to cause localized dystrophic calcification. More widespread dystrophic cutaneous calcification (calcinosis universalis) can be seen in dermatomyositis, scleroderma, pseudoxanthoma elasticum, Ehlers-Danlos syndrome, and systemic lupus erythematosus.

Metastatic calcinosis cutis occurs in undamaged tissue in conditions with an abnormality of calcium and/or phosphorus metabolism. Examples include chronic renal failure, milk-alkali syndrome, vitamin D intoxication, parathyroid neoplasms, and sarcoidosis.

Idiopathic calcinosis cutis occurs without a metabolic abnormality or regional soft tissue defect. Usually these are localized tiny nodules in the skin found on the face or ears of neonates and small children. Idiopathic calcinosis of the skin of the scrotum or labia may also occur.

OSTEOMA CUTIS

Spontaneous new bone formation may occur in the skin and is termed *osteoma cutis* (Fig. 1). This may be primary or secondary. Primary osteoma cutis occurs without an underlying skin lesion and is either an isolated condition or seen with Albright hereditary osteodystrophy and the associated pseudohypoparathyroidism or pseudopseudohypoparathyroidism. Secondary osteoma cutis arises in cutaneous neoplasms (similar to calcinosis cutis) or areas of inflammation, most notably in acne vulgaris treated with tetracycline compounds.

Osteoma cutis may occur at any age. Isolated or multiple hard, raised nodules measuring 1 to 5 mm are found, most commonly on the face. The lesion(s) may be painful. The overlying skin might vary from normal to ulcerated. Laboratory values are typically normal unless the patient has pseudohypoparathyroidism with decreased serum calcium and elevated serum phosphorus. The treatment of choice is surgical excision.

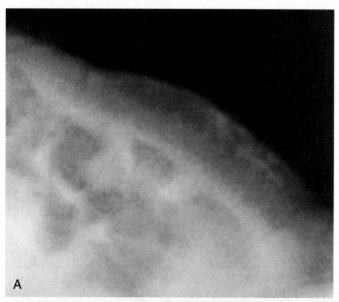
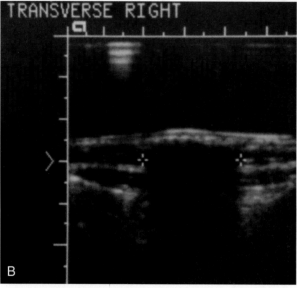
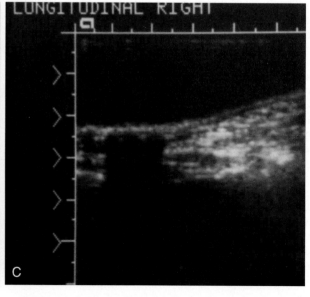

FIGURE 1. Osteoma cutis. Localized firm plaque was observed on the lower abdomen at 1 month; there was no birth trauma or hypothermia, and calcium and phosphorus concentrations were normal. The plaque increased in size, and a biopsy specimen was obtained at 4 months. **A,** Radiograph at 4 months shows low anterior abdominal wall calcification. **B,** On transverse ultrasound scan through area of abnormality, the calcification is superficial to the rectus muscles and demonstrates acoustic shadowing. **C,** A longitudinal midline ultrasound scan also shows shadowing; the urinary bladder below is partially distended. Sonograms were performed with a "water bath" to improve the image of superficial skin. (Courtesy of Dr. Diane Babcock, Cincinnati, OH.)

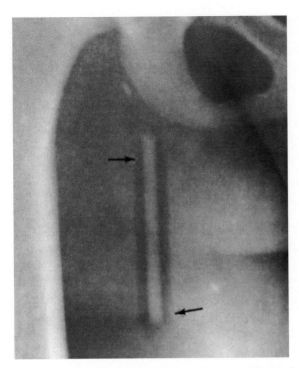

FIGURE 2. Fragment of a standard lead pencil in the right buttock of a boy of 6 years who was said to have "sat down on a sharp pencil" that penetrated his clothing and skin and left this unsharpened fragment. Because of its higher content of gas, the soft wood of the pencil *(arrows)* casts a more radiolucent tubular image around the central core of the graphite cylinder, which approximates the density of water in the heavy muscles. "Lead" pencils, of course, contain no lead.

FOREIGN BODY

Suspected foreign body is a relatively common indication for imaging evaluation of the soft tissues in children. Foreign bodies include any substance that may penetrate the skin. These vary from inert materials such as glass and metal to organic materials such as thorns, cactus needles, and sea urchin spines. Once present, a significant foreign body reaction may occur in the surrounding soft tissues, with a local inflammatory response particularly with organic materials. Some foreign bodies are clinically obvious, whereas others are occult. The occult foreign body with surrounding soft tissue granuloma may produce adjacent bone changes and simulate a neoplasm. More severe reactions can occur if the offending agent enters a joint.

Evaluation of any suspected foreign body should begin with conventional radiographs of the area of concern using soft tissue technique (lower kilovoltage peak). Two views obtained in planes at 90 degrees to each other with the entry site indicated are usually adequate to screen for radiopaque or radiolucent foreign bodies. Any foreign body that contains gas will produce a radiolucent appearance. The most common example is a lead pencil, in which the "lead" is actually water-density graphite. The surrounding soft wood has a higher gas content, which casts a radiolucent shadow around the graphite core in the acute stage, making it

visible on radiography (Fig. 2). As the gas is resorbed and soft tissue reaction occurs, the pencil fragment will become invisible on radiographs, as are most organic foreign bodies.

Most published studies find sonography is very valuable for reliably detecting radiographically occult foreign bodies as small as 2.5 mm in live patients as well as cadaveric specimens. Detection of a foreign body on sonography requires meticulous attention to detail with high-resolution transducers, stand-off pads as necessary, and methodical scanning of the area in question. Most foreign bodies will appear as hyperechoic foci with varying degrees of posterior acoustic shadowing depending on the composition of the foreign substance (Fig. 3). Sonography has also proven valuable in guiding foreign body removal. However, attempts to localize a nonradiopaque foreign body for removal may be compromised if a large amount of air is introduced in the surrounding soft tissues by extensive dissection prior to scanning.

In cases where foreign body penetration is not recognized, the clinical picture is more puzzling. If the foreign body is not removed, it becomes surrounded by fibrous tissue, forming a localized granuloma. The child may present with a new soft tissue mass with or without systemic findings of infection. Radiographs might demonstrate the foreign body if radiopaque. Often, foreign bodies are not visible, and the radiographs may present a confusing picture of reactive changes in the adjacent bone that could mimic neoplasm. In this setting, MRI becomes the study most frequently requested for evaluation. CT might be useful in localizing some foreign bodies (Fig. 4) but does not offer the soft tissue contrast and marrow evaluation necessary in those confusing cases where bone and soft tissue tumors are under diagnostic consideration. MRI provides this type of evaluation and may well demonstrate the foreign body as an area of signal void, often surrounded by a

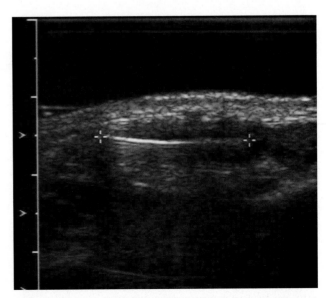

FIGURE 3. Foreign body (glass) in the cheek of a 15-year-old struck in the face with a bottle. Calipers mark the well-defined 2-cm subcutaneous foreign body.

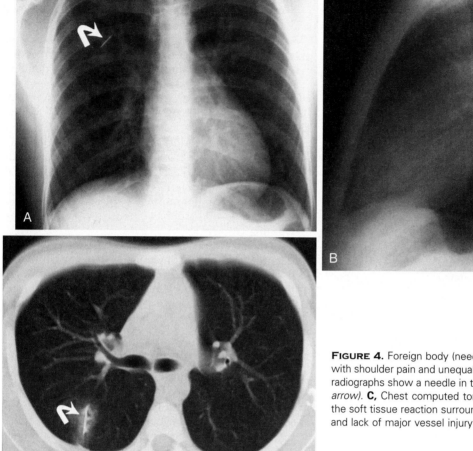

FIGURE 4. Foreign body (needle). This 10-year-old presented with shoulder pain and unequal breath sounds. **A** and **B,** Chest radiographs show a needle in the posterior right chest *(curved arrow).* **C,** Chest computed tomography better demonstrates the soft tissue reaction surrounding the needle *(curved arrow)* and lack of major vessel injury or pneumothorax.

high-T_2-signal mass or fluid collection with varying degrees of contrast enhancement (Fig. 5). Histologically, foreign body giant cells with an inflammatory reaction are seen. Most fluid collections are sterile. In cases where a foreign body is discovered in close proximity to a joint, MRI might be useful for preoperative joint evaluation. Foreign body removal with antibiotic therapy as needed is usually curative.

MYOSITIS OSSIFICANS

Myositis ossificans is an uncommon benign mass characterized by ectopic bone formation in the soft tissues, most commonly in skeletal muscle. It may mimic a true neoplasm on both imaging and histologic examination. This entity is known by several other names, including myositis ossificans traumatica, myositis ossificans circumscripta, and pseudomalignant myositis ossificans. A history of local trauma is common but is not recognized in approximately one third of patients. This disorder is

most frequent in young adults, though up to 25% of patients are not skeletally mature. Of the skeletally immature group, most are teenagers, with a few reported cases in young childhood and infants. This entity is one of a larger spectrum of ectopic ossification in various tissues from different causes that may share pathogenetic mechanisms. Although the cells of origin of myositis ossificans are not fully understood, Illes et al. suggested that bone marrow-derived myofibroblasts are responsible for bone formation in the damaged muscle.

Myositis ossificans undergoes a maturation process, and the imaging findings change as the histology of the lesion evolves. Biopsy in the early stages of the process may lead to a false diagnosis of osteosarcoma. Acute myositis ossificans consists of central fibroblastic proliferation. Peripheral organization leads to new bone formation in 6 to 8 weeks. Radiographs and CT images will typically show faint calcification within 2 to 6 weeks after the onset of symptoms, followed by development of a curvilinear or circular rim of peripheral calcification

(Fig. 6A, B). Intense radioactivity may be seen on bone scintigrams (Fig. 6C), with a ring-like pattern in some patients. By about 6 months, the lesion consists of dense compact bone surrounding a central zone of lamellar bone. Periosteal reaction and cortical thickening of adjacent bones may also be seen on radiographs and on CT images. As the myositis ossificans shrinks away from the bone, a cleavage zone results. Differential diagnosis in the late stage of the process includes parosteal and extraosseous osteosarcoma (see Section IX, Part XII, Table 6, page 2401).

MRI is generally not necessary or helpful in making the diagnosis. If an MRI exam is performed, the findings will vary depending on the stage of the myositis ossifi-

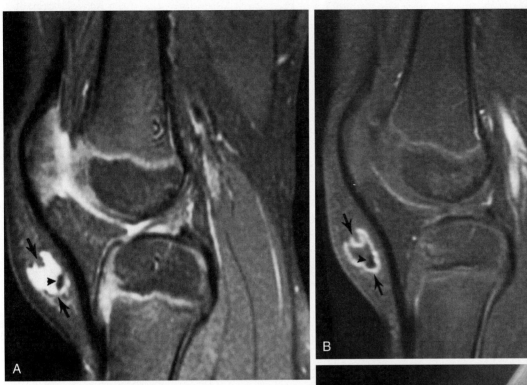

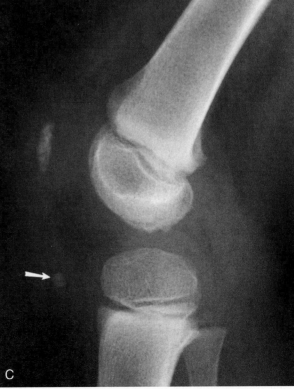

FIGURE 5. Foreign body reaction. This 5-year-old had a palpable infrapatellar mass without a history of trauma. On magnetic resonance imaging sagittal T_2-weighted fast spin-echo **(A)** and gadolinium-enhanced T_1-weighted **(B)** images, both with fat suppression, show a high-T_2-signal mass *(arrows)* with peripheral enhancement and a focal area of persistent signal void inferiorly *(arrowhead)*. **C,** This proved on radiography to represent a radiopaque foreign body *(arrow)*.

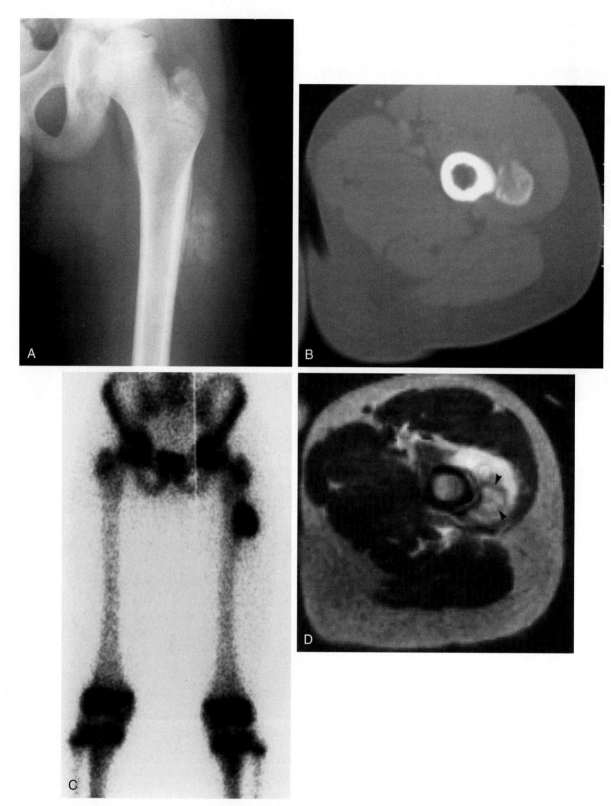

FIGURE 6. Myositis ossificans in an 11-year-old boy with a 3-week history of thigh pain. **A,** An anteroposterior radiograph of the thigh shows a well-defined, calcified soft tissue lesion with periosteal new bone formation involving the adjacent femur. (From Hanna SL, Fletcher BD, Parham DM, et al: Muscle edema in musculoskeletal tumors: MR imaging characteristics and clinical significance. J Magn Reson Imaging 1991;1:445. ©John Wiley & Sons. Reprinted by permission of Wiley-Liss, Inc., a subsidiary of John Wiley & Sons, Inc.) **B,** Computed tomography image shows peripheral calcification. There is no cortical bone involvement. **C,** Marked activity is seen in the mass on a technetium-99m methylene diphosphonate bone scintigram. **D,** A transverse T_2-weighted magnetic resonance image shows hyperintense signal in the muscle superficial to the hypointense, calcified rim *(arrowheads).* (**B** and **D** from Fletcher BD, Hanna SL: Pediatric musculoskeletal lesions simulating neoplasms. Magn Reson Imaging Clin N Am 1996;4:741, with permission.)

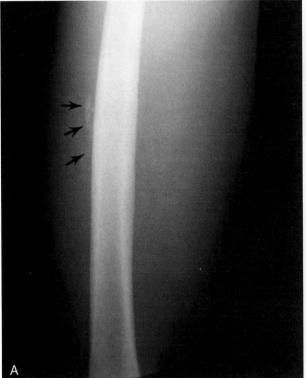

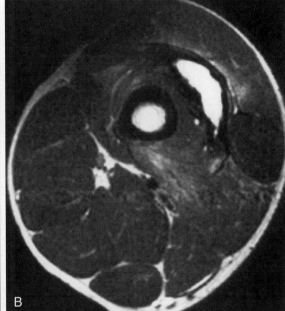

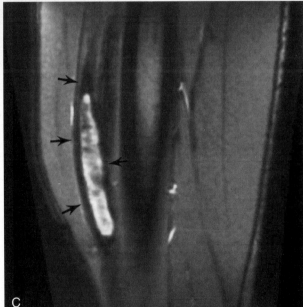

FIGURE 7. Myositis ossificans. A 16-year-old soccer player kicked in the right thigh 6 weeks earlier had a palpable "knot" that has calcification *(arrows)* on radiography **(A)** appearing separate from the femur. **B,** Axial T_2-weighted magnetic resonance image shows a high-signal-intensity mass in the quadriceps with a very low-signal-intensity rim corresponding to calcification. **C,** Sagittal T_2-weighted gradient-echo image highlights the calcified rim *(arrows)* and the heterogeneous low-signal center, likely due to aging blood products (i.e., hemosiderin).

cans. Early lesions (3 to 6 weeks) have a central core of proliferating fibroblasts and myofibroblasts with minimal bone formation at the periphery. The central proliferating core is minor and the peripheral rim of osteoid and mature lamellar bone becomes more prominent in intermediate lesions (6 to 8 weeks). Late lesions (several months to years) are composed almost entirely of mature lamellar bone. A heterogeneously high-T_2-signal mass is evident centrally with surrounding edema in early and intermediate lesions (Fig. 7). The lesion may enhance with gadolinium. Hyaline cartilage, myxoid stroma, hemorrhagic components, and fluid–fluid levels may be present. The peripheral ring of ossification that is so well seen on CT is much less conspicuous as a low-signal-intensity rim on MRI. Plain radiographs are very helpful in this setting. In late lesions, a heterogeneous, well-defined mass lacking edema is seen with signal intensity that approximates fat, reflecting adipose tissue in the intertrabecular spaces of the mature lamellar bone.

Treatment is rest and analgesia with nonsteroidal anti-inflammatory agents. Partial or total involution of the lesion over time is common. Excision is rarely necessary for functional reasons and is usually delayed until the lesion matures.

HEMATOMA

Hemorrhage involving the muscle itself or the fascial planes is a frequent component of muscle strains, and may also result from direct trauma, including injections.

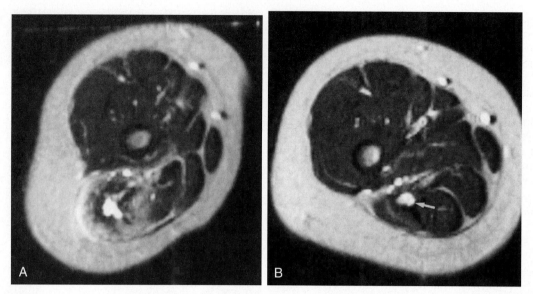

FIGURE 8. Hematoma of uncertain duration in the biceps femoris muscle of a 2-year-old girl. **A,** T_2-weighted transverse magnetic resonance image of the thigh at the time of presentation shows a hyperintense muscle edema with a very hyperintense center. **B,** Two months later, only a small hyperintense focus (arrow) remains. (**B** from Fletcher BD, Hanna SL: Pediatric musculoskeletal lesions simulating neoplasms. Magn Reson Imaging Clin N Am 1996;4:743, with permission.)

The presence of an intramuscular hematoma may simulate tumor. In the case of complete muscle tears, a mass may also form as the muscle retracts.

Hematomas may be imaged by ultrasonography or CT, but MRI provides the best contrast and characterization of the injury. However, the findings, although distinctive, can be confusing because of alterations in signal intensity that occur as hematomas age.

Acute hematomas (1 to 6 days after injury) may be isointense, hypointense, or hyperintense to normal muscle on T_1-weighted images, but most of these acute lesions are markedly hypointense on T_2-weighted images. This hypointensity probably corresponds to the formation of deoxyhemoglobin. Subacute hematomas (7 to 49 days after injury) become hyperintense on both T_1- and T_2-weighted images because of the formation of methemoglobin as a blood degradation product. The liquefied center may be markedly hyperintense (Fig. 8). In some patients, a thin, well-defined peripheral rim is seen that is hypointense on T_1- and T_2-weighted images. On CT images, this rim may be seen as a soft tissue–density capsule. With further aging (15 to 48 days after injury), the lesions become uniformly hyperintense. Hematomas usually reabsorb in 6 to 8 weeks but may occasionally persist as seromas.

INFLAMMATORY MUSCLE DISEASES

Inflammatory muscle disorders in children are either acute or chronic. Acute muscular symptoms other than those associated with trauma or overuse are most commonly associated with an infectious agent, either bacterial, viral, or parasitic. Other environmental triggers of myositis include drugs, vaccines, growth hormone, and bone marrow transplants that may induce

graft-versus-host myositis. The subgroup of chronic myositis is a diverse collection of rare syndromes sharing the common finding of chronic muscle inflammation of as yet undetermined pathophysiology, leading to damaged function of smooth and striated muscle. The juvenile idiopathic inflammatory myopathies include a variety of syndromes, the most common being dermatomyositis, polymyositis, and overlap myositis (myositis with another connective tissue disease in which vasculitis is a component, such as lupus or mixed connective tissue disease).

DERMATOMYOSITIS

Juvenile dermatomyositis is the most common form of idiopathic inflammatory myopathy in childhood, with a more prominent vasculitis component than other myopathic syndromes. It occurs 10 to 20 times more frequently than polymyositis and has a peak age distribution between 5 and 14 years of age. No definite genetic link has been documented, though various genetic components may be associated with disease expression and susceptibility. Children typically present with the symptom of persistent and progressive symmetric proximal muscle weakness that may be insidious in onset. The characteristic rash is violaceous, involving the eyelids and nasal bridge, and is photosensitive (heliotropic), perhaps accounting in part for the increased occurrence in the springtime. Scaly erythematous papules (Gottron's papules) are another common cutaneous finding most frequently seen over the small joints on the dorsum of the hands. One or more of the muscle-associated enzymes, including creatine phosphokinase, aldolase, lactate dehydrogenase, and the transaminases, are typically elevated. Evidence of inflammatory myopathy is sought by electromyography (EMG) and histopathology. The muscle biopsy shows chronic inflammatory infiltrates of perivascular or interstitial mononuclear cells with myocyte degeneration, necrosis, and regeneration. Demonstration of the characteristic rash with three of the other four criteria (proximal muscle weakness, elevated muscle-associated enzymes, EMG findings of inflammatory myopathy, and/or characteristic muscle biopsy findings) is necessary for diagnosis. Polymyositis is similar but lacks cutaneous involvement and has a different histologic picture. The vasculopathy that characterizes dermatomyositis may also cause gastrointestinal dysfunction (mainly swallowing and esophageal abnormalities), pulmonary fibrosis, and reversible cardiac conduction abnormalities.

MRI has proven to be very helpful in the diagnosis and management of adult and pediatric patients with dermatomyositis. The inflammatory changes in muscle and fascia, while not visible on T_1-weighted images, are exquisitely demonstrated as high signal areas on fat-saturated, T_2-weighted, and short tau inversion–recovery (STIR) sequences (Fig. 9). Although very sensitive, the MRI findings are not specific and may be seen following traumatic denervation, in rhabdomyolysis, with infection, and in necrotizing fasciitis. Exercise alone has been shown to visibly increase the muscle signal intensity on STIR sequences for approximately 30 minutes in patients with known inflammatory myopathy. If fat suppression is not used with T_2 weighting, a pronounced chemical shift artifact is often seen as a high-signal band along the frequency-encoding gradient at the muscle–fat interface of involved regions. Reticulated areas of increased T_2 signal may be seen in the subcutaneous fat in patients with skin involvement.

Soft tissue calcification is reported to occur in 30% to 70% of patients and may be related to disease duration and severity. Calcium deposition in the soft tissues typically occurs at sites exposed to trauma (buttocks, elbows, and knees). The calcinosis is dystrophic and

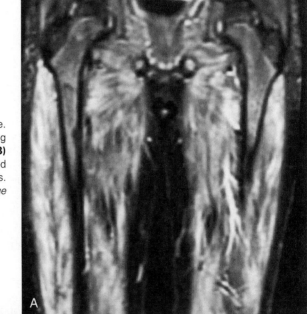

FIGURE 9. Dermatomyositis in an 8-year-old male. T_2-weighted fast spin-echo magnetic resonance imaging with fat suppression in the coronal **(A)** and axial **(B)** planes at diagnosis show diffusely abnormal increased signal intensity throughout the muscles of both thighs.
Illustration continued on following page

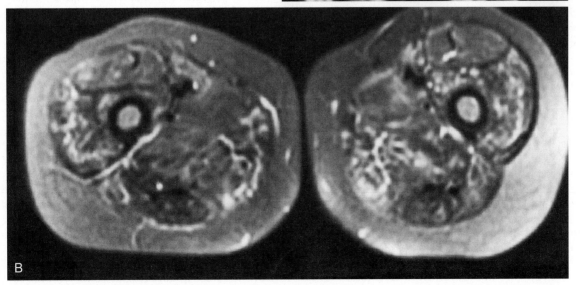

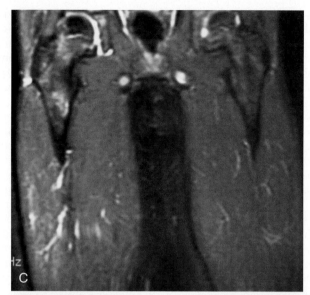

FIGURE 9. *Continued.* **C** and **D,** Same sequence of images after 10 months of therapy now show normal muscle signal intensity.

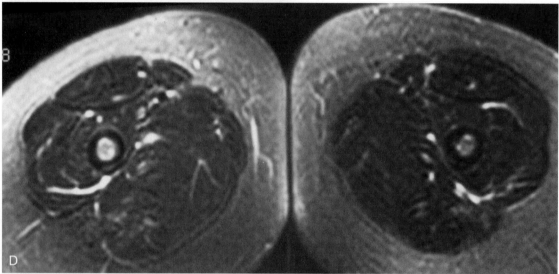

believed to be the end result of scarring from microvascular destruction and tissue necrosis. Five patterns have been described: superficial plaques on the extremities (calcinosis cutis), deep tumorous deposits in proximal muscles (calcinosis circumscripta), intermuscular fascial plane deposits (calcinosis universalis), subcutaneous reticular exoskeleton-like deposits, and mixed forms. In patients with severe forms of calcinosis, milk of calcium fluid collections have also been described in the soft tissues. Although readily visible on radiography and CT, areas of calcinosis are much less conspicuous on MR images (Fig. 10). They appear as areas of signal void on T_1- and T_2-weighted images, but may be enhanced on gradient-echo sequences. When chronic muscle atrophy develops, fatty muscle infiltration will be apparent on T_1-weighted images.

The distribution of muscle involvement is often symmetric and may be patchy. Because of the patchy distribution, EMG and muscle biopsy may be falsely negative as a result of sampling error. Occasionally, muscle enzymes are deceptively normal, as they may be at disease onset, after therapy initiation, during remission, or in those patients with severe muscle atrophy. MRI is very helpful in confirming or excluding muscle abnormality noninvasively, particularly in patients with atypical clinical and laboratory findings (Fig. 11). The results of MRI are useful to optimize biopsy location or EMG lead placement. In one study in adults, Schweitzer and Fort showed MRI to be cost effective for patients with polymyositis by reducing the number of false-negative biopsies. For patients who are difficult to assess clinically, MRI may be useful as a monitor of disease progress or return to normalcy with steroid or other immunosuppressive therapy. Whether the use of intravenous gadolinium is warranted remains unanswered by any controlled study. It may be helpful to exclude abscess formation in patients in whom infection is in the differential. Our clinicians appreciate gadolinium enhancement to confirm areas of active inflammation prior to biopsy.

MR spectroscopy (MRS) utilizing phosphorus-31 may provide a more quantitative assessment of the metabolic abnormalities in dermatomyositis and can be performed at the time of the MRI study. Lower than normal levels of adenosine triphosphate and phosphocreatine have been demonstrated at rest that are accentuated with exercise. Most of the data are in adults, and future work in this area is needed in children to determine the potential utility of MRS in patient management.

PYOMYOSITIS

Pyomyositis is a localized, primary infection of muscle that can mimic tumor, osteomyelitis, hematoma, cellulitis, and thrombophlebitis. This disorder is endemic in Africa, South America, Indochina, and the South Pacific. It is being reported more frequently in temperate zones in otherwise healthy children as well as in those suffering from debilitating diseases, including human immunodeficiency virus infection. *Staphylococcus aureus* is the causative organism in 95% of cases.

Clinically, the gluteal muscles, thighs, and calves are more commonly affected than the upper extremities, trunk, and chest wall. Usually, only a single muscle is involved. Early in the course of the illness, patients experience localized pain and tenderness, often in the absence of fever. The involved area lacks cutaneous erythema and has a "woody," nonfluctant feel. Fever usually occurs as the infection advances, and, in the absence of treatment, the entire muscle may become suppurant.

Ultrasonography, CT, and gallium-67 scintigraphy are helpful in localizing the abscess. The CT findings are indicative of abscess, with enlargement of the involved muscle, a central low-attenuation fluid collection, and a peripheral rim that enhances with the administration of intravenous contrast agents (Fig. 12). MRI appears to be

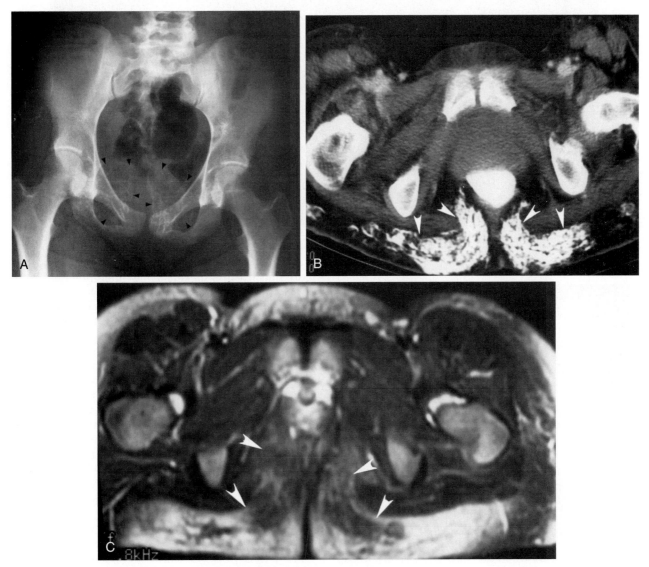

FIGURE 10. Dermatomyositis. The extensive soft tissue calcifications, predominately in the subcutaneous gluteal fat *(arrowheads)*, in this 19-year-old female with severe multisystemic involvement are much more conspicuous on radiography **(A)** and computed tomography **(B)** than on T$_2$-weighted magnetic resonance imaging **(C)**.

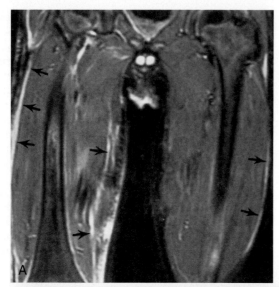

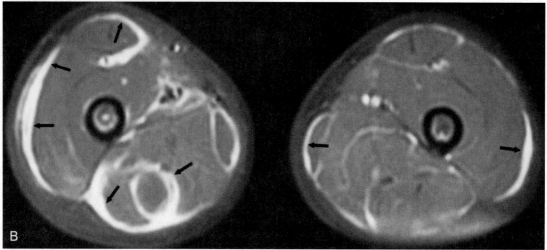

FIGURE 11. Eosinophilic fasciitis. This 3-year-old male presented with pain and swelling of the lower extremities with joint contractures. On magnetic resonance imaging, coronal T_2-weighted fast spin-echo **(A)** and axial postgadolinium T_1-weighted **(B)** images, both with chemical fat suppression, the abnormal increased signal and enhancement are limited to the superficial and deep fascial planes of both thighs *(arrows)*, right worse than left, with sparing of the adjacent muscles.

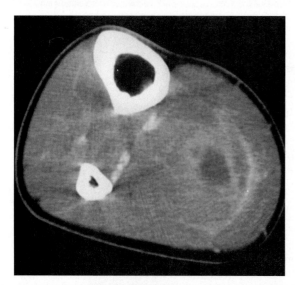

FIGURE 12. An abscess in the lower leg of a 16-year-old boy with leukemia. A contrast-enhanced computed tomography scan section shows a central low-attenuation fluid collection with an ill-defined enhanced periphery.

more sensitive and specific. On T_1-weighted images, the signal intensity of some abscesses is homogeneously greater than that of the involved muscle. The abscess wall enhances with gadolinium. On T_2-weighted MR images, the abscess shows high signal intensity with a hypointense rim and less well-defined hyperintensity of adjacent muscles. Patients may have changes associated with cellulitis, including skin thickening, stranding of subcutaneous fat, and swelling of fascial planes with high T_2-weighted signal intensity. A sympathetic effusion may also be seen in the joint distal to the infection. Drainage of the abscess and appropriate antibiotic therapy are usually curative. Muscle abscesses show avidity for gallium-67– and indium-111–labeled leukocytes.

Focal Myositis

Focal myositis is a rare pseudotumor of muscle sometimes seen in children. It is characterized histologically by lymphocytic infiltration, necrotic and regenerating muscle fibers, and interstitial fibrosis. The lesion is painful and causes fever, weakness, myalgia, and weight loss. The affected muscle is enlarged with hypoattenua-

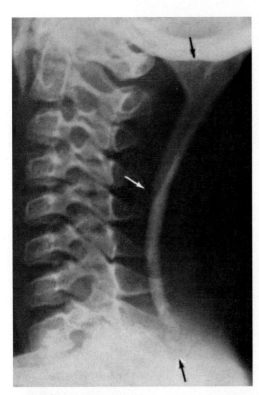

FIGURE 13. Juvenile progressive fibrodysplasia ossificans in a girl 9 years of age who had had swellings in the neck and back since age 4. A tubular mass of calcium density is seen in the position of the ligamentum nuchae *(arrows)* on this radiograph. The texture and shape of the calcareous mass resemble those of a tubular bone with cortex, medullary cavity, and spongiosa.

tion on CT images and produces an increased T_2-weighted signal on MR images, which may also show a focal mass surrounded by more intense edema. Occasionally, the lesions are multiple, and they may be a precursor of polymyositis.

FIBRODYSPLASIA OSSIFICANS PROGRESSIVA

Fibrodysplasia ossificans progressiva is a rare heritable disorder characterized by hypoplasia of the bases of the great toe and thumb associated with progressive development of heterotopic ossification in connective tissue and striated muscle, resulting in disabling ankylosis and muscle fixation.

Most cases of this disease represent spontaneous mutations, though an autosomal dominant mode of inheritance has been confirmed. Affected individuals are normal at birth with the exception of the digital abnormalities, most commonly microdactyly of the great toe with hallux valgus. Sometime during infancy or young childhood, patients will develop a soft tissue nodule(s) or mass(es), often painful and erythematous, typically over the upper trunk or neck, that may be associated with trauma. The swellings will resolve or ossify (Fig. 13). Heterotopic ossification begins at a mean of 5 years of age, with the course of the disease

being that of exacerbations of nodular swellings with progressive ossification of the muscle and connective tissue proceeding from the posterior neck and shoulder girdle distally, caudally, and anteriorly. Involvement of the chest wall and muscles of mastication contribute to the nutritional deficiencies, restrictive pulmonary disease, and pneumonia that commonly lead to death in adulthood.

Prior to ossification, cross-sectional imaging may simply demonstrate nonspecific soft tissue mass(es) on CT that have high T_2 signal on MRI (Fig. 14). Recognition of the characteristic digital changes, which occur in 70% to 90% of patients, can obviate biopsy, which is known to aggravate the condition. Once the lesions begin to ossify, they can be recognized on CT and by radionuclide bone scan even before the band-like areas of heterotopic bone formation are visible on conventional radiographs. Additional radiographic findings include narrow anteroposterior cervical and lumbar vertebral body diameter (possibly explained by hypotonia).

Biopsy of fibrodysplasia ossificans progressiva typically reveals different phases of normal endochondral osteogenesis at heterotopic sites. Early lesions demonstrate infiltrating loose myxoid fibrous tissue that may be misinterpreted as fibromatosis or sarcoma, hence the importance of recognizing the characteristic findings in the great toe(s) seen in nearly all patients, which obviate the need for biopsy. The coexistence of the pathologic changes with the congenital malformations of the great toes implies that defective induction of endochondral osteogenesis may underly this disorder.

Surgical therapy is not indicated in this disorder. Diphosphonates may be given to inhibit the ossification process, possibly with steroids to diminish the inflammation, though the results are inconsistent. Nutritional supplementation, prevention of pressure sores, and devices to assist with mobility are often necessary.

TUMORAL CALCINOSIS

Tumoral calcinosis is a relatively rare, benign condition characterized by mass-like calcific deposits of hydroxyapatite crystals in the soft tissues near major joints. The idiopathic variety tends to occur in otherwise healthy adolescents and young adults. There are a number of recorded cases of tumoral calcinosis in infants. Secondary tumoral calcinosis is a variation occurring in patients with a high calcium-phosphorus product and metastatic calcification (as in renal failure and secondary hyperparathyroidism).

Although the precise pathogenesis of the idiopathic form is unknown, an inborn error of phosphorus metabolism is considered likely, relating to abnormal phosphate reabsorption and 1,25-dihydroxyvitamin D formation in the proximal renal tubule. An autosomal dominant mode of genetic transmission has been identified in this condition, which occurs more frequently in blacks. Serum calcium levels are normal, but hyperphosphatemia and elevated serum 1,25-dihydroxyvitamin D may be found. Despite these abnormalities present in

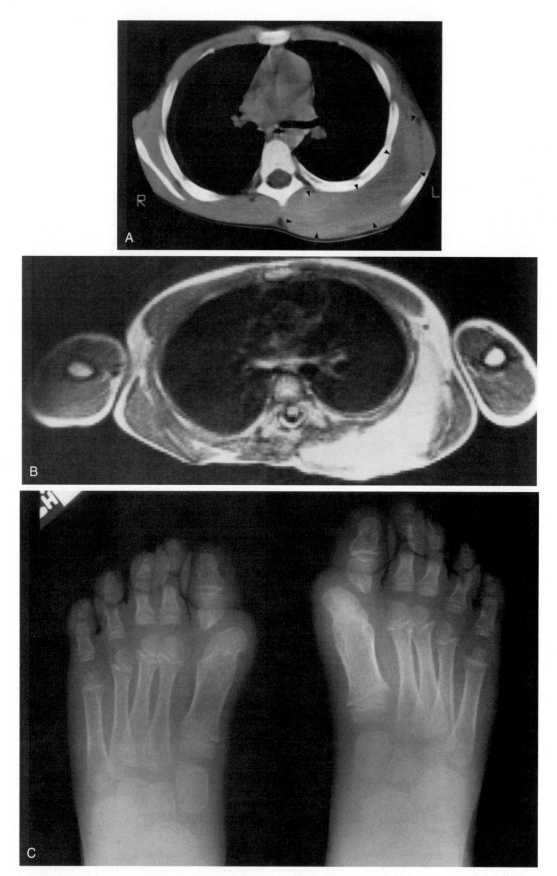

FIGURE 14. Fibrodysplasia ossificans progressiva prior to calcification in a 5-year-old boy. **A,** A nonenhanced computed tomography scan of the chest demonstrates a noncalcified soft tissue mass in the left posterior chest wall *(arrowheads)*. **B,** T$_2$-weighted magnetic resonance image shows diffuse high signal throughout the mass, possibly representing neoplasm. **C,** Skeletal survey revealed short first metacarpals and hallux valgus deformity bilaterally. Biopsy findings of a fibrous lesion in association with these characteristic skeletal findings was diagnostic of the disorder and directed conservative management. (From Caron KH, DiPietro MA, Aisen AM, et al: MR imaging of early fibrodysplasia ossificans progressiva. J Comput Assist Tomogr 1990;14:318–321, with permission.)

some individuals, the normal serum phosphorus and vitamin D levels in others and the juxta-articular predilection and morphology of these calcific masses remain unexplained.

Patients typically present with a painless mass or masses in juxta-articular locations. The most common sites of involvement include the shoulder, hip, and elbow, though the knee, hands, and feet can be involved. On conventional radiographs, tumoral calcinosis is usually a well-defined mass having a lobulated appearance, with fibrous septae giving a cobblestone or "chicken wire" appearance (Fig. 15). If semifluid calcific material is present within, the mineral portion will pool dependently, creating fluid–calcium levels (the "sedimentation sign") on radiographs, CT, or MRI. Other entities that may present with individual lesions with calcifications include hyperparathyroidism, hypervitaminosis D, chronic renal disease, milk-alkali syndrome, and soft tissue chondromas.

Less commonly, patchy areas of marrow calcification (calcific myelitis) may be seen in the diaphyses of long bones, with associated periostitis that may resemble bone marrow infarcts, osteomyelitis, or neoplasm. Despite the calcified appearance of the marrow lesions, high signal on T_2-weighted images is present and likely attributable to an inflammatory response to the pathologic calcification. Radionuclide bone scintigraphy will typically demonstrate increased uptake in both the soft tissue masses and marrow lesions.

Pathologically, multiple irregular cysts separated by dense fibrous tissue are present that contain pasty white to yellow material sometimes mistaken for pus, though no organisms are present. Chronic inflammatory changes surrounding the calcified central material in the active phase are lacking in the inactive phase. The exact anatomic origin of these calcific masses remains unclear. Some authors believe that the masses occur in synovial bursae around joints based on their locations on CT and the early pattern of calcification resembling bursitis. However, there is conspicuous absence of bursal or synovial tissue on histologic examination, which is attributed by some to destruction of the synovial tissue in the bursa by progressive growth of the mass(es).

The appropriate therapy in the skeletally immature patient remains unclear. The phosphate restrictions used in adults may be, in theory, rachitogenic in children, though such restrictions might still be attempted. Resection of symptomatic lesions is sometimes necessary and curative but may lead to skin ulceration and infection if excision is incomplete.

SUBCUTANEOUS FAT NECROSIS

Fat necrosis of the subcutaneous tissues is an uncommon entity that may result in soft tissue calcification. It has been described in association with local trauma and in newborns who have suffered difficult deliveries.

Subcutaneous fat necrosis of the newborn presents 1 to 6 weeks after birth in a full-term or post-term neonate as firm, red to violaceous nodules measuring several millimeters to centimeters on the cheeks, shoulders, back, buttocks, or thighs. It is usually associated with stressful delivery and hypothermia, but the exact etiology is not known. Newborns with subcutaneous fat necrosis can develop potentially fatal hypercalcemia and should have serum calcium levels monitored. Although the reason for the association is not completely clear, unregulated production of 1,25-dihydroxyvitamin D by granulomatous cells involved in fat necrosis might be involved. Elevated prostaglandin E levels may also be identified in some hypercalcemic infants with fat necrosis.

On histology, lobular panniculitis with fat crystallization is seen that may have deposits of calcium. Calcification may be visible on radiographs (Fig. 16). These infants might undergo MRI if the diagnosis is not recognized clinically and there is concern for other soft tissue masses or malignancy. Linear areas of increased T_2 signal in the subcutaneous fat without a discrete mass have been seen both in traumatic and neonatal forms of subcutaneous fat necrosis (Fig. 17). CT can demonstrate

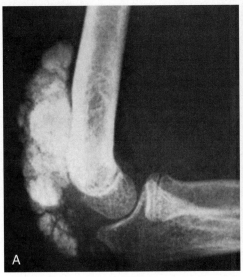
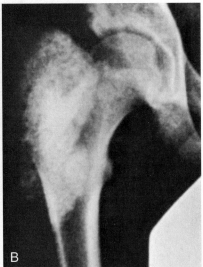

FIGURE 15. Tumoral calcinosis as seen radiographically. **A,** Lobulated mass of calcium density behind the elbow of a boy 4 years of age. **B,** Lobulated mass of calcium density below the right hip around the greater trochanter of a boy 15 years of age. (From Harkess JW, Peters HJ: Tumoral calcinosis. A report of six cases. J Bone Joint Surg Am 1967;49:721–731, with permission.)

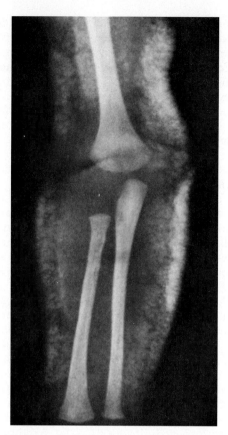

FIGURE 16. Generalized subcutaneous fat necrosis in an infant 5 months of age who was thriving otherwise. Subcutaneous fat of the right arm and forearm is extensively calcified in a diagnostically lobulated pattern on this radiograph. Similar changes were present in the skin of both arms, both legs, the abdomen, and the pelvis. (Courtesy of Dr. R. Parker Allen, Denver, CO.)

nonspecific subcutaneous nodules or fullness. With hypercalcemia, venous calcifications may be identified, and nephrocalcinosis and nephrolithiasis have been described, on sonography.

These lesions will typically resolve without specific therapy during the first few months of life. If calcified, nodules may persist. Complicating hypercalcemia must be actively treated to avoid a potentially fatal outcome.

NEUROMUSCULAR DISORDERS

The size, shape, and density of muscle groups may be altered by a wide range of neuromuscular disorders, most commonly cerebral palsy and myelodysplasia. Other less common neuromuscular abnormalities that also cause muscle atrophy include the muscular dystrophies, spinal muscular atrophy, Friedreich's ataxia, hereditary sensorimotor neuropathies, and poliomyelitis.

The muscular dystrophies are a group of inherited disorders causing progressive degeneration and weakness of skeletal muscle. They are not associated with inflammation, and no central or peripheral nervous system cause is present. Duchenne's muscular dystrophy, a sex-linked recessive trait, is the most common form. In spinal muscular atrophy, muscular weakness and atrophy is the result of degeneration of the anterior horn cells of the spinal cord. These disorders are classified by age of onset and severity, though they have considerable overlap, with acute Werdnig-Hoffmann disease being the most recognizable and severe form. Friedreich's ataxia is the most common form of the group of spinocerebellar degenerative diseases with

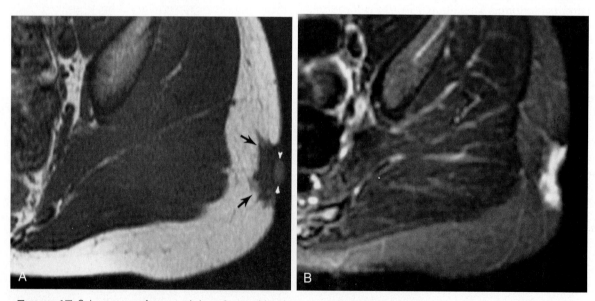

FIGURE 17. Subcutaneous fat necrosis in an 8-year-old male as seen on magnetic resonance imaging. **A,** T_1-weighted image shows a stellate area of low signal limited to the subcutaneous fat of the left buttock *(arrows)* *(arrowheads* indicate a vitamin E capsule). **B,** T_2-weighted fast spin-echo image with fat suppression shows the mass to be of high signal. No significant enhancement occurred after gadolinium administration (not pictured).

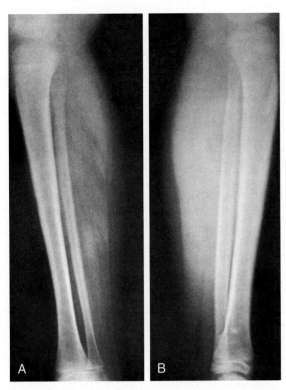

FIGURE 18. Postpoliomyelitic fatty replacement and radiolucent striping on radiographs of the gastrocnemius–soleus group of the right leg of a girl 8½ years of age who had had acute poliomyelitis 6 years before. **A,** The bones and muscles in the right shank are hypoplastic and atrophic. **B,** Normal muscles in the left leg.

autosomal dominant inheritance. Hereditary sensorimotor neuropathies, of which Charcot-Marie-Tooth disease is the prototype, are a group of variably inherited peripheral neuropathic disorders causing skeletal muscle weakness and atrophy. Poliomyelitis, while largely eradicated by routine vaccination in this country, remains a health problem in developing nations. The poliovirus enters via the gastrointestinal tract and settles in the anterior horn cells of the spinal cord and several brain stem nuclei, resulting in denervation atrophy and fatty infiltration most commonly of muscles supplied by the cervical and lumbar segments (Fig. 18).

All of these groups of disorders result in varying degrees of skeletal muscle atrophy and fatty infiltration that can be observed on conventional radiographs but are more readily detected on CT scans and MRI. Acquired muscular atrophy, such as with immobilization in a cast, may demonstrate similar findings. Associated scoliosis, contractures, and foot deformities are common in the neuromuscular disorders and the major reasons for therapeutic intervention.

SUBCUTANEOUS FAT EXCESS/DEFICIENCY

Childhood obesity has become a recognized problem in the United States and other industrialized countries around the world and may potentially cause multiple health problems. A number of syndromes aside from excessive caloric intake and limited physical activity may cause obesity and excessive adipose tissue that is evident on imaging studies. Examples include endogenous and exogenous Cushing's syndrome, Prader-Willi syndrome, Stein-Leventhal syndrome (polycystic ovaries), Bardet-Biedl syndrome, and pickwickian syndrome. Newborn infants of diabetic mothers often demonstrate excess subcutaneous fat, especially over the shoulders. Excessive fat may also accumulate in patients with neuromuscular disorders with limited physical activity and muscular atrophy (Fig. 19).

Subcutaneous fat deficiency is encountered less frequently. It is seen in infants with insufficient fat stores, most commonly premature infants or, less commonly, markedly postmature infants who have consumed their fat stores. Malnourished children may have severely depleted subcutaneous fat. Syndromic forms of lipodystrophy or lipoatrophy are associated with diffuse and localized absence of subcutaneous fat. Congenital total lipodystrophy (Berardinelli-Seip syndrome) is associated with total absence of subcutaneous fat, prominent musculature, hirsuitism, and insulin-resistant diabetes mellitus. Localized forms of lipodystrophy are seen at insulin injection sites in patients with diabetes mellitus.

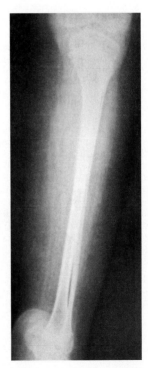

FIGURE 19. Severe infantile muscular atrophy (Werdnig-Hoffmann disease) in a boy 6 years of age. Practically all of the shrunken muscular mass has been replaced by fat so that the atrophic muscles are barely visible on this radiograph. Subcutaneous fat is greatly increased, and it is obvious that external measurements of the leg circumference would give a misleading idea of the amount of muscular tissue actually present, owing to compensatory thickening of the fat.

SUGGESTED READINGS

Cutaneous Calcification/Ossification

Bernardo BD, Huettner PC, Merritt DF, Ratts VS: Idiopathic calcinosis cutis presenting as labial lesions in children: report of two cases with literature review. J Pediatr Adolesc Gynecol 1999;12:157–160

Dehner L, Kaye, V: The skin. *In* Stocker J, Dehner LP (eds): Pediatric Pathology, 2nd ed. Philadelphia, JB Lippincott, 1992:1157–1158

Evans MJ, Blessing K, Gray ES: Subepidermal calcified nodule in children: a clinicopathologic study of 21 cases. Pediatr Dermatol 1995;12:307–310

Mallory SB: Infiltrative diseases. *In* Schachner LA, Hansen RC (eds): Pediatric Dermatology, 2nd ed. New York, Churchill Livingstone, 1995:848–851

Moritz DL, Elewski B: Pigmented postacne osteoma cutis in a patient treated with minocycline: report and review of the literature [see comments]. J Am Acad Dermatol 1991;24(5 Pt 2):851–853

Prendiville JS, Lucky AW, Mallory SB, et al: Osteoma cutis as a presenting sign of pseudohypoparathyroidism. Pediatr Dermatol 1992;9:11–18

Rodriguez-Cano L, Garcia-Patos V, Creus M, et al: Childhood calcinosis cutis. Pediatr Dermatol 1996;13:114–117

Sell EJ, Hansen RC, Struck-Pierce S: Calcified nodules on the heel: a complication of neonatal intensive care. J Pediatr 1980;96 (3 Pt 1):473–475

Wright S, Navsaria H, Leigh IM: Idiopathic scrotal calcinosis is idiopathic [see comments]. J Am Acad Dermatol 1991;24(5 Pt 1): 727–730

Foreign Body

Bodne D, Quinn SF, Cochran CF: Imaging foreign glass and wooden bodies of the extremities with CT and MR. J Comput Assist Tomogr 1988;12:608–611

Borgia CA: An unusual bone reaction to an organic foreign body in the hand. Clin Orthop 1963;30:188–193

Butler WP: Plant thorn granuloma. Mil Med 1995;160:39

Jacobson JA, Powell A, Craig JG, et al: Wooden foreign bodies in soft tissue: detection at US. Radiology 1998;206:45–48

Laor T, Barnewolt CE: Nonradiopaque penetrating foreign body: "a sticky situation." Pediatr Radiol 1999;29:702–704

Leung A, Patton A, Navoy J, Cummings RJ: Intraoperative sonography-guided removal of radiolucent foreign bodies. J Pediatr Orthop 1998;18:259–261

Manthey DE, Storrow AB, Milbourn JM, Wagner BJ: Ultrasound versus radiography in the detection of soft-tissue foreign bodies. Ann Emerg Med 1996;28:7–9

Maylahn D: Thorn-induced "tumors" of bone. J Bone Joint Surg Am 1952;34:386–388

Shiels WED, Babcock DS, Wilson JL, Burch RA: Localization and guided removal of soft-tissue foreign bodies with sonography. AJR Am J Roentgenol 1990;155:1277–1281

Sponseller P: Localized disorders of bone and soft tissue. *In* Morrissy RT, Weinstein SL (eds): Lovell & Winter's Pediatric Orthopaedics, 4th ed. Philadelphia, Lippincott–Raven Publishers, 1996:334–337

Myositis Ossificans

Ackerman L: Extra-osseous localized non-neoplastic bone and cartilage formation (so-called myositis ossificans). J Bone Joint Surg Am 1958;40:279–298

Amendola MA, Glazer GM, Agha FP, et al: Myositis ossificans circumscripta: computed tomographic diagnosis. Radiology 1983;149: 775–779

Carlson WO, Klassen RA: Myositis ossificans of the upper extremity: a long-term follow-up. J Pediatr Orthop 1984;4:693–696

Cushner FD, Morwessel RM: Myositis ossificans in children. Orthopedics 1995;18:287–291

De Smet AA, Norris MA, Fisher DR: Magnetic resonance imaging of myositis ossificans: analysis of seven cases. Skeletal Radiol 1992;21: 503–507

Gindele A, Schwamborn D, Tsironis K, et al: Myositis ossificans traumatica in young children: report of three cases and review of the literature. Pediatr Radiol 2000;30:451–459

Howard CB, Porat S, Bar-On E, et al: Traumatic myositis ossificans of the quadriceps in infants. J Pediatr Orthop B 1998;7:80–82

Illes T, Dubousset J, Szendroi M, Fischer J: Characterization of bone forming cells in posttraumatic myositis ossificans by lectins. Pathol Res Pract 1992;188:172–176

Kransdorf MJ, Meis JM: Extraskeletal osseous and cartilaginous tumors of the extremities. Radiographics 1993;13:853–884

Kransdorf MJ, Meis JM, Jelinek JS: Myositis ossificans: MR appearance with radiologic-pathologic correlation. AJR Am J Roentgenol 1991;157:1243–1248

Ogilvie-Harris DJ, Fornasier VL: Pseudomalignant myositis ossificans: heterotopic new-bone formation without a history of trauma. J Bone Joint Surg Am 1980;62:1274–1283

Shirkhoda A, Armin A-R, Bis KG, et al: MR imaging of myositis ossificans: variable patterns at different stages. J Magn. Reson Imaging 1995;5:287–292

Sponseller P: Localized disorders of bone and soft tissue. *In* Morrissy RT, Weinstein SL (eds): Lovell & Winter's Pediatric Orthopaedics, 4th ed. Philadelphia, Lippincott–Raven Publishers, 1996:332–334

Thickman D, Bonakdar-pour A, Clancy M, et al: Fibrodysplasia ossificans progressiva. AJR Am J Roentgenol 1982;139:935–941

Hematoma

El-Khoury GY, Brandser EA, Kathol MH, et al: Imaging of muscle injuries. Skeletal Radiol 1996;25:3–11

Rubin JI, Gomori JM, Grossman RI, et al: High-field MR imaging of extracranial hematomas. AJR Am J Roentgenol 1987;148:813–817

Unger EC, Glazer HS, Lee JKT, et al: MRI of extracranial hematomas: preliminary observations. AJR Am J Roentgenol 1986;146:403–407

Inflammatory Muscle Diseases

Dermatomyositis

Adams EM, Chow CK, Premkumar A, Plotz PH: The idiopathic inflammatory myopathies: spectrum of MR imaging findings. Radiographics 1995;15:563–574

Bowyer SL, Blane CE, Sullivan DB, Cassidy JT: Childhood dermatomyositis: factors predicting functional outcome and development of dystrophic calcification. J Pediatr 1983;103:882–888

Fleckenstein JL, Burns DK, Murphy FK, et al: Differential diagnosis of bacterial myositis in AIDS: evaluation with MR imaging. Radiology 1991;179:653–658

Fleckenstein JL, Watumull D, Conner KE, et al: Denervated human skeletal muscle: MR imaging evaluation. Radiology 1993;187: 213–218

Gordon BA, Martinez S, Collins AJ: Pyomyositis: characteristics at CT and MR imaging. Radiology 1995;197:279–286

Hernandez RJ, Keim DR, Chenevert TL, et al: Fat-suppressed MR imaging of myositis. Radiology 1992;182:217–219

Hernandez RJ, Sullivan DB, Chenevert TL, Keim DR: MR imaging in children with dermatomyositis: musculoskeletal findings and correlation with clinical and laboratory findings. AJR Am J Roentgenol 1993;161:359–366

Hesla RB, Karlson LK, McCauley RG: Milk of calcium fluid collection in dermatomyositis: ultrasound findings. Pediatr Radiol 1990;20: 344–346

Kransdorf MJ, Temple HT, Sweet DE: Focal myositis. Skeletal Radiol 1998;27:283–287

Lam WW, Chan H, Chan YL, et al: MR imaging in amyopathic dermatomyositis. Acta Radiol 1999;40:69–72

Lamki L, Willis RB: Radionuclide findings of pyomyositis. Clin Nucl Med 1982;7:465–467

Lamminen AE, Hekali PE, Tiula E, et al: Acute rhabdomyolysis: evaluation with magnetic resonance imaging compared with computed tomography and ultrasonography. Br J Radiol 1989;62: 326–330

Loh N-N, Ch'en IY, Cheung LP, Li KCP: Deep fascial hyperintensity in soft tissue abnormalities as revealed by T_2-weighted imaging. AJR Am J Roentgenol 1997;168:1301–1304

Pachman LM: Juvenile dermatomyositis: pathophysiology and disease expression. Pediatr Clin North Am 1995;42:1071–1098

Park JH, Olsen NJ, King L Jr, et al: Use of magnetic resonance imaging and P-31 magnetic resonance spectroscopy to detect and quantify muscle dysfunction in the amyopathic and myopathic variants of dermatomyositis. Arthritis Rheum 1995;38:68–77

Park JH, Vital TL, Ryder NM, et al: Magnetic resonance imaging and P-31 magnetic resonance spectroscopy provide unique quantitative data useful in the longitudinal management of patients with dermatomyositis. Arthritis Rheum 1994;37:736–746

Raphael SA, Wolfson BJ, Parker P, et al: Pyomyositis in a child with acquired immunodeficiency syndrome. Am J Dis Child 1989;143:779–781

Rider LG, Miller FW: Classification and treatment of the juvenile idiopathic inflammatory myopathies. Rheum Dis Clin North Am 1997;23:619–655

Samson C, Soulen RL, Gursel E: Milk of calcium fluid collections in juvenile dermatomyositis: MR characteristics. Pediatr Radiol 2000;30:28–29

Schmid MR, Kossmann T, Duewell S: Differentiation of necrotizing fasciitis and cellulitis using MR imaging. AJR Am J Roentgenol 1998;170:615–620

Schweitzer ME, Fort J: Cost-effectiveness of MR imaging in evaluating polymyositis [see comments]. AJR Am J Roentgenol 1995;165:1469–1471

Shintani S, Shiigai T: Repeat MRI in acute rhabdomyolysis: correlation with clinicopathological findings. J Comput Assist Tomogr 1993;17:786–791

Sirinavin S, McCracken GH Jr: Primary suppurative myositis in children. Am J Dis Child 1979;133:263–265

Steinbach LS, Tehranzadeh J, Fleckenstein JL, et al: Human immunodeficiency virus infection: musculoskeletal manifestations. Radiology 1993;186:833–838

Stock KW, Helwig A: MRI of acute exertional rhabdomyolysis—in the paraspinal compartment. J Comput Assist Tomogr 1996;20:834–836

Stonecipher MR, Jorizzo JL, Monu J, et al: Dermatomyositis with normal muscle enzyme concentrations: a single-blind study of the diagnostic value of magnetic resonance imaging and ultrasound. Arch Dermatol 1994;130:1294–1299

Summers RM, Brune AM, Choyke PL, et al: Juvenile idiopathic inflammatory myopathy: exercise-induced changes in muscle at short inversion time inversion-recovery MR imaging. Radiology 1998;209:191–196

Yousefzadeh DK, Schumann EM, Mulligan GM, et al: The role of imaging modalities in diagnosis and management of pyomyositis. Skeletal Radiol 1982;8:285–289

Yuh WTC, Schreiber AE, Montgomery WJ, et al: Magnetic resonance imaging of pyomyositis. Skeletal Radiol 1988;17:190–193

Fibrodysplasia Ossificans Progressiva

Brantus JF, Meunier PJ: Effects of intravenous etidronate and oral corticosteroids in fibrodysplasia ossificans progressiva. Clin Orthop 1998;Jan(346):117–120

Caron KH, DiPietro MA, Aisen AM, et al: MR imaging of early fibrodysplasia ossificans progressiva. J Comput Assist Tomogr 1990;14:318–321

Cohen RB, Hahn GV, Tabas JA, et al: The natural history of heterotopic ossification in patients who have fibrodysplasia ossificans progressiva: a study of forty-four patients. J Bone Joint Surg Am 1993;75:215–219

Fang MA, Reinig JW, Hill SC, et al: Technetium-99m MDP demonstration of heterotopic ossification in fibrodysplasia ossificans progressiva. Clin Nucl Med 1986;11:8–9

Kaplan FS, McCluskey W, Hahn G, et al: Genetic transmission of fibrodysplasia ossificans progressiva: report of a family. J Bone Joint Surg Am 1993a;75:1214–1220

Kaplan FS, Tabas JA, Gannon FH, et al: The histopathology of fibrodysplasia ossificans progressiva: an endochondral process. J Bone Joint Surg Am 1993b;75:220–230

Mahboubi S, Glaser DL, Shore EM, et al: Fibrodysplasia ossificans progressiva. Pediatr Radiol 2001;31:307–314

Reinig JW, Hill SC, Fang M, et al: Fibrodysplasia ossificans progressiva: CT appearance. Radiology 1986;159:153–157

Tumoral Calcinosis

Ballina-Garcia FJ, Queiro-Silva R, Fernandez-Vega F, et al: Diaphysitis in tumoral calcinosis syndrome. J Rheumatol 1996;23:2148–2151

Clarke E, Swischuk LE, Hayden CK Jr: Tumoral calcinosis, diaphysitis, and hyperphosphatemia. Radiology 1984;151:643–646

Cofan F, Garcia S, Combalia A, et al: Uremic tumoral calcinosis in patients receiving longterm hemodialysis therapy. J Rheumatol 1999;26:379–385

Greenberg SB: Tumoral calcinosis in an infant. Pediatr Radiol 1990;20:206–207

Harkess JW, Peters HJ: Tumoral calcinosis. A report of six cases. J Bone Joint Surg Am 1967;49:721–731

Heydemann JS, McCarthy RE: Tumoral calcinosis in a child. J Pediatr Orthop 1988;8:474–477

Kolawole TM, Bohrer SP: Tumoral calcinosis with "fluid levels" in the tumoral masses. Am J Roentgenol Radium Ther Nucl Med 1974;120:461–465

Kozlowski K, Barylak A, Campbell J, et al: Tumoral calcinosis in children (report of 13 cases). Australas Radiol 1988;32:448–457

Lyles KW, Burkes EJ, Ellis GJ, et al: Genetic transmission of tumoral calcinosis: autosomal dominant with variable clinical expressivity. J Clin Endocrinol Metab 1985;60:1093–1096

Martinez S, Vogler JBD, Harrelson JM, Lyles KW: Imaging of tumoral calcinosis: new observations. Radiology 1990;174:215–222

Metzker A, Eisenstein B, Oren J, Samuel R: Tumoral calcinosis revisited—common and uncommon features: report of ten cases and review. Eur J Pediatr 1988;147:128–132

Pakasa NM, Kalengayi RM: Tumoral calcinosis: a clinicopathological study of 111 cases with emphasis on the earliest changes. Histopathology 1997;31:18–24

Prince MJ, Schaeffer PC, Goldsmith RS, Chausmer AB: Hyperphosphatemic tumoral calcinosis: association with elevation of serum 1,25-dihydroxycholecalciferol concentrations. Ann Intern Med 1982;96:586–591

Richardson PH, Yang YM, Nimityongskul P, Brogdon BG: Tumoral calcinosis in an infant. Skeletal Radiol 1996;25:481–484

Rodriguez-Peralto JL, Lopez-Barea F, Torres A, et al: Tumoral calcinosis in two infants. Clin Orthop 1989;May(242):272–276

Steinbach LS, Johnston JO, Tepper EF, et al: Tumoral calcinosis: radiologic-pathologic correlation. Skeletal Radiol 1995;24:573–578

Steinherz R, Chesney RW, Eisenstein B, et al: Elevated serum calcitriol concentrations do not fall in response to hyperphosphatemia in familial tumoral calcinosis. Am J Dis Child 1985;139:816–819

Zaleske DJ: Metabolic and endocrine abnormalities. In Morrissy RT, Weinstein SL (eds): Lovell and Winter's Pediatric Orthopaedics, 4th ed. Philadelphia, Lippincott–Raven, 1996:178

Subcutaneous Fat Necrosis

Anderson DR, Narla LD, Dunn NL: Subcutaneous fat necrosis of the newborn. Pediatr Radiol 1999;29:794–796

Burden AD, Krafchik BR: Subcutaneous fat necrosis of the newborn: a review of 11 cases. Pediatr Dermatol 1999;16:384–387

Cunningham K, Atkinson SA, Paes BA: Subcutaneous fat necrosis with hypercalcemia. Can Assoc Radiol J 1990;41:158–159

Fretzin DF, Arias AM: Sclerema neonatorum and subcutaneous fat necrosis of the newborn. Pediatr Dermatol 1987;4:112–122

Gu LL, Daneman A, Binet A, Kooh SW: Nephrocalcinosis and nephrolithiasis due to subcutaneous fat necrosis with hypercalcemia in two full-term asphyxiated neonates: sonographic findings. Pediatr Radiol 1995;25:142–144

Hicks MJ, Levy ML, Alexander J, Flaitz CM: Subcutaneous fat necrosis of the newborn and hypercalcemia: case report and review of the literature. Pediatr Dermatol 1993;10:271–276

Kruse K, Irle U, Uhlig R: Elevated 1,25-dihydroxyvitamin D serum concentrations in infants with subcutaneous fat necrosis. J Pediatr 1993;122:460–463

Norton KI, Som PM, Shugar JM, et al: Subcutaneous fat necrosis of the newborn: CT findings of head and neck involvement. AJNR Am J Neuroradiol 1997;18:547–550

Prendiville JS: Diseases of the dermis and subcutaneous tissues: nodular diseases. In Schachner LA, Hansen RC (eds): Pediatric Dermatology, 2nd ed. New York, Churchill Livingstone, 1995:821–822

Sharata H, Postellon DC, Hashimoto K: Subcutaneous fat necrosis, hypercalcemia, and prostaglandin E. Pediatr Dermatol 1995;12:43–47

Tsai TS, Evans HA, Donnelly JF, et al: Fat necrosis after trauma: a benign cause of palpable lumps in children [see comments]. AJR Am J Roentgenol 1997;169:1623–1626

Neuromuscular Disorders

Hawley RJ Jr, Schellinger D, O'Doherty DS: Computed tomographic patterns of muscles in neuromuscular diseases. Arch Neurol 1984; 41:383–387

Iannaccone ST, Browne RH, Samaha FJ, Buncher CR: Prospective study of spinal muscular atrophy before age 6 years. DCN/SMA Group. Pediatr Neurol 1993;9:187–193

Murphy WA, Totty WG, Carroll JE: MRI of normal and pathologic skeletal muscle. AJR Am J Roentgenol 1986;146:565–574

Pearn J: Classification of spinal muscular atrophies. Lancet 1980;1: 919–922

Serratrice G, Salamon G, Jiddane M, et al: Results of muscular x-ray computed tomography in 145 cases of neuromuscular disease [in French]. Rev Neurol (Paris) 1985;141:404–412

Stern LM, Caudrey DJ, Clark MS, et al: Carrier detection in Duchenne muscular dystrophy using computed tomography. Clin Genet 1985;27:392–397

Strebel PM, Sutter RW, Cochi SL, et al: Epidemiology of poliomyelitis in the United States one decade after the last reported case of indigenous wild virus-associated disease. Clin Infect Dis 1992;14: 568–579

Thompson G: Neuromuscular disorders. In Morrissy RT, Weinstein SL (eds): Lovell and Winter's Pediatric Orthopaedics, 4th ed. Philadelphia, Lippincott–Raven, 1996:537–577

Subcutaneous Fat Excess/Deficiency

Kakourou T, Dacou-Voutetakis C, Kavadias G, et al: Limited joint mobility and lipodystrophy in children and adolescents with insulin-dependent diabetes mellitus. Pediatr Dermatol 1994;11: 310–314

Kuhns LR, Berger PE, Roloff DW, et al: Fat thickness in the newborn infant of a diabetic mother. Radiology 1974;111:665–671

Must A, Strauss RS: Risks and consequences of childhood and adolescent obesity. Int J Obes Relat Metab Disord 1999;23 (Suppl 2):S2–S11

Smevik B, Swensen T, Kolbenstvedt A, Trygstad O: Computed tomography and ultrasonography of the abdomen in congenital generalized lipodystrophy. Radiology 1982;142:687–689

Strauss R: Childhood obesity. Curr Probl Pediatr 1999;29:1–29

Taybi HL, Lachman RS: Radiology of Syndromes, Metabolic Disorders, and Skeletal Dysplasias, 3rd ed. Chicago, Year Book Medical Publishers, 1990

Chapter 2

SOFT TISSUE NEOPLASMS

BARRY D. FLETCHER

The role of diagnostic imaging in the assessment of soft tissue masses has expanded due to the superior soft tissue contrast afforded by magnetic resonance imaging (MRI). The ability to obtain multiplanar displays offers a further advantage for treatment planning, and tumors adjacent to bone can be visualized without the beam-hardening artifacts inherent in computed tomography (CT) images. However, MRI is limited by its inability to accurately depict calcifications or gas within soft tissues, and, except in a few instances, no imaging methods can accurately differentiate between benign and malignant neoplasms.

Despite the advantages of MRI, radiographs have retained an important role in the initial evaluation of soft tissue masses, especially in detecting secondary changes in the configuration of the adjacent bones and the presence of cortical bone erosion, periosteal reaction, and soft tissue calcifications. Occasionally, radiolucency will indicate the presence of a fat-containing tumor. Ultrasonography may be useful in demonstrating smaller superficial tumors, and color Doppler ultrasound can be used to demonstrate tumor vascularity. Many soft tissue sarcomas are detected by gallium-67 and thallium-201 scintigraphy. Patients with suspected ma-

lignant soft tissue tumors should undergo technetium-99m–methylene diphosphonate (MDP) bone scintigraphy to detect local bone involvement and distant skeletal metastases, although these findings are uncommon in the absence of pulmonary metastases.

Magnetic resonance (MR) images should include the entire tumor so as to demonstrate its margins and, in the case of suspected malignancy, should include any needle biopsy tracks that must be excised at the time of surgical resection. In the case of large tumors, a body coil may be required to cover the entire lesion and important adjacent structures. However, signal:noise ratio and spatial resolution will be increased by using coils of smaller volume, such as those designed for head and knee imaging, or by applying flexible coils especially designed for extremity imaging. Surface coils receive signals in a nonuniform manner, with excess signal in the tissues close to the coil and gradual loss of signal in the deeper tissues. A head coil will frequently accommodate both lower extremities of infants or small children.

The tissues containing the tumor should be imaged in at least two orthogonal planes. T_1-weighted and T_2-weighted images can be obtained with either spin-echo, fast spin-echo, or gradient-echo techniques. Spin-echo imaging is more time consuming but avoids signal loss associated with magnetic field inhomogeneity that occurs with gradient-echo sequences. Newer fast spin-echo sequences save imaging time but are characterized by loss of contrast because of higher fat intensity and slight loss of detail or blurring. Short tau inversion–recovery (STIR) sequences are frequently used for oncologic imaging because this method renders the tumor high in intensity while suppressing signal from nearby fat. However, STIR images tend to overestimate the tumor margins because they also accentuate the signal of adjacent edema. Similar contrast is produced by fat-saturated T_2-weighted images. Gadolinium-enhanced T_1-weighted images add information about tumor vascularization and are helpful in guiding percutaneous biopsy because viable tumor can be differentiated from areas of necrosis. Furthermore, cystic lesions can be identified by their lack of central enhancement. To better define the tumor margin, chemical shift fat-suppression pulses should be included to improve the contrast between the intense signal of the contrast-enhanced mass and that of the adjacent fat. MR angiography is also useful in planning the surgical approach when large vessels may be involved.

MR images of soft tissue tumors have low specificity and are only occasionally helpful in differentiating between benign and malignant masses with certainty (Table 1). However, benign tumors tend to be well marginated and do not usually invade bone or encase neurovascular structures. Most soft tissue tumors have low signal intensity, similar to that of muscle on T_1-weighted images, and heterogeneous high signal intensity, greater than that of fat on T_2-weighted images. Tumors that produce intense signal on T_1-weighted images are likely to contain fat, methemoglobin blood products, or abundant proteinacious material. Tumor hypointensity on T_2-weighted images suggests relative acellularity and abundant collagen formation. Hemosiderin resulting from previous hemorrhage is hypointense to muscle on both T_1- and T_2-weighted images, and calcifications are also usually hypointense. Although, in general, biopsy is necessary to determine tumor type, familiarity with the imaging characteristics and the clinical presentation of common soft tissue tumors allows one to offer a focused differential diagnosis (Tables 2 and 3).

BENIGN SOFT TISSUE TUMORS

HEMANGIOMAS

Hemangiomas, unlike vascular malformations, are considered to be true neoplasms, and they account for 7% to 10% of all benign soft tissue tumors. They may be localized or diffuse and, despite being histically benign, are capable of insidious or even aggressive growth causing coagulopathy, bone deformity, fracture, and regional gigantism. Extrahepatic hemangiomas may involve the mucocutaneous, cutaneous, and subcutaneous tissues as well as the skeletal muscles, in which they mimic malignant tumors. Capillary (usually cutaneous), cavernous, venous, and mixed types of hemangiomas have been described and classified according to the apparent origin of their vascular channels. Hemangiomas also contain variable amounts of nonvascular tissue and other elements, including fat, smooth muscle, fibrous tissue, myxoid stroma, hemosiderin, thrombus, and even bone. Spindle cell hemangiomas are more recently characterized lesions containing thin-walled cavernous vascular spaces and spindle cells resembling Kaposi's sarcoma. They are slowly progressive, frequently invasive, recurrent neoplasms that usually involve the dermis and subcutaneous tissue. Intramuscular hemangiomas are relatively rare but are the vascular lesions most likely to be confused with malignant tumors.

A number of imaging methods, including radiography, CT, MRI, and radiolabeled red cell scintigraphy, can facilitate preoperative diagnosis (see Table 2). Recently, Doppler sonography has shown high vessel density and peak arterial Doppler shift in hemangiomas; these findings may be useful in distinguishing hemangiomas from other soft tissue masses. Radiographs are important for detecting associated osseous abnormality, and the finding of calcified phleboliths on radiographs or CT images is an indication of a venous hemangioma (Fig. 1). The highly vascular nature of intramuscular hemangiomas can be determined on a properly timed dynamic contrast-enhanced CT scan. MRI provides excellent contrast and is better than CT in determining a tumor's extent and its relationship to contiguous structures. Hemangiomas also frequently demonstrate typical features on MR images. On T_1-weighted images, hemangiomas are either isointense or, when they contain sufficient fat, hyperintense to muscle (Figs. 1 and 2). On T_2-weighted images, the lesions are well defined and markedly hyperintense with serpiginous high-signal zones that correlate with torturous vascular channels interlaced with lower intensity fibrous or fatty septal tissue. Tubular structures within the mass that have low T_1-weighted signal and high T_2-weighted signal correlate with thrombi. Phleboliths are hypointense on both T_1- and T_2-weighted sequences.

Hemangiomas are often confused with vascular mal-

Table 1 ■ MUSCULOSKELETAL SOFT TISSUE TUMORS: MAGNETIC RESONANCE IMAGING FEATURES OF MALIGNANCY	
Neurovascular encasement	Highly suggestive
Adjacent bone/joint involvement	Highly suggestive
Marrow abnormality	Highly suggestive
Homogeneous T1W, heterogeneous T2W pattern	Suggestive
Necrosis	Suggestive
Poorly defined, irregular margins	Suggestive
Peritumoral edema	Not helpful

T1W = T_1-weighted; T2W = T_2-weighted.
From Hanna SL, Fletcher BD: MR imaging of malignant soft tissue tumors. Magn Imaging Clin N Am 1995;3:629–650, with permission.

Table 2 ■ IMAGING FEATURES OF BENIGN SOFT TISSUE TUMORS

BENIGN	COMMON LOCATION	X-RAY/CT	MRI*	OTHER
Hemangioma	Muscle	Phleboliths Marked CT enhancement	Isointense to hyperintense on T1W images Hyperintense on T2W images Serpiginous vessels Flow voids	Bone erosion
Hemangiopericytoma	Subcutaneous	Calcifications Marked CT enhancement	Nonspecific	Bone erosion Angiogram: tumor vessels, draining veins
Desmoid tumor	Deep tissue Head and neck Trunk Extremities	Mild hyperattenuation	Variably hyperintense on T2W images with signal voids	
Peripheral nerve sheath tumor	Peripheral nerve	Calcification in degenerating tumors Hypoattenuated	Hypointense on T1W images Hyperintense on T2W images with target-like appearance	Muscle atrophy Associated with NF1
Lipoblastoma	Extremities Head and neck Trunk	Mixed attenuation Fat, myxoid tissue	Hyperintense on T1W images Isointense on T2W images	Hyperechoic fat signal on ultrasound

CT = computed tomography; MRI = magnetic resonance imaging; NF1 = neurofibromatosis type 1; T1W = T_1-weighted; T2W = T_2-weighted.
*T_1-weighted signal intensity relative to that of muscle; T_2-weighted signal intensity relative to that of subcutaneous fat.

formations, which, according to Mulliken and Glowacki, can be distinguished from hemangiomas by a number of characteristic features (Fig. 3). Vascular malformations can be venous, arterial, or lymphatic or contain a combination of vascular elements. They are usually present at birth and grow proportionally with the child. Unlike hemangiomas, endothelial cell proliferation does not account for their growth and they are not true neoplasms. Vascular malformations are discussed in Section IX, Part IV, page 2099.

Table 3 ■ IMAGING FEATURES OF MALIGNANT SOFT TISSUE TUMORS

MALIGNANT	COMMON LOCATION	X-RAY/CT	MRI*	OTHER
Rhabdomyosarcoma	20% extremities	Bone erosion	Nonspecific	Bone erosion
PPNET	Trunk, paravertebral space, extremities	No calcification	Nonspecific	Askin's tumor involves chest wall
Synovial sarcoma	Lower extremities	Calcification in 30% Bone erosion	Nonspecific or fluid levels	Vessel involvement
MPNST	Lower extremity (thigh)	Nonspecific	Nonspecific	Gallium-avid; associated with NF1
Fibrosarcoma	Lower extremity	Nonspecific	Nonspecific	Bone erosion Vascular
Liposarcoma	Lower extremity (thigh)	Differentiated: low attenuation	Differentiated: Hyperintense on T1W images Isointense on T2W images Myxoid: Nonspecific	Fat in differentiated tumors
ASPS	Lower extremity (thigh)	Marked CT enhancement Necrotic center Draining veins	Hyperintense on both T1W and T2W images	Highly vascular Draining veins
MFH	Lower extremity	Bone erosion Calcifications in 5%–20%	Nonspecific	Gaillium avid
Epithelioid sarcoma	Upper extremity (forearm)	Rare calcification	Nonspecific or hemorrhagic, hyperintense on T1W and T2W images	Subcutaneous lymphatic spread Muscle atrophy
Lymphoma	Muscle, skin	Diffuse muscle enlargement Density similar to that of muscle	Nonspecific	Gallium avid

ASPS = alveolar soft part sarcoma; CT = computed tomography; MFH = malignant fibrous histocytoma; MPNST = malignant peripheral nerve sheath tumor; MRI = magnetic resonance imaging; NF1 = neurofibromatosis type 1; PPNET = peripheral primitive neuroectodermal tumor; T1W = T_1-weighted; T2W = T_2-weighted.
*T_1-weighted signal intensity relative to muscle; T_2-weighted signal intensity relative to subcutaneous fat.

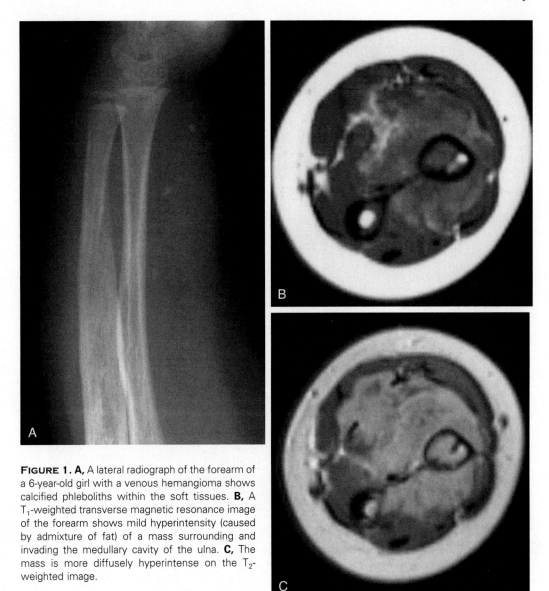

FIGURE 1. A, A lateral radiograph of the forearm of a 6-year-old girl with a venous hemangioma shows calcified phleboliths within the soft tissues. **B,** A T_1-weighted transverse magnetic resonance image of the forearm shows mild hyperintensity (caused by admixture of fat) of a mass surrounding and invading the medullary cavity of the ulna. **C,** The mass is more diffusely hyperintense on the T_2-weighted image.

HEMANGIOPERICYTOMA

Hemangiopericytoma is a rare soft tissue tumor of low but unpredictable malignant potential that is believed to arise from vascular endothelial pericytes. These tumors are usually located in the thigh or the pelvic retroperitoneum but can arise in any part of the body.

Approximately 10% of hemangiopericytomas occur during childhood, and about one third of these are congenital. The congenital tumors are considered a distinct clinical entity because of their benign behavior despite microscopic evidence of mitotic activity and focal necrosis. Congenital hemangiopericytomas can exhibit rapid initial growth, but spontaneous regression has also been reported. Microscopically, these tumors show endothelial proliferation with some similarity to hemangioma. The congenital tumors occur more commonly in the subcutaneous tissues, where they appear clinically as firm, usually solitary swellings. They can become very large and hemorrhagic.

Most descriptions of the imaging features of heman-giopericytoma are based on tumors in adult patients. Calcifications may be detected radiographically or by CT, and the tumors are well circumscribed. There may be partial destruction of adjacent bone (Fig. 4A). No specific features are demonstrated by radiography, CT, or ultrasonography. However, hemangiopericytomas are very vascular lesions and show marked enhancement and, frequently, central necrosis on contrast-enhanced CT images. Like most soft tissue sarcomas, hemangio-pericytomas are isointense to muscle on T_1-weighted images and exhibit high signal intensity on T_2-weighted and STIR images (Fig. 4B, C) and they enhance moderately with gadolinium (Fig. 4D). Angiograms show dense staining of tumor vasculature and early-draining veins (Fig. 5).

DESMOID TUMORS

Desmoid tumors are rare quasi-neoplastic lesions that are included in the group of disorders termed *fibromato-*

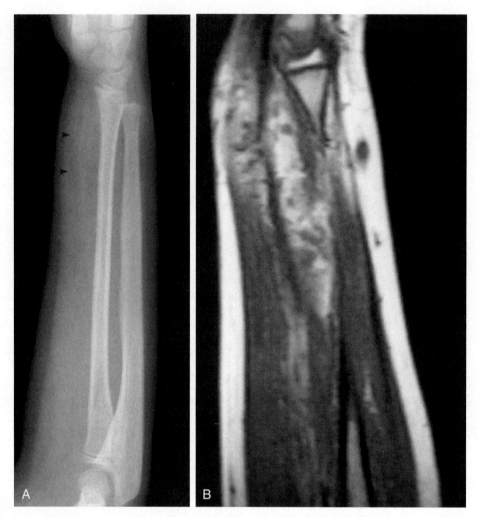

FIGURE 2. Hemangioma in an 8-year-old boy. **A,** A lateral radiograph of the forearm shows poorly defined lucencies in the soft tissues anteriorly corresponding to fat within the lesion *(arrowheads)*. **B,** A sagittal T_1-weighted magnetic resonance image shows inhomogeneous hyperintensity consistent with fat and hypointense foci representing vascular flow voids or thrombi. Microscopic examination showed capillaries within a matrix of adipose tissue.

ses. Unlike juvenile fibromatoses, they are more prevalent in adults than in children. Extra-abdominal desmoid tumors are usually solitary and arise from the fascial sheaths and aponeuroses of striated muscle. Histologically, they consist of benign fibrous tissues containing spindle cells and abundant collagen. Although they do not metastasize, they can infiltrate contiguous structures, including bone, despite their benign microscopic appearance. In children, extra-abdominal desmoid tumors are more common than the abdominal type. However, most desmoid tumors in patients with Gardner's syndrome are found in the abdomen.

Extra-abdominal desmoid tumors are deep seated. In the series of tumors studied at St. Jude Children's Research Hospital, they involved the head and neck, trunk, and extremities with approximately equal frequency. These tumors are variably echogenic on ultrasound, and their borders may be smooth or irregular. On contrast-enhanced CT images, most desmoid tumors appear more attenuated than striated muscle. On MR images, their appearance is also variable, with a

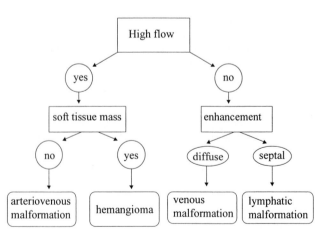

FIGURE 3. Magnetic resonance imaging features of hemangiomas and vascular malformations. (Modified from Laor T, Burrows PE: Congenital anomalies and vascular birthmarks of the lower extremities. Magn Reson Imaging Clin North Am 1998;6:510. Copyright 1998 Elsevier Science [USA]. All rights reserved.)

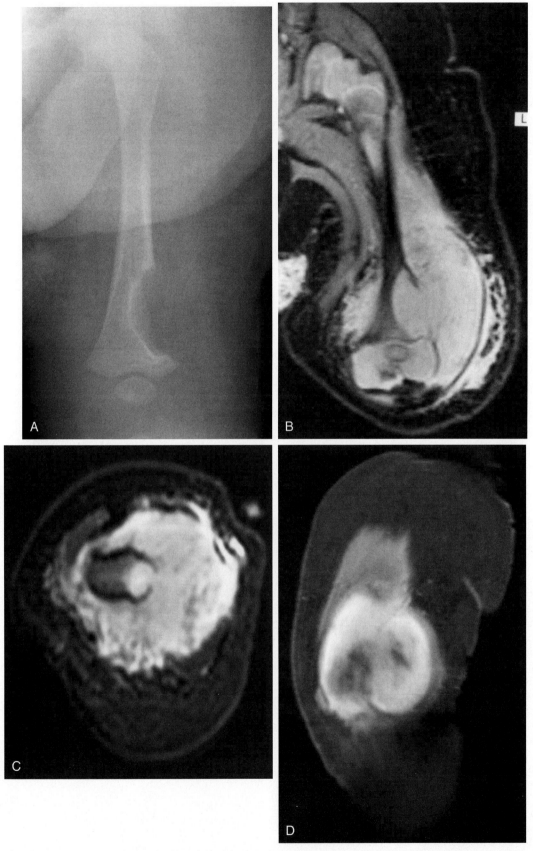

FIGURE 4. A 2-month-old infant with hemangiopericytoma. **A,** An anteroposterior radiograph of the femur demonstrates a well-defined erosion of the distal femur. Coronal short tau inversion–recovery **(B)** and transverse T_2-weighted **(C)** magnetic resonance images show a hyperintense soft tissue mass eroding the bony cortex and extending into the medullary space. **D,** The central hypointensities demonstrated on a coronal contrast-enhanced, fat-suppressed T_1-weighted image are consistent with pathologic findings of necrosis.

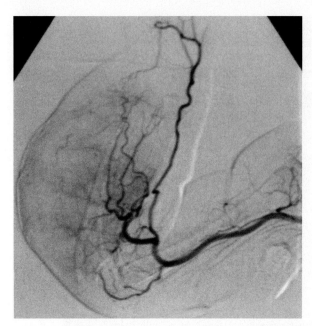

FIGURE 5. An arteriogram of the upper extremity of a 6-month-old girl with hemangiopericytoma shows a highly vascular mass involving the forearm, with numerous tumor vessels.

signal that is isointense or slightly hyperintense when compared with that of muscle on T_1-weighted images and either intermediate (between muscle and fat) or high signal on T_2-weighted images (Fig. 6). Occasionally, these tumors may be hypointense on T_2-weighted im-

ages. This variability in signal may be due to differences in the relative proportions of collagen, spindle cells, and mucopolysaccharides within the lesion. Linear and curvilinear signal voids, probably caused by deposits of dense collagen, were found in 86% of the cases reported by the Armed Forces Institute of Pathology.

Desmoid tumors are related histologically to generalized fibromatosis (congenital fibromatosis, juvenile fibromatosis, infantile myofibromatosis), and some have histologic features suggesting hemangiopericytoma. Other fibrous tumors of infants and children include fibrous hamartoma, fibromatosis coli, digital fibromatosis, calcifying aponeurotic fibroma, and hyaline fibromatosis.

BENIGN PERIPHERAL NERVE SHEATH TUMORS

Benign neurofibromas and, less commonly, schwannomas are frequently multiple and associated with neurofibromatosis type 1 (NF1). However, both tumors may be solitary and occur sporadically. They are similar histologically, composed primarily of Schwann cells, and therefore they exhibit similar imaging characteristics. Microscopic examination reveals a dense central core of Schwann cells surrounded by a peripheral zone of myxoid tissue. Peripheral nerve sheath tumors have a low incidence of malignant degeneration.

A tumor can be suspected to be of neurogenic origin if it is located along the distribution of a periph-

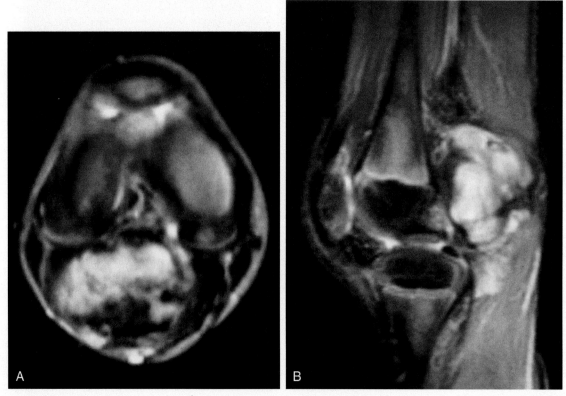

FIGURE 6. On magnetic resonance imaging, transverse T_2-weighted **(A)** and sagittal short tau inversion–recovery **(B)** images of the knee of a 6-year-old boy with a desmoid tumor show heterogeneously high signal intensity with peripheral ill-defined hypointense foci.

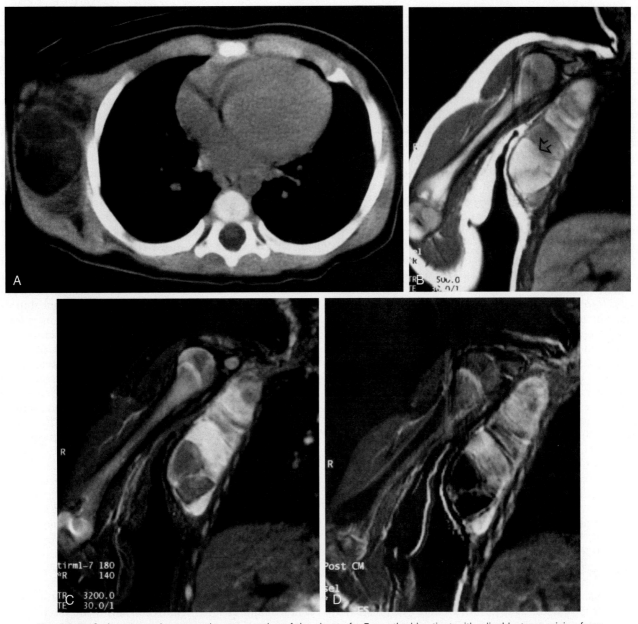

FIGURE 7. A, A computed tomography scan section of the chest of a 5-month-old patient with a lipoblastoma arising from the right axilla shows a low-attenuation mass. **B,** On a coronal T_1-weighted magnetic resonance image, the inferior portion of the mass *(arrow)* is markedly hyperintense as a result of adipose tissue. The low signal in this portion of the mass shown in short tau inversion–recovery **(C)** and fat-suppressed contrast-enhanced T_1-weighted **(D)** images is also characteristic of fat.

eral nerve. Calcification in degenerating ("ancient") schwannomas may be visible radiographically, and these tumors have been observed to take up technetium-99m MDP on bone scintigrams. Peripheral nerve sheath tumors may be accompanied by subtle atrophy of surrounding or distally innervated muscle. Most of these tumors are well-defined spherical or fusiform masses. On CT images, they tend to be hypoattenuated, possibly because of lipids in their Schwann cells, adipocytes, and perineural tissues. Unlike fat, however, on MRI the bulk of the tumor is low in intensity on T_1-weighted sequences and high in intensity on T_2-weighted sequences. Typically, the central zone consisting of collagen and neurofibroma cells is hypointense on T_2-

weighted images, lending a "target" appearance to the lesion that helps distinguish these benign tumors from their less well-organized malignant counterparts (see Fig. 10*B* below). This sign is also exhibited on contrast-enhanced T_1-weighted images.

Plexiform neurofibromas arise from the axis of a primary nerve and form torturous cord-like tumors along its axis. They are considered to be indicators of neurofibromatosis even if they are the sole manifestation of this disease. Like solitary neurofibromas, these tumors are also usually hyperintense on T_2-weighted images and often have well-defined, central, tubular, hypointense structures or form large masses resembling a "bag of worms" on transverse images.

LIPOBLASTOMA

Lipoblastoma and lipoblastomatosis are benign mesenchymal tumors of immature fat that occur primarily in infants and young children, most often in boys less than 8 years of age. Collins and Chatten reported that the average age of patients at the time of presentation is 3.6 years. Lipoblastomas are usually painless superficial tumors that are most commonly located in the extremities and the head and neck region, but they may also involve the trunk and deeper structures such as the mediastinum and retroperitoneum. The tumor consists of lobules of immature adipose tissue with a variable amount of myxoid stroma separated by richly vascularized septa composed of connective tissue. The discrete form, lipoblastoma, is a well-circumscribed lesion that mimics lipoma. Lipoblastomatosis refers to the diffuse type that often infiltrates adjacent deeper tissues such as muscle and has a tendency to recur locally. In one patient of Cowling et al., with recurrent lipoblastoma radiographs and CT images showed expansion of ribs adjacent to the tumor, a feature also associated with lymphangiomas, hemangiomas, and arteriovenous malformations.

Imaging features reflect the amount of fatty tissue present. On ultrasound images, the hyperechoic fat can be clearly delineated from the myxoid component, and CT images show a similar combination of hypoattenuated fat and denser myxoid tissue (Fig. 7A). On MR images, the signal is often heterogeneous (Fig. 7B–D), with lipomatous elements appearing hyperintense to muscle on T_1-weighted images and isointense to subcutaneous fat on T_2-weighted images, whereas the nonfatty tissues produce lower signal intensity than fat on T_1-weighted images and are more intense than fat on T_2-weighted images.

The differential diagnosis includes lipoma, which is much more prevalent in adults than in children; hibernoma, a rare tumor analogous to brown fat; and myxoid liposarcoma. Histologically, liposarcoma is nearly indistinguishable from lipoblastoma, but it is rare in children less than 5 years of age. Recent evidence suggests that lipoblastoma and liposarcoma can be differentiated on the basis of specific molecular and cytogenetic markers.

MALIGNANT SOFT TISSUE TUMORS

Almost all musculoskeletal malignancies of childhood are sarcomas that arise from primitive mesenchymal cells that normally mature into supportive tissues. The presumed origin of these tumors is based on the histologic finding of a specific differentiated cell line within the tumor. Of the fewer than 6000 soft tissue sarcomas diagnosed annually in the United States, about 15% occur in patients younger than 15 years of age. Rhabdomyosarcomas (RMS) comprise slightly more than half of pediatric soft tissue sarcomas. Unlike RMS, nonrhabdomyosarcomatous tumors of the musculoskeletal system are more common in adults and are quite rare in children. Nonrhabdomyosarcomatous neoplasms consist of fibrosarcoma, neurofibrosarcoma, malignant fibrous histiocytoma (MFH), synovial sarcoma, alveolar soft part sarcoma (ASPS), and liposarcoma, as well as peripheral primitive neuroectodermal tumors (PPNETs) that are histologically and cytogenetically closely related to Ewing's sarcoma.

Diagnosis of soft tissue sarcoma is complex and depends on histologic, cytologic, histochemical, and molecular genetic studies. Imaging is usually nonspecific and contributes less to the tissue diagnosis than in the case of bone sarcomas but is essential for staging and surgical management. Imaging should be performed before biopsy so that the tumor does not become obscured by tracking of edema and blood into the adjacent tissues. MRI has largely superceded CT and ultrasonography in this clinical setting. Most malignant masses are either isointense or hypointense to muscle on T_1-weighted images and hyperintense to fat and muscle on T_2-weighted and STIR images, and they enhance with gadolinium. Imaging techniques, especially MRI, can resolve important issues in local staging, such as the anatomic location of the tumor, its relationship to important nerves and blood vessels, and the local involvement of bone or lymph nodes. Infiltration of adjacent soft tissue structures is a hallmark of malignancy that can affect prognosis, because patients with completely resected tumors have a better outcome. However, malignant soft tissue tumors are frequently accompanied by considerable adjacent or surrounding soft tissue edema that displays a high T_2-weighted signal and therefore may be impossible to distinguish from tumor. Involvement of contiguous bony structures is not common and is usually better defined on CT images. Coronal and sagittal MR images are particularly helpful because the surgical approach to soft tissue sarcomas of the extremities is usually longitudinal rather than transverse. In addition to CT or MRI of the primary tumor, CT of the chest and radionuclide bone scintigraphy should be performed at the time of diagnosis. In the case of tumors involving the lower extremities, CT of the abdomen and pelvis is recommended to assess inguinal and retroperitoneal lymph node involvement. Some clinical and imaging features of soft tissue sarcomas are shown in Table 3.

RHABDOMYOSARCOMA

RMS, the most common soft tissue sarcoma of the pediatric age group, contains a mixture of rhabdomyoblasts, which are recognized by their typical cross striations, and undifferentiated cells. The head and neck and genitourinary tract are the most frequent locations of RMS. Fewer than 20% of these tumors affect the extremities, followed by the trunk and retroperitoneum. Most extremity tumors are alveolar or undifferentiated histologic types, as opposed to the embryonal or botryoid types found in the face and neck and genitourinary system. Prognosis is less favorable for patients with RMS of the extremities than for those with tumors arising from the genitourinary system or the head and neck region. In the extremities, the tumors are deep and tend to spread along fascial planes. There are no specific imaging characteristics. Most RMS take up

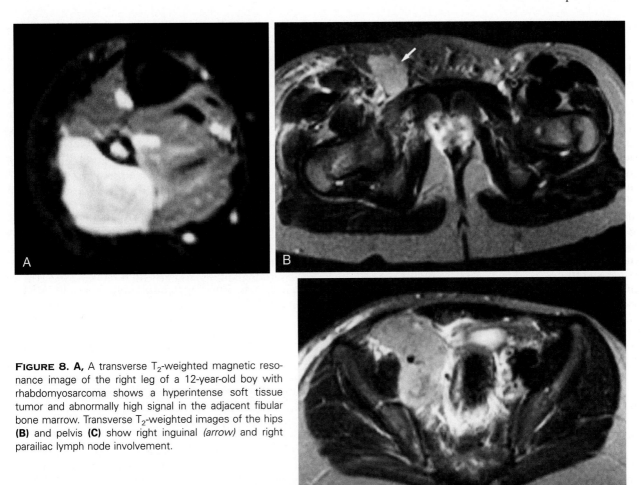

FIGURE 8. A, A transverse T$_2$-weighted magnetic resonance image of the right leg of a 12-year-old boy with rhabdomyosarcoma shows a hyperintense soft tissue tumor and abnormally high signal in the adjacent fibular bone marrow. Transverse T$_2$-weighted images of the hips **(B)** and pelvis **(C)** show right inguinal *(arrow)* and right parailiac lymph node involvement.

gallium. There may be metastatic lymph node involvement (Fig. 8) and erosion of adjacent bone. Bone marrow metastases also carry a poor prognosis. Bone metastases resemble those occurring with neuroblastoma and have been reported even in the absence of detectable primary tumor. The lungs are also frequent sites of distant metastases; less commonly, the liver, breasts, and brain may be involved.

Primitive Peripheral Neuroectodermal Tumor and Extraosseous Ewing's Sarcoma

PPNET and extraosseous Ewing's sarcoma (EOES) are small round cell neoplasms belonging to the Ewing's sarcoma family of tumors that can arise in either soft tissue or bone. They are related histogenically and share a common cytogenetic characteristic, the translocation of bands 24 and 12 of the short arms of chromosomes 11 and 22, but are often indistinguishable histologically. PPNET, also known as peripheral neuroepithelioma, has a higher degree of neural differentiation than Ewing's sarcoma; thus, these two tumors can be distinguished on the basis of immunohistochemical markers. The distinc-

tion is important, because disease-free survival is poorer for patients with PPNET than for those with EOES.

Both tumors occur most commonly in truncal and paravertebral soft tissues (50% to 60% of cases) and the extremities (25% of cases), although PPNET occurs less commonly in the extremities than EOES. Patients with EOES are generally younger; both tumors are rare in black children. Askin's tumors are thoracic PPNETs that involve the chest wall (see Section IV, Part IV, page 817 and Section IV, Part VII, Chapter 8, page 1128).

The tumors can be very large at the time of presentation and tend to be poorly circumscribed. The soft tissue mass does not calcify. These tumors usually enhance on CT images. On MRI, they are isointense to muscle on T$_1$-weighted images and inhomogeneously hyperintense on T$_2$-weighted and STIR images, and they show variable enhancement. They may erode adjacent bone. Distant spread is to bone, lung, liver, and brain. However, distant metastases are uncommon in Askin's tumors.

Synovial Sarcoma

Synovial sarcomas typically occur between the ages of 16 and 25 years and are the most common nonrhabdomyosarcomatous soft tissue sarcomas in children. These tumors arise from undifferentiated mesenchymal cells and, despite their name, are nearly always para-articular rather than intra-articular. The monophasic variety is composed of spindle cells, and the biphasic type consists of both spindle cells and epithelial elements. These tumors are considerably more common in the lower extremities than in the upper extremities, head and neck, retroperitoneum, and mediastinum. They may spread to regional lymph nodes, and the lungs are the most common site of distant metastases.

Radiographically visible calcifications are present in 30% of cases. On MRI, synovial sarcomas are often lobulated, well-defined, deep-seated lesions, although they can also be infiltrative and can encase major blood vessels. Femoral vein invasion has been described, and erosion of the cortex of adjacent bones is present in up to 20% of patients (Fig. 9A).

MR signal characteristics do not distinguish monophasic from biphasic tumors. They are usually isointense to muscle on T_1-weighted images, with occasional foci of high T_1-weighted signal caused by hemorrhage (Fig. 9B). Synovial sarcoma generally demonstrates internal septa and inhomogeneous hyperintensity on T_2-weighted images (Fig. 9C). In a large series by Jones et al. of patients with synovial sarcoma from the Armed Forces Institute of Pathology, 35% of the tumors showed a triple signal pattern on T_2-weighted images; these findings are consistent with high (fluid) signal intensity, intermediate signal intensity similar to that of fat, and low signal intensity resembling that of fibrous tissue. Some synovial sarcomas simulate cysts because of their homogeneous signal intensity on T_1- and T_2-weighted images and their well-defined borders. However, the degree of specificity of this finding is uncertain. A multilocular appearance with fluid–fluid levels may be seen in 18% to 25% of these tumors.

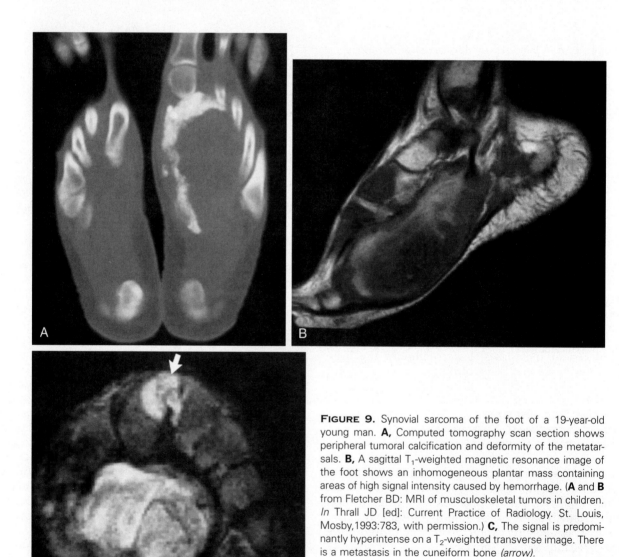

FIGURE 9. Synovial sarcoma of the foot of a 19-year-old young man. **A,** Computed tomography scan section shows peripheral tumoral calcification and deformity of the metatarsals. **B,** A sagittal T_1-weighted magnetic resonance image of the foot shows an inhomogeneous plantar mass containing areas of high signal intensity caused by hemorrhage. (**A** and **B** from Fletcher BD: MRI of musculoskeletal tumors in children. *In* Thrall JD [ed]: Current Practice of Radiology. St. Louis, Mosby, 1993:783, with permission.) **C,** The signal is predominantly hyperintense on a T_2-weighted transverse image. There is a metastasis in the cuneiform bone *(arrow).*

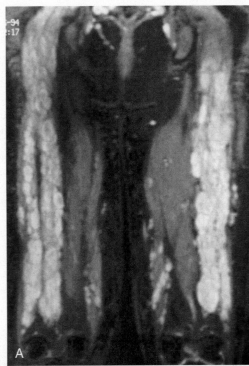

FIGURE 10. **A,** A coronal short tau inversion–recovery magnetic resonance image of the thighs shows multiple neurofibromas distributed along the sciatic nerves of a young woman first seen at the age of 16 with a malignant peripheral nerve sheath tumor. **B,** Transverse T$_2$-weighted images show multiple discrete high-intensity neurofibromas. A characteristic target sign is present *(arrow)*. The larger lesion in the posterior left thigh had shown recent growth and was a low-grade malignant peripheral nerve sheath tumor.

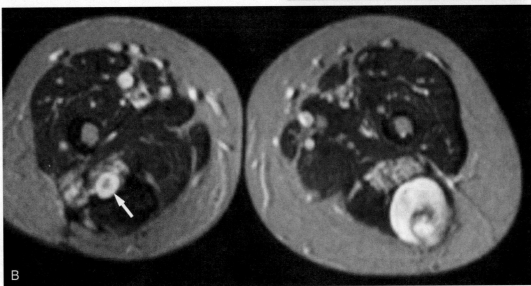

MALIGNANT PERIPHERAL NERVE SHEATH TUMOR

Malignant peripheral nerve sheath tumor (MPNST) is a designation that has replaced many formerly used terms, including malignant schwannoma, neurofibrosarcoma, neurogenic sarcoma, and malignant neural neoplasm. A "triton" tumor is an MPNST containing both neural and rhabdomyosarcomatous elements; the tumor was named after a salamander in which transplantation of the sciatic nerve induces growth of a supernumerary limb. MPNSTs account for about 10% of soft tissue sarcomas and are the malignancy most commonly associated with NF1. Half of these tumors occur in patients with NF1; conversely, 2% to 29% of patients with NF1 develop MPNST, a much higher incidence than in the general population. Patients with NF1 who have

MPNSTs are usually younger than those in whom the tumor arises without association with NF1. Furthermore, in NF1 patients, MPNSTs tend to arise in pre-existing benign neurofibromas and are high-grade tumors with a tendency to local recurrence and metastasis. MPNSTs may also arise at previously irradiated sites.

Like benign neurofibromas, MPNSTs are deep soft tissue lesions often associated with primary nerves, especially those of the thigh and lower extremity. The appearance of these tumors on CT and MR images is nonspecific. They may be well or poorly defined, homogeneous or inhomogeneous; they occasionally erode bone. Malignant transformation of benign neurofibromas should be considered in patients in whom the mass is painful or enlarging and when the typical target appearance of benign neurofibroma is absent (Fig. 10). Tumor uptake on gallium scintigrams may indicate malignant transformation or progressive growth of neurofibromas. However, biopsy is usually necessary.

FIBROSARCOMA

Fibrosarcoma is primarily a neoplasma of adults, but a histologically indistinguishable form is also found in children, for whom the prognosis is more favorable. In nearly 40% of cases, the tumor is present at birth and is then called congenital fibrosarcoma. The neoplasm is composed of anaplastic spindle-shaped cells. Previously, well-differentiated fibrosarcomas in children were grouped with aggressive fibromatosis because of histologic similarities. The currently accepted term is *congenital-infantile fibrosarcoma.*

The extremities, particularly the lower limbs, are the most frequent sites of fibrosarcoma. Unlike adult fibrosarcomas, those found in young children are usually low-grade malignancies that seldom metastasize but may recur locally.

Clinically, fibrosarcomas present as enlarging, sometimes painful masses that rarely erode bone. Because of their high degree of vascularization, they may be confused with hemangiomas on physical and imaging examinations. However, the CT attenuation and MRI signal intensity of fibrosarcomas are less homogeneous than those of hemangiomas (Fig. 11). Angiography may reveal tumor vasculature. No specific characteristics have been identified by MRI. Fibrosarcomas are usually isointense to muscle on T_1-weighted images and hyperintense on T_2-weighted images. They may contain hypointense foci, which correlate with fibrosis.

LIPOSARCOMA

Liposarcoma is one of the more common soft tissue tumors of adults but is rare in children, especially those under the age of 5 years, in whom a benign counterpart, lipoblastoma, is prevalent. The lower extremities, particularly the thigh, are the most common sites of liposarcoma. These tumors may also involve the retroperitoneum, mediastinum, neck, back, axilla, buttocks, and forearm. In the extremities, the tumors can be subcutaneous or intramuscular, or they can involve fascial planes.

The two main histologic types are myxoid and well differentiated. Myxoid liposarcomas are by far the more common type in children, accounting for 76% of 17 cases studied by Shmookler and Enzinger. These lobular, partially encapsulated neoplasms contain primitive mesenchymal cells, lipoblasts, and capillaries in a myxoid matrix. Distinguishing liposarcoma from lipoblastoma is difficult.

Well-differentiated liposarcoma has imaging characteristics similar to those of fat, with high T_1-weighted signal and intermediate intensity on T_2-weighted images. Enhancement is slight and best shown on subtraction or fat-suppressed images. The more common

myxoid liposarcomas are isointense with muscle on T_1-weighted images and have homogeneously high signal intensity on T_2-weighted images with linear septa. In children, both the well-differentiated and myxoid types appear to have only low-grade malignant potential, but local recurrence is possible.

ALVEOLAR SOFT PART SARCOMA

ASPS is a very rare tumor, accounting for only 0.5% to 1.0% of all soft tissue sarcomas, with the highest incidence in adolescents and young adults. It has no benign counterpart, and its possibly myogenic histogenesis is unproven. The tumor is usually found in the muscles of the lower extremities, especially those of the thigh, although isolated cases have involved many other sites. There may be destruction of adjacent bone. Despite slow growth, ASPS is highly malignant, and metastasis to lymph nodes, lungs, bones, and brain can occur either early or late.

The tumor consists of alveolar arrangements of large granular cells separated by vascular channels. Because of its high vascularity, it may present as a pulsatile mass with a bruit that may lead to an erroneous diagnosis of vascular malformation.

On noncontrast CT images, the tumor is less attenuated than muscle and punctate calcification may be visible. As with hemangiomas, there may be marked enhancement with contrast. However, unlike most hemangiomas, ASPS is low in attenuation at its center, a finding consistent with necrosis. CT may also demonstrate bone erosion. The highly vascular nature of ASPS may account for a MRI appearance similar to that of hemangioma but different from that of other soft tissue sarcomas in that the signal intensity of ASPS is usually higher than that of muscle on T_1-weighted images. Intensity on T_2-weighted images may be very high. Tubular flow voids at the margins and in the substance of the tumors are consistent with enlarged vessels.

Despite the vascularity of the tumor, flow within it is slow, and the angiographic demonstration of delayed contrast washout can help distinguish ASPS from arteriovenous malformation. Prominent draining veins may be demonstrated angiographically and by CT or MRI (Fig. 12).

MALIGNANT FIBROUS HISTIOCYTOMA

MFH is the most common soft tissue sarcoma of adults, but fewer than 5% of these tumors occur in children. MFH may occur in almost any anatomic location, but the extremities are involved in 75% of cases, and 50% arise in the muscle or fascia of the lower limbs. Metastases are to lung, bone, liver, and regional lymph nodes. Local recurrence is common.

The most common form of the tumor is composed mainly of spindle cells arranged in a "storiform" (woven) pattern surrounding blood vessels. Other types contain mucoid tissue (myxoid MFH) or giant cells

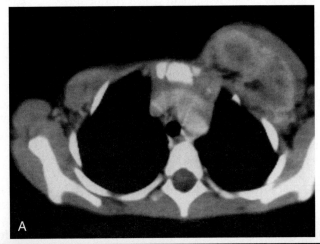

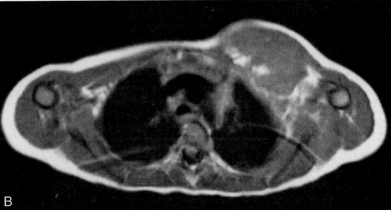

FIGURE 11. Fibrosarcoma in a 3-year-old girl. **A,** Contrast-enhanced computed tomography scan section demonstrates a large, enhanced mass involving the muscles of the left anterior chest wall. On magnetic resonance imaging, the lesion is isointense to muscle on a T_1-weighted image **(B)** and mainly less intense than fat on a T_2-weighted image **(C). D,** It enhances on a fat-suppressed, contrast-enhanced T_1-weighted image. The lesions recurred 1 year after initial surgical resection, and the mass, initially diagnosed as an aggressive myofibroma, was then considered to be a fibrosarcoma. The accompanying enlarged axillary lymph nodes were negative for tumor. (From Hanna SL, Fletcher BD: MR imaging of malignant soft-tissue tumors. Magn Reson Imaging Clin N Am 1995;3:642–643. Copyright 1995 Elsevier Science [USA]. All rights reserved.)

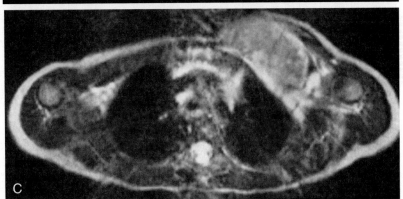

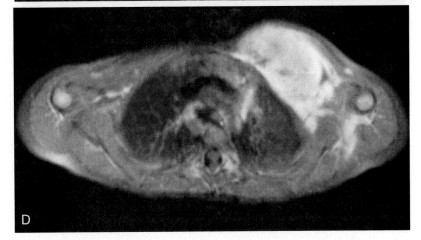

(malignant giant cell tumor of soft parts). A fourth rare type that occurs in children and young adults is the angiomatoid MFH. This is a locally invasive tumor that spreads along fascial planes and encases neurovascular structures. MFH tends to recur but not to metastasize. On CT images, tumor density is similar to that of muscle, and necrotic areas of lower attenuation may be present. Poorly defined calcifications are occasionally visible.

On MRI, MFH, like most other soft tissue sarcomas, is isointense to muscle on T_1-weighted images, and its intensity is equal to or greater than that of subcutaneous fat on T_2-weighted images. MRI may be helpful in differentiating intratumoral hemorrhage with high T_1-weighted signal from tumor progression in patients whose tumors show enlargement during preoperative chemotherapy. Lin et al. reported intense gallium-67 uptake by almost all MFHs studied.

EPITHELIOID SARCOMA

Epithelioid sarcoma is a soft tissue tumor of uncertain histogenesis in which there is epithelial differentiation. The tumor is sometimes difficult to differentiate from chronic inflammation, necrotizing granuloma, and squamous cell carcinoma. This neoplasm comprised only 7% of 112 nonrhabdomyosarcomatous soft tissue sarcomas treated at St. Jude Children's Research Hospital during an 11-year period as reported by Gross et al. Two of the eight children with epithelioid sarcoma died of early progressive disease. About half of these sarcomas involve the upper extremity; the volar aspect of the forearm is a typical location (Fig. 13). Epithelioid sarcoma may be either subcutaneous in location, presenting as single or multiple firm, sometimes ulcerating nodules; or deep-seated, involving tendons, tendon sheaths, and fascia. The tumor spreads along neurovas-

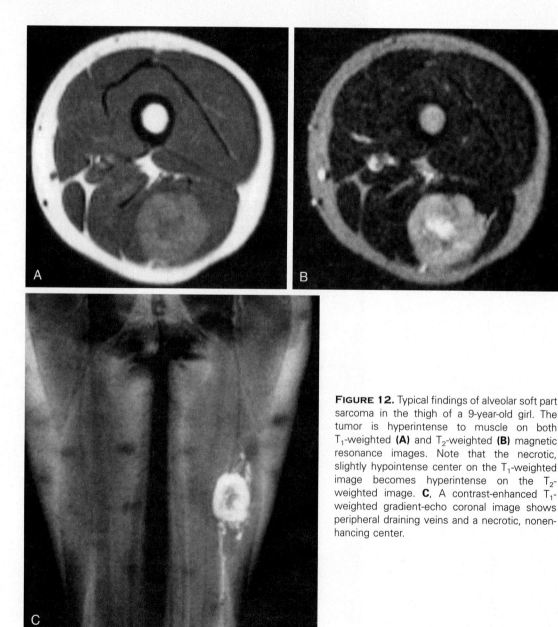

FIGURE 12. Typical findings of alveolar soft part sarcoma in the thigh of a 9-year-old girl. The tumor is hyperintense to muscle on both T_1-weighted **(A)** and T_2-weighted **(B)** magnetic resonance images. Note that the necrotic, slightly hypointense center on the T_1-weighted image becomes hyperintense on the T_2-weighted image. **C,** A contrast-enhanced T_1-weighted gradient-echo coronal image shows peripheral draining veins and a necrotic, nonenhancing center.

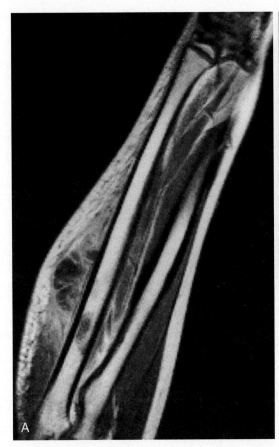

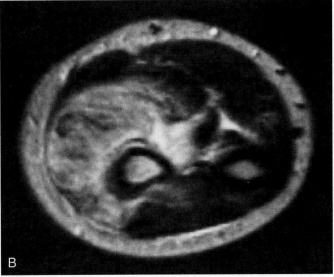

FIGURE 13. Coronal contrast-enhanced T_1-weighted **(A)** and transverse T_2-weighted **(B)** magnetic resonance images of the forearm of an 11-year-old boy shows an epithelioid sarcoma in a typical location. The unenhanced, hypointense areas in **A** are consistent with necrosis. Note involvement of the marrow of the proximal ulna. (From Hanna SL, Kaste S, Jenkins JJ, et al: Epithelioid sarcoma: clinical, MR imaging and pathologic findings. Skeletal Radiol 2002;31:403, with permission.)

cular bundles and may invade vascular structures, but it rarely involves bone. Metastases, which may occur late, are mainly to the lung.

Epithelioid sarcomas rarely calcify, but one tumor with radiographically visible bone formation has been reported. Several interesting MRI patterns have been observed. Of 12 patients examined by Romero et al., 10 had nonhemorrhagic neoplasms isointense to muscle on T_1-weighted images and hyperintense to muscle on T_2-weighted images. However, two patients' tumors were hemorrhagic and thus hyperintense on both T_1- and T_2-weighted images. Both hemorrhagic lesions resulted in early metastases. Another unusual presentation consisted of honeycombing of subcutaneous fat as the result of lymphatic involvement and denervation-induced muscle atrophy, with high T_2-weighted signal in the large muscles of the arm. These findings occurred before humeral involvement and soft tissue tumor nodules became evident.

DISSEMINATED DISEASE OF SOFT TISSUES

LYMPHOMA

Muscle involvement by non-Hodgkin lymphoma is usually due to metastatic spread via lymphatic and hematogenous routes or to direct extension from primary bone lymphoma. Much less commonly, muscle lymphoma occurs as a primary extranodal tumor. Muscle involvement results in solitary or multiple masses that are detectable by CT and MRI as well as by gallium-67 scintigraphy and 2-[^{18}F]fluoro-2-deoxy-D-glucose (FDG) positron emission tomography (PET). The disease can cross compartmental boundaries or invade the subcutaneous tissues. Involvement of adjacent bone and bone marrow may also be demonstrated. Mycosis fungoides is a primary T-cell lymphoma of the skin. Typical findings are focal thickening caused by dermal and epidural infiltrates with lymphadenopathy in advanced-stage disease.

On CT images, muscles affected by lymphoma appear diffusely enlarged with or without obliteration of normal fat planes. The tumor may be poorly defined, and its attenuation is either equal to or slightly less than that of normal muscle on either contrast-enhanced or noncontrast CT images.

On MRI, the masses are isointense or slightly hypointense to normal muscle on T_1-weighted images and hyperintense on T_2-weighted images. They are markedly hyperintense on STIR images and enhance homogeneously with gadolinium. Abnormal activity in the masses on gallium-67 and FDG PET scintigrams correlates well with MRI findings.

METASTASES

Despite its proportionally large mass, muscle is not a frequent host of metastatic disease. Muscle metastases occur at various locations and on CT images produce

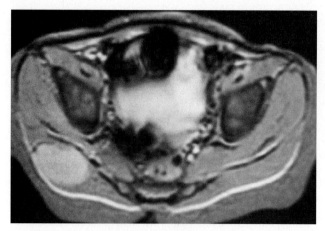

FIGURE 14. A transverse T_2-weighted magnetic resonance image of the pelvis of a 2-year-old girl with stage 4 neuroblastoma shows a large metastasis in the right gluteal muscle.

low-attenuation masses with loss of normal muscle planes. On MRI, metastases are similar in intensity to muscle on T_1-weighted images and are hyperintense on T_2-weighted images. Contrast-enhanced T_1-weighted images show high signal intensities of masses with focal necrosis. Muscle metastases have been identified in adults with a variety of primary neoplasms; we have seen both intramuscular and subcutaneous metastases in children with neuroblastoma (Fig. 14).

SUGGESTED READINGS

Soft Tissue Tumors—General

Bitran JD, Bekerman C, Golomb HM, Simon MA: Scintigraphic evaluation of sarcomata in children and adults by Ga^{67} citrate. Cancer 1978;42:1760–1765

Chang AE, Matory YL, Dwyer AJ, et al: Magnetic resonance imaging versus computed tomography in the evaluation of soft tissue tumors of the extremities. Ann Surg 1987;205:340–348

Crim JR, Seeger LL, Yao L, et al: Diagnosis of soft-tissue masses with MR imaging: can benign masses be differentiated from malignant ones? Radiology 1992;185:581–586

Dwyer AJ, Frank JA, Sank VJ, et al: Short-TI inversion-recovery pulse sequence: analysis and initial experience in cancer imaging. Radiology 1988;168:827–836

Enzinger FM, Weiss SW: Soft Tissue Tumors, 3rd ed. St. Louis, Mosby–Year Book, 1995

Hanna SL, Fletcher BD: MR imaging of malignant soft-tissue tumors. Magn Reson Imaging Clin N Am 1995;3:629–650

Howman-Giles R, Uren RF, Shaw PJ: Thallium-201 scintigraphy in pediatric soft-tissue tumors. J Nucl Med 1995;36:1372–1376

Kransdorf MJ, Jelinek JS, Moser RP Jr, et al: Soft-tissue masses: diagnosis using MR imaging. AJR Am J Roentgenol 1989;153:541–547

Kransdorf MJ, Murphey MD: Imaging of Soft Tissue Tumors. Philadelphia, WB Saunders, 1997

May DA, Good RB, Smith DK, et al: MR imaging of musculoskeletal tumors and tumor mimickers with intravenous gadolinium: experience with 242 patients. Skeletal Radiol 1997;26:2–15

Munk PL, Poon PY, Chhem RK, et al: Imaging of soft-tissue sarcomas. Can Assoc Radiol J 1994;45:438–446

Petasnick JP, Turner DA, Charters JR, et al: Soft-tissue masses of the locomotor system: comparison of MR imaging with CT. Radiology 1986;160:125–133

Pettersson H, Eliasson J, Egund N, et al: Gadolinium-DTPA enhancement of soft tissue tumors in magnetic resonance imaging—
preliminary clinical experience in five patients. Skeletal Radiol 1988;17:319–323

Pizzo PA, Poplack DG: Principles and Practice of Pediatric Oncology, 2nd ed. Philadelphia, JB Lippincott, 1993

Sundaram M, McGuire MH, Herbold DR, et al: High signal intensity soft tissue masses on T1 weighted pulsing sequences. Skeletal Radiol 1987;16:30–36

Sundaram M, McGuire MH, Schajowicz F: Soft-tissue masses: histologic basis for decreased signal (short T2) on T2-weighted MR images. AJR Am J Roentgenol 1987;148:1247–1250

Totty WG, Murphy WA, Lee JKT: Soft-tissue tumors: MR imaging. Radiology 1986;160:135–141

Weinberger E, Shaw DWW, White KS, et al: Nontraumatic pediatric musculoskeletal MR imaging: comparison of conventional and fast-spin echo short inversion time inversion-recovery technique. Radiology 1995;194:721–726

Hemangiomas

Buetow PC, Kransdorf MJ, Moser RP, et al: Radiologic appearance of intramuscular hemangioma with emphasis on MR imaging. AJR Am J Roentgenol 1990;154:563–567

Cohen EK, Kressel HY, Perosio T, et al: MR imaging of soft-tissue hemangiomas: correlation with pathologic findings. AJR Am J Roentgenol 1988;150:1079–1081

Dubois J, Garel L: Imaging and therapeutic approach of hemangiomas and vascular malformations in the pediatric age group. Pediatr Radiol 1999;26:879–893

Dubois J, Patriquin HB, Garel L, et al: Soft-tissue hemangiomas in infants and children: diagnosis using Doppler sonography. AJR Am J Roentgenol 1998;171:247–252

Hawnaur JM, Whitehouse RW, Jenkins JPR, et al: Musculoskeletal haemangiomas: comparisons of MRI with CT. Skeletal Radiol 1990;19:251–258

Kaplan PA, Williams SM: Mucocutaneous and peripheral soft-tissue hemangiomas: MR imaging. Radiology 1987;163:163–166

Laor T, Burrows PE: Congenital anomalies and vascular birthmarks of the lower extremities. Magn Reson Imaging Clin N Am 1998;6:497–519

Levine E, Wetzel LH, Neff JR: MR imaging and CT of extrahepatic cavernous hemangiomas. AJR Am J Roentgenol 1986;147:1299–1304

Mulliken JB, Glowacki J: Hemangiomas and vascular malformations in infants and children: a classification based on endothelial characteristics. Plast Reconstr Surg 1982;69:412–422

Steinbach LS, Ominsky SH, Shpall S, et al: MR imaging of spindle cell hemangioendothelioma. J Comput Assist Tomogr 1991;15:155–157

Yuh WTC, Kathol MH, Sein MA, et al: Hemangiomas of skeletal muscle: MR findings in five patients. AJR Am J Roentgenol 1987;149:765–768

Hemangiopericytoma

Auguste L-J, Razack MS, Sako K: Hemangiopericytoma. J Surg Oncol 1982;20:260–264

Chen KTK, Kassel SH, Medrano VA: Congenital hemangiopericytoma. J Surg Oncol 1986;31:127–129

Enzinger FM, Smith BH: Hemangiopericytoma: an analysis of 106 cases. Hum Pathol 1976;7:61–82

Grant EG, Grønvall S, Sarosi TE, et al: Sonographic findings in four cases of hemangiopericytoma. Radiology 1982;142:447–451

Kumar R, Corbally M: Childhood hemangiopericytoma. Med Pediatr Oncol 1998;30:294–296

Lorigan JG, David CL, Evans HL, et al: The clinical and radiologic manifestations of hemangiopericytoma. AJR Am J Roentgenol 1989;153:345–349

Desmoid Tumors

Casillas J, Sais GJ, Greve JL, et al: Imaging of intra- and extraabdominal desmoid tumors. Radiographics 1991;11:959–968

Eich GF, Hoeffel J-C, Tschäppeler H, et al: Fibrous tumours in children: imaging features of a heterogeneous group of disorders. Pediatr Radiol 1998;28:500–509

Kransdorf MJ, Jelinek JS, Moser RP, et al: Magnetic resonance appearance of fibromatosis: a report of 14 cases and review of the literature. Skeletal Radiol 1990;19:495–499

Rao BN, Horowitz ME, Parham DM, et al: Challenges in the treatment of childhood fibromatosis. Arch Surg 1987;122:1296–1298

Romero JA, Kim EE, Kim C-G, et al: Different biologic features of desmoid tumors in adult and juvenile patients: MR demonstration. J Comput Assist Tomogr 1995;19:782–787

Peripheral Nerve Sheath Tumors

Bhargava R, Parham DM, Lasater OE, et al: MR imaging differentiation of benign and malignant peripheral nerve sheath tumors: use of the target sign. Pediatr Radiol 1997;27:124–129

Burk DL Jr, Brunberg JA, Kanal E, et al: Spinal and paraspinal neurofibromatosis: surface coil MR imaging at 1.5 T. Radiology 1987;162:797–801

Ducatman BS, Scheithauer BW, Piepgras DG, et al: Malignant peripheral nerve sheath tumors. Cancer 1986;57:2006–2021

Knapp TR, Struk DW, Munk PL, et al: Tumour of a peripheral nerve sheath with invasion of the lumbar spine. Can Assoc Radiol J 1994;45:469–472

Kuman AJ, Kuhajda FP, Martinez CR, et al: Computed tomography of extracranial nerve sheath tumors with pathological correlation. J Comput Assist Tomogr 1983;7:857–865

Levine E, Huntrakoon M, Wetzel LH: Malignant nerve-sheath neoplasms in neurofibromatosis: distinction from benign tumors by using imaging techniques. AJR Am J Roentgenol 1987;149:1059–1064

Lin F, Martel W: Cross-sectional imaging of peripheral nerve sheath tumors: characteristic signs on CT, MR imaging, and sonography. AJR Am J Roentgenol 2001;176:75–82

Mandell GA, Herrick WC, Harcke HT, et al: Neurofibromas: location by scanning with Tc-99m DTPA. Work in progress. Radiology 1985;157:803–806

Ros PR, Eshaghi N: Plexiform neurofibroma of the pelvis: CT and MRI findings. Magn Reson Imaging 1991;9:463–465

Schultz E, Sapan MR, McHeffey-Atkinson B, et al: Case report 872: "ancient" schwannoma (degenerated neurilemoma). Skeletal Radiol 1994;23:593–595

Stull MA, Moser RP, Kransdorf MJ, et al: Magnetic resonance appearance of peripheral nerve sheath tumors. Skeletal Radiol 1991;20:9–14

Suh J-S, Abenoza P, Galloway HR, et al: Peripheral (extracranial) nerve tumors: correlation of MR imaging and histologic findings. Radiology 1992;183:341–346

Varma DGK, Moulopoulos A, Sara AS, et al: MR imaging of extracranial nerve sheath tumors. J Comput Assist Tomogr 1992;16:448–453

Lipoblastoma and Liposarcoma

Al-Qattan MM, Weinberg M, Clarke HM: Two rapidly growing fatty tumors of the upper limb in children: lipoblastoma and infiltrating lipoma. J Hand Surg Am 1995;20:20–23

Arkun R, Memis A, Akalin T, et al: Liposarcoma of soft tissue: MRI findings with pathologic correlation. Skeletal Radiol 1997;26:167–172

Castleberry RP, Kelly DR, Wilson ER, et al: Childhood liposarcoma: report of a case and review of the literature. Cancer 1984;54:579–584

Chung EB, Enzinger FM: Benign lipoblastomatosis: an analysis of 35 cases. Cancer 1973;32:482–492

Collins MH, Chatten J: Lipoblastoma/lipoblastomatosis: a clinicopathologic study of 25 tumors. Am J Surg Pathol 1997;21:1131–1137

Cowling MG, Holmes SJK, Adam EJ: Benign chest wall lipoblastoma of infancy producing underlying bone enlargement. Pediatr Radiol 1995;25:54–55

Dewit L, Albus-Lutter CE, De Jong ASH, et al: Malignant schwannoma with a rhabdomyoblastic component, a so-called triton tumor. Cancer 1986;58:1350–1356

Fisher MF, Fletcher BD, Dahms BB, et al: Abdominal lipoblastomatosis: radiographic, echographic, and computed tomographic findings. Radiology 1981;138:593–596

Gilbert TJ, Goswitz JJ, Teynor JT, et al: Lipoblastoma of the foot. Skeletal Radiol 1996;25:283–286

Katz DS, Merchant N, Beaulieu CF, et al: Lipoblastoma of the thigh: MR appearance. J Comput Assist Tomogr 1996;20:1002–1003

Miller GG, Yanchar NL, Magee JF: Tumor karyotype differentiates lipoblastoma from liposarcoma. J Pediatr Surg 1997;32:1771–1772

Shmookler BM, Enzinger FM: Liposarcoma occurring in children: an analysis of 17 cases and review of the literature. Cancer 1983;52:567–574

Rhabdomyosarcoma

Arndt CAS, Crist WM: Common musculoskeletal tumors of childhood and adolescence. N Engl J Med 1999;341:342–352

Cogswell A, Howman-Giles R, Bergin M: Bone and gallium scintigraphy in children with rhabdomyosarcoma: a 10-year review. Med Pediatr Oncol 1994;22:15–21

Gehan EA, Glover FN, Maurer HM: Prognostic factors in children with rhabdomyosarcoma. Natl Cancer Inst Monogr 1981;56:83–92

Maurer HM: The intergroup rhabdomyosarcoma study: update, November 1978. Natl Cancer Inst Monogr 1981;56:61–68

Shapeero LG, Couanet D, Vanel D, et al: Bone metastases as the presenting manifestation of rhabdomyosarcoma in childhood. Skeletal Radiol 1993;22:433–438

Primitive Peripheral Neuroectodermal Tumor

Askin FB, Rosai J, Sibley RK, et al: Malignant small cell tumor of the thoracopulmonary region in childhood: a distinctive clinicopathologic entity of uncertain histogenesis. Cancer 1979;43:2438–2451

Dehner LP: Primitive neuroectodermal tumor and Ewing's sarcoma. Am J Surg Pathol 1993;17:1–13

Ibarburen C, Haberman JJ, Zerhouni EA: Peripheral primitive neuroectodermal tumors: CT and MRI evaluation. Eur J Radiol 1996;21:225–232

Kushner BH, Hajdu SI, Gulati SC, et al: Extracranial primitive neuroectodermal tumors: the Memorial Sloan-Kettering Cancer Center experience. Cancer 1991;67:1825–1829

Schmidt D, Herrmann C, Jürgens H, et al: Malignant peripheral neuroectodermal tumor and its necessary distinction from Ewing's sarcoma. Cancer 1991;68:2251–2259

Synovial Sarcoma

Blacksin MF, Siegel JR, Benevenia J, et al: Synovial sarcoma: frequency of non-aggressive MR characteristics. J Comput Assist Tomogr 1997;21:785–789

Cadman NL, Soule EH, Kelly PJ: Synovial sarcoma: an analysis of 134 tumors. Cancer 1965;18:613–627

Jones BC, Sundaram S, Kransdorf MJ: Synovial sarcoma: MR imaging findings in 34 patients. AJR Am J Roentgenol 1993;161:827–830

Mahajan H, Lorigan JG, Shirkhoda A: Synovial sarcoma: MR imaging. Magn Rason Imaging 1989;7:211–216

Morton MJ, Berquist TH, McLeod RA, et al: MR imaging of synovial sarcoma. AJR Am J Roentgenol 1991;156:337–340

Scully RE, Mark EJ, McNealy WF, et al: Case records of the Massachusetts General Hospital: weekly clinicopathological exercises. case 1-2001: a 26-year-old man with a mass in the knee. N Engl J Med 2001;344:124–131

Fibrosarcoma

Boon LM, Fishman SJ, Lund DP, et al: Congenital fibrosarcoma masquerading as congenital hemangioma: report of two cases. J Pediatr Surg 1995;30:1378–1381

Dahlin DC: Case report 189: infantile fibrosarcoma (congenital fibrosarcoma-like fibromatosis). Skeletal Radiol 1982;8:77–78

Exelby PR, Knapper WH, Huvos AG, et al: Soft-tissue fibrosarcoma in children. J Pediatr Surg 1973;8:415–420

Lee MJ, Cairns RA, Munk PL, et al: Musculoskeletal radiology: congenital-infantile fibrosarcoma: magnetic resonance imaging findings. Can Assoc Radiol J 1996;47:121–125

Lilleng PK, Monge OR, Walløe A, et al: Fibrosarcoma in children. Acta Oncol 1997;36:438–440

Ninane J, Gosseye S, Panteon E, et al: Congenital fibrosarcoma: preoperative chemotherapy and conservative surgery. Cancer 1986; 58:1400–1406

Soule EH, Pritchard DJ: Fibrosarcoma in infants and children: a review of 110 cases. Cancer 1977;40:1711–1721

Alveolar Soft Part Sarcoma

Aluigi P, Sangiorgi L, Picci P: Alveolar soft part sarcoma. Skeletal Radiol 1996;25:400–402

Foschini MP, Eusebi V: Alveolar soft-part sarcoma: a new type of rhabdomyosarcoma? Semin Diagn Pathol 1994;11:58–68

Iwamoto Y, Morimoto N, Chuman H, et al: The role of MR imaging in the diagnosis of alveolar soft part sarcoma: a report of 10 cases. Skeletal Radiol 1995;24:276–270

Lorigan JG, O'Keeffe FN, Evans HL, et al: The radiologic manifestations of alveolar soft-part sarcoma. AJR Am J Roentgenol 1989;153: 335–339

Pang LM, Roebuck DJ, Griffith JF, et al: Alveolar soft-part sarcoma: a rare soft-tissue malignancy with distinctive clinical and radiological features. Pediatr Radiol 2001;31:196–199

Temple HT, Scully SP, O'Keefe RJ, et al: Clinical presentation of alveolar soft-part sarcoma. Clin Orthop 1994;300:213–218

Sciot R, Cin PD, De Vos R, et al: Alveolar soft-part sarcoma: evidence for its myogenic origin and for the involvement of 17q25. Histopathology 1993;23:439–444

Malignant Fibrous Histiocytoma

Lin WY, Kao CH, Hsu CY, et al: The role of Tc-99m MDP and Ga-67 imaging in the clinical evaluation of malignant fibrous histiocytoma. Clin Nucl Med 1994;19:996–1000

Mahajan H, Kim EE, Wallace S, et al: Magnetic resonance imaging of malignant fibrous histiocytoma. Magn Reson Imaging 1989;7: 283–288

Munk PL, Sallomi DF, Janzen DL, et al: Malignant fibrous histiocytoma of soft tissue imaging with emphasis on MRI. J Comput Assist Tomogr 1998;22:819–826

Panicek DM, Casper ES, Brennan MF, et al: Hemorrhage simulating tumor growth in malignant fibrous histiocytoma at MR imaging. Radiology 1991;181:398–400

Raney RB Jr, Allen A, O'Neill J, et al: Malignant fibrous histiocytoma of soft tissue in childhood. Cancer 1986;57:2198–2201

Ros PR, Viamonte M Jr, Rywlin AM: Malignant fibrous histiocytoma: mesenchymal tumor of ubiquitous origin. AJR Am J Roentgenol 1984;142:753–759

Tracy T Jr, Neifeld JP, DeMay RM, et al: Malignant fibrous histiocytomas in children. J Pediatr Surg 1984;19:81–83

Epithelioid Sarcoma

Gross E, Rao BN, Pappo A, et al: Epithelioid sarcoma in children. J Pediatr Surg 1996;31:1663–1665

Hanley SD, Alexander N, Henderson DW, et al: Epithelioid sarcoma of the forearm. Australas Radiol 1996;40:254–256

Hanna SL, Kaste S, Jenkins JJ, et al: Epithelioid sarcoma: clinical, MR imaging and pathologic findings. Skeletal Radiol 2002;31:400–412

Romero JA, Kim EE, Moral IS: MR characteristics of epithelioid sarcoma. J Comput Assist Tomogr 1994;18:929–931

von Hochstetter AR, Cserhati MD: Epithelioid sarcoma presenting as chronic synovitis and mistaken for osteosarcoma. Skeletal Radiol 1995;23:636–638

Yamato M, Nishimura G, Yamaguchi T, et al: Epithelioid sarcoma with unusual radiological findings. Skeletal Radiol 1997;26:606–610

Disseminated Disease of Soft Tissue

Eustace S, Winalski CS, McGowen A, et al: Skeletal muscle lymphoma: observations at MR imaging. Skeletal Radiol 1996;23:425–430

Lee VS, Martinez S, Coleman RE: Primary muscle lymphoma: clinical and imaging findings. Radiology 1997;203:237–244

Malloy PC, Fishman EK, Magid D: Lymphoma of bone, muscle, and skin: CT findings. AJR Am J Roentgenol 1992;159:805–809

Metzler JP, Fleckenstein JL, Vuitch F, et al: Skeletal muscle lymphoma: MRI evaluation. Magn Reson Imaging 1992;10:491–494

Schultz SR, Bree RL, Schwab RE, et al: CT detection of skeletal muscle metastases. J Comput Assist Tomogr 1986;10:81–83

Williams JB, Youngberg RA, Bui-Mansfield LT, et al: MR imaging of skeletal muscle metastases. AJR Am J Roentgenol 1997;168: 555–557

PART III

THE BONES: NORMAL AND VARIANTS

THEODORE E. KEATS
BARRY D. FLETCHER

Chapter 1

NORMAL ANATOMY, GROWTH AND DEVELOPMENT

THEODORE E. KEATS

NORMAL STRUCTURE

In the limbs, there are three kinds of bones: the long and short tubular bones; the round bones in the wrists and ankles; and the sesamoids, small bones in the tendons and articular capsules. Functionally, a growing tubular bone is made up of four segments: the diaphysis, the epiphysis, the physis, and the metaphysis (Fig. 1). Long bones have epiphyses at both ends; short tubular bones have epiphyses at one end, generally where the greater joint motion of the individual bone occurs. Apparent epiphyseal ossification centers at the ends of short bones where their occurrence is not expected are termed *pseudoepiphyses* (see Section IX, Part III, Chapter 2, Fig. 8, page 2057). Bones provide a rigid support for the body and sites of insertion for muscles, to which they respond as levers. They are active physiologically in the infant

2035

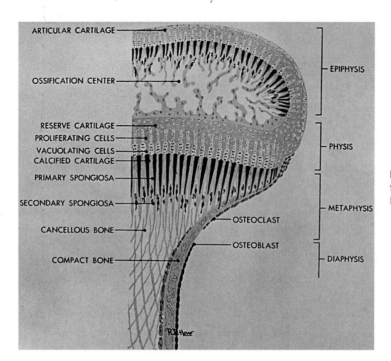

ARTICULAR CARTILAGE

OSSIFICATION CENTER

RESERVE CARTILAGE
PROLIFERATING CELLS
VACUOLATING CELLS
CALCIFIED CARTILAGE
PRIMARY SPONGIOSA
SECONDARY SPONGIOSA
CANCELLOUS BONE
COMPACT BONE

OSTEOCLAST
OSTEOBLAST

EPIPHYSIS
PHYSIS
METAPHYSIS
DIAPHYSIS

FIGURE 1. Functional components of the growing end of a tubular bone and their anatomic substrate, according to Rubin.

and child, changing size and shape with growth and in response to mechanical stresses, and at all ages serve as a reservoir of calcium for body needs.

The diaphysis, or shaft, of a tubular bone consists of a central cavity and a cortical wall. The central cavity (medullary cavity) contains blood-forming marrow during growth; cancellous bone (spongiosa) closes the medullary cavity at the epiphyseal ends, and a thin layer of spongy bone lines the inner surface of the cortex. The diaphysis is covered externally by a cellular and fibrous envelope, the periosteum. This is composed of an inner layer of osteoblasts and an outer layer of densely packed collagenous fibers parallel to its long axis. The inner layer deposits subperiosteal bone on the outer surface of the cortex, increasing the girth of the diaphysis. The periosteum is bound to the cortex by its perpendicular fibers (Sharpey's fibers), which are less numerous and shorter in children than in adults and are thus less effective as binding agents in young bones. Resorption of the internal surface of the cortex accounts for expansion of the medullary cavity during growth. The balance between subperiosteal apposition of bone and endosteal resorption is largely responsible for the thickness of the cortex. Except during adolescence, when endosteal apposition contributes to cortical thickness and narrows the medullary cavity, the medullary cavity widens progressively during childhood.

The epiphyses are terminal remnants of the original cartilaginous models of the bone. They are bounded by articular cartilage where a bone articulates with an adjacent bone, and by the physis, which unites the epiphysis to the metaphysis. Longitudinal growth takes place at the junction of the physis and metaphysis by proliferation of cartilage cells in the physis, calcification of their surrounding matrix, and transformation to bone through the activity of metaphyseal vessels and accompanying osteoblasts and osteoclasts. Ossification

centers develop within the epiphyses; growth ceases when these secondary centers fuse, through the physis, with the metaphysis.

Apophyses are outgrowths of a bone that have never been entirely separated from the bone of which they form a part; they frequently arise where muscle tendons insert and develop ossification centers within them that fuse with the main body of the bone, but they do not contribute to the longitudinal growth as do the epiphyses.

The components of a long tubular bone are shown in Figure 2.

RADIOGRAPHIC APPEARANCE

Calcified portions of growing bone cast opaque shadows of calcium density; noncalcified components cast shadows of lesser density comparable to that of other noncalcified tissues apart from fat (Fig. 3). The overall density of a bone is provided almost exclusively by the cortical bone; the medullary spicules (spongiosa) are poorly visible except in the ends of the bones or in disorders in which there is excess trabecular bone. Their visibility is increased in the presence of osteomalacia, in which thick trabeculae remain faintly visible while thin trabeculae become invisible, as in rickets. Channels in bone for nutrient vessels may present as focal defects in specific areas (Figs. 4 and 5).

GROWTH AND MATURATION

Near the end of the second month of fetal life, the embryonal cartilaginous skeleton has already been subdivided into its principal segments, which are the forerunners of the bones of the limbs. Primary ossification centers are formed by deposition of calcium in the cartilaginous matrix following hypertrophy and vacuolization of local cartilage cells. In the tubular bones, this occurs at approximately the midpoint of the shaft and is followed by central resorption, giving rise to the primary marrow cavity. The calcified disks proximal and distal to the primary cavity become the preparatory zones of calcification and follow the development of the advancing, proliferating shaft during growth. Cartilage proximal and distal to the zones of calcification becomes the epiphyses. A layer of cells in the epiphyses near the shaft produces new cells that are interposed between the resting cartilage of the epiphysis and the older cells and calcified cartilage adjacent to the shaft. The matrix around the old cells calcifies and becomes invaded by capillaries and bone cells from the marrow. Bone is formed on the calcified cartilage and both new bone and cartilage undergo remodeling by osteoclasts and osteoblasts so that the length of the bone is increased

(Fig. 6). The girth of the bone and the thickness of the cortex are increased by subperiosteal accretion resulting from activity of subperiosteal osteoblasts. Peripheral resorption of bone at the advancing ends of the shaft maintains the gentle flaring that characterizes a normal tubular bone and is the mechanism responsible for what is termed *modeling*. Disproportionate osteoclastic activity within the shaft of the bone reams out a marrow cavity. Continued, balanced activity of all these processes permits a small tubular bone to become a large tubular bone while maintaining the same functional shape and relations with adjacent structures.

Secondary ossification centers appear in the cartilaginous epiphyses and enlarge by similar but much slower processes than those enlarging the shaft. Tubular bones that have secondary centers at both ends are, by convention, known as "long bones" and those with a center at only one end are known as "short bones." In the hands and feet, secondary ossification centers

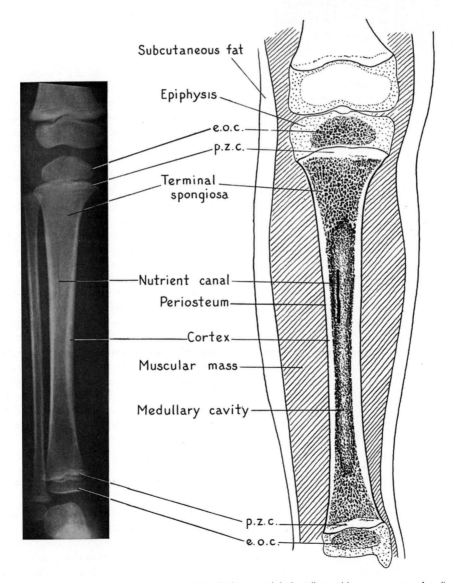

Subcutaneous fat
Epiphysis
e.o.c.
p.z.c.
Terminal spongiosa
Nutrient canal
Periosteum
Cortex
Muscular mass
Medullary cavity
p.z.c.
e.o.c.

FIGURE 2. The macroscopic components of a normal tubular bone and their radiographic counterparts. A radiograph and the longitudinal section of the right tibia of a child 2 years of age. *e.o.c.* = epiphyseal ossification center; *p.z.c.* = provisional zone of calcification and cartilage plate.

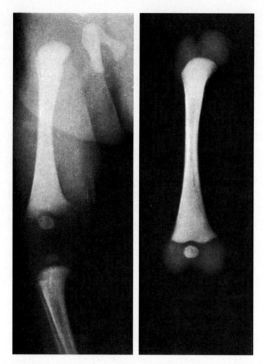

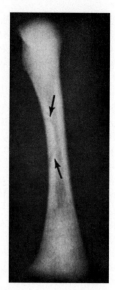

FIGURE 5. Double canals through the posteromedial cortical wall of the femur carry the nutrient arteries in a normal newly born infant.

FIGURE 3. Femur of a stillborn term infant in situ and surrounded by air following dissection. The water-density cartilage is clearly delineated when surrounded by air, although it is obscured by the contiguous water-density soft tissue structures in situ. The four basic densities in conventional radiographs are, in increasing order, air, fat, water, and bone.

appear in the bases of the phalanges and in the distal ends of metacarpals and metatarsals 2 through 5. The epiphyses for the first metacarpal and first metatarsal are found in the proximal ends of the bones. The location of the secondary centers appears to be related to the sites of maximal joint motion of the individual bones. In marine mammals with flippers, secondary ossification centers occur at both ends of the metacarpals and phalanges. Irregularities of density and discontinuities of structure are normally frequent during mineralization of these centers and simulate the features of disease. The ages of children at first appearance of these ossification centers are known within limits and serve as indicators of physical maturation (Table 1).

During the period of growth, in addition to its constant increase in length and breadth, the shaft is being continuously molded or reshaped to produce its final form. The mechanism responsible for these changes in shape has been called modeling or tubulation. One of the most conspicuous features of modeling is the progressive concentric contraction of the shaft behind the wider advancing terminal segment (Fig. 7) that results in the flared ends of the bones. Significant disturbances in configuration of the shafts occur in many of the diseases affecting the growing skeleton.

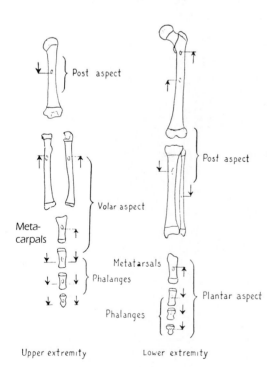

FIGURE 4. Schematic representation of the position of nutrient canals in the long bones. (Modified from Hodges PC: Am J Roentgenol Radium Ther 1933;30:800–810.)

VELOCITY OF GROWTH AND DEVELOPMENT

Ultrasound measurement of the fetal femur during pregnancy is usually reliable for estimation of fetal age (Table 2), and can be supplemented by demonstration of ossification centers in the fetal calcaneus (24th week), talus (26th week), distal femur (32nd week), and proximal tibia (37th week), as well as by biparietal diameters. If gestational age is known, the measurements may identify growth disturbances such as dwarfism. Abnormal fetal dimensions and configurations may help identify specific skeletal dysplasias, such as achondroplasia or osteogenesis imperfecta, as well as malformation syndromes. In the former, bones may be abnormally short, or initially only mildly short with subsequent inappropriate growth. During infancy and childhood, serial examinations are necessary to ascertain velocity of growth and development, but evaluation of films of the limbs is adequate to identify the state of development of the skeletal structures, which reflect, fairly accurately, the general status of the child. Hernandez and associates reported a method for assessment in the first 2 years of life with a single lateral radiograph of the foot and ankle, evaluating five separate centers for both size and shape. If the reliability they observed can be confirmed by

other studies, the technique may provide a relatively simple means of bone age assessment in early life. Lengths of tubular bones, on films obtained by use of techniques developed for these purposes, can be evaluated from tables listing age standards (Table 3). The values are sex dependent. The observations of bone lengths are useful for identification of growth disturbances, in planning surgery in cases of limb length discrepancy, and in many other circumstances. Moseley converted standards from orthoroentgenograms (scanograms) to a nomogram on which measurements from serial lower limb scanograms can be plotted. Optimal times for epiphyseodesis to correct a discrepancy are easily determined using his straight-line graph. Bone age rather than chronologic age is used as a reference point for surgical procedures.

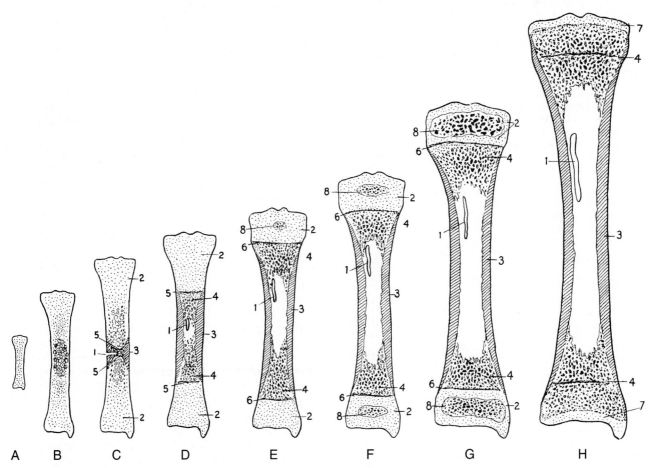

FIGURE 6. Schema of the progressive stages in the growth and maturation of the tibia. **A,** The mass of embryonal cartilage that is the anlage of the tibia. **B,** Initial enlargement and multiplication of the central cartilage cells and an increase in cartilaginous matrix, the chondrification center that is the forerunner of the primary ossification center. **C,** The early primary ossification center showing the formation of a central belt of subperiosteal bone (early cortex) and penetration of the cartilaginous matrix by the periosteal elements; the channel of this penetration persists as the nutrient canal. **D,** Extension of ossification toward both ends of the shaft, with central resorption to form the medullary cavity. **E,** The tibia at birth, with a secondary ossification center in the proximal epiphyseal cartilage. **F,** At approximately the fourth postnatal month, there are ossification centers in both of the epiphyseal cartilages. **G,** Juvenile tibia showing the growth of all components and enlargement of the epiphyseal secondary ossification centers. **H,** Adult tibia, with complete fusion of the shaft and both epiphyses. The narrow plates of articular cartilage that cap each end of the bone persist throughout life. *1,* nutrient canal; *2,* epiphyseal cartilage; *3,* corticalis; *4,* spongiosa; *5* and *6,* provisional zones of calcification or epiphyseal plates; *7,* articular cartilages; *8,* secondary epiphyseal ossification centers. (Modified from an original drawing by W.M. Rogers, M.D.)

Table 1 ■ AGE-AT-APPEARANCE PERCENTILES FOR MAJOR POSTNATAL OSSIFICATION CENTERS

| | PERCENTILES* | | | | | |
| | Boys | | | Girls | | |
OSSIFICATION CENTER	5th	50th	95th	5th	50th	95th
Head of humerus	37g	2w	4m	37g	2w	3m3
Proximal epiphysis of tibia	34g	2w	5w	34g	1w	2w
Coracoid process of scapula	37g	2w	4m2	37g	2w	5m
Cuboid of tarsus	37g	3w	3m3	37g	3w	2m
Capitate of carpus	—	3m	7m	—	2m	7m
Hamate of carpus	2w	3m3	10m	2w	2ml	7m
Capitulum of humerus	3w	4m	13m	3w	3m	9ml
Head of femur	3w	4ml	7m3	2w	4m	7m2
Third cuneiform of tarsus	3w	5m2	19m	—	2m3	14m3
Greater tubercle of humerus	3m	10m	2y4	2m2	6ml	13m3
Primary center, middle segment of 5th toe	—	12m2	3y10	—	9m	2y1
Distal epiphysis of radius	6m2	12m1	2y4	4m3	10m	20m2
Epiphysis, distal segment of 1st toe	8m2	12m3	2y1	4m3	9m2	20m1
Epiphysis, middle segment of 4th toe	5m	14m3	2y11	5m	11m	3y
Epiphysis, proximal segment of 3d finger	9m1	16m2	2y5	5m	10m1	19m2
Epiphysis, middle segment of 3d toe	5m	17m	4y3	2m3	12m1	2y6
Epiphysis, proximal segment of 2d finger	9m2	17m	2y2	5m	10m2	19m3
Epiphysis, proximal segment of 4th finger	9m3	18m	2y5	5m	11m	20m
Epiphysis, distal segment of 1st finger	9m	17m1	2y8	5m	12m	20m3
Epiphysis, proximal segment of 3d toe	11m	19m	2y6	6m1	12m3	22m3
Epiphysis of 2d metacarpal	11m1	19m2	2y10	7m3	13m	20m1
Epiphysis, proximal segment of 4th toe	11m2	19m3	2y8	7m2	15m	2y1
Epiphysis, proximal segment of 2d toe	11m3	21m	2y8	7m3	14m2	2y1
Epiphysis of 3d metacarpal	11m2	21m2	3y	8m	13m2	23m1
Epiphysis, proximal segment of 5th finger	12m	22m1	2y10	8m	14m2	2y1
Epiphysis, middle segment of 3d finger	12m1	2y	3y4	7m3	15m2	2y4
Epiphysis of 4th metacarpal	13m	2y	3y7	9m	15m2	2y2
Epiphysis, middle segment of 2d toe	10m3	2y1	4y1	6m	14m1	2y3
Epiphysis, middle segment of 4th finger	12m	2y1	3y3	7m3	15m	2y5
Epiphysis of 5th metacarpal	15m1	2y2	3y10	10m2	16m2	2y4
First cuneiform of tarsus	10m3	2y2	3y9	6m	17m1	2y10
Epiphysis of 1st metatarsal	16m3	2y2	3y1	11m3	19m	2y3
Epiphysis, middle segment of 2d finger	15m3	2y2	3y4	8m	17m2	2y7
Epiphysis, proximal segment of 1st toe	17m2	2y4	3y4	10m3	18m3	2y5
Epiphysis, distal segment of 3d finger	15m3	2y5	3y9	8m3	17m3	2y8
Triquetrum of carpus	6m	2y5	5y6	3m2	20m2	3y9
Epiphysis, distal segment of 4th finger	16m2	2y5	3y9	8m3	18m1	2y10
Epiphysis, proximal segment of 5th toe	18m2	2y6	3y8	11m3	20m3	2y8
Epiphysis of 1st metacarpal	17m2	2y7	4y4	11m	19m1	2y8
Second cuneiform of tarsus	14m2	2y8	4y3	9m3	21m3	3y
Epiphysis of 2d metatarsal	23m1	2y10	4y4	14m3	2y2	3y5
Greater trochanter of femur	23m	3y	4y4	11m2	22m1	3y
Epiphysis, proximal segment of 1st finger	22m1	3y	4y7	11m1	20m2	2y10
Navicular of tarsus	13m2	3y	5y5	9m1	23m1	3y7
Epiphysis, distal segment of 2d finger	21m3	3y2	5y	12m3	2y6	3y4
Epiphysis, distal segment of 5th finger	2y1	3y4	5y	12m	23m3	3y6
Epiphysis, middle segment of 5th finger	23m1	3y5	5y10	10m3	23m3	3y7
Proximal epiphysis of fibula	22m2	3y6	5y3	16m	2y7	3y11
Epiphysis of 3d metatarsal	2y4	3y6	5y	17m1	2y6	3y8
Epiphysis, distal segment of 5th toe	2y4	3y11	6y4	14m1	2y4	4y1
Patella of knee	2y6	4y	6y	17m3	2y6	4y
Epiphysis of 4th metatarsal	2y11	4y	5y9	21m1	2y10	4y1
Lunate of carpus	18m2	4y1	6y9	13m	2y8	5y8
Epiphysis, distal segment of 3d toe	3y	4y4	6y2	16m2	2y9	4y1
Epiphysis of 5th metatarsal	3y1	4y5	6y4	2y1	3y3	4y11
Epiphysis, distal segment of 4th toe	2y11	4y5	6y5	16m2	2y7	4y1
Epiphysis, distal segment of 2d toe	3y3	4y8	6y9	18m	2y11	4y6
Capitulum of radius	3y	5y3	8y	2y3	3y11	6y3
Scaphoid of carpus	3y7	5y8	7y10	2y4	4y1	6y
Greater multangular of carpus	3y7	5y11	9y	23m1	4y1	6y4
Lesser multangular of carpus	3y1	6y3	8y6	2y5	4y2	6y
Medial epicondyle of humerus	4y3	6y3	8y5	2y1	3y5	5y1
Distal epiphysis of ulna	5y3	7y1	9y1	3y4	5y5	7y8

Table continued on opposite page

Table 1 ■ AGE-AT-APPEARANCE PERCENTILES FOR MAJOR POSTNATAL OSSIFICATION CENTERS *Continued*

OSSIFICATION CENTER	Boys 5th	Boys 50th	Boys 95th	Girls 5th	Girls 50th	Girls 95th
Epiphysis of calcaneus	5y2	7y7	9y7	3y7	5y5	7y4
Olecranon of ulna	7y9	9y8	11y11	5y8	8y	9y11
Lateral epicondyle of humerus	9y3	11y3	13y8	7y2	9y3	11y3
Tubercle of tibia	9y11	11y10	13y5	7y11	10y3	11y10
Adductor sesamoid of 1st finger	11y	12y9	14y8	8y8	10y9	12y8
Acetabulum	11y11	13y7	15y4	9y7	11y6	13y5
Acromion	12y2	13y9	15y6	10y4	11y11	13y10
Epiphysis, iliac crest of hip	12y	14y	15y11	10y10	12y10	15y4
Accessory epiphysis, coracoid process of scapula	12y9	14y4	16y4	10y5	12y3	14y5
Ischial tuberosity	13y7	15y3	17y1	11y9	13y11	16y

*g = gestational week; w = week; m = month; y = year. Number following m or y refers to next smaller time unit (e.g., 9y4 = 9 years, 4 months).
From Garn SM, et al: Med Radiogr Photogr 1967;43:45–66, with permission.

It is well established that the quantities of longitudinal growth derived from the two ends of a tubular bone are unequal. In the arm, the ends of the bones at the elbow grow less than their counterparts at the shoulder and wrist; in the leg, those at the knee grow more than those at the hip and ankle. It is not certain that the rates of growth at specific sites maintain constant relations throughout childhood.

Growth in girth of tubular bones, and thickness in flat bones, takes place through a process that involves addition and removal of bone at the external and internal surfaces, respectively. Garn and associates have provided considerable data with respect to cortical bone thickness and medullary width of the second metacarpal bone as an indication of bone gain and loss in the remainder of the skeleton (Table 4). Measurement is made at midshaft with a pinpoint micrometer caliper or a 6× to 8×

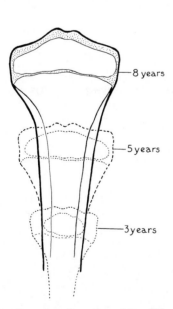

FIGURE 7. Growth and configuration of the tibia with advancing age. The progressive concentric constriction of the shaft away from the wider epiphyseal plate is shown schematically in superimposed tracings of radiographs.

8 years

5 years

3 years

magnifier eye-piece with a scale calibrated to 0.1 mm (Fig. 8). The cortical thickness (C) is obtained by subtracting the medullary width (M) from the total width (T) at the level measured. Cortical area $(0.785[T^2 - M^2])$ and percent cortical area $([T^2 - M^2]/[T^2] \times 100)$ are more sensitive indicators of the bone thickness. These techniques are adequate for clinical use, but much more exact information on bone density is provided by dual-energy x-ray absorptiometry and quantitative computed tomography methods. This subject is discussed in Section IX, Part VII, Chapter 1, page 2232.

Measurement of metacarpal and phalangeal lengths (metacarpophalangeal pattern profile analysis), as described by Poznanski et al., may be useful in the diagnosis of dysmorphic syndromes. The plus or minus deviations of the measurements from the mean values for age and sex are displayed on a graph (Figs. 9 and 10). The shape of the curve thus formed tends to be consistent in certain disorders and can be diagnostic in cases equivocal by other criteria. Standards for metacarpal and phalangeal lengths are shown in Table 5.

Evaluation of the number, size, and configuration of secondary ossification centers (bone age) is used to estimate biologic maturation relative to chronologic age. Various techniques and standards are available and are generally in agreement, but the procedure to follow for each must be adhered to carefully at each examination and, especially, in sequential examinations. The range of values is great even in premature infants (Table 6).

The possibility of evaluating maturity by radiographic techniques was explored in the first years after the discovery of x-rays, both by Lambertz and by other investigators in Europe and America. Subsequently, longitudinal growth studies were mounted in the United States and elsewhere. With the increased realization, in the mid-1950s, that medically unnecessary radiation should be avoided, serial radiographic examinations of study populations were discontinued, and later studies of skeletal maturation have utilized cross-sectional methods. Thus, current standards for sequential skeletal maturation in individual children are based on exami-

Table 2 ■ MEAN PRENATAL FEMORAL LENGTH (MM) IN RELATION TO GESTATIONAL AGE

GESTA-TIONAL AGE (WK)	O'BRIEN & QUEENAN	JEANTRY ET AL.	HADLOCK ET AL.*	
			A	B
14	17	16	19	15
15	20	19	21	18
16	22	23	23	21
17	25	26	26	24
18	30	30	28	27
19	32	33	30	30
20	35	36	33	33
21	38	39	35	36
22	41	42	38	39
23	44	45	40	42
24	46	48	42	44
25	48	51	45	47
26	51	54	47	49
27	53	57	49	52
28	54	59	52	54
29	57	62	54	56
30	59	65	57	58
31	62	67	59	61
32	63	70	61	63
33	65	72	64	65
34	66	74	66	66
35	68	77	69	68
36	70	79	71	70
37	71	81	73	72
38	72	83	76	73
39	74	85	78	75
40	75	87	80	76

*Calculated from raw data by two separate methods.
Data from O'Brien and Queenan (1981), Jeantry et al. (1981), and Hadlock et al. (1982).

nations dating from approximately 25 to more than 50 years earlier, and do not address secular trends, which have been in the direction of earlier maturity and larger size. The patients whose hand films were used for the Todd and the Greulich and Pyle atlases were born between 1917 and 1942, according to Roche. The continued reliability of the Greulich and Pyle standards derives from the fact that the children in the Cleveland Brush Foundation Study came from above-average socioeconomic environments and therefore were advanced in relation to other children not so fortunately situated. The British children studied by Acheson were born between 1946 and 1953. The standardizing group of Tanner and Whitehouse and associates included approximately 2200 children studied cross-sectionally dating from the 1950s and 1960s, and 500 children studied longitudinally between 1952 and 1972. Other cross-sectional investigations, such as the Health Examination Surveys of 1963–1965 and 1966–1970, have provided more recent data. The unisex standards of Pyle, Waterhouse, and Greulich used to evaluate bone age in this study, however, were drawn from the same Brush Foundation material as were the Todd and Greulich and Pyle atlases. Notwithstanding the limitations related to sex, race, geographic location, and socioeconomic factors, serial evaluation of bone maturation with the use of appropriate standards, in a consistent fashion, can provide helpful information in the evaluation of children with medical problems affecting growth and development. None of the standards apply to patients with skeletal dysplasias.

The hand, with its numerous secondary centers in

Text continued on page 2052

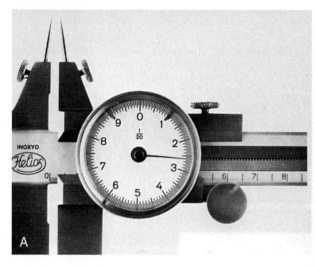

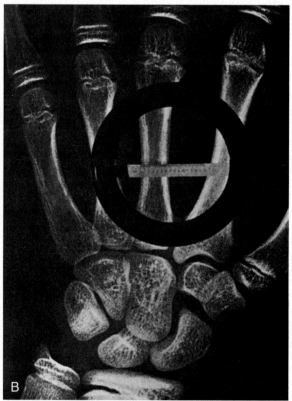

FIGURE 8. Apparatus used to measure cortical thickness of metacarpal bones. **A,** Caliper (Garn). **B,** Calibrated magnifying lens (Bonnard).

Table 3 ■ LINEAR GROWTH OF LONG BONES OF LIMBS FROM INFANCY THROUGH ADOLESCENCE

BOYS—SMOOTHED PERCENTILES AND OBSERVED RANGE FOR ROENTGENOGRAPHIC BONE LENGTHS (CM)
A. ARM BONES

Age (yr-mo)	Humerus 10%	25%	50%	75%	90%	Range	Radius 10%	25%	50%	75%	90%	Range	Ulna 10%	25%	50%	75%	90%	Range

Measurements Between Epiphyseal Plates

Age (yr-mo)	Humerus 10%	25%	50%	75%	90%	Range	Radius 10%	25%	50%	75%	90%	Range	Ulna 10%	25%	50%	75%	90%	Range
0-2	6.68	7.02	7.28	7.47	7.65	6.3–7.9	5.54	5.68	5.85	6.16	6.30	5.4–6.4	6.29	6.48	6.66	6.89	7.04	6.1–7.2
0-4	7.43	7.78	8.05	8.29	8.52	7.3–9.0	6.14	6.29	6.52	6.70	6.95	6.1–7.0	6.82	7.04	7.22	7.42	7.61	6.8–7.8
0-6	8.13	8.50	8.80	9.06	9.33	7.8–9.4	6.60	6.76	7.02	7.24	7.51	6.4–7.9	7.31	7.55	7.71	7.95	8.22	7.0–8.7
1-0	9.91	10.25	10.48	10.77	11.20	9.4–11.6	7.68	7.86	8.17	8.42	8.73	7.6–9.3	8.63	8.85	9.08	9.35	9.69	8.5–10.3
1-6	11.25	11.58	11.84	12.12	12.58	11.0–12.8	8.53	8.73	9.06	9.34	9.67	8.4–10.2	9.55	9.80	10.06	10.37	10.69	9.4–11.4
2-0	12.29	12.72	12.97	13.26	13.71	12.1–14.1	9.23	9.45	9.80	10.10	10.44	9.0–11.0	10.35	10.62	10.90	11.22	11.55	10.1–12.3
2-6	13.12	13.56	13.84	14.13	14.58	12.9–15.0	9.90	10.13	10.47	10.76	11.12	9.6–11.8	11.05	11.33	11.63	11.96	12.29	10.6–13.0
3-0	13.92	14.42	14.65	14.96	15.41	13.6–16.1	10.55	10.78	11.09	11.38	11.75	10.1–12.4	11.70	11.99	12.30	12.64	12.98	11.2–13.6
3-6	14.68	15.21	15.44	15.75	16.21	14.3–16.9	11.13	11.38	11.69	11.97	12.35	10.7–13.0	12.30	12.60	12.93	13.27	13.65	11.8–14.2
4-0	15.41	15.97	16.21	16.52	17.00	15.0–18.0	11.68	11.96	12.26	12.54	12.94	11.1–13.8	12.88	13.19	13.54	13.88	14.30	12.2–15.1
4-6	16.12	16.70	16.95	17.28	17.79	15.8–18.5	12.21	12.51	12.80	13.09	13.51	11.6–14.2	13.44	13.76	14.13	14.48	14.92	12.8–15.5
5-0	16.80	17.39	17.66	18.03	18.57	16.1–19.4	12.73	13.04	13.32	13.61	14.06	11.9–15.0	13.98	14.32	14.70	15.06	15.52	13.1–16.4
5-6	17.47	18.07	18.35	18.76	19.32	17.3–20.3	13.23	13.55	13.82	14.12	14.59	12.8–15.5	14.50	14.86	15.25	15.62	16.08	14.1–17.0
6-0	18.14	18.73	19.03	19.47	20.05	17.4–21.2	13.72	14.01	14.32	14.63	15.12	13.3–16.1	15.00	15.38	15.77	16.15	16.63	14.9–17.6
6-6	18.81	19.38	19.69	20.17	20.76	18.6–22.0	14.19	14.47	14.79	15.13	15.65	13.8–16.8	15.48	15.87	16.27	16.66	17.17	15.2–18.2
7-0	19.46	20.00	20.34	20.86	21.44	19.0–22.9	14.64	14.93	15.26	15.63	16.18	14.1–17.4	15.95	16.35	16.76	17.16	17.71	15.6–18.9
7-6	20.06	20.61	20.97	21.53	22.10	19.6–23.6	15.08	15.38	15.72	16.12	16.69	14.5–18.0	16.41	16.81	17.24	17.66	18.24	16.0–19.5
8-0	20.64	21.19	21.59	22.19	22.75	19.9–24.6	15.50	15.82	16.18	16.60	17.19	14.9–18.6	16.86	17.26	17.70	18.15	18.76	16.3–20.1
8-6	21.19	21.74	22.21	22.83	23.40	20.6–24.4	15.91	16.25	16.63	17.08	17.70	15.5–18.0	17.29	17.71	18.15	18.64	19.28	17.0–19.5
9-0	21.74	22.28	22.81	23.45	24.05	21.2–25.7	16.32	16.68	17.08	17.56	18.21	15.8–19.5	17.72	18.15	18.60	19.13	19.80	17.5–21.2
9-6	22.28	22.82	23.40	24.06	24.69	21.8–26.5	16.72	17.10	17.53	18.04	18.72	16.1–20.0	18.14	18.59	19.05	19.62	20.32	17.8–21.7
10-0	22.79	23.37	23.98	24.67	25.33	22.0–26.9	17.11	17.50	17.97	18.52	19.20	16.9–20.4	18.56	19.03	19.50	20.10	20.84	18.3–22.1
10-6	23.30	23.91	24.56	25.27	25.96	22.6–27.4	17.50	17.90	18.39	18.97	19.68	17.1–20.9	18.97	19.47	19.95	20.58	21.35	18.6–22.5
11-0	23.79	24.44	25.13	25.87	26.59	23.4–28.1	17.88	18.30	18.79	19.40	20.18	17.5–21.4	19.38	19.90	20.39	21.06	21.85	19.0–23.2
11-6	24.27	24.97	25.70	26.48	27.22	22.4–28.5	18.25	18.69	19.19	19.83	20.67	17.8–21.8	19.79	20.31	20.83	21.54	22.35	19.3–23.0
12-0	24.74	25.49	26.28	27.09	27.84	22.8–29.5	18.60	19.07	19.60	20.26	21.15	18.2–22.2	20.20	20.72	21.26	22.01	22.85	19.8–24.0

Measurements Including Epiphyses

Age (yr-mo)	Humerus 10%	25%	50%	75%	90%	Range	Radius 10%	25%	50%	75%	90%	Range	Ulna 10%	25%	50%	75%	90%	Range
10-0	24.67	25.31	25.87	26.83	27.58	23.6–29.2	18.42	18.90	19.28	19.85	20.60	18.0–22.2	19.26	19.72	20.27	20.89	21.67	18.9–23.2
10-6	25.12	25.78	26.40	27.37	28.13	24.3–29.8	18.85	19.30	19.71	20.32	21.10	18.4–22.7	19.74	20.21	20.78	21.44	22.27	19.1–23.8
11-0	25.59	26.29	26.98	27.98	28.78	25.0–30.7	19.28	19.71	20.14	20.84	21.63	18.9–23.1	20.23	20.71	21.31	22.01	22.89	19.5–24.4
11-6	26.09	26.83	27.60	28.63	29.48	24.0–31.0	19.73	20.13	20.60	21.39	22.23	19.0–23.7	20.74	21.23	21.86	22.62	23.55	19.8–24.8
12-0	26.62	27.40	28.26	29.33	30.23	24.2–33.3	20.18	20.60	21.11	21.97	22.86	19.4–24.5	21.26	21.76	22.43	23.28	24.32	20.5–26.6
12-6	27.20	28.00	28.98	30.08	31.03	26.8–33.7	20.66	21.09	21.66	22.58	23.53	20.1–25.1	21.81	22.32	23.05	23.99	25.15	20.6–26.9
13-0	27.88	28.70	29.75	30.88	31.88	27.5–34.0	21.16	21.63	22.26	23.23	24.23	20.5–25.0	22.38	22.94	23.71	24.76	25.93	21.6–26.4
13-6	28.69	29.53	30.58	31.75	32.80	27.6–35.1	21.68	22.22	22.96	23.96	24.98	20.7–25.6	22.98	23.63	24.43	25.56	26.68	22.5–27.4
14-0	29.55	30.47	31.48	32.70	33.80	28.5–36.1	22.23	22.90	23.74	24.77	25.80	21.2–26.3	23.62	24.34	25.18	26.33	27.40	22.8–28.2
14-6	30.45	31.43	32.42	33.62	34.59	28.9–36.6	22.85	23.63	24.45	25.39	26.47	21.7–27.1	24.30	25.07	25.94	27.05	28.09	23.5–29.0
15-0	31.40	32.30	33.20	34.38	35.30	30.0–36.6	23.53	24.30	25.13	25.93	27.03	23.4–27.5	25.05	25.82	26.64	27.65	28.72	24.8–29.6
15-6	32.00	32.87	33.87	34.95	35.93	31.0–36.7	24.14	24.84	25.62	26.35	27.46	23.5–27.8	25.68	26.45	27.18	28.10	29.18	25.8–29.8
16-0	32.40	33.33	34.42	35.45	36.43	31.7–37.2	24.52	25.20	25.97	26.66	27.78	23.5–28.4	26.08	26.80	27.57	28.45	29.54	25.3–29.9
16-6	32.72	33.65	34.79	35.84	36.82	29.8–37.8	24.79	25.45	26.20	26.90	27.99	24.5–28.9	26.36	27.05	27.87	28.68	29.82	26.0–30.6
17-0	32.92	33.87	35.02	36.12	37.10	30.4–38.3	24.95	25.59	26.32	27.05	28.14	24.5–29.6	26.50	27.22	28.05	28.85	30.01	26.0–31.1
17-6	33.07	34.04	35.16	36.33	37.28	30.4–38.3	25.00	25.64	26.38	27.14	28.25	24.5–29.6	26.55	27.30	28.14	28.95	30.12	26.0–31.1
18-0	33.17	34.15	35.28	36.46	37.42	31.0–38.7	25.02	25.66	26.42	27.20	28.32	24.5–30.1	26.58	27.34	28.20	29.00	30.17	26.0–31.6

Table continued on following page

Table 3 ■ LINEAR GROWTH OF LONG BONES OF LIMBS FROM INFANCY THROUGH ADOLESCENCE CONTINUED

BOYS—SMOOTHED PERCENTILES AND OBSERVED RANGE FOR ROENTGENOGRAPHIC BONE LENGTHS (CM)

B. LEG BONES

Age (yr-mo)	Femur 10%	25%	50%	75%	90%	Range	Tibia 10%	25%	50%	75%	90%	Range	Fibula 10%	25%	50%	75%	90%	Range
Measurements Between Epiphyseal Plates																		
0–2	7.76	8.18	8.58	8.85	9.20	7.2–9.6	6.28	6.65	6.90	7.25	7.67	6.0–8.3	5.94	6.36	6.65	7.04	7.44	5.6–8.0
0–4	9.16	9.60	10.00	10.25	10.55	8.8–10.9	7.46	7.75	7.98	8.32	8.73	7.1–8.8	7.16	7.46	7.70	8.00	8.33	6.8–8.6
0–6	10.45	10.87	11.21	11.46	11.72	10.2–12.3	8.44	8.70	8.91	9.22	9.63	8.1–10.1	8.03	8.30	8.54	8.84	9.13	7.8–9.8
1–0	12.75	13.19	13.56	13.96	14.28	12.8–14.9	10.32	10.63	10.87	11.20	11.62	9.9–12.2	9.90	10.21	10.57	10.92	11.26	9.6–11.7
1–6	14.62	15.08	15.50	15.92	16.30	14.5–16.8	11.92	12.26	12.55	12.90	13.34	11.5–13.7	11.48	11.84	12.24	12.61	13.04	11.3–13.5
2–0	16.24	16.73	17.17	17.61	18.03	15.8–18.5	13.22	13.60	13.97	14.35	14.82	13.0–15.1	12.86	13.24	13.68	14.08	14.55	12.7–15.1
2–6	17.66	18.21	18.67	19.13	19.62	16.9–20.0	14.37	14.80	15.22	15.61	16.12	14.0–16.5	14.09	14.50	14.97	15.39	15.88	13.8–16.4
3–0	18.93	19.52	20.00	20.50	21.05	18.2–21.3	15.43	15.87	16.32	16.73	17.26	14.8–17.7	15.22	15.66	16.14	16.58	17.07	14.8–17.6
3–6	20.09	20.70	21.20	21.75	22.35	19.2–22.8	16.43	16.88	17.35	17.78	18.32	16.1–18.9	16.26	16.71	17.20	17.64	18.14	15.9–18.7
4–0	21.23	21.85	22.36	22.97	23.64	19.9–24.8	17.37	17.84	18.33	18.78	19.34	16.8–20.9	17.18	17.65	18.15	18.62	19.15	16.5–20.9
4–6	22.34	22.98	23.51	24.16	24.92	21.0–25.3	18.28	18.77	19.28	19.74	20.31	17.6–21.0	18.08	18.57	19.08	19.58	20.12	17.4–20.7
5–0	23.44	24.10	24.65	25.34	26.18	21.9–27.6	19.15	19.65	20.18	20.66	21.25	18.2–23.0	18.96	19.46	19.98	20.52	21.08	17.9–23.0
5–6	24.52	25.20	25.77	26.51	27.42	23.9–28.3	19.99	20.51	21.06	21.57	22.18	19.6–24.2	19.80	20.31	20.84	21.44	22.03	19.6–24.0
6–0	25.58	26.27	26.87	27.66	28.62	24.7–29.6	20.79	21.34	21.92	22.46	23.10	20.4–25.0	20.62	21.14	21.68	22.33	22.96	20.4–25.0
6–6	26.62	27.33	27.96	28.79	29.78	26.0–30.7	21.57	22.14	22.75	23.35	24.01	21.1–26.4	21.42	21.95	22.50	23.21	23.87	21.0–26.1
7–0	27.64	28.37	29.02	29.90	30.92	26.9–32.9	22.33	22.94	23.57	24.23	24.91	21.6–27.5	22.19	22.74	23.30	24.07	24.77	21.4–27.3
7–6	28.62	29.37	30.06	30.98	32.03	28.2–33.5	23.08	23.73	24.39	25.10	25.81	22.0–28.6	22.94	23.52	24.09	24.92	25.67	22.0–28.4
8–0	29.58	30.35	31.09	32.02	33.10	29.4–35.1	23.83	24.52	25.20	25.96	26.71	23.0–29.6	23.67	24.28	24.87	25.75	26.56	22.9–29.3
8–6	30.52	31.31	32.06	33.03	34.14	30.4–34.6	24.57	25.30	26.01	26.82	27.61	24.1–28.1	24.38	25.02	25.63	26.57	27.44	23.9–28.1
9–0	31.42	32.23	33.02	34.02	35.15	31.3–37.3	25.31	26.05	26.80	27.67	28.50	24.6–31.6	25.07	25.74	26.38	27.37	28.32	24.6–31.0
9–6	32.30	33.12	33.95	35.00	36.14	31.5–38.5	26.03	26.78	27.59	28.50	29.38	24.6–32.5	25.74	26.44	27.12	28.17	29.19	24.8–31.9
10–0	33.16	33.99	34.86	35.96	37.11	33.1–39.2	26.74	27.51	28.37	29.31	30.26	26.2–33.3	26.38	27.13	27.86	28.96	30.06	26.0–32.5
10–6	34.00	34.85	35.76	36.91	38.07	33.3–40.2	27.45	28.23	29.14	30.10	31.13	26.0–34.0	27.01	27.82	28.59	29.75	30.92	26.2–33.2
11–0	34.84	35.70	36.64	37.85	39.03	34.6–41.0	28.15	28.95	29.90	30.89	32.00	27.6–35.2	27.64	28.51	29.31	30.53	31.77	27.1–34.2
11–6	35.67	36.55	37.52	38.79	39.98	33.0–42.0	28.84	29.66	30.66	31.67	32.85	27.0–35.9	28.27	29.19	30.02	31.30	32.61	27.1–35.0
12–0	36.50	37.40	38.40	39.73	40.93	33.7–43.3	29.52	30.37	31.42	32.45	33.70	28.4–36.4	28.90	29.86	30.73	32.06	33.44	27.9–35.3
Measurements Including Epiphyses																		
10–0	37.10	37.70	38.52	39.72	40.95	36.3–43.8	30.28	31.05	32.10	33.11	34.35	29.2–37.9	29.42	30.15	31.05	32.22	33.66	28.8–35.9
10–6	37.85	38.58	39.44	40.67	41.94	36.9–45.3	30.95	31.80	32.92	34.01	35.33	29.6–38.6	30.02	30.80	31.68	32.90	34.36	29.0–36.7
11–0	38.64	39.46	40.39	41.67	43.00	38.0–45.7	31.70	32.59	33.80	34.96	36.34	30.8–39.8	30.65	31.50	32.44	33.68	35.16	30.2–37.6
11–6	39.46	40.35	41.37	42.70	44.10	36.5–46.8	32.50	33.45	34.72	35.96	37.37	31.0–40.6	31.34	32.26	33.27	34.53	36.03	30.0–38.7
12–0	40.32	41.26	42.40	43.80	45.26	37.2–48.0	33.35	34.38	35.70	36.99	38.42	32.2–41.3	32.08	33.06	34.16	35.44	36.97	30.7–38.9
12–6	41.22	42.19	43.44	44.95	46.45	40.7–48.8	34.27	35.35	36.73	38.04	39.50	33.2–42.0	32.87	33.91	35.10	36.43	38.00	32.1–39.7
13–0	42.15	43.15	44.50	46.18	47.67	41.0–49.3	35.25	36.38	37.80	39.13	40.64	34.2–42.7	33.73	34.83	36.10	37.51	39.15	33.0–40.7
13–6	43.12	44.18	45.60	47.45	48.97	40.5–50.9	36.36	37.57	39.00	40.40	41.93	34.5–43.5	34.64	35.81	37.25	38.72	40.43	33.1–41.2
14–0	44.10	45.27	46.77	48.70	50.22	41.3–51.9	37.55	38.70	39.95	41.37	43.03	36.8–44.5	35.70	36.89	38.25	39.79	41.57	35.1–42.6
14–6	45.18	46.43	47.96	49.80	51.36	41.9–52.5	38.53	39.57	40.80	42.25	43.95	35.9–45.2	36.70	37.89	39.15	40.74	42.57	34.8–43.1
15–0	46.30	47.60	49.00	50.65	52.23	44.8–53.7	39.17	40.25	41.50	42.98	44.72	38.5–45.9	37.55	38.65	39.94	41.56	43.43	36.6–44.2
15–6	47.25	48.45	49.83	51.32	52.90	46.4–54.2	39.61	40.75	42.10	43.62	45.39	37.9–47.0	38.08	39.20	40.54	42.20	44.11	37.0–45.6
16–0	47.67	48.83	50.21	51.82	53.38	45.3–54.9	39.82	41.07	42.50	44.05	45.90	38.6–48.2	38.36	39.50	40.95	42.66	44.63	36.7–46.3
16–6	47.95	49.07	50.40	52.15	53.75	47.1–56.5	39.95	41.20	42.75	44.33	46.21	39.4–48.7	38.43	39.62	41.22	42.99	45.03	38.2–46.3
17–0	48.10	49.14	50.45	52.38	54.02	47.0–57.0	40.04	41.27	42.90	44.51	46.42	39.1–49.1	38.47	39.66	41.37	43.22	45.33	37.9–46.8
17–6	48.17	49.19	50.48	52.52	54.20	47.0–57.0	40.08	41.30	42.98	44.60	46.51	39.1–49.1	38.49	39.69	41.46	43.36	45.54	37.9–46.8
18–0	48.20	49.22	50.50	52.60	54.30	48.1–57.4	40.10	41.33	43.03	44.66	46.60	39.0–49.6	38.50	39.70	41.50	43.45	45.68	37.9–47.5

GIRLS—SMOOTHED PERCENTILES AND OBSERVED RANGE FOR ROENTGENOGRAPHIC BONE LENGTHS (CM)

A. ARM BONES

Age (yr-mo)	Humerus						Radius						Ulna					
	10%	25%	50%	75%	90%	Range	10%	25%	50%	75%	90%	Range	10%	25%	50%	75%	90%	Range
	Measurements Between Epiphyseal Plates																	
0-2	6.72	6.91	7.12	7.30	7.50	6.0-7.7	5.43	5.58	5.72	5.88	6.05	5.2-6.5	6.08	6.30	6.50	6.65	6.82	5.8-7.2
0-4	7.52	7.73	8.00	8.17	8.38	7.4-8.8	5.93	6.11	6.28	6.46	6.64	5.7-7.0	6.59	6.84	7.05	7.21	7.38	6.4-7.9
0-6	8.22	8.44	8.74	8.89	9.12	7.7-9.5	6.37	6.56	6.74	6.95	7.14	6.0-7.5	7.09	7.35	7.58	7.75	7.92	6.7-8.2
1-0	9.77	10.04	10.38	10.60	10.86	8.8-11.4	7.42	7.64	7.85	8.10	8.31	7.1-8.6	8.27	8.56	8.82	9.06	9.32	7.9-9.7
1-6	11.02	11.32	11.70	11.98	12.27	10.6-12.7	8.22	8.48	8.74	9.00	9.24	7.9-9.7	9.24	9.55	9.84	10.11	10.41	8.8-10.9
2-0	12.07	12.40	12.80	13.10	13.42	11.5-14.0	8.92	9.20	9.50	9.77	10.04	8.5-10.4	10.00	10.34	10.66	10.95	11.27	9.3-11.6
2-6	12.94	13.32	13.75	14.09	14.44	12.6-14.9	9.55	9.85	10.18	10.47	10.75	8.7-11.1	10.69	11.05	11.39	11.70	12.04	9.8-12.4
3-0	13.73	14.13	14.58	14.99	15.39	13.2-15.7	10.12	10.45	10.80	11.12	11.41	9.9-11.8	11.32	11.70	12.07	12.39	12.75	11.0-13.2
3-6	14.49	14.91	15.38	15.84	16.28	13.8-16.7	10.66	11.01	11.39	11.73	12.05	10.3-12.5	11.90	12.31	12.71	13.04	13.42	11.6-13.9
4-0	15.21	15.66	16.15	16.66	17.14	14.3-17.4	11.18	11.55	11.95	12.33	12.68	10.8-12.9	12.45	12.88	13.32	13.67	14.06	12.1-14.4
4-6	15.90	16.37	16.89	17.44	17.97	15.0-18.5	11.68	12.06	12.48	12.91	13.30	11.3-13.8	12.98	13.43	13.90	14.29	14.69	12.6-15.2
5-0	16.56	17.05	17.60	18.21	18.77	15.8-19.5	12.16	12.55	12.99	13.47	13.90	11.8-14.9	13.49	13.96	14.45	14.89	15.30	13.1-16.5
5-6	17.19	17.71	18.29	18.94	19.54	16.1-20.1	12.62	13.02	13.48	14.01	14.48	12.3-15.0	13.99	14.47	14.98	15.46	15.90	13.5-16.5
6-0	17.80	18.35	18.95	19.64	20.29	16.8-20.7	13.06	13.49	13.97	14.53	15.03	12.7-15.4	14.47	14.96	15.50	16.02	16.48	14.0-17.0
6-6	18.40	18.98	19.60	20.32	21.01	17.4-22.2	13.49	13.95	14.45	15.05	15.55	13.1-16.5	14.94	15.45	16.01	16.56	17.05	14.6-18.4
7-0	18.99	19.60	20.25	20.99	21.71	18.2-23.3	13.91	14.41	14.92	15.56	16.06	13.6-17.2	15.41	15.94	16.51	17.09	17.60	15.0-19.1
7-6	19.56	20.21	20.89	21.65	22.40	18.6-23.1	14.33	14.86	15.39	16.05	16.56	13.9-16.9	15.87	16.42	17.01	17.62	18.13	15.5-18.6
8-0	20.12	20.82	21.51	22.30	23.07	19.4-24.4	14.74	15.29	15.86	16.53	17.04	14.5-18.1	16.32	16.90	17.50	18.14	18.65	15.9-20.1
8-6	20.66	21.42	22.13	22.94	23.73	19.8-24.4	15.15	15.71	16.33	17.00	17.51	14.9-18.1	16.77	17.38	17.99	18.66	19.16	16.4-19.6
9-0	21.19	22.01	22.75	23.58	24.40	20.3-25.1	15.55	16.13	16.80	17.47	18.00	15.1-18.5	17.20	17.85	18.47	19.18	19.68	16.8-20.4
9-6	21.71	22.59	23.38	24.24	25.08	20.8-26.5	15.96	16.54	17.26	17.96	18.50	15.6-19.7	17.62	18.30	18.94	19.70	20.22	17.2-21.7
10-0	22.23	23.17	24.03	24.91	25.78	21.4-26.4	16.38	16.97	17.72	18.45	19.02	16.0-19.7	18.04	18.73	19.44	20.23	20.79	17.7-21.5
10-6	22.77	23.76	24.70	25.60	26.51	21.7-28.2	16.81	17.42	18.20	18.95	19.55	16.4-21.4	18.50	19.20	19.99	20.78	21.40	18.0-23.8
11-0	23.32	24.36	25.38	26.31	27.25	22.0-28.0	17.25	17.89	18.70	19.48	20.13	16.7-21.1	18.97	19.69	20.57	21.37	22.03	18.5-23.6
11-6	23.88	24.98	26.07	27.03	28.01	22.4-29.5	17.72	18.39	19.23	20.03	20.77	17.0-21.9	19.46	20.24	21.17	21.98	22.68	19.1-24.5
12-0	24.45	25.62	26.78	27.76	28.78	22.8-30.0	18.22	18.93	19.80	20.63	21.44	17.5-22.3	19.98	20.82	21.80	22.60	23.33	19.6-25.1
	Measurements Including Epiphyses																	
10-0	23.80	24.66	25.80	26.73	27.50	23.0-28.2	17.50	18.32	19.03	19.87	20.62	17.0-21.0	18.95	19.75	20.50	21.40	22.20	18.6-22.9
10-6	24.55	25.52	26.73	27.73	28.66	23.6-30.7	17.94	18.85	19.65	20.61	21.39	17.5-23.0	19.53	20.36	21.28	22.20	23.07	19.0-25.1
11-0	25.28	26.31	27.60	28.64	29.68	23.8-30.9	18.41	19.38	20.28	21.33	22.12	17.8-23.0	20.12	20.97	22.00	22.94	23.83	19.7-24.6
11-6	25.98	27.06	28.38	29.46	30.60	24.2-32.0	18.93	19.92	20.90	21.99	22.78	18.2-23.7	20.70	21.58	22.65	23.60	24.51	20.2-25.4
12-0	26.65	27.75	29.09	30.19	31.43	24.8-32.9	19.45	20.48	21.50	22.59	23.39	18.8-24.5	21.28	22.18	23.24	24.20	25.12	20.5-26.8
12-6	27.28	28.38	29.72	30.86	32.18	25.4-33.2	19.97	21.06	22.07	23.10	23.89	19.3-24.8	21.85	22.77	23.75	24.70	25.62	21.0-26.9
13-0	27.87	28.97	30.30	31.46	32.85	26.1-33.8	20.49	21.57	22.55	23.54	24.29	19.9-24.8	22.40	23.28	24.18	25.13	26.04	21.5-27.2
13-6	28.42	29.51	30.82	32.00	33.40	26.6-34.5	21.00	22.03	22.98	23.89	24.60	20.5-24.9	22.92	23.73	24.57	25.48	26.40	22.1-27.2
14-0	28.92	30.00	31.30	32.40	33.77	27.7-35.2	21.50	22.45	23.34	24.12	24.80	20.9-25.4	23.36	24.13	24.89	25.76	26.69	22.6-27.2
14-6	29.37	30.42	31.70	32.66	33.95	28.0-35.9	21.88	22.80	23.62	24.28	24.94	21.4-25.9	23.69	24.47	25.16	25.92	26.90	22.9-27.5
15-0	29.72	30.74	32.00	32.79	34.06	28.5-36.1	22.13	23.02	23.82	24.38	25.03	21.6-26.1	23.95	24.76	25.37	26.04	27.03	23.0-27.7
15-6	29.92	30.92	32.15	32.88	34.10	28.8-36.5	22.22	23.12	23.92	24.45	25.08	21.8-26.2	24.12	24.98	25.51	26.14	27.12	23.4-28.1
16-0	30.02	31.01	32.20	32.92	34.10	28.8-36.5	22.25	23.15	23.98	24.48	25.10	21.8-26.2	24.22	25.10	25.60	26.21	27.16	23.4-28.1

Table continued on following page

Table 3 ■ LINEAR GROWTH OF LONG BONES OF LIMBS FROM INFANCY THROUGH ADOLESCENCE CONTINUED

GIRLS—SMOOTHED PERCENTILES AND OBSERVED RANGE FOR ROENTGENOGRAPHIC BONE LENGTHS (CM)
B. LEG BONES

Age (yr–mo)	Femur 10%	25%	50%	75%	90%	Range	Tibia 10%	25%	50%	75%	90%	Range	Fibula 10%	25%	50%	75%	90%	Range
Measurements Between Epiphyseal Plates																		
0-2	8.20	8.50	8.72	9.00	9.28	7.8-9.7	6.32	6.67	7.00	7.28	7.58	6.0-8.0	6.06	6.30	6.55	6.86	7.16	5.7-7.5
0-4	9.43	9.78	10.00	10.25	10.50	9.4-10.9	7.35	7.69	8.03	8.30	8.60	7.0-8.8	7.02	7.36	7.67	7.90	8.21	6.7-8.4
0-6	10.57	10.91	11.15	11.36	11.58	9.8-12.0	8.20	8.60	8.87	9.17	9.48	7.3-9.8	7.74	8.16	8.52	8.78	9.00	6.9-9.4
1-0	12.67	13.06	13.36	13.80	14.18	12.3-14.8	10.12	10.50	10.77	11.10	11.51	9.6-12.0	9.67	10.13	10.52	10.86	11.15	9.3-11.6
1-6	14.44	14.88	15.26	15.80	16.30	14.2-16.7	11.64	12.05	12.37	12.73	13.20	11.2-13.5	11.23	11.73	12.17	12.56	12.90	10.6-13.4
2-0	16.00	16.47	16.89	17.48	18.02	15.8-18.7	12.92	13.39	13.75	14.14	14.65	12.4-15.2	12.55	13.08	13.54	13.96	14.36	12.0-15.1
2-6	17.39	17.89	18.37	19.00	19.58	17.0-20.1	14.03	14.54	15.00	15.42	15.95	13.7-16.4	13.74	14.29	14.78	15.22	15.67	13.3-16.3
3-0	18.64	19.19	19.74	20.40	21.02	17.8-21.4	14.99	15.56	16.10	16.57	17.15	14.0-17.8	14.82	15.40	15.93	16.40	16.88	14.1-17.7
3-6	19.80	20.39	21.01	21.73	22.41	19.1-22.9	15.87	16.52	17.14	17.67	18.30	15.0-19.1	15.83	16.45	17.02	17.51	18.02	15.1-18.8
4-0	20.90	21.54	22.24	23.02	23.76	20.1-24.2	16.71	17.46	18.15	18.73	19.43	15.7-20.0	16.76	17.42	18.03	18.58	19.12	15.8-19.8
4-6	21.96	22.66	23.44	24.27	25.07	21.2-25.8	17.55	18.38	19.12	19.75	20.54	16.7-21.1	17.58	18.30	18.96	19.62	20.20	16.6-21.0
5-0	23.00	23.76	24.63	25.50	26.35	22.4-27.1	18.38	19.28	20.06	20.74	21.62	17.5-22.6	18.35	19.15	19.85	20.62	21.26	17.4-22.4
5-6	24.02	24.84	25.79	26.71	27.60	23.3-28.2	19.20	20.16	20.96	21.71	22.63	18.3-23.1	19.12	19.97	20.73	21.59	22.29	18.3-23.1
6-0	25.02	25.92	26.94	27.89	28.81	24.2-30.0	20.00	21.01	21.83	22.67	23.61	19.3-24.3	19.88	20.78	21.60	22.52	23.27	19.6-24.0
6-6	26.02	26.99	28.07	29.04	29.98	25.2-30.8	20.77	21.84	22.70	23.60	24.57	20.0-25.7	20.64	21.59	22.46	23.41	24.21	19.9-25.3
7-0	27.01	28.06	29.16	30.15	31.10	26.0-32.2	21.54	22.67	23.56	24.51	25.51	20.7-26.7	21.39	22.39	23.32	24.27	25.09	20.6-26.3
7-6	27.99	29.11	30.22	31.22	32.18	26.8-34.0	22.31	23.50	24.41	25.42	26.45	21.5-27.5	22.13	23.19	24.18	25.10	25.91	21.3-27.2
8-0	28.94	30.11	31.25	32.25	33.21	27.8-34.3	23.07	24.32	25.25	26.32	27.38	22.3-28.4	22.87	23.98	25.04	25.91	26.74	22.1-27.9
8-6	29.84	31.06	32.25	33.26	34.24	28.8-34.9	23.80	25.12	26.09	27.22	28.28	23.1-29.2	23.58	24.76	25.88	26.74	27.58	22.7-28.6
9-0	30.69	31.95	33.22	34.24	35.26	29.6-36.2	24.50	25.91	26.93	28.12	29.18	23.7-30.1	24.26	25.52	26.70	27.62	28.52	23.4-29.5
9-6	31.50	32.80	34.14	35.18	36.28	30.5-38.1	25.19	26.67	27.77	29.02	30.10	24.4-31.3	24.92	26.25	27.48	28.60	29.60	24.1-30.7
10-0	32.28	33.62	35.02	36.17	37.30	31.3-38.3	25.87	27.42	28.59	29.93	31.05	25.3-31.9	25.61	26.99	28.28	29.54	30.65	24.8-31.4
10-6	33.03	34.47	35.96	37.20	38.35	32.2-41.6	26.54	28.17	29.40	30.85	32.01	25.9-33.8	26.31	27.77	29.12	30.46	31.67	25.4-33.0
11-0	33.78	35.36	36.95	38.28	39.45	33.2-43.2	27.28	28.95	30.26	31.80	32.98	26.5-35.0	27.02	28.56	29.90	31.31	32.61	25.9-33.9
11-6	34.60	36.29	38.05	39.40	40.60	34.0-44.1	28.10	29.77	31.18	32.77	33.99	27.3-35.8	27.72	29.32	30.60	32.08	33.45	26.7-35.0
12-0	35.50	37.35	39.32	40.55	41.85	35.2-44.9	29.02	30.71	32.18	33.80	35.10	28.1-36.6	28.40	30.02	31.26	32.80	34.30	27.3-35.7
Measurements Including Epiphyses																		
10-0	35.57	37.05	39.03	40.15	41.50	34.6-42.0	29.51	31.10	32.55	34.12	35.22	28.4-35.9	28.47	30.12	31.55	32.70	33.75	27.6-34.6
10-6	36.39	37.93	40.02	41.50	43.15	35.5-46.3	30.34	32.00	33.64	35.30	36.60	29.2-37.8	29.13	30.82	32.28	33.88	35.12	28.3-36.1
11-0	37.32	38.90	41.02	42.72	44.41	36.6-47.8	31.18	32.92	34.64	36.35	37.76	30.3-39.0	29.87	31.58	33.04	34.86	36.12	28.9-37.3
11-6	38.33	40.04	42.08	43.85	45.49	37.5-48.7	32.03	33.86	35.52	37.28	38.70	31.1-40.4	30.68	32.42	33.90	35.74	37.03	29.7-38.4
12-0	39.40	41.21	43.30	44.90	46.48	38.9-49.3	32.91	34.80	36.30	38.13	39.49	32.0-41.0	31.47	33.26	34.75	36.53	37.83	30.4-39.2
12-6	40.34	42.22	44.37	45.83	47.35	39.8-48.4	33.74	35.66	37.00	38.88	40.14	32.7-41.0	32.25	34.06	35.55	37.22	38.56	31.2-39.4
13-0	41.18	43.10	45.27	46.62	48.09	39.9-51.0	34.50	36.39	37.66	39.47	40.67	33.6-42.1	33.01	34.83	36.28	37.80	39.18	32.0-40.6
13-6	41.95	43.90	46.03	47.24	48.67	41.5-49.1	35.21	37.02	38.28	39.93	41.08	34.3-42.8	33.63	35.46	36.87	38.26	39.65	32.6-41.3
14-0	42.65	44.58	46.65	47.69	49.10	41.7-52.1	35.80	37.55	38.78	40.28	41.39	34.6-43.4	34.13	35.94	37.33	38.61	39.98	33.1-41.8
14-6	43.31	45.09	47.05	48.03	49.42	42.3-50.1	36.21	37.92	39.17	40.51	41.58	34.9-43.3	34.51	36.30	37.70	38.86	40.20	33.3-41.7
15-0	43.86	45.41	47.22	48.27	49.58	42.2-52.0	36.50	38.15	39.36	40.66	41.67	34.8-41.9	34.82	36.60	37.94	39.00	40.32	33.5-40.6
15-6	44.17	45.60	47.28	48.37	49.65	42.2-52.0	36.69	38.30	39.45	40.75	41.70	34.8-42.0	35.05	36.83	38.06	39.07	40.36	33.4-40.7
16-0	44.35	45.66	47.28	48.40	49.65	42.2-52.0	36.78	38.37	39.50	40.78	41.70	34.8-42.0	35.20	36.98	38.10	39.10	40.36	33.4-40.7

From Maresh MM: Linear growth of the long bones of the extremities from infancy through adolescence. Am J Dis Child 1955;89:735-742, with permission.

Table 4 ■ METACARPAL LENGTHS AND CORTICAL DIAMETERS (MM) IN WHITES, BLACKS, AND MEXICAN-AMERICANS IN THE UNITED STATES

Age	n	LENGTH Mean	LENGTH SD	TOTAL Mean	TOTAL SD	MEDULLARY Mean	MEDULLARY SD	CORTICAL Mean	CORTICAL SD
					White Males				
1	15	24.62	2.30	4.59	0.52	2.85	0.67	1.74	0.47
2	45	30.19	2.71	5.09	0.52	3.20	0.73	1.88	0.47
3	95	34.22	2.49	5.33	0.58	3.33	0.70	2.00	0.48
4	123	37.02	2.70	5.41	0.45	3.10	0.63	2.31	0.47
5	158	39.99	2.89	5.57	0.51	3.12	0.61	2.54	0.43
6	169	42.72	3.02	5.83	0.54	3.23	0.63	2.61	0.43
7	216	45.59	3.14	6.02	0.60	3.20	0.69	2.82	0.52
8	214	47.84	3.43	6.34	0.68	3.34	0.75	3.00	0.49
9	207	50.37	3.25	6.60	0.61	3.42	0.70	3.18	0.50
10	224	52.06	3.84	6.83	0.58	3.47	0.68	3.35	0.52
11	202	54.43	3.89	7.11	0.67	3.63	0.78	3.47	0.57
12	212	57.19	4.40	7.52	0.73	3.83	0.82	3.69	0.65
13	209	61.33	4.98	7.87	0.78	3.77	0.77	4.10	0.69
14	144	63.96	5.19	8.21	0.90	3.90	0.75	4.31	0.84
15	144	66.86	4.58	8.56	0.78	3.81	0.82	4.75	0.77
16	108	68.36	4.35	8.84	0.78	3.92	0.81	4.92	0.77
					Black Males				
1	17	26.79	2.99	4.83	0.41	3.35	0.49	1.48	0.44
2	20	32.41	3.30	5.21	0.52	3.35	0.62	1.86	0.37
3	42	35.64	2.96	5.37	0.53	3.21	0.79	2.16	0.48
4	55	39.60	3.35	5.84	0.57	3.52	0.71	2.32	0.46
5	97	43.03	3.34	5.97	0.56	3.45	0.70	2.52	0.42
6	105	45.40	3.12	6.31	0.57	3.62	0.68	2.68	0.41
7	131	47.99	3.45	6.46	0.61	3.55	0.68	2.90	0.50
8	124	50.60	3.77	6.71	0.66	3.65	0.70	3.05	0.44
9	136	52.46	3.76	6.91	0.64	3.77	0.72	3.14	0.46
10	119	54.76	3.76	7.14	0.67	3.81	0.69	3.33	0.43
11	126	57.38	4.32	7.49	0.72	4.03	0.70	3.46	0.51
12	136	59.63	4.42	7.72	0.61	4.18	0.73	3.54	0.54
13	134	62.90	4.93	8.08	0.82	4.18	0.83	3.89	0.69
14	130	66.16	5.17	8.44	0.80	4.31	0.83	4.13	0.72
15	104	68.33	5.08	8.68	0.91	4.30	0.87	4.39	0.75
16	96	71.51	4.12	9.03	0.85	4.22	0.85	4.81	0.72
					Mexican-American Males				
1	1	31.60	0.00	5.30	0.00	3.30	0.00	2.00	0.00
2	6	31.93	2.82	5.08	0.83	3.20	1.07	1.88	0.45
3	9	36.08	2.45	5.41	0.61	3.08	0.49	2.33	0.36
4	15	38.21	2.73	5.63	0.55	3.15	0.64	2.47	0.28
5	20	40.28	2.96	5.50	0.60	2.97	0.62	2.53	0.33
6	25	43.59	2.70	5.90	0.61	3.12	0.59	2.78	0.35
7	28	45.79	2.88	6.20	0.56	3.32	0.71	2.88	0.35
8	27	47.91	3.65	6.33	0.49	3.36	0.61	2.96	0.41
9	20	48.61	3.04	6.45	0.61	3.46	0.61	2.99	0.34
10	27	51.77	3.11	6.84	0.69	3.57	0.75	3.28	0.49
11	24	53.48	3.41	6.94	0.57	3.40	0.74	3.54	0.46
12	27	55.78	4.64	7.37	0.75	3.60	0.76	3.77	0.48
13	23	59.00	4.25	7.62	0.98	3.64	1.03	3.98	0.57
14	24	62.41	4.98	7.83	0.70	3.54	0.79	4.30	0.72
15	11	66.46	4.41	8.46	0.63	3.92	0.69	4.55	0.48
16	9	65.87	4.46	8.77	0.73	3.88	0.97	4.89	0.59

Table continued on following page

Table 4 ■ METACARPAL LENGTHS AND CORTICAL DIAMETERS (MM) IN WHITES, BLACKS, AND MEXICAN-AMERICANS IN THE UNITED STATES CONTINUED

Age	n	LENGTH Mean	LENGTH SD	TOTAL Mean	TOTAL SD	MEDULLARY Mean	MEDULLARY SD	CORTICAL Mean	CORTICAL SD
					White Females				
1	25	25.96	3.52	4.34	0.57	2.72	0.48	1.62	0.31
2	35	31.77	2.23	4.76	0.42	2.91	0.61	1.85	0.41
3	61	34.68	2.60	4.99	0.49	2.97	0.69	2.01	0.45
4	124	37.63	3.55	5.21	0.59	2.91	0.68	2.30	0.45
5	142	40.66	3.02	5.38	0.56	2.92	0.60	2.46	0.47
6	171	43.13	3.10	5.54	0.50	2.86	0.61	2.68	0.44
7	188	45.81	2.91	5.83	0.58	2.95	0.64	2.88	0.46
8	198	48.22	3.27	6.07	0.67	2.96	0.67	3.11	0.54
9	205	50.38	3.87	6.26	0.60	3.00	0.68	3.27	0.55
10	213	53.36	3.89	6.57	0.62	3.13	0.67	3.43	0.51
11	205	56.20	4.08	6.89	0.62	3.17	0.70	3.72	0.64
12	192	58.81	4.13	7.19	0.66	3.21	0.74	3.98	0.65
13	184	61.20	4.55	7.43	0.65	3.07	0.73	4.36	0.66
14	143	62.82	3.83	7.64	0.75	2.92	0.88	4.72	0.73
15	149	63.13	3.34	7.74	0.64	2.88	0.74	4.86	0.64
16	129	63.78	3.58	7.85	0.60	3.00	0.83	4.85	0.64
					Black Females				
1	14	25.39	4.69	4.11	0.50	2.57	0.29	1.54	0.51
2	30	32.83	2.09	4.88	0.60	2.99	0.73	1.90	0.38
3	29	36.91	2.72	5.38	0.51	3.17	0.66	2.21	0.49
4	64	40.63	4.46	5.56	0.64	3.08	0.69	2.49	0.60
5	79	42.83	3.49	5.68	0.61	3.08	0.78	2.60	0.46
6	123	45.66	3.72	5.93	0.62	3.12	0.72	2.81	0.48
7	139	48.12	3.48	6.09	0.60	3.13	0.67	2.96	0.48
8	128	50.81	3.31	6.42	0.58	3.24	0.62	3.18	0.47
9	153	53.45	4.12	6.78	0.73	3.47	0.77	3.31	0.55
10	146	56.46	4.22	6.97	0.70	3.48	0.73	3.50	0.59
11	161	59.93	4.53	7.36	0.70	3.50	0.79	3.86	0.71
12	141	62.32	4.49	7.71	0.74	3.62	0.83	4.09	0.65
13	130	64.65	4.57	7.84	0.66	3.48	0.83	4.36	0.69
14	122	65.52	4.04	8.16	0.67	3.53	0.93	4.63	0.70
15	102	65.95	3.99	8.24	0.69	3.48	0.82	4.76	0.63
16	97	66.40	3.76	8.14	0.78	3.33	0.90	4.79	0.58
					Mexican-American Females				
1	0	0.00	0.00	0.00	0.00	0.00	0.00	0.00	0.00
2	4	31.83	4.49	4.73	0.13	2.78	0.36	1.95	0.40
3	10	34.33	2.38	4.99	0.49	2.86	0.53	2.13	0.33
4	16	37.51	3.00	5.01	0.47	2.73	0.44	2.28	0.33
5	22	40.39	2.91	5.47	0.45	2.92	0.41	2.55	0.33
6	18	44.14	3.61	5.56	0.53	2.79	0.54	2.76	0.47
7	30	45.90	3.83	5.92	0.61	2.93	0.57	2.99	0.47
8	43	47.61	3.29	6.12	0.66	3.06	0.66	3.06	0.52
9	28	48.82	4.05	6.09	0.66	2.83	0.72	3.26	0.53
10	27	53.20	3.94	6.45	0.53	3.11	0.61	3.34	0.40
11	32	55.37	3.52	6.74	0.70	2.92	0.69	3.82	0.60
12	25	59.11	3.63	7.19	0.68	2.91	0.92	4.28	0.78
13	24	61.60	4.30	7.54	0.79	2.95	0.75	4.59	0.49
14	18	62.56	3.09	7.68	0.58	3.08	0.66	4.61	0.55
15	17	61.16	3.86	7.60	0.59	2.94	0.65	4.66	0.70
16	12	60.93	2.99	7.51	0.59	2.63	1.00	4.88	0.77

Data from Garn SM, Poznanski AK, Larson K: Metacarpal lengths, cortical diameters and areas from the 10-state survey. In Jaworski ZFG (ed): Proceedings of the First Workshop on Bone Morphometry. Ottawa, University of Ottawa Press, 1976:367–391.

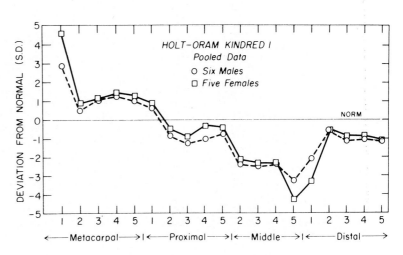

FIGURE 9. Metacarpophalangeal pattern profile analysis of Holt-Oram syndrome. The graph, constructed by connecting the deviations from the mean of each bone measured, has a consistent pattern that differs from the normal pattern and from patterns in other conditions. (From Poznanski AK, Garn SM, Nagy J, et al: Metacarpophalangeal pattern profiles in the evaluation of skeletal malformation. Radiology 1972;104: 1–11, with permission.)

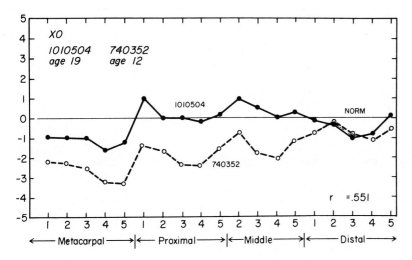

FIGURE 10. Metacarpophalangeal pattern profile in Turner syndrome. Note the difference between this pattern and that for the Holt-Oram syndrome in Figure 9. (From Poznanski AK, Garn SM, Nagy J, et al: Metacarpophalangeal pattern profiles in the evaluation of skeletal malformation. Radiology 1972;104:1–11, with permission.)

Table 5 ■ STANDARDS FOR METACARPAL AND PHALANGEAL LENGTHS AND VARIABILITY*

BONES		2 Mean	2 SD	3 Mean	3 SD	4 Mean	4 SD	5 Mean	5 SD	6 Mean	6 SD	7 Mean	7 SD	8 Mean	8 SD	9 Mean	9 SD	10 Mean	10 SD
Children Ages 2 to 10 Years																			
A. Males																			
Distal	5	8.8	...	8.4	0.6	9.0	0.7	9.9	0.7	10.7	0.6	11.4	0.8	12.2	0.9	12.6	1.0	13.5	0.9
	4	9.2	0.7	9.9	0.8	10.5	0.8	11.5	0.9	12.3	0.9	13.1	1.0	13.9	1.0	14.4	1.0	15.3	1.2
	3	8.7	0.9	9.5	0.8	10.2	0.8	11.1	0.8	11.8	0.8	12.7	1.0	13.4	1.0	14.0	1.0	14.8	1.2
	2	8.2	0.5	8.8	1.1	9.1	1.1	10.1	0.9	10.8	0.9	11.6	1.0	12.4	1.0	13.0	1.0	13.7	1.1
	1	11.1	0.6	12.3	0.8	13.2	1.0	14.4	0.9	15.4	0.9	16.5	1.0	17.4	1.1	17.9	1.2	19.0	1.2
Middle	5	8.8	0.9	9.8	0.8	10.6	1.0	11.2	1.0	12.0	1.0	12.7	1.1	13.5	1.1	14.3	1.2	15.0	1.2
	4	13.5	0.9	14.5	1.0	15.8	0.9	16.7	0.9	17.7	1.0	18.7	1.1	19.8	1.2	20.9	1.3	21.6	1.4
	3	14.1	0.8	15.1	1.0	16.5	1.0	17.6	1.0	18.7	1.0	19.8	1.2	20.9	1.3	22.0	1.4	22.9	1.4
	2	11.2	0.8	12.3	1.1	13.5	1.1	14.4	0.9	15.3	1.1	16.1	1.1	17.1	1.1	18.1	1.2	18.8	1.2
Proximal	5	16.1	0.7	17.8	0.9	19.2	1.0	20.6	1.0	21.8	1.0	23.0	1.0	24.2	1.3	25.2	1.5	26.4	1.5
	4	20.5	0.9	22.8	1.0	24.7	1.2	26.4	1.2	27.9	1.3	29.5	1.4	31.0	1.6	32.3	1.9	33.9	1.8
	3	21.8	1.0	24.2	1.1	26.3	1.1	28.1	1.4	29.8	1.4	31.5	1.6	33.2	1.8	34.7	2.2	36.1	1.9
	2	19.5	1.0	21.9	1.2	23.7	1.2	25.4	1.4	26.8	1.5	28.3	1.6	29.7	1.8	31.4	1.9	32.5	1.9
	1	15.2	...	15.9	1.1	17.2	1.1	18.3	1.2	19.6	1.2	20.8	1.3	21.8	1.3	23.1	1.5	24.2	1.4
Metacarpal	5	23.9	1.0	26.3	1.5	28.9	1.9	32.1	2.2	34.6	2.2	36.7	2.1	38.8	2.5	40.6	2.5	42.7	2.9
	4	25.5	1.1	28.9	1.5	31.7	2.1	35.0	2.5	37.9	2.7	40.1	2.5	42.2	3.1	44.1	2.8	46.5	3.5
	3	28.6	1.3	32.3	1.8	35.6	2.3	39.3	2.8	42.6	2.9	45.3	2.8	47.6	3.5	49.8	3.0	52.3	3.7
	2	30.6	1.5	34.5	1.7	37.9	2.3	41.6	2.7	44.9	2.9	47.7	2.8	50.2	3.4	52.6	3.0	55.0	3.9
	1	19.6	1.3	22.0	1.3	24.1	1.6	26.7	1.6	29.0	1.7	30.9	1.8	32.7	2.1	34.4	2.1	36.3	2.3
B. Females																			
Distal	5	7.8	0.6	8.4	0.6	9.1	0.7	9.9	0.7	10.6	0.8	11.4	0.9	12.1	1.0	12.7	1.1	13.5	1.2
	4	9.1	0.7	9.9	0.7	10.6	0.8	11.5	0.9	12.4	1.0	13.2	1.1	14.0	1.1	14.4	1.2	15.5	1.4
	3	8.8	0.7	9.9	0.8	10.2	0.8	11.1	0.9	12.2	1.3	12.7	1.1	13.5	1.1	14.1	1.1	15.0	1.4
	2	8.0	0.8	8.6	0.7	9.4	0.7	10.1	0.8	10.9	0.9	11.7	1.0	12.3	1.1	13.1	1.1	13.8	1.4
	1	11.3	0.8	12.5	0.8	13.2	0.8	14.4	1.0	15.4	1.1	16.3	1.2	17.3	1.3	17.8	1.3	19.0	1.6
Middle	5	9.0	1.2	9.8	1.1	10.5	1.1	11.2	1.1	12.2	1.2	12.9	1.3	13.6	1.4	14.2	1.4	15.2	1.6
	4	13.5	0.9	14.9	1.0	15.8	1.0	16.9	1.2	18.1	1.3	19.1	1.4	20.1	1.4	20.9	1.5	22.2	1.7
	3	14.2	0.9	15.6	1.1	16.6	1.1	17.9	1.2	19.2	1.3	20.3	1.4	21.4	1.4	22.1	1.6	23.6	1.8
	2	11.6	0.9	12.8	1.0	13.6	1.0	14.8	1.1	16.0	1.4	16.8	1.3	17.8	1.4	18.1	1.5	19.6	1.7
Proximal	5	16.3	1.0	17.9	1.1	19.1	1.1	20.6	1.3	22.0	1.7	23.1	1.6	24.4	1.6	25.2	1.6	27.1	2.0
	4	20.7	1.1	22.9	1.3	24.6	1.3	26.3	1.5	28.2	1.9	29.7	1.9	31.2	2.0	32.4	2.0	34.5	2.4
	3	22.2	1.2	24.5	1.3	26.4	1.4	28.3	1.8	30.4	1.8	32.1	2.0	33.7	2.2	35.0	2.2	37.3	2.6
	2	20.1	1.2	22.3	1.3	24.0	1.8	25.8	1.7	27.7	1.7	29.2	1.9	30.7	2.0	31.5	2.4	34.0	2.4
	1	14.9	1.0	16.3	1.1	17.2	1.3	18.8	1.3	20.2	1.5	21.4	1.5	22.7	1.6	23.5	2.0	25.5	2.1
Metacarpal	5	23.7	1.5	26.9	2.1	29.4	1.8	32.6	2.0	35.1	2.1	37.2	2.4	39.4	2.5	40.8	2.5	43.8	2.8
	4	26.0	1.9	29.6	2.7	32.2	2.0	35.6	2.5	38.4	2.7	43.1	2.8	44.3	3.0	44.3	2.8	47.5	3.5
	3	29.4	2.1	33.4	2.9	36.3	2.2	40.3	2.7	43.3	3.1	45.8	3.1	48.7	3.2	49.9	3.2	53.6	3.8
	2	31.3	1.9	35.2	2.7	38.2	2.3	42.2	2.7	45.6	3.2	48.1	3.3	51.2	3.3	52.6	3.4	56.6	4.1
	1	19.9	1.6	22.7	1.6	24.8	1.7	27.3	1.8	29.6	1.9	31.5	2.0	33.5	2.1	34.8	2.4	37.4	2.6

Children Ages 11 Years to Adult

A. Males

Bone	Digit	Mean	SD	Mean	SD	Mean	SD	Mean	SD	Mean	SD	Mean	SD	Mean	SD	Mean	SD
Distal	5	14.2	0.9	15.0	0.9	15.8	0.9	16.8	1.0	17.6	1.1	17.9	1.0	18.1	1.0	18.7	1.3
	4	16.1	1.2	17.0	1.3	17.8	1.3	18.8	1.3	19.6	1.4	20.0	1.3	20.3	1.3	20.5	1.2
	3	15.6	1.2	16.4	1.2	17.1	1.2	18.2	1.3	19.0	1.4	19.3	1.3	19.4	1.3	20.1	1.2
	2	14.3	1.1	15.0	1.0	15.7	1.0	16.7	1.2	17.5	1.2	17.8	1.4	18.1	1.4	18.8	1.4
	1	19.7	1.2	20.6	1.3	21.7	1.3	22.8	1.3	24.1	1.4	24.5	1.4	24.8	1.4	24.2	1.5
Middle	5	15.7	1.4	16.5	1.5	17.5	1.5	18.9	1.6	19.9	1.6	20.5	1.7	21.0	1.4	21.6	1.6
	4	22.6	1.5	23.6	1.5	24.8	1.7	26.5	1.6	27.7	1.8	28.4	1.6	29.1	1.5	29.6	1.6
	3	24.0	1.4	24.9	1.4	26.3	1.6	28.0	1.5	29.2	1.6	30.0	1.6	30.6	1.8	31.1	1.8
	2	19.8	1.8	20.4	1.8	21.6	1.6	23.2	1.5	24.3	1.5	25.0	1.8	25.6	1.7	26.1	1.6
Proximal	5	27.6	1.7	28.9	2.0	30.5	2.0	32.9	2.4	34.7	2.0	35.6	1.8	35.9	1.8	36.3	2.0
	4	35.3	2.0	37.0	2.4	38.8	2.4	41.6	2.8	43.7	2.6	44.9	2.3	45.2	2.2	45.5	2.3
	3	37.8	2.3	39.5	2.6	41.5	2.6	44.4	2.8	46.6	2.5	47.8	2.4	48.2	2.3	48.5	2.6
	2	33.9	2.1	35.5	2.4	37.2	2.4	39.8	2.6	41.8	2.2	42.8	2.0	43.4	2.1	43.7	2.2
	1	25.4	1.6	26.7	2.0	28.5	2.0	30.9	2.2	32.9	1.8	33.8	1.5	34.7	2.6	35.0	1.9
Metacarpal	5	44.6	2.8	47.1	3.2	49.1	3.2	52.2	3.6	55.4	3.9	57.1	2.8	57.5	2.5	58.0	3.0
	4	48.4	3.1	51.0	3.7	53.1	3.7	56.4	4.1	59.5	4.5	61.5	3.7	61.7	3.1	62.1	3.5
	3	54.6	3.4	57.3	4.0	59.5	4.0	63.1	4.4	66.7	4.9	68.7	4.1	69.0	3.3	69.0	3.8
	2	57.3	3.5	60.6	3.9	63.3	3.9	67.1	4.3	70.6	4.8	73.2	3.8	73.9	2.9	73.7	3.8
	1	38.2	2.4	40.2	2.7	42.5	2.7	45.1	2.6	47.6	2.8	48.8	2.3	49.4	2.1	49.6	2.9

B. Females

Bone	Digit	Mean	SD	Mean	SD	Mean	SD	Mean	SD	Mean	SD	Mean	SD	Mean	SD	Mean	SD
Distal	5	14.2	1.3	15.0	1.3	15.4	1.3	15.6	1.3	15.9	1.4	15.9	1.3	16.0	1.3	16.2	1.2
	4	16.2	1.4	17.1	1.4	17.6	1.2	17.9	1.4	18.0	1.4	18.0	1.4	17.9	1.4	18.0	1.3
	3	15.8	1.3	16.6	1.3	17.1	1.4	17.3	1.3	17.6	1.5	17.5	1.4	17.4	1.5	17.7	1.3
	2	14.4	1.3	15.2	1.5	15.7	1.5	15.8	1.5	16.1	1.6	16.0	1.6	16.2	1.5	16.6	1.3
	1	20.0	1.7	20.9	1.7	21.4	1.6	21.7	1.6	22.0	1.7	22.0	1.7	22.0	1.8	22.1	1.6
Middle	5	16.2	1.7	17.2	1.7	17.9	1.8	18.1	1.8	18.4	1.6	18.5	1.7	18.6	1.9	18.7	1.7
	4	23.4	1.8	24.7	1.8	25.7	1.9	25.9	1.9	26.3	1.8	26.4	1.8	26.3	1.9	26.4	1.7
	3	24.9	1.9	26.2	1.9	27.2	2.0	27.5	2.0	28.1	1.8	28.0	1.9	27.8	1.8	27.9	1.7
	2	20.6	1.8	21.8	1.9	22.7	1.8	23.0	1.8	23.5	1.8	23.4	1.9	23.1	1.9	23.2	1.6
Proximal	5	28.7	2.1	30.5	2.2	31.9	2.2	32.3	2.2	32.9	2.1	32.8	2.3	32.5	2.3	32.5	2.0
	4	36.5	2.5	38.8	2.6	40.3	2.6	40.9	2.5	41.5	2.3	41.6	2.6	41.1	2.6	40.8	2.4
	3	39.5	2.7	41.7	2.8	43.5	2.8	44.1	2.6	44.8	2.6	44.8	2.7	44.2	2.5	44.0	2.3
	2	35.9	2.6	38.0	2.6	39.5	2.6	39.9	2.6	40.6	2.4	40.7	2.6	39.9	2.6	40.0	2.3
	1	27.2	2.3	29.2	2.4	30.6	2.4	31.1	2.2	31.8	2.0	31.9	2.1	31.3	2.2	31.4	2.0
Metacarpal	5	46.3	2.9	48.7	2.9	50.8	2.8	52.1	2.8	52.6	3.0	52.8	2.7	53.0	2.7	51.9	3.6
	4	50.2	3.8	52.8	3.7	55.1	3.6	56.2	3.6	56.9	3.6	57.2	3.5	57.2	3.5	56.0	3.5
	3	56.5	4.0	59.5	4.2	62.1	4.0	63.4	4.0	63.9	3.9	64.3	4.0	64.5	4.1	62.6	4.0
	2	59.9	4.3	63.2	4.4	66.2	4.2	67.4	4.2	68.1	4.2	68.6	4.3	68.9	4.1	66.9	4.3
	1	39.7	3.0	42.0	3.0	43.8	2.7	44.4	2.5	45.3	2.4	45.0	2.8	45.0	2.6	44.2	2.6

*For each sex, n ≡ 150 at age 4, 124 at age 9, 78 in adulthood, and 30 to 85 at intermediate ages. All values are in millimeters.
Data from Garn SM, Hertzog KP, Poznanski AK, et al: Metacarpophalangeal lengths in the evaluation of skeletal malformation. Radiology 1972;105:375–381.

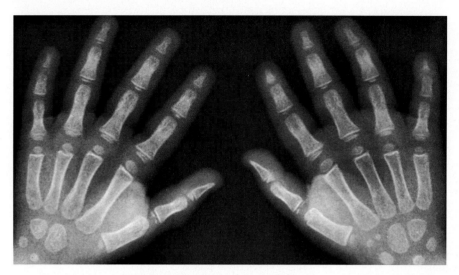

FIGURE 11. Disparity in maturation of round bones in the left and right wrists of a healthy boy 3 years of age in whom maturation of the epiphyseal ossification centers in the tubular bones of the same hands is identical. There are four centers in the left wrist and seven in the right. The four carpal centers in the left wrist agree with the boy's chronologic age and with maturation of the tubular bones in both hands. These findings demonstrate the principle that carpal bones are much more erratic in development than tubular bones in some patients, as has been shown repeatedly in large groups of healthy infants and children.

Table 6 ■ EPIPHYSEAL OSSIFICATION IN THE FETUS AND NEONATE— 5TH AND 95TH PERCENTILES

CENTER	5TH PERCENTILE	95TH PERCENTILE
Humeral head	37th week	16 postnatal weeks
Distal femoral	31st week	39th week (female) 40th week (male)
Proximal tibial	34th week	2 postnatal weeks (female) 5 postnatal weeks (male)
Calcaneus	22d week	25th week
Talus	25th week	31st week
Cuboid	37th week	8 postnatal weeks (female) 16 postnatal weeks (male)

Data from Kuhns LR, Finnstrom O: New standards of ossification of the newborn. Radiology 1976;119:655–660.

phalanges and metacarpals, and the wrist, with its tightly packed primary centers, are used most frequently as an index of total skeletal maturation. Genetic variability in the timing of ossification in the carpal bones accounts for their elimination from some types of evaluation (Fig. 11). Racial variation also occurs, but the differences are well within the normal range for any well-studied population.

SUGGESTED READINGS

Acheson RM: A method of assessing skeletal maturity from radiographs: a report from the Oxford Child Health Survey. J Anat 1954;88:498–508

Anderson M, Messner MB, Green WT: Distribution of lengths of the normal femur and tibia in children from 1 to 18 years of age. J Bone Joint Surg Am 1964;46:1197–1202

Bonnard D: Cortical thickness and diaphyseal diameter of the metacarpal bones from the age of 3 months to 11 years. Helv Paediatr Acta 1968;23:445–463

Clark WEL: The Tissues of the Body, 2nd ed. Oxford, Clarendon Press, 1945

Garn SM: The Earlier Gain and the Later Loss of Cortical Bone in Nutritional Perspective. Springfield, IL, Charles C Thomas, 1970

Garn SM, Hertzog KP, Poznanski AK, et al: Metacarpophalangeal lengths in the evaluation of skeletal malformation. Radiology 1972;105:375–381

Garn SM, Poznanski AK, Larson K: Metacarpal lengths, cortical diameters and areas from the 10-state survey. In Jaworski ZFG (ed): Proceedings of the First Workshop on Bone Morphometry. Ottawa, University of Ottawa Press, 1976:367–391

Gilsanz V, Gibbens DT, Roe TF, et al: Vertebral bone density in children: effect of puberty. Radiology 1988;166:847–850

Greulich WW, Pyle SI: Radiographic Atlas of Skeletal Development of the Hand and Wrist, 2nd ed. Stanford, CA, Stanford University Press, 1959

Hadlock FP: Computer-assisted, multiple-parameter assessment of fetal age and growth. Semin Ultrasound CT MR 1989;10:383–385

Hadlock FP, Harrist RB, Deter RL, et al: Fetal femur length as a predictor of menstrual age: sonographically measured. AJR Am J Roentgenol 1982;138:875–878

Hashimoto BE, Filly RA, Callen PW: Sonographic diagnosis of clubfoot in utero. J Ultrasound Med 1986;5:81–83

Hernandez M, Sanchez E, Sobradillo B, et al: A new method for assessment of skeletal maturity in the first 2 years of life. Pediatr Radiol 1988;18:484–489

Jeantry P, Kirkpatrick C, Dramaix-Wilmet M, et at: Ultrasonic evaluation of fetal limb growth. Radiology 1981;140:165–168

Johnson LC: The kinetics of skeletal remodeling: A further consideration of theoretical biology of bone. Birth Defects Orig Artic Ser 1966;2:66–142

Kuhns LR, Finnstrom O: New standards of ossification of the newborn. Radiology 1976;119:655–660

Kurtz AB, Filly RA, Wagner RJ, et al: In utero analysis of heterozygous achondroplasia: variable time onset as detected by femur length measurements. J Ultrasound Med 1986;5:137–140

Lambertz: Die Entwicklung des menschlichen Knochengerüstes während des fötalen Lebens. In Atlas der normalen und pathologischen Anatomie in typischen Röntgenbildern. Hamburg, Lucas Gräfe & Sillem, 1900

Maresh MM: Linear growth of the long bones of the extremities from infancy through adolescence. Am J Dis Child 1955;89:735–742

Moseley CF: A straight line graph for leg-length discrepancies. J Bone Joint Surg Am 1977;59:174–179

O'Brien GD, Queenan JT: Growth of the ultrasound fetal femur length during normal pregnancy. Part I. Am J Obstet Gynecol 1981;141:833–837

Ogden JA, Conlogue GJ, Rhodin AGJ: Roentgenographic indicators of skeletal maturity in marine mammals (Cetaea). Skeletal Radiol 1981;7:119–123

Poznanski AK, Garn SM, Nagy J, et al: Metacarpophalangeal pattern profiles in the evaluation of skeletal malformation. Radiology 1972;104:1–11

Pyle SI, Waterhouse AM, Greulich WW: A Radiographic Standard of Reference for the Growing Hand and Wrist. Prepared for the National Health Examination Survey. Cleveland, OH, Case Western Reserve University Press, 1971

Roche AF: Skeletal Maturity of Children 6–11 years; Racial, Geographic and Socioeconomic Differentials. DHEW Publication No (HRA) 76-1631. Bethesda, MD, U.S. National Center for Health Statistics, 1975

Rubin P: Dynamic Classification of Bone Dysplasias. St. Louis, Mosby–Year Book, 1964

Seeds JW, Cefalo RC: Relationship of fetal limb lengths to both

parietal diameter and gestational age. Obstet Gynecol 1982;60: 580–585

Siffert RS, Gilbert MD: Anatomy and physiology of the growth plate. *In* Rand M (ed): The Growth Plate and Its Disorders. Baltimore, Williams & Wilkins, 1969

Sontag LW, Snell D, Anderson M: Rate of appearance of ossification centers from birth to the age of five years. Am J Dis Child 1939;58:949–956

Tanner JM, Whitehouse RH, Marshall WA, et al: Assessment of Skeletal Maturity and Prediction of Adult Height (TW2 Method). London, Academic Press, 1975

■ C h a p t e r   2

ANATOMIC VARIANTS

THEODORE E. KEATS

Numerous anatomic variants in the growing skeleton closely simulate the productive and destructive lesions caused by disease. Caffey was convinced that many so-called cases of osteochondrosis or osteochondritis described in the literature were normal variations in the bones rather than the result of ischemic necrosis. However, Lawson has pointed out that "all that varies is not necessarily normal, and there is nothing to exempt a normal variant from harboring a pathologic process that may be symptomatic." Bone scintigraphy has been helpful in evaluation of questionable cases. Figure 1 illustrates common sites of irregular mineralization in the skeleton; examples of anatomic variation are described below.

Projection artifacts may also simulate disease. The Mach effect is a visual perception phenomenon in which an abrupt change in the interface between dark and light zones enhances the edge of the interface. Its presence at the margin of superimposed structures (Fig. 2) may simulate fracture. Similarly, overlap of adjacent bony structures may cause local areas of pseudosclerosis that may be eye catching (Figs. 3 and 4).

HAND AND WRIST

Sclerotic epiphyseal ossification centers of the phalanges are often termed "ivory epiphyses" when they are large enough to be trabeculated but are not (Fig. 5). They are found typically in distal phalanges and in the middle phalanx of the fifth digit. They may also occur in association with cone epiphyses in dysplastic syndromes. Cone-shaped epiphyses (CSE) of the phalanges (Fig. 6) occur most frequently, singly or in combination, in the distal phalanx of the first digit or the middle phalanx of

the fifth in normal children and are frequently associated with shortening of the latter, especially in girls. They are seen only in disease states in the proximal phalanges and in the middle phalanges of the third and fourth digits, but occur in the second through fifth middle phalanges and the second middle phalanx in both normal and diseased children. Giedion described 38 types of CSE and indicated those most commonly seen in both groups. Dysplastic renal disease has been noted in association with his types 28, 37, and 38; he has designated disease entities showing the association as "conorenal syndromes."

Extra and false epiphyseal ossification centers may appear in the proximal cartilaginous portion of the growing second through fifth metacarpal bones and in the distal cartilage of the first (Fig. 7). They are formed from a thin rod of osteogenic tissue that invades the proximal cartilage from the shaft. The end of the rod enlarges to form a mushroom-shaped mass of bone that appears radiographically as the "pseudoepiphysis." Unlike true epiphyses, there is bony continuity with the shaft from the beginning of their development and they contribute little or nothing to longitudinal growth. The site of fusion of the bone mass with the shaft is often indicated by a notch (Fig. 8); notches have been found in the base of the second metacarpal in up to 60% of normal children, and in the distal end of the first metacarpal in up to 85%. Pseudoepiphyses are frequent in children with hypothyroidism and in cleidocranial dysplasia.

Irregularity of mineralization occasionally occurs in the carpal bones during development. These result from the onset of ossification in several centers, which is generally followed by coalescence to a single center. The pisiform is the bone most frequently affected (Fig. 9).

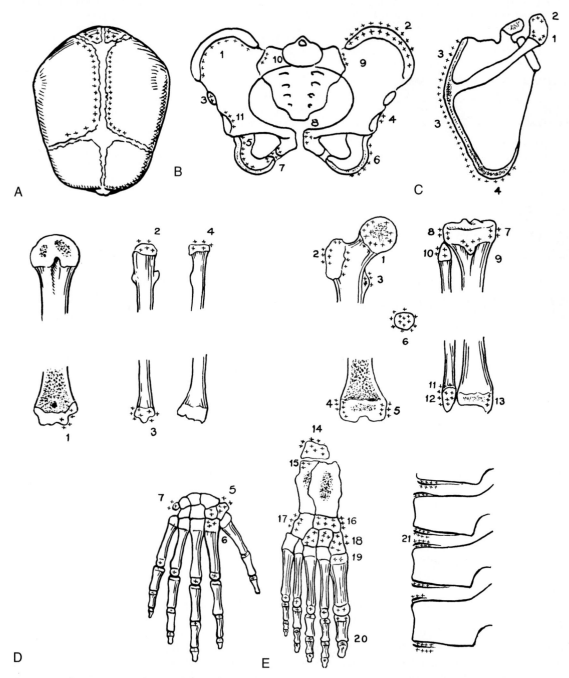

FIGURE 1. Common sites of normally irregular mineralization in the growing skeleton are marked by *crosses*. **A,** Cranium. During the first weeks of life and continuing for several months, edges of the bones at the great sutures are commonly irregular, and in many infants deep fissures extend from the sutures into the bodies of the bones. Irregularities are also common on the edges of the temporal suture (not shown). **B,** Pelvis: *1,* crest of ilium; *2,* secondary center in crest of ilium; *3,* secondary center of anterosuperior spine; *4,* os acetabuli marginalis; *5,* body of the ischium; *6,* secondary center of ischium; *7,* ischium and pubis at the ischiopubic synchondrosis; *8,* body of pubis; *9,* ilium at sacroiliac joint; *10,* sacrum at sacroiliac joint; *11,* iliac edge and roof of the acetabular cavity. **C,** Scapula: *1* and *2,* secondary centers of acromion process; *3,* secondary center of vertebral edge; *4,* secondary center of inferior angle. **D,** Upper limb: *1,* secondary center of trochlea, always irregular; *2* and *3,* proximal and distal epiphyseal centers of ulna; *4,* proximal epiphyseal center of radius; *5,* greater and lesser multangulars; *6,* inconstant center of second metacarpal (pseudoepiphysis); *7,* pisiform. **E,** Lower limb and spine; *1,* proximal metaphysis of femur; *2* and *3,* secondary center and edges of shaft at the greater and the lesser trochanter; *4* and *5,* lateral and medial edges of distal epiphyseal center of femur; *6,* patella; *7* and *8,* medial and lateral edges of proximal epiphyseal center of tibia; *9,* secondary center in anterior tibial process; *10,* proximal epiphyseal center of fibula; *11* and *12,* distal metaphysis and distal epiphyseal center of fibula; *13,* internal malleolus of distal epiphyseal center of tibia; *14,* apophysis of calcaneus; *15,* primary center of calcaneus; *16,* navicular; *17,* cuboid; *18,* cuneiform; *19,* proximal epiphyseal center of first metatarsal; *20,* epiphyseal centers of phalanges; *21,* marginal centers of spine.

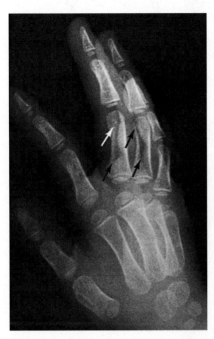

FIGURE 2. Mach effect on the volar margins of the fourth and fifth digits in this oblique projection of the hand simulates fracture lines on the superimposed third and fourth proximal phalanges. The patient was an asymptomatic girl 2 years of age.

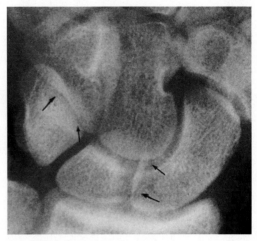

FIGURE 3. Pseudosclerotic marginal strips on the edges of the carpal bones caused by projection and superimposition of the edges of the scaphoid and lunate *(arrows at right)* and the triquetrum and the hamate *(arrows at left)* of a boy 16 years of age. Note the Mach effect adjacent to the pseudosclerosis.

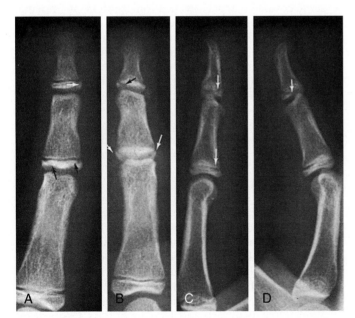

FIGURE 4. Pseudofractures of the epiphyseal ossification centers *(arrows)*. The curved epiphyseal plates of the middle and distal phalanges, best seen in the lateral projections, are superimposed on the secondary ossification centers in frontal projection and produce an effect simulating fractures at the lateral margins. The features are altered by minor degrees of flexion or extension. **A** and **C,** Straight index finger. **B** and **D,** Middle finger slightly flexed at proximal interphalangeal joint.

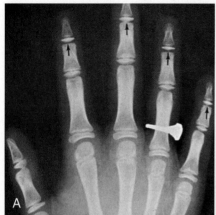
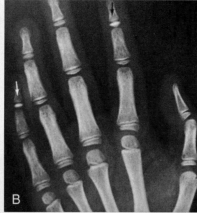
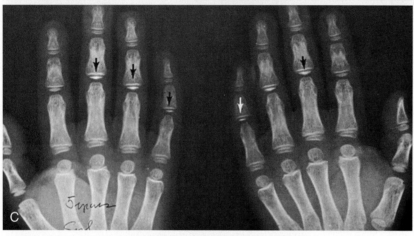

FIGURE 5. Physiologic sclerosis of the epiphyseal ossification centers in the phalanges of asymptomatic children. **A,** Sclerosis in the distal phalanges of digits 2, 3, 4, and 5 of a girl 8 years of age. **B,** Sclerosis in the terminal phalanges of digits 2 and 5 of a boy 6 years of age. **C,** Symmetric sclerosis in both hands, digits 3, 4, and 5 of the middle phalanges, of a girl 5 years of age.

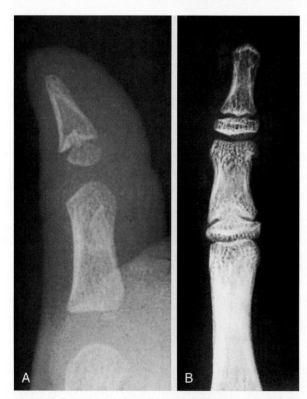

FIGURE 6. Cone epiphyses as incidental findings in healthy children. **A,** Distal phalanx of the thumb. **B,** Middle phalanx of the fifth digit. (From Poznanski AK: The Hand in Radiologic Diagnosis, 2nd ed. Philadelphia, WB Saunders, 1984, with permission.)

Approximately 25 separate, well-defined bones appear as accessory carpal ossification centers in normal persons (Fig. 10), and others occur in certain dysplastic disorders. In the normal person, the ossicles can simulate (and be simulated by) sequelae of injury. Fusions of ossification centers of adjacent carpal bones probably result from segmentation errors in early embryonic development. Lunatotriquetral "fusion" is the most common, particularly in persons of black African origin (Fig. 11); capitate–hamate "fusion" is next in frequency. "Fusions" of any pair of adjacent carpal bones, and even of adjacent carpal and metacarpal bones, have been observed. Most are isolated anomalies, but some are associated with malformation or dysplastic syndromes.

Named for their resemblance to sesame seeds, sesamoid bones in the hands are found on the palmar surface of the distal ends of the metacarpal bones and, less frequently, in the regions of the interphalangeal joints. They lie within the insertions of tendons, articulating with the palmar surface of the adjacent bone. They appear at the first metacarpophalangeal joint at about 11 years in girls and 13 years in boys. Ossification may occur from multiple centers; failure of these centers to unite is probably responsible for partite sesamoid bones. Fractures of the sesamoids are rare in the hands. The number and distribution of the sesamoids of the hand are shown in Figure 12.

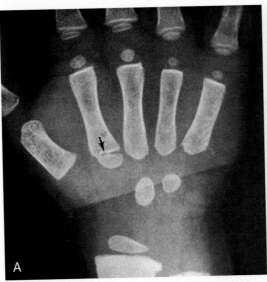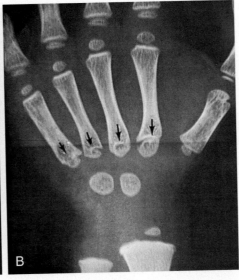

FIGURE 7. Accessory and false secondary ossification centers in the proximal cartilage of the metacarpals of normal infants. **A,** Accessory center in the second metacarpal of an infant 12 months of age; a similar center was present in the other hand. **B,** False centers in the second, third, fourth, and fifth metacarpals of a child 2 years of age; similar false centers were present in the other hand.

FOREARM

Separate ossification centers may appear in the regions of the ulnar (Fig. 13) and radial (Fig. 14) styloid processes before uniting smoothly with the main ossification center. During the latter half of childhood, the shafts of the radius and ulna may terminate in wavy, irregular surfaces (Fig. 15) in normal children whose other bones show normally smooth metaphyseal ends. In the shafts of the bones, the interosseous ridges may produce external cortical thickening encroaching on the interosseous space; this may simulate pathologic productive bone reaction. The radial tuberosity projected en face may simulate a destructive lesion (Fig. 16).

ELBOW

The several secondary epiphyseal centers in the elbow cannot be satisfactorily identified with a single projection; their positions are indicated in Figure 17. In frontal projections, the ulnar centers are superimposed on the supracondylar portions of the humerus. Like the center for the trochlea of the humerus (Fig. 18), the olecranon centers tend to be grossly irregular during the early years after their appearance and may simulate fractures (Figs. 19 and 20). The lateral epicondyle does not fuse directly with the humeral shaft, as the medial epicondyle does, but fuses first with the neighboring epiphyseal ossification center (capitulum); their fused mass then joins with the end of the humeral shaft (Fig. 21). Accessory ossification centers for the named centers may persist ununited even into adult life (Figs. 22 and 23). The radial head center frequently originates with two moieties that subsequently unite. In all projections and

positions of the normal elbow, the radial head and its subjacent shaft should be in line with the capitulum. The humeral centers appear in a sequence that can be remembered with the acronym CITE—*c*apitulum, *i*nternal (medial) epicondyle, *t*rochlea, and *e*xternal (lateral)

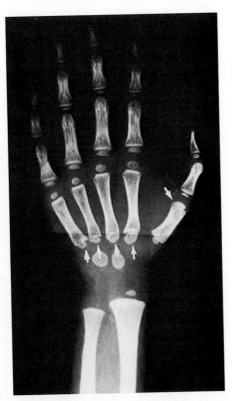

FIGURE 8. Notches at the proximal end of metacarpal bones where pseudoepiphyses had been present previously and have recently united with the shafts.

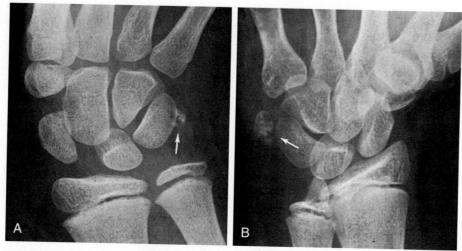

FIGURE 9. Normal irregular mineralization of the pisiform. **A,** Fine multiple bony foci in the pisiform of an asymptomatic boy 9 years of age. **B,** Granular pisiform in an asymptomatic boy 12 years of age.

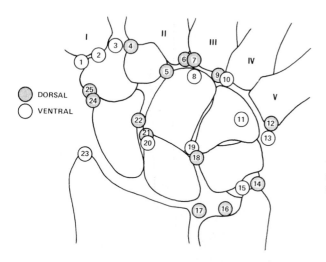

FIGURE 10. Schematic diagram of sites for best known accessory ossicles of the wrist: *1,* paratrapezium; *2,* praetrapezium; *3,* trapezium secundarium; *4,* trapezoideum secundarium; *5,* metastyloideum; *6,* parastyloideum; *7,* styloideum; *8,* subcapitatum; *9,* capitatum secundarium; *10,* os Gruberi; *11,* ununited hamulus; *12,* vesalianum; *13,* ulnare externum; *14,* ulnostyloideum; *15,* pisiforme secundarium; *16,* triangulare; *17,* small radioulnar ossicle; *18,* epitriquetrum; *19,* hypotriquetrum; *20,* hypolunatum; *21,* epilunatum; *22,* os centrale; *23,* radiostyloideum; *24,* radiale externum; *25,* epitrapezium.

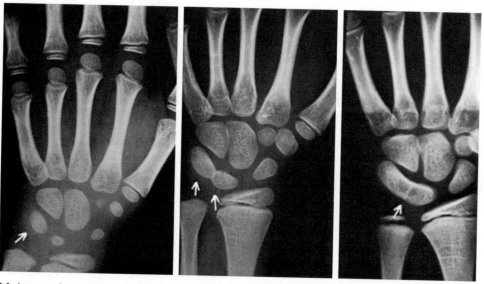

FIGURE 11. Lunatrotriquetral "fusion" *(arrows)* observed in serial films of a black child with sickle cell anemia at, *from left,* ages 6, 7, and 8 years.

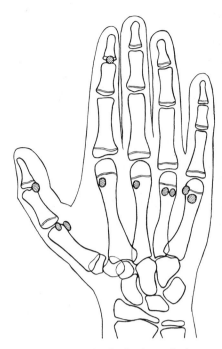

FIGURE 12. Location and distribution of the constant and inconstant sesamoid bones of the hands. Five sesamoids are of almost constant occurrence: the pair at the base of the thumb that appears just before adolescence, the single sesamoid more distal in the thumb, and the solitary sesamoids at the bases of the second and fifth digits. Five additional sesamoids are shown.

epicondyle. If a bony density is seen in one area when an earlier appearing center is lacking, a traumatic fragment is very likely the cause. The sequence of appearance is the same on the two sides but the actual timing is not always the same (Fig. 24). Rarely, a sesamoid bone develops in the triceps tendon (patella cubiti). Schwarz indicated that there are rare anomalous ossicles in the

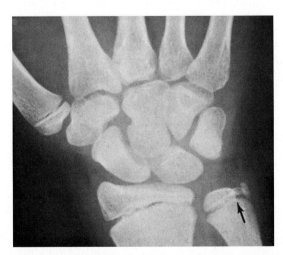

FIGURE 13. Separate secondary epiphyseal ossicles *(arrow)* for the styloid in the distal epiphyseal cartilage of the ulna of an asymptomatic boy 11 years of age. Ossicles of this type should not be mistaken for fracture fragments in case of injury. Such separate ossification centers may later fuse with the main epiphyseal ossification center or may persist throughout life as separate ossicles.

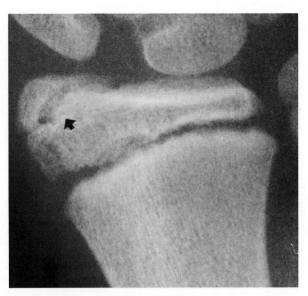

FIGURE 14. A large accessory ossification center *(arrow)* in the styloid process of the radial epiphyseal ossification center of a healthy boy 13 years of age simulates a fracture fragment.

elbows—the antecubital bone, the paratrochlear bone, and the accessory coracoid (Fig. 25). The absence of a history and injury and of symptoms differentiates them from identical osteochondral loose bodies that can follow injury.

In the distal end of the humerus, the bony septum that separates the olecranon fossa behind from the coronoid fossa in front varies in thickness and casts a shadow of variable density. Extraradiolucency in this area is usually caused by absence of this septum (supratrochlear foramen) rather than by pathologic destruction.

The supracondylar process of the humerus is a vestigial structure that projects from the medial aspect of the anterior surface of the humeral shaft (Figs. 26 and 27). It may be connected by a tendinous band, which may become calcified, to the medial epicondyle. In occasional cases, median nerve neuralgia can be associated. It is best demonstrated in slightly oblique, internally rotated projections of the humerus.

SHOULDER

At the upper end of the humerus, two and occasionally three secondary ossification centers can be observed. The first to appear develops in the medial half of the epiphysis at about 2 weeks of age; because of its eccentric location, it shifts to a factitious lateral position when the arm is rotated (Fig. 28). The second center appears laterally in the greater tuberosity during the second half of the first year. The rare third center occurs in the lesser tuberosity during the third year and fuses with the humeral head during the sixth to seventh years. It may be seen in axillary views of the shoulder and may simulate a fracture fragment.

The radiolucent cartilaginous plate at the upper end of the humerus is "tented," with the apex well above the

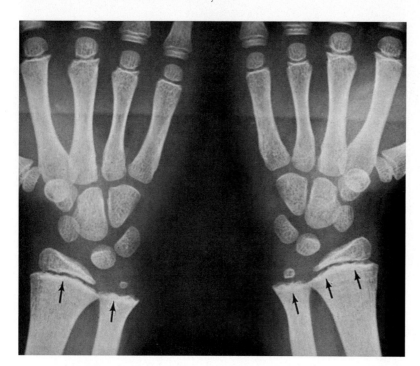

FIGURE 15. Physiologic wavy irregularities *(arrows)* in the distal metaphyses of the radii and ulnae in an asymptomatic girl 9 years of age; none of the other bones showed similar changes.

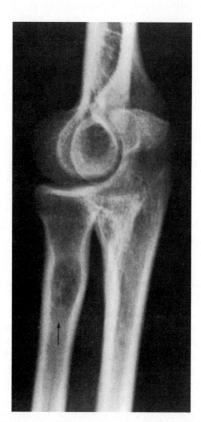

FIGURE 16. Slightly oblique projection of the elbow with the forearm extended in a teenage boy. The bicipital tuberosity of the radius is projected en face and simulates a destructive lesion in the proximal shaft just distal to the neck *(arrow)*. The cortical bone of the tuberosity is projected parallel to the direction of the x-ray beam and provides a contrasting dense margin for the portion of the medullary cavity that extends into the tuberosity. (From Keats TE: An Atlas of Normal Roentgen Variants That May Simulate Disease, 7th ed. St. Louis, Mosby, 2001, with permission.)

pitched anterior and posterior segments (Fig. 29). In rotated positions of the humerus, these segments are projected at different levels and may simulate fracture. Similarly, the eccentric position of the early-appearing medial ossification center for the humeral head may suggest, on rotation of the arm, malposition at the shoulder joint. The bicipital groove in the anterior surface of the humerus may simulate local bone destruction or production (Fig. 30), and local cortical thickening, resembling a pathologic periosteal reaction, occurs frequently at sites of insertion of major muscles of the upper arm, possibly resulting from minor trauma of heavy muscular efforts in physically active children. The medial cortical wall of the surgical neck may be notched in the absence of disease. When the humeral head is well ossified, the region of the greater tuberosity is so radiolucent as to suggest a destructive lesion (Fig. 31); it has been called pseudocyst of the humerus.

PELVIS

NORMAL ANATOMY

The pelves of fetus, infant, and child are conspicuously small and funnel-shaped; during the neonatal period, the vertical diameter is elongated in proportion to the lateral and sagittal diameters. At birth, the acetabular cavities are relatively larger and shallower than in older children and the obturator foramina are proportionately smaller and situated nearer together. The sacrum makes up a larger segment of the pelvic girdle during the early years and is situated higher in relation to the ilia than later. The infantile sacral promontory is less marked than in the adult until the infant assumes an erect posture, when the sacrum descends between the

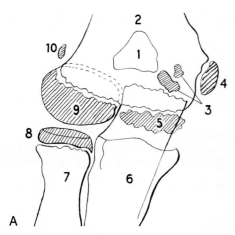 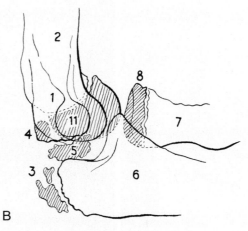

FIGURE 17. Normal secondary epiphyseal ossification centers at the elbow in frontal **(A)** and lateral **(B)** projections: *1,* olecranon fossa; *2,* shaft of the humerus; *3,* centers of the olecranon process; *4,* medial epicondyle; *5,* trochlea; *6,* shaft of the ulna; *7,* shaft of the radius; *8,* capitulum of the radius; *9,* capitulum of the humerus; *10,* lateral epicondyle; *11,* lateral projection of the diaphyseal end below the olecranon fossa.

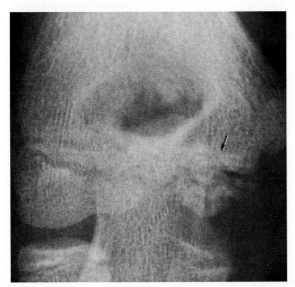

FIGURE 18. Normal irregular ossification center *(arrow)* of the trochlea of a healthy boy 13 years of age. This irregular ossification of the trochlea persists throughout the growth period and should always be recognized as a normal variant; actually it is the norm. The capitulum, in contrast, ossifies uniformly as it expands during the growth period.

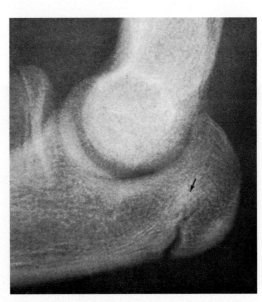

FIGURE 19. Synchondrosis of a partially fused single normal secondary ossification center of the olecranon that simulates an incomplete fracture line *(arrow).* The patient was a healthy boy 13½ years of age.

FIGURE 20. Multiple ossification centers in the olecranon epiphysis *(arrow)* that simulate multiple fracture fragments at the elbow. The patient was a healthy boy 11 years of age.

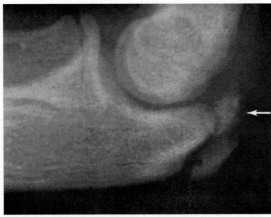

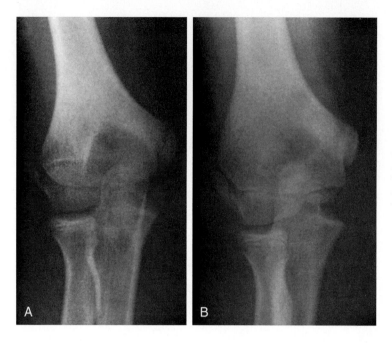

FIGURE 21. The lateral epicondyle center is independent of both the capitulum and the shaft at 11 years **(A);** it has already fused with the capitulum at 12½ years **(B),** and these combined ossification centers will later fuse with the shaft. The medial epicondyle center is fusing directly with the shaft in **A** and **B.** In **B,** the trochlea is normally irregular.

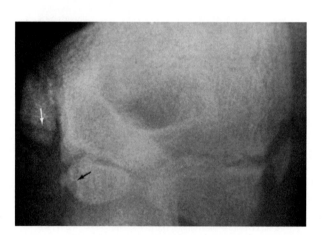

FIGURE 22. False fracture line and fragment at the lower pole of the medial epicondyle of the humerus *(white arrow)* of a healthy boy, 10 years of age, cast by an accessory ossification center and its radiolucent synchondrosis at the lower pole. The *black arrow* points to an accessory center of the trochlea.

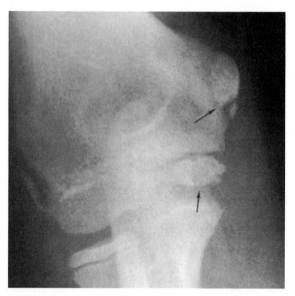

FIGURE 23. Accessory ossification center *(proximal arrow)* at the lower pole of the medial epicondyle of a healthy boy 12 years of age, which simulates a fracture fragment. *Distal arrow* points to the normal irregular edges of the trochlear center of the humerus.

FIGURE 24. Frontal projections of the right **(A)** and left **(B)** elbows of an asymptomatic girl 11 years of age. The ossification center for the right lateral epicondyle *(arrows)* is large and has been present for several months. On the left, this ossification center has not yet appeared.

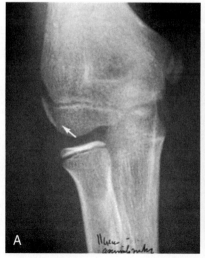

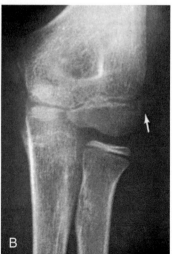

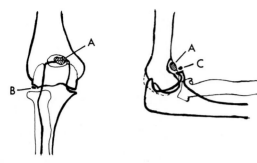

FIGURE 25. Rare accessory ossicles at the elbow. *A,* antecubital bone; *B,* paratrochlear bone; *C,* accessory coronoid. (From Schwarz GS: Bilateral antecubital ossicles [fabella cubiti] and other rare accessory bones of the elbow: with a case report. Radiology 1965;69:730–734, with permission.)

ilia and tilts forward. Pelvic growth is rapid during the first 2 years, after which growth is slow until puberty.

Anatomists claim that sexual differences in pelves can be recognized as early as the fourth fetal month but, from the radiographic standpoint, the pelves of young boys and girls are practically indistinguishable. Later, the male pelves tend to be larger but the major sexual differences are not obvious until after puberty. In girls, the ossification centers for the iliac crests usually appear within 6 months of menarche. It is possible that similar changes in the ilia of boys represent an analogous level of maturation.

RADIOGRAPHIC APPEARANCE

NORMAL SOFT TISSUES

In frontal projections, overlapping of the buttocks may be responsible for a vertical spindle-shaped shadow of

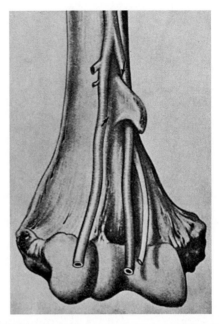

FIGURE 26. Drawing of the supracondylar process on the anterior surface of the humerus that shows the relation of the process to the brachial artery and its branches and to the median nerve. (From Barnard LB, McCoy SM: The supracondyloid process of the humerus. J Bone Joint Surg Am 1946;28:845–850, with permission.)

increased opacity which is superimposed on the symphysis pubis at or near the midsagittal pelvic plane (Fig. 32*A*). Axial projection of the shaft and glans of the penis results in a surprisingly opaque, rounded shadow (Fig. 32*B*), which may suggest to the inexperienced observer a foreign body in the rectum or bladder, or even an intrapelvic calcification. Superimposition of the glans on the bones of the pubic arch may suggest localized osteosclerosis.

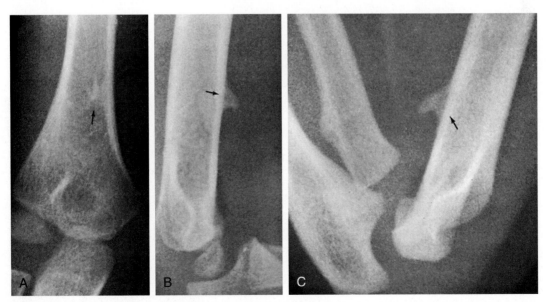

FIGURE 27. A and **B,** The supracondylar process in a healthy child 5 years of age. **A,** In the frontal projection, the process superimposed on the humeral shaft casts a small, opaque, formless image *(arrow)*. **B,** In lateral projection, a short, thick, hook-like bony mass *(arrow)* extends ventrad off the ventral edge of the humeral shaft. **C,** The supracondylar process *(arrow)* is often bilateral and varies little in its longitudinal position on the humeral shaft in different individuals; this boy was 3½ years of age.

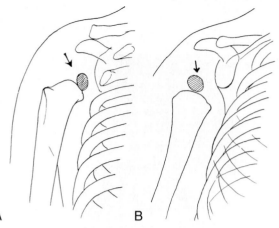

FIGURE 28. Tracings of radiographs showing factitious shift in position of the normally eccentric proximal ossification center of the humerus caused by rotation of the bone. **A,** Anatomic position of the humerus with the ossification center in the medial segment of the epiphysis. **B,** With the humerus in internal rotation, the ossification center appears to be displaced laterad. The patient was 8 months of age.

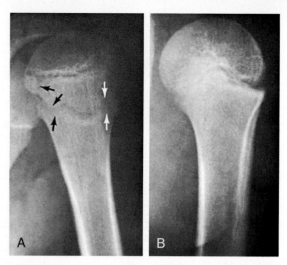

FIGURE 29. A, False fracture *(arrows)* of the humeral neck on internal rotation to 90 degrees. **B,** There is no fracture line in the anatomic position. The anterior pitch of the upper end of the humeral shaft is wider and deeper than the posterior, and it is the image of the segment below the posterior end of the shaft that casts the factitious fracture line.

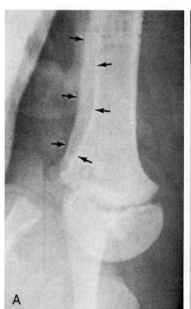
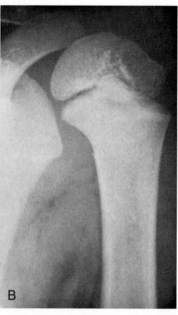

FIGURE 30. The normal shadow of the bicipital groove in the proximal end of the humerus. **A,** The humerus in full abduction and external rotation; the groove *(arrows)* appears as a shadow of diminished density. **B,** The same humerus in anatomic position; the groove is invisible because it is superimposed on the heavy shadow of the humeral shaft.

FIGURE 31. Normal shallow notching of the humeral cortical wall at the surgical neck *(arrow)*. This healthy girl was 14 years of age. Note the normal radiolucency of the greater tuberosity.

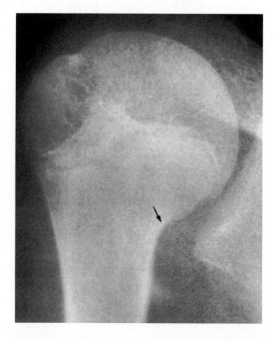

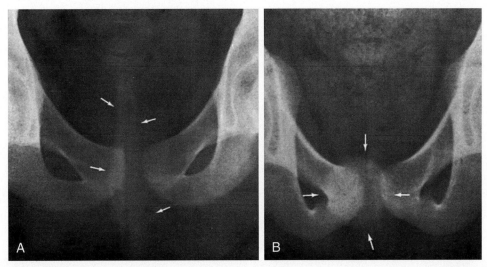

FIGURE 32. A, Spindle-shaped shadow of increased density in the midpelvic plane caused by overlapping buttocks. **B,** Heavy circular shadow cast by the penis projected in its axial plane.

Inconstant radiolucencies seen in the pelvis due to gas in the small intestine, colon, or rectum can simulate lytic lesions or bony defects. Residual barium from earlier contrast examinations, foreign bodies and fecaliths can simulate abnormal calcifications. After procedures utilizing intravenous or intraluminal contrast enhancement, partial filling of the bowel or bladder can produce confusing opacities in the pelvis.

ABNORMAL SOFT TISSUES

Dermoids are not infrequently located in the buttocks, and teratomas occur in that region as well as in the ovaries. Their skeletal components may be visualized but not clearly identified and lead to diagnostic concern during evaluation of pelvic radiographs. Opaque appendicent fecaliths, urinary tract stones and various medications should be considered when small, discrete, rounded, or oval opacities are encountered. Old granulomatous infection can cause calcification of pelvic lymph nodes. Pelvic phleboliths are rare in children but are occasionally seen in association with pelvic hemangiomas.

NORMAL AND VARIANT SKELETAL STRUCTURES

The normal pelvis at three different ages, and some of the normal secondary ossification centers, are shown in Figures 33 and 34. Grooves or channels for vascular structures can be seen in the ilium and ischium (Fig. 35A, B). The crestal center of the ilium often develops from several foci that fuse with one another before fusing with the ala (Fig. 36). Irregular extension of ossification into the cartilaginous roof of the acetabulum is a normal phenomenon during growth (Fig. 37); the regularly smooth configuration of the roof develops

from confluence of individual bony foci near the end of the first decade. Accessory centers of ossification may develop in cartilage in the spine of the ischium, and also in the rim of the acetabulum (the radiographic "os acetabuli"); they usually become visible between the 14th and 18th year (Figs. 38 and 39), after which they fuse with the main body of the ischium and ilium, respectively. Rarely, the radiographic os acetabuli persists as a separate ossicle. The anatomical os acetabuli is an ossification center, or group of centers, that appears during puberty in the anterior segment of the Y cartilage in the wall of the acetabulum.

Ossification of the cartilage in the ischiopubic synchondrosis is extremely variable in both velocity and pattern. Caffey and Ross (1956) found that bilateral fusion of the ischiopubic synchondrosis is complete in about 6% of children at 4 years of age, and in 83% at 12 years. Unilateral swelling at the synchondrosis (Fig. 40) was present in 18% of children at 7 years, and bilateral swelling in 47%. In some girls, the ischiopubic synchondrosis may close as early as the third year. They concluded that swelling preceded closure of the synchondrosis in most, and perhaps all, cases. The swellings lasted from 1 to 3 years. Irregular mineralization was present in about 42% of all subjects between ages 4 and 11, it was never present without swelling and tended to develop in the more pronounced examples of swelling. Occasionally, an independent supernumerary ossification center may develop in the ischiopubic synchondrosis (Fig. 41). Kaufmann observed a similar center in an infant aged 6 months. Cawley and associates found accumulation of radionuclide to vary in intensity and, frequently, to be asymmetric in the ischiopubic synchondrosis area in healthy children during the period of beginning, but incomplete, fusion.

Cases have been reported in which regional pain and tenderness and impaired locomotion were associated with irregular mineralization and swelling of the ischiopubic synchondrosis; this clinical picture and the associ-

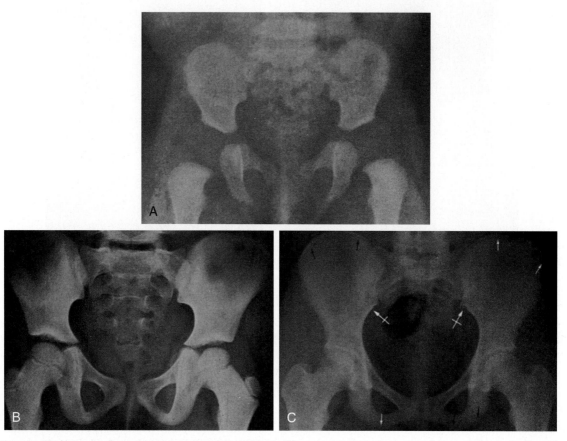

FIGURE 33. Normal radiographic appearance of the pelvis at different ages. **A,** At 3 months of age in a girl, the ischiopubic synchondroses are widely opened. The symphysis pubis is normally wide. The ossification centers in the femoral epiphyses have not yet appeared. **B.** At 5 years, the ilia are still separated from the ischia and pubic bones, but the ischiopubic synchondroses are almost completely closed; the lateral masses of the sacrum have fused with their bodies; the acetabula are proportionately smaller and deeper than in **A. C,** At 14 years, the innominate bone is completely fused, and secondary centers are now visible in the crests of the ilia and in the inferior margins of the ischia *(arrows)*. A small paraglenoid fossa indents the top of each sciatic notch *(crossed arrows)*.

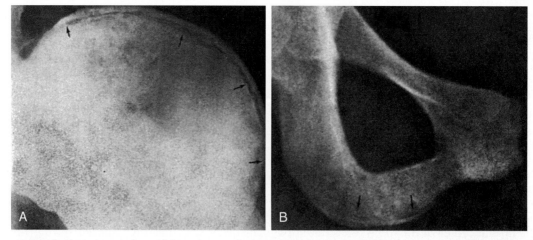

FIGURE 34. A, Normal secondary epiphyseal center in the crest of the ilium of a girl 12 years of age. The edges of the striplike crestal center and the contiguous edge of the ilium are both normally irregular—often more irregular than in this normal patient. **B,** Apophyseal center on the inferior ramus of the ischium of an asympatomatic girl 15 years of age.

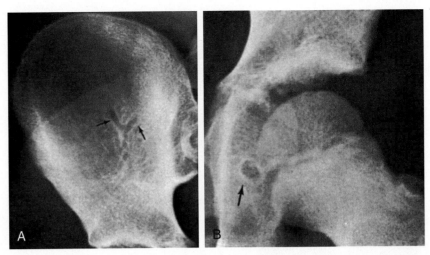

FIGURE 35. Normal vascular markings in the pelvic bones. **A,** Y-shaped tubular shadow *(arrows)* in the ilium of a boy 4 years of age. **B,** Circular vascular foramen *(arrow)* in the body of the ischium of an asymptomatic girl 4 years of age. Sometimes several small circular foramina are present in the same site instead of a single large foramen, as in this patient.

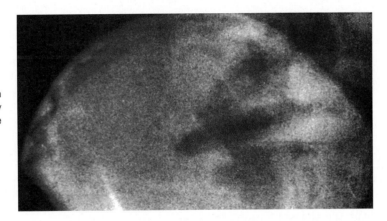

FIGURE 36. Multiple independent ossification centers in the apophyseal cartilage of the crest of the ilium of a healthy girl 15 years of age, which simulate comminuted fracture fragments.

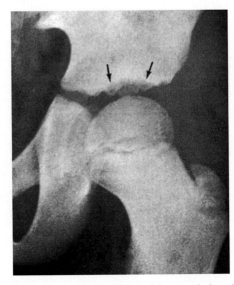

FIGURE 37. Normal irregular margins of the acetabulum *(arrows)* in a boy 6 years of age.

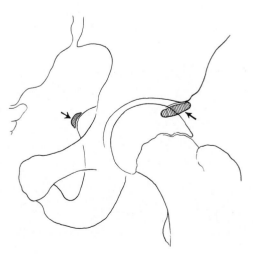

FIGURE 38. Accessory secondary pelvic ossification centers; tracing of a radiograph. Ossicle in the rim of the acetabulum and in the tip of the ischial spine in a patient 14 years of age.

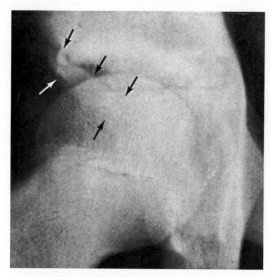

FIGURE 39. Os acetabuli marginalis superior in the cartilaginous rim of the acetabulum of a girl 11 years of age. These normal separate marginal ossicles should not be mistaken for fracture fragments or calciferous foci in the soft tissues.

ated roentgen findings have been called ischiopubic osteochondrosis (van Neck disease) in the belief that it is analogous anatomically and pathogenetically to ischemic necrosis of the skeleton, such as Perthes disease in the head of the femur and Köhler disease in the navicular bone. Junge and Heuck noted the considerable frequency with which the radiographic changes occur in asymptomatic school children, beginning about the age of 5 years. These authors, as well as Byers, report no evidence of inflammation or other pathologic change in material removed from a "swollen" ischiopubic synchondrosis. Apparently, the prognosis has always been favorable. Osteochondrosis is believed to arise, near the time of fusion, from microtrauma resulting from excessive or repeated activity of the adductor muscles that insert into the region of the synchondrosis. This region is also a classic site of stress fracture in the adult, and the lesion has been considered a pediatric equivalent of this in an appropriate clinical setting of local pain and progressive radiographic signs.

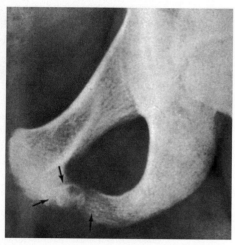

FIGURE 41. Independent supernumerary circular ossification center in the ischiopubic synchondrosis of an asymptomatic boy 8 years of age.

The diagnosis of osteomyelitis has also been made in some children with swelling of the ischiopubic junction. It is supported by positive blood cultures, elevated erythrocyte sedimentation rates, change from normal radiographs to focal irregularity before healing, and scintigraphic findings that differed from those in normal ischiopubic synchondroses. Histologic proof has not been demonstrated. In these cases, too, the prognosis has always been favorable following antibiotic treatment of 4½ to 12 weeks' duration.

Notwithstanding the above, it would seem that for the incidental observation of radiographic features, the normal irregular mineralization and variable scintigraphic features in this site should be kept in mind when the question of osteochondrosis or early osteomyelitic or neoplastic destruction at the ischiopubic synchondrosis is raised.

Irregularities in the posterolateral edge of the ischium may also be observed; occasionally during preadolescence, the lateral borders of the body of the ischium

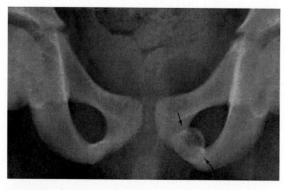

FIGURE 40. Irregular mineralization and swelling of the left ischiopubic synchondrosis *(arrows)* in an asymptomatic boy 7 years of age. The osteoporotic swollen synchondrosis projects into the obturator foramen.

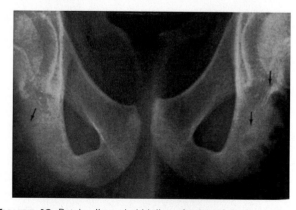

FIGURE 42. Patchy, "soap-bubble" rarefaction of the ischial ramus and tuberosity on the left, with similar but much less marked changes at the same site on the right ischium of an asymptomatic boy 12 years of age. The possibility of prior, self-induced injury during play cannot be excluded. (Courtesy of Dr. R. Parker Allen, Denver, CO.)

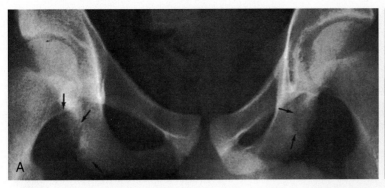
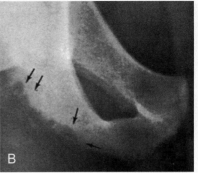

FIGURE 43. Irregularities in both ischia of asymptomatic boys 12 and 11 years of age. In **A,** the right ischium is irregularly rarefied at the tuberosity and slightly caudad into the ramus. The tuberosity of the left ischium is evenly rarefied. In **B,** there is "bubbly" rarefaction in the right tuberosity and caudad into the ramus.

and its inferior ramus show marked irregularity both in the margin and in density (Fig. 42); the two sides may be unequally affected (Fig. 43). During growth and before fusion of the body of the ischium to its scalelike epiphysis along its under edge, this ischial edge is a provisional zone of calcification and is analogous to the provisional zones of calcification in the metaphyses of all the long bones; it is not cortical lamellar bone. The ischial spine, projecting posteriorly, usually is not visible in frontal radiographs of the pelvis. The lesser sciatic notch lies below it and sometimes appears as an indentation on the lateral margin of the ischium (Fig. 44), at the region where the ischial irregularities are most common.

Some of the "variations" in mineralization are almost certainly sequelae to the normal vigorous activity of children and the response to minor tendon avulsions from sites where cartilage has yet to change to bone; they are comparable to minor epiphyseal separations. A few weeks of clinical observation during limited activity serves to resolve the significance of the observations when local symptoms were the reason for examination. The response to avulsions in more heavily muscled older children is illustrated in Figure 45.

Delayed and irregular mineralization of the pubic rami may be present at birth with subsequent mineralization from several ossification centers (Fig. 46). Vertical, radiolucent clefts occasionally noted as incidental findings in pelvis radiographs (Fig. 47) probably represent bars of nonossified cartilage between expanding

ossification centers. The medial edges of the bodies of the pubic bones are often irregularly mineralized during the growth period.

Failure of segmentation between the lateral masses of the first sacral and the fifth lumbar segments occurs in the variant known as sacralization of the fifth lumbar vertebra (Fig. 48); it can be unilateral or bilateral and may be associated with narrowing of the lumbosacral interspace.

Defects in mineralization of the sacral neural arches are common in apparently normal infants and children. The neural arches of the fourth and fifth lumbar segments are often similarly affected. These "defects" are not necessarily actual anatomical defects of the neural arches and, consequently, the term "spina bifida occulta" is often a misleading one. The arch is usually intact anatomically and the image defect represents a localized deficiency of ossification in cartilage rather

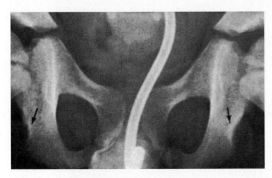

FIGURE 44. Conspicuously deep and large lesser sciatic notches with sclerotic edges *(arrows)* in an asymptomatic boy 4 years of age.

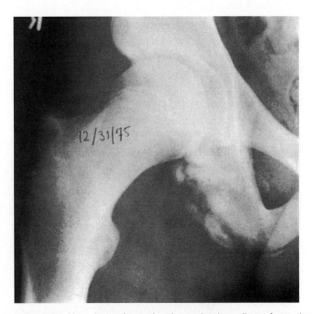

FIGURE 45 New bone formation in avulsed cartilage from the ischium in a teen-age athlete who had been active in spite of moderate pain for over 6 months following an acute episode. (From Silverman FN: Problems in pediatric fractures. Semin Roentgenol 1978;13:167–176, with permission.)

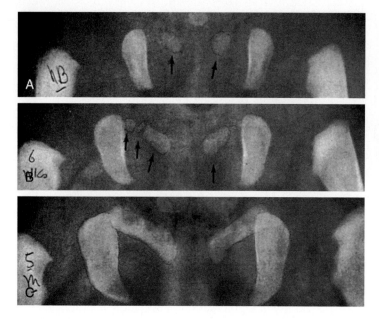

FIGURE 46. Retarded and irregular mineralization of both superior pubic rami. **A,** Neonatal. In the pubic rami, ossification is confined on each side to a round center; most of the superior pubic rami are entirely radiolucent because ossification has not yet occurred. **B,** At 6 weeks. Ossification is now increased in both superior rami, but it is still incomplete and irregular. On the right side there are at least three large independent ossification centers with radiolucent clefts between them. **C,** At 5 months. The superior rami are evenly and extensively ossified, but there is still cartilage between the dorsal ends of the rami and their ischial bodies. The changes in the pubic bones are chance findings in a patient who also had bilateral dysplasia and dislocation of the hips. (From Ribbing S: Acta Radiol 1944;25:732–755.)

FIGURE 47. Congenital "strip" defect in the superior ramus of the pubis; these lesions may be unilateral or bilaterally symmetric. **A,** At birth, there is a vertical band of diminished density in the middle third of the pubic ramus. **B,** At 6 months, at the same site there is a narrower radiolucent band, which is now bordered by strips of increased density. The patient was always asymptomatic, and palpation disclosed no signs of fracture at this site.

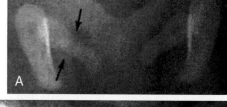

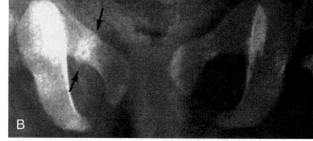

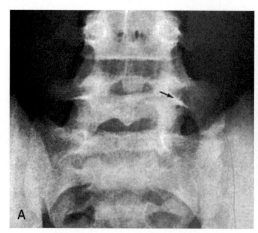
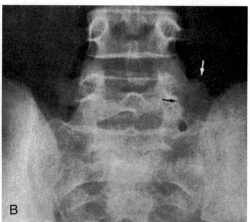

FIGURE 48. Unilateral sacralization of the fifth lumbar vertebra. **A,** In a boy 6 years of age. **B,** In a boy 11 years of age.

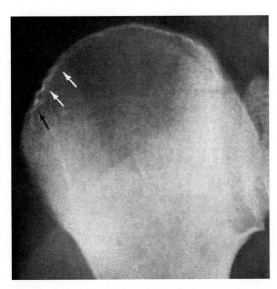

FIGURE 49. Normal marginal scalloping in the ventral segment of the iliac crest of an asymptomatic girl 6 years of age.

than a gap in the arch itself. In many cases, the defects seen during the early years of life disappear in later childhood owing to ossification of the cartilaginous segment.

The iliac crest is smooth at birth but often becomes wavy and irregular after the second or third year (Fig. 49). The ventral segment of the crest is always the most affected, and in many instances the scalloping of the crest is confined to the anterior portions. Such crestal irregularities may persist until puberty, after which they are obliterated by fusion of the crest of the ilium with the epiphyseal center.

FEMUR

The ossification center for the head of the femur appears at about 4 months of age and enlarges with time. As it fills in the hemispheric cartilage of the head, the center may exhibit irregularities of form and density during the first decade in the absence of disease (Fig. 50). Ossification may begin with coarse stippling and progress, as the size increases, to irregularities along the margin. The variations may occur unilaterally, but generally they are bilateral so that comparison with the asymptomatic side, in questions of disease, may avoid misdiagnosis. Before the ossification center has rounded out fully, some flattening of the contour may be observed where subsequently the fovea can be recognized (Fig. 51). Consideration must always be given to density changes caused by superimposition of components of the bone constituting the acetabular cavity; channels for nutrient vessels in the ischium can simulate destructive lesions in the femoral head when superimposition occurs.

FIGURE 50. Factitious splitting of the femoral head in an asymptomatic girl 4 years of age. **A,** In frontal projection, the femoral head image is normal. **B,** In lateral externally rotated position, the femoral head image is divided longitudinally into two unequal segments by a strip of decreased density that represents the synchondrosis between the two ossification centers that developed one behind the other ventrodorsally.

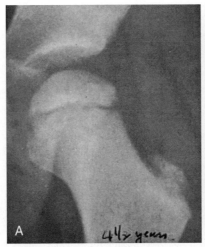
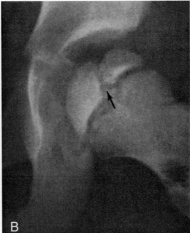

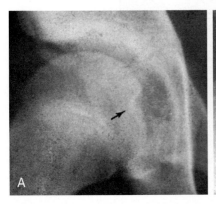
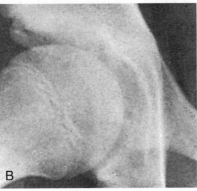

FIGURE 51. The fovea capitis femoris *(arrow)* is characteristically visible in standard frontal projection **(A)** but is not visible when the femur is externally rotated and abducted into the frog position **(B).** The patient was a healthy boy 15 years of age.

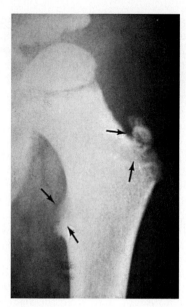

FIGURE 52. Normal irregularities *(arrows)* in density of the shaft adjacent to the trochanters and the secondary center in the greater femoral trochanter in an asymptomatic boy 5 years of age.

The femoral neck has an anterior deviation from the coronal plane (the angle of anteversion) that is greatest in early infancy and diminishes to approximately 23 degrees in late childhood. Ambulation plays a role in this change just as it does in diminishing the angle

between the neck and the shaft in frontal projection from almost 180 degrees at birth to 120 to 140 degrees over a similar time frame. Consequently, a child who is non–weight bearing from infancy usually retains large angles between the shaft and the neck of the femur (coxa valga). Internal rotation of the femur during examination decreases this angle and external rotation increases it because of geometric projection. A decrease in the normal angle at any time is termed *coxa vara*. Occasionally, radiolucent defects with sclerotic borders are observed incidentally in the femoral neck; some that have been followed radiographically have resolved much as those of benign cortical defects. The centers for the greater and lesser trochanters are frequently irregularly mineralized (Fig. 52).

The shaft of the femur is usually regular in health. Cortical defects, radiolucent or sclerotic, may occur in the upper or middle portions (Fig. 53) and are thought to have the same significance or lack of it as benign cortical defects in the region of the knee. Foramina and canals for the nutrient arteries are often visible in several projections (Fig. 54). Although the veins for the cancellous tissue run separately from the arteries, one or two may accompany the main nutrient artery. The others leave the bone through apertures near the ends of the bone and may contribute to some of the irregularities of cortex in these regions.

Benign fibrous cortical defects occur frequently in the distal metaphysis of the femur and are more common on the medial than the lateral portion. The lesions are

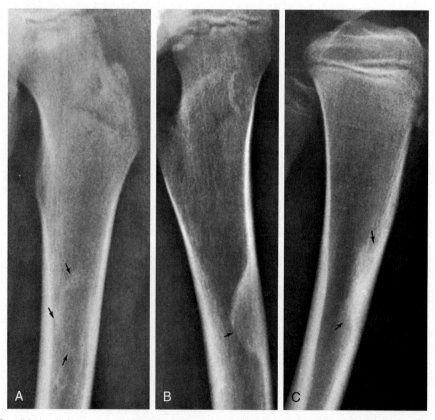

FIGURE 53. Possible healed opaque cortical defect *(arrows)* in the proximal third of the left femur in frontal **(A)** and lateral **(B)** projections. **C,** Similar healed opaque cortical defects *(arrows)* through the ventral cortical wall of the tibia in lateral projection.

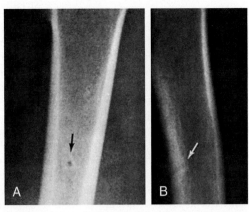

FIGURE 54. Superior foramina for femoral nutrient arteries in frontal **(A)** and lateral **(B)** projections. **A,** The foramen casts a small circular radiolucent image. **B,** The canal perforates the anterior cortical wall and could be interpreted as a cortical fracture line. Similar foramina and canals were present in the other femur at the same level in this asymptomatic boy 3½ years of age.

almost always posteriorly located; they are extremely rare ventrally. They first occur after 1½ years of age and usually are best developed after the fifth and sixth years. The frequency of these defects in normal children (up to 40% or greater) indicates that they will be found in children suffering from a variety of diseases associated with destructive lesions of bone. Generally, their benign nature can be recognized by the radiographic characteristics and location. Magnetic resonance imaging may provide more definitive information about their nature. However, in rare instances when the significance of a lesion cannot be evaluated satisfactorily, biopsy diagnosis may be necessary.

The defects have a round or oval radiolucent cyst-like appearance when projected en face; when projected in profile, they appear most frequently as shallow superfi-

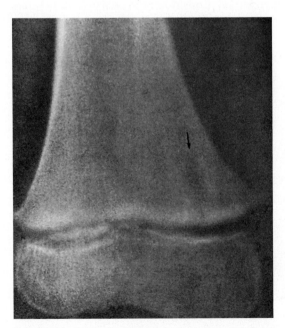

FIGURE 55. Small, poorly defined cortical defect in the medial segment of the femoral metaphysis of a healthy boy 5 years of age. A small, benign cortical defect was also present in the medial cortical wall of the tibia.

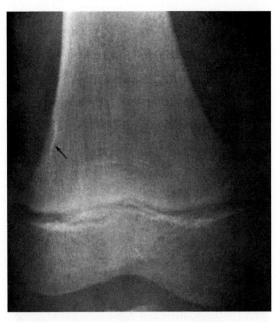

FIGURE 56. Early superficial benign cortical defect in the lateral cortical wall of the right femur of an asymptomatic boy 10 years of age. (Modified from Köhler A, Zimmer EA: Borderlands of the Normal and Early Pathologic in Skeletal Roentgenology. New York, Grune & Stratton, 1993.)

cial defects in the cortex extending into it from the outer surface (Figs. 55 and 56). During their earliest phase, they are usually small and poorly defined, and located near the end of the shaft, often extending to the primary zone of calcification. Most defects gradually shift away from the end of the shaft with advancing age and shrink until they become invisible. Some become more opaque, first in their shaftward segments and later in toto (Figs. 57 and 58). Others may persist in the site of origin for many years or completely disappear only to reappear in the same site several times over a period of years. Rarely, they may enlarge progressively to develop the radiographic characteristics of nonossifying fibromas. Microscopically, the two conditions are similar, if not identical, with whorls of connective tissue and frequent multinuclear giant cells. Although their greatest frequency is in the distal metaphysis of the femur, they occur in other tubular bones such as the tibia.

Local external thickenings with irregular margins are common findings in the posterior aspect of the distal femoral metaphysis in healthy adolescents (Fig. 59), particularly along the medial extension of the linea aspera. Sometimes the thickenings are present on both sides. They are probably the result of repetitive, vigorous, muscular activity but have been the object of undue concern for neoplastic change when the frequency of their occurrence has been overlooked, as has the absence of any adjacent soft tissue swelling. Bufkin found the lesion to be a localized segment of periosteal thickening embedded within the cortical wall. It was made up of proliferating fibrous tissue that merged imperceptibly with the overlying thickened periosteum. Small fragments of resorbing bone were often present in the proliferating mass of fibrous tissue near the periosteum. He concluded that the pathogenic mechanism responsible for the lesion was repeated microavulsions

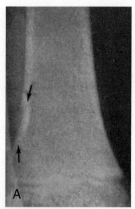

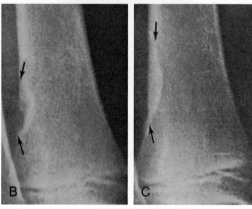

FIGURE 57. Concurrent migration shaftward and opacification of a tibial cortical defect at 7 years **(A)**, 8 years **(B)**, and 9 years **(C)**. In the evolution of these defects, opacification always begins in the segment farthest from the epiphyseal cartilage.

of cortical fragments at the site of insertion of a portion of the tendon of the adductor magnus muscle. This opinion has been supported by others. In any case, this finding is of no clinical significance.

In the epiphyseal ossification center that is present at the lower end of the femur in almost all term infants at birth, extension in width occurs rapidly between the second and sixth years. As a result, the lateral and medial margins are commonly irregular and ragged (Fig. 60). In lateral projection, normal centers may present a rough, fringe-like margin (Fig. 61*A*). Accessory ossification centers may persist at the margins of cartilage–shaft junctions when ossification is almost complete (Fig. 61*B*). Rarely, an accessory ossification center develops in the epiphyseal cartilage contiguous to the medial edge of the epiphyseal ossification center (Fig. 62). In older children, marginal mineralization of the femoral condyles is characteristically uneven and is often associated with independent ossification centers beyond the edge of the main bony mass (Fig. 63). Their radiographic appearance simulates that of osteochondritis dissecans. Caffey et al. found this variant in approximately 30% of healthy children when the knees were examined in tunnel and lateral projections. The pattern and distribution of these extra, normal, independent ossification centers in the distal femoral epiphyseal cartilage is shown schematically in Figure 64. This defect is much more common on the lateral than on the medial condyle, in contradistinction to the findings in osteochondritis dissecans. In addition, these irregularities are seen in children younger than the usual age for this disease.

The popliteal groove is a normal marginal defect that appears on the posterolateral aspect of the outer condyle in the prepubertal period (Fig. 65); at times it may be very prominent. This groove carries the tendon of the popliteal muscle and is never visible during infancy or early childhood. The nutrient foramen of the distal femoral epiphysis is often clearly visible in frontal projections in children older than 4 years (Fig. 66); bilateral symmetry may not be present. During late childhood, when the intercondylar fossa becomes deeper, lateral projection of the distal femoral epiphysis shows the anterior segment to be more radiolucent than

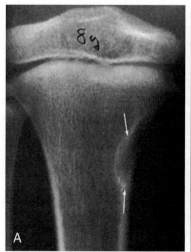

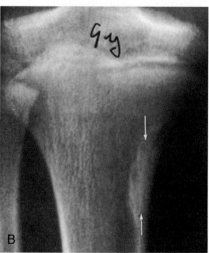

FIGURE 58. A, Radiolucent defect *(arrows)* in the medial cortical wall of the tibia of an asymptomatic girl of 8 years. **B,** At 9 years, the defect *(arrows)* has become opaque as a result of either generalized ossification or calcification. The microscopic changes in the healed opaque defect have not been studied. Healing consistently begins at the shaftward end of the defect and proceeds toward the epiphysis.

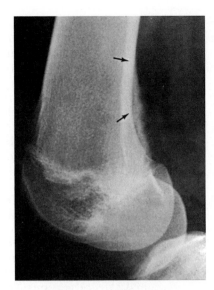

FIGURE 59. Normal long, thick, irregular overgrowth of the planum popliteum femoris *(arrows)* of a healthy boy 14 years of age. This external thickening has raised the question of osteosarcoma in some patients. In three such patients, biopsy study showed normal bone.

the remainder (Fig. 67). This reflects the fact that the posterior portion of the epiphysis is wider than the anterior, and the radiant energy also has to traverse four layers of cortex (the lateral and medial walls of each of the two condyles) instead of only two anteriorly. The lateral condyle can be differentiated from the medial in lateral projections of the knee because it is relatively flat in comparison with the rounded configuration of the latter.

KNEE

Additional variants occur in the region of the distal part of the femur that also can be considered in relation to the knee joint. Several sesamoid bones occur in this region: the patella, fabella, and cyamella. The patella is the largest sesamoid bone of the body, lying within the tendon of the quadriceps muscle. Ossification normally develops from several foci. The patella is often granular early, and its edges may be irregular during childhood

(Fig. 68). Following fusion of the focal centers, another center may develop in the superolateral portion of the bone and may persist as a distinct ossicle (Fig. 69). Focal defects occasionally occur in asymptomatic children, most commonly indenting the posterior aspect of the patella and presenting as clear radiolucent defects in frontal projection (Fig. 70). These also occur in the superolateral portion of the bone, and both are currently believed to be variants related to aberrant traction by the vastus lateralis muscle, which inserts into the patella in the upper and outer quadrant. Both may become symptomatic. Alexander and associates observed one such defect in association with a knee effusion and believed it to be a Brodie abscess. Additional centers may also appear, but most usually unite with the main body of the patella by late adolescence. Segmentation of the patella into anterior and posterior components has been described in multiple epiphyseal dysplasia and also has been reported without reference to any associated skeletal abnormalities.

The fabella is an inconstant sesamoid bone in the lateral head of the gastrocnemius muscle that is visible in lateral projections of the knee in adolescents (Fig. 71). It is difficult to see in frontal projection. The cyamella is a rare ossicle in the popliteal tendon, partially buried in the edge of the lateral condyle of the femur and in the popliteal groove (Figs. 65 and 72).

TIBIA AND FIBULA

Anatomic variants are more common in the tibia than in the fibula at the knee. Irregular mineralization along the margins of the tibial ossification center is similar to that in the distal femoral epiphysis during periods of rapid transformation of cartilage to bone. A step-like defect appears in the upper anterior border of the tibia in lateral projection before ossification proceeds into the cartilaginous anterior tibial tubercle from the main proximal tibial ossification center. The tubercle may also be ossified from accessory centers that, before union, may simulate avulsed fragments of bone. When ossification of the anterior tibial process is complete, the radiolucent cartilage still separating the process from the shaft may appear as a notch or a horizontal strip depending on the projection used (Figs. 73 and 74).

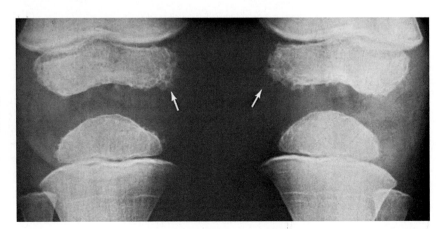

FIGURE 60. Normal irregular mineralization on the margins of the ossification centers in the distal epiphyses of the femora of a boy 3 years of age.

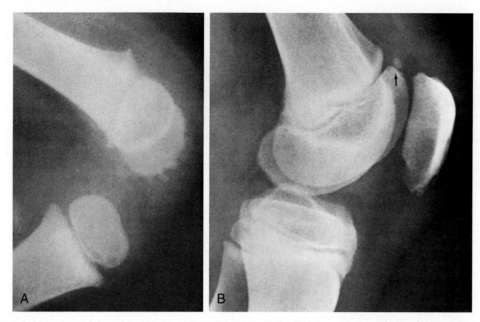

FIGURE 61. A, Lateral projection of the left knee of an asymptomatic boy 3½ years of age. The femoral condyle has a rough, fringe-like edge as a result of partial fusion with several marginal accessory ossification centers in the contiguous epiphyseal cartilage. Similar marginal centers were present at both ends of the ossification center in the frontal projection. **B,** Small triangular independent accessory ossification center at the proximal ventral edge of the greater condyle *(arrow)* of an asymptomatic boy 13 years of age. Smaller scale accessory centers are also visible at the ventral edge of the lower pole of the patella.

Asymmetry of development on the two sides is common. External rotation tends to superimpose the thick cortex, extending to the anterior tibial crest onto the lateral aspect of the bone (Fig. 75). Benign cortical defects may occur in the proximal ends of the tibia and fibula; their radiographic characteristics are comparable to those of the femoral ones.

In the distal ends of the bones, the Achilles tendons and overlying skin are often visible in frontal projection (Fig. 76). The cephalad notching of the distal tibial physis in its medial aspect is a normal phenomenon (Krump's hump). Separate accessory ossification centers are common in the cartilages of the medial malleoli of the tibias and less common in the lateral malleoli of the fibulas (Figs. 77 and 78). The provisional zone of calcification in the distal fibular metaphysis may be notched shaftward, and a tiny extra ossicle may develop

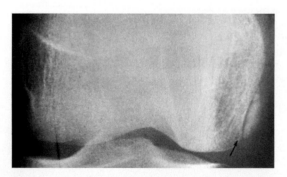

FIGURE 62. Accessory medial ossification center *(arrow)* contiguous to the medial edge of the epiphyseal ossification center of the right femur of an asymptomatic girl 13 years of age.

in the notch (Fig. 79); the notching is usually bilateral. Benign cortical defects or nonossifying fibromas may occur in this level as in the upper ends of the tibia and fibula (Figs. 80 and 81).

FEET

The bones of the foot are assigned to three anatomic divisions: the forefoot, which includes the metatarsals and phalanges; the midfoot, which includes the three cuneiform bones, the cuboid, and the navicular; and the hindfoot, which includes the talus and calcaneus. The forefoot and the midfoot are separated by the distal row of tarsal joints, while the proximal row separates the midfoot from the hindfoot. A middle row of tarsal joints extends transversely between the navicular and the three cuneiform bones. The cuboid bone extends between the proximal and distal rows of tarsal joints, blocking lateral or medial movement through the middle row of tarsal joints.

Accessory ossification centers may occur in the epiphyses of phalanges and metatarsal bones and are common in the great toes, where examination before fusion of the centers is complete may simulate fracture (Fig. 82). Incompletely fused pseudoepiphyses of metatarsal bones may do so also (Fig. 83); as in the metacarpals, the pseudoepiphyses are located distally in the first metatarsal and proximally in the second through fifth. The pedal phalanges, especially the middle group, frequently lack epiphyseal centers in healthy children; this absence is often associated with symphalangism at the affected joints. CSE of the pedal phalanges are shown in

Text continued on page 2083

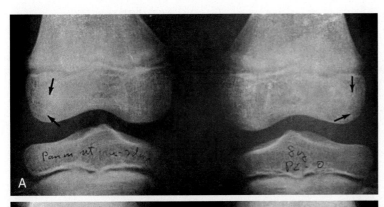

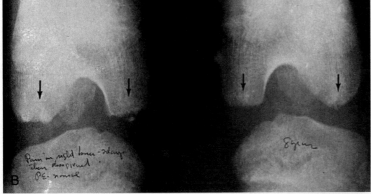

FIGURE 63. Knees of a boy 10 years of age in frontal **(A)**, "tunnel" **(B)**, and lateral **(C and D)** projections. The right knee had been slightly and indefinitely painful for 2 days only. The left was always asymptomatic. In the frontal projection the condylar margins are smooth, but their texture is slightly irregular *(arrows)*. In both tunnel and lateral projections, there are deep marginal irregularities in the dorsal edges of the condyles. Independent marginal ossification centers can be seen in the cartilage, well beyond the edge of the main condylar mass.

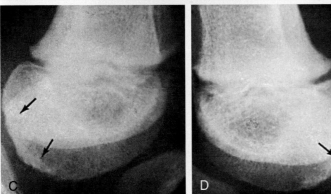

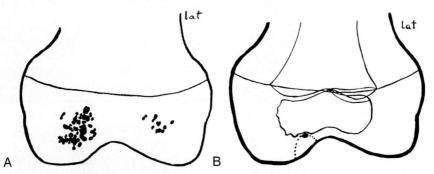

FIGURE 64. A, Sites of focal extraossification centers in the left distal femoral epiphyseal cartilages of 291 children recorded on tracings of an adult femur. **B,** Tracing of the distal ends of a child's femur superimposed on a tracing of the distal end of an adult femur that shows an accessory ossification center *(black dot)* in the cartilage of the epiphysis just beyond the caudal edge of the main ossification center. The *dotted line* indicates projected growth of the accessory center. (From Ribbing S: Zur ätlologie der osteochondrosis dissecans. Acta Radiol 1944;25:732–755, with permission.)

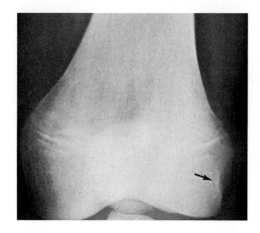

FIGURE 65. Normal popliteal groove *(arrow)* in the posterolateral wall of the lateral femoral condyle of an asymptomatic girl 11 years of age.

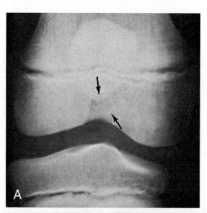

FIGURE 66. Normal radiolucent shadow of the nutrient foramen of the distal femoral epiphysis *(arrows)* on the posterior wall of the intercondylar fossa. **A,** Poorly defined foramen in a boy 7 years of age. **B,** Sharply defined foramen in a girl 11 years of age. **C,** Long transverse foramen in a girl 10½ years of age. **D–F,** Photographs of nutrient foramina in adult femora.

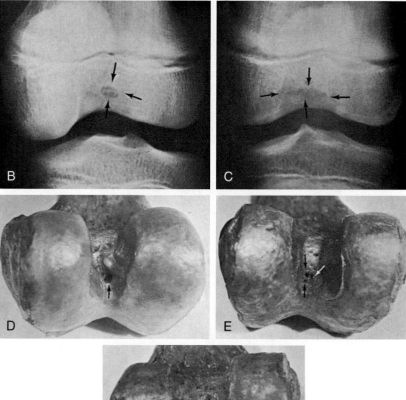

FIGURE 67. Normal radiolucent anterior segment of the distal femoral epiphysis of a girl 5 years of age, as seen in frontal **(A)** and lateral **(B)** projections. It is more radiolucent than the posterior segment because the rays traverse only two opaque walls: the medial wall of the medial condyle and the lateral wall of the lateral condyle. Posteriorly, where the intercondylar notch is deeper, the rays traverse four opaque walls: the lateral and medial walls of both condyles. The *arrows* point to an opaque sclerotic band cast by the floor of the intercondylar notch.

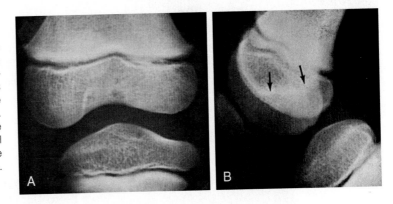

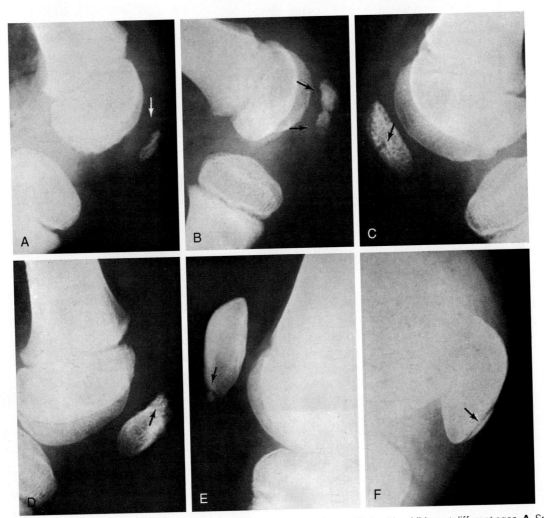

FIGURE 68. Normal variations in size, shape, and density of the patella *(arrows)* in healthy children at different ages. **A,** Small irregular patella of a boy 5 years of age. **B,** Multiple irregular centers in a girl 6 years of age. **C,** Generalized granular texture with partial segmentation in a girl 8 years of age. **D,** Irregularity in density of the superior third of the patella in a boy 8 years of age. **E,** Small separate ossicle at the inferior pole of the patella of a boy 11 years of age. **F,** Scale-like marginal ossicle on the anterior edge of the patella in a girl 9 years of age.

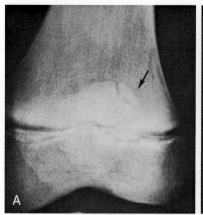
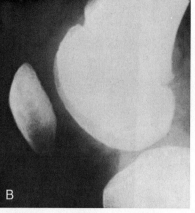

FIGURE 69. Marginal segmentation of the patella of an asymptomatic boy 10 years of age. The separate ossicle is clearly visible in frontal projection (**A,** *arrow*), but is invisible in lateral projection **(B)** because it is superimposed on the main mass of the patella.

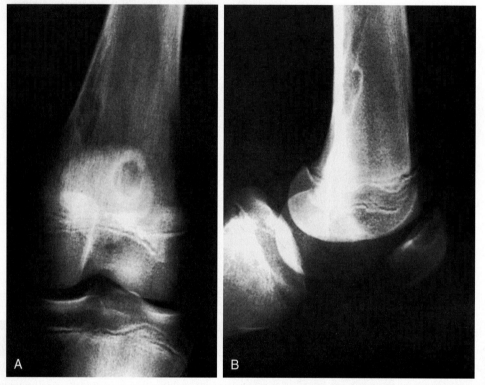

FIGURE 70. Posterior radiolucent defect in the patella in an asymptomatic child with a benign cortical defect as well. These defects usually fill in with mildly sclerotic bone and subsequently reconstitute to normal bone in a normally configured patella.

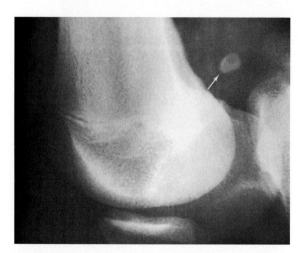

FIGURE 71. Fabella *(arrow)* in the lateral head of the gastrocnemius in its normal position, well separated from the femur itself.

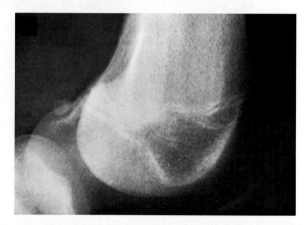

FIGURE 72. Sesamoid (cyamella). Small, partially embedded ossicle in the edge of the lateral femoral condyle of an asymptomatic boy 16 years of age. This ossicle appears to be in the position of the head of the popliteal muscle near its site of origin on the lateral femoral condyle. This is the normal position for this rare sesamoid of the popliteus.

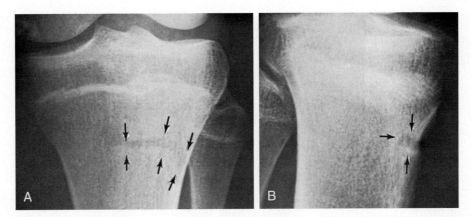

FIGURE 73. Radiolucent shadow of the notch on the anterior surface of the tibia that the anterior tibial process overlies *(arrows).* The peripheral portions of this depression in the tibial shaft that are not covered by the opaque anterior tibial process appear as a strip of diminished density in the anteromedial segment of the tibia. This shadow is never visible in infants and younger children. Frontal **(A)** and lateral **(B)** projections of the tibia of a boy 13 years of age.

FIGURE 74. Normal variations in the size and configuration of the anterior tibial process. (Modified from Köhler A, Zimmer EA: Borderlands of the Normal and Early Pathologic in Skeletal Roentgenology, 4th ed. New York, Grune & Stratton, 1993.)

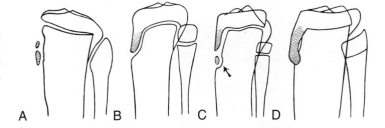

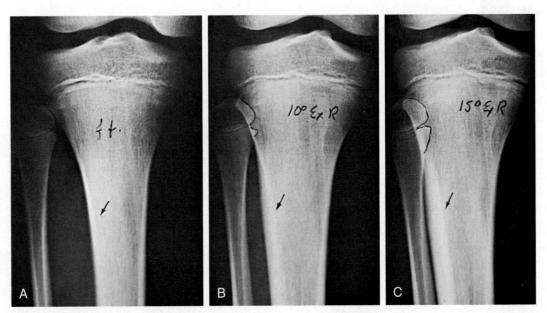

FIGURE 75. Spurious thickening of the lateral cortical wall of the tibia due to external rotation of the leg of a boy 10 years old. **A,** Full frontal projection; the lateral and medial cortical walls are approximately equal in thickness. **B** and **C,** Ten and 15 degrees of rotation, respectively; the lateral cortical wall becomes progressively thicker *(arrows)* as external rotation is increased. The thickening is due to the fact that the anterior tibial crest comes progressively more into profile on the lateral edge of the shaft as the tibia is rotated externally. This phenomenon cannot be demonstrated radiographically during the first years of life.

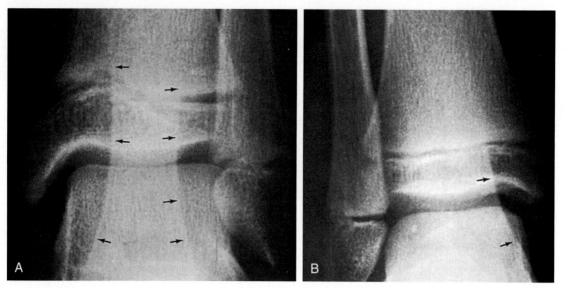

FIGURE 76. A, Demonstration of the skin over both edges *(arrows)* of the Achilles tendon of a healthy girl 10 years of age. **B,** Demonstration of the medial edge only *(arrows)* of the Achilles tendon of an asymptomatic boy 9 years of age.

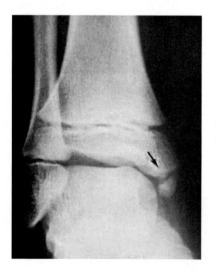

FIGURE 77. Separate ossification center *(arrow)* in the medial malleolus of the distal tibial epiphyseal cartilage of an asymptomatic girl 9 years of age. There was an analogous ossicle in the other foot. This ossicle must not be mistaken for a fracture fragment.

FIGURE 78. "Inset" accessory center in the distal epiphysis of the fibula whose superior radiolucent synchondrosis suggests a transverse fracture in the frontal projection **(A)** but is seen to be a smooth, rounded center in a deep, smooth notch *(arrow)* in the lateral oblique projection **(B).** This patient was a boy 10 years of age.

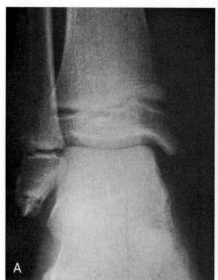
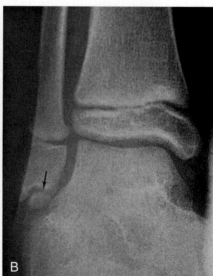

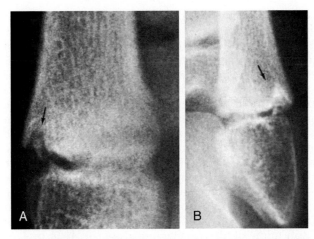

FIGURE 79. A, Extra ossicle in a notched marginal recess *(arrow)* in the lateral segment of the distal fibular metaphysis in an asymptomatic boy 9 years of age. Similar changes were present in the right fibula. In case of injury, this little variant ossicle must not be mistaken for a fracture fragment or osteochondrosis dissecans. **B,** Similar ossicle with a notch *(arrow)* in an asymptomatic boy 10 years of age.

Figure 84. They are more frequent than CSE of the hands but apparently do not have the association with specific disorders that occurs with similar findings in the hands. Premature fusion and shortening of the affected bones probably occurs in both locations.

During puberty, a scale-like secondary center appears on the proximal apophyseal cartilage of the fifth metatarsal (Fig. 85). This may persist throughout life as a separate ossicle, in which case it is designated the os vesalianum; usually, it fuses with the shaft after a few years and completely disappears. Sesamoid bones are present in the foot as in the hand. Bipartite sesamoids are not uncommon (Figs. 86 and 87). In general, there is an absence of local complaints when the separation is a variant; in the case of local injury, it is helpful to know

that a bipartite sesamoid is larger than a fractured normal sesamoid. Sesamoids are the most common of normal supernumerary ossicles of the foot (Fig. 88).

The ossification center for the calcaneus is present at birth. Occasionally, the body of the calcaneus may ossify from two or more independent centers (Fig. 89), but this observation must be suspected of being a manifestation of systemic disease because accessory centers of this type have been noted in Down syndrome, mucolipidosis, and Larsen's syndrome. The ossification centers for the apophysis of the calcaneus appear in the cartilage behind its normally irregular border about the middle of the first decade and maintain their fragmented or sclerotic character well into the second decade until fusion with the body of the calcaneus is complete (Fig. 90). Sclerosis is diminished or lacking only in the case of nonuse or absence of weight bearing. The calcaneus secondarius (Fig. 91; also see Fig. 88) may simulate a fracture fragment. A pseudocystic triangular area of radiolucency is present in the anterior half of the laterally imaged calcaneus because of a normal deficiency of spongy bone and has no clinical significance (Fig. 92). Enosteomas (bone islands) are focal accumulations of excess amounts of cancellous bone and are common in the calcaneus. They have no known clinical significance.

The primary ossification center for the talus is also present at birth. A secondary center appears in the dorsal process during the 5th and 6th postnatal years and fuses with the body of the talus between the 16th and 20th years. Before fusion, it may simulate pathologic changes (Figs. 93 and 94); if it fails to fuse, it is called the os trigonum. The os supratalare on the crest of the head of the talus may simulate, or be simulated by, response to injury (Fig. 95).

The center for the navicular bone is frequently irregular up to about 5 years of age, and occasionally later (Fig. 96). The os supranaviculare (Fig. 97) is an accessory ossicle that can be confused with an accessory

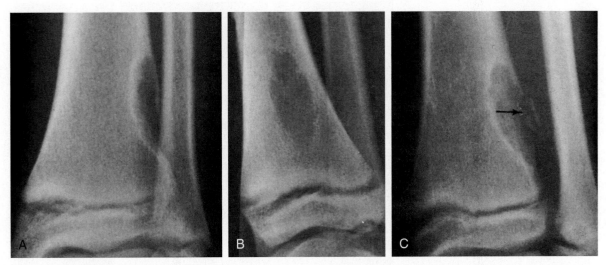

FIGURE 80. Comminuted marginal fracture fragments in the edge of a tibial cortical defect after traumatic injury *(arrow* in **C**). The cartilage plate space is deepened in all three projections, which suggests Salter type I cartilage plate injury as well. This boy, age 14 years, had pain and swelling at the ankle following a football injury. Frontal **(A),** lateral **(B),** and lateral oblique **(C)** projections of the left ankle.

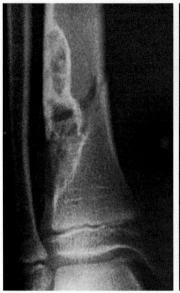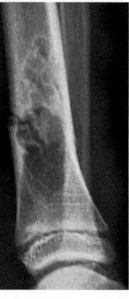

FIGURE 81. Large multiloculated benign cortical defect or nonossifying fibroma with a pathologic fracture in a girl 8 years of age. Injury was denied. This fracture healed rapidly with abundant callus.

ossification center before the latter fuses with the parent bone, and both must be differentiated from fracture. Here, as elsewhere, the tendency for bilaterality of anatomic variants is helpful. The os tibiale externum is the best known and one of the most important variants in the foot. Two types have been described: type I is a true sesamoid bone that lies within the tendon of the posterior tibial muscle and is anatomically separate from the navicular bone (Fig. 98); type II is united to the navicular by a cartilaginous or fibrocartilaginous bridge and represents an accessory ossification center for the tubercle of the navicular. Fusion with the navicular bone occurs in the great majority of these cases. The first type accounts for approximately 10% to 15% of cases in children and up to 30% in adults because of delay in ossification of the cartilaginous anlage. It is oval or rounded and is rarely symptomatic. When pain and local tenderness occur, they are almost always associated with the second type, which is triangular in shape. Females are affected four times as frequently as males; symptoms generally develop in the second decade. Bilateral ossicles are present in slightly more than half of patients. Lawson et al. suggested that bone scanning is useful to

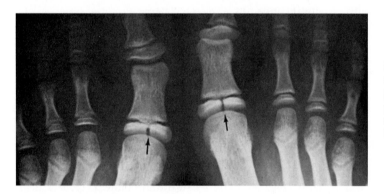

FIGURE 82. Symmetric fissures of the secondary ossification centers *(arrows)* in proximal epiphyses of the basal phalanges of the great toes of an asymptomatic boy 11 years of age. Radiolucent synchondroses between the segments of each center must not be mistaken for fracture lines.

FIGURE 83. Incomplete synchondrosis of a false accessory epiphyseal ossification center that simulates a transverse fracture at the distal end of the left first metatarsal *(arrows)*. There were similar findings in the right metatarsal of this asymptomatic boy 11 years of age. Frontal **(A)**, oblique **(B)**, and lateral **(C)** projections. (From Koo WW, Oestreich AE, Sherman R, et al: Radiological case of the month: osteopenia, rickets, and fractures in preterm infants. Am J Dis Child 1985;139:1045–1046.)

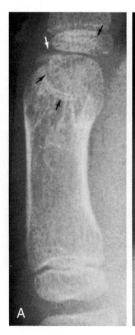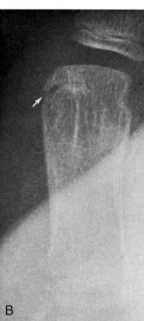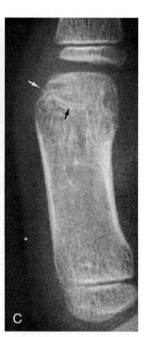

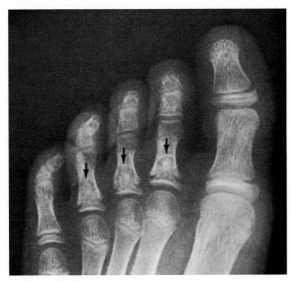

FIGURE 84. Symmetric bilateral conical or bell-shaped epiphyseal ossification centers *(arrows)* in the proximal phalanges of the second, third, and fourth toes of both feet of an asymptomatic girl 8 years of age. The contiguous distal end of each shaft is recessed to receive its elongated ossification center. The epiphyseal ossification centers in basal phalanges of the first and fifth toes are the normal, flat, shallow, transverse disks usually present in all of the phalanges. In the middle and distal phalanges of toes 2, 3, 4, and 5, the primary and secondary ossification centers have fused in single bony masses.

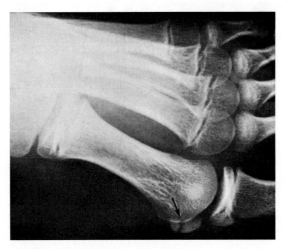

FIGURE 86. Normal bipartite sesamoid *(arrow)* at the base of the great toe of an asymptomatic girl 13 years of age. This normal developmental variant should not be mistaken for a fracture of the sesamoid in the case of local injury. The companion sesamoid superimposed on the shaft of the first metatarsal appears as an opaque circular mass that is not fissured.

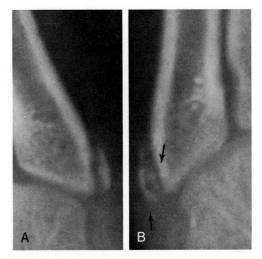

FIGURE 85. Normal scale-like ossification centers in the apophyses at the proximal ends of the fifth metatarsals in a boy 10½ years old who injured one foot 2 years earlier. **A,** The injured foot. **B,** The uninjured foot.

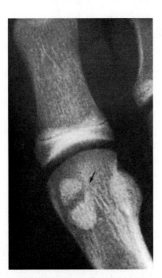

FIGURE 87. Bipartite sesamoid *(arrow)* superimposed on the distal end of the first metatarsal of an asymptomatic boy 13 years of age. The facing edges of the two parts of the sesamoid are irregular and are highly suggestive of a fracture with distraction, but the parts had never been injured, and there were no local signs or disability.

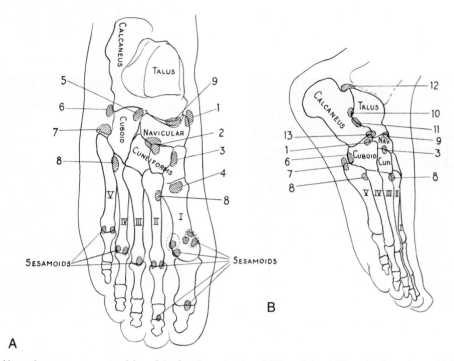

FIGURE 88. Normal supernumerary ossicles of the feet in ventrodorsal **(A)** and lateral **(B)** projections: *1*, os tibiale externum; *2*, processus uncinatus; *3*, os intercuneiforme; *4*, pars peronea metatarsalia; *5*, os cuboideum secundarium; *6*, os peroneum; *7*, os vesalianum pedis; *8*, os intermetatarseum; *9*, accessory navicular; *10*, talus accessorius; *11*, sustentaculum tali; *12*, os trigonum tarsi; *13*, calcaneus secundarius.

evaluate painful feet in the presence of ossicles because increased activity occurs in the site when one or both types are responsible for the symptoms. Histologically, resected surgical specimens resemble those of experimental epiphyseal separations.

The cuboid during the earliest phases of its ossification is often composed of multiple fine ossification centers (Fig. 99) that later slowly fuse to form a single bony mass. The three cuneiforms may also ossify irregularly in children who are healthy and have no clinical evidence of local disease in the feet. In evaluation of the significance of irregular mineralization in a single area, it is often helpful to remember that normal irregularities of the type under discussion are often accompanied by similar changes in other areas.

GENERALIZED AND MULTIPLE SCATTERED NORMAL VARIANTS

The long tubular bones of fetuses, premature infants, and newborn mature infants often appear sclerotic radiographically in comparison with the bones of older children because of proportionately thicker cortical bone and more abundant spongiosa during fetal and neonatal periods. The sclerotic features disappear gradually during the first weeks of life. External cortical thickening is a common finding in premature infants (Fig. 100); these features are probably related to the physical manipulation of the infants, but an element of rickets is very likely in some because parenteral nutri-

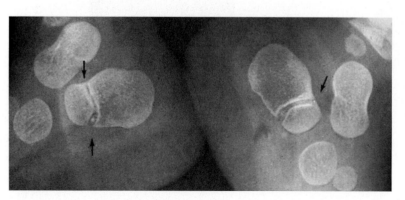

FIGURE 89. Double ossification centers *(arrows)* in the body of the calcaneus on each side of an infant 20 months of age. The infant was normal, and films were made only because of an injury to the left ankle a few hours before. We have seen similar double ossification centers in the body of the calcaneus in patients with Down syndrome and in mucolipidosis type I.

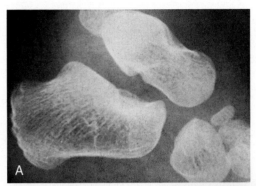

FIGURE 90. Normal radiographic features of the growing calcaneus and its apophysis in asymptomatic children. **A,** Irregular dorsal margin in a boy 3 years of age before the appearance of the apophyseal ossification center. **B,** Irregular but sclerotic apophyseal center in a boy 10 years of age; the normal dorsal margin of the calcaneal mass is deeply jagged *(arrow)*. **C,** Normally sclerotic apophyseal center in a girl 10 years of age; the margins of the calcaneal body and of its apophysis are relatively smooth.

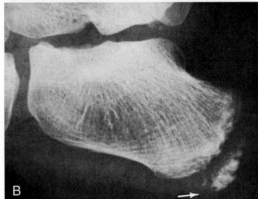

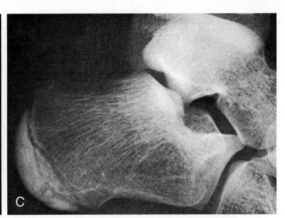

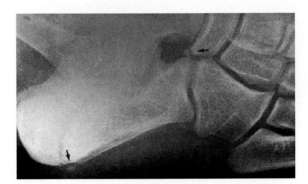

FIGURE 91. Small, round, smooth calcaneus secundarius *(arrow at right)* in the center of the space between the calcaneus, cuboid, navicular, and talus; lateral oblique projection. The patient was an asymptomatic boy 12 years of age. The *posterior arrow* points to a center in the apophysis. Similar ossicles were present in the other foot.

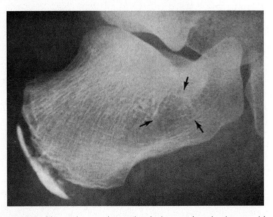

FIGURE 92. Normal pseudocystic circle or triangle *(arrows)* in the calcaneus of a healthy boy 10 years of age. The segmental radiolucency is due to local normal deficiency of spongy bone.

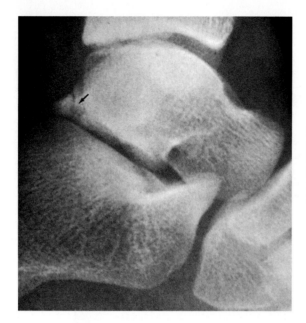

FIGURE 93. Normal apophyseal ossification center *(arrow)* in the dorsal process of the talus in a healthy boy 11 years of age. The radiolucent strip between the body of the talus and the ossification center is a normal synchondrosis, not a fracture line. When the synchondrosis persists after the normal age for its fusion with the body of the talus, the persistent ossification center is called the os trigonum.

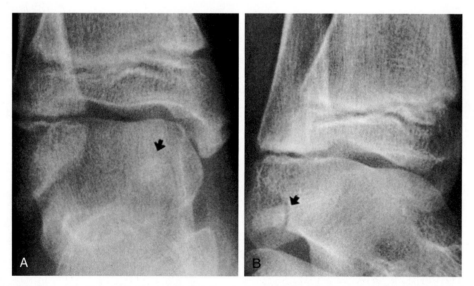

FIGURE 94. Normal ossification center *(arrows)* in the dorsal process of the talus that simulates an enostosis in the frontal projection **(A)** and a fracture fragment in the lateral projection **(B)**. This boy, 9 years of age, was asymptomatic.

FIGURE 95. Os supratalare *(arrows)* on the dorsal edge of the talus just proximal to the talonavicular joint at 13 years **(A)** and at 18 years **(B)** in an asymptomatic girl.

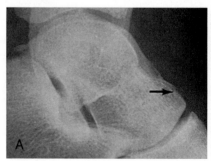
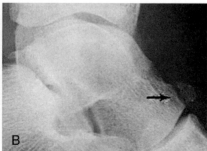

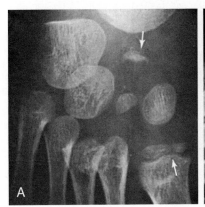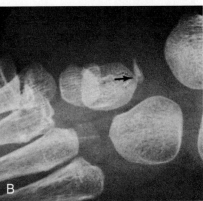

FIGURE 96. Normal irregular mineralization and flat appearance of the navicular *(upper arrows)* of an asymptomatic boy 3 years of age. The *lower arrow* is directed at the fissure shadow between separate ossification centers in the proximal epiphysis of the first metatarsal. Frontal **(A)** and lateral **(B)** projections.

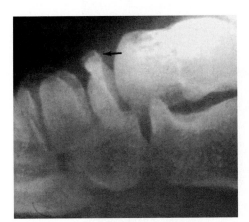

FIGURE 97. Large supranavicular bone *(arrow)* that seems to be partially fused with the main mass of the navicular itself. This appears to be an accessory ossification center in the periphery of the navicular cartilage; similar changes were present in the other foot. The asymptomatic boy was 8 years of age.

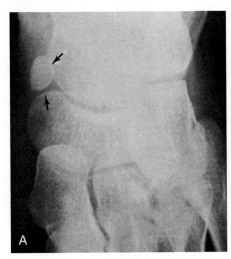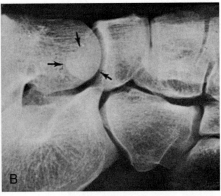

FIGURE 98. Os tibiale externum *(arrows)* in an asymptomatic boy 11 years of age in frontal **(A)** and lateral **(B)** projections.

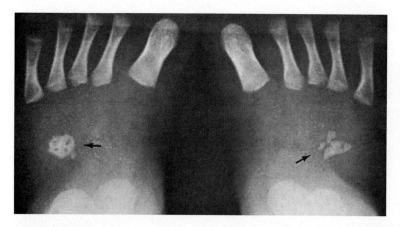

FIGURE 99. Normal bilateral irregular mineralization of the cuboids *(arrows)* of an asymptomatic infant 3 days of age. The left cuboid contains nine or ten separate small bony centers; the right cuboid is a single, relatively large bony mass of irregular density and rough edges.

tion is not optimal in the very small premature infant. The diagnosis of rickets radiographically is difficult because the productive cortical changes are often present when there is no radiographic evidence of the condition in the metaphyses. Trace elements, such as copper, may be less than adequate, complicating any vitamin D deficiencies. The features most indicative of rickets are usually found about the third month in the intensive care nursery and consist of, in addition to subperiosteal new bone formation, osteopenia, unsuspected rib fractures, and widened rib ends (Fig. 101). An alkaline phosphatase level 10 or more times greater than the adult maximal level in a given laboratory is said to confirm the diagnosis of rickets in premature infants. There is some evidence that the periosteal reaction,

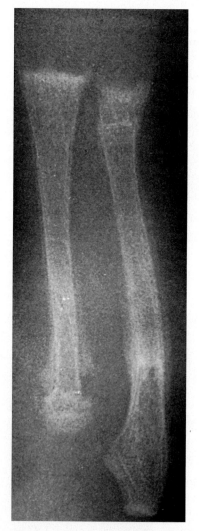

FIGURE 101. Cortical thickening of rickets in an infant with very low birth weight (26 weeks' gestation, 680 g) 15 weeks after delivery. Osteomalacia, fractures, and metaphyseal irregularities are present as well. (From Koo WW, Oestreich AE, Sherman R, et al: Radiological case of the month: osteopenia, rickets, and fractures in preterm infants. Am J Dis Child 1985;139:1045–1046, with permission.)

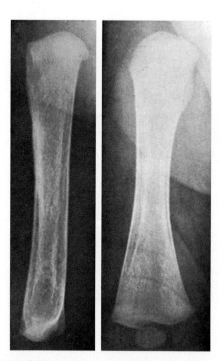

FIGURE 100. Diffuse thickenings of prematurity in a nonsyphilitic premature infant 6 months of age. The blood of both parents and of the infant gave negative reactions to Wassermann and Kahn tests on several occasions. It is noteworthy that there is no radiographic evidence of recent or old rickets in the metaphysis.

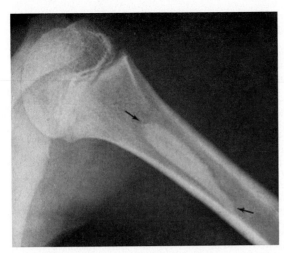

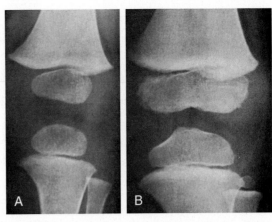

FIGURE 104. Normal absolute and relative increase, with advancing age, in depth of the metaphyseal bands that represents normal primary zones of calcification and their normal, contiguous, tightly meshed cartilaginous and bony spongiosa. **A,** Normal bands in a child at 9 months. **B,** Normally wider bands in the same child at 37 months.

FIGURE 102. An elongated sclerotic strip *(arrows)* in the humerus that, in a single projection, suggests an enostosis of the cancellous bone in the center of the medullary cavity. In two projections, however, this proved to be attached to the inner edge of the dorsal cortical wall of the humerus over a long distance. A second and better explanation of this image is that it represents the late calcified stage of a fibrous cortical defect that was radiolucent earlier. The patient, 11 years of age, had never had clinical signs at this site.

which often raises the question of congenital syphilis, is a manifestation of an accelerated growth rate. The reaction can be sufficiently marked in infants treated with prostaglandin to simulate infantile cortical hyperostosis. The role of endogenous prostaglandin is unknown.

Round and oval, small, and occasionally large, shadows of opaque bone density occur in various sites in round, tubular, and flat bones (Figs. 102 and 103). They are usually denoted "bone islands." The larger islands are generally observed in tubular bones and appear to be produced by persistence of what have been considered hamartomatous foci of cancellous structure that usually are resorbed but may occasionally enlarge. The persistence of thick, intersecting, marginal trabeculae in

the smaller lesions are believed to help distinguish bone islands from infarcts or tumors. Bone islands and individual lesions of osteopoikilosis have been said to show similar histologic features. Rarely, pain may occur in the region of a bone island and, when associated with a positive bone scan, may be worrisome. Scans are usually negative, but a third of large lesions tend to be positive. A typical benign histologic finding of a bone island has been reported in a case with a positive scan involving the capitate bone.

The thickness of the provisional zone of calcification at the ends of the shafts of long bones, and in metaphyseal-equivalent regions of flat and round bones, is extremely variable in healthy children (Fig. 104). They are most prominent between the second and fifth years, possibly reflecting the flattening of the growth curve at that time, and simulate the dense lines of lead poisoning.

SUGGESTED READINGS

Keats TE: An Atlas of Normal Roentgen Variants That May Simulate Disease, 7th ed. St. Louis, Mosby, 2001
Köhler A, Zimmer EA: Borderlands of the Normal and Early Pathologic in Skeletal Roentgenology, 4th ed. New York, Grune & Stratton, 1993
Lawson JP: Symptomatic radiographic variants in extremities. Radiology 1985;157:625–631

Hand and Wrist

Carlson DH: Coalition of the carpal bones. Skeletal Radiol 1981;7: 125–127
Cockshott WP: Carpal fusions. Am J Roentgenol Radium Ther Nucl Med 1963;89:1260–1271
Giedion A: Zapfenepiphysen: Naturgeschichte und diagnostiche Bedeutung einer Störung des enchondralen Wachstums. *In* Glauner R, Rüttimann A, Thurn P, et al (eds): Ergebnisse der medizinischen Radiologie, vol 1. Stuttgart, Georg Thieme, 1968
Giedion A: Phalangeal cone-shaped epiphyses of the hands (PhCSEH) and chronic renal disease—the conorenal syndromes. Pediatr Radiol 1979;8:32–38
Hubay CA: Sesamoid bones of the hands and feet. Am J Roentgenol Radium Ther 1949:61:493–505

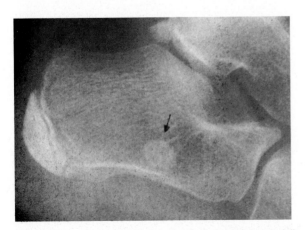

FIGURE 103. An oval mass of bone density *(arrow)* in the medullary cavity of the body of the calcaneus of an asymptomatic boy 9 years of age. Such masses are known as "bone islands" or enosteomas and have no clinical significance. The calcaneal apophysis is normally sclerotic.

O'Rahilly R: Developmental deviations in the carpus and the tarsus. Clin Orthop 1957;10:9–18

Poznanski AK: The Hand in Radiologic Diagnosis, 2nd ed. Philadelphia, WB Saunders, 1984

Forearm, Elbow, and Shoulder

Barnard LB, McCoy SM: The supracondyloid process of the humerus. J Bone Joint Surg Am 1946;28:845–850

Levine MA: Patella cubiti. J Bone Joint Surg Am 1950;32:686–687

Resnick D, Cone RO III: The nature of humeral pseudocysts. Radiology 1984;150:27–28

Schwarz GS: Bilateral antecubital ossicles (fabella cubiti) and other accessory bones of the elbow. Radiology 1965;69:730–734

Pelvis

Bernard C, Sirinelli D, Timores A, et al: Ostéochondrose ischiopublienne (cas radiologique du mois). Arch Fr Pediatr 1986;43:505–506

Byers PD: Ischiopubic "osteochondritis": A report of a case and a review: J Bone Joint Surg [Br] 1963;45:694–702

Caffey J, Madell SH: Ossification of the pubic bones at birth. Radiology 1956;67:346–350

Caffey J, Ross SE: The ischiopubic synchondrosis in healthy children: Some normal roentgenographic findings. Am J Roentgenol 1956;76:488–494

Caffey J, Ross SE: Pelvic bones in infantile mongoloidism: Radiographic features. Am J Roentgenol 1958;80:458–467

Cawley KA, Dvorak AD, Wilmot MD: Normal anatomic variant: Scintigraphy of the ischiopubic synchondrosis. J Nucl Med 1983;24:14–16

Fawcitt J: Some radiological aspects of congenital anomalies of the spine in childhood and infancy. Proc R Soc Med 1959;52:331–333

Freedman E: Os acetabuli. Am J Roentgenol 1934;32:492–495

Jarvis J, McIntyre W, Udjus K, et al: Osteomyelitis of the ischiopubic synchondrosis. J Pediatr Orthop 1985;5:163–166

Junge H, Heuck F: Die Osteochondropathia ischiopubica (gleichzeitig ein Beitrag zur normalen Entwicklung der Scham-Sitzbeingrenze in Wachstumsalter). Fortschr Geb Rontgenstr 1953;78:656–668

Kaufmann HJ: Röntgenbefunde am kindlichen Becken bei angeborenen Skelettaffektionen und chromosomalen Aberrationen. Stuttgart, Georg Thieme Verlag, 1964

Kloiber R, Udjus K, McIntyre W, et al: The scintigraphic and radiographic appearance of the ischiopubic synchondroses in normal children and in osteomyelitis. Pediatr Radiol 1988;18:57–61

Reynolds EL: The bony pelvic girdle in early infancy: A roentgenometric study. Am J Phys Anthropol 1945;3:321–354

Sutow WW, Pryde AW: Incidence of spina bifida occulta in relation to age. Am J Dis Child 1956;91:211–217

Van Neck M: Ostéochondrite du pubis. Arch Franco-Belge Chir 1924;27:238-240

Zander G: "Os acetabuli" and other bone nuclei: Periarticular calcifications at hip-point. Acta Radiol 1943;24:317–327

Femur, Knee, Tibia, Fibula, Feet, and Generalized and Multiple Scattered Normal Variants

Alexander JE, Seibert JJ, Aronson J: Dorsal defect of the patella and infection. Pediatr Radiol 1987;30:325–327

Araki S, Otani T, Watanabe K, et al: Positive bone scan in a bone island: a histologically verified case in os capitatum. Acta Orthop Scand 1989;60:369–370

Bufkin WJ: The avulsive cortical irregularity. Am J Roentgenol Radium Ther Nucl Med 1971;112:487–492

Caffey J, Madell SH, Royer C, et al: Ossification of the distal femoral epiphysis. J Bone Joint Surg Am 1958;40:647–654

DeLuca SA, Rhea JT, Sheehan J: Radiographic anatomy of the carpal bones. Med Radiogr Photogr 1985;61:10–13

Gold RH, Mirra JM, Remotti B, et al: Case report 527: Giant bone island of tibia. Skeletal Radiol 1989;18:129–132

Greulich WW, Pyle SI: Radiographic Atlas of Skeletal Development of the Hand and Wrist, 2nd ed. Stanford, CA, Stanford University Press, 1959

Griscom NT, Craig JN, Neuhauser EBD: Systemic bone disease developing in small premature infants. Pediatrics 1071;48:883–895

Hubay CA: Sesamoid bones of the hands and feet. Am J Roentgenol Radium Ther 1949;61:493–505

Keats TE: An Atlas of Normal Roentgen Variants That May Simulate Disease, 7th ed. St. Louis, Mosby, 2001

Kim SK, Barry WF Jr: Bone islands. Radiology 1968;90:77–78

Köhler A, Zimmer EA: Borderlands of the Normal and Early Pathologic in Skeletal Roentgenology, 4th ed. New York, Grune & Stratton, 1993

Lagier R, Nussle D: Anatomy and radiology of a bone island. ROFO 1978;128:261–264

Lawson JP: Symptomatic radiographic variants in extremities. Radiology 1985;157:625–631

Lawson JP, Ogden JA, Sella E, et al: The painful accessory navicular. Skeletal Radiol 1984;12:250–262

O'Rahilly R: Developmental deviations in the carpus and tarsus. Clin Orthop 1957;10:9–18

Poznanski AK, Fernbach SK, Berry TE: Bone changes from prostaglandin therapy. Skeletal Radiol 1985;14:20–25

Poznanski AK, Garn SM, Nagy JM, et al: Metacarpophalangeal pattern profiles in the evaluation of skeletal malformations. Radiology 1972;104:1–11

Simon K, Mulligan ME: Growing bone islands revisited. J Bone Joint Surg Am 1985;67:809–811

Tanner JM, Whitehouse RH, Marshall WA, et al: Assessment of Skeletal Maturity and Prediction of Adult Height (TW2 Method). London, Academic Press, 1975

van Holsbeeck M, Vandamme B, Marchal G, et al: Dorsal defect of the patella: concept of its origin and relationship with bipartite and multipartite patella. Skeletal Radiol 1987;16:304–311

Chapter 3

NORMAL BONE MARROW

BARRY D. FLETCHER

Magnetic resonance imaging (MRI) provides a method of directly visualizing the gross anatomic structure of the bone marrow and observing changes in its signal induced by a variety of physiologic and pathologic alterations of marrow composition. In children, evaluation of bone marrow is complicated by age-related changes in the relative content of red (hematopoietic) and yellow (fatty) marrow. Although efforts have been made to assess these changes by quantitative MRI techniques, most information has been derived from observations made using T_1-weighted images obtained for clinical purposes. Knowledge of normal bone marrow maturation is necessary to differentiate developmental phenomena from pathologic conditions associated with hematologic disease, neoplasia, and other causes of marrow infiltration.

NORMAL MARROW FUNCTION AND COMPOSITION

Bone marrow is one of the largest, most diffuse, and most dynamic organs in the body. Its functions include the production of red and white blood cells and platelets for tissue oxygenation, as well as regulation of cellular immunity and blood coagulation. Marrow occupies approximately 85% of the medullary cavity and is supported by a latticework of trabeculae. In addition to hematopoietic elements, it contains stromal cells, collagen, nerves, and a variable amount of fat. Red marrow is rich in vascular sinusoids, whereas yellow marrow is considerably less vascular. Hematopoietically active red marrow contains approximately 40% water, 40% fat, and 20% protein, whereas yellow marrow consists of 15% water, 5% protein, and twice the amount of fat (80%) as red marrow (Fig. 1).

MARROW DISTRIBUTION AND CONVERSION

During early intrauterine life hematopoiesis occurs in the yolk sac, and later in gestation it shifts to the liver. By the sixth month of gestation, the marrow becomes entirely responsible for hematopoietic activity, and, by then, it is distributed throughout the bony portion of the fetal skeleton. Shortly before birth, conversion from red to yellow marrow begins in the distal phalanges and procedes in a centripetal fashion from the distal to the

more proximal portions of the appendicular skeleton. Within the individual long bones, conversion procedes from mid-diaphysis to the distal metaphysis and then to the proximal metaphysis. By early adult life, red marrow is mainly confined to the pelvis, ribs, sternum, and skull.

MRI OF MARROW CONVERSION

Conversion from red to yellow marrow is readily detected by MRI because of the high sensitivity of T_1-weighted images to even small increases in fat content. On T_1-weighted images, signal intensity of red marrow is similar to that of muscle (hypointense) while the intensity of yellow marrow approaches that of hyperintense subcutaneous fat. Early in the conversion process, marrow signal may be intermediate in intensity and/or heterogeneous in appearance. There is less contrast between red and yellow marrow on T_2-weighted images. On these images, red marrow is higher in signal intensity than yellow marrow, the signal intensity of which parallels that of subcutaneous fat. Imaging sequences incorporating chemical shift fat saturation or short-inversion-time inversion-recovery pulses null the fat signal of yellow marrow and maximize the intensity of red marrow. Gradient-echo sequences are highly sensitive to magnetic field inhomogeneities such as those caused by trabecular bone, leading to a reduction in signal intensity. Consequently, T_1-weighted spin-echo sequences have been the most widely used technique for the study of bone marrow conversion (Table 1).

EXTREMITIES

The most thorough MRI studies of the long bone marrow cavities have involved the femur. These investigations have shown an orderly change from red to yellow marrow beginning in early infancy. Fatty marrow, seen as heterogeneous high-intensity T_1-weighted signal, is present in the diaphysis as early as 3 months of age and is commonly observed in this location by age 12 months. After 5 years of age, the diaphyseal fat signal becomes homogeneous and extensive while the low-signal-intensity red marrow in the distal metaphysis is replaced almost entirely by high-signal-intensity yellow marrow. However, the relatively low signal of red marrow in the proximal femoral metaphysis persists (Fig. 2).

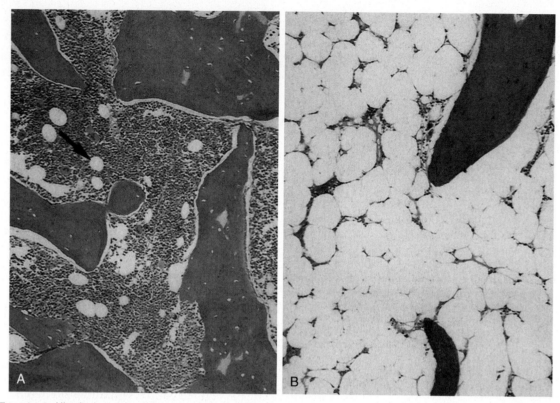

FIGURE 1. Histologic sections of normal bone marrow (hematoxylin-eosin, ×75). **A,** Hematopoietic elements and bony trabeculae of red marrow with few fat cells *(arrow).* **B,** Yellow marrow containing numerous fat cells. (From Babyn PS, Ranson M, McCarville ME: Normal bone marrow: signal characteristics and fatty conversion. Magn Reson Imaging Clin N Am 1998;6:474, with permission.)

Table 1 ■ T$_1$-WEIGHTED SIGNAL INTENSITIES ASSOCIATED WITH BONE MARROW CONVERSION

	SIGNAL INTENSITY[†]				
MARROW SITE*	**0–1 yr**	**1–5 yr**	**6–10 yr**	**11–15 yr**	**15+ yr**
Femur[‡]					
Diaphysis	L–H	M–H	H	H	H
PM	L	V	M	M	M
DM	L	H	H	H	H
Epiphyses	L–H	H	H	H	H
Sternum	L	L	M	M	M
Clavicle	L	L	M	M	M
Humerus[‡]					
PE	M	H	H	H	H
PM	L	M	M	M	M
Diaphysis	M	H	H	H	H
DM	L	M	M	M	H
Pelvis	L,M	M	M	M	M
Vertebrae	L,I	I,H	H	H	H
Skull					
Clivus	L	L,M	M,H	H	H
Calvarium	L	L,M	M,H	H	H

*Intensity of vertebral bodies compared to intervertebral disks. All other marrow sites compared to muscle (hypointense) and fat (hyperintense).
[†]H = hyperintense; I = isointense; L = hypointense; M = intermediate and/or heterogeneous signal intensity; V = variable signal intensity.
[‡]DM = distal metaphysis; PE = proximal epiphysis; PM = proximal metaphysis.

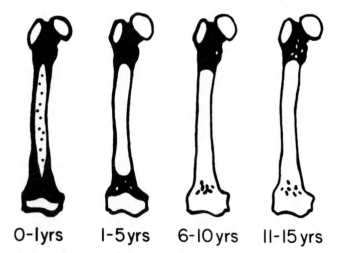

0-1 yrs   1-5 yrs   6-10 yrs   11-15 yrs

FIGURE 2. Diagrammatic representation of changes in MRI appearance of femoral marrow with increasing age. *Black areas* represent red marrow, *white areas* represent yellow marrow or cartilage, and *stippled areas* indicate heterogeneous marrow. (From Waitches G, Zawin JK, Poznanski AK: Sequence and rate of bone marrow conversion in the femora of children as seen on MR imaging: are accepted standards accurate? AJR Am J Roentgenol 1994;162:1401, with permission.)

Conversion of marrow in the bones of the forearm and foreleg lags slightly behind the more proximal bones of the arm and thigh. Conversion to yellow marrow begins in the diaphyses between 1 and 5 years of age and is complete in all portions of the forearm and foreleg bones by 11 to 15 years of age.

Under normal circumstances, the secondary ossification centers do not participate in hematopoiesis to any appreciable degree. In early infancy they are cartilaginous and produce a signal of intermediate intensity on T_1-weighted images. The recently ossified epiphyses of infancy may be hypointense for a brief period of time (up to 1 year). After it ossifies, the greater trochanter usually exhibits hyperintense yellow marrow. The round bones such as the patella also show evidence of yellow marrow content soon after they ossify.

Bone marrow conversion in the humerus follows a similarly predictable pattern. Conversion to fatty marrow with high T_1-weighted signal intensity is nearly complete in the proximal epiphysis, the diaphysis, and the distal metaphysis by age 6 years. Conversion occurs less rapidly in the proximal humeral metaphysis but is nearly complete in patients older than 15 years. However, low signal may be retained in the medial aspect of the humeral head of teenage children. In the clavicle, marrow is uniformly hypointense for the first 5 years after birth and then becomes inhomogeneously hypointense.

FLAT BONES

In the first year after birth, the pelvis exhibits low signal intensity except for the triradiate cartilage of the acetabulum, the symphysis pubis, and the cartilaginous apophyses, which are of intermediate intensity. The low signal intensity of the pelvis persists except for the anterior ilium and the bony acetabulum, in which moderately high signal intensity can be seen as early as 2 years of age (Fig. 3). In the second decade of life, the remainder of the pelvic marrow increases to intermediate signal intensity while the slightly higher signal of the acetabulum and pubis persists into adult life.

High signal intensity may be seen in the scapula as early as the first year of life. The sternum is homoge-

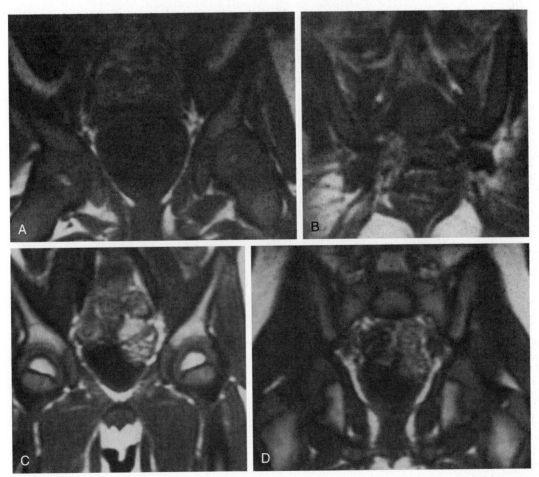

FIGURE 3. Coronal T_1-weighted MRI sections of the pelvis. **A** and **B,** Seven-month-old girl. **C** and **D,** Three-year-old boy. Note conversion from low-signal-intensity red marrow to high-signal-intensity yellow marrow in the acetabulae, anterior ilia, proximal femoral epiphyses, and diaphyses. (From Babyn PS, Ranson M, McCarville ME: Normal bone marrow: signal characteristics and fatty conversion. Magn Reson Imaging Clin N Am 1998;6:488, with permission.)

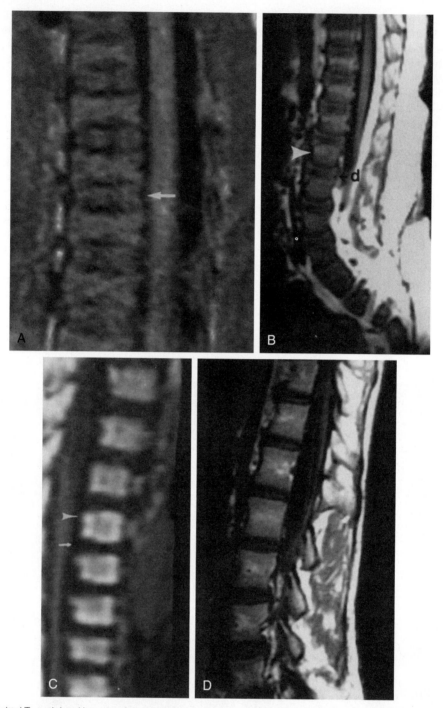

FIGURE 4. Sagittal T_1-weighted images of the lumbar spine show gradual increase in signal intensity of vertebral bodies with age. **A,** Two-week-old infant. *Arrow* indicates vertebral body. **B,** Eight-month-old girl. *Arrowhead* indicates slightly asymmetric increase in signal intensity of vertebral body. **C,** Three-year-old boy. Superior *(arrowhead)* and inferior ossification centers are hyperintense compared to hypointense intervertebral disks *(arrow)*. **D,** Seven-year-old boy. Note central vertebral band-like foci of high signal intensity. (From Babyn PS, Ranson M, McCarville ME: Normal bone marrow: signal characteristics and fatty conversion. Magn Reson Imaging Clin N Am 1998;6:492, with permission.)

neously hypointense during the first 5 years of life and then has increasingly heterogeneous, higher signal thereafter. However, the sternum remains hematopoietic into adulthood. Signal generated by the ribs increases from low or intermediate intensity to high signal intensity by 7 to 10 years of age.

AXIAL SKELETON

Autopsy studies of vertebral marrow indicate that the proportion of red marrow declines from 60% to 30% between the first and fifth decades, whereas fat content increases from 20% to 50%. T_1-weighted imaging during childhood reflects these changes. During the first year after birth, the vertebral marrow of most infants appears to lack fat and produces a uniformly lower signal than the adjacent cartilaginous disks. Signal intensity of the ossified portions of the vertebral bodies then increases to become equal to or greater than that of the disks (Fig. 4). In addition, a triangular focus of high fat signal is often visible posteriorly in the region of the basivertebral vein. In some children, a horizontal band of fat can be seen in the central portion of the vertebral body (Fig. 4D).

SKULL

Because most MRI studies are obtained to investigate potential disorders of the head, it is important to differentiate between normal and abnormal marrow. In the clivus and calvarium, T_1-weighted signal intensity is uniformly low (isointense to muscle) in most patients less than 1 year of age. Signal intensity in the clivus increases rapidly thereafter. By 3 to 4 years of age, some areas of high signal intensity are seen in the clivus of almost all patients, with gradually increasing intensity to 15 years of age or older (Fig. 5).

Conversion from red to yellow marrow occurs more slowly in the calvarium. In a substantial number of children, the calvarium retains low signal intensity until 6 years of age. However, in a small percentage of patients, high signal intensity can be seen in the frontal bone within the first year after birth, a finding that is more common in older children. In the great majority of patients, the calvarium shows uniformly intense signal by age 15 years. As a general rule, homogeneously low signal intensity in the clivus and calvarium is an abnormal finding after age 7 years.

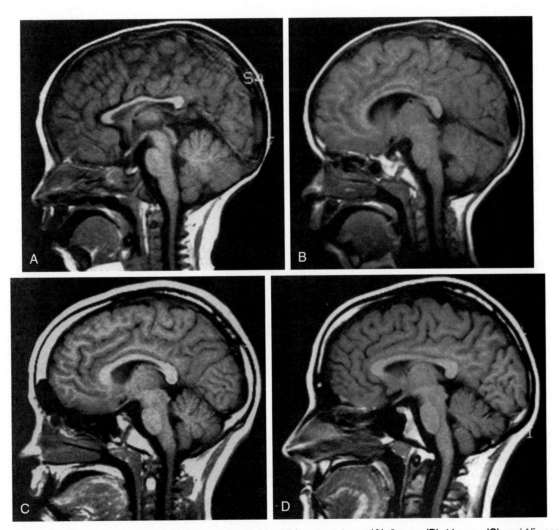

FIGURE 5. Sagittal T_1-weighted MRI sections of the skull in children ages 1 year **(A)**, 3 years **(B)**, 11 years **(C)**, and 15 years **(D)**. Note minimal high signal intensity of presphenoid in **A** *(arrow)*. In older children **(B–D)**, the clivus is of mainly high signal intensity, indicating conversion to yellow marrow. The calvarium is hypointense at 1 year of age **(A)** and gradually increases in intensity with advancing age. (From Babyn PS, Ranson M, McCarville ME: Normal bone marrow: signal characteristics and fatty conversion. Magn Reson Imaging Clin N Am 1998;6:490, with permission.)

MARROW RECONVERSION

Reconversion is a process in which established yellow marrow is replaced by red marrow in response to conditions that create a demand for increased hematopoiesis. These conditions include chronic anemias such as thalassemia and sickle cell disease, marrow replacement disorders, and chronic cyanosis associated with congenital heart disease. In addition, physiologic marrow response to increased erythrocyte requirements in endurance athletes and iatrogenic phenomena such as administration of hematopoietic growth factors can lead to reconversion from yellow to red marrow.

Reconversion occurs in the reverse order of normal marrow conversion, beginning in the axial skeleton and flat bones and proceding sequentially to the proximal metaphyses, distal metaphyses, and diaphyses of the femurs and humeri. The more distal long bones are the last to undergo this process. The epiphyses are usually spared but undergo reconversion in response to unusually high hematopoietic demand.

On T_1-weighted images, reconverted marrow is hypointense and tends to involve the appendicular skeleton in a symmetric fashion. The newly formed red marrow may be distributed in either a homogeneous or patchy pattern and can mimic diffuse pathologic processes including metastases, hematologic malignancies, myeloid hyperplasia associated with glycogen storage disease, myelofibrosis, Gaucher's disease, and transfusional hemosiderosis. Although MRI is very sensitive to changes in marrow fat content, specificity is low. Therefore, the distinction between reconverted and diseased marrow often requires knowledge of the patient's clinical status.

SUGGESTED READINGS

Babyn PS, Ranson M, McCarville ME: Normal bone marrow: Signal characteristics and fatty conversion. Magn Reson Clin N Am 1998;6:473–495

Dawson KL, Moore SG, Rowland JM: Age-related marrow changes in the pelvis: MR and anatomic findings. Radiology 1992;183:47–51

Fletcher BD, Wall JE, Hanna SL: Effect of hematopoietic growth factors on MR images of bone marrow in children undergoing chemotherapy. Radiology 1993;189:745–751

Jaramillo D, Laor T, Hoffer FA, et al: Epiphyseal marrow in infancy: MR imaging. Radiology 1991;180:809–812

Kricun ME: Red-yellow marrow conversion: its effect on the location of some solitary bone lesions. Skeletal Radiol 1985;14:10–19

Mirowitz SA: Hematopoietic bone marrow within the proximal humeral epiphysis in normal adults: investigation with MR imaging. Radiology 1993;188:689–693

Moore SG, Bisset GS, Siegel MJ, et al: Pediatric musculoskeletal imaging. Radiology 1991;179:345–360

Moore SG, Dawson KL: Red and yellow marrow in the femur: age-related changes in appearance at MR imaging. Radiology 1990;175:219–223

Okada Y, Aoki SA, Barkovitch AJ, et al: Cranial bone marrow in children: assessment of normal development with MR imaging. Radiology 1989;171:161–164

Sebag GH, Dubois J, Tabet M, et al: Pediatric spinal bone marrow: assessment of normal age-related changes in the MRI appearance. Pediatr Radiol 1993;23:515–518

Steiner RM, Mitchell DG, Rao VM, et al: Magnetic resonance imaging of diffuse bone marrow disease. Radiol Clin North Am 1993;31:383–409

Taccone A, Oddone M, Occhi M, et al: MRI "road map" of normal age-related bone marrow. I. Cranial bone and spine. Pediatr Radiol 1995;25:588–595

Taccone A, Oddone M, Dell'Acqua A, et al: MRI "road map" of normal age-related bone marrow. II. Thorax, pelvis and extremities. Pediatr Radiol 1995;25:596–606

Vande Berg BC, Malghem J, Lecouvet FE, et al: Magnetic resonance imaging of normal bone marrow. Skeletal Radiol 1998;27:471–483

Vogler JB, Murphy WA: Bone marrow imaging. Radiology 1988;168:679–693

Waitches G, Zawin JK, Poznanski AK: Sequence and rate of bone marrow conversion in the femora of children as seen on MR imaging: are accepted standards accurate? AJR Am J Roentgenol 1994;162:1399–1406

Zawin JK, Jaramillo D: Conversion of bone marrow in the humerus, sternum and clavicle: changes with age on MR images. Radiology 1993;188:159–164

CONGENITAL MALFORMATIONS

TAL LAOR

The most obvious congenital malformations of the skeleton are those of size, shape, and number of bones. These malformations are frequently accompanied by soft tissue abnormalities. Occasionally, a soft tissue abnormality may be an isolated finding. Most limb malformations are classified as reduction (deficiency), excess, and fusion (malsegmentation) deformities. The last group often occurs in association with reduction deformities. Congenital malformations that result in abnormalities of limb size, configuration, and segmentation are reviewed here.

ABNORMAL SIZE: SMALL LIMBS

Congenital deficiencies are more common than acquired amputations in children. Frantz and O'Rahilly developed a system of classification that is still commonly used to evaluate congenital anomalies of the extremities. Each malformation is defined by the part that is deficient. For example, the fibula is deficient in fibular hemimelia. The abnormality is considered *terminal* if the deformity extends to the distal aspect of the extremity, or *intercalary* if the limb distal to the deformity is normal. For example, in fibular hemimelia, if the foot is abnormal, the deficiency is terminal, and if the foot is normal, it is intercalary. Likewise, a defect can be classified as *longitudinal (paraxial)* or *transverse*. The malformation is paraxial if only the fibular side is affected. If both the tibia and fibula are affected, the deformity is considered transverse.

Aplasia and hypoplasia of the long bones occur in the following descending order of frequency: fibula, radius, femur, ulna, and humerus. Deficiencies of the tibia are very uncommon. The etiology of reduction malformations is known in only a small number of cases. There are a few inheritable abnormalities, but most are sporadic. Environmental factors are infrequently implicated. A drug firmly associated with anomalies is thalidomide.

This drug, introduced as an antipyretic and sedative, had potential teratogenic effects on the human embryo if ingested by the mother early in the pregnancy. The induced malformations were usually reduction deformities that ranged from severe amelias to mild muscular hypoplasia. Most malformations were preaxial (deformities of the radial or tibial side), affecting the upper limbs more often than the lower extremities. Infrequently, excess deformities such as polydactyly were observed. Deprivation of factors necessary for normal development may also result in reduction deformities, as demonstrated by Warkany and Nelson in the case of maternal riboflavin deficiency. Paraxial congenital malformations of the extremities also have been attributed to early compromise of embryonic vascular structures.

Regardless of etiology, abnormal limb development tends to fall into patterns that can be recognized clinically and radiographically (Fig. 1). Most classification systems of congenital malformations are based on osseous structures, but it is well recognized that anomalous conditions of the surrounding soft tissues are certain to be present. Although one deficiency is usually dominant, the dysplasia often involves the entire limb. Deficiencies may involve both the lower and upper extremities.

LOWER EXTREMITY DEFICIENCIES

Congenitally Short Femur

Femoral shortening can be unilateral or bilateral, and is often associated with reduction defects elsewhere in the same limb. The abnormality ranges from mild hypoplasia to complete absence of the femur. Most cases are sporadic, but several external factors have been implicated in the more complex deformities. Known etiologies include drugs (such as thalidomide), trauma, irradiation, infection, and focal ischemia.

Anterolateral bowing and medial cortical thickening

TRANSVERSE LIMB DEFICIENCIES

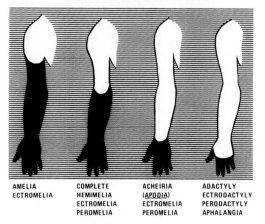

| AMELIA ECTROMELIA | COMPLETE HEMIMELIA ECTROMELIA PEROMELIA | ACHEIRIA (APODIA) ECTROMELIA PEROMELIA | ADACTYLY ECTRODACTYLY PERODACTYLY APHALANGIA |

LONGITUDINAL LIMB DEFICIENCIES

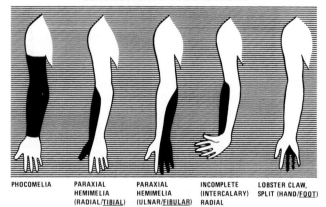

| PHOCOMELIA | PARAXIAL HEMIMELIA (RADIAL/TIBIAL) | PARAXIAL HEMIMELIA (ULNAR/FIBULAR) | INCOMPLETE (INTERCALARY) RADIAL HEMIMELIA | LOBSTER CLAW, SPLIT (HAND/FOOT) |

FIGURE 1. Skeletal deformities of the limbs. The *blackened areas* indicate deficient parts. Terms used both currently and previously are listed. (Modified from O'Rahilly R: Morphologic patterns in limb deficiencies and duplications. Am J Anat 1951;89:135–193. Reprinted by permission of Wiley-Liss, Inc., a subsidiary of John Wiley & Sons, Inc.)

manifest hypoplasia of the femur. The femoral and tibial condyles are flattened (Fig. 2). The knee joint often is lax and may have an accentuated valgus alignment. Unlike proximal femoral focal deficiency (PFFD) (see below), the hip is stable. A coxa vara alignment of the femoral neck may be present. The hypoplastic femur grows at the same rate as or a slower rate than the contralateral normal femur, so that the leg length discrepancy persists or increases. The degree of hypoplasia of the femur and instability of the knee joint guide therapy. Leg lengthening can be performed if the shortening is less than 20 cm.

Proximal Femoral Focal Deficiency

PFFD refers to abnormalities that range from mild shortening and hypoplasia of the femur to severe deficiency of the bone and dysplasia of the acetabulum. The defect is thought to be due to altered proliferation and maturation of the chondrocytes of the proximal femoral physis in utero, which in turn result in underdevelopment of the ipsilateral acetabulum. The child with PFFD usually presents in infancy with a short

extremity. A well-formed acetabulum implies the presence of a femoral head, which might be cartilaginous, and therefore not apparent radiographically early in life. Most cases are sporadic; however, the combination of bilateral femoral deficiencies and abnormal facies, known as the femoral hypoplasia–unusual facies syndrome, is thought to be an autosomal dominant disorder.

There are numerous attempts to classify PFFD, all based on radiographic findings. The most commonly used classification is that of Aitken (Fig. 3). The least severe type is class A, which refers to an adequate or only mildly dysplastic proximal femur and acetabulum. The femoral head is present but is separated from the shortened distal femoral segment. With age, a fibrous connection between the head and distal femoral segment ossifies, but usually not completely. A subtrochanteric varus deformity is invariably present. In the most severe form, class D, most of the femur and ipsilateral acetabulum are absent (Fig. 4).

PFFD is associated with other ipsilateral deformities that include fibular hemimelia (in more than 50% of affected children), shortening of the tibia, equinovalgus deformity of the foot (more often than equinovarus deformity), and deficiency of the lateral rays of the foot. PFFD is bilateral in 15% of affected children.

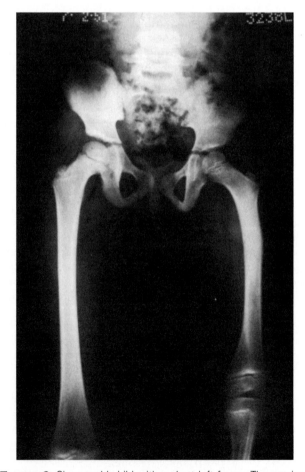

FIGURE 2. Six-year-old child with a short left femur. The proximal and distal femoral epiphyses are hypoplastic and there is mild bowing.

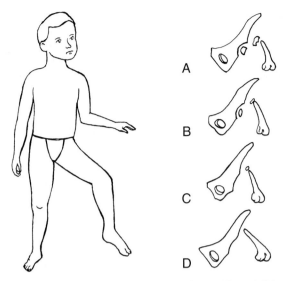

FIGURE 3. Aitken classification of proximal femoral focal deficiency. (Modified from Aitken G [ed]: Proximal femoral focal deficiency—definition, classification, and management. *In* Proximal Femoral Focal Deficiency: A Congenital Anomaly. Washington, DC, National Academy of Sciences, 1969:1–22.)

Sonography can be used to delineate radiographically inapparent structures at an early age. If a cartilaginous femoral head and its connection to the femoral shaft can be shown, the stability of the hip joint is likely more than that implied from radiographs. Like sonography, magnetic resonance imaging (MRI) is useful to define the anatomy of the hip joint and the associated deformities of the limb (Fig. 5). It also allows for appropriate early classification of a child, when structures may be radiographically inapparent. Most muscles about the affected hip are hypoplastic when compared to the contralateral normal side, with the exception of the sartorius muscle, which is often hypertrophied. This results in the characteristic flexion deformity of the hip and knee. MRI also defines the anatomy of the soft tissues that can guide surgical exposure and preparation of the limb stump for fitting of a prosthesis.

Therapy for children with PFFD is based on severity of the deficiency and projection of growth and final limb length discrepancy at maturity. Objectives for treatment are to maximize the length of the extremity; to promote stability of the hip, knee, and ankle; and to optimize anatomic alignment. Mild deformities may not require surgery. Stabilization of the upper femoral defect is controversial and usually is indicated if a deformity is progressive. Children with more severe deformities benefit from amputation of the foot and fusion of the knee. Rotationplasty of the tibia, in which the foot is rotated 180 degrees (so that the toes face posteriorly and the ankle now serves as a knee joint) allows the ankle

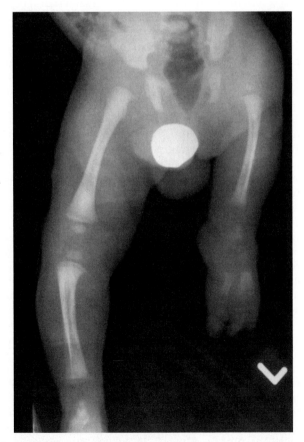

FIGURE 4. Two-month-old boy with severe proximal femoral focal deficiency, Aitken type D. There is radiographic absence of the left femur and associated ipsilateral acetabular hypoplasia. The left ankle joint is located at approximately the same level as the right knee joint.

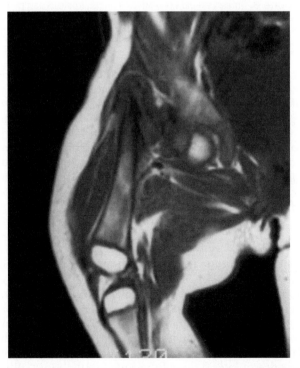

FIGURE 5. Coronal T$_1$-weighted magnetic resonance image of a girl with proximal focal femoral deficiency. The femoral head is ossified and the acetabulum is well developed. There is marked angulation at the site of a proximal femoral fibrous pseudarthrosis. The distal femoral condyle is well developed.

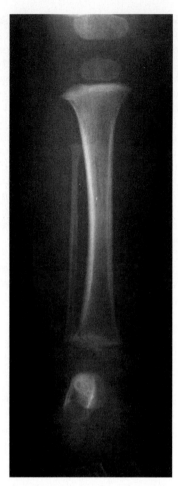

FIGURE 6. Three-year-old boy with fibular hemimelia. The fibula is short, predominantly at its proximal end.

and foot to control a distal prosthesis. Intact sensory feedback from the foot provides proprioceptive control of the knee. Thus it is imperative to assess the morphology of the proximal femur and acetabulum as well as the cartilaginous epiphyses of the knee and the supporting soft tissue structures. For example, instability of the knee can result from absence of the anterior cruciate ligament. In the rare case of bilateral PFFD, amputation is contraindicated and therapy is based on extension prostheses that improve the child's height.

Fibular Hemimelia

Deformities of the fibula range from mild deficiency of the proximal end of the bone (Fig. 6) to complete absence accompanied by multiple malformations of the neighboring structures. Unilateral absence is more frequent than bilateral deformity. A band of strong connective tissue may replace all or most of the fibula. Fibular hemimelia is associated with a short, bowed tibia; absence of lateral rays of the foot; tarsal abnormalities (particularly coalitions); and femoral shortening or deficiency in 15% of patients. Other associations include small, subluxed, or dislocated patellae; hypoplastic femoral condyles; and absent cruciate ligaments.

MRI can document these associated abnormalities, particularly if surgery is contemplated.

The talipes equinovalgus deformity of the foot and severe shortening of the limb associated with fibular hemimelia result in poor function of the limb. Children with extensive abnormalities involving the fibula, ipsilateral tibia, femur, and foot benefit the most from early amputation of the foot and often the more proximal structures. If the deformity is less severe, lengthening of the affected side, realignment of the talotibial articulation, and epiphysiodesis of the contralateral limb are often undertaken. Attempts at lengthening a severely dysplastic limb are often unsatisfactory.

Vascular anomalies associated with congenital malformations of the extremities, including fibular hemimelia, can be delineated with magnetic resonance (MR) arteriography. Preoperative knowledge of the vascularity of the limb can help to avoid ischemic complications related to vascular injury during surgery.

Tibial Hemimelia

Most cases of tibial hemimelia are sporadic, although there are reported forms (particularly bilateral deformities) that display an autosomal dominant inheritance pattern. Jones and coworkers classified the spectrum of tibial dysplasia into four groups. In type I, which is the most severe form, the tibia is not recognized radiographically at birth. Lack of ossification of the distal femoral epiphysis implies that no proximal tibia is present. The least severe form, type IV, includes congenital tibial diastasis. In these children, the tibia is short and diverges from the fibula at the ankle. The talus is displaced proximally. No normal distal tibial articulation surface is present (Fig. 7).

As with other deformities of the extremities, radiography is insensitive to unossified structures, and the true extent of the malformation can be overestimated. An unossified tibial remnant may not be recognized. Sonography can be used to document a tibial anlage and the integrity of the patellar tendon. MRI may identify a tibial remnant and associated osteocartilaginous abnormalities. The patella can be absent or hypoplastic. The epiphyses of the knee are often dysplastic, and tarsal bone abnormalities that include coalition may be present. Other associated deformities include foot malalignment, muscular hypoplasia (especially of the quadriceps muscle), fibular displacement, and vascular anomalies.

Treatment of tibial hemimelia varies with the severity of the deformity. A knee disarticulation is recommended for complete tibial absence. Brown pioneered centralization of the fibula with a Syme amputation of the foot in children with complete tibial hemimelia. This produces adequate results in the rare cases where the quadriceps muscles are well developed. Knee instability and flexure contracture caused by unopposed hamstring pull as a result of hypoplastic quadriceps muscles are complications of knee salvage procedures. When the quadriceps mechanism is abnormal, the patella is often absent. MRI can be useful to assess the deficiencies preoperatively and thus discern who will function better with a primary knee disarticulation (the majority) rather than a knee reconstruction.

If the tibial deficiency is partial (Jones type II deformity), fusion of the proximal fibula to the proximal tibial remnant can provide excellent function. In these cases, the foot is amputated to alleviate the accompanying distal instability. This usually is performed after the proximal tibia has ossified.

UPPER EXTREMITY DEFICIENCIES

Radial Deficiency

Congenital radial deficiency, also referred to as *radial clubhand,* ranges from hypoplasia of the thumb to various degrees of radial hypoplasia. Complete absence is the most common longitudinal deficiency. This deformity usually is accompanied by radial and volar deviation of the hand, in part resulting from the unopposed pull by the flexor carpi radialis and brachioradialis muscles. In most cases of radial aplasia, the forearm is bowed to the radial side and the distal ulna is prominent (Fig. 8). The forearm is short (usually approximately two thirds the length of the normal contralateral side),

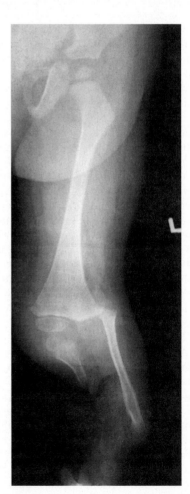

FIGURE 7. Two-year-old girl with tibial hemimelia. There is a dysplastic proximal tibial remnant, fibular deformity, and absence of multiple tarsal bones.

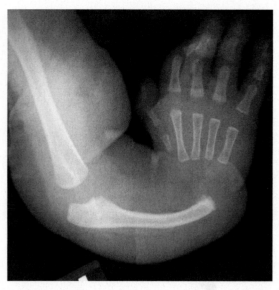

FIGURE 8. Radial clubhand in a 10-month-old boy with complete absence of the radius. The ulna is short and bowed. The thumb is hypoplastic and displaced proximally.

and remains proportionately so throughout growth. Often only the capitate, hamate, and triquetral bones and the metacarpals and phalanges of the four ulnar rays are present and normal. The trapezium, scaphoid, and first ray often are deformed or absent. If a remnant of the radius is present proximally, it usually is fused to the ulna, which is curved, shortened, and thickened. Bilateral deficiency occurs in approximately 50% of affected children. The degree of deformity of the hand is related to the severity of deficiency of the forearm. Conditions associated with radial dysplasia are listed in Table 1. Usually the entire limb is involved to some degree, often resulting in joint dysfunction of the shoulder, elbow, wrist, carpus, and small joints of the hand. Associated muscular deficiencies also are proportional to the degree of skeletal abnormality. Neurovascular abnormalities include an absent radial artery and superficial radial nerve.

Table 1 ■ CONDITIONS ASSOCIATED WITH RADIAL DYSPLASIA

Syndromes associated with congenital heart disease
  Holt-Oram syndrome
Syndromes associated with blood dyscrasias
  Fanconi's anemia (pancytopenia–dysmelia syndrome)
  Thrombocytopenia–absent radius syndrome
Syndromes associated with mental retardation
  Cornelia de Lange's (Brachmann-de Lange's) syndrome
  Seckel's syndrome
Syndromes associated with chromosomal abnormalities
  Trisomy 13
  Trisomy 18
Syndromes associated with teratogens
  Thalidomide embryopathy
  Varicella embryopathy
Other: VATER association

Modified from Goldberg MJ, Bartoshevsky LE: Congenital hand anomaly: etiology and associated malformations. Hand Clin 1985;1:405–415.

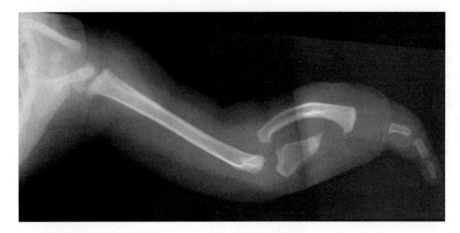

FIGURE 9. Ulnar deficiency. There is partial formation of the proximal ulna with aplasia of the distal portion. The radius is bowed, and only a single digit of the hand is present. The humerus is normal.

Whether the radial dysplasia is isolated or associated with a syndrome, the primary malformation is likely the result of a vascular abnormality in the embryo that occurred prior to differentiation of mesenchyme into muscle and bone. In humans, the critical time for radial development occurs between the fifth and sixth post-ovulatory weeks. Most cases are sporadic, but some autosomal dominant and autosomal recessive inheritance patterns are reported. Other cases are likely the result of various environmental insults from viruses, chemicals, radiation, and drugs during limb bud development.

Treatment of a longitudinal radial deficiency begins with serial casting and splinting intended to improve the radial deviation by stretching the soft tissues. This often is followed by surgical centralization of the hand over the ulna to improve function and appearance. Thumb reconstruction and pollicization of the index finger are often indicated. Experimental work with vascularized epiphyseal transplantation has shown promising results and may become part of the established therapy.

Ulnar Deficiency

Deficiency occurring along the ulnar or postaxial border of the upper extremity is known as *ulnar clubhand*. This is a relatively uncommon disorder, occurring much less frequently than radial clubhand. Approximately 25% of cases are bilateral. Most cases are sporadic, but associations with many other syndromes have been reported, one of the most common being Cornelia de Lange's syndrome.

In ulnar hypoplasia or aplasia, abnormalities are almost always present in the ulnar carpal, metacarpal, and phalangeal rays. The pisiform is always absent. The hamate frequently is not detected. Syndactyly, carpal fusion, and radiohumeral fusion are also seen. The forearm is shortened and bowed, with a concavity to the ulnar side. The hand is deviated in an ulnar direction (Fig. 9). Elbow abnormalities are common.

Teatment for ulnar deficiency includes early correction of the ulnar deviation of the hand with serial casting. Surgical treatment is reserved for those cases with significant limitation of function. Forearm instability and associated hand deformities must be addressed.

GENERALIZED DEFICIENCIES

Congenital Constriction Bands

Constricting rings around limbs present at birth are known as *Streeter's bands, congenital constriction bands,* or *amniotic bands.* These bands occasionally are associated with loss of the limb distal to the constriction. Various theories have attempted to explain these malformations. Streeter proposed one of the most popular early theories. He believed that ring contractions of the limbs, often associated with intrauterine amputations, were the result of local dysplasias occurring early in fetal life. This dysplasia caused the soft tissue to slough and eventually heal, resulting in the constricting ring. This ring tissue was unable to expand while the tissue on each side of the ring continued to grow.

Now evidence strongly suggests that the bands result from intrauterine rupture of the amnion, with subsequent mechanical constriction of fetal limbs. Various body parts become entangled in the amnion as it separates from the surrounding chorion. In some instances, adjacent structures are pulled together by the bands and ultimately become fused, producing a soft tissue syndactyly. Bony syndactyly is very rare. The earlier the rupture of the amnion, the more severe the malformations. Limb abnormalities range from slight soft tissue grooves to transverse intrauterine amputations (Fig. 10). Acrosyndactyly, craniofacial and visceral anomalies, and fetal death are part of the spectrum of congenital constriction band syndrome (see also Section IX, Part VI, Fig. 1, page 2182).

Radiography may underestimate the degree of soft tissue compromise, and associated anomalous vascular anatomy may go unrecognized. MRI can be used to evaluate the depth of the constriction band, the degree of resultant lymphedema, and the integrity of the involved musculature. Delineating the vascular anatomy using MR arteriography may help to prevent injury to the vessels during surgery.

Surgical treatment is usually cosmetic, although it may be needed to relieve massive edema distal to a constriction band, or to improve neurovascular function. Intervention for patients with acrosyndactyly may allow for partial correction of the deformity and improved longitudinal growth.

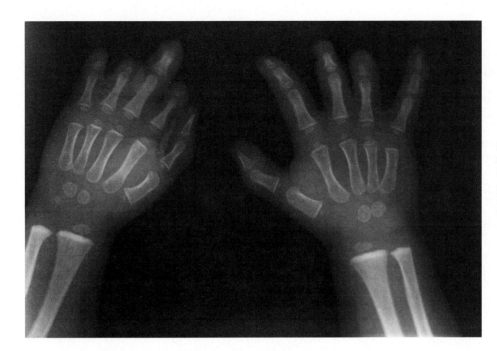

FIGURE 10. Two-year-old girl with absence of several distal phalanges bilaterally as a result of amniotic band syndrome. Several small middle phalangeal remnants are seen. The thumbs are nearly normal.

Arthrogryposis

Multiple congenital contractures presenting in infants was termed *arthrogryposis multiplex congenita* early in the century. *Arthrogryposis,* derived from the Greek for crooked or curved joint, is also referred to as *amyoplasia congenita fetalis deformans, multiple congenital articular rigidities,* and *multiple congenital contractures.* However, the term is a descriptive diagnosis and does not specify an etiology. It is used loosely to refer to any condition that results in congenital contractures, such as conditions that limit intrauterine movement of joints. The earlier in gestation the movement is limited, and the longer the duration of the restriction, the more severe the contractures will be at birth. Normal in utero motion is necessary for normal development of joints.

Most cases of multiple congenital contractures are the result of abnormal muscles (such as myopathies), abnormal nerve function or innervation, abnormal connective tissues, or mechanical limitation of movement (such as oligohydramnios or multiple fetuses). Other causes include mutagenic agents, mitotic abnormalities, and toxic chemicals or drugs. Over 150 different conditions have been reported in association with multiple congenital contractures. Arthrogryposis is also associated with genetic syndromes and other malformations. There is an increased incidence of clubfeet, dysplastic hips, and hyperextensibility in the families of children with arthrogryposis.

Radiography is used to evaluate the skeleton for bony anomalies. The contractures that are present at birth are often symmetric and most commonly affect distal parts of limbs. The lower extremities are usually involved, but over half of patients have upper limb abnormalities as well. Rigid joints and hypotonia contribute to frequent perinatal fractures. Soft tissue samples may be seen over the affected joints, and muscle mass is decreased in affected limbs (Fig. 11). Affected muscles are partially or completely replaced by fatty or fibrous tissue.

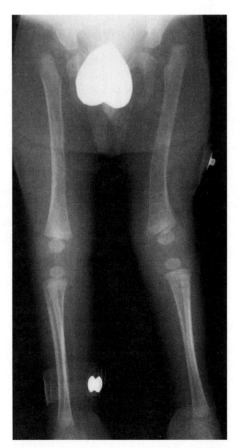

FIGURE 11. Lower extremities of a child with arthrogryposis. The bones are gracile and demineralized, and there is reduced muscle mass. The proximal femurs are dislocated and the acetabula are dysplastic. Femoral bowing on the left is the result of prior fractures.

Coalitions and ankylosis of various bones, pterygia, and shortened digits may be present. Many children will eventually develop a scoliosis. MRI can be used to assess joint integrity when surgery to maximize joint function is planned.

The long-term prognosis for most children with arthrogryposis is good. However, children with associated central nervous system abnormalities usually have a limited lifespan. A neuromuscular work-up is recommended for all children with arthrogryposis.

ABNORMAL SIZE: LARGE LIMBS

Overgrowth of the body ranges from involvement of a whole side (hemihypertrophy) to involvement of a limb (macromelia) or only a digit (macrodactyly). Abnormal growth may be confined to a single tissue, or involve all tissues of the affected body part. Children with asymmetry resulting from hemihypertrophy are predisposed to develop neoplasms, most commonly within the abdomen. The various congenital causes of localized or general body asymmetry include idiopathic, vascular disorders (vascular birthmarks and combined vascular lesions), phakomatoses, asymmetry associated with neoplasia, and bone dysplasias.

VASCULAR DISORDERS

Historically, the nomenclature applied to congenital vascular lesions has resulted in a poor understanding of their pathophysiology, natural history, and appropriate therapy. A classification of vascular lesions in infants and children based on their biologic activity and endothelial characteristics was proposed by Mulliken and Glowacki, and accepted by the International Society for the Study of Vascular Anomalies (ISSVA). This classification differentiates *hemangiomas* (characterized by rapid growth and proliferation of endothelial cells in the neonatal period followed by slow involution) from *vascular malformations* (dysplastic vessels without cellular proliferation or regression). Vascular malformations are further subdivided based on the type of anomalous channels present and rate of flow. Vascular malformations are present at birth, although occasionally recognized later in life. Most lesions are sporadic, but genetic defects for some have been reported. The lesions are named for their components, such as abnormal veins, lymphatics, arteries, or capillaries.

Hemangiomas

The most common vascular tumor of infancy is the hemangioma. Although this benign neoplasm is present at birth, it usually is not recognized until the infant is several weeks of age. This neoplasm typically shows a rapid proliferative stage followed by a slower involutional stage. Most lesions regress by adolescence.

Hemangiomas that involve the skin have a strawberry-like appearance. Multiple cutaneous hemangiomas are associated with concomitant visceral lesions. Large draining veins of a deep hemangioma may produce a deep, bluish hue. Both Doppler sonography and MRI document the high-flow component of a hemangioma (Fig. 12; see also Section IX, Part II, Chapter 2, Fig. 3, page 2020). The soft tissue component and extent of the lesion are clearly seen with MRI. The mass is usually focal, well marginated, and of low T_1-weighted and high T_2-weighted signal intensity. Following intravenous contrast, there is diffuse enhancement. Dilated feeding arteries and draining veins are seen as bright signal intensity on gradient-recalled echo images, and as flow voids on spin-echo images. With involution, there is progressive deposition of fibrofatty tissue. The differential diagnosis of a hemangioma includes an infantile fibrosarcoma. This latter lesion, however, usually enhances more heterogeneously following intravenous contrast administration than does a hemangioma. Biopsy of a lesion is indicated if there is any suspicion of malignancy.

In larger hemangiomas or those with severe ulceration, therapy with systemic or intralesional corticosteroids or subcutaneous interferon-alpha is indicated. Infrequently, a large hemangioma results in congestive heart failure, and arterial embolization or surgical resection is indicated. The Kasabach-Merritt syndrome is a life-threatening thrombocytopenia (and consumption of fibrinogen and clotting factors) associated with platelet trapping in vascular tumors. It has been associated with the Kaposiform hemangioendothelioma and tufted angioma but is not seen with large common infantile hemangiomas. These rare lesions require more aggressive chemotherapy. The mortality rate in children with Kasabach-Merritt syndrome can be as high as 30%.

Vascular Malformations

Vascular malformations are errors in developmental morphology, resulting in dysplastic vessels. Most vascular malformations grow proportionately with the child,

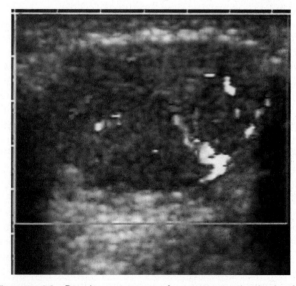

FIGURE 12. Doppler sonogram of a mass on the back of a 4-month-old girl with multiple cutaneous hemangiomas elsewhere. This solid, well-circumscribed lesion with prominent arterial vessels is another hemangioma.

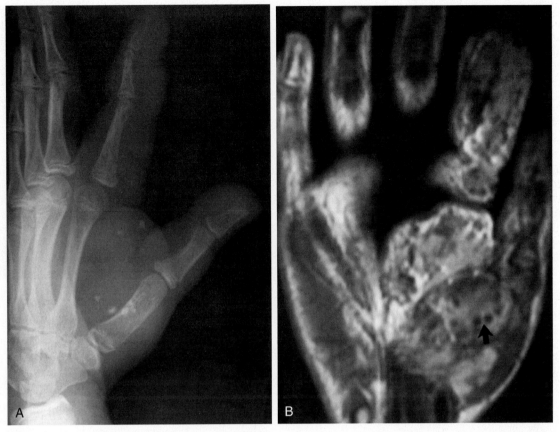

FIGURE 13. A, Soft tissue mass with phleboliths in the hand of a girl with a venous malformation. **B,** Coronal T₁-weighted magnetic resonance image following contrast enhancement of the same girl shows the enhancing tissue of the venous malformation and phleboliths *(arrow)* in the thenar region.

but they may grow more rapidly at times of hormonal change, such as puberty and pregnancy. Vascular malformations are named based on their composition and flow characteristics. Lesions with slow flow are composed of veins, lymphatics, and capillaries. The fast-flow malformations include arterial malformations, arteriovenous malformations (AVMs), and arteriovenous fistulas. Vascular malformations may also be of mixed composition. Many of these mixed lesions have eponyms, such as the Klippel-Trénaunay or Parkes Weber syndromes (see below).

Venous Malformations

Venous malformations are the most common vascular malformations of childhood. The confusing term *cavernous hemangiomas* often has been applied to these lesions. Venous malformations may be localized unifocal or multifocal masses, or represent diffuse dilatation and varicosities of major draining veins. Venous malformations enlarge when a limb is dependent and often decompress with elevation or compression.

Sonography reveals a lesion of mixed echogenicity with occasional phleboliths. Doppler tracings range from no flow to monophasic, low-flow patterns. A biphasic Doppler sample is due to mixed composition of vessels in the lesion (such as capillaries and lymphatics). Venous malformations are compressible, which helps to distinguish them from soft tissue neoplasms. Angiography is not needed for diagnosis of a venous malformation. It may be normal or show only venous stasis.

MRI is useful for diagnosis and management of venous malformations. They usually are multilocular, multiseptated masses that can be superficial or deep. They are bright on T₂-weighted images and enhance diffusely following intravenous contrast administration. Small hypointense foci on both T₁- and T₂-weighted sequences represent thrombi or phleboliths (Fig. 13). Gradient-recalled echo images may show dilatation and anomalies of the venous system. No enlarged arteries are seen. MR venography in pure venous lesions is usually normal.

Venous malformations of the synovium deserve special mention. They have been mistakenly referred to as *synovial hemangiomas* in the literature. Although usually isolated, they may also be associated with diffuse venous malformations. On MRI, features typical of venous malformations are seen within the knee joint, usually within the suprapatellar pouch. The affected child may complain of recurrent, painful knee swelling. There is a high incidence of hemosiderin arthropathy from repeated episodes of bleeding into the joint. This results in significant loss of articular cartilage and formation of subchondral cysts (Fig. 14). Synovectomy is recommended to minimize articular damage.

Extensive pure venous malformations that involve an

entire upper or lower limb and adjacent trunk are rare. These malformations worsen over time, causing painful deformity and loss of function of the limb. Diffuse pure venous malformations are associated with a local coagulopathy that must be recognized prior to surgical intervention to avoid unexpected hemorrhage.

Lymphatic Malformations

Lymphatic malformations are slow-flow lesions that present as a localized mass or diffuse limb enlargement. Deep lymphatic malformations may extend to the skin and result in superficial vesicles. Like venous malformations, lymphatic anomalies grow commensurate with the child but can enlarge acutely from hemorrhage, infection, or obstruction. Cystic lymphatic malformations result from sequestered primitive lymphatic tissue that fails to communicate with peripheral drainage pathways.

The cystic lesions can be divided into macrocystic, microcystic, and mixed malformations. Sonography of lymphatic malformations shows multilocular architecture with flow present only in the septa. Microcystic lesions are hyperechoic as a result of the numerous interfaces. Lymphatic malformations do not show flow with Doppler interrogation.

On MRI, macrocystic lymphatic malformations are typically septated masses of low T_1- and high T_2-weighted signal intensity. Variable signal intensity and

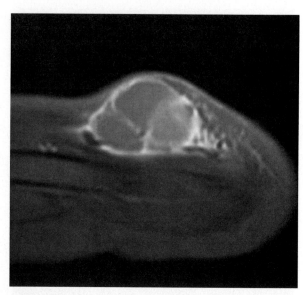

FIGURE 15. Oblique T_1-weighted image with fat suppression following contrast enhancement of the forearm of a girl with a lymphatic malformation. A multilocular mass in the soft tissues shows enhancement of the septa only.

fluid–fluid levels are due to hemorrhage or infection. Only the septa enhance following intravenous gadolinium (Fig. 15). No flow voids are seen on spin-echo sequences, and gradient-recalled echo images do not show signal from high flow. Occasionally, adjacent veins may be enlarged or anomalous. MR lymphangiography may be useful to distinguish varicose lymphatic channels from interstitial leakage resulting from lymphatic hypoplasia.

Arteriovenous Malformations

A vascular malformation composed of channels that bypass the capillary bed with connections between feeding arteries and draining veins is termed an *arteriovenous malformation*. AVMs are high-flow lesions that can result in tissue overgrowth and limb hypertrophy. Unlike a hemangioma, which also has high flow, an AVM has no endothelial cell proliferation.

Like the slow-flow lesions, AVMs may be localized or diffuse. On physical examination, an affected limb may demonstrate an increase in temperature, a palpable thrill, or pulsations. Most AVMs are in the skin, but they can occur anywhere. Large lesions, such as those in the liver, may be complicated by congestive heart failure.

Sonographic evaluation of AVMs shows a heterogeneous lesion with large feeding vessels. Doppler interrogation shows pulsatile tracings with high systolic flow and multiple sites of arteriovenous shunting. MRI can be used to evaluate the extent of the lesion and the extent of soft tissue overgrowth. High-flow enlarged channels are seen as flow voids on spin-echo images (Fig. 16), and as vessels of high signal on gradient-recalled echo sequences. No surrounding mass is seen. Contrast angiography can be combined with interventional embolization therapy.

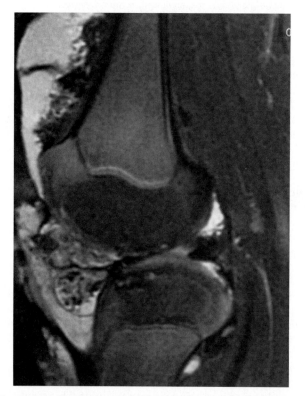

FIGURE 14. Sagittal T_2-weighted magnetic resonance image of the knee of a 4-year-old boy with a synovial venous malformation. Repeated hemarthrosis has resulted in hemosiderin deposition (dark signal intensity) and significant loss of articular cartilage of the distal femur.

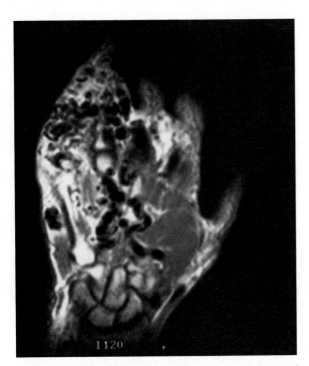

FIGURE 16. Coronal T$_1$-weighted magnetic resonance image of an arteriovenous malformation of the hand. The fast-flow vessels produce the flow voids seen throughout the lesion.

Complex-Combined Lesions

Various eponyms have been assigned to vascular malformations composed of mixed channel types. *Klippel-Trénaunay syndrome* refers to a capillary–lymphaticovenous malformation associated with limb gigantism. This syndrome includes a dermal capillary stain with lymphatic vesicles; varicosities of superficial veins and abnormal, often valveless channels; deep venous malformations; and variable soft tissue lymphatic malformations. Affected children usually develop a leg length discrepancy.

MRI is useful to evaluate the components and extent of the vascular malformation. MR venography is particularly useful to document patency of the deep venous system, because it frequently may be hypoplastic or absent (Fig. 17). Intervention of abnormal superficial or collateral veins may result in more varicosities and edema. Conventional venography to opacify the deep venous structures is difficult. A hallmark of the diffuse combined vascular malformations is the persistence of embryonic channels, most often the superficial primitive lateral marginal vein of Servelle. This is readily demonstrated with MR venography. It is speculated that the Klippel-Trénaunay syndrome is due to a somatic mutation in a factor critical to vasculogenesis and angiogenesis in embryonic development.

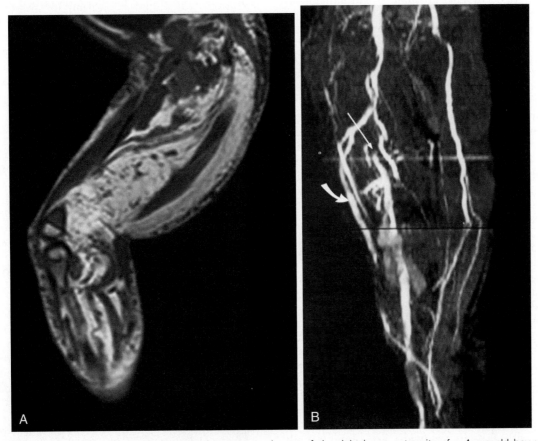

FIGURE 17. A, Sagittal T$_1$-weighted magnetic resonance image of the right lower extremity of a 4-year-old boy with Klippel-Trénaunay syndrome following contrast enhancement. The limb is markedly enlarged from the diffuse capillary–lymphaticovenous malformation. **B,** Magnetic resonance venography of the lower extremities in the same boy shows enlarged draining veins on the right. The deep femoral venous system is discontinuous *(arrow)*, and a large primitive lateral vein of Servelle is present *(curved arrow)*.

Parkes Weber syndrome is similar to Klippel-Trénaunay syndrome in that a combined vascular malformation is associated with limb gigantism. However, the vascular anomaly includes high-flow vessels within a capillary–lymphaticoarteriovenous lesion. Diffuse arteriovenous shunting can result in ischemic skin lesions and congestive heart failure, particularly in neonates. The lower limb is involved more often than the upper extremity.

Proteus Syndrome

Cohen and Hayden in 1979 first described a disorder characterized by tissue overgrowth, connective tissue nevi, epidermal nevi, and hyperostosis in two patients. It was then termed *Proteus syndrome* by Weidemann and coworkers in 1983. The name refers to the variability of clinical expression of this congenital hamartomatous syndrome that includes partial gigantism of the hands and feet, pigmented nevi, hemihypertrophy, subcutaneous hamartomatous tumors, macrocephaly, and bony exostoses. The syndrome, named after the Greek god Proteus (the polymorphous), has since been expanded to include many other anomalies. In 1998, a workshop on Proteus syndrome was held at the National Institutes of Health to develop recommendations for diagnostic criteria and guidelines for evaluation of these patients. The mosaic distribution of lesions, progressive course, and infrequent occurrence are mandatory for diagnosis.

John Merrick who was known as the "Elephant Man," originally thought to have neurofibromatosis, was subsequently diagnosed as having Proteus syndrome. Proteus syndrome has been reported as a sporadic occurrence, whereas other hamartomatous disorders usually display a dominant inheritance pattern. Proteus syndrome involves developmental dysplastic changes of all three germ layers. Two essential features that help make the diagnosis include regional gigantism and lymphangiomatous hamartomas or malformations. Other manifestations of Proteus syndrome include macrodactyly, macrocephaly or other skull abnormalities, lipomas, lymphatic and other vascular malformations (often with a diffuse cutaneous purpuric staining), subcutaneous tumors, exostoses, and scoliosis.

The gigantism is a result of overgrowth of epidermis, connective tissue, endothelium, fat, and bone. Asymmetric growth of the extremities is almost always present. Conventional radiography is used to characterize the bony abnormalities, and MRI is helpful to evaluate the mesodermal malformations. MRI can be used to delineate the extensive fatty and lymphomatous lesions prior to surgical excision. This is particularly useful in the abdomen and pelvis, where the extent of the malformations may be underestimated. Vascular abnormalities such as AVMs are frequent and should be recognized prior to resection. In order to avoid postoperative lymphatic leakage and recurrence, the entire lymphatic malformation must be removed.

Patients with Proteus syndrome are often initially misdiagnosed with another hamartomatous disorder. The differential diagnosis of Proteus syndrome includes neurofibromatosis type 1 (NF1), Klippel-Trénaunay syndrome, Parkes Weber syndrome, macrodystrophia lipomatosa, Maffucci's syndrome, epidermal nevus syndrome (Solomon syndrome), and the Bannayan-Riley-Ruvalcaba syndrome.

NEUROFIBROMATOSIS

This hamartomatous disorder involves the neuroectoderm, the mesoderm, and the endoderm throughout the body, occasionally resulting in an enlarged limb. It is discussed in detail in Section III. NF1 is the peripheral form caused by a disorder of chromosome 17. The multiple musculoskeletal abnormalities associated with NF1 are likely due to a mesodermal dysplasia. The most common osseous abnormality is scoliosis, which can be of varying severity. Spinal deformities may be due to osteomalacia, a localized neurofibroma, an endocrine disturbance, or mesodermal dysplasia. Other findings, particularly in the lower extremity, include bone lengthening with thinned shafts, anterolateral bowing of the tibia often associated with a pseudarthrosis, and multiple nonosseous fibromas. Well-circumscribed benign peripheral nerve sheath tumors (neurofibromas) are associated with NF1. These may be solitary or multifocal. A plexiform neurofibroma is pathognomonic for NF1 (Fig. 18). This lesion presents as an interdigitating, convoluted mass that travels about the axis of a nerve. The gross appearance has been described as a "bag of worms." Plexiform neurofibromas may cause massive enlargement of an extremity, called *elephantiasis neuromatosa*. The hyperemia of the limb can result in bony

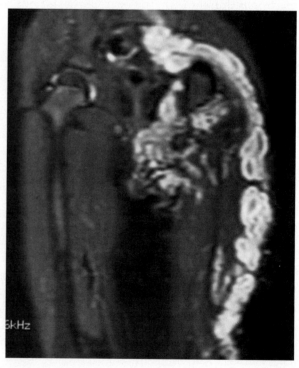

FIGURE 18. Enlargement of the left lower extremity in a 4-year-old girl with neurofibromatosis type 1 and a large plexiform neurofibroma is seen on this coronal T_2-weighted magnetic resonance image.

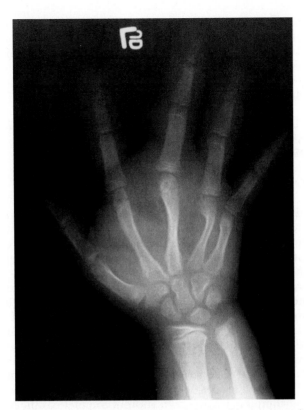

FIGURE 19. Soft tissue enlargement of the hand in a patient with macrodystrophia lipomatosis. Note the increased lucency from overgrowth of fatty tissue affecting the second, third, and fourth digits.

hypertrophy. Infrequently, the neurofibromas undergo malignant degeneration.

MRI is used to show tumor extent and relationship to the neurovascular bundle and to plan resection. A neurofibroma usually is of intermediate T_1-weighted and high T_2-weighted signal intensity. MRI cannot differentiate between a benign lesion and a neurofibrosarcoma. A "target-like" appearance on T_2-weighted sequences is suggestive of benignity (see Section IX, Part II, Chapter 2, Fig. 10*B*, page 2027).

MACRODYSTROPHIA LIPOMATOSA

Macrodystrophia lipomatosa is a congenital, nonhereditary disorder that results in localized limb enlargement, usually recognized at birth. It is characterized by an increase in all of the mesenchymal elements, with proportionally more fibroadipose tissue. Both upper and lower extremities can be involved. There may be unilateral enlargement of one or two digits, most often the second and third (Fig. 19). Enlargement of the digits follows the distribution of a nerve. The median nerve in the upper extremity and plantar nerves in the lower extremity are commonly affected. Infiltration of the nerve sheath by fibroadipose tissue can result in neural enlargement. It can be difficult to distinguish between macrodystrophia lipomatosa and neurofibromatosis based on clinical evaluation alone, because neurofibro-

matosis can also affect mesenchymal elements in a neural distribution and result in limb enlargement.

The cause of localized hypertrophy can be determined based on signal characteristics on MRI. Proliferation of fat (high T_1 signal intensity), which is characteristic of macrodystrophia lipomatosa, can be differentiated from the high T_2 signal intensity of a neurofibroma or lymphatic malformation.

ABNORMAL CONFIGURATION

PHYSIOLOGIC LOWER EXTREMITY BOWING

Physiologic bowing, or bowleggedness, in an infant is considered normal (Fig. 20). The alignment between the femur and the tibia, or the tibiofemoral angle, follows a predictable pattern of development from bowleggedness to knock-knee alignment as a child grows. A longitudinal axis is drawn through the femur and the tibia. The angle made by the intersection of these two axes is the tibiofemoral angle. Newborns and infants show a tibiofemoral angle that averages 17 degrees of varus early in life and decreases to approximately 9 degrees by 1 year of age. Between the ages of 18 months and 3 years, the tibiofemoral angle changes into a valgus alignment of approximately 2 degrees at 2 years of age and 11 degrees at 3 years, and diminishes to 6 degrees up to 6 to 7 years of age. The valgus alignment diminishes further as the child grows to adolescence.

Physiologic bowing of the lower extremities is typified by thickening of the medial femoral and tibial cortices, and prominent medioposterior metaphyseal beaks of the distal femur and proximal tibia. No bony fragmentation like that seen in Blount disease is present. Generalized bowing of the long bones is a nonspecific manifestation of many conditions, including skeletal dysplasias and metabolic abnormalities such as osteogenesis imperfecta, hypophosphatasia, achondroplasia, camptomelic dysplasia, and thanatophoric dysplasia.

UNILATERAL CONGENITAL TIBIAL BOWING AND CONGENITAL PSEUDARTHROSIS OF THE TIBIA

Posteromedial congenital bowing is also referred to as *kyphoscoliosis tibia*. This congenital deformity affects the tibia, fibula, and soft tissues of the lower extremity. Both the tibia and fibula show marked posteromedial bowing. The foot is held in a calcaneovalgus position. The etiology remains uncertain and may be related to abnormal early embryologic development rather than abnormal fetal positioning or intrauterine fracture. As the child grows, there often is partial resolution of the tibial bowing and shortening. Treatment is conservative, such as corrective casts or splints to hold the foot and support the leg during remodeling. If there is a severe persistent deformity beyond toddler age, surgical correction may be needed.

Anterolateral bowing of the tibia has been termed *congenital pseudarthrosis*. This is a misnomer because the pseudarthrosis or fracture is rarely congenital. The deformity is almost always unilateral. The preferred term is *congenital tibial dysplasia* (CTD). It is a rare anomaly (1 in 140,000 live births), but occurs in 1% to 2% of children with NF1. However, at least 70% of children with CTD have NF1. This may be an underestimation because clinical features of NF1 may appear only later in life. CTD presents as anterolateral bowing or fracture of the tibia, often before other manifestations of NF1 present. Lack of involvement of the fibula suggests that the bowing will resolve spontaneously. In anterolateral bowing associated with NF1, the fracture and refracture rate is very high. Limb length inequality is frequent as a result of both disuse atrophy and abnormal growth at the distal tibial physis. There often is a valgus deformity at the ankle. Surgical management can be frustrating because nonunion or pseudarthrosis following osteotomy is frequent.

The radiographic changes seen with CTD are variable. These include anterolateral bowing of the tibia, fracture, pseudarthrosis, hourglass-like constriction of the midshaft of the tibia, cystic changes usually at the junction of the upper and middle thirds of the tibia, sclerosis that narrows the medullary canal, and, infrequently, involvement of the fibula alone (Fig. 21). Several classifications of CTD have been proposed, all of which include sclerotic, cystic and dysplastic types.

Pathologic studies show that there is abnormal, highly cellular fibrovascular tissue with variable amounts of fibrocartilage and hyaline cartilage within the tibia. Bone growth and repair is abnormal. The pattern of abnormal fibrous tissue results in the dysplastic or cystic changes characteristic of the disorder.

ABNORMAL SEGMENTATION (FUSION DEFORMITIES)

TARSAL COALITION

Tarsal coalition is a congenital failure of segmentation of the primitive mesenchyme that results in union of two or more tarsal bones. Intertarsal bridges have been found in fetal tissue. A preadolescent or adolescent child with pain in the midfoot and hindfoot that is associated with lack of motion in the subtalar region should be suspected of having a tarsal coalition. The prevalence in the U.S. population is approximately 1% or less. At least 50% of patients with coalitions have bilateral findings. An autosomal dominant inheritance pattern with a high level of penetrance is reported, although the coalition need not involve the same joint.

Tarsal coalition is defined based on anatomic location and completeness of ossification. A complete ossific bar

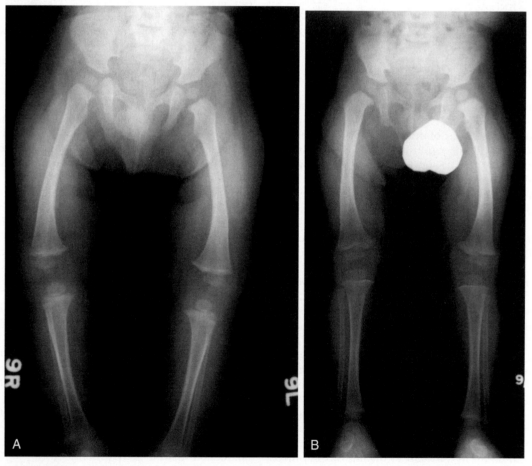

FIGURE 20. A, Sixteen-month-old boy with physiologic bowing of the lower extremities. The proximal tibias are normal, and no fragmentation is seen to suggest Blount disease. **B,** Seven months later, the bowing has diminished.

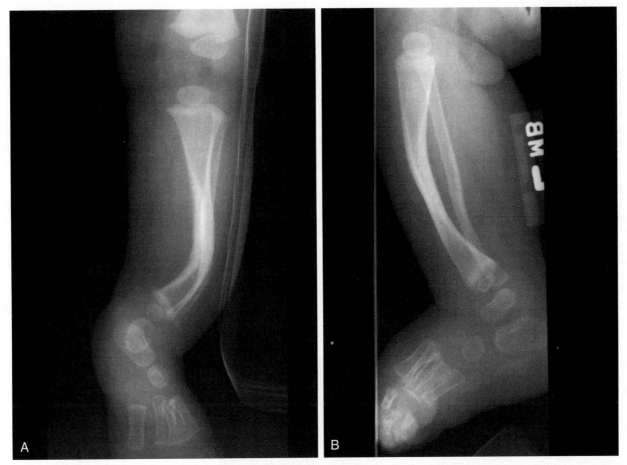

FIGURE 21. Anterolateral tibial bowing in a child with congenital tibial dysplasia and neurofibromatosis type 1. The medullary canal is nearly obliterated, but there is no fracture.

forms a *synostosis*, a cartilaginous bar forms a *synchondrosis*, and a fibrous union is termed a *syndesmosis*. The most common of fusions are talocalcaneal and calcaneonavicular. Talonavicular and calcaneocuboid coalitions are much less common. Synostoses can occur between other bones of the foot, but frequently are associated with other limb abnormalities, such as fibular hemimelia or short femur, or syndromes, such as Apert's syndrome.

Symptoms from a tarsal coalition present when the union ossifies. Pain with activity usually is the presenting symptom. The child may have a peroneal spastic flatfoot, which includes pain and rigid valgus deformity of the hindfoot and forefoot, and peroneal muscle spasm. However, any abnormality of the subtalar joint that restricts motion, such as a fracture, arthritis, or tumor, also can result in a peroneal spastic flatfoot.

Imaging evaluation of all children suspected of having a tarsal coalition should begin with conventional radiographs. Anteroposterior (AP), lateral, and 45-degree lateral oblique views should be obtained. Although the AP view rarely directly delineates a coalition, it can be used to exclude other causes of a peroneal spastic foot. A "ball-and-socket" articulation of the distal tibia and talus is an uncommon association with tarsal coalition. This configuration at the ankle joint is nonspecific and may be associated with congenital long bone deficien-

cies. The lateral radiograph is useful to show secondary signs of tarsal coalition. These include a hypoplastic talar head, a talar beak, and broadening or rounding of the lateral talar process. An "anteater nose" on a lateral radiograph, which represents an anterior prolongation of the superior calcaneus, is a consistent sign of a calcaneonavicular coalition. A "C-line" formed by the medial outline of the talar dome and the inferior aspect of the sustentaculum tali is suggestive of a talocalcaneal coalition.

The oblique radiograph is used to demonstrate a calcaneonavicular bar (Fig. 22*A*). The axial or Harris-Beath view is used to evaluate for a talocalcaneal coalition. In this projection, the normal middle and posterior talocalcaneal facets are parallel to each other. Because most subtalar coalitions involve the middle facet, most abnormalities are seen medially. A frank bony bridge may be seen. In nonosseous fusions, the facet surfaces may be irregular and angled inferomedially. Because the axial view may be difficult to angle correctly for optimal visualization of the subtalar joint, children suspected of having subtalar fusions are commonly referred for cross-sectional imaging (Fig. 22*B*).

Computed tomography (CT) and MRI help to define the nature and cross-sectional area of a fusion. Either modality can be used, with a high percentage of agreement between imaging findings on both. CT is more cost-effective if the clinical suspicion for coalition is high. However, if other etiologies for pain and limited hindfoot mobility are entertained, then MRI may be indicated.

Casting is often the initial treatment for symptomatic children. If symptoms are not relieved and there are no degenerative changes, then surgical resection of the abnormal tarsal bridging is often attempted. Subtalar fusion or triple arthrodesis may be indicated in refractory cases.

CARPAL FUSION

Fusion of the carpal bones is a normal variant that is seen in approximately 0.1% of the population (Fig. 23). The most frequently seen carpal fusion is between the lunate and triquetrum bones. A fusion between bones of the proximal and distal carpal rows usually is associated with a syndrome. Fusions also may be acquired, such as in juvenile rheumatoid arthritis.

SYNDACTYLY

Fusion between adjacent digits resulting from an intra-uterine failure to separate is termed *syndactyly*. These fusions can involve only soft tissue (simple syndactyly) (Fig. 24) or also involve bone (complex syndactyly). If the entire length of the digit is involved, it is termed *complete*, and if only partial length is bridged, it is *incomplete*. Syndactyly is easily diagnosed at birth. The fusion may be unilateral or bilateral, and most often involves the third and fourth digits. Syndactyly may be isolated or associated with congenital syndromes such as Poland's, Apert's, and Carpenter's syndromes. Surgery is performed early in life to improve function and appearance.

SYMPHALANGISM

Symphalangism is an uncommon autosomal dominant disorder of fusion of the interphalangeal joints of the

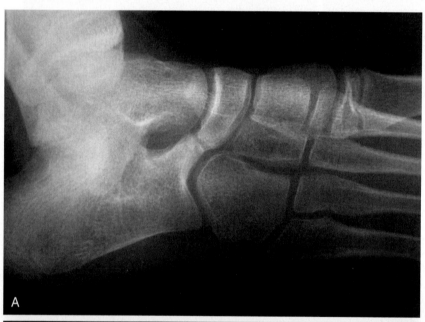

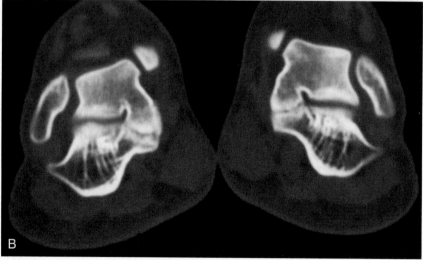

FIGURE 22. Tarsal coalition. **A,** Calcaneonavicular incomplete osseous coalition is seen on an oblique view of the foot. **B,** Direct coronal computed tomography images of both feet show bilateral calcaneotalar coalitions of the middle facet.

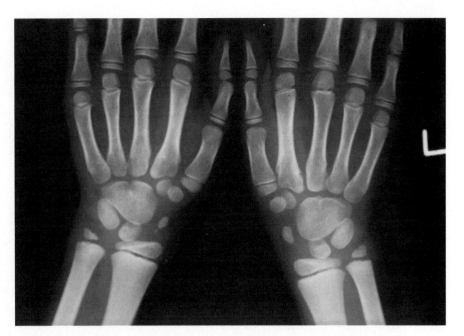

FIGURE 23. Fusion of the hamate and capitate bones bilaterally.

hands and feet (Fig. 25). Although proximal interphalangeal joint fusion is more common, fusion can also be more distal. The anomaly is usually bilateral. The little finger is affected most often. Fusion may not be recognized radiographically until later in childhood. Despite the radiographic appearance of the digits, seldom is there disability or loss of function of the hand. Symphalangism may be associated with other skeletal abnormalities, various digit deformities (e.g., brachydactyly, clinodactyly, camptodactyly), radioulnar fusion, hip dislocation, tarsal coalitions, and spinal anomalies.

RADIOULNAR SYNOSTOSIS

Congenital radioulnar synostosis anomaly is due to failure of longitudinal segmentation between the radius and ulna. In utero, the cartilaginous anlages of the humerus, radius, and ulna are connected. During the course of normal separation, which progresses from the distal end of the forearm to the proximal end, there is a time when the proximal ends of the radius and ulna

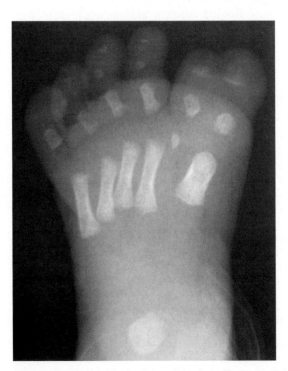

FIGURE 24. Newborn with six digits of the foot. The extra digit is hypoplastic, while the great toe is only slightly small. There is simple syndactyly between the first two digits.

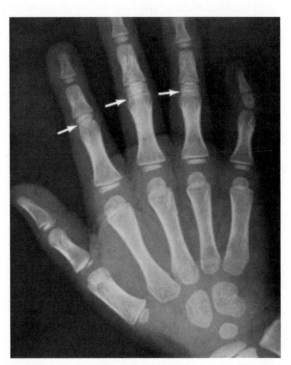

FIGURE 25. Symphalangism, or absence of joints, in the hands of a 5-year-old girl with stiff fingers and toes since birth. There is fusion of the proximal and middle phalanges of the second, third, and fourth digits. There also is carpal fusion. Fusion of the metatarsals and cuneiforms was present in the foot. (Courtesy of Dr. R. Parker Allen, Denver, CO.)

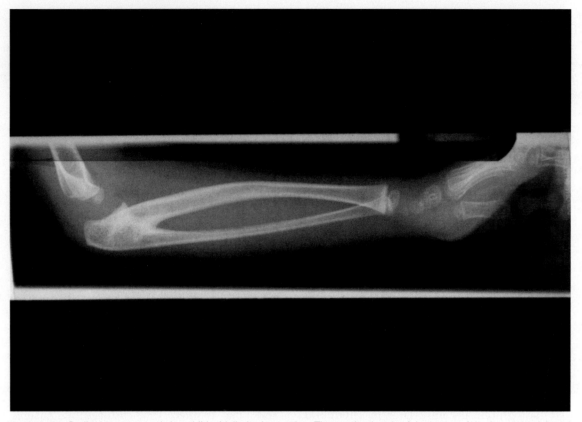

FIGURE 26. Radioulnar synostosis in a child with limited pronation. The proximal ends of the bones of the forearm are fused. There is a mild bowing deformity.

are connected by a common perichondrium. An insult to segmentation during early in utero development can lead to bony or fibrous synostosis (Fig. 26). Radioulnar synostosis is associated with syndromes such as Apert's and Carpenter's syndromes, as well as other upper extremity abnormalities such as polydactyly, syndactyly, and carpal coalition.

On clinical examination, the child has a fixed degree of pronation and a mild degree of flexion at the elbow. Pain usually occurs during the teen years, when progressive and symptomatic radial head subluxation can be seen. Surgical treatment is usually reserved for patients with a severe pronation deformity or symptomatic radial head subluxation. A derotation osteotomy through the fusion mass must take the degree of associated soft tissue contracture and neurovascular bundle compromise into consideration.

MISCELLANEOUS CONGENITAL MALFORMATIONS

DIGITS

Clinodactyly

Clinodactyly is a curvature of the finger in a radial or ulnar direction (in the mediolateral plane). Although it can involve any digit, it most often refers to radial curvature of the distal interphalangal joint of the fifth digit (Fig. 27). Clinodactyly is associated with a short

middle phalanx and is often bilateral. It may be seen in the normal population as a sporadic variant, but also can be inherited in an autosomal dominant pattern. It has been described in numerous syndromes, in bone dysplasias, following trauma, and in many miscellaneous conditions. It frequently is seen in Down syndrome. Treatment is undertaken for cosmesis or excessive scissoring of the digits.

Camptodactyly

Camptodactyly refers to a congenital or acquired flexion contracture of the finger. It usually is located at the proximal interphalangeal joint of the fifth finger, but also can involve the second through fourth digits (Fig. 28). The cause remains unknown, but may relate to abnormal insertion of the lumbrical muscles or the flexor digitorum superficialis tendon. Like clinodactyly, camptodactyly may be sporadic or show an autosomal dominant inheritance pattern. It occasionally is associated with a chromosomal abnormality, a bony dysplasia, or other syndrome. Treatment includes bracing or, infrequently, a surgical release.

Kirner Deformity

Palmar bending of the distal phalanx of the fifth digit is termed *Kirner deformity*. It usually is an isolated abnormality that is bilateral and symmetric. The long axis of the distal phalanx is bent toward the palm, while the

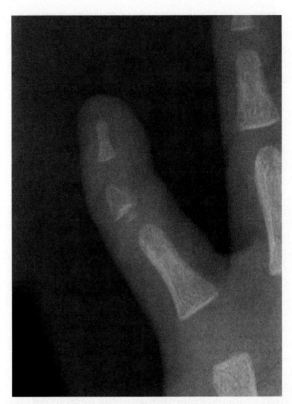

FIGURE 27. One-year-old girl with clinodactyly of the fifth digit. There is medial bending of the finger and a short middle phalanx.

epiphysis is normally oriented (Fig. 29). The physis is widened. Like the other digit deformities, Kirner deformity can be a sporadic or autosomal dominant inherited anomaly.

Longitudinal Epiphyseal Bracket

Abnormal longitudinal development of the diaphyseal–metaphyseal segment of a phalanx, metacarpal or metatarsal that often results in a triangular shape has been termed a *delta phalanx*. However, because a metatarsal or metacarpal may be involved, this term is not entirely correct. The phrase *longitudinal epiphyseal bracket* is more accurate to describe the pathologic anatomy.

This congenital deformity affects the short tubular bones that normally develop a proximal epiphyseal ossification center (e.g., phalanges, first metacarpal or metatarsal). The involved bone is trapezoid or triangular in shape. The diaphyseal–metaphyseal osseous unit is bracketed along the longitudinal side by a physis and an epiphysis. The physis is arc-like, extending from the medial proximal surface along the longitudinal margin of the bone to the distal medial surface, similar in configuration to a bracket. The thumb most commonly is affected. Other anomalies of the digits are frequently associated with the longitudinal epiphyseal bracket. The deformity may be sporadic, but also is found in the Rubinstein-Taybi syndrome and fibrodysplasia ossificans progressiva. The cause is likely incomplete development of the primary ossification center of the bone during embryonic or early fetal growth. The growth distur-

bance relates to the longitudinally oriented cartilaginous bracket that causes growth to follow a "C-shaped" curve (Fig. 30). MRI can be helpful to delineate the size and location of the bracket when it is not yet ossified. Early surgical intervention, often a wedge osteotomy, is recommended for better remodeling.

Duplication

Duplication of digits may result from an insult in utero to the apical ectodermal ridge during development. The deformity is more likely of a "splitting" nature, with the resultant parts being mildly or severely hypoplastic rather than truly duplicated. Polydactyly or supernumerary digits is a common congenital anomaly seen most often of the thumb or small finger. Extra digits may be bilateral and may involve both fingers and toes (see Fig. 24). The malformation may be isolated or be associated with a syndrome. Duplication can be of soft tissue alone, or soft tissue and bone. An anomaly on the radial or thumb side is termed *preaxial,* and on the ulnar side, *postaxial.* Prexial polydactyly is more frequently seen in Caucasians, and is associated with various syndromes, such as Holt-Oram syndrome, Fanconi's anemia, and the VATER association.

DUPLICATION OF THE FEMUR

Duplication of the femur is a rare anomaly, occurring more often in the distal portion of the bone. Bifurcation

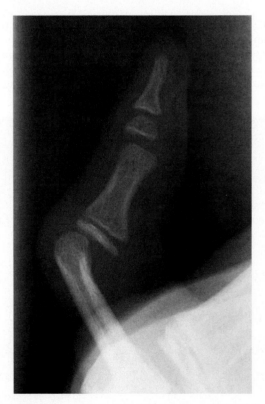

FIGURE 28. Flexion of the proximal interphalangeal joint of the fifth digit is seen in this child with camptodactyly. No skin crease is seen, and there is palmar subluxation of the middle phalanx.

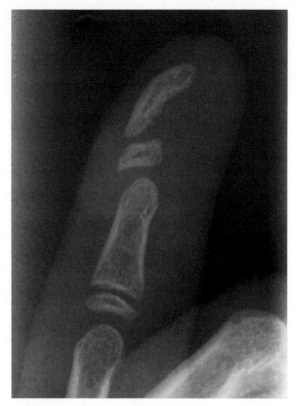

FIGURE 29. There is palmar bending of the distal phalanx of the fifth digit in this girl with Kirner deformity. The epiphysis is in a normal position. (From Oestreich AE, Crawford AH: Atlas of Pediatric Orthopedic Radiology. New York, Thieme, 1985;166, with permission.)

of the femur is associated with tibial dysplasia (partial or complete hemimelia). The femur is Y-shaped, with the anteromedial limb forming a protuberance in the medial thigh. At birth, the limb can resemble an exostosis, but, with growth, it may become the longer of the two limbs. The lateral limb usually forms an unstable articulation with the proximal fibula. There is no true knee joint. The patella may be absent, and complex foot deformities can be seen. An autosomal recessive form of this complex limb deformity has been reported.

CONGENITAL RADIAL HEAD DISLOCATION

Congenital radial head dislocation is the most commonly identified congenital abnormality of the elbow. More than half of cases are associated with other conditions, such as anomalies of the lower extremities, scoliosis, and various syndromes (e.g., Klippel-Feil). Whether it is an isolated abnormality or associated with other conditions, congenital radial head dislocation is believed to have an autosomal dominant inheritance pattern. The deformity can be unilateral or bilateral.

Congenital radial head dislocation is associated with a small, underdeveloped forearm; a flattened and hypoplastic capitellum; and a short ulna. The radial head is elongated and thinned or rounded, and most commonly dislocated in a posterior direction (Fig. 31). Radiographs should be carefully evaluated for concomitant radioulnar synostosis. In the young child, the deformity is painless, but motion is usually limited.

Asymptomatic dislocations are not treated. If the child has pain, the radial head can be excised. However, excision of the radial head frequently is accompanied by pain from abnormal mechanics at the wrist. Recent work suggests that open reduction of the proximal radius at an early age may be beneficial.

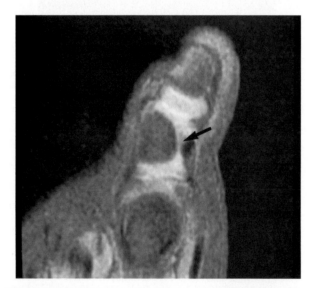

FIGURE 30. Coronal proton density–weighted magnetic resonance image of the first toe of a boy with a longitudinal epiphyseal bracket. The ossified portion of the middle phalanx is trapezoidal. An arc or bracket of high-signal-intensity cartilage *(arrow)* is seen along the medial aspect of the phalanx.

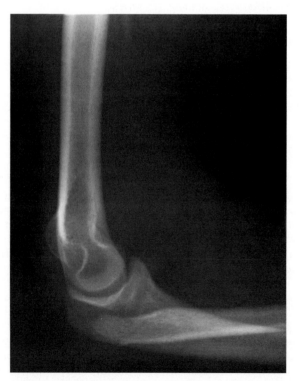

FIGURE 31. Congenital dislocation of the proximal radius. The radial head is rounded and dislocated in a posterior direction. Similar findings were present in the contralateral elbow.

VATER Association

In 1965, Kirkpatrick and coworkers described an association of congenital anomalies in newborns that included gastrointestinal, osseous, and cardiac abnormalities. In 1971, the term *VATER* was coined to refer to an association of *v*ertebral defects, *a*nal atresia or other anorectal malformations, *t*racheoesophageal fistula, and *e*sophageal atresia, and *r*adial and renal dysplasia that occur more often than would be expected with a random tendency. The *VATER* term has been expanded to include *c*ardiovascular and additional *l*imb anomalies (*VACTERL* association). The orthopedic aspects of the VATER association include a congenital scoliosis, sacral agenesis, radial hypoplasia or aplasia, and thumb abnormalities (polydactyly, hypoplasia, or absence). Rib anomalies, hip dislocation, PFFD, absence of the tibia and fibula, and congenital vertical talus also have been described. Anomalies of the hand, such as hypoplasia of the thumb, clinodactyly, and polydactyly, appear to be more common than other extremity anomalies. Children with the VATER association have normal intelligence, and management should be directed toward enhancing the quality of their lives.

SUGGESTED READINGS

Achterman C, Kalamchi A: Congenital deficiency of the fibula. J Bone Joint Surg Br 1979;61:133–137

Aitken G (ed): Proximal femoral focal deficiency—definition, classification, and management. *In* Proximal Femoral Focal Deficiency: A Congenital Anomaly. Washington, DC, National Academy of Sciences, 1969:1–22

Anton CG, Applegate KE, Kuivila TE, Wilkes DC: Proximal femoral focal deficiency (PFFD): more than an abnormal hip. Semin Musculoskelet Radiol 1999;3:215–226

Askins G, Ger E: Congenital constriction band syndrome. J Pediatr Orthop 1988;8:461–466

Barnes JC, Smith WL: The VATER association. Radiology 1978;126:445–449

Bayne LG, Klug MS: Long-term review of the surgical treatment of radial deficiencies. J Hand Surg Am 1987;12:169–179

Beals RK, Rolfe B: VATER association: a unifying concept of multiple anomalies. J Bone Joint Surg Am 1989;71:948–950

Berry SA, Peterson C, Mize W, et al: Klippel-Trenaunay syndrome. Am J Med Genet 1998;79:319–326

Bhargava R, Parham DM, Lasater OE, et al: MR imaging differentiation of benign and malignant peripheral nerve sheath tumors: use of the target sign. Pediatr Radiol 1997;27:124–129

Biesecker LG, Happle R, Mulliken JB, et al: Proteus syndrome: diagnostic criteria, differential diagnosis, and patient evaluation. Am J Med Genet 1999;84:389–395

Blacksin M, Barnes FJ, Lyons MM: MR diagnosis of macrodystrophia lipomatosa. AJR Am J Roentgenol 1992;158:1295–1297

Boden SD, Fallon MD, Davidson R, et al: Proximal femoral focal deficiency: evidence for a defect in proliferation and maturation of chondrocytes. J Bone Joint Surg Am 1989;71:1119–1129

Botto LD, Khoury MJ, Mastroiacovo P, et al: The spectrum of congenital anomalies of the VATER association: an international study. Am J Med Genet 1997;71:8–15

Brown FW: Construction of a ball joint on congenital absence of the tibia (paraxial hemimelia tibia). J Bone Joint Surg (Am) 1965;47:695–704

Burrows PF, Robertson RL, Barnes PD: Angiography and the evaluation of cerebrovascular disease in childhood. Neuroimaging Clin N Am 1996;6:561–588

Christini D, Levy EJ, Facanha FA, Kumar SJ: Fibular transfer for congenital absence of the tibia. J Pediatr Orthop 1993;13:378–381

Clark MW: Autosomal dominant inheritance of tibial meromelia: report of a kindred. J Bone Joint Surg Am 1975;57:262–264

Cohen MM Jr, Hayden PW: A newly recognized hamartomatous syndrome. Birth Defects Orig Artic Ser 1979;15:291–296

Cornah MS, Dangerfield PH: Reduplication of the femur: report of a case. J Bone Joint Surg Br 1974;56:744–745

Cowell HR: Tarsal coalition—review and update. Instr Course Lect 1982;31:264–271

Crawford AH Jr, Bagamery N: Osseous manifestations of neurofibromatosis in childhood. J Pediatr Orthop 1986;6:72–88

Crawford AH, Schorry EK: Neurofibromatosis in children: the role of the orthopaedist. J Am Acad Orthop Surg 1999;7:217–230

Cremin BJ, Viljoen DL, Wynchank S, Beighton P: The Proteus syndrome: the magnetic resonance and radiological features. Pediatr Radiol 1987;17:486–488

Czeizel A, Ludanyi I: VACTERL-association. Acta Morphol Hung 1984;32:75–96

Daentl DL, Smith DW, Scott CI, et al: Femoral hypoplasia–unusual facies syndrome. J Pediatr 1975;86:107–111

Davidson R, Drummond D: Arthrogryposis. *In* Drennan JC (ed): The Child's Foot and Ankle. New York, Raven Press, 1992:253–266

Davidson WH, Bohne WH: The Syme amputation in children. J Bone Joint Surg Am 1975;57:905–909

D'Costa H, Hunter JD, O'Sullivan G, et al: Magnetic resonance imaging in macromelia and macrodactyly. Br J Radiol 1996;69:502–507

Dubois J, Garel L: Imaging and therapeutic approach of hemangiomas and vascular malformations in the pediatric age group. Pediatr Radiol 1999;29:879–893

Dubois J, Garel L, David M, Powell J: Vascular soft-tissue tumors in infancy: distinguishing features on Doppler sonography. AJR Am J Roentgenol 2002;178:1541–1545

Emery KH, Bisset GS 3rd, Johnson ND, Nunan PJ: Tarsal coalition: a blinded comparison of MRI and CT. Pediatr Radiol 1998;28:612–616

Enjolras O, Ciabrini D, Mazoyer E, et al: Extensive pure venous malformations in the upper or lower limb: a review of 27 cases. J Am Acad Dermatol 1997a;36:219–225

Enjolras O, Wassef M, Mazoyer E, et al: Infants with Kasabach-Merritt syndrome do not have "true" hemangiomas. J Pediatr 1997b;130:631–640

Ezekowitz RA, Mulliken JB, Folkman J: Interferon alfa-2a therapy for life-threatening hemangiomas of infancy. N Engl J Med 1992;326:1456–1463

Fernbach SK, Glass RB: The expanded spectrum of limb anomalies in the VATER association. Pediatr Radiol 1988;18:215–220

Fisher RM, Cremin BJ: Limb defects in the amniotic band syndrome. Pediatr Radiol 1976;5:24–29

Fishman SJ, Mulliken JB: Hemangiomas and vascular malformations of infancy and childhood. Pediatr Clin North Am 1993;40:1177–1200

Fishman SJ, Mulliken JB: Vascular anomalies: a primer for pediatricians. Pediatr Clin North Am 1998;45:1455–1477

Fordham LA, Applegate KE, Wilkes DC, Chung CJ: Fibular hemimelia: more than just an absent bone. Semin Musculoskelet Radiol 1999;3:227–238

Frantz C, O'Rahilly R: Congenital limb deficiencies. J Bone Joint Surg Am 1961;43:1202–1224

Gillespie R, Torode IP: Classification and management of congenital abnormalities of the femur. J Bone Joint Surg Br 1983;65:557–568

Goldberg MJ, Bartoshesky LE: Congenital hand anomaly: etiology and associated malformations. Hand Clin 1985;1:405–415

Goldman AB, Kaye JJ: Macrodystrophia lipomatosa: radiographic diagnosis. AJR Am J Roentgenol 1977;128:101–105

Grissom LE, Harcke HT: Sonography in congenital deficiency of the femur. J Pediatr Orthop 1994;14:29–33

Grissom LE, Harcke HT, Kumar SJ: Sonography in the management of tibial hemimelia. Clin Orthop 1990:266–270

Gupta SK, Sharma OP, Sharma SV, et al: Macrodystrophia lipomatosa: radiographic observations. Br J Radiol 1992;65:769–773

Hall BD, Spranger J: Congenital bowing of the long bones: a review and phenotype analysis of 13 undiagnosed cases. Eur J Pediatr 1980;133:131–138

Hall JG: An approach to congenital contractures (arthrogryposis). Pediatr Ann 1981;10:15–26

Hall JG: Arthrogryposis. Am Fam Physician 1989;39:113–119

Hamanishi C: Congenital short femur: clinical, genetic and epidemiologic comparison of the naturally occurring condition with that caused by thalidomide. J Bone Joint Surg Br 1980;62:307–320

Hand JL, Frieden IJ: Vascular birthmarks of infancy: resolving nosologic confusion. Am J Med Genet 2002;108:257–264

Harris RI: Retrospect—personeal spastic flat foot (rigid valgus foot). J Bone Joint Surg Am 1965;47:1657–1667

Hefti F, Bollini G, Dungl P, et al: Congenital pseudarthrosis of the tibia: history, etiology, classification, and epidemiologic data. J Pediatr Orthop B 2000;9:11–15

Herring A, Cummings DR: The limb deficient child. In Morrissy RT, Weinstein SL (eds): Lovell and Winter's Pediatric Orthopaedics, 4th ed. Philadelphia, Lippincott–Raven, 1996:1137–1176

Hillmann JS, Mesgarzadeh M, Revesz G, et al: Proximal femoral focal deficiency: radiologic analysis of 49 cases. Radiology 1987;165:769–773

Hochman M, Reed MH: Features of calcaneonavicular coalition on coronal computed tomography Skeletal Radiol 2000;29:409–412

Hootnick DR, Levinsohn EM, Randall PA, Packard DS Jr: Vascular dysgenesis associated with skeletal dysplasia of the lower limb. J Bone Joint Surg Am 1980;62:1123–1129

Ippolito E, Corsi A, Grill F, et al: Pathology of bone lesions associated with congenital pseudarthrosis of the leg. J Pediatr Orthop B 2000;9:3–10

Jayakumar SS, Eilert RE: Fibular transfer for congenital absence of the tibia. Clin Orthop 1979;97–101

Jones D, Barnes J, Lloyd-Roberts GC: Congenital aplasia and dysplasia of the tibia with intact fibula: classification and management. J Bone Joint Surg Br 1978;60:31–39

Kalamchi A, Cowell HR, Kim KI: Congenital deficiency of the femur. J Pediatr Orthop 1985;5:129–134

Kirkpatrick JA, Wagner ML, Pilling GF: Complex of anomalies associated with tracheoesophageal fistula and esophageal atresia. Am J Roentgenol Radium Ther Nucl Med 1965;95:208–211

Kirks DR, Shackelford GD: Idiopathic congenital hemihypertrophy with associated ipsilateral benign nephromegaly. Radiology 1975;115:145–148

Klatte EC, Franken EA, Smith JA: The radiographic spectrum in neurofibromatosis. Semin Roentgenol 1976;11:17–33

Kohn G, el Shawwa R, Grunebaum M: Aplasia of the tibia with bifurcation of the femur and ectrodactyly: evidence for an autosomal recessive type. Am J Med Genet 1989;33:172–175

Kritter AE: Tibial rotation-plasty for proximal femoral focal deficiency. J Bone Joint Surg Am 1977;59:927–934

Kulik SA Jr, Clanton TO: Tarsal coalition. Foot Ankle Int 1996;17:286–296

Laor T, Burrows PE: Congenital anomalies and vascular birthmarks of the lower extremities. Magn Reson Imaging Clin N Am 1998;6:497–519

Laor T, Burrows PE, Hoffer FA: Magnetic resonance venography of congenital vascular malformations of the extremities. Pediatr Radiol 1996a;26:371–380

Laor T, Hoffer FA, Burrows PE, Kozakewich HP: MR lymphangiography in infants, children, and young adults. AJR Am J Roentgenol 1998a;171:1111–1117

Laor T, Jaramillo D, Hoffer FA, Kasser JR: MR imaging in congenital lower limb deformities. Pediatr Radiol 1996b;26:381–387

Laor T, Jaramillo D, Oestreich AE: Musculoskeletal system. In Kirks D, Griscom N (eds): Practical Pediatric Imaging: Diagnostic Imaging of Infants and Children, 3rd ed. Philadelphia, Lippincott–Raven, 1998b:327–510

Lateur LM, Van Hoe LR, Van Ghillewe KV, et al: Subtalar coalition: diagnosis with the C sign on lateral radiographs of the ankle. Radiology 1994;193:847–851

Lawhon SM, MacEwen GD, Bunnel WP: Orthopaedic aspects of the VATER association. J Bone Joint Surg Am 1986;68:424–429

Lenz W: Malformations caused by drugs in pregnancy. Am J Dis Child 1966;112:99–106

Leonard MA: The inheritance of tarsal coalition and its relationship to spastic flat foot. J Bone Joint Surg Br 1974;56:520–526

Letts M, Davidson D, Beaule P: Symphalangism in children: case report and review of the literature. Clin Orthop 1999:178–185

Levine C: The imaging of body asymmetry and hemihypertrophy. Crit Rev Diagn Imaging 1990;31:1–80

Levinson ED, Ozonoff MB, Royen PM: Proximal femoral focal deficiency (PFFD). Radiology 1977;125:197–203

Lie RT, Wilcox AJ, Skjaerven R: A population-based study of the risk of recurrence of birth defects. N Engl J Med 1994;331:1–4

Light TR, Ogden JA: The longitudinal epiphyseal bracket: implications for surgical correction. J Pediatr Orthop 1981;1:299–305

Loder RT, Herring JA: Fibular transfer for congenital absence of the tibia: a reassessment. J Pediatr Orthop 1987;7:8–13

Lourie GM, Lins RE: Radial longitudinal deficiency: a review and update. Hand Clin 1998;14:85–99

Mahboubi S, Davidson R: MR imaging in longitudinal epiphyseal bracket in children. Pediatr Radiol 1999;29:259–261

McCarthy JJ, Glancy GL, Chang FM, Eilert RE: Fibular hemimelia: comparison of outcome measurements after amputation and lengthening. J Bone Joint Surg Am 2000;82-A:1732–1735

McCredie J: Sclerotome subtraction: a radiologic interpretation of reduction deformities of the limbs. Birth Defects Orig Artic Ser 1977;13:65–77

McGuirk CK, Westgate MN, Holmes LB: Limb deficiencies in newborn infants. Pediatrics 2001;108:E64

Metry DW, Hebert AA: Benign cutaneous vascular tumors of infancy: when to worry, what to do. Arch Dermatol 2000;136:905–914

Meyer JS, Hoffer FA, Barnes PD, Mulliken JB: Biological classification of soft-tissue vascular anomalies: MR correlation. AJR Am J Roentgenol 1991;157:559–564

Mulliken JB, Glowacki J: Hemangiomas and vascular malformations in infants and children: a classification based on endothelial characteristics. Plast Reconstr Surg 1982;69:412–422

Murphey MD, Smith WS, Smith SE, et al: From the archives of the AFIP. Imaging of musculoskeletal neurogenic tumors: radiologic-pathologic correlation. Radiographics 1999;19:1253–1280

Naudie D, Hamdy RC, Fassier F, et al: Management of fibular hemimelia: amputation or limb lengthening. J Bone Joint Surg Br 1997;79:58–65

Newman JS, Newberg AH: Congenital tarsal coalition: multimodality evaluation with emphasis on CT and MR imaging. Radiographics 2000;20:321–332; quiz 526–527, 532

Oestreich AE, Crawford AH: Atlas of Pediatric Orthopedic Radiology. New York, Thieme, 1985:166

Oestreich AE, Mize WA, Crawford AH, Morgan RC Jr: The "anteater nose": a direct sign of calcaneonavicular coalition on the lateral radiograph. J Pediatr Orthop 1897;7:709–711

Ogden JA, Light TR, Conlogue GJ: Correlative roentgenography and morphology of the longitudinal epiphyseal bracket. Skeletal Radiol 1981:6:109–117

O'Rahilly R: Morphologic patterns in limb deficiencies and duplications. Am J Anat 1951;89:135–193

Ozonoff M: Pediatric Orthopedic Radiology, 2nd ed. Philadelphia, WB Saunders, 1992

Pachuda NM, Lasday SD, Jay RM: Tarsal coalition: etiology, diagnosis, and treatment. J Foot Surg 1990;29:474–88

Pappas AM: Congenital abnormalities of the femur and related lower extremity malformations: classification and treatment. J Pediatr Orthop 1983;3:45–60

Pappas AM: Congenital posteromedial bowing of the tibia and fibula. J Pediatr Orthop 1984;4:525–531

Patel M, Paley D, Herzenberg JE: Limb-lengthening versus amputation for fibular hemimelia. J Bone Joint Surg Am 2002;84-A:317–319

Pfister RC, Weber AL, Smith EH, et al: Congenital asymmetry (hemihypertrophy) and abdominal disease: radiological features in 9 cases. Radiology 1975;116:685–691

Pirani S, Beauchamp RD, Li D, Sawatzky B: Soft tissue anatomy of proximal femoral focal deficiency. J Pediatr Orthop 1991;11:563–570

Poznanski A: The Hand in Radiologic Diagnosis, 2nd ed. Philadelphia, WB Saunders, 1984:204–208

Poznanski AK, La Rowe PC: Radiographic manifestations of the arthrogryposis syndrome. Radiology 1970;95:353–358

Poznanski AK, Pratt GB, Manson G, Weiss L: Clinodactyly, camptodactyly, Kirner's deformity, and other crooked fingers. Radiology 1969;93:573–582

Price NJ, Cundy PJ: Synovial hemangioma of the knee. J Pediatr Orthop 1997;17:74–77

Ritter R, Siafarikas K: Hemihypertrophy in a boy with renal polycystic disease: varied patterns of presentation of renal polycystic disease in his family. Pediatr Radiol 1976;5:98–102

Robinow M, Schatzman ER, Oberheu K: Peromelia, ipsilateral subclavian atresia, coarctation, and aneurysms of the aorta resulting from intrauterine vascular occlusion. J Pediatr 1982;101:84–87

Roux MO, Carlioz H: Clinical examination and investigation of the cruciate ligaments in children with fibular hemimelia. J Pediatr Orthop 1999;19:247–251

Sachar K, Akelman E, Ehrlich M: Radioulnar synostosis. Hand Clin 1994;10:399–404

Sachar K, Mih A: Congenital radial head dislocations. Hand Clin 1998;14:39–47

Sakellariou A, Claridge RJ: Tarsal coalition. Orthopedics 1999;22:1066–1073; discussion 1073–1074; quiz 10

Salenius P, Vankka E: The development of the tibiofemoral angle in children. J Bone Joint Surg Am 1975;57:259–261

Sanpera I Jr, Sparks LT: Proximal femoral focal deficiency: does a radiologic classification exist? J Pediatr Orthop 1994;14:34–38

Sarkar M, Mulliken JB, Kozakewich HP, et al: Thrombocytopenic coagulopathy (Kasabach-Merritt phenomenon) is associated with kaposiform hemangioendothelioma and not with common infantile hemangioma. Plast Reconstr Surg 1997;100:1377–1386

Shapiro F, Specht L: The diagnosis and orthopaedic treatment of childhood spinal muscular atrophy, peripheral neuropathy, Friedreich ataxia, and arthrogryposis. J Bone Joint Surg Am 1993;75:1699–1714

Simmons ED Jr, Ginsburg GM, Hall JE: Brown's procedure for congenital absence of the tibia revisited. J Pediatr Orthop 1996;16:85–89

Smith JG, Weiss AP, Weiss YS: Congenital anomalies of the hand. Clin Pediatr (Phila) 1998;37:459–467

Sodergard J, Ryoppy S: The knee in arthrogryposis multiplex congenita. J Pediatr Orthop 1990;10:177–182

Soltan HC, Holmes LB: Familial occurrence of malformations possibly attributable to vascular abnormalities. J Pediatr 1986;108:112–114

Stern WA: Arthrogryposis multiplex congenita. JAMA 1923;81:1507–1510

Stormont DM, Peterson HA: The relative incidence of tarsal coalition. Clin Orthop 1983:28–36

Streeter G: Focal deficiencies in fetal tissues and their relation to intra-uterine amputation. Contrib Embryol 1930;22:1–44

Stricker S: Musculoskeletal manifestations of Proteus syndrome: report of two cases with literature review. J Pediatr Orthop 1992;12:667–674

Stull MA, Moser RP Jr, Kransdorf MJ, et al: Magnetic resonance appearance of peripheral nerve sheath tumors. Skeletal Radiol 1991;20:9–14

Suh JS, Abenoza P, Galloway HR, et al: Peripheral (extracranial) nerve tumors: correlation of MR imaging and histologic findings. Radiology 1992;183:341–346

Swinyard CA, Bleck EE: The etiology of arthrogryposis (multiple congenital contracture). Clin Orthop 1985:15–29

Takakura Y, Tamai S, Masuhara K: Genesis of the ball-and-socket ankle. J Bone Joint Surg Br 1986;68:834–837

Temtamy SA, Miller JD: Extending the scope of the VATER association: definition of the VATER syndrome. J Pediatr 1974;85:345–349

Tibbles JA, Cohen MM Jr: The Proteus syndrome: the Elephant Man diagnosed. Br Med J 1986;293:683–685

Trop I, Dubois J, Guibaud L: Soft-tissue venous malformations in pediatric and young adult patients: diagnosis with Doppler US. Radiology 1999;212:841–845

Tuncay IC, Johnston CE 2nd, Birch JG: Spontaneous resolution of congenital anterolateral bowing of the tibia. J Pediatr Orthop 1994;14:599–602

Van Allen MI, Hoyme HE, Jones KL: Vascular pathogenesis of limb defects. I. Radial artery anatomy in radial aplasia. J Pediatr 1982;101:832–838

Van Heest AE: Congenital disorders of the hand and upper extremity. Pediatr Clin North Am 1996;43:1113–1133

VanNes C: Rotation-plasty for congenital defects of the femur: making use of the ankle of the shortened limb to control the knee joint of a prosthesis. J Bone Joint Surg Br 1950;32:32

Vaughn RY, Selinger AD, Howell CG, et al: Proteus syndrome: diagnosis and surgical management. J Pediatr Surg 1993;28:5–10

Vincent KA: Tarsal coalition and painful flatfoot. J Am Acad Orthop Surg 1998;6:274–281

Warkany J, Nelson R: Skeletal abnormalities induced in rats by maternal nutritional deficiency. Arch Pathol 1942;34:375–384

Westin GW, Sakai DN, Wood WL: Congenital longitudinal deficiency of the fibula: follow-up of treatment by Syme amputation. J Bone Joint Surg Am 1976;58:492–496

Whimster IW: The pathology of lymphangioma circumscriptum. Br J Dermatol 1976;94:473–486

Wiedemann HR, Burgio GR, Aldenhoff P, et al: The Proteus syndrome: partial gigantism of the hands and/or feet, nevi, hemihypertrophy, subcutaneous tumors, macrocephaly or other skull anomalies and possible accelerated growth and visceral affections. Eur J Pediatr 1983;140:5–12

Wiedrich TA: Congenital constriction band syndrome. Hand Clin 1998:14:29–38

Wolfgang GL: Complex congenital anomalies of the lower extremities: femoral bifurcation, tibial hemimelia, and diastasis of the ankle. Case report and review of the literature. J Bone Joint Surg Am 1984;66:453–458

Wood BP, Putnam TC, Chacko AK: Infantile hepatic hemangioendotheliomas associated with hemihypertrophy. Pediatr Radiol 1977;5:242–245

Yetkin H, Cila E, Bilgin Guzel V, Kanatli U: Femoral bifurcation associated with tibial hemimelia. Orthopedics 2001;24:389–390

PART V

SKELETAL DYSPLASIAS

RALPH S. LACHMAN

The skeletal dysplasias (bone dysplasias, osteochondrodysplasias) are a group of over 200 well-defined disorders of which about 70 are often lethal in the perinatal period. Therefore, the thrust of this text will be to acquaint the reader with an approach to the skeletal dysplasias, and deal with about 45 of the most important and common of these disorders. The dysplasias covered here are those that the pediatric radiologist is most likely to encounter in his or her practice and therefore needs to know about.

Most of the bone dysplasias result in clinically disproportionate short-stature individuals. Therefore, one cannot consider the imaging evaluation of these disorders without first considering the radiologic assessment of all significant short stature. When one is faced with the problem of short stature in the pediatric age group, the clinical determination of whether one is dealing with proportionate or disproportionate short stature is crucial.

When the clinician has determined that the patient has *proportionate short stature,* the differential diagnosis as a general rule consists of constitutional delay, familial short stature, a small group of endocrinopathies, and some dysmorphology syndromes. The beginning clinical imaging assessment usually warrants a left hand and wrist radiograph for bone age determination. A complete "genetic skeletal survey" is not necessary in those cases and perhaps even contraindicated given our determination to keep ionizing radiation doses to pediatric patients as low as possible. However, should the patient in question have normal proportions and be dysmorphic or manifest multiple congenital anomalies on clinical evaluation, then one is dealing with one of the dysmorphology syndromes, and a modified genetic skeletal survey may be appropriate.

TERMINOLOGY

Certain terms are very important in the assessment of the skeletal dysplasias. Aside from the truncal shortening ("spine shortening"), extremity shortening may occur in total and/or in parts. This shortening may be radiologic and/or clinical. *Rhizomelia* (short upper arms/humeri and thighs/femurs), *mesomelia* (short middle segments, radii and ulnas, and tibias and fibulas), and *acromelia* (short hands and feet) play a major role in not only clinical and radiologic assessment, but also in nomenclature. We are all aware of the key areas in growing bone, so that abnormal development of epiphyses, metaphyses, and diaphyses have given rise to nomenclature using those site names (Fig. 1). The term *micromelic* should be reserved for very severe shortening of all four limbs and their limb parts. Abnormal development of the vertebral bodies signifies a *spondylo . . .* abnormality.

RADIOLOGIC ASSESSMENT

The history of the delineation and classification of many of the specific skeletal dysplasias reveals that the radiologic assessment has played a major role up to and including the present time. This is apparent because most of the skeletal dysplasias may have distinctive radiographic features (i.e., stippled ossification centers), are dense or osteopenic bone disorders, or have pathophysiologic abnormalities at or near the developing growth plates. An organized evaluation of the radiographs in the skeletal dysplasia survey includes the following steps.

STEP I: ASSESSMENT OF DISPROPORTION

An assessment is made again as to whether or not there is disproportion, this time from a radiographic point of view. A quick look at the films will decide whether or not there is significant generalized *platyspondyly* present, contributing to shortness of the trunk. Then a look at the extremities to try to ascertain whether rhizomelia, mesomelia, and/or acromelia are present will be helpful. It should be noted that clinical rhizomelia, mesome-

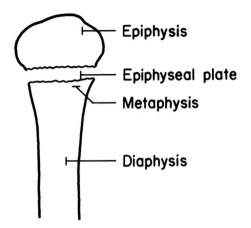

FIGURE 1. Key areas of the growing bone.

Epiphysis

Epiphyseal plate

Metaphysis

Diaphysis

lia, and acromelia are not always confirmed by the radiographic findings because the clinical visual evaluation is guided by the skin creases and folds rather than the underlying bone length. A significantly curved long bone may appear much shorter externally than radiographically. If the femurs and humeri are very shortened compared to the other segments, this constitutes *rhizomelia,* which, for example, is very important to confirm the specific diagnosis of the rhizomelic form of chondrodysplasia punctata. Very significant *mesomelia,* alone, suggests a group of specific disorders loosely classified as the mesomelic dysplasias. *Acromelia* is found in many disorders but is important to recognize because, for example, if it is associated with a particular form of vertebral abnormality, then one can make the rather specific diagnosis of the most common form of spondyloperipheral dysplasia. Of course, acromelia may be present by itself, and one might be dealing with a variety of disorders including skeletal dysplasias such as acro-

dysostosis and acromicric dysplasia or nonskeletal dysplasia; brachydactyly of any sort, especially brachydactyly type E; pseudohypoparathyroidism with cyclic AMP or GMP abnormalities; or even a chromosomal disorder (Turner's syndrome). Acromelia is found as part of other shortening in many specific skeletal dysplasias (i.e., achondroplasia), whereas the lack of significant hand and foot shortening is very important in spondyloepiphyseal dysplasia congenita.

STEP II: ASSESSMENT OF EPIPHYSEAL OSSIFICATION

Next, an overall assessment of epiphyseal ossification is made. If the *ossified epiphyses* are very small and/or irregular for age, then an epiphyseal dysplasia of some sort is present. Should the *metaphyses* be widened, flared, and/or irregular, the diagnosis of a metaphyseal chondrodysplasia is entertained. Finally, if *diaphyseal* abnormalities are present, such as widening and/or cortical thickening or marrow space expansion, the implication is that this represents a diaphyseal dysplasia of some sort. Early on, combinations of the aforementioned abnormalities with or without platyspondyly were ascribed not only to specific disorders but also nonspecific types of disorders such as congenital forms of spondyloepiphyseal dysplasia and the nonspecific group of spondyloepi(meta)physeal dysplasias [SE(M)Ds]. This rough estimation of type of disorder helps one to narrow down the diagnosis to a specific (well-described) entity. Figure 2 shows a crude depiction of these radiographic manifestations. If only the vertebral bodies are affected, with no significant changes in any of the growth plate regions, then one is dealing with a patient manifesting brachyolmia. Which one of the three well-described

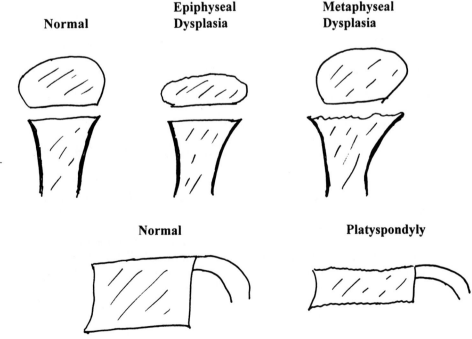

FIGURE 2. Radiographic manifestations of the dysplasias.

Normal

Epiphyseal Dysplasia

Metaphyseal Dysplasia

Normal

Platyspondyly

types of brachyolmia is present will be ascertained by the type of vertebral involvement and other clinical findings, as described by Shohat et al. At this point, it is important to re-emphasize that, although the radiology may play a major role in the diagnosis, other *clinical manifestations* are often very important to make a correct and complete diagnosis.

More precise evaluation of all the skeletal structures available in the skeletal dysplasia survey should then be performed. This may result in the recognition of a specific, well-described skeletal dysplasia from a previous broad categorization into a nonspecific group. This is crucial for genetic counseling. Another possibility from this precise evaluation is that a single pathognomonic finding will give a precise diagnosis (i.e., snail-shaped iliac bones of Schneckenbecken dysplasia).

STEP III: DIFFERENTIATION OF NORMAL VARIANTS FROM PATHOLOGIC ABNORMALITIES

This next step is more difficult and requires someone with at least some quite significant radiologic experience, preferably in the pediatric portion of radiologic imaging. It is necessary to recognize normal variations from pathologic abnormalities in the growing skeleton. An assessment needs to be made of *all* the skeletal structures. I personally believe this is best performed in an organized fashion, dealing with each one separately. Although every portion of every structure is looked at for any possible abnormal features, one should concentrate especially on certain abnormalities that specifically relate to the skeletal dysplasias. One must also recognize pathognomonic and other singular findings that suggest a specific diagnosis or a narrow group of differential diagnostic possibilities that in turn may lead to a specific diagnosis by other features.

DIAGNOSIS

After all the pathologic findings in every area have been established, then a gamut search of some or all of these abnormalities, in conjunction with the clinical findings, may lead to the specific diagnosis. If the "group" of dysplasias has been established, then often the specific disorder diagnosis can be made by referring to a differential diagnosis table, such as that developed by Taybi and Lachman.

MOLECULAR NOMENCLATURE

Recently there have been remarkable breakthroughs in the genetics of the skeletal dysplasias. These new findings are primarily molecular in nature. These molecular abnormalities now govern a new nomenclature, as reviewed by Lachman in 1998. In this text, I follow that molecular nomenclature in presenting the 40 odd specific bone dysplasias. The presentation is primarily

focused on the radiology rather than other clinical findings. For completeness regarding any entity described one, must turn to other more complete texts (i.e., Taybi and Lachman).

ACHONDROPLASIA GROUP

In the achondroplasia group of disorders, three specific entities are important: thanatophoric dysplasia, achondroplasia, and hypochondroplasia. They all have the same chromosomal locus (4p16.3). The gene/protein abnormality in all of them is a different mutation or group of mutations in *FGFR3* (fibroblast growth factor receptor 3).

THANATOPHORIC DYSPLASIA

Thanatophoric dysplasia, or thanatophoric dwarfism, actually represents at least two molecularly distinct disorders that have been termed *thanatophoric dysplasia types I* and *II*. They share common radiographic features except for straight, not quite as short femurs and a kleeblattschädel (cloverleaf skull) in thanatophoric dysplasia type II (Fig. 3). This delineation may not be that important because both types are new autosomal dominant mutations and are almost invariably lethal. This dysplasia perhaps represents the most common lethal bone dysplasia.

Radiologic Findings*

- Skull: proportionately large skull in relation to the body, narrow skull base, *kleeblattschädel*
- Thorax: long, narrow trunk; very short ribs; handlebar clavicles
- Spine: *flat, small vertebral bodies with round anterior ends; U, H, and upside-down U vertebrae in the anteroposterior projection*
- Pelvis: *small, flared iliac bones; very narrow sacrosciatic notches; flat, dysplastic acetabula*
- Extremities: generalized micromelia; *French telephone receiver femurs*, round proximal femoral metaphyses with medial spike

ACHONDROPLASIA

Achondroplasia is by far the most common form of nonlethal skeletal dysplasia. Presentation for most cases is at birth. Patients with this disorder have the combination of rhizomelia, mesomelia, and acromelia radiographically but more rhizomelia at clinical inspection (Fig. 4). This is an autosomal dominant condition with a spontaneous mutation rate of about 80%.

---

*Throughout the text, pathognomonic radiologic findings are in italics.

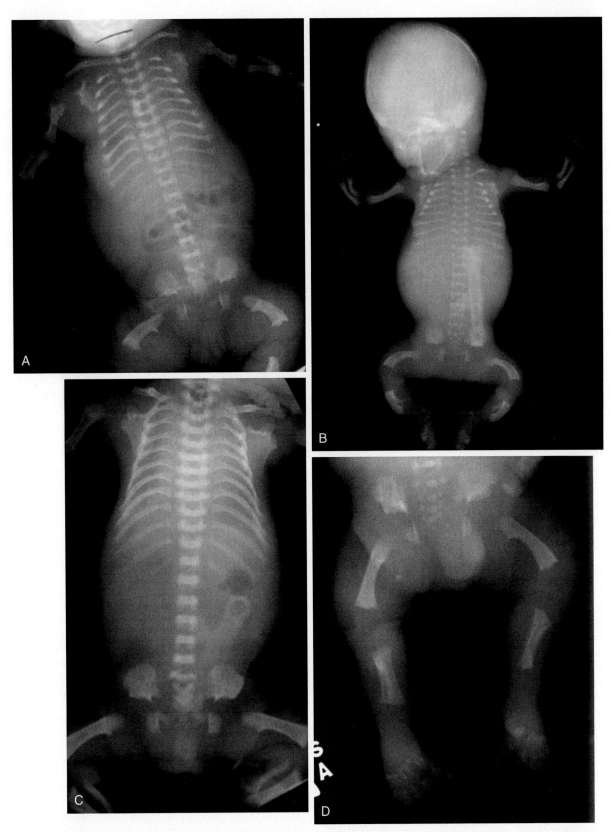

FIGURE 3. **A** and **B,** Radiologic findings in thanatophoric dysplasia type I. In a fetus of 30 weeks' gestation **(A),** there is a long, narrow trunk; very short ribs; U- and H-shaped vertebral bodies; small, flared iliac wings; narrowed sacrosciatic notches; dysplastic (trident) acetabular roofs; and French telephone receiver femurs. At 22 weeks' gestation in another fetus **(B),** there is a proportionally large skull, micromelia, and other findings similar to those in **A. C–F,** Radiologic findings in thanatophoric dysplasia type II. A preterm gestation **(C)** shows findings similar to those in type I except for higher vertebral bodies and straighter femurs. Another case **(D)** also shows the same findings as in type I but straighter femurs.

Illustration continued on following page

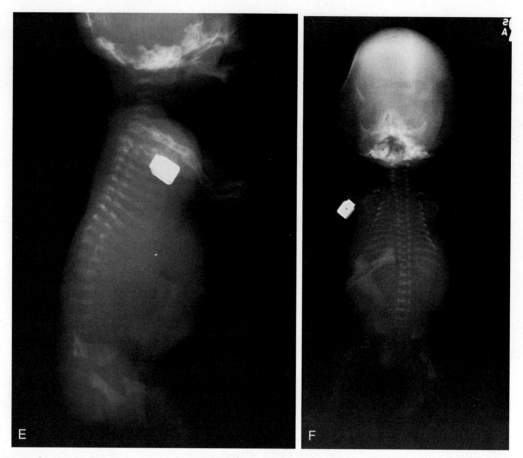

FIGURE 3. *Continued.* **E,** Infant with severe platyspondyly, anteriorly rounded vertebrae, straight femurs, and severely constricted skull base. **F,** Case showing cloverleaf skull and almost straight femurs; otherwise, radiographic findings are similar to those in **C.**

Radiologic Findings

- Skull: enlarged, with significant midface hypoplasia; hydrocephalus rarely present, small skull base with tight foramen magnum
- Thorax: small; shortened and anteriorly splayed ribs
- Spine: vertebral bodies only slightly flattened, short and slightly round anteriorly, but normalize from late childhood on; very short pedicles with *decreased interpediculate distance* most marked in lumbar spine; *posterior vertebral scalloping* that persists through life
- Pelvis: *elephant ear–shaped iliac wings* (flared, superiorly and laterally flattened ilia), *narrow sacrosciatic notches, flat acetabular roofs*
- Extremities: *rhizo-, meso-, and acromelia*
  - Hands: brachydactyly, metacarpal metaphyseal cupping, phalangeal metaphyseal widening
  - Knees: *Chevron and upside-down chevron deformity* (tibia/femur)
  - Hips: *proximal femoral fade-out* (infancy); *hemispheric capital femoral epiphyses,* short femoral necks
  - Legs: prominent tibial tubercle apophyseal region, *proximal and distal fibula overgrowth*
  - Arms: very prominent deltoid insertion area

HYPOCHONDROPLASIA

Hypochondroplasia, also a very common disorder, is allelic with achondroplasia, and they share many features. It is often difficult to distinguish severe hypochondroplasia from mild achondroplasia. Ninety-seven percent of molecularly proven cases of achondroplasia have an identical gene abnormality; however, multiple different molecular changes in *FGFR3* have been noted in hypochondroplasia. Hypochondroplasia usually presents after 2 years of age (Fig. 5). One should be *very wary* of making this diagnosis in a newborn. The diagnosis is often a clinical one in mild cases.

Radiologic Findings

The imaging findings of hypochondroplasia are identical to those of achondroplasia but to a milder degree of abnormality. The overall experience with this disorder suggests that all cases, no matter how mild, exhibit *interpediculate narrowing in the lumbar spine.* There may be some brachydactyly, fibula overgrowth, and even short femoral necks. Other "achondroplasia-like" changes may or may not be present.

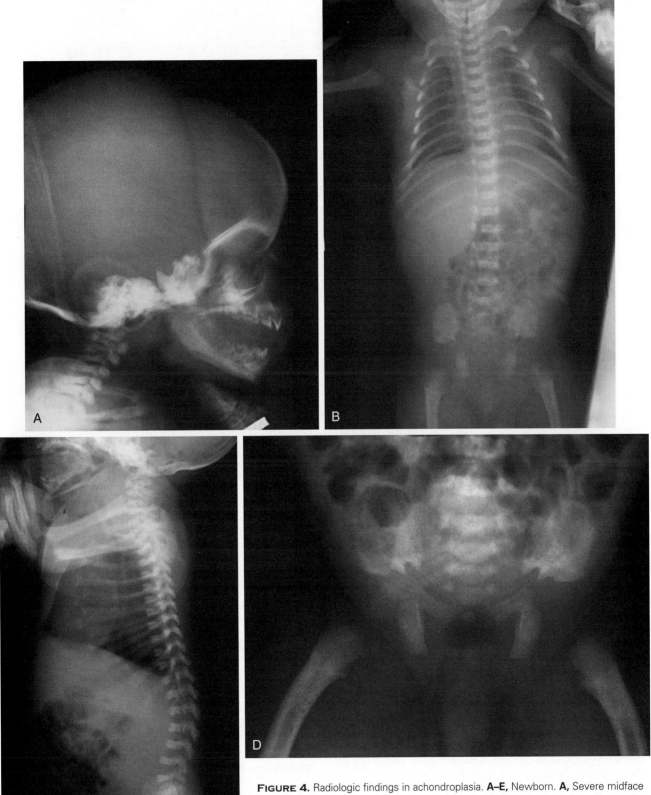

FIGURE 4. Radiologic findings in achondroplasia. **A–E,** Newborn. **A,** Severe midface hypoplasia. **B,** Thorax: small thorax and short ribs. **C,** Thorax: short ribs with anterior scalloping and bullet-shaped vertebrae. **D,** Pelvis: elephant ear–shaped iliac bones, narrow sacrosciatic notches, flat acetabular roof, and proximal femoral fadeout.

Illustration continued on following page

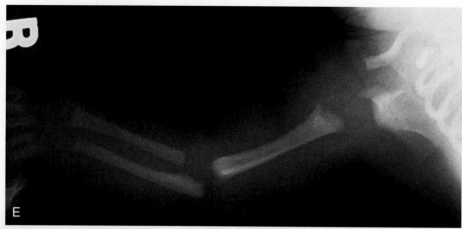

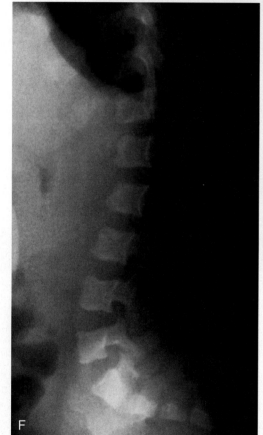

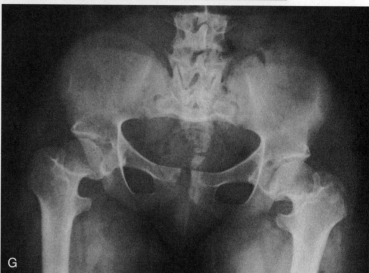

FIGURE 4. *Continued.* **E,** Extremities: rhizo- and mesomelia. **F,** A 1½–year-old with classical vertebrae with short pedicles, posterior scalloping, and somewhat short vertebral bodies. **G,** Adult female with flat acetabular roofs, "elephant ear" iliac wings, and short femoral necks (compare with **D**). (**G** from Silverman FN: Achondroplasia. Prog Pediatr Radiol 1973;4:94–124. Karger, Basel, with permission.)

METATROPIC DYSPLASIA GROUP

The metatropic dysplasia group has several disorders that appear to be linked because of their similar clinical and radiographic findings. Thus far no molecular breakthrough has occurred. The important disorder in this group is metatropic dysplasia.

METATROPIC DYSPLASIA

Metatropic dysplasia, or metatropic dwarfism, is discoverable in the newborn with a relatively long trunk and markedly shortened limbs (Fig. 6). This "changing" dysplasia with time produces a short trunk/short limb form of dwarfism (severe scoliosis) with a *tail.* Although heterogeneous, most cases are nonlethal and are autosomal dominant.

Radiologic Findings

- Thorax: small; short ribs
- Spine: *dense wafer vertebral bodies* (newborn), reconstituted platyspondyly (child and adult), *scoliosis* (adult)
- Pelvis and hips: *short, squared iliac wings;* flat, irregular acetabular roof; narrow sacrosciatic notches; *halberd (hunting ax)–shaped proximal femurs*

- Extremities: *trumpet-shaped metaphyses* (newborn), dumbbell-shaped short tubular bones of hands and feet

SCHNECKENBECKEN (SNAIL PELVIS) DYSPLASIA

This dysplasia, although relatively uncommon, has a very interesting radiographic feature, as the name of this disorder implies (Fig. 7). It is a lethal skeletal dysplasia, but can be diagnosed as short limbed and with a small thorax on second-trimester ultrasound, which is especially valuable in this autosomal recessive disorder.

Radiologic Findings

- Thorax: small; short, anteriorly cupped ribs; handlebar clavicles; hypoplastic scapulas
- Vertebrae: small, *round vertebral body ossification* (unossified posterior portion)
- Pelvis: *snail-shaped iliac bones (Schneckenbecken)*
- Extremities: micromelia, *dumbbell-shaped* long bones, especially *femurs*

SHORT RIB–POLYDACTYLY GROUP

The short rib dysplasia (with or without)–polydactyly (SRP) group of disorders is a rather diverse group, but they are linked at least radiologically. The chromosomal locus for at least one of this group has been located at 4p16 (chondroectodermal dysplasia). The entire group is important and rather common in occurrence. The group consists of all the SRPs (types I through IV), asphyxiating thoracic dysplasia (ATD), and chondroectodermal dysplasia. They are all autosomal recessive.

SHORT RIB (WITH OR WITHOUT)– POLYDACTYLY DYSPLASIA

SRP is a subgroup of disorders that are typed largely on radiographic grounds (Fig. 8). Types I and III are quite similar, as are types II and IV. The important role for the pediatric radiologist is to make the diagnosis of this subgroup as separate from ATD and chondroectodermal dysplasia. This usually can be done rather easily because the SRPs have the shortest ribs of any of the skeletal dysplasias.

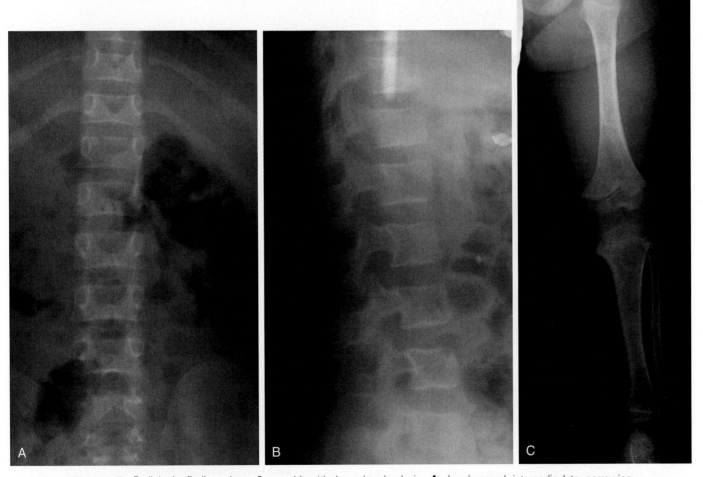

FIGURE 5. Radiologic findings in a 3-year-old with hypochondroplasia. **A,** Lumbosacral interpediculate narrowing. **B,** Posterior vertebral body scalloping with normal pedicles. **C,** Proximal and distal fibular overgrowth. There are mild beginning chevron deformity changes in distal femur.

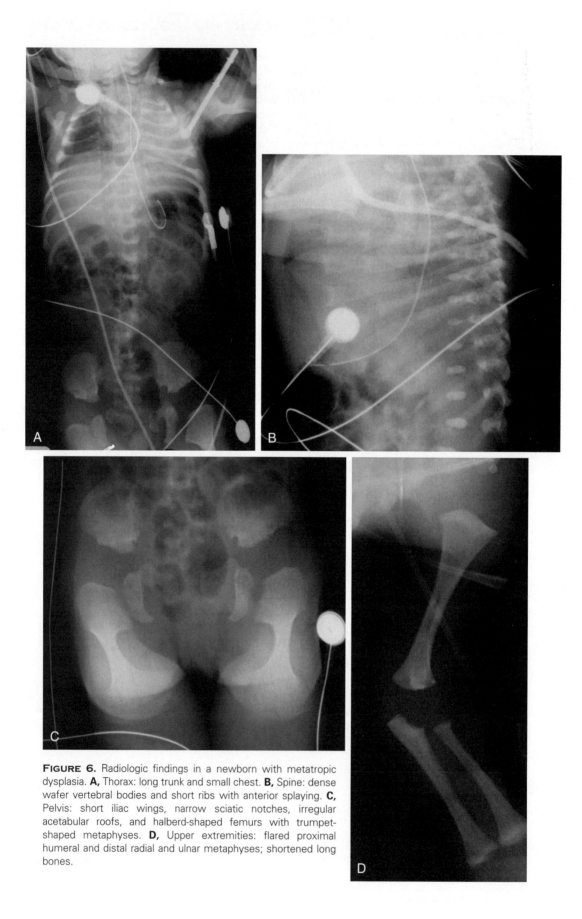

FIGURE 6. Radiologic findings in a newborn with metatropic dysplasia. **A,** Thorax: long trunk and small chest. **B,** Spine: dense wafer vertebral bodies and short ribs with anterior splaying. **C,** Pelvis: short iliac wings, narrow sciatic notches, irregular acetabular roofs, and halberd-shaped femurs with trumpet-shaped metaphyses. **D,** Upper extremities: flared proximal humeral and distal radial and ulnar metaphyses; shortened long bones.

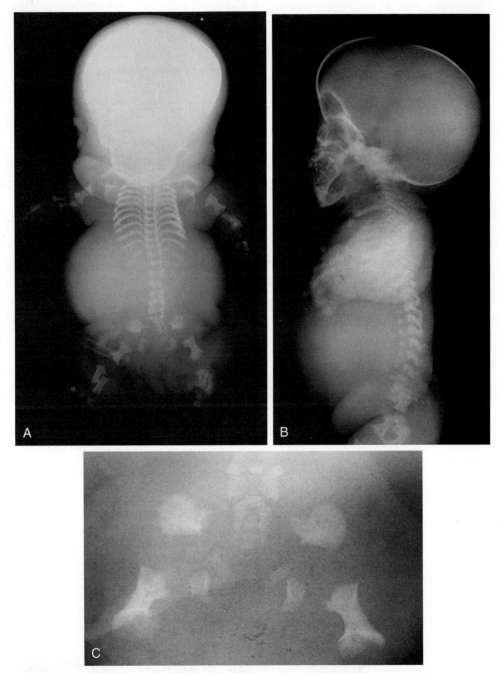

FIGURE 7. Radiologic findings in Schneckenbecken dysplasia. **A,** Stillborn fetus with large head; short trunk; micromelia; small, barrel-shaped thorax; snail-shaped iliac bones; and dumbbell femurs and humeri. **B,** Stillborn fetus with round vertebral bodies with posterior ossification failure; the hands are proportionally large. **C,** Artistic rendering of "schneckenbecken" (snail-shaped iliac bones). (**C** courtesy of A. Giedion, Zurich, Switzerland.)

Radiologic Findings

- Thorax: small; *very, very short horizontal ribs*
- Spine: relatively normally shaped
- Pelvis: small, dysplastic ilia
- Extremities: *micromelia; rolling pin–shaped or round-ended or metaphyseal-spiked femora; ovoid* or tiny, normal-shaped *tibias;* severe brachydactyly with hypoplastic middle and distal phalanges; *polydactyly commonly present*

ASPHYXIATING THORACIC DYSPLASIA (JEUNE'S SYNDROME)

ATD is a disorder with a mixed prognosis. Many patients die in the perinatal period from respiratory complications (small chest) (Fig. 9). Survivors may succumb from renal complications (progressive nephropathy) in later life. Other internal organs may also be involved. Uncommonly, polydactyly may be present. There are definite radiographic (but not clinical) similarities to

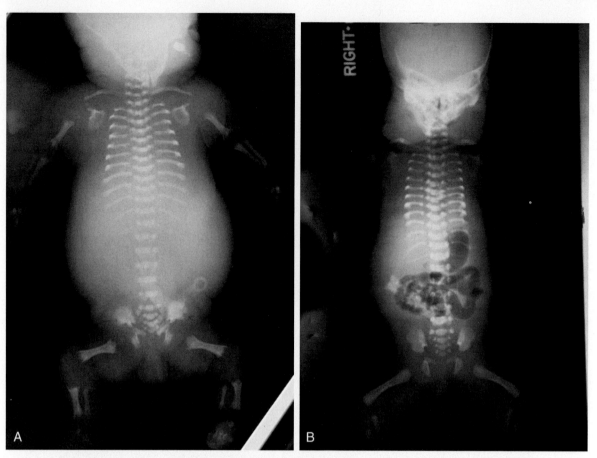

FIGURE 8. Radiologic findings in short rib–polydactyly dysplasia. **A,** Stillborn fetus with type I/III form demonstrating very short ribs, handlebar clavicles, hypoplastic pelvis with notched acetabula, and metaphyseal-spiked femora. **B,** Stillborn fetus with short rib–polydactyly dysplasia type II. Findings are similar to those in type I/III but with round-ended femora and hypoplastic acetabula.

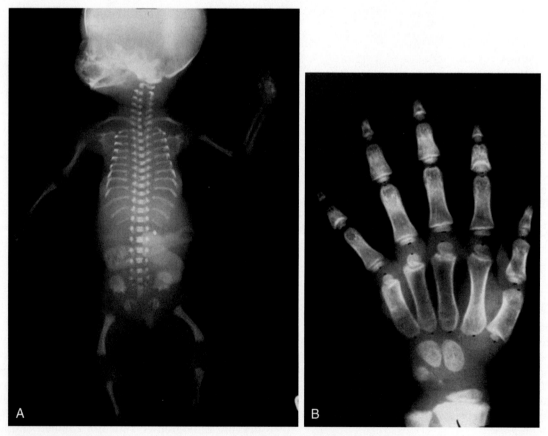

FIGURE 9. Radiologic findings in asphyxiating thoracic dysplasia. **A,** Preterm stillborn fetus with small thorax, short ribs, trident acetabula, narrow sacrosciatic notches, and normal spine. **B,** Infant of 26 months with cone-shaped epiphyses in the hand, especially involving the second and fifth middle phalanges. (**B** courtesy of T. Coburn, Memphis, TN.)

chondroectodermal dysplasia (Ellis-van Creveld syndrome [EvC]), a possible allelic disease. Some cases are so alike radiologically that they are best termed ATD/EvC complex.

Radiologic Findings

- Thorax: long and *barrel shaped,* handlebar clavicles, short horizontal ribs with bulbous anterior ends
- Spine: normal
- Pelvis: small; short, flared iliac wings; *trident acetabular roof; narrowed sacrosciatic notches*
- Extremities: generalized shortening, *precocious proximal femoral epiphyseal ossification,* cone-shaped epiphyses in hands

CHONDROECTODERMAL DYSPLASIA (ELLIS VAN CREVELD SYNDROME)

EvC is a nonlethal skeletal dysplasia. The nonskeletal involvement in this disorder is extremely important in defining this condition. Signs include hair, nail, and teeth abnormalities, as well as congenital heart disease. Polydactyly is almost invariably present. The radiologic findings are very similar to those of ATD (Fig. 10). Recently, the gene has been identified in this autosomal recessive condition. The chromosome location of this gene is 4p16.

Radiologic Findings

- Thorax: small; moderately short ribs
- Pelvis: small; short, flared iliac wings; *trident acetabulas; narrowed sacrosciatic notches*
- Spine: almost normal
- Extremities: generalized shortening with more meso- and acromelia; premature ossification of capital femoral epiphyses, delayed ossification of proximal tibial epiphyses, humeral and femoral bowing, *exostosis of proximal/medial portion of tibia*
  - Hands: characteristic—*postaxial polydactyly, capitate/hamate* (and other carpal) *fusions, extra carpal bone, cone-shaped epiphyses*
  - Feet: *polydactyly*

DIASTROPHIC DYSPLASIA GROUP

The diastrophic dysplasia group is a molecularly defined group of disorders with a defect on chromosome 5 in *DTDST,* a sulfate transporter gene. This group is of course composed of diastrophic dysplasia, as well as achondrogenesis IB and atelosteogenesis type II. This reveals how sometimes the radiology does not point to molecular grouping, because achondrogenesis IA, with radiographic changes almost identical to those of IB, does not have a *DTDST* gene abnormality, nor do the other forms of atelosteogenesis. For radiographic clarity, I will discuss both forms of achondrogenesis I together.

DIASTROPHIC DYSPLASIA

Diastrophic dysplasia, as are all the other members of this group of disorders, is an autosomal recessive condition. It is commonly identifiable at birth and usually nonlethal. Early on it was called "achondroplasia with clubbed feet," alluding to some of its distinctive clinical findings: severe foot abnormalities (talipes equinovarus), neonatal cauliflower ear development, hitchhiker thumb, and cleft or high-arched palate. The chondro-osseous morphology (resting chondrocyte death and fibro-ossification) explains some of the characteristic clinical and radiographic findings (Fig. 11).

Radiologic Findings

- Head: *Ear pinna calcification*
- Thorax: moderately small
- Spine: *progressive scoliosis, kyphosis,* upper cervical subluxation (odontoid hypoplasia), *cervical kyphosis, posterior process clefting* (cervical and sacral)
- Extremities: often micromelia; *short, thick tubular bones;* generalized brachydactyly—*short ovoid first metacarpal, twisted metatarsals, accessory and irregular carpal bones;* joint regions—epiphyseal dysplasia (especially hips), joint dislocations
- Other sites: *precocious* costochondral and laryngeal area *cartilage calcification;* multiple sternal and patella centers

ACHONDROGENESIS I

Achondrogenesis I is actually two separate disorders that appear almost identical radiographically (Fig. 12). Achondrogenesis IB belongs in this diastrophic dysplasia (molecular) group. Achondrogenesis IA has not yet been assigned a molecular or gene abnormality. Clinically they appear identical: proportionately large skull; lethal, micromelic, hydropic, pear-shaped trunk; and polyhydramnios.

Radiologic Findings

- Skull: decreased ossification
- Thorax: *tiny; very short ribs with anterior splaying*
- Spine: *absent or minimal vertebral body ossification*
- Pelvis: *short iliac bones with concave acetabular roofs, absent pubic (ischial) ossification*
- Extremities: *severe micromelia* with broadened ends of limbs, *trapezoidal or wedge-shaped femurs*
  Note: Achondrogenesis IA: *multiple fractured, beaded ribs; wedged femurs*
  Achondrogenesis IB: *no rib fractures or beading; trapezoidal femurs*

TYPE II COLLAGENOPATHIES

The type II collagenopathies are a heterogeneous group of disorders all of which show some relationship to each other not only molecularly but clinically and radiographically. Although they range from invariably lethal to mildly affected, they have in common involvement of the spine (platyspondyly/deficiency of vertebral ossification) and epiphyseal (epiphyseal equivalent) ossification delay/dysplasia. Clinically, normal type II collagen is important not only for the development of the epiphyseal plate region of developing bone but also hyaline cartilage, nucleus pulposus, and even the vitreous of the eye (myopia). The type II collagenopathies range from lethal and severe achondrogenesis II/hypochondrogenesis through spondyloepiphyseal dysplasia congenita (SEDC), Kniest dysplasia, and Strudwick type SE(M)D to more mildly affected Stickler dysplasia (some Stickler cases are a type XI collagenopa-

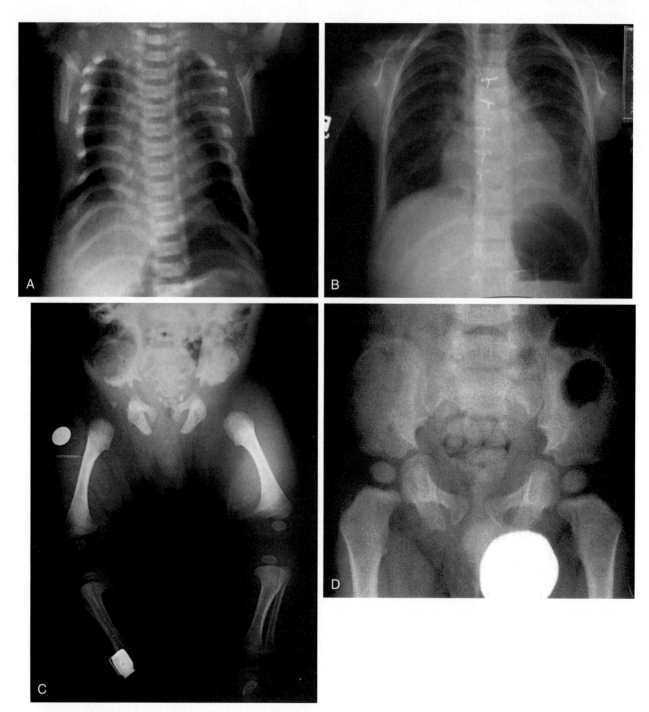

FIGURE 10. Radiologic findings in chondroectodermal dysplasia (Ellis-van Creveld syndrome). **A,** A 3-month-old infant with narrow thorax, short ribs, anterior rib flaring and a normal spine. **B,** A 5-year-old with similar chest configuration; there is cardiomegaly with sternal sutures from a primum defect repair. **C,** A 3-month-old with short, flared iliac wings; trident acetabula; and meso- and rhizomelia. **D** and **E,** A child at 2½ **(D)** and 12 years of age **(E)** showing normalization of pelvis with residual "red wine glass" configuration.
Illustration continued on opposite page

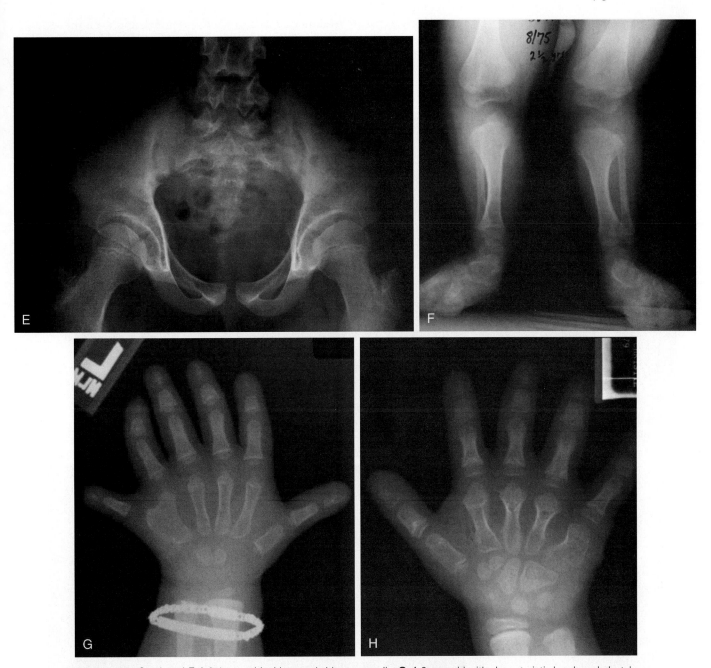

FIGURE 10. *Continued.* **F,** A 2½-year-old with remarkable mesomelia. **G,** A 2-year-old with characteristic hands: polydactyly, middle and distal phalangeal hypoplasia, cone-shaped epiphyses of middle phalanges, and beginning carpal coalition. **H,** The same child as in **G** at 6 years of age. Following polydactyly repair, there is a residual wide fifth metacarpal; other findings are similar except there is no carpal coalition.

thy). All these disorders are autosomal dominant and, in lethal conditions, new mutations with very little likelihood of recurrence.

ACHONDROGENESIS II / HYPOCHONDROGENESIS

Achondrogenesis II is invariably lethal. Clinically, these stillborns and fetuses appear very similar to achondrogenesis IA and IB patients. However, radiographically they are easily diagnosed correctly (Fig. 13). The clinical appearance is a micromelic dwarf, somewhat hydropic,

with a nuchal cystic hygroma. A cleft palate is not uncommon, as in other type II collagenopathies.

Hypochondrogenesis is just a slightly milder rendition of achondrogenesis II and, by definition, affected infants survive the immediate perinatal period but often cannot be extubated and will invariably die from respiratory complications in the first month or two of life. Obviously this is a spectrum of severity, but this diagnosis is important to both family and physician to try to prognosticate for them. Patients who survive beyond these time periods are given the diagnosis of SEDC. The pediatric radiologist can be helpful by analyzing the chest film(s) for thoracic size, lung volume, and rib length.

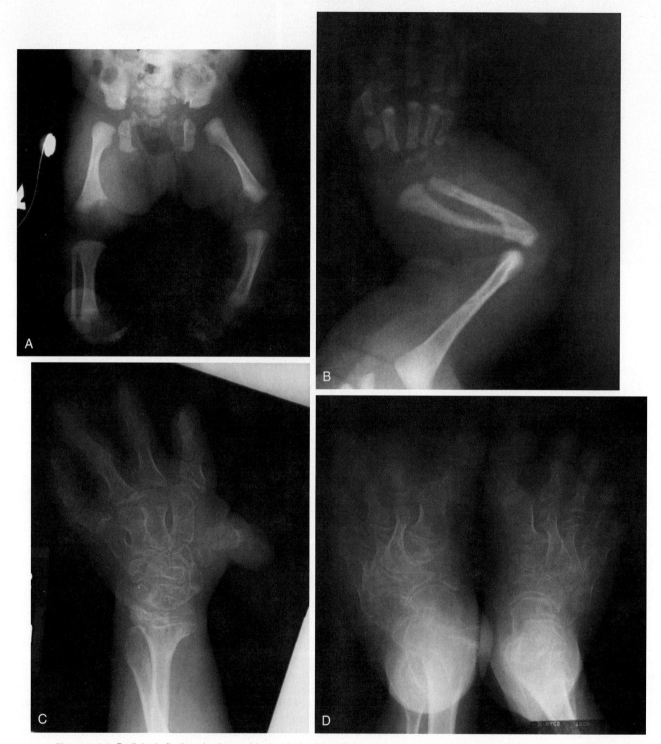

FIGURE 11. Radiologic findings in diastrophic dysplasia. **A** and **B,** Newborn. **A,** Lower extremities: rhizo- and mesomelia and severe clubbed feet. **B,** Upper extremity: elbow dislocation and short, ovoid first metacarpal. **C** and **D,** A 12-year-old. **C,** Upper extremity: hitchhiker thumb, ovoid first metacarpal, brachydactyly, and irregular and extra carpal bones. **D,** Lower extremities: unusual clubbed foot and twisted metatarsals.

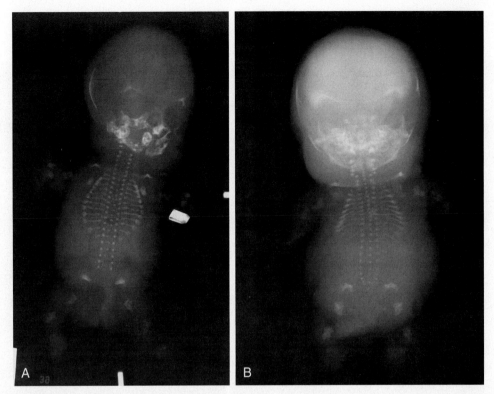

FIGURE 12. Radiologic findings in achondrogenesis. **A,** Stillborn fetus with type IA achondrogenesis demonstrates a tiny thorax; short, anteriorly cupped ribs with *beading;* micromelia; wedged femurs; and poor to absent vertebral body ossification. **B,** Stillborn fetus with type IB achondrogenesis. Findings are similar to those in type IA but with arched iliac wings, no rib beading, and trapezoidal femurs.

Radiologic Findings

Achondrogenesis II

- Skull: proportionately large
- Thorax: *very small; very short ribs*
- Spine: *almost complete lack of mineralization of most vertebral bodies; cervical and sacral posterior elements also often unossified*
- Pelvis: small iliac wings with concave inferior and medial margins; absent ischia, pubic bones, and sacral elements
- Extremities: *micromelia, mostly rhizo- and mesomelia, with relative sparing of hands and feet;* almost normally modeled long bones with metaphyseal flare, *absent talus and calcaneal ossification* (epiphyseal equivalents)

Hypochondrogenesis

- Thorax: larger, with longer ribs
- Spine: more vertebral body ossification *(hypoplasia and platyspondyly)*
  Note: Otherwise similar to achondrogenesis II

SPONDYLOEPIPHYSEAL DYSPLASIA CONGENITA

Most cases of spondyloepiphyseal dysplasia with a congenital onset are type II collagenopathies. SEDC is part of the previously discussed spectrum and is not lethal (respiratory death). The clinical presentation in the newborn is that of a severely short-trunked, short-limbed dwarf with normal hands and feet and skull. There may be major problems with the upper cervical spine (Fig. 14). Degenerative arthrosis of the hips can be a significant concern in the adult.

Radiologic Findings

- Thorax: small; short ribs
- Spine: *pear-shaped or oval vertebral bodies* (newborn), anteriorly rounded *platyspondyly* (later)
- Pelvis: *absent pubic ossification* (newborn and infancy)
- Extremities: normally modeled but *shortened long bones, significant generalized ossification delay* (early) and *hypoplastic-appearing/dysplastic epiphyses* (later), *unossified talus/calcaneus* in the newborn, normal hands and feet with ossification delay (epiphyses/carpal, tarsal)

KNIEST DYSPLASIA

This uncommon entity presents in the newborn almost identically to SEDC, again as a nonlethal dysplasia. With the passage of time, however, radiographic (and clinical) changes occur to help diagnose this condition (Fig. 15). Salient clinical findings include cleft palate,

Text continued on page 2142

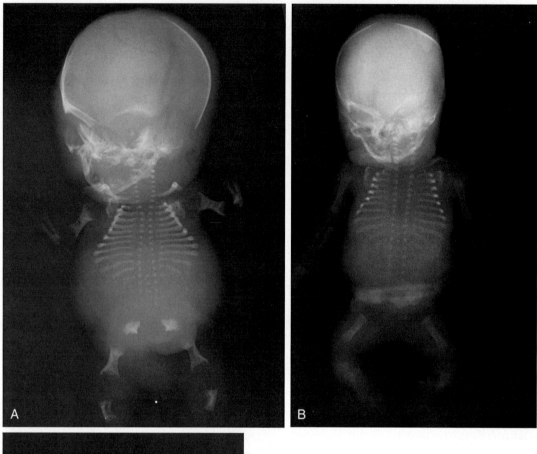

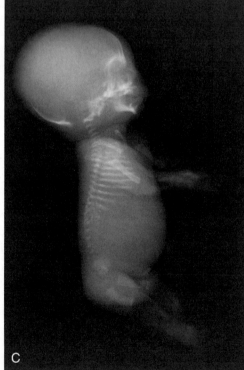

FIGURE 13. A, Radiologic findings in a stillborn fetus with achondrogenesis II. Findings include: a proportionately enlarged skull; tiny thorax with short ribs; almost no vertebral body ossification with lower pedicle ossification deficiency; small wide ilia, notched acetabular roofs, and absent ischial and pubic ossification; micromelia; and normally modeled femurs with metaphyseal flare and cupping. **B** and **C,** Radiologic findings in a fetus of 21 weeks' gestation with hypochondrogenesis showing better vertebral ossification, with more and better long bone modeling.

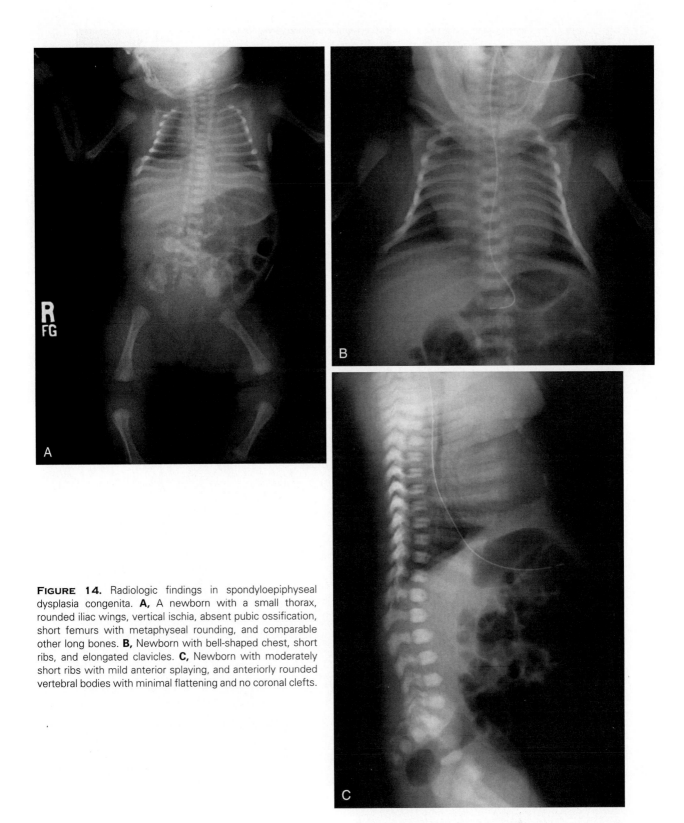

FIGURE 14. Radiologic findings in spondyloepiphyseal dysplasia congenita. **A,** A newborn with a small thorax, rounded iliac wings, vertical ischia, absent pubic ossification, short femurs with metaphyseal rounding, and comparable other long bones. **B,** Newborn with bell-shaped chest, short ribs, and elongated clavicles. **C,** Newborn with moderately short ribs with mild anterior splaying, and anteriorly rounded vertebral bodies with minimal flattening and no coronal clefts.

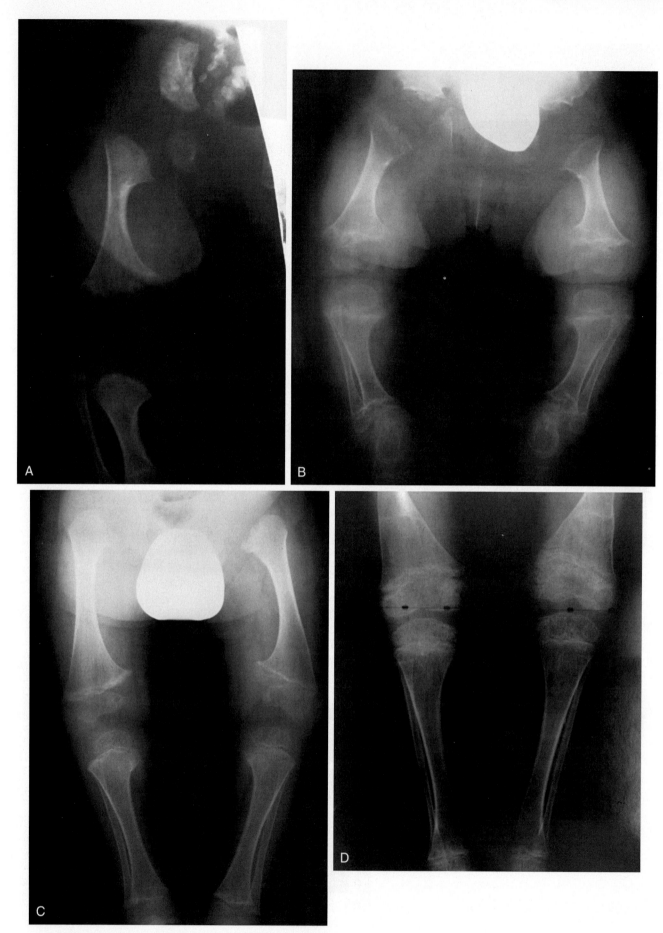

FIGURE 15. Radiologic findings in Kniest dysplasia. In two infants at 5 months **(A)** and 1 year of age **(B),** there are shortened femurs and tibias with metaphyseal widening, absent femoral head ossification, knee epiphyseal ossification delay in the 5-month-old **(A)** beginning megaepiphyses in the 1-year-old **(B),** and fibular overgrowth. In three other children at 1½ years **(C),** 5 years **(D),** and 4 years of age **(E),** there is no femoral head ossification and beginning woolly metaphyseal calcification with enlarging knee ossification.

Illustration continued on opposite page

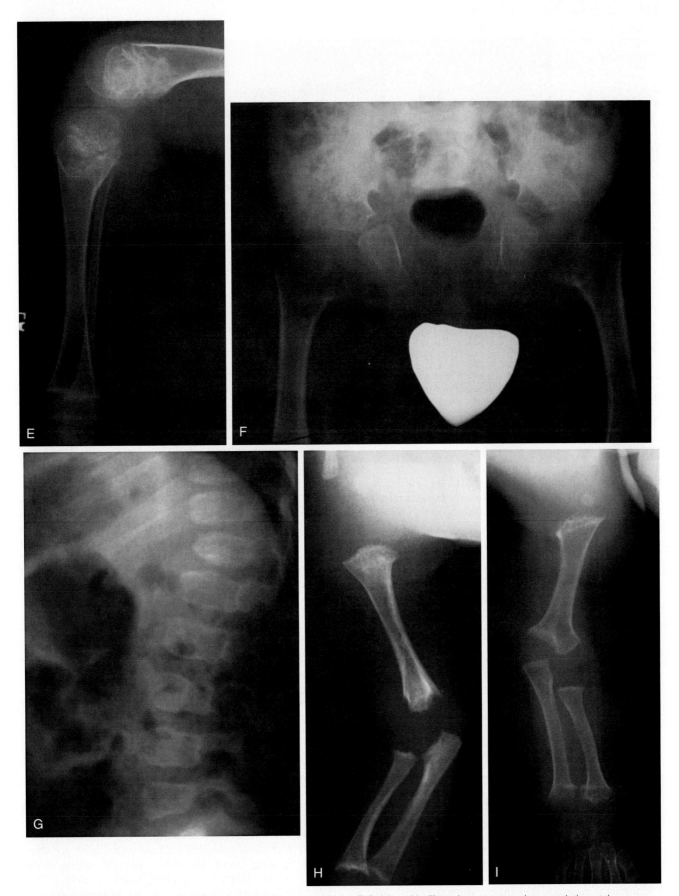

FIGURE 15. *Continued.* **F** and **G,** Another 1½–year-old child. **F,** Pelvis: wide iliac wings, narrowed sacrosciatic notches, downward-angled pubic bones, and small femoral heads. **G,** Spine: platyspondyly and end plate indentations (residua of coronal clefts). In a newborn **(H)** and the same patient at 1 year **(I),** there is progression from metaphyseal rounding to metaphyseal flaring and irregularity, with proximal humeral ossification delay.

Illustration continued on following page

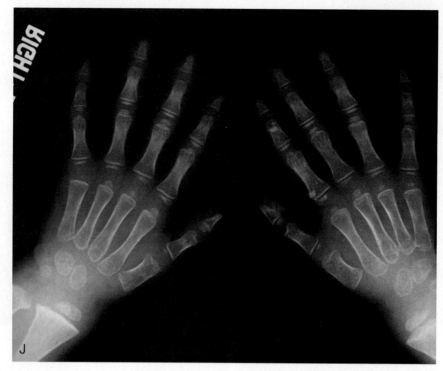

FIGURE 15. *Continued.* **J,** Hands: in a 6-year-old, there are small epiphyses, widened metaphyses (bulbous joints), and no significant brachydactyly.

myopia (retinal detachment), deafness, limited joint motion with enlarged and painful joints, occipitoatlantal instability, and progressive kyphoscoliosis.

Radiologic Findings

- Thorax: small to normal
- Spine: *coronal clefts* (newborn/infancy), *platyspondyly with end plate irregularity* (later)
- Extremities: *dumbbell femurs;* generalized ossification delay, epiphyses becoming hypoplastic/dysplastic then even *megaepiphyses, fluffiness/irregular calcification (cloud effect) in physeal plate regions* (late childhood/young adult); hands—bulbous joints (*metaphyseal flare/epiphyseal fragmentation*) mimicking rheumatoid arthritis.
  Note: In the newborn, Kniest syndrome is radiographically identical to SEDC except for *coronal clefts and dumbbell femurs.*

OTHER SPONDYLOEPI(META)PHYSEAL DYSPLASIAS

The other SE(M)Ds are an indistinctly classified group of disorders that are not completely worked out molecularly. As the name of the group implies, some have metaphyseal changes and others do not. There are at least two members of this group that are important or interesting: spondyloepiphyseal dysplasia tarda (SEDT) and Dyggve-Melchior-Clausen syndrome (DMC).

SPONDYLOEPIPHYSEAL DYSPLASIA TARDA

This is an X-linked disorder. The *SEDL* gene's location is on the p arm of the X chromosome (Xp22). SEDT is often diagnosed in an adolescent or in a young adult (Fig. 16) with nonsevere short stature, especially a short trunk. There is early-onset degenerative arthrosis of the hips.

Radiologic Findings

- Spine: mild platyspondyly with *centrally humped end plates* with intervertebral disk space narrowing
- Extremities: *mild to moderate "epiphyseal dysplasia" (small and irregular epiphyseal centers),* sparing of hands and feet

DYGGVE-MELCHIOR-CLAUSEN SYNDROME

This autosomal recessive disorder is uncommon but rather interesting. The alternative eponym *pseudo-Morquio syndrome* explains why. DMC is usually diagnosed in the first year of life. These individuals are short trunked and short limbed, with all three limb-components affected, including hands and feet (Fig. 17). Although 80% have severe psychomotor retardation and the rest have normal mentation (*Smith-McCort syndrome),* one suspects they will all turn out to be a single entity.

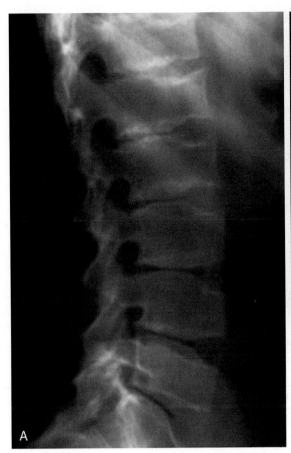

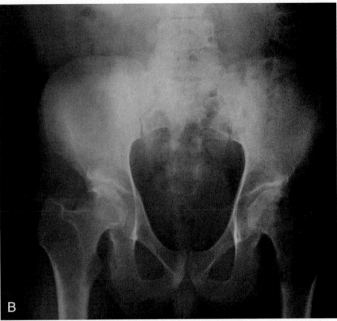

FIGURE 16. Radiologic findings in a 24-year-old with spondyloepiphyseal dysplasia tarda. **A,** Platyspondyly and centrally humped end plates. **B,** Dysplastic capital femoral epiphyses and degenerative arthrosis (joint space narrowing).

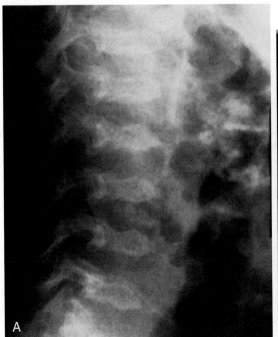

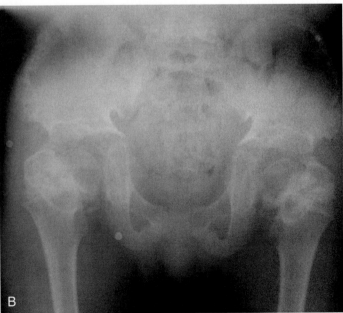

FIGURE 17. Radiologic findings in Dyggve-Melchior-Clausen syndrome. **A,** A 3-year-old with severe platyspondyly with residual double-humped end plates and anterior beaking. **B,** A 10-year-old with rounded iliac wings, lacy iliac crests, narrow sciatic notches, flat acetabular roofs, and epi/metaphyseal hip changes.

Radiologic Findings

- Skull: *microcephaly*
- Thorax: broad; anterior rib widening
- Spine: *double-humped vertebral bodies* with end plate notching and posterior scalloping
- Pelvis: small iliac wings with *irregularly calcified apophyseal regions (lacy iliac crests)*
- Extremities: moderate shortening with epi/metaphyseal changes, generalized brachydactyly with cone-shaped epiphyses and small carpal bones (*no proximal metacarpal pointing* as in mucopolysaccharidosis [MPS]).

MULTIPLE EPIPHYSEAL DYSPLASIA AND PSEUDOACHONDROPLASIA GROUP

The multiple epiphyseal dysplasia (MED) and pseudoachondroplasia group is rather well delineated molecularly and shows that radiology does not play the definitive role in every disorder. Pseudoachondroplasia and many cases of typical MED are cartilage oligomeric protein *(COMP)* gene defects on chromosome 19 and share some commonality of radiographic findings. However, some cases of MED (with the same apparent radiologic abnormalities) represent type IX collagen defects on chromosome 1. It appears that all the described entities within this group are autosomal dominant disorders.

MULTIPLE EPIPHYSEAL DYSPLASIA

MED has by custom been divided into two types: the Fairbanks and Ribbing forms (Figs. 18 and 19). Molecularly this has turned out to be incorrect. Ribbing MED, the milder type, may have only hip involvement and can be confused with bilateral Legg-Calvé-Perthes disease and Meyer dysplasia. Differentiation from these entities is possible because clinically MED always has significant short stature. Many patients with MED later go through an asymptomatic phase of avascular necrosis of their capital femoral epiphyses. The Fairbanks form has involvement of all the "long bone" epiphyses to a greater or lesser degree. MED presents after about 2 years of age but is most commonly diagnosed in an adolescent or young adult. Involvement is always bilateral and symmetrical. The shortening is quite mild.

Radiologic Findings

- Spine: young adult—disc herniations into vertebral end plates (*Schmorl nodes*)
- Extremities: *small, irregular, flattened ossification centers (epiphyses);* small, irregular carpal (and tarsal) centers

PSEUDOACHONDROPLASIA

This short-limbed, short-trunked form of skeletal dysplasia was referred to early on as "achondroplasia with a normal face." In actuality, the facial appearance in affected individuals is usually the most beautiful or most handsome in the family. There is often mild to moderate brachydactyly (Fig. 20).

Radiologic Findings

- Skull: normal
- Thorax: mild anterior rib widening
- Spine: *superiorly and inferiorly rounded vertebral bodies, anterior central tongue (exaggerated ring epiphyses),* normalization of vertebrae (later)
- Pelvis: *rounded iliac wings; hypoplastic, poorly formed acetabular roofs*
- Extremities: *mini-epiphyses in the hips,* moderate to severe generalized epiphyseal "dysplasia" (small, irregular, poorly ossified), metaphyseal widening and irregularity in the knees, *proximally rounded metacarpals* with mini-epiphyses in the hands, *irregular carpal* (tarsal) *bones*

CHONDRODYSPLASIA PUNCTATA GROUP

The chondrodysplasia punctata (CP; stippled epiphyses) group is very diverse, united by the radiographic commonality of epiphyseal stippling. Several but not all of these entities are related to each other. The rhizomelic form of CP is a peroxisomal enzyme abnormality, Conradi-Hünermann type is X-linked on the q arm of the X chromosome, and the brachytelephalangic type is on the p arm. Because of their different genetics, it is very important to make a correct and complete diagnosis.

RHIZOMELIC CHONDRODYSPLASIA PUNCTATA

This is a distinct form of CP and has an autosomal recessive inheritance pattern. This is a symmetric rhizomelic skeletal dysplasia presenting in the newborn period (Fig. 21). Affected infants usually die in the first year of life. Associated clinical findings include cataracts, skin lesions and alopecia, and joint contractures. Later manifestations are severe psychomotor retardation and spasticity. These infants appear to be in constant pain. This abnormality represents a peroxin-7 defect found on chromosome 4p.

Radiologic Findings

- Spine: *coronal clefting,* anteriorly rounded vertebral bodies
- Extremities: *stippling, symmetric bilateral shorting of femurs* (and humeri) with less severe shortening of all the remaining long bones

CONRADI-HÜNERMANN SYNDROME/
DYSPLASIA

This is a *specific entity* within the group of CP disorders! It is incorrect to label just any dysplasia with stippling, Conradi's disease. Conradi-Hünermann type of CP is an X-linked dominant disorder. The facies show midface hypoplasia and a high-arched palate. Cataracts and other ocular abnormalities may occur, as well as skin lesions. Asymmetric shortening of limbs (one side versus other) is an important diagnostic feature (Fig. 22). This dysplasia is compatible with a normal life span.

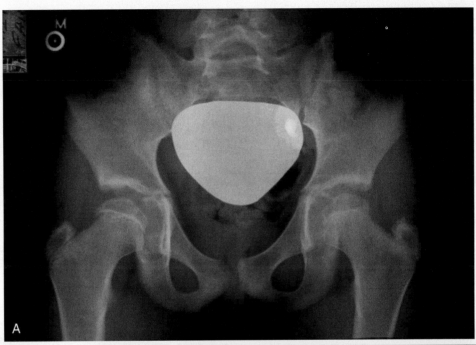

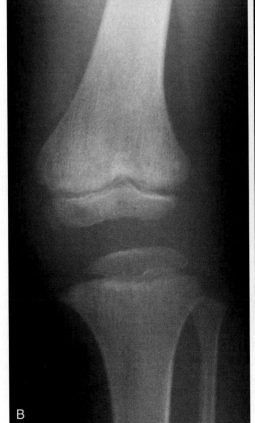

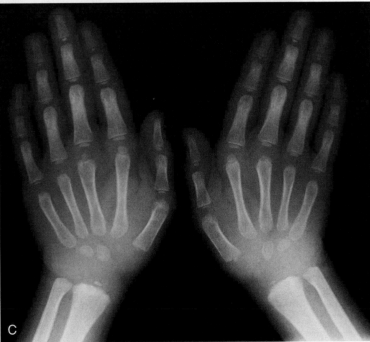

FIGURE 18. Radiologic findings in Fairbanks-type multiple epiphyseal dysplasia. **A,** A 10-year-old with small ossified proximal femoral epiphyses (ossification defect). **B** and **C,** A 6-year-old. **B,** Similar epiphyseal ossification defects in the knee. **C,** Small epiphyses of the short tubular bones of the hands and carpal ossification delay (epiphyseal equivalents), but no brachydactyly.

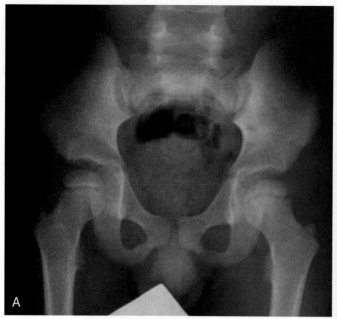

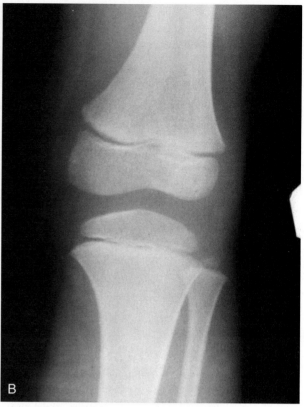

FIGURE 19. Radiologic findings in a 7-year-old with Ribbing-type multiple epiphyseal dysplasia include small-appearing hip epiphyses **(A)** and relatively normal-sized knee epiphyses **(B)**.

Radiologic Findings

- Spine: *diffuse stippling*, scoliosis in childhood, abnormal vertebral body formation
- Extremities: mild symmetric or *asymmetric* shortening, diffuse generalized stippling in epiphyseal (and epiphyseal-equivalent) areas as well as periarticular and other locations; hands and feet—normal aside from stippling

  Note: *Stippling resolves* during infancy to develop into *normal or malformed epiphyseal centers.*

BRACHYTELEPHALANGIC CHONDRODYSPLASIA PUNCTATA

This distinctive disorder with characteristic hand changes is also an X-linked disorder but is recessively inherited. It is far less common than the previously described disorders but quite easily diagnosed. These patients manifest severe midface hypoplasia with short hands and feet, as the dysplasia's name suggests (Fig. 23).

Radiologic Findings

- Spine: *hypoplastic vertebral bodies with posterior scalloping and anterior rounding; stippling, especially in the sacrococcygeal area; sagittal clefting*
- Extremities: normal length (mild shortening), *distinctive brachydactyly with hypoplastic tufts and deformed*

hypoplastic proximal phalanx of the second digit in the hand and the first metatarsal of the foot

METAPHYSEAL CHONDRODYSPLASIA GROUP

The metaphyseal chondrodysplasias (MCDs) are also a heterogeneous group of disorders that have radiologic features in common. This is a rather large group, and I will only cover several important (common) and interesting entities. Two have had their molecular defect worked out. All members of this group should have normal spines, but recently it has been shown that transient but significant spine changes occur in Schmid-type MCD.

JANSEN-TYPE METAPHYSEAL CHONDRODYSPLASIA

This MCD was described in 1934, with a follow-up report on the same patient by Silverthorn et al. It represents the severest form of MCD. The presentation is in the newborn or during infancy, with marked short stature and a waddling gait. This is a distinct autosomal dominant disorder with an abnormality in a parathyroid receptor gene *(PTHR)*, which explains the findings of hypercalcemia and its complications. The radiographic findings in the skeleton are *not* those of typical hyper/hypoparathyroidism (Fig. 24).

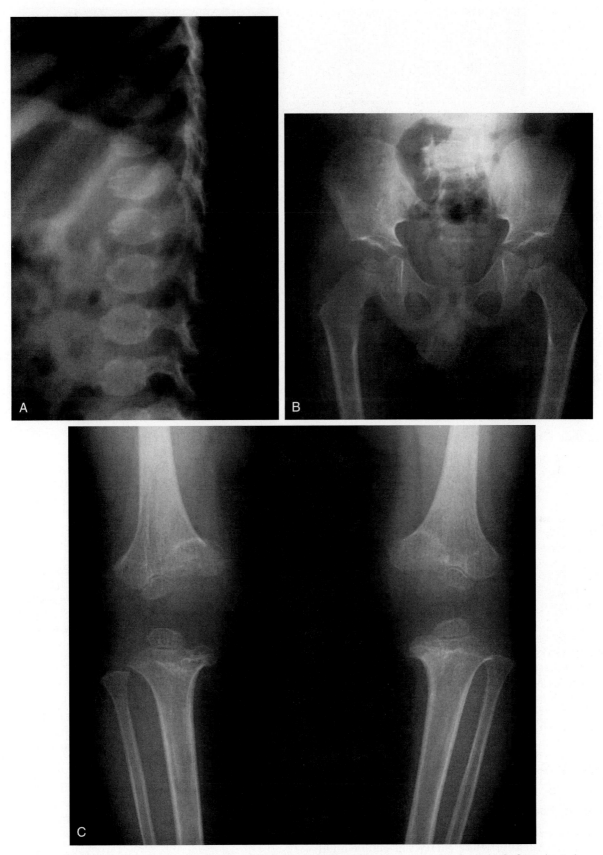

FIGURE 20. Radiologic findings at 3 years (**A** and **C**) and 4 years (**B** and **D**) with pseudoachondroplasia. **A,** Central anterior tonguing and superior and inferior rounding of vertebral bodies. **B,** Acetabular roof hypoplasia and mini-epiphyses. **C,** Small knee epiphyses and metaphyseal widening with ossification defects.

Illustration continued on following page

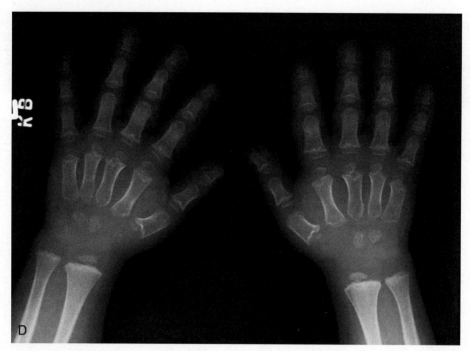

FIGURE 20. *Continued.* **D,** Proximal metacarpal rounding, small epiphyseal centers, metaphyseal widening and irregularity, and carpal ossification delay.

Radiologic Findings

- Skull: brachycephaly, platybasia, underdeveloped mandible
- Thorax: normal size; expanded irregular anterior rib ends
- Extremities: *extensive irregularity of markedly expanded metaphyses involving all metaphyseal regions; hands— wide separation of epiphyses from metaphyses*
  Note: As in other parathyroid abnormalities, pathologic fractures (45%) and subperiosteal bone resorption (50%) are common.

SCHMID-TYPE METAPHYSEAL CHONDRODYSPLASIA

This form of MCD is also a specific disorder. It is an autosomal dominant condition and represents a defect in collagen type X, the gene for which is located on chromosome 6. This disorder is the mildest condition in the MCD group. Presentation is usually at about 2 years of age or later with a waddling gait and/or bowed legs (Fig. 25). Mild short stature is present.

Radiologic Findings

- Thorax: *widened anterior rib ends*
- Spine: transient vertebral changes in middle childhood
- Extremities: *metaphyseal flaring, especially at the knees; rounded capital femoral epiphysis with widened growth plate;* usually *no hand involvement*

MCKUSICK-TYPE METAPHYSEAL CHONDRODYSPLASIA

Cartilage–hair hypoplasia, as this entity is also known, is an autosomal recessive disorder, and, although the chromosome site has been established at the 9p region, the molecular defect is not yet clear. It has a high frequency in the Amish ("Pennsylvania Dutch") and Finnish populations. The presentation is of variable short-limbed dwarfism in early childhood (Fig. 26). There are significant clinical features that help make the diagnosis and are important for management: sparse, thin, light-colored hair; Hirschprung's disease; immune mechanism problems; and increased incidence of malignancy.

Radiologic Findings

- Thorax: anterior rib widening/flaring
- Spine; slightly small *square* vertebral bodies
- Extremities: *flaring cupping* fragmentation *of metaphyses (especially knees), hips usually spared;* hands— *marked shortening with metacarpal and phalangeal cupping* and coning

SHWACHMAN-DIAMOND SYNDROME/ DYSPLASIA

This rare autosomal recessive disorder, also known as MCD with pancreatic insufficiency (see Section IX, Part VI, Fig. 47, page 2215) and cyclic neutropenia, has helpful diagnostic clinical clues of malabsorption and

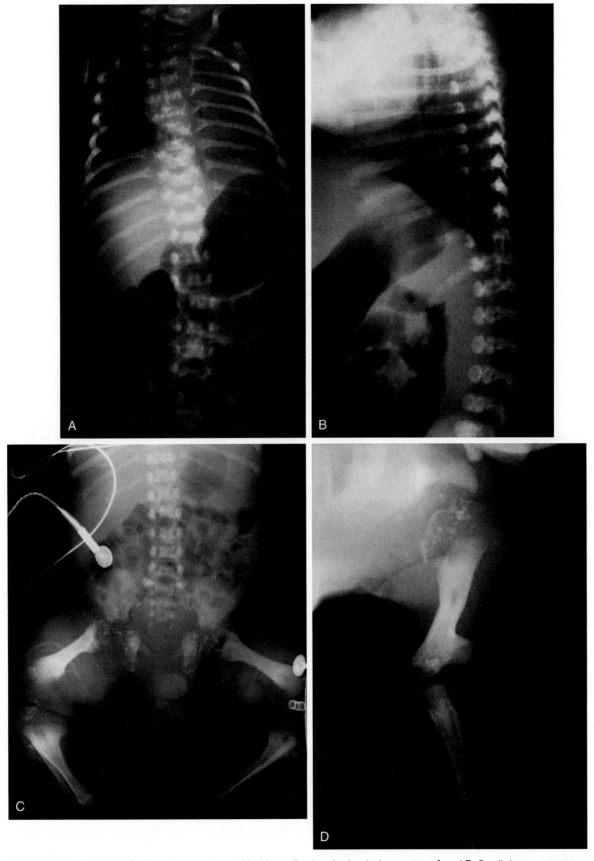

FIGURE 21. Radiologic findings in a newborn with rhizomelic chondrodysplasia punctata. **A** and **B,** Small thorax, punctate vertebral body ossification, and coronal clefting. **C** and **D,** Diffuse stippling in epiphyseal regions and exaggerated rhizomelia (femurs and humeri).

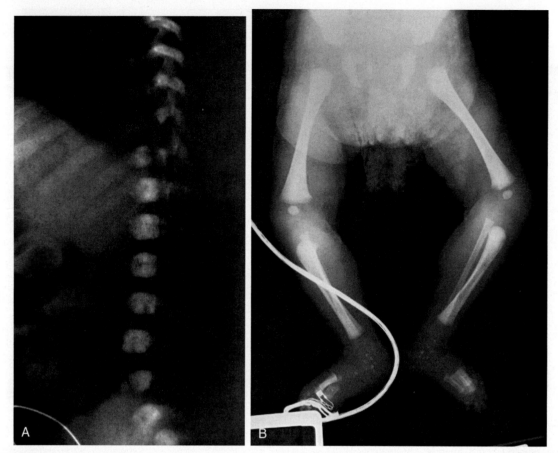

FIGURE 22. Radiologic findings in a newborn with Conradi-Hünermann dysplasia. **A,** Mildly hypoplastic vertebral bodies and stippling (residua of coronal clefts). **B,** Stippling of ankles and hips, normal knee epiphyses, no rhizomelia.

recurrent infections. It presents in infancy, but its radiographic features are quite mild (Fig. 27).

Radiologic Findings

- Thorax: *anterior rib irregularity/splaying*
- Extremities: *metaphyseal changes (irregularity and sclerosis),* especially at knees (hips)
- *Malabsorption pattern* on small bowel examination
- *Lipomatosis of pancreas* on computed tomography

SPONDYLOMETAPHYSEAL DYSPLASIA GROUP

Spondylometaphyseal dysplasia (SMD) denotes a group of disorders that of course have the appropriate spine and metaphyseal changes to warrant that terminology. Although this is a very large and diverse group, the only important and relatively common member is Kozlowski-type SMD.

KOZLOWSKI-TYPE SPONDYLOMETAPHYSEAL DYSPLASIA

This bone dysplasia is an autosomal dominant disorder presenting usually in early childhood. Clinical manifes-

tations include moderate dwarfism, progressive kyphoscoliosis, and limited joint mobility (Fig. 28).

Radiologic Findings

- Spine: *severe platyspondyly, anteriorly rounded/wedged vertebral bodies, increased intervertebral disk spaces, overfaced (close-set) pedicles, "open staircase spine"*
- Pelvis: short, flared iliac wings; *irregular hypoplastic acetabular roofs*
- Extremities: widening, sclerosis and irregularity of metaphyses; *hemispheric capital femoral epiphysis and widened proximal femoral growth plate with irregularity on both sides;* hands—mild shortening *with metaphyseal cupping* and irregularity, disharmonious ossification (*marked carpal ossification delay,* i.e., bone age at 5 or 6 years without carpal ossification)

MESOMELIC DYSPLASIA GROUP

The mesomelic dysplasia (mesomelic dwarfism) group consists of a large number of disorders that have shortening of their middle segment bones in common. Milder shortening of other segments may also be noted. The single most common entity by far in this group is dyschondrosteosis.

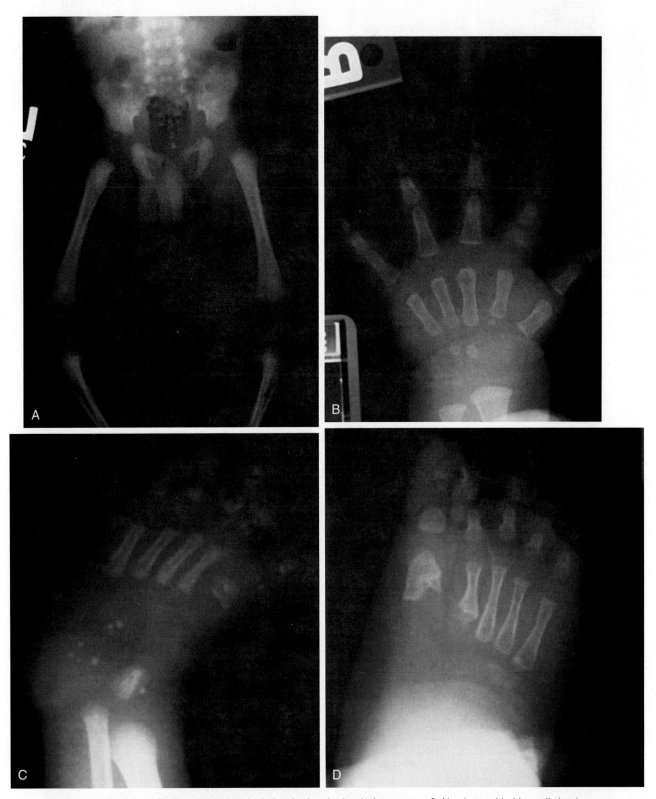

FIGURE 23. Radiologic findings in brachytelephalangic chondrodysplasia punctata. **A,** Newborn with rhizomelia but intense sacral stippling. **B,** A 5-month-old with characteristic hand, demonstrating hypoplastic malformed proximal phalanx of second digit with hypoplastic tufts. **C,** Newborn with foot stippling and hypoplastic deformed metatarsals of great and other toes. **D,** Older infant with characteristically shaped first metatarsal and stippling.

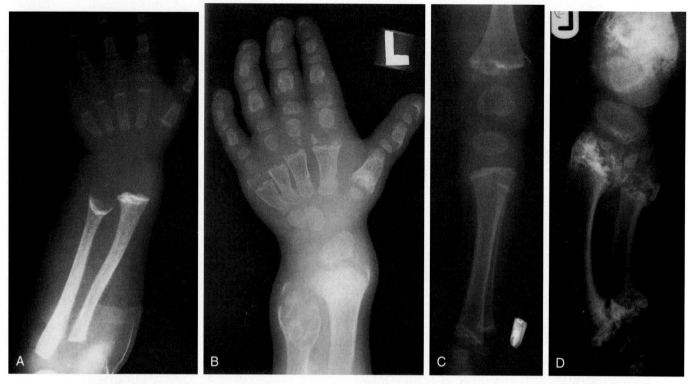

FIGURE 24. Radiologic findings in a child with Jansen-type metaphyseal chondrodysplasia. **A,** At 1 year, there is severe metaphyseal cupping and splaying at the wrists and also in the hand bones. **B,** At 7 years, there is increasing metaphyseal change at the wrists with enlarged epiphysis; enlarged epiphyses with wide epiphyseal plates are also present in the hands. **C,** At 1 year, there are severe metaphyseal irregularities at knees and ankles (femur, tibia, and fibula) and enlarged, rounded epiphyses. **D,** At 7 years, there are severely fragmented, sclerotic metaphyses, wide epiphyseal plates, and enlarged epiphyses.

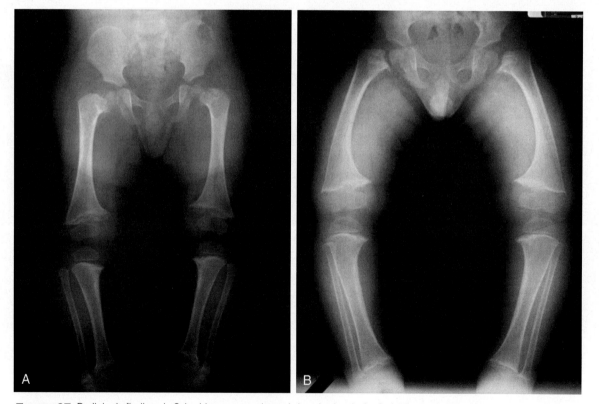

FIGURE 25. Radiologic findings in Schmid-type metaphyseal chondrodysplasia. **A,** A 19-month-old with severe coxa vara and moderate metaphyseal changes (cupping irregularity, widening) at the knees (and ankles). **B,** A 3-year-old with coxa vara, genu varum, and moderate metaphyseal changes at hips and knees (widening, irregularity).

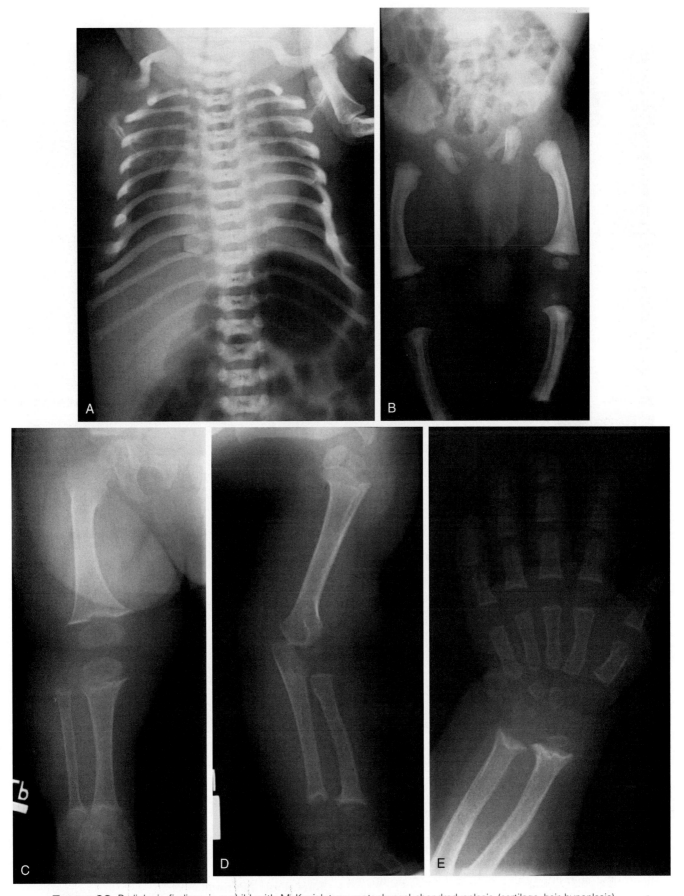

FIGURE 26. Radiologic findings in a child with McKusick-type metaphyseal chondrodysplasia (cartilage–hair hypoplasia). **A** and **B,** Newborn. **A,** Thorax: anterior rib end widening and cupping. **B,** Lower extremities: mild femoral bowing with minimal distal femoral flare. **C** and **D,** Late infancy. **C,** Lower extremity: metaphyseal flaring and irregularity at the knees (and ankles), but the hips are spared. **D,** Upper extremity: similar metaphyseal changes at the wrists (the shoulders are spared). **E,** At 6 months of age, there is metaphyseal widening and cupping of the short tubular bones of the hand, with similar metaphyseal changes in the wrist.

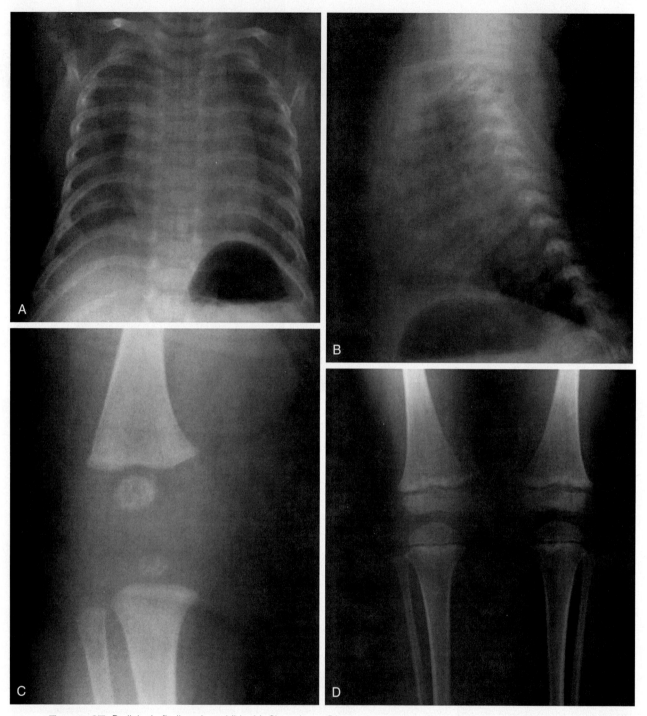

FIGURE 27. Radiologic findings in a child with Shwachman-Diamond syndrome. **A** and **B,** At 2 months, there is a narrow thorax with anterior rib splaying. **C,** At 2 months, the knees are normal. **D,** At 4 years, there are sclerotic, irregular, widened metaphyses in the knees.

DYSCHONDROSTEOSIS

This skeletal dysplasia, also known as Leri-Weill syndrome, is an apparent dominant condition. Recently Belin et al. identified the molecular defect producing this genetically strange condition. It consists of a pseudoautosomal homeobox gene (*SHOX* gene) found on the p arm of the X chromosome. Dyschondrosteosis presents with mild to moderate short stature, usually with both forearm and shank shortening. A clinical Madelung's deformity may be present (Fig. 29).

Radiologic Findings

- Extremities: *symmetrical bowing and shortening of both radii, shortened ulnae, radiographic Madelung's deformity changes, variable tibial and fibular shortening*

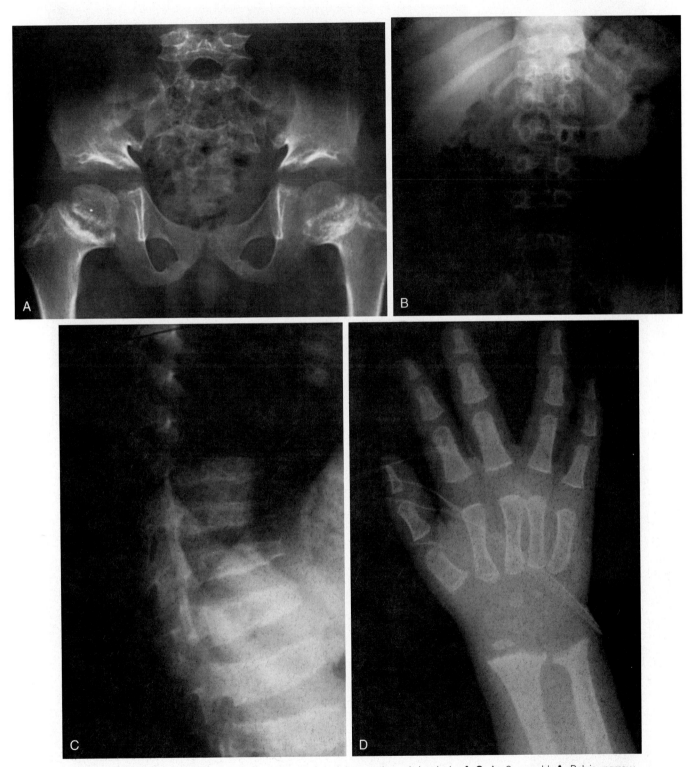

FIGURE 28. Radiologic findings in Kozlowski-type spondylometaphyseal dysplasia. **A–C,** An 8-year-old. **A,** Pelvis: narrow sacrosciatic notches, ossification defect (acetabular roofs), and widened epiphyseal plates. **B** and **C,** Spine: overfaced vertebral bodies (open staircase, or closely set pedicles) and flattened, irregular vertebral bodies (platyspondyly). **D,** In a 2-year-old, there is metaphyseal widening and irregularity at the wrist and short tubular bones of the hands, with almost no carpal bone ossification.

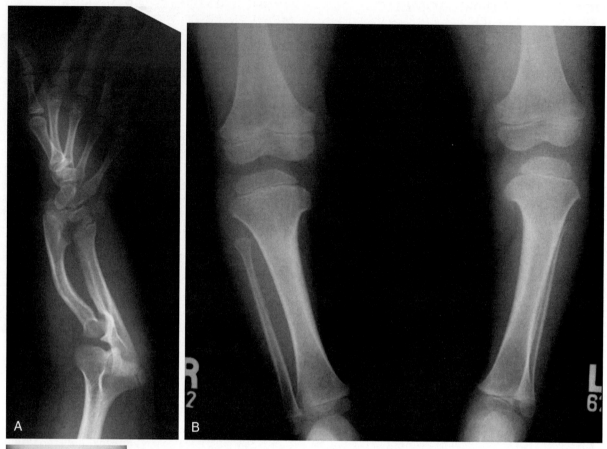

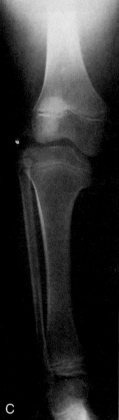

FIGURE 29. Radiologic findings in dyschondrosteosis. **A,** A 12-year-old with severe mesomelia and Madelung's deformity. **B** and **C,** Two children of 4 years **(B)** and 9 years **(C)** with mesomelia (short tibia and fibula).

ACROMELIC/ACROMESOMELIC DYSPLASIA GROUP

The acromelic/acromesomelic dysplasia group consists of a large, heterogeneous collection of disorders all of which have those types of shortening of their limbs. A number of these dysplasias have their molecular defect delineated but are too rare to discuss here. Only trichorhinophalangeal syndrome (TRP) types I and II and the interesting acromesomelic dysplasia (acromesomelic dwarfism) are detailed.

TRICHORHINOPHALANGEAL SYNDROME TYPES I AND II

Both of these disorders have been located on the long (q) arm of chromosome 8. The gene implicated in TRP I is *TRPS1*. TRP II is slightly more complicated. TRP II, also known as Langer-Giedion syndrome, is the result of a contiguous gene abnormality resulting from the loss of not only *TRPS1* but also *EXT1*, an exostosis gene distal to *TRPS1*. TRP I is autosomal dominant, whereas most cases of TRP II are sporadic. The clinical manifestations of both disorders include mild short stature; sparse, slow-growing hair; pear-shaped nose ("hose nose"); and short, crooked fingers (Fig. 30). The contiguous gene abnormality explains the added features in TRP II, which include multiple exostoses and mental retardation.

Radiologic Findings

- Extremities: Perthes-like changes at the hips, *cone-shaped epiphyses in the phalanges of both hands*
  Note: *Multiple exostoses* in TRP II

ACROMESOMELIC DYSPLASIA OF MAROTEAUX

This skeletal dysplasia is actually a misnomer in that the changes in this disorder are hardly just acro- and mesomelic. There are significant spinal abnormalities (Fig. 31). This is an autosomal recessive disorder for which the gene/molecular defect is not known but maps to chromosome 9q. Abnormalities are discoverable at birth but are quite significant by 1 year of age. Clinical findings include moderate short stature, short forearms, stubby hands and feet, and short shanks.

Radiologic Findings

- Spine: oval vertebral bodies (early), anterior beaking and posterior wedging (later), *gibbus and/or kyphoscoliosis* ultimately
- Extremities: shortening of all tubular bones, *especially radius/ulna and tibia/fibula; very short tubular bones of hands and feet with cone-shaped epiphyses* and large great toes

DYSPLASIAS WITH PROMINENT MEMBRANEOUS BONE INVOLVEMENT

Among the dysplasias with prominent membraneous bone involvement, only cleidocranial dysplasia is important for us to diagnose.

CLEIDOCRANIAL DYSPLASIA

This autosomal dominant disorder has its chromosome locus at 6p and a gene called *CBFA1* (core binding factor alpha-1). This dysplasia is quite common, with marked clinical variability. Often diagnosable at birth, the clinical findings include enlarged skull with large, late-closing fontanelles; dental abnormalities; drooping, hypermobile shoulders; mild short stature; and narrow chest (Fig. 32).

Radiologic Findings

- Skull: large, brachycephalic; *wormian bones;* wide sutures; *persistently open anterior fontanelle*
- Thorax: *absence/hypoplasia of clavicles,* mildly shortened ribs with downward slope, 11 ribs
- Spine: *significant posterior wedging of thoracic vertebrae*
- Pelvis: *high narrow iliac wings, absence/hypoplasia of pubic bones*
- Extremities: numerous pseudoepiphyses of metacarpals and *tapered distal phalanges* in the hands

BENT BONE DYSPLASIA GROUP

The bent bone dysplasia group of disorders is a rather small group with an important and not uncommon entity, campomelic dysplasia (campomelic dwarfism), that is well worked out molecularly. These dysplasias have been grouped together because of their radiographic expression.

CAMPOMELIC DYSPLASIA

This unusual entity is an autosomal dominant disorder diagnosable at birth, presenting with bent thighs, clubbed feet, respiratory distress, and unusual small facies (Fig. 33). Sex reversal is often present. All the extremities are moderately short. Neonatal/perinatal death occurs in most cases. The molecular defect is a homeobox gene abnormality called *SOX9,* found on chromosome 17.

RADIOLOGIC FINDINGS

- Skull: enlarged, narrow with a small face
- Thorax: mildly short ribs, *numbering 11; severe hypoplasia of the bodies of the scapulae*

- Spine: *nonossification of thoracic pedicles, cervical kyphosis,* hypoplasia of cervical vertebral bodies
- Pelvis: *narrow, tall iliac wings*
- Extremities: *proportionately long, bowed femurs with shortened bowed tibiae;* shortened upper extremity long bones

DYSOSTOSIS MULTIPLEX GROUP

The dysostosis multiplex group contains all the MPSs, mucolipidoses (MLs), and multiple other "storage diseases" that produce a skeletal dysplasia. The abnormalities in this entire group consist of well-described

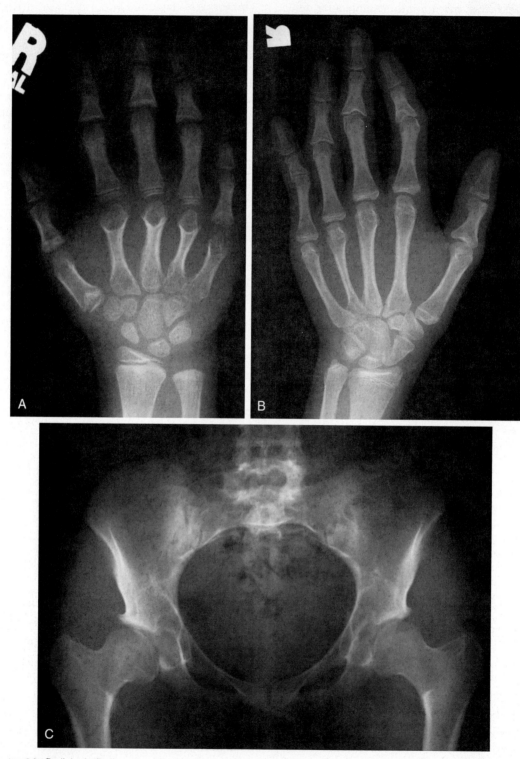

FIGURE 30. Radiologic findings in trichorhinophalangeal syndrome. **A,** In an 8-year-old, there are cone-shaped epiphyses involving the first metacarpal, the proximal fifth phalanx, and all middle phalanges and metacarpals in digits 2 through 5 (early fusion). **B,** Radiograph in an 18-year-old shows result of similar changes. **C,** In a young adult, there are coxa vara and small capital femoral epiphyses (residua of avascular necrosis).

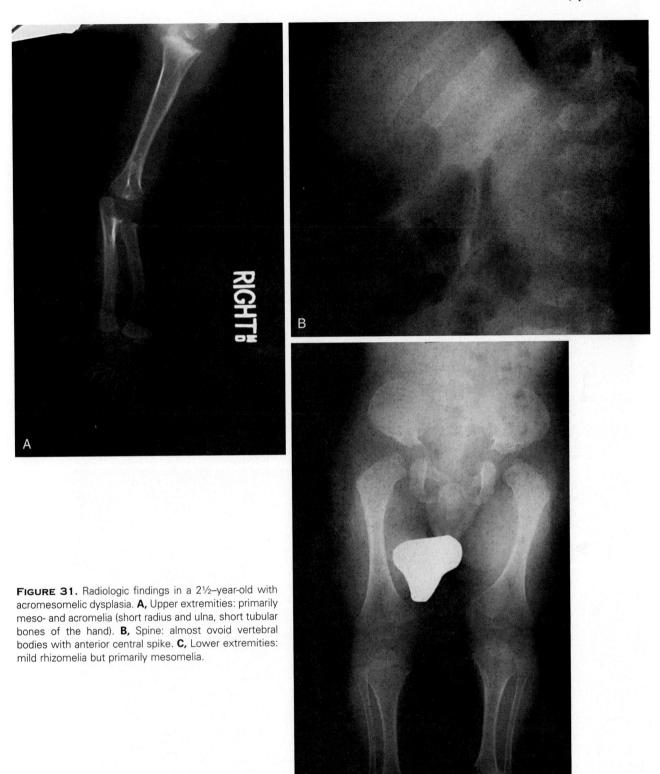

FIGURE 31. Radiologic findings in a 2½–year-old with acromesomelic dysplasia. **A,** Upper extremities: primarily meso- and acromelia (short radius and ulna, short tubular bones of the hand). **B,** Spine: almost ovoid vertebral bodies with anterior central spike. **C,** Lower extremities: mild rhizomelia but primarily mesomelia.

enzymatic defects that can be rather easily diagnosed by appropriate urine, blood, and/or fibroblast culture analyses. They have in common the ability to act similarly on the skeleton to produce a dysostosis multiplex picture to a greater or lesser degree. The term *dysostosis multiplex* was coined for the radiology of this group of conditions. Therefore, the real role of the

radiologist is to suggest the likelihood of one of these disorders, leaving it to the geneticist to biochemically determine which exact dysplasia it is. I shall use Hurler's syndrome (MPS IH) as the stereotypical example of this group. Morquio's syndrome (MPS IVA, B) has some slightly different abnormalities and thereby can often be differentiated from the other MPS entities radiographically. Separately, I discuss the unusual findings in I-cell disease (ML II).

HURLER'S SYNDROME (MPS IH)

The enzyme abnormality in this specific form of MPS is in α_1–iduronidase, located on chromosome 4p. As with all the other members of this group, the inheritance pattern is recessive. Most of the MPS entities present clinically in late infancy or early childhood (Fig. 34).

Radiologic Findings (Dysostosis Multiplex)

- Skull: enlarged neurocranium, *abnormal J-shaped sella*

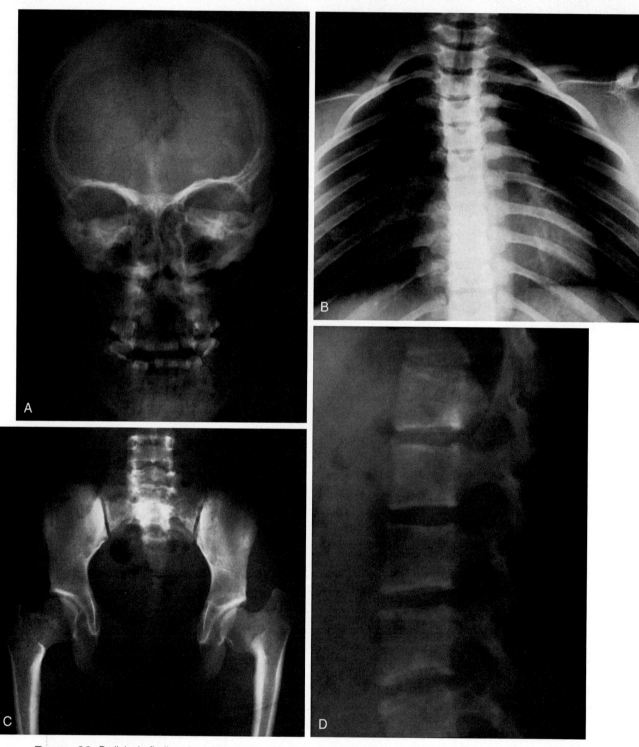

FIGURE 32. Radiologic findings in a 15-year-old with cleidocranial dysplasia. **A,** Skull: large open anterior fontanelle and multiple wormian bones. **B,** Thorax: asymmetric hypoplastic/absent clavicles and downward-sloping ribs. **C,** Pelvis: tall, narrow ilia and hypoplastic pubic bones. **D,** Spine: posteriorly wedged but otherwise normal vertebral bodies.

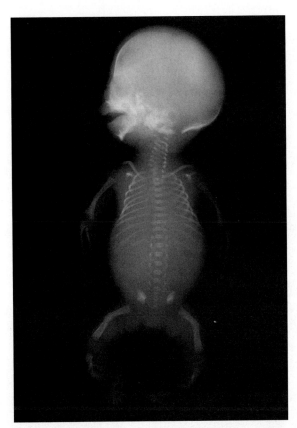

FIGURE 33. Radiologic findings in a fetus of 21 weeks' gestation with campomelic dysplasia. Findings include a large skull with a small face; hypoplastic/absent scapular bodies; 11 ribs; poorly ossified thoracic pedicles; tall, narrow iliac wings; and short extremities with proportionately long, bent femurs.

- Thorax: *short, thick clavicles; paddle (oar)–shaped ribs;* hypoplastic glenoid
- Spine: gibbus, *superior notched (inferior beaked)* thoracolumbar vertebral bodies, upper cervical subluxation
- Pelvis: *flared, small iliac wings with inferior tapering; steep acetabular roofs*
- Extremities: *diaphyseal widening of long bones ("marrow expansion"); dysplastic epiphyses;* characteristic hands—brachydactyly, *proximal metacarpal "pointing," diaphyseal widening of metacarpals* and proximal/middle phalanges, small irregular carpal bones

MORQUIO'S SYNDROME (MPS IVA, B)

MPS IVA has an enzyme abnormality in galactose 6-sulfatase, resulting in the accumulation of excess MPS material in multiple organ systems, including the skeletal system (Fig. 35). This is the most common form of Morquio's syndrome, and there are radiographically and clinically rare mild cases. There is some unpublished evidence that suggests that Morquio chondrocytes do not grow normally in vitro, perhaps alluding to the cause of the skeletal abnormalities differing from those of other forms of MPS.

Radiologic Findings (Differentiating Features from Other MPSs)

- Skull: *no J-shaped sella*
- Thorax: *widened,* not oar-shaped, *ribs*
- Spine: *middle tonguing,* not inferior beaking
- Pelvis: no tapering of ileum
- Extremities: *proximal metacarpal rounding,* not pointing, of hands

MUCOLIPIDOSIS II (I-CELL DISEASE)

ML II is another enzyme abnormality, of *N*-acetylglucosamine phosphotransferase, found on chromosome 4q. It clinically (and radiographically) presents in the newborn (and prenatally). Most patients die in infancy. Certain radiographic features are quite unique (Fig. 36).

Radiologic Findings

- Extremities: *severe osteopenia, poorly defined corticies, "periosteal cloaking"* (newborn)
  Note: The changes of "dysostosis multiplex" occur later.

DYSPLASIAS WITH DECREASED BONE DENSITY

The dysplasias with decreased bone density are primarily represented by *osteogenesis imperfecta (OI)*, a very large group of disorders all of which have a type I collagen abnormality. The affected genes are called *COLA1* and *COLA2* and are found on chromosomes 17q and 7q, respectively. The clinical classification is not well corroborated by the molecular findings. The radiographic findings help to delineate mild and severe cases for management and prognosis. OI type II is almost the most common lethal skeletal dysplasia.

OSTEOGENESIS IMPERFECTA TYPE II

This disorder is a specific autosomal dominant condition and occurs as a spontaneous new mutation, but has a high rate of germ cell mosaicism (6% to 8%), resulting in the potential for other affected fetuses in the same family. Those affected can be picked up on second-trimester ultrasonography. OI type II is specific radiographically as an invariable lethal disorder with no significant intrafamilial variability (Fig. 37).

Radiologic Findings

- Skull: *very poor to no ossification*
- Thorax: small, narrow chest; *beaded ribs*

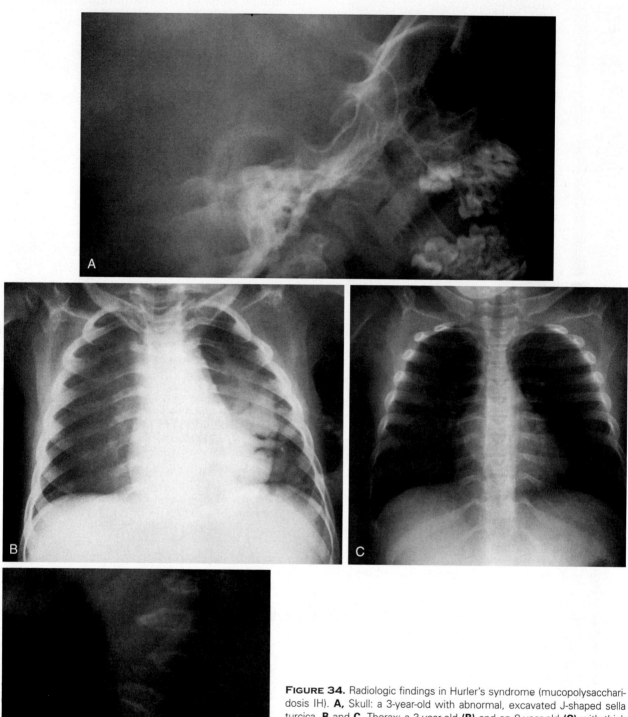

FIGURE 34. Radiologic findings in Hurler's syndrome (mucopolysaccharidosis IH). **A,** Skull: a 3-year-old with abnormal, excavated J-shaped sella turcica. **B** and **C,** Thorax: a 3-year-old **(B)** and an 8-year-old **(C)** with thick clavicles and paddle-shaped ribs (thin posteriorly and thick anteriorly). **D,** Spine: an 8-year-old with superiorly notched (inferiorly beaked) vertebral bodies.   *Illustration continued on opposite page*

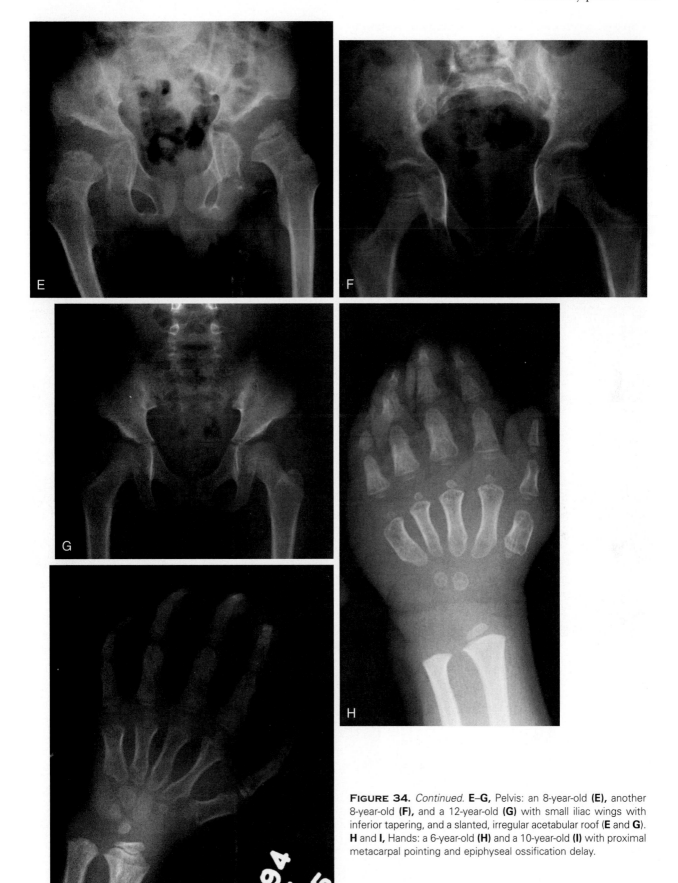

FIGURE 34. *Continued.* **E–G,** Pelvis: an 8-year-old **(E)**, another 8-year-old **(F)**, and a 12-year-old **(G)** with small iliac wings with inferior tapering, and a slanted, irregular acetabular roof (**E** and **G**). **H** and **I,** Hands: a 6-year-old **(H)** and a 10-year-old **(I)** with proximal metacarpal pointing and epiphyseal ossification delay.

- Spine: severe deossification, collapsed vertebral bodies
- Extremities: generalized osteoporosis with or without fractures; shortened, widened long bones with thin cortices; *"accordion femurs"*

Osteogenesis Imperfecta—Other Types

It is difficult to type OI radiographically. From the radiologic point of view, one can suggest this diagnosis and ascertain if it is mild or severe. This is the important role for the pediatric radiologist to play, letting the typing be determined on associated clinical grounds.

Radiologic Findings

- Skull: *abnormal number of wormian bones (>8 to 10),* variable decreased ossification
- Spine: wedged or collapsed vertebrae
- Remaining skeleton: *at least some osteoporosis,* variable number of fractures (*especially pathologic fractures*)

DYSPLASIAS WITH DEFECTIVE MINERALIZATION

Among the dysplasias with defective mineralization, the important entity for us to recognize and deal with is hypophosphatasia. Hyperparathyroidism and rickets are covered elsewhere in this book.

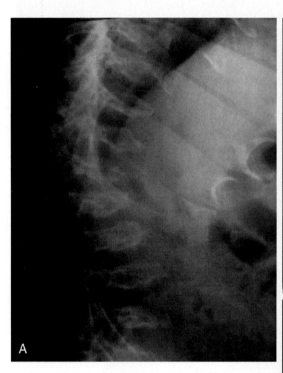

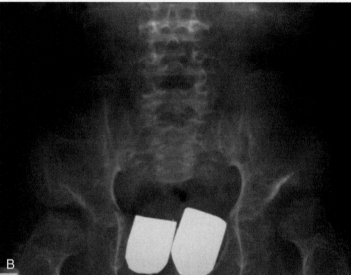

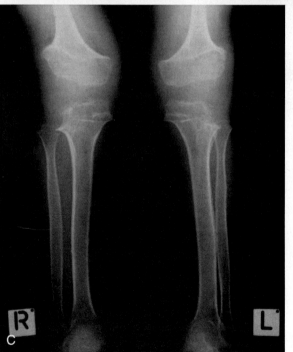

FIGURE 35. Radiologic findings in Morquio's syndrome (mucopolysaccharidosis IVA, B). **A,** A 7-year-old with platyspondyly with central beaking (tongue). **B,** An 18-year-old with severe capital femoral epiphyseal and acetabular dysplasia but no inferior iliac tapering. **C,** A 15-year-old with lateral distal femoral and proximal tibial epiphyseal ossification defects with genu varum.

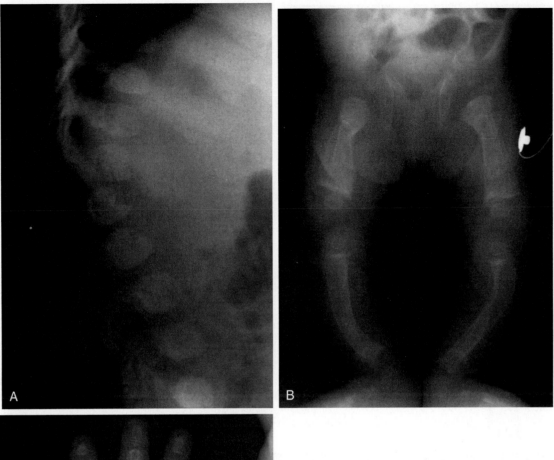

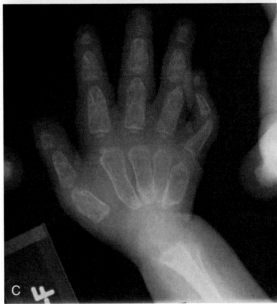

FIGURE 36. Radiologic findings in mucolipidosis II (I-cell disease). **A,** Several hypoplastic superiorly notched vertebral bodies (mucopolysaccharidosis-like). **B,** Characteristic periosteal cloaking. **C,** Proximal metacarpal pointing and expanded short tubular bones with thin cortices.

HYPOPHOSPHATASIA

There are two distinct genetic forms of hypophosphatasia, the autosomal recessive perinatal lethal/infantile type and a later-onset autosomal dominant "adult" type (Fig. 38). These conditions represent an enzyme abnormality. The chromosome loci for both conditions lie at 1p at or close to each other. The gene and the genetics of the perinatal lethal/infantile disorder are clear, but the adult-form gene is not clearly identified, and the genetics suggest either dominant or recessive inheri-

tance patterns (see also Section IX, Part VII, Chapter 2, page 2242).

Radiologic Findings

Perinatal Lethal/Infantile

- Skull: decreased ossification with *single island-like centers* for frontal occipital and parietal bones
- Thorax: poorly ossified ribs; *sporadic dropout of ribs;* thin, wavy, fractured ribs

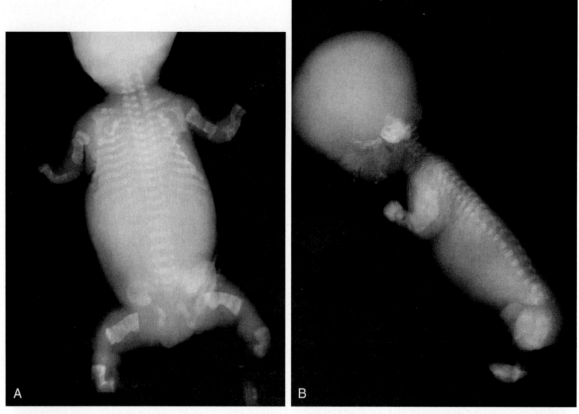

FIGURE 37. A and **B,** Radiologic findings in a stillborn term fetus with osteogenesis imperfecta type II include generalized osteoporosis, absent skull ossification, beaded ribs, and crumpled long bones, including accordion femurs.

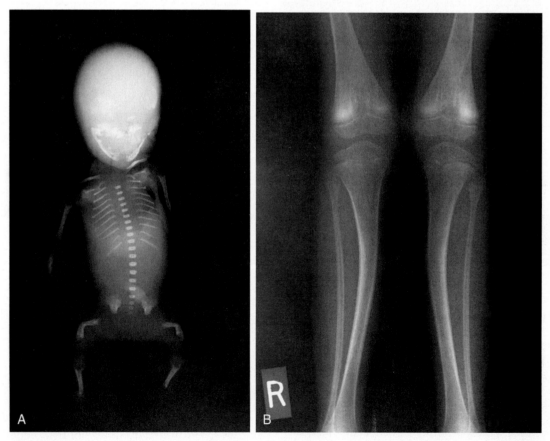

FIGURE 38. Radiologic findings in hypophosphatasia. **A,** Fetus with perinatal lethal type demonstrates island-like skull ossification (parietal); thin, wavy ribs; platyspondyly and missing cervical vertebrae ossification; no pedicles; and bent femurs. **B,** A 7-year-old with adult-type hypophosphatasia, demonstrates osteopenia, bent tibias, and punched-out metaphyseal lesions.

- Spine: *sporadic unossified vertebral bodies, dense and osteopenic vertebrae, sporadic platyspondyly, butterfly-shaped vertebral bodies, sporadic missing pedicles*
- Extremities: *generalized decreased ossification, chromosome-shaped femurs, metaphyseal cupping* and irregularity, central lucent defect, "campomelic femurs," *sporadic "missing" short tubular bones of hands and feet*
  Note: Clavicles are not affected; *infantile form is less severe.*

Adult

- Generalized osteopenia
- Extremities: *metaphyseal widening* (rickets-like changes), *punched-out metaphyseal lesions,* pathologic fractures

INCREASED BONE DENSITY WITHOUT MODIFICATION OF BONE SHAPE GROUP

The increased bone density without modification of bone shape group contains several members of interest. These disorders are still grouped by their radiographic expression. The osteopetrosis subgroup contains at least three separate entities. Pycnodysostosis is a rare but fascinating dysplasia.

OSTEOPETROSIS

Osteopetrosis is a subgroup of disorders the members of which appear to have their chromosomal loci on several different chromosomes. The very severe *precocious type,* which is autosomal recessive, is located on chromosome 11q, and has a suspect gene called CSF1 ("mouse osteopetrosis gene"). The *delayed type,* which is autosomal dominant, is located at chromosome 1p, but its gene to date is unknown. The condition known as *osteopetrosis with renal tubular acidosis (carbonic anhydrase II deficiency)* is well clarified as to chromosomal locus (8q), and gene (*CA2*—carbonic anhydrase II). Although the latter dysplasia is a rare entity, certain radiographic findings suggest the correct diagnosis (Figs. 39 and 40).

Radiologic Findings

- *Generalized increased bone density*
- Skull: *thick and dense, especially at the base*
- Thorax: splayed anterior ribs
- Spine: *"sandwich" vertebral bodies, "picture frame" vertebral bodies*
- Extremities: *splayed metaphyses,* bone-within-bone configuration, *dense metaphyseal bands*
  Note: Pathologic fractures, rickets, and osteomyelitis can be seen.
  Carbonic anhydrase II deficiency has *diffuse dense cerebral calcifications.*

PYKNODYSOSTOSIS

This appears to represent the malady of the painter *Toulouse-Lautrec.* This is an autosomal recessive disorder that often presents in infancy. Clinical findings include short-limbed dwarfism, micrognathia, fractures, and short fingertips (Fig. 41).

Radiologic Findings

- Generalized osteosclerosis
- Skull: *marked delay in closure of fontanelles and sutures, wormian bones, obtuse or absent mandibular angle,* dense skull
- Thorax: *resorbed acromial ends of clavicles*
- Extremities: *resorbed phalangeal tufts*

CRANIOTUBULAR DYSPLASIAS

The *craniotubular dysplasias* are actually found in two separate nomenclature groups: increased bone density with diaphyseal involvement and increased bone density with metaphyseal involvement. Within these two groups, I shall only cover craniodiaphyseal dysplasia, craniometaphyseal dysplasia, and Pyle dysplasia.

CRANIODIAPHYSEAL DYSPLASIA

This rather rare autosomal recessive condition presents in early infancy with *progressive facial and calvarial thickening* (Fig. 42). Sudden death is frequent as the result of cranial foraminal narrowing.

Radiologic Findings

- Skull: *marked thickening and sclerosis of calvarium and facial bones, obliteration of foramina* and sinuses
- Thorax: *diffusely widened, sclerotic ribs and clavicles*
- Extremities: *straightened, undermodeled long bone diaphyses* with metaphyseal sparing; *"flame" sclerosis (cortical thickening) of the short-tubular bones (hands)*

CRANIOMETAPHYSEAL DYSPLASIA

This is also an autosomal recessive craniotubular bone dysplasia. There is cranial and facial thickening, often with *nasal obstruction* (Fig. 43). There can be improvement with age. Cranial encroachment–induced neurologic abnormalities may develop.

Radiologic Findings

- Skull: diffuse *hyperostosis of cranial vault base and facial bones,* obliterated paranasal sinuses
- Extremities: sclerosis of diaphyses (early), *undermodeled flared metaphyses* of long bones (later)

Text continued on page 2173

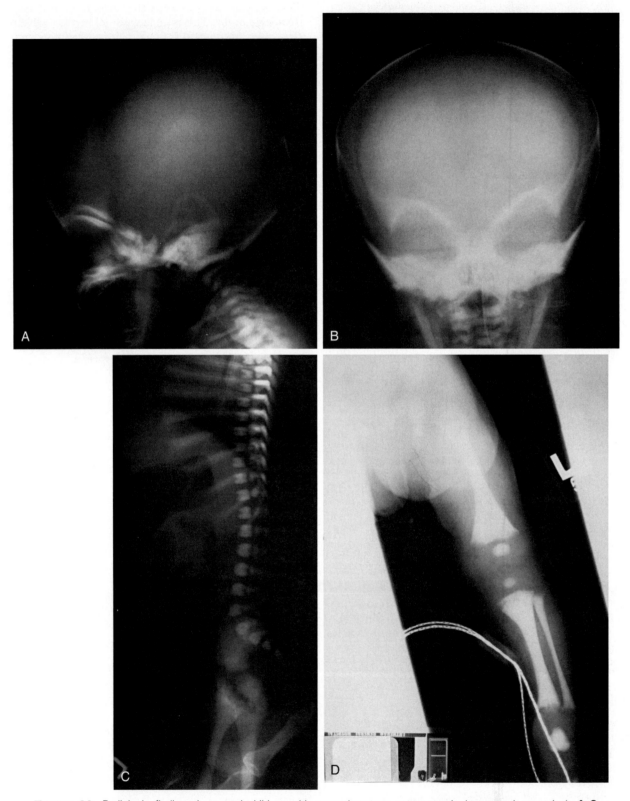

FIGURE 39. Radiologic findings in several children with precocious-type osteopetrosis (autosomal recessive). **A–C,** Newborn. **A** and **B,** Dense skull and face, especially skull base. **C,** Dense spine and ribs. **D,** At 3 months, there are very dense long bones, medullary obliteration, and frayed metaphyses (rickets).

Illustration continued on opposite page

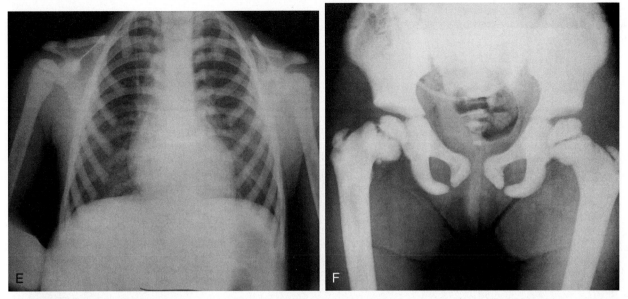

FIGURE 39. *Continued.* **E** and **F,** Four years. **E,** Dense thorax (ribs, clavicles, scapulas) and upper extremity long bones (*note:* less medullary obliteration). **F,** Dense pelvis and lower extremity long bones (including capital femoral epiphyses), and bilateral pathologic femoral neck fractures.

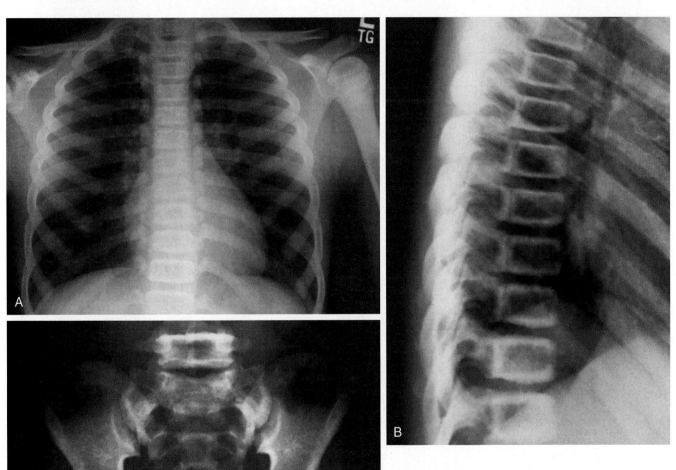

FIGURE 40. Radiologic findings in an 8-year-old with delayed-type osteopetrosis (autosomal dominant). **A,** Dense thoracic bones without medullary encroachment of left humerus. **B,** "Sandwich," almost "picture frame" vertebral bodies (dense outer borders). **C,** Increased bone density outlining ileum, including supraacetabular regions, and pubic symphysis region, as well as dense proximal femoral epiphyses and femoral necks with sparing of lower medullary space.

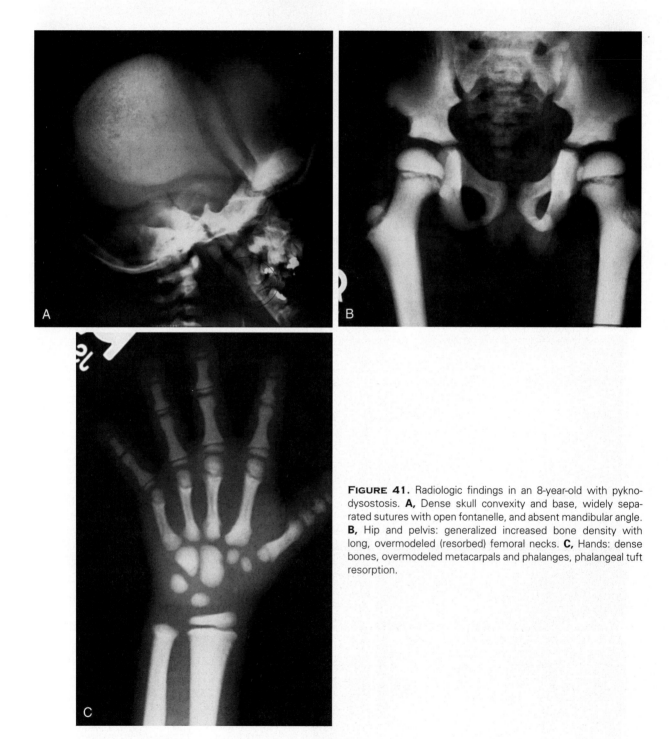

FIGURE 41. Radiologic findings in an 8-year-old with pykno-dysostosis. **A,** Dense skull convexity and base, widely separated sutures with open fontanelle, and absent mandibular angle. **B,** Hip and pelvis: generalized increased bone density with long, overmodeled (resorbed) femoral necks. **C,** Hands: dense bones, overmodeled metacarpals and phalanges, phalangeal tuft resorption.

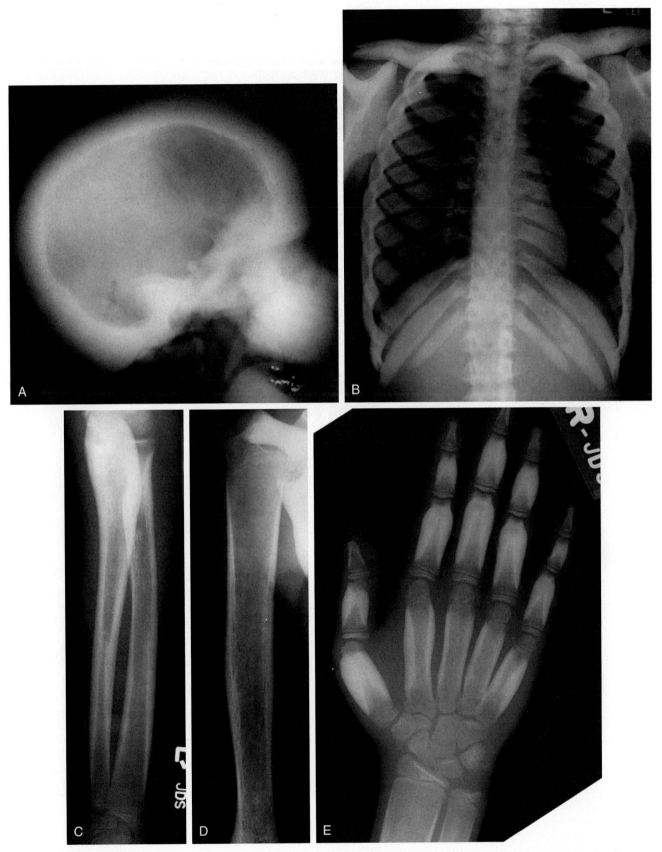

FIGURE 42. Radiologic findings in a 13-year-old with craniodiaphyseal dysplasia. **A,** Extremely dense bone filling in the facial region and thickening the diploic space. **B,** Diffusely dense, thickened ribs and clavicles. **C** and **D,** Diffuse cortical long bone diaphyseal thickening and diaphyseal undermodeling. **E,** "Flame" sclerosis (cortical thickening) of the tubular bones of the hand.

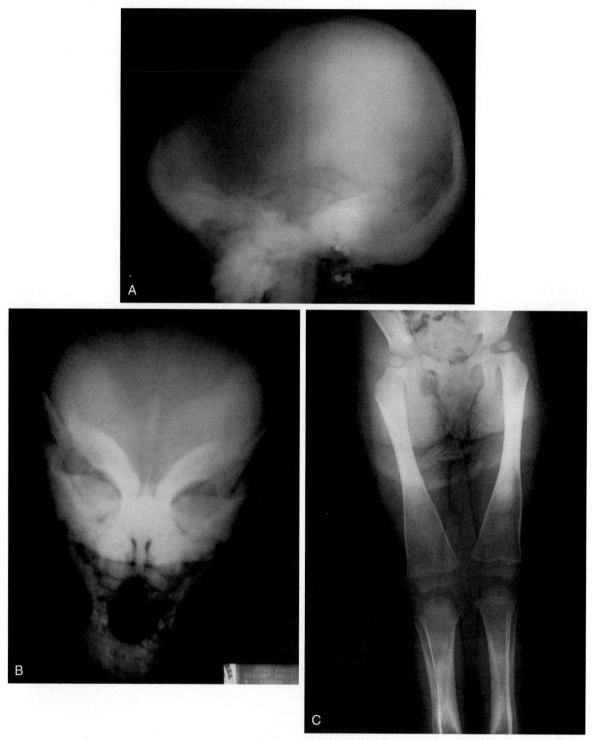

FIGURE 43. Radiologic findings in a 2-year-old with craniometaphyseal dysplasia. **A** and **B,** Marked increased bone density of cranial base and vault, and dense facial bones with obliteration of sinuses. **C,** Undermodeled flared metaphyses (Erlenmeyer flask deformity) of distal femurs, especially with sparing of diaphyses.

PYLE DYSPLASIA

This entity, also known as familial metaphyseal dysplasia, is somewhat similar to craniometaphyseal dysplasia but differs in its minimal craniofacial involvement. Patients are often asymptomatic or develop knock-knees. This is also an autosomal recessive condition.

Radiologic Findings

- Skull: *mild skull and facial involvement,* minimal base-of-skull sclerosis, prominent supraorbital ridging
- Thorax: mildly thickened clavicles and ribs
- Pelvis: thickened ischium and pubis
- Extremities: marked undertubulation of long bones, *especially distal femurs (Erlenmeyer flask deformity); distal flaring of metacarpals and proximal flaring of phalanges*

DISORGANIZED DEVELOPMENT OF CARTILAGENOUS AND FIBROUS COMPONENTS OF THE SKELETON

The group known as disorganized development of cartilaginous and fibrous components of the skeleton contains many important entities that are covered elsewhere in this text, including multiple exostosis, enchondromatosis, and fibrous dysplasia. However, there are two members of this group that we also need to be aware of that consist of entities with significant spine involvement: spondyloenchondromatosis and dysspondyloenchondromatosis.

SPONDYLOENCHONDROMATOSIS

This autosomal recessive disorder is also known as spondyloenchondrodysplasia. There is low-normal or mild short stature, with kyphosis and/or lordosis (Fig. 44). Prominent joints may be apparent.

Radiologic Findings

- Spine: *severe platyspondyly with end plate irregularity*
- Extremities: *typical enchondromata*
  Note: Enchondromas may be present in all enchondral bone areas but rarely involve the hands and feet

DYSSPONDYLOENCHONDROMATOSIS

This entity is also called dysspondylochondromatosis. The patients have short stature, kyphoscoliosis, and abnormal facies (Fig. 45).

Radiologic Findings

- Spine: vertebral anomalies, *hemivertebrae, anisospondyly,* and end plate irregularity
- Extremities: *typical enchondromata,* including hand and foot involvement, with *long bone asymmetry*

OSTEOLYSIS GROUP

The osteolysis group of disorders is a very large and diverse one that lacks significant clarification. No molecular identification has occurred in this group, and only one chromosome site has been found in a rather rare member. Only one interesting entity in this group is discussed here.

MULTICENTRIC CARPAL/TARSAL OSTEOLYSIS WITH OR WITHOUT NEPHROPATHY

This is an autosomal dominant condition. The onset of symptoms is in early childhood with progressive arthritic complaints in the wrists and ankles (Fig. 46). A chronic progressive nephropathy may ensue. Two forms have been identified on the basis of variability in the onset of the nephropathy, but, because of the difficulty in distinguishing between them, it is unclear if this variability really represents two separate conditions.

Radiologic Findings

- Extremities (wrists and ankles): *deossification of carpal bones,* loss of carpal/tarsal contours, *bone resorption and collapse,* sclerosis, at times extension into adjacent short tubular bones ("*sucked candy*" *appearance)*

PATELLAR DYSPLASIA GROUP

The patellar dysplasia group contains only two members: the newly described scyphopatellar dysplasia and the not uncommon and important nail–patella syndrome.

NAIL–PATELLA SYNDROME

This autosomal dominant disorder is also known by a variety of synonyms, including Fong disease and onycho-osteodysplasia, among several others. The gene for this disorder *(NPS1)* has been identified and is located on chromosome 9q. The major clinical manifestations include dysplastic nails, small or absent patellae on palpation, and a nephropathy with onset in childhood or in the young adult and characteristic electron microscopic changes. The "iliac horns" (Fig. 47) are sometimes palpable (see Section IX, Part VI, Fig. 31, page 2204).

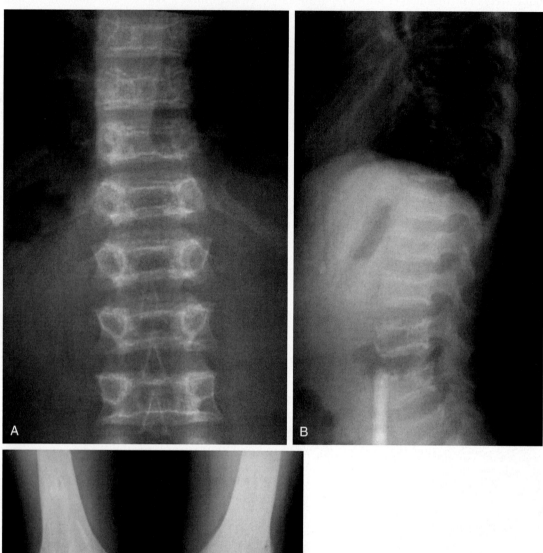

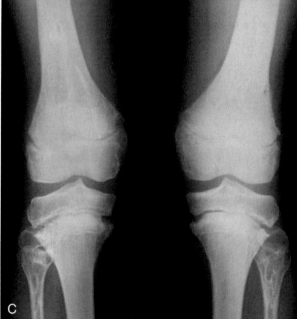

FIGURE 44. Radiologic findings in a 14-year-old with spondyloenchondromatosis. **A** and **B,** Platy-spondyly with end plate irregularity. **C,** Multiple enchondromata in the long bones.

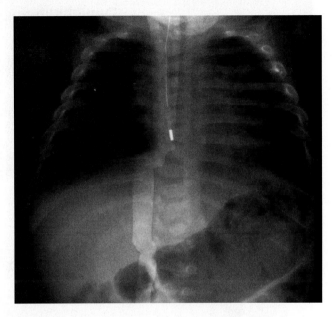

FIGURE 45. Radiologic findings in a 6-month-old with dysspondyloenchondromatosis include multiple hemivertebrae in thoracolumbar junctional area. (Patient also manifested many enchondromata in his appendicular skeleton.)

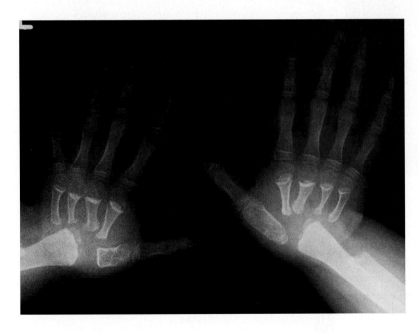

FIGURE 46. Radiologic findings in a 9-year-old with multicentric carpal/tarsal osteolysis include complete resorption of the carpal bones, loss of the carpal joint space, and resorption/remodeling shortening of the adjacent metacarpals.

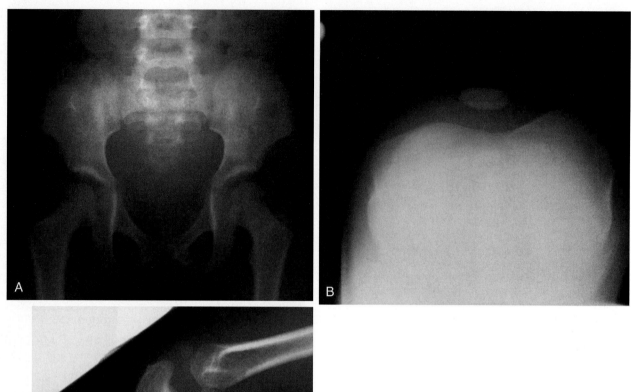

FIGURE 47. Radiologic findings in a 5-year-old with nail–patella syndrome. **A,** Iliac horn in the center of each iliac wing. **B,** Tiny (hypoplastic) patella in this sunrise view of the knee. **C,** Congenital elbow (radial head) dislocation.

Radiologic Findings

- Pelvis: *iliac horn* in the center of the iliac wing extending posteriorly
- Extremities (knees and elbows): *hypoplastic or absent patellas,* radial head and capitellum hypoplasia/elbow dislocation

SUGGESTED READINGS

General

Lachman RS: International nomenclature and classification of the osteochondrodystrophies (1997). Pediatr Radiol 1988;28: 737–744

Shohat M, Lachman R, Gruber HE, Rimoin DL: Brachyolmia: clinical, radiographic and genetic evidence of heterogeneity. Am J Med Genet 1989;33:209

Taybi H, Lachman RS: Radiology of Syndromes, Metabolic Disorders, and Skeletal Dysplasias, 4th ed. St. Louis, Mosby, 1996

Thanatophoric Dysplasia

Brodie SG, Kitoh H, Lachman RS, et al: Platyspondylic lethal skeletal dysplasia, San Diego type is caused by FGFR III mutations. Am J Med Genet 1999;84:476

Langer LO Jr, Spranger JW, Greinacher I, Herdman RC: Thanatophoric dwarfism: a condition confused with achondroplasia in the neonate, with brief comments on achondrogenesis and homozygous achondroplasia. Radiology 1969;92:285

Langer LO Jr, Yang SS, Hall JG, et al: Thanatophoric dysplasia and cloverleaf skull. Am J Med Genet Suppl 1987;3:167

Norman AM, Rimmer S, Landy S, Donnai D: Thanatophoric dysplasia of the straight bone type (type 2). Clin Dysmorphol 1992;1:115

Wilcox WR, Tavormina PL, Krakow D, et al: Molecular, radiologic, and histopathologic correlations in thanatophoric dysplasia. Am J Med Genet 1998;78:274

Achondroplasia

Caffey J: Achondroplasia of pelvis and lumbosacral spine: some roentgenographic features. Am J Roentgenol Radium Ther Nucl Med 1958;80:449

Langer LO Jr, Baumann PA, Gorlin RJ: Achondroplasia. Am J Roentgenol Radium Ther Nucl Med 1967;100:12

Lemyre E, Azouz EM, Teebi AS, et al: Bone dysplasia series. Achondroplasia, hypochondroplasia and thanatophoric dysplasia: review and update. Can Assoc Radiol J 1999;50:185

Hypochondroplasia

Hall BD, Spranger J: Hypochondroplasia: clinical and radiological aspects in 39 cases. Radiology 1979;133:95

Le Merrer M, Rousseau F, Legeai-Mallet L, et al: A gene for achondroplasia-hypochondroplasia maps to chromosome 4p. Nature Genet 1994;6:318

Maroteaux P, Falzon P: Hypochondroplasia: review of 80 cases [in French]. Arch Fr Pediatr 1988;45:105

Metatropic Dysplasia

Beck M, Roubicek M, Rogers JG, et al: Heterogeneity of metatropic dysplasia. Eur J Pediatr 1983;140:231

Shohat M, Lachman R, Rimoin DL: Odontoid hypoplasia with cervical spine subluxation and ventriculomegaly in metatropic dysplasia. J Pediatr 1989;114:239

Schneckenbecken (Snail Pelvis) Dysplasia

Borochowitz Z, Jones KL, Silbey R, et al: A distinct lethal neonatal chondrodysplasia with snail-like pelvis: Schneckenbecken dysplasia. Am J Med Genet 1986;25:47

Giedion A, Biedermann K, Briner J, et al: Case report 693: Schneckenbecken dysplasia. Skeletal Radiol 1991;20:534

Short Rib (With or Without)–Polydactyly Dysplasia

Beemer FA, Langer LO Jr, Klep-de Pater JM, et al: A new short rib syndrome: report of two cases. Am J Med Genet 1982;14:115

Lungarotti MS, Martello C, Marinelli I, Falasca L: Lethal short rib syndrome of the Beemer type without polydactyly. Pediatr Radiol 1993;23:325

Naumoff P, Young LW, Mazer J, Amortegui AJ: Short rib-polydactyly syndrome type 3. Radiology 1977;122:443

Saldino RM, Noonan CD: Severe thoracic dystrophy with striking micromelia, abnormal osseous development, including the spine, and multiple visceral anomalies. Am J Roentgenol Radium Ther Nucl Med 1972;114:257

Sillence D, Kozlowski K, Bar-Ziv J, et al: Perinatally lethal short rib-polydactyly syndromes. 1. Variability in known syndromes. Pediatr Radiol 1987;17:474

Spranger J, Grimm B, Weller M, et al: Short-rib-polydactyly (SRP) syndromes, types Majewski and Saldino-Noonan. Z Kinderheilkd 1974;116:73

Asphyxiating Thoracic Dysplasia (Jeune's Syndrome)

Langer LO: Thoracic-pelvic-phalangeal dystrophy: asphyxiating thoracic dystrophy of the newborn, infantile thoracic dystrophy. Radiology 1968;91:447

Chondroectodermal Dysplasia (Ellis–van Creveld Dysplasia)

Caffey J: Chondroectodermal dysplasia (Ellis–van Creveld syndrome): report of three cases. Am J Roentgenol Radium Ther Nucl Med 1952;68:875

McKusick VA: The Amish. Endeavour 1980;4:52

McKusick VA: Ellis-van Creveld syndrome and the Amish. Nature Genet 2000;24:203

Diastrophic Dysplasia

Horton WA, Rimoin DL, Lachman RS, et al: The phenotypic variability of diastrophic dysplasia. J Pediatr 1978;93:609

Lachman R, Sillence D, Rimoin D, et al: Diastrophic dysplasia: the death of a variant. Radiology 1980;140:79

Taybi H: Diastrophic dwarfism. Radiology 1963;80:1

Achondrogenesis I

Borochowitz Z, Lachman R, Adomian GE, et al: Achondrogenesis type 1: delineation of further heterogeneity and identification of two distinct subgroups. J Pediatr 1988;112:23

Achondrogenesis II/Hypochondrogenesis

Borochowitz Z, Ornoy A, Lachman R, Rimoin DL: Achondrogenesis II–hypochondrogenesis: variability versus heterogeneity. Am J Med Genet 1986;24:273

Eyre DR, Upton MP, Shapiro FD, et al: Nonexpression of cartilage type II collagen in a case of Langer-Saldino achondrogenesis. Am J Hum Genet 1986;39:52

Lachman RS, Tiller GE, Graham JM Jr, Rimoin DL: Collagen, genes and the skeletal dysplasias on the edge of a new era: a review and update. Eur J Radiol 1992;14:1

Saldino RM: Lethal short-limbed dwarfism: achondrogenesis and thanatophoric dwarfism. Am J Roentgenol Radium Ther Nucl Med 1971;112:185

Spondyloepiphyseal Dysplasia Congenita

Harding CO, Green CG, Perloff WH, Pauli RM: Respiratory complications in children with spondyloepiphyseal dysplasia congenita. Pediatr Pulmon 1990;9:49

Lachman RS: Fetal imaging in the skeletal dysplasias: overview and experience. Pediatr Radiol 1994;24:413

Spranger J, Langer LO Jr: Spondyloepiphyseal dysplasia congenita. Radiology 1970;94:313

Spranger J, et al: Dysplasia spondyloepiphysaria congenita. Helv Paediatr Acta 1966;21:598

Tiller GE, Rimoin DL, Murray LW, Cohn DH: Tandem duplication within a type II collagen gene (COL2A1) exon in an individual with spondyloepiphyseal dysplasia. Proc Natl Acad Sci USA 1990;87:3889

Kniest Syndrome

Kniest W: Zur Abgrenzung der Dysostosis enchondralis von der Chondrodystrophie. Z Kinderheilkd 1952;70:633

Lachman RS, Rimoin DL, Hollister DW, et al: The Kniest syndrome. Am J Roentgenol Radium Ther Nucl Med 1975;123:805

Spranger J, Menger H, Mundlos S, et al: Kniest dysplasia is caused by dominant collagen II (COL2A1) mutations: parental somatic mosaicism manifesting as Stickler phenotype and mild spondyloepiphyseal dysplasia. Pediatr Radiol 1994;24:431

Wilkin DJ, Bogaert R, Lachman RS, et al: A single amino acid substitution (G103D) in the type II collagen triple helix produces Kniest dysplasia. Hum Mol Genet 1994;3:1999

Spondyloepiphyseal Dysplasia Tarda

Gedeon AK, Colley A, Jamieson R, et al: Identification of the gene (SEDL) causing X-linked spondyloepiphyseal dysplasia tarda. Nature Genet 1999;22:400

Langer LO: Spondyloepiphyseal dysplasia tarda, hereditary chondrodysplasia with characteristic vertebral configuration in the adult. Radiology 1964;82:833

Dyggve-Melchior-Clausen Syndrome

Beighton P: Dyggve-Melchior-Clausen syndrome. J Med Genet 1990; 27:512

Dyggve HV, Melchior JC, Clausen J: Morquio-Ulrich's disease. Arch Dis Child 1962;37:525

Schorr S, Legum C, Ochshorn M, et al: The Dyggve-Melchior-Clausen syndrome. Am J Roentgenol 1977;128:107

Multiple Epiphyseal Dysplasia

Deere M, Sanford T, Francomano CA, et al: Identification of nine novel mutations in cartilage oligomeric matrix protein in patients with pseudoachondroplasia and multiple epiphyseal dysplasia. Am J Med Genet 1999;85:486

Hulvey JT, Keats T: Multiple epiphyseal dysplasia: a contribution to the problem of spinal involvement. Am J Roentgenol Radium Ther Nucl Med 1969;106:170

Lohiniva J, Paassilta P, Seppanen U, et al: Splicing mutations in the COL3 domain of collagen IX cause multiple epiphyseal dysplasia. Am J Med Genet 2000;90:216

Pseudoachondroplasia

Heselson NG, Cremin BJ, Beighton P: Pseudoachondroplasia: a report of 13 cases. Br J Radiol 1977;50:473

Rimoin DL, Rasmussen IM, Briggs MD: A large family with features of pseudoachondroplasia and multiple epiphyseal dysplasia: exclusion of seven candidate gene loci that encode proteins of the cartilage extracellular matrix. Hum Genet 1994;93:236

Wynne-Davies R, Hall CM, Young ID: Pseudoachondroplasia: clinical diagnosis at different ages and comparison of autosomal dominant and recessive types. A review of 32 patients (26 kindreds). J Med Genet 1986;23:425

Chondrodysplasia Punctata

Brites P, Motley A, Hoganhout E, et al: Molecular basis of rhizomelic chondrodysplasia punctata type 1: high frequency of the Leu-292 stop mutation in 38 patients. J Inherit Metab Dis 1998;21:306

Gilbert EF, Opitz JM, Spranger JW, et al: Chondrodysplasia punctata—rhizomelic form: pathologic and radiologic studies of three infants. Eur J Pediatr 1976;123:89

Maroteaux P: Brachytelephalangic chondrodysplasia punctata: a possible X-linked recessive form. Hum Genet 1989;82:167

Silengo MC, Luzzati L, Silverman FN: Clinical and genetic aspects of Conradi-Hünermann disease. J Pediatr 1980;97:911

Spranger JW, Bidder U, Voelz C: Chondrodysplasia punctata (chondrodystrophia calcificans). II: The rhizomelic type [in German]. Forschr Geb Rontgenstr Nuklearmed 1971;114:327

Wells TR, Landing BH, Bostwick FH: Studies of vertebral coronal cleft in rhizomelic chondrodysplasia punctata. Pediatr Pathol 1992; 12:593

Jansen-Type Metaphyseal Chondrodysplasia

de Haas WHD, de Boer W, Griffioen F: Metaphyseal dysostosis: a late follow-up of the first reported case. J Bone Joint Surg Br 1969;51:290

Kruse K, Schute C: Calcium metabolism in the Jansen type of metaphyseal dysplasia. Eur J Pediatr 1993;152:912

Nazará Z, Hernandez A, Corona-Rivera E, et al: Further clinical and radiological features in metaphyseal chondrodysplasia Jansen type. Radiology 1981;140:697

Ozonoff MB: Metaphyseal dysostosis of Jansen. Radiology 1969;93: 1047

Schipani E, Langman CB, Parfitt AM, et al: Constitutively activated receptors for parathyroid hormone and parathyroid hormone-related peptide in Jansen's metaphyseal chondrodysplasia. N Engl J Med 1996;335:708

Silverthorn KG, Houston CS, Duncan BP: Mark Jansen's metaphyseal chondrodysplasia with long-term follow-up. Pediatr Radiol 1987; 17:119

Schmid-Type Metaphyseal Chondrodysplasia

Lachman RS, Rimoin DL, Spranger J: Metaphyseal chondrodysplasia, Schmid type: clinical and radiographic delineation with a review of the literature. Pediatr Radiol 1988;18:93

McIntosh I, Abbott MH, Warman ML, et al: Additional mutations of type X collagen confirm COL10A1 as the Schmid metaphyseal chondrodysplasia locus. Hum Mol Genet 1994;3:303

McKusick-Type Metaphyseal Chondrodysplasia

Mäkitie O, Marttinen E, Kaitila I: Skeletal growth in cartilage-hair hypoplasia: a radiological study of 82 patients. Pediatr Radiol 1992;22:434

Mäkitie O, Kaitila I: Cartilage-hair hypoplasia—clinical manifestations in 108 Finnish patients. Eur J Pediatr 1993;152:211

van der Burgt I, Haraldsson A, Oosterwijk JC, et al: Cartilage hair hypoplasia, metaphyseal chondrodysplasia type McKusick: description of seven patients and review of the literature. Am J Med Genet 1991;41:371

Shwachman-Diamond Syndrome

McLennan TW, Steinbach HL: Shwachman's syndrome: the broad spectrum of bony abnormalities. Radiology 1974;112:167

Robberecht E, Nachtegaele P, Van Rattinghe R, et al: Pancreatic lipomatosis in the Shwachman-Diamond syndrome: identification by sonography and CT-scan. Pediatr Radiol 1985;15:348

Shwachman H, Diamond L: The syndrome of pancreatic insufficiency and bone marrow dysfunction. J Pediatr 1964;65:645

Taybi H, Mitchell AD, Friedman GD: Metaphyseal dysostosis and associated syndrome of pancreatic insufficiency and blood disorders. Radiology 1969;93:563

Kozlowski-Type Spondylometaphyseal Dysplasia

Kozlowski K, Maroteaux P, Spranger JW: La dysostose spondylo-métaphysaire. Presse Med 1967;75:2769

Lachman R, Zonana J, Khajavi A, Rimoin D: The spondylometaphyseal dysplasias: clinical, radiologic and pathologic correlation [in French]. Ann Radiol (Paris) 1979;22:125

Dyschondrosteosis

Belin V, Cusin V, Viot G, et al: SHOX mutations in dyschondrosteosis (Leri-Weill syndrome). Nature Genet 1998;19:67

Carter AR, Currey HL: Dyschondrosteosis (mesomelic dwarfism)—a family study. Br J Radiol 1974;47:634

Young LW, Goldberg EE, Morrison J: Radiological case of the month: Dyschondrosteosis. Am J Dis Child 1978;132:1038

Trichorhinophalangeal Syndrome Types I and II

Fryns JP, Logghe N, van Eygen M, Van den Berghe H: Langer-Giedion syndrome and deletion of the long arm of chromosome 8. Hum Genet 1981;58:231

Giedion A: Das tricho-rhino-phalangeale syndrome. Helv Paediatr Acta 1966;21:475

Hamers A, Jongbloet P, Peeters G, et al: Severe mental retardation in a patient with tricho-rhino-phalangeal syndrome type I and 8q deletion. Eur J Pediatr 1990;149:618

Ludecke HJ, Wagner MJ, Nardmann J, et al: Molecular dissection of a contiguous gene syndrome: localization of the genes involved in Langer-Giedion syndrome. Hum Mol Genet 1995;4:31

Momeni P, Glockner G, Schmidt O, et al: Mutations in a new gene, encoding a zinc-finger protein, cause tricho-rhino-phalangeal syndrome type I. Nature Genet 2000;24:71

Parizel PM, Dumon J, Vossen P, et al: The tricho-rhino-phalangeal syndrome revisited. Eur J Radiol 1987;7:154

Zaletaev DV, Kuleshov NP, Lur'e IV, Marincheva GS: Langer-Giedion syndrome and a deletion in the long arm of chromosome 8 [in Russian]. Genetika 1987;213:907

Acromesomelic Dysplasia of Maroteaux

Borrelli P, Fasanelli S, Marini R: Acromesomelic dwarfism in a child with an interesting family history. Pediatr Radiol 1983;13:165

Kant SG, Polinkovsky A, Mundlos S: Acromesomelic dysplasia Maroteaux type maps to human chromosome 9. Am J Hum Genet 1998;63:155

Langer LO Jr, Beals RK, Solomon IL, et al: Acromesomelic dwarfism: manifestations in childhood. Am J Med Genet 1977;1:87

Langer LO, Garrett RT: Acromesomelic dysplasia. Radiology 1980; 137:349

Maroteaux P, Martinelli B, Campailla E: Le nanisme acromésomélique. Presse Med 1971;79:1839

Cleidocranial Dysplasia

Keats TE: Cleidocranial dysostosis: some atypical roentgen manifestations. Am J Roentgenol Radium Ther Nucl Med 1967;100:71

Mundlos S: Cleidocranial dysplasia: clinical and molecular genetics. J Med Genet 1999;36:177

Campomelic Dysplasia

Khajavi A, Lachman R, Rimoin D, et al: Heterogeneity in the campomelic syndromes: long and short bone varieties. Radiology 1976;120:641

Macpherson RI, Skinner SA, Donnenfeld AE: Acampomelic campomelic dysplasia. Pediatr Radiol 1989;20:90

Tommerup N, Schempp W, Meinecke P, et al: Assignment of an autosomal sex reversal locus (SRA1) and campomelic dysplasia (CMPD1) to 17q24.3-q25.1. Nature Genet 1993;4:170

Mucopolysaccharidoses

Nelson J, Broadhead D, Mossman J: Clinical findings in 12 patients with MPS IV A (Morquio's disease): further evidence for heterogeneity. Part I: Clinical and biochemical findings. Clin Genet 1988; 33:111

Schmidt H, Ullrich K, von Lengerke HJ, et al: Radiological findings in patients with mucopolysaccharidosis I H/S (Hurler-Scheie syndrome). Pediatr Radiol 1987;17:409

Spranger J: Mini review: inborn errors of complex carbohydrate metabolism. Am J Med Genet 1987;28:489

van der Horst GTJ, Kleijer WJ, Hoogeveen AT, et al: Morquio B syndrome: a primary defect in β-galactosidase. Am J Med Genet 1983;16:261

Mucolipidosis II (I-Cell Disease)

Babcock DS, Bove KE, Hug G, et al: Fetal mucolipidosis II (I-cell disease): radiologic and pathologic correlation. Pediatr Radiol 1986;16:32

Lemaitre L, Remy J, Farriaux JP, et al: Radiological signs of mucolipidosis II or I-cell disease: a study of nine cases. Pediatr Radiol 1978;7:97

Osteogenesis Imperfecta

Byers PH, Wallis GA, Willing MC: Osteogenesis imperfecta: translation of mutation to phenotype. J Med Genet 1991;28:433

Lachman RS: Fetal imaging in the skeletal dysplasias: overview and experience. Pediatr Radiol 1994;24:413

Sillence DO, Barlow KK, Garber AP, et al: Osteogenesis imperfecta type II: delineation of the phenotype with reference to genetic heterogeneity. Am J Med Genet 1984;17:407

Tabor EK, Curtin HD, Hirsch BE, May M: Osteogenesis imperfecta tarda: appearance of the temporal bones at CT. Radiology 1990; 175:181

Hypophosphatasia

Oestreich AE, Bofinger MK: Prominent transverse (Bowdler) bone spurs as a diagnostic clue in a case of neonatal hypophosphatasia without metaphyseal irregularity. Pediatr Radiol 1989;19:341

Shohat M, Rimoin DL, Gruber HE, Lachman RS: Perinatal lethal hypophosphatasia: clinical, radiologic and morphologic findings. Pediatr Radiol 1991;21:421–427

Osteopetrosis

Andersen PE Jr, Bollerslev J: Heterogeneity of autosomal dominant osteopetrosis. Radiology 1987;164:223

el-Tawil T, Stoker BJ: Benign osteopetrosis: a review of 42 cases showing two different patterns. Skeletal Radiol 1993;22:587

Horton WA, Schimke RN, Iyama T: Osteopetrosis: further heterogeneity. J Pediatr 1980;97:580

Kaibara N, Katsuki I, Hotokebuchi T, Takagishi K: Intermediate form of osteopetrosis with recessive inheritance. Skeletal Radiol 1982;9:47

Kaplan FS, August CS, Fallon MD, et al: Osteopetrorickets: the paradox of plenty. Pathophysiology and treatment. Clin Orthop 1993;Sep[294]:64

Otsuka N, Fukunaga M, Ono S, et al: Bone marrow scintigraphy and MRI in a patient with osteopetrosis. Clin Nucl Med 1991;16:443

Rao VM, Dalinka MK, Mitchell DG, et al: Osteopetrosis: MR characteristics at 1.5 T. Radiology 1986;161:217

Schroeder RE, et al: Longitudinal follow-up of malignant osteopetrosis by skeletal radiographs and RLFP analysis after bone marrow transplantation. Pediatr 1992;88:986

Pyknodysostosis

Currarino G: Primary spondylolysis of the axis vertebra (C_2) in three children, including one with pyknodysostosis. Pediatr Radiol 1989; 19:535

Maroteaux P, Lamy M: La pycnodysostose. Presse Med 1962;70:999

Yousefzadeh DK, Agha AS, Reinertson J: Radiographic studies of upper airway obstruction with cor pulmonale in a patient with pycnodysostosis. Pediatr Radiol 1979;8:45

Craniodiaphyseal Dysplasia

Brueton LA, Winter RM: Craniodiaphyseal dysplasia. J Med Genet 1990;27:701

Tucker AS, et al: Craniodiaphyseal dysplasia: evolution over a five-year period. Skeletal Radiol 1976;1:47

Craniometaphyseal Dysplasia

Carnevale A, Grether P, del Castillo V, et al: Autosomal dominant craniometaphyseal dysplasia: clinical variability. Clin Genet 1983; 23:17

Holt JF: The evolution of cranio-metaphyseal dysplasia. Ann Radiol 1966;9:209

Penchaszadeh VB, Gutierrez ER, Figueroa E: Autosomal recessive craniometaphyseal dysplasia. Am J Med Genet 1980;5:43

Pyle Dysplasia

Heselson NG, Raad MS, Hamersma H: The radiological manifestations of metaphyseal dysplasia (Pyle disease). Br J Radiol 1979; 52:431

Shibuya H, Suzuki S, Okuyama T, Yukawa Y: The radiological appearances of familial metaphyseal dysplasia. Clin Radiol 1982; 33:439

Spondyloenchondromatosis

Frydman M, Bar-Ziv J, Preminger-Shapiro R, et al: Possible heterogeneity in spondyloenchondrodysplasia: quadraparesis, basal ganglia calcifications, and chondrocyte inclusions. Am J Med Genet 1990; 36:279

Menger H, Kruse K, Spranger J: Spondyloenchondrodysplasia. J Med Genet 1989;26:93

Schorr S, Legum C, Ochshorn M: Spondyloenchondrodysplasia: enchondromatosis with severe platyspondyly in two brothers. Radiology 1976;118:133

Dysspondyloenchondromatosis

Azouz EM: Case report 418: multiple enchondromatosis (Ollier disease) with severe vertebral changes. Skeletal Radiol 1987;16:236

Freisinger P, Finidori G, Maroteaux P: Dysspondylochondromatosis. Am J Med Genet 1993;45:460

Kozlowski K, Brostrom K, Kennedy J, et al: Dysspondyloenchondromatosis in the newborn: report of four cases. Pediatr Radiol 1994; 24:311

Osteolysis

Macpherson RI, Walker RD, Kowall MH: Essential osteolysis with nephropathy. J Can Assoc Radiol 1973;24:98

Tuncbilek E, Besim A, Bakkaloglu A, et al: Carpal-tarsal osteolysis. Pediatr Radiol 1985;15:255

Nail–Patella Syndrome

Dreyer SD, Morello R, German MS, et al: LMX1B transactivation and expression in nail-patella syndrome. Hum Mol Genet 2000;9:1067

Guidera KJ, Satterwhite Y, Ogden JA, et al: Nail patella syndrome: a review of 44 orthopaedic patients. J Pediatr Orthop 1991;11:737

Reed D, Nichols DM: Computed tomography of "iliac horns" in hereditary osteo-onychodysplasia (nail-patella syndrome). Pediatr Radiol 1987;17:168

■
■

P A R T   V I

SELECTED SYNDROMES AND CHROMOSOMAL DISORDERS

WILLIAM H. McALISTER

THOMAS E. HERMAN

KEITH A. KRONEMER

There has been a remarkable expansion of our knowledge base in the realm of developmental biology and pathobiology of inherited and acquired conditions. In this part, we describe some syndromes and chromosomal disorders (Table 1) that we believe would be of greatest interest and usefulness to radiologists.

SYNDROMES

ACRORENAL SYNDROME

The acrorenal syndrome is a familial condition characterized by hand anomalies, foot anomalies, and renal dysgenesis. The inheritance is most often autosomal dominant, although recessive inheritance does occur. The most frequent hand and foot anomalies are ectrodactyly, oligodactyly, syndactyly, brachydactyly, and anomalous tarsal and carpal bones. Oligomeganephronic renal hypoplasia is the most common renal anomaly, although collecting system duplications, hydronephrosis, and bladder outlet obstruction also occur. In patients with oligomeganephronic renal hypoplasia, renal failure is common. Cryptorchidism and hypospadias occur in 50% of males with acrorenal syndrome.

AMNIOTIC BAND SYNDROME

Amniotic band syndrome is a collection of mechanical injuries to the fetus arising from entanglement by bands of ruptured amnion. Findings include limb reductions or constrictions and craniofacial and body wall clefts. Radiographic findings in the hands and feet include partial or complete amputation of digits, single or multiple soft tissue constriction bands, and soft tissue fusions (Fig. 1). Bands can result in pseudoarthrosis and bowing or angulation deformities

Table 1 ■ SELECTED SYNDROMES AND CHROMOSOMAL DISORDERS	
Syndromes	
Acrorenal	Marfan
Amniotic band	Marshall-Smith
Bardet-Biedl	Mayer-Rokitansky-Küster-
Beckwith-Wiedemann	Hauser sequence
Brachmann-de Lange	Meckel's (Meckel-Gruber)
(Cornelia de Lange's)	Nail–patella
Cerebrocostomandibular	Nevoid basal cell carcinoma
Cerebrohepatorenal	(Gorlin's)
(Zellweger)	Noonan's
Cockayne's	Occipital horn
Congenital contractural	Opitz (G/BBB)
arachnodactyly	Oral-facial-digital
Congenital insensitivity to	Osteolysis
pain	Oropalatodigital
Currarino's triad	Pena-Shokeir I and II
Diamond-Blackfan	Poland's
Ehlers-Danlos	Progeria
Epidermolysis bullosa	Proteus
Fanconi's anemia	Rubinstein-Taybi
Fibrodysplasia ossifications	Russell-Silver
progressiva	Shwachman-Diamond
Freeman-Sheldon	Smith-Lemli-Opitz
(whistling face)	Sotos'
Goldenhar's	Thrombocytopenia–absent
Hadju-Cheney	radius (TAR)
Hallermann-Streiff	VACTERL (VATER)
Holt-Oram	association
Homocystinuria	Warfarin embryopathy
Kaufman-McKusick	Weill-Marchesani
Klippel-Trénaunay	Werner's
Larsen's	Williams
Chromosomal Disorders	
Cri du chat	Trisomy 21 (Down)
Trisomy 13 (Patau's)	Turner's
Trisomy 18 (Edwards')	Wolf-Hirschhorn

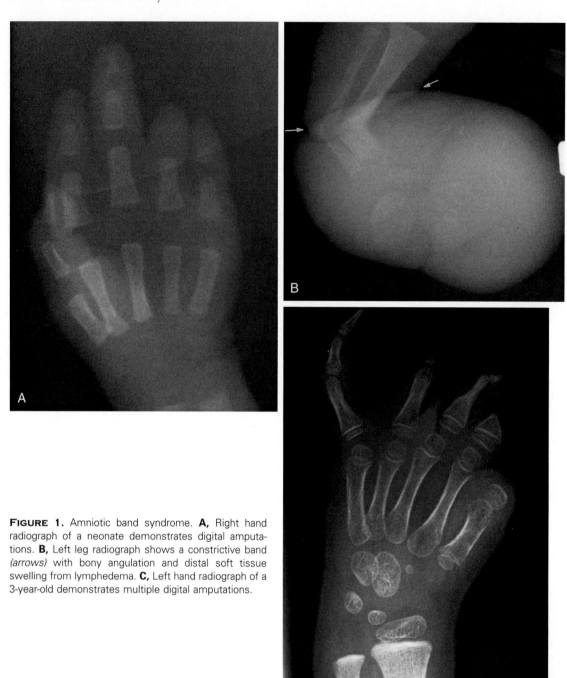

FIGURE 1. Amniotic band syndrome. **A,** Right hand radiograph of a neonate demonstrates digital amputations. **B,** Left leg radiograph shows a constrictive band *(arrows)* with bony angulation and distal soft tissue swelling from lymphedema. **C,** Left hand radiograph of a 3-year-old demonstrates multiple digital amputations.

of the long bones, and can deform any portion of the head, neck, or trunk. This syndrome's occurrence is sporadic; however, a possible association has been suggested with chorionic villus biopsy. Other authors suggest that somatic damage occurs as early as the first month of gestation. Prenatal sonography is helpful in evaluating limb, trunk, and craniofacial defects, as well as visualizing the bands. Spontaneous resolution of amniotic bands has been documented by sonography (see also Section IX, Part IV, Fig. 10, page 2105).

BARDET-BIEDL SYNDROME

Bardet-Biedl syndrome is an autosomal recessive condition now separated from the Laurence-Moon syndrome, a very rare condition with some features of Bardet-Biedl syndrome but characterized additionally by progressive spastic paralysis and ataxia. However, the Bardet-Biedl syndrome remains genetically heterogeneous, with linkage to at least five loci. Characteristic features of the Bardet-Biedl syndrome are obesity (92%), retinitis pigmentosa (92%), mental retardation (82%), polydactyly (72%), hypogenitalism (67%), and renal disease (approximately 100%). Other occasional features include heart disease (7%), diabetes mellitus (32% of patients by age 55 years), hearing loss, speech impairment, hepatic fibrosis, situs inversus, and Hirschsprung disease. In infancy, before obesity (at a mean age of 2 years) and retinitis pigmentosa (at a mean age of 8 years) develop, Bardet-Biedl syndrome may be confused with the Kaufman-McKusick syndrome.

Complications of the Bardet-Biedl syndrome are often severe. Almost all patients are blind by age 30 years. Approximately 25% of patients die before 44 years of age, with renal failure frequently being the cause of death.

Calyceal clubbing and blunting in the absence of reflux, fetal lobulation, small kidneys with parenchymal thinning, multiple renal calyceal diverticula (multidiverticular renal dysplasia) (Fig. 2), and a histologic glomerulopathy and tubulointerstitial nephropathy are the most frequent renal findings. Urinary tract infection and stone formation are common complications of multidiverticular renal dysplasia. One of the earliest clinical manifestation of renal disease is polydipsia and polyuria caused by a reduced concentrating ability resulting from decreased responsiveness to vasopressin. In some cases this may progress to nephrogenic diabetes insipidus.

Multidiverticular renal dysplasia is characteristically a stable congenital anomaly not related to reflux. Radiographically, similar cavities may be seen in renal tuberculosis, isolated calyceal diverticula, and renal papillary necrosis. The congenital nature and multiplicity of the diverticula excludes these diagnoses in Bardet-Biedl syndrome.

Hypogonadism is more obvious in male patients with Bardet-Biedl syndrome than in female patients. How-

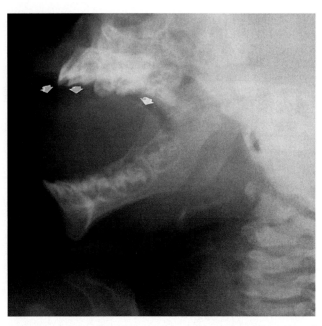

FIGURE 3. Beckwith-Wiedemann syndrome as seen on lateral facial radiograph. A massively enlarged tongue *(arrows)* is present in the oral cavity, holding the mouth open. In addition, the child had an omphalocele and a birth weight of over 4 kg.

ever hydrocolpos and vaginal atresia are common in females with this syndrome.

BECKWITH-WIEDEMANN SYNDROME

Beckwith-Wiedemann syndrome is an imprinted autosomal dominant condition characterized by exomphalos (anterior abdominal wall defects), macroglossia, hemihypertrophy, nephromegaly, islet cell hyperplasia, nephroblastomatosis, adrenal cytomegaly, neonatal adrenal macrocysts, linearly grooved ear lobes, intestinal malrotation, and an increased incidence of benign and malignant tumors. Beckwith-Wiedemann syndrome is usually associated with mutations at 11p15.5, the locus of the insulin-like growth factor-II (IGF-II) gene. In fact, cells that express IGF-II most abundantly are those that most frequently give rise to tumors in the Beckwith-Wiedemann syndrome. However, the inheritance of the syndrome may be complex because imprinting is common. Imprinting is the functional difference between maternal- and paternal-derived chromosomes. The paternal mutation is associated with an excess of growth promoter and the maternal mutation with a deficiency of growth suppression.

Originally Beckwith-Wiedemann syndrome was described as a triad of exomphalos, macroglossia, and gigantism. The most characteristic of these abnormalities is macroglossia, occurring in 99% of patients and often requiring surgical reduction because of feeding and respiratory difficulties (Fig. 3). Gigantism (defined as postnatal size over the 90th percentile) is present in 87% of patients. Anterior abdominal wall defects occur in 50% to 70% of patients. Hemihypertrophy is found in 25% and is the only clinical feature highly associated

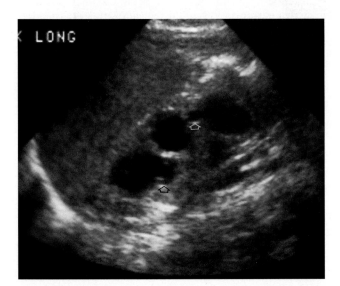

FIGURE 2. Bardet-Biedl syndrome as seen on longitudinal right renal sonogram. Caliectasis is present, with cortical thinning and a small calyceal diverticulum from a lower pole calyx and a larger one from an upper pole calyx, consistent with multidiverticular renal dysplasia seen in this syndrome. *Arrows* indicate diverticulae.

with the development of malignancy. Neonatal neph-romegaly is a feature that may also be associated with an increased risk of Wilms' tumor. Neonatal hypoglycemia is most often transient, but in severe cases may be prolonged and associated with neurologic damage if not appropriately treated.

The risk of malignant tumor is approximately 7%. The most common malignant tumors found are Wilms' tumor, adrenal carcinoma, and hepatoblastoma and neuroblastoma. Other tumors that may occur include rhabdomyosarcoma, pancreatoblastoma, breast fibroad-enoma, gastric teratoma, hepatic hemangioendotheli-oma, and splenic hemangioma. Most patients have been found to have favorable-outcome tumors. Although controversial, tumor surveillance screening in Beckwith-Wiedemann syndrome is widely practiced, with current recommendations including abdominal sonography to evaluate renal, adrenal, pancreatic, and hepatic masses every 3 to 6 months at least to the age of 6 years and possibly to 12 years of age.

BRACHMANN-DE LANGE (CORNELIA DE LANGE'S) SYNDROME

The Brachmann-de Lange syndrome is characterized by mental retardation, a low birth weight, postnatal growth retardation, a characteristic facies (synophrys, low anterior hairline, long eyelashes, microbrachycephaly, a short upturned nose, and carp mouth), and upper limb anomalies. Clinical findings vary considerably, and there is no known genetic or biochemical basis for the syndrome.

The radiographic changes in the upper limbs may be severe and variable and include micromelia, phocomelia, dislocation and deformity of the radial heads, and ulnar dysgenesis. Severe cases have reduction deformities of the ulna and ulnar portion of the hand (Fig. 4). Most other syndromes have a radial rather than an ulnar deficiency. The digital findings are also variable and include proximal placed thumbs, short and broad first metacarpals, syndactyly, clinodactyly, oligodactyly, ectrodactyly, abnormal metacarpophalangeal pattern profile, small digits, and delayed skeletal maturation. Findings in the chest are increased anteroposterior diameter, short sternum with reduced number of ossification centers and premature fusion, slender and sloping ribs, fusion of the first two ribs, clavicles that are hooked laterally, and tracheomegaly. Gastrointestinal problems are common and can be severe, and include reflux esophagitis, aspiration pneumonia, esophageal stenosis, and Sandifer's syndrome. Miscellaneous findings include clubfoot, flat acetabula, Legg-Perthes disease, large anterior fontanelle, small brachycephalic skull, and supracondylar spurs.

Based on the clinical variability of Brachmann-de Lange syndrome, the following classification has been proposed:

Type I (classical form)—characteristic and skeletal changes, growth deficiency, and severe psychomotor retardation

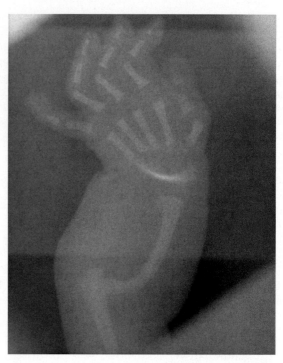

FIGURE 4. Radiograph of upper extremity in a child with Brachmann-de Lange (Cornelia de Lange's) syndrome shows absent ulna with dislocated elbow and flexion deformities of the hand.

Type II—milder clinical manifestations
Type III (phenocopy type)—causally related to chromosomal aneuploidies or teratogenic exposures

There are no biochemical/genetic tests that can make the diagnosis; the diagnosis is based on the characteristic facial features, prenatal and postnatal growth retardation, mental retardation, and the deficiency defects of the upper limbs.

CEREBROCOSTOMANDIBULAR (RIB-GAP) SYNDROME

Cerebrocostomandibular syndrome, also called rib-gap syndrome, is characterized by features of the Pierre-Robin syndrome (small mandible, cleft palate, glossoptosis) and posterior rib gaps (usually the third through the seventh, although all rib levels have been reported) (Fig. 5). Neonatal respiratory distress is the usual presenting sign. Eventually the rib gaps, which can be symmetric, will partially heal and may give rise to pseudoarthrosis (Fig. 5C). Mental retardation is seen in one half of the patients and microcephaly in 20%. Miscellaneous findings include stippled epiphyses, clubfoot, elbow dysplasia, scoliosis, multiple ossification centers of the calcaneus, vesicoureteral reflux, and renal cysts. The disease is likely autosomal recessive, but evidence of autosomal dominant inheritance has also been reported.

CEREBROHEPATORENAL (ZELLWEGER) SYNDROME

Cerebrohepatorenal, or Zellweger, syndrome is the result of mutation of genes involved in peroxisome biogenesis. Knowing the PEX1 gene mutation helps predict the course of the disease. A characteristic flat facies with a high forehead, severe hypotonia, seizures, mental retardation, liver enlargement and dysfunction, stippled epiphyses, and renal cysts can be found in this syndrome. The infants, because of the facies, have been confused with those with Down syndrome. The most helpful radiographic findings include stippled calcifications, typically of the patellas and the Y cartilages of the pelvis. The calcifications can involve many areas and can be periarticular (Fig. 6A, B). The renal cysts tend to be small and in the periphery of the kidneys (Fig. 6C). Extremity abnormalities include contractures, clubfoot, and retarded skeletal maturation. There are dysmyelination and neuronal migration derangements resulting in microgyria, pachygyria,

heterotopic dysplasia of the inferior olivar nucleus, ventricular dilatation, widened cranial sutures, and dolichocephaly. Death in infancy is typical, but some patients have lived into the teenage years. There is a mouse model for Zellweger syndrome.

COCKAYNE'S SYNDROME

This syndrome's manifestations usually start at birth with a progressive growth failure. Microcephaly, mental retardation, sun sensitivity, premature aging (Fig. 7), sensorineural hearing loss, abnormal nerve conduction, disproportionally long limbs with large hands and feet, flexion contractures, and eye abnormalities (including enophthalmos, retinal pigmentation and degeneration, optic atrophy, and cataracts) can be seen. Exposure of cells to ultraviolet light in this syndrome results in chromosomal breakage. The disease is autosomal recessive. The dwarfing is proportional, and the radiographic

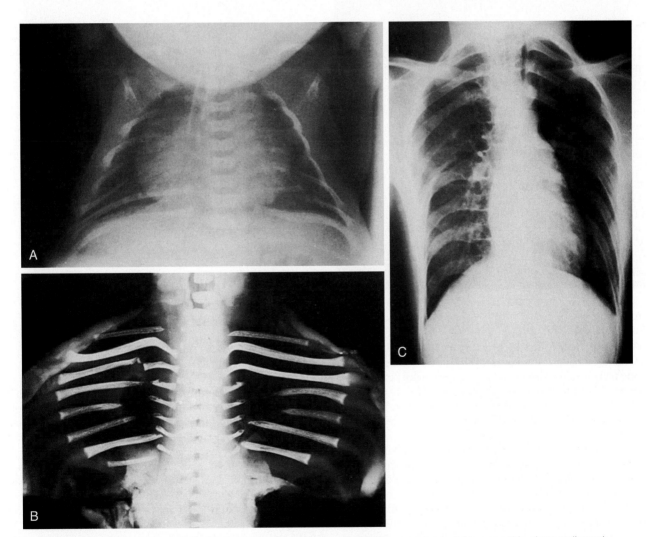

FIGURE 5. Cerebrocostomandibular syndrome. **A,** Posterior rib defects are seen in infancy on this chest radiograph. **B,** Outfolded chest wall at necropsy shows multiple rib gaps after removal of the thoracic contents. **C,** In survivors, the chest radiograph shows that some of the defects may fill in, resulting in a deformed but intact thoracic cage. (From Silverman FN, Strefling AM, Stevenson DK, et al: Cerebro-costo-mandibular syndrome. J Pediatr 1980;97:408–416, with permission.)

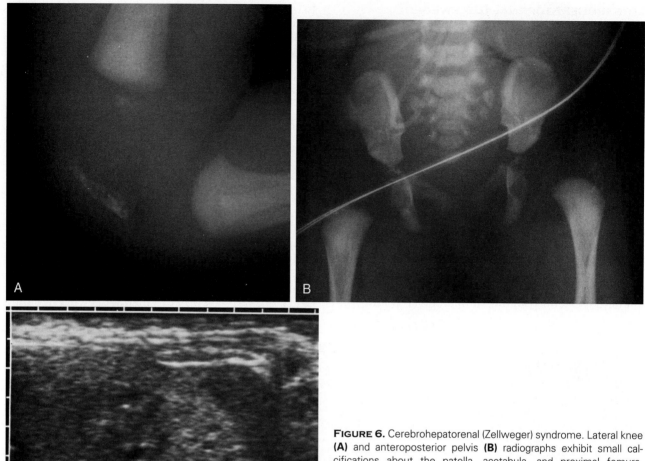

FIGURE 6. Cerebrohepatorenal (Zellweger) syndrome. Lateral knee **(A)** and anteroposterior pelvis **(B)** radiographs exhibit small calcifications about the patella, acetabula, and proximal femurs. **C,** Transverse sonogram of left kidney illustrates cysts, the largest of which is indicated by an *arrow.*

findings include microcephaly, thin long bones with narrow medullary cavities and flared metaphyses, large-appearing ossification centers, large carpal and tarsal bones, hypoplasia of the iliac wings and acetabular roofs, brachydactyly, ivory epiphyses in the distal phalanges, thin ribs (Fig. 8), coxa valga, and abnormal vertebral bodies with anterior notching with resultant kyphosis or posterior scalloping. Other findings that have been seen include short and broad metacarpals and metatarsals, fibular bowing, slender clavicles, and progressive osteolysis.

In addition to microcephaly, the sella is small and the calvaria are thick. Calcification in the cerebral cortex and basal ganglia, ventricular dilatation, demyelination, leukodystrophy, and atrophy are common. The classical form of the disease is called type I; an early-onset, more severe form associated with early death is called type II; and there is a mild form of the disease called type III.

CONGENITAL CONTRACTURAL ARACHNODACTYLY

Congenital contractural arachnodactyly is an autosomal dominant disorder of connective tissue that is characterized by arachnodactyly, multiple congenital flexion contractures, external ear malformations (crumpled ears), and progressive kyphoscoliosis. It is phenotypically related to Marfan syndrome. Mutations in the fibrillin-2 *(FBN2)* gene cause this disorder. This gene has been mapped to the 5q23-31 region of chromosome 5 and this has been used in prenatal diagnosis of the condition.

The imaging findings consist of arachnodactyly (Fig. 9), camptodactyly, and flexion contractures that are usually symmetric and affect the knees most severely. As the contractures improve during childhood, scoliosis or kyphoscoliosis appears, although it may be present in

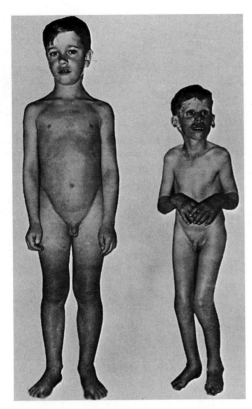

FIGURE 7. Normal boy **(left)** and boy with Cockayne's syndrome **(right)**, both age 10 years. Patient with Cockayne's syndrome manifests short stature, shriveled facies, microcephaly, large ears and lower jaw, and disproportionately large hands and feet. (From MacDonald WB, Fitch KD, Lewis IC: Cockayne's syndrome: an heredofamilial disorder of growth and development. Pediatrics 1960;25:997–1007, with permission.)

infancy. Kyphoscoliosis is progressive and usually starts before age 5 years. The long bones are long and narrow, and, along with normal-width epiphyses, make the joints appear prominent. Slight long bone bowing is also present. Skeletal adaptive changes are seen in the joints secondary to contractures. Congenital limb deficiencies have also been seen, as have heart abnormalities, especially mitral valve prolapse and aortic root dilatation. The gastrointestinal abnormalities found include duodenal atresia, esophageal atresia, and intestinal malrotation.

CONGENITAL INSENSITIVITY TO PAIN

Congenital insensitivity to pain is an autosomal recessive disorder characterized by decreased sensitivity to pain without affecting touch or proprioception. Early radiographic changes include subperiosteal hemorrhages in neonates, with later development of fractures and epiphyseal separations near weight-bearing joints. Progression to neuropathic joints with destruction, especially periarticular; focal bony sclerosis; and fragmentation can be seen (Fig. 10). Osteomyelitis can also occur. Congenital insensitivity to pain has been misdiagnosed as child abuse.

CURRARINO'S TRIAD

The autosomal dominant Currarino's triad, or hereditary sacral agenesis syndrome, consists of congenital anal stenosis or low imperforate anus, sickle or scimitar

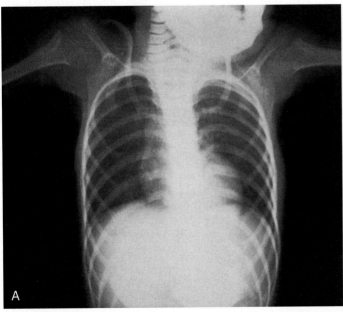

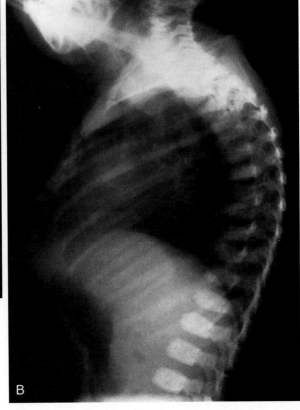

FIGURE 8. Frontal **(A)** and lateral **(B)** radiographs of the chest on an extremely small 5-year-old with Cockayne's syndrome show thin, sclerotic ribs and clavicles and proximal humeri, along with osteopenia and an increased anteroposterior diameter of the chest.

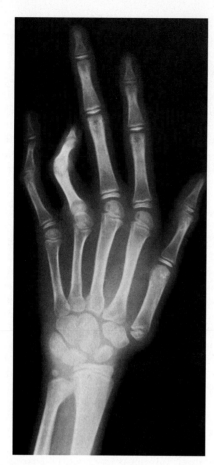

FIGURE 9. Posteroanterior radiograph of right hand of a 9-year-old girl with contractural arachnodactyly demonstrates the arachnodactyly and flexion deformities of fourth and fifth digits and mild osteopenia.

hemisacrum (Fig. 11*A*) and a presacral mass, either teratoma (two thirds of cases), lipoma, dermoid cyst, enteric cyst, or anterior meningocele (Fig. 11*B*). An intact first sacral segment and a sickle-shaped sacrum are distinctive to this syndrome. Myelodysplasia with tethered cord and intradural lipoma also occurs frequently. Malignant presacral teratomas are uncommon, but careful follow-up after resection of teratoma is required to exclude recurrence and malignant degeneration. The syndrome is linked to 7q36 deletions and is familial in 50% of patients. Approximately one third of patients with anal stenosis have Currarino's triad. In these patients, spinal magnetic resonance imaging MRI is helpful to exclude Currarino's triad lesions such as tethered cord or meningomycele. Meningoceles should be repaired prior to anorectoplasty because of the risk of meningitis. Asymptomatic affected patients are at risk for malignancies, especially if they have a typical sacral deformity.

DIAMOND-BLACKFAN SYNDROME

Diamond-Blackfan anemia is a constitutional erythroblastopenia characterized by absent or decreased erythroid precursors that usually presents in the first year of life. Most cases are sporadic, but autosomal dominant and recessive inheritance have been reported. The disease, previously mapped to chromosome 19q13, is frequently associated with a variety of malformations. Physical abnormalities are seen in about a third of patients and are more likely in boys (50%) than girls (25%). Thumb abnormalities, especially the triphalangeal thumb, are the most characteristic radiographic feature but were found in only 18% of the patients (Fig. 12). Other findings in the thumb that are more common include hypoplasia, duplication, subluxation, absence, and flat thenar eminence. Radial ray anomalies, Klippel-Feil syndrome, and Sprengel's deformity can be seen along with some renal findings that include horseshoe kidneys, renal dysplasia, and hypoplasia. Abnormal facial features are many and include snub nose, thick upper lips, widely separated eyes, and cleft palate.

EHLERS-DANLOS SYNDROME

Ehlers-Danlos syndrome (EDS) is a heterogeneous group of inherited anomalies of connective tissue characterized by varying degrees of skin hyperextensibility, joint hypermobility, and connective tissue fragility. Mutations in genes that deal with collagen seem to be the cause of EDS. Variable expression of the features, different modes of inheritance, and distinctive associated manifestations distinguish the 11 types of the syndrome. Joint laxity, hypermobility, and dislocation are most often seen with types I, III, VI, VII, and XI, while scoliosis is associated with types I, VI, and XI, being most severe in type VI. Aneurysms and spontaneous arterial rupture are typically associated with type IV, and vessel rupture (either arterial or venous) can be a hazard when performing angiography. Supporting structures of the colon, bladder, and uterus can be weakened by defective collagen and spontaneously rupture, especially in types I and IV. Recurrent inguinal hernias should raise the possibility of EDS, as should unexplained bladder or bowel diverticula in children.

Joint dislocation or subluxation can involve any joint and be acute, chronic, or repetitive (Fig. 13). The hip may be dislocated at birth, especially in type VII. Premature polyarticular arthritis may result from the dislocations. The affected joints can be large (e.g., hip, knee, and shoulder) or small (e.g., in the thumb). Flatfoot, clubfoot, and hallux valgus are common. Subcutaneous round soft tissue calcifications are characteristic of EDS. The joint laxity, especially in children, may be associated with pain, and a suspicion of arthritis will arise.

In addition to scoliosis or kyphoscoliosis (types I, VI, and XI), there may be spondylolisthesis and a wide spinal canal. A lateral upper spine radiograph may show the cervical and upper thoracic vertebrae because of the downward-sloping shoulders. In the chest, there may be recurrent pneumothorax, cystic lung disease (Fig. 14), and mitral valve prolapse.

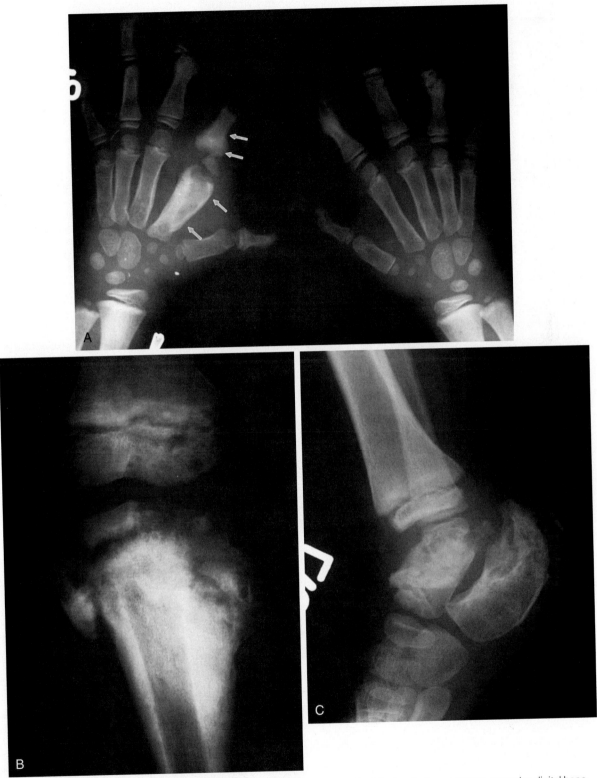

FIGURE 10. Congenital insensitivity to pain. **A,** Posteroanterior radiograph of the hands demonstrates extensive digital bone loss, with marked periostitis involving the right second metacarpal and the remaining portion of the proximal phalanx *(arrows)*. Anteroposterior knee **(B)** and lateral ankle **(C)** radiographs demonstrate fragmentation and irregularity typical of neuropathic joints.

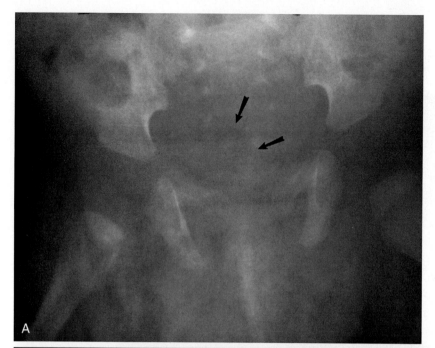

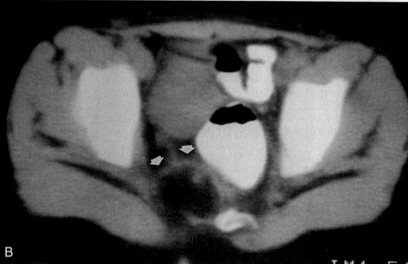

FIGURE 11. Currarino's triad. **A,** Anteroposterior radiograph of the pelvis. A crescentic defect is present in the right inferior sacrum *(arrows),* producing a so-called scimitar sacrum. **B,** Computed tomography scan of the pelvis at the level of the sacral defect in a patient with anal stenosis demonstrates a small fat-containing mass *(arrows)* at the level of the sacral defect. This was surgically removed and proved to be a teratoma.

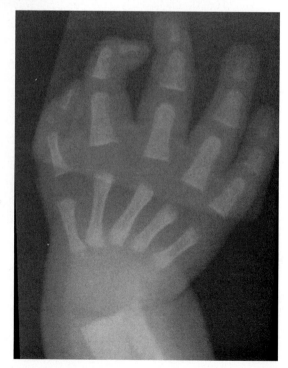

FIGURE 12. Posteroanterior hand radiograph in a 1-week-old with Diamond-Blackfan syndrome shows a triphalangeal thumb.

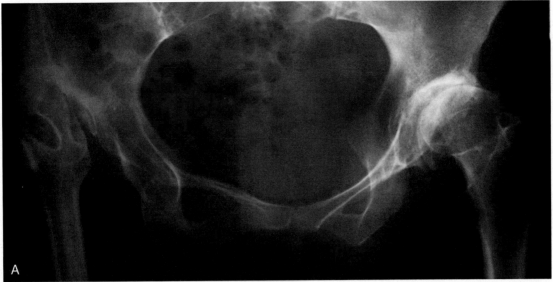

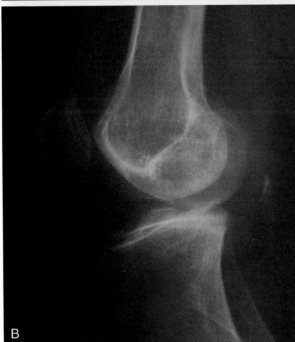

FIGURE 13. Ehlers-Danlos syndrome. **A,** Radiograph of the pelvis shows the end result of a congenital dislocation of the right hip, with absorption of much of the femoral head and neck, soft tissue calcification, and secondary acetabular dysplasia. There is lateral subluxation and joint space narrowing on the left. **B,** Lateral knee radiograph demonstrates anterior subluxation of the tibia on the femur.

EPIDERMOLYSIS BULLOSA

Epidermolysis bullosa (EB) is the name given to several conditions in which there is extreme fragility of the skin because of breakdown of tissues at the junction between the epidermis and dermis. Three familial varieties are recognized:

1. Autosomal dominant EB simplex, in which no gastrointestinal manifestations are usually present.
2. Autosomal recessive junctional EB, which is associated with pyloric atresia.
3. Autosomal recessive and dominant varieties of EB dystrophica in which, particularly in the recessive forms, severe esophageal involvement may occur.

Acquired EB is an autoimmune disease sometimes associated with Crohn's disease and ulcerative colitis.

Pyloric atresia in junctional EB is due to fibrous tissue, although its etiology is uncertain. Junctional EB is almost uniformly fatal and often referred to as EB lethalis. Recessive EB dystrophica is associated with esophageal strictures, predominantly in the upper esophagus, that may be multiple and lead to complete esophageal obstruction (Fig. 15). In addition, anal stricturing may lead to constipation or obstipation, and vaginal and periurethral stricturing may lead to bladder and vaginal obstruction.

FANCONI'S ANEMIA

Fanconi's anemia is a rare autosomal recessive disease characterized by multiple congenital abnormalities, pancytopenia, and cancer susceptibility, especially to leukemia, although an increased incidence of malignancies occurs in many organs. There is evidence for at least eight Fanconi genes. The mean age of onset is 8 years, and the mean survival is 16 years. About 50% have radial ray abnormalities ranging from bilateral absent thumbs and radii to unilateral hypoplastic thumb or bifid thumb (Fig. 16). Renal abnormalities occur in about one third of the patients and include absence of one kidney, horseshoe kidney, hypoplasia, double ureters, and hydronephrosis. Microcephaly, mental retardation, mild hearing loss, ear malformations, café au lait spots, brown pigmentation of the skin, and short stature are features of this condition.

Syndactyly, brachydactyly, pseudoepiphysis of the first metacarpal, retarded bone age, hooked clavicles, Sprengel's deformity, clubfoot, hip dislocation, scoliosis, kyphosis, and sacral agenesis can be seen. Gastrointestinal findings are occasionally seen and include tracheoesophageal fistula, duodenal atresia and stenosis, malrotation, and anorectal malformations. Central nervous system abnormalities include brain tumors, Arnold-Chiari malformation, hydrocephalus, microcephaly, and moyamoya disease.

FIBRODYSPLASIA OSSIFICANS PROGRESSIVA

Fibrodysplasia ossificans progressiva is a rare disorder of connective tissue characterized by congenital malformations of the great toes and intermittently progressive heterotopic ossification of the striated muscles and soft tissue, especially over the spine and shoulder, leading to progressive disability. Most cases arise by spontaneous mutation, but autosomal dominant inheritance has been demonstrated. Linkage of the fibrodysplasia ossification progressiva phenotype was found to the 4q27-q31 region. Altered expression of bone morphogenic proteins may be a contributing cause.

The disease is manifested at birth by shortened great toes, which are found in most instances and evidenced on radiographs as a short monophalangeal digit, often with hallux valgus (Fig. 17A; see also Section IX, Part II, Chapter 1, Fig. 14, page 2010). A short proximal first phalanx subluxed laterally on the first metatarsal is also typical. The sesamoids associated with the first metatarsophalangeal joints are absent. The terminal phalanges

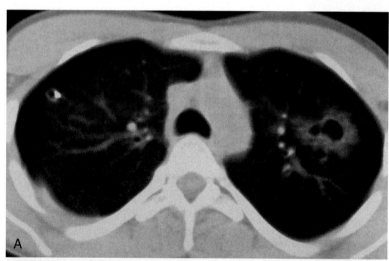

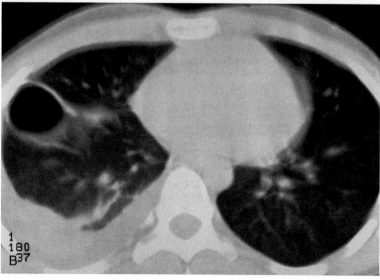

FIGURE 14. Chest computed tomography scans (**A** and **B**) in a teenager with Ehlers-Danlos syndrome who presented with a spontaneous right pneumothorax. The scans, taken at different levels, show multiple cystic areas in the lung, in addition to a right pneumothorax and right pleural reaction.

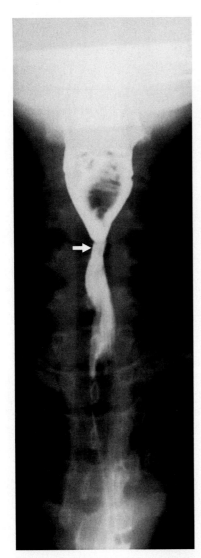

FIGURE 15. Barium swallow in teenager with epidermolysis bullosa shows a cervical esophageal stricture *(arrow)*.

of the thumbs are short and pointed, as are some of the phalanges.

Other skeletal findings include broad short femoral necks, small cervical vertebral bodies, variable vertebral fusion, narrow spinal canal in the lumbar region, exostoses on many bones from ossification of ligamentosus insertions, polydactyly, synovial chondromatosis, and metaphyseal irregularities.

The soft tissue changes often start as cystic soft tissue swellings in the subcutaneous tissues of the neck, back, and shoulders (see Section IX, Part II, Chapter 1, Fig. 13, page 2009), and the ossification can evolve a few months later (Fig. 17*B, C*). The average age to first identify ossification is 5 years (range, birth to 25 years). By age 15 years, a majority of patients will have restricted mobility of the arms. Large sheets of bones with cortex and medullary cavities can immobilize joints (Fig. 17*C*). Heterotopic ossification proceeds from axial to appendicular, cranial to caudal, and proximal to distal.

Computed tomography (CT) nicely demonstrates the extent of ectopic ossification, while MRI may be useful in assessing soft tissue changes.

FREEMAN-SHELDON (WHISTLING FACE) SYNDROME

Freeman-Sheldon syndrome, also known as whistling face syndrome, is an uncommon entity characterized clinically by its characteristic facies and lip protrusion, with the lips held as if whistling. Brain anomalies and hearing loss have been reported. Radiologic findings include craniofacial disproportion with brachycephaly, ulnar deviation of the hands, disharmonic maturation of the carpals compared with the phalanges, mild vertebral abnormalities including scoliosis, hip and radial head dislocations, equinovarus of the feet, digital contractures, and delayed skeletal maturity. The syndrome can be inherited with genetic heterogeneity,

FIGURE 16. Posteroanterior radiograph of the hand and forearm of a child with Fanconi's anemia shows an absent first ray, radius, and some carpal bones. The ulna is shortened and bowed. The patient also had only one kidney.

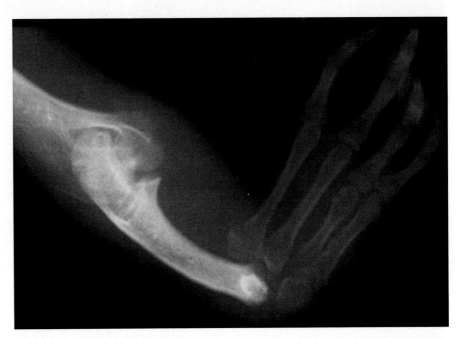

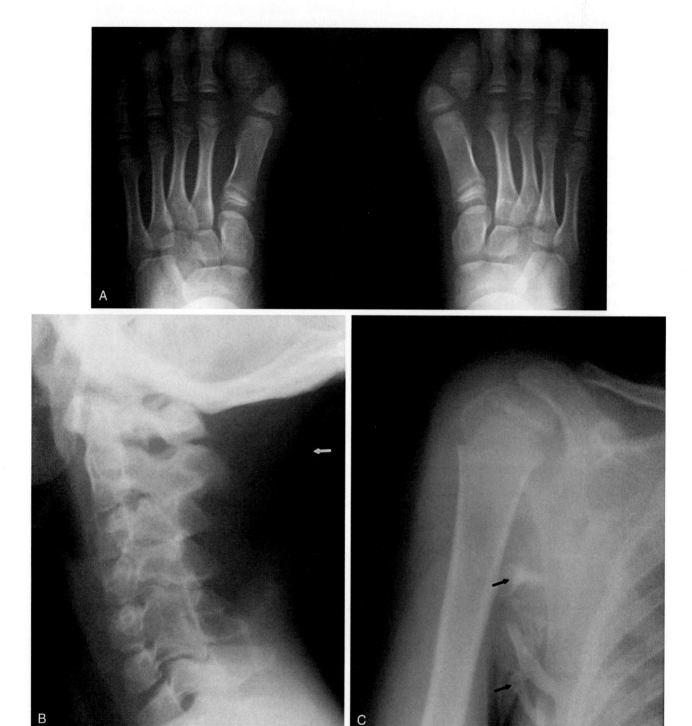

FIGURE 17. Fibrodysplasia ossifications progressiva. **A,** Radiograph of the feet of a 9-year-old boy showing the deformity of the great toes. **B,** Lateral neck radiograph in the same patient shows soft tissue ossification *(arrow).* Fusion has developed in the facet joints, with underdevelopment of the vertebral bodies. **C,** Soft tissue calcifications and ossifications *(arrows)* between the chest wall and right humerus are seen in this 5-year-old boy.

and has been diagnosed on prenatal sonography in an affected family.

GOLDENHAR'S SYNDROME

Goldenhar's syndrome, or oculoauriculovertebral syndrome (OAVS), is a sporadically occurring complex developmental field defect of unknown etiology, infrequently familial and caused by an event occurring at 30 to 45 days of gestation. The phenotype has been reported in association with other conditions, including trisomy 18 and maternal thalidomide, primidone, and retinoic acid use. The hallmarks of OAVS are epibulbar dermoids, preauricular appendages, mandibular hypoplasia, microtia, and vertebral anomalies. Most frequently the orbital lesions, mandibular hypoplasia (Fig. 18*A*) and microtia are unilateral and on the same side. Colobomas of the upper eyelid also occur in 60% of patients; they may be large and require immediate repair to prevent corneal ulceration. Colobomas and facial anomalies create some overlap between OAVS and CHARGE association (*c*oloboma of the eye, *h*eart defect, *a*tresia of the choanae, *r*etarded growth and development, *g*enital anomalies, and *e*ar defect with deafness). Deafness is not uncommon because of associated anomalies of the middle and inner ear.

Vertebral anomalies occur in 60% of patients and are most often cervical, including basilar invagination, occipitalization of the atlas, cervical synostosis, and hemivertebra (Fig. 18*B*). Vertebral anomalies below the cervical spine are found in only 10% of patients. However, they may be severe and associated with costal malformations similar to those of Jarcho-Levin syndrome.

Hemifacial microsomia consisting of macrostomia, unilateral microtia, and ipsilateral hypoplasia of the mandibular ramus and condyle is believed to characterize a well-defined subgroup of patients with Goldenhar's syndrome. A wide variety of additional anomalies have been described in OAVS patients, including renal anomalies; radial anomalies; clubfoot; vascular anomalies such as congenital absence of the portal vein; cerebral anomalies, including Arnold-Chiari malformation, lipoma, and/or agenesis of the corpus callosum; and cardiovascular anomalies, primarily ventricular septal defects, atrial septal defects, and pulmonic stenosis.

HAJDU-CHENEY SYNDROME

Hajdu-Cheney syndrome, or serpentine fibula–polycystic kidney syndrome, is an autosomal dominant disorder with characteristic facial features, osteolysis of the distal phalanges of the hands and feet, and multiple wormian bones. The face is broad, with low-set ears, bushy eyebrows, course hair, enlarged outer supraorbital ridges, long philtrum, hypoplastic midface, receding chin, early tooth loss, and prominent occiput. Craniofacial findings include multiple wormian bones, bathrocephaly, cranial suture persistence, hypoplastic sinuses, an elongated sella, progressive basilar impression, absorption of the anterior nasal spine, and anteriorly positioned mandibular condyles (Fig. 19). In over 90% of the patients, the hands and feet show band-like osteolysis in the middle of the distal phalanges, especially the former, that can start as early as age 3 to 4 years but typically occurs in late childhood (Fig. 20). Occa-

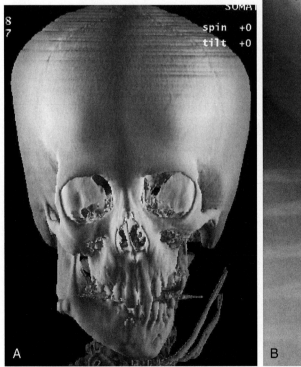
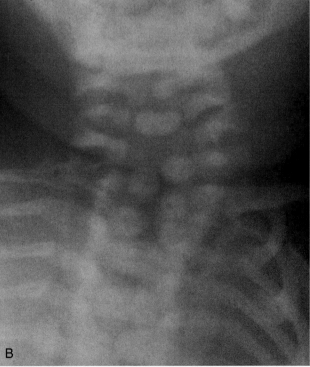

FIGURE 18. Goldenhar's syndrome (hemifacial microsomia). **A,** Marked left hemimandibular hypoplasia is present on this three-dimensional computed tomography scan. **B,** Cervical spine radiograph shows formation and segmentation errors.

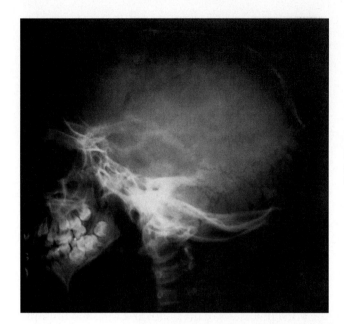

FIGURE 19. In Hajdu-Cheney syndrome, the skull is large, with prominence and bowing of the occipital bone. The lambdoid suture contains multiple wormian bones, and there is basilar impression.

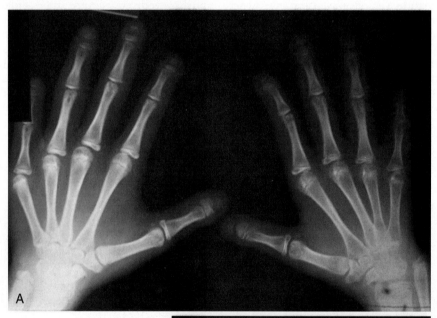

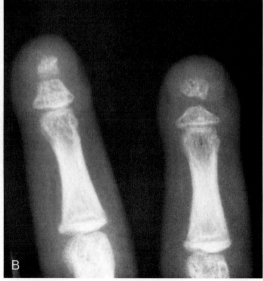

FIGURE 20. Hajdu-Cheney syndrome. **A,** Posteroanterior radiographs of the hands demonstrate osteolysis of the midportions of the distal phalanges. There is some irregularity and decreased size of the carpal bones, with elongation and displacement of the right distal ulna. **B,** Radiograph of the distal third and fourth digits shows the band-like osteolysis through the midportions of the distal phalanges.

sionally the middle phalanges are involved. Osteolysis may also be seen in the radial heads.

Other skeletal findings include osteoporosis, scolioses, kyphosis, vertebral body variation in height including biconcave vertebral flattening, coxa valga, dislocated hips and elbows, joint laxity, bowing of the bones, and short stature. Cystic kidney disease resembling adult polycystic disease can be seen in up to 10% of the patients, as can intestinal or renal malrotation.

The central nervous system findings include Arnold-Chiari malformation, hydrocephalus, and changes associated with the progressive basilar impression. Cardiovascular abnormalities include valvular disease and heart block.

HALLERMANN-STREIFF SYNDROME

Hallermann-Streiff syndrome is a sporadic condition associated with malformations of the face, skull, and eyes. Radiographic findings include a thin calvarium, small mandible, wide sutures, delayed fontanelle closure, dental abnormalities, and brachycephaly (Fig. 21). The appendicular skeleton demonstrates gracile bones with thinning of the cortex, while the axial skeleton is involved with scoliosis, lordosis, and platyspondyly. Other findings include osteopenia, decreased sternal ossification centers, and hip dislocation. Respiratory obstruction, particularly involving the upper airway, may lead to respiratory compromise, pulmonary hypertension, and death, especially in infancy. MRI may be useful in evaluating ocular changes, including microphthalmia and congenital cataracts.

HOLT-ORAM SYNDROME

Holt-Oram syndrome is a high-penetrant autosomal dominant condition in which anomalies of the upper extremities and shoulders are associated with congenital heart disease. The gene locus for this condition is on chromosome 12q24, at the T-box gene *TBX5*. The common limb anomalies range from phocomelia with absent or hypoplastic humerus (10% of patients in some series) to triphalangeal thumbs. The most common limb anomalies are radial ray anomalies (Fig. 22), including triphalangeal thumb, hypoplastic thumb, abnormal carpal scaphoid (bipartite or hypoplastic), extra carpal bones, absent or hypoplastic radii, and laterally hooked clavicles. The limb anomalies tend to be bilateral and asymmetric, usually more severe on the left. Cardiac anomalies occur in 76% to 95% of patients. The most common cardiac anomalies are secundum atrial septal defect, ventricular septal defect, and first-degree atrioventricular block. However, more severe heart disease, such as tetralogy of Fallot and atrioventricular canal, may occur.

HOMOCYSTINURIA

Homocystinuria is a metabolic disorder caused by cystathionine β-synthetase deficiency and is inherited as an autosomal recessive trait. The clinical manifestations are related to the central nervous system, eyes, skeleton, and vascular systems. Affected individuals are tall and thin. The central nervous system abnormality most often seen is mental retardation, which may result from vascular occlusions in the brain or in the carotid arteries,

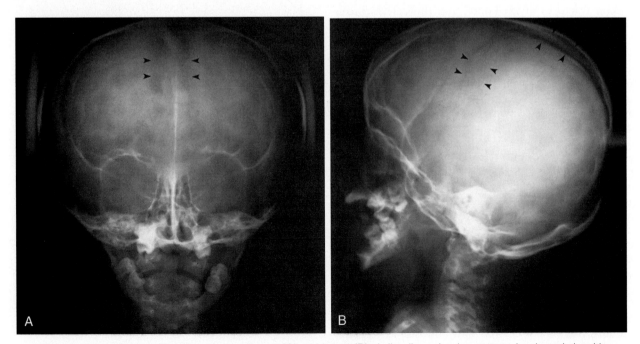

FIGURE 21. Hallermann-Streiff syndrome. Frontal **(A)** and lateral **(B)** skull radiographs demonstrate brachycephaly with sutural widening *(arrowheads)*, hypotelorism, micrognathia, and calvarial thinning.

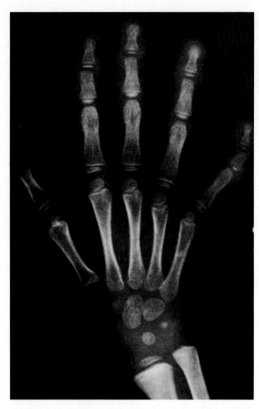

FIGURE 22. Radiograph of right hand in a patient with a known family history of Holt-Oram syndrome and a ventricular septal defect. Hypoplasia of first ray and adjacent carpal bones are shown, along with a triphalangeal thumb. Clinodactyly of the fifth digit is shown.

infarctions, and atrophy. The most common skeletal manifestation is osteoporosis, which may become severe and can result in biconcave vertebral bodies, compression fractures of the spine, and thoracic kyphosis (Fig. 23). There are long and slender bones, mild arachnodactyly not as severe as in Marfan syndrome, knock-knees, humerus varus, bony spicules in the distal radial and ulnar epiphyseal lines, cupped metaphyses, short fourth metacarpals, malformed and enlarged carpal bones, relative epiphyseal and metaphyseal enlargement resulting in part from the slender long bones, advanced skeletal maturation, and pes cavus. The skull is small but has large paranasal sinuses. Chest deformities are common, usually pectus excavatum or carinatum. The typical eye finding is ectopia lentis, but myopia and glaucoma can be seen. Thrombosis and embolism are the life-threatening complications, and they can involve any vessel in the body, either artery or vein. Coronary artery occlusions, renal artery stenoses with hypertension, and arterial thrombosis have the greatest clinical importance. Corrugated arterial walls can be seen on angiography, in addition to the occlusions.

A specific diagnosis is made by the typical pattern of amino acid disturbances in the blood: elevated methionine and homocystine levels and abnormally low cysteine levels. The vitamin B_6-responsive patients do better than the B_6-nonresponsive patients.

KAUFMAN-McKUSICK SYNDROME

Kaufman-McKusick syndrome is an autosomal recessive condition consisting of hydrometrocolpos usually due to vaginal atresia, anorectal malformation, mesoaxial or postaxial polydactyly, and congenital heart disease. The disease is frequently found in old-order Amish families in the United States. Males with the syndrome are diagnosed if there are affected female siblings, although postaxial polydactyly and hypospadias occur. Imperforate anus, often with a rectovaginal fistula, occurs in approximately 50% of patients. The congenital heart disease is often ventriculoseptal defect, atrioseptal defect, and single atria. There appears to be an increased incidence of long-segment Hirschsprung's disease in patients with this syndrome. The diagnosis of Kaufman-McKusick syndrome in mentally retarded patients should be made with care because of the overlap of findings of this syndrome with those of Bardet-Biedl syndrome.

KLIPPEL-TRÉNAUNAY SYNDROME

The triad of congenital varicosities, cutaneous hemangioma (port-wine nevus), and hypertrophy of bone and soft tissues in a limb typify Klippel-Trénaunay syndrome. Limb asymmetry is seen in 65% to 90% of the patients. There is a broad spectrum of cutaneous malformations.

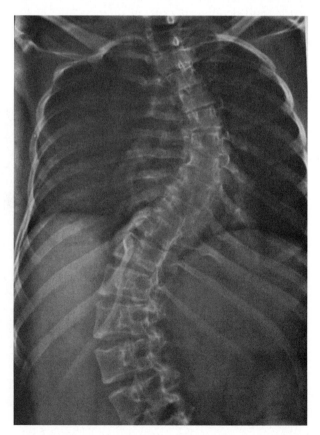

FIGURE 23. Anteroposterior radiograph of the spine of a teenager with homocystinuria shows osteopenia and scoliosis.

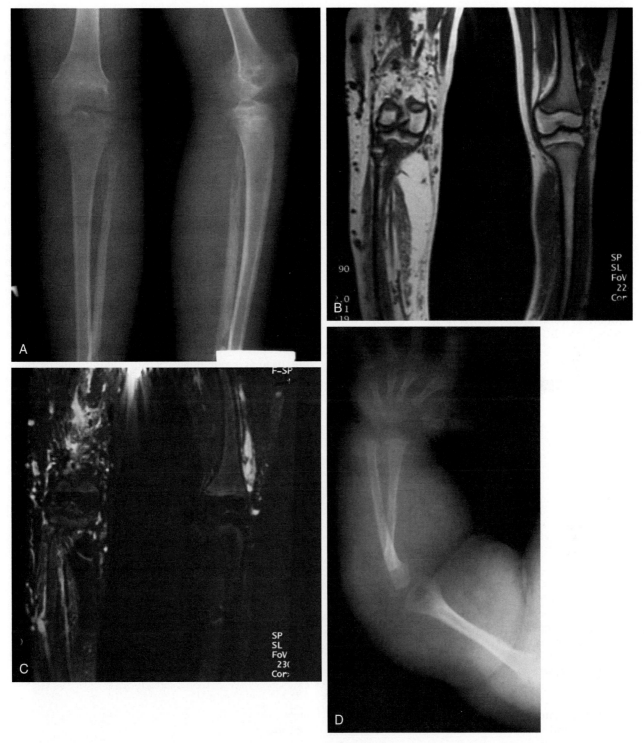

FIGURE 24. Klippel-Trénaunay syndrome. **A,** Leg radiograph demonstrates soft tissue fullness with multiple tortuous channels seen in the tibia and fibula secondary to osseous vascular malformations. **B** and **C,** Magnetic resonance imaging findings in another patient using T_1-weighted (TR: 512, TE: 12) **(B),** and T_2-weighted fat-suppressed TSE (TR: 3585, TE:85) **(C)** techniques. (TR = recovery time; TE = echo-delay time; TSE = turbo spin echo.) **D,** Upper extremity of a third patient shows marked hypertrophy of the soft tissues.

Venous involvement varies from massive varicositis to absence of deep venous structures. Polydactyly, syndactyly, and clinodactyly have been seen. It has also been associated with hemangiomas or vascular malformations that can be intracranial, spinal, hepatic, and splenic (Fig. 24). Hematuria, rectal bleeding, and pulmonary embolism can occur. Congenital hip dislocation has been associated. Findings may be documented prenatally on ultrasound or postnatally using multiple imaging modalities (see Section IX, Part IV, Fig. 17, page 2109).

LARSEN'S SYNDROME

Larsen's syndrome is characterized by multiple joint dislocations, especially of the knees, hips, and elbows; clubfoot; and a typical facies of prominent forehead, flat nasal bridge, and hypertelorism. In knee dislocations, which are the most frequent, the tibia is displaced anteriorly. Considerable epiphyseal deformity can occur secondary to the dislocations (Fig. 25A). Other osseous abnormalities include accessory carpal bones (Fig. 26), bifid calcaneus (Fig. 25B), short terminal phalanges of the hands, irregular shortening of some metacarpals, abnormal pattern profile analysis, kyphoscoliosis, delayed epiphyseal ossifications, coronal vertebral clefts, and retarded bone age.

Cervical kyphosis can be seen as a result of dysplastic cervical vertebrae, usually at C4 and C5. Although not common, kyphosis can be life-threatening because of cord compression. Other findings include cleft palate, tracheomalacia, genital anomalies, aortic dilatation and valvular insufficiency, and mitral valve prolapse. The condition is usually autosomal recessive, but dominant inheritance is also seen. A gene cytogenetically maps to 3p21.1-p14.1.

MARFAN SYNDROME

Marfan syndrome is a connective tissue disorder inherited as autosomal trait with almost complete penetration. The locus is chromosome 15 (q15-q21). It seems that Marfan's syndrome is caused by mutation in a fibrillin gene (FBN1) causing patients to lack fibrillin, a component of elastin. The typical patient is tall, with disproportionate long, slim limbs and digits. Commonly the cardiovascular, ocular, and skeletal systems are involved, with pectus deformities (excavatum or carinatum), joint laxity, ocular problems (usually ectopia lentis from lax suspensory ligaments and myopia), and spinal deformity (scoliosis, thoracolumbar, kyphosis, and flat back).

Cardiovascular manifestations, seen in about one third of patients, result from loss of tensile strength of the supporting tissue of the aortic and cardiac valves. These are the most devastating aspect of Marfan syndrome, leading to aortic dilatation, regurgitation, and dissection along with mitral valve prolapse (Fig. 27). A measurement of aortic root growth may have prognostic value for aortic complications. Serious cardiovascular abnormalities may be seen at birth.

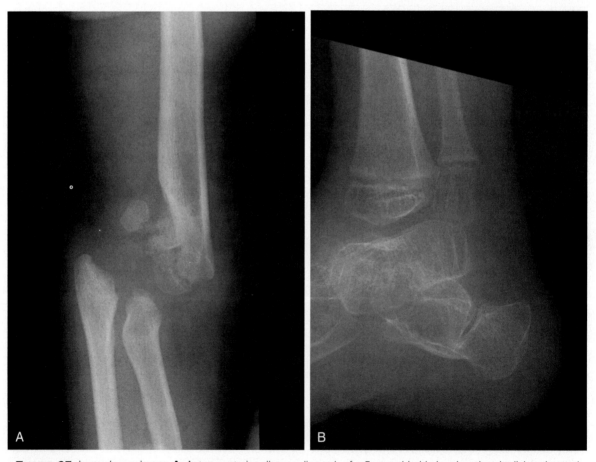

FIGURE 25. Larsen's syndrome. **A,** Anteroposterior elbow radiograph of a 5-year-old girl showing chronic dislocation and secondary deformities of the bones. **B,** Lateral radiograph of an ankle in a 5-year-old boy demonstrates a bifid calcaneus and deformity of the distal tibial epiphysis and talus.

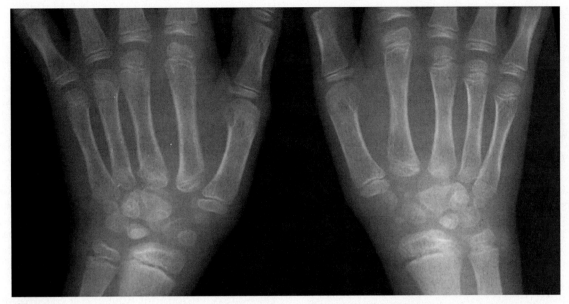

FIGURE 26. Posteroanterior radiograph of the hands of an 8-year-old girl with Larsen's syndrome shows multiple extra carpal bones with minimal deformity of the distal head of the second metacarpals. An accessory ossification center is seen at the base of the second metacarpals.

Gastrointestinal tract complications are few but include diaphragmatic and intestinal hernias, diverticulosis coli, and Zenker's diverticulum. Other findings include high-arched palate, crowding of teeth, dural ectasia, spinal arachnoid cysts or diverticula, pulmonary

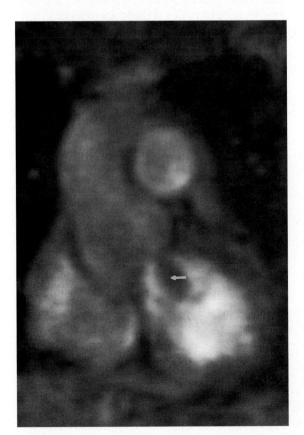

FIGURE 27. Gradient-echo cardiac magnetic resonance image (left anterior oblique equivalent) of a child with Marfan syndrome shows enlarged sinuses of Valsalva and jet of aortic insufficiency *(arrow)*.

blebs, and recurrent pneumothoraces. The joint laxity can result in joint dislocations, arachnodactyly (Fig. 28) with an abnormal metacarpal index greater than 9 (sum of lengths of metacarpals 2 through 5 divided by the sum of width of the same bones), middle digit 50% longer than its metacarpal, and abnormal metacarpophalangeal pattern profile, with a long first metacarpal and short first distal phalanx.

MARSHALL-SMITH SYNDROME

Marshall-Smith syndrome is characterized by accelerated skeletal maturation associated with failure to thrive. In addition to prenatal development of ossification centers, radiologic findings include "bullet-shaped" proximal and middle phalanges with narrow distal phalanges (Fig. 29A), narrow vertebral bodies with anterior wedging, and hypoplasia of the dens with prominence of the supraoccipital bone above the foramen magnum (Fig. 29B) and the posterior arch of C1. Hypoplastic mandibular rami and shallow orbits can also be seen. Clinically patients often do poorly, with death in infancy common as a result of respiratory compromise. However, long-term survival has been reported.

MAYER-ROKITANSKY-KÜSTER-HAUSER SEQUENCE

The Mayer-Rokitansky-Küster-Hauser sequence (MRKHS) is a congenital müllerian duct malformation characterized by vaginal and uterine hypoplasia/aplasia. Two varieties of the malformation occur. In the typical or classical variety, a small muscular uterine fundal remnant, normal fallopian tubes, and normal ovaries are present. Asymmetry of the fallopian tubes

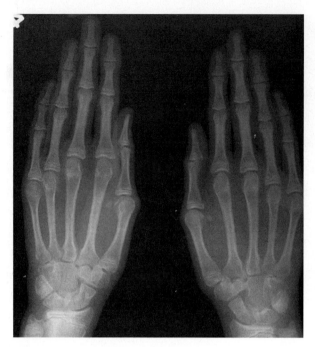

FIGURE 28. Posteroanterior radiograph of the hand of a child with Marfan syndrome shows arachnodactyly.

and the presence of ovarian malformations differentiate the nonclassical variety. The Mayer-Rokitansky-Küster-Hauser sequence (MRKHS) has been described in several genetic syndromes; the most frequent association is with the MURCS syndrome (see below), the hereditary urogenital adysplasia syndrome, and other malformations including limb anomalies.

MURCS Syndrome

MURCS is an acronym for a congenital syndrome consisting of müllerian duct aplasia, especially MRKHS; renal agenesis, and cervical spine anomalies. This syndrome has cervical spine anomalies of the Klippel-Feil variety and a high incidence of deafness. An autosomal dominant inheritance pattern is most likely. In a male, the anomalies are often of the wolffian system, and the acronym WORCS is occasionally used for male patients. Differentiation of cases without all the typical features of MURCS syndrome from VACTERL association, Turner's syndrome, Goldenhar's syndrome, and the hereditary urogenital adysplasia syndrome may be difficult.

Hereditary Urogenital Adysplasia Syndrome

This is a syndrome of probable autosomal dominant inheritance characterized by bilateral renal agenesis (Potter's syndrome) or dysgenesis. There is a high association with müllerian malformations, including MRKHS. Although bilateral renal agenesis/dysgenesis may be sporadic, increasing evidence indicates that many of cases are expressions of the hereditary urogenital adysplasia syndrome. In males, anomalies of the wolffian system occur, often leading to azospermia. Anomalies seen in males include agenesis or cyst of the

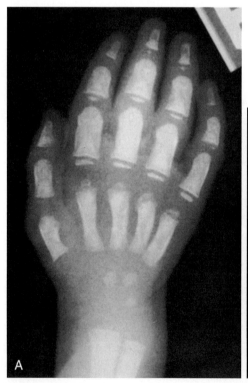

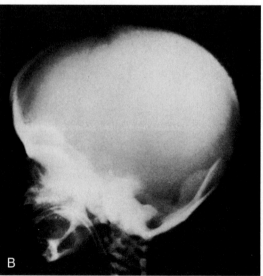

FIGURE 29. Marshall-Smith syndrome. **A,** Hand radiograph shows bullet-shaped proximal and middle phalanges and accelerated skeletal maturation. **B,** Lateral skull radiograph shows a hypoplastic mandible, prominent supraoccipital bone, and shallow orbits. (Courtesy of Dr. A. H. Felman, Jacksonville, FL.)

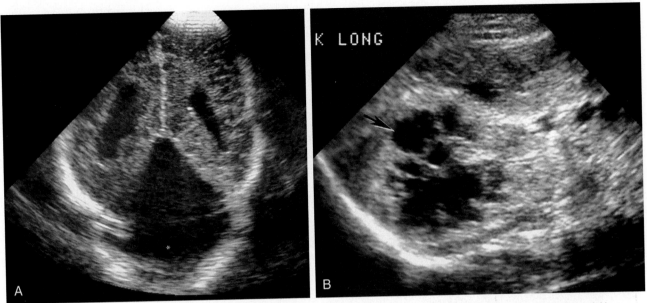

FIGURE 30. Meckel's syndrome. **A,** Cranial sonogram of the head demonstrates a large occipital encephalocele *(asterisk).* **B,** Transverse renal sonogram demonstrates a cyst *(arrow)* in the right kidney. Normal neonatal increased cortical echogenicity is seen with sonolucent pyramids.

seminal vesicles, wolffian paravesical cyst, atresia of the ejaculatory duct, cyst of müllerian remnant, and prostatic utricle. Limb anomalies may also occur in this syndrome, possibly, as suggested by Opitz, because of poor production of limb inductor by the mesonephros. It is uncertain whether some cases of MURCS syndrome are due to a similar genetic abnormality. The better definition of this syndrome is hindered partly by the failure to recognize müllerian anomalies such as MRKHS as possibly part of a larger syndrome.

MECKEL'S (MECKEL-GRUBER) SYNDROME

Meckel's syndrome, also known as Meckel-Gruber syndrome, is an autosomal recessive lethal malformation syndrome characterized by occipital encephalocele (Fig. 30A), renal abnormalities including cysts (Fig. 30B), and dysplasia, dysplastic kidneys, and postaxial polydactyly. Other visceral changes include fibrosis and hamartomas of visceral organs, cleft lip and palate, and visceral heterotaxias. Other skeletal changes include dysplastic hips, micrognathia, limb bowing, short limbs, and vertebral anomalies. Prenatal sonographic evaluation demonstrates oligohydramnios and typical morphologic findings in the second trimester.

NAIL–PATELLA SYNDROME

The nail–patella syndrome has as cardinal features dysplastic nails, absent or hypoplastic patellas, prominent iliac horns, elbow dysplasia, and in some patients nephropathy. It is a disorder caused by mutations of in the LIM-homeodomain protein *LMX1*B, and the gene has been localized to chromosome 17q21-22.

Patellas may be absent (Fig. 31A) or hypoplastic and subject to dislocation or subluxation. Also seen are undeveloped distal femoral epiphyses, subluxation and flexion contractures of the knee joint, and osteochondritis dissecans of the distal femora. The radial heads are hypoplastic, as are the capitellae, and are associated with limitation of elbow motion and dislocation (Fig. 31B).

Iliac horns, spike-like projections from the upper posterior surface of the iliac wings (Fig. 31C), are bilateral and found in 80% of patients (see Section IX, Part V, Fig. 47, page 2176). The iliac wings flare and the acetabular angles are low. Other findings include a clavicular horn, an underdeveloped and slightly deformed scapula, sternal and rib deformities, scoliosis, and foot deformities. The renal disease resembles glomerulonephritis and is not usually fatal. An in utero diagnosis of nail–patella syndrome can be made.

NEVOID BASAL CELL CARCINOMA (GORLIN'S) SYNDROME

Nevoid basal cell carcinoma syndrome (NBCCS), or Gorlin's syndrome, is an autosomal dominant condition characterized by basal cell skin carcinomas, odotogenic keratocysts of the jaw (Fig. 32), palmar and plantar pits, and lamellar calcifications in the falx cerebri (Fig. 33), diaphragma sellae, and tentorium cerebelli. In addition to basal cell carcinoma, there is increased incidence of multiple neoplastic conditions, including medulloblastoma, Hodgkin's disease, fibrosarcoma, bilateral calcified ovarian fibromas, intra-abdominal lymphangiomas, and cardiac fibroma. Skeletal malformations include anterior bifid ribs, cervical spine segmentation anomalies, Sprengel's deformity, spotty sclerotic skeletal lesions, and phalangeal lucent lesions.

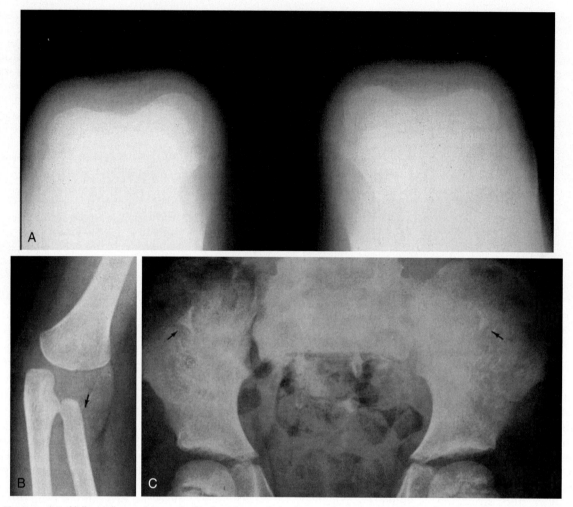

FIGURE 31. Nail–patella syndrome. **A,** Skyline views of the knees show absent patellas. **B,** Radiograph of the elbow demonstrates hypoplasia of the radial head *(arrow)* and olecranon fossa. **C,** Anteroposterior radiograph of the pelvis shows the iliac horns *(arrows)*.

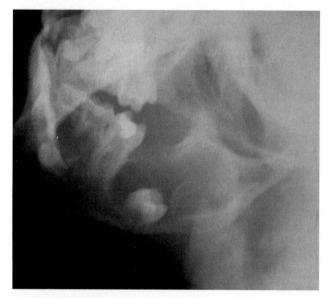

FIGURE 32. Oblique mandible radiograph of a child with nevoid basal cell nevus syndrome shows a lucent lesion of a keratocyst with distortion of surrounding teeth.

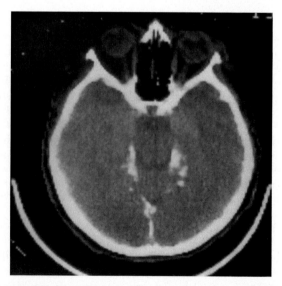

FIGURE 33. Nevoid basal cell nevus syndrome, as seen on noncontrast computed tomography scan of the brain. Extensive dural calcifications are present along the falx cerebri and the edges of the tentorium cerebelli.

The genetic locus of the syndrome is the *PTCH* tumor suppressor gene, mapped to 9q22. Basal cell carcinomas, often occurring in great numbers, are found in over 90% of patients over 40 years of age but are rare before 20 years of age. The basal cell carcinomas in this syndrome are related to ultraviolet radiation and are uncommon in blacks with the syndrome. It is also known that patients with NBCCS who have had spinal radiation for medulloblastoma may develop hundreds or thousands of scalp basal cell carcinomas. It has been suggested that, if a patient with a medulloblastoma has NBCCS, chemotherapy should be considered in lieu of radiation therapy. Odontogenic keratocysts are much more common in the mandible than the maxilla, are infrequently symptomatic, and begin to appear between the ages of 7 and 40 years.

NOONAN'S SYNDROME

Noonan's syndrome is a sporadic autosomal dominant condition associated with short stature, lymphedema, lymphatic dysplasia (especially pulmonary lymphangiectasia), webbed neck, mild mental retardation, cryptorchidism in males, pectus deformities, and congenital heart disease, especially pulmonary stenosis and left ventricular asymmetric hypertrophy. The similarity of the phenotype to Turner's syndrome has long been recognized.

There is also a subpopulation of Noonan's syndrome patients whose disease more closely resembles Turner's syndrome. These patients have left ventricular obstructing lesions, especially aortic coarctation, and frequent renal anomalies. This contrasts with the pulmonic stenosis and infrequent renal anomalies in classical Noonan's syndrome. It is thought that a putative lymphogenic gene on the Xp chromosome may cause this type of Noonan's syndrome, accounting for the close resemblance to Turner's syndrome.

In addition to classical Noonan's syndrome, there are several Noonan-like syndromes. The best defined is the Noonan phenotype associated with café au lait spots, referred to as Noonan-neurofibromatosis syndrome. Two similar conditions that are difficult to differentiate from Noonan's syndrome are LEOPARD syndrome (multiple lentigines, electrocardiographic conduction abnormalities, ocular hypertelorism, pulmonary stenosis, retardation of growth and sensorineural deafness), in which pulmonary valve dysplasia and left ventricular hypertrophy occurs with multiple lentigines, and cardiofaciocutaneous syndrome, in which valvular pulmonic stenosis, and unusual facies occurs associated with hyperkeratosis.

The gene locus for autosomal dominant classical Noonan's syndrome is on chromosome 12, although the gene is not further characterized. Patients may also have cerebral vascular dysplasia and arteriovenous malformations resulting in stroke, factor XI deficiency, and an increased incidence of malignancy, including malignant schwannoma, pheochromocytoma, leukemia, and rhabdomyosarcoma.

OCCIPITAL HORN SYNDROME

The occipital horn syndrome (OHS), previously called X-linked cutis laxa and type IX Ehlers-Danlos syndrome, is an X-linked recessive condition associated with a pathognomonic skeletal dysplasia, chronic diarrhea, obstructive uropathy, bladder diverticula, hypermobile fingers and joints, characteristic facies, and soft, velvety, easily bruised skin. OHS is thought to be due to a disorder of copper metabolism, with elevated copper levels in fibroblasts and decreased serum copper and ceruloplasmin levels. The major manifestations may be due to the copper-dependent enzyme lysyl oxidase, which is required to produce cross-links in collagen. The pathognomonic radiographic features of this condition include occipital horns (Fig. 34) and short, broad clavicles with hammer-shaped ends (Fig. 35A). Occipital horns are bilateral parasagittal ectopic bone within the trapezium and sternocleidomastoid insertions that extend caudally from the occiput and probably increase in size with age. Other radiographic manifestations include abnormal elbows (Fig. 35B), capitate–hamate fusion, mild platyspondyly, undulating thickness of long bone cortices, and flat acetabular roofs. The facies are also said to be characteristic, with a narrow face, high forehead, and long neck. The

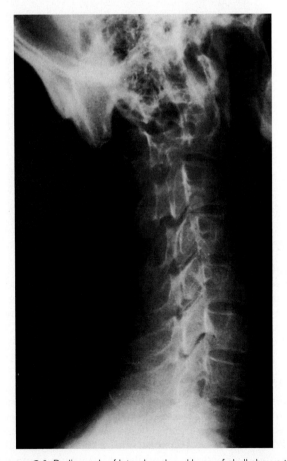

FIGURE 34. Radiograph of lateral neck and base of skull shows the occipital horn in a child with occipital horn syndrome. (Courtesy of Dr. D. Sartoris, Stanford, CA.)

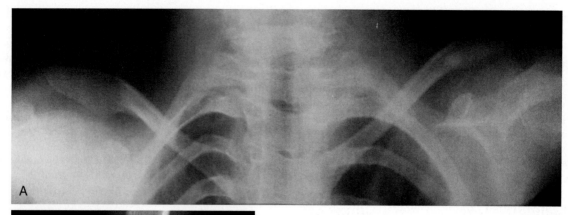

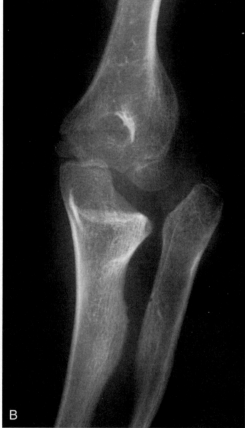

FIGURE 35. Occipital horn syndrome. **A,** Anteroposterior (AP) radiograph of the clavicles show their abnormally shaped outer ends. **B,** AP elbow radiograph demonstrates lateral radial head dislocation and bulbous distal humerus, proximal ulna, and radius.

etiology of the chronic diarrhea is not known. Obstructive uropathy and bladder diverticula may lead to recurrent infections and require surgical reconstruction of the urinary tract. Vascular ectasia and aneurysms also occur.

OPITZ (G/BBB) SYNDROME

Opitz (G/BBB) syndrome is a heterogeneous malformation disorder characterized by hypertelorism, hypospadias, characteristic facies, swallowing dysfunction, and stridor caused by laryngeal abnormalities, including hypoplastic epiglottis, hypoplastic larynx, and congenital laryngotracheoesophageal cleft (Fig. 36). There are two identified forms: X-linked recessive (type I) and

autosomal dominant (type II). The laryngeal abnormalities are limited to type I, occurring only in males, and are associated with a high morbidity resulting from aspiration pneumonia and airway obstruction. Female carriers most frequently manifest only hypertelorism or are normal. Imperforate anus has been reported occasionally both in males and female carriers. Cardiac lesions occur in approximately 20% of patients, but are not characteristic; reported lesions include atrioseptal defect, partial anomalous pulmonary venous return, and patent ductus arteriosus. Characteristic facial anomalies of Opitz (G/BBB) syndrome include cleft lip, palate, or uvula in 40%; broad, high nasal bridge; and short, posteriorly angled ears. Midline central nervous system anomalies include agenesis/hypoplasia of the corpus callosum, large cisterna magna, and cerebellar

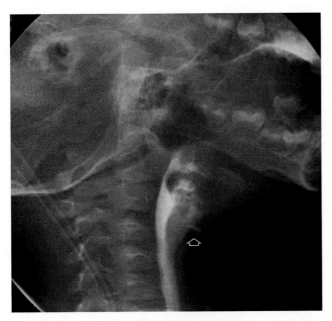

FIGURE 36. Lateral view of cervical esophagus as seen with barium swallow. A type 1 laryngotracheoesophageal cleft is present *(arrow)*, with barium entering the larynx directly, in this child with known Opitz (G/BBB) syndrome.

vermian atrophy. The gene locus for the autosomal dominant type II disease is at the 22q11.2 locus, a locus similar to those of DiGeorge and velocardiofacial syndromes.

ORAL-FACIAL-DIGITAL SYNDROMES

The oral-facial-digital (OFD) syndromes are a heterogeneous group. All have facial anomalies, oral findings (cleft or lobulated tongue, oral frenula, and/or cleft palate) (Fig. 37A), and digital anomalies (brachy-, syn-, clino-, and polydactyly). We discuss types I and II here.

OFD syndrome type I has dominant X-linked inheritance and a distinctive facies. Malformations of the fingers are seen in 50% to 70% and also include some slightly malformed wide short tubular bones, Y-shaped metatarsals, and cone epiphyses (Fig. 37B, C). Irregular mineralization is seen in the metacarpals, metatarsals, and proximal and middle phalanges, and spiculated areas on the middle parts of some phalanges are seen largely in type I. Toe malformations (25%) also include preaxial polydactyly.

Central nervous system findings include neuronal migration defects, intracerebral cysts and porencephaly or arachnoid cysts, hydrocephalus, vermis hypoplasia, Dandy-Walker malformation, and agenesis of the corpus callosum. The nasion–sella–basion angle is increased from a normal of 133 degrees (1 SD = 4.5) to 144 degrees. Renal abnormalities include polycystic kidneys, which look like those in adult polycystic disease except that the cysts form from the tubules and glomeruli, whereas, in adult polycystic kidney disease, the cysts are from the tubules.

OFD syndrome type II is distinguished from type I in that it is autosomal recessive, is seen in females, does not have hyperplastic frenula, may have absent lower central incisors, and may have a conductive hearing loss and tibial pseudoarthrosis (Fig. 38A). Polydactyly, which is postaxial in the hands and preaxial in the feet, is more common in OFD syndrome type II (Fig. 38B).

OSTEOLYSIS SYNDROMES

The osteolysis syndromes are difficult to classify but can be roughly divided into five forms based on the areas of bone absorption and associated malformations:

1. Multicentric, affecting predominantly the carpal and tarsal bones with and without nephropathy
2. Multicentric, predominantly carpal, tarsal, and interphalangeal forms (François, Winchester, Torg, Whyte-Hemingway)
3. Forms affecting primarily the distal phalanges (Hajdu-Cheney syndrome, mandibular-acral form)
4. Forms involving the diaphyses and metaphyses (familial expansile osteolysis, juvenile hyaline fibromatosis)
5. Massive osteolysis of Gorham

Hereditary multicentric osteolysis involving the carpal and tarsal bones starts in early childhood, usually by age 3 or 4 years, with arthritis-like symptoms of the wrists and feet. There develops a progressive absorption of the carpal and tarsal bones that become crenated and eventually disappear, with marked narrowing of the carpal and tarsal areas (Fig. 39). The adjacent metacarpals and metatarsals are often involved, showing erosions and pencilling. Unlike in rheumatoid arthritis, the mineral content of the bones remains good. Despite severe wrist and foot deformities, there may be few symptoms related to these areas.

The lesions are bilateral but not necessarily symmetric. The ankles (Fig. 40), elbows (Fig. 41), and knees may be involved, but the phalanges are generally spared. The metatarsophalangeal and the metacarpophalangeal joints can be involved. The disease becomes quiescent in adulthood. Both autosomal dominant and recessive forms can be seen. When associated with nephropathy, the disease can be fatal in the third decade. The pathogenesis is unknown, and on biopsy the tissues have fibrous elements and increased vascularity with little inflammation.

The forms principally involving the distal phalanges are also progressive and can be called acro-osteolysis. The lesions may stabilize in adult life. The more proximal phalanges can also exhibit absorption. (Hajdu-Cheney syndrome is discussed elsewhere in this chapter.) Some cases are difficult to classify.

Gorham's syndrome or vanishing bone disease, is a condition usually starting gradually or abruptly before the age of 40 years and has striking radiographic findings of massive osteolysis. In the first stage of this disease, there is patchy osteoporosis with intramedullary and subcortical radiolucent foci. These foci enlarge with the development of new foci in the second stage. The third stage is cortical erosion and invasion of an angiomatous mass into surrounding tissues. Finally, the bone disappears with lack of new bone formation. The remaining osseous tissue is tapered, and the destructive process may involve a whole region (i.e., shoulder or hip), with the adjacent bones being severely affected.

OTOPALATODIGITAL SYNDROME

Two types of otopalatodigital syndrome are described, and there are many similarities in facial features and radiologic findings. Type II is more severe. The syn-

drome's main features are abnormal facies, thumb and great toe deformity, cleft palate, and conductive hearing loss. There is some support for mapping the OPD gene to Xq28.

In type I, the typical face has prominent supraorbital ridges, a broad nasal root, poorly formed ears, and small nose and mouth, all giving the impression of a prize fighter. The skull radiographs show thickening of the frontal and occipital regions, sclerotic skull base, large anterior fontanelle, unpneumatized sinuses and mastoids, and a small mandible. The deformities of the fingers and toes include shortening of the thumb and big toe and wide spacing between the first and second toes, give the foot a resemblance to that of a tree frog. Broad shortening of the first toes and thumbs associated

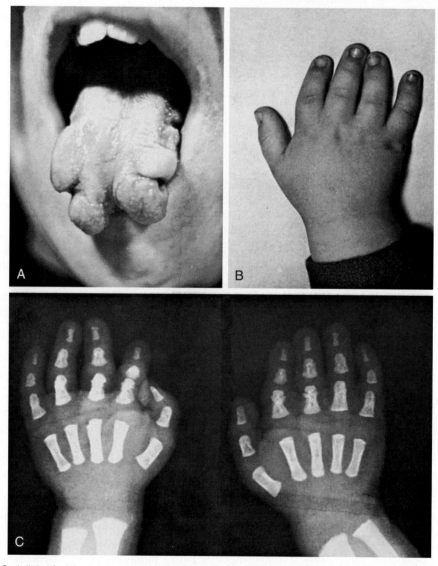

FIGURE 37. Oral-digital-facial syndrome, type I. **A,** Longitudinal and lateral clefts and fibrous swellings in the tongue of a 14-year-old girl. **B,** The fingers and the hand are broad and short, and some of the fingers are bent. The fourth and fifth fingers are relatively long in this 10-year-old girl. (**A** and **B** from Gorlin RJ, Psaume J: Orodigitofacial dysostosis—a new syndrome. A study of 22 cases. J Pediatr 1962;61:520–530, with permission.) **C,** Posteroanterior radiograph of the hands shows shortening and bending of the proximal and middle phalanges of the second and third digits and relative elongation of the fourth and fifth fingers despite some deformity of these proximal phalanges. (From Schwarz E, Fish A: Roentgenographic features of a new congenital dysplasia. Am J Roentgenol Radium Ther Nucl Med 1960;84:511–517. Reprinted with permission from the American Journal of Roentgenology.)

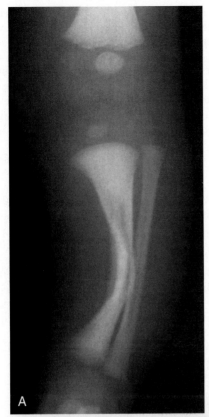

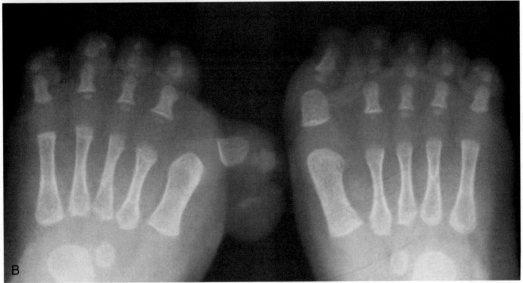

FIGURE 38. Oral-facial-digital syndrome, type II. **A,** Radiograph of a newborn shows marked lateral bowing of the left tibia. **B,** Anteroposterior foot radiographs at 11 months demonstrate preaxial polydactyly of the first digit on the left.

with fusions of accessory ossification centers of the second metacarpals and metatarsals with adjacent carpal and tarsal bones is characteristic (Fig. 42). Other radiographic findings in the hands and feet include relatively long second and fifth metacarpals, clinodactyly, duplication of the terminal phalanges of the index finger and second toe, cone-shaped epiphyses of the terminal phalanges of the thumbs, carpal fusions, comma-shaped trapezoid, transverse capitate, tarsal fusions, and extra carpal and tarsal bones. Other radiographic findings include dislocation of radial

heads, pectus excavatum, thin undulating posterior ribs, and hip subluxation.

Type II is X-linked recessive and has more severe changes in the face, hands, and feet. The latter two show hypoplastic metacarpals and metatarsals, hypoplasia of the phalanges (especially the first), and camptodactyly. The ribs show more marked waviness and angulation, sloping clavicles, and fused sternal segments. The long bones are dense, undermodeled, and bowed and may have irregular surfaces, and there may be hypoplastic fibulas. The ilia are flared, the acetabula flat, and the fibulas may be hypoplastic. Coronal cleft vertebra, dislocated hips, and postaxial polydactyly can be seen. There may be an overlap of OPD type II and Melnick-Needles syndrome.

PENA-SHOKEIR SYNDROME I (FETAL AKINESIA SEQUENCE)

Pena-Shokeir syndrome I, or the fetal akinesia sequence, is a phenotype and not a nosological entity. Because of the decreased fetal movement involved, it belongs to the overall category of arthrogryposis multiplex congenita (AMC) syndromes. AMC is characterized by multiple joint contractures at birth with an intact skeleton. The major findings of Pena-Shokeir syndrome I include pulmonary hypoplasia (Fig. 43), maternal polyhydramnios, micrognathia, thin ribs, arthrogryposis, clubfoot, camptodactyly, fetal growth retardation, and short umbilical cord. Moessinger has demonstrated that the findings of the Pena-Shokeir syndrome I can be produced by fetal akinesia in experiments with curarized fetal rats. Neuropathologic studies have demonstrated many abnormalities of the spinal motor neurons,

pyramid tracts, and muscles and of the central nervous system, including reactive gliosis, multicystic encephalopathy, polymicrogyria, persistent meningeal vascularization, agenesis of septum pellucidum, and hydranencephaly. These cerebral lesions probably play a role in the development of the spinal muscular atrophy, which in turn leads to fetal akinesia.

PENA-SHOKEIR SYNDROME II (CEREBRO-OCULOFACIOSKELETAL SYNDROME)

Pena-Shokeir syndrome II is an autosomal recessive condition of microcephaly, cataracts, microphthalmia, blepharophimosis, characteristic facies, camptodactyly, kyphoscoliosis, joint contractures of the elbows and knees, failure to thrive, and progressive central nervous system demyelination. Frequently associated findings include hypoplasia or agenesis of the corpus callosum and hypoplasia of the second tarsal cuneiform with a proximally positioned second metatarsal. Intracranial basal ganglia calcifications may occur, and other features of the phenotype suggest some relationship to Cockayne's syndrome.

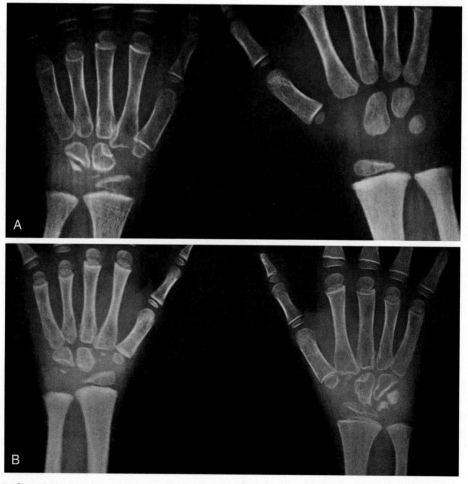

FIGURE 39. Osteolysis syndrome (tarsocarpal osteolysis) in a patient whose left hand had been caught in a washing machine wringer. **A,** The deformity of the carpal bones noted 10 months after injury had been attributed to the accident. **B,** The development of similar changes in the right hand 18 months after **A** indicates the intrinsic nature of the changes.

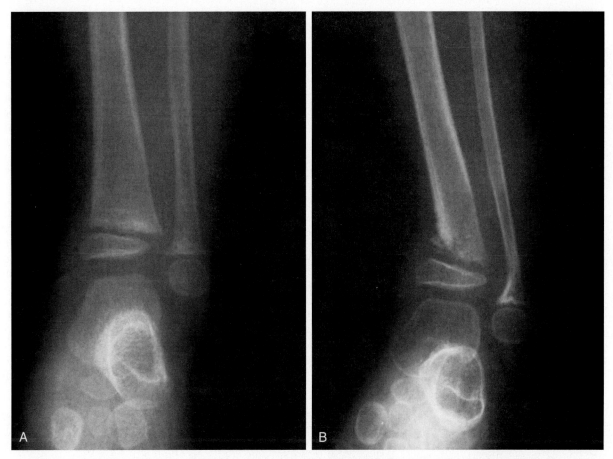

FIGURE 40. Left ankle radiographs of a child with osteolysis syndrome at ages 15 months **(A)** and 18 months **(B).** There has been significant progressive absorption of the metaphyseal area on the distal tibia, with bowing of the distal fibula.

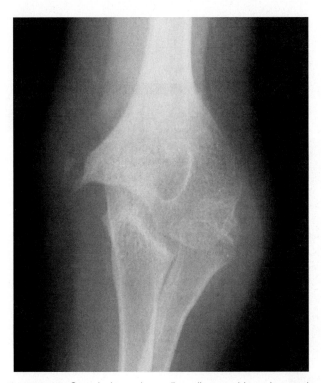

FIGURE 41. Osteolysis syndrome (hereditary multicentric osteolysis) as seen on an elbow radiograph of a 7-year-old boy. Destructive changes are seen about the elbow, most notably in the distal medial aspect of the humerus.

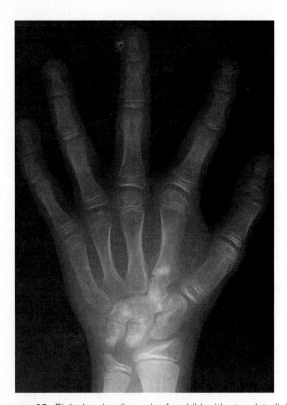

FIGURE 42. Right hand radiograph of a child with otopalatodigital syndrome shows typical findings of fusion of the accessory ossification center of the second metacarpal with the adjacent deformed carpal bones. There is widening or abnormal tubulation of the metacarpals. The distal phalanx of the thumb is shortened, with a coned-shaped epiphysis. Clinodactyly is also noted.

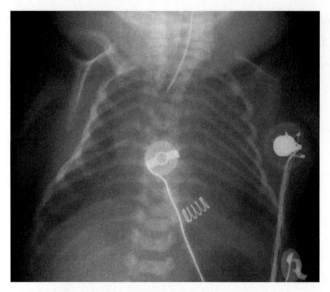

FIGURE 43. Chest radiograph of newborn with Pena-Shokeir syndrome I shows hypoplastic lungs, hypoplastic glenoid fossas, and dislocated proximal humerii.

POLAND'S SYNDROME

Poland's syndrome is characterized by partial or complete absence of the pectoral muscles associated with anomalies of the ipsilateral upper extremity. It is occasionally associated with neoplasm and may have familial inheritance. Extremity changes range from syndactyly, polydactyly, or phalangeal hypoplasia to radial ray anomalies and shoulder girdle anomalies (Fig. 44A). Other reported anomalies include scoliosis, rib anomalies, and renal hypoplasia/agenesis. Plain radiographs demonstrate relative thoracic hyperlucency as well as skeletal extremity changes (Fig. 44B). CT and MRI better demonstrate the musculoskeletal anomalies and possible breast hypoplasia (Fig. 44C). Poland's syndrome is thought to arise from subclavian arterial compromise in fetal life.

PROGERIA

Progeria is a rare condition causing premature aging. There is growth retardation and accelerated degen-

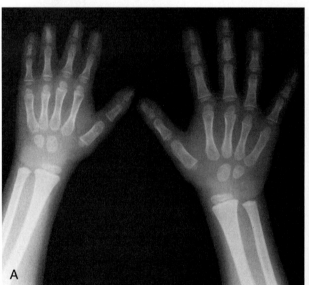

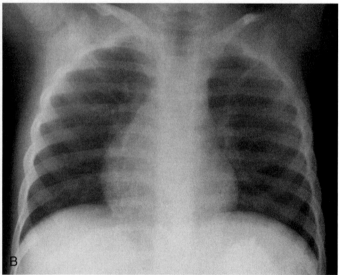

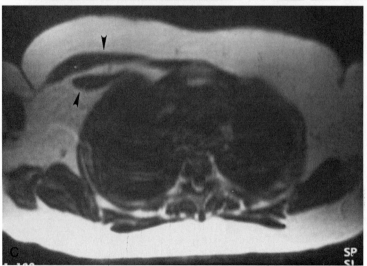

FIGURE 44. Poland's syndrome. **A,** Hand radiograph demonstrates generalized hypoplasia on the left with cutaneous syndactyly affecting the second through fourth digits. **B,** Anteroposterior chest radiograph in a different patient demonstrates relative lucency of the left hemithorax with loss of the pectoral shadow. **C,** Axial T$_1$-weighted magnetic resonance image (800/45) demonstrates absence of the left anterior chest wall musculature (*arrowheads* indicate normal musculature on the right).

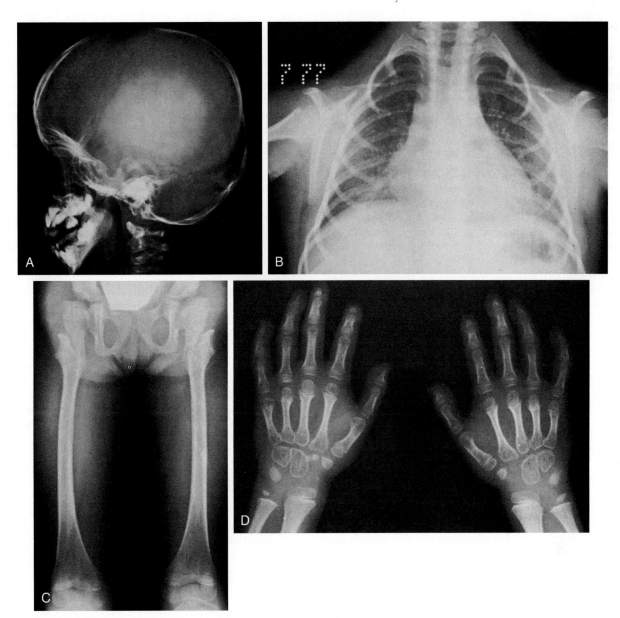

FIGURE 45. Progeria in a 7¾–year-old girl. **A,** Lateral skull film shows small facial structures in relation to the neurocranium, with a persistent open anterior fontanelle. The ascending rami of the mandible are very short. **B,** The clavicles are miniscule, in part as a result of osteolysis of the lateral portions, which are remote from the acromion processes bilaterally. The ribs are abnormally gracile. **C,** Coxa valga deformity is marked, with the necks continuing in the axis of the femoral shafts; the femoral heads are only partially within their acetabular fossas. The greater trochanters are bizarre in shape and position. **D,** Acro-osteolysis is prominent in the terminal phalanges. Some carpal ossification centers are sclerotic, while others participate in the general osteopenia. Skeletal maturation is appropriate for the age.

erative changes in the cutaneous, cardiovascular, and musculoskeletal system. The infant is normal at birth, but the changes are evident by the first or second year of life when progressive signs of aging appear, such as alopecia, craniofacial disproportion, beak-like nose, atrophic skin, decreased subcutaneous tissue, prominent eyes, and horse-riding stance.

The radiographic findings include osteopenia, fish-mouth vertebrae, coxa valga, thin long bones with widened metaphysis, genu valgus, hypoplastic mandible with tooth loss, thin diploic space in the skull, open fontanelles, thin and sloping ribs, small thoracic cage,

hip subluxation or aseptic necrosis, and cerebrovascular occlusions (Fig. 45). An unusual feature is that certain parts of the skeleton undergo progressive osteolysis. This occurs in the clavicles, distal phalanges, upper ribs, and proximal humeri. In the clavicle, the absorption progresses from lateral to medial, and the clavicle can completely resorb. The distal phalanges of fingers and toes can disappear, leaving only the proximal phalanges. The ribs most commonly involved are the posterior portions of ribs 2 and 3. Most patients die by their teenage years, but the condition can be lethal at birth.

PROTEUS SYNDROME

Proteus syndrome falls into a category of congenital hamartomatous disorders that may be autosomant dominant. There is asymmetric overgrowth and malformations of different parts of the body in association with various cutaneous abnormalities, including connective tissue nevi and epidermal nevi. The tissue overgrowth is progressive but tends to plateau after puberty.

There may be marked craniofacial abnormalities with facial and ocular asymmetry. A hyperplastic plantar overgrowth called "moccasin lesion" is characteristic in the feet. The hands and feet are large and often have macrodactyly (see Section IX, Part IV, page 2099).

The radiographic findings reflect what is seen clinically, namely overgrowth of limbs and digits from both bone and soft tissues. The hands and feet are particularly involved. There may be postaxial polydactyly. The skull may be large, may have sclerotic bone, and may be dolichocephalic. Hydrocephaly and hemimeganencephaly can be seen. The spine can show large vertebral bodies and neural arches, asymmetric vertebral bodies, and scoliosis. There are many unusual types of tumors associated with the Proteus syndrome: ovarian cystadenoma, various testicular tumors, central nervous system tumors (especially meningiomas), and monomorphic adenoma of the parotid.

RUBINSTEIN-TAYBI SYNDROME

Rubinstein-Taybi syndrome is a sporadic condition caused by a mutation on chromosome 16, characterized by facial dysmorphism, mental retardation, and broadening of the thumbs and great toes. Characteristic broadening of the distal phalanges of the thumb and great toe is a diagnostic marker for the syndrome and is seen in about one third of the cases (Fig. 46). Additional radiographic findings include delayed skeletal maturation and dislocations, flared iliac wings, large foramen magna, and cervical instability with odontoid malformation. Visceral malformations, including malrotation and vesicoureteral reflux, as well as intracranial lesions, including agenesis of the corpus callosum and Dandy-Walker malformation, have been reported. Congenital heart defects, usually ventricular septal defect or patent ductus arteriosus, are seen in about 25% of the patients.

RUSSELL-SILVER SYNDROME

Russell-Silver syndrome is characterized by body asymmetry, low birth weight, and variable dysmorphic features with both autosomal dominant and X-linked inheritance described. Additional features include intrauterine growth retardation, postnatal retardation of height and weight (hence the occasional reference to Russell-Silver dwarfism), clinodactyly, toe syndactyly, retarded bone age, triangular facies, and urogenital anomalies. Body asymmetry with leg length discrepancy is found in approximately 50% of patients. Discrepancies of up to 6 cm may occur. The bone age is delayed in childhood (69% of chronologic age) but at puberty is approximately 95% of the chronologic age. Hand anomalies include ivory epiphyses of distal phalanges, brachymesophalangy of the fifth digit, and clinodactyly. Genitourinary anomalies include ureteropelvic junction obstruction, reflux, renal ectopia, renal fusion anomalies, hypospadias, cryptorchidism (42% of males), posterior urethral valves, hydroceles, and scrotal hypoplasia. There may be an increased incidence of Legg-Perthes disease, which, like Russell-Silver syndrome, is associated with delayed bone age, and of malignancies, which interestingly also occur in some other syndromes of growth disturbance and asymmetric growth, such as the Beckwith-Weidemann syndrome.

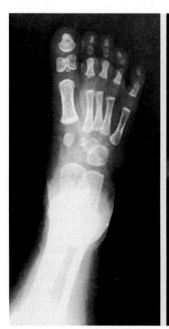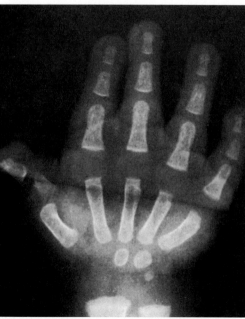

FIGURE 46. Radiographs of hand and foot in patient with Rubinstein-Taybi syndrome. The thumb and first toe demonstrate short, wide phalanges with partial complete duplication of the proximal phalanx of the toe.

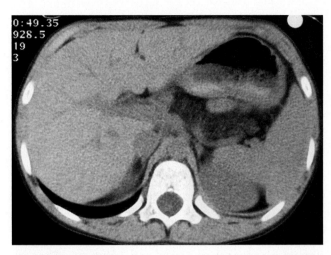

FIGURE 47. Abdominal computed tomography scan at the level of the pancreas reveals a virtually completely fat-replaced pancreas in this child with immune deficiency consistent with Shwachman-Diamond syndrome.

SHWACHMAN-DIAMOND SYNDROME

Shwachman-Diamond syndrome is a presumed autosomal recessive condition associated with exocrine pancreatic insufficiency with fat replacement of the pancreas, short stature, bone marrow dysfunction with neutropenia, and metaphyseal chondrodysplasia. Skeletal manifestations include delayed bone age with marked carpal delay, broad cup-like anterior ribs, metaphyseal irregularities, and coxa vara with short femoral necks (see Section IX, Part V, Fig. 27, page 2154). CT or MRI demonstration of a fat-replaced pancreas may be useful in establishing the diagnosis (Fig. 47). Variable bone marrow dysfunction is present, often with anemia and thrombocytopenia in addition to frequently cyclic neutropenia. Recurrent infections are related to neutropenia, chemotactic defect, impaired neutrophil mobility, and impaired complement activation. Patients with Shwachman-Diamond syndrome have an increased incidence of leukemia, especially acute myelogenous leukemia. This increased incidence of leukemia correlates with an increased frequency of spontaneous chromosomal breakage in Shwachman-Diamond syndrome. The disease maps to a locus at 7q11.

SMITH-LEMLI-OPITZ SYNDROME

Smith-Lemli-Opitz syndrome, or RSH/Smith-Lemli-Opitz syndrome, is an autosomal recessive condition with two phenotypes. The classical, or type I, phenotype is associated with microcephaly; mental retardation; growth delay; characteristic facies with anteverted nostrils, ptosis, and high-arched palate; hypotonia; cryptorchidism; and syndactyly of the second and third toes. The type II or lethal phenotype is characterized by features of the type I phenotype but also male pseudohermaphrodism with complete sex reversal, postaxial polydactyly of the hands and/or feet, small

tongue, Hirschsprung's disease or total colonic aganglionosis, and high lethality. Other anomalies described in type II Smith-Lemli-Opitz syndrome include unilobar lungs, renal hypoplasia, and testicular dysgenesis with diminished number of Leydig cells. Malformations of the central nervous system include agenesis of the corpus callosum, cerebellar hypoplasia, fusion of the cerebral hemispheres, arhinencephaly, and holoprosencephaly.

Cardiovascular malformations have included atrioventricular canal defects and anomalous pulmonary venous return. Interestingly, conotruncal anomalies do not occur in this syndrome. An increased incidence of pyloric stenosis has been described. Both type I and type II are associated with markedly reduced activity of the enzyme converting 7-dehydrocholesterol to cholesterol. This deficiency is more marked in the type II patients. The higher the level of plasma cholesterol, the greater the chance of survival of the infant; the lower the level, the greater the number of malformations present. Because of the marked variability of expression, including very mild forms, it is suggested that children with mental retardation, developmental delay, any degree of cleft palate, micrognathia, and second/third toe syndactyly should have plasma cholesterol levels drawn to exclude Smith-Lemli-Opitz syndrome.

SOTOS' SYNDROME

Sotos' syndrome, or cerebral gigantism, is an autosomal dominant condition associated with somatic gigantism, with height, weight, and head circumference all greater than the 97th percentile for age; advanced bone age with the phalanges being more advanced than the carpals; abnormal metacarpophalangeal pattern profile; large hands and feet; craniofacial anomalies, usually a large dolichocephalic skull with frontal bossing; and mental retardation. A risk of malignancy is present and is between 1.8% and 7%. Tumors reported have included Wilms' tumor, hepatocellular carcinoma, small cell carcinoma of the lung, leukemia, neuroblastoma, and lymphoma. Haploinsufficiency of NSD1 is the major cause of Sotos' syndrome.

THROMBOCYTOPENIA—ABSENT RADIUS (TAR) SYNDROME

Thrombocytopenia with absent radius is a rare autosomal recessive disorder. The thrombocytopenia has an early onset but is usually transient, and may be associated with a marked leukemoid reaction. A distinguishing feature from other absent radius conditions is the presence of the thumb (Fig. 48). Phocomelia simulating thalidomide embryopathy may be seen.

There may be very significant lower extremity abnormalities, including absent fibula; dislocated knees, ankles, and hips; fusion of the femur and tibia; and short long bones. Approximately 30% have congenital heart disease, primarily tetralogy of Fallot and septal defects. A patient was reported with hypoplasia of the vermis

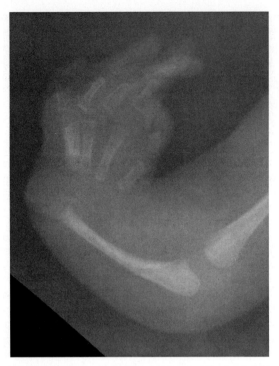

FIGURE 48. Radiograph of right upper extremity in a child with thrombocytopenia–absent radius syndrome shows an absent radius with five digits and shortening and bowing of the ulna.

and corpus callosum along with delay in myelination. A prenatal diagnosis at 11 weeks is possible, and early diagnosis and treatment of the thrombocytopenia is the key to preventing death from internal bleeding, which can be intracerebral.

VACTERL (VATER) Association

The acronym VATER was first used in 1973 by Quan and Smith to describe the anomalies in multiple organ systems believed to arise from mesodermal defects occurring by the fifth week of fetal life, probably from a defect in blastogenesis. The VACTERL association, as it is now known, is believed to be a primary, polytopic, developmental field defect that is causally heterogeneous and rarely familial. The acronym delineates the following: *v*ertebral anomalies, *a*tresia of colon or duodenum, *c*ardiac lesions, *t*racheo*e*sophageal anomalies (especially esophageal atresia), *r*enal anomalies, and *l*imb anomalies (especially radial ray anomalies).

Many infants are initially evaluated for VACTERL association because of either esophageal atresia or imperforate anus. The vertebral anomalies may occur in any part of the spine, although sacral anomalies are most common in patients with imperforate anus (Fig. 49). Thirteen rib-bearing vertebral bodies is the most common anomaly in some series of esophageal atresia patients. Hemivertebra and hypoplastic vertebra are the next most common (Fig. 49). Limb anomalies are variable, including radial segment hypoplasia, proximal focal femoral deficiency, fibular hemimelia, and amelia. The VATER association is present in 4% of infants with

limb reduction defects. Renal anomalies include agenesis, dysplasia, hypoplastic kidneys, horseshoe kidney, and pelvic kidney.

Cardiovascular anomalies include isolated ventriculoseptal defect most frequently, followed by atrial septal defect, tetralogy of Fallot, and transposition of the great arteries. Central nervous system anomalies are not included in the VACTERL acronym but are not uncommon. As many as 34% of imperforate anus patients have spinal dysraphism, including tethered cord, intradural lipoma, and lipomeningocele. Hydrocephalus associated with the VACTERL association is known to have a high rate of recurrence in subsequent pregnancies. This is sometimes referred to as VACTERL-H association, in order to include hydrocephalus in the acronym. Defects in at least three organ systems of the VACTERL acronym should be present in order to confirm the diagnosis and to avoid misdiagnosing other conditions, such as Goldenhar's syndrome or Holt-Oram syndrome.

WARFARIN EMBRYOPATHY

Warfarin, an anticoagulant in common use, can have marked teratogenic effects when taken during the first trimester of pregnancy. Common findings include nasal hypoplasia, epiphyseal calcifications, stippled calcification of the axial skeleton, and mental retardation (Fig. 50). Other skeletal changes include shortening of the long bones, especially the phalanges. Occipital prominence and frontal bossing can be seen. Other less commonly reported findings include dextrocardia and situs inversus, asplenia, intracranial hemorrhage, and diaphragmatic hernia. Recently, prenatal sonography

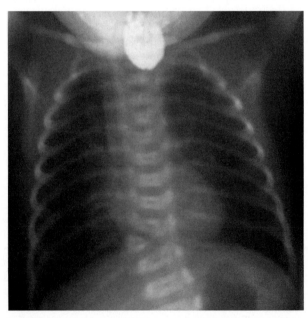

FIGURE 49. VATER or VACTERL association: chest radiograph of newborn with esophageal atresia and tracheoesophageal fistula (contrast media in upper esophageal pouch) and a hemivertebra. Patient also had a pelvic kidney.

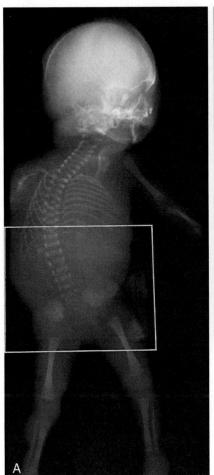

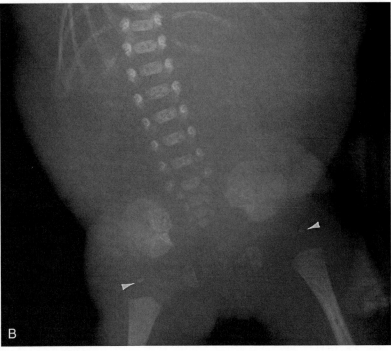

FIGURE 50. Warfarin embryopathy. Fetal radiograph **(A)** and detailed photograph of the pelvis **(B)** demonstrate early ossification in area of femoral head epiphyses *(arrowheads).*

has demonstrated the nasal hypoplasia and epiphyseal calcifications. The radiographic findings can be confused with those of chondrodysplasia punctata.

WEILL-MARCHESANI SYNDROME

Weill-Marchesani syndrome has both autosomal recessive and autosomal dominant modes of inheritance and is characterized by short stature, brachydactyly, and misshapen small lenses. Radiographs demonstrate brachycephaly with hypotelorism; shortened metacarpals, metatarsals, and phalanges; and a delayed bone age (Fig. 51). Undertubulation of bones with thinning of the cortices, widened ribs, rounding of vertebral bodies, and osteoporosis have also been reported.

WERNER'S SYNDROME

Werner's syndrome, or progeria adultorum, is a syndrome of premature aging that begins sometime after puberty. It results from mutations in the WRN DNA helicase/exonuclease gene. It is an autosomal recessive syndrome most common in Japan. Typical radiographic features include generalized osteopenia with osteosclerosis of the phalanges. Generalized muscle atrophy and

osteoarthritis are often seen, as well as markedly advanced coronary atherosclerosis. Advanced brain atrophy is also associated. There is an increased incidence of sarcomas and other tumors of mesenchymal origin.

WILLIAMS SYNDROME

Williams syndrome is a sporadic genetic condition associated with distinctive facial appearance, mental retardation, distinctive behavioral phenotype with gregarious personality, cardiovascular anomalies (especially supravalvar aortic stenosis), peripheral pulmonic stenosis, pulmonary artery hypoplasia (Fig. 52), infantile hypercalcemia, and hyperacusis. This condition is due to submicroscopic deletions in the 7q11.23 chromosome at the elastin gene. Idiopathic hypercalcemia syndrome of infancy is of unknown etiology but resolves by 18 to 24 months of age. Other problems encountered in infancy include frequent crying, constipation, rectal prolapse, and inguinal hernias. Cardiovascular lesions are seen in about three quarters of patients. In addition, a vasculopathy may be present, which can affect the carotid, cerebral, and vertebral arteries, resulting in stroke. Increased cortical gyrification may be shown by three-dimensional MR imaging methods. Similar stenotic lesions in the coronary arteries associated with

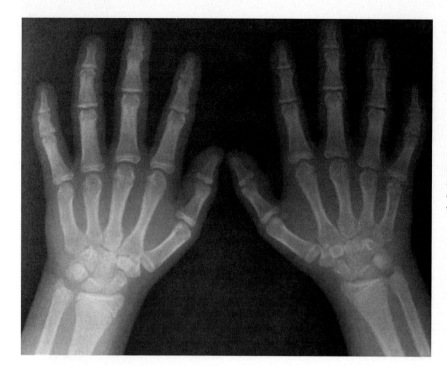

FIGURE 51. Hand radiograph demonstrates shortened metacarpals and phalanges with delayed bone age in this 18-year-old female with Weill-Marchesani syndrome.

supravalvar aortic stenosis predispose to myocardial infarction and sudden death. Renal lesions have also been described, especially renal artery stenosis and nephrocalcinosis. The nephrocalcinosis may relate to the hypercalcemia seen in infancy, for which the cause is not yet known. Radioulnar fusion is encountered in 10% of patients with Williams syndrome. Other orthopedic problems include scoliosis, joint contractures, and recurrent patellar dislocation.

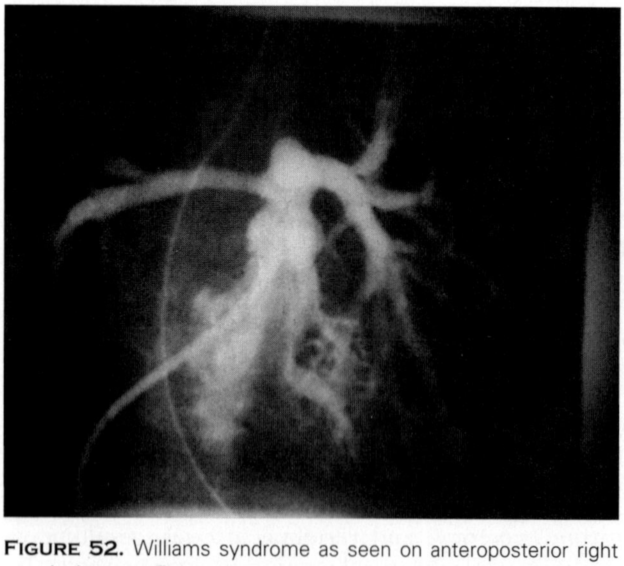

FIGURE 52. Williams syndrome as seen on anteroposterior right ventriculogram. There is hypoplasia of the right main pulmonary artery and stenosis of the takeoff of the artery to the right upper lobe in this child with characteristic facies of Williams syndrome.

CHROMOSOMAL DISORDERS

CRI DU CHAT SYNDROME

Cri du chat syndrome is a chromosomal syndrome caused by partial deletion of the short arm of chromosome 5, and characterized clinically by severe growth and mental retardation associated with a classic "cat-like" cry. Radiographic findings include microcephaly with hypertelorism, micrognathia, gracile bones, and shortened metacarpals with elongated proximal phalanges. Hirschsprung's disease, malrotation, and developmental dysplasia of the hip have also been seen.

TRISOMY 13 (PATAU'S) SYNDROME

Trisomy 13, also known as Patau's syndrome, is a chromosomal syndrome characterized by low birth weight, craniofacial dysmorphism, and mental retardation. Radiographic findings include microcephaly, a sloping forehead, hypotelorism, and possible facial clefts (Fig. 53). Other skeletal findings include thin ribs (Fig. 53C), pelvic hypoplasia, and hand and foot abnormalities, including overlapping fingers, polydactyly, syndactyly, and rocker-bottom feet. Eighty percent of patients present with holoprosencephaly; other intracranial complications include agenesis of the corpus callosum and Dandy-Walker malformation. Other findings include congenital heart disease, diaphragmatic hernia, polydactyly, cystic hygroma, and webbed neck. Prenatal sonography can detect many of the morphologic findings of trisomy 13, suggesting further evaluation or karyotyping.

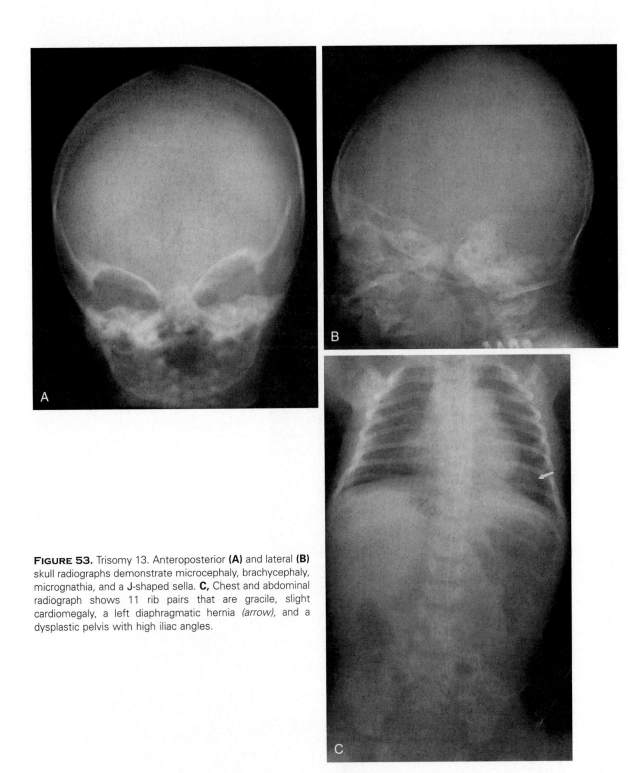

FIGURE 53. Trisomy 13. Anteroposterior **(A)** and lateral **(B)** skull radiographs demonstrate microcephaly, brachycephaly, micrognathia, and a J-shaped sella. **C,** Chest and abdominal radiograph shows 11 rib pairs that are gracile, slight cardiomegaly, a left diaphragmatic hernia *(arrow),* and a dysplastic pelvis with high iliac angles.

TRISOMY 18 (EDWARDS') SYNDROME

Trisomy 18, also known as Edwards' syndrome, is a chromosomal syndrome characterized by low birth weight, hypotonia followed by hypertonia, craniofacial dysmorphism, and mental retardation. Common radiographic findings include gracile ribs, congenital heart disease, and a small pelvis with a narrow iliac crest and wide acetabular angles (Fig. 54*A*). Other findings include thinning of the calvarium with hypoplasia of the mandible and maxilla, dolichocephaly, aplasia of the medial thirds of the clavicles, rocker-bottom feet, and changes of the hand, including short first metacarpal, ulnar deviation of the digits, flexion contractures (Fig. 54*B*), and V-shaped deformity between the second and third digits. Intracranial complications include gyral and lobar dysplasia, often involving the hippocampus, cerebellum, and midbrain. Neonatal hepatitis and

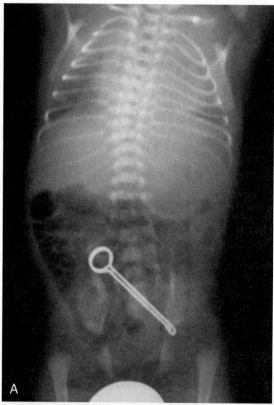

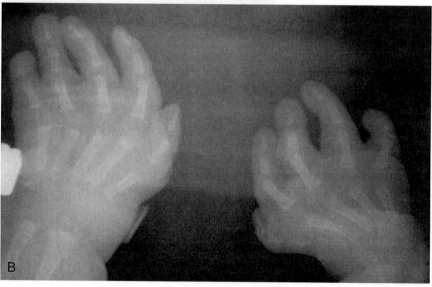

FIGURE 54. Trisomy 18. **A,** Chest and abdominal radiograph demonstrates cardiac enlargement from complex heart disease with a transverse liver associated with asplenia, and a small pelvis with dysplastic hips and high iliac angles. **B,** Posteroanterior hand radiographs show ulnar deviation of the digits, flexion deformities, and some hypoplastic phalanges. The first right metacarpal is hypoplastic.

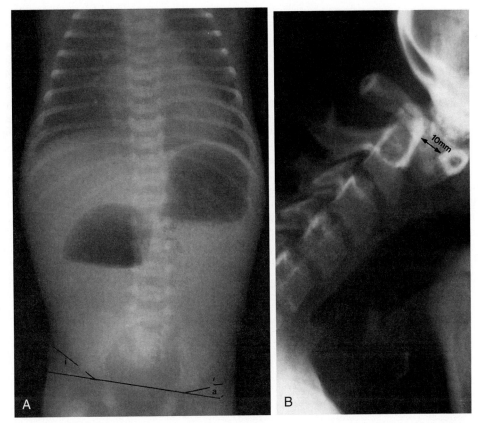

FIGURE 55. Trisomy 21. **A,** This newborn chest and abdomen radiograph demonstrates many findings typical of trisomy 21, including pulmonary overcirculation resulting from the patient's atrioventricular canal, "double bubble" sign typical of duodenal atresia, lack of widening of the intrapedicular distances in the lumbar region, and a decreased iliac index. The iliac index is the sum of the acetabular angle *(a)* and the iliac angle *(i)*. **B,** Flexion radiograph of cervical spine demonstrates widening of the predens interval *(arrows)*.

biliary atresia have also been reported. Prenatal sonography can detect many of the morphologic findings of trisomy 18, suggesting further evaluation or karyotyping.

TRISOMY 21 (DOWN) SYNDROME

Trisomy 21, also known as Down syndrome, is the most common chromosomal syndrome. It is characterized by mental retardation, low birth weight, craniofacial dysmorphism, and a host of anomalies involving virtually all organ systems.

Pelvis radiographs demonstrate Down syndrome characteristics early in life. Flaring of the iliac wings and flattening of the acetabular roofs are seen and can be quantified by measuring the iliac index (Fig. 55A). The iliac index is the sum of the acetabular angle (the angle between the roof of the acetabulum and a line drawn through the triradiate cartilage) and the iliac angle (the angle between the iliac wing and a line drawn through the triradiate cartilage). In trisomy 21 patients, this index is less than 60 degrees.

Skeletal changes include brachycephaly with micrognathia, short hard palate, hypoplastic atlas, occipitoatlantal and atlantoaxial instability (greater than 5 to 7 mm translation on spontaneous flexion and extension seen in 12% to 20% of patients) (Fig. 55B), hypersegmentation of the sternum, 11 rib pairs, gracile ribs, bell-shaped thorax, congenital hip dislocation, and absence of widening of the interpediculate distance of the lumbar spine. Other radiographic findings include congenital heart disease (often endocardial cushion defect), duodenal atresia (Fig. 55A), and congenital megacolon. Prenatal sonography may be helpful in screening, demonstrating a thickened nuchal fold, limb shortening, and echogenic bowel among other findings.

TURNER'S SYNDROME

Turner's syndrome, or isochromosome X, was initially described as a triad of infertility, webbing of the neck, and cubitus valgus deformity of the elbow. Since that time, a multitude of associated findings have been described involving most organ systems. Hand radiographs demonstrate typical changes of osteopenia, shortening of the fourth and fifth metacarpals, delayed maturation, phalangeal predominance, a V-shaped deformity of the distal radioulnar joint, and drumstick-shaped distal phalanges (Fig. 56A). In addition to the classical valgus deformity of the elbow, skeletal findings include brachycephaly, hypoplasia of the clavicles and sacrum, pectus carinatum, platyspondyly, overtubulation of long bones, and flattening of the medial tibial condyle with associated patellar dislocation and proximal tibial spur (Fig. 56B). A shortened bi-iliac distance may be seen prenatally. Cardiovascular findings include aortic coarctation and cardiac septal defects. Renal anomalies, including horseshoe kidney and multicystic dysplastic kidney, may be seen in up to one third of patients. Genital abnormalities, best evaluated with pelvic ultrasound, include ovarian and uterine absence or hypoplasia.

WOLF-HIRSCHHORN SYNDROME

Wolf-Hirschhorn syndrome is a chromosomal syndrome caused by partial deletion of the short arm of chromosome 4, and characterized clinically by mental retardation and severe craniofacial anomalies. Cranial findings include microcephaly with hypertelorism and micrognathia with proportionately small maxilla. The axial skeleton demonstrates dysplastic cervical vertebrae (Fig. 57A), 13 rib pairs (Fig. 57B), scoliosis, vertebral segmentation anomalies, and poorly ossified or widely separated pubic rami (Fig. 57C). The appendicular skeleton shows gracile long bones with a tendency toward radioulnar synostosis, hip dysplasia, and clubfoot. Visceral changes include various malformations of the heart and great vessels as well as diaphragmatic hernia. Intracranial malformations include agenesis of the corpus callosum and other midline defects, as well as cerebellar disorders, disorders in gyration, and multifocal white matter lesions.

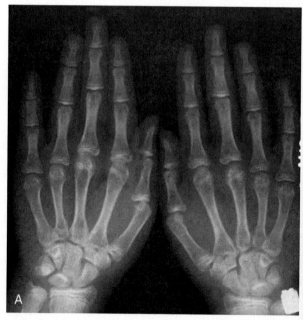

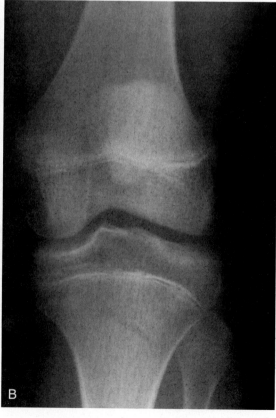

FIGURE 56. Turner's syndrome. **A,** Hand radiograph demonstrates shortening of the fourth and fifth metacarpals with phalangeal predominance typical of Turner's syndrome. **B,** Knee radiograph demonstrates flattening of the medial tibial condyle.

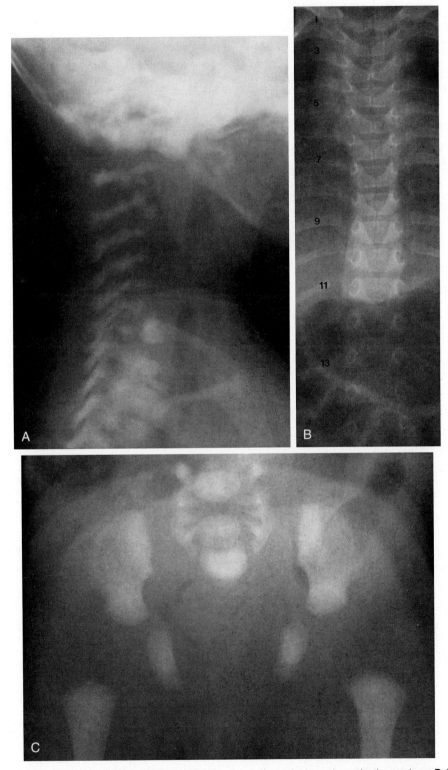

FIGURE 57. Wolf-Hirschhorn syndrome. **A,** Lateral cervical spine radiograph shows hypoplastic vertebrae. **B,** Thoracic spine in an older patient demonstrates 13 rib pairs and spina bifida occulta in some of the upper thoracic vertebrae. **C,** Pelvic radiograph demonstrates poorly ossified, widely separated pubic bones, small iliac bones, and a hypoplastic sacrum.

SUGGESTED READINGS

Acrorenal Syndrome

Al Salloum AA, Al Rasheed SA, Al Husain MA, et al: Acrorenal syndrome associated with visual defect. Pediatr Nephrol 1996;10: 759–760

Miltenyi M, Balogh L, Schmidt K, et al: A new variant of the acrorenal syndrome associated with bilateral oligomeganephronic hypoplasia. Eur J Pediatr 1984;142:40–43

Miltenyi M, Czeizel AE, Balogh L, et al: Autosomal recessive acrorenal syndrome. Am J Med Genet 1992;43:789–790

Amniotic Band Syndrome

Bamforth JS: Amniotic band sequence: Streeter's hypothesis reexamined. Am J Med Genet 1992;44:280–287

Boyd PA, Keeling JW, Selinger M, et al: Limb reduction and chorion villus sampling. Prenatal Diagn 1990;10:437–441

Burton DJ, Filly RA: Sonographic diagnosis of the amniotic band syndrome. AJR Am J Roentgenol 1991;156:555–558

Foulkes GD, Reiner K: Congenital constriction band syndrome: a seventy-year experience. J Pediatr Orthop 1994;14:242–248

Pedersen TK, Thomsen SG: Spontaneous resolution of amniotic bands. Ultrasound Obstet Gynecol 2001;18:673-674

Bardet-Biedl Syndrome

Beales PL, Elcioglu N, Woolf AS, et al: New criteria for improved diagnosis of Bardet-Biedl syndrome: results of a population survey. J Med Genet 1999;36:437–446

Bitoun DA, Lacombe D, Lambert JC, et al: Hydrometrocolpos and polydactyly: a common neonatal presentation of Bardet-Biedl and McKusick-Kaufman syndromes. J Med Genet 1999;36:599–603

Cramer B, Green J, Harnett J, et al: Sonographic and urographic correlation in Bardet-Biedl syndrome. Urol Radiol 1988;10:176–180

Fralick RA, Leichter HE, Sheth KJ: Early diagnosis of Bardet-Biedl syndrome. Pediatr Nephrol 1990;4:264–265

Katsanis N, Lewis RA, Stockton DW, et al: Delineation of the critical interval of Bardet-Biedl syndrome 1 (BBS1). Am J Hum Genet 1999;65:1672–1679

Lorda-Sanchez I, Ayuso C, Ibanez A: Situs inversus and Hirschsprung disease: two uncommon manifestations in Bardet-Biedl syndrome. Am J Med Genet 2000;90:80–81

Mehrota N, Taub S, Covert TF: Hydrometrocolpos as a neonatal manifestation of the Bardet-Biedl syndrome. Am J Med Genet 1997; 69:220

Michel JR, Labrune M, Moreau JF, et al: Une nouvelle entité radio-clinique: la dysplasia rénal multidiverticulaire: rapports avec le syndrome de Laurence-Moon-Bardet-Biedl. Ann Radiol (Paris) 1975;18:533–541

O'Dea D, Parfrey PS, Harnett JD, et al: The importance of renal impairment in the natural history of Bardet-Biedl syndrome. Am J Kidney Dis 1996;6:776–783

Stoler JM, Herrin JT, Holmes LB: Genital abnormalities in females with Bardet-Biedl syndrome. Am J Med Genet 1995;55:276–278

Tieder M, Levy M, Gulber MC: Renal abnormalities in the Bardet-Biedl syndrome. Int J Pediatr Nephrol 1982;3:193–203

Ucar B, Yakut A, Kural N: Renal involvement in the Laurence-Moon-Bardet-Biedl syndrome: report of 5 cases. Pediatr Nephrol 1997;11: 31–37

Young TL, Penny L, Woods MO: A fifth locus for Bardet-Biedl syndrome maps to a chromosome 2q31. Am J Hum Genet 1999;64: 901–904

Beckwith-Wiedemann Syndrome

Andrews MW, Ampar EG: Wilms tumor in a patient with Beckwith Wiedemann syndrome: onset detected with 3 months serial sonography. AJR Am J Roentgenol 1992;159:835–836

Azouz EM, Larsen EJ, Patel J, et al: Beckwith Wiedemann syndrome: development of nephroblastoma during the surveillance period. Pediatr Radiol 1990;20:550–552

Biljoen D, Ramesar R: Evidence for paternal imprinting in familial Beckwith Wiedemann syndrome. J Med Genet 1992;29:221–225

DeBaun MR, Tucker MA: Risk of cancer during the first four years of life in children from the Beckwith Wiedemann Syndrome Registry. J Pediatr 1998;132:398–400

Drut R, Celina Jones M: Congenital pancreatoblastoma in Beckwith Wiedemann syndrome: an emerging association. Pediatr Pathol 1988;8:331–339

Elliott M, Maher ER: Beckwith Wiedemann syndrome. J Med Genet 1994;31:560–564

Hedborg F, Holmgren L, Sandstedt B, et al: Cell type specific IGF2 expression during early human development correlates to the pattern of overgrowth and neoplasia with the Beckwith Wiedemann syndrome. Am J Pathol 1994;145:802–817

McCauley RGK, Becwith JB, Elias ER, et al: Benign hemorrhagic adrenocortical macrocysts in Beckwith Wiedemann syndrome. AJR Am J Roentgenol 1991;157:549–552

Vaughn WG, Sanders DW, Grosfeld JL, et al: Favorable outcome in children with Beckwith-Wiedemann syndrome and intraabdominal malignant tumors. J Pediatr Surg 1995;30:1042–1045

Worth LL, Slopis JM, Herzog CE: Congenital hepatoblastoma and schizencephaly in an infant with Beckwith Wiedemann syndrome. Med Pediatr Oncol 1999;33:591–593

Brachmann-de Lange (Cornelia de Lange's) Syndrome

Allanson JE, Hennekam RCM, Ireland M: De Lange syndrome: subjective and objective comparison of the classical and mild phenotypes. J Med Genet 1997;34:645–650

Braddock SR, Lachman RS, Stoppenhagen CC, et al: Radiological features in Brachmann-de Lange syndrome. Am J Med Genet 1993;47:1006–1013

Butler MG, Dahir GA, Gale DD, et al: Metacarpophalangeal pattern profile analysis in Brachmann-de Lange syndrome. Am J Med Genet 1993;47:1003–1005

Grunebaum M, Kornreich L, Horev G, et al: Tracheomegaly in Brachmann-de Lange syndrome. Pediatr Radiol 1996;26:184–187

Ireland M, Donnai D, Burn J: Brachmann-de Lange syndrome: delineation of the clinical phenotype. Am J Med Genet 1993;47: 959–964

Cerebrocostomandibular Syndrome

Burton EM, Oestreich AE: Cerebro-costo-mandibular syndrome with stippled epiphysis and cystic fibrosis. Pediatr Radiol 1988;18: 365–367

Ibba RM, Corda A, Zoppi MA, et al: Cerebro-costo-mandibular syndrome: early sonographic prenatal diagnosis. Ultrasound Obstet Gynecol 1997;10:142–144

Merlob P, Schonfeld A, Grunebaum A, et al: Autosomal dominant cerebro-costo-mandibular syndrome: ultrasonographic and clinical findings. Am J Med Genet 1987;26:195–202

Plotz FB, van Essen AJ, Bosschaart F, et al: Cerebro-costo-mandibular syndrome. Am J Med Genet 1996;62:286–293

Cerebrohepatorenal (Zellweger) Syndrome

Kelley RI: Review: the cerebrohepatorenal syndrome of Zellweger, morphologic and metabolic aspects. Am J Med Genet 1983;16: 503–517

Luisiri A, Sotelo-Avila C, Silberstein MJ, et al: Sonography of the Zellweger syndrome. J Ultrasound Med 1988;7:169–173

Nakai A, Shigematsu Y, Nishida K, et al: MRI findings of Zellweger syndrome. Pediat Neurol 1995;13:346–348

Poznanski AK, Nosanchuk JS, Baublis J, et al: The cerebro-hepato-renal syndrome (CHRS) (Zellweger's syndrome). Am J Roentgenol Radium Ther Nucl Med 1970;109:313–322

Preuss N, Brosius U, Biermanns M, et al: PEX1 mutations in complementation group 1 of Zellweger spectrum patients correlate with severity of disease. Pediatr Res 2002;51:706–714

Weese-Mayer DE, Smith KM, Reddy JK, et al: Computerized tomography and ultrasound in the diagnosis of cerebro-hepato-renal syndrome of Zellweger. Pediatr Radiol 1987;17:170–172

Cockayne's Syndrome

Cleaver JE, Thompson LH, Richardson AS, et al: A summary of mutations in the UV-sensitive disorders: xeroderma pigmentosum, Cockayne syndrome, and trichothiodystrophy. Hum Mutat 1999; 14:9–22

Dabbagh O, Swaiman KF: Cockayne syndrome: MRI correlates of hypomyelination. Pediatr Neurol 1988;4:113–116

Nance MA, Berry SA: Cockayne syndrome: review of 140 cases. Am J Med Genet 1992;42:68–84

Nishio H, Kodama S, Matsuo T, et al: Cockayne syndrome: magnetic resonance images of the brain in a severe form with early onset. J Inherit Metab Dis 1988;11:88–102

Silengo MC, Franceschini P, Bianco R, et al: Distinctive skeletal dysplasia in Cockayne syndrome. Pediatr Radiol 1986;16:264–266

Congenital Contractural Arachnodactyly

Courtens W, Tjalma W, Messiaen L, et al: Prenatal diagnosis of a constitutional interstitial deletion of chromosome 5 (q15q31.1) presenting with features of congenital contractural arachnodactyly. Am J Med Genet 1998;77:188–197

Currarino G, Friedman JM: A severe form of congenital contractural arachnodactyly in two newborn infants. Am J Med Genet 1986;25: 763–773

Ramos Arroyo MA, Weaver DD, Beals RK: Congenital contractural arachnodactyly: report of four additional families and review of literature. Clin Genet 1985;27:570–581

Congenital Insensitivity to Pain

Bar-On E, Weigl D, Parvari R, et al: Congenital insensitivity to pain. Orthopedic manifestations. J Bone Joint Surg Br 2002;84:252–257

Rosenberg S, Marie SK, Kliemann S: Congenital insensitivity to pain with anhidrosis (hereditary sensory and autonomic neuropathy type IV). Pediatr Neurol 1994;11:50–56

Spencer JA, Grieve DK: Congenital indifference to pain mistaken for non-accidental injury. Br J Radiol 1990;3:308–310

Currarino's Triad

Currarino G, Coln D, Votteler T: Triad of anorectal, sacral and presacral anomalies. AJR Am J Roentgenol 1981;137:395–398

Gudinchet F, Maeder P, Laurent T, et al: Magnetic resonance detection of myelodysplasia in children with Currarino triad. Pediatr Radiol 1997;27:903–907

Kirks DA, Merten DF, Filston HC, et al: Currarino triad: complex of anorectal malformation, sacral bony abnormality and presacral mass. Pediatr Radiol 1984;14:220–225

Lee SC, Chun YS, Jung SE, et al: Currarino triad: anorectal malformation, sacral bony abnormality and presacral mass—a review of 11 cases. J Pediatr Surg 1997;32:58–61

Masuno M, Imaizumi K, Aida N, et al: Currarino triad with terminal deletion 7q35 and 7q634. J Med Genet 1996;33:877–878

Ross AJ, Ruiz Perez V, Wang Y, et al: A homeobox gene HLXB9 is the major locus for dominantly inherited sacral agenesis. Nat Genet 1998;20:358–361

Tander B, Bashkin D, Bulut M: A case of incomplete Currarino triad with malignant transformation. Pediatr Surg Int 1999;15:409–410

Diamond-Blackfan Syndrome

Ball SE, McGuckin CP, Jenkins G, et al: Diamond-Blackfan anaemia in the U.K.: analysis of 80 cases from a 20-year birth cohort. Br J Haematol 1996;94:645–653

Draptchinskaia N, Gustavsson P, Andersson B, et al: The gene encoding ribosomal protein S19 is mutated in Diamond-Blackfan anaemia. Nat Genet 1999;21:169–175

Ehlers-Danlos Syndrome

Beighton P: The Ehlers-Danlos syndromes. *In* McKusick VA (ed): McKusick's Heritable Disorders of Connective Tissue, 5th ed. St. Louis, Mosby–Year Book, 1993:189–251

Giunta C, Superti-Furga A, Spranger S, et al: Ehlers-Danlos syndrome type VII: clinical features and molecular defects. J Bone Joint Surg Am 1999;81:225–238

Herman TE, McAlister WH: Cavitary pulmonary lesions in type IV Ehlers-Danlos syndrome. Pediatr Radiol 1994;24:263–265

Pepin M, Schwarze U, Superti-Furga A, Byers PN: Clinical and genetic features of Ehlers-Danlos syndrome type IV, the vascular type. N Engl J Med 2000;342:673–680

Epidermolysis Bullosa

Castillo RO, Davies YK, Lin YC, et al: Management of esophageal strictures in children with recessive dystrophic epidermolysis bullosa. J Pediatr Gastroenterol Nutr 2002;34:535–541

Dolan CR, Smith LT, Sybert VP: Prenatal detection of EB letalis with pyloric atresia. Am J Med Genet 1993;47:395–400

Lin AN, Carter DM: Epidermolysis bullosa. J Pediatrics 1989;114: 349–355

Orlando RC, Bozymski EM, Birggman RA, et al: Epidermolysis bullosa: gastrointestinal manifestations. Ann Intern Med 1974;81:203–206

Smith PK, Davidson GP, Moore L, et al: Epidermolysis bullosa and severe ulcerative colitis in an infant. J Pediatr 1993;122:600–603

Fanconi's Anemia

Ahmad SI, Hanaoka F, Kirk SH: Molecular biology of Fanconi anemia: an old problem, a new insight. Bioessays 2002;24:439–448

Alter BP: Fanconi's anaemia and its variability. Br J Haematol 1993;85:9–14

dos Santos CC, Gavish H, Buchwald M: Fanconi anemia revisited: old ideas and new advances. Stem Cells 1994;12:142–153

Joenje H, Oostra AB, Wijker M, et al: Evidence for at least eight Fanconi anemia genes. Am J Hum Genet 1997;61:940–944

Rogers PC, Desai F, Karabus CD, et al: Presentation and outcome of 25 cases of Fanconi's anemia. Am J Pediatr Hematol Oncol 1989;11: 141–145

Fibrodysplasia Ossificans Progressiva

Buyse G, Silberstein J, Goemans N, et al: Fibrodysplasia ossificans progressiva: still turning to wood after 300 years? Eur J Pediatr 1996;154:694–699

Caron KH, DiPietro MA, Aisen AM, et al: MR imaging of early fibrodysplasia ossificans progressiva. J Comput Assist Tomogr 1990; 14:318–321

Cohen RB, Hahn GV, Tabas JA, et al: The natural history of heterotopic ossification in patients who have fibrodysplasia ossificans progressiva: a study of forty-four patients. J Bone Joint Surg Am 1993;75:215–219

Smith R, Athanasou NA, Vipond SE: Fibrodysplasia (myositis) ossificans progressive: clinicopathological features and natural history. Q J Med 1996;89:445–456

Virdi AS, Shore EM, Oreffo ROC, et al: Phenotypic and molecular heterogeneity in fibrodysplasia ossificans progressiva. Calcif Tissue Int 1999;65:250–255

Freeman-Sheldon (Whistling Face) Syndrome

Burton BK, Sumner T, Langer LO Jr, et al: A new skeletal dysplasia: clinical, radiologic, and pathologic findings. J Pediatr 1986;109: 642–648

Robbins-Furman P, Hecht JT, Rocklin M, et al: Prenatal diagnosis of Freeman-Sheldon syndrome (whistling face). Prenatal Diagn 1995; 15:179–182

Zampino G, Conti G, Balducci F, et al: Severe form of Freeman-Sheldon syndrome associated with brain anomalies and hearing loss. Am J Med Genet 1996;62:293–296

Goldenhar's Syndrome

Beltinger C, Saule H: Imaging of lipoma of the corpus callosum and intracranial dermoids in the Goldenhar syndrome. Pediatr Radiol 1988;18:72–73

Gibson JNA, Sillence DO, Taylor TKF: Abnormalities of the spine in Goldenhar syndrome. J Pediatr Orthop 1996;16:344–349

Gosain AK, McCarthy JG, Pinto RS: Cervicovertebral anomalies and basilar impression in Goldenhar syndrome. Plastic Reconstr Surg 1994;93:498–507

Johnson KA, Fairhurst J, Clarke NMP: Oculo-auriculo-vertebral spectrum: new manifestations. Pediatr Radiol 1995;25:446–448

Kaye CI, Rollnick BR, Hauck WW, et al: Microtia and associated anomalies. Am J Med Genet 1989;34:574–578

Lasram L, Gmar R, Ouertani A, et al: Syndrome de Goldenhar. J Fr Ophthalmol 1992;15:419–422

Morrison PJ, Mulholland HC, Craig BG, et al: Cardiovascular abnormalities in the oculo-auriculo-vertebral spectrum. Am J Med Genet 1992;44:425–428

Rodriguez JI, Palacios J, Lapunzina P: Severe axial anomalies in the oculo-auriculo-vertebral (Goldenhar) complex. Am J Med Genet 1993;47:69–73

Schrander-Stumpel CTRM, de Die-Smulders CE, Hennekam RC: Oculo-auriculo-vertebral spectrum and cerebral anomalies. J Med Genet 1992;29:326–331

Van Meter TD, Weaver DD: Oculo auriculo vertebral spectrum and the CHARGE association: clinical evidence for a common pathogenetic mechanism. Clin Dysmorphol 1996;5:187–196

Hadju-Cheney Syndrome

Kaplan P, Ramos F, Zackai EH, et al: Cystic kidney disease in Hajdu-Cheney syndrome. Am J Med Genet 1995;56:25–30

Kawamura J, Miki Y, Yamazaki S, et al: Hajdu-Cheney syndrome: MR imaging. Neuroradiology 1991;33:441–442

O'Reilly MAR, Shaw DG: Hajdu-Cheney syndrome. Ann Rheum Dis 1994;53:276–279

Ramos FJ, Kaplan BS, Bellah RD, et al: Further evidence that the Hajdu-Cheney syndrome and the "serpentine fibula-polycystic kidney syndrome" are a single entity. Am J Med Genet 1998;78:474–481

Hallermann-Streiff Syndrome

Bitoun P, Timsit JC, Trang H, et al: A new look at the management of the oculo-mandibulo-facial syndrome. Ophthalmic Pediatr Genet 1992;13:19–26

Christian CL, Lachman RS, Aylsworth AS, et al: Radiological findings in Hallermann-Streiff syndrome: report of five cases and a review of the literature. Am J Med Genet 1991;41:508–514

Cohen MM Jr: Hallermann-Streiff syndrome: a review. Am J Med Genet 1991;41:488–499

Robinow M: Respiratory obstruction and cor pulmonale in the Hallermann-Streiff syndrome. Am J Med Genet 1991;41:515–516

Holt-Oram Syndrome

Basson CT, Huant T, Lin RC, et al: Different TBX235 interactions in heart and limb defined by Holt Oram syndrome mutations. Proc Natl Acad Sci U S A 1999;96:2919–2924

Hurst JA, Hall CM, Baraister M: The Holt Oram syndrome. J Med Genet 1991;28:406–410

Newbury-Ecob RA, Leanage R, Raeburn JA, et al: Holt Oram syndrome: a clinical genetic study. J Med Genet 1996;33:300–307

Poznanski AK, Gall JC, Stern AM: Skeletal anomalies of the Holt Oram syndrome. Radiology 1970;94:45–53

Sletten LJ, Pierpont MEM: Variation in severity of cardiac disease in Holt Oram syndrome. Am J Med Genet 1996;65:128–132

Spranger S, Ulmer H, Troger J, et al: Muscular involvement in Holt Oram syndrome. J Med Genet 1997;34:978–981

Homocystinuria

Brill PW, Mitty HA, Gaull GE: Homocystinuria due to cystathionine synthase deficiency: clinical roentgenologic correlations. Am J Roentgenol Radium Ther Nucl Med 1974;121:45–54

Morreels CL Jr, Fletcher BD, Weilbaecher RG, Dorst JP: The roentgenographic features of homocystinuria. Radiology 1968;90:1150–1158

Mudd SH, Skovby F, Levy HL, et al: The natural history of homocystinuria due to cystathionine beta-synthase deficiency. Am J Hum Genet 1985;37:1–31

Ruano MM, Castillo M, Thompson JE: MR imaging in a patient with homocystinuria. AJR Am J Roentgenol 1998;171:1147–1149

Kaufman-McKusick Syndrome

Davenport M, Taitz LS, Dickson JAS: The Kaufman-McKusick syndrome: another association. J Pediatr Surg 1989;24:1192–1194

David A, Bitou P, Lacombe D, et al: Hydrometrocolpos and polydactyly: a common neonatal presentation of Bardet-Biedl and McKusick-Kaufman syndromes. J Med Genet 1999;36:599–603

Kaufman RL, Hartmann HF, McAlister WH: Family studies in congenital heart disease II: a syndrome of hydrometrocolpos, post axial polydactyly and congenital heart disease. Birth Defects Orig Artic Ser 1972;8:85–87

Robinow M, Shaw A: The McKusick-Kaufmann syndrome. J Pediatr 1979;94:776–778

Stone DL, Agarwala R, Schaffer AA, et al: Genetic and physical mapping of the McKusick-Kaufman syndrome. Hum Mol Genet 1998;7:475–481

Klippel-Trénaunay Syndrome

Anlar B, Yalaz K, Erzen C: Klippel-Trenaunay-Weber syndrome: a case with cerebral and cerebellar hemihypertrophy. Neuroradiology 1988;30:360

Gianlupi A, Harper RW, Dwyre DM, et al: Recurrent pulmonary embolism associated with Klippel-Trenaunay-Weber syndrome. Chest 1999;115:1199–1201

James CA, Allison JW, Waner M: Pediatric case of the day: Klippel-Trenaunay syndrome. Radiographics 1999;19:1093–1096

Roberts RV, Dickenson JE, Hugo PJ, et al: Prenatal sonographic appearances of Klippel-Trenaunay-Weber syndrome. Prenatal Diagn 1999;19:369–371

Roebuck DJ, Howlett DC, Frazer CK, et al: Pictorial review: the imaging features of lower limb Klippel-Trenaunay syndrome. Clin Radiol 1994;49:346–350

Wang Q, Timur AA, Szafranski P, et al: Identification and molecular characterization of de novo translocation t(8;14) (q22.3;q13) associated with a vascular and tissue overgrowth syndrome. Cytogenet Cell Genet 2001;95:183–188

Larsen's Syndrome

Forese LL, Berdon WE, Harcke HT, et al: Severe mid-cervical kyphosis with cord compression in Larsen's syndrome and diastrophic dysplasia: unrelated syndromes with similar radiologic findings and neurosurgical implications. Pediatr Radiol 1995;25:136–139

Houston CS, Reed MH, Desansch JEL: Separating Larsen's syndrome from the "arthrogryposis basket." J Canad Assoc Radiol 1981;32:206–214

Laville JM, Lakermance P, Limouzy E: Larsen's syndrome: review of the literature and analysis of thirty-eight cases. J Pediatr Orthop 1994;14:63–73

Vujic M, Hallstensson K, Wahlstrom J, et al: Localization of a gene for autosomal dominant Larsen syndrome to chromosome region 3p21.1-14.1 in the proximity of, but distinct from, the COL7A1 locus. Am J Hum Genet 1995;57:1104–1113

Marfan Syndrome

Bresters D, Nikkels PGJ, Meijboom EJM, et al: Clinical, pathological and molecular genetic findings in a case of neonatal Marfan syndrome. Acta Paediar 1999;88:98–101

De Paepe A, Devereux RB, Dietz HC, et al: Revised diagnostic criteria for the Marfan syndrome. Am J Med Genet 1996;62:417–426

Dijkstra PF, Cole TR, Oorthuys JW, et al: Metacarpophalangeal pattern profile analysis in Sotos and Marfan syndrome. Am J Med Genet 1994;51:55–60

Fattori R, Nienaber CA, Descovich B, et al: Importance of dural ectasia in phenotypic assessment of Marfan's syndrome. Lancet 1999;354:910–913

Groenink M, Rozendaal L, Naeff MS, et al: Marfan syndrome in children and adolescents: predictive and prognostic value of aortic root growth for screening for aortic complications. Heart 1998;80: 163–169

Sponseller PD, Hobbs W, Riley LH III, et al: The thoracolumbar spine in Marfan syndrome. J Bone Joint Surg Am 1995;77:867–876

Marshall-Smith Syndrome

Eich GF, Silver MM, Weksberg R, et al: Marshall-Smith syndrome: new radiographic, clinical, and pathologic observations. Radiology 1991;181:183–188

Marshall RE, Graham CB, Scott CR, et al: Syndrome of accelerated skeletal maturation and relative failure to thrive: a newly recognized clinical growth disorder. J Pediatr 1971;78:95–101

Williams DK, Carlton DR, Green SH, et al: Marshall-Smith syndrome: the expanding phenotype. J Med Genet 1997;34:842–845

Yoder CC, Wiswell T, Cornish JD, et al: Marshall-Smith syndrome: further delineation. South Med J 1988;81:1297–1300

Mayer-Rokitansky-Küster-Hauser Sequence

Bau CHD, Ribeiro CA, Ribeiro SA, et al: Bilateral femoral hypoplasia associated with Rokitansky sequence: another example of a mesodermal malformation spectrum. Am J Med Genet 1994;49:205–206

Biedl CW, Pagon RA, Zapata JO: Mullerian anomalies and renal agenesis: autosomal dominant urogenital adysplasia. J Pediatr 1984;104:861–864

Braun Quentin C, Billes C, Bowing B, et al: MURCS association: case report and review. J Med Genet 1996;33:618–620

Buchta RM, Viseskul C, Gilbert EF, et al: Familial bilateral renal agenesis and hereditary renal adysplasia. Z Kinderheilkd 1973;115: 111–129

Dieker H, Opitz JM: Associated acral and renal malformations. Birth Defects Orig Artic Ser 1969;5:68–77

Lin HJ, Cornford ME, Hu B, et al: Occipital encephalocele and MURCS association: case report of central nervous system anomalies in MURCS patients. Am J Med Genet 1996;61:59–61

Moermann P, Fryns JP, Sastrowijoto SH, et al: Hereditary renal adysplasia: new observations and hypothesis. Pediatr Pathol 1994; 14:405–410

Moore WB, Matthews TJ, Rabinowitz R: Genitourinary anomalies associated with Klippel Feil syndrome. J Bone Joint Surg Am 1975;57:355–357

Strubbe EH, Willemsen WNP, Lemmens JAM, et al: Hauser syndrome: distinction between two forms based on excretory urographic, sonographic and laparoscopic findings. AJR Am J Roentgenol 1993;160:331–334

Trigaux JP, van Beers B, Del Chambre F: Male genital tract malformations associated with ipsilateral renal agenesis: sonographic findings. J Clin Ultrasound 1991;19:3–10

Wellesley DG, Slaney SF: MURCS in a male? J Med Genet 1995;32: 314–315

Meckel's (Meckel-Gruber) Syndrome

Kjaer KW, Fischer HB, Keeling JW, et al: Skeletal malformations in fetuses with Meckel syndrome. Am J Med Genet 1999;84:469–475

Nyberg DA, Hallesy D, Mahony BS, et al: Meckel-Gruber syndrome: importance of prenatal diagnosis. J Ultrasound Med 1990;9: 691–696

Rapola J, Salonen R: Visceral anomalies in the Meckel syndrome. Teratology 1985;31:193–201

Salonen R, Paavola P: Meckel syndrome. J Med Genet 1998;35: 497–501

Shen-Schwarz S, Dave H: Meckel syndrome with polysplenia: case report and review of the literature. Am J Med Genet 1988;31: 349–355

Nail–Patella Syndrome

Guidera KJ, Satter White Y, Ogden JA, et al: Nail patella syndrome: a review of 44 orthopaedic patients. J Pediatr Orthop 1991;11: 737–742

Mangino M, Sanchez O, Torrente I, et al: Localization of a gene for familial patella aplasia-hypoplasia (PTLAH) to chromosome 17q21-22. Am J Hum Genet 1999;54:441–447

Pinette MG, Ukleja M, Blackstone J: Early prenatal diagnosis of nail-patella syndrome by ultrasonography. J Ultrasound Med 1999; 18:387–389

Yarali HN, Erden GA, Karaarslan F, et al: Clavicular horn: another bony projection in nail-patella syndrome. Pediatr Radiol 1995;25: 549–550

Nevoid Basal Cell Carcinoma (Gorlin's) Syndrome

Evans DGR, Ladusans EJ, Rimmer S, et al: Complications of nevoid basal cell carcinoma syndrome. J Med Genet 1993;30: 460–464

Gorlin RJ: Nevoid basal-cell carcinoma syndrome. Medicine 1987;66: 98–113

Gorlin RJ: Nevoid basal cell carcinoma (Gorlin) syndrome: unanswered issues. J Lab Clin Med 1999;134:551–552

Hermann G, Som P: Multiple basal cell nevus syndrome. Skeletal Radiol 1981;6:62–64

Kimonis VE, Goldstein AM, Pastakia B, et al: Clinical manifestations in 105 persons with nevoid basal cell carcinoma syndrome. Med Genet 1997;369:299–308

Korczak JF, Brahim JS, DiGiovanna JJ, et al: Nevoid basal cell carcinoma syndrome with medulloblastoma: a rare case illustrating gene-environment interaction. Am J Med Genet 1997;69:309–314

Mortele KJ, Hoier MR, Mergo PJ, et al: Bilateral adrenal cystic lymphangiomas in nevoid basal cell carcinoma (Gorlin Goltz) syndrome: US, CT and MR findings. J Comp Assist Tomogr 1999;23:562–564

Noonan's Syndrome

Baltaxe HA, Levin AR, Ehlers KH, et al: Appearance of the left ventricle in Noonan syndrome. Radiology 1973;109:155–159

Bieden LC, Schneeweiss A, Shemtov A, et al: Unifying link between Noonan and Leopard syndromes. Pediatr Cardiol 1983;4: 168–169

Digilio MC, Barino B, Giannotti A, et al: Noonan syndrome with cardiac left-sided obstructive lesions. Hum Genet 1997;99:289

Hagekawa T, Ogata T, Hasegawa Y, et al: Coarctation of the aorta and renal hypoplasia in a boy with Turner/Noonan surface anomalies and a 46 XY karyotype: a clinical model for the possible impairment of a putative lymphogenic gene for Turner somatic stigmata. Hum Genet 1996;97:564–567

Khan S, McDowel H, Upadhyaya P, et al: Vaginal rhabdomyosarcoma in a patient with Noonan syndrome. J Med Genet 1995;32:743–745

Noonan JA: Noonan syndrome: an update and review for the primary pediatrician. Clin Pediatr 1994;33:548–555

Raymond G, Holmes LB: Cardio-facio-cutaneous syndrome. Dev Med Child Neurol 1993;35:727–741

Schorry EK, Lovell AM, Milatovich A, et al: Ullrich-Turner syndrome and neurofibromatosis. Am J Med Genet 1996;66:423–425

Tanaka Y, Masuno M, Kwamoto H, et al: Noonan syndrome and cavernous hemangioma of the brain. Am J Med Genet 1999;82: 212–214

Vander Burgt I, Thoonen G, Roosenboom N, et al: Patterns of cognitive functioning in school-aged children with Noonan syndrome associated with variability in phenotypic expression. J Pediatr 1999;135:707–713

Occipital Horn Syndrome

Beighton P, dePaepe A, Danks D, et al: International nosology of heritable disorders of connective tissue, 1986. Am J Med Genet 1988;29:581–594

Dagenais SL, Adam AN, Innis JW, et al: A novel frameshift mutation in exon 23 of ATP7A (MNK) results in occipital horn syndrome and not in Menkes disease. Am J Hum Genet 2001;69:420–427

Herman TE, McAlister WH, Boniface A: Occipital horn syndrome: additional radiographic findings in two new cases. Pediatr Radiol 1992;22:363–365

Mentzel HJ, Seidel J, Vogt S, et al: Vascular complications (splenic and hepatic artery aneurysms) in the occipital horn syndrome: report of a patient and review of the literature. Pediatr Radiol 1999;29:19–22

Sartoris DJ, Luzzatti L, Weaver DD, et al: Type IX Ehlers Danlos syndrome. Radiology 1984;152:665–670

Tsukahara M, Kmaizumi K, Kawai S, et al: Occipital horn syndrome: report of a patient and review of the literature. Clin Genet 1994;45:32–35

Opitz (G/BBB) Syndrome

Cote GB, Katsantoni A, Papadakou-Lagoyanni S, et al: The G syndrome. Clin Genet 1981;19:473–478

de Silva EO: The hypertelorism-hypospadias syndrome. Clin Genet 1983;23:30–34

Funderburk SJ, Stewart R: The G and BBB syndromes: case presentations, genetics and nosology. Am J Med Genet 1978;2:131–144

MacDonald MR, Olney AH, Kolodziej P: Opitz syndrome (G/BBB). Ear Nose Throat J 1998;77:528–529

MacDonald MR, Schaefer GB, Olney A, et al: Brain magnetic resonance imaging findings in the Opitz G/BBB syndrome: extension of the spectrum of midline brain anomalies. Am J Med Genet 1993;46:706–711

Schrander J, Schrander-Stumpel C, Berg J, et al: Opitz BBBG syndrome: new family with late-onset serious complication. Clin Genet 1995;48:76–79

Oral-Facial-Digital Syndromes

Anneren G, Arvidson B, Gustavson KH, et al: Oro-facio-digital syndromes I and II: radiological methods of diagnosis and the clinical variations. Clin Genet 1984;26:178–186

Gorlin RJ: Branchial arch and oro-acral disorders. In Gorlin RJ, Cohen MM Jr, Levin LS (eds): Syndromes of the Head and Neck, 3rd ed. New York, Oxford University Press, 1990:676–686

Hsieh YC, Hou JW: Oral-facial-digital syndrome with Y-shaped fourth metacarpals and endocardial cushion defect. Am J Med Genet 1999;86:278–281

Odent S, Le Marec B, Toutain A, et al: Central nervous system malformations and early end-stage renal disease in oro-facio-digital syndrome type I: a review. Am J Med Genet 1998;75:389–394

Osteolysis Syndromes

Chung C: Gorham syndrome of the thorax and cervical spine: CT and MRI findings. Skeletal Radiol 1997;26:55–59

Pai GS, Macpherson RI: Idiopathic multicentric osteolysis: report of two new cases and a review of the literature. Am J Med Genet 1988;29:929–936

Urlus M, Roosen P, Lammens J, et al: Carpo-tarsal osteolysis: case report and review of the literature. Genet Couns 1993;4:25–36

Otopalatodigital Syndrome

Brewster TG, Lachman RS, Kushner DE, et al: Oto-palato-digital syndrome, type II—an X-linked skeletal dysplasia. Am J Med Genet 1985;20:249–254

Corona-Rivera JR: Infant with manifestations of oto-palato-digital syndrome type II and of Melnick-Needles syndrome. Am J Med Genet 1999;85:79–81

Gendall PW, Kozlowski K: Oto-palato-digital syndrome type II: report of two related cases. Pediatr Radiol 1992;22:267–269

Langer LO Jr: The roentgenographic features of the oto-palato-digital (OPD) syndrome. Am J Roentgenol Radium Ther Nucl Med 1967;100:63–70

Pena-Shokeir Syndrome I (Fetal Akinesia Sequence)

Agapitos M, Theodoropoulou M, Kouselinis A, et al: Athrogryposis multiplex congenita, Pena Shokeir phenotype with gastroschisis and agenesis of the leg. Pediatr Pathol 1988;8:409–413

Choi BH, Ruess WR, Kim RC: Disturbances in neuronal migration and laminar cortical formation with multicystic encephalopathy in Pena Shokeir syndrome. Acta Neuropathol 1986;69:177–183

Hageman G, Willemse J, van Ketel BA, et al: The heterogeneity of the Pena Shokeir syndrome. Neuropediatrics 1987;18:45–50

Moessinger AC: Fetal akinesia deformation sequence: an animal model. Pediatrics 1983;72:857–863

Porter HJ: Lethal arthrogryposis multiplex congenita. Pediatr Pathol Lab Med 1995;15:617–637

Pena-Shokeir Syndrome II (Cerebro-oculofacioskeletal Syndrome)

Gorlin RJ, Cohen MM, Hennekam RCM: Syndromes with contractures. In Gorlin RJ, Cohen MM, Levin LS (eds): Syndromes of the Head and Neck, 4th ed. New York, Oxford University Press, 2001:767–769

Linna SL, Finni K, Simila A, et al: Intracranial calcifications in cerebro-oculo-facial-skeletal (COFS) syndrome. Pediatr Radiol 1982;79:282–284

Pena SDJ, Shokeir MHK: Autosomal recessive cerebro-oculo-facial-skeletal (COFS) syndrome. Clin Genet 1974;5:285–293

Poland's Syndrome

Al-Quattan MM: Classification of hand anomalies in Poland syndrome. Br J Plast Surg 2001;54:132–136

Azouz EM, Oudjhane K: Disorders of the upper extremity in children. Magn Reson Imaging Clin N Am 1998;63:677–695

Bavinck JN, Weaver DD: Subclavian artery supply disruption sequence: hypothesis of a vascular etiology for Poland, Klippel-Feil, and Mobius anomalies. Am J Med Genet 1986;234:903–918

Darian VB, Argenta LC, Pasyk KA: Familial Poland's syndrome. Ann Plast Surg 1989;236:531–537

Wright AR, Milner RH, Bainbridge LC, et al: MR and CT in the assessment of Poland syndrome. J Comput Assist Tomogr 1992;163:442–447

Progeria

Ackerman J, Gilbert-Barness E: Hutchinson-Gilford progeria syndrome: a pathologic study. Pediatr Pathol Mol Med 2002;21:1–13

Hogan PA, Krafchik BR: Hutchinson-Gilford syndrome. Pediatr Dermatol 1990;7:317–319

Rodriquez JI, Perez-Alonso P, Funes R, et al: Lethal neonatal Hutchinson-Gilford progeria syndrome. Am J Med Genet 1999;82:242–248

Proteus Syndrome

Azouz EM, Cost T, Fitch N: Radiologic findings in the Proteus syndrome. Pediatr Radiol 1987;17:481–485

Cohen MM Jr: A comprehensive and critical assessment of overgrowth and overgrowth syndromes: Proteus syndrome. Adv Hum Genet 1989;18:274–281

Cremin BJ, Vilihoen DL, Wynchank S, et al: The Proteus syndrome: the magnetic resonance and radiological features. Pediatr Radiol 1987;17:486–488

Stricker S: Musculoskeletal manifestations of Proteus syndrome: report of two cases with literature review. J Pediatr Orthop 1992;12:667–674

Rubinstein-Taybi Syndrome

Cirillo RL Jr: Pediatric case of the day: Rubinstein-Taybi syndrome. Radiographics 1997;176:1604–1605

Mazzone D, Milana A, Practico G, et al: Rubinstein-Taybi syndrome associated with Dandy-Walker cyst: case report in a newborn. J Perinatal Med 1989;175:381–384

Petrij F, Giles RH, Dauwerse HG, et al: Rubinstein-Taybi syndrome caused by mutations in the transcriptional co-activator CBP. Nature 1995;376:348–351

Rubinstein JH: Broad thumb-hallux Rubinstein-Taybi syndrome 1957–1988. Am J Med Genet Suppl 1990;6:3–16

Stevens CA: Patellar dislocation in Rubinstein-Taybi syndrome. Am J Med Genet 1997;72:188–190

Russell-Silver Syndrome

Al Fifi S, Teebi AS, Shevell M: Autosomal dominant Russell Silver syndrome. Am J Med Genet 1996;61:96–972

Bruckheimer E, Abrahamov A: Russell Silver syndrome and Wilms tumor. J Pediatr 1993;122:165–166

Herman TE, Crawford JD, Cleveland RJ, et al: Hand radiographs in Russell Silver syndrome. Pediatrics 1987;79:743–744

Hotokebuchi T, Miyahara H, Sugioka Y: Legg Calve Perthes' disease in Russell Silver syndrome. Int Orthop 1994;18:32–37

Nakabayashi K, Fernandez BA, Teshima I, et al: Molecular genetic studies of human chromosome 7 in Russell-Silver syndrome. Genomics 2002;79:186–196

Ortiz C, Cleveland RH, Jaramillo D: Urethral valves in Russell Silver syndrome. J Pediatr 1991;119:776–778

Patton MA: Russell Silver syndrome. J Med Genet 1988;25:557–560

Saal HM, Pagon RA, Pepin MG: Reevaluation of the Russell Silver syndrome. J Pediatr 1985;107:733–778

Specht EE, Hazelrig PE: Orthopaedic considerations of Silver's syndrome. J Bone Joint Surg Am 1973;55:1502–1510

Tanner JM, LeJarraga H, Cameron N: Natural history of the Silver Russell syndrome: a longitudinal study of 39 cases. Pediatr Res 1975;9:611–623

Weiss GR, Garnick MB: Testicular cancer in Russell Silver dwarf. J Urol 1981;126:836–837

Shwachman-Diamond Syndrome

Bom EP, vander Sande FM, Tjonatham RTO, et al: Shwachman syndrome: CT and MRI diagnosis. J Comput Assist Tomogr 1993;17:474–476

Hershkovitz BS, Dagan J, Freier S: Increased spontaneous chromosomal breakage in Shwachman syndrome. J Pediatr Gastroenterol Nutr 1999;28:449–450

Popovic M, Goobie S, Morrison J, et al: Fine mapping of the locus for Shwachman-Diamond syndrome at 7q11, identification of shared disease haplotypes, and exclusion of TPST1 as a candidate gene. Eur J Hum Genet 2002;10:250–258

Sacchi F, Maggiore G, Marseglia G, et al: Association of neutrophil and complement defects in two twins with Shwachman syndrome. Helv Pediatr Acta 1982;37:177–181

Stanley P, Sutcliffe J: Metaphyseal chondrodysplasia with dwarfism, pancreatic insufficiency and neutropenia. Pediatr Radiol 1973;1:119–126

Woods WG, Roloff JS, Lukens JN, et al: Occurrence of leukemia in patients with the Shwachman syndrome. J Pediatr 1981;99:425–428

Smith-Lemli-Opitz Syndrome

Curry CJR, Carey JC, Holland JS, et al: Smith Lemli Opitz syndrome type II. Am J Med Genet 1987;26:45–57

Herman TE, Siegel MJ, Lee BCP, et al: Smith Lemli Opitz syndrome type II: report of a case with additional radiographic findings. Pediatr Radiol 1993;23:37–40

Kelly RI, Roessler E, Hennekam RCM, et al: Holoprosencephaly in RSH/Smith Lemli Opitz syndrome. Am J Med Genet 1996;66:478–484

Kratz LE, Kelly RI: Prenatal diagnosis of the RSH/Smith-Lemli-Opitz syndrome. Am J Med Genet 1999;82:376–381

LeMerrer M, Briard ML, Girard S, et al: Lethal acrodysogenital dwarfism: a severe lethal condition resembling Smith Lemli Opitz syndrome. J Med Genet 1988;25:88–95

Lin AE, Ardinger HH, Ardinger RH, et al: Cardiovascular malformations in Smith Lemli Opitz syndrome. Am J Med Genet 1997;68:270–278

Nowaczyk MJM, Whelan DT, Hill RE: Smith Lemli Opitz syndrome. Am J Med Genet 1998;78:419–423

Patterson K, Toomey KE, Chandra RS: Hirschsprung disease in a 46 XY

phenotypic infant girl with Smith Lemli Opitz syndrome. J Pediatr 1983;103:425–427

Tint GS, Salen G, Batta A, et al: Correlation of severity and outcome with plasma sterol levels in variants of the Smith Lemli Opitz syndrome. J Pediatr 1995;127:82–87

Sotos' Syndrome

Cole TRP, Hughes HE: Sotos syndrome. J Med Genet 1994;31:20–32

Cole TRP, Hughes HE, Jeffreys MJ, et al: Small cell lung carcinoma in a patient with Sotos syndrome. J Med Genet 1992;29:338–341

Hersh HM, Cole TRP, Bloom AS, et al: Risk of malignancy in Soto syndrome. J Pediatr 1992;120:572–574

Kurotaki N, Imaizumi K, Harada N, et al: Haploinsufficiency of NSD1 causes Soto syndrome. Nat Genet 2002;30:365–366

Thrombocytopenia–Absent Radius (TAR) Syndrome

Boute O, Depret-Mosser S, Vinatier D, et al: Prenatal diagnosis of thrombocytopenia-absent radius syndrome. Fetal Diagn Ther 1996;11:224–230

Hall JG: Thrombocytopenia and absent radius (TAR) syndrome. J Med Genet 1987;24:79–83

MacDonald MR, Schaefer GB, Olney AH, et al: Hypoplasia of the cerebellar vermis and corpus callosum in thrombocytopenia with absent radius syndrome on MRI studies. Am J Med Genet 1994;50:46–50

Schoenecker PL, Cohn AK, Sedgwick WG, et al: Dysplasia of the knee associated with the syndrome of thrombocytopenia and absent radius. J Bone Joint Surg Am 1984;66:421–427

VACTERL (VATER) Association

Appignani BA, Jaramillo D, Barnes PD, et al: Dysraphic myelodysplasia associated with urogenital and anorectal anomalies: prevalence and types seen with MRI imaging. AJR Am J Roentgenol 1994;163:1199–1203

Bendon RW, Dungy-Poythress L: Perinatal pathology of interhemispheric cyst with thinned posterior corpus callosum. Pediatr Pathol Lab Med 1996;16:299–317

Day DL: Aortic arch in neonates with esophageal atresia. Radiology 1985;155:99–100

Louhimo I, Lindahl H: Esophageal atresia: primary results of 500 consecutively treated patients. J Pediatr Surg 1983;18:217–229

Martinez-Frias ML, Frias JL: VACTERL as primary, polytopic developmental field defects. Am J Med Genet 1999;83:13–16

Muraji T, Majour GH: Surgical problems in patients with VATER associated anomalies. J Pediatr Surg 1984;19:550–554

Nezarati MM, McLeod DR: VACTERL manifestation in two generations of a family. Am J Med Genet 1999;82:40–42

Quan L, Smith DW: The VATER association. J Pediatr 1973;28:104–107

Van Hewin LW, Cheng W, DeVries B, et al: Anomalies associated with esophageal atresia in Asians and Europeans. Pediatric Surg Int 2002;18:241–243

Warfarin Embryopathy

Barker DP, Konje JC, Richardson JA: Warfarin embryopathy with dextrocardia and situs inversus. Acta Paediatr 1994;83:411

Becker MH, Genieser NB, Finegold M, et al: Chondrodysplasia punctata: is maternal warfarin therapy a factor? Am J Dis Child 1975;129:356–359

Cotrufo A, DeFeo M, DeSanto LS, et al: Risk of warfarin during pregnancy with mechanical valve prosthesis. Obstet Gynecol 2002;99:35–40

Normann EK, Stray-Pedersen B: Warfarin-induced fetal diaphragmatic hernia. Br J Obstetr Gynaecol 1989;96:729–730

Tongsong T, Wanapirak C, Piyamongkol W: Prenatal ultrasonographic findings consistent with fetal warfarin syndrome. J Ultrasound Med 1999;18:577–580

Zakzouz MS: The congenital warfarin syndrome. J Laryngol Otol 1986;100:215–219

Weill-Marchesani Syndrome

Faivre L, Megarbane A, Alsward A, et al: Homozygosity mapping of a Weill-Marchesani syndrome locus to chromosome 19q13.3—p13.2. Hum Genet 2002;110:366–370

Giordano N, Senesi M, Battisti E, et al: Weill-Marchesani syndrome: report of an unusual case. Calcif Tissue Int 1997;60:358–360

Gorlin RJ: Spherophakia-brachymorphia syndrome (Weill-Marchesani). Semin Roentgenol 1973;8:236

Haik GM Sr, Terrell WL III, Haik GM Jr: The Weill-Marchesani syndrome: report of two cases and a review. J Louisiana State Med Soc 1990;142:25–28, 30–32

McGavic JS: Weill-Marchesani syndrome: brachymorphism and ectopia lentis. Am J Ophthalmol 1966;62:820–823

Werner's Syndrome

Goto M, Kindynis P, Resnick D, et al: Osteosclerosis of the phalanges in Werner's syndrome. Radiology 1989;172:841–843

Kakigi R, Endo C, Neshige R, et al: Accelerated aging of the brain in Werner's syndrome. Neurology 1992;42:922–924

Laroche M, Ricq G, Cantagrel A, et al: Bone and joint involvement in adults with Werner's syndrome. Rev Rhum Engl Ed 1997;64:843–846

Poot M, Gollahon KA, Emond MJ, et al: Werner syndrome diploid fibroblasts are sensitive to 4-nitroquinoline-N-oxide and 8-methoxypsoralen: implication for the disease phenotype. FASEB J 2002;16:757–758

Zackai AH, Weber D, Noth R: Cardiac findings in Werner's syndrome. Geriatrics 1974;29:141–148

Williams Syndrome

Bird LM, Billman GF, Lacro RV, et al: Sudden death in Williams syndrome. J Pediatr 1996;129:926–931

Cammareri V, Vignati G, Nocera G, et al: Thyroid hemiagenesis and elevated thyrotropin levels in a child with Williams syndrome. Am J Med Genet 1999;85:491–494

Charvat KA, Hornstein L, Oestreich AE: Radioulnar synostosis in Williams syndrome. Pediatr Radiol 1991;21:508–510

Ingelfinger JR, Newburger JW: Spectrum of renal anomalies patients with Williams syndrome. J Pediatr 1991;119:771–773

Joyce CA, Zorich B, Pike SJ, et al: Williams Beuren syndrome. J Med Genet 1996;33:986–992

Kaplan P, Levinson M, Kaplan BS: Cerebral artery stenosis in Williams syndrome causes strokes in childhood. J Pediatr 1995;126:943–945

Kruse K, Pankau R, Gosch A, et al: Calcium metabolism in Williams Beuren syndrome. J Pediatr 1992;121:902–907

Metcalfe K: Williams syndrome: an update on clinical and molecular aspects. Arch Dis Child 1999;81:198–200

Schmitt JE, Watts K, Eliez S, et al: Increased gyrification in Williams syndrome: evidence using 3D MRI methods. Dev Med Child Neurol 2002;44:292–295

Cri du Chat Syndrome

Fenger K, Niebuhr E: Measurements on hand radiographs from 32 cri-du-chat probands. Radiology 1978;129:137–141

James AE Jr, Atkins L, Feingold M, et al: The cri du chat syndrome. Radiology 1969;92:50–52

Levy B, Dunn TM, Kern JH, et al: Delineation of dup 5q phenotype by molecular cytogenetic analysis in a patient with dup 5q/del5p (cri du chat). Am J Med Genet 2002;108:192–197

Niebuhr E: The cri du chat syndrome: epidemiology, cytogenetics, and clinical features. Hum Genet 1978;44:227–275

Trisomy 13 (Patau's) Syndrome

James AE Jr, Merz T, Janower ML, et al: Radiological features of the most common autosomal disorders: trisomy 21-22 (mongolism or Down's syndrome), trisomy 18, trisomy 13-15, and the cri du chat syndrome. Clin Radiol 1971;22:417–433

Kumar AJ, Naidich TP, Stetten G, et al: Chromosomal disorders: background and neuroradiology. AJNR Am J Neuroradiol 1992;13:577–593

Lehman CD, Nyberg DA, Winter TC, et al: Trisomy 13 syndrome: prenatal ultrasound findings in a review of 33 cases. Radiology 1995;194:217–222

Patau K, Smith D, Thernan E, et al: Multiple congenital anomaly caused by an extra autosome. Lancet 1960;1:790–793

Shipp TD, Benacerraf BR: Second trimester ultrasound screening for chromosomal abnormalities. Prenat Diagn 2002;22:296–307

Trisomy 18 (Edwards') Syndrome

Alpert LI, Strauss L, Hirschhorn K: Neonatal hepatitis and biliary atresia associated with trisomy 17-18 syndrome. N Engl J Med 1969;280:16–20

Edwards JH, Harnden DG, Cameron AH, et al: A new trisomic syndrome. Lancet 1960;1:787–790

James AE Jr, Merz T, Janower ML, et al: Radiological features of the most common autosomal disorders: trisomy 21-22 (mongolism or Down's syndrome), trisomy 18, trisomy 13-15, and the cri du chat syndrome. Clin Radiol 1971;22:417–433

Kumar AJ, Naidich TP, Stetten G, et al: Chromosomal disorders: background and neuroradiology. AJNR Am J Neuroradiol 1992;13:577–593

Kurjak A, Kos M, Stipoljev F, et al: Ultrasonic markers of fetal chromosomal abnormalities. Eur J Obstet Gynecol Reprod Biol 1999;85:105–108

Singleton EB, Rosenberg HS, Yang SJ: The radiographic manifestations of chromosomal abnormalities. Radiol Clin North Am 1964;2:281–295

Trisomy 21 (Down) Syndrome

Caffey J, Ross SE: Pelvic bones in infantile mongoloidism: radiographic features. Am J Roentgenol Radium Ther Nucl Med 1958;80:458–467

Edwards DK 3rd, Berry CC, Hilton SW: Trisomy 21 in newborn infants: chest radiographic diagnosis. Radiology 1988;167:317–318

Hayes A, Batshaw ML: Down syndrome. Pediatr Clin North Am 1993;40:523–535

James AE Jr, Merz T, Janower ML, et al: Radiological features of the most common autosomal disorders: trisomy 21-22 (mongolism or Down's syndrome), trisomy 18, trisomy 13-15, and the cri du chat syndrome. Clin Radiol 1971;22:417–433

Kriss VM: Down syndrome: imaging of multiorgan involvement. Clin Pediatr (Phila) 1999;38:441–449

Kumar AJ, Naidich TP, Stetten G, et al: Chromosomal disorders: background and neuroradiology. AJNR Am J Neuroradiol 1992;13:577–593

Nyberg DA, Luthy DA, Resta RG, et al: Age-adjusted ultrasound risk assessment for fetal Down's syndrome during the second trimester: description of the method and analysis of 142 cases. Ultrasound Obstet Gynecol 1998;12:8–14

Turner's Syndrome

Haber HP, Ranke MB: Pelvic ultrasonography in Turner syndrome: standards for uterine and ovarian volume. J Ultrasound Med 1999;18:271–276

Hall JG, Gilchrist DM: Turner syndrome and its variants. Pediatr Clin North Am 1990;37:1421–1440

Hartling UB, Hansen BF, Keeling JW, et al: Short bi-iliac distance in pre-natal Ullrich-Turner syndrome. Am J Med Genet 2002;108:290–294

Singleton EB, Rosenberg HS, Yang SJ: The radiographic manifestations of chromosomal abnormalities. Radiol Clin North Am 1964;2:281–295

Subramaniam PN: Turner's syndrome and cardiovascular anomalies: a case report and review of the literature. Am J Med Sci 1989;297:260–262

Turner HH: A syndrome of infantilism, congenital webbed neck, and cubitus valgus. Endocrinology 1938;23:566–574

Wolf-Hirschhorn Syndrome

De Keersmaecker B, Albert M, Hillion Y, et al: Prenatal diagnosis of brain abnormalities in Wolf-Hirschhorn (4p-) syndrome. Prenat Diagn 2002;22:366–370

Johnson VP, Mulder RD, Hosen R: The Wolf-Hirschhorn 4p– syndrome. Clin Genet 1976;10:104–112

Kumar AJ, Naidich TP, Stetten G, et al: Chromosomal disorders: background and neuroradiology. AJNR Am J Neuroradiol 1992;132:577–593

Magill HL, Shackelford GD, McAlister WH: 4p– Wolf-Hirschhorn syndrome. AJR Am J Roentgenol 1980;1352:283–288

Sergi C, Schulze BR, Hager HD, et al: Wolf-Hirschhorn syndrome: case report and review of the chromosomal aberrations associated with diaphragmatic defects. Pathologica 1998;903:285–293

PART VII

BONE FORMATION AND METABOLIC BONE DISEASE

SAMBASIVA R. KOTTAMASU

Chapter 1

CHANGES IN BONE STRUCTURE AND DENSITY

SAMBASIVA R. KOTTAMASU

STRUCTURE AND COMPOSITION OF BONE

Bone is a specialized connective tissue of mesodermal origin that consists of bone matrix, mineral, and water. Bone matrix is composed of 95% collagen and 5% ground substance, which includes mucopolysaccharides and other substances. The mineral portion of bone contains 99% of the total body calcium, predominantly in the form of hydroxyapatites and small quantities of other minerals, such as magnesium, sodium, and strontium. The skeleton is composed of two different types of bone: compact cortical bone, which constitutes 80% of the bone mass but only 20% of the bone volume; and spongy trabecular bone, which comprises 20% of the bone mass but 80% of the bone volume. Bones in the axial skeleton, such as the vertebrae, ribs, skull, and iliac bones, as well as ends of the long bones, have a greater proportion of trabecular bone.

Microscopically, newly formed bone is primarily of two types: lamellar and woven. Lamellar bone is formed in an orderly sequential manner during the process of normal modeling and remodeling and consists of alternating layers of cross-linked collagen fibers. Woven bone (primitive bone) is formed on existing bone surfaces during normal bone remodeling or in areas of fibrous tissue condensation by osteoblasts that rapidly deposit collagen fibers in a haphazard fashion. Matrix calcification follows in a diffuse but spotty manner in woven bone. Woven bone, with its loose collagen meshwork, is able to accumulate a larger amount of mineral, and as a result it may appear denser than lamellar bone on radiographs.

Throughout life, the skeleton is continuously renewed by bone remodeling, a process which serves the purpose of repairing damaged bone and adapting the skeleton to changes in physical load. In this process, old bone is removed by osteoclastic resorption and new bone is laid down by osteoblastic formation. Bone mass increases with growth in the first decades of life, and peaks at about the age of 30 years. Bone modeling, remodeling, and calcium homeostasis are modulated predominantly by osteoblasts, osteocytes, and osteoclasts. Osteoblasts form bone matrix. The multinucleated osteoclasts resorb bone, and osteocytes play a role in the calcium homeostasis.

Despite the fact that osteocytes are the most abundant cells in bone, their role in bone metabolism is still poorly understood. During bone formation, some of the osteoblasts lining the surface of bone are incorporated into the newly formed osteoid matrix and become osteocytes. Osteocytes are contained within lacunae and are connected with each other in bone and with osteoblasts on the bone surface through canaliculi, forming cellular networks. Osteocyte lacunar density and size may cause significant gender- and age-related variations in apparent stiffness of bone matrix.

Several functions of osteocytes in bone have been proposed:

1. Osteocytes are actively involved in bone turnover.
2. Osteocytes, through their large cellular network, participate in calcium transport from bone matrix to tissue fluid, via the process of "osteocytic osteolysis."
3. Osteocytes play an important role in sensing mechanical stress, and the signals mediated by osteocytes may regulate the overall metabolism of cells in bone tissue.

Between the plasma membrane of osteocytes and the bone matrix is the periosteocytic space, filled with extracellular fluid. The changes in flow of fluid through the lacunar-canalicular system as a result of mechanical loading results in activation of signals mediated by the osteocytes.

Osteocytes do not have a direct blood supply, and their metabolic needs are met by a combination of passive and enhanced diffusion, arising when the tissue is loaded during functional activity. Some investigators hypothesize that depriving a bone of mechanical loading (and thus eliminating diffusion enhanced by loading) would induce osteocyte hypoxia and brief mechanical stress would rescue osteocytes from ischemia.

BONE MODELING AND REMODELING

Bone modeling is a dynamic process resulting from spatial drifts of individual bone surfaces that undergo continuous bone formation, resorption, and reshaping. The end result is the normal shape of a tubular bone, narrowest in the shaft and widened toward the ends. The normal modeling process can be disturbed by various pathologic processes. Excessive narrowing of the shaft (overtubulation) occurs in longstanding paralytic conditions (Fig. 1; Table 1) excessive width of the shaft and metaphyses (undertubulation) (Fig. 2; Table 2) is encountered frequently in metabolic, systemic, and storage disorders and skeletal dysplasias.

Throughout life, cortical and trabecular bone are remodeled in small packets of coordinated cellular activity causing removal of existing bone and by varying amounts of new lamellar bone. Normal bone remodeling helps maintain mechanical strength of the skeleton and contributes to calcium homeostasis.

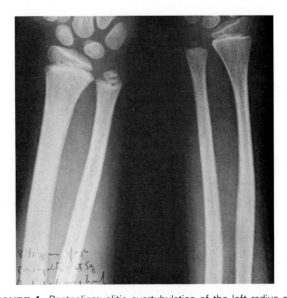

FIGURE 1. Postpoliomyelitic overtubulation of the left radius and ulna of a girl 8 years of age who had contracted acute poliomyelitis at age 5. Comparison of analogous bones in the two forearms shows that the left radius and ulna are of smaller caliber than their counterparts on the right and flare more at the ends. The loss of volume of these bones is due almost entirely to loss of volume of the medullary cavities; the cortical thickness of the bones is practically the same on the two sides.

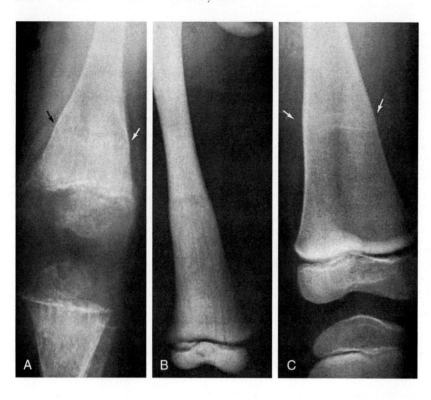

FIGURE 2. Undertubulation *(arrows)* of long tubular bones in healing rickets **(A)**, in osteopetrosis **(B)**, and after recovery from lead poisoning **(C)**.

Table 1 ■ PATHOLOGIC PROCESSES CAUSING OVERTUBULATION OR OVERCONSTRICTION OF LONG BONES

Neuromuscular diseases (e.g., poliomyelitis, arthrogryposis)
Congenital pseudarthrosis
Disuse atrophy
Neurofibromatosis
Epidermolysis bullosa
Osteogenesis imperfecta
Marfan syndrome
Homocystinuria

Table 2 ■ PATHOLOGIC PROCESSES CAUSING UNDERTUBULATION OR UNDERCONSTRICTION OF LONG BONES

Chronic severe anemia (e.g., thalassemia, sickle cell anemia)
Fibrous dysplasia
Mucopolysaccharidosis
Gaucher's disease
Healing rickets
Biliary atresia
Multiple enchondromatosis (Ollier's disease)
Multiple heriditary osteochondromatosis
Chronic lead poisoning
Metaphyseal dysplasia (Pyle's disease)
Osteopetrosis
Engelmann's disease
Pyknodysostosis

TRANSVERSE LINES OF PARK

Opaque transverse lines in the metaphyses of growing long bones are found in healthy and sick children at all ages and may persist in the bones of adults, although they cannot form after growth is completed (Fig. 3). Marginal lines of increased density are their counterparts in the round and flat bones (Fig. 4). Usually, those in the long bones are distributed symmetrically through-

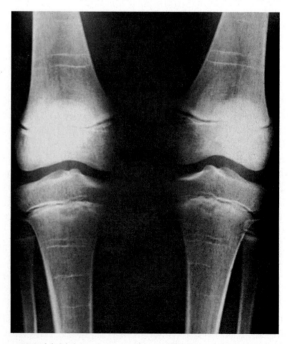

FIGURE 3. Multiple transverse lines of Park in a patient 11 years of age who was, and apparently had been, healthy.

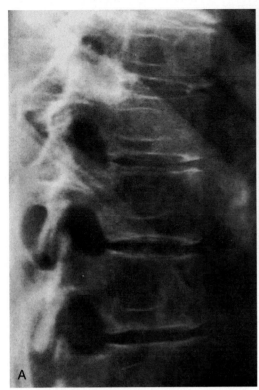

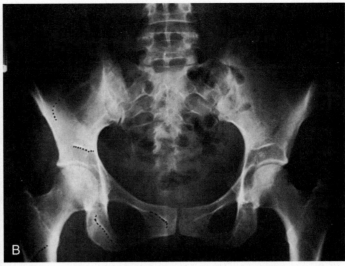

FIGURE 4. Transverse lines in a 50-year-old woman indicate the approximate sizes of the vertebral bodies **(A)** and bones of the pelvis **(B)** at the time of severe scarlet fever at the age of 9 years. The *dotted lines* on the right side in **B** correspond to the "transverse" lines on the *left* and provide an "exploded" sketch of the metaphyseal-equivalent regions at the earlier age. (Courtesy of Dr. Harold Schneider, Cincinnati, OH.)

out the skeleton and occupy identical sites in corresponding bones on both sides of the body. During formation, they are thickest closer to the ends of the bones where they are formed and in bones where growth is most rapid. The transverse lines are almost exactly parallel to the contours of provisional zones of calcification that they underlie and are parallel to one another when several are present.

The exact cause of the lines is uncertain, but they appear to form whenever there is stress of sufficient degree and duration, such as that associated with starvation or severe illness (Fig. 5). Their development, however, is often unassociated with any recognized stress. In experimentally produced lines in animals, it appears that an initial period of growth depression and subsequent recovery are required. During the period of growth inhibition, bone formation continues transversely at the cartilage–shaft junction and is manifested by thickening of the dense line at the junction. With recovery of longitudinal growth, vertical trabeculae reappear in the most recently formed bone between the cartilage and the transversely oriented bone that remains buried in the shaft as further growth moves the epiphysis–shaft junction away from it (Fig. 6). The dense, transversely oriented bone is more radiopaque than the normal bone on each side of it and produces

FIGURE 5. The generation of transverse lines of Park *(arrows)* under the proliferating cartilage whose growth was accelerated by chronic hyperemia incidental to osteomyelitis of the left tibia. Transverse lines developed at all cartilage–shaft junctions. The line is deeper in the shaft in the left tibia than in the right tibia (5 mm compared to 3 mm), which proves that growth of the left tibia was accelerated, The left tibial line is thicker than the line in the right tibia, which indicates that longitudinal growth of the bone was accelerated during generation of the transverse lines. The lines in the two femora are each 7 mm from the physes.

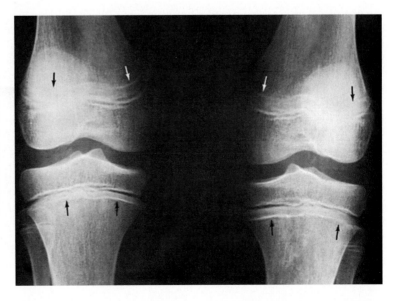

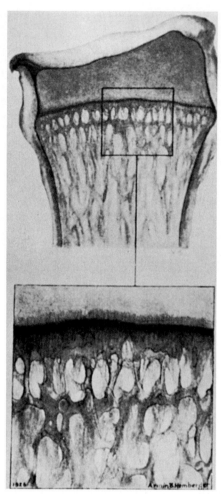

FIGURE 6. View of Park's transverse line (TL) made in a study with a binocular dissecting microscope from a preparation cleared with wintergreen, according to the method of Spalteholz. The TL is composed entirely of bone in transversely disposed trabeculae, which is identical with the bone in the normal longitudinally disposed trabeculae above and below it. This transversely disposed trabecular bone is formed independently of the action of the proliferative cartilage in the physis. (Courtesy of Dr. E. A. Park, Baltimore, MD.)

the transverse line, or the growth alteration line of Park, on the radiograph. With the passage of time, the lines tend to disappear.

Dense transverse lines develop following exposure to lead and other heavy metals, and their incidental finding often is the first clue that a child has toxic levels of the element in his or her body (Fig. 7). In the case of lead, the lines are not the result of absorption of x-rays by the lead, but rather by a very tight spongiosa formed under its influence. Similar lines may be found following exposure to other heavy metals, so that undue specific diagnostic significance cannot be given to the lines, which should nevertheless serve as an indication for more specific diagnostic tests in an appropriate clinical setting. Drugs given to pregnant mothers may result in the presence of transverse lines in the newborn infant. Antimetabolites and cytotoxic drugs used to treat malignant disease may cause dense transverse lines resembling heavy metal lines. Radiolucent lines or

bands at the ends of the shafts of the long bones in a growing child may also indicate stress during the period that the undermineralized portions were growing (Fig. 8). They are seen in many acute diseases, including leukemia, and are prominent in premature infants during their stay in intensive care units.

MEASUREMENT OF BONE MASS IN CHILDREN

Dual-energy x-ray absorptiometry (DXA), with its short scan time, low radiation dose, and high precision and accuracy, is particularly suitable for measuring total body bone mineral density in infants and children. X-rays at two discrete energy levels are collimated and directed into the body. The attenuation of the x-rays by the various tissues in the body can be quantitated. The apparatus detects the bone mineral content (BMC) and bone mineral density (BMD), and compares the measured values with the average values in the healthy population. Using a World Health Organization report published in 1994, osteoporosis can be diagnosed from the patient's T-score value (difference of BMD from young adult mean, normalized to the population standard deviation [SD]). However, there are limitations relating to the use of T scores in infants, children, and the elderly, and decisions about treatment in these age groups are generally best made on the basis of the Z-score value (difference of BMD from age- and sex-matched mean, normalized to the population SD) because this measures the patient's fracture risk relative to his or her peers. Lapillonne et al. reported that very small amounts of mineral can be measured accurately by whole-body DXA. Quantitative x-ray computed tomography, though less widely used than DXA, has the advantage of being able to determine three-dimensional bone density of a lumbar vertebral body, which cannot be done with DXA.

Koo, Walters, and Bush investigated various clinical and experimental parameters that could interfere with DXA-based BMC and BMD measurements in infants. They found that movement artifact, radiographic contrast media, plaster cast, and variations in operator-dependent data analysis significantly interfered with regional DXA BMC and BMD measurement in neonates and infants. A minor adjustment of the step phantom during data analysis may result in almost a 30% difference in apparent BMC and BMD. It is suggested that a single measurement of BMD should not be used in isolation to assign a given patient to a specific diagnostic category.

Tsukahara et al. measured lumbar spine BMD in 40 preterm infants by DXA. During the first several months of life, their BMD was considerably lower than that of normal term infants, and osteopenia was more pronounced in the more premature and smaller infants. Inverse correlation was found between the BMD and urinary calcium:creatinine ratio. A follow-up study was performed in 10 preterm infants. In three of the four who underwent the last DXA between 8 and 12 months, BMD had improved remarkably. Salle et al. used DXA to assess the BMC and BMD of the lumbar spine in newborns (on day 1 to 2) and infants (1 to 24 months of age). In newborns, BMC and BMD correlated positively with birth weight, body area, length, and gestational age. In infants, both BMC and BMD were highly correlated with weight, age, length, and body area.

Koo et al. studied bone mineral status in 150 singleton newborn infants with birth weights of 1002 to 3990 g and gestational ages of 27 to 42 weeks using DXA. Data showed a highly significant correlation with gestational age, birth weight, study weight, and study length. The best single determinant of bone mineral status was body weight. Sievanen et al. performed DXA twice on left forearms of newborn preterm and term babies. They concluded that DXA provides adequate reliability for in vivo determinations of BMC and areal BMD in the distal and midforearm in term and preterm infants and thus strongly supports the clinical utility of DXA in the diagnosis and monitoring of metabolic disease of prematurity. Movements during

scanning decrease the precision considerably. Therefore, every effort must be made to prevent movement artifacts.

Yeste et al. reported normative DXA data for BMD at the lumbar spine in a normal population of children with ages ranging from the neonatal period to 4 years. BMD increased progressively from birth to 4 years, and values were similar in both sexes. A statistically significant correlation was found between BMD values and age. Lumbar BMD increased annually, with the most rapid increase observed during the first 2 years of life. Southard et al. used DXA to study the lumbar vertebral bone mass in 218 healthy children ages 1 to 19 years. Vertebral bone mass increased with weight, age, and pubertal Tanner stage. Results of multiple regression analyses showed that Tanner stage and weight were the best predictive indicators of bone mass and BMD. These data provide a tool for the study and follow-up of pediatric populations at risk for low bone mineralization.

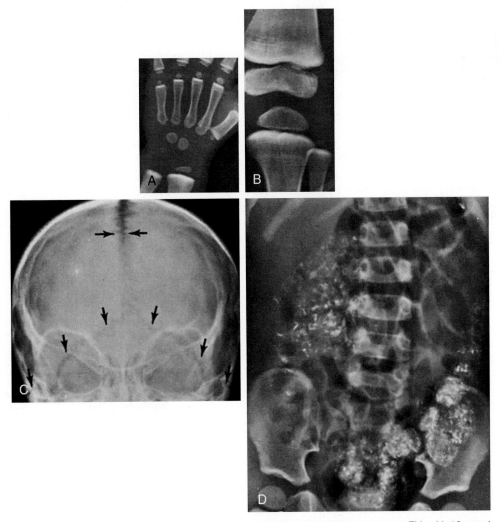

FIGURE 7. Radiographic changes of lead poisoning in growing bones and the alimentary tract. This girl, 16 months of age, had been eating dry paint from the walls of her home for many months. Transverse bands of increased density are seen in the metaphyses of the bones of the hands **(A)** and the knees **(B)**. The distal end of the femoral shaft is underconstricted. **C,** The cranial sutures *(arrows)* are widened as a result of increased intracranial pressure. **D,** Opaque lead particles are present in the lumen of the colon.

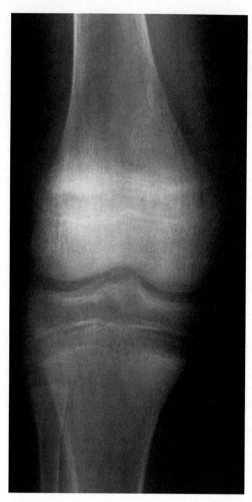

FIGURE 8. Transverse radiolucent metaphyseal bands in the distal femur and proximal tibia of a nonambulatory patient with vitamin D dependent rickets and severe myopathy.

OSTEOPENIA

OSTEOMALACIA

Generalized decrease in bone density (osteopenia) may result from decreased mass of normally mineralized bone (osteoporosis) or from a relative excess of uncalcified osteoid tissue (osteomalacia). Osteomalacia in children is associated with rickets, of which there are several pathogenetic types. Osteomalacia produces a coarsening of the trabecular markings because the larger, poorly mineralized trabeculae, containing excess uncalcified osteoid, are still visible on the film, while the smaller ones are not. In addition, cortical bone margins are unsharp. Furthermore, the newly formed bone at the metaphyseal ends of the shafts in growing children fails to mineralize, and the ends of the bones fade out toward the apparently remote epiphyseal centers (Fig. 9) without the sharp demarcation of the zone of provisional calcification that is normally present.

OSTEOPOROSIS

Osteoporosis is a systemic bone disease with reduced bone mass, altered bone architecture, and increased fracture rate. In children with osteoporosis, the zone of provisional calcification is preserved and may be exaggerated by decreased density of the adjacent bone. Osteoporosis is characterized by thinning of the cortex and a disappearance of trabecular bone markings together with a distinct diminution of total bone density. Bone mineral density in later life largely depends on the peak bone mass achieved in adolescence or young adulthood. A reduced bone density is associated with increased fracture risk; therefore, it is important to make a diagnosis early and treat childhood osteoporosis.

The varied forms of osteoporosis in childhood can be classified as those secondary to a chronic disease or its treatment and primary forms of the disorder, which include the genetically determined osteogenesis imperfecta types and idiopathic forms of osteoporosis. Osteogenesis imperfecta is discussed in Section IX, Part V, page 2122. *Osteoporosis* is seen in many conditions and has no specific etiologic significance. *Generalized osteopenia* develops in chronic undernutrition, gastrointestinal disorders associated with diarrhea or malabsorption, and various metabolic disorders in which protein matrix formation is disturbed. Premature infants, even at the postconceptual age of 40 weeks, are osteopenic in comparison with full-term infants. *Regional bone atrophy* follows such conditions as fracture, osteomyelitis, arthritis, and others in which there is localized hyperemia or disuse of a part of the skeleton for a long period of time.

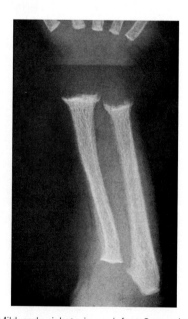

FIGURE 9. Mild early rickets in an infant 3 months of age. The provisional zones of calcification at the distal ends of the ulna and radius are irregularly mineralized and frayed. The distal end of the ulna is cupped. Slight widening of the distal ends of both bones is evident. The shafts are diffusely osteopenic, and demonstrate coarse trabeculations. There are no visible changes in the proximal end of either bone, where growth is slower than at the distal end.

Reflex Sympathetic Dystrophy

Reflex sympathetic dystrophy is a rare condition of unknown cause characterized by pain, swelling, tenderness, and vasomotor alterations in a limb, frequently following mechanical injury, and manifests as pronounced decreased density of bone distal to the injury. It is less frequent and of shorter duration in children than in adults. Radiographs are normal, and bone scans serve to exclude other causes of bone and joint pain.

Regional Migratory Osteoporosis

Regional migratory osteoporosis (RMO) is a disorder of unknown etiology characterized by successive episodes of severe periarticular lower limb pain accompanied by localized and migratory osteoporosis that may be oligoarticular or disseminated. The region of the foot, knee, or hip is frequently involved. Each episode usually lasts several months and is followed by spontaneous recovery. Recurrence of symptoms in an adjacent joint is a distinguishing feature. An early clinical and radiographic diagnosis of RMO can be difficult. There are no specific laboratory features of RMO. Diagnosis is made after exclusion of more common entities. A three-phase bone scan is very helpful in the diagnosis of suspected cases before the development of radiographic stigmata.

Tannenbaum et al. described four patients with RMO, all of whom had at least two episodes of periarticular osteoporosis. The interval between attacks ranged from 5 months to 11 years, and attacks lasted from 3 months to 2 years. In two cases septic arthritis was initially suspected. The ankle joints were affected in three patients, hips in two, and knees in two. Involvement of the small joints of the foot was demonstrated in two patients by ^{99m}Tc-methylene diphosphonate skeletal imaging. Bone scans corroborated the clinical diagnosis in two patients before regional osteoporosis was visible radiologically. Bone biopsy revealed severe osteopenia with accelerated bone resorption. Knowledge of the features of RMO can prevent unnecessary invasive procedures.

Santori et al. described RMO in eight patients who belonged to two families. The high familial incidence appears to indicate the existence of a predisposition to local disturbances of bone turnover in the periarticular bone tissues. A precipitating factor, which is often clearly evident, then causes the disease to become clinically manifest. It has been suggested that traumatic ischemia may be the pathogenic basis of RMO. In view of overlapping features, some investigators suggested that RMO, reflex sympathetic dystrophy, and transient osteoporosis may be examples of a spectrum of the same disease, rather than being distinct entities.

Transient Osteoporosis of the Hip

Pain in the hip area and functional disability of the affected limb are the main clinical features of transient osteoporosis of the hip. The etiology is still unclear, yet, in view of similarities to RMO and reflex sympathetic dystrophy, vascular and neurologic disturbances have been proposed as possible pathogenic mechanisms.

Diagnosis is supported by regional osteopenia on radiographs and increased uptake on three-phase skeletal scintigraphy. Gradual return to normal radioactivity parallels the spontaneous recovery. Magnetic resonance imaging, computed tomography, and other imaging methods are supplementary diagnostic tools. Exclusion of more common entities is required. Awareness of the presence of this condition may prevent unnecessary invasive procedures and treatment.

Idiopathic Juvenile Osteoporosis

Idiopathic juvenile osteoporosis (IJO) is a term reserved for acute osteoporosis with onset in the prepubertal or pubertal age. The initial complaint is pain in the extremities and difficulty walking, followed by multiple fractures of the spine and lower extremities. Radiologically, a severe generalized decrease in bone density is noted. Diagnosis of IJO is based on clinical and radiographic studies and exclusion of other causes of osteoporosis, other diseases of bones, and renal, metabolic, and endocrine disorders. Usually the disease remits spontaneously after the onset of puberty. Milder forms of IJO may remain undiagnosed because of the self-limited course and the pain being confused with a variety of rheumatic disorders. The basic strategy of treatment of currently affected adolescents involves activity restriction to protect the spine and other skeletal structures until remission occurs.

Osteoporosis in Homocystinuria

Homocystinuria caused by cystathionine synthase deficiency is an autosomal recessive error of amino acid metabolism characterized by dislocation of the lens, mental retardation, skeletal abnormalities and thromboembolic phenomena. Generalized osteoporosis (see Section IX, Part VI, Fig. 23, page 2198) is the most significant finding and is associated with vertebral compression fractures and fractures of long tubular bones. Other skeletal findings include arachnodactyly and disproportionate skeleton (pubis–heel length greater than crown–pubis length). Calcified distal radial and ulnar physeal and metaphyseal spicules are also characteristic of this inherited disease.

OSTEOSCLEROSIS AND HYPEROSTOSIS

The term *osteosclerosis* is used to denote an increase in radiodensity of trabecular bone, and the term *hyperostosis* is used to describe an increase in the width of the cortex of tubular bones or flat bones with or without an increase in their external diameter. Osteosclerosis and/or hyperostosis can result from a reduction in bone resorption, an increase in bone formation, or changes in the ratio of these two determinants of bone modeling and remodeling, with net bone formation exceeding bone resorption. The conditions associated with osteosclerosis and hyperostosis include metabolic disorders, infiltrative and neoplastic disorders of the bone and

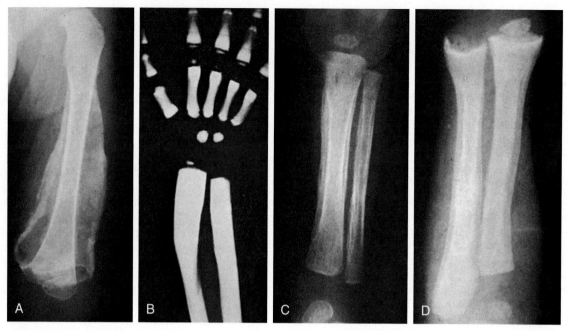

FIGURE 10. Examples of hyperostosis and osteosclerosis. **A,** Large calcifed subperiosteal hematoma in healing scurvy. **B,** Diffuse sclerosis of bones in osteopetrosis. Periosteal new bone formation in syphilitic osteitis **(C)** and healing rickets **(D).**

bone marrow, endocrine disorders, hypervitaminoses, osteonecrosis, chronic and healed osteomyelitis, articular disorders, and sclerosing bone dysplasias (Fig. 10; Table 3).

Generalized osteosclerosis in the newborn may be physiologic and is characterized by a transient increase in bone density that resolves spontaneously in 2 to 3 months. Physiologic osteosclerosis of the newborn is not associated with anemia, granulocytopenia, thrombocytopenia, or hepatosplenomegaly. Other causes of diffuse osteosclerosis in the newborn include infantile ostopetrosis, osteopetrosis associated with carbonic anhydrase II deficiency, pyknodysostosis, idiopathic hypercalcemia (Williams syndrome), intrauterine infections such as rubella and syphilis, and erythroblastosis fetalis.

The variations in shape and density of the bones as noted on the imaging studies reflect the response of the skeleton to various physiologic and pathologic alterations. They may provide the first indication of an aberration of health or a confirmation of a pathologic process suggested by physical examination or laboratory observations.

Table 3 ■ CONDITIONS ASSOCIATED WITH OSTEOSCLEROSIS

Physiologic osteosclerosis of the newborn
Fibrous dysplasia
Renal osteodystrophy
Primary hyperparathyroidism
Congenital hyperphosphatasia (juvenile Paget's disease)
Hypervitaminosis D
Idiopathic hypercalcemia of infancy (Williams syndrome)
Hypoparathyroidism
Lymphoma
Systemic mastocytosis
Metaphyseal dysplasia (Pyle's disease)
Craniometaphyseal dysplasia
Frontometaphyseal dysplasia
Osteopetrosis
Pyknodysostosis
Osteopoikilosis
Osteopathia striata
Melorrheostosis
Osteosarcomatosis
Endosteal hyperostosis
van Buchem's syndrome
Endemic flurorosis
Engelmann's disease (progressive diaphyseal dysplasia)
Ribbing's disease
Erythroblastosis fetalis
Myelofibrosis and myelosclerosis
Hypophosphatemic rickets and osteomalacia
Chronic lead poisoning
Radiation therapy
Neuropathic arthropathy
Neurofibromatosis

SUGGESTED READINGS

Structure and Composition of Bone

Aarden EM, Burger EH, Nijweide PJ: Function of osteocytes in bone. J Cell Biochem 1994;55:287–299

Bernstein BH, Singsen BH, Kent JT, et al: Reflex neurovascular dystrophy in childhood. J Pediatr 1978;93:211–215

Blake GM, Fogelman I: Interpretation of bone densitometry studies. Semin Nucl Med 1997;27:248–260

Burger EH, Klein-Nulend J, van der Plas A, Nijweide PJ: Function of osteocytes in bone—their role in mechanotransduction. J Nutr 1995;125(7 Suppl):2020S–2023S

Dodd JS, Raleigh JA, Gross TS: Osteocyte hypoxia: a novel mechanotransduction pathway. Am J Physiol 1999;277:c598–602

Follis RG Jr, Park EA: Some observations on bone growth with particular respect to zones and transverse lines of increased density in the metaphysis. Am J Roentgenol Radium Ther Nucl Med 1952;68:709–724

Frisancho AR, Garn SM, Ascoli W: Subperiosteal and endosteal bone apposition in adolescence. Hum Biol 1970;42:639–664

Garn SM, Silverman FN, Hertzog KP, et al: Lines and bands of increased density: their implications to growth and development. Med Radiogr Photogr 1968;44:5889

Hakeda Y, Arakawa T, Ogasawara A, Kumegawa M: Recent progress in studies on osteocytes—osteocytes and mechanical stress. Kaibogaku Zasshi 2000;75:451–456

Hoekman K, Papapoulos SE, Peters AC, et al: Characteristics and bisphosphonate treatment of a patient with juvenile osteoporosis. J Clin Endocrinol Metab 1985;61:952–955

Honasoge M, Frame B, Kottamasu SR: Pathophysiology of osteosclerosis and hyperostosis. In Osteosclerosis, Hyperostosis and Related Disorders. New York, Elsevier Science Publishing Company, 1987:1–21

James JR, Congdon PJ, Truscott J, et al: Osteopenia of prematurity. Arch Dis Child 1986;61:871–876

Jowsey J, Johnson KA: Juvenile osteoporosis: bone findings in seven patients. J Pediatr 1972;81:511–517

Koo WW, Walters J, Bush AJ: Technical considerations of dual-energy X-ray absorptiometry-based bone mineral measurements for pediatric studies. J Bone Miner Res 1995;10:1998–2004

Koo WW, Walters J, Bush AJ, et al: Dual-energy X-ray absorptiometry studies of bone mineral status in newborn infants. J Bone Miner Res 1996;11:997–1002

Kottamasu SR, Honasoge M, Frame B: Physical and chemical agents associated with osteosclerosis. In Osteosclerosis, Hyperostosis and Related Disorders. New York, Elsevier Science Publishing Company, 1987:165–196

Kottamasu SR, Rao DS, Meema HE, Genant HK: Radiology of metabolic bone disease. Henry Ford Hosp Med J 1983;31:239–243

Lapillonne A, Braillon PM, Claris O, et al: Use of dual-energy X-ray absorptiometry for the measurements of small quantities of mineral. Biol Neonate 1997;71:198–201

Meema HE: Recognition of cortical bone resorption in metabolic disease in vivo. Skeletal Radiol 1977;2:11–19

Nadvi SZ, Kottamasu SR, Bawle E, Abella E: Physiologic osteosclerosis versus osteopetrosis of the newborn. Clin Pediatr 1999;38:235–238

Ozawa H, Amizuka N: Structure and function of bone cells. Nippon Rinsho 1994;52:2246–2254

Park EA: The imprinting of nutritional disturbances on growing bone. Pediatrics 1964;33(Pt 2 Suppl):815–862

Salle BL, Braillon P, Glorieux FH, et al: Lumbar bone mineral content measured by dual energy X-ray absorptiometry in newborns and infants. Acta Paediatr 1992;81:953–958

Sartain P, Whitaker JA, Martin J: Absence of lead lines in bones of children with early lead poisoning. Am J Roentgenol Radium Ther Nucl Med 1964;91:597–601

Sherrard DJ, Maloney NA: Single-dose tetracycline labeling for bone histomorphometry. Am J Clin Pathol 1989;91:682–687

Sievanen H, Backstrom MC, Kuusela AL, et al: Dual energy x-ray absorptiometry of the forearm in preterm and term infants: evaluation of the methodology. Pediatr Res 1999;45:100–105

Silber TJ, Majd M: Reflex sympathetic dystrophy in children and adolescents: report of 18 cases and review of the literature. Am J Dis Child 1988;142:1325–1330

Silverman FN: Treatment of leukemia and allied disorders with folic acid antagonists: effect of aminopterin on skeletal lesions. Radiology 1950;54:665–677

Southard RN, Morris JD, Mahan JD, et al: Bone mass in healthy children: measurement with quantitative DXA. Radiology 1991;179:735–738

Steichen JJ, Asch PA, Tsang AC: Bone mineral content measurement in small infants by single-photon absorptiometry: current methodologic issues. J Pediatr 1988;113:181–187

Teitelbaum SL, Bullough PG: The pathophysiology of bone and joint disease. Am J Pathol 1979;96:283–364

Tsukahara H, Sudo M, Umezaki M, et al: Measurement of lumbar spinal bone mineral density in preterm infants by dual-energy X-ray absorptiometry. Biol Neonate 1993;64:96–103

Warrier RP, Waisanen J, Sultana S, et al: Childhood lead poisoning. Henry Ford Hosp Med J 1986;34:32–34

Webber CE: Uncertainties in bone mineral density T scores. Clin Invest Med 1998;21:94–96

Yeni YN, Vashishth D, Fyhrie DP: Estimation of bone matrix apparent stiffness variation caused by osteocyte lacunar size and density. J Biomech Eng 2001;123:10–17

Yeste D, del Rio L, Gussinye M, Carrascosa A: Bone mineral density in nursing infants and young children (0–4 years old) at the level of the lumbar spine: the normal patterns. An Esp Pediatr 1998;49:248–252

Osteoporosis

Regional Migratory Osteoporosis, Reflux Sympathetic Dystrophy, Transient Osteoporosis of the Hip

Banas MP, Kaplan FS, Fallon MD, Haddad JG: Regional migratory osteoporosis: a case report and review of the literature. Clin Orthop 1990;250:303–309

Bray ST, Partain CL, Teates CD, et al: The value of the bone scan in idiopathic regional migratory osteoporosis. J Nucl Med 1979;20:1268–1271

Kim SM, Desai AG, Krakovitz M, et al: Scintigraphic evaluation of regional migratory osteoporosis. Clin Nucl Med 1989;14:36–39

Klier I, Zoldan J, Yosipovitch Z, Gadoth N: Transient regional and migratory osteoporosis: a possible neural mechanism. Isr J Med Sci 1989;25:279

Major GA: Regional migratory osteoporosis. Postgrad Med J 1984;60:420–423

Mavichak V, Murray TM, Hodsman AB, et al: Regional migratory osteoporosis of the lower extremities with vertebral osteoporosis. Bone 1986;7:343–349

Naides SJ, Resnick D, Zvaifler NJ: Idiopathic regional osteoporosis: a clinical spectrum. J Rheumatol 1985;12:763–768

Roig-Escofet D, Rodriguez-Moreno J, Ruiz Martin JM: Concept and limits of the reflex sympathetic dystrophy. Clin Rheumatol 1989;8(Suppl 2):104–108

Santori FS, Calvisi V, Manili M, Gambini A: Regional migratory osteoporosis. Ital J Orthop Traumatol 1985;11:371–380

Schapira D: Transient osteoporosis of the hip. Semin Arthritis Rheum 1992;22:98–105

Shier CK, Ellis BI, Kleerekoper M, Jurisson ML: Disseminated migratory osteoporosis: an unusual pattern of osteoporosis. Can Assoc Radiol J 1987;38:56–59

Tannenbaum H, Esdaile J, Rosenthall L: Joint imaging in regional migratory osteoporosis. J Rheumatol 1980;7:237–244

Idiopathic Juvenile Osteoporosis

Bartal E, Gage JR: Idiopathic juvenile osteoporosis and scoliosis. J Pediatr Orthop 1982;2:295–298

Dent CE: Osteoporosis in childhood. Postgrad Med J 1977;53:450–457

Grubbauer HM, Stogmann W, Wendler H: Differential diagnosis and course of the idiopathic juvenile osteoporosis. Klin Pediatr 1976;188:353–359

Kauffman RP, Overton TH, Shiflett M, Jennings JC: Osteoporosis in children and adolescent girls: case report of idiopathic juvenile osteoporosis and review of the literature. Obstet Gynecol Surv 2001;56:492–504

Kitajima I, Une F, Kuriyama M, Igata A: An adult case of idiopathic juvenile osteoporosis. Nippon Naika Gakkai Zasshi 1986;75:753–758

Krassas GE: Idiopathic juvenile osteoporosis. Ann N Y Acad Sci 2000;900:409–412

Smith R: Idiopathic osteoporosis in the young. J Bone Joint Surg Br 1980;62:417–427

Teotia M, Teotia SP, Singh RK: Idiopathic juvenile osteoporosis. Am J Dis Child 1979;133:894–900

van der Sluis IM, de Muinck Keizer-Schrama SM: Osteoporosis in childhood: bone density of children in health and disease. J Pediatr Endocrinol Metab 2001;14:817–832

Villaverde V, De Inocencio J, Merino R, Garcia-Consuegra J: Difficulty walking: a presentation of idiopathic juvenile osteoporosis. J Rheumatol 1998;25:173–176

Osteoporosis in Homocystinuria

Brenton DP: Skeletal abnormalities in homocystinuria. Postgrad Med J 1977;53:488–496

MacCarthy JM, Carey MC: Bone changes in homocystinuria. Clin Radiol 1968;19:128–134

Tamburrini O, Bartolomeo-De Iuri A, Andria G, et al: Bone changes in homocystinuria in childhood. Radiol Med (Tornio) 1984;70:937–942

Thomas PS, Carson NA: Homocystinuria: the evolution of skeletal changes in relation to treatment. Ann Radiol (Paris) 1978;21:95–104

Chapter 2

METABOLIC BONE DISEASES

SAMBASIVA R. KOTTAMASU

RICKETS

Rickets is the best known metabolic bone disease (MBD), and various types of rickets (Table 1) share several common radiographic patterns. A description of radiographic abnormalities in vitamin D–deficiency rickets serves as a standard for other forms of the condition manifesting similar findings.

VITAMIN D–DEFICIENCY RICKETS

Vitamin D–deficiency rickets is a disease of infancy and childhood characterized by the failure of calcification of growing cartilage and bone. It is a disease caused by deprivation of the short ultraviolet radiations of sunlight and deficiency of vitamin D in the diet. Constitutional factors probably play an important causal role in individual susceptibility to rickets and in the vitamin D requirement for its cure. Contributory causal factors include the quantities and ratios of calcium and phosphorus available to the body, the velocity of growth of the individual, and the ultraviolet ray–filtering power of the atmosphere. Prematurity is an important predisposing factor. The bone mineral content of premature infants measured by photon absorptiometry at 40 weeks postgestational age is significantly lower than that of full-term infants. Vitamin D–deficient rickets is rare today and seen most commonly in breast-fed infants who have limited exposure to sunlight.

The classical physiologic functions of vitamin D are to maintain calcium homeostasis and prevent rickets and osteomalacia. Vitamin D is synthesized endogenously in the skin from its precursor, 7-dehydrocholesterol, following adequate exposure to sunlight. The lack of adequate sunlight exposure resulting from geographic location or personal or cultural habit may predispose to vitamin D deficiency. Vitamin D synthesis may be relatively less in individuals with dark skin pigmentation than in lightly pigmented individuals, predisposing these individuals to vitamin D deficiency. Dietary vitamin D from plants is known as ergocalciferol or vitamin D_2 and that from animals is known as cholecalciferol or vitamin D_3. Both vitamins D_2 and D_3 must be further metabolized in the liver and the kidney to generate their respective physiologically active metabolites. In general, both sources of vitamin D undergo the same metabolism and provide the same physiologic function, thus the numeric suffix is usually dropped unless a specific source of vitamin D is indicated. In the liver, vitamin D is metabolized to 25-hydroxyvitamin D (25-OHD), the most abundant vitamin D metabolite in the circulation. In the kidney, 25-OHD is further metabolized to 1,25-dihydroxyvitamin D [1,25-(OH)2D]. There are over 30 metabolites of vitamin D, some of which have documented physiologic function; 1,25-(OH)2D is the most potent metabolite physiologically. Its action in conjunction with the classic calciotropic hormones parathyroid hormone and calcitonin maintains calcium homeostasis. It increases intestinal absorption and renal retention of calcium and phosphorus, and modulates osteoblastic function. The formation of 1,25-(OH)2D is stimulated by parathyroid hormone, and its deficiency in the blood stimulates parathyroid hyperplasia and function. The skeletal changes in rickets result from failure of calcification of the growing skeleton owing to an insufficient supply of inorganic components of bone, primarily calcium and phosphorus, in the blood and body fluids.

Radiographic Findings

In the earliest stage, specific changes of rickets are not detectable radiographically; histologic changes are evident in the bones and chemical abnormalities develop

---

Table 1 ■ CLINICAL CONDITIONS ASSOCIATED WITH RICKETS AND OSTEOMALACIA

Vitamin D deficiency
Renal disease
Intestinal malabsorption
Hepatic disease
Anticonvulsant medication
Vitamin D resistance
Fanconi's syndrome
Vitamin D dependence—type I and type II
Congenital disorders
Prematurity
Breast feeding
Oncogenic condition
Renal dialysis
Aluminum toxicity
Copper deficiency
Hypophosphatasia
Congenital hyperphosphatasia
Osteopetrosis

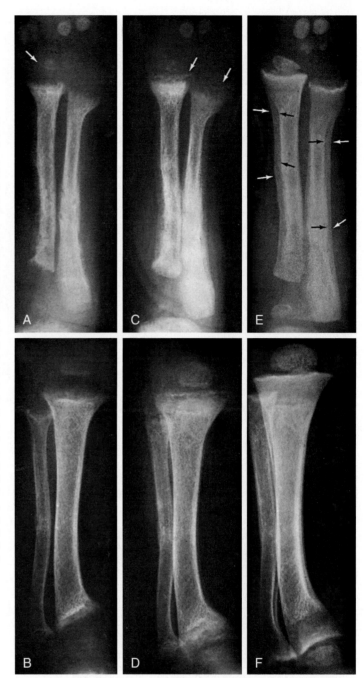

FIGURE 1. Advanced rickets showing active and healing stages in the forearms (**A, C,** and **E**) and legs (**B, D,** and **F**). **A,** Active stage before treatment. The shafts are diffusely osteopenic and coarse in texture and demonstrate fractures. The distal metaphyses of both bones are widened, frayed, and cupped. Provisional zones of calcification are invisible. The radial epiphyseal center is small and barely visible *(arrow)*. The zone between the ossification center and the visible end of the shaft is deepened. The shafts appear to be short because the terminal rachitic metaphyses are invisible. **B,** Active stage in the tibia and fibula. The changes are analogous to those in the radius and ulna. The middle third of the fibula exhibits a fracture. Both ends of the fibula are cupped. The deep intermediate rachitic zone between the proximal end of the tibia and its epiphyseal center is well shown. Deformity and change in inclination of the distal tibial metaphysis are evident, and growth is proceeding in a plane oblique to the long axis of the shaft. **C** and **D,** Healing after 34 days of treatment. **C,** In the forearm, the provisional zones of calcification are partially recalcified and located well beyond the ends of the shafts, where they appear as transverse lines of increased density *(arrows)*. **D,** In the tibia and fibula, findings are similar to those in **C.** Apparent increase in length of the shafts in comparison with **B** is due to recalcification of the rachitic metaphyses in each end of the bones, which were invisible during the active phase. **E** and **F,** Healing after 63 and 94 days of treatment, respectively. **E,** In the forearm, previously rachitic metaphyses are completely recalcified and radiolucent intermediate rachitic zones have disappeared. Ossification centers are sharply defined and in normal close proximity to the ends of the shafts. Recalcification of the subperiosteal osteoid has produced a thick opaque envelope of cortex that surrounds the shafts *(arrows)*. **F,** The tibia and fibula exhibit changes similar to those in **E,** except that the subperiosteal cloaking is not so conspicuous.

in the blood serum several weeks prior to the appearance of conclusive radiographic changes. The rapidly growing ends of the long tubular bones, such as distal femur, proximal tibia, proximal humerus, and distal ulna and radius are the optimal sites for the demonstration of the earliest lesions. The principal diagnostic features are the rarefaction and irregular fraying of the zone of provisional calcification. The normally sharply defined provisional zone of calcification fades out indistinctly into the soft tissue density of the adjacent epiphyseal cartilage. The affected metaphyses may be concave and slightly widened. Cupping of the distal end of the ulna in younger infants is not necessarily abnormal because it has been observed in some nonrachitic

infants during the first months of life. The shaft often appears normal when changes are first detected in the metaphysis; rarefaction of the shaft becomes evident a few weeks later.

In more advanced stages, the radiographic findings are pathognomonic and the diagnosis can be made immediately on inspection of the films. The diagnostic signs are similar to those in the early stage but are more marked. The sclerotic zone of provisional calcification is absent and the terminal segment of the shaft—the rachitic metaphysis—is partially or totally invisible (Fig. 1). Owing to the nonvisualization of the uncalcified rachitic metaphyses at each end of the shaft, the visible calcified portion of the shaft is shortened longitudinally;

for the same reason, the space between the visible end of the shaft and its neighboring epiphyseal ossification center is deepened. The abnormal large radiolucent zone between the epiphyseal ossification center and the irregularly frayed end of the shaft is pathognomonic of rickets.

The end of the shaft may be straight or hollowed out into a concave, cup-like central depression. Cupping is common in both ends of the fibula and in the distal ends of the ulna and tibia. Metaphyseal cupping is never found in the bones of the elbows. Cupping and widening of the ends of the shafts are absent in some of the severest cases of rickets—the atrophic type in which poor muscular power permits little activity of the limbs. In well-nourished rachitic infants with relatively good muscular power who crawl and walk, cupping and flaring of the ends of the shafts are common features. In many cases, metaphyseal cupping and widening become more conspicuous radiographically when rickets is partially healed (Fig. 2).

The changes in the shaft lag slightly behind those in the metaphyses. The entire shaft shows a diffuse rarefaction caused by the loss of mineral content. The cortex is thin and its texture coarsens. The mesh of the spongiosa coarsens owing to the decalcification and disappearance of the finer secondary trabeculae; when the cortex is markedly thin, the underlying spongiosa is more conspicuous. Greenstick fractures of the cortex are not uncommon. Sometimes sharply defined radiolucent transverse bands, also known as Looser's zones, are found in the shafts (Fig. 3). Looser's zones initially manifest as hairline infractions and are often bilateral and symmetric. The sites of the radiolucent transverse

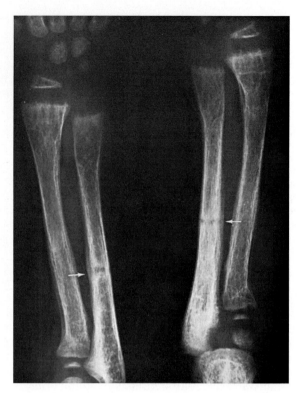

FIGURE 3. Symmetric transverse radiolucent bands in ulnar shafts.

bands are often related to sites of circumflex arteries whose local pulsating character may result in erosion of the partially demineralized bone. These symmetric "stress fractures" occur in children and adults with osteomalacia and disappear when the osteomalacic bone disease heals.

The epiphyseal ossification centers in the carpal and tarsal bones show radiographic changes similar to those in the tubular bones. The margins of these rounded bones, which are analogous to the zones of provisional calcification of the tubular bones, disappear, and changes of osteomalacia develop in the spongiosa. In severe cases, the ossification centers may become invisible during the active stage of rickets and reappear when they are recalcified during healing, erroneously suggesting a rapid advance in skeletal maturation. In the adolescent with rickets, the growth plate between the primary and secondary iliac and ischial ossification centers may appear abnormally wide when most other epiphyses have fused.

The first evidence of healing is the reappearance of the zone of provisional calcification. The recalcified zone of provisional calcification casts a transverse linear shadow of increased density in rachitic metaphyses beyond the visible ends of the shaft. The radiolucent rachitic metaphysis, interposed between the newly calcified zone of provisional calcification and the visible end of the shaft, is still not mineralized and is of soft tissue density. As healing continues, the new zone of provisional calcification thickens into a transverse band; at the same time, the metaphyseal spongiosa is gradually recalcified and fills in the previously radiolucent intermediate rachitic zone, fusing with that of the zone of

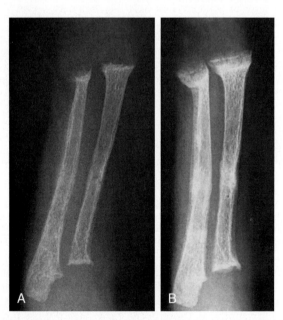

FIGURE 2. Exaggeration of cupping and widening during the healing stage of rickets. **A,** Typical atrophic rickets prior to treatment and healing. **B,** Sixteen days after inception of treatment. The partially recalcified healing metaphyses show marked increase in cupping and spreading. The length of the shafts also appears to be increased because the previously invisible metaphyseal areas have now become visible.

provisional calcification. This recalcification of the terminal segments of the shaft produces a false appearance of rapid increase in length of the shaft. In the shaft, the spongiosal mesh becomes more sharply defined and more delicate. Healing of the cortical bone is usually slower and less conspicuous radiographically. However, when thick layers of osteoid have been deposited under the periosteum, recalcification of this osteoid discloses a diffuse cortical envelope that may be of uniform density or lamellated. Deposition of calcium in the zone of provisional calcification on the floor of the cup near the end of the shaft may occasionally give the factitious appearance of "diaphyseal" healing (Fig. 4). Widening, cupping, and irregularity of anterior ends of the ribs is a classical manifestation of severe rickets and is commonly refered to as a "rachitic rosary" (Fig. 5).

Rachitic Sequelae

Complete healing and restoration of normal structures are the rule in dietary deficiency rickets, even when severe changes are present during the active stage. Distortion and sclerosis of the spongiosa in the bones affected during active disease may be visible after healing (Fig. 6) and remain evident in the same level of the shaft for years. Central rarefaction of the ossification centers also persists in many cases but not to the degree noted in scurvy. Cortical thickening of the segments of the bone involved during the active stage may remain evident for years after healing is completed, particularly on the concave surface of bowed long bones. Most of the bowing and angulation deformities result from displacement of the epiphyseal cartilage during the active stage. This gives rise to a change in inclination of the physis and a resultant change in the direction of subsequent longitudinal growth that proceeds in the direction of the deformity instead of in the direction of the longitudinal axis of the shaft (Fig. 7). Angulation deformities may also be secondary to pathologic fractures during the active stage. The most common deformities in the lower limbs are knock-knee and bowleg.

Findings suggestive of rickets are observed in premature infants, particularly those with additional deficiency of trace metals such as copper, and in infants receiving prolonged periods of total parenteral nutrition. In premature infants, rickets may be recognized by osteopenia and osteomalacia as well as by fractures. The typical metaphyseal lesions may be difficult to identify because of lack of adjacent epiphyseal centers. Rib fractures may also occur from ordinary manipulation and be recognized belatedly only by healing callus.

OTHER FORMS OF RICKETS

Renal Rickets

Damage to the renal parenchyma can interfere with the formation of 1,25(OH)2D and, together with phosphate retention, can result in rickets and osteomalacia with secondary hyperparathyroidism (SHPT). Thus renal osteodystrophy (ROD) is a consequence of two major hormonal changes: a deficiency of 1,25-(OH)2D and an excess of parathyroid hormone.

Low calcium and high phosphorus serum levels are frequently observed in patients with chronic renal failure. Higher serum levels of parathyroid hormone and alkaline phosphatase (ALP) have been noted in patients with osteosclerosis than those without it. An excess of partially calcified osteoid, hyperphosphatemia, SHPT, and periosteal neostosis contribute to osteosclerosis in ROD.

The term *renal osteodystrophy* refers to the osseous manifestations of chronic renal insufficiency. Radiographic findings include osteopenia and patchy and generalized osteosclerosis in addition to characteristic findings of rickets, osteomalacia, and hyperparathyroidism (Fig. 8). Osteosclerosis is commonly observed in the spine, but also occurs in the pelvis, ribs, skull, and tubular bones (Fig. 9). In the spine, osteosclerosis may be predominantly noted along the vertebral margins, commonly referred to as "rugger jersey spine" because of its resemblance to the striped jersey worn by rugby

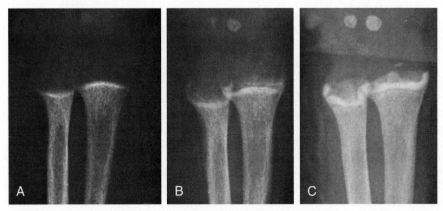

FIGURE 4. Healing of rachitic metaphyses. The recalcification appears to spread from the end of the shaft toward the epiphyseal plate instead of from the epiphyseal plate toward the end of the shaft. **A,** Before treatment. **B,** Thirteenth day of healing. **C,** Thirty-fourth day of healing. The apparent reversal of the direction of healing is actually due to cupping of the epiphyseal plate in this case. Deposition of calcium in the provisional zone of calcification on the floor of the cup near the end of the shaft is responsible for the factitious appearance of "diaphyseal" healing.

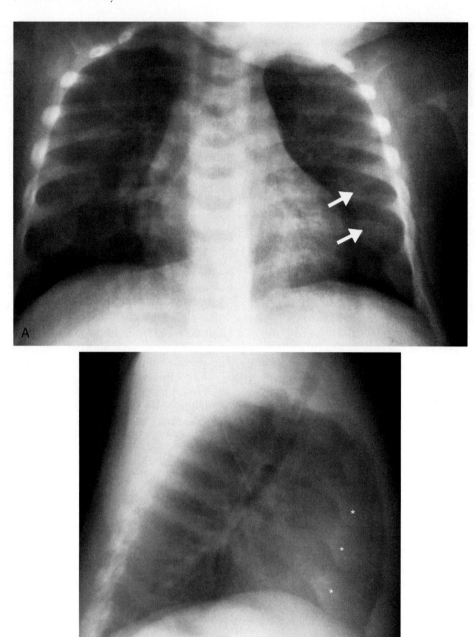

FIGURE 5. Rachitic rosary: Cupping and widening of sternal ends of the ribs (**A** *[arrows]* and **B** *[*]*) are classical manifestations of severe rickets.

players. Metaphyseal sclerosis may manifest as bands of increased density. Subperiosteal resorption is the most common radiographic abnormality in patients with uremic SHPT; however, periosteal new bone formation is noted in some patients. Periosteal neostosis refers to new bone formation under the periosteum elevated by proliferation of fibrous tissue at the sites of subperiosteal bone resorption. In periosteal neostosis, a radiolucent stripe of fibrous tissue separates new periosteal bone from the underlying cortex. Aseptic necrosis of the femoral head and less commonly of the femoral condyles, humeral head, and talus has been noted. Arterial calcification and chondrocalcinosis are frequent manifestations of ROD. Young et al. reviewed radiographs of the hands and wrists of 33 children with chronic renal disease. In addition to various radiographic manifestations of ROD, including osteopenia, subperiosteal resorption, distal tuft resorption, osteosclerosis, and soft tissue calcification, they noted that 13 patients (39%) exhibited metaphyseal sclerosis adjacent to the growth plates. Five of these 13 showed persistent sclerosis years after the growth plates had fused.

Rickets in Intestinal Malabsorption

The widened zone between the end of the shaft and the epiphyseal ossification center with loss of the zone of provisional calcification is also seen in rickets associated

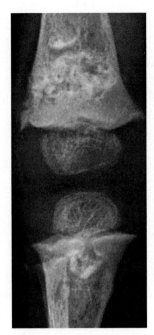

FIGURE 6. "Chambering" of the ends of rachitic shafts as a result of recalcification of distorted and deformed spongiosa following healing.

with malabsorption states such as celiac disease and cystic fibrosis of the pancreas. Osteosclerosis is rare in patients with osteomalacia secondary to intestinal malabsorption.

Hepatic Rickets

In some forms of hepatobiliary disease, such as biliary atresia, decreased intestinal absorption of fat-soluble vitamin D secondary to absence of bile in the gut and inability of hepatocytes to form adequate amounts of

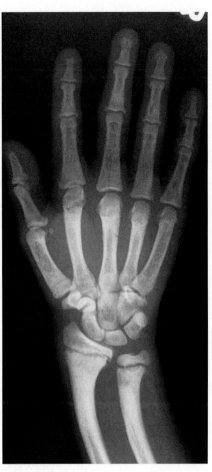

FIGURE 8. Patchy osteosclerosis and osteopenia, subperiosteal resorption along middle phalanges, resorption of tufts of distal phalanges, metaphyseal irregularity, and bowing of the radius and ulna characterize renal rickets and osteomalacia.

FIGURE 7. Pathogenesis of curvature deformities of the long bones in rickets (drawings of radiographs). **A,** Active rickets in a patient 20 months of age. The distal halves of the shafts appear to be straight. The middle third of the ulna is bowed at the site of the fractures. **B,** Healing stage 60 days after **A.** Angulation deformities are now evident at the junction of the calcifying metaphyses and the shaft; before calcification, the angulations were present but were invisible. The bowing deformity in the middle third of the ulna persists.

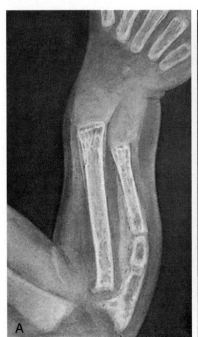
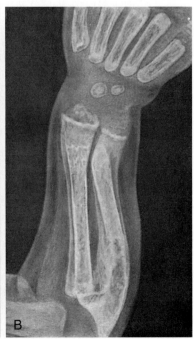

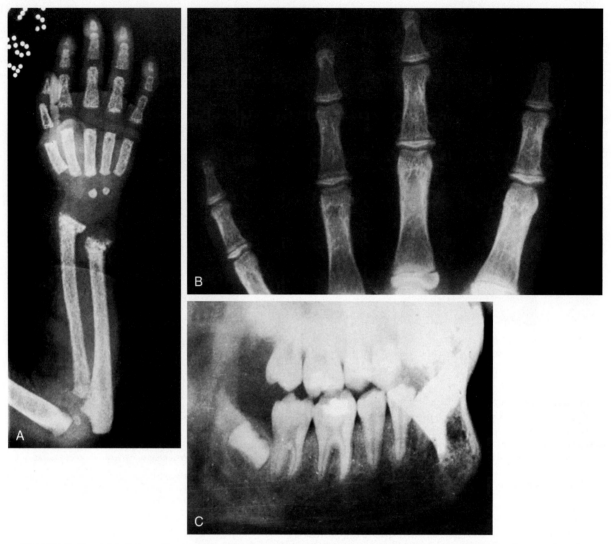

FIGURE 9. Renal rickets in an 8-year-old girl. **A,** In addition to the metaphyseal changes, there is generalized osteosclerosis, which is frequently characteristic of renal osteodystrophy. **B,** Subperiosteal resorption of bone on the radial aspect of the middle phalanges. **C,** Loss of lamina dura.

25-OHD contribute to the development of rickets and osteomalacia. There is also associated deficiency of other fat-soluble vitamins (A, E, and K). Deficiency of vitamin K leads to recurrent hemarthrosis, which frequently occurs in the knee joints. The unusual combination of clubbing of the digits, evidence of hemarthrosis, rickets, and osteomalacia is characteristic of hepatic osteodystrophy (Fig. 10).

Anticonvulsant Rickets

The administration of anticonvulsive agents has an effect on liver cells that limits its production of 25-OHD and can result in rickets and osteomalacia. Other factors that may contribute to MBD in children undergoing treatment with anticonvulsant drugs include malnutrition, lack of exposure to sunlight, lack of physical activity, number and dosage of anticonvulsant drugs used, and duration of treatment. The skeletal manifestations include severe osteopenia, metaphyseal widen-

ing and irregularity, lacy periarticular bone resorption, subperiosteal resorption along the shafts, and pathologic fractures with more severe involvement of the lower extremities (Fig. 11). We observed one patient with severe osteomalacia and SHPT. The fibulas were barely visible on pretherapy radiographs, but the phantom fibulas reappeared following therapy with 25-OHD and calcium and reduction in dosages of anticonvulsant medictions.

HEREDITARY RICKETS

Vitamin D–Resistant Rickets

Vitamin D–resistant rickets (VDRR), also known as hereditary primary hypophosphatemic rickets, results from a genetic defect of the renal tubules limiting reabsorption of phosphate ions. Because of its relatively late clinical onset, it is sometimes called juvenile rickets (Fig. 12). There are several variations of hypophosphatemic rickets based largely on inheritance, but the most common is the X-linked dominant form (XLHR). The gene causing XLHR was isolated in 1996 and named *PEX* (phosphate-regulating endopeptidase on X chromosome).

VDRR is generally associated with short stature and prominent bowing deformities together with rachitic changes that are marked in the most rapidly growing ends of the long bones. Premature closure of cranial sutures may be an associated manifestation. Cortical thickening along the concave aspect of bowed long tubular bones appears to be a compensatory response to the increased curvature and is often referred to as "buttressing." Looser's zones characteristic of osteomalacia have been reported (Fig. 13). Generalized and patchy osteosclerosis is noted in some children with hypophosphatemic rickets and osteomalacia after a prolonged period of observation and therapy. Even though the mineral content per unit volume of bone is decreased, an overabundance of partially mineralized

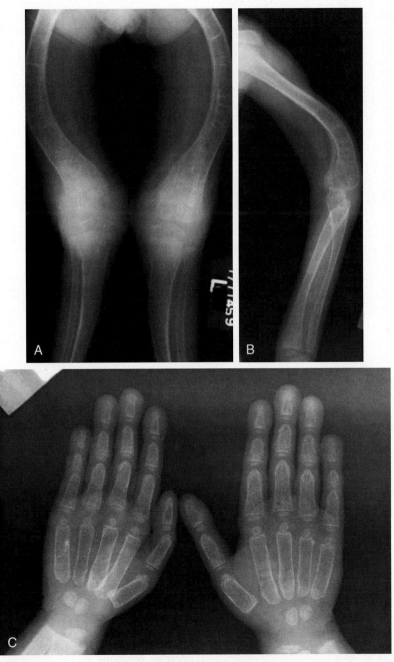

FIGURE 10. Hepatic rickets and osteomalacia. A 15-year-old boy who had a Kasai operation for extrahepatic biliary atresia during perinatal period. Severe generalized osteopenia, bowing of the long tubular bones, slight irregularities of the metaphyses and swelling of both knees secondary to hemarthroses (**A** and **B**) caused by associated vitamin K deficiency and clubbing of the digits (**C**) are characteristic of hepatic osteodystrophy. In infants and children with poor muscular power and decreased activity, cupping and flaring of the metaphyses may be less evident or absent.

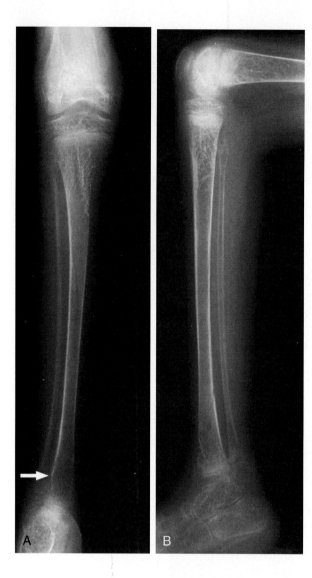

FIGURE 11. Rickets and osteomalacia with secondary hyperparathyroidism associated with anticonvulsant therapy. Severe osteopenia, resorption of medial tibial cortex, lacy resorption of ends of the long bones, irregularities of the metaphyses, slight bowing of the tibia and fibula, a pathologic fracture of the distal tibial shaft *(arrow),* and soft tissue atrophy are noted in a patient with cerebral palsy and seizures who has been on long-term therapy with phenobarbitol and dilantin.

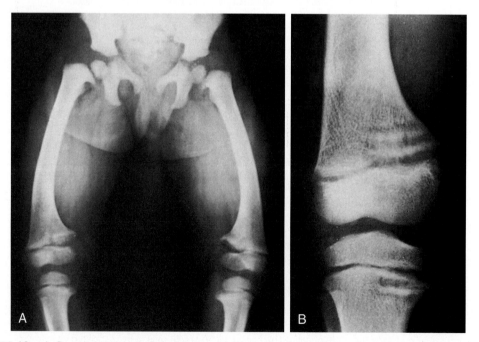

FIGURE 12. Vitamin D–resistant rickets. **A,** In a 3-year-old girl, the bowing and metaphyseal lesions resemble changes in metaphyseal chondrodysplasia (see Section IX, Part V, Figs. 24 and 25, page 2152). **B,** Same patient at 6 years. The transverse bands in the distal femoral metaphyses indicate periods of healing and relapse. (From Silverman FN, Currarino G: Metabolism 1960;9:248-283, with permission.)

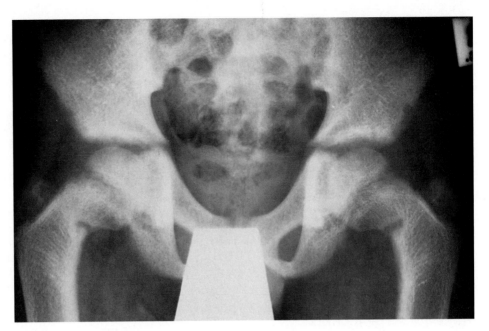

FIGURE 13. Looser's zones in hypophosphatemic rickets and osteomalacia. Symmetric transverse lucent areas in medial aspect of the femoral necks, patchy increased density, coarse trabeculations, and irregularity of the metaphyses are noted in a child with X-linked hypophosphatemia.

osteoid may be responsible for increased radiodensity observed in some patients with VDRR. Mild hyperparathyroidism noted in some patients with hypophosphatemic rickets and osteomalacia during phosphate therapy may play a role in the occurrence of osteosclerosis.

Enthesopathy characterized by calcification and ossification at the sites of muscle, ligament, joint capsule, or tendon insertions to bone has been observed; they are more common in adults. Common sites of involvement are the hands, sacroiliac joints, spine, hips, and shoulders. Spinal stenosis secondary to ossification of intervertebral ligaments associated with backache and radiculopathy in lower extremities has been described. Dental manifestations are frequent and include caries, periapical abscesses, and fractured teeth. Nephrocalcinosis has been found by ultrasound in some cases. This complication may be a consequence of vitamin D therapy.

Minamitani et al. reported a prospective study in three neonates born to mothers with hypophosphatemic vitamin D–resistant MBD. At birth, despite a low maternal serum inorganic phosphorus level, the serum phosphorus level was normal. At 3 months, their serum phosphorus levels, percentages of tubular reabsorption of phosphate, and renal tubular maximal rates of phosphate reabsorption in relation to the glomerular filtration rate were low. Radiographic changes of rickets were not apparent at birth but were evident at age 3 months in all three infants. The authors reported healing of the rickets and a normal increase in height following early detection and treatment before manifestation of physical signs of bowlegs and short stature.

Some increase in longitudinal growth has been obtained with vitamin D and oral phosphate therapy, but nephrocalcinosis was found in 79% of one group so treated. Treatment with calcitrol [1,25-(OH)2D], however, resulted in distinctly improved growth without complications.

Conventional treatment of XLHR, oral phosphate and calcitriol, is often unable to normalize serum phosphate concentration fully, and many patients fail to reach normal adult height. Wilson summarized seven trials of growth hormone (GH) treatment for XLHR. These trials range in size from 5 to 30 patients; they represent the largest studies to date of GH in this disorder. The studies reviewed report increased growth velocity when exogenous GH is added to conventional therapy, although the independent effect of GH is difficult to evaluate. Younger patients appear to respond better to GH than do older patients. However, little is known about the impact of GH on adult height.

Fanconi's Syndrome

A related inherited form of hereditary primary hypophosphatemic rickets occurs in Fanconi's syndrome. In this condition, phosphaturia of tubular origin is associated with glycosuria and various aminoacidurias. Tyrosinosis and Wilson's disease may present with comparable metabolic and radiographic features.

Vitamin D–Dependent Rickets

Two forms of rare hereditary rickets, often called vitamin D–dependent rickets (VDDR) to differentiate them from VDRR (see above), involve problems with the formation or function of 1,25-(OH)2D. In type I VDDR (VDDR-1), there is a selective defect in the renal 1α-hydroxylase enzyme that converts 25-OHD to 1,25-(OH)2D the active form of the vitamin. VDDR-1 is an autosomal recessive disorder, and the gene responsible for the disease has been mapped to the long arm of chromosome 12 on segment q14. Serum levels of 1,25-(OH)2D are undetectable or low in untreated patients, in spite of normal or slightly elevated 25-OHD. Serum 1,25-(OH)2D concentrations may remain low even after treatment with high doses of vitamin D or

25-OHD. This disorder is also known as pseudo-vitamin D–deficiency rickets, because patients with this condition respond to large doses of vitamin D or physiologic doses of 1,25-(OH)2D with resolution of the clinical, biochemical, and radiographic abnormalities.

VDDR type II, also known as calcitriol-resistant rickets (CRR), is a rare autosomal recessive disorder that results in failure of end organs to respond to physiologic levels of the 1,25-(OH)2D. The main features of CRR are severe rickets and osteomalacia from early infancy, growth retardation, severe dental changes, and alopecia of the entire body hair. Because maternal calcium crosses the placenta and reaches the fetus, the newborn does not develop bone disease for the first 3 to 6 months. The diagnosis should be suspected from the unusual association of severe rickets and alopecia. The hallmark of CRR is the high serum levels of 1,25-(OH)2D. Serum 25-OHD levels are normal.

RARE FORMS OF RICKETS

Congenital Rickets

Congenital rickets has been described in infants of mothers with severe malnutrition, malabsorption syndromes, pre-eclampsia, hypoparathyroidism, and chronic renal failure. It is now uncommon. Fetal calcium is derived from the mother, hence a baby born to a mother with hypocalcemia from various causes runs an increased risk of having a low calcium reserve. Eighty percent of fetal calcium acquisition from the mother occurs during the third trimester of pregnancy; hence preterm neonates are at a higher risk of developing metabolic bone disease. Various reports have described newborn infants in whom congenital rickets was associated with advanced maternal nutritional osteomalacia, maternal vitamin D deficiency, and untreated maternal chronic renal insufficiency.

Rickets of Prematurity

MBD in infants predominantly affects very-low-birth-weight preterm infants, although there are reports of gestationally more mature babies with congenital rickets secondary to maternal causes. Calcium and phosphorus deficiency are primarily responsible for MBD in preterm infants. It usually occurs during the period of "catch-up" growth after recovery from acute illness and nutritional deprivation. This often coincides with 36 to 40 weeks' corrected gestation and is observed around the time of hospital discharge. Radiographic manifestations include osteopenia, rickets, and/or fractures (Fig. 14). Radionuclide bone scanning may detect unsuspected fractures of clinical or medicolegal significance. The fractures are frequently under-reported, and, if discovered after hospital discharge, are frequently mistakenly diagnosed as child abuse, particularly if the infant presents with swelling of an extremity associated with a fracture.

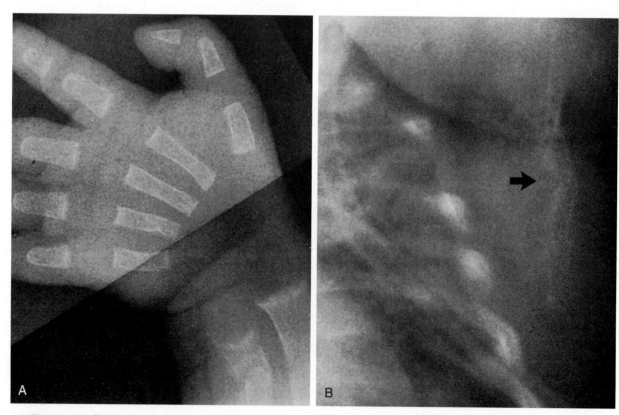

FIGURE 14. Rickets in a premature infant. **A,** In the hand and wrist, metaphyseal changes and osteopenia are associated with a fracture of the distal end of the ulna. **B,** Osteopenia, widening of costochondral junctions, and fractures of the scapula. (From Koo WW, Oestreich AE, Sherman R, et al: Radiologic case of the month: Osteopenia, rickets and fractures in preterm infants. Am J Dis Child 1985;139:1045-1046, with permission.)

Rickets Among Breast-Fed Infants

Vitamin D–deficiency rickets occurs as a result of low vitamin D intake and decreased exposure to sunlight. Although today rickets occurs primarily in underdeveloped countries, it remains a risk for breast-fed infants and children, particularly those with dark skin or decreased exposure to sunlight. Deeply pigmented infants and children require higher exposure levels to ultraviolet radiation for vitamin D synthesis than do children with less pigment. Human breast milk will not prevent rickets among infants and children who do not have sufficient exposure to sunlight. The American Academy of Pediatrics recommends vitamin D supplementation for breast-fed infants who are deeply pigmented or who do not have adequate exposure to sunlight, while the Canadian Pediatric Society recommends that vitamin D supplementation be provided for all infants in northern communities.

Oncogenic Rickets and Osteomalacia

Oncogenic rickets and osteomalacia is a rare syndrome associated with some skeletal and soft tissue tumors of mesenchymal origin, and is characterized by hypophosphatemia, phosphaturia, and low or undetectable plasma concentrations of 1,25-(OH)2D. Serum calcium and parathyroid hormone concentrations are normal in most patients. Many investigators postulate that the tumors secrete a phosphaturic factor responsible for renal phosphate wasting and osteomalacia and that the same or another factor inhibits 25-OHD 1α-hydroxylase activity in the proximal renal tubules. The symptoms resolve and phosphaturia ceases after total excision of the tumor/lesion, and the phosphate content of the serum returns to normal. Several investigators demonstrated phosphaturia and hypophosphatemia following injection of tumor extract into dogs, mice, and rats.

Although most tumors associated with oncogenic rickets and osteomalacia are benign, malignant tumors have also been reported. A wide variety of both bone and soft tissue tumors, including hemangiopericytoma, giant cell tumor, osteoid osteoma, osteoblastoma, osteogenic sarcoma, chondrosarcoma, angiosarcoma, ossifying fibroma, nonossifying fibroma, fibrous dysplasia, schwannoma, and neurofibromatosis have been noted. Epidermal nevus syndrome and McCune-Albright syndrome (polyostotic fibrous dysplasia) have also been reported as rare causes of oncogenic rickets.

Patients with oncogenic rickets and osteomalacia present with chronic vague symptoms including generalized pain and muscle weakness. The clinical presentation can be mistaken for a variety of other conditions, including rheumatoid arthritis, muscular dystrophy, and psychiatric disorder. Oncogenic rickets remains one of the few endocrine syndromes in which the abnormally produced hormone is not known. Oncogenic rickets presents a diagnostic problem because of difficulties in locating what may be a small, slow-growing tumor, and a treatment problem if the tumor cannot be found or completely resected. A search for the tumor should begin with a thorough physical examination followed by a skeletal survey. Computed tomography and magnetic resonance imaging (MRI) of any clinically suspicious area, as well as technetium-labeled blood pool scanning, have been successfully used to locate the tumor. Despite diligent searching, the tumor may not be located. It is possible that some patients diagnosed as sporadic cases of hypophosphatemic rickets and osteomalacia may in fact have oncogenic osteomalacia. However, dental abscesses, common in patients with XLHR, have not been described in oncogenic rickets. In addition, 1,25-(OH)2D levels are low or undetectable in oncogenic rickets and osteomalacia, whereas they are normal in XLHR.

Rickets in Osteopetrosis

Rickets is a common and paradoxic feature of infantile malignant osteopetrosis and results from the inability to maintain a normal calcium–phosphorus balance in the extracellular fluid. Despite a markedly positive total body calcium balance, rickets arises when the serum calcium–phosphorus product is insufficient to mineralize newly formed chondroid and osteoid. Kaplan et al. reported five children with malignant infantile osteopetrosis who manifested clinical, radiographic, biochemical, and histologic findings of rickets. Characteristic biochemical abnormalities included hypocalcemia, hypophosphatemia, and elevated levels of alkaline phosphatase (ALP) and C-terminal parathyroid hormone. The serum calcium–phosphorus product was below 30 in all children at the time the rickets was diagnosed, and above 40 by the time the rickets had resolved. Baseline bone density measurements were markedly elevated in all children and increased significantly when the rickets was treated with vitamin D and calcium. The children showed marked clinical improvement, decreased lethargy, increased mobility and activity, and stimulation of appetite, without any additional adverse hematologic or neurologic effects. The rickets was reversible in all children, in one by human leukocyte antigen–identical sibling bone marrow transplantation and in four by physiologic doses of vitamin D and calcium. The parathyroid and renal responses to hypocalcemia were appropriate, but glucocorticoids, used in treating the hematologic complications of the disease, may have blunted the intestinal response to maximal vitamin D stimulation. This latter blockade can be overcome by increasing dietary calcium. By liberalizing rather than restricting calcium and phosphorus intake, hypocalcemia can be minimized, phosphorus metabolism can be improved, and rickets can be cured.

UNUSUAL CAUSES OF MBD

MBD in Children on Renal Dialysis

Patients on renal dialysis may have skeletal manifestations of rickets, osteomalacia, osteitis fibrosa, aluminum osteopathy, or amyloidosis; these changes are often present simultaneously. Aluminum bone disease is a severe disorder leading to low turnover bone disease and osteomalacia (see MBD in Aluminum Toxicity below). Renal transplantation is the treatment of choice for normalizing serum aluminum and reducing aluminum bone content. Amyloidosis is responsible for several tendon and skeletal complications in dialysis patients, such as carpal tunnel syndrome and destructive arthropathies.

MBD in Aluminum Toxicity

Aluminum intoxication is an iatrogenic disease caused by the use of aluminum compounds for phosphate binding and by the contamination of parenteral fluids. Aluminum toxicity causes encephalopathy, MBD, and microcytic anemia. Andreoli et al. reported two children with chronic renal failure who developed aluminum intoxication as a result of long-term ingestion of aluminum hydroxide for the control of hyperphosphatemia. In each child, bone biopsy confirmed severe osteomalacia, absence of features of hyperparathyroid bone disease, and massive aluminum deposition at the bone–osteoid junction. Radiographs during the period of aluminum intoxication demonstrated osteopenia, pathologic fractures, fraying of the metaphyses of the long bones, and widening of the physes. When aluminum hydroxide therapy was discontinued and aluminum was removed with chelation therapy, radiographs demonstrated calcification of the long bones beginning at the most recently formed osteoid, which then proceeded toward the diaphysis. Pivnick et al. presented two infants with growth failure and generalized osteomalacia and rickets caused by phosphate depletion from prolonged administration of an aluminum-containing antacid given for intestinal colic. Aluminum-containing antacids should be used with caution in infants and young children, particularly those with renal failure.

Copper Deficiency

The bone abnormalities of copper deficiency are indistinguishable from those seen in MBD because of bone mineral deficiency in preterm neonates. Additional skeletal features of copper deficiency include subperiosteal new bone formation. Clinical features include neutropenia and anemia. All of these findings can occur in preterm neonates for several other reasons, although neutropenia seems more specific for copper deficiency.

SCURVY (VITAMIN C DEFICIENCY)

Scurvy is caused by deficiency of vitamin C (ascorbic acid). Historically, infantile scurvy occurs almost exclusively in babies who are fed pasteurized or boiled milk. It is the heating of cow's milk to reduce the bacterial content that destroys enough vitamin C to lead to clinical scurvy. The addition of orange juice or ascorbic acid to the diet prevents scurvy easily and effectively. In nearly all cases of scurvy, the appearance of manifest disease is preceded by a prodromal asymptomatic interval of 4 to 6 months. Authentic cases of scurvy in infants younger than 3 months are so rare that the diagnosis

should be questioned in every case considered during the first 6 months of life. During the first weeks of life, skeletal syphilis has been misinterpreted as skeletal scurvy on radiographs.

The basic skeletal changes are due to the suppression of normal cellular activity in the growing bones. Mineral deposition in the zone of provisional calcification and resorption of previously formed bone are not disturbed. Lack of intercellular cement substance in the endothelial layer of the capillaries is supposedly the cause of a hemorrhagic tendency; the blood clotting mechanism is not significantly altered. This disruption of the normal balance of bony productive and resorptive forces results in generalized atrophy of the cortex and spongiosa.

At the cartilage–shaft junction, the proliferating cartilage cells are markedly diminished in number, and their mitoses and growth are reduced. On the epiphyseal side of the zone of provisional calcification, mineral deposition continues in the cartilaginous matrix, while on the diaphyseal side, destruction of the provisional zone is diminished or stops. Radiographs show a thickened zone of provisional calcification that is not as strong physically as its width suggests. Actually, it is brittle and often presents with fissures and fractures. The trabeculae just beneath the thickened provisional zone are irregularly disposed in a random network, having lost much of their normally longitudinal parallel pattern. These trabeculae, like the provisional zone, are brittle and fracture easily. Transverse fractures through the brittle zone of provisional calcification and the metaphyseal region lead to epiphyseal displacement and separation.

When the heavy zones of provisional calcification project peripherally beyond the usual limits of the shaft, they form spurs and provide one of the most diagnostic radiographic features of scurvy. Early ossification under the raised periosteum, in the angle between the zone of provisional calcification and the periosteal attachment, is another cause of spur formation. The trabeculae just beneath the provisional zone are sparse. This atrophic layer, between the sclerotic provisional zone and a heavier spongiosa deeper in the shaft, casts a transverse band of diminished density in the radiograph that has been called the "scurvy line." Defects in the spongiosa and cortex just below the zone of provisional calcification may permit incomplete separation of the plate from the shaft with subepiphyseal marginal clefts. These clefts appear as the "corner" or "angle" sign of scurvy (Fig. 15). All of these metaphyseal changes appear earliest and are most marked at the sites of most rapid growth and most active endochondral bone formation, especially at the distal end of the femur, the proximal end of the humerus, both ends of the tibia and fibula, and the distal ends of the radius and ulna.

In the ossification centers, the changes are analogous to those in the metaphyses. The persistence and thickening of the zone of provisional calcification produce a thickened peripheral shell of calcified cartilage in the ossification center. Atrophy of the spongiosa is responsible for central rarefaction and heightens the contrast between the two components. Proportionately, the apparent rarefaction of the ossification center is greater

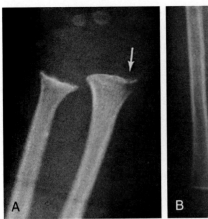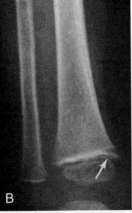

FIGURE 15. Peripheral metaphyseal clefts in scurvy. The cortical and spongiosal defects in the angle between the provisional zone of calcification and the cortex *(arrows)* are responsible for this radiographic change, called the "corner sign" of scurvy. The peripheral segment of the provisional zone is tilted off the shaft toward the epiphyseal cartilage. **A,** Distal end of the radius in an infant 11 months of age. **B,** Distal end of the tibia in an infant 14 months of age.

than that in the shafts and the small round bones of the wrists and ankles. The marked central rarefaction with intensification of the margin of the ossification center is one of the most characteristic radiographic findings in active scurvy and is known as Wimberger's sign.

In the shaft, the spongiosa becomes atrophic, causing a "ground-glass" texture in the radiograph (osteoporosis). The ground-glass appearance is also found in many types of bone atrophy of nonscorbutic origin. In the terminal segments of the shaft, where the cortex is normally exceedingly thin, the cortex may disappear on radiographs. Notwithstanding severe cortical atrophy in scurvy, diaphyseal cortical fractures are rare; in contrast, fractures of the calcified cartilage in the metaphysis are common.

Subperiosteal hemorrhages are a frequent manifestation; they are most common in the larger tubular bones such as the femur, tibia, and humerus. Occasionally, subperiosteal hematomas form on the flat bones of the calveria, orbit, and shoulder girdle. Intraorbital hematoma may be a cause of proptosis. The hemorrhages vary greatly in size; they may extend the entire length of the shaft from one epiphyseal plate to the other. Subperichondrial hemorrhages over the epiphyses are said never to occur in scurvy; hemarthrosis is also exceedingly rare during infancy and childhood. Large subperiosteal hemorrhages present as areas of increased opacity in the soft tissues surrounding the bone and may spread apart two bones that normally lie close together in parallel, such as the tibia and fibula (Fig. 16) or the radius and ulna. Subperiosteal hemorrhage is actually not as large as it appears; much of the regional swelling is due to edema and hemorrhage external to the periosteum in the overlying soft tissues.

The optimal sites for the detection of scurvy in the skeleton are the bones of the lower extremities; diagnostic changes may be demonstrable at the knees when minimal changes are present at the wrists. The mildest and probably the earliest radiographic changes in human scurvy are generalized bone atrophy and thickening of the provisional zones of calcification. These findings are, of course, not diagnostic of scurvy because they are found in many nonscorbutic types of bone atrophy. In more severe cases, several other radiographic signs may be added to the basic atrophic changes and thus give rise to a variety of pictures pathognomonic of scurvy. The combination of diffuse bone atrophy and multiple spurs at the cartilage–shaft junctions occurs only in scurvy but, rarely, may be simulated in patients under treatment with methotrexate. The transverse band of diminished density on the shaftward border of the zone of provisional calcification (scurvy line) favors the diagnosis of scurvy but is not diagnostic without spur formation (Table 2). Fractures through the thickened provisional zone and deformities secondary thereto are diagnostic of scurvy (Fig. 17) when syphilis can be excluded.

The radiographic signs of healing scurvy are easy to recognize. With the onset of healing, the cortex be-

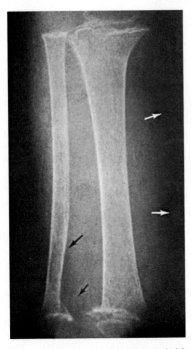

FIGURE 16. Fresh subperiosteal hematoma *(white arrows)* surrounding the distal half of the tibia and spreading apart the distal ends of the tibia and fibula. Transverse fractures are present in the terminal segments of the shafts of the tibia and fibula *(black arrows).*

Table 2 ■ CAUSES OF RADIOLUCENT METAPHYSEAL BANDS
Leukemia
Metastatic neuroblastoma
Systemic illness in infancy or in utero
Transplacental infection (e.g., toxoplasmosis, cytomegalic inclusion disease, rubella, herpes, syphilis)
Scurvy

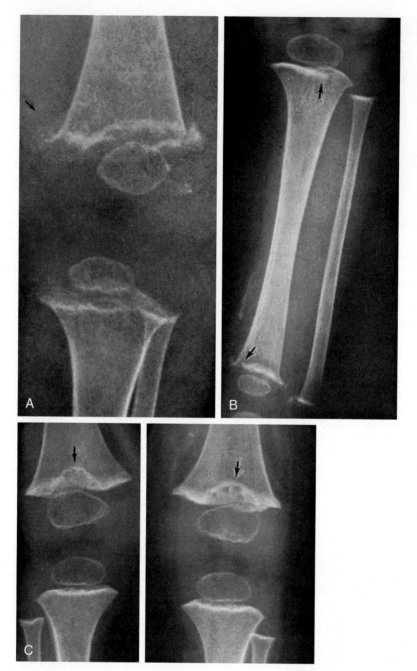

FIGURE 17. Advanced scurvy with fractures of thickened, brittle provisional zones of calcification. **A,** Multiple infractions in the provisional zone, with peripheral spurring *(arrow)* and beginning subperiosteal ossification of the terminal segment of the shaft by the externally displaced periosteum. The osteogenetic layer is lifted by hemorrhage and continues to form new cortical bone. The bones generally are rarefied, but the provisional zones of the femur, tibia, and of the femoral and tibial ossification centers are thickened. **B,** Longitudinal fractures of provisional zones and distal ends of the tibia *(arrows).* **C,** Crumpling fractures of proximal and distal provisional zones of the ends of the femora, with incomplete cupping of ends of the shafts *(arrows).*

comes thicker and the spongiosa more clearly defined. The transverse band of diminished density in the metaphysis regains its normal density and disappears. As growth proceeds, the thickened provisional zone of calcification (Fig. 18) is buried within the shaft as a "transverse line" (Fig. 19C, D). When a subperiosteal hematoma is present, the raised periosteum begins to layer the periphery of the hematoma with a new shell of subperiosteal bone. Concurrent with resorption of a

hematoma, this new layer of bone thickens and shrinks down onto the shaft to become the new cortex (Fig. 19). Residues of these cortical thickenings may persist for years. In the event of epiphyseal displacement, the longitudinal growth after healing proceeds from the displaced proliferating cartilage; the shaft and the marrow cavity shift to this new position and adapt to the new axis of longitudinal growth. The healed epiphyseal ossification center may exhibit a central inset of rarefaction that

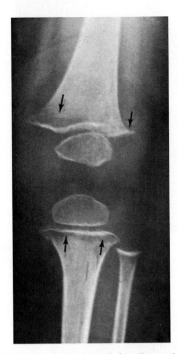

FIGURE 18. Advanced scurvy in an infant 7 months of age. Deep transverse bands of diminished density *(arrows)*, so-called scurvy lines, are adjacent to the thickened provisional zones of calcification. Atrophy of the cortex and spongiosa is also evident. Small lateral spurs project from the cartilage–shaft junctions at the distal ends of the femur and proximal end of the tibia. This combination of findings is pathognomonic of scurvy.

persists for years after the inception of healing (Fig. 20); these rarefied insets are identical in size and contour with the rarefied epiphyseal centers that are present during the active stage of the disease. Rarely, segmental central cupping of the metaphysis and epiphyseal invagination may occur following epiphyseal fracture and indicate premature fusion. Despite initial shortening, almost complete catch-up growth is noted in some children (Fig. 21).

The risk of vitamin C deficiency is underestimated in industrialized countries, and clinical diagnosis of low-grade vitamin C deficiency can be difficult. The biochemical analysis requires special care in sample collection and transport. Campistol Plana et al. presented six children with scurvy in whom symptoms included irritability, skin hemorrhages, and swollen gums, scorbutic rosary, swelling and tenderness of the lower limbs. Radiographic manifestations were generalized osteopenia, corner sign, Wimberger's sign, and in some cases subperiosteal hemorrhages with calcification. Ascorbic acid levels were below normal values in all cases. Boulinguez et al. reported three cases of scurvy presenting with ecchymotic purpura and hemorrhagic ulcerations of the lower limbs. Vitamin C supplementation led to rapid improvement of the skin lesions.

Although textbook descriptions of manifestations of avitaminoses are presented as if a profound single deficiency is present, multiple deficiencies are the rule and may modify the radiographic appearance of the skeletal response. Differences in the time of onset of

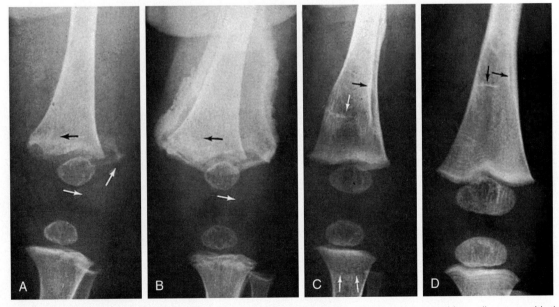

FIGURE 19. Healing scurvy in an infant 6 months of age shows formation of a new cortex and its realignment with the displaced epiphyses of the left femur. **A,** Active stage: the provisional zone of calcification of the femur is fractured *(vertical arrow)* and the epiphysis displaced laterally *(horizontal white arrow)*. **B,** Fourteen days after the administration of ascorbic acid, a heavy shell of subperiosteal bone has formed around the subperiosteal hematoma. **C,** Four months after **A,** the shell of bone around the subperiosteal hematoma has shrunk and now forms the new cortex. The old cortex and provisional zone are still visible *(arrows)*; they are buried in the new shaft and are being gradually resorbed. The new shaft is now aligned with the displaced epiphyses. **D,** One year after **A.** The old cortex *(horizontal arrow)* is barely visible, and the old provisional zone is buried deeply in the shaft as a "transverse line" *(vertical arrow)*. The new shaft is in perfect alignment with its distal epiphysis, which in turn is in normal relation to the tibial epiphysis across the knee joint.

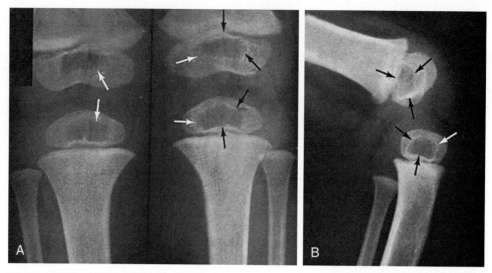

FIGURE 20. Frontal **(A)** and lateral **(B)** projections of healed scurvy, showing the epiphyseal insets of central rarefaction *(arrows),* 20 months after the active stage of the disease, in distal ossification centers of the femora and proximal centers of the tibias.

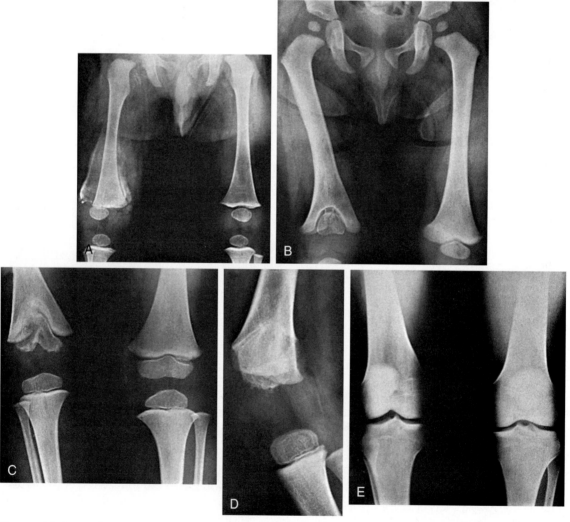

FIGURE 21. Successive changes in scurvy resulting from unrecognized epiphyseal plate injury. **A,** Epiphyseal displacement and associated subperiosteal hematoma in a 6-month-old boy. **B,** At 19 months, the femoral metaphysis is deeply cupped and the distal ossification center is invaginated into the metaphysis because of fusion and failure of growth in the central portion of the epiphyseal growth cartilage. The ossification center is also deformed by the central tethering. **C,** At 4 years, there is shortening of the femur with increasing invagination of the epiphysis that, nevertheless, appears to be undergoing ossification distally into the cartilaginous condyles. **D,** Lateral projection at 4 years demonstrates central continuity of bone across the epiphyseal plate. **E,** At 22 years, only mild length discrepancy of the femurs is seen, with slight persistent tenting of the articular surface on the affected side. The patient had no complaints and walked without a limp. This result suggests corrective overgrowth to an unusual degree, very likely in response to stresses of use. Compare with Figure 26.

individual deficiencies, as well as periods of remission and relapse, may also affect the classical description. When scurvy and rickets are both present, the scurvy features usually predominate because of the diminished osteoblastic activity. The consequent low ALP levels contrast with the high levels in rickets that are associated with excessive osteoid production.

HYPERVITAMINOSES

Accurate diagnosis and successful treatment, both prophylactic and curative, of disorders caused by vitamin deficiency stand high among the major triumphs of modern medicine. Early vitamins were used in natural form in foodstuffs, where they occurred in such dilute concentrations that they could be safely sold without restriction for uncontrolled use at home. The belief has long prevailed and generally persists that all vitamin preparations are harmless. This belief has not been tenable for some years. Substantial experience demonstrates clearly that prolonged feedings of excessive amounts of highly potent concentrates of fat-soluble vitamins A and D are seriously, and in the case of vitamin D sometimes fatally, toxic. As a result, manmade diseases have appeared in humans—the hypervitaminoses.

Hypervitaminosis D can develop in patients being treated with high doses of vitamin D; parental enthusiasm for vitamins has also been at fault. Most recorded cases of vitamin A poisoning in children have resulted from prolonged daily feeding of excessive amounts of vitamin A concentrates by adult custodians who either increased the dose to toxic levels on their own initiative, in ignorance of the potential danger, or misunderstood the directions of their physicians, although the correct dosage is clearly stated on the manufacturer's label. Because there is a time lapse between the onset of excessive dosage and the development of symptoms and signs, it is possible that radiographic manifestations may provide the first clue to the reason for this disturbing undiagnosed illness in a child.

VITAMIN A POISONING

Chronic vitamin A poisoning was recognized in 1944. Three years later a second example was recorded when radiographically detectable hard swellings in the limbs and bone changes were first described. The skeletal changes were described in detail and the clinical picture confirmed by subsequent reports. In a patient reported by Woodward et al., who was poisoned during the first weeks of life from the administration of 70,000 IU/day from birth, the anterior fontanelle bulged at 2 months of age and the child then suffered from hyperirritability, hyperesthesia, alopecia, and tender hyperostoses of the clavicles and one parietal bone. Most infants with vitamin A poisoning do not develop cortical hyperostoses until the second half of the first year, in contradistinction to infantile cortical hyperostosis, in which the clinical onset is usually prior to the fifth month.

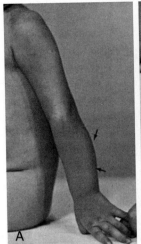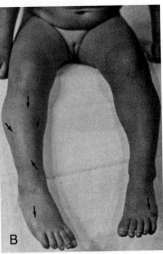

FIGURE 22. Soft tissue swellings in a 21-month-old girl with hypervitaminosis A 5 weeks after onset. **A,** Swelling of the left forearm *(arrows);* there was a similar swelling in the right forearm. **B,** Pretibial swelling on the right shank and symmetric swelling over the fifth metatarsals in both feet *(arrows).*

The early clinical features in infants and children are not distinctive; they include such common complaints as loss of appetite, itching, and irritability. Many weeks or months after the onset of these early signs, the clinical picture becomes diagnostic when hard, tender lumps appear in the limbs (Fig. 22) and the underlying bones show cortical thickening. At this stage, the blood vitamin A content is markedly elevated. Additional findings in some patients include fissures in the lips, loss of hair, dry skin, jaundice, and enlargement of the liver. In most cases, 6 months or more elapse between the beginning of excessive vitamin A intake and the appearance of swelling in the limbs. In some cases, the latent period has continued for as long as 15 months. Complete recovery follows rapidly on withdrawal of the vitamin. The clinical signs often subside in 72 hours, and the high vitamin A level falls to normal within about 6 weeks. The cortical hyperostoses are gradually and slowly resorbed over a period of several weeks to several months.

Radiographic examination of the skeleton has played an important role both in the recognition of vitamin A poisoning as an entity and in the diagnosis of individual cases. In every case, some of the tubular bones are thickened (Figs. 23 and 24). Both ulnas and some of the metatarsals are consistently affected. The basic skeletal change is external thickening of the cortical wall that is often wavy in outline when first seen. These cortical thickenings usually stop short of the ends of the shafts; the metaphyses and the epiphyseal ossification centers are characteristically normal. The microscopic structure of the cortical hyperostoses shows only an excess of normal subperiosteal bone, with fibrous marrow in the neighboring spongiosa. Radionuclide bone scans are positive, demonstrating increased uptake over the diaphyses, before radiographic changes are observed. Bony erosion of the sella secondary to increased intracranial pressure has been described (Fig. 25).

Permanent sequelae to vitamin A poisoning have

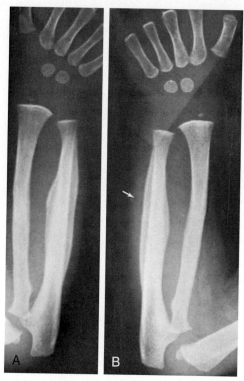

FIGURE 23. Symmetric cortical hyperostosis *(arrow)* of the right **(A)** and left **(B)** ulnas in poisoning due to vitamin A, 5 weeks after onset of clinical signs.

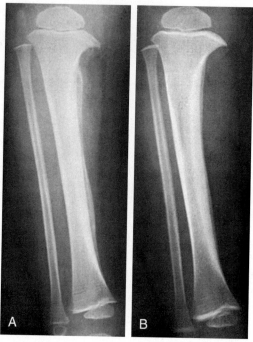

FIGURE 24. Tibial cortical hyperostosis in the same patient as in Figure 23. **A,** Five weeks after onset of clinical signs. **B,** Ten weeks after onset and 5 weeks after stopping vitamin A intake. The patient had been well for 4 weeks.

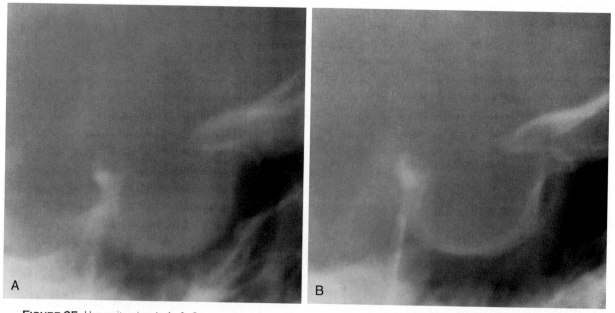

FIGURE 25. Hypervitaminosis A. **A,** Severe resorption of floor of the sella in a patient with vitamin A poisoning. **B,** Marked improvement in density of floor of the sella in a few months after the patient discontinued ingesting large amounts of vitamin A.

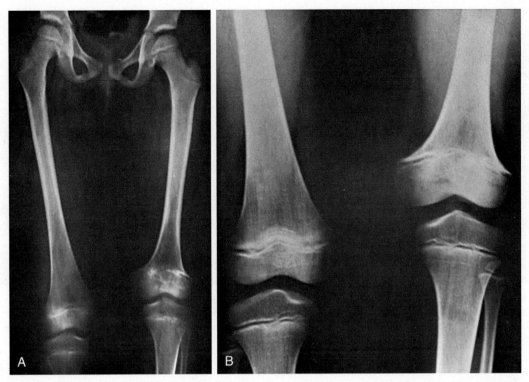

FIGURE 26. Residual changes from vitamin A poisoning. **A,** Three years after acute poisoning, the left femur is shortened several centimeters, and its distal end flares to join with a greatly enlarged epiphyseal ossification center. **B,** Frontal projection of the knees of another patient shows enlargement of the distal end of the femur and premature fusion of the shaft with the enlarged epiphyseal ossification center. The other bones were normal radiographically. (Courtesy of Dr. Charles N. Pease, Chicago, IL.)

been found in several patients (Fig. 26). Arrest in growth of the long bones may occur because of premature fusion of epiphyses with shafts and cone epiphysis formation. In one girl who was acutely poisoned at 2 years of age, Pease found that the left femur was shortened by 5 cm at age 18. In two patients described by Pickup, the clinical and biochemical manifestations of vitamin A poisoning were severe, but there were no radiographic changes in the skeleton, although both patients had pain in the arms and legs. In the first patient, a boy 6 years of age, large doses of vitamin A had been given for only 6 weeks; in the second, a girl 4 years of age, 350,000 IU/day of vitamin A had been given over 2 years for treatment of ichthyosis.

In contrast to the many cases of chronic poisoning by vitamin A concentrate described in the literature, acute poisoning from this source is uncommon. It causes hydrocephalus with bulging of the anterior fontanelle in infants. Acute poisoning usually follows a single massive dose of vitamin A of several hundred thousand units. Bulging of the fontanelle is evident within 12 hours and usually has disappeared after 36 hours. Vomiting is the principal clinical disturbance. Ocular fundi and cerebral electroencephalograms are normal. In one infant said to have ingested large amounts of vitamin A, films of the skull showed widening of the coronal suture. Three girls, ages 14, 15, and 16 years, studied by Morrice and associates, took 90,000 to 200,000 units of vitamin A daily for the treatment of acne and developed signs of increased intracranial pressure, bone pain, alopecia,

and hypomenorrhea, all of which disappeared when vitamin A intake was stopped. Other examples of pseudotumor cerebri have been recorded.

Native people and experienced travelers in the Arctic have long believed that livers of polar bears are toxic to man and other animals. The highest hepatic concentrations of vitamin A in Arctic animals are found in polar bears. There is convincing experimental evidence that the toxic effect of polar bear liver is due to its richness in vitamin A. The liver of the bearded seal, the principal food of the polar bear, also has an exceedingly high vitamin A content.

High-potency synthetic analogs of vitamin A (e.g., isotretinoin), used in prolonged treatment of keratinizing disorders such as icthyosis and keratoderma, have produced changes similar to those of diffuse idiopathic skeletal hyperostosis and premature epiphyseal closure. The retinoid-induced hyperostoses are different from those seen with vitamin A toxicity and may be subtle. The common sites of involvement include the cervical, thoracic, and lumbar spine. The anterior longitudinal ligament, other spinal ligaments, and ileolumbar ligaments may be ossified. Beak-like ossifications occur at margins of the vertebral bodies, at the calcaneus, and near ends of the long bones. Vitamin A–induced periosteal new bone formation, by contrast, involves diaphyseal and metaphyseal regions of short and long tubular bones. The costal cartilages may be diffusely calcified. Exposure during pregnancy can result in what has been called the "isotretinoin dysmorphic syn-

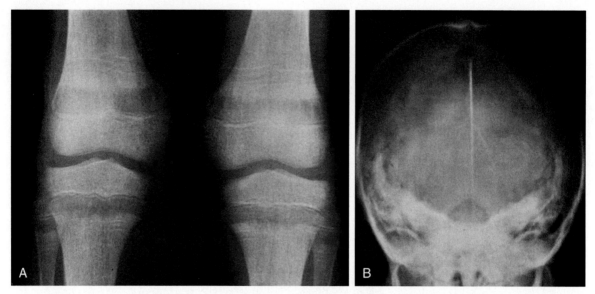

FIGURE 27. Fatal vitamin D poisoning in a boy 9 years of age who had diabetes mellitus and had been on a high-vitamin diet as part of his general treatment. **A,** In the metaphyses of all of the bones at the knees are series of radiolucent and radiopaque transverse bands. The epiphyseal ossification centers are not affected. **B,** Towne projection of the skull. The falx cerebri and tentorium cerebelli are calcified.

drome" in the fetus, characterized by anomalies of the ears, face, central nervous system, and heart. Caffey's warning bears repetition, namely, that vitamin A concentrates are probably superfluous, certainly expensive, and potentially toxic preparations.

VITAMIN D POISONING

Vitamin D poisoning may be acute or chronic. Most symptoms and signs are associated with manifestations of hypercalcemia. Massive dosage (4 to 18 million U/day) may cause severe illness or even death within 3 to 9 days. Vomiting followed by dehydration and high fever are common in the severely ill; other manifestations in some patients include coma, convulsions, abdominal cramps, and "bone pain." In chronic poisoning, the common early symptoms are lethargy, thirst, anorexia, and urinary urgency, with or without polyuria. Later symptoms are vomiting, diarrhea, and abdominal discomfort. Renal damage with renal calcification is due to increased urinary excretion of calcium. The blood levels of calcium and phosphate are increased, and the urine contains albumin, casts, blood, and an excess of calcium. The radiographic changes include metastatic calcifications in the media of blood vessels, kidneys (especially the tubules), heart, gastric wall, alveoli of the lungs, bronchi, adrenals, and even the falx cerebri; renal ultrasound may demonstrate medullary nephrocalcinosis. In the long bones, the initial change is an increase in depth of the zones of provisional calcification, followed by cortical thickening and, later, osteoporosis with deep zones of diminished density in the ends of the shafts and, often, alternating bands of increased and diminished density (Fig. 27).

IDIOPATHIC HYPERCALCEMIA OF INFANCY AND WILLIAMS SYNDROME

Idiopathic hypercalcemia of infancy was described by Lightwood and subsequently by Fanconi and associates. In 1963, Black and Bonham-Carter associated the facial features with those described previously by Williams et al. in relation to children with supravalvular aortic stenosis. Later reports appeared to confirm and expand the clinical picture (see Section IX, Part VI, Fig. 52, page 2218). There is current support for distinguishing idiopathic hypercalcemia and Williams syndrome from an autosomal dominant form of isolated supravalvular aortic stenosis although they have several features in common. Not all are in agreement with the distinction, and some consider the Williams syndrome to be a more severe expression of the gene that causes the isolated disorder. Patients affected with Williams syndrome usually demonstrate a facial appearance that has been described as "elfin," with broad epicanthal folds, short palpebral fissures, ocular hypotelorism, a depressed nasal bridge, and a prominent upper lip with a long philtrum. Mental retardation is common. Some children are autistic and some are hyperactive, with a short attention span and poor motor coordination. Most patients have cardiac defects. In addition to aortic stenosis, peripheral pulmonary stenosis has been observed. Mild and severe forms were explained by variable expression of the trait.

Not all patients have hypercalcemia. The etiology of hypercalcemia is uncertain, but several investigators postulate hypersensitivity to the effects of vitamin D. Some patients have been reported to have excessive intestinal absorption of calcium. Many patients have hypercalciuria. There are no reports of parathyroid hypersecretion as a causative factor. Some investigators postulate that impaired secretion of calcitonin may be responsible for manifestations of the syndrome. The vitamin D metabolite profile in Williams syndrome patients reported in the literature has a variety of patterns. Many patients have normal serum 25-OHD and 1,25-(OH)2D values, except during periods of hypercalcemia, when 1,25-(OH)2D values are reduced. Elevated 1,25-OHD has also been documented in children with typical features of Williams syndrome, suggesting that hypercalcemia could result from abnormal synthesis or degradation of the active vitamin compound in affected patients.

The radiographic features in the skeleton initially are those of a generalized osteosclerosis. With time, transverse bands of both increased and diminished density develop at the ends of the shafts; and peripheral radio-lucent zones occur in the round bones and epiphyseal ossification centers (Fig. 28). The skeletal changes simulate those of vitamin D poisoning. Premature closure of cranial sutures as well as nephrocalcinosis have been observed; also reported are calcifications in the blood vessels, intermuscular septa, and other soft tissues (Fig. 29). Sonography has disclosed increased renal medullary echogenicity in 20% of children with the disease.

Several cerebral anomalies have been noted in patients with Williams syndrome. Schmidt et al. measured the area of corpus callosum using high-resolution MRI in 20 individuals with Williams syndrome (13 females and 7 males). Total midsagittal corpus callosum area was reduced, and the area of the splenium and isthmus were disproportionately reduced. There was also decreased volume of parieto-occipital lobes. Subjects with Williams

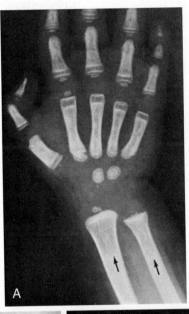

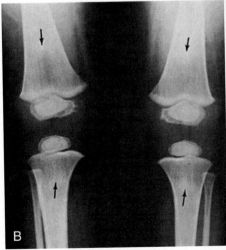

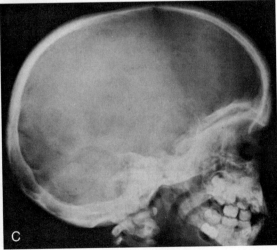

FIGURE 28. Chronic idiopathic hypercalcemia with generalized sclerosis of the skeleton and transverse bands in the metaphyses in a boy 4 years of age who had failed to grow and gain weight, with retardation of motor development; serum calcium value was 13.8 mg/100 ml when these films were made. **A,** There are deep transverse radiolucent bands in the metaphyses of the tubular bones *(arrows)* and peripheral radiolucent zones in the round bones of the wrists. **B,** Similar changes are evident in the bones at the knees, although the terminal radiolucent bands are much deeper in these larger and more rapidly growing metaphyses *(arrows).* **C,** All parts of the skull (calvarium, base, and facial segment) are sclerotic. Both renal regions were stippled with fine foci of calcium density.

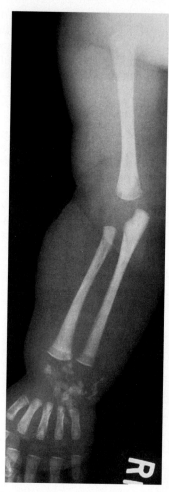

FIGURE 29. Idiopathic infantile hypercalcemia. Generalized osteosclerosis and soft tissue calcifications in the wrist are noted in an infant with Williams syndrome.

syndrome also have significantly different cerebral shape from normal controls, perhaps as a result of decreased parieto-occipital lobe volumes relative to frontal regions. Compared to controls, subjects with Williams syndrome were noted to have decreased overall brain and cerebral volumes, relative preservation of cerebellar volume, and disproportionate volume reduction of the parieto-occipital lobes and brainstem. Individuals with Williams syndrome have relative preservation of cerebral gray matter volume and disproportionate reduction in cerebral white matter volume.

Calcium homeostasis is altered in patients with Williams syndrome. Mathias reported a 4-week-old infant with Williams syndrome who presented with hypercalcemia, hypercalciuria, and medullary nephrocalcinosis. This infant was treated with a low-calcium/vitamin D–deficient infant formula that resulted in rickets. Replacement of the low-calcium/vitamin D–deficient formula with standard formula led to resolution of the rickets.

VITAMIN C POISONING

Vitamin C poisoning is believed to be a reality by Gordonoff, and the overingestion of vitamin C danger-

ous. He found guinea pigs especially prone to scurvy if they had been previously maintained on high-intake levels of vitamin C. In the siege of Leningrad, those who formerly had large intakes of vitamin C developed scurvy in greater numbers than those who had not. Repasky et al. suggest that the mobilization of calcium and phosphorus may be increased when vitamin C is given in large amounts and may contribute to the fractures observed in children with myelomeningocele who are treated with large doses of vitamin C. Because vitamin C is water soluble and excesses are excreted via the kidney, conclusive proof of adverse affects of increased intake have not been forthcoming.

HYPOPHOSPHATASIA

Hypophosphatasia (HP) is an inborn error of bone metabolism characterized by reduced serum and tissue ALP, which plays a major role in normal skeletal mineralization. The childhood and adult forms of HP represent clinical expressions of the heterozygous state for ALP deficiency. Homozygosity results in the clinically severe, autosomal recessive, infantile form. Histochemical and direct enzyme analysis of osseous tissue from 23 patients with hypophosphatasia revealed that all clinical forms of this inherited metabolic bone disease are characterized by deficiency of ALP activity in bone. In general, the severity of the clinical expression of HP reflects the magnitude of the deficiency of ALP in bone. The severe infantile form has the most profound deficiency.

Recognition of the marked clinical and radiographic variability in perinatal (lethal) HP is important for accurate genetic counseling and prenatal diagnosis. The clinical manifestations of perinatal HP include soft calvarium, large fontanelle, extremely wide cranial sutures, low-set ears, a depressed nasal bridge, funnel chest, and short and bowed distal limbs. Shohat et al. analyzed clinical and radiographic manifestations in 19 cases of perinatal HP. Three families each had two affected offsprings. All of the patients had lethal short limb dwarfism with very soft calvaria. Other clinical findings included polyhydramnios and blue sclerae. Radiographically, in addition to widened sutures and poor ossification of the skull, findings included marked variability in the amount of bone ossification; variability between patients as to which bones were most severely affected; dense, round, or flattened vertebral bodies with sagittal clefts; femoral bowing and shortening with or without metaphyseal cupping or irregularities (Fig. 30); modeling defects in the long bones; and spurs in the midportion of the ulnas and fibulas.

Girshick et al. measured bone mineral density (BMD) in 6 boys with childhood HP (ages 2 to 13 years). BMD of the total body or spine, measured by dual-energy x-ray absorptiometry, was in the lower normal range. BMD of the distal metaphyses of the radius, measured by peripheral quantitative computed tomography, was normal. However, trabecular BMD of both radius and femur was grossly elevated. Increased mineralization and sclerosis of trabecular bone might serve as a compensation for an impaired mineralization of cartilage caused by the genetic deficiency of ALP.

Lundgren et al. retrospectively analyzed dental and biochemical abnormalities in 17 Swedish children with HP. The first clinical sign of HP may be a premature loss of deciduous teeth. A case of HP presenting with prenatal bowing of long bones and spontaneous postnatal improvement of bowing and a subsequent benign course has been reported. Robinow observed a patient with hypophosphatasia from age 20 months to 21 years. Her height has followed the third percentile track. The skeletal deformities improved during early childhood, while the more striking radiographic anomalies disappeared during puberty, but her osteopenia has shown minimal improvement, indicating persistence of the basic defect in bone formation. Chodirker et al. investigated 20 carriers of infantile HP. Relative HP, decreased serum ALP activity, increased urinary phosphoethanolamine excretion and relative hyperphosphatemia were documented in all.

CONGENITAL HYPERPHOSPHATASEMIA

Chronic idiopathic hyperphosphatasemia, or juvenile Paget's disease (JPD), is a very rare syndrome character-ized by short stature, fragile bones, undertubulation of bones with coarse trabeculations, cortical thickening, periosteal new bone formation, bowing deformities, large head, widened bones of the skull, and premature loss of teeth. Increased levels of serum ALP and increased levels of urinary total hydroxyproline are notable.

Golob et al. investigated a 21-year-old white woman with mild JPD and mental retardation. Progressive bowing deformitiy of her lower limbs began at age 1½ years. Nontraumatic fractures of both femora and both tibias occurred between ages 9 and 14 years. During adulthood, cortical thickening, osteosclerosis, and bowing affected these bones. Serum ALP activity was persistently elevated. Histologic examination of the iliac crest at ages 14 and 21 years showed wide cortices and enhanced skeletal remodeling, yet the bone was exclusively lamellar. Features of classical Paget's bone disease, such as hypermultinucleated osteoclasts, peritrabecular fibrosis, and mosaic or woven bone, were absent. Six months of daily synthetic human calcitonin therapy reduced her lower limb pain, but radiographs, biochemical parameters of skeletal turnover, and bone scintigraphy were unaltered. Lamellar bone has been reported in JPD but accompanied by excessive amounts of woven bone. These findings suggest that the presence of lamellar bone without features of classical Paget's disease may characterize the skeletal histopathology of mild JPD.

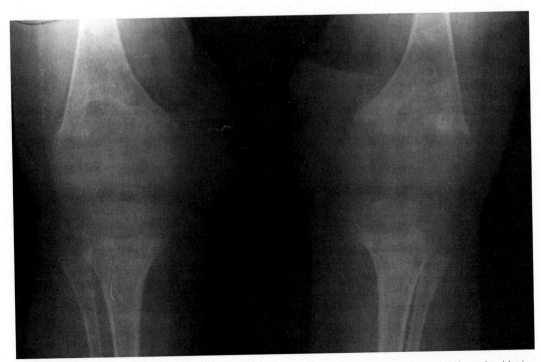

FIGURE 30. Infant with congenital hypophosphatasia. Severe decreased bone density, metaphyseal widening and irregularity. There is apparent widening of the growth plates of the distal femur and proximal tibia resembling rickets. Note the punched out areas of decreased ossification in the central portions of the distal femoral metaphyses, a characteristic finding in hypophosphatasia.

SUGGESTED READINGS

Rickets

Vitamin D–Deficiency Rickets, Renal Rickets, Anticonvulsant Rickets Vitamin D–Resistant Rickets, Fanconi's Syndrome, Vitamin D–Dependent Rickets, Congenital Rickets, Rickets of Prematurity, Rickets Among Breast-Fed Infants

Arico M, Bianchi E, Del Curto E, et al: Radiological aspects of a case of rickets during therapy with anticonvulsant agents. Radiol Med (Torino) 1984;70:996–998

Asnes RS, Berdon WE, Bassett CA: Hypophosphatemic rickets in an adolescent cured by excision of a nonossifying fibroma. Clin Pediatr 1981;20:646–648

Begum R, Coutinho ML, Dormandy TL, Yudkin S: Maternal malabsorption presenting as congenital rickets. Lancet 1968;1:1048–1052

Blond MH, Gold F, Pierre F, et al: Nutritional fetal rickets: a case report. J Gynecol Obstet Biol Reprod (Paris) 1997;26:834–836

Burnstein MI, Lawson JP, Kottamasu SR, et al: The enthesopathic changes of hypophosphatemic osteomalacia in adults: radiologic findings. AJR Am J Roentgenol 1989;153:785–790

Cartwright DW, Latham SC, Masel JP, et al: Spinal canal stenosis in adults with hypophosphataemic vitamin D-resistant rickets. Aust N Z J Med 1979;9:705–708

Evans A, Caffey J: Metaphyseal dysostosis resembling vitamin D-refractory rickets. Am J Dis Child 1958;95:640–648

Fadavi S, Fowold E: Familial hypophosphatemic vitamin D-resistant rickets: review of the literature and report of a case. ASDC J Dent Child 1990;57:212–215

Friedman AL, Trygstad CW, Chesney RW: Autosomal dominant Fanconi syndrome with early renal failure. Am J Med Genet 1978;2:225–232

Gessner BD, deSchweinitz E, Peterson KM, Lewandowski C: Nutritional rickets among breast-fed black and Alaska native children. Alaska Med 1997;39:72–74

Glorieux FH: Calcitriol treatment in vitamin D-dependent and vitamin D-resistant rickets. Metabolism 1990;39(Suppl 1):10–12

Glorieux FH: Pseudo-vitamin D deficiency rickets. J Endocrinol 1997;154:575–578

Gradus D, LeRoith D, Karplus M, Zmora E: Congenital hyperparathyroidism and rickets: secondary to maternal hypoparathyroidism and vitamin D deficiency. Isr J Med Sci 1981;17:705–708

Greer FR: Osteopenia of prematurity. Annu Rev Nutr 1994;4:169–185

Gupta PC, Patwari AK, Mullick DN: Alopecia with rickets—an endogenous unresponsiveness to 1,25 dihydroxy vitamin D_3: a case report. Indian J Med Sc 1990;44:239–245

Harrison HE: Vitamin D, the parathyroid and the kidney. Johns Hopkins Med J 1979;144:180–191

Hillman LS, Hoff N, Salmons S, et al: Mineral homeostasis in very premature infants: serial evaluation of serum 25-hydroxyvitamin D, serum minerals, and bone mineralization. J Pediatr 1985;106:970–980

Hillman LS, Hollis B, Salmons S, et al: Absorption, dosage and effect on mineral homeostasis of 25-hydroxycholecalciferol in premature infants: comparison with 400 and 800 IU vitamin D_2 supplementation. J Pediatrics 1985;106:981–989

Honasoge M, Kottamasu SR, Frame B: Hypervitaminoses, hypovitaminoses and related disorders. *In* Frame B, Honasoge M, Kottamasu SR (eds): Osteosclerosis, Hyperostosis and Related Disorders. New York, Elsevier Science Publishing Company, 1987:197–213

Hunter GJ, Schneidau A, Hunter JV, Chapman M: Rickets in adolescence. Clin Radiol 1984;35:419–421

James JR, Congdon PJ, Truscott J, et al: Osteopenia of prematurity. Arch Dis Child 1986;61:871–876

Jequier S, Cramer B, Goodyer P, et al: Renal ultrasound in metabolic bone disease. Pediatr Radiol 1986;16:135–139

Koo WW, Oestreich AE, Sherman R, et al: Radiologic case of the month: Osteopenia, rickets and fractures in preterm infants. Am J Dis Child 1985;139:1045–1046

Kottamasu SR, Honasoge M, Frame B: Osteosclerosis in disorders associated with impaired bone mineralization. *In* Frame B, Honasoge M, Kottamasu SR (eds): Osteosclerosis, Hyperostosis and Related Disorders. New York, Elsevier Science Publishing Company, 1987:146–164

Kottamasu SR, Rao DS, Meema HE, Genant HK: Radiology of metabolic bone disease. Henry Ford Hosp Med J 1983a;31:239–243

Kottamasu SR, Rao DS, Meema HE, Genant HK: Workshop on Radiology of Metabolic Bone Disease: Clinical Disorders of Bone and Mineral Metabolism. Amsterdam, Excerpta Medica, 1983b:529–535

Laing IA, Glass EJ, Hendry GMA, et al: Rickets of prematurity: calcium and phosphorus supplementation. J Pediatr 1985;106:265–268

Le May M, Blunt JW Jr: A factor determining the location of pseudofractures in osteomalacia. J Clin Invest 1949;28:521–525

Levin TL, States L, Greig A, Goldman HS: Maternal renal insufficiency: a cause of congenital rickets and secondary hyperparathyroidism. Pediatr Radiol 1992;22:315–316

Marel G, Kleerekoper M, Kottamasu SR, et al: Unusual radiographic appearance of osteomalacia in an adolescent. *In* Norman AW (ed): Vitamin D—Chemical, Biochemical and Clinical Endocrinology of Calcium Metabolism. New York, Walter de Gruyter and Company, 1982:111–185

Mason RS, Rohl PG, Lissner D, Posen S: Vitamin D metabolism in hypophosphatemic rickets. Am J Dis Child 1982;136:909–913

Meema HE, Oreopoulos DG, Rabinovich S, et al: Periosteal new bone formation (periosteal neostosis) in renal osteodystrophy. Radiology 1974;110:513–522

Minamitani K, Minagawa M, Yasuda T, Nimi H: Early detection of infants with hypophosphatemic vitamin D resistant rickets. Endocr J 1996;43:339–343

Moncrieff M, Fadahunsi T: Congenital rickets due to maternal vitamin D deficiency. Arch Dis Child 1974;49:810–811

Moser CR, Fessel WJ: Rheumatic manifestations of hypophosphatemia. Arch Intern Med 1974;134:674–678

Ozsoylu S, Gurgey A, Coskun T: Congenital rickets. Eur J Pediatr 1995;154:915–918

Polisson RP, Marinez S, Khoury M, et al: Calcification of entheses associated with X-linked hypophosphatemic osteomalacia. N Engl J Med 1985;313:1–6

Rosen JF, Fleishman AR, Feinberg L, et al: Rickets with alopecia: an inborn error of vitamin D metabolism. J Pediatr 1979;94:729–735

Ryan S: Nutritional aspects of metabolic bone disease in the newborn. Arch Dis Child 1996;74:F145–F148

Saul PD, Lloyd DJ, Smith FW: The role of bone scanning in neonatal rickets. Pediatr Radiol 1983;13:89–91

Sebes JI, Rothschild BM: Rickets due to chronic anticonvulsant therapy. Ill Med J 1981;160:28–30

Sills IN, Skuza KA, Horlick MN, et al: Vitamin D deficiency rickets: reports of its demise are exaggerated. Clin Pediatr (Phila) 1994;33:491–493

Steinbach HL, Kolb FO, Gilfillon A: A mechanism of the production of pseudofractures in osteomalacia (Milkman's syndrome). Radiology 1954;62:388–395

Teotia M, Teotia SP, Nath M: Metabolic studies in congenital vitamin D deficiency rickets. Indian J Pediatr 1995;62:55–61

Tsuchiya Y, Matsuo N, Cho H, et al: An unusual form of vitamin D-dependent rickets in a child: alopecia and marked end-organ hyposensitivity to biologically active vitamin D. J Clin Endocrinol Metab 1980;51:685–690

Verge CF, Lam A, Simpson JM, et al: Effects of therapy in x-linked hypophosphatemic rickets. N Engl J Med 1991;325:1843–1848

Vohra P: Metaphyseal chondrodysplasia—a differential diagnosis of rickets. Indian J Pediatr 1996;63:127–128

Walters AG, Murphy JF, Henry P, et al: Plasma alkaline phosphatase activity and its relation to rickets in pre-term infants. Ann Clin Biochem 1986;23:653–656

Wang DC, Kottamasu SR, Karvelis KC: Scintigraphy in metabolic bone disease. *In* Favus MJ (ed): Primer on the Metabolic Bone Diseases and Disorders of Mineral Metabolism, 3rd ed. Philadelphia, Lippincott–Raven, 1996:142–151

Wang LY, Hung HY, Hsu CH, et al: Congenital rickets—a patient report. J Pediatr Endocrinol Metab 1997;10:437–441

Weinstein RS, Sappington LJ: Qualitative bone defect in uremic osteosclerosis. Metabolism 1982;31:805–811

Weisman Y, Hochberg Z: Genetic rickets and osteomalacia. Curr Ther Endocrinol Metab 1994;5:527–529

Wilson DM: Growth hormone and hypophosphatemic rickets. J Pediatr Endocrinol Metab 2000;13(Suppl 2):993–998

Yamamoto T: Diagnosis of X-linked hypophosphatemic vitamin D resistant ricket. Acta Paediatr Jpn 1997;39:499–502

Young LW, Forbes GB, Borgstedt AD, et al: "Antiepileptic therapy" rickets: roentgenologic implications. Ann Radiol 1974;17:375–383

Young W, Sevcik M, Tallroth K: Metaphyseal sclerosis in patients with chronic renal failure. Skeletal Radiol 1991;20:197–200

Zeidan S, Bamford M: Congenital rickets with maternal pre-eclampsia. J R Soc Med 1984;77:426–427

Oncogenic Rickets and Osteomalacia

Avila NA, Skarulis M, Rubino DM, Doppman JL: Oncogenic osteomalacia—lesion detection by MR skeletal survey. AJR Am J Roentgenol 1996;167:343–345

Crockard I-IA: Oncogenic osteomalacia associated with a meningeal phosphaturic mesenchymal tumor—case report. J Neurosurg 1996; 84:288–292

Drezner D, Revesz T, Path MRC, et al: The pathogenesis and treatment of tumor-induced osteomalacia. *In* Norman AW, Schaefer K, Herrath DV, Grigoleit HG (eds): Vitamin D: Chemical, Biochemical and Clinical Endocrinology of Calcium Metabolism. Berlin, Walter de Gruyter & Co., 1982:949–954

Drezner MK: Tumor-induced rickets and osteomalacia. *In* Favus M (ed): Primer on the Metabolic Bone Diseases and Disorders of Mineral Metabolism. New York, Raven Press, 1996:319–325

Econs MJ, Drezner MK: Tumor-induced osteomalacia—unveiling a new hormone [editorial; comment]. N Engl J Med 1994;330: 1679–1681

Eyskens B, Proesmans W, Vandamme B, et al: Tumour-induced rickets—a case report and review of the literature [review]. Eur J Pediatr 1995;154:462–468

Gonzalez-Compta X, Manos-Pujol M, Foglia-Fernandez M, et al: Oncogenic osteomalacia: case report and review of head and neck associated tumors. J Audiol Otol 1998;112:389–392

Harvey IN, Gray C, Belchetz PE: Oncogenous osteomalacia and malignancy. Clin Endocrinol 1992;37:379–382

Lee HK, Sung WW, Solodnik P, Shimshi M: Bone scan in tumor-induced osteomalacia. J Nucl Med 1995;36:247–249

McClure J, Smith PS: Oncogenic osteomalacia. J Clin Pathol 1987;40: 446–453

Miyauchi A, Fukase M, Tsutsumi M, Fujita T: Hemangiopericytoma-induced osteomalacia: tumor transplantation in nude mice causes hypophosphatemia and tumor extracts inhibit renal 25-hydroxyvitamin D 1-hydroxylase activity. J Clin Endocrinol Metab 1988;67:46–53

Nelson AE, Robinson BG, Mason RS: Oncogenic osteomalacia: is there a new phosphate regulating hormone? Clin Endocrinol 1997;47: 635–642

Nuovo MA, Dorfman HD, Sun CC, et al: Tumor-induced osteomalacia and rickets. Am J Surg Pathol 1989;13:588–599

Olivares JL, Ramos FJ, Carapeto FJ, Bueno M: Epidermal naevus syndrome and hypophosphataemic rickets: description of a patient with central nervous system anomalies and review of the literature. Eur J Pediatr 1999;158:103–107

Renton P, Shaw DG: Hypophosphatemic osteomalacia secondary to vascular tumors of bone and soft tissue. Skeletal Radiol 1976;1:21–24

Rowe PSN: Molecular biology of hypophosphataemic rickets and oncogenic osteomalacia. Hum Genet 1994;94:457–467

Ryan EA, Reiss E: Oncogenous osteomalacia: review of the world literature of 42 cases and report of two new cases. Am J Med 1984;77:501–512

Schapira D, Benizhak O, Nachtigal A, et al: Tumor-induced osteomalacia. Semin Arthritis Rheum 1995;25:35–46

Seshadri MS, Cornish CJ, Mason RS, Posen S: Parathyroid hormone-like bioactivity in tumours from patients with oncogenic osteomalacia. Clin Endocrinol 1985;23:689–697

Tanaka T, Suwa S: A case of McCune-Albright syndrome with hyperthyroidism, and vitamin D-resistant rickets. Helv Paediatr Acta 1977;32:263–273

Tokatli A, Ccoskun T, Ozalp I: Hypophosphatemic vitamin-D resistant rickets associated with epidermal nevus syndrome. Turk J Pediatr 1997;39:247–251

Weidner N, Santa Cruz D: Phosphaturic mesenchymal tumors: a polymorphous group causing osteomalacia or rickets. Cancer 1987;59:1442–1454

Weiss D, Bar RS, Weidner N, et al: Oncogenic osteomalacia: strange tumours in strange places. Postgrad Med J 1985;61:349–355

Wilkins GE, Granleese S, Hegele RG, et al: Oncogenic osteomalacia: evidence for a humoral phosphaturic factor. J Clin Endocrinol Metab 1995;80:1628–1634

Yoshikawa S, Nakamura T, Michito T, et al: Benign osteoblastoma as a cause of osteomalacia: a report of 2 cases. J Bone Joint Surg Br 1977;59:279–286

Rickets in Osteopetrosis

Datta V, Prajapati NC, Kamble M, Pathak S: Osteopetrorickets. Indian Pediatr 2000;37:98–99

Di Rocco M, Buoncompagni A, Loy A, Dellacqua A: Osteopetrorickets: case report. Eur J Pediatr 2000;159:579–581

Donnelly LF, Johnson JF 3rd, Benzing G: Infantile osteopetrosis complicated by rickets. AJR Am J Roentgenol 1995;164:968–970

Kaplan FS, August CS, Fallon MD, et al: Osteopetrorickets: the paradox of plenty. Pathophysiology and treatment. Clin Orthop 1993;294:64–78

Milhaud G, Labat ML, Litwin I, et al: Osteopetro-rickets: a new congenital bone disorder. Metab Bone Dis Relat Res 1981;3:91–97

Oliveira G, Boechat MI, Amaral SM, Young LW: Osteopetrosis and rickets: an intriguing association. Am J Dis Child 1986;140:377–378

Ozdirim E, Altay C, Pirnar T: Osteopetrosis with rickets in infancy. Turk J Pediatr 1981;23:211–218

Ozsoylu S: Malignant osteopetrosis with rickets. Eur J Pediatr 2000; 159:412–415

Metabolic Bone Disease in Aluminum Toxicity

Andreoli SP, Smith JA, Bergstein JM: Aluminum bone disease in children: radiographic features from diagnosis to resolution. Radiology 1985;156:663–667

Chesney RW: A new form of rickets during infancy: phosphate depletion-induced osteopenia due to antacid ingestion. Arch Pediatr Adolesc Med 1998;152:1243–1245

Pivnick EK, Kerr NC, Kaufman RA, et al: Rickets secondary to phosphate depletion: a sequela of antacid use in infancy. Clin Pediatr (Phila) 1995;34:73–78

Salusky IB, Coburn JW, Paunier L, et al: Role of aluminum hydroxide in raising serum aluminum levels in children undergoing continuous ambulatory peritoneal dialysis. J Pediatr 1984;105:717–720

Sedman A: Aluminum toxicity in childhood. Pediatr Nephrol 1992;6: 383–393

Scurvy

Allen JI, Naas PL, Pern RT: Scurvy: bilateral lower extremity ecchymoses and paraparesis. Ann Emerg Med 1982;11:446–448

Allue Bellosta L, Vives Vila P, Grau Bartomeu J, Pevn Rev J: Scurvy: a diagnosis that should be remembered. Rev Clin Esp 1990;187: 431–432

Bhat BV, Srinivasan S: Neonatal scurvy. Indian Pediatr 1989;26: 1258–1260

Boeve WJ, Martijn A: Case report 406: scurvy. Skeletal Radiol 1987;16:67–69

Boulinguez S, Bouyssou-Gauthier M, De Vencay P, et al: Scurvy presenting with ecchymotic purpura and hemorrhagic ulcers of the lower limbs. Ann Dermatol Venereol 2000;127:510–512

Campistol Plana J, Pou Fernandez J, Rissech Payret M, et al: Scurvey: presentation of six cases. An Esp Pediatr 1979;12:745–752

Faber-Niiholt R, van Loon JK: Scurvy in a Dutch child. Ned Tijdschr Geneeskd 1986;130:2351–2353

Fain O, Mathieu E, Thomas M: Scurvy in patients with cancer. BMJ 1998;316:1661–1662

Gomez-Carrasco JA, Lopez-Herce Cid J, Bernabe de Frutos C, et al: Scurvy in adolescence. J Pediatr Gastroenterol Nutr 1994;19: 118–120

Grewar O: Infantile scurvy. Clin Pediatr 1965;4:82–89

Haraguchi G, Yamada S, Tanaka M, et al: A case of scurvy rarely encountered in Japan. Vasc Med 1997;2:143–146

Hess AF: Scurvy, Past and Present. Philadelphia, JB Lippincott, 1920

Maroscia D, Negrini AP, Salsano G, Merola S: Scurvy: a disease that has not yet disappeared. [Apropos a case]. Radiol Med (Torino) 1992;83:462–464

McKenna KE, Dawson JF: Scurvy occurring in a teenager. Clin Exp Dermatol 1993;18:75–77

Oeffinger KC: Scurvy: more than historical relevance [review]. Am Fam Physician 1993;48:609–613

Onorato J, Lynfield Y: Scurvy. Cutis 1992;49:321–322

Park EA, Guild HG, Jackson D: Recognition of scurvy with especial reference to early x-ray changes. Arch Dis Child 1935;10:265–294

Paul DK, Lahiri M, Garai TB, Chatterjee MK: Scurvy persists in the current era. Indian Pediatr 1999;36:1067

Ruffa G, Cottafava F, Bonioli E, et al: Confirmed scurvy in childhood: two more cases. Minerva Pediatr 1983;35:885–889

Schwartz AM, Leonidas JC: Methotrexate osteopathy. Skeletal Radiol 1984;11:13–16

Silverman FN: Recovery from epiphyseal invagination: sequel to an unusual complication of scurvy. J Bone Joint Surg Am 1970;52:384–390

Sprague PL: Epiphyseo-metaphyseal cupping following infantile scurvy. Pediatr Radiol 1976;4:122–123

Sthoeger ZM, Sthoeger D: Scurvy from self-imposed diet. Harefuah 1991;120:332–333

Hypervitaminoses

Vitamin A Poisoning

Caffey J: Chronic poisoning due to excess of vitamin A. Am J Roentgenol Radium Ther 1951;65:12–26

Knudson AG Jr, Rothman PE: Hypervitaminosis A: a review with discussion of vitamin A. Am J Dis Child 1953;85:316–334

Miller JH, Hayon II: Bone scintigraphy in hypervitaminosis A. AJR Am J Roentgenol 1985;144:767–768

Morrice G Jr, Havener WH, Kapetansky F: Vitamin A intoxication as a cause of pseudotumor cerebri. JAMA 1960;173:1802–1805

Pease CN: Focal retardation and arrestment of growth of bones due to vitamin A intoxication. JAMA 1962;182:980–985

Pickup JD: Hypervitaminosis A. Arch Dis Child 1956;31:229–232

Rosa FW, Wilk AL, Kelsey FO: Environmentally induced birth defect risks. In Sever JL, Brent AL (eds): Teratogen Update: Environmentally Induced Birth Defect Risks. New York, Alan R Liss, 1986:61–70

Toomey JA, Morissette RA: Hypervitaminosis A. Am J Dis Child 1947;73:473–480

Woodward WK, Miller U, Legant O: Acute and chronic hypervitaminosis in a 4-month-old infant. J Pediatr 1961;59:260–264

Vitamin D Poisoning, Idiopathic Hypercalcemia of Infancy, and Williams Syndrome

Aarskog D, Akanes L, Markistad T: Vitamin D metabolism in idiopathic infantile hypercalcemia. Am J Dis Child 1981;135:1021–1024

Besbas N, Oner A, Akhan O, et al: Nephrocalcinosis due to vitamin D intoxication. Turk J Pediatr 1989;31:239–244

Black JA, Bonham-Carter RE: Association between aortic stenosis and facies of severe infantile hypercalcemia. Lancet 1963;2:745–749

Fanconi G, Girdardet P, Schlesinger B, et al: Cronische Hypercalcämie, kombiniert mit Osteosklerose, Hyperazotämie, Minderwuchs, und congenitalen Missbildungen. Helv Paediatr Acta 1952;7:314–347

Fraser D, Kidd BSL, Kooh SW, et al: A new look at infantile hypercalcemia. Pediatr Clin North Am 1966;13:503–525

Garabedian M, Jacqz E, Guillozo H, et at: Elevated plasma 1,25-dihydroxyvitamin D concentrations in infants with hypercalcemia and elfin facies. N Engl J Med 1985;312:948–952

Greenberg F: Williams syndrome. Pediatrics 1989;84:922–923

Jernigan IL, Bellugi U: Anomalous brain morphology on magnetic resonance images in Williams syndrome and Down syndrome. Arch Neurol 1990;47:29–33

Lightwood A: Idiopathic hypercalcemia in infants with failure to thrive. Arch Dis Child 1932;27:302–303

Mathias RS: Rickets in an infant with Williams syndrome. Pediatr Nephrol 2000;14:489–492

Schmidt MA, Ensing GJ, Michels VV, et al: Autosomal dominant supravalvular aortic stenosis: large three-generation family. Am J Med Genet 1989;32:384–389

Williams JCP, Barratt-Boyes BG, Lowe JB: Supravalvular aortic stenosis. Circulation 1961;24:1311–1318

Vitamin C Poisoning

Gordonoff T: Sur Ia vitaminothérapie abusive: essais avec Ia vitamine C. Therapie 1960;15:623–628

Pauling L, Moertel C: A proposition: megadoses of vitamin C are valuable in the treatment of cancer. Nutr Rev 1986;44:28–32

Repasky I, Rickard K, Lindseth A: Ascorbic acid and fractures in children with myelomeningocele. J Am Diet Assoc 1976;69:511–513

Hypophosphatasia

Chodirker BN, Evans JA, Seargeant LE, et al: Hyperphosphatemia in infantile hypophosphatasia. Am J Hum Genet 1990;46:280–285

Currarino G: Hypophosphatasia. Prog Pediat Radiol 1973;4:469–494

Fraser D: Hypophosphatasia. Am J Med 1957;22:730–746

Girshick et al: Treatment of childhood hypophosphatasia with nonsteroidal antiinflammatory drugs. Bone 1999;25:603–607

Kousseff BG, Mulivor RA: Prenatal diagnosis of hypophosphatasia. Obstet Gynecol 1981;57(Suppl 6):9S–12S

Kozlowski K, Sutcliffe J, Barylak A, et al: Hypophosphatasia: review of 24 cases. Pediatr Radiol 1976;5:103–117

Lundgren T, Westphal O, Bolme P, et al: Retrospective study of children with hypophosphatasia with reference to dental changes. Scand J Dent Res 1991;99:357–364

Mulivor RA, Mennuti M, Zackai EH, et al: Prenatal diagnosis of hypophosphatasia: genetic, biochemical and clinical studies. Am J Hum Genet 1978;30:271–281

Oestreich AE, Bofinger MS: Prominent transverse (Bowdler) bone spurs as a diagnostic clue in a case of neonatal hypophosphatasia without metaphyseal irregularity. Pedratr Radiol 1989;19:341–342

Robinow M: Twenty-year follow-up of a case of hypophosphatasia. Birth Defects 1971;7:86–93

Scriver C, Cameron P: Pseudohypophosphatasia. N Engl J Med 1969;281:604–606

Shohat M, Rimoin DL, Gruber HE, Lachman RS: Perinatal lethal hypophosphatasia; clinical, radiologic and morphologic findings. Pediatr Radiol 1991;21:421–427

Silver MM, Vilos GA, Milne KJ: Pulmonary hypoplasia in neonatal hypophosphatasia. Pediatr Pathol 1988;8:483–493

Sumner TE, Volberg FM, Kerstaedt N, et al: Hypophosphatasia and nephrocalcinosis demonstrated by ultrasound and CT. Clin Nephrol 1984;22:317–319

van Dongen PW, Hamel BC, Nijhuis JG, et al: Prenatal follow-up of hypophosphatasia by ultrasound: case report. Eur J Obstet Gynecol Reprod Biol 1990;34:293–299

Congenital Hyperphosphatasia (Juvenile Paget's Disease)

Eroglu M, Taneli NN: Congenital hyperphosphatasia (juvenile Paget's disease): eleven years follow-up of three sisters. Ann Radiol (Paris) 1977;20:145–150

Golob DS, McAlister WH, Mills BG, et al: Juvenile Paget disease: life-long features of a mildly affected young woman. J Bone Miner Res 1996;11:1041

Jett S, Frost HM: Tetracycline-based measurements of the bone dynamics in the rib of a girl with hyperphosphatasia. Henry Ford Hosp Med J 1968;16:325–338

Thompson RC Jr, Gaull GE, Horwitz SJ, Schenk RK: Hereditary hyperphosphatasia: studies of three siblings. Am J Med 1969;47:209–219

PART VIII

TRAUMA TO THE GROWING SKELETON

H. THEODORE HARCKE
GERALD A. MANDELL
BRADLEY A. MAXFIELD

FRACTURES AND FRACTURE HEALING

Fractures in children's bones generally result from abnormal stresses in normal bone or normal stresses in abnormal bone. They differ from fractures in adults because there is more elasticity to bone and the process of growth is active, especially in otherwise healthy children; this favors rapid repair and remodeling. Growth, however, may be compromised if the injury adversely affects the growth cartilage that is responsible for endochondral ossification. This can result in overgrowth, undergrowth, and/or progressive angular deformity. However, children's fractures are also "forgiving" to those providing treatment. The potential correction is greater if the child is younger because the fracture site is closer to the physis, and there is usually presentation of alignment in the normal plane of motion of the joint. Rotational deformities do not correct spontaneously. Remodeling may be expected in children with 2 or more years of skeletal growth; however, every effort should be made to obtain as much anatomic reduction as possible. Films of a fractured bone should show the relative orientation of the two ends to evaluate rotation.

IMAGING TECHNIQUES

Plain radiographs in orthogonal views are the standard first imaging technique. Oblique and special views depend on location and injured structure. Contralateral views of the unaffected side can be obtained for paired structures to distinguish developmental changes from pathologic ones. Developmental variations that simulate pathology are discussed in Section IX, Part III, Chapter 2, page 2053.

Scintigraphy has traditionally been utilized to detect occult skeletal trauma when radiographs are normal. Pathologic alterations of the skeleton can be detected within 24 to 48 hours after the initiating event. One disadvantage of bone scintigraphy is its lack of specificity.

Use of cross-sectional imaging with computed tomography (CT) and magnetic resonance imaging (MRI) has progressively increased in cases of musculoskeletal trauma. CT is employed to optimize the delineation of fracture fragments and their relationships. MRI defines nonosseous trauma, particularly to cartilage and ligaments.

Growing use of ultrasound in musculoskeletal trauma is focused on specific instances in which visualization of cartilage, muscle, and tendons is desired to augment radiographic findings. When the operator has suitable experience and skill, ultrasound has been found to be very effective for several pediatric trauma applications.

MECHANISMS OF FRACTURE

During parturition, and most frequently in breech deliveries, fractures and dislocations can occur. The most common obstetric fractures are those in the skull and clavicles. Femur fractures have been observed with cesarean section. During the first postnatal year, fractures are relatively rare; their occurrence warrants exclusion of child abuse. Most willful assaults on children occur during the first 2 years of life and are included in the battered-child syndrome, in which radiographic examination of the skeleton often offers the first diagnostic lead. After age 2, the radius is the most commonly fractured single large bone; fractures of the phalanges and metacarpals also are common. "Toddler's fracture" of the distal half of the tibia is

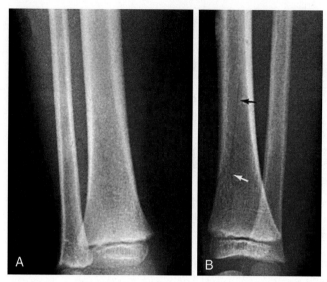

FIGURE 1. Toddler's fracture in a boy, 4½ years of age, who had refused to walk or bear weight on the right foot after twisting the right leg 24 hours before. **A,** In frontal projection, the findings are normal. **B,** In lateral projection, there is a long oblique hairline fracture *(arrows)* in the distal third of the tibial shaft. Such fractures are easily missed radiographically, and oblique views should be obtained when clinical evidence suggests toddler's fracture.

common during the period between the second and fifth years (Fig. 1). The incidence of fractures increases until adolescence, many of them involving sports participation. At all ages, the most severe skeletal injuries to children result from vehicular accidents.

Fatigue stress fractures occur in children as in adults as a result of excessive, repetitive muscle forces acting across the affected bone. They present with persistent, focal, activity-related pain. Among young athletes, girls are affected almost as frequently as boys. The tibia is most frequently affected, with the majority of its lesions in the upper third. Fibulas and metatarsal bones are next in frequency. Initially, there may be no radiographic changes, but, with healing (usually after rest), local sclerosis or subperiosteal new bone, or both, may be noted (Fig. 2). In compact bone, a linear radiolucency may be noted; focal sclerosis is the usual initial sign in cancellous bone. Bone scans are usually positive before radiographic changes are visible. Stress (insufficiency) fractures also occur in abnormal bone under normal activity, as in rickets.

Plastic bowing fractures occur in tubular bones that have an inherent curve and are subjected to compression forces (Fig. 3). The increased curvature is a form of greenstick fracture in which microfractures are present on the concave side without disruption on the convex side, so that the deformity becomes fixed. With continued growth at the ends of the bone, the curve may become exaggerated to the point of interfering with function. Conversion of the incomplete fracture to a complete one, as in some greenstick fractures, may be necessary to permit satisfactory alignment for healing.

FRACTURE HEALING

Children experience more rapid healing of fractures than adults, with younger children showing faster bone union than older ones. Healing time is also related to the fracture location, with physeal and metaphyseal fractures healing faster than diaphyseal fractures. The mechanism of healing in a simple fracture is illustrated

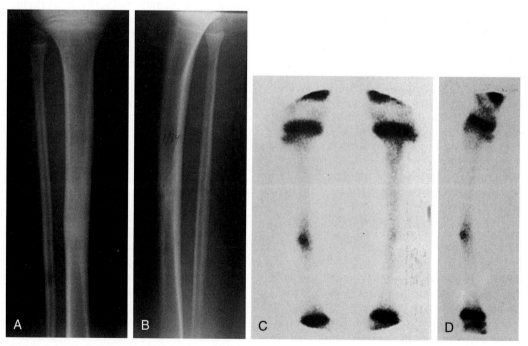

FIGURE 2. Stress fracture of tibia. **A,** Anteroposterior projection demonstrates sclerosis and slight periosteal reaction. **B,** Lateral projection shows a defect in the anterior cortex at the level of the reactive sclerosis. The fracture is also evident on coronal **(C)** and lateral **(D)** scintigrams.

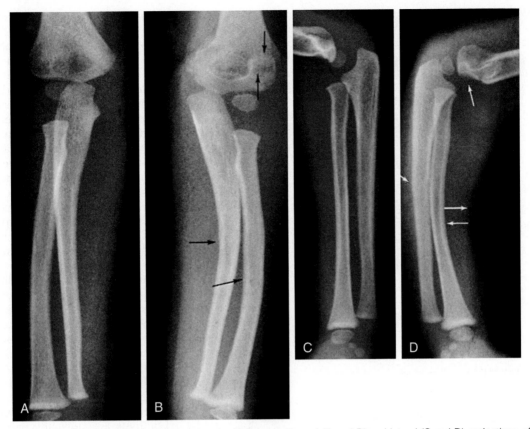

FIGURE 3. A 3-year-old child fell on the outstretched left hand. Frontal (**A** and **B**) and lateral (**C** and **D**) projections of the elbows and forearms show traumatic bowings of the left radial shaft in lateral and dorsal directions (**B** and **D**). The left ulnar shaft is broken in the lateral direction only (**B**). The left humeral shaft is broken transversely at a supracondylar level (**B** and **D**). There is no radiographic evidence of either fractures or microfractures in the bowed left radius or ulna.

in Figure 4. When a fracture occurs in a tubular bone, disruption occurs in both the bone and its periosteum and is usually accompanied by damage of adjacent muscle and numerous blood vessels. The periosteum in children is more durable and usually sustains less damage, with more remaining intact. A hematoma is formed between the broken ends of the bone, assuming they are not widely separated, and extends out into the surrounding soft tissues. Clotting of the hematoma incorporates dead bone that has lost its blood supply, necrotic marrow, and damaged muscle cells. An inflammatory response occurs locally because of the necrotic material, and hyperemia of the entire area develops. The hematoma begins to organize; stem cells from the periosteum, endosteum, marrow, and haversian systems form osteoblasts and chondroblasts with the good blood flow and increased cellular activity of childhood. Rapid ingrowth of capillary buds occurs, mainly from periosteal vessels. Osteoid and chondroid material formed by the specialized cells gradually envelops the bone ends, stabilizing the fracture. Cartilage and, slightly later, primary woven bone develop (callus). Subsequently, the primary bone remodels, adapting to the pressure and tension forces exerted on it by muscular activity and gravity stresses. Excess callus is removed and replaced with new bone that can ultimately blend almost imperceptibly with the uninjured portion. Capacity to remodel depends on longitudinal growth

potential. Consequently, remodeling is maximal in younger patients and in the end of a bone, which contributes most to its length.

Besides growth plate damage (discussed below under Injuries to the Cartilage Plate), complications of fracture include vascular and other soft tissue injuries during the trauma and delayed union, malunion, or nonunion afterward. Infection is a frequent cause of malunion. Pseudarthroses rarely develop unless there is gross failure of immobilization or underlying dysplasia of bone, particularly neurofibromatosis. Severe secondary deformities may follow injury to the blood supply of growing bone when the bone itself is not injured.

INJURIES TO THE CARTILAGE PLATE

The Salter and Harris classification of epiphyseal injuries has provided a useful radiographic and prognostic approach to their identification and management (Fig. 5). The zone of calcified cartilage and its subjacent, newly formed bone are apparently the weak points when growing bones are subjected to combined tension and shearing forces. A line of discontinuity develops and is propagated through one or the other, or both, often in an irregular fashion. Periosteal attachments to the epiphysis may or may not be disrupted, but the proliferating growth cartilage remains with the separated epiphysis and is most susceptible to damage if a fracture line extends through it, as in types III and IV, or if there is crush injury, as postulated for type V. It should also be noted that types III and IV fractures are intra-articular, and prognosis relates to the ability to restore anatomic alignment. Orthopedic surgeons add a type VI fracture (described by Rang), which is damage to the

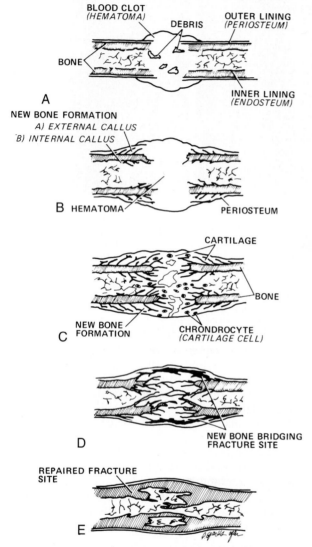

FIGURE 4. Stages in healing of a fracture. **A,** Hematoma under the periosteum surrounding the fracture, communicating through the fracture with blood clot within the medullary cavity. **B,** Subperiosteal and endosteal cellular proliferation encroaching on the hematoma. Islands of cartilage may be present. Bone at the margins of the fracture has been devitalized. **C,** Callus formation from osteoblastic cells in the proliferating cellular masses. The intercellular substance produced becomes calcified to form woven bone. The dead bone at the margins of the fracture undergoes resorption. **D,** Replacement of woven bone by lamellar bone with bony continuity across the fractured area. **E,** Remodeling. Cortical bone is organized to conform to the cortex. Resorption of excess bone results in recanalization of the medullary cavity. (From Bleck EE, Nagel DA: Physically Handicapped Children. New York, Grune & Stratton, 1982, with permission.)

peripheral perichondrial ring at the margin of the physis.

As a result of physeal damage, growth plate arrest can occur. Early closure results in a bridge of bone joining the metaphysis and epiphysis. The effect of this bridge or bony bar depends on location, extent, and how much growth remains. Even a partial closure can inhibit growth across the plate by creating a tethering effect. Peripheral bars produce angular deformity. A central bar induces cupping of the metaphysis and central epiphyseal invagination. Beside direct injury of the cartilage, there are other conditions that result in vascular injury in the terminal vessels that supply the proliferating cartilage and may not be recognized until long after the original insult (Fig. 6). Cupping occurs because the central segment of the bone grows slower longitudinally than its peripheral segment or fuses earlier and ceases growing entirely. The epiphyseal center often undergoes compensatory changes and becomes cone shaped or horseshoe shaped. Vascular injury from catheterization has caused cupping, as have infections, vitamin A poisoning, and, very rarely, epiphyseal separation in scurvy. Severe cupping has followed vascular injury in meningococcemia.

Partial growth arrest is not usually apparent radiographically for 3 to 6 months after injury. An early sign is asymmetric migration of growth recovery lines (also called growth arrest or Harris lines). These sclerotic lines in the metaphysis are normally parallel to the physis. Obliquity, slow migration, and absence can be indicative of growth disturbance.

Bone scintigraphy is an excellent indicator of physiologic growth plate activity after fractures have healed. A band of increased tracer activity is evident in active physes on both tissue-phase (blood pool) and delayed bone images. Growth plate disturbances are reflected scintigraphically by decreased uptake when plates are inactive and closing (Fig. 7). Occasionally, plates can be stimulated by healing of adjacent fractures; in such cases, plate activity increases over normal and overgrowth occurs.

To anatomically delineate the presence and extent of physeal bar formation, linear tomography and CT have been utilized to "map" the growth plate. Sagittal and coronal plane sections (acquired or reconstructed) are used. MRI is now also used to assess growth plate closure. Pulse sequences that enhance cartilage make it possible to see defects and identify localized growth disturbances (invaginations into the adjacent metaphysis). Physeal bars can be mapped in the same manner as with CT (Fig. 8).

There are many treatment options for partial growth plate damage. These depend on location, size, and patient age. More than 50% of a plate must be undamaged for bar resection to be considered. Even after successful resection, full growth potential may not be restored.

EPIPHYSEAL SEPARATIONS

Epiphyseal separations of the major long bones, comparable to Salter-Harris fractures, may occur in the new-

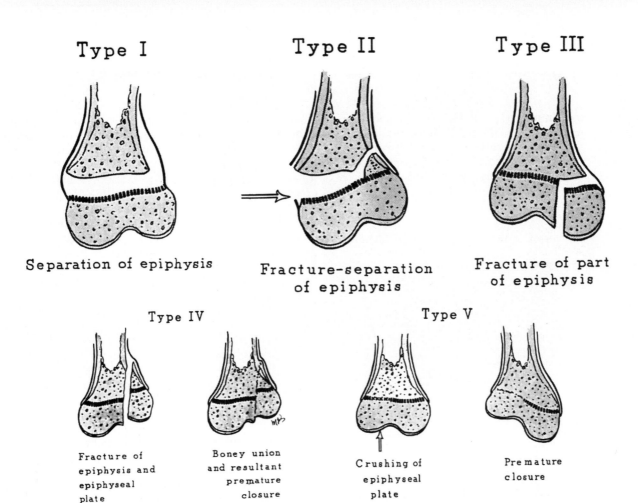

Type I

Separation of epiphysis

Type II

Fracture-separation
of epiphysis

Type III

Fracture of part
of epiphysis

Type IV

Fracture of
epiphysis and
epiphyseal
plate

Boney union
and resultant
premature
closure

Type V

Crushing of
epiphyseal
plate

Premature
closure

FIGURE 5. Injuries to the cartilage plate classified according to Salter and Harris. **Type I,** Complete transverse laceration of the cartilage plate with longitudinal distraction and some transverse displacement of the epiphysis. The bone itself is not broken. **Type II,** Incomplete transverse laceration of the cartilage through a variable distance is associated with an oblique fracture of the contiguous shaft with a triangular tag of shaft attached to the displaced epiphysis. The prognosis is good. **Type III,** Short incomplete transverse laceration of the cartilage plate with a longitudinal fracture extending through the epiphyseal ossification center toward the joint. This usually occurs in cartilage plates of the tibia. The prognosis is bad if the epiphyseal fracture is not reduced with smooth joint surfaces. **Type IV,** Oblique longitudinal fracture extending from the articular cartilage through the epiphyseal ossification center, across the cartilage plate, and through a short segment of the metaphysis through the cortical wall. This type is most frequently seen at the lateral condyle of the humerus. Perfect reduction is essential for a good prognosis. **Type V,** Segmental crushing of the cartilage plate, often followed by closure of the plate prematurely and stoppage of growth. (From Salter RE, Harris WR: Injuries involving the epiphyseal plate. J Bone Joint Surg Am 1963;45:587–622, with permission.)

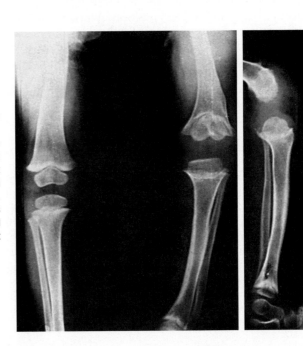

FIGURE 6. Traumatic epiphyseal cupping of the knees and shanks in frontal **(left)** and lateral **(right)** projections. This girl, 18 months of age, had multiple fractures of both femurs and the left tibia at 5 months of age when abused and beaten by her mother. Residual metaphyseal cupping is present in both bones at the left knee and at the distal end of the left tibia. At the left knee, the femur and tibia are shortened and splayed and the joint space is deepened. In the femur and proximal end of the tibia, the epiphyseal ossification centers are enlarged and the cartilage plates are thinner and appear to be fusing with their shafts in the central segments of the cupped cartilaginous plate. The deformities are greatest at the distal end of the femur and least at the distal end of the tibia.

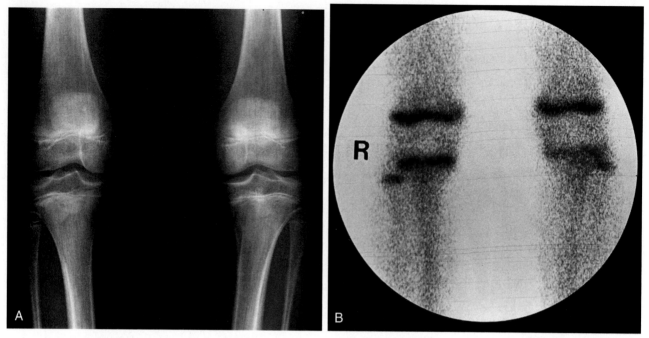

FIGURE 7. Post-traumatic partial growth plate arrest in a 13-year-old boy. **A,** Anteroposterior views of the knees show a healing proximal left tibial fracture. The growth plate appears open. **B,** Anterior tissue-phase (blood pool) bone scan shows decreased uptake in the proximal left tibial physis, indicating it is closing medially.

born as a result of birth trauma. In the absence of secondary ossification centers, the separations are difficult to diagnose radiographically. Ultrasound has been used (Fig. 9).

"BASEBALL FINGER"

The so-called baseball finger (Fig. 10) results from sudden flexion of the distal interphalangeal joint when the common extensor tendon is under tension. The fragment of the epiphysis and shaft is avulsed and pulled back by unopposed action of this tendon as the flexor tendon on the volar surface pulls the distal phalanx into the "dropped finger" position. Avulsions of bone and cartilage from margins of other epiphyses may occur. The attached bony fragment, separated from its blood supply, may become sclerotic. In epiphysis-equivalent regions such as in the pelvis, scapulas, and spinous processes of vertebrae, avulsions may also occur (Fig. 11).

OSGOOD-SCHLATTER DISEASE

Osgood-Schlatter disease is probably the best-known form of avulsion injury, although previously classified among the osteochondroses (aseptic necroses). It is encountered most frequently in children between 10 and 15 years of age who complain of local pain, tenderness, and swelling over the anterior tibial tubercle, with limp and disability in running and climbing stairs. Even though Osgood-Schlatter disease is suspected clinically, a lateral knee radiograph is recommended to exclude a possible tumor or infection. The

roentgen signs are fragmentation of the tubercle, displacement of the fragments away from the shaft, and swelling of the overlying soft tissues (Fig. 12). This condition should not be confused with normal irregular mineralization of the anterior tibial tubercle, which is not associated with pain and swelling. Comparable injury before the anterior tibial tubercle is mineralized (Fig. 13) shows only the soft tissue swelling.

SINDING-LARSEN-JOHANSSON DISEASE

Sinding-Larsen-Johansson disease is very likely comparable to Osgood-Schlatter disease but involves the proximal attachment of the patellar ligament to the inferior pole of the patella. It is occasionally associated with Osgood-Schlatter disease and occurs most frequently in physically active children. It has also been observed in spastic cerebral palsy patients. Clinical signs are similar, including knee pain that is accentuated on climbing stairs, running, or kneeling. Local tenderness and swelling may be found at the lower border of the patella. Radiologically, soft tissue swelling may be noted; serial films often demonstrate transient irregular mineralization of the affected portion of the patella and calcification in the juxtapatellar portion of the ligament. Spontaneous resolution of the symptoms and the radiologic signs is the rule, with little or no deformity. Localization of the bony irregularity to the inferior portions of the patella helps differentiate the condition from developmental irregular mineralization. The latter also is more frequently bilateral than is the avulsion disorder. The pathogenesis is believed to be analogous to that of the painful bipartite patella.

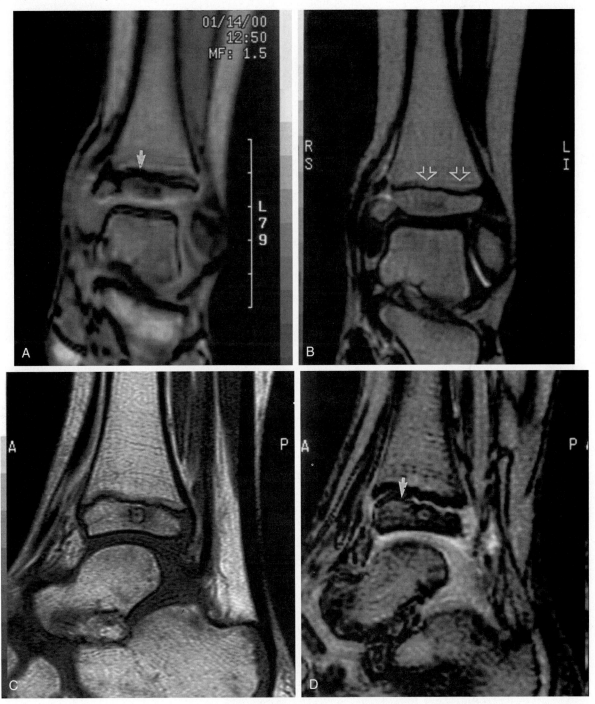

FIGURE 8. Growth plate closure in the distal tibia of a 6-year-old female following a Salter-Harris type IV fracture. Screw fixation of the epiphysis was done as part of the treatment. **A** and **B,** Coronal magnetic resonance images. **A,** Fat-suppressed, gradient-echo image shows loss of high-signal physeal cartilage medially *(solid arrow).* **B,** Fat-suppressed T$_2$-weighted image shows asymmetric migration of growth arrest line *(open arrows).* This indicates lack of growth medially. **C** and **D,** Sagittal magnetic resonance images. **C,** Medial T$_1$-weighted image shows absence of growth arrest line. **D,** Fat-suppressed, gradient-echo image shows loss of high-signal physeal cartilage *(arrow). Note:* All images show some screw artifact in the epiphysis.

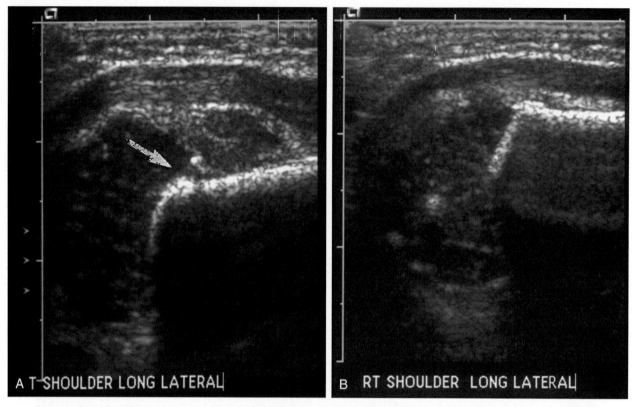

FIGURE 9. Proximal left humeral fracture in a 16-day-old female with decreased arm movement and a normal radiograph. Sonographic images of the shoulders were made in a coronal plane with lateral transducer positioning. **A,** In the left shoulder, the cartilage epiphysis is displaced laterally from the metaphysis *(arrow).* There is soft tissue swelling at the fracture site. **B,** Normal right shoulder for comparison.

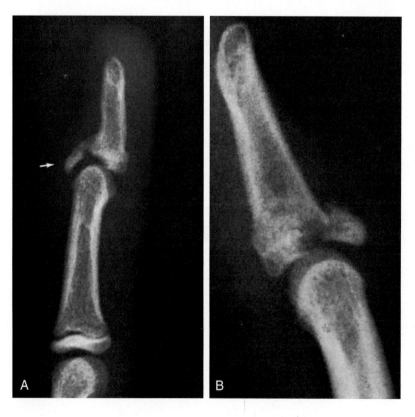

FIGURE 10. A, Transverse hyperextension fracture of the cartilage plate at the proximal end of the distal phalanx of the third digit in a 12-year-old girl, with longitudinal fracture of the epiphyseal ossification center and dorsad avulsion of the epiphyseal fragment, which also has a tag on the end of the shaft attached to it. **B,** Avulsion hyperextension fracture of the dorsal segment of the fused epiphyseal ossification center of the distal phalanx, third digit, left hand of a 13-year-old boy.

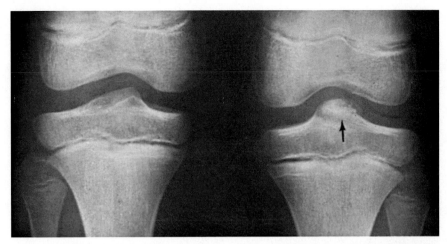

FIGURE 11. Fracture and sclerosis of the tibial spines in a 12-year-old boy who had intermittent pain in the knee for several weeks.

SLIPPED CAPITAL FEMORAL EPIPHYSIS

Slipping of the capital femoral epiphysis (SCFE) is the most common adolescent hip disorder and is rare in children younger than 9 years of age. There are three recognized presentations: chronic, acute, and acute on chronic. The most common is chronic, with a gradual onset and progression of symptoms. SCFE is more common in boys than girls and occurs earlier in girls

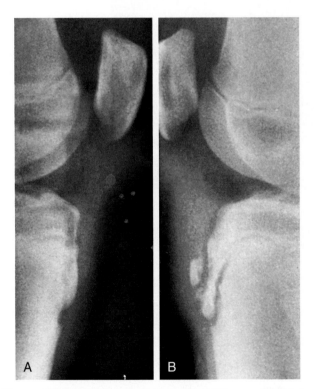

FIGURE 12. Osgood-Schlatter lesion in a boy, 13 years of age, 1 day after injury to the left knee. The right **(A)** and left **(B)** knees are shown for comparison. An avulsed fragment of the tibial tubercle lies loose in the swollen soft tissues in front of the anterior tibial process. Its presence 1 day after injury indicates that it is a fracture fragment, not heterotopic bone in the swollen patellar tendon.

because of its relation to puberty. African-Americans are at a higher risk for the disorder than whites. Mechanical and endocrine factors have been advanced as causal; the fact that most patients are distinctly overweight favors the first, and the common occurrence during the changing endocrine environment of early adolescence, the latter. Slipping is associated with established endocrine deficiencies such as primary hypothyroidism, pituitary dysfunction, and hypogonadism. Renal rickets, radiation therapy, and chemotherapy have also been identified as causes of SCFE. Bilateral disease is frequent and may be seen at presentation in about 20% of cases. When this occurs, a search for the conditions noted above is warranted.

Later contralateral slip is found in 18% to 36% of cases, and nearly all occur within 18 months. The epiphysis slips posteriorly and medially; the progression of a mild slip to a severe one can be very sudden (acute on chronic). In most cases, limp, pain, and limitation of motion at the hip begin during such ordinary activity as walking or running. Pain may be referred to the anterior thigh or knee. Radiographic examination of the pelvis discloses widening of the epiphyseal plate with varying degrees of displacement of the femoral head dorsad and mediad (Figs. 14 and 15). Mild displacement is often best appreciated on the lateral view. Widening of the epiphyseal plate without displacement, considered a preslipping phase, should be looked for in patients with hip pain and also on the asymptomatic side of patients with slips because it may be the first indication of bilateral disease. The Klein line (Fig. 15) will transect a normal amount of physis in this case and when a slip is posterior only.

Treatment is directed toward prevention of further slippage and closure of the physis. Pinning in situ is presently the treatment of choice. Complications of treatment include pin penetration/extrusion, avascular necrosis, and chondrolysis. The radiographic signs of avascular necrosis in the femoral head are very similar to those of Perthes' disease. Joint space narrowing is a late manifestation of chondrolysis. Bone scintigraphy is useful in the diagnosis of complications because the

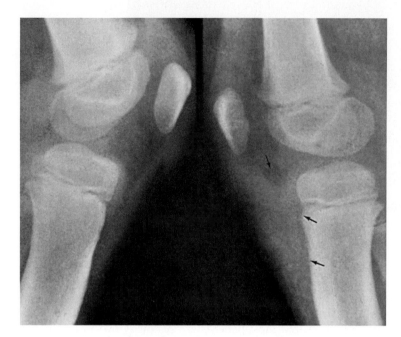

FIGURE 13. Probable Osgood-Schlatter injury prior to ossification of the anterior process of the left tibia of a 6-year-old girl. The pretibial soft tissues and caudal end of the patellar ligament are thickened. Local pain and swelling followed injury to the left knee several days before. It is possible that swelling of the inferior infrapatellar bursa contributes to thickening of the pretibial soft tissues.

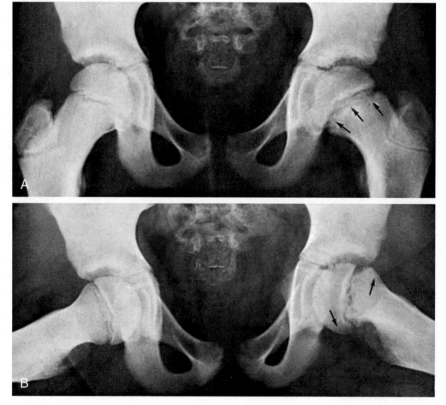

FIGURE 14. Slipped femoral epiphysis of a 10-year-old boy who sprained his foot 1 year before. Pain became much worse and he began to limp a few weeks before this study. **A,** Frontal projection with the femurs in adduction. The epiphyseal plate of the left femur is widened *(arrows)* in a pattern that at one time suggested the "preslipping phase" of a slipped femoral epiphysis. **B,** With the femurs abducted and rotated externally, the head of the left femur is slipped caudad and dorsad in relation to the femoral neck *(arrows)* but is still in normal relationship with the acetabular cavity. It is clear in these films that the diagnosis of "preslipping phase" should never be based on films made with femurs in adduction alone.

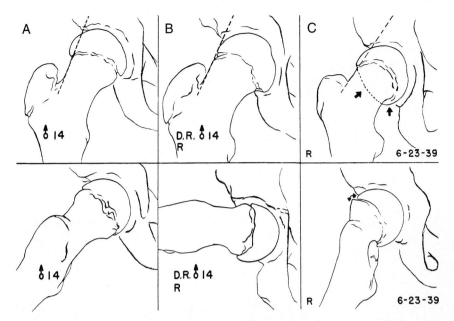

FIGURE 15. Klein's method of differentiating medial and dorsal slipping of the femoral head. **A,** Normal femur. **B,** Medial slipping of the femoral head in relation to a line that is the prolongation of the lateral edge of the femoral neck as seen in frontal projection. **C,** Posterior slipping, which is often invisible in frontal projection but is clearly visible in lateral projection (see *arrow* at cartilage–shaft junction). (From Klein A, Joplin RJ, Reidy JA, et al: Roentgenographic features of slipped capital femoral epiphysis. Am J Roentgenol Radium Ther 1951;66:361–373, with permission.)

presence of metal may limit the value of CT and MRI (Fig. 16).

TYPES OF PEDIATRIC FRACTURES

BONES OF THE HANDS

Fractures of bones of the hands and wrists most commonly involve the epiphyses and juxtaepiphyseal regions of phalanges and metacarpal bones (Figs. 10 and 17). The distal phalanges may also suffer crush fractures, as shown in Figure 18. The Salter-Harris II type of epiphyseal fracture seems to be most common (Figs. 17, 19, and 20). Occasionally, a small "flake" of bone is observed adjacent to a swollen finger joint, and a marginal defect can be noted in a nearby phalanx. The fragment may be attached to a collateral ligament that has been torn off, causing instability that can lead to painful, longstanding dysfunction and deformity unless clinically recognized and properly treated. In all cases of flake fractures of the phalanges, careful tests of joint function should be made. Fracture of the proximal end of the shaft of the first metacarpal and its cartilage plate is occasionally seen, but associated disruption of the metacarpotrapezial joint (Bennett's fracture) is extremely rare.

Carpal bones are rarely broken prior to adolescence because, during early childhood, these ossification centers are surrounded and protected by thick cushions of cartilage. The scaphoid bone is occasionally fractured transversely in older children; it may be difficult to demonstrate initially but can be recognized in its healing state (Fig. 21). As in adults, the proximal

fragment may become necrotic if its blood supply is damaged (Fig. 22).

BONES OF THE FOREARM

Bones of the forearm are much more frequently fractured than those of the hands, with the distal end of the radius being the most common site. Epiphyseal displacements (Fig. 23), distal cortical buckling with or without impaction (Fig. 24), and distal shaft fractures are common. Associated fractures of the ulna may be present. Figures 25 and 26 illustrate the importance of examination in two planes for evaluation of the anatomy of a fracture. Midshaft fracture may be manifested as plastic deformation (see Fig. 3). When the radius is broken in its middle or distal third and shortened, the distal radioulnar joint can be dislocated (Galeazzi's fracture) when the triangular fibrocartilage complex is disrupted.

Breaks in the proximal part of the ulna are often accompanied by dislocation of the radius at the elbow (Monteggia's fracture–dislocation). When the injury occurs with the elbow in extension and ventral dislocation occurs, this is the classical type. When it occurs in flexion, the radius is dislocated dorsad (reversed Monteggia's fracture) (Figs. 27 and 28). The radial head and neck should line up exactly with the capitellum of the humerus in any projection of the elbow if there is no radiohumeral dislocation. There are several variations of this injury that are typed as "Monteggia-equivalent lesions." These are fracture–dislocation combinations involving the proximal radius and ulna (Fig. 29).

Rarely, a temporary dorsal dislocation of the radius and ulna at the elbow is followed by separation of the radial head, which is rotated 90 degrees from its normal position and displaced dorsad (Figs. 30 and 31).

Subluxation of the radial head (a common clinical diagnosis known as nursemaid's elbow or pulled elbow syndrome) occurs chiefly in children between 2 and 6 years of age (peak incidence 2 to 3 years). This injury most commonly occurs when a longitudinal pull is applied to the upper extremity. Usually the forearm is pronated. There is a partial tear in the orbicular ligament, allowing it to subluxate into the radiocapitel-lar joint. It is rarely demonstrable radiographically and may be reduced unintentionally in the course of positioning to obtain films.

HUMERUS

Fractures of the distal humerus are very common in growing children, especially those between 5 and 10 years of age. The supracondylar type is by far the most common, followed by the lateral dicondylar and medial epicondylar injuries (Fig. 32). The ossification centers,

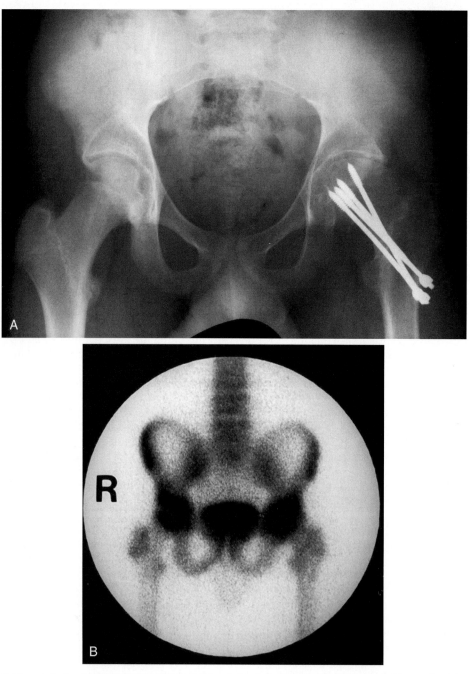

FIGURE 16. Chondrolysis of the left hip in a 12-year-old boy following pinning of a slipped capital femoral epiphysis. **A,** The radiograph shows multiple pins traversing the femoral neck. There is marked bony demineralization on both sides of the joint, and the joint space is narrowed. **B,** Delayed bone scan images show increased uptake on both sides of the left hip joint.

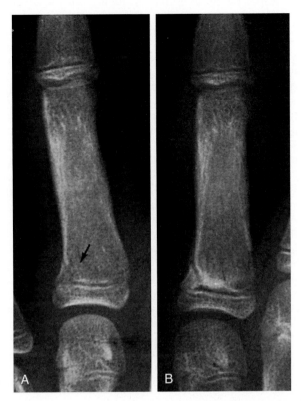

FIGURE 17. Angle fracture at the base of the shaft of the middle phalanx, fourth digit. The epiphyseal ossification center is also displaced slightly laterad as a result of transverse laceration of its cartilage plate. **A,** Immediately after the injury. **B,** Twenty days later, when distraction of the cartilage plate and also the shaft fracture fragment are more clearly seen (Salter-Harris type II cartilage plate injury).

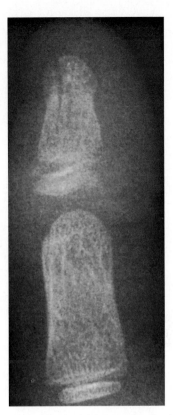

FIGURE 18. Comminuted crush injury to the distal phalanx of the thumb. The shaft has two long longitudinal fracture lines. The cartilage plate is lacerated transversely, and the epiphyseal ossification center is impacted on one side of the shaft. An automobile door was slammed on the thumb of this 6-year-old boy.

FIGURE 19. Frontal **(A)** and lateral **(B)** projections of an impacted fracture at the distal end of the shaft of the second metacarpal in a 12-year-old boy. This appears to be an angle fracture at the end of the shaft, with a tag of the shaft attached to the slightly displaced epiphyseal ossification center.

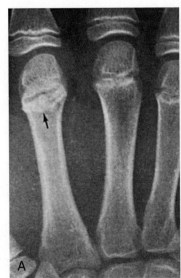
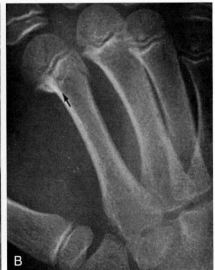

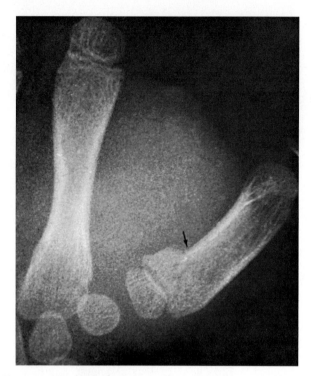

FIGURE 20. Angle fracture at the proximal end of the first metacarpal that appears to run into the cartilage plate. This might have developed into a Bennett's fracture with disruption of the trapeziometacarpal joint in an adult. In this 11-year-old girl, it is probably a Salter-Harris type II injury of the cartilage plate.

which appear at different ages, become important reference structures for determining fracture extent and displacement. A general guideline for the developmental pattern is capitellum (1 year), medial epicondyle (7 years), trochlea (9 years), and lateral epicondyle (11 years). In most cases, fractures are of the "flexion type," in which the distal fragment is displaced dorsad (Fig. 33). Even if there is little or no displacement, a fracture can be suspected in the proper clinical setting if displacement of the extracapsular olecranon fat pad is observed in a lateral film (Fig. 34). The anterior fat pad may be visible normally. The displacement indicates acutely increased intra-articular fluid, most commonly blood, as a concomitant of fracture. Avulsion fractures of the medial epicondyle are recognized when their ossification centers are abnormally remote from the expanded supracondylar portion of the distal humerus (Fig. 35). This lesion is one of the manifestations of self-induced trauma and is categorized as an example of "little leaguer's elbow" resulting from excessive use in childhood sports. It could equally be discussed under injuries to the cartilaginous plate or osteochondroses. Prior to appearance of the ossification center for the condyles, only marked soft tissue swelling is observed (Fig. 36). Rarely, a displaced medial epicondyle is drawn into the joint space and simulates normal trochlear mineralization (Fig. 37). Recognition of this complication is facilitated by reference to the crisscross sequence of appearance of the ossification centers of the humerus

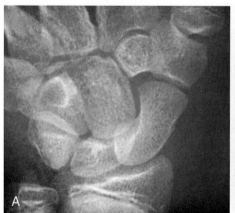
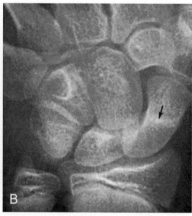

FIGURE 21. Fracture of the scaphoid in a boy 13½ years of age that is invisible immediately after the injury **(A)** but is marked by a sclerotic band *(arrow)* of opaque internal callus 21 days later **(B).** Both films were made with the hand in ulnar deviation.

FIGURE 22. Schematic drawing of the different types of breaks in relation to arterial circulation in scaphoid fractures. **A,** Fracture between the two sources of arterial blood, with good prognosis because each fragment has a satisfactory arterial supply. **B** and **C,** Fractures at the central and proximal levels, in which the blood supply of the proximal fragment is impaired or lost. (From Cave EF: Fractures and Other Injuries. St. Louis, Mosby, 1958, with permission.)

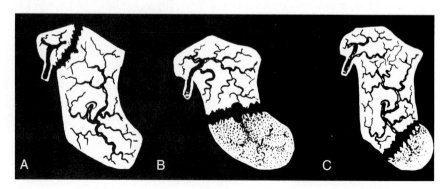

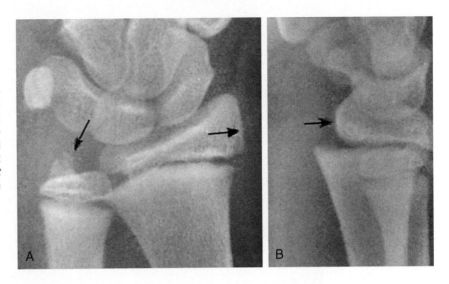

FIGURE 23. Cartilage plate injury (Salter-Harris type I) at the distal end of the radius in an 8-year-old boy. There is lateral dorsal displacement of the radial epiphyseal ossification center in the frontal (**A,** *right arrow*) and lateral (**B,** *arrow*) projections. An independent bone at the tip of the ulnar styloid (**A,** *left arrow*) could be a fracture fragment or an accessory ossification center.

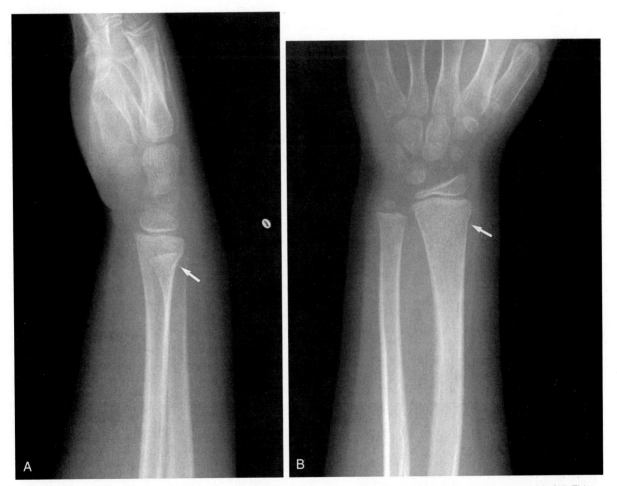

FIGURE 24. Buckle fracture of the distal radius in a 7-year-old boy who fell with the arm outstretched to break his fall. This common occurrence results in buckling of the dorsal cortex. **A,** The subtle cortical change is best seen in the lateral radiograph *(arrow).* **B,** The posteroanterior projection can be normal with these fractures. In this case, the lateral cortex is minimally involved *(arrow).*

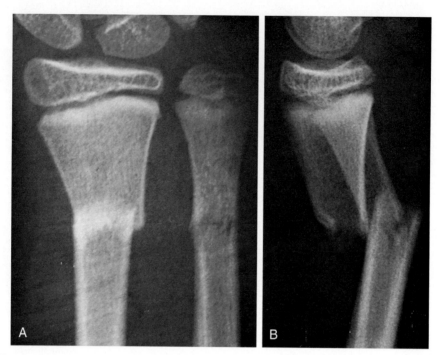

FIGURE 25. Transverse fracture of the radial and ulnar shafts at the same level. In frontal projection **(A),** there is no fracture line at the junction of the radial fragments, but there is a deep transverse sclerotic band caused by overlap of the radial fragments, which is clearly seen on the lateral projection **(B).** In the ulna, the distraction fracture causes the standard transverse band of diminished density between the fragments because there is no overlap and the fragments are distracted from each other.

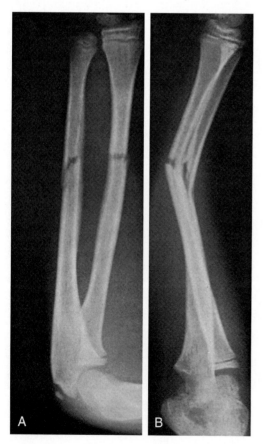

FIGURE 26. Frontal **(A)** and lateral **(B)** projections showing a fracture in the middle thirds of the radius and ulna, with dorsiflexion of the distal fragments, in a 10-year-old girl.

at the elbow. Apparent trochlear calcification cannot be normal in the absence of a center in the medial epicondyle. In incomplete fractures of the distal humerus in which bony deformity is not obvious, the anterior humeral line (Fig. 38) can be useful except when the ossification center for the capitellum is very small. Nonrotated lateral projections are mandatory for this evaluation.

Proximal humeral fractures are often Salter-Harris type I in infants and children under 5 years of age (see Fig. 9). They are metaphyseal between 5 and 10 years of age and tend to be the Salter-Harris type II in adolescence. Deformity after fractures at the proximal end of the humerus depends on the level of fracture relative to the levels of insertions of the deltoid muscle (abduction), pectoralis major muscle (adductor and internal rotator), and abduction and rotation muscles of the rotator cuff (Figs. 39 and 40). Avulsion fractures of the lesser tuberosity of the humerus are not common but may be missed if an axillary view is not obtained in appropriate instances (Fig. 41). They are believed to result from sudden forceful traction by the subscapularis tendon when the shoulder is in hyperextension and hyperexternal rotation. Little leaguer's shoulder is a term applied to fracture of the proximal cartilage plate of the humerus in similar circumstances. Radiographically, there is widening of the proximal cartilaginous plate of the humerus and rarefaction of the contiguous metaphysis in comparison with the unaffected shoulder. Actual separation can take place. Proximal humeral epiphysiolysis has been noted in adolescent baseball pitchers. The radiographic features resemble those in the hip.

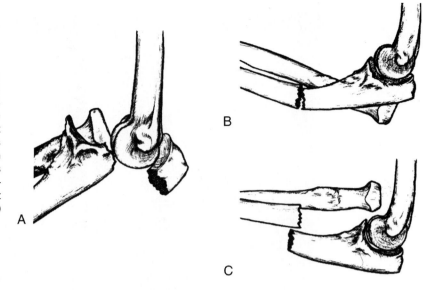

FIGURE 27. Fracture–dislocations at the elbow. **A,** Transverse fracture of the olecranon process with forward dislocation of the unfractured radius and the distal ulnar fragment. **B,** Fracture of the shaft of the ulna with dorsal displacement of the unfractured radius (reversed Monteggia's fracture). **C,** Fracture of the ulnar shaft with forward displacement of the unfractured radius (standard Monteggia's fracture). (From Keon-Cohen BT: Fractures at the elbow. J Bone Joint Surg Am 1966;48:1623–1639, with permission.)

The supracondylar process is rarely fractured. When it is, evaluation for signs of compression of the neighboring median nerve are in order. Oblique spiral fractures of the midshaft of the humerus may occur when there are strong twisting forces.

PELVIC FRACTURES

Fractures of the pelvis may be single or multiple (Figs. 42 and 43); multiple fractures are common in automobile accidents (Fig. 44) and injuries to pelvic soft tissues, especially bladder and urethra, should not be overlooked. Athletic injuries in the pelvis are most commonly stress fractures and apophyseal avulsions. Secondary epiphyses in the region of the iliac crests, ischial tuberosities, ischial spine, and the rims of the acetabula can be mistaken for fracture fragments in adolescents. Breaks in one portion of the bony ring surrounding the obturator foramen are usually accompanied by a fracture on another segment of the ring; a similar situation may be present in the pelvic ring as well. Traumatic separation of the symphysis or sacroiliac joints may accompany fractures. If there is little separation of the fragments and the plane of a fracture is oblique to the projection of the x-ray beam, it may be necessary to examine the pelvis in several projections before the fracture is visualized. Stereoscopic films are helpful in clarifying the problem, but CT is the preferred method to demonstrate complex fractures and the position of the component parts. Various pathologic processes that are uncertain or even invisible on conventional exami-

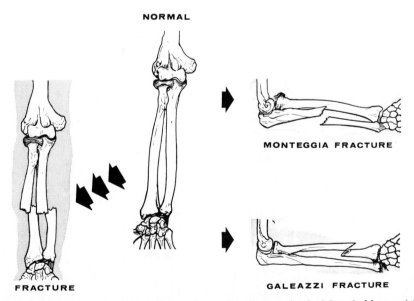

FIGURE 28. Effect of midshaft fracture of the radius or ulna on the elbow and wrist joints. In Monteggia's fracture of the ulna, the radial head is dislocated at the elbow. In Galeazzi's fracture of the radius, the ulna is dislocated at the wrist. When the radius and ulna are fractured simultaneously, these dislocations do not occur. (From Reckling FW, Cordell ID: Unstable fracture-dislocations of the forearm: the Monteggia and Galeazzi lesions. Arch Surg 1968;96:999–1007. © 1968 American Medical Association.)

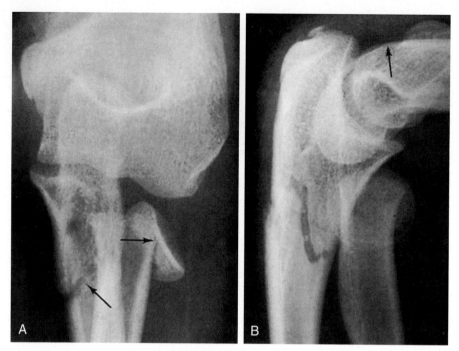

FIGURE 29. Impaction injury to the radial head with rotation of the head, and oblique fracture of the ulnar shaft (*arrows* on **A**) with longitudinal distraction of the fragments. Frontal **(A)** and lateral **(B)** projections in an 11-year-old girl. *Arrow* in **B** points to the dorsally displaced fat pad.

nations may be clearly defined with CT. For example, it has demonstrated subchondral fractures previously unrecognized in sacroiliac joint trauma in children. Furthermore, CT demonstrates associated soft-tissue abnormalities, such as hematoma, not clinically obvious, within the bony pelvis or in the deep muscles of the upper thigh, and with three-dimensional reconstruction can demonstrate relations that are of importance for the orthopedic surgeon. Subtle diastasis and intra-articular fragments are best delineated by coronal reconstructions, sometimes coupled with sagittal reconstructions.

The ununited epiphyseal ossification centers of the pelvic bones may be torn away from the main mass during ordinary athletic activities, such as jumping and in sprinting races (Figs. 45 and 46). Avulsion fractures of the ilia and ischia occur in a variety of patterns (Figs. 47 and 48). The clinical features are not markedly different from those of slipped capital femoral epiphysis, toxic synovitis, or pathologic fractures, all of which must be considered. In some instances, the avulsed osteocartilaginous mass undergoes a proliferative reaction but ultimate spontaneous resorption is the rule although it may be prolonged.

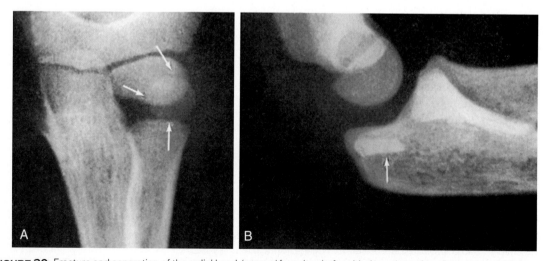

FIGURE 30. Fracture and separation of the radial head *(arrows)* from its shaft, with dorsad rotation of the head of 90 degrees, so that the displaced head appears to be an erect disk in frontal projection **(A)** and a recumbent disk in lateral projection **(B)**, superimposed on the olecranon of the ulna (see also Fig. 31). (From Cave EF: Fractures and Other Injuries. St. Louis, Mosby, 1958, with permission.)

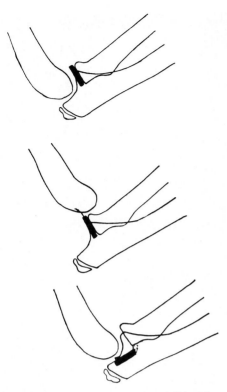

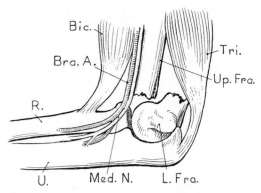

FIGURE 33. Morbid anatomy of supracondylar fracture of the humerus; semi-schematic drawing. The proximal fragment displaced forward may puncture the brachial vessels or injure the median nerve. *Bic.* = biceps; *Bra. A.* = brachial artery; *R.* = radius; *Tri.* = triceps; *Up. Fra.* = upper fragment; *L. Fra.* = lower fragment; *Med. N.* = median nerve; *U.* = ulna.

IMAGING OF ACETABULAR INJURY IN CHILDHOOD*

Fracture of the acetabulum is a rare injury in childhood, reported in only 2–9% of pediatric pelvic fractures. Despite the relative rarity of acetabular fractures, they often develop late sequelae or require open reduction and fixation. The rate and pattern of injury in adoles-

*This section written by Dr. Bradley Maxfield.

FIGURE 31. The pattern and course of dorsal dislocation of the ulna on the humerus, in which the radial head is separated and rotated 90 degrees and displaced dorsad. (From Jeffrey CC: Fractures of the neck of the radius in children. J Bone Joint Surg Br 1972;54:717–719, with permission.)

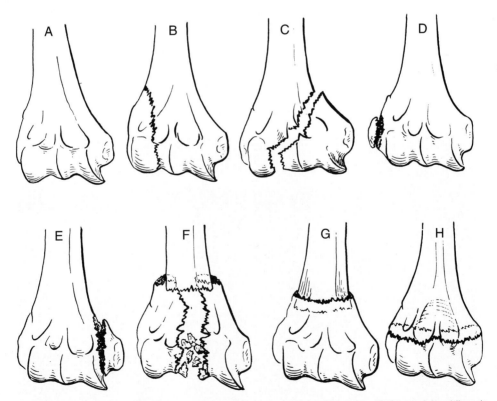

FIGURE 32. Patterns of fractures of the distal end of the humerus. **A,** Normal humerus. **B,** Diacondylar oblique-longitudinal fracture of the lateral epicondyle and capitellum. **C,** Diacondylar oblique fracture of the medial epicondyle and trochlea. **D,** Longitudinal fracture of the lateral epicondyle. **E,** Longitudinal fracture of the medial epicondyle. **F,** T transverse fracture of the shaft and longitudinal diacondylar fracture with comminution. **G,** Simple impacted supracondylar fracture of the shaft. **H,** Transverse diacondylar fracture. (From Cave EF: Fractures and Other Injuries. St. Louis, Mosby, 1958, with permission.)

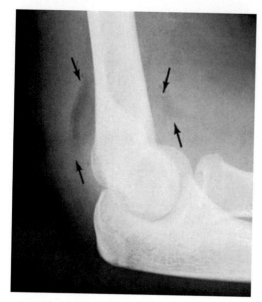

FIGURE 34. Displacement of the olecranon fat pad dorsad out of the olecranon fossa and the coronoid fat pad ventrad out of the coronoid fossa after injury and acute swelling at the elbow. The bones are normal. Acute distention of the elbow joint resulting from acute traumatic hemarthrosis is the probable cause of displacement of the fat pads.

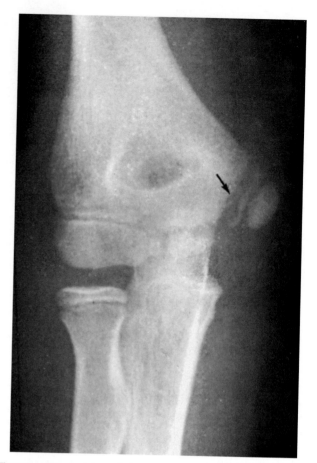

FIGURE 35. Avulsion of the ossification center of the medial epicondyle with a strip of attached shaft (type II Salter-Harris injury to the cartilage plate). This 12-year-old boy had sharp pain and regional swelling at the elbow while pitching baseball ("little leaguer's elbow").

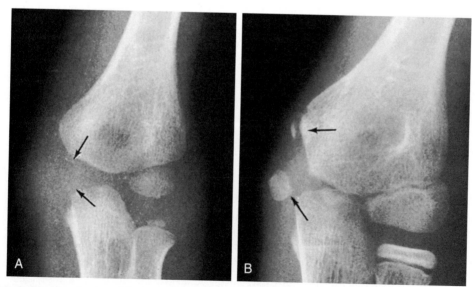

FIGURE 36. A, Frontal projection of the left elbow of a 5-year-old boy prior to the appearance of the ossification center for the medial epicondyle, with pronounced soft tissue local swelling medial to the elbow. **B,** Five years later, the displaced ossification center for the medial epicondyle is now evident *(lower arrow)* and a second accessory center is also visible *(upper arrow)* in the normal portion of the medial epicondyle.

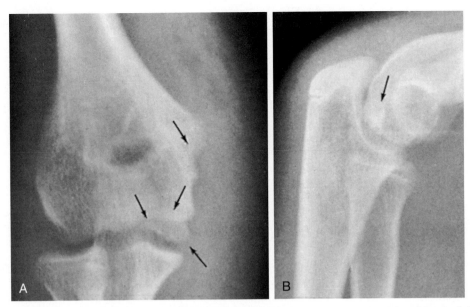

FIGURE 37. Frontal **(A)** and lateral **(B)** projections in a 13-year-old girl showing fracture and avulsion of the medial epicondyle (*upper arrow* in **A**), with the fracture fragment enfolded in the joint (*lower three arrows* in **A** and *single arrow* in **B**).

cents, with closed triradiate cartilage, are comparable to adults, but distinctly different in children with open triradiate cartilage. The pediatric pelvis is more pliable and elastic than is the mature pelvis. Thus the pediatric pelvis has a greater capacity for absorption and dispersal of impact injury, resulting in fewer fractures. This results in an acetabular fracture rate of 6.6% in the immature pelvis patients, at mean age of 5.7 years. Patients with a mature pelvis had a 44% rate of acetabular injury at an average age of 14 years. The relatively higher energy required for pediatric pelvic fracture results in a higher

rate of associated solid organ and CNS injury. Unlike adults, exsanguination directly related to pelvic fracture is extremely rare in children. Due to the high energy required to induce pediatric acetabular injury, the vast majority of injuries are due to vehicular trauma. Vehicle versus pedestrian injuries are implicated more commonly than automobile passenger injuries.

Acute and subacute imaging of the injured pelvis should be directed to detect the injuries that place the child most at risk for complications or those that require operative management. Important risk factors include; fracture dislocation, triradiate cartilage injury, and displacement of acetabular fragments (Figs. 49 through 51). Open fractures and penetrating injury to the joint space require operative management. An AP film of the pelvis is recommended in all blunt trauma patients. Trauma patients are likely to undergo CT of the abdomen and pelvis to evaluate for viscous and solid organ injury. Careful review of the bony pelvis is necessary in all trauma CT evaluations. Acetabular and triradiate cartilage injuries are better detected with CT and can change clinical management (Figs. 49 through 51). Volumetric acquisition using multi-detector scanners makes 2D reconstruction techniques available with routine trauma protocols. 3D reformation is used less frequently in children than in the adult population and is not part of the routine evaluation of pediatric pelvis fractures. 3D techniques are useful for rapid evaluation of comminuted fracture geometry.

BONES OF THE LOWER LIMBS

Bones in the lower limbs are broken less frequently than those in the upper limbs, but their treatment and healing are complicated by weight bearing. Pedal phalanges may be fractured by falls of heavy objects on them and by stubbing the toes when barefoot. Occult compound fracture may occur with subsequent osteomyelitis

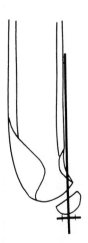

FIGURE 38. The anterior humeral line is drawn parallel to the anterior border of the humeral cortex in true lateral projection. Another line is constructed perpendicular to it, of a length equivalent to the anteroposterior dimension of the ossification center in the capitellum, and is divided into thirds. If the anterior humeral line does not pass through the middle third of this second line, anterior or posterior displacement must be suspected. Exceptions may occur if the ossification center is very small and eccentrically located. (Modified from Rogers LF, Malave S Jr, White H, Tachdjian MO: Plastic bowing, torus and greenstick supracondylar fractures of the humerus: radiographic clues to obscure fractures of the elbow in children. Radiology 1978;128:145–150.)

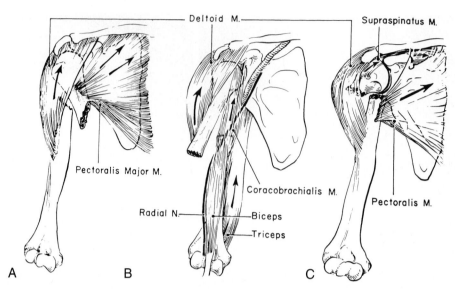

FIGURE 39. Fractures at the proximal end of the humerus, with characteristic deformities. **A,** Adduction of the proximal fragment as a result of pull of the pectoralis major and deltoid muscles. **B,** Abduction of the proximal fragment when the fracture is distal to the insertion of the deltoid muscle. **C,** Abduction and rotation of the proximal fragment when the fracture is proximal to the insertion of the pectoralis major and the rotator cuff. (From Cave EF: Fractures and Other Injuries. St. Louis, Mosby, 1958, with permission.)

when the base of the distal phalanx of the hallux is injured adjacent to the germinal matrix of the nail, where the skin is directly attached to the periosteum. Reduction of proximal phalangeal fractures is more important than reduction of those of middle or distal phalanges because of possible disabling flexion deformities in the former. A common fracture in older children is a transverse metaphyseal–diaphyseal one at the base of the fifth metatarsal called the Jones fracture (Fig. 52). Avulsion fractures also occur at the base of the fifth metatarsal and must be differentiated from the secondary ossification center. Typical stress fractures occur also in the shafts of the other metatarsal bones (Figs. 53 and 54).

Fractures of the tarsal bones (Figs. 55 through 57) may be difficult to recognize in conventional surveys. If clinically warranted, the bone scan may be used to identify occult fractures (Fig. 58). Abnormal areas can be more closely scrutinized with nonroutine x-ray projections or CT. The calcaneus is the most frequently fractured tarsal bone in childhood. CT has become the preferred method for imaging calcaneal fractures, particularly to assess displacement. Occult fractures of the calcaneus and cuboid bones are described as variants of the "toddler's fracture" (spiral fracture of the tibia). These fractures may present with unexplained reluctance to walk, and confirmation is found as focal sclerosis during healing. Osteomyelitis of the talus also may produce similar clinical features. Fractures of the talus are subject to vascular complications as well as traumatic arthritis. Avulsion fractures may occur in tarsal bones at sites of tendon attachments.

Fractures of the distal tibial and fibular epiphyses are common; Salter-Harris types I and II are most frequent. Attention must be given to subtle differences in epiphyseal cartilage thickness for their identification, and exposures in two planes are indicated for initial examination of patients with ankle injury and swelling

(Fig. 59). Transepiphyseal fractures (Salter-Harris type III) may occur medially (Fig. 60) or laterally (Fig. 61) in the tibial epiphysis. Because the distal tibial physis closes asymmetrically in early adolescence, ankle injuries can produce fracture patterns not seen in younger children

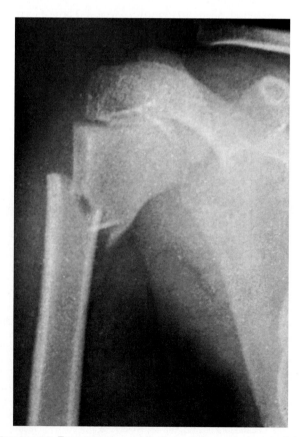

FIGURE 40. Transverse jagged fracture of the surgical neck of the humerus of a 6-year-old girl. The fracture line is at the level of the insertion of the pectoralis major.

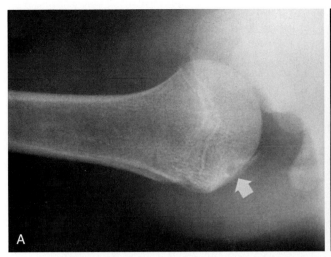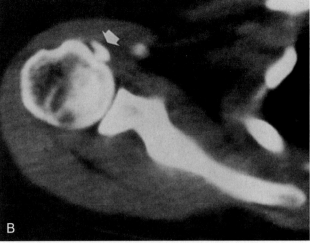

FIGURE 41. Adolescent girl with shoulder pain after injury. Initial radiologic examination showed a small avulsion fragment from the lesser tuberosity on axillary films only. Symptoms subsided after 3 months. **A,** Follow-up examination in the identical axillary view 2 years and 4 months after injury showed some enlargement of the fragment with no further displacement. **B,** Computed tomography scan at that time corresponds to the radiograph. (From Shibuya S, Ogawa K: Isolated avulsion fracture of the lesser tuberosity of the humerus: a case report. Clin Orthop 1986;211:215–218, with permission.)

with completely open physes. The juvenile Tilleaux fracture is an avulsion fracture of the anterolateral portion of a distal tibial epiphysis that has undergone fusion of all but that portion (Fig. 61). An external rotational force operating through the anterior tibiofibular ligament, which links the tibial epiphysis to the fibular metaphysis, dislodges the ununited lateral third. The displaced fragment may become locked between the tibia and fibula and widen the mortise. The distal tibiofibular syndesmotic complex is almost invariably disrupted. The triplane fracture results from supination–eversion forces producing coronal, transverse, and sagittal fractures in a combination of Salter-Harris types II and III. The classical three major fragments are the following: (1) the anterolateral quadrant of the distal tibial epiphysis, (2) the medial and

posterior portions of the epiphysis with a posterior metaphyseal spike, and (3) the tibial metaphysis. CT is commonly employed to evaluate multiplane fractures because displacement of fragments by more than 2 mm after closed reduction usually prompts internal fixation (Fig. 62). The most common serious injury to the ankle is sprain of the lateral ligaments, usually from inversion forces. Soft tissue swelling without bone injury is the usual manifestation, and evaluation of films with stress applied may demonstrate abnormal motion in comparison with that of the uninjured limb.

Fractures of the tibial and fibular shafts are also common. The child with unexplained refusal to bear weight or limping often will have a spiral (more correctly, helical), nondisplaced fracture of the tibia that may be visible to examination in the lateral projection but not in the anteroposterior (see Fig. 1). These usually heal well because the intact fibula acts as an internal splint. Other fractures are more obvious, but it is important to examine the knees and ankles in addition to the shafts, because a fracture in the distal segment of the tibia may be associated with a companion fracture in the proximal segment of the fibula (Fig. 63). Stress fractures are commonly located in the proximal segments of the tibial shaft (Fig. 64). Their features are the same as those of stress fractures at other levels and in other bones. They result from repeated slight overloading of the bone. Pain may precede the radiographic signs by several weeks. Adjacent periosteal reaction may simulate inflammatory or malignant tumors. The fracture line is usually obscured by the internal and external productive reaction. Painful limp is the common complaint; pain increases with activity and disappears with rest. After complete immobilization, stress fractures in long bones usually heal in 8 to 12 weeks, a feature that is reassuring in relation to the conditions in the original differential diagnosis.

Fractures of the femur are less common than those in the lower leg and usually involve significant force. In

FIGURE 42. Multiple fractures of the pelvis. *Arrows* indicate bilateral pubic fractures and sacroiliac separation as manifestations of the rule that the pelvic ring usually fractures in more than one site. Note the separation of the pubic bones at the synchondrosis.

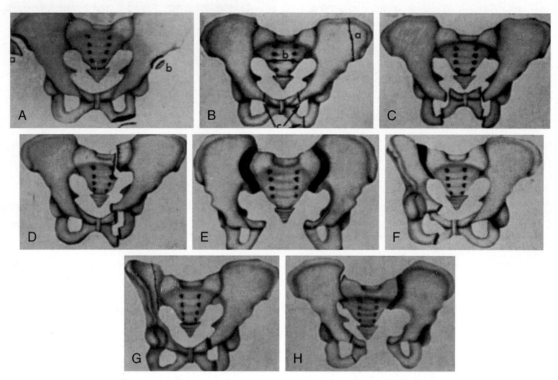

FIGURE 43. Examples of pelvic fractures. **A,** Avulsion fracture of the anterosuperior iliac spine *(a)*, anteroinferior iliac spine *(b)*, and ischial tuberosity *(c)*. **B,** Stable fractures of the wing of the ilium *(a)*, body of the sacrum *(b)*, and in the pubic rami *(c)*. **C,** Straddle fractures of the pubic rami with distraction of the fragments. **D,** Longitudinal unilateral shear fractures of the lateral process of the sacrum and pubic rami on the left side. **E,** Widening of both sacroiliac joints and separation of the symphysis pubis. **F,** Lateral compression injury with fracture of the pubic rami on the side of the impact and widening of the sacroiliac joint on the same side. **G,** Fracture (longitudinal) of the right iliac wing on the side of the impact and of the pubic rami on the opposite side. **H,** Total pelvic disruption with stable fractures of the pubic rami on the side of the impact. (From Dunn AW, Morris HD: Fractures and dislocations of the pelvis. J Bone Joint Surg [Am] 1968;50:1639–1648, with permission.)

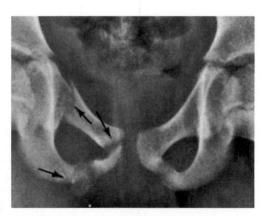

FIGURE 44. Fractures of the right pubic and ischial bones of a boy 7 years of age who was injured in an automobile accident. A substantial fragment is avulsed from the ischium *(lowest arrow)*. (Courtesy of Dr. John Dorst, Baltimore, MD.)

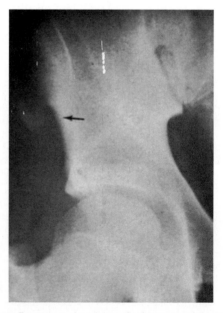

FIGURE 45. Fracture and avulsion of a fragment of the ilial wing in a healthy boy 16 years of age who felt a sharp pain above his right hip as he left the starting block in a sprint.

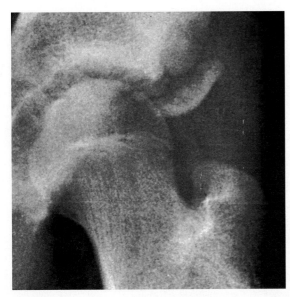

FIGURE 46. Segmental avulsion fracture of the ilium at the site of the anteroinferior spine of a boy 13 years of age.

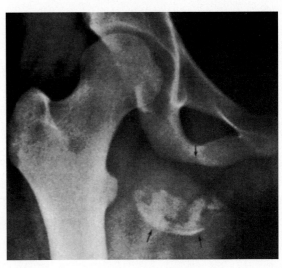

FIGURE 48. Avulsion of the ischial apophysis *(upper arrow)* with a large comminuted fracture fragment widely displaced *(lower arrows)*. The patient was a girl 15 years of age.

adolescent football players, sudden valgus stress applied to the knee when a player is tackled or blocked while his ipsilateral foot is firmly implanted in the turf may lead to epiphyseal separation at the knee because the ligaments are stronger than the epiphyseal cartilage at that age (Fig. 65). Shaft fractures generally result from vehicular accidents, falls from a tree, or accidents involving forces of similar magnitude. In the absence of such history, primary abnormalities within the bone have to be considered and sought, and, if not found, nonaccidental trauma has to be suspected. Injury to adjacent nerves and vessels should not be overlooked with femoral fractures, because the position of the

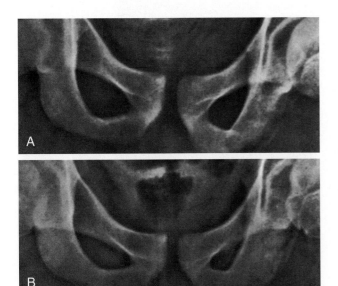

FIGURE 47. Avulsion fracture of the apophysis of the ischium. **A,** This boy, 14 years of age, felt a sharp pain in the left buttock while jumping hurdles in a gymnasium. **B,** Ten days later, he tripped and fell and again had sharp pain in the left buttock.

broken ends of the bone in the radiographs does not indicate their movement in the soft tissues at the time of injury.

TRAUMA FROM PHYSICAL AGENTS

ELECTRICAL INJURY

Electrical trauma to bone involves several possible mechanisms. Tetanic convulsions and muscular contractions result in fractures more frequently in adults than in children because of differences in muscle development and strength. Focal and regional bone necrosis and soft tissue changes are related to the course and duration of the electrical discharge and the conductivity of the various tissues. Soft tissues are said to be better conductors than bone, but experimental studies suggest that resistance of skeletal muscle is high, resulting in a large temperature rise that heats adjacent tissues and accounts for deep tissue loss. Direct overheating, therefore, causes much of the damage; small vessel occlusion contributes to it. Secondary renal damage may occur from myoglobin and hemoglobin products. Destruction of epiphyseal growth areas results in premature fusion of epiphyses and shafts and retarded growth. Cortical thickenings may form, similar to those occurring after severe thermal burns. Delayed soft tissue contractures and bone necrosis may be secondary to vascular injury; neurologic damage and secondary infection probably contribute to deformities. Late changes are similar to those seen in severe burns.

THERMAL INJURY

Regional radiographic changes in bones injured by excessive heat include rarefaction, cortical thickening, destruction of the epiphyses, and the formation of osteophytes. Necrotic para-articular and juxtaosteal soft

Text continued on page 2298

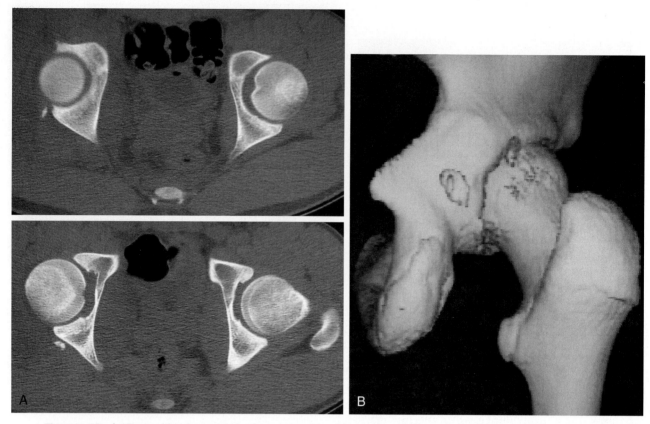

FIGURE 49. A 15-year-old male unrestrained passenger injured in a motor vehicle vs. tree collision. A right hip dislocation was reduced in the emergency room. **A,** Post-reduction CT shows the mildly displaced posterior rim fracture. No intra-articular fragments were present. **B,** 3D CT of the right hip shows the relationship of the multiple fracture fragments.

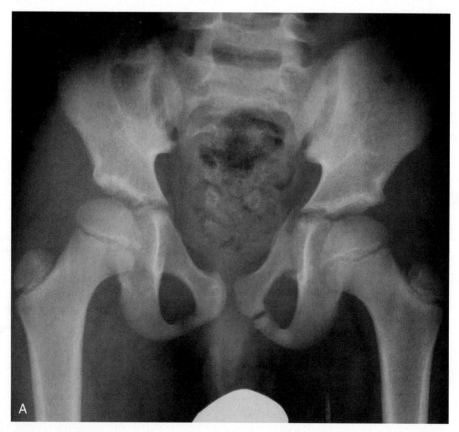

FIGURE 50. An 8-year-old male struck by an automobile. **A,** AP radiograph of the pelvis shows left pubic fractures. The left triradiate cartilage is widened.

Illustration continued on opposite page

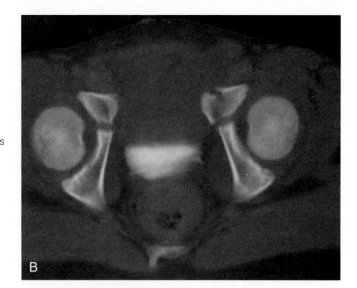

FIGURE 50. *Continued.* **B,** Axial CT shows the pubic fractures involve the triradiate cartilage but not the articular surface.

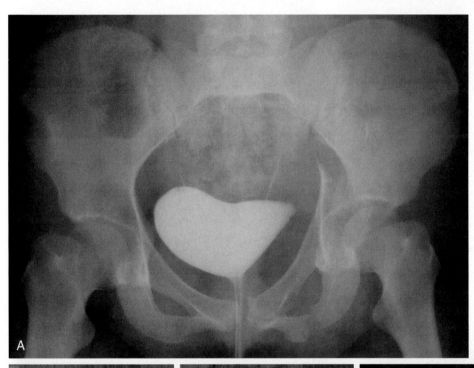

FIGURE 51. A 17-year-old female restrained passenger injured in a rollover motor vehicle collision. Mature pelvis. **A,** AP radiograph of the pelvis shows displaced left pubic, iliac and acetabular fractures. **B,** Coronal (right) and sagittal (left) reformations show the complex geometry of multiple fracture fragments. **C,** 3D CT images following extensive open reduction and internal fixation. (Courtesy of Dr. Lloyd Morris, Adelaide, South Australia.)

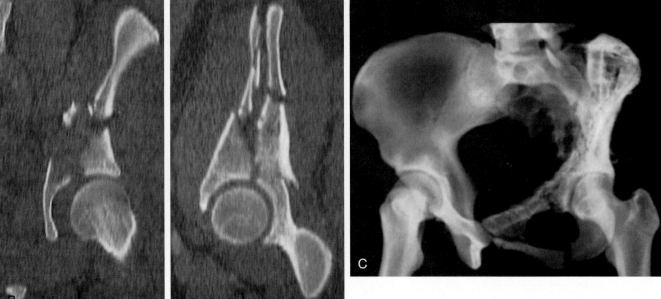

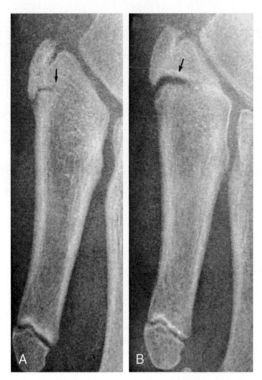

FIGURE 52. Transverse fracture at the proximal end of the fifth metatarsal of a 10-year-old girl. **A,** In a radiograph taken immediately after a twsting injury, the *arrow* is directed at the incomplete transverse fracture. The independent small mass of bone lateral to the end of the shaft is the normal apophyseal center. **B,** Thirty-four days later, the fracture line is widened and the apophyseal center is more completely fused. Fusion has probably been accelerated by the local chronic hyperemia induced by the fracture. This is known as the Jones dancing fracture.

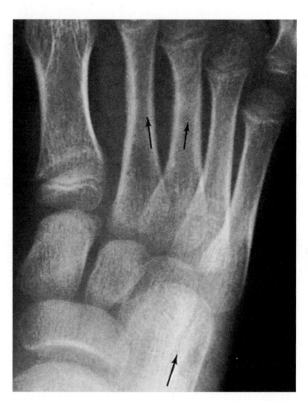

FIGURE 54. Early stress fractures of the second and third metatarsals without fracture lines but with early slight cortical thickenings *(distal arrows).* This boy of 8 years was a cross-country runner who averaged about 5 miles/day running and had developed pain and swelling in these metatarsals. The *proximal arrow* points to a false fracture line in the cuboid bone caused by the overlap of the radiolucent articular cartilages of the lateral cuneocuboid joint.

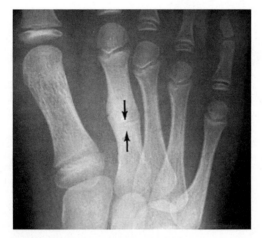

FIGURE 53. "March" or fatigue stress fracture in the second metatarsal of a 5-year-old girl.

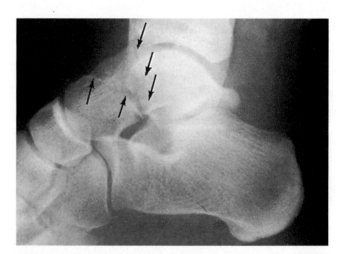

FIGURE 55. Fresh, large ventral fracture fragment of the talus *(arrows),* broken when this 17-year-old girl jumped down from a horse. The large triangular fragment is displaced cephalad. (Courtesy of Dr. L.F. Rogers and Associates, Departments of Radiology and Orthopedic Surgery, Hermann Hospital, Houston, TX.)

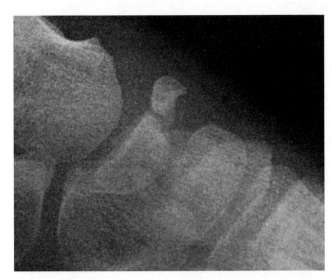

FIGURE 56. Fracture of the navicular with distraction of the superior fragment dorsad. The larger inferior segment is not dislocated. This boy, 7½ years of age, fell from his bicycle and the foot was struck by the pedal.

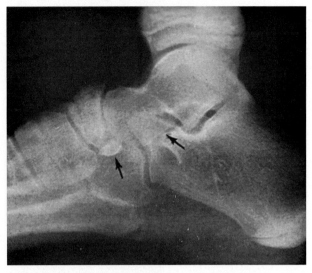

FIGURE 57. Multiple fractures of the tarsal bones of a 13-year-old boy. The *posterior arrow* is directed at a fracture line at the base of the sustentaculum of the calcaneus. The *anterior arrow* points to the fracture fragment of the tuberosity of the navicular. The large fragment of the navicular is also fractured and compressed. (Courtesy of Dr. K. Kozlowski, Royal Alexandra Hospital for Children, Sydney, Australia.)

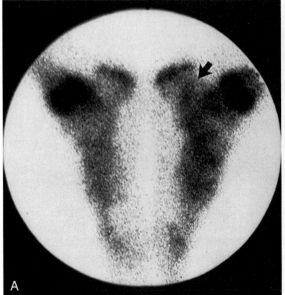

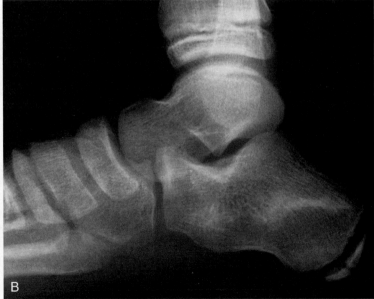

FIGURE 58. Calcaneal fracture in an 8-year-old boy required scintigraphy for diagnosis after foot radiographs were found to be normal. **A,** The lateral view of the feet shows more uptake in the right foot when compared with the left. In the right calcaneus, there is a linear increase in tracer uptake *(arrow)*. **B,** A follow-up radiograph taken 4 weeks after the bone scan shows sclerosis in the fracture line corresponding to bone scan abnormality.

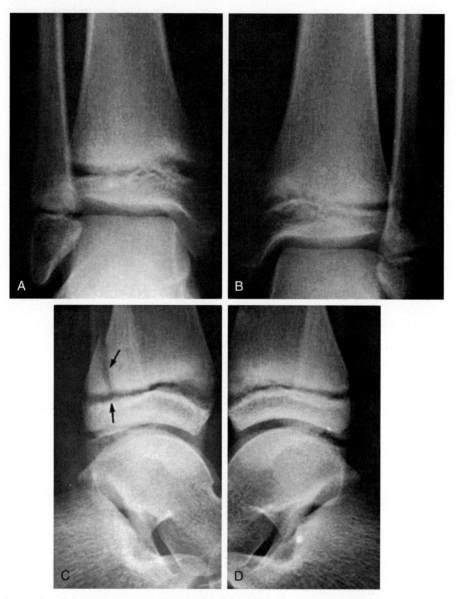

FIGURE 59. Laceration of the cartilage plate with a dorsal longitudinal fracture at the end of the tibial shaft of an 11-year-old girl who had fallen on her right ankle. Frontal **(A)** and lateral **(C)** projections of the injured right ankle show that the tibial cartilage plate is deepened as a result of longitudinal distraction of the fragments. **C,** The dorsal fragment of the tibial shaft, which was not visible in the frontal projection, is also clearly delineated (Salter-Harris type II injury to the cartilage plate). Frontal **(B)** and lateral **(D)** projections of the uninjured left ankle are presented for comparison.

tissues may calcify, and ankylosis of joints may follow destruction of articular cartilage. Osteoporosis after burns probably results from reflux vasomotor response and immobilization and disuse. It occurs within weeks to months following injury. Occasionally, acceleration of growth occurs in the burned area, possibly as a result of secondary hyperemia, but usually somatic growth in children is profoundly retarded during the first year after burns affecting more than 40% of the body surface. Recovery to normal rates takes place after another 2 years or more.

Bone lesions resulting from excessive cold are seen more often in the fingers and are due to frostbite. Vasoconstrictive reaction to cold is believed to lead to

hypoxic injury. Direct cellular damage may result from the development of ice crystals; in addition, microvascular damage probably plays a role in the tissue changes. The epiphyses of growth bones are especially vulnerable and may be completely destroyed and disappear. The terminal phalanges are customarily the most exposed to cold and most frequently injured by it (Fig. 66). The epiphyses of the thumbs are usually protected by flexion of the thumbs into the palms of the hands and flexion of the fingers over them. Triple-phase bone scans performed by Mehta and Wilson within 48 hours of frostbite injury showed the following three patterns: (1) hyperemic blood flow with normal early blood pool and normal delayed bone images; (2) absent blood flow

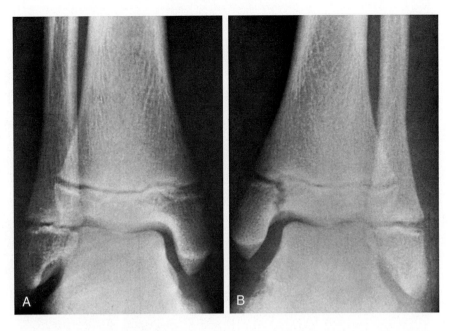

FIGURE 60. Fracture at the base and medial side of the medial malleolus of the left tibia of a 14-year-old boy who "wrenched" his ankle and foot. **A,** Normal right ankle in frontal projection. **B,** Injured left ankle. The medial segment of the left cartilage plate is deepened and the malleolar fragment displaced mediad as a result of distraction. The mortise at the ankle is enlarged and weakened (Salter-Harris type III injury to the cartilage plate).

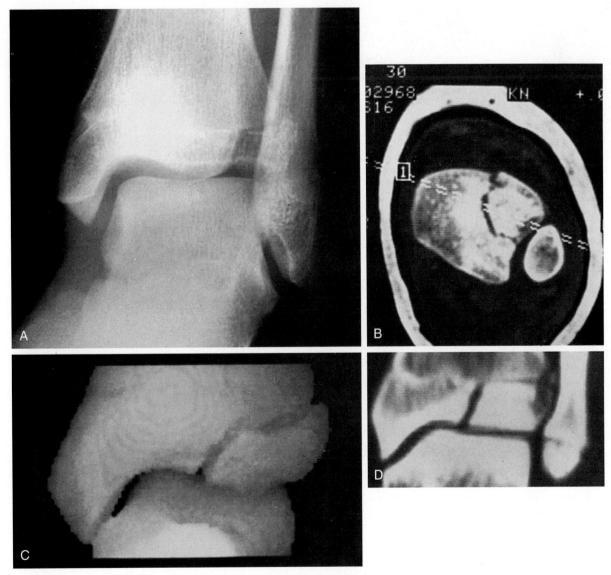

FIGURE 61. Tillaux fracture of the distal tibial epiphysis. **A,** Conventional radiograph. **B,** Computed tomography (CT) scan. **C,** Reconstructed three-dimensional coronal CT scan. **D,** Reconstructed coronal CT scan. (Courtesy of Dr. Lloyd Morris, Adelaide, South Australia.)

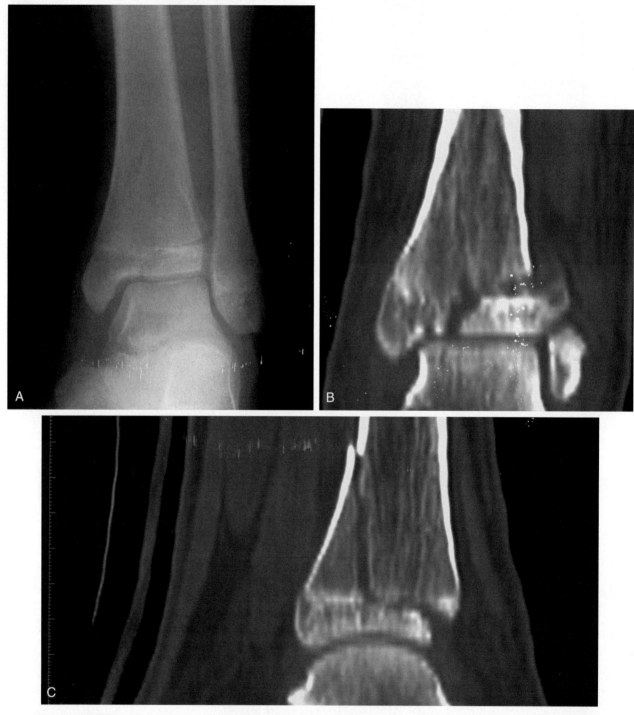

FIGURE 62. Triplane fracture of the left distal tibia in a 6-year-old boy. **A,** A radiograph in the oblique (mortise) view indicates there are three planes involved. To best determine separation and position of fragments, 2-mm computed tomography sections were reconstructed in coronal **(B)** and sagittal **(C)** planes. Fragment separations of 4 mm necessitated open reduction and screw fixation to restore anatomic position.

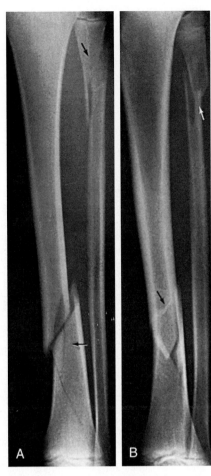

FIGURE 63. Frontal **(A)** and lateral **(B)** projections in a 14-year-old boy showing a comminuted oblique spiral fracture of the distal third of the left tibial shaft with a comminuted oblique fracture of the proximal third of the left fibular shaft.

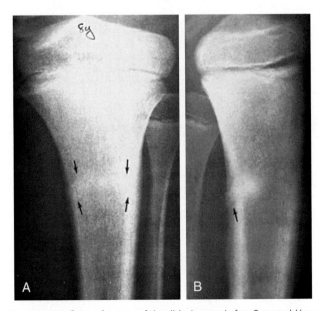

FIGURE 64. Stress fracture of the tibia *(arrows)* of an 8-year-old boy. **A,** In frontal projection, a transverse band of increased density marks the site of fracture. **B,** In lateral projection, the dorsal cortical wall only appears to be affected. This fracture appears to be incomplete.

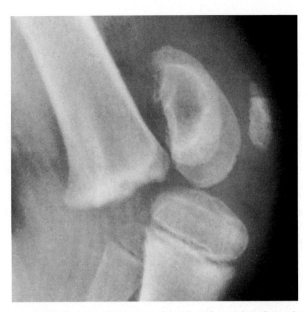

FIGURE 65. Complete laceration of the distal femoral cartilage plate with separation, forward displacement, and counterclockwise rotation of the epiphyseal ossification center. The femoral shaft is displaced dorsad. This adolescent boy incurred a "clipping" injury while playing football. The immature adolescent femur is especially vulnerable to such stresses. (Courtesy of Dr. L. F. Rogers and associates, Departments of Radiology and Orthopedic Surgery, Hermann Hospital, Houston, TX.)

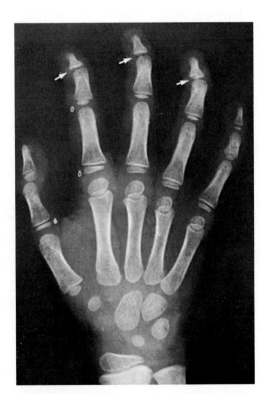

FIGURE 66. Destruction of the epiphyseal cartilages of the terminal phalanges of fingers 2 through 4 of a 5-year-old boy who had severe frostbite 2 years earlier. Similar changes were present in the bones of the other hand. (Courtesy of Dr. K. Kozlowski, Royal Alexandra Hospital for Children, Sydney, Australia.)

and absent early blood pool but delayed bone images; and (3) absent perfusion and blood pool depiction, as well as no delayed bone uptake. The first pattern was interpreted as mild ischemia; the second, ischemia with some superficial tissue infarction requiring minor débridement; and the third, deep tissue and bone infarction requiring amputation.

Necrosis of epiphyseal ossification centers is said to occur in about 30% of cases of frostbite, often without cutaneous changes. Angulation deformities of involved digits usually begin several months after the acute episode. Growth disturbances of phalanges, abnormal angulations, and absence of epiphyseal ossification centers in children should raise the question of prior frostbite exposure. Degenerative arthritis often develops after varying periods of time.

RADIATION INJURY

The epiphyses and epiphyseal-equivalent regions are the most sensitive to radiation injury, so that the predominant effect of radiation in children is growth hindrance. The degree of change is dose dependent. With high doses, premature epiphyseal fusion may occur as well as hypoplasia of the bone. In the hip, SCFE may take place. Reduction of vertebral body height, irregularities of the end plates, and abnormalities of contour may follow irradiation of the spine as in the treatment of abdominal tumors. Scoliosis was frequent in the past but has been reduced by careful selection of portals to avoid partial irradiation of growth plates. Neoplasia induction may develop after radiation therapy in childhood. Osteochondromas are the most frequent tumors occurring; they tend to appear at the

margins of the radiation field after intervals of 17 months to 9 years (Fig. 67). Malignant bone tumors include osteosarcoma, fibrosarcoma, and chondrosarcoma in order of decreasing frequency. Genetic factors may play a role in their development, as in the case of radiation therapy of retinoblastoma.

SUGGESTED READINGS

Fractures and Fracture Healing

Borden S IV: Roentgen recognition of acute plastic bowing of the forearm in children. Am J Roentgenol Radium Ther Nucl Med 1975;125:524–530

Conway JJ: Radionuclide bone scintigraphy in pediatric orthopedics. Pediatr Clin North Am 1986;33:1313–1334

Harcke HT, Grissom LE, Finkelstein MS: Evaluation of the musculoskeletal system with sonography. AJR Am J Roentgenol 1988;150:1253–1261

Keats TE (ed): Atlas of Normal Roentgen Variants That May Simulate Disease, 6th ed. St. Louis, Mosby–Year Book, 1996

Ogden JA: The uniqueness of growing bones. In Rockwood CA Jr, Wilkins KE, King RE (eds): Fractures in Children, vol 3, 3rd ed. Philadelphia, JB Lippincott, 1991:1–86

Oppenheim WL, Davis A, Growdon WA, et al: Clavicle fractures in the newborn. Clin Orthop 1990;250:176–180

Schmidt H, Schmidt JF: Borderlands of Normal and Early Pathologic Findings in Skeletal Radiography, 4th ed. New York, Thieme Medical Publishers, 1993

Injuries to the Cartilage Plate

Brenkel IJ, Dias JJ, Davies TG, et al: Hormone status in patients with slipped capital femoral epiphysis. J Bone Joint Surg Br 1989;71:33–38

Grogan DP, Love SM, Ogden JA, et al: Chondro-osseous growth abnormalities after meningococcemia: a clinical and histopathological study. J Bone Joint Surg Am 1989;71:920–928

Hagglund G, Hansson LI, Ordeberg G, et al: Bilaterality in slipped upper femoral epiphysis. J Bone Joint Surg Br 1988;70:179–181

Jaramillo D, Hoffer FA, Shapiro F, et al: MR imaging of fractures of the growth plate. AJR Am J Roentgenol 1990;155:1261–1265

Kaye JJ, Nance EP Jr: Pain in the athlete's knee. Clin Sports Med 1987;6:873–883

Kelsey JL, Keggi KJ, Southwick WO: The incidence and distribution of slipped capital femoral epiphysis in Connecticut and the Southwestern United States. J Bone Joint Surg Am 1970;52:1203–1216

Klein A, Joplin RJ, Reidy JA, et al: Roentgenographic features of slipped capital femoral epiphysis. Am J Roentgenol Radium Ther 1951;66:361–373

Loder AT, Aronson DD: Epidemiology of bilateral slip of the capital femoral epiphysis. J Bone Joint Surg 1993;75:1141

Mandell GA, Keret D, Harcke HT, Bowen JR: Chondrolysis: detection by bone scintigraphy. J Pediatr Orthop 1992;12:80–85

McAfee PC, Cady RB: Endocrinologic and metabolic factors in atypical presentations of slipped capital femoral epiphysis: report of four cases and review of the literature. Clin Orthop 1983;180:188–197

Medlar RC, Lyne ED: Sinding-Larsen-Johansson disease: its etiology and natural history. J Bone Joint Surg Am 1978;60:1113–1116

Morrissy RT (ed): Slipped capital femoral epiphysis. In Pediatric Orthopedics, vol 2, 3rd ed. Philadelphia, JB Lippincott, 1990:881–904

Ogden JA, Faney TM, Ogden DA: The biological aspects of children's fractures. In Rockwood CA Jr, Wilkins JE, Beaty JH (eds): Fractures in Children, 4th ed. Philadelphia, Lippincott–Raven, 1996:19–52.

Ogden JA, McCarthy SM, Jokl P: The painful bipartite patella. J Pediatr Orthop 1982;2:263–269

Rang M: Children's Fractures. Philadelphia, JB Lippincott, 1974

Salter RB, Harris WR: Injuries involving the epiphyseal plate. J Bone Joint Surg Am 1963;45:587–622

Young JW, Bright RW, Whitley NO: Computed tomography in the evaluation of partial growth plate arrest in children. Skeletal Radiol 1986;15:530–535

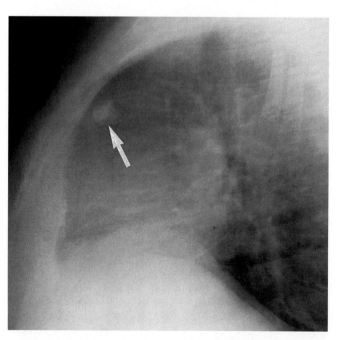

FIGURE 67. Osteochondroma of an anterior rib *(arrow)* in a 20-year-old male who received mediastinal irradiation for Hodgkin's disease.

Types of Pediatric Fractures

Bledsoe RE, Izenmark IL: Displacement of fat pads in disease and injury at the elbow. Radiology 1959;73:717–724

Blumberg K, Patterson RJ: The toddler's cuboid fracture. Radiology 1991;179:93–94

Borden S IV: Roentgen recognition of acute plastic bowing of the forearm in children. Am J Roentgenol Radium Ther Nucl Med 1975;125:524–530

Brogden BG, Crow NE: Little Leaguer's elbow. Am J Roentgenol Radium Ther Nucl Med 1963;83:671–675

Bryan WJ, Tullos HS: Pediatric pelvic fractures: review of 52 patients. J Trauma 1979;19:799–805

Grattan-Smith JD, Wagner ML, Barnes DA: Osteomyelitis of the talus: an unusual cause of limping in childhood. AJR Am J Roentgenol 1991;156:785–789

Junkins EP, Furnival RA, Bolte RG: The clinical presentation of pediatric pelvic fractures. Pediatr Emerg Care 2001;17:15–18

Magid D, Fishman EK, Sponseller PD, Griffin PP: 2D and 3D computed tomography of the pediatric hip. Radiographics 1988;8: 901–933

Penrose JH: The Monteggia fracture with posterior dislocation of the radial head. J Bone Joint Surg Br 1951;33:65–72

Pinckney LE, Currarino G, Kennedy LA: The stubbed great toe: a cause of occult compound fracture and infection. Radiology 1981;138:375–377

Reckling FW, Cordell LD: Unstable fracture-dislocation of the forearm: the Monteggia and Galeazzi lesions. Arch Surg 1968;96:999–1007

Rieger H, Brug E: Fractures of the pelvis in children. Clin Orthop 1997;336:226–239

Rogers LF, Jones S, Davis AR, et al: "Clipping injury" fracture of the epiphysis in the adolescent football player: an occult lesion of the knee. Am J Roentgenol Radium Ther Nucl Med 1974;121:69–78

Salter RB, Zaltz C: Anatomic investigations of the mechanism of injury and pathologic anatomy of "pulled elbow" in young children. Clin Orthop 1971;77:134–143

Shibuya S, Ogawa K: Isolated avulsion fracture of the lesser tuberosity of the humerus: a case report. Clin Orthop 1986;211:215–218

Silber JS, Flynn JM: Changing patterns of pediatric pelvic fractures with skeletal maturation: implications for classification and management. J Pediatr Orthop 2002;22:22–26

Silber JS, Flynn JM, Koffler KM, et al: Analysis of the cause, classification, and associated injuries of 166 consecutive pediatric pelvic fractures. J Pediatr Orthop 2001;21:446–450

Spiegel PG, Mast JW, Cooperman DR, et al: Triplane fractures of the distal tibial epiphysis. Clin Orthop 1984;188:74–89

Starshak RJ, Simons GW, Sty JR: Occult fracture of the calcaneus—another toddler's fracture. Pediatr Radiol 1984;14:37–40

Stefanich RJ, Lozman J: The juvenile fracture of Tillaux. Clin Orthop 1986;210:219–227

Trauma from Physical Agents

Bingham H: Electrical burns. Clin Plast Surg 1986;13:75–85

Brown HC: Current concepts of burn pathology and mechanisms of deformity in the burned hand. Orthop Clin North Am 1973;4: 987–999

Carrera GF, Kozin F, Flaherty L, et al: Radiographic changes in the hands following childhood frostbite injury. Skeletal Radiol 1981;6: 33–37

Dalinka MK, Neustadter LM: Radiation changes. In Resnick D, Niwayama G (eds): Diagnosis of Bone and Joint Disorders, vol 5, 2nd ed. Philadelphia, WB Saunders, 1988:3024–3055

Lee RC, Kolodney MS: Electrical injury mechanisms: dynamics of the thermal response. Plast Reconstr Surg 1987;80:663–671

Mehta RC, Wilson MA: Frostbite injury: prediction of tissue viability with triple-phase bone scanning. Radiology 1989;170:511–514

Oeconomopoulos CT: Electrical burns in infancy and early childhood: a review of the current literature. Am J Dis Child 1962;103:35–38

Ogden JA, Southwick WO: Electrical injury involving the immature skeleton. Skeletal Radiol 1981;6:187–192

Riseborough EJ, Grabias SL, Burton RI, et al: Skeletal alterations following irradiation for Wilms' tumor: with particular reference to scoliosis and kyphosis. J Bone Joint Surg Am 1976;58:526–536

Rutan RL, Herndon DN: Growth delay in postburn pediatric patients. Arch Surg 1990;125:392–395

Wenzl JE, Burke EC, Bianco AJ Jr: Epiphyseal destruction from frostbite of the hands. Am J Dis Child 1967;114:668–670

PART IX

CHILD ABUSE

DANIELLE K. B. BOAL

OVERVIEW

In the decades since the landmark articles by Caffey in 1946 and by Kempe and Silverman, the medical community, law enforcement, and child protective services (CPS) have developed a much greater awareness of and sensitivity to the diagnosis of child abuse, and a more aggressive approach toward the identification and prosecution of offending individuals. While reports of various agencies vary somewhat, according to the most recent survey from Peddle and Wang in 1999, a total of 3,224,000 children were reported to CPS as alleged victims of child abuse, and approximately 1 million of these reports were confirmed. Thus 46 out of every 1000 children in the United States were reported and 15 out of every 1000 children were confirmed as abused or neglected in 1999. Neglect accounts for 51% of confirmed cases, physical abuse 26%, sexual abuse 10%, emotional maltreatment 4%, and other forms of maltreatment 9%. Young children are at greatest risk for fatality, with 78% under the age of 5 years at time of death and 38% less than 1 year of age at death as reported by Wang and Daro. In neglect and physical abuse cases, female perpetrators predominate at 60%. More than 70% of all confirmed perpetrators have a parental relationship to the victim (mother, father, stepparent, paramour of parent), with some studies reporting as high as 80% of all child victims being abused by one or both parents. Neglect and abuse remain a difficult and emotionally charged topic. Occurring behind closed doors, it is unobserved and confessions are rare. There are varied presentations, and abuse and neglect may mimic other disease processes.

Although there is significant morbidity and mortality, the diagnosis and treatment of child abuse are intertwined with legal issues of parental rights and family preservation. Lack of research support further impairs progress in finding practical solutions that will protect children at risk and at the same time avoid erroneous accusations. As reported in SCAN, according to the National Institutes of Health, the amount of funded research devoted to abuse, at $3.33 for each new confirmed case per year, is less than that devoted to all other funded pediatric diseases, such as pediatric acquired immunodeficiency syndrome, which is funded at $6,346.15 per year for each new case diagnosed. The current system of CPS is overwhelmed, underfunded, and understaffed. Approximately 41% of the children who die as a result of abuse are known to CPS agencies as current or prior clients at the time of death. Abuse and neglect are truly societal issues. These dismal statistics will not improve until the risk factors, such as poverty, drugs, ignorance, and isolation, are identified and addressed.

ROLE OF IMAGING

Radiologic imaging has evolved to play a major role in the diagnosis of physical abuse, and, with the advent of nuclear medicine, ultrasonography, computed tomography (CT), and magnetic resonance imaging (MRI), its usefulness is no longer limited to the identification of bony trauma. CT and MRI are the primary diagnostic modalities in the diagnosis of abusive head trauma, including shaken baby syndrome with or without impact. The role of diagnostic imaging is threefold:

1. Recognition of physical abuse, supporting the diagnosis in suspected cases, and recognizing characteristic lesions when the possibility of child abuse has not been suspected
2. As evidence in the prosecution or defense of offenders by understanding the mechanism, pattern of healing (dating), and likelihood of such injuries with a reasonable degree of medical certainty
3. Exclusion of the diagnosis of child abuse in cases of true accidental trauma or variants of normal and disease processes that may mimic abuse.

IMAGING FINDINGS

Abused infants and children are rarely brought to medical attention with an accurate history. Often the radiologist will be the first to suggest the possibility of child abuse when characteristic lesions are identified on imaging studies. With the possible exception of the classic metaphyseal lesion and multiple rib fractures in infancy, it is risky to state unequivocally that certain patterns or types of fractures are pathognomonic of abuse. Each case must be considered individually with respect to the history provided and the possibility of underlying abnormalities that would predispose to fracture, such as history of prematurity, metabolic disease, or dysplasia. With that proviso, certain patterns and types of skeletal injury occur more or less commonly as a result of abuse (Table 1). When a child presents with an injury, it is necessary to consider whether the explanation offered for that injury is plausible, and if the developmental level of the child is consistent with that history.

Multiple fractures at variable locations in different stages of healing are well described and continue to be highly specific for child abuse, unless an underlying bone dysplasia or metabolic abnormality is diagnosed (Figs. 1 and 2). Patterns of injury, including distribution and characteristic traumatic lesions unique to abuse, have been studied and reported by various authors. It is now recognized that fractures to the rib cage, metaphyseal fractures, and skull fractures predominate in infants under 1 year of age, whereas the diaphyseal fracture is more common in the older infant and child. The appropriateness of the history in relationship to the mechanism of injury(s) is the first and most important clue to the diagnosis of nonaccidental or abuse injuries. Infants who cannot walk do not normally incur fractures from unintentional injury events. A fall from 3 to 4 feet to a hard surface may result in a linear parietal skull fracture, but rarely do long bones fracture or central nervous system (CNS) injuries occur in this circum-

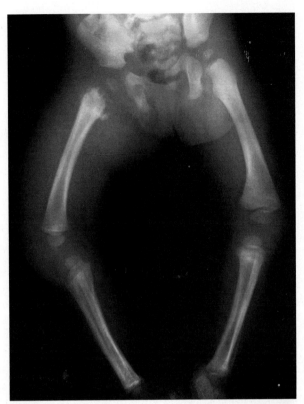

FIGURE 1. A 7-month-old female brought to the emergency room for swelling of thigh. Skeletal survey revealed 54 fractures, including 35 rib fractures and 19 fractures of long bones. Anteroposterior film of pelvis and lower extremities reveals chronic traumatic epiphysiolysis at the proximal right femur. Well-organized periosteal healing bone is seen about shaft of both femurs. Abnormal modeling of proximal right tibia is the result of healed injury. Classic metaphyseal lesions are seen at proximal left femur, both distal femurs, proximal left tibia, and both distal tibias, and the infant has a swollen right thigh.

stance. Midshaft transverse, spiral, and oblique diaphyseal fractures of the femur and humerus in a young infant are almost always inflicted, as are rib fractures and the classical metaphyseal fracture.

DIAPHYSEAL FRACTURES

Solitary long bone fractures may occur following nonintentional trauma in the older infant and child; however, factors that increase the likelihood of an abuse injury include association with another fracture or other clinical features with a high suspicion for abuse, inappropriate clinical history, failure to seek medical attention, and discovery of the fracture in a healing state. Diaphyseal fractures may be transverse, oblique, or spiral, and it is risky to assign significance to the type of fracture because all occur with unintentional or true accidental trauma as well as abuse.

Particular note is made of the spiral diaphyseal fracture, because this fracture has erroneously become synonymous with abuse. The spiral nature of the fracture indicates that torque was a component of the stress applied resulting in fracture. The fracture is thought to

---

**Table 1 ■ SKELETAL INJURIES
FROM ABUSE**

Common
Multiple fractures (unsuspected and/or varying in age)
Classic metaphyseal lesions*
Multiple rib fractures*
Diaphyseal fractures (nonambulatory infant/child)
Skull fractures
Subperiosteal new bone formation

Less Common
Spinal fractures
Fractures of small bones of hands and feet
Clavicular fractures
Dislocations and epiphyseal separations

Uncommon
Scapular fractures*
Pelvic fractures
Sternal fractures
Facial and mandibular fractures

*High specificity for abuse in infants.

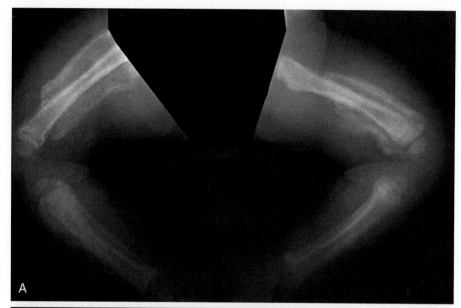

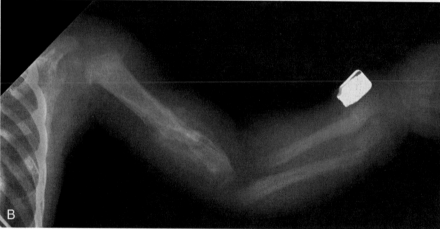

FIGURE 2. A 3-month-old female with 30 fractures of long bones and ribs. **A,** Frog lateral projection of lower extremities shows extensive proliferation of callus and subperiosteal new bone with metaphyseal fractures. Callus extends into physeal regions. Traumatic epiphysiolysis was evident at proximal right hip (not included on radiograph). Subsequent growth arrest at multiple sites required surgical intervention. **B,** Anteroposterior film of left upper extremity shows transverse fractures of distal diaphyses of radius and ulna, classic metaphyseal lesion of proximal humerus, and mid-humeral diaphyseal healed oblique fracture.

occur when an infant is grabbed or shaken, using the extremity as a handle. However, spiral fractures do occur in a child who is ambulatory, and we now know that they may occur accidentally in younger infants. One mechanism was graphically illustrated and reported by Hymel when a 5-month-old infant was videotaped lying prone; the extended upper extremity was unable to adduct as the baby was rolled from the prone to the supine position. What is most important to consider, when presented with a spiral fracture, is the explanation offered and developmental level of the child, in addition to the age of the fracture at presentation and whether or not there are other injuries.

Nonaccidental fractures of the hands and feet occur in abused infants and toddlers. These fractures are often subtle, are frequently torus fractures, and may be better appreciated on oblique views.

in 1986 using detailed histopathologic and radiographic studies. He determined that this traumatic lesion seen in infancy as a result of shaking abuse is indeed a complete shearing or planar fracture extending through the primary spongiosa of the metaphysis, not an avulsion injury as described by Caffey. Depending on the amount of metaphyseal bone that is included in the fracture fragment and the radiographic projection, this highly specific metaphyseal lesion for abuse may project as a corner or bucket-handle fracture (Fig. 3).

The *classic metaphyseal lesion,* as coined by Kleinman, occurs with violent shaking as the infant is held by the trunk or extremities (Figs. 4 through 8). Typically there is no bruising or outward sign of injury. The same can be said for rib fractures, the most common fracture from abuse in infants under 1 year of age.

METAPHYSEAL FRACTURES

The classic metaphyseal lesion first described by Caffey in 1974 and commonly referred to as a corner or bucket-handle fracture was re-examined by Kleinman

RIB FRACTURES

Kleinman, Marks, Nimkin, and colleagues found that 51% of all fractures in 31 infants who died from abuse involved the rib cage. Rib fractures from abuse are

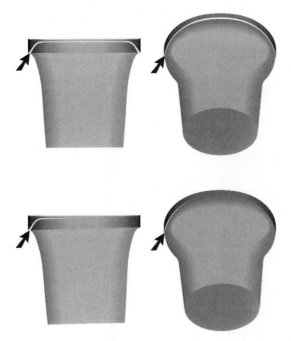

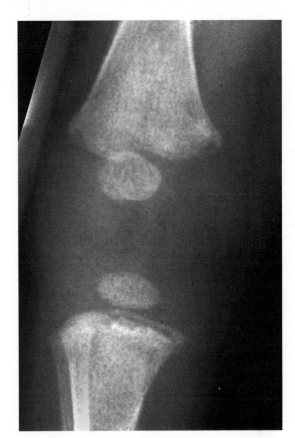

FIGURE 3. General diagram of the corner fracture and bucket-handle patterns of a classic metaphyseal lesion (CML). Fractures *(arrows)* extend adjacent to the chondro-osseous junction *(COJ)* and then veer toward the diaphysis to undercut the larger peripheral segment that encompasses the subperiosteal bone collar. When the physis is viewed tangentially, the CML appears as a corner fracture pattern (**left** images). When a view is obtained with beam angulation, a bucket-handle pattern results (**right** images). **Top images,** Diffuse injury. **Bottom images,** localized injury. (From Kleinman PK: Diagnostic Imaging of Child Abuse, 2nd ed. St. Louis, Mosby, 1998:18, with permission. Originally modified from Kleinman PK, Marks SC Jr: Relationship of the subperiosteal bone collar to metaphyseal lesions in abused infants. J Bone Joint Surg Am 1995;77:1471–1476.)

FIGURE 4. A 2½–month-old male infant with acute-on-chronic subdural hematoma and 18 fractures. Anteroposterior radiograph of right knee shows classic metaphyseal lesions at distal femur and proximal tibia.

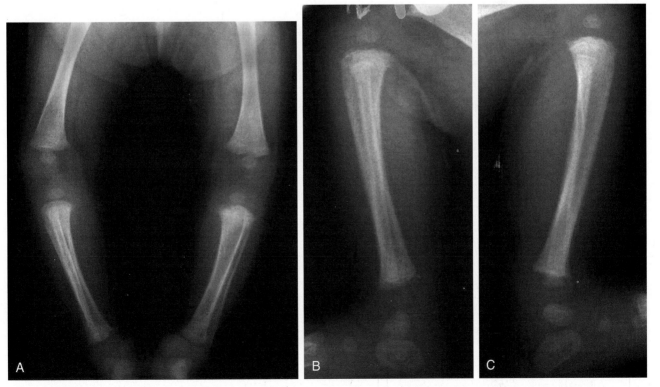

FIGURE 5. A 1-month-old female infant presented with bruising and swelling of buttocks. Her father confessed to aggravated assault. **A,** Anteroposterior radiograph of lower extremities. **B,** Lateral radiograph of right lower leg. **C,** Lateral radiograph of left lower leg shows classic metaphyseal lesions at distal femurs and both proximal and distal tibias.

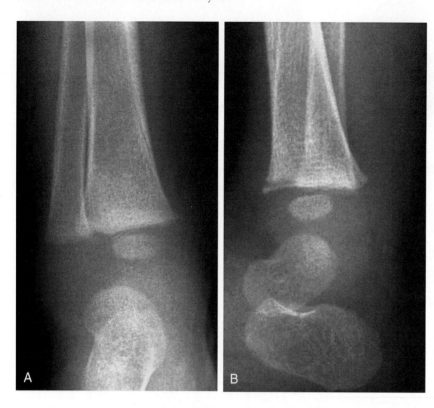

FIGURE 6. Anteroposterior **(A)** and lateral **(B)** radiographs of an 11-month-old infant sustained severe closed head injury with retinal hemorrhages from shaken baby syndrome while in the care of a babysitter. The only other injury is a classic metaphyseal lesion of the distal left tibia.

occult; the astute clinician may palpate callus with healing, but otherwise there is typically no physical sign of injury. Moreover, acute rib fractures are easily overlooked on radiographs and frequently not appreciated until there is evidence of healing (Fig. 9). Rib fractures may occur at any point along the arc of the rib (costovertebral, posterior, lateral, anterior, and costo-

chondral) but frequently involve the posterior rib. There is excellent scientific evidence that posterior rib fractures at the costovertebral junction have a high specificity for abuse. Boal, in a roundtable discussion, noted that, if one compares individual sites along the rib arc, costovertebral junction fractures outnumbered each other individual site in a large population of 141

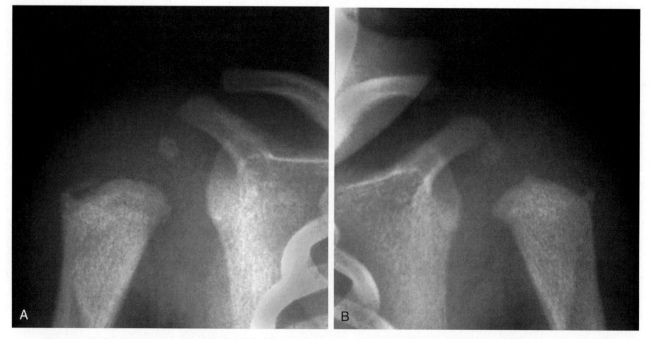

FIGURE 7. Anteroposterior right **(A)** and left **(B)** shoulders of a 5-month-old female infant, deceased, cause of death unknown; both parents are drug abusers. Eight fractures were identified at postmortem skeletal survey, including bilateral proximal humeral classic metaphyseal lesion.

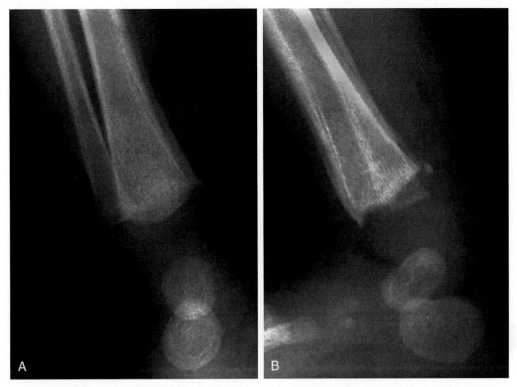

FIGURE 8. Anteroposterior **(A)** and lateral **(B)** radiographs of a 2-month-old female, one of identical twins. Her twin was the index case, with severe bruising, torn frenulum, and multiple fractures. Screening skeletal survey on this twin revealed spine and metaphyseal fractures and a classic metaphyseal lesion of the distal right tibia.

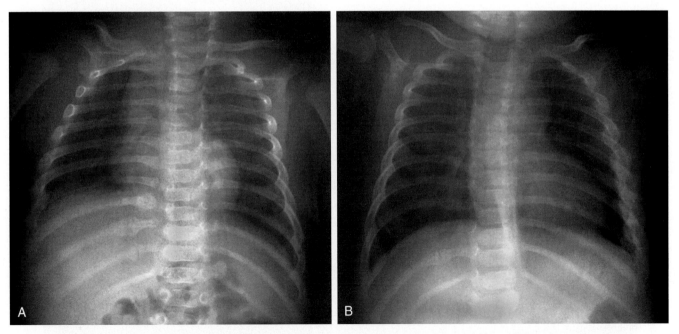

FIGURE 9. A 6-week-old male infant who was sent for upper gastrointestinal series to evaluate colicky pain was found to have healing rib fractures. **A,** Initial chest x-ray identifies healing fractures at the right 9th, 10th, and 11th ribs. **B,** Follow-up chest film 2 weeks later shows additional acute fractures, now healing, at the lateral aspect of the left third through ninth ribs. Father admitted to shaking the infant.

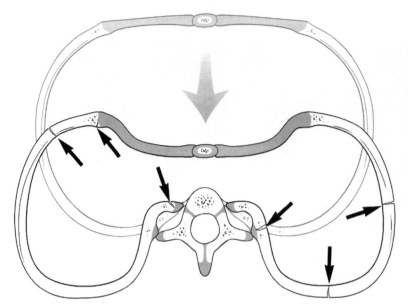

FIGURE 10. Diagram of mechanism of injury to ribs. With anteroposterior compression of the chest, there is excessive leverage of the posterior ribs over the fulcrum of the transverse processes. This places tension along the inner aspects of the rib head and neck regions, resulting in fractures at these sites *(arrows)*. This mechanism is also consistent with the morphologic patterns of injury occurring at other sites along the rib arcs and at the costochondral junctions *(arrows)*. (From Kleinman PK: Diagnostic Imaging of Child Abuse, 2nd ed. St. Louis, Mosby, 1998:116, with permission.)

abused patients with 1463 rib fractures. However, if one looks at the costovertebral junction site as compared to all other fracture sites collectively, the costovertebral junction represented only 33% of the total number of rib fractures in this abuse population.

A squeezing, shaking injury with compression of the sternum posteriorly results in levering of the posterior rib arc over the transverse process and abnormal impaction and distraction forces to the lateral and anterior rib arc and the metaphyseal equivalent at the costovertebral junction of the posterior rib (Figs. 10 and 11). Multiple fractures may involve a single rib

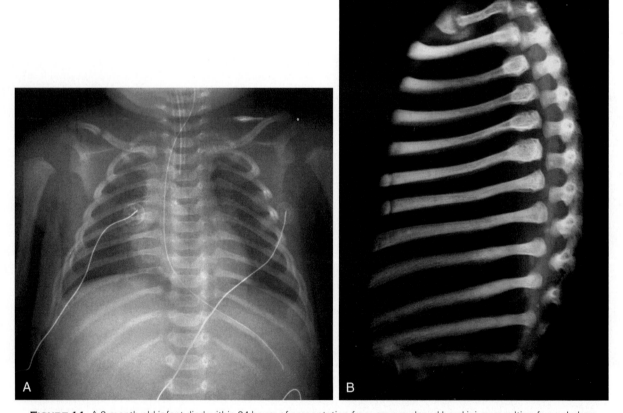

FIGURE 11. A 2-month-old infant died within 24 hours of presentation from severe closed head injury resulting from shaken baby syndrome. There were 33 fractures of ribs and long bones. **A,** Portable anteroposterior chest radiograph taken prior to death reveals multiple bilateral costovertebral junction rib fractures and fractures of both first ribs, as well as midshaft fracture of the right clavicle. **B,** Faxitron image of postmortem right ribs better demonstrates classical clubbing and callus at the costovertebral junction of the first through sixth ribs, and posterolateral fracture of right first rib.

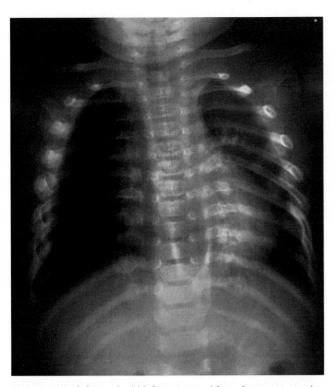

FIGURE 12. A 3-month-old infant returned from foster care to the mother and boyfriend was found 6 weeks later to have 26 rib fractures and a linear skull fracture. Anteroposterior chest radiograph shows multiple lateral and posterior costovertebral junction rib fractures bilaterally.

(Fig. 12). Nuclear scintigraphy will aid in the detection of rib fractures and plays a complimentary role to radiography (Fig. 13). Oblique views of the chest and CT also provide increased sensitivity. Unlike the adult rib, fractures do not occur in the infant rib following cardiopulmonary resuscitation, and there are numerous reports in the literature to support that finding. Although there are several case reports of rib fractures occurring as a result of birth trauma, confirmed by personal experience, rib fractures in infants under the age of 12 months without a predisposing condition such as prematurity or bronchopulmonary dysplasia, like the classic metaphyseal lesion, are highly specific for the diagnosis of abuse.

FRACTURE OF THE SCAPULA

Any part of the skeleton may be traumatized from abuse. Although uncommon, fracture of the scapula, in particular the acromion, is highly specific for abuse (Fig. 14). It results from abnormal indirect forces applied during shaking and is usually accompanied by other bony thoracic trauma. A normal anatomic variant in the ossification of the acromion may present a diagnostic dilemma. Follow-up films to assess whether or not there is healing will allow discrimination between fracture and ossification variant (see Section IX, Part III, Chapter 2, Fig. 1, page 2054).

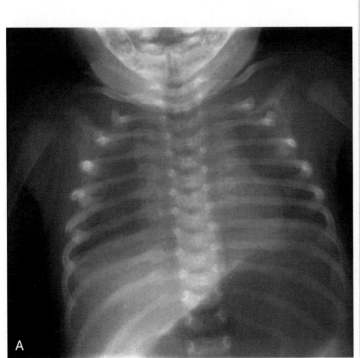

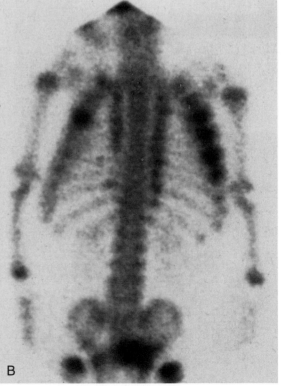

FIGURE 13. A 17-day-old infant presented with hemothorax and flail chest. The mother's paramour admitted throwing the baby against a wall after shaking. **A,** Anteroposterior chest radiograph taken 6 days after injury reveals multiple fractures at costovertebral junction and lateral ribs bilaterally. **B,** Posterior image from bone scintigraphy performed the same day shows multiple posterior and lateral rib fractures.

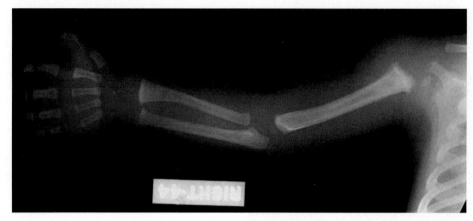

FIGURE 14. Anteroposterior radiograph of right upper extremity in a 4-month-old male infant whose father confessed to abuse reveals fracture of acromion, classic metaphyseal lesion of proximal humerus, and buckle fracture of the distal second metacarpal.

SPINAL FRACTURES

Also rare, spinal fractures in infants and young children are highly associated with abuse (Fig. 15). The mechanism is thought to be hyperextension, hyperflexion, and/or axial loading. Radiographically, the injuries manifest as compression deformities of the vertebral body, often with associated end plate defects and avulsive injuries of the spinous processes. Commonly involving multiple vertebral bodies, the injury is often located near the thoracolumbar junction. More severe fracture–dislocations have been described in addition to the classical hangman's fracture of the C2 vertebral body (Fig. 16). Although spinal cord injury is uncommon, severe spinal cord injury without radiographic

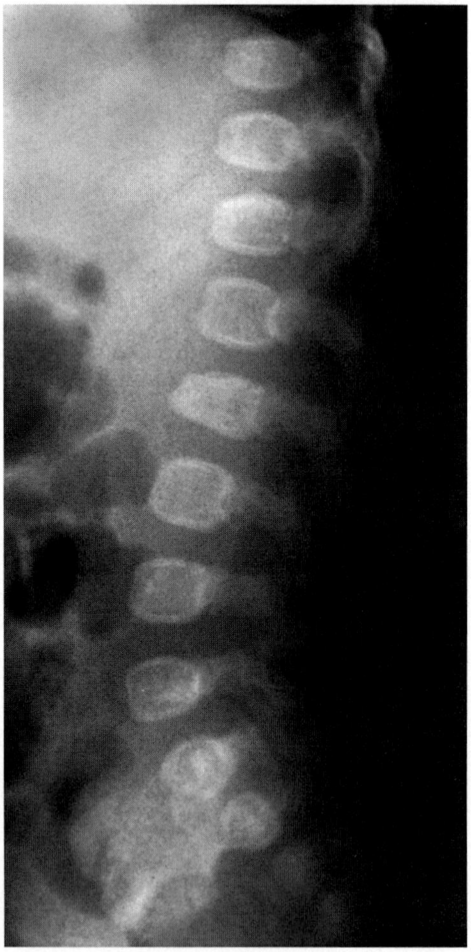

FIGURE 15. Lateral radiograph of the spine in a 2-month-old female infant (same patient as Fig. 8) shows a compression fracture of the L2 vertebral body.

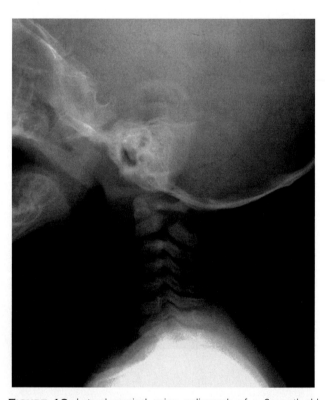

FIGURE 16. Lateral cervical spine radiograph of a 6-month-old infant who presented with bruising over left neck. Although the infant is neurologically intact, there are 14 fractures, including a hangman's fracture of C2. Four months later, computed tomography showed complete healing of bilateral pedicle fractures of C2 vertebral body.

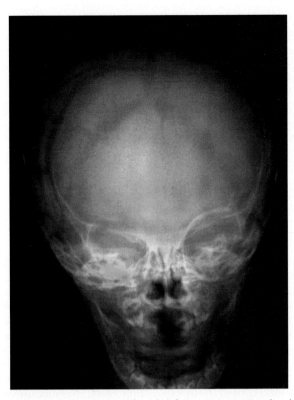

FIGURE 17. In a 5-month-old female infant, an anteroposterior skull radiograph shows a diastatic stellate right parietal fracture with diastasis of sutures and extension across the sagittal suture into the left parietal bone. There are associated right frontal and posterior interhemispheric subdural hematomas. The mother's paramour pleaded guilty to reckless endangerment.

abnormality (SCIWORA) has been described in the shaken infant.

SKULL FRACTURES

Skull fractures are frequent in abuse and always indicative of an impact injury to the head, but there is poor correlation between the presence of fracture and associated intracranial injury. Several authors have tried to characterize specific patterns of injury occurring in abuse and thus distinguish abuse skull fractures from true accidental skull fractures. There is some agreement that multiple fractures, bilateral fractures, diastasis of

fractures and sutures, and fractures that cross suture lines are significantly associated with abuse (Fig. 17). However, no particular pattern of skull fracture is diagnostic of abuse. Bilateral complex fractures crossing the sagittal suture may result from a single high-impact blow to the midline, and simple linear fractures are seen in both abuse and accidental trauma. One must consider the appropriateness of the history with respect to the type of injury in trying to make the distinction of abuse versus accidental trauma. Anteroposterior (AP) and lateral skull films should always be part of the radiographic skeletal survey in suspected abuse; additional views may be necessary. CT alone is inadequate because skull fractures may be overlooked in the axial plane.

DATING OF FRACTURES

Dating of fractures is dependent on many variables, including age of the child, state of nutrition, immobilization of fracture and/or possibility of repetitive injury, and fracture location. Fractures of the skull and spine cannot be satisfactorily dated, and the classic metaphyseal lesion is also difficult to date with any degree of precision. In general, a young infant will develop subperiosteal new bone much earlier and form callus more quickly. The range for the appearance of subperiosteal new bone is 4 days to several weeks. Soft tissue swelling resolves during this same time period, with subsequent loss of fracture line definition and the appearance of soft callus followed by hard callus. Remodeling of fractures occurs over a span of months to years. Precise dating of fractures is not possible, but some general guidelines are provided in Table 2.

RADIOGRAPHIC EVALUATION

In all cases of suspected physical abuse in children less than 2 years of age, a skeletal survey is mandatory (Table 3). A "babygram," a single or several films of the entire infant, is unsatisfactory. High-detail film used without a grid is recommended; the American College of Radiology recommends imaging systems with a spatial resolution of 10 line pairs/mm and film speed of no more than 200. There are limited data at present

Table 2 ■ TIMETABLE OF RADIOLOGIC CHANGES IN CHILDREN'S FRACTURES*

CATEGORY	EARLY	PEAK	LATE
1: Resolution of soft tissues	2–5 days	4–10 days	10–21 days
2: SPNBF†	4–10 days	10–14 days	14–21 days
3: Loss of fracture line definition	10–14 days	14–21 days	
4: Soft callus	10–14 days	14–21 days	
5: Hard callus	14–21 days	21–24 days	42–90 days
6: Remodeling	3 mo	1 yr	2 yr to physeal closure

*Repetitive injuries may prolong categories 1, 2, 5, and 6.
†Subperiosteal new bone formation.
From Kleinman PK: Diagnostic Imaging of Child Abuse, 2nd ed. St. Louis, Mosby, 1998:176, with permission.

Table 3 ■ SKELETAL SURVEY*

Anteroposterior (AP) and lateral of skull
AP and lateral of spine
AP and both obliques (right posterior, left posterior) of chest
AP of pelvis and hips
AP and frog lateral of lower extremities
AP of upper extremities (shoulder through wrist)
Posteroanterior of hands
AP of feet
Lateral of sternum

*Additional collimated projections are recommended for all questioned abnormalities. Follow-up survey films in 10 to 14 days often confirm or refute questionable findings.

comparing the efficacy of filmless or digital radiography to that of conventional radiography.

The initial survey should include AP and lateral views of the skull and spine with AP and lateral views of the extremities to include hands and feet. Additional views of any suspected abnormality must be obtained (Fig. 18). In addition to an AP view of the chest, it is now recognized that oblique views increase the screening sensitivity for rib fractures (Fig. 19). A follow-up skeletal survey performed 2 weeks after the initial exam frequently adds additional information (see Fig. 9). As noted by Kleinman, the follow-up survey can also (1) detect additional fractures, (2) differentiate fractures from normal developmental variants, and (3) assist in dating injuries. In the child older than 5 years, skeletal scintigraphy may be substituted, but neither radiographic nor scintigraphic screening have proven utility

in the older child. For infants and children under 2 years, nuclear scintigraphy should be viewed as a complimentary modality to x-ray evaluation. The imaging evaluation of children between 2 and 5 years in age must be assessed individually.

CT and/or MRI of the brain is necessary for any infant with suspected CNS injury. CT is adequate for the emergent work-up, but follow-up MRI in select cases identifies injuries not appreciated on CT and provides greater detail and understanding of the pathophysiology of abusive head injuries. Contrast-enhanced CT is indicated in any child with suspected blunt trauma to the abdomen or pelvis.

DIFFERENTIAL DIAGNOSIS

True accidental injury is not the only consideration in the differential for child abuse. Unrecognized obstetric trauma, normal metaphyseal variants, physiologic new bone formation, variation in acromion ossification, accessory skull sutures, and other conditions may all, on first inspection, initially suggest an abuse lesion. Rickets of prematurity may result in multiple rib fractures. Other disease processes, including inherited bone dysplasias, copper deficiency, congenital syphilis, neurologic disorders, and osteogenesis imperfecta, in particular, may have radiographic features that overlap with those of abuse (Table 4). Kleinman's text presents an excellent overview of the differential diagnosis and review of diseases simulating abuse. Fortunately, it is almost always possible to make an accurate determina-

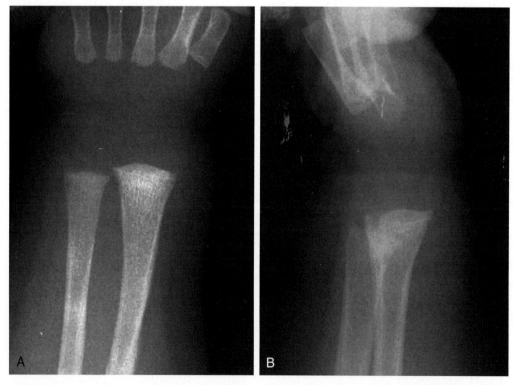

FIGURE 18. Radiologic evidence of abuse in a 2-month-old female infant. **A,** Anteroposterior view of the right wrist demonstrates a subtle irregularity of the radial metaphysis. **B,** Lateral view confirms healing classic metaphyseal lesion.

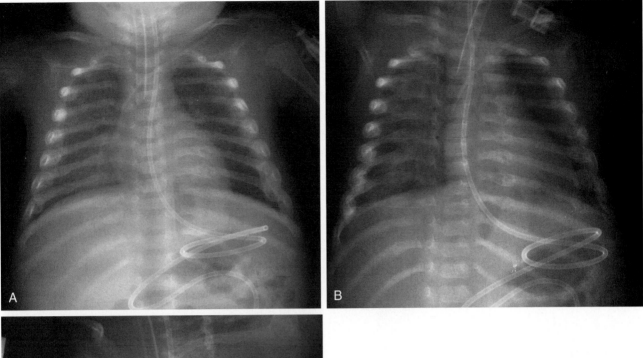

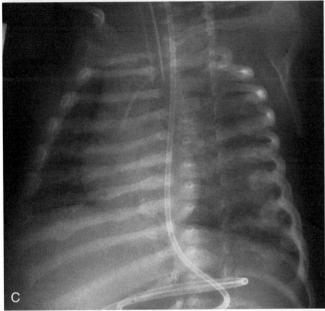

FIGURE 19. A, Anteroposterior radiograph of a 4-month-old female infant with 41 rib fractures. (Older sibling of this patient previously removed to foster care for abuse.) Fractures are better depicted with aid of left posterior oblique **(B)** and right posterior oblique **(C)** chest x-rays.

tion as to the presence or absence of genetic disease based on clinical and radiographic examination, and review of family and social history.

A well-publicized controversy with respect to accidental versus nonaccidental fractures in infancy is that of temporary brittle bone disease (TBBD). This was proposed as a variant of osteogenesis imperfecta by Patterson and colleagues, who identified a group of young infants thought to have diminished bone strength, possibly on the basis of a temporary deficiency of a metalloenzyme such as copper. Supporting evidence for the existence of TBBD has been listed as caregivers deny wrongdoing, no episode of trauma to explain fractures, no bruising, no systemic injuries, radiographs reveal normal bones, and laboratory studies are normal. This particular diagnosis has been

refuted by other researchers, and to date there is no definitive scientific proof as to its existence.

MORBIDITY AND MORTALITY

The morbidity and mortality associated with nonaccidental or abusive head injury has been recognized for some time. Caffey coined the term *whiplash shaken baby* over 20 years ago. Unlike in true accidental head injury, the neurologic deficits that occur in shaken baby syndrome are out of proportion to both the degree of physical trauma and changes present on CT and MRI. Retinal hemorrhages are present in 80% to 85% of shaken babies, in addition to intracranial injury and often skeletal trauma. There is debate as to whether or

Table 4 ■ DIFFERENTIAL DIAGNOSTIC CONSIDERATIONS

Trauma
True accidental
Birth trauma

Variants of Ossification and Maturation
Acromion
Metaphyseal
Accessory skull sutures
Physiologic periosteal new bone

Metabolic
Bone disease of prematurity
Copper deficiency (Menkes' syndrome)
Rickets
Vitamin A toxicity

Dysplasia
Osteogenesis imperfecta
Metaphyseal and spondylometaphyseal dysplasias

Drug Induced
Prostaglandin E_1 therapy

Neurogenic
Spina bifida
Congenital insensitivity to pain

Miscellaneous
Caffey's disease
Congenital syphilis
Neoplastic-metastatic round cell tumors

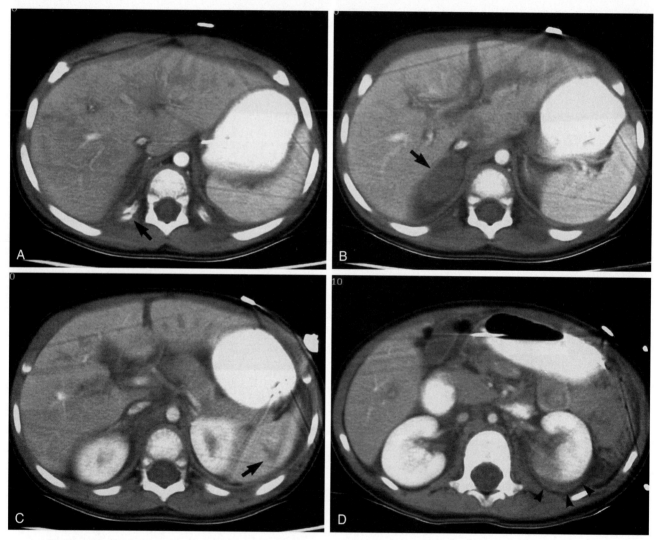

FIGURE 20. A 24-month-old female beaten and abandoned by her mother presented with subdural hemorrhage, retinal hemorrhages, and skeletal and abdominal trauma. Computed tomography of abdomen with oral and intravenous contrast was used to assess her injuries. **A,** Axial image shows subtle liver laceration in the right lobe and fracture of the twelfth rib *(arrow)*. **B,** Right adrenal hemorrhage *(arrow)*. **C,** Splenic laceration *(arrow)*. **D,** Contusion of the medial cushion of the left kidney with perinephric urinoma *(arrowheads)*.

not shaking alone is sufficient to result in brain injury or whether an impact injury must accompany the shaking event. Using models equipped with accelerometers, Duhaime et al. provided experimental evidence that shaking with impact of the head increases the magnitude of angular deceleration forces by 50 times. Whether shaking is done alone or accompanied by impact, it is the abnormal movement of the infant brain within the skull that results in diffuse axonal injury, subdural and subarachnoid hemorrhages, and apnea leading to cerebral hypoxia. Shaking an infant is a violent act, and blows to the head with or without skull fractures are frequent. The critical question is whether or not the head injury is inflicted or accidental. The baby may be shaken alone; shaken and impacted; or shaken, choked, and impacted. The outcome for each is often fatal. Neuroimaging is necessary in all infants with suspected shaken and/or shaken–impact injury, using CT emergently and MRI for more detailed evaluation of the brain.

The other major cause of morbidity and mortality in child abuse is visceral injury from thoracoabdominal trauma. In contrast to CNS injury from abuse, which occurs more commonly in infants under 12 months, abdominal/pelvic and thoracic injury is more common in the toddler and young child. Blunt trauma from physical assault results in contusion and laceration of the solid viscera and mesentery and perforation and/or hematoma of the bowel (Fig. 20). The fatality rate may be as high as 50%, usually the result of shock from hemorrhage or peritonitis, compounded by delay in seeking medical treatment. CT with intravenous contrast is the most readily available and efficacious way to evaluate suspected abusive trauma of the abdomen/pelvis and chest.

SUGGESTED READINGS

Ablin DS, Greenspan A, Reinhart M, et al: Differentiation of child abuse from osteogenesis imperfecta. AJR Am J Roentgenol 1990;154:1035–1046

Ablin DS, Sane SM: Non-accidental injury: confusion with temporary brittle bone disease and mild osteogenesis imperfecta. Pediatr Radiol 1997;27:111–113

American Academy of Pediatrics, Section on Radiology: Diagnostic Imaging of Child Abuse. Pediatrics 2000;105:1345–1348

American Academy of Pediatrics: News Letter of the section of child abuse and neglect (SCAN). 1999;2:6

American College of Radiology: ACR standards for skeletal surveys in children. Resolution 22. Reston, VA: Am Coll Radiol 1997;23

Billmire ME, Myers PA: Serious head injury in infants: accident or abuse? Pediatrics 1985;75:340–342

Boal DKB: Child abuse roundtable discussion: controversial aspects of child abuse. 43rd Annual Meeting of the Society for Pediatric Radiology. Pediatr Radiol 2001;31:760–774

Brown JK, Minns RA: Non-accidental head injury, with particular reference to whiplash shaking injury and medico-legal aspects. Dev Med Child Neurol 1993;35:849–869

Caffey J: Multiple fractures in the long bones of infants suffering from chronic subdural hematoma. Am J Roentgenol Radium Ther 1946;56:163–173

Caffey J: The whiplash-shaken-infant syndrome: manual shaking by the extremities with whiplash-induced intracranial and intraocular bleedings, linked with residual permanent brain damage and mental retardation. Pediatrics 1974;54:396–403

Carty HML: Fractures caused by child abuse. J Bone Joint Surg Br 1993;75:849–857

Chadwick DL, Chin S, Salerno C, et al: Deaths from falls in children: how far is fatal? J Trauma 1991;31:1353–1355

Cohen RA, Kaufman RA, Myers PA, et al: Cranial computed tomography in the abused child with head injury. AJR Am J Roentgenol 1986;146:97–102

Conway EE: Non-accidental head injury in infants: the shaken-baby syndrome revisited. Pediatr Ann 1998;27:677–690

Duhaime AC, Christian CW, Rorke LB, et al: Non-accidental head injury in the infants—the "shaken-baby syndrome." N Engl J Med 1998;338:1822–1829

Duhaime AC, Gennarelli TA, Thibault LE: The shaken baby syndrome. J Neurosurg 1987;66:409–415

Feldman KW, Brewer KD: Child abuse, cardiopulmonary resuscitation, and rib fractures. Pediatrics 1984;73:339–342

Feldman KW, Brewer DK, Shaw DW: Evolution of the cranial computed tomography scan in child abuse. Child Abuse Negl 1995;19:307–314

Han KB, Towbin RB, DeCourten-Myers G, et al: Reversal sign of CT: effect of anoxic/ischemic cerebral injury in children. AJR Am J Roentgenol 1990;154:361–368

Helfer RE, Slovis TL, Black M: Injuries resulting when small children fall out of bed. Pediatrics 1977;60:533–535

Hobbs CJ: Skull fracture and the diagnosis of abuse. Arch Dis Child 1984;59:246–252

Hymel KP: Abusive spiral fractures of the humerus: a videotaped exception. Arch Dis Child 1996;150:226–227

Johnson DL, Boal D, Baule R: Role of apnea in nonaccidental head injury. Pediatr Neurosurg 1995;23:305–310

Kempe CH, Silverman FN, Steele BF, et al: The battered child syndrome. JAMA 1962;181:17–24

Kleinman PK: The metaphyseal lesion in abused infants: a radiologic-histopathologic study. AJR Am J Roentgenol 1986;146:895–905

Kleinman PK: Diagnostic imaging in infant abuse. AJR Am J Roentgenol 1990;155:703–712

Kleinman PK: Diagnostic Imaging of Child Abuse, 2nd ed. St. Louis, Mosby, 1998

Kleinman PK, Belanger PL, Karellas A, et al: Normal metaphyseal radiologic variants not to be confused with findings of infant abuse. AJR Am J Roentgenol 1991;156:781–783

Kleinman PK, Marks SC, Adams VI, et al: Factors affecting visualization of posterior rib fractures in abused infants. AJR Am J Roentgenol 1988;150:635–638

Kleinman PK, Marks SC, Nimkin K, et al: Rib fractures in 31 abused infants: postmortem radiologic-histopathologic study. Radiology 1996;200:807–810

Kleinman PK, Marks SC, Richmond JM, et al: Inflicted skeletal injury: a postmortem radiologic-histopathologic study in 31 infants. AJR Am J Roentgenol 1995;165:647–650

Kleinman PK, Marks SC, Spevak MR, et al: Fractures of the rib head in abused infants. Radiology 1992;185:119–123

Krugman RD, et al: Shaken baby syndrome: inflicted cerebral trauma. American Academy of Pediatrics Committee on Child Abuse and Neglect. Pediatrics 1993;92:872–875

Leventhal JM, Thomas SA, Rosenfield NS: Fractures in young children: distinguishing child abuse from unintentional injuries. Am J Dis Child 1993;147:87–92

Lyons TJ, Oates RK: Falling out of bed: a relatively benign occurrence. Pediatrics 1993;92:125–127

Merten DF, Radkowski MA, Leonidas JC: The abused child: a radiological reappraisal. Radiology 1983;146:377–381

Meservy CJ, Towbin R, McLaurin RL, et al: Radiographic characteristics of skull fractures resulting from child abuse. AJNR Am J Neuroradiol 1987;8:455–457

Mogbo KI, Slovis TL, Canady AI, et al: Appropriate imaging in children with skull fractures and suspicion of abuse. Radiology 1998;208:521–524

Newsletter of the Section on Child Abuse and Neglect (1999). Am Acad Ped (sept) vol II, no 3, p 6

Patterson CR, Burns J, McAllison SJ: Osteogenesis imperfecta: the distinction from child abuse and the recognition of a variant form. Am J Med Genet 1993;45:187–192

Peddle N, Wang CT: Current trends in child abuse reporting and fatalities: the results of the 1999 Annual Fifty State Survey. Chicago:

Prevent Child Abuse America. 2001, Apr. www.preventchildabuse.org

Sane SM, et al: Diagnostic imaging of child abuse. Section on Radiology of the American Academy of Pediatrics. Pediatrics 2000;105:1345–1348

Sato Y, Yuh WTC, Smith WL, et al: Head injury in child abuse: evaluation with MR imaging. Radiology 1989;173:653–657

Silverman FN: Unrecognized trauma in infants, the battered child syndrome, and the syndrome of Amboise Tardieu. Rigler Lecture. Radiology 1972;104:337–353

Spevak MR, Kleinman PK, Belanger PL, et al: Cardiopulmonary resuscitation and rib fractures in infants: a postmortem radiologic-pathologic study. JAMA 1994;272:617–618

Wang CT, Daro D: Current Trends in Child Abuse Reporting and Fatalities: The Results of the 1997 Annual Fifty State Survey. Chicago: National Committee to Prevent Child Abuse, 1998

Worlock P, Stower M, Barbor P: Patterns of fractures in accidental and non-accidental injury in children: a comparative study. Br Med J 1986;293:100–102

Zimmerman RA, Bilanluk LT, Genneralli T: Computed tomography of shearing injuries of the cerebral white matter. Radiology 1978;127:393–396

PART X

OSTEOCHONDROSES AND MISCELLANEOUS ALIGNMENT DISORDERS

H. THEODORE HARCKE
GERALD A. MANDELL

OSTEOCHONDROSES

The osteochondroses are a heterogeneous group of idiopathic conditions characterized by disordered endochondral ossification that reflect both abnormal chondrogenesis and osteogenesis. They occur almost exclusively in the growing skeleton. Well over 75 bones, or portions of bones, have been documented as sites of these growth disturbances. Osteochondroses affect either chondro-osseous junctions or ovoid ossification centers within cartilage and are characterized radiographically by sclerosis, fragmentation, and collapse. The end result may be permanent deformity or reconstitution of the affected bone. Most of the osteochondroses fall into one of three categories: developmental variations, growth disturbances without evidence of necrosis, and osteonecrosis. Some osteochondroses (Osgood-Schlatter disease, Blount disease, etc.) may be associated with mechanical stress, but the precise etiology is often speculative and the categorization arbitrary. Most of these conditions maintain their eponyms with the names of the original observers, even when a pathologic etiology such as avascular or aseptic necrosis has been determined (Fig. 1). The conditions discussed here overlap with those discussed elsewhere, such as little leaguer's elbow, which is discussed in Section IX, Part VIII, page 2269, under Injuries to the Cartilaginous Plate. Developmental irregularities of mineralization, which are not clinically significant, occur in many of the same sites (see Section IX, Part III, Chapter 2, page 2053). Osteochondroses, such as Sever disease of the calcaneal apophysis and Van Neck disease of the ischiopubic synchondrosis, were originally believed to be secondary to a primary interruption of the local arterial supply. They are now believed to be variations of ossification. Köhler's disease of the navicular bone is a rare entity that simulates, and may be simulated by, the normal irregular sclerosis and hypoplasia of this bone. The best known example of osteochondrosis is Legg-Calvé-Perthes disease.

LEGG-CALVÉ-PERTHES DISEASE

Legg-Calvé-Perthes disease is avascular necrosis (AVN) of the capital femoral epiphysis. It develops in children between the ages of 3 and 12 years, with peak incidence at 6 to 8 years. Boys are affected four to five times as frequently as girls, and skeletal maturation is usually retarded. African-American children are rarely affected. In about 10% to 13% of cases, there is bilateral disease that is usually sequential rather than concurrent (a clue to the diagnosis of epiphyseal dysplasia). The principal clinical signs are limp, pain, and limitation of motion in the affected hip. Differential diagnosis includes any findings of synovitis, septic arthritis, and early osteomyelitis. Symptoms may lag behind the onset of AVN by weeks to months. Radiographs may be normal; the earliest changes begin with mild lateral displacement of the femoral head, previously presumed to be secondary to synovial thickening and joint effusion. Magnetic resonance imaging (MRI) studies have indicated that appreciable thickening of the femoral head cartilage occurs, so that fluid and synovial thickening are only partially responsible. Ancillary imaging studies may be required for diagnosis because the early changes are nonspecific.

Radiographic diagnosis is usually made when some flattening, sclerosis, and irregularity of mineralization, which comprise the characteristic triad of changes, are

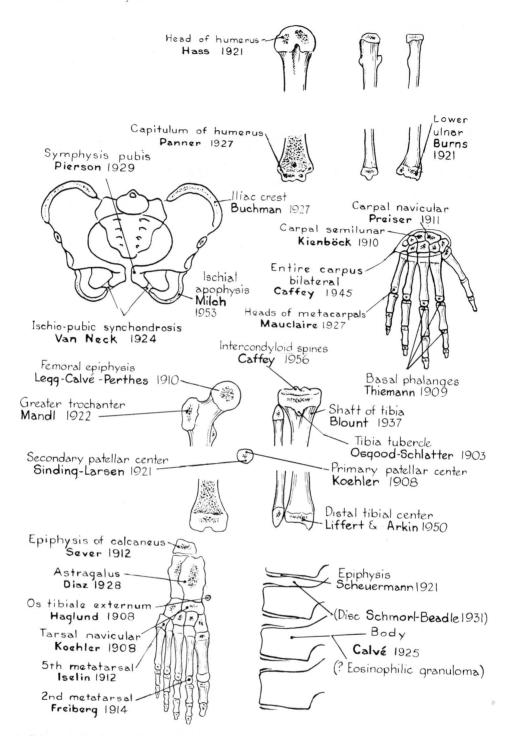

FIGURE 1. Schematic drawing of the growing skeleton with the supposed sites of the juvenile osteochondroses (focal ischemic necroses), names of the discoverers of the different lesions, and the year that each lesion was first reported. These sites are also regions where irregularity of mineralization occurs as a normal anatomic variant in growing children.

noted in the ossification center. Caffey emphasized the early occurrence of a subchondral fracture, which is best seen as a curvilinear fissure in films exposed with the leg in abduction and external rotation (Figs. 2 and 3). Frequently, the fissure is so radiolucent that it appears to be filled with gas liberated by the stresses of maintaining the limb in the abducted–externally rotated position. Subsequently, the triad develops and progresses as

a result of the infarcted trabeculae. Radionuclide diagnosis can predate radiographic changes, with decreased uptake affecting part or all of the femoral head by 4 to 6 weeks. To make a correct assessment of femoral head perfusion, magnification images (electronic or pinhole collimator) are mandatory. At the time of obvious radiographic findings, radionuclide studies demonstrate either decreased uptake, usually in the anterolateral portion of the head, where a subchondral fracture may be observed on conventional films, or a mixed pattern of decreased and increased uptake related to ongoing reconstitution of the femoral head. Revascularization or increased activity on scintigraphy also can predate radiologic evidence of new bone formation by an average of 5.5 months.

An effective alternative method of early diagnosis is MRI. The sensitivity of MRI may be enhanced by use of contrast. MRI examinations demonstrate variable degrees of loss of the normal high signal intensity from the epiphyseal marrow resulting from circulatory changes (Fig. 4). These examinations show loss of containment of the head in the acetabulum resulting from the previously noted swelling of its cartilage. They also demonstrate infarcted areas of the femoral head. MRI changes can occur in the course of intensive steroid therapy for various diseases, in sickle cell disease, and in other hemoglobinopathies.

The usual course of Legg-Calvé-Perthes disease includes three successive periods of about 18 months each: a destructive phase, a relatively stable phase, and a remineralization and healing phase. With progression, there is collapse and fragmentation of the sclerotic head and shortening and widening of the femoral neck, often with development of a focal, metaphyseal, radiolucent cystic detect (Fig. 5) and, ultimately, a coxa vara deformity. The radiolucent femoral neck defect *may* simulate neoplastic destruction. Ponseti found that these defects contain uncalcified fibrillated cartilage. Healing may result in complete reconstitution, but more frequently ends in varying degrees of coxa plana–coxa

magna deformity of the femoral head and neck. Results are better in patients whose onset was between 3 and 5 years of age than in those with later onsets.

An issue in prognosis is femoral head–acetabular congruence. This issue can be studied by conventional arthrography or by cross-sectional imaging with three-dimensional reconstruction. Lack of congruity of the femoral head and the acetabular cavity leads to painful osteoarthritis in the third and fourth decades of life because of progressive destruction of the articular cartilage of the components of the hip joint. To prevent or ameliorate this complication, surgical procedures for containment, such as femoral derotational osteotomies and acetabular reconstructions, are used sometimes to redirect the femoral head and deepen the effective acetabular cavity. Demonstration of the degree of containment of the femoral head may have some therapeutic implications.

MEYER DYSPLASIA (FEMORAL EPIPHYSEAL DYSPLASIA)

Meyer dysplasia probably represents a mild epiphyseal dysplasia limited to the proximal femoral epiphyses. It occurs almost exclusively in boys, frequently in those with a family history of hip disease. Of the patients originally described by Meyer, 42% had bilateral disease. Clinical signs in this limited dysplasia are usually mild or absent. The onset of complications (AVN or synovitis) is usually heralded by the onset of severe pain, or a change in the pattern of pain, and decreased range

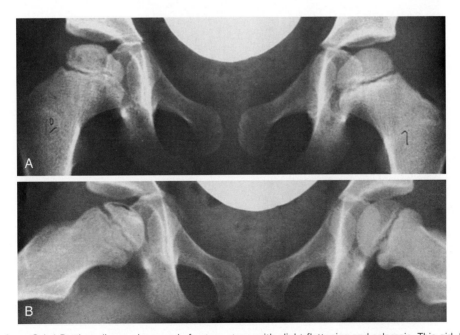

FIGURE 2. Legg-Calvé-Perthes disease in an early fracture stage with slight flattening and sclerosis. This girl, 5½ years of age, had limped and had pain in the right hip for "some weeks." **A,** In standard projection, there is no fracture. The epiphyseal ossification center, however, is displaced laterad 3 mm (note the discrepancy in overlap of the femoral heads on the ischial acetabular edge in this nonrotated film). **B,** A clear submarginal fracture line parallels the superior anterolateral edge of the epiphyseal ossification center. Its bright black density suggests that there may be gas between the edges of the fracture fragments. This is an example of segmental fracture prior to flattening and sclerosis that is invisible in the standard position **(A)** but clearly visible when the femora are abducted and externally rotated, throwing the anterior portion of the head in relief **(B).**

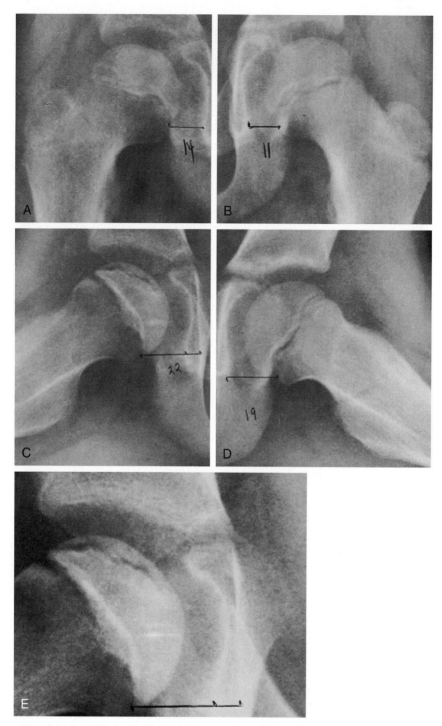

FIGURE 3. A and **B,** Frontal projection of the pelvis with the femora in normal adducted anatomic position. The right femoral head is slightly displaced laterad (3 mm) but shows no evidence of fracture or flattening. **C** and **D,** With the femora abducted and externally rotated about 45 degrees (Lauenstein position), a long, distracted, submarginal fracture is clearly visible in the anterior segment of the epiphyseal ossification center with no evidence of flattening. **E,** Enlargement of the right femur in **C,** which demonstrates the fracture without evidence of flattening.

of motion. In some cases, the radiographic signs are discovered by chance in patients whose hips were included in radiographic exposures for examination of other systemic problems. Sometimes, the proximal femoral epiphyseal dysplasia is a mild expression of the more diffuse involvement of multiple epiphyseal dyspla-

sia. Schlesinger et al. described measurements of the height and width of distal femoral epiphyses that are helpful in differentiating a local, limited dysplasia or normal variation from an inherited autosomal dominant disorder with complete penetrance but variable expression.

Patients with multiple epiphyseal dysplasia constitute a heterogeneous population. The radiographic features of Meyer epiphyseal dysplasia, however, resemble those of Legg-Calvé-Perthes disease (Fig. 6), and, according to Meyer, AVN may actually develop in about 20% of affected patients. As in Legg-Calvé-Perthes disease, a generalized retardation of skeletal maturation is present. The ossification centers for the femoral heads are late in appearance and are generally multiple, small, and granular. Focal scleroses may be mimicked by superimposition of several of the individual centers, but also may indicate the onset of AVN. If serial radiographs are not available for comparison and sclerosis of the epiphysis is present, bone scintigraphy with pinhole imaging or MRI can be performed to confirm avascularity in the dysplastic proximal femoral epiphysis of a symptomatic individual (Fig. 7). Fusion of the separate

ossification centers occurs gradually with more uniform mineralization, and, unless AVN supervenes, the appearance becomes normal in 3 to 4 years. Occasionally, Legg-Calvé-Perthes changes develop after the head has become normal radiographically. When this happens, there are accompanying clinical signs. The chief distinguishing features of Meyer dysplasia are the occurrence of the radiographic signs without clinical signs and progressive improvement to healing without much residual deformity. This is in contrast to Legg-Calvé-Perthes disease, in which a normally mineralized femoral head undergoes sclerosis, flattening, fragmentation, and varying degrees of subsequent recovery. It has been suggested that the original description of Meyer dysplasia may have included several related disorders because of the variable clinical features in some patients with similar radiographic changes.

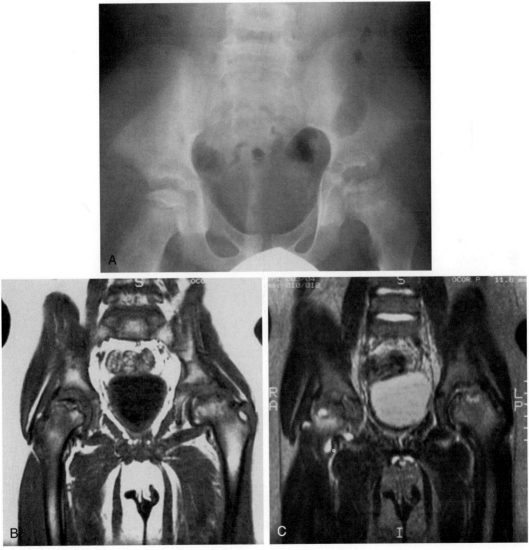

FIGURE 4. Advanced bilateral Legg-Calvé-Perthes disease in a 6-year-old boy. **A,** Conventional film of pelvis. On T_1- **(B)** and T_2-weighted **(C)** magnetic resonance images, both femoral heads are flattened and irregular, with lateral subluxation of the left hip, and hypertrophy of the cartilage of the femoral heads and also of the adjacent acetabula. A metaphyseal "cyst" appears as a small area of increased signal intensity below the growth plate on the right in **B**. The low signal intensity of both femoral epiphyses in **A** contrasts with the normal high signal intensity of marrow in the ossification center of the greater trochanter as well as in the bodies of the ilia. (Courtesy of Dr. Sheila Moore, Stanford, CA.)

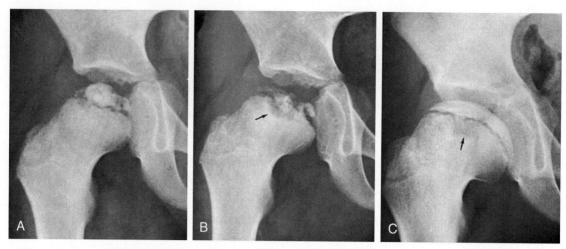

FIGURE 5. This boy with Legg-Calvé-Perthes disease had limped and had pain in the right knee for about 4 months. **A,** Eight months after onset, flattening of the epiphyseal ossification center is marked, and its medial and lateral parts are radiolucent because they are being replaced by radiolucent vascular fibrous tissue. The metaphysis is normal. **B,** Eighteen months after onset, a radiolucent patch is evident in the metaphysis *(arrow)* directly below the cartilage plate. The multiple bony patches of the epiphyseal ossification center are made up of residual shreds of sclerotic bone and new bony centers, which indicate beginning reossification. **C,** Four and one-half years after onset, a large radiolucent patch is still evident in the metaphysis *(arrow)*. The neck has widened progressively since **A,** and the flattened epiphyseal ossification center is completely healed and widened to fit onto the widened neck. The acetabular cavity is enlarged.

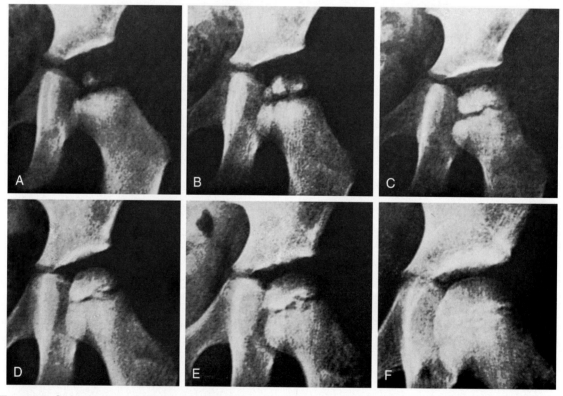

FIGURE 6. Serial changes in Meyer dysplasia from 2 to 10 years of age. At ages 2 **(A)** and 3 **(B),** the femoral epiphyseal ossification center is small and irregularly mineralized and is made up of multiple ossification centers. **C,** At 3 years and 10 months, the multiple centers have fused into a single, slightly flattened mass. At ages 4 **(D),** 6 **(E),** and 9 **(F),** the flattened center has rounded into a roughly hemispherical center with normal density and texture. This patient was not treated. (From Meyer J: Dysplasia epiphysealis capitis femoris: a clinical-radiological syndrome and its relationship to Legg-Calvé-Perthes disease. Acta Orthop Scand 1964;34:183-197, with permission.)

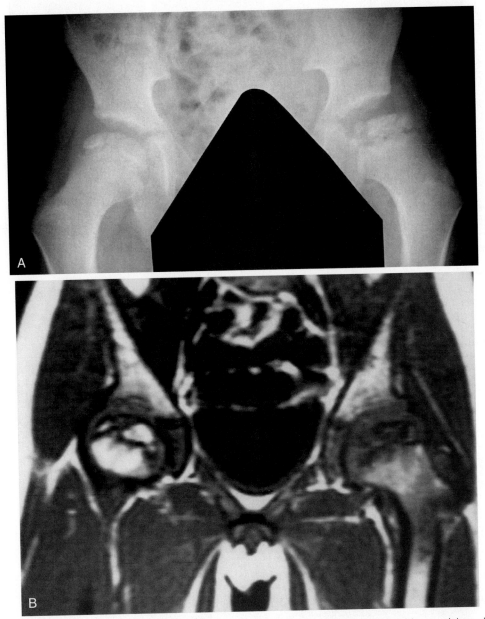

FIGURE 7. Avascular necrosis of the left proximal femoral epiphysis in a 7-year-old male with Meyer epiphyseal dysplasia. **A,** Radiographic changes in the epiphyses are similar. There is flattening and fragmentation. **B,** T$_1$-weighted magnetic resonance image shows low signal intensity in the left capital femoral epiphysis in contrast with high signal in the right ossification center and marrow.

KÖHLER'S DISEASE

A limp is usually the first clinical sign of the focal sclerosis of the tarsal navicular bone that characterizes Köhler's disease. Local pain and tenderness and sometimes swelling are found on examination. The condition occurs with a greater frequency in boys than in girls. As in Legg-Calvé-Perthes disease, flattening and irregular sclerosis are present and the bone is photopenic ("cold") on scintigraphy (Fig. 8). The diagnosis of Köhler's disease cannot be made by radiographic signs alone. Developmental dysplastic changes are observed in the navicular bone as a manifestation of what has been called "Karp dysplasia." This condition is characterized by late appearance of the bony nucleus, slow growth, flatness, and irregular sclerosis in the affected bone with little or no relation to clinical symptoms. The dysplastic changes are often found in the foot contralateral to an injury when a control film is obtained, or in the course of examination for trauma or skeletal survey. Radiographic improvement occurs with advancing age. Problems arise when pain or limp from an unrelated cause leads to discovery of the small, dense, irregular ossification center. The radiographic diagnosis of Köhler's disease can be assured only with serial examinations in which progressive destruction is demonstrated, as in Figure 9, or when radioisotopic studies are in accord. The type and length of treatment do not affect the final outcome.

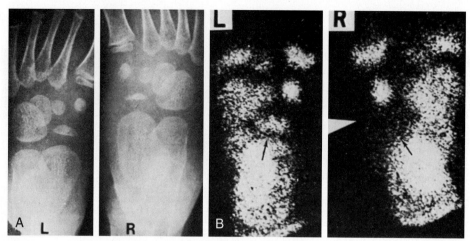

FIGURE 8. Köhler's disease. **A,** Flattening and sclerosis of the right tarsal navicular in a girl of 29 months. **B,** Polyphosphate scintigram; there is lack of uptake in the flattened sclerotic right navicular *(arrows).* In a similar scan 6 months later, the uptake was normal in the right navicular. (From McCauley RG, Kahn PC: Osteochondritis of the tarsal navicular: radioisotopic appearance. Radiology 1977;123:705, with permission.)

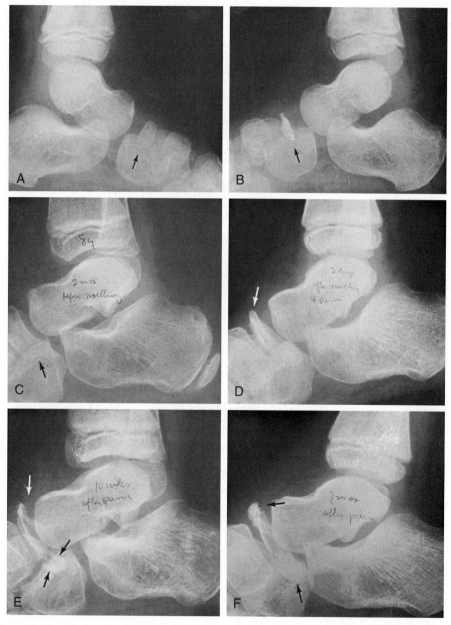

FIGURE 9. A and **B,** Hypoplasia and sclerosis of the left navicular (*arrow* in **B**) in an asymptomatic girl 3 years of age with Karp benign dysplasia. **C,** The navicular in a girl of 8 years with dysautonomia and reduced sensitivity to pain is normal 2 months before the onset of regional painful swelling with limp. Two days **(D)** 2 months **(E)** and 7 months **(F)** after the onset of true Köhler's disease, there is progressive flattening and sclerosis of the navicular without loss of the cartilage spaces at the joints.

PANNER'S DISEASE

This eponym refers to pathologic, symptomatic or asymptomatic, irregular mineralization of the capitellum of the humerus, often with associated changes in the radial head. Panner's disease is a rare lesion that usually follows known trauma to the elbow with local persistent pain and moderate limitation of movement (Fig. 10). Average age of onset is 8 years. It is likely that prior trauma has been forgotten in patients who have typical clinical and radiographic changes apparently arising de novo. Some instances may be the result of necrotic change after very distal, lateral condylar fractures of the humerus. Adams considered the condition an exaggerated form of little leaguer's elbow. Most patients with acute presentation recover without sequelae. Late-developing cases often show arrested growth and collapse of the capitellum from osteonecrosis. In addition, the radial head may overgrow because of hyperemia, resulting in joint incongruity and secondary osteoarthritis.

FREIBERG'S DISEASE

Freiberg's "ischemic necrosis," or infarction of the head of the second metatarsal bone, generally occurs in girls between the ages of 8 and 17 years. A similar lesion can occur in the heads of other metatarsals (Fig. 11). The predilection for female patients may be related to the wearing of high-heeled shoes. The etiology is thought to be ischemia producing AVN secondary to repeated trauma. Freiberg's disease is commonly found in association with stress fractures of the same or the other foot and results from a superficial fissure fracture in the edge of the epiphyseal ossification center followed by sclerosis, fragmentation, and then repair. The radiographic signs are similar to those of Legg-Calvé-Perthes disease, with initial widening of the contiguous joint space followed by flattening, sclerosis, and fragmentation. Pinhole bone scintigraphy can demonstrate initial photopenia of the epiphysis followed by increased uptake of reconstitution and revascularization. MRI findings depend on the stage of the disease, with marrow defects as in AVN. The head of the affected metatarsal eventually becomes squared and flat. The adjacent metaphyses widen to contain the flattened epiphysis. Loose fragments may perpetuate symptoms; their removal reportedly has been followed by clinical improvement.

VAN NECK DISEASE

Van Neck disease is the normal appearance of the ischiopubic synchondrosis seen in children just prior to fusion. At this time, there is swelling and uneven mineralization at the synchondrosis. Fusion often occurs asymmetrically. Fifty-seven percent of children at age 7 years and 17% of children at age 12 years still have a unilateral, unfused ischiopubic synchondrosis. Its irregular bubbly appearance, which may or may not be associated with regional clinical signs, should not be interpreted as ischemic necrosis. Painful swelling of the synchondrosis is usually indicative of significant

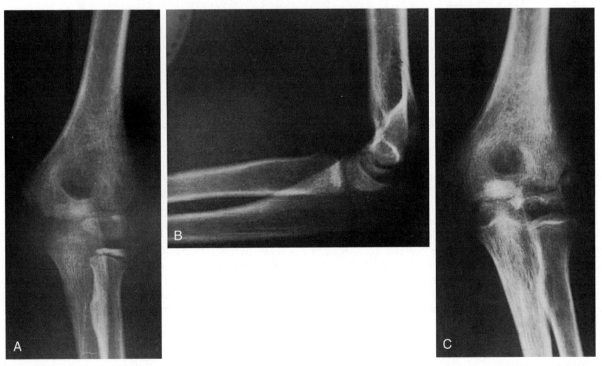

FIGURE 10. Panner's disease in a 10-year-old girl. Anteroposterior **(A)** and lateral **(B)** projections of the elbow immediately after injury showing the normal capitellum of the humerus. **C,** Disappearance of the distal two thirds of the capitellum 1 year after injury. Patient had only mild complaints of discomfort on full extension. The sclerosis and irregularities in mineralization in the trochlea are most likely an anatomic variant.

FIGURE 11. Freiberg's disease of the second right metatarsal in a 12-year-old child. **A,** Initial radiograph shows questionable increase in density of the metatarsal head. **B,** Magnification scintigraphic images of the feet. The head of the second right metatarsal is photopenic *(arrows).* Adjacent growth plate and metaphyseal uptake is increased. **C,** Radiograph done 6 months after **A** shows flattening and sclerosis of the metatarsal head.

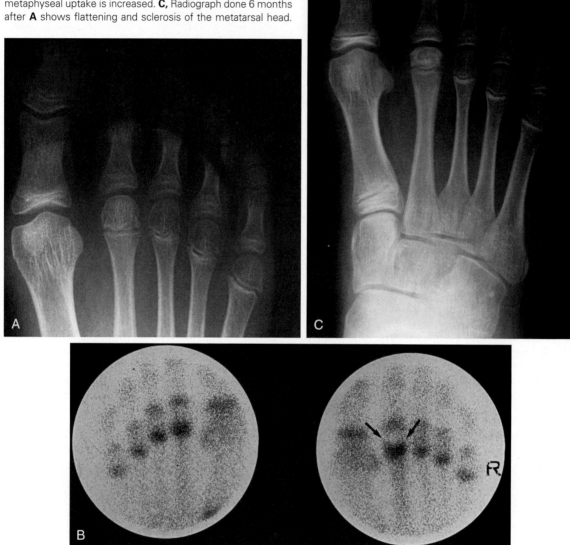

underlying pathology. Fractures and osteomyelitis that occur in this region may require bone scintigraphy or MRI for differentiation. The normal ischiopubic synchondrosis will be either photopenic or show focal, well-marginated, mildly increased uptake. A pathologic process is more active than the uptake in the area surrounding the triradiate cartilage; there is poor margination and extension of activity into the ipsilateral superior and inferior pubic rami. MRI would demonstrate soft tissue and marrow edema in the region of the pathologic process.

SEVER'S DISEASE

The original description of this disease by Sever was of the normal irregular, dense apophysis of the calcaneus.

This configuration is seen in all healthy children, including those with painful heels. The appearance of the secondary ossification center of the os calcis occurs between 7 and 9 years of age. It is now believed that Sever incorrectly described tendonitis and bursitis as "apophysitis." Posterior heel pain near the insertion of the Achilles tendon can be due to retrocalcaneal bursitis in otherwise healthy, active children and adolescents. Repeated dorsiflexion of the foot in flat-heeled athletic shoes results in compression and irritation of the soft tissues of the posterior heel. The characteristic pain is related to inflammation of regional soft tissues rather than an abnormality of the os calcis itself. Contusion or partial rupture of the Achilles tendon and alvulsion injuries at the tendon insertion may mimic retrocalcaneal bursitis. If, in addition to the retrocalcaneal bursitis, erosions of the posterosuperior cortex of the os calcis are noted, an inflammatory disorder such as juvenile rheumatoid arthritis, ankylosing spondylitis, psoriasis, Reiter's syndrome, or infection should be considered. Retrocalcaneal bursitis is indicated when the sharp definition of the retrocalcaneal recess is lost, and the lucency of the pre-Achilles fat pad is replaced by soft tissue density. Ultrasonography or MRI can confirm the presence of fluid in the bursa in most instances.

SCHEUERMANN'S DISEASE

Scheuermann's disease (vertebral osteochondrosis) is a growth disturbance affecting the spine in 3% to 5% of healthy adolescents. The kyphotic involvement of the thoracic spine (juvenile kyphosis) represents 75% of patients with this condition. Diagnostic criteria include dorsal spine kyphosis of greater than 35 degrees, with anterior wedging of greater than 5 degrees of at least one vertebral body. Usually, three to five contiguous vertebral bodies are involved. This structural deformity is usually painless and develops between the ages of 13 and 17 years. The incidence is slightly greater in males than females. The pathogenesis of Scheuermann's kyphosis is not definitively known. Schmorl's theory of herniation of disk material through the vertebral end plates during the adolescent growth spurt is the most widely accepted. The lumbar form is referred to as "atypical," or lumbar Scheuermann's disease because of the presenting feature of low back pain. Radiographic features of the lumbar type of the disease include involvement of one or more vertebrae (from T11 to L5), with radiographs showing "scooped" defects in the anterosuperior or anteroinferior end plates (herniated Schmorl's nodes), end plate irregularities, and disk space narrowing. There is an increased incidence of idiopathic scoliosis in the lumbar form of Scheuermann's disease (43% to 70%). Adolescents with lumbar Scheuermann's disease tend to be more athletic and have a history suggesting increased axial stress to the spine.

Traditionally, bone scintigraphy has been used to diagnose other osseous etiologies causing low back pain in adolescence, the most common being spondylolysis. In the lumbar form of Scheuermann's disease, when one or two levels are involved, the clinical picture can be confused with infection or neoplastic disease. In these instances, bone scintigraphy has been utilized effectively. The bone scan findings in lumbar Scheuermann's disease consist of either normal or mildly increased vertebral activity on planar scintigraphy and single-photon emission computed tomography (Fig. 12). The characteristic subtle accumulation of the radiotracer differentiates Scheuermann's disease from the more intense uptake of acute infectious and traumatic events. MRI can demonstrate the presence of disk material in the region of the anterior end plate herniation as well as associated disk space narrowing and disk degeneration related to decreased signal intensity. This condition is usually self-limiting and benign, and differentiation from other pathologic entities of the spine will prevent overtreatment.

KIRNER DISEASE

Kirner disease is manifested by bilateral swelling and bending of the tips of the fifth fingers and their terminal phalanges. The cause is unknown; familial and sporadic cases have been recorded. The clinical features are generally noted in preadolescence. Slight redness and interference with manual activities, such as sewing or typing, have been the major complaints. Soft tissue swellings preceded skeletal changes in affected members of a family reported by Blank and Girdany. Biopsy, in a case reported by Kaufmann and Taillard, showed only irregularity at the cartilage–shaft junction with diminished trabecular bone and a decrease in thickness of the zone of provisional calcification. Clinical and radiographic features are shown in Figures 13 and 14. In familial cases, autosomal dominant inheritance appears to be involved. One instance of abnormalities in several fingers of both hands has been offered as the likely result of homozygosity for the gene.

OSTEOCHONDROSIS DISSECANS

Often called "osteochondritis dissecans," this condition can be considered a marginal fracture of subchondral bone, adjacent cartilage, or both, located directly under the articular cartilage. A fragment of the involved cartilage and bone may loosen and separate from the articular margin and become a loose body. Local necrosis of bone and cartilage is secondary to the fracture and the complete or incomplete separation of a fragment. Localized pain, tenderness, and limitation of motion are mild, inconstant, and intermittent. The femoral condyles are most commonly involved, especially the weight-bearing medial condyle, but bones at other joints also may be affected.

The radiographic feature supporting the diagnosis is a marginal defect in the subchondral bone on the edge of the ossification center near the joint surface (Fig. 15). An independent particle of normal-looking or sclerotic bone may be seen in the crater-like marginal defect or loose in the articular cavity. In proven cases, osteochondrosis of the femoral condyles has almost always been located on the anteromedial edge of the medial condyle. When similar lesions are observed on the dorsal edges, and especially on the lateral condyle, they are much more likely to represent anatomic variation in normal children (see Section IX, Part III, Chapter 2, page 2053). However, true instances of osteochondrosis dissecans affecting the lateral condyle have been documented. Tunnel views of the knee best demonstrate both types of lesions. Similar features are present when the lesion occurs in other joints, such as in the tibiotalar or metatarsophalangeal joints (Fig. 16). In the former site, the radiographic changes are located on the superior curved edge of the talus, either medial or lateral, and consist of marginal indentations that may or may not contain a bone fragment. In the latter, the destructive lesion is in the end of the shaft, not in a secondary epiphyseal center as in most of the osteochondroses. In a sense, this lesion resembles the features

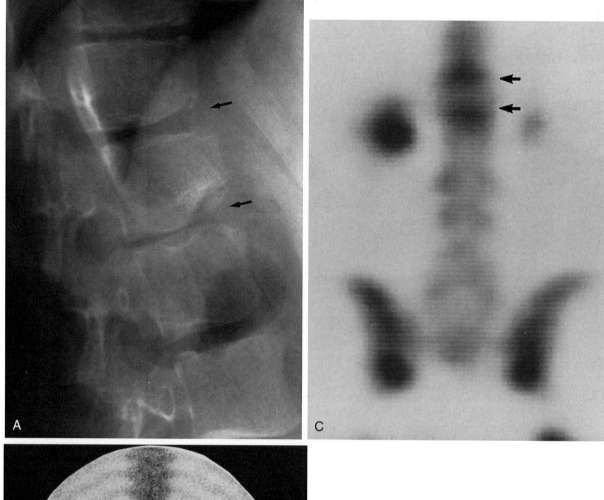

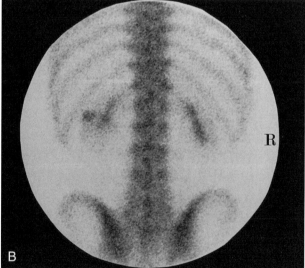

FIGURE 12. Scheuermann's disease of the lower dorsal and upper lumbar spine. **A,** Coned-down lateral radiograph showing end plate defects *(arrows)* and narrowing of the disk spaces. **B,** Bone scintigraphy (posterior delayed image). **C,** Single-photon emission computed tomography image reveals mildly increased upper lumbar uptake and bands of increased uptake in the dorsal spine.

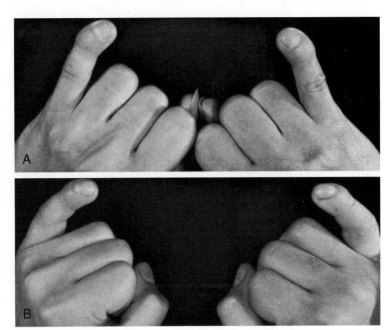

FIGURE 13. Bilateral idiopathic swelling of the terminal segments of the fifth fingers with radial and ventral deviation (Kirner disease) in sibling girls ages 14 **(A)** and 19 **(B)** years. These swellings were painless, were not inflammatory, and had appeared gradually over the last half of childhood. (Courtesy of Dr. Eugene Blank, Portland, OR.)

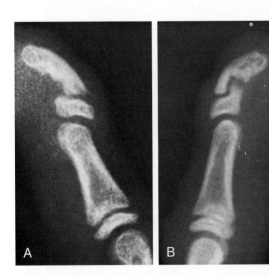

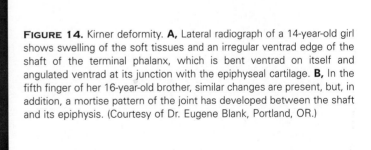

FIGURE 14. Kirner deformity. **A,** Lateral radiograph of a 14-year-old girl shows swelling of the soft tissues and an irregular ventrad edge of the shaft of the terminal phalanx, which is bent ventrad on itself and angulated ventrad at its junction with the epiphyseal cartilage. **B,** In the fifth finger of her 16-year-old brother, similar changes are present, but, in addition, a mortise pattern of the joint has developed between the shaft and its epiphysis. (Courtesy of Dr. Eugene Blank, Portland, OR.)

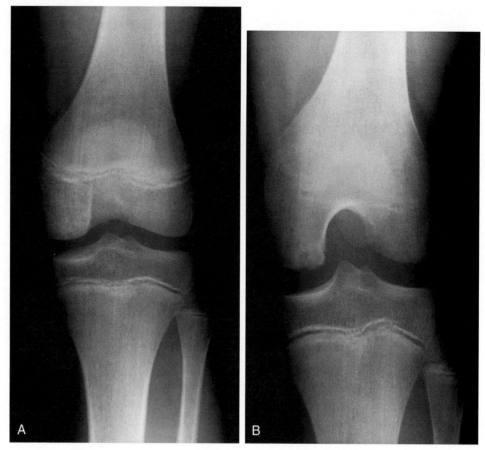

FIGURE 15. Osteochondrosis dissecans of the distal femur in a 12-year-old male. The defect in the lateral aspect of the medial femoral condyle is barely visible on the anteroposterior **(A)** radiograph, and better seen on tunnel (notch) view **(B)**.

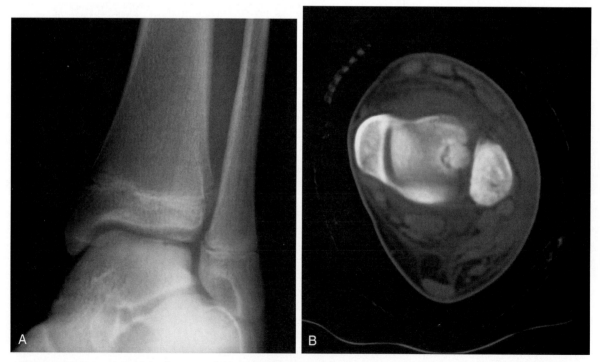

FIGURE 16. Osteochondrosis dissecans of the talus. **A,** Oblique radiograph of the ankle shows an elevated bone fragment off the articular margin of the lateral talus. **B,** Axial computed tomography image through the talus shows a rounded fragment of sclerotic bone that has separated from the talar dome. Such fragments may become loose bodies within a joint.

in talar lesions. The traumatic basis is probably involved in instances in which steroid therapy has preceded the osteochondrosis and made the bone more vulnerable.

In most instances, bone scintigraphy shows a focal increase in activity at the site of the osteochondritis on delayed images. CT and MRI should be relegated to confirming loosening and evaluating displacement, size, and location of a fragment in instances in which radiography and/or scintigraphy are equivocal.

MISCELLANEOUS ALIGNMENT DISORDERS

The bones of the extremities are aligned to best serve the functions required of them by evolutionary change. Malalignment of bony components of limbs may be congenital or acquired. The defect creating malalignment can be primary to bone or to soft tissue.

BOWLEG

Bowleg deformity, also referred to as genu varum, is manifested by separation of the knees when the legs are placed in anatomic position. A radiograph is obtained to differentiate developmental or physiologic bowing from bowing that reflects underlying pathology. There are a variety of pathologic causes: rickets, skeletal dysplasias, prenatal bowing, Blount disease, and occasionally growth plate trauma. Both clinician and radiologist should remember that most lateral bowing in otherwise normal infants and young children less than 2 years of

age is developmental and resolves without treatment. Radiographically, the femur and tibia are intrinsically bowed laterally and often ventrally (Fig. 17). The medial and posterior cortices of the shafts are thickened. There can be spurring and beaking of the medial and posterior aspects of the metaphyses at the knee. The medial halves of the tibial and femoral ossification centers are incompletely ossified, giving a wedge shape to the epiphyses. The varus deformity is common in normal infants and converts into valgus between 18 and 36 months of age (Fig. 18). Degree of valgus reduces spontaneously by age 6 to 7 years to a mild degree that remains throughout life. Bowing is usually more marked in the tibias, but, occasionally, the bowing may almost exclusively result from lateral bowing of the distal femur (Fig. 19). Radiographs should be obtained with the patient bearing weight as soon as he or she is able to stand (Fig. 20). The clue to pathologic causes is found principally in the distal ends of the long bones, where changes of rickets are manifested in the growth plate and changes of dysplasia are reflected by abnormal metaphyseal and/or epiphyseal development. Serial radiographs are frequently necessary to determine a pathologic condition, particularly if progressive deformity is due to Blount disease.

BLOUNT DISEASE

Tibia vara, referred to as Blount disease or osteochondroses deformens tibiae, is a progressive deformity relating to changes in the proximal tibia. The infantile form develops in children between 1 and 3 years of age and must be differentiated from developmental bowing

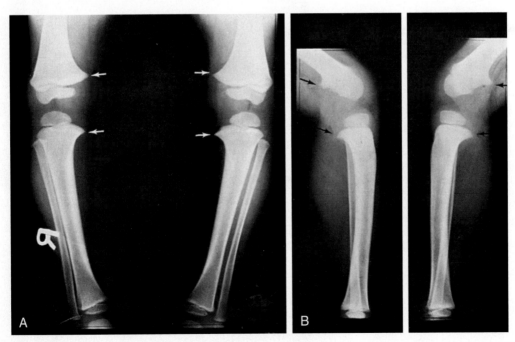

FIGURE 17. A, Bilateral idiopathic bowed legs (frontal projection) in a boy 22 months of age. *Arrows* point to the mediad and dorsad breaking of the femoral and tibial metaphyses at the knees. The increased stress of weight bearing has also thickened the medial and dorsal cortical walls of the tibias inward. The femoral epiphyseal ossification centers are much too small, especially in their medial halves, which are under a greater stress of weight bearing when the legs are bowed. **B,** Lateral projection. After correction of bowed legs, these "stress" phenomena disappear after several months.

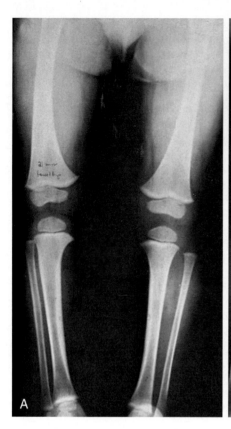
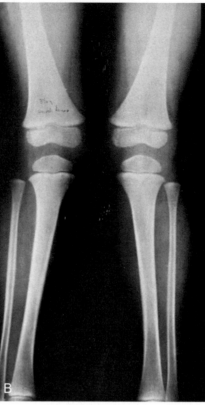

FIGURE 18. Spontaneous conversion of bowed legs to knock-knees. **A,** At 21 months, both femora and both tibias are bowed laterad. **B,** The same patient at 42 months exhibits symmetric knock-knees with wide spreading at the ankles.

FIGURE 19. Femoral bowed legs (femora vara): endogenous stress trauma at the knees without weight bearing. **A,** Frontal projection shows marked bowlegs, in which the tibias are straight and both femora are bowed abruptly laterad near their distal ends (femora vara). The femoral epiphyseal ossification centers are small and flattened on their medial halves. **B,** On lateral projection, the right tibia is straight, but the femur is bowed ventrad near its distal end and a spur projects dorsad from the same level of the femoral shaft. When possible, a frontal projection of the leg should be obtained with the patient standing and the ankles in apposition.

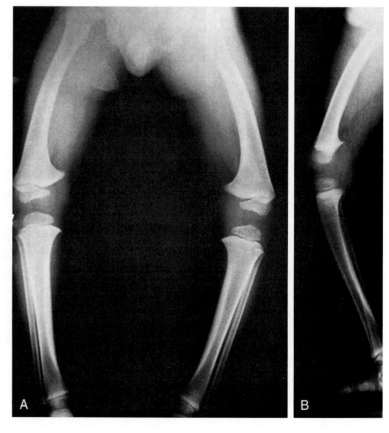

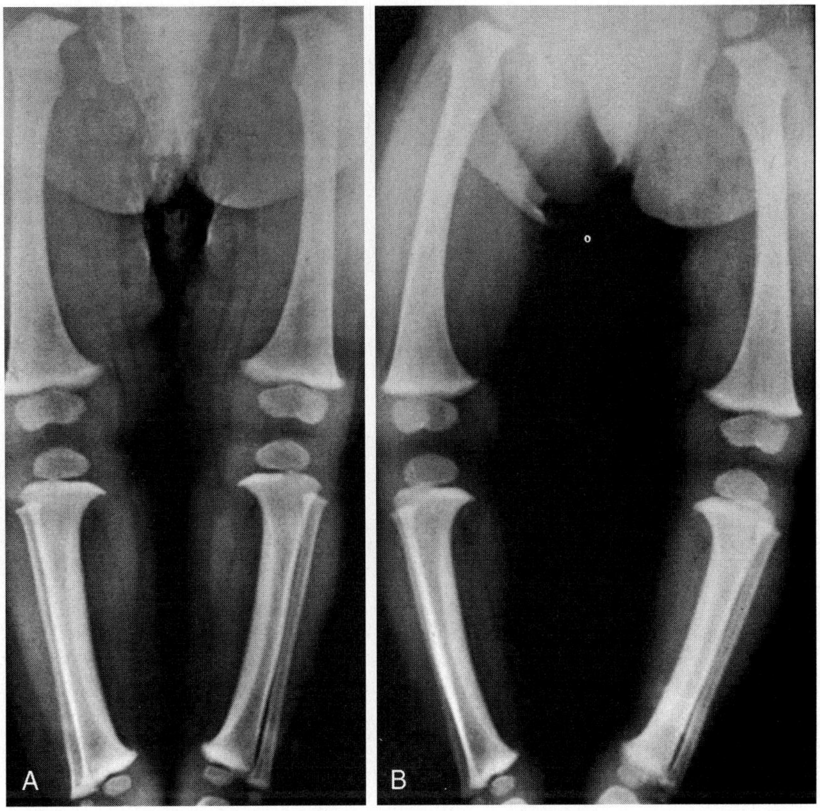

FIGURE 20. Bowed legs of a girl 12 months of age who started to walk at 8 months. **A,** In recumbent position, the tibias and femora are bowed, but the legs are not bowed because the knees and ankles are in apposition. **B,** In erect position during weight bearing and with ankles in apposition, the legs are bowed, with a gap of 12 cm at the knees. The real clinical deformity of bowed legs is shown most accurately radiographically when the patient is erect and bearing weight.

(Fig. 21). The disease is typically bilateral but can be unilateral. There is often a family history. Blount disease was initially considered an osteochondrosis or a result of ischemic necrosis of the medial aspect of the proximal tibial epiphysis. Later evidence, however, indicates that excessive compressive stress at the proximal medial tibial physis alters endochondral bone formation. Pathologic changes are not limited to the growth plate but include abnormalities in growth in the metaphysis, epiphyseal cartilage, and osseous epiphysis. Occasionally, changes can be observed in the opposing femur at the knee (Fig. 22).

Adolescent tibia vara is a separate entity from the infantile form. It occurs in children 8 to 14 years of age, with obese African-American males of normal height at particular risk (Fig. 23). Adolescent tibia vara is commonly unilateral but may be bilateral. It is slowly progressive and probably results from the repetitive trauma of weight bearing on the medial physis of the proximal tibia. Differential diagnosis of unilateral tibial vara includes growth plate injury secondary to trauma, fibrocartilaginous dysplasia of the proximal tibia, osteochondroma, or enchondroma of the proximal tibia or distal femur.

The characteristic radiographic feature of Blount disease is change in the medial metaphysis of the proximal tibia (Fig. 24). Irregularity with a more vertically oriented growth plate creates a beak-like appearance. The severity of radiographic changes has been characterized by the six-stage Langenskiöld classification. The medial portion of the epiphyseal ossification center is often smaller than the lateral portion. Prior to

the development of the tibial metaphyseal changes, it is often impossible to distinguish Blount disease from physiologic bowing. The metaphyseal–diaphyseal angle measurement by Levine and Drennan has been proposed as one method. A metaphyseal–diaphyseal angle of more than 11 degrees suggests Blount disease.

Although spontaneous resolution of infantile Blount disease is reported in some instances (Fig. 25), treatment with bracing is begun usually between ages 18 and 24 months and continued during waking hours for an average of 2 years. Failure of conservative management leads to a realignment osteotomy, which is most effective when performed before 5 years of age. For adolescent Blount disease, the customary surgical procedure is a proximal tibial valgus osteotomy to produce normal alignment.

Cross-sectional modalities and scintigraphy are occasionally employed in the assessment of bowleg. One use is to provide cross-sectional mapping of the physis if there is concern about segmental growth plate closure. In severe tibia vara, coronal CT images can be used like linear tomograms to assist with preoperative planning.

KNOCK-KNEE

In knock-knee, or genu valgum, the lower legs deviate laterally when the knees are placed in anatomic position. There is a wide separation at the ankles (Fig. 26). As noted in the discussion of bowleg deformity, genu valgum is a developmental phase that is most apparent at 3 to 4 years of age in normal children and follows the

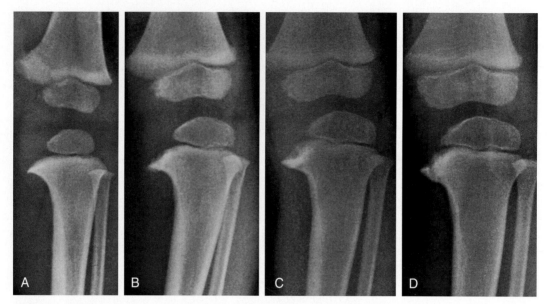

FIGURE 21. Progressive changes in Blount tibia vara. **A,** At 17 months, the medial segment of the tibial metaphysis is widened and sharpened into a short beak or spur that is bent slightly caudad. **B,** At 26 months, the spur is longer, sharper, and more bent; a radiolucent strip on its upper edge represents noncalcified cartilage. **C,** At 32 months, the amount of cartilage is increased and the spur thickened. **D,** At 38 months, the beak of the spur is displaced caudad, possibly owing to trauma; the medial edge of the ossification center is flattened, and the femur has shifted mediad in relation to the tibia.

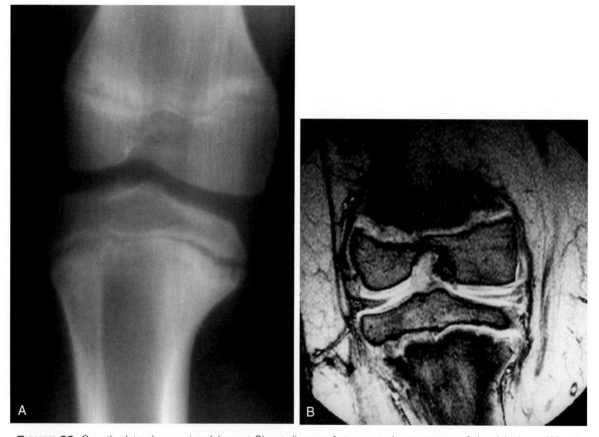

FIGURE 22. Growth plate changes in adolescent Blount disease. Anteroposterior tomogram of the right knee **(A)** and gradient-echo coronal magnetic resonance image **(B)** show widening and irregularity of the proximal tibial growth plate both medially and laterally. Note that the distal femoral growth plate shows changes of a similar nature.

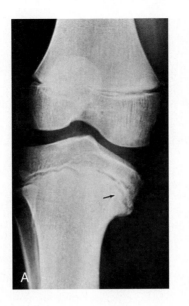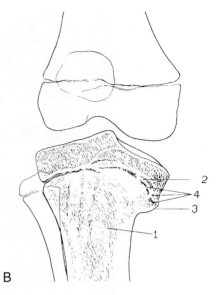

FIGURE 23. A, Sharp bending of the medial segment of the tibial metaphysis caudad and mediad in tibia vara. The medial segment of the tibial ossification center has followed the metaphysis caudad. The medial femoral condyle is hypertrophied in compensation for the tibial deformity. This girl, 10 years of age, was bowlegged on the right side. The straight lateral cortical wall of the tibia is noteworthy. **B,** A tracing of **A** showing *1*, medially bowed shaft; *2* and *3*, medially and caudally bent tibial ossification center and tibial metaphysis; and *4*, irregular ossification and early closure of the medial segment of the bent cartilaginous plate.

physiologic bowing seen earlier. Persistent knock-knee can be related to pathologic causes such as skeletal dysplasia, metabolic disease, or laxity of muscles and ligaments. Knock-knee may also be secondary to a foot or ankle deformity. With genu valgum, there may also be external tibial torsion so that, when the patella is placed straight ahead, there is external rotation of the feet.

Unilateral tibia valga may be found following tibial metaphyseal fracture. Even when the fracture does not involve the growth plate, progressive valgus deformity develops despite adequate postreduction alignment. Many mechanisms have been postulated relating to both growth plate effects and soft tissue changes.

LEG LENGTH DISCREPANCY

A leg length discrepancy of less than 1 cm is a normal variant. The presence of a leg length discrepancy may reflect overgrowth of the long limb or decreased size or growth of the short limb. Leg length discrepancy is often of clinical significance because of alteration of gait and a resultant pelvic tilt. With significant pelvic tilt, a secondary compensatory scoliosis can develop.

The differential diagnoses for overgrowth and undergrowth are too numerous to list here. Overgrowth is associated with a number of syndromes. It can also be found in association with vascular abnormalities. At times, overgrowth secondary to a fracture accounts for the discrepancy; in many cases, the cause cannot be found. The small or short limb occurring at birth is associated with a variety of congenital conditions linked to hypoplasia or aplasia of a segment of the limb. Acquired shortening can be linked to either slowing or accelerated closure of the growth plate. This process can occur not only following trauma but also in association with vascular insufficiency or infection, and as a result of changes occurring with any focal lesion of the extremities, to include the osteochondroses.

Radiographic techniques seek to determine lengths in a manner that minimizes magnification and other technical factors. A standard method should be used to assess leg length inequality. The technique of orthoroentgenography utilizes three separate exposures collimated to the hip, knee, and ankle made on a single film containing a radiopaque ruler. The digital scout or pilot image for computed tomography (CT) has been utilized to measure bone length. This is limited by the field size and is subject to errors in cursor placement on a small image.

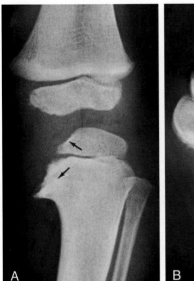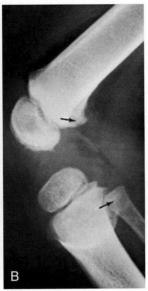

FIGURE 24. Blount tibia vara in a girl, 2½ years of age, who had pronounced lateral bowing of the left leg. **A,** In frontal projection, the medial end of the tibial ossification center is flattened into a slope in place of the normal convex curve at this site. This is a hypoplasia of the medial segment of the bony nucleus rather than destruction by ischemic necrosis. The metaphysis is widened mediad by a broad horizontal spur that is roughened on its medial edge where the previously bony terminal segment of the spur has been replaced by a radiolucent cartilage. The lateral cortical wall is not bent at the level of the medial wall. **B,** In lateral projection, spurs project dorsad from the dorsal walls of the femoral and tibial shafts.

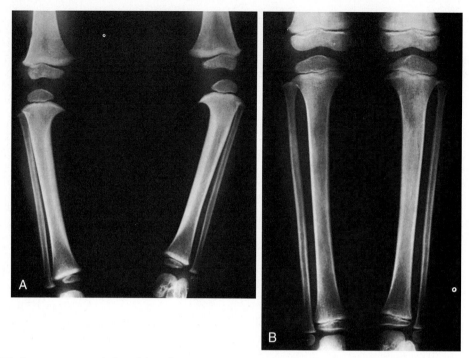

FIGURE 25. Spontaneous resolution of the infantile form of Blount disease. **A,** A 21-month-old girl with bowing of the left leg. Medial metaphyseal changes on the left are much more marked than on the right. The thickened medial cortex of the tibia may indicate an ongoing corrective response to abnormal compression stresses. **B,** Same patient at 57 months with practically complete regression of the bowing deformity. The patient had worn a left shoe with lateral lifts during the period of observation.

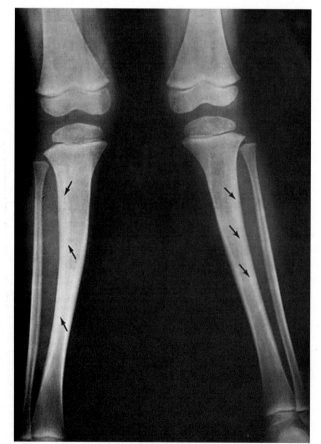

FIGURE 26. Bilateral idiopathic knock-knee in a girl 4 years of age. The lower halves of the tibias are bent laterad owing to the medial bowing of their upper halves. There is a wide gap between the ankles when the thighs and knees are in anatomic position. The lateral cortical walls of both tibias, through which the principal lines of force are transmitted in this deformity, are thickened *(arrows)*. This is the converse of the cortical thickenings in bowleg.

CLUBFOOT

Talipes equinovarus, or clubfoot, is a common congenital anomaly that is clinically obvious at birth. The principle components of the deformity are plantar flexion of the ankle (equinus), inversion of the heel (varus), and adduction of the forefoot (varus) (Fig. 27). Abnormal intrauterine pressures contribute to the development of clubfoot. Genetics also appears to play a role, with a higher than normal incidence of the deformity in first-degree relatives. The majority of congenital clubfeet are supple and managed conservatively by serial casting. Very stiff, inflexible clubfeet and those that fail to respond to conservative treatment require operative reduction.

Radiographic assessment of clubfoot is done to detect congenital anomalies and to assess the relationships of the visualized osseous structures. It is common to position the foot in a simulated weight-bearing position with an attempt to passively correct the deformity as much as possible. These anteroposterior (AP) and lateral views then permit determination of the talocalcaneal angulation, which is a common method for grading the extent of deformity and monitoring treatment (Fig. 28). An AP radiograph shows superimposition of the talus on the calcaneus. Parallelism of the talus and calcaneus are seen on a lateral view. CT has been employed principally to evaluate residual hindfoot deformity in clubfeet refractive to treatment. A short-axis or coronal examination allows the relationship of the talus and calcaneus to be assessed. Relationships of the hindfoot to the ankle can also be evaluated.

Anatomic deformities persist after treatment of club-

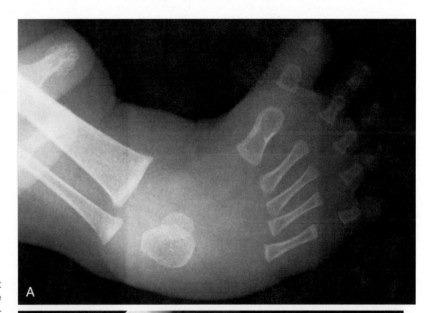

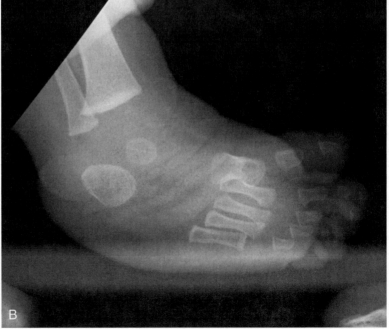

FIGURE 27. Radiographs of congenital clubfoot obtained with simulated weight bearing. **A,** Note inversion and forefoot adduction in the anteroposterior view. **B,** Inversion on the lateral view shows "laddering" of the metatarsals. There is equinus of the hindfoot and parallelism of the talus and calcaneus.

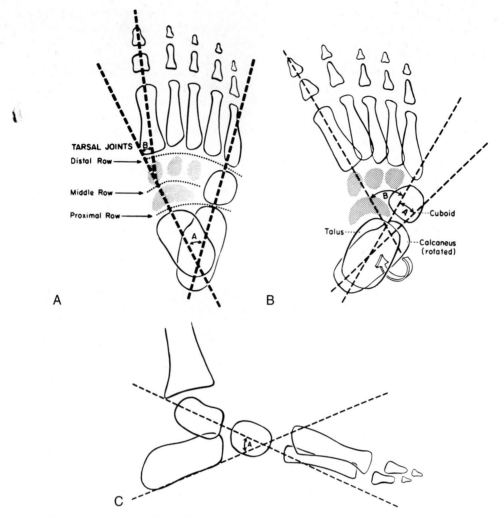

FIGURE 28. Drawings of a normal foot with lines commonly used to evaluate clubfoot and flatfoot deformities. **A,** Antero-posterior projection. The talocalcaneal angle *(A)* is measured by the lines representing the estimated longitudinal axes of the two bones. The range of normal for young children is 20 to 40 degrees. The talo–first metatarsal angle *(B)* is defined by the talar axis line and a line in the axis of the first metatarsal bone; the range of normal is 0 to −20 degrees. **B,** Anteroposterior projection of a foot with hindfoot varus. Rotation of the calcaneus under the talus decreases the talocalcaneal angle below the normal range, and talonavicular subluxation with forefoot adduction is indicated by the positive talo–first metatarsal angle. A lateral projection would show the talocalcaneal angle to be less than 35 degrees, with the axes approaching parallelism. **C,** Lines for angles in a lateral projection of the foot. The talocalcaneal angel *(A)* is subtended by the axial line of the talus and a line along the plantar margin of the calcaneus. Its range of normal is 35 to 55 degrees. (From Simons GW: Analytical radiography of club feet. J Bone Joint Surg Br 1977;59:485–489, with permission.)

foot and should be recognized as children grow. Many clubfeet have small, flattened talar heads; decreased talocalcaneal angles, subtalar joint changes; and medial displacement of the navicular.

In the differential diagnosis of foot deformity, congenital vertical talus exists both as an isolated condition and in association with various syndromes (e.g., the trisomy syndromes) or other systemic abnormalities (e.g., central nervous system defects, arthrogryposis, and neurofibromatosis). The talus is almost completely vertical in this condition (parallel with the longitudinal axis of the tibia), and the calcaneus is plantar flexed. The navicular dislocates dorsally, and, clinically, a pronated,

rocker-bottom foot is present. After the navicular ossifies, its abnormal position helps to distinguish congenital vertical talus from severe planovalgus or flatfoot deformity.

METATARSUS VARUS (ADDUCTUS)

A "toeing in" gait or stance is a common problem in young children. The forefoot adduction differs from clubfoot in that the midfoot and hindfoot relationships are normally maintained. This condition commonly disappears with normal maturation and no treatment. Forefoot adduction can also occur as a result of excessive internal tibial torsion or increased femoral neck anteversion. Radiographically, the forefoot is adducted on AP films done with simulated weight bearing. Mild or moderate amounts of inversion correct with the plantar pressure, and the forefoot and hindfoot are aligned.

FLATFOOT

Variable degrees of hindfoot valgus, plantar arch flattening, and forefoot pronation occur. These are usually categorized as planovalgus foot or flatfoot deformity. The pathology is thought to involve increased ligamentous laxity, allowing the calcaneus to shift into a valgus position under the talus. Abduction and eversion results from loss of calcaneal support.

The differential diagnosis of planovalgus feet includes hindfoot valgus secondary to neuromuscular conditions such as cerebral palsy, peroneal spastic or (rigid) flatfoot, congenital vertical talus (Fig. 29), and congenital calcaneovalgus foot. On weight-bearing radiographs, the AP projection shows the talocalcaneal angle to be increased secondary to abduction of the calcaneus. The midtalar line passes medial to the first metatarsal. On the lateral projection, hindfoot valgus causes the talus to be more vertical than normal. The calcaneus and metatarsals are horizontal, with loss of the plantar arch. The common flatfoot deformity is flexible and painless; with a rigid or painful flatfoot, Harris-Beath views and/or CT may be performed to detect subtalar coalition or other abnormality.

CAVUS FOOT

In pes cavus, the longitudinal plantar arch is deepened. The anterior calcaneus is abnormally dorsiflexed and the metatarsals are plantar flexed. Although an idiopathic congenital form of cavus foot exists, more commonly the finding is secondary to neuromuscular

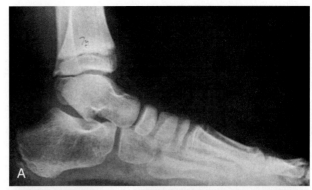

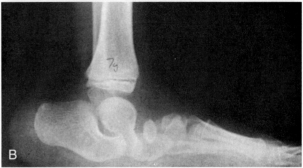

FIGURE 29. Severe congenital flatfoot with plantar flexion of the talus. **A,** Normal foot at 7 years of age. **B,** Rocker-bottom flatfoot at 7 years of age. The calcaneus is rotated clockwise on its transverse axis with the ventral end down and the dorsal tuberosity (heel) up; the talus is rotated into a vertical position with its ventral end down and the dorsal end up. The navicular has not followed the end of the talus caudad, but articulates with the ventral edge of the ectopic talus. The metatarsals are lifted slightly into a shallow equinus position. The longitudinal arch not only is flattened but has gone beyond flatness into a convex plane.

abnormalities. MRI of the spinal cord or central nervous system may be indicated. Differential diagnoses include peroneal muscular atrophy (Charcot-Marie-Tooth disease) (Fig. 30), Friedreich's ataxia, myelomeningocele, poliomyelitis, and other paralytic conditions.

FIGURE 30. Marked pes cavus in Charcot-Marie-Tooth peroneal muscular atrophy. The talocalcaneal angle is increased, and there is an elevated longitudinal arch. The metatarsophalangeal joints are extended, and the interphalangeal joints are flexed (hammer toe deformity).

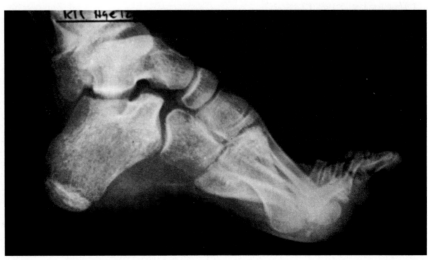

SUGGESTED READINGS

Osteochondroses

Adams JE: Injury to the throwing arm: a study of traumatic changes in the elbow joints of boy baseball players. Calif Med 1965;102:127–132

Barker DJP, Hall AJ: The epidemiology of Perthes disease. Clin Orthop 1986;209:89–94

Bensahel H, Bok B, Cavailloles F, et al: Bone scintigraphy in Perthes disease. J Pediatr Orthop 1983;3:302–305

Blank E, Girdany BR: Symmetric bowing of the terminal phalanges of the fifth fingers in a family (Kirner's deformity). Am J Roentgenol Radium Ther Nucl Med 1965;93:367–373

Blumenthal SL, Roach J, Herring JA: Lumbar Scheuermann's: a clinical series and classification. Spine 1987;12:929–932

Bradford DS: Vertebral osteochondrosis (Scheuermann's kyphosis). Clin Orthop 1981;158:83–90

Brower AC: The osteochondroses. Orthop Clin North Am 1983;14:99–117

Byers PD: Ischio-pubic "osteochondritis": a report of a case and a review. J Bone Joint Surg Br 1963;45:694–702

Caffey J: The early roentgenographic changes in essential coxa plana: their significance in pathogenesis. Am J Roentgenol Radium Ther Nucl Med 1968;103:620–634

Caffey J, Madell SH, Royer C, et al: Ossification of the distal femoral epiphysis. J Bone Joint Surg Am 1958;40:647–654

Caterall A: Legg-Calve-Perthes syndrome. Clin Orthop 1981;158:41–52

Cawley K, Dvorak A, Wilmot M: Normal anatomic variant: scintigraphy of ischiopubic synchrondoses. J Nucl Med 1983;24:14–16

Conway JJ: A scintigraphic classification of Legg-Calve-Perthes disease. Semin Nucl Med 1993;23:274–295

Daniel WW: Panner's disease. Arthritis Rheum 1989;32:341–342

Ducou le Pointe H, Haddad S, Silberman B, et al: Legg-Perthes-Calvé disease: staging by MRI using gadolinium. Pediatr Radiol 1994;24:88–91

Emmery L, Timmermans J, Leroy JG: Dysplasia epiphysealis capitis femoris? A longitudinal observation. Eur J Pediatr 1983;140:345–347

Flick AB, Gould N: Osteochondritis dissecans of the talus (transchondral fractures of the talus): review of the literature and new surgical approach for medial dome lesions. Foot Ankle 1985;5:165–185

Freiberg A, Forrest C: Kirner's deformity: a review of the literature and case presentation. J Hand Surg 1986;11:28–32

Heneghan MA, Wallace T: Heel pain due to retrocalcaneal bursitis—radiographic diagnosis (with an historical footnote on Sever's disease). Pediatr Radiol 1985;15:119–122

Hoskinson J: Freiberg's disease: a review of the long-term results. Proc R Soc Med 1974;67:106–107

Kaniklides C, Lonnerholm T, Moberg A, et al: Legg-Calve-Perthes disease: comparison of conventional radiography, MR imaging, bone scintigraphy and arthrography. Acta Radiol 1995;36:434–439

Karp MG: Köhler's disease of the tarsal scaphoid: an end result study. J Bone Joint Surg 1937;19:84–96

Kaufmann HJ, Taillard WF: Bilateral incurving of the terminal phalanges of the fifth fingers, An isolated lesion of the epiphyseal plate. Am J Roentgenol Radium Ther Nucl Med 1961;86:490–495

Mandell GA, Harcke HT: Scintigraphic manifestations of infraction second metatarsal (Freiberg's disease). J Nucl Med 1987;28:249–251

Mandell GA, MacKenzie WG, Scott CI Jr, et al: Identification of avascular necrosis in the dysplastic proximal femoral epiphysis. Skeletal Radiol 1989;18:273–281

Mandell GA, Morales RW, Harcke HT, et al: Bone scintigraphy in patients with atypical lumbar Scheuermann's disease. J Pediatr Orthop 1993;13:622–627

McCauley RG, Kahn PC: Osteochondritis of the tarsal navicular: radioisotopic appearance. Radiology 1977;123:705–706

Mesgarzadeh M, Sapega AA, Bonakdarpout A, et al: Osteochondritis dissecans: analysis of mechanical stability with radiography, scintigraphy, and MR imaging. Radiology 1987;165:775–780

Meyer J: Dysplasia epiphysealis capitis femoris: a clinical-radiological syndrome and its relationship to Legg-Calve-Perthes disease. Acta Orthop Scand 1964;34:183–197

Milgram JW: Radiological and pathological manifestations of osteo-chondritis dissecans of the distal femur: a study of 50 cases. Radiology 1978;126:305–311

Mitchell DG, Rao VM, Dalinka MK, et al: Femoral head avascular necrosis: correlation of MR imaging, radiographic staging, radionuclide imaging and clinical findings. Radiology 1987;162:709–715

Ponseti IV: Legg-Perthes disease. J Bone Joint Surg Am 1956;38:739–750

Rush BH, Bramson RT, Ogden JA: Legg-Calve-Perthes disease: detection of cartilaginous and synovial change with MR imaging. Radiology 1988;167:473–476

Schlesinger AE, Poznanski AK, Pudlowski RM, et al: Distal femoral epiphysis: normal standards for thickness and application to bone dysplasias. Radiology 1986;159:515–519

Scoles PV, Yoon YS, Makley JT, et al: Nuclear magnetic resonance imaging in Legg-Calve-Perthes disease. J Bone Joint Surg Am 1984;66:1357–1363

Sever JW: Apophysitis of the os calcis. N Y Med J 1912;95:1025

Siffert RS: Classification of the osteochondroses. Clin Orthop 1981;158:10–18

Stulberg SD, Cooperman DR, Wallensten R: The natural history of Legg-Calve-Perthes disease. J Bone Joint Surg Am 1981;63:1095–1108

Uno A, Hattori T, Noritake K, et al: Legg-Calve-Perthes disease in the evolutionary period: comparison of magnetic resonance imaging with bone scintigraphy. J Pediatr Orthop 1995;15:362–367

Yulish BS, Mulopolos GP, Goodfellow DB, et al: MR imaging of osteochondral lesions of talus. J Comput Assist Tomogr 1987;11:296–301

Miscellaneous Alignment Disorders

Bathfield CA, Beighton PH: Blount disease: a review of etiological factors in 110 patients. Clin Orthop 1978;135:29–33

Bell SN, Campbell PE, Cole WG, et al: Tibia vara caused by focal fibrocartilaginous dysplasia: three case reports. J Bone Joint Surg Br 1985;67:780–784

Chmell M, Dvonch VM: Adolescent tibia vara. Orthopedics 1989;12:295–297

Conway JJ, Cowell HR: Tarsal coalition: clinical significance and roentgenographic demonstration. Radiology 1969;92:799–811

Drennan JC (ed): Congenital Vertical Talus in the Child's Foot and Ankle. New York, Raven Press, 1992:155–168

Holt JF, Latourette HB, Watson EH: Physiological bowing of the legs in young children. JAMA 1954;154:390–394

Kling TF Jr: Angular deformities of the lower limbs in children. Orthop Clin North Am 1987;18:513–526

Langenskiöld A: Tibia vara: a critical review. Clin Orthop 1988;246:195–207

Langenskiöld A, Riska EB: Tibia vara (osteochondrosis deformans tibiae): a survey of seventy-one cases. J Bone Joint Surg Am 1964;46:1405–1420

Lee MS, Harcke HT, Kumar SJ, Bassett GS: Subtalar joint coalition in children: new observations. Radiology 1989;172:635–639

Levine AM, Drennan JC: Physiological bowing and tibia vara: the metaphyseal-diaphyseal angle in the measurement of bowleg deformities. J Bone Joint Surg Am 1982;64:1158–1163

Loder RT, Johnston CE II: Infantile tibia vara. J Pediatr Orthop 1987;7:639–646

MacEwan DW, Dunbar JS: Radiologic study of physiologic knock knee in childhood. J Can Assoc Radiol 1958;10:59–63

Ponseti IV, El-Khoury GY, Ippolito E, et al: A radiographic study of skeletal deformities in treated clubfeet. Clin Orthop 1981;160:30–42

Salenius P, Vankka E: The development of the tibiofemoral angle in children. J Bone Joint Surg Am 1975;57:259–261

Schoenecker PL, Meade WC, Pierron RL, et al: Blount's disease: a retrospective review and recommendations for treatment. J Pediatr Orthop 1985;5:181–186

Simons GW: Analytical radiography of club feet. J Bone Joint Surg Br 1977;59:485–489

Zionts LE, Harcke HT, Brooks KM, et al: Posttraumatic tibia valga: a case demonstrating asymmetric activity at the proximal growth plate on technetium bone scan. J Pediatr Orthop 1987;7:458–462

PART XI

INFECTIONS IN BONE

E. MICHEL AZOUZ

OSTEOMYELITIS

In spite of the availability of new diagnostic methods and a broad armamentarium of antibiotics, infections in bone remain a diagnostic and therapeutic medical challenge. With early diagnosis, rapid initiation of medical treatment with the appropriate antibiotic should be curative. Hematogenous osteomyelitis is preponderantly a disease of the growth period; infantile and even neonatal cases are not uncommon. Bacteria are the common inflammatory agents, but growing bones may also be invaded by other pathogens, including viruses, spirochetes, and fungi. Rarely, osteomyelitis in children is post-traumatic, including postsurgery or after accidental penetrating trauma, wound, or foreign body. Nonaccidental trauma (battered child) may also result in bone, joint, or soft tissue infection. The radiographic changes may be similar regardless of the infecting agent. The diagnosis is established by identification of the causative organism by blood and tissue culture, but may be suggested by radiographs after early soft tissue changes, such as soft tissue swelling and deep soft tissue edema, develop in an appropriate clinical setting.

- Bone infection source
  - Hematogenous
  - Adjacent infection
  - Direct implantation
    - Trauma
    - Foreign body
    - Surgery

Radionuclide imaging is more sensitive than plain radiographs in the early detection of bone infection. It can also identify additional foci of disease not clinically apparent at the time of examination. Vascular-phase images of the bone scan done within the first 5 minutes

following injection, delayed images with pinhole collimators, and special attention to the affected area have proved of great value. Osteomyelitis appears as an area of increased tracer activity reflecting the hyperemia and bone turnover induced by the infectious process. Park found that the sensitivity and specificity of three-phase bone scans for acute osteomyelitis were 84% and 97%, respectively, in 100 children with acute limb pain. Sensitivity and specificity for acute septic joint disease and cellulitis were even higher. Errors arose from simulation of infection by fracture and obscuration of osteomyelitis by septic arthritis, prior antibiotic treatment, and "cold" defects resulting from ischemia. It may be difficult to detect infection close to the growth plate because both the region of the growth plate and the nearby area of bone infection show increased activity on the bone scan. Newer cameras, magnification, digital imaging, and better positioning of the infant or child allow better differentiation between the metaphysis and the growth plate.

- Diagnosis of bone infection
  - Blood culture
  - Tissue culture
  - Imaging
    - Radionuclide scanning
    - Plain radiography
    - ± Sonography
    - ± Computed tomography
    - ± Magnetic resonance imaging

Computed tomography (CT) is very sensitive with respect to identification of marrow changes, and specificity is good in the appropriate clinical circumstances. CT is of limited clinical value in acute osteomyelitis. It is more useful in advanced disease to detect cortical destruction and delineate bone cavities and sequestra. Magnetic resonance imaging (MRI) is as sensitive as scintigraphy and delineates the anatomy and extent of

2343

marrow involvement to better advantage, providing more specificity in diagnosis. Its ability to define soft tissue and its multiplanar capabilities further enhance its value. Because of cost and possible delay of definitive diagnosis and treatment, we do not advocate that CT or MRI be used routinely for the study of osteomyelitis. Imaging should aim at guiding or modifying treatment, if necessary.

PYOGENIC HEMATOGENOUS OSTEOMYELITIS

Bone can be infected with a variety of organisms by extension from contiguous soft tissue infection or joint infection, or via the bloodstream from a remote source; the last is most frequent in the pediatric age group, and results in what is known as hematogenous osteomyelitis, a true infection of the bone marrow with early extension to other bony components and severe, systemic symptoms. Hematogenous osteomyelitis usually involves the highly vascularized metaphyses of the fastest growing bones, such as the distal femur, proximal tibia, proximal humerus, and distal radius. Organisms lodge most frequently in the terminal capillary loops of the metaphyses, but can locate initially in the epiphyses or in the cortex (Fig. 1). In the usual case, a small abscess forms in the marrow of the metaphysis, followed by local decalcification and destruction of the adjacent bone. When multiple focal abscesses are generated, multiple foci of bone destruction develop and later coalesce. Inflammatory swelling increases the intraosseous pressure because of the rigid bony walls of the marrow cavity, and can force extension of the infected exudate into several sites, as indicated in Figure 2. The most common route is via the haversian canals of the cortex to the subperiosteal space, where a subperiosteal abscess is formed. Simultaneously, spread also occurs further within the

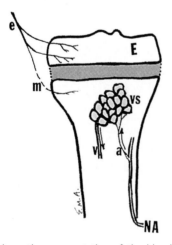

FIGURE 1. Schematic representation of the blood supply to the metaphysis and epiphysis of a child and the arterial channels through which invading organisms enter the growing bone. *NA* = nutrient artery; *a* = arteriole; *vs* = venous sinuses in the metaphysis; *v* = venule. An epiphyseal artery *(e)* supplies the epiphysis *(E)* and may branch to give (minor) metaphyseal vessels *(m)*. The major blood supply of the metaphysis comes from the nutrient artery.

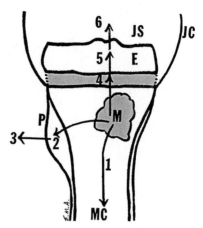

FIGURE 2. Schematic representation of the pathways of infection after hematogenous implantation in the metaphysis and formation of a metaphyseal focus *(M)* of bone infection (bone abscess). *1* = spread to the medullary canal *(MC)*; *2* = formation of a subperiosteal abscess; *3* = penetration of the periosteum *(P)* and spread to the adjacent soft tissues; *4, 5,* and *6* = spread across the growth plate to the epiphysis *(E)*, and eventually to the joint space *(JS)*. *JC* = joint capsule.

medullary cavity. Rupture of the periosteal abscess is responsible for extension of infection into the adjacent soft tissues. Inflammation and rapidly increased intraosseous pressure cause thrombosis of the vascular channels. Very early bone scans may therefore demonstrate a cold metaphyseal lesion as a result of compression or occlusion of the metaphyseal vessels. In these cases, increased activity is observed toward the diaphysis, beyond the cold metaphyseal area, which subsequently becomes "hot" and merges with the adjacent increased activity. The multiphase bone scan is very sensitive and is usually positive after 24 to 48 hours from the onset of symptoms. It can identify silent foci of bone infection as well as extension of metaphyseal osteomyelitis into the epiphysis through the growth plate (Fig. 3).

The earliest plain radiographic changes do not involve the bone. The deep soft tissues are swollen and edematous, obliterating the deep intermuscular fat septa. This occurs within the first 48 to 72 hours after infection and before the subcutaneous fat becomes edematous. Recognizable changes in bone are seldom present radiographically until the second week of the disease, but scintigraphy is very helpful in the early stages. CT and, better still, MRI can demonstrate the marrow alterations and extent of disease in bone, soft tissues, or adjacent joint at the same time (Fig. 4). Subperiosteal abscess formation is an early sonographic finding in osteomyelitis, preceding radiographic bony changes (Fig. 5). Needle puncture of the abscess can be carried out under sonographic control and the fluid sent for microscopic and bacteriologic analysis. Subperiosteal abscess may also be visualized with other cross-sectional modalities, such as CT (Fig. 6) and MRI (Fig. 7), even before visible plain radiographic changes. The early bone changes in conventional films are one or more small radiolucencies, usually in the metaphyseal region, where necrosis and destruction of bone has occurred (Fig. 8). On serial examinations, these may enlarge and become confluent.

With continuing appropriate antibiotic therapy, the periosteum begins to produce new bone on its undersurface after the second or third week. The resumption of osteogenic function by the periosteum suggests that the infectious process has been at least partly controlled at that site. Subsequent healing may involve remodeling of the cortical new bone and reconstitution of the underlying bone or, if damage has been extensive,

increase in the amount of periosteal reaction to form an involucrum around the fragments of the old devitalized diaphyseal bone (Fig. 9). Dead bone is relatively sclerotic and is called sequestrum. A sequestrum may be demonstrated on plain radiography, conventional tomography (Fig. 10), CT, or MRI; the best demonstration is usually achieved with CT. Sequestration has become rare since effective anti-infectious agents have been available. Although the mortality and morbidity of bone infection have decreased significantly, permanent sequelae do

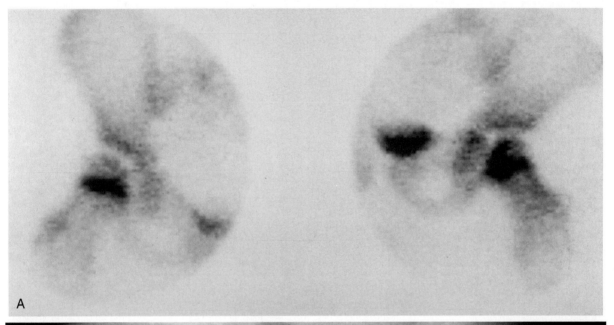

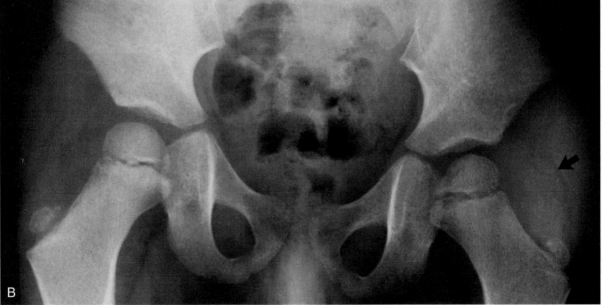

FIGURE 3. A 4-year-old boy with fever and "inability" to walk or move the left lower extremity for 6 days. **A,** Bone scan shows increased uptake in the femoral neck and head on the left side, likely resulting from extension of an initial metaphyseal focus of infection into the epiphysis. The right hip shows normal increased uptake in the region of the growth plate. **B,** Plain radiograph of the hips 2 weeks after the beginning of symptoms shows osteopenia on the left side, ill-defined medial metaphyseal and epiphyseal bone lucencies on each side of the growth plate, and indirect evidence of left hip joint effusion. *Arrow* points to the fat line displaced laterally by the joint fluid. Adjacent deep soft tissues are also swollen and edematous. Compare with the normal right side.

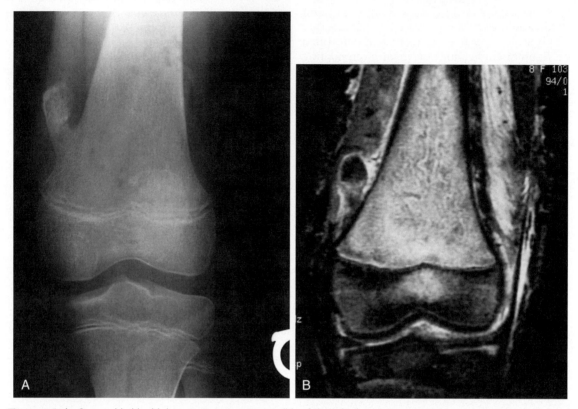

FIGURE 4. An 8-year-old girl with hematogenous osteomyelitis of the left distal femur. **A,** Anteroposterior plain radiograph shows generalized osteopenia of the left distal femur and proximal tibia. Note an incidental osteochondroma of the distal femoral metaphysis. **B,** Coronal short tau inversion–recovery magnetic resonance image (repetition time: 4000; echo delay time: 44; inversion time: 160) showing abnormal (high) bone marrow signal in the diaphysis, the metaphysis, and the central part of the epiphysis of the distal femur. There are also extensive changes in the soft tissues, especially laterally, again showing as high-signal-intensity areas on this inversion–recovery sequence.

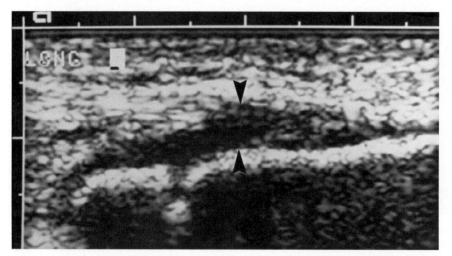

FIGURE 5. A 2-year-old girl with fever and anterior tibial swelling for 4 days. Plain radiographs (not shown) revealed soft tissue swelling and edema anterior to the proximal tibia. Bone appearance was normal. Longitudinal sonogram showed anterior subperiosteal fluid collection (between *arrowheads*).

occur, largely as a result of delay in diagnosis or inadequate treatment. Complications of bone infection include pathologic fracture through regions of bone destruction; adjacent infectious arthritis and destruction of joints (Fig. 11); and premature union of an epiphysis with the metaphysis across the growth plate, with resulting growth disturbance and discrepancy of limb length.

■ **Radiographic diagnosis of bone infection**
- Deep soft tissue edema
- Bone destruction (usually metaphyseal if hematogenous)
- Periosteal reaction
- Later: bone sclerosis, cavity, sequestrum, involucrum

■ **Complications of bone infection**
- Premature and asymmetric epiphyseal plate closure
- Joint destruction
- Pathologic fracture
- Growth disturbance
- Limb length discrepancy

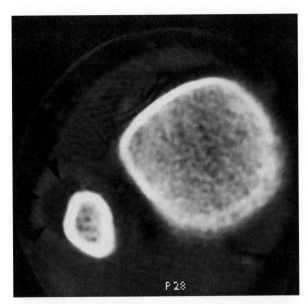

FIGURE 6. A 6-year-old boy with subperiosteal abscess formation demonstrated on plain axial computed tomography scan. Note that the fluid collection (between *arrowheads*) is of low attenuation. Adjacent bone (fibula) is normal.

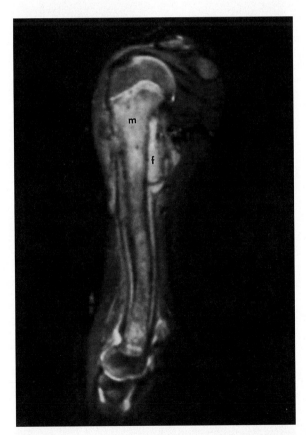

FIGURE 7. A 13-month-old boy with osteomyelitis of the proximal humerus. Magnetic resonance imaging shows no bone destruction. There is, however, abnormal increase of the bone marrow signal *(m)* on this short tau inversion–recovery image (repetition time: 4500; echo delay time: 44; inversion time: 160), extensive linear periosteal reaction along the whole humeral diaphysis, and proximal medial subperiosteal fluid collection *(f)*. The proximal and distal humeral epiphyses are normal.

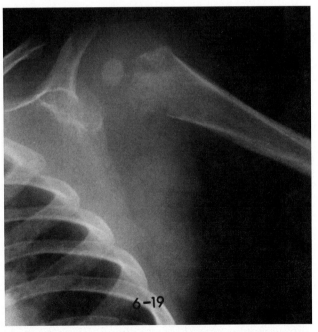

FIGURE 8. Early plain radiographic changes of osteomyelitis in the proximal metaphysis of the left humerus in a 9-month-old boy with fever and local signs and symptoms for 12 days. Metaphyseal areas of bone destruction are visualized as irregular, ill-defined lucencies. There is adjacent deep soft tissue swelling and edema, but there is no visible periosteal reaction.

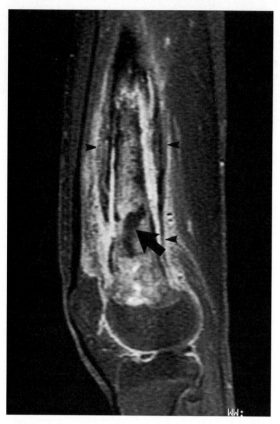

FIGURE 9. T$_1$-weighted sagittal magnetic resonance image (repetition time: 566; echo delay time: 11) with fat suppression, taken after gadolinium administration, in a 16-year-old boy with chronic osteomyelitis of the left femur shows a newly formed periosteal thick sheath or envelope called the involucrum *(arrowheads).* A separate large, nonenhancing devitalized piece of bone *(arrow)* represents a sequestrum. Extensive areas of high signal intensity are seen in soft tissues and bone marrow.

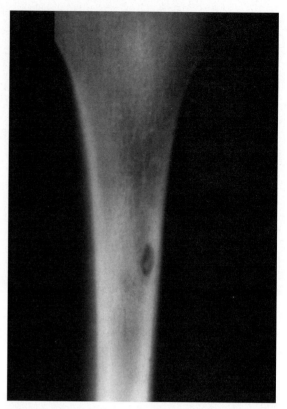

FIGURE 10. Anteroposterior tomography of the tibia in a 17-year-old girl with chronic osteomyelitis. Diaphyseal sclerosis is seen, as well as an eccentric oval bone cavity (bone abscess) in which lies a small fragment of dead bone: the sequestrum. *Staphylococcus aureus* was found in culture material from the abscess cavity.

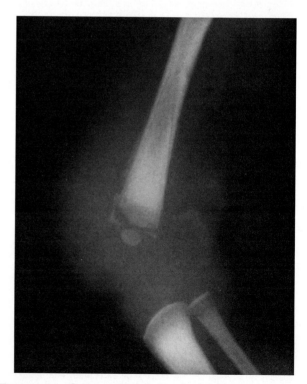

FIGURE 11. Osteomyelitis of the distal femur in a newborn showing metaphyseal destructive bone changes and periosteal reaction, as well as extensive adjacent soft tissue swelling and edema, cellulitis, and infectious arthritis of the knee joint.

In infants, the disease is generally milder and the recovery more rapid, because extension to form a subperiosteal abscess is more rapid and spontaneous rupture into the soft tissues more common. The high incidence of staphylococcal disease in older children is not seen in infant osteomyelitis, in which is found a large variety of organisms, many of which do not carry the tissue-disruptive enzymes that the staphylococci do. Various organisms of low pathogenicity may be responsible for low-grade, chronic sclerosing osteomyelitis in immunosuppressed children. Bone-production reaction greater than bone destruction is common in such cases. Osteomyelitis in the acquired immunodeficiency syndrome (AIDS) population is most often caused by common organisms such as *Staphyloccus aureus. Salmonella* and *Escherichia coli* have also been reported as etiologic agents of osteomyelitis in AIDS. In chronic granulomatous disease of childhood, which is an X-linked recessive disorder of leukocyte function, repeated infections occur in lymph nodes, skin, and lungs. Osteomyelitis is seen in approximately one third of patients. Cat-scratch disease, which is now known to be bacterial in origin *(Bartonella henselae),* is an infectious lymphadenitis frequently occurring in children and adolescents. Osteolytic lesions have on rare occasions been reported in this disease.

■ Likely causative organisms in hematogenous osteomyelitis
1. Neonatal period
   • Group B streptococcus
   • *Escherichia coli*
2. Infancy
   • Staphylococcus aureus
   • *Haemophilus influenzae*
3. Childhood
   • *Staphylococcus aureus*
4. In acquired immunodeficiency and sickle cell disease
   • *Staphylococcus aureus*
   • *Salmonella*
   • *Escherichia coli*

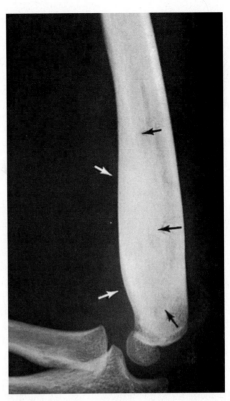

FIGURE 13. Chronic sclerosing (Garré's) osteomyelitis in the distal end of the humerus of a boy 4 years of age. The anterior cortex is thickened internally and externally *(arrows)*. Changes of this nature should also raise the question of an osteoid osteoma, in which the lucent nidus is concealed in the surrounding dense bone.

Brodie's Abscess

Occasionally, in nonimmunologically compromised children, a focus of subacute or chronic osteomyelitis is sharply localized and minimally active, presumably because of low virulence of the infecting organism. The initial purulent exudate is replaced by granulation tissue and the clinical manifestations are mild, consisting mainly of local pain. The lesion is generally in a metaphysis, commonly in the tibia (Fig. 12). It is characterized radiographically by a variable zone of sclerosis with a central or eccentric round, oval, or serpiginous radiolucency that not infrequently crosses the growth plate into the epiphysis. The growth plate is only a partial barrier against the spread of infection. The cavity may contain a small, dense sequestrum visible on plain radiographs or CT. Periosteal new bone formation may be present. Material removed from the abscess may disclose an organism of low virulence or none at all.

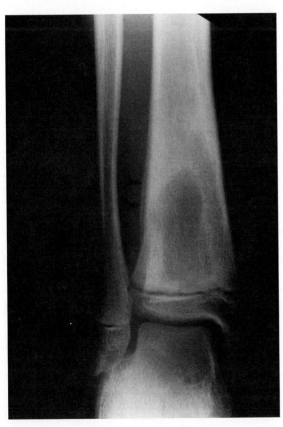

FIGURE 12. An 11-year-old boy with a 6-week history of pain and swelling of the right ankle. Patient was afebrile and had no leukocytosis. The erythrocyte sedimentation rate was 63 mm/hr. A large "active" Brodie's abscess cavity is seen in the distal tibial metaphysis. There is no sequestrum and no visible extension into the epiphysis. There is, however, linear periosteal reaction *(arrowheads)* along the lateral cortex of the distal tibia. Surgical incision and drainage were performed. *Staphylococcus aureus* was cultured. In most cases, cultures of the contents of Brodie's abscesses are sterile.

Garré's Sclerosing Osteomyelitis

This sclerosing form of chronic osteomyelitis affects children and young adults. Onset is insidious. Pain is the presenting symptom, but systemic signs are mild or absent. The diagnosis is made by the radiographic picture of diffuse bone production with little or no bone destruction or sequestrum formation (Fig. 13) in the absence of other causes for the finding. Mild bowing may be present (Fig. 14). The diaphysis of tubular bones is the most common localization. Osteoid osteoma is clinically and radiographically similar. CT helps for the search of the small lucent nidus in osteoid osteoma. Biopsy is often necessary for differentiation. The cause of Garré's osteomyelitis is believed to be a low-grade infection.

Epiphyseal Bone Infection

In tubular bones, the early changes of pyogenic hematogenous osteomyelitis are usually localized to the metaphysis, where capillary vascularization is very rich and blood flow is slow on the venous side of the loops. In children, a purely epiphyseal location of infection is possible but very rare. Epiphyseal osteomyelitis and septic arthritis occur more freely in infants less than 15 months of age because metaphyseal vessels cross the growth plate and enter the epiphysis.

Plain radiography usually demonstrates a focus of bone destruction localized to the epiphysis. In subacute and chronic cases, a small round or oval epiphyseal abscess cavity with well-defined borders is seen. CT is useful for imaging of the bone cavity, detecting the presence of a sequestrum or an associated joint effusion. Suspected spread of infection to the adjacent soft tissues is best imaged by MRI. This will reveal the epiphyseal focus of infection as low signal on T_1-weighted images and high signal on T_2-weighted images. Gadolinium

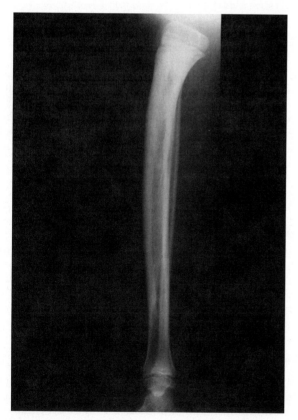

FIGURE 14. An 8-year-old boy with chronic sclerosing (Garré's) osteomyelitis. Note the increased bone density, the diffuse cortical thickening, and the mild anterior bowing of the proximal tibia.

injection helps outline the abscess cavity (Fig. 15). The differential diagnosis of an epiphyseal (or apophyseal) lucent lesion mainly includes infection and chondroblastoma. Epiphyseal infection may also be tuberculous or fungal.

Late epiphysiometaphyseal changes are sometimes seen in children months or years after severe meningococcal sepsis, likely as a result of occlusion of small blood vessels by microthrombi or septic emboli during the acute phase of the meningococcemia. Irregular ball-and-socket deformities or triangular-shaped epiphyses are seen at the ends of long bones (Fig. 16), with secondary shortening, bowing, and limb length discrepancy.

OSTEOMYELITIS RESULTING FROM UNUSUAL ORGANISMS OR UNKNOWN CAUSES

Fungal infections of bone are becoming more common as the immunosuppressed population increases. The radiographic changes are similar to those of chronic pyogenic osteomyelitis or tuberculosis—destruction of bone and periosteal reaction, with areas of cortical thickening and trabecular sclerosis. *Candida, Histoplasma, Blastomyces,* and others have been implicated. In musculoskeletal *Candida* infections, predisposing factors include multiple broad-spectrum antibiotic administration, hyperalimentation with indwelling vascular lines, immunosuppressive therapy, prematurity, and, in the newborn, maternal vaginal candidiasis. Sepsis may be present for several weeks before the skeletal complications arise. Arthritis usually precedes adjacent osteitis, in contradistinction to staphylococcal infections, in which septic arthritis generally extends from contiguous bone infection. The knee is most frequently affected, but multiple joint involvement is common. Clinical findings are primarily soft tissue swelling and effusions with pain and tenderness but little or no increase in local heat. Bone involvement is infrequent in classic histoplasmosis, although patchy rarefaction of the skull, metaphyseal bone destruction, and periosteal reaction have been reported. It is commonplace and prominent in African histoplasmosis caused by *Histoplasma duboisii*, in which bone and joint involvement is associated with large soft tissue abscesses. Bone lesions are frequent in actinomycosis, coccidioidomycosis, and more so in blastomycosis. Actinomycosis is a very rare cause of osteomyelitis in long bones. Skeletal coccidioidomycosis is frequently multicentric, and the lesions are usually well demarcated. In Latin America, children infected by *Para-coccidioides braziliensis* may have bone involvement, usually in the clavicle, ribs, and forearm bones. Blastomycosis may be focal or diffuse. The focal lesions tend to have a sclerotic margin, whereas the bone lesions of diffuse blastomycosis tend to show rapid destruction with penetration into adjacent joints. Long bones and ribs are frequently involved, followed by carpal and tarsal bones. Chest wall aspergillosis is usually secondary to contiguous spread of pulmonary aspergillosis (Fig. 17). Multifocal hematogenous peripheral *Aspergillus* osteomyelitis is very rare. Most of the patients with

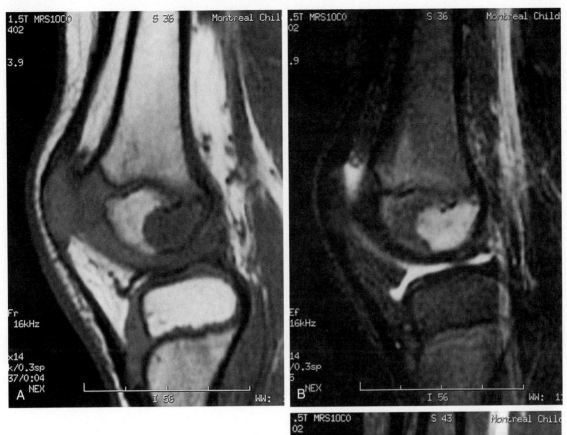

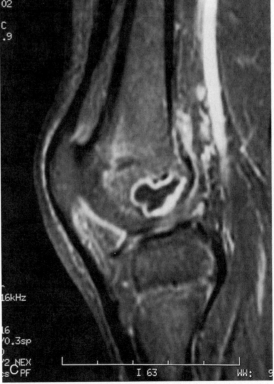

FIGURE 15. Magnetic resonance imaging in a 5-year-old boy with a primary epiphyseal focus of osteomyelitis. **A,** T_1-weighted image (repetition time [TR]: 466; echo delay time [TE]: 12) shows low-signal-intensity area in the distal femoral epiphysis. **B,** That same area shows high signal on the fat-suppressed T_2-weighted image (TR: 3300, TE: 102). **C,** T_1-weighted fat-suppressed image (TR: 416, TE: 11) after intravenous injection of gadolinium chelate clearly outlines the enhancing wall of the abscess cavity.

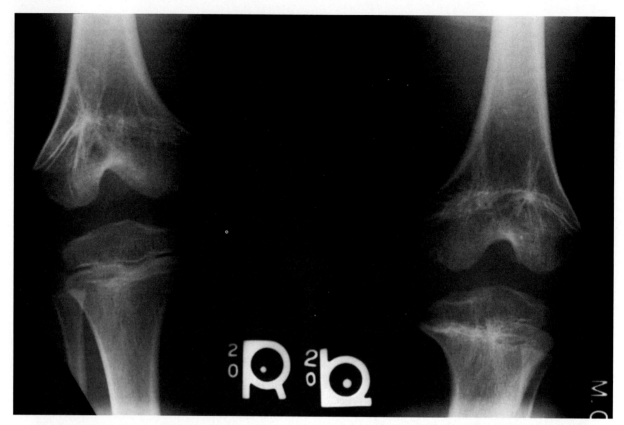

FIGURE 16. Late sequelae of infantile meningococcemia in an 8-year-old boy with severe changes seen in both knees. Early central fusion of the growth plates is seen in the distal femurs and left tibia, with metaphyseal cupping and secondary abnormal shape of the related epiphyses.

invasive aspergillosis have an underlying debilitating primary problem.

Viruses, such as those of rubella (Fig. 18), cytomegalic inclusion disease, chickenpox (varicella), and smallpox (Fig. 19), have been associated with bone lesions. In smallpox (variola), bizarre shortening of metacarpal bones has been observed (Fig. 20) mimicking brachy-dactylies of the types seen in skeletal dysplasias and

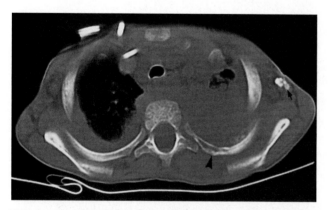

FIGURE 17. Axial image of a computed tomography scan of the upper chest of a 4-year-old boy with left rib destructive changes *(arrowhead)* and periosteal reaction, the result of contiguous spread from invasive pulmonary and pleural aspergillosis. Pleural disease with significant pleural thickening is seen on the right. Note the calcified left anterior axillary lymph nodes *(arrow).*

endocrinopathies. Varicella can produce cutaneous and bone lesions in fetuses of mothers infected during the first trimester. Limb hypoplasia is the most common osseous manifestation, and is regularly associated with cutaneous scarring in a pattern corresponding to a dermatome distribution that is believed to indicate a neuropathic effect of the virus on the fetus. The tibia has been affected in several cases (Fig. 21). Rubella (German measles) and cytomegalic inclusion disease may show very similar metaphyseal and metadiaphyseal changes in infected newborns with longitudinal linear sclerosis and lucencies.

Parasitic diseases are uncommon in Western countries and are seldom considered in the differential diagnosis of bone lesions; consequently, they may be easily over-looked in immigrants. Hydatid disease can cause bone lesions, although this location is rare in comparison with other sites (e.g., liver and lung). Gharbi et al. reported involvement of a phalanx of the big toe in one case and another case with vertebral involvement in a series of 13 carefully studied children with hydatid disease. In both cases, the bone lost its normal architecture and devel-oped irregular cystic expansions. Other instances of lesions in the ilium, vertebral column, and femur have been observed in children. No cases of bone hydatidosis have been observed in children under 2½ years, suggest-ing that a lengthy period of infestation is necessary for disease of bone to declare itself. O'Connor et al. reported a lytic lesion in the talus of an 8-year-old boy

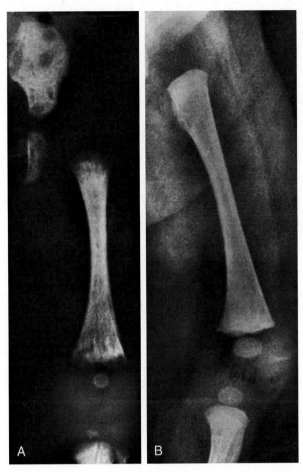

FIGURE 18. Radiographic changes in the bones of a newborn caused by transplacental rubella infection. **A,** On the third postnatal day, the ilium, ischium, femur, tibia, and fibula are irregularly mineralized, with large and small scattered patches of rarefaction. Deep transverse terminal bands of rarefaction, longitudinally streaked, occupy the metaphyseal zones. The absence of cortical thickening is noteworthy. The mother had typical clinical rubella during the first trimester of the pregnancy. The infant, born after gestation of 40 weeks, had thrombocytopenic purpura. Rubella virus was isolated from throat swabs. Serologic tests for syphilis were negative for infant and mother. **B,** On the 62nd postnatal day, the bones are normal radiographically. (Courtesy of Dr. Aaron R. Rausen, Elmhurst, NY.)

from which granulation tissue containing calcifying hookworm larvae was removed.

CHRONIC RECURRENT MULTIFOCAL OSTEOMYELITIS

This condition is seen mostly in children and adolescents. It is a bone-destructive and bone-productive inflammatory disorder of, as yet, unknown cause. Recurrent episodes of local swelling and pain, low-grade fever, leukocytosis, and elevated sedimentation rate are associated with focal lytic lesions usually seen in the metaphyses of tubular bones (Fig. 22). Pustular lesions of the palms and soles (pustulosis palmoplantaris), often associated with exacerbations of the disease, have been noted in several instances. The tibia has been affected

most frequently, followed by the clavicle, fibula, spine, and femur. The upper limb bones and the flat bones are less frequently affected. Lesions may be bilateral and symmetric. Vertebral lesions resembling those of diskitis have been observed. Not all lesions are symptomatic. Mild to moderate progressive sclerosis may surround the lesions. Cavities and sequestra are not seen in chronic recurrent multifocal osteomyelitis.

Biopsies demonstrate only a nonspecific chronic inflammatory reaction, often with numerous plasma cells, hence the name *plasma cell osteomyelitis*. Cultures are negative. The course of the disease may extend over several years with exacerbations and remissions. Complete resolution may occur, but some patients are left with residual bone changes such as sclerosis and expansion. Epiphyseal extension across the growth plate may occasionally cause premature physeal fusion and secondary degenerative arthritis.

The differential diagnosis is with subacute osteomyelitis, Langerhans' cell histiocytosis, and neoplasm (e.g., osteosarcoma, Ewing's sarcoma, leukemic bone changes, bone lymphoma, and metastases). A similar condition, sternocostoclavicular hyperostosis, occurs more commonly in adults, is limited to the chest wall, and has a frequent association with pustulosis palmoplantaris. Some affected individuals have the human leukocyte antigen allele B27 tissue type and may also have features of a seronegative spondyloarthropathy (psoriatic arthritis). SAPHO (*s*ynovitis, *a*cne, *p*ustulosis, *h*yperostosis, and *o*steitis) is now a frequently used acronym that unifies these idiopathic inflammatory or infectious disorders of bone and skin.

> ■ Differential diagnosis of chronic recurrent multifocal osteomyelitis
> • Subacute osteomyelitis
> • Langerhans' cell histiocytosis
> • Primary bone malignancy
> • Metastases

Diagnosis is based on plain radiographic appearance. Scintigraphy with ^{99m}Tc-methylene diphosphonate demonstrates intense focal increased activity at affected sites and may also detect clinically silent lesions. MRI, as expected with inflammatory processes, will show low signal intensity on T_1-weighted images and high signal on T_2-weighted images. With chronicity and intense sclerosis, there is decreased signal on the T_2-weighted images also.

> ■ Diagnosis of chronic recurrent multifocal osteomyelitis
> • Plain radiography
> • Radionuclide scanning
> • ± Computed tomography
> • ± Magnetic resonance imaging
> • Biopsy

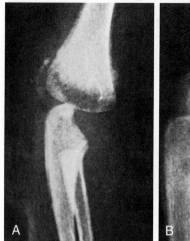
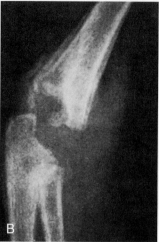
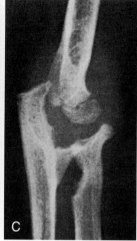

FIGURE 19. Serial changes in the elbow in osteomyelitis variolosa. **A,** Acute phase. **B,** Further disorganization of the joint 3 weeks later. **C,** Flail joint 2 years later. (From Cockshott WP: Osteomyellitis variolosa [in German]. Z Tropenmed Parasitol 1965;16: 199–206, with permission.)

TUBERCULOSIS

With AIDS epidemic, there has been a significant increase in cases of tuberculosis (TB) worldwide. Although bone TB is a relatively rare condition today, cases are still encountered that are not diagnosed until an extensive and expensive work-up has been completed. Hematogenous metastases of tubercle bacilli to the skeleton may take place early during the active phase of the primary complex in the thorax or later from postprimary tuberculous foci. After implantation in the bone, an immediate active inflammatory reaction may develop, or the bacilli may be dormant for years until activated by local factors such as trauma to the bone or joint. The synovial surface may be infected before the bones are involved; the infection may then spread from the joint into the contiguous epiphysis and metaphysis. In Cremin's experience in South Africa, the distribution of childhood skeletal TB is 60% to 70% vertebral, 20% to 25% large joints, and 10% to 15% tubular and flat bones.

TB produces a chronic inflammatory reaction in the bones that is similar in its macroscopic aspects to

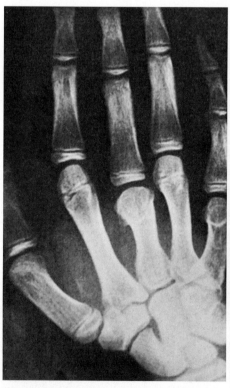
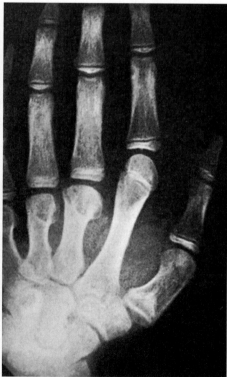

FIGURE 20. Late bizarre brachymetacarpia secondary to premature epiphyseal union as a complication of osteomyelitis variolosa affecting the hands. (From Cockshott WP: Osteomyelitis variolosa [in German]. Z Tropenmed Parasitol 1965; 16:199-206, with permission.)

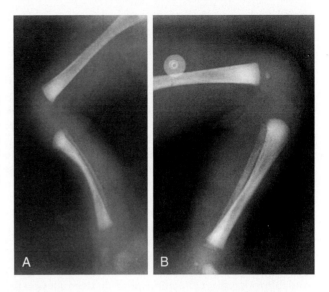

FIGURE 21. Hypoplasia of the lower limb in the congenital varicella syndrome. **A,** The tibia and fibula are most affected and are bowed. The soft tissues are also affected; a deep cutaneous scar was present over the anterior aspect of the tibia and extended onto the foot. **B,** The normal opposite limb is shown for comparison. The patient was born at 37 weeks' gestation complicated by polyhydramnios and had chorioretinitis, cortical atrophy, and gastroesophageal reflux. The infant died at 6 months of recurrent aspiration pneumonia.

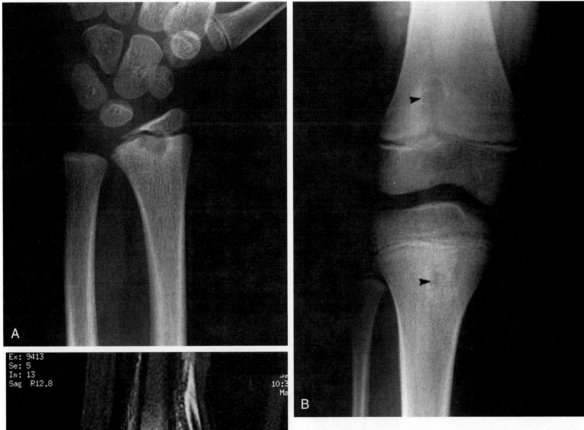

FIGURE 22. An 8-year-old girl with recurrent knee pain and swelling and biopsy-proven chronic recurrent multifocal osteomyelitis. There was simultaneous bone involvement in the left wrist and right knee. **A,** A plain radiograph of the wrist shows a metaphyseal lucent focus in the distal radius, abutting the central part of the growth plate. **B,** Anteroposterior radiograph of the right knee shows irregular lucencies in the distal femoral and in the proximal tibial metaphyses *(arrowheads)*. **C,** Sagittal T_2-weighted, fat-suppressed magnetic resonance image (repetition time: 5000; echo delay time: 108) reveals relatively well-defined areas of increased signal intensity in the distal femur and proximal tibia. These are areas of active inflammation. The wrist lesion was clinically silent and was discovered after a total-body bone scan revealed an area of increased uptake in that specific region.

chronic pyogenic osteomyelitis. Local necrosis of the intraosseous tissues develops at the site of implantation and is then followed by regional decalcification and bone destruction. Spread of infection from the focus in the bone takes place through the same pathways as those described in the pathogenesis of pyogenic osteomyelitis. During infancy and early childhood, when the epiphyseal cartilages are relatively thick, direct transfer of the infection from the joint to the bone, or infection across joints, is not common. The articular cartilages are preserved longer in tuberculous osteitis and arthritis than in pyogenic arthritis because of the lack of a destructive proteolytic enzyme in tuberculous exudates. Sinus formation and cold abscesses are common in tuberculous osteitis; involucrum formation and sequestration are very rare. With the antituberculous agents available today, direct needle aspiration from a lesion for diagnosis may be done without danger of chronic sinus formation.

The radiographic findings also are similar to those of chronic pyogenic osteomyelitis in all of the principal features, so that TB should be added regularly to the differential diagnosis of focal bone disease just as are neoplasms, neurofibromatosis, and osteomyelitis. Kozlowski and Lipson reported a 7-year-old child with both neurofibromatosis and metacarpal TB. Certain features do occur that can suggest the diagnosis of TB. In the metaphyses and epiphyses, destruction of bone is more prominent than is production (Figs. 23 and 24). The epiphysis is a site of predilection in primary skeletal TB. Nevertheless, Gardner and Azouz found 40% of solitary radiolucent epiphyseal lesions in a series of 15 children to represent nontuberculous osteomyelitis. The joint space is characteristically preserved in the early phases of tuberculous arthritis. In the diaphyses of tubular bones, long segments may exhibit destructive and productive changes while metaphyseal regions are unaffected (Fig. 25). Sometimes, sharply defined rarefactions are present that gave rise to the term *cystic tuberculosis of bone*. In the short bones of the hands and feet, tuberculous lesions may cause bone expansion and are called *spina ventosa* (Figs. 26 and 27). Skeletal TB

may affect multiple sites, and a bone scan is recommended to detect the presence of quiescent lesions. MRI is useful in certain cases and clearly demonstrates the full extent of the bone marrow, subperiosteal, and soft tissue involvement as well as any extension into the adjacent joint (Fig. 28).

■ Imaging signs of tuberculosis in bone
1. Common
   • Osteopenia
   • Bone destruction
   • Sinus formation
   • Cold abscesses
2. Rare
   • Bone sclerosis
   • Cyst/cavity formation
   • Bone expansion
   • Involucrum
   • Sequestration

Growth disturbances of affected bones are not uncommon and may result from premature fusion of growth plates. Disuse osteopenia is a constant feature of the bones when movement has been limited for more than a few weeks. Limitation of movement may contribute to the occasional premature fusion of the growth plates on both sides of a joint with subsequent limb shortening.

ATYPICAL MYCOBACTERIAL INFECTION

Atypical mycobacterial infection in humans is caused by organisms that are not *Mycobacterium tuberculosis* but are closely related to it. The best known is *Mycobacterium bovis*, causing TB in cattle and transmitted to humans through unpasteurized milk. Several other nontuberculous acid-fast organisms have been found to cause focal and disseminated infections in children and are called

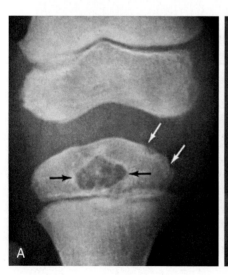 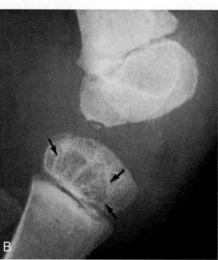

FIGURE 23. Destructive tuberculous epiphysitis of the tibia and arthritis of the knee in a boy 3 years of age. On frontal **(A)** and lateral **(B)** projections. Note that both central *(black arrows)* and marginal *(white arrows)* destructive changes are visible in the ossification center. Tuberculous tissue was found at biopsy.

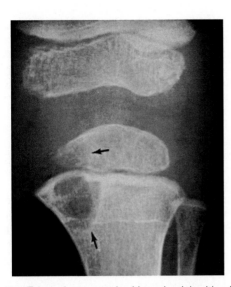

FIGURE 24. Tuberculous metaphysitis and epiphysitis of the tibia and arthritis of the knee in a boy 3 years of age. Large areas of destruction are present in the medial aspects of the metaphysis and the epiphyseal ossification center *(arrows)*. The large metaphyseal lesion suggests that the bone was infected independently of the joint and possibly prior to synovial involvement.

atypical tubercle bacilli; they are identified and categorized by microbiologic techniques. Bone lesions produced by these organisms are indistinguishable from those of TB, but, although they are characterized clinically by chronicity and recurrent breakdown of tissue, healing usually occurs with little relation to therapy. Frequent association with skin and lymph node lesions is a helpful clue in recognizing this form of infection.

Focal, TB-like bone lesions have occurred in a few infants and young children inoculated with bacille Calmette-Guérin (BCG) vaccine (Fig. 29), and the attenuated organism has been recovered from some lesions. These children were not seriously ill, unlike immunodeficient children, who may develop a generalized disease with widespread, predominantly metaphyseal osteopenic lesions following BCG inoculation.

BRUCELLOSIS

Brucellosis is a zoonosis, seen all over the world. It is caused by gram-negative bacilli of the genus *Brucella*. *Brucella melitensis* is the most common cause of brucello-

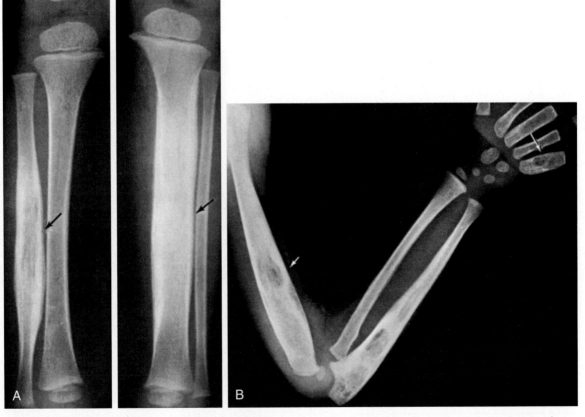

FIGURE 25. Benign multiple tuberculous diaphysitis in a boy 18 months of age, with cold abscesses on the dorsal surfaces of the hands. **A,** Lower extremities. The left tibia and right fibula are swollen; the medullary canals are expanded, and the overlying cortex is thickened *(arrows)*. **B,** Left upper extremity. The distal half of the humerus is swollen into a sausage-shaped contour and the cortex is thickened; the medullary canal is expanded and exhibits cystic rarefaction *(short arrow)*. The proximal half of the ulna is swollen, dilated, and irregularly cystic; its cortex is thickened. The fifth left metacarpal is expanded and irregularly lytic and osteoporotic *(long arrow)*. All of these lesions healed slowly but completely. In films made 2 years later, the skeleton appeared to be normal.

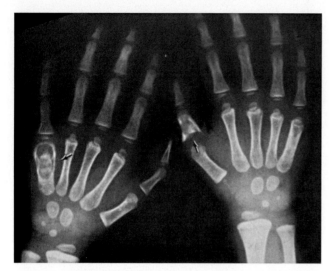

FIGURE 26. Tuberculous dactylitis (spina ventosa) in a boy 2 years of age. Cystic swelling of the fifth metacarpal and destructive changes in the proximal phalanx of the first digit are evident *(arrows)*. Spina ventosa is of historical interest because it was the first lesion described roentgenographically in a child.

sis. In a series of 96 Saudi patients, Madkour et al. found the spine to be most frequently involved (101 spinal sites showed increased uptake on the bone scan), followed by the joints (53 joints); only 3 long bones were involved. *Brucella* osteomyelitis of tubular bones was osteolytic, with only minimal periosteal reaction. Ruyssen et al. reported the case of a French child (from Yvelines), with *B. melitensis* osteomyelitis of the second metatarsal.

SARCOIDOSIS

This chronic granulomatous disease very rarely involves the bones of children. Skin, lungs, and lymphatic structures are often affected. In the skeleton, small, destructive cystic areas or a coarse lace-like reticulated pattern occur in the tubular bones of the hands and feet (Fig. 30). There is no periosteal reaction. There may be acro-osteolysis, but there is usually no osteopenia. Well-defined lytic lesions may occur in long bones or vertebral bodies, reminiscent of TB or metastatic disease. Redman et al. reported a case of sarcoidosis of the femur in a child who presented with a pathologic fracture. Occasionally, joint manifestations are present and simulate rheumatoid arthritis clinically. There is no radiologic evidence of joint involvement in sarcoidosis. Concomitant involvement of salivary glands and eyes may suggest the diagnosis. Biopsy of skin lesions may establish the diagnosis. A causal agent has not been established.

CONGENITAL SYPHILIS

There is now an increased incidence of this transplacental infection caused by *Treponema pallidum*. Congenital syphilis causes hepatosplenomegaly, lymphadenopathy, skin rash, and anemia. Bones are often involved but may not become clinically or radiologically manifest in the

first weeks of life. Bone pain in one or more extremities may be severe and may result in lack of movement of those extremities, a condition termed *Parrot's pseudoparalysis*. Syphilis of bone can be suggested on the basis of radiologic signs when it has not been considered on clinical grounds. The diagnosis, however, still rests on appropriate serologic tests. Two main forms are observed, infantile and juvenile, and their radiographic features are different.

The outstanding characteristic of infantile syphilis is multiple bone involvement with almost selective localization in the metaphyses. Broad bands of metaphyseal radiolucency were considered evidence of "metaphysitis" but are now known to be nonspecific responses to the stress of disseminated infection. Syphilitic granulation tissue can occur in these regions (Fig. 31). Radiographically, the two causes cannot be distinguished, but, when there is associated metaphyseal serration (the so-called sawtooth metaphysis) (Fig. 32), the diagnosis of congenital syphilis is practically assured. Similar diagnostic "specificity" is provided by Wimberger's sign after the newborn period, when focal destructive foci are found in the medial tibial metaphyses at the knee (Fig. 33). These lesions are not pathognomonic of congenital syphilis. They may be seen with ordinary osteomyelitis, hyperparathyroidism, and skeletal infantile myofibromatosis. The epiphyses are generally spared. Diaphyseal involvement, especially with periosteal new bone formation, also tends to occur after the

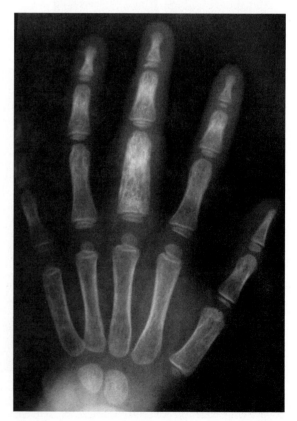

FIGURE 27. Tuberculous dactylitis (spina ventosa) in the proximal phalanx of the third finger of a 2-year-old girl. The whole diaphysis is involved. The epiphysis is spared. There is expansion of the rest of the phalanx, which shows mixed areas of bone destruction and sclerosis.

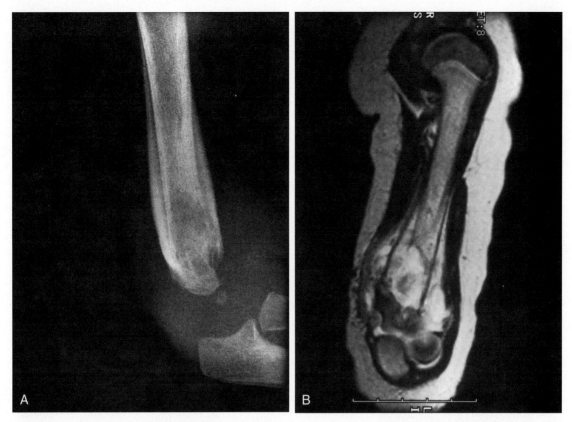

FIGURE 28. A 7-month-old Inuit boy presented with left elbow swelling. **A,** Lateral plain radiograph of the distal humerus and elbow shows an ill-defined lytic lesion in the distal humerus and thick periosteal reaction parallel to the cortex. There is also soft tissue swelling and edema. **B,** Sagittal T_2-weighted magnetic resonance image (repetition time: 3050; echo delay time: 92) shows with exquisite detail the abnormal high-signal bone marrow involvement of the distal humerus, the large subperiosteal inflammatory masses, and the extension into the elbow joint. Needle aspiration material from the distal humeral lesion grew *Mycobacterium tuberculosis*.

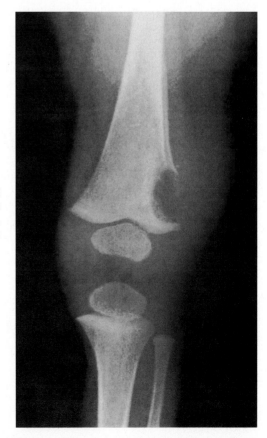

FIGURE 29. Bacille Calmette-Guérin osteomyelitis in a 7-month-old boy who had been immunized in the first week of life. Swelling and tenderness began 16 days prior to taking this film. Only focal demineralization was visible radiographically. (From Mortensson W, Eklof O, Jorulf H: Radiologic aspects of BCG osteomyelitis in infants and children. Acta Radiol 1976;17:845–855, with permission.)

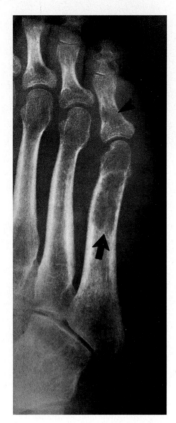

FIGURE 30. Lytic bone lesions of sarcoidosis in the foot of a 17-year-old girl. There is a definitely lytic destructive lesion in the distal half of the fifth metatarsal *(arrow),* and foamy rarefaction of the base of its proximal phalanx *(arrowhead).*

first month and may be associated with some destructive foci (Fig. 34) and even scattered focal cortical destruction and expansion of the medullary cavity (Fig. 35). Healing of the bone lesions in the infantile form of the disease occurs with or without therapy, usually without deformity. Metaphyseal destructive lytic lesions may lead to pathologic fractures, and battered baby syndrome is in the differential diagnosis.

■ Imaging signs of bone involvement in syphilis
  (Treponema pallidum)
  1. Congenital—infantile
     • Multiple bone involvement
     • Metaphyseal lucent bands
     • Metaphyseal serration (sawteeth)
     • Metaphyseal bone destruction:
       Wimberger's sign
     • Diaphyseal involvement
     • Periosteal reaction
  2. Congenital—juvenile
     • Periosteal and cortical thickening:
       saber shin
     • Focal destructive lesions
  3. Acquired
     • Gumma

Juvenile syphilis is observed radiographically in childhood and is manifested by diffuse or localized subperiosteal thickening of the cortex (Fig. 36). Associated focal destructive lesions, resembling cystic TB, occasionally are present. Thickening of the anterior cortex of the tibia is responsible for the "saber shin" deformity of congenital syphilis that appears in late childhood.

The above discussion relates to congenital syphilis. However, acquired syphilis does occur very rarely in children, and its clinical manifestations are comparable to those in adults.

Yaws is a nonvenereal spirochetal disease caused by *Treponema pertenue.* Bone pain and active osteoperiostitis are common. Thick, irregular bony outlines may be clinically palpable. New bone formation may be massive, simulating a tumor. In later stages, bone destruction with sequestration and fistula formation may occur.

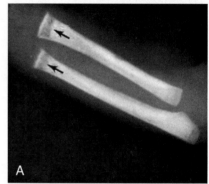

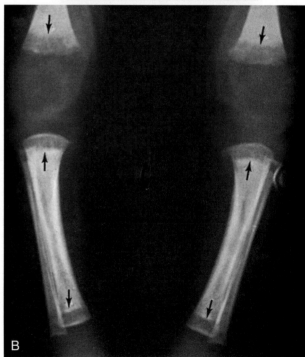

FIGURE 31. Radiographs of syphilic metaphysitis in a premature infant 1 month of age, showing deep segments of diminished density *(arrows).* The spongiosa in these segments has been replaced by radiolucent syphilitic granulation tissue. **A,** Upper limb. **B,** Lower limbs.

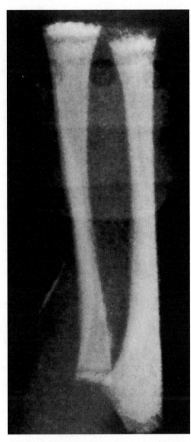

FIGURE 32. Sawtooth metaphysis in a newborn infant with congenital syphilis. This patient had a rash and mucocutaneous lesions characteristic of the disease.

INFANTILE CORTICAL HYPEROSTOSIS

Infantile cortical hyperostosis (ICH) is a disorder affecting the skeleton and some of its contiguous fasciae and muscles. The cause is unknown and the pathogenesis obscure. For the last two decades, the incidence of ICH has been declining, and it is now a rare disease. It carries the eponymic designation Caffey's disease as a result of Caffey's in-depth report of the condition in 1945, when he coined the descriptive term, as well as of his subsequent publications. One of Caffey's original patients was first reported by him in 1939 in a paper on the nonspecificity of the roentgen signs of syphilis. Descriptions of individual cases, unknown to Caffey, preceded his initial report and were subsequently acknowledged. These include those of DeToni and Roske.

Since ICH was first clearly recognized and named in 1945, it has been widely reported, especially in the United States, where several cases have been observed in almost every large hospital and clinic. It has occurred in all manner of circumstances—in cities and rural communities, in all kinds of climates in all seasons of the year, in all races, in poverty and luxury, among the primitive and the cultured. The incidence in boys and girls is approximately equal, but there is a striking age limitation. Caffey believed that there were no valid cases

in which the onset occurred later than the fifth to seventh month of life. Occasional reports now indicate initial onsets up to the middle of the first decade in patients in whom the diagnosis is acceptable by all other standards. Although several cases have been recognized in utero, most patients have been well for several weeks after birth. In some of these patients who had radiographs, the skeleton was normal before the disease appeared clinically. The average age at onset is about 9 weeks.

CLINICAL FINDINGS

There are but three manifestations common to all patients: hyperirritability, swellings of the soft tissues, and cortical thickenings of the underlying bones. The soft tissue swellings appear suddenly at the onset and present a painful wooden hardness during the active phases of the disease. They are always deeply situated and do not extend into the subcutaneous fat; early, the swellings may be exquisitely tender but are not overly warm or discolored (Figs. 37 and 38). In rare cases, local redness has been described. Massive deep swelling in the muscular masses probably represents the extension of the primary intraperiosteal reaction into the overlying connective tissues. The swellings appear clinically before the hyperostoses become visible roentgenographically; they subside and lose their tenderness long

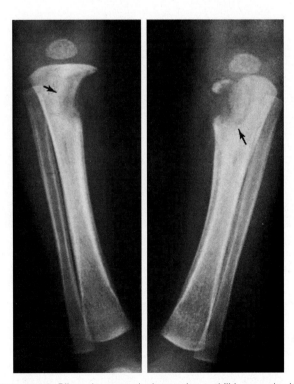

FIGURE 33. Bilateral symmetric destructive syphilitic metaphysitis of the proximal ends of the tibias (Wimberger's sign) in an infant 2 months of age. On the medial aspects of the tibias *(arrows)* are large areas of destruction of the spongiosa and its overlying cortex. In the left tibia, the medial segment of the epiphyseal plate is partially destroyed. Note also the diffuse periosteal thickening of the diaphyses.

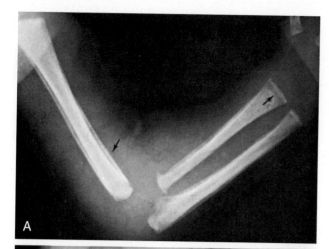

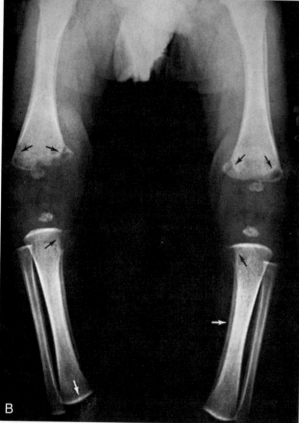

FIGURE 34. Syphilitic panosteitis in an infant 5 weeks of age. **A,** Upper limb. **B,** Lower limbs. Focal destructive changes are visible in the metaphyses, and the diaphyses show diffuse periosteal thickening. The main radiographic differential diagnosis here is non-accidental trauma (battered child syndrome).

before the hyperostoses resolve. The swellings involute slowly without suppuration; sometimes they recur suddenly in their original sites or in new sites either during or after the subsidence of the swellings that appeared at the onset of the disease. Edema and swellings around the orbits and even unilateral proptosis have been described. Although most swellings are accompanied by fever, the temperature was carefully measured in all stages of the disease in two of Caffey's patients and fever was never found. Other clinical features, present in some patients but lacking in others, have been pallor,

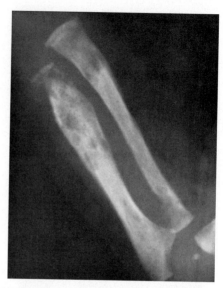

FIGURE 35. Expansion and destructive metaphyseal and diaphyseal changes in a syphilitic infant 3 months of age.

painful pseudoparalysis, and pleurisy. The condition has been found in asymptomatic persons in the course of family surveys or radiographic examination for other causes.

The uneven, protracted clinical course of the disease, with unpredictable remissions and relapses, is one of

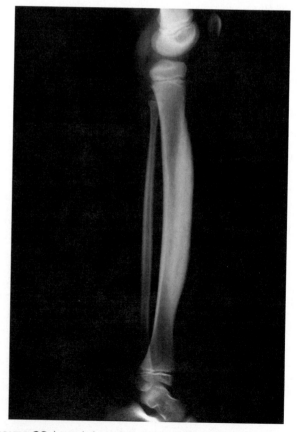

FIGURE 36. Lateral view of the lower leg in an 8-year-old boy with saber shin due to congenital syphilis. There is extensive anterior cortical and periosteal thickening of the tibial diaphysis.

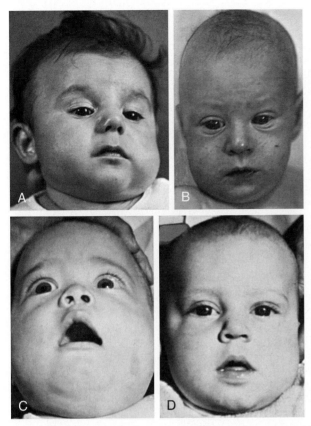

FIGURE 37. Facies in infantile cortical hyperostosis. In almost all cases, the changes have appeared before the fifth month of life. **A,** Unilateral swelling of the left cheek and left side of the jaw in an infant 12 weeks of age, 5 weeks after its first appearance. **B,** Unilateral swelling of the right cheek and right side of the jaw in an infant 15 weeks of age, 8 weeks after its first appearance. **C,** Bilateral swelling of the cheeks and jaw in an infant 6 months of age, 5 weeks after their first appearance. **D,** Bilateral swelling of the cheeks and jaw in an infant 12 weeks of age, 4 days after their first appearance; hyperostosis of the mandible was not visible in films made at this time but became visible in later films. The cervical lymph nodes were not enlarged.

the most characteristic features and one that makes the evaluation of therapeutic agents uncertain.

The disease is usually self-limited, with severe symptoms lasting from 2 to 3 weeks to 2 or 3 months. Swellings may persist even longer, but generally disability is limited to the early acute phase. Occasionally, active disease may persist and recur intermittently for years, with crippling deformities in the limbs and markedly delayed muscular and motor development. In one case, the disease persisted recurrently in the mandible and the soft tissues of the jaw from early infancy into the seventh year of life; other patients demonstrated late recurrences at 12 and 15 years. A patient with a clinical onset at 4½ years had recurrences persisting for 5 years associated with a slight overgrowth of one lower limb; in another, recurrences occurred from the 4th month of life until the 19th year. Hyperostoses are usually gone within 12 months (Fig. 39), but several cases have indicated persistence of cortical thickening and bowing even into adult life. The few deaths that have been recorded appear to result from intercurrent infection rather than from the primary disease.

Complications include pseudoparalyses, particularly of the upper limb with scapular involvement, and pleural effusion with costal involvement. Ipsilateral diaphragmatic elevation has been observed in several instances of scapular involvement. Torticollis has been associated with clavicular hyperostosis. Dysphagia has occurred in the presence of mandibular reaction. Sequelae are rare but include mandibular asymmetry, bowing deformities of the lower limbs, and bony fusions between adjacent bones such as ribs or bones of the arm or leg (Figs. 40 and 41).

LABORATORY FINDINGS

The most constant positive laboratory findings in ICH are increased sedimentation rate of erythrocytes and increased alkaline phosphatase activity of the blood serum. During active phases of the swellings and fever, these two laboratory findings are usually present. Hemoglobin level and the number of red blood cells are frequently reduced. Thrombocytosis has occurred in several instances and has been associated with thromboses in some infants. An increase in immunoglobulins has been noted in some cases. The results of serologic tests for both bacterial and viral infections have been consistently negative. All attempts to culture bacteria from the tissues and fluids of these patients have failed. In several infants, the disease has been associated with the Wiskott-Aldrich syndrome, a rare X-linked recessive immunodeficiency characterized by

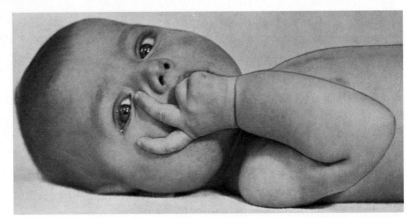

FIGURE 38. Swelling of the forearm and recurrent swelling of the right side of the face in an infant 5 months of age. The facial swelling first appeared at age 2 months; the forearm became swollen at age 3 months. The mandible and both bones in the forearm showed massive hyperostoses at the time this photograph was made (see Fig. 44B). All cervical, axillary, and epitrochlear lymph nodes were normal.

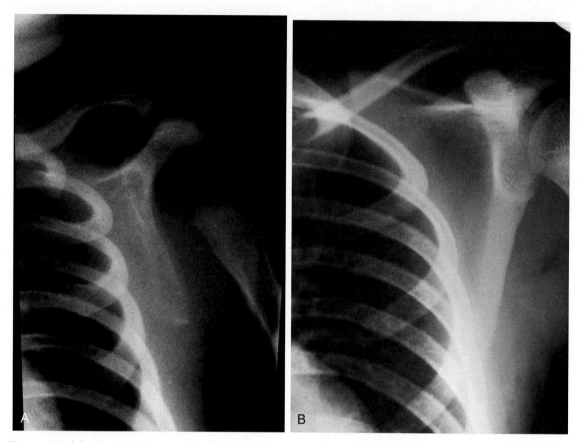

FIGURE 39. Infantile cortical hyperostosis (ICH) of the scapula. **A,** Periosteal thickening is seen along the lateral cortex of the left scapula. **B,** Film taken 13 years later shows a completely normal left scapula. In ICH, periosteal thickening is usually completely gone within 12 months.

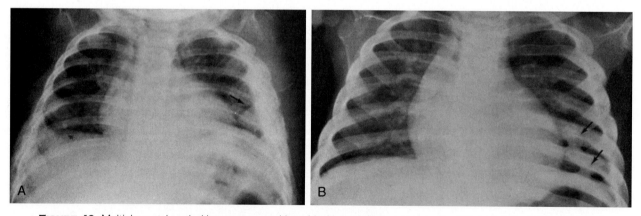

FIGURE 40. Multiple costal cortical hyperostoses with residual bony bridges between the fifth and sixth and the sixth and seventh left ribs. **A,** At 4½ months, 4 weeks after onset, during the active phase, there are multiple bilateral hyperostoses in the ribs and a longitudinal strip of water density *(arrow)* along the inner edges of the ribs that suggests pleural reaction. **B,** At 9 months, after subsidence of all general and local manifestations, there is still some expansion of the ribs, and bridges of bone have formed *(arrows)*.

a triad of eczema, infections, and bleeding caused by thrombocytopenia.

IMAGING FINDINGS

The radiographic features of the disease are a sine qua non for diagnosis and consist of stages in the appearance, development, and regression of hyperostotic lesions throughout the skeleton. Hyperostoses develop in contact with the external cortical surface, expand, and then remodel by resorption externally or expansion from the internal aspect of the bone. In the latter case, the affected bone may show an expanded medullary cavity and thin cortex for months or longer.

Bone and gallium scans have been positive even prior to the development of radiographic signs; Katz D et al. suggested a bone scan to seek other lesions if only one bone has radiographic abnormalities suggesting the diagnosis. MRI has demonstrated the marked soft tissue reaction surrounding the affected bones with increased signal on T_2-weighted images (Fig. 42). Diffuse enhancement after gadolinium administration has been described.

Cortical hyperostoses have been demonstrated in all of the tubular bones of the skeleton except the phalanges (Fig. 43). Vertebral bodies have also been spared. Of all the bones, the mandibles, clavicles, and ulnas have been involved the most frequently, the first in approxi-

mately 75% of cases. In the tubular bones, the lesions of ICH are confined to the dyaphyses and metaphyses. Epiphyseal ossification centers are normal roentgenographically. In the lower limbs, distribution of lesions is asymmetric; the larger hyperostoses of the limb bones often present conspicuous marginal irregularities (Fig. 44). Involvement may be very marked in one of a pair of adjacent bones while the other remains conspicuously normal.

Of the flat bones, the mandibles, scapulas, ilia, parietals, and frontals have all shown alterations (Figs. 45 and 46). Scapular lesions have usually been unilateral and have always appeared during the first half of the first year. In a few instances, the scapular hypertrophy and sclerosis of ICH have been mistaken for malignant neoplasm.

Fauré et al. reported four cases with exclusively orbital and facial involvement. Thickenings in the calvaria have been identified in several patients, and it seems likely that many inconspicuous lesions in the calvaria have been overlooked. Focal radiolucent lesions of the flat bones of the skull also have been observed. Cortical hyperostoses are usually most prominent in the lateral arcs of the ribs, possibly as a result of projection factors, because both vertebral and costochondral portions of the ribs may be affected (Fig. 47).

The distribution of the bone lesions is one of the most diagnostic features of ICH. If the disease were ever confined to one bone, other than the mandible, it

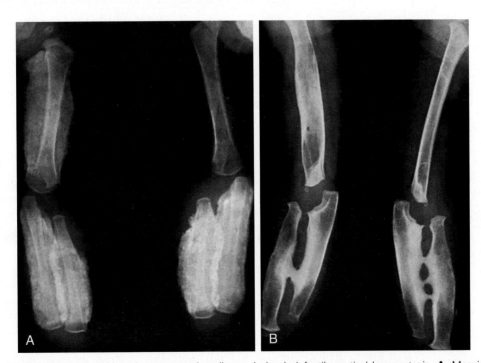

FIGURE 41. Residual bony bridges between each radius and ulna in infantile cortical hyperostosis. **A,** Massive cortical thickenings of the radii and ulnas at 4½ months of age. Pressure from the external thickenings has forced the radial heads laterad out of the elbows. **B,** At 12½ months, 9 months after onset, all affected bones are still greatly swollen, owing largely to expansion of the medullary cavities, although there are still residues of the earlier cortical thickening. The radial heads are still dislocated, and the radial diaphyses are now anchored in this ectopic position by solid bony bridges between them and the ulnar diaphyses—a single bridge on the right and three on the left. At 32 months, these bridges were still intact, although they had diminished slightly in caliber. It is possible that these bony bridges represent ossification of parts of the interosseous membrane.

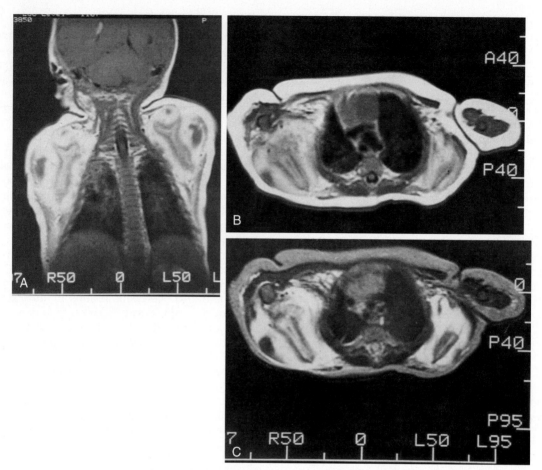

FIGURE 42. Magnetic resonance (MR) images of scapular involvement in infantile cortical hyperostosis. This 7-week-old boy with firm masses overlying the scapulae, bilateral Erb's palsy, irritability, and generalized hypotonia was sent to the neurologist because of paralysis, and MR imaging was requested. Skull and cervical spine were normal. Shoulders show increased marrow signal and cortical thickening of scapulas bilaterally; an extensive area of high signal completely surrounds both scapulas. **A,** Coronal contrast-enhanced T_1-weighted image (repetition time [TR]: 760; echo delay time [TE]: 20). **B,** Axial contrast-enhanced T_1-weighted image (TR: 800; TE: 20). **C,** Axial T_2-weighted image (TR: 2000; TE: 80). The severity of the edema surrounding the affected bones is clearly shown, especially on the T_2-weighted image, and, although the brachial plexus was not clearly identified, it seemed reasonable that compression by the large swellings was responsible for the Erb's palsy. (Courtesy of Dr. Drew Sullivan, San Jose, CA.)

would be impossible to identify it with certainty. It is possible, even probable, that most of the mild cases of ICH are overlooked clinically and are never examined radiographically. After a short course of mild fever, these patients recover without a satisfactory diagnosis. Slight swellings of the mandible are exceedingly difficult to palpate in the deep subcutaneous fat of the infantile jaw, as are deep, slight swellings of the ribs and long bones in the limbs. Many of the unexplained cortical hyperostoses encountered radiographically in healthy infants may be residuals of earlier and mild unrecognized ICH. Their presence has been instrumental in case finding in several of the studies on familial disease.

DIFFERENTIAL DIAGNOSIS

From the standpoint of differential diagnosis, the clinical course, laboratory findings, and radiographic features differentiate ICH from the most common diseases of infants with skeletal manifestations. Moreover, the serial changes in the formation of the hyperostoses are quite different from those of scurvy, osteomyelitis, and trauma. In the last-named lesions, a thin shell of bone forms first over the soft tissue swelling, separated from the bone diaphysis by a deep strip of relative radiolucency. In ICH, new bone formation begins in the soft tissue swelling, directly contiguous to the original cortex; becomes progressively more dense; and then is capped by a dense shell of limiting bone. Eversole et al. confirmed this feature in microscopic sections of biopsy specimens. The periosteal reaction of congenital syphilis develops later than that of ICH, and the serologic test for syphilis is positive. The hyperostosis of vitamin A intoxication appears only after many months of excessive ingestion of large amounts of vitamin A; the mandible is not involved, and the degree of hyperostosis is relatively mild. Two of the six

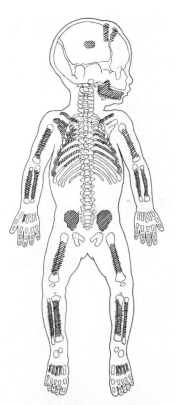

FIGURE 43. Schematic drawing of distribution of the skeletal lesions in infantile cortical hyperostosis. The sites of hyperostosis are shaded. The mandible, clavicles, and ulnas are affected most frequently. Hyperostoses in the vertebrae, round bones of the wrists and ankles, and phalanges have not been observed.

additional cases reported by Caffey in his second communication (1946) were subsequently accepted by him as probable examples of vitamin A intoxication, partly because of the late onset. As mentioned above, neoplasm has been considered in instances of isolated scapular involvement; the infrequency of primary bone neoplasms in infants is an important diagnostic consideration.

TREATMENT

Heyman et al. treated patients with typical ICH and increased prostaglandin serum levels with indomethacin, a prostaglandin synthetase inhibitor, and reported clinical improvement within 48 hours and progressive decrease of soft tissue swelling subsequently. Investigation of levels of endogenous prostaglandin may be of value in typical cases of ICH. If prostaglandin is involved in the disorder, the role of treatment of undiagnosed illnesses with aspirin in the ascertainment of cases may merit study.

Because the disease is generally self-limited, no therapy has been necessary in the great majority of cases. Caffey advocated the use of steroids for severe cases, and generally a prompt clinical response was observed, although recurrence was not infrequent following withdrawal of the drug. Steroids are contraindicated when thrombocytosis is present because of their tendency to induce thrombosis.

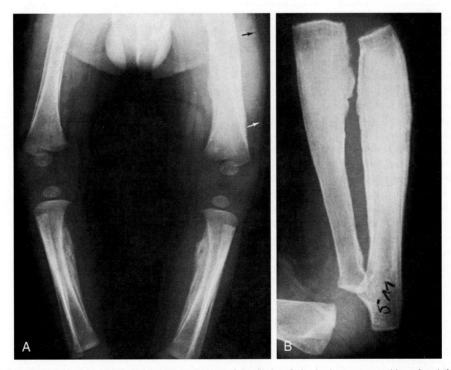

FIGURE 44. Massive cortical hyperostoses in tubular bones of the limbs. **A,** In the lower extremities of an infant 14 weeks of age, the *arrows* point to thick swellings in the soft tissues of the thigh. **B,** In the forearm of an infant 5 months of age, note the coarse and deep marginal irregularities in the distal radius.

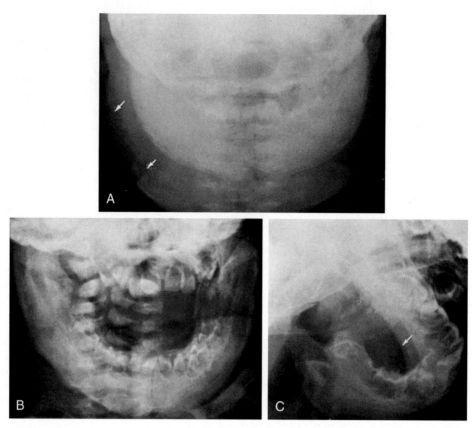

FIGURE 45. A and **B,** Massive cortical thickenings of the mandible in an infant 6 months of age whose facial swellings (*arrows* in **A**) first appeared during the fourth week of life. **A,** Mouth closed. **B,** Mouth open. **C,** Massive mandibular hyperostosis in an infant 7 weeks of age whose facial swelling *(arrow)* first appeared during the fourth week of life.

OTHER CONDITIONS ASSOCIATED WITH HYPEROSTOTIC LESIONS

Other conditions associated with hyperostotic lesions have been described in children older than those usually affected with ICH. Goldbloom et al. observed cortical hyperostoses in long tubular bones and the mandible associated with dysproteinemia in two unrelated children, 10 and 14 years of age, who had fever, pain, and tenderness in bones and who were unable to walk. The serum gamma globulin content in one patient was increased, with an increase in the immunoglobulin G fraction. Plasma cells were overabundant in the bone marrow. These radiographic changes subsided gradually over several months after the fever subsided. Melhem and associates reported more prominent cortical hyperostoses in association with hyperphosphatemia in a 5½-year-old boy with migrating swellings of the limbs and face of several months' duration. A less severely affected 13-year-old girl had similar clinical and laboratory findings. Grégoire et al. reported older patients with a prolonged clinical course who demonstrated hyperphosphatemia and also increased immunoglobulin G and M. These older children, with protracted disease and biochemical alterations not, or rarely, observed in ICH, most likely represent cases of other diseases. They are of interest, however, in relation to the reports of

otherwise acceptable cases of ICH with clinical features extending into adolescence.

> ■ **Types of cortical hyperostosis and periosteal reaction**
> - Trauma
> - Osteomyelitis
> - Vitamin A intoxication
> - Scurvy
> - Congenital syphilis
> - Primary bone tumor
> - Infantile cortical hyperostosis (DeToni-Caffey disease)
> - Goldbloom disease
> - Hyperphosphatemia
> - Prostaglandin administration

The occurrence of ICH in siblings, in twins, and in cousins raises the question of familial and possibly genetic transmission. Veller and Laur reported the disease in an infant 9 weeks of age whose father had productive periostitis of unknown origin when he was 4 weeks of age in 1929. The father was the patient described by Roske in 1930. Several large family studies

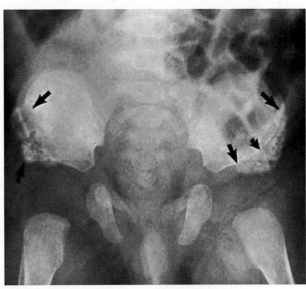

FIGURE 46. Massive marginal hyperostoses on the lateral edges of the iliac wings *(arrows)*. The lesions stop short of the faces of the acetabular cavities and crests of the ilia. The patient, 6 weeks of age, had classical signs of infantile cortical hyperostosis, with thick hyperostoses in the mandible and several long bones. (Courtesy of Dr. W. P. Yarbrough, Greene, MI.)

have been reported, supporting an autosomal dominant transmission with incomplete penetrance. Saul et al. have illustrated 26 pedigrees with over 100 persons affected to support this conclusion. Additional familial cases have been reported. There can be no question now that hereditary factors are involved, but the pathogenesis remains obscure. Some authors suggest that there are two major types of ICH: a common autosomal dominant form and a rare sporadic form. Among the factors that have been postulated as possible causes are allergy, viral infections, and collagen disorder. An animal model for the disease has been suggested by Thornburg in the condition known as craniomandibular osteopathy in the canine. This condition is occasionally familial in animals.

Prostaglandin administration in neonates with cyanotic congenital heart disease commonly used to maintain patency of the ductus arteriosus, has been associated with periostitis. This type of cortical/periosteal hyperostosis has been experimentally duplicated in dogs in response to long-term prostaglandin infusions. Bone changes have been observed as early as the ninth day of treatment (Fig. 48) and may increase and persist for weeks to months; they ultimately resolve without sequelae. In contrast with the features in ICH, the productive reactions tend to be symmetric (Fig. 49) and usually fail to affect the mandible. Ribs, clavicles, and scapulas may be affected. Gallium scan showed increased uptake in affected areas in one patient as reported by Poznanski et al.

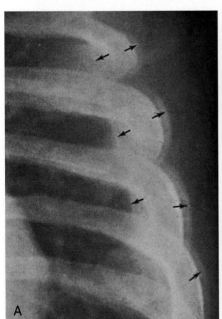
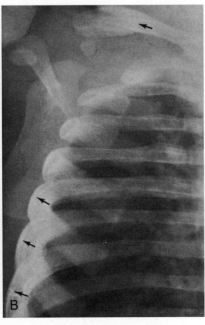

FIGURE 47. Costal hyperostoses. **A,** Early bilateral multiple thickenings of the ribs with underlying pleural thickening in an infant 14 weeks of age. **B,** Older multiple costal hyperostoses in an infant 5 months of age. The lamellations are a sign that the hyperostoses are old and beginning to involute.

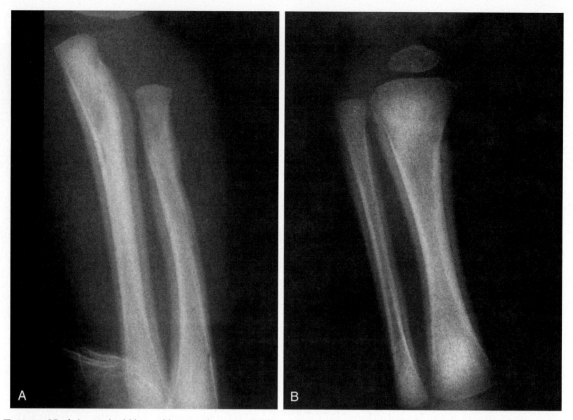

FIGURE 48. A 1-month-old boy with cyanotic congenital heart disease on prostaglandin E therapy. Forearm **(A)** and lower leg **(B)** radiographs show periosteal reaction along the entire length of the diaphyses of the radius, ulna, tibia, and fibula. Both sides were similarly affected.

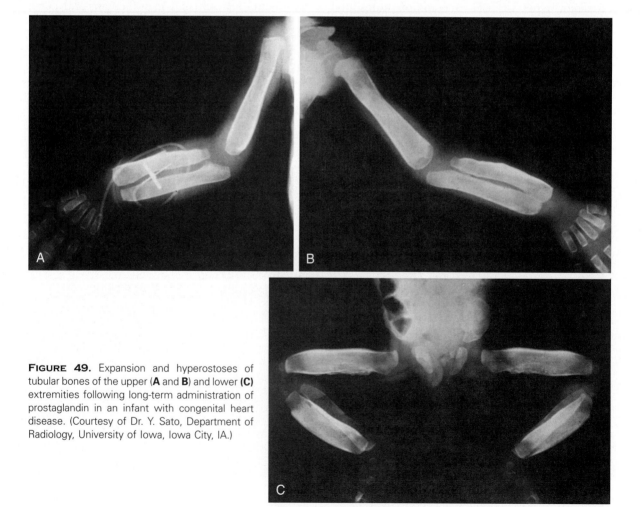

FIGURE 49. Expansion and hyperostoses of tubular bones of the upper **(A** and **B)** and lower **(C)** extremities following long-term administration of prostaglandin in an infant with congenital heart disease. (Courtesy of Dr. Y. Sato, Department of Radiology, University of Iowa, Iowa City, IA.)

SUGGESTED READINGS

Osteomyelitis

Alazraki NP: Radionuclide imaging in the evaluation of infections and inflammatory disease. Radiol Clin North Am 1993;31:783–793

André C, Badoual J, Kalifa G, et al: Histoplasmose africaine. Arch Fr Pediatr 1984;41:429–431

Azouz EM, Greenspan A, Marton D: CT evaluation of primary epiphyseal bone abscesses. Skeletal Radiol 1993;22:17–23

Azouz EM, Jurik AG, Bernard C: Sternocostoclavicular hyperostosis in children: a report of eight cases. AJR Am J Roentgenol 1998;171:461–466

Barron BJ, Dhekne RD: Cold osteomyelitis: radionuclide bone scan findings. Clin Nucl Med 1984;9:292–383

Barter SJ, Hennessy O: Actinomycetes as the causative organism of osteomyelitis in sickle cell disease. Skeletal Radiol 1984;11:271–273

Borzyskowski M, Harris RF, Jones RWA: The congenital varicella syndrome. Eur J Pediatr 1981;137:335–338

Boutin RD, Resnick D: The SAPHO syndrome: an evolving concept for unifying several idiopathic disorders of bone and skin. AJR Am J Roentgenol 1998;170:585–591

Bray H, Stringer DA, Poskitt K, et al: Maple tree knee: a unique foreign body—value of ultrasound and CT examination. Pediatr Radiol 1991;21:457–458

Brown T, Wilkinson RH: Chronic recurrent multifocal osteomyelitis. Radiology 1988;166:493–496

Bureau NJ, Chhem RK, Cardinal E: Musculoskeletal infections: US manifestations. Radiographics 1999;19:1585–1592

Carithers HA: Cat-scratch disease associated with an osteolytic lesion. Am J Dis Child 1983;137:968–970

Cockshott P, MacGregor M: Natural history of osteomyelitis variolosa. J Fac Radiol 1969;10:57–63

Cohen MD, Cory DA, Kleiman M, et al: Magnetic resonance differentiation of acute and chronic osteomyelitis in children. Clin Radiol 1990;41:53–56

Cotten A, Flipo RM, Mentre A, et al: SAPHO syndrome. Radiographics 1995;15:1147–1154

Dadi-Benmoussa F: L'hydatidose osseuse: à propos de 9 observations. Rev Maroc Méd Santé 1979;1:165–236

Damry N, Schurmans T, Perlmutter N: MRI evaluation and follow-up of bone necrosis after meningococcal infection and disseminated intravascular coagulation. Pediatr Radiol 1993;23:429–431

Dangman BC, Hoffer FA, Rand FF, et al: Osteomyelitis in children: gadolinium-enhanced MR imaging. Radiology 1992;182:743–747

Dargouth M, Essadam H, Ben Hamida H, et al: The value of ultrasound in acute osteomyelitis. Fr J Orthop Surg 1989;3:174–180

Davies AM, Marino AJ, Evans N, et al: SAPHO syndrome: 20-year follow-up. Skeletal Radiol 1999;28:159–162

Demharter J, Bohndorf K, Michl W, et al: Chronic recurrent multifocal osteomyelitis: a radiological and clinical investigation. Skeletal Radiol 1997;26:579–588

Doria AS, Taylor GA: Bony involvement in paracoccidioidomycosis. Pediatr Radiol 1997;27:67–69

Gaisie G, Bowen A, Quattromani FL, et al: Chest wall invasion by aspergillus in chronic granulomatous disease of childhood. Pediatr Radiol 1981;11:203–206

Gamble JG, Rinsky LA: Chronic recurrent multifocal osteomyelitis: a distinct entity. J Pediatr Orthop 1986;6:579–584

Gehweiler JA, Capp MP, Chick EW: Observations on the roentgen patterns in blastomycosis of bone. Am J Roentgenol Radium Ther Nucl Med 1970;108:497–510

Gharbi HA, Ben Cheikh M, Hamza R, et al: Les localisations rares de l'hydatidose chez l'enfant. Ann Radiol (Paris) 1977;20:151–157

Gill PJ, Goddard E, Beatty DW: Chronic granulomatous disease presenting with osteomyelitis: favorable response to treatment with interferon-γ. J Pediatr Orthop 1992;12:398–400

Girschick HJ, Krauspe R, Tschammler A, et al: Chronic recurrent osteomyelitis with clavicular involvement in children: diagnostic value of different imaging techniques and therapy with non-steroidal anti-inflammatory drugs. Eur J Pediatr 1998;157:28–33

Gylys-Morin V: MR imaging of pediatric musculoskeletal inflammatory and infectious disorders. Magn Reson Imaging Clin N Am 1998;6:537–559

Hamdan J, Asha M, Malloun A, et al: Technetium bone scintigraphy in the diagnosis of osteomyelitis in children. Pediatr Infect Dis J 1987;5:529–532

Hernandez RJ: Visualization of small sequestra by computerized tomography: report of six cases. Pediatr Radiol 1985;15:238–241

Hoffer FA, Emans J: Percutaneous drainage of subperiosteal abscess: a potential treatment for osteomyelitis. Pediatr Radiol 1996;26:879–881

Jaramillo D, Hoffer FA: Cartilaginous epiphysis and growth plate: normal and abnormal MR imaging findings. AJR Am J Roentgenol 1992;158:1105–1110

Jaramillo D, Treves ST, Kasser JR, et al: Osteomyelitis and septic arthritis in children: appropriate use of imaging to guide treatment. AJR Am J Roentgenol 1995;165:399–403

Jurik AG, Egund N: MRI in chronic recurrent multifocal osteomyelitis. Skeletal Radiol 1997;26:230–238

Kozlowski K: Brodie's abscess in the first decade of life. Pediatr Radiol 1980;10:33–37

Kuhn JP, Berger PE: Computed tomographic diagnosis of osteomyelitis. Radiology 1979;130:503–506

Laasonen LS, Karvonen SL, Reunala TL: Bone disease in adolescents with acne fulminans and severe cystic acne: radiologic and scintigraphic findings. AJR Am J Roentgenol 1994;162:1161–1165

Lachman RS, Yamauchi T, Klein J: Neonatal systemic candidiasis and arthritis. Radiology 1972;105:631–632

Lagard D, Dupont S, Boutry N, et al: Ostéite corticale septique. J Radiol 2000;81:54–58

Laxer RM, Shore AD, Manson D, et al: Chronic recurrent multifocal osteomyelitis and psoriasis—a report of a new association and review of related disorders. Semin Arthritis Rheum 1988;17:260–270

Mah ET, LeQuesne GW, Gent RJ, et al: Ultrasonic features of acute osteomyelitis in children. J Bone Joint Surg Br 1994;76:969–974

Majd M: Radionuclide imaging in detection of childhood osteomyelitis and its differentiation from cellulitis and bone infarction. Ann Radiol (Paris) 1977;20:9–18

Manson D, Wilmot DM, King S, et al: Physeal involvement in chronic recurrent multifocal osteomyelitis. Pediatr Radiol 1989;20:76–79

Marti-Bonmati L, Aparisi F, Poyatos C, et al: Brodie abscess: MR imaging appearance in 10 patients. J Magn Reson Imaging 1993;3:543–546

Modic MT, Pflanze W, Feiglin DH, et al: Magnetic resonance imaging of musculoskeletal infections. Radiol Clin North Am 1986;24:247–278

Morrissy RT, Shore SL: Bone and joint sepsis. Pediatr Clin North Am 1986;33:1551–1564

Mortensson W, Edeburn G, Fries M, et al: Chronic recurrent multifocal osteomyelitis in children: a roentgenologic and scintigraphic investigation. Acta Radiol 1988;29:565–570

Nilsson BE, Uden A: Skeletal lesions in palmarplantar pustulosis. Arch Orthop Scand 1984;55:366–370

O'Connor RI, Luedke DC, Harkess JW: Hookworm lesion of bone. J Bone Joint Surg Am 1971;53:362–364

Park HM: Scintigraphic evaluation of extremity pain in children: its efficacy and pitfalls. AJR Am J Roentgenol 1985;145:1079–1084

Paryani SG, Arvin AM: Intrauterine infection with varicella-zoster virus after maternal varicella. N Engl J Med 1986;314:1542–1546

Patriquin HB, Trias A, Jecquier S, et al: Late sequelae of infantile meningococcemia in growing bones of children. Radiology 1981;141:77–82

Pauli SL, Valkeakari T, Räsänen L, et al: Osteomyelitis-like bone lesions in acne fulminans. Eur J Pediatr 1989;149:110–113

Piddo C, Reed MH, Black GB: Premature epiphyseal fusion and degenerative arthritis in chronic recurrent multifocal osteomyelitis. Skeletal Radiol 2000;29:94–96

Pope TL Jr: Pediatric Candida albicans arthritis: case report of hip involvement with a review of the literature. Prog Pediatr Surg 1982;15:271–283

Probst FP, Björksten B, Gustavson KH: Radiological aspects of chronic recurrent multifocal osteomyelitis. Ann Radiol (Paris) 1978;21:115–125

Ratner LM, Kesack A, McCauley TR, et al: Disseminated Bartonella henselae (cat-scratch disease): appearance of multifocal osteomyelitis with MR imaging. AJR Am J Roentgenol 1998;171:1164–1165

Riebel TW, Nasir R, Nazarenko O: The value of sonography in the detection of osteomyelitis. Pediatr Radiol 1996;26:291–297

Rosenbaum DN, Blumhagen JD: Acute epiphyseal osteomyelitis in children. Radiology 1985;156:89–92

Roukoz S, Kahwaji A, Haddad-Zebouni S, et al: Ostéomyélite chronique multifocale récurrente : scintigraphie ou IRM: a propos de deux cas. J Radiol 1999;80:469–472

Schlesinger AE, Hernandez RJ: Diseases of the musculoskeletal system in children: imaging with CT, sonography and MR. AJR Am J Roentgenol 1992;158:729–741

Silverman FN: Virus diseases of bone: do they exist? AJR Am J Roentgenol 1976;126:677–703

Sonozaki H, Azuma A, Okai K, et al: Clinical features of 22 cases with inter-sterno-costo-clavicular ossification: a new rheumatic syndrome. Arch Orthop Trauma Surg 1979;95:12–22

Steinbach LS, Tehranzadeh J, Fleckenstein JL, et al: Human immunodeficiency virus infection: musculoskeletal manifestations. Radiology 1993;186:833–838

Sugimoto H, Tamura K, Fujii T: The SAPHO syndrome: defining the radiologic spectrum of diseases comprising the syndrome. Eur Radiol 1998;8:800–806

Sundaram M, McDonald D, Engel E, et al: Chronic recurrent multifocal osteomyelitis: an evolving clinical and radiological spectrum. Skeletal Radiol 1996;25:333–336

Tang JS, Gold RH, Bassett LW, et al: Musculoskeletal infection of the extremities: evaluation with MR imaging. Radiology 1988;166:205–209

Torricelli P, Martinelli C, Biagini R, et al: Radiographic and computed tomography findings in hydatid disease of bone. Skeletal Radiol 1990;19:435–439

Unger E, Moldofsky P, Gatenby R, et al: Diagnosis of osteomyelitis by MR imaging. AJR Am J Roentgenol 1988;160:605–610

Urso S, Pacciani E, Fariello G, et al: Osteomieliti aspecifiche dell'infanzia e dell'adolescenza: contributo della diagnostica per immagini. Radiol Med 1995;90:212–218

Yousefzadeh DK, Jackson JH: Neonatal and infantile candidal arthritis with or without osteomyelitis: a clinical and radiographical review of 21 cases. Skeletal Radiol 1980;5:77–90

Zeppa MA, Laorr A, Greenspan A, et al: Skeletal coccidioidomycosis: imaging findings in 19 patients. Skeletal Radiol 1996;25:337–343

Tuberculosis, Brucellosis, Sarcoidosis, and Syphilis

Adler DD, Blane CE, Holt JF: Case report 220: osseous sarcoidosis of left 5th digit in a young child with systemic sarcoidosis. Skeletal Radiol 1983;9:205–207

Cockshott WP, Davies AGM: Tumoural gummatous yaws. J Bone Joint Surg Br 1960;42:785–787

Cremin BJ: Tuberculosis: the resurgence of our most lethal infectious disease—a review. Pediatr Radiol 1995;25:620–626

Diard F, Kozlowski K, Masel J, et al: Multifocal, chronic, nonstaphylococcal osteomyelitis in children (report of four cases—aspergillosis, klebsiella, tuberculosis). Australas Radiol 1983;27:39–44

Engeset A, Eek S, Giljie O: On the significance of growth in the roentgenological skeletal changes of early congenital syphilis. Am J Roentgenol Radium Ther Nucl Med 1953;69:542–556

Gardner DJ, Azouz EM: Solitary lucent epiphyseal lesions in children. Skeletal Radiol 1988;17:497–504

Grossman H, Merten DF, Spock A, et al: Radiographic features of sarcoidosis in pediatric patients. Semin Roentgenol 1985;20:393–399

Hugosson C, Harfi H: Disseminated BCG-osteomyelitis in congenital immunodeficiency. Pediatr Radiol 1991;21:384–385

Kozlowski K, Lipson A: Bony tuberculosis misinterpreted—a cautionary tale. Australas Radiol 1993;37:119–121

Madkour MM, Sharif HS, Abed MY, et al: Osteoarticular brucellosis: results of bone scintigraphy in 140 patients. AJR Am J Roentgenol 1988;150:1101–1105

McClean S: Osseous lesions of congenital syphilis: summary and conclusions in one hundred and two cases. Am J Dis Child 1931;41:1411–1418

Mortensson W, Eklof O, Jorulf H: Radiologic aspects of BCG osteomyelitis in infants and children. Acta Radiol 1976;17:845–855

Pace JL: Treponematoses in Arabia. Saudi Med J 1983;4:211–220

Rasool MN, Govender S, Naidoo KS: Cystic tuberculosis of bone in children. J Bone Joint Surg Br 1994;76:113–117

Redman DS, McCarthy RE, Jimenez JF: Sarcoidosis in the long bones of a child: a case report and review of the literature. J Bone Joint Surg Am 1983;65:1010–1014

Robinson RJ, Olinsky A: Sarcoidosis in children. Aust Paediatr J 1986;22:291–293

Ruyssen S, Le Pennec MP, Perreau M, et al: Ostéite à brucelles chez l'enfant. Arch Fr Pediatr 1983;40:803–805

Salzman AL, Hoffer FA, Burns JC: Infectious disease rounds: chronic hip pain and limp in a 3 year old girl. Rev Infect Dis 1989;11:341–348

Shannon FB, Moore M, Houkom JA, et al: Multifocal cystic tuberculosis of bone. J Bone Joint Surg Am 1990;72:1089–1092

Solomon A, Rosen E: Focal osseous lesions in congenital lues. Pediatr Radiol 1978;7:36–39

Vanthournout I, Quinet B, Neuenschwander S: Pediatric yaws osteoperiostitis. Pediat Radiol 1991;21:303

Wessels G, Hesseling PB, Beyers N: Skeletal tuberculosis: dactylitis and involvement of the skull. Pediatr Radiol 1998;28:234–236

Infantile Cortical Hyperostosis and Other Conditions Associated with Hyperostotic Lesions

Abinum M, Mikuska M, Filipovic B: Infantile cortical hyperostosis associated with the Wiskott-Aldrich syndrome. Eur J Pediatr 1988;147:518–519

Beluffi G, Chirico G, Colombo A, et al: Report of a new case of neonatal cortical hyperostosis: histological and ultrastructural study. Ann Radiol 1984;27:79–88

Boyd RDH, Shaw DG, Thomas BM: Infantile cortical hyperostosis with lytic lesions in the skull. Arch Dis Child 1972;47:471–472

Caffey J: Infantile cortical hyperostoses. J Pediatr 1946;29:541–559

Caffey J: Infantile cortical hyperostosis: a review of the clinical and radiographic features. Proc R Soc Med 1957;50:347–354

Caffey J, Silverman WA: Infantile cortical hyperostoses: preliminary report on a new syndrome. Am J Roentgenol Radium Ther 1945;54:1–16

Claesson I: Infantile cortical hyperostosis: report of a case with late manifestation. Acta Radiol 1976;17:594–600

Clemett R, Williams JH: The familial occurrence of infantile cortical hyperostosis. Radiology 1963;80:409–416

DeToni G: Una nuova malattia dell'apparato ossea: la poliosteopatia deformante connatale regressive. Policlin Infant 1943;11:1–32

Eversole SL Jr, Holman GH, Robinson RA: Hitherto undescribed characteristics of the pathology of infantile cortical hyperostosis (Caffey's disease). Bull Johns Hopkins Hosp 1957;101:80–89

Fauré C, Beyssac J-M, Montagne J-P: Predominant or exclusive orbital and facial involvement in infantile cortical hyperostosis (DeToni-Caffey's disease). Pediatr Radiol 1977;6:103–106

Gentry RR, Rust RS, Lohr JA, et al: Infantile cortical hyperostosis of the ribs (Caffey's disease) without mandibular involvement. Pediatr Radiol 1983;13:236–238

Gerscovich EO, Greenspan A, Lehman WB: Idiopathic periosteal hyperostosis with dysproteinemia—Goldbloom's syndrome. Pediatr Radiol 1990;20:208–211

Goldbloom RB, Stein PB, Eisen A, et al: Idiopathic periosteal hyperostosis with dysproteinemia: a new clinical entity. N Engl J Med 1966;274:873–878

Grégoire A, Combes JC, Hornung H, et al: Périostose multifocale récurrente de l'enfant: problèmes nosologiques. Pediatrie 1978;33:491–496

Heyman E, Laver J, Beer S: Prostaglandin synthetase inhibitor in Caffey disease [Letter]. J Pediatr 1982;101:314

Jorgensen HR, Svanholm H, Host A: Bone formation induced in an infant by systemic prostaglandin-E2 administration. Acta Orthop Scand 1988;59:464–466

Katz D, Eller DJ, Bergman G, et al: Caffey's disease of the scapula: CT and MR findings. AJR Am J Roentgenol 1997;168:286–287

Katz JM, Kirkpatrick JA, Papanicolaou N, et al: Case report 139: infantile cortical hyperostosis (Caffey disease). Skeletal Radiol 1981;6:77–80

Keeton BR: Vitamin E deficiency and thrombocytosis in Caffey's disease. Arch Dis Child 1976;51:393–395

Leung VC, Lee KE: Infantile cortical hyperostosis with intramedullary lesions. J Pediatr Orthop 1985;5:354–357

Maclachlan AK, Gerrard JW, Houston CS, et al: Familial infantile cortical hyperostosis in a large Canadian family. Can Med Assoc J 1984;130:1172–1174

Matzinger MA, Briggs VA, Dunlap HJ, et al: Plain film and CT observations in prostaglandin-induced bone changes. Pediatr Radiol 1992;22:264–266

Melhem RE, Najjar SS, Khachadurian AK: Cortical hyperostosis with hyperphosphatemia: new syndrome? J Pediatr 1970;77:986–990

Neuhauser EBD: Infantile cortical hyperostosis and skull defects. Postgrad Med 1970;48:57–59

Newberg AH, Tampas JP: Familial infantile cortical hyperostosis: an update. AJR Am J Roentgenol 1981;137:93–96

Pazzaglia UE, Byers PD, Beluffi G, et al: Pathology of infantile cortical hyperostosis (Caffey's disease): report of a case. J Bone Joint Surg Am 1985;67:1417–1426

Poznanski AK, Fernbach SK, Berry TE: Bone changes from prostaglandin therapy. Skeletal Radiol 1985;14:20–25

Ringel RE, Haney PJ, Brenner JI, et al: Periosteal changes secondary to prostaglandin administration. J Pediatr 1983;103:251–253

Roske G: Eine eigenartige Knochenerkrankung im Säugling-salter. Montasschr Kinderheilkd 1930;25:385–400

Saatci I, Brown JJ, McAlister WH: MR findings in a patient with Caffey's disease. Pediatr Radiol 1996;26:68–70

Saul RA, Lee WH, Stevenson RE: Caffey's disease revisited: further evidence for autosomal dominant inheritance with incomplete penetrance. Am J Dis Child 1982;136:56–60

Sheppard JJ, Pressman H: Dysphagia in infantile cortical hyperostosis (Caffey's disease): a case study. Dev Med Child Neurol 1988;30:111–114

Sone K, Tashiro M, Fujinaka T, et al: Long-term low-dose prostaglandin E1 administration [Letter]. J Pediatr 1980;97:866–867

Swerdloff BA, Ozonoff MB, Gyepes MT: Late recurrence of infantile cortical hyperostosis (Caffey's disease). Am J Roentgenol Radium Ther Nucl Med 1970;108:461–467

Thornburg LP: Animal model of human disease: infantile cortical hyperostosis (Caffey-Silverman syndrome). Craniomandibular osteopathy in the canine. Am J Pathol 1979;95:575–578

Ueda K, Saito A, Nakano H, et al: Cortical hyperostosis following long-term administration of prostaglandin E1 in infants with cyanotic congenital heart disease. J Pediatr 1980;97:834–836

Veller K, Laur A: Zur Ätiologie der infantilen kortikalen hyperostose (Caffey-Syndrom). Fortschr Geb Roentgenstr 1953;79:446–452

Williams JL: Periosteal hyperostosis resulting from prostaglandin therapy. Eur J Pediatr 1986;6:231–232

Yousefzadeh DK, Brosnan P, Jackson JH Jr: Infantile cortical hyperostosis, Caffey's disease, involving two cousins. Skeletal Radiol 1979;4:141–147

BENIGN AND MALIGNANT BONE TUMORS

BARRY D. FLETCHER

BENIGN BONE TUMORS

Approximately 50% of all childhood bone neoplasms are benign. It is important that radiologists recognize the typical benign tumors so that appropriate therapy can be initiated and so that the patient can avoid unnecessary diagnostic procedures. Although it is not always possible to differentiate between benign and malignant lesions, this determination will significantly affect the course of subsequent imaging evaluations, the approach to biopsy, and the choice of definitive treatment. Furthermore, the pathologist frequently takes into account the results of the imaging examination in reaching a histologic diagnosis.

Plain film radiographs remain the primary tool for evaluating bone tumors. However, other imaging methods, particularly magnetic resonance imaging (MRI) and in some cases computed tomography (CT) and nuclear studies, provide support for initial diagnoses by demonstrating specific features. Table 1 summarizes the clinical and imaging features of the benign bone tumors discussed in this chapter.

CARTILAGINOUS TUMORS

Osteochondroma

Osteochondromas are common lesions of the growing skeleton, occurring in approximately 1% of the general population. Rather than a true tumor, osteochondromas are thought to be a developmental defect of growing bone in which an injury to the perichondrium causes bone growth in an aberrant direction. The metaphysis from which the osteochondroma arises is usually widened because of the absence of normal modeling. Although the shape of osteochondromas can vary on radiographs, these tumors are usually either pedunctulated or sessile (Figs. 1 and 2). The long axis of

the osteochondroma pedicle or stalk is almost always directed away from the adjacent joint. The direct communication between the osteochondroma and the cortex and marrow cavity of the bone from which it arises is a distinctive feature that is particularly well demonstrated on CT and magnetic resonance (MR) images. T_2-weighted MR images also demonstrate an intense cartilaginous cap that is, in essence, a recapitulation of the physis. Consequently, the cap can be quite thick in early childhood and, like the normal physis, becomes narrower with age. After epiphyseal closure, growth of the osteochondroma ceases.

Many osteochondromas are radiation induced and have been found in 6% to 12% of patients who received radiation at a young age. Latent periods vary from 3 to 16 years. Osteochondromas can occur even after low doses of radiation therapy and often occur in bones that were in the periphery of the radiation field. Multiple osteochondromas have been found in patients who received total-body irradiation as preparation for bone marrow transplantation at a young age.

Because most osteochondromas are asymptomatic, they are usually discovered incidentally. However, mechanical irritation of adjacent soft tissues or nerves, vascular injuries, fracture of the stalk, or malignant transformation can produce symptoms. When one of a pair of adjacent bones is affected, the osteochondroma can cause pressure deformity of the other bone. Multiple exostoses of the forearm may cause ulnar shortening and angular deformation of the distal radius that results in a pseudo-Madelung's deformity at the wrist. Dysplasia epiphysealis hemimelica (Trevor's disease) may be a manifestation of epiphyseal osteochondroma.

Malignant transformation of solitary osteochondromas, even those that are radiation induced, is rare. However, transformation to chondrosarcoma may occur in as many as 10% of cases of multiple osteochondromas. Malignant transformation should be considered when the osteochondroma grows after epiphyseal clo-

Table 1 ■ CHARACTERISTIC FEATURES OF BENIGN BONE TUMORS

TUMOR TYPE	SPECIAL FEATURES
Cartilaginous Tumors	
Surface	
Osteochondroma	Has cartilage cap; may be multifocal
Periosteal chondroma	Has frequent calcifications and no cartilage cap
Central	
Enchondroma	Often associated with Ollier's disease or Maffucci's syndrome
Chondroblastoma	Often located in epiphysis
Chondromyxoid fibroma	Lytic, often eccentric metaphyseal location
Cysts	
Simple cyst	Often contains bone fragments detectable on radiographs
Aneurysmal bone cyst	Fluid–fluid levels detectable on magnetic resonance images
Giant cell tumor	Located in diametaphyses of children; is precursor of aneurysmal bone cyst
Fibrous Tumors	
Nonossifying fibroma	Located in posterior cortex of metaphyses
Fibrous dysplasia	Polyostotic form often associated with McCune-Albright syndrome
Osteofibrous dysplasia	Often found in anterior cortex of tibia
Adamantinoma	Is possible precursor of osteofibrous dysplasia
Langerhans' Cell Histiocytosis	Occurs in local form as eosinophilic granuloma
Osseous Tumors	
Osteoid osteoma	Associated with characteristic pain pattern and nidus
Osteoblastoma	Is larger than osteoid osteoma; is usually located in vertebra

sure. Malignancy occurs in the cartilaginous cap, which becomes thickened. The cap of an osteochondroma usually measures less than 1 cm in thickness, whereas that of a chondrosarcoma often exceeds 2 cm.

A rare case of osteosarcoma arising in a longstanding osteochondroma has been described in a 17-year-old boy. Unlike chondrosarcoma, which arises in the periphery of an osteochondroma, in this case CT and MRI showed marrow, cortical, and soft tissue involvement.

Periosteal Chondroma

This variant of an enchondroma arises from the periosteal surface of the cortex of the large and small tubular bones and tends to occur in the proximal humerus and the phalanges of the hand. Although periosteal chondroma may bear superficial similarity to a sessile osteochondroma, it is associated with sclerosis and saucerized erosion of the adjacent cortex and frequent focal calcifications in the matrix of the lesion. Cross-sectional imaging shows that the cortex clearly separates the tumor from the medulla and that a cartilaginous cap is absent (Fig. 3). Histologically, the lesion consists of normal cartilage arranged in a lobular fashion. This tumor does not have malignant potential, but biopsy

may be advisable to distinguish periosteal chondroma from juxtacortical chondrosarcoma and periosteal osteosarcoma.

Enchondroma

Enchondromas, tumors of cartilage cells derived from the neighboring epiphysis, are most frequently located in the large and small tubular bones of the limbs, particularly those of the hand. Like other cartilaginous tumors, enchondromas exhibit a loblulated growth pattern that results in asymmetric expansion of the medullary cavity and endosteal scalloping. Focal calcifications of variable size are often visible in the otherwise radiolucent mass, and the tumor may exhibit a characteristic cartilaginous ring-and-arc pattern on radiographs and CT images. The tumor is isointense with muscle on T_1-weighted MR images and exhibits a heterogeneous, predominantly high T_2-weighted signal. Gadolinium enhancement of T_1-weighted images may demonstrate a pattern of thin arcs and rings.

Ollier's disease is a nonheritable disorder of cartilage proliferation in which enchondromas involve multiple bones, especially those of the hands. Onset during infancy or early childhood usually eventually results in severe skeletal deformity. The lesions of Ollier's disease are expansile and lucent or trabeculated, usually with a shell of thin cortex (Fig. 4). In the long bones, longitudinal lucent columns or streaks may be present.

Enchondromatosis accompanied by multiple hemangiomas is known as Maffucci's syndrome. Calcified phleboliths may be demonstrated radiographically in the hemangiomatous soft tissue masses of patients with Maffucci's syndrome. Recent evidence of an association between spindle cell hemangioendothelioma and enchrondromatosis suggests that some of the vascular lesions of Maffucci's syndrome are actually spindle cell hemangioendotheliomas and that the two entities may be a form of mesodermal dysplasia. Lesions associated with both Ollier's disease and Maffucci's syndrome carry a significant risk of malignant degeneration to chondrosarcoma: 30% to 50% of lesions undergo transformation. Approximately 5% of patients with chondrosarcoma have Ollier's disease.

Enchondroma protuberans is a cartilaginous tumor that can resemble either a periosteal chondroma or a sessile osteochondroma. Like its precursor, enchondroma, this tumor arises in the medulla and expands eccentrically in the cortex so that the tumor eventually protrudes beyond it.

Chondroblastoma

Chondroblastoma, an uncommon tumor composed of primitive cartilage cells, usually occurs in the second decade of life. Its most specific feature is its location in the epiphysis of a long bone, most often the proximal humerus, distal femur, or proximal tibia. Apophyseal chondroblastomas have also been reported, and involvement of the adjacent metaphysis may occur, especially in skeletally mature persons. Chondroblastomas can give rise to secondary aneurysmal bone cysts.

Radiographically, a chondroblastoma is an eccentric, lucent, well-defined lesion with sclerotic borders (Fig. 5A). Periosteal reaction distant from the lesion is another common feature suggesting an accompanying inflammatory process. Approximately one third of chondroblastomas have a calcified matrix. These features are well demonstrated by CT, which may also show cortical destruction.

On MR images (Fig. 5B–D) the tumor typically exhibits signal intensity similar to that of muscle; however, the rim of the tumor has a lower intensity, and some foci give no signal because of calcification. On T_2-weighted images, the signal intensity of the tumor is low to intermediate in comparison with that of fat. In contrast, on both T_2-weighted and short tau inversion–recovery (STIR) images, the signals of adjacent soft tissues are usually hyperintense because of edema associated with periosteal new bone formation. Intense

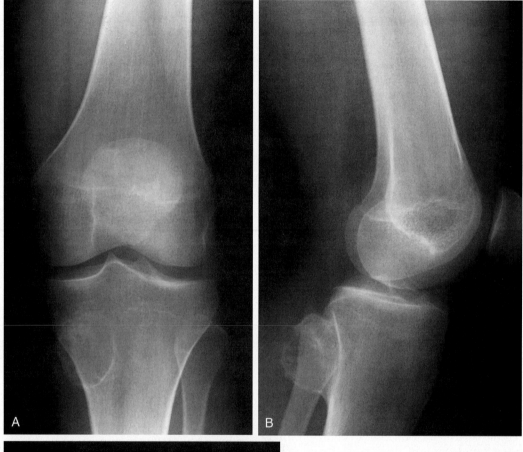

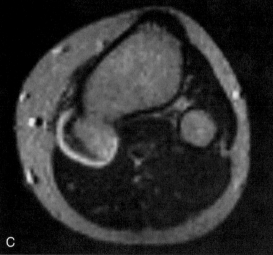

FIGURE 1. Anteroposterior **(A)** and lateral **(B)** views of the knee of a 17-year-old boy show a large osteochondroma arising from the medial aspect of the proximal tibia. **C,** T_2-weighted transverse magnetic resonance image shows a short, broad pedicle. Note the thin, hyperintense cartilaginous cap and the continuity of the marrow cavity of the tibia with that of the osteochondroma. This patient had multiple osteochondromas of the long bones 10 years after undergoing total-body irradiation before bone marrow transplantation for leukemia. (**B** from Fletcher BD, Crom DB, Krance RA, Kun LE: Radiation-induced bone abnormalities after bone marrow transplantation in childhood leukemia. Radiology 1994;191:233, with permission.)

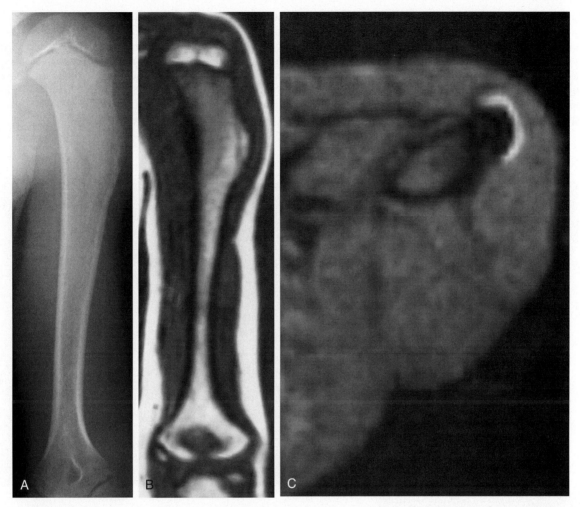

FIGURE 2. A, Radiograph of the arm of an 8-year-old boy shows a broad-based sessile osteochondroma of the proximal humerus. **B,** Coronal T_1-weighted magnetic resonance image of the humerus shows normal bone marrow signal extending into the tumor base. **C,** Transverse short tau inversion–recovery image shows a thin, hyperintense cartilaginous cap.

activity on the blood pool phase of skeletal scintigrams is consistent with hyperemia.

Chondromyxoid Fibroma

Chondromyxoid fibroma is a less common tumor than chondroblastoma, affecting predominantly males in the second or third decade of life. The ilium and the bones of the knee and the foot are the most common sites of this tumor. Unlike chondroblastoma, chondromyxoid fibroma involves the metaphysis and apparently does not cross an open growth plate.

The tumor contains a variable amount of chondroid, fibrous, and myxoid tissue. Its characteristic but nonspecific radiographic appearance is that of a central or eccentric lucent lesion with sclerotic margins and cortical expansion. Half of the lesions in the series of patients reported by Wilson et al. were elongated and oriented parallel to the long axis of the involved bone. Matrix calcification and periosteal new bone formation usually do not occur.

CYSTS

Simple Bone Cyst

Although pathologists do not consider simple bone cysts to be true neoplasms, radiologists include them in the differential diagnosis of bone-replacing tumors. The lesion is a fluid-filled cavity that is mainly found within the metaphysis of a large tubular bone (usually the upper end of the humerus or femur) of teenaged boys (Fig. 6). However, these cysts can occur at other sites, including the axial skeleton and pelvis (Fig. 7). A simple bone cyst is also referred to as a solitary or unicameral cyst, although the latter term is a misnomer because these cysts may be septated.

During the cyst's so-called active phase, when its size is increasing, it remains in close proximity to the epiphyseal cartilaginous plate. The "inactive" phase follows separation of the cyst from the physis as a result of normal metaphyseal bone growth. The cyst, which has a membrane of loose vascular connective tissue and contains osteoclast-like giant cells and accumulations of fibrinoid-like material, is most frequently detected as an incidental finding or when its wall is fractured by a relatively minor injury. A common feature is the presence within the cyst cavity of a fragment from the thin wall. The fragment has been observed to change position on radiographs obtained in upright and recumbent positions ("fallen fragment" sign). Spontaneous healing may result, but these cysts are generally treated with curettage and introduction of bone chips. Aspiration and the injection of corticosteroids provide results comparable to those of surgery. Inactive, relatively small, and monolocular lesions respond best to both types of treatment. Selective embolization has also been used successfully. Malignancy in a solitary unicameral bone cyst has been reported, but there is general agreement that such malignancies are extremely rare.

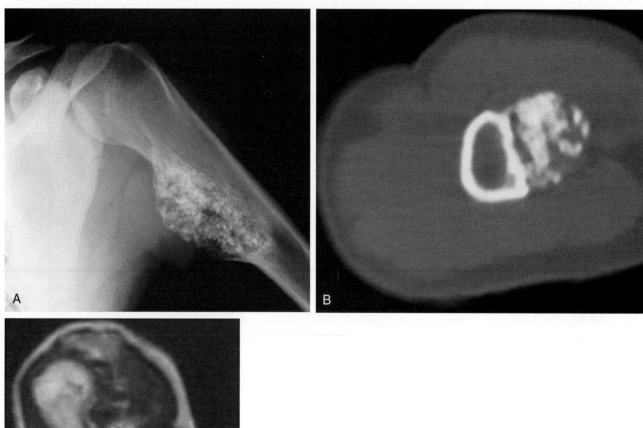

FIGURE 3. Periosteal chondroma in a 19-year-old young woman. **A,** Anteroposterior view of the humerus shows a broad-based tumor with a lobular mineralized matrix. **B,** Computed tomography scan shows the superficial nature of the lesion, which is separated from the medulla by cortical bone. **C,** Sagittal T_2-weighted magnetic resonance image shows the lobular organization of the inhomogeneous cartilaginous matrix. Unlike osteochondroma (see Figs. 1 and 2), there is no cartilaginous cap.

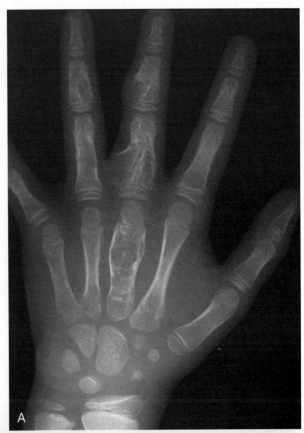

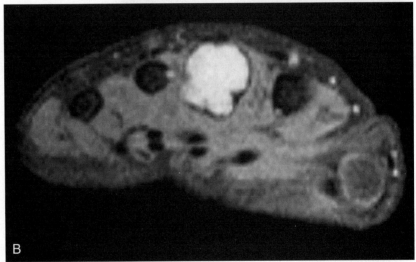

FIGURE 4. A, Multiple enchondromatosis (Ollier's disease) involving multiple phalanges and the third metacarpal of the hand of a 10-year-old boy. **B,** Transverse T_2-weighted magnetic resonance image shows uniformly high signal in the expansile cartilaginous tumor of the third metacarpal.

Solitary unicameral bone cysts have been found in the calcanei of pediatric patients 5 to 15 years of age and in adults. Often these cysts are painless and are first detected by radiography of acute injuries to the feet. Radiolucent cysts are located at practically the same site in all cases: near the base of the neck of the calcaneus. The thin, overlying lateral cortical wall of the calcaneus forms a well-defined bony border that allows differentiation from the "physiologic" pseudocystic radiolucent areas observed in the same region of normal bones (see Section IX, Part III, Chapter 2, Fig. 92, page 2087).

The cyst space is usually filled with yellow, sometimes bloody fluid. The cyst wall consists of proliferat-ing fibrous tissue containing hemosiderin, cholesterol clefts, and a foreign body giant cell reaction. Van Linthoudt and Lagier consider calcaneal cysts to be the result of organizing hemorrhages. In atypical cases, CT and MRI may disclose the cystic nature of the lesion. The fluid contents are usually of low intensity on T_1-weighted images and of uniform hyperintensity on T_2-weighted images. Contrast-enhanced T_1-weighted images reveal enhancement of the fibrous lining and no change in the intensity of the cyst contents (see Fig. 7D). However, hemorrhage into the cyst can alter the signal characteristics; fluid–fluid levels representing settled, degraded blood products have been observed.

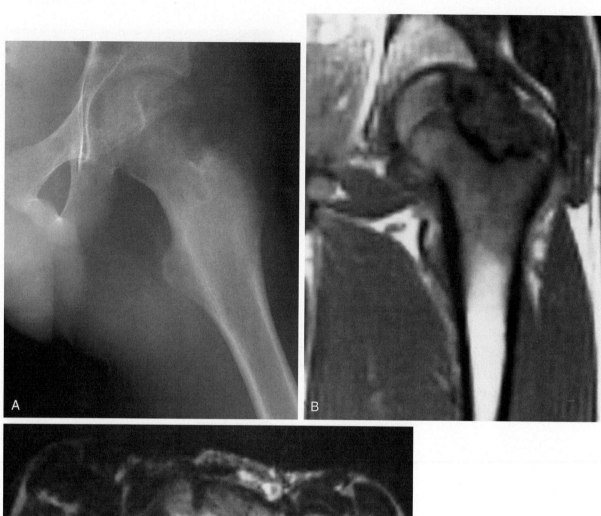

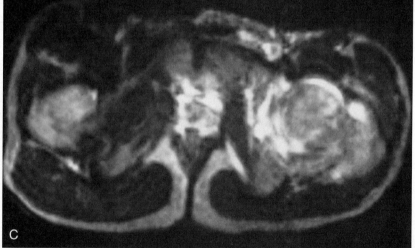

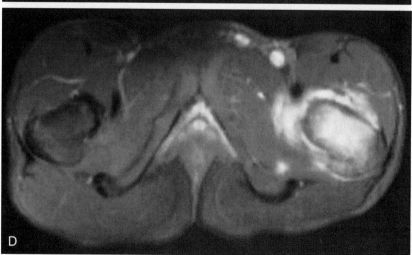

FIGURE 5. Chondroblastoma in a 14-year-old boy. **A,** There is an ill-defined lucent lesion involving the lateral aspect of the femoral head and the adjacent metaphysis. The epiphyseal portion of the tumor is delineated medially by a sclerotic border. **B,** Coronal T_1-weighted magnetic resonance (MR) image shows a well-defined medial tumor border and hypointensity of the femoral head and metaphyseal marrow, probably caused by edema. The hypointense medial tumor border is clearly defined. Transverse T_2-weighted **(C)** and fat-saturated, contrast-enhanced T_1-weighted **(D)** MR images show extensive, hyperintense soft tissue reaction.

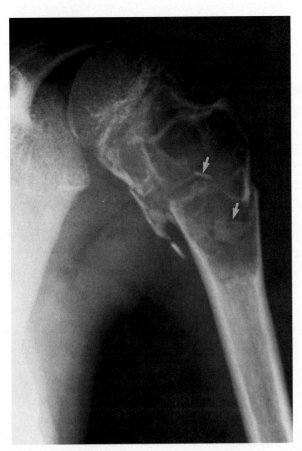

FIGURE 6. Radiograph of the shoulder of a 6-year-old boy with a simple bone cyst shows an expansile, lucent lesion containing multiple septations and several bony fragments *(arrows)*.

Aneurysmal Bone Cyst

Aneurysmal bone cysts are complex lesions that can be radiographically and histologically difficult to differentiate from telangiectatic osteosarcoma. Although Kransdorf et al. stated that aneurysmal bone cysts reflect "a pathophysiologic change rather than a unique entity," Dorfman and Czerniak divide aneurysmal bone cysts into primary and secondary categories and list a number of precursor lesions (Table 2). Whether primary or secondary, the lesions are most frequently discovered in patients in the first to third decades of life and often appear in the craniofacial bones, the vertebral column, or the metaphyses of the bones of the lower extremities. Most aneurysmal bone cysts are thought to be reactive lesions.

Radiographically, aneurysmal bone cysts appear as lucent, eccentric, expansile, "blowout" lesions with thin, smooth, bony walls that may or may not produce periosteal reaction (Figs. 8 and 9). A common distinguishing feature is the presence of fluid–fluid levels that may be visible on CT images and both T_1- and T_2-weighted MR images (Figs. 8*B* and 9*C*). These levels are formed by sedimentation of degraded blood products, especially methemoglobin, which has a much shorter T_1 relaxation time than that of hemoglobin. The fluid–fluid levels may be single or multiple and may be contained within numerous loculations. The signal characteristics of the cyst contents are quite variable and are probably dependent on the relative age and concentration of the blood components. We have also observed an aneurysmal bone cyst in which the presence of abundant hemosiderin resulted in a complete lack of signal on T_1- and T_2-weighted images. The cyst contents, which are contained within a thin, hypointense rim, do not enhance with the administration of paramagnetic contrast agents. Fluid–fluid levels are not unique to aneurysmal bone cysts and have been identified in numerous benign and malignant bone lesions, including fibrous dysplasia, chondroblastoma, giant cell tumor, myositis ossificans, nonossifying fibroma, simple bone cyst, and osteosarcoma.

Small aneurysmal bone cysts may be incidental findings in otherwise typical primary lesions. However, if the cysts are large, they may entirely obscure the diagnostic features of a primary tumor. Differentiating between aneurysmal bone cyst and telangiectatic osteosarcoma is particularly difficult and, at times, cannot be achieved by imaging methods. It should also be noted that a secondary aneurysmal bone cyst may develop in a conventional osteosarcoma (see also Fig. 20 below).

An unusual solid variant of aneurysmal bone cyst with radiographic features similar to those of the typical aneurysmal bone cyst has also been reported. This solid variant lacks cavernous, blood-containing spaces but is characterized histologically by the solid elements (proliferating fibrous tissue, benign giant cells, and newly formed osteoid matrix) found in the typical aneurysmal bone cysts. Solid aneurysmal bone cysts are histologically indistinguishable from extragnathic giant cell reparative granuloma.

GIANT CELL TUMOR

Giant cell tumor is an uncommon neoplasm, and, until recently, there has been some doubt about its occurrence before skeletal maturity has been achieved. In adults, giant cell tumor appears as an eccentric radiolucent lesion involving the metaphysis and the former

---

Table 2 ■ PRECURSORS OF SECONDARY ANEURYSMAL BONE CYST

Giant cell tumor
Chondroblastoma
Osteoblastoma
Nonossifying fibroma
Fibrous dysplasia
Giant cell reparative granuloma
Chondromyxoid fibroma
Fibrous histiocytoma
Solitary bone cyst
Eosinophilic granuloma
Hemangioma
Myositis ossificans
Osteosarcoma
Malignant fibrous histocytoma

Modified from Dorfman HD, Czerniak B: Bone Tumors. St. Louis, Mosby, 1998:879.

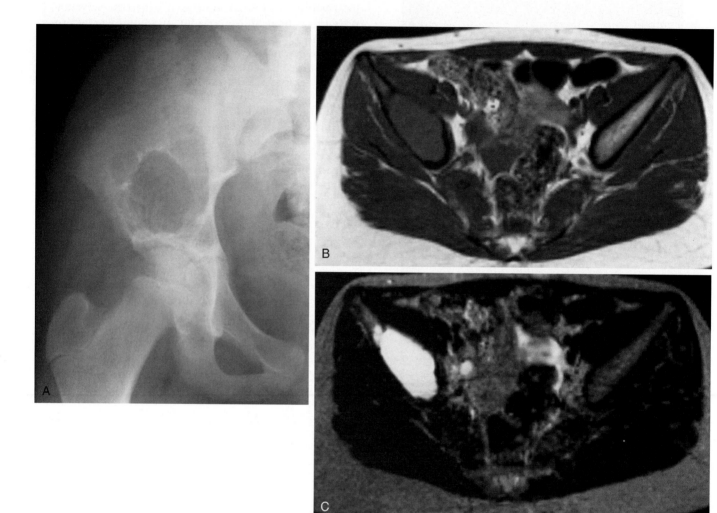

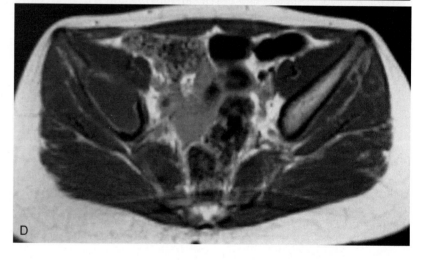

FIGURE 7. Simple bone cyst of the ilium of a 9-year-old boy. **A,** On a radiograph, there is a lucent bony defect with slightly sclerotic, scalloped borders. **B,** On a transverse T_1-weighted magnetic resonance image, the cyst contents show homogeneous intermediate signal intensity. **C,** On a T_2-weighted image, the signal is homogeneously hyperintense. **D,** On a contrast-enhanced T_1-weighted image, there is enhancement of the inner margin of the cyst and no increase in intensity of the contents of the lesion. The magnetic resonance imaging findings are consistent with those associated with a fluid-filled lesion. (From Fletcher BD, Hanna SL: Pediatric musculoskeletal lesions simulating neoplasms. Magn Reson Imaging Clin N Am 1996;4: 722–723, with permission.)

epiphysis of long bones. In skeletally immature patients, these tumors are located in the diaphysis or metaphysis rather than in the epiphysis.

In children and adolescents, giant cell tumors tend to be centrally located lesions that expand concentrically and can be either sclerotic or ill-defined (Fig. 10A). There may be associated periosteal reaction and pathologic fracture. In one series, the tibia was the most commonly affected bone; the next most common sites were other tubular bones, including those of the hands and feet. The histologic findings of giant cell tumors in skeletally immature patients are similar to those of the tumors of adults: the tumors consist of osteoclast-like, multinucleated giant cells distributed in a stroma of spindle-shaped cells. MRI signal characteristics may be nonspecific (low to intermediate T_1-weighted signal and inhomogeneous T_2-weighted signal with hyperintense areas). However, accumulation of hemosiderin resulting from the phagocytosis of extravasated erythrocytes by tumor cells may cause variably shaped foci of low signal intensity (Fig. 10B, C) that is sometimes intermixed with high T_2-weighted signal resulting from hemorrhage or cyst formation. Aneurysmal bone cysts, a secondary feature of as many as 20% of adult giant cell tumors, may also contain blood products such as

hemosiderin, thus altering the image of the primary lesion (see earlier).

Although giant cell tumors are considered benign, they can metastasize to the lungs. This biologic behavior cannot be predicted by histologic findings. The pulmonary "implants" usually have a self-limited growth potential, but recurrence and disease progression are possible.

FIBROUS TUMORS

Nonossifying Fibroma

Nonossifying fibroma (fibroxanthoma), a benign fibroblastic mass that occurs most frequently in the major long bones of children, represents continuation of growth of a fibrous cortical defect (see Part IX, Section III, Chapter 2, Fig. 70, page 2080) into the medullary cavity (Fig. 11A, B). No symptoms are usually associated with the mass, but slight pain or swelling can occur with large lesions. Generally found in the posterior surface of the metaphysis of a large bone, the nonossifying fibroma is eccentric, with a thin, bulging cortex. Its inner border is often sclerotic. Trabeculae-like corrugations, which

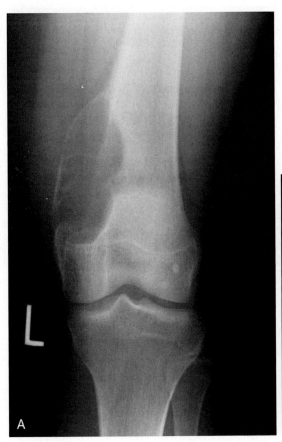
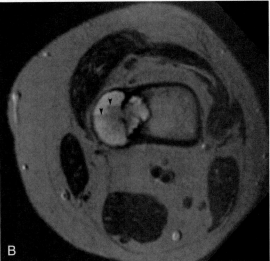

FIGURE 8. Aneurysmal bone cyst. **A,** Radiograph of the knee of a 13-year-old girl shows an eccentric, expansile lucent lesion with a thin, bony shell involving the medial aspect of the distal femur. **B,** On a transverse T_2-weighted magnetic resonance image, the lesion is seen to penetrate the cortex of the femur and extend into the adjacent soft tissues. Several fluid–fluid levels are demonstrated *(arrowheads)*.

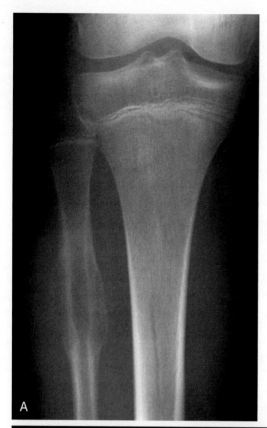

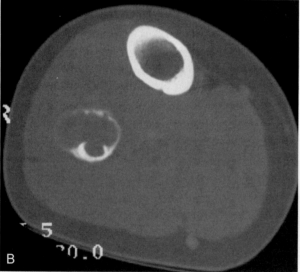

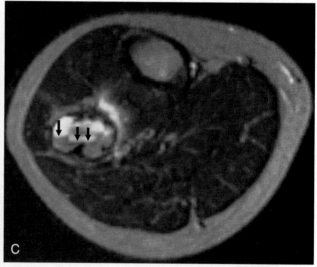

FIGURE 9. Aneurysmal bone cyst of the proximal fibula of a 14-year-old boy. **A,** Anteroposterior radiograph shows an expansile, lucent lesion. **B,** Computed tomography scan shows a thin, bony shell containing the cyst. **C,** T$_2$-weighted magnetic resonance image shows multiple loculations within the lesions; these loculations contain fluid–fluid levels (*arrows* in **C**). Mild soft tissue reaction appears as ill-defined hyperintense signal in **C.**

may be present on the inner surface of the cavity, give the lesion a multilocular appearance. In thin bones, such as the fibula, the entire width of the bone may be involved. The radiographic appearance is frequently so typical that biopsy can be avoided for many patients. However, large lesions should be observed closely because of the risk of pathologic fracture. Spontaneous resolution with associated ossification is the usual outcome of these lesions. Differential diagnosis includes unicameral bone cyst, aneurysmal bone cyst, fibrous dysplasia, and chondromyxoid fibroma.

Disseminated nonossifying fibromas are occasionally associated with cystic lesions of the jaw and café au lait skin lesions in the absence of signs of neurofibromatosis. This combination has been given the eponym Jaffe-Campanacci syndrome.

Nonossifying fibroma is composed of highly cellular stromal tissue with a few multinucleated giant cells and xanthomatous reaction with histocytes. As a result, the intensity of most of these lesions is equal to or lower than muscle on T$_1$-weighted MR images (Fig. 11C), and on T$_2$-weighted images the lesions are usually hypointense to fat. Very-low-intensity signals on T_2-weighted images may be due to hemosiderin deposition. After administration of paramagnetic contrast agent, the lesions enhance intensely throughout or in their margins or septa (Fig. 11*D*).

Fibrous Dysplasia

Fibrous dysplasia can be monostotic, polyostotic, monomelic, or polymelic. It is more common in females than in males and most patients are young adults. It is occasionally seen in the first decade of life. In a small

percentage of cases (2% to 3%), fibrous dysplasia is associated with endocrine disorders, especially precocious puberty in girls (McCune-Albright syndrome). Mazabraud syndrome, which is usually characterized by polyostotic fibrous dysplasia and intramuscular myxoma, has been observed in adults. Although it is not a true neoplasm, fibrous dysplasia involving a long bone may mimic a bone tumor or cyst, especially when it causes localized expansion of the bone and is monostotic.

The most common form of fibrous dysplasia is monostotic and affects craniofacial bones, a rib, or a

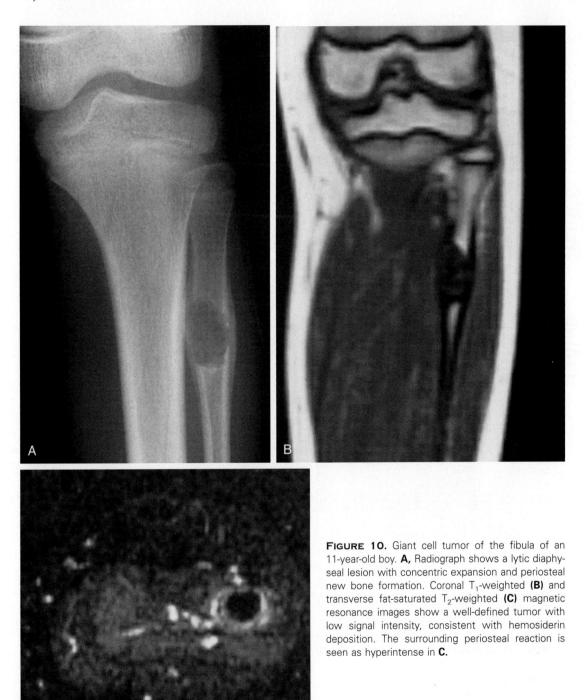

FIGURE 10. Giant cell tumor of the fibula of an 11-year-old boy. **A,** Radiograph shows a lytic diaphyseal lesion with concentric expansion and periosteal new bone formation. Coronal T_1-weighted **(B)** and transverse fat-saturated T_2-weighted **(C)** magnetic resonance images show a well-defined tumor with low signal intensity, consistent with hemosiderin deposition. The surrounding periosteal reaction is seen as hyperintense in **C.**

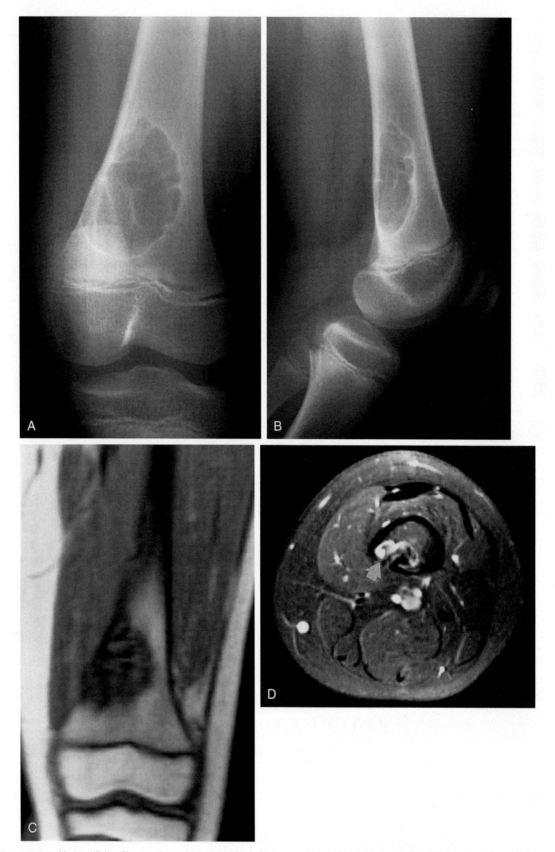

FIGURE 11. Nonossifying fibroma in an 11-year-old boy. Anteroposterior **(A)** and lateral **(B)** radiographs of the distal femur show a large radiolucent lesion with thin, well-defined borders and apparent septa involving the cortex and medulla of the posterior aspect of the metaphysis. **C,** Coronal T_1-weighted magnetic resonance image demonstrates that the signal intensity of the lesion is predominantly low. **D,** Transverse fat-saturated, contrast-enhanced T_1-weighted image shows partial enhancement of the lesion. Note the discontinuity of the cortex *(arrow)*.

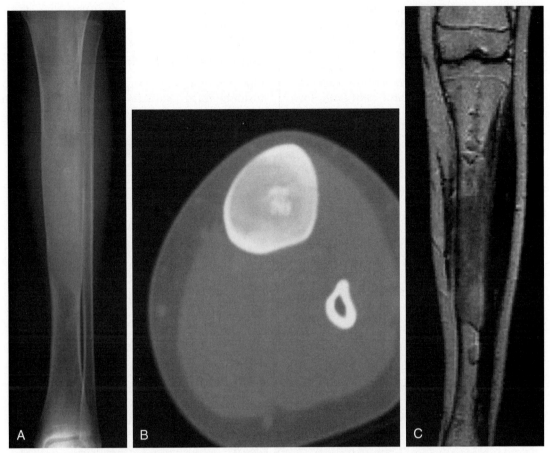

FIGURE 12. Fibrous dysplasia of the tibia of a 14-year-old girl. **A,** Radiographically, the lower leg shows an expanded medullary cavity with a ground-glass appearance, faint calcific foci, and cortical thinning. **B,** A similar appearance is demonstrated by computed tomography. **C,** Coronal T$_2$-weighted magnetic resonance image shows mainly low signal in the dysplastic medulla. This patient's left femur was also involved. (From Fletcher BD, Hanna SL: Pediatric musculoskeletal lesions simulating neoplasms. Magn Reson Imaging Clin N Am 1996;4:729, with permission.)

long bone (usually the diaphysis of the femur). The tibia is affected in nearly 20 percent of cases. This type of fibrous dysplasia causes expansion of the medullary cavity of tubular bones, endosteal scalloping, and trabeculation; it frequently has sclerotic margins or "rind." Bowing of the affected bone may occur; when the affected bone is the femur, the resulting deformity is called a "shepherd's crook." The radiographic density depends on the relative amount of dysplastic bone and fibrous material within the lesion; therefore, the lesion's appearance can vary from "ground glass" to radiolucent. Small cartilaginous nodules within the lesion may eventually calcify (Fig. 12). Focal or multifocal thinning and destruction of the bony cortex may also be seen on CT or MR images. Soft tissue extension of the lesion is unusual.

On T$_1$-weighted MR images, the intensity of fibrous dysplasia is similar to that of skeletal muscle. Although the signal of pure fibrous tissue is hypointense on T$_2$-weighted images, the signal of fibrous dysplasia is variable and frequently hyperintense to fat. This seeming inconsistency is probably due to the inhomogeneous nature of the lesion, which consists of spindle cells, trabeculae of immature woven bone with osteoid seams, and small cysts. A fluid–fluid level has been described in one instance of fibrous dysplasia that had a large cystic component. After gadolinium administration, central or, less frequently, peripheral enhancement may occur.

Osteofibrous Dysplasia

Osteofibrous dysplasia, also called ossifying fibroma of long bones or intracortical fibrous dysplasia, is a rare lesion that is usually confined to the tibia but can also involve the fibula. In some patients, the tibia and ipsilateral fibula are affected synchronously. Most cases occur during the first decade of life, although some tumors have been found in newborn infants. Usually painless, osteofibrous dysplasia is characterized by deformity that can progress until epiphyseal fusion occurs. Fracture or even pseudoarthrosis may complicate its course. Osteofibrous dysplasia is histologically similar to fibrous dysplasia in that it contains well-differentiated fibroblasts, collagen, and bony trabeculae. The main differentiating feature is the presence of active osteoblasts in osteofibrous dysplasia.

The radiographic appearance is that of an eccentric, lucent, solitary or multiloculated lesion involving the anterior aspect of the tibia; the lesion is associated with cortical thickening and anterior bowing of the bone. Cross-sectional imaging is very helpful in determining its intracortical location, an important feature in distinguishing osteofibrous dysplasia from fibrous dysplasia (Fig. 13). This finding in young patients strongly suggests the correct diagnosis of osteofibrous dysplasia. Surgical excision and perhaps biopsy should be avoided because of the self-limiting nature of the tumor and its tendency to recur after surgical intervention. Especially in the second decade, radiologic and even pathologic

differentiation between osteofibrous dysplasia and adamantinoma is difficult. This subject is discussed below.

Long Bone Adamantinoma

On the basis of clinical, radiologic, histologic, and histochemical characteristics, long bone adamantino-

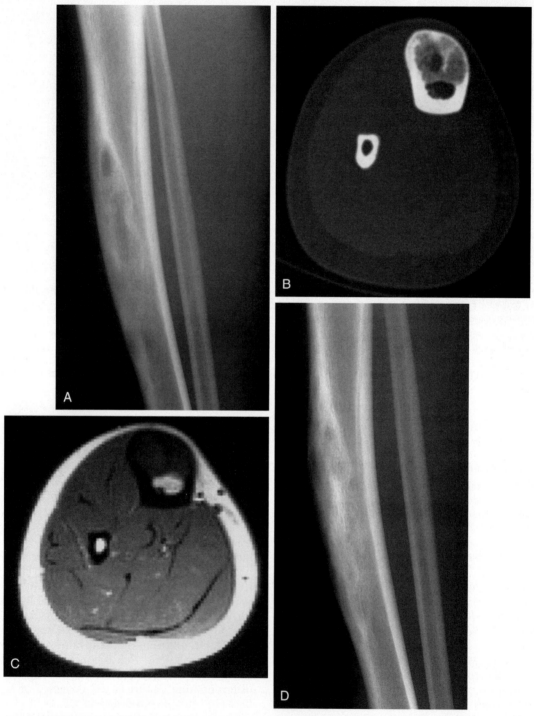

FIGURE 13. A, Lateral radiograph of the leg of a 10-year-old girl with osteofibrous dysplasia shows a partially lucent lesion of the anterior tibia with cortical thickening. There is mild anterior tibal bowing. Computed tomography scan **(B)** and transverse T$_1$-weighted magnetic resonance image **(C)** show the intracortical location of the lesion. **D,** Two years later, a radiograph of the leg shows further healing of the tumor, as the formerly lucent areas have undergone ossification. **(A–C** from Fletcher BD, Hanna SL: Pediatric musculoskeletal lesions simulating neoplasms. Magn Reson Imaging Clin N Am 1996;4:730, with permission.)

Table 3 ■ FEATURES OF FIBROUS DYSPLASIA–LIKE LESIONS

LESION	LOCATION*	HISTOLOGIC FEATURES
Fibrous dysplasia	*Medulla*, long bones, face, ribs	Immature bone, fibroblasts present
Osteofibrous dysplasia	*Cortex*, anterior tibia	Like those of fibrous dysplasia
Adamantinoma	*Cortex*, anterior tibia, fibula	Like those of osteofibrous dysplasia; epithelial elements present

*Italics indicate the bone region that is the primary site of each tumor.

mas, which are unrelated to the jaw lesion of the same name, have recently been divided into two groups: classical and differentiated (osteofibrous dysplasia–like). Both types involve the tibia, the fibula, or both, but the classical form occurs almost exclusively in adults, is located in either the cortex or the medulla, and can expand through the cortex and periosteum. The differentiated form is seen in children and young adults up to 20 years of age and has been reported in newborn infants. The tumor is limited to the bony cortex, and has a radiographic appearance identical to that of osteofibrous dysplasia. Osteofibrous dysplasia and adamantinoma are pathologically distinct: epithelial and mesenchymal cells are present in adamantinomas, which express immunoreactive cytokeratin and vimentin.

The concept of differentiation implies a continuum between osteofibrous dysplasia and adamantinoma and suggests that osteofibrous dysplasia is a regressive phase of adamantinoma. Czerniak et al. suggested that patients with the differentiated type have a more favorable prognosis than those with classical adamantinoma—no differentiated tumors have been known to metastasize—and that long bone adamantinoma could be included among the few neoplasms that are capable of spontaneous regression.

One study analyzed and compared the radiographic features of adamantinoma (no distinction was made between the classical and differentiated forms) and osteofibrous dysplasia. The most important features suggesting a diagnosis of osteofibrous dysplasia rather than adamantinoma were a ground-glass matrix, the absence of periosteal reaction and "moth-eaten" destruction, and the presence of anterior bowing of the tibia. MRI of adamantinoma was nonspecific: the T_1- and T_2-weighted signal characteristics were similar to those of other tumors. Table 3 lists distinguishing features of fibrous dysplasia, osteofibrous dysplasia, and adamantinoma.

LANGERHANS' CELL HISTIOCYTOSIS OF BONE

Like the cells of monocyte–macrophage lineage, the Langerhans' cell originates from CD34+ stem cells of the bone marrow. Knowledge of the derivation of these cells has made the term *histiocytosis X* obsolete; *Langerhans' cell histiocytosis* is the nomenclature currently used to encompass the clinical disorders of eosinophilic granuloma, Hand-Schüller-Christian disease, and Letterer-Siwe disease. Eosinophilic granuloma refers to localized skeletal disease and is one of the most commonly occurring bone tumors of boys in the first decade of life. The

average age of patients at the onset of eosinophilic granuloma is 10 to 12 years. The skull is the most frequent location, followed by the femur, mandible, pelvis, ribs, and spine, where vertebra plana is the usual manifestation. The lesions are usually located in the medulla of the diaphysis or metaphysis. The cortex and epiphysis are rare sites of eosinophilic granuloma. Multiple lesions occur in about 25% of cases, and affected patients experience local pain, tenderness, and palpable masses. Langerhans' cell histiocytosis localized to the skeleton carries a favorable prognosis.

Histologically, the tumors are composed of Langerhans' histiocytes containing their characteristic cleaved nuclei, and electron microscopy reveals Birbeck granules in the cytoplasm adjacent to the cell membrane. The lesions also contain ordinary histocytes and eosinophils.

Radiographically, eosinophilic granuloma of the calvarium typically appears as a lytic bone lesion with well-defined, scalloped, and beveled borders and sometimes a button sequestrum. In the extremities, most lesions are purely osteolytic, with well-defined, minimally sclerotic borders. Some eosinophilic granulomas are permeative, and periosteal new bone formation may occur, giving them an aggressive appearance (Fig. 14). (See also Section IX, Part XIII, Chapter 1, Fig. 23, page 2430.)

MRI is a very sensitive but nonspecific method of detecting eosinophilic granuloma. Beltran et al. observed low T_1-weighted and high T_2-weighted signals, as detected for many other tumors. Half of the lesions described by De Schepper et al. were hyperintense to muscle on T_1-weighted images. Marked enhancement with gadolinium was noted. An important feature of eosinophilic granuloma is the presence of extensive bone marrow and soft tissue edema, which produces high signals on T_2-weighted images (Fig. 14D). This reactive edema lends an aggressive appearance to MR images of these lesions, suggesting a malignant process. Occasionally, the granulomas disrupt the cortex, forming extracortical soft tissue masses.

Because multiple skeletal lesions may coexist in any one patient, skeletal imaging is necessary at the time of diagnosis and for purposes of follow-up. Controversy exists about the relative accuracy of radiographic skeletal surveys and radionuclide bone scintigraphy. However, because nuclear studies may detect lesions not seen on radiographs and because some eosinophilic granulomas may not be detected on bone scintigrams, both examinations are recommended at the time of diagnosis. Anecdotal evidence suggests that thallium-201 scintigraphy is useful in detecting these lesions.

OSSEOUS TUMORS

Osteoid Osteoma

Osteoid osteoma is fairly common, accounting for approximately 12% of all benign skeletal neoplasms. These tumors occur predominantly in boys, usually those in the second decade of life. Most patients complain of pain that is especially severe at night and in many cases is relieved by aspirin or other nonsteroidal anti-inflammatory agents.

The single most common location of osteoid osteoma is the femur, especially its neck. Osteoid osteomas occur less frequently in the upper extremities than in the lower extremities. Osteoid osteomas frequently affect the tubular bones of the hands and feet. They are less common in the flat bones and in the spine, where they affect the posterior arches of the vertebrae; in such cases, patients usually present with painful scoliosis. Osteoid osteomas are difficult to distinguish from the usually larger osteoblastomas. Their differentiation is discussed under Osteoblastoma below.

Pathologically, the lesion consists of a nidus that is usually surrounded by dense sclerotic bone. The nidus contains interlacing trabeculae at various stages of

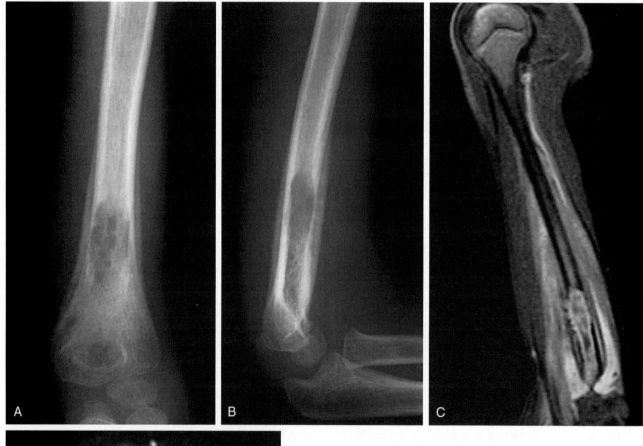

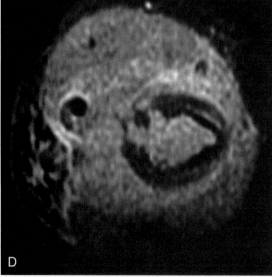

FIGURE 14. Solitary eosinophilic granuloma of the humerus of a 9-year-old boy. Anteroposterior **(A)** and lateral **(B)** radiographs show a lytic lesion with periosteal reaction. **C,** The lesion and surrounding soft tissues appear hyperintense on sagittal short tau inversion–recovery image. **D,** Transverse T_2-weighted magnetic resonance (MR) image shows permeation of the cortex in several locations and moderately hyperintense signal in the marrow and swollen soft tissues, findings consistent with reactive edema. Both the radiographic and MR imaging appearances of this benign tumor suggest an aggressive, even malignant neoplasm.

ossification within a stroma of loose, vascular connective tissue. Three types of osteoid osteoma are recognized: cortical (the most common type), cancellous or medullary, and subperiosteal. The latter two types produce less sclerotic bone than those in the cortex do, making radiologic diagnosis difficult. Kayser et al. proposed that osteomas originate subperiosteally and gradually become incorporated in the cortex by continual remodeling, periosteal new bone formation, and endosteal resorption.

Radiographically, the nidus may be purely radiolucent or contain a dense center. In cortical osteoid osteomas, the nidus is encased by a broad zone of dense bone (Fig. 15). Intra-articular osteoid osteomas may be either cancellous or periosteal and have little reactive bone or periosteal new bone formation. This type of osteoid osteoma most frequently affects the hip, where it causes osteopenia and joint effusion.

CT is valuable in showing the lesion, especially the nidus, which can vary in its degree of ossification, and in determining the location of the lesion before percutaneous or surgical excision. CT appears to display the nidus better than MRI; signals of low intensity are often seen on both T_1- and T_2-weighted images, depending on the relative amount of ossification and fibrovascular tissue. Although there is no signal from the sclerotic bone, the inherent contrast available with MRI provides precise definition of potentially extensive reactive changes in the bone marrow and adjacent soft tissues. In one report, the high T_2-weighted signal of reactive tissue in several patients suggested the presence of a soft tissue mass and malignancy. The findings correlated with atrophy and myxomatous changes in the muscle, and with replacement of the marrow elements with proteinacious material (serous atrophy). Both the nidus and the reactive tissue enhance with gadolinium. Intra-articular osteoid osteomas produce joint effusions and synovial proliferation that also appear intense on T_2-weighted images.

Angiography and radionuclide bone scans have been used for many years to help diagnose and locate osteoid osteomas. Angiography shows increased vascularity in the region of the lesion and contrast enhancement of the nidus. A feeding vessel may also be identified. Bone scintigraphy, a highly sensitive method of detecting osteoid osteoma, typically shows increased flow to the lesion on immediate images and a focus of increased activity on skeletal equilibrium images. On bone scintigrams, a "double density" pattern representing localization of the radiotracer in the nidus surrounded by less intense activity in the reactive bone is considered to be a characteristic finding of osteoid osteoma.

The traditional treatment has been surgical excision. However, a number of imaging-guided procedures have recently been developed to remove the tumor percutaneously or perform laser coagulation.

Osteoblastoma

Osteoblastoma most commonly occurs in patients in the second and third decades of life. According to the files of the Netherlands Committee on Bone Tumors, osteoblastomas accounted for 6% of all benign bone tumors

and were more common in males than in females. Osteoblastomas are closely related to osteoid osteomas and have, in the past, been considered a larger version of that tumor (giant osteoid osteoma). Size is an important consideration in distinguishing between the two types of tumors: tumors less than 1.5 cm in diameter are considered to be osteoid osteomas, whereas tumors larger than 1.5 cm are usually osteoblastomas. Unlike osteoid osteomas, osteoblastomas are not associated with a typical pattern of pain. Moreover, the two types of tumors can be distinguished by differences in anatomic location and imaging features.

Histologically, osteoblastoma consists of numerous osteoblast-lined trabeculae containing osteoid; these trabeculae are less organized than those in osteoid osteoma. Osteoblastoma may cause the periosteum to expand, but the tumor often lacks the wide, dense rim of sclerosis that is typical of osteoid osteoma. Clinically, many osteoblastomas are found in the posterior elements of the vertebrae, where they can cause scoliosis and neurologic deficits. Nearly half of these tumors occur in the appendicular skeleton, primarily in the proximal femoral diaphysis and metaphysis. This tumor may also involve the dorsal aspect of the neck of the talus.

In the long bones, osteoblastomas appear radiologically as round or oval lucent tumors with frequent mineralization of the matrix and an eccentric location in the medulla. Periosteal reaction is common. Talar lesions may expand into the soft tissues, and osteoporosis of the talus and other bones of the foot may be an associated finding. The calcified or ossified matrix and the tumor's thin, bony outer shell are especially well seen on CT images. Edema in the soft tissues or marrow may give highly intense T_2-weighted signals on MRI, but the signal characteristics are not specific. Radionuclide imaging may help in determining the location of the lesion. Angiography may reveal a dense capillary blush. Treatment is by surgical excision or curettage, but there is a moderate recurrence rate after those procedures.

MALIGNANT BONE TUMORS

Approximately 50% of all bone tumors in the pediatric age group are malignant; nearly two thirds of these are osteosarcomas. Ewing's sarcomas of bone comprise most of the remainder. Other types of osseous malignancies, such as chondrosarcoma, are extremely rare in children, although non-Hodgkin's lymphoma occasionally presents as a primary bone neoplasm.

Osteosarcomas and Ewing's sarcomas differ sufficiently both in their clinical and imaging presentation that they can usually be distinguished from one another. Their characteristic features, to be discussed in this chapter, are summarized in Table 4.

OSTEOSARCOMA

The peak incidence of osteosarcoma is in patients 15 to 25 years of age, but the youngest patient described to

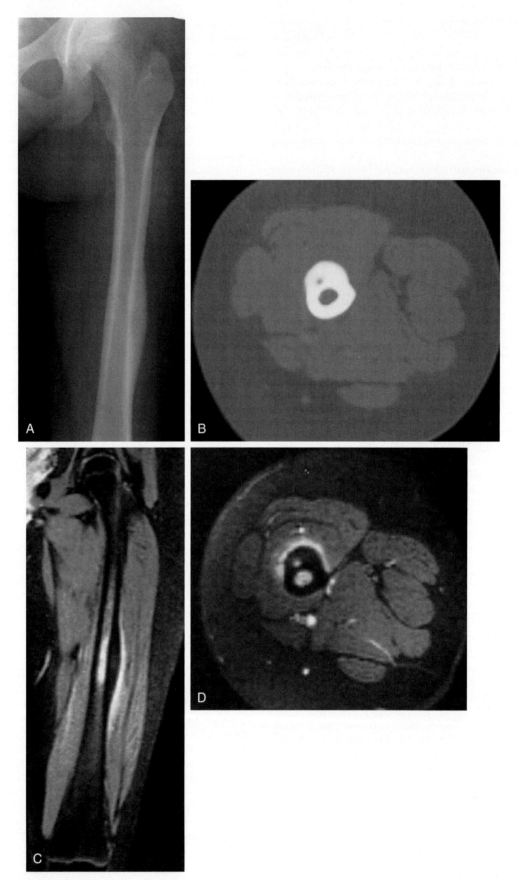

FIGURE 15. Osteoid osteoma in a 13-year-old boy. **A,** Radiograph of the femur shows dense sclerosis and focal cortical thickening of the lateral aspect of the midshaft. There is slight periosteal new bone formation on the outer margin of the lesion. A nidus is not visible. **B,** Computed tomography scan shows a lucent nidus within the thickened cortex. **C,** Bone marrow and local soft tissue edema are shown as hyperintense signal on a coronal short tau inversion–recovery image. **D,** Hyperintense nidus is shown within the thickened cortex on a transverse fat-saturated T_2-weighted image.

Table 4 ■ DIFFERENTIATING FEATURES OF OSTEOSARCOMA (OS) AND EWING'S SARCOMA (ES)

	OSTEOSARCOMA	EWING'S SARCOMA
Age range	15–25 years	0–25 years
Incidence	More common than ES	Less common Rare in nonwhites
Location	Metaphyses of long bones	Metadiaphysis of long bones Axial, flat bone involvement more common than OS
Matrix	Usually "cloud-like" mineralization	Not mineralized or sclerotic
Periosteal reaction	"Sunburst" Codman's triangles	"Onion-skin"
Metastases	Lung (80%) Bone (20%)	Lung, rarely bone, marrow, lymph nodes
Other	Occasional multi-focal disease Association with retinoblastoma	11:22 translocation Radiation sensitive

date with osteosarcoma was a 19-month-old girl. The tumors are slightly more common in males.

Most osteosarcomas are single, primary neoplasms that arise from the medullary cavity of the metaphyses of the long bones. The diaphyses alone are less commonly involved, and epiphyseal origin of osteosarcoma is extremely rare. Often referred to as conventional osteosarcomas, most are considered to be high grade because of their degree of cellular atypia and anaplasia. Other much less common categories of this tumor include well-differentiated medullary osteosarcoma, telangiectatic osteosarcoma, and surface osteosarcomas, including intracortical osteosarcoma and parosteal, periosteal, and high-grade surface osteosarcomas. Secondary osteosarcomas, which are rare in children, are usually associated with previous radiation therapy. Osteosarcoma can also arise in patients with inherited (usually bilateral) retinoblastoma who have a defect in the *RB* gene or in patients in whom there has been a spontaneous mutation of the gene. Osteosarcoma unassociated with other malignancies is occasionally familial and has been identified in siblings.

The long bones are affected in approximately 70% of cases; more than half of these neoplasms are distributed about the bones of the knee. The face, mandible, cranium, and axial skeleton are among the less commonly affected sites. Osteosarcomas can involve multiple skeletal sites synchronously; this condition is known as osteosarcomatosis. Extremely rare in children, extraskeletal osteosarcomas are found in various organs or the soft tissues of the extremities of adults. Because osteosarcomas are not radiosensitive, treatment consists of preoperative chemotherapy, extirpation of resectible lesions and usually limb-sparing surgery, and postoperative chemotherapy. Prognosis is influenced by response to initial chemotherapy, which is evaluated postoperatively by histologic estimation of necrosis within the treated tumor. Little change in tumor size is expected even in tumors that respond well to chemotherapy. Imaging methods of assessing the effects of therapy include thallium-201 scintigraphy and dynamic contrast-enhanced MRI.

Long-term follow-up of osteosarcoma and other malignant bone tumors in children is essential and involves many imaging methods over a long period of time. A sample imaging protocol for osteosarcoma is shown in Table 5.

Intramedullary Osteosarcoma

Conventional Osteosarcoma

The histologic hallmark of osteosarcoma is the presence of an osteoid matrix produced by sarcoma cells. In most cases, there is extensive immature bone formation. However, other tissues may predominate in the tumor matrix. The three main types of osteosarcoma, which are based on matrix type, are osteoblastic, chondroblastic, and fibroblastic. These tumors have differing mineral content.

Plain film radiography remains the primary method

Table 5 ■ TIMELINE FOR IMAGING EVALUATION OF PATIENTS WITH OSTEOSARCOMA AT ST. JUDE CHILDREN'S RESEARCH HOSPITAL

TIME	TREATMENT	EVALUATIONS	IMAGING METHODS*,†
Week 1	Begin preoperative chemotherapy	Diagnosis and pretreatment	Primary tumor: XR, CT, MRI, BS, TI Metastases: CXR, Chest CT, BS
Week 6	Continue chemotherapy	Interim response	Primary tumor: CT, MRI Metastases: CXR, Chest CT
Week 9	Surgical resection	Preoperative response	Primary tumor: XR, CT, MRI, BS, TI Metastases: CXR, Chest CT, BS
Week 11	Begin postoperative chemotherapy	Postoperative monitoring	CXR: every 2 mo Chest CT at wk 18–20
Week 37	End chemotherapy	Off therapy	XR primary site, CXR, Chest CT, BS
Week 37–month 60	Off therapy	Long-term follow-up	CXR every 6 months Chest CT, BS every 6 mo for 24 mo

*BS = technetium-99m MDP scintigram; CT = computed tomography; CXR = chest radiograph; MRI = magnetic resonance imaging; TI = thallium-201 scintigram; XR = radiograph.
†*Notes:* MRI includes dynamic contrast-enhanced study (DEMRI). Bone scintigraphy is three phase in weeks 1 through 9, then single phase (skeletal equilibrium) after resection.
From Fletcher BD: Imaging pediatric bone sarcomas: diagnosis and treatment related issues. Radiol Clin N Am 1997;35:1478, with permission.

of diagnosis. Other imaging methods are used mainly for staging purposes and to help the surgeon plan an en bloc resection of the tumor. Typical osteosarcomas present as fairly large, mixed sclerotic–lytic masses with a "cloud-like" matrix involving the long-bone metaphyses. The tumors cause cortical erosion and destruction rather than expansion. Resultant periosteal new bone formation, often of the spiculated "sunburst" variety, and elevation are often observed, frequently with Codman's triangles at the tumor extremities (Fig. 16*A*, *B*). However, occasionally conventional osteosarcomas are purely lytic and do not exhibit periosteal reaction.

CT images illustrate the same features in a cross-sectional plane. In addition, CT is the most sensitive method for detecting subtle mineralization of the osteoid matrix. In contrast to the normally hypoattenuated fatty marrow, abnormally high marrow attenuation caused by the tumor is observed on CT images (Fig. 16*C*).

MRI is used extensively to evaluate osteosarcoma. The longitudinal extent of marrow involvement, an important determinant of surgical therapy, is accurately shown as well-defined hypointense signals on T_1-weighted images obtained in either coronal or sagittal planes. Normal yellow marrow is hyperintense. It is important to obtain a longitudinal T_1-weighted image of the entire bone to measure intramedullary tumor length (Fig. 16*D*); to assess possible epiphyseal involvement, which can occur in as many as 80% of metaphyseal tumors; and to detect skip metastases that occur in a small percentage of cases (see Fig. 18*C* below).

On T_2-weighted images, the tumor-containing marrow can be either hyperintense or, if there is sufficient bone formation, hypointense to normal fat. The soft tissue component usually produces heterogeneous, mainly high-intensity signals that contrast greatly with those of the surrounding muscles (Fig. 16*E*). STIR images are very sensitive to the water content of tumors, making most osteosarcomas very conspicuous. Contrast-enhanced T_1-weighted images, preferably made with fat saturation, provide similar contrast and better signal-to-noise ratios than T_2-weighted images. Furthermore, contrast-enhanced T_1-weighted images are especially useful in determining the relationship between the tumor and the major blood vessels, in detecting joint involvement in the presence of effusion, and in estimating the amount of necrosis within the tumor (Fig. 16*G*). Osteosarcoma is frequently accompanied by edema of the adjacent soft tissues that is hyperintense to muscle on T_2-weighted, STIR, and contrast-enhanced T_1-weighted images. This edema can be localized to the tumor periphery (paratumoral or peritumoral) or can involve whole muscle groups, as in the case of larger tumors (Fig. 16*F*).

Between 10% and 20% of patients with osteosarcoma will have metastases, mainly in the lungs, at the time of diagnosis. Therefore, chest radiography and chest CT are essential in the search for pulmonary lesions at this time. Like the primary tumor, these metastases can be calcified and, therefore, difficult to distinguish from calcified granulomas (Fig. 17). Pleura-based lung metastases can also produce a pneumothorax, hemothorax,

or malignant pleural effusion. Bone metastases are much less frequent, but radionuclide bone scans are justified to detect these lesions and to assess the extent of the primary tumor (see Fig. 24). Skip metastases, which can occur in the same bone as the primary tumor or can be transarticular in location, may also be detected (Fig. 18). Bone scintigraphy and chest CT should also be performed periodically after treatment with chemotherapy and surgery, especially within the subsequent 2 years. Eighty percent of relapses occur in the lung only, and 20% in the skeleton. Local or distant lymph node involvement is extremely rare.

Telangiectatic Osteosarcoma

Telangiectatic osteosarcoma is now considered to be a specific type of osteosarcoma, comprising about 2% of all osteosarcomas. Like conventional osteosarcomas, telangiectatic osteosarcoma tends to occur in the long bones adjacent to the knee and is seen more frequently in boys than in girls. These tumors contain little osteoid and do not form bone but are composed of single or multiple cavities containing blood or necrotic tumor with septa of anaplastic cells. Radiographically, they appear as lytic rather than sclerotic lesions, often having a nonaggressive appearance in that they tend to expand, rather than destroy, the cortex (Fig. 19). There is often little or no periosteal new bone formation. They may be associated with a soft tissue mass.

Except for the presence of malignant cells that are often at the periphery of the cavity, the pathologic appearance of telangiectatic osteosarcoma mimics that of an aneurysmal bone cyst. Indeed, on MR images the appearance of telangiectatic osteosarcoma and aneurysmal bone cyst may be identical; both may have single or multiple fluid–fluid levels produced by blood products of differing ages that are best demonstrated on T_2-weighted images (Fig. 20). According to Murphey et al., telangiectatic osteosarcomas are characterized by enhancing soft tissue in the periphery and septations of the tumor, a feature that is absent in aneurysmal bone cysts. The prognosis of patients with telangiectatic osteosarcoma is similar to that of patients with conventional osteosarcoma.

Well-Differentiated Medullary Osteosarcoma

Unlike most medullary osteosarcomas, which display histologic features of a high-grade malignancy, this unusual variant of osteosarcoma (fewer than 2% of osteosarcoma patients in the Mayo Clinic files) is a low-grade and usually clinically indolent entity. The peak incidence is during the third decade of life, but well-differentiated medullary osteosarcoma has been found in several teenaged patients. Unlike conventional osteosarcoma, the well-differentiated variety occurs more often in females than in males. The skeletal distribution of the tumor is similar to that of conventional osteosarcoma: the most common location is the diametaphyseal region of the long bones about the knee, especially the distal femur.

Histologically, this tumor contains well-differentiated

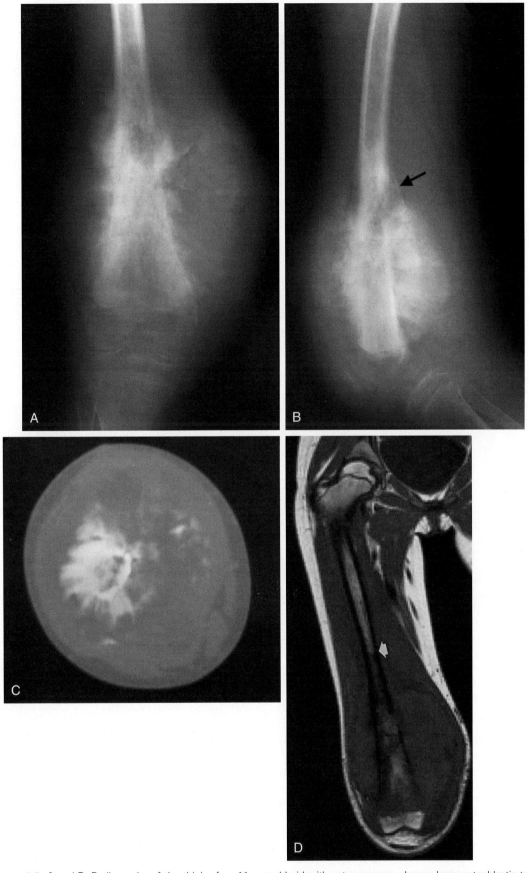

FIGURE 16. **A** and **B,** Radiographs of the thigh of an 11-year-old girl with osteosarcoma show a large osteoblastic tumor arising from the distal femoral diametaphysis. The epiphysis appears to be spared. "Sunray" periosteal new bone formation and cloud-like tumor mineralization are seen in the soft tissue mass. Codman's triangles are present superiorly (*arrow* in **B**). **C,** Radiating periosteal new bone and amorphous mineralization of the medulla and the soft tissue mass are demonstrated on a contrast-enhanced computed tomography scan. **D,** Coronal T$_1$-weighted magnetic resonance (MR) image shows medullary involvement extending proximally to the midshaft of the femur *(arrow)*.

Illustration continued on following page

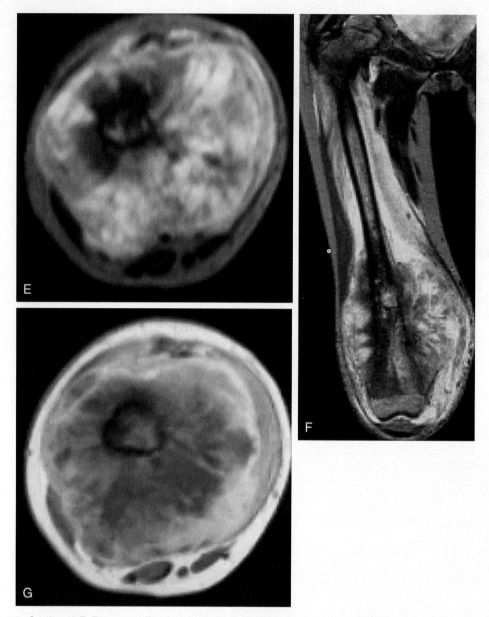

FIGURE 16. *Continued.* **E,** Transverse T$_2$-weighted MR image demonstrates a heterogeneously hyperintense soft tissue mass. Relatively little signal is seen from the medulla and radiating periosteal new bone. **F,** Coronal T$_2$-weighted MR image shows extensive hyperintensity of the edematous thigh muscles adjacent and proximal to the tumor. **G,** Transverse contrast-enhanced T$_1$-weighted image shows extensive hypointensity consistent with necrosis.

fibroblastic and osteoblastic components similar to those seen in parosteal osteosarcoma (see Surface Osteosarcomas below). Well-differentiated medullary osteosarcoma can be mistaken for fibrous dysplasia on both pathologic and radiologic examinations. Its radiographic appearance is quite variable and ranges from that of a well-defined lesion with sclerotic margins (Fig. 21) to that of an expansile, poorly defined tumor with periosteal reaction and soft tissue invasion. The tumor matrix varies from dense trabecular bone to homogeneous "cloud-like" mineralization. Less often, the tumor is osteolytic. Patients with this variant of osteosarcoma have a favorable prognosis, although dedifferentiation and metastasis can occur.

Intracortical Osteosarcoma

Intracortical osteosarcoma is the rarest of all osteosarcomas; only 13 cases have been reported since 1960, when the lesion was first defined histologically. It is a high-grade tumor that occurs in the diaphysis of the tibia or femur and typically may be as large as 4 cm in diameter. Radiographs show a deep or superficial cortical lucency with cortical thickening. The radiographic differential diagnosis includes osteoblastoma, osteoid osteoma, and osteomyelitis. Cross-sectional CT and MR images reveal an expanded sclerotic cortex and no medullary involvement. However, edema of the marrow and adjacent soft tissues may be seen as high signal on T$_2$-weighted

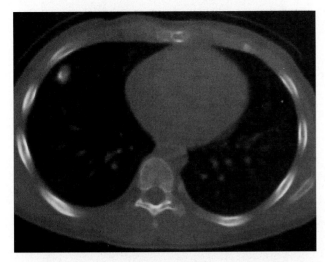

FIGURE 17. A computed tomography (CT) scan section of the chest of a 13-year-old boy with femoral osteosarcoma shows a partially calcified metastasis in the right lung. On other CT scan sections, several other calcified and noncalcified metastases were demonstrated in both lungs.

MRI. One reported case was associated with oncogenic rickets.

Surface Osteosarcomas

There are two main categories of surface osteosarcomas: parosteal (juxtacortical) osteosarcoma and the less common periosteal osteosarcoma. Parosteal osteosarcoma is thought to arise from the outer layer of periosteum, whereas periosteal osteosarcoma probably arises from the deep layers of periosteum or the outer cortex. The more superficial origin of parosteal osteosarcoma permits exophytic growth from the surface of the bone, usually the posterior aspect of the distal femoral metaphysis. Periosteal elevation and new bone formation are lacking. Parosteal osteosarcoma is more common in males than in females and tends to occur after skeletal maturity has been achieved. These osteosarcomas are considered to be low-grade tumors, but they may have dedifferentiated elements. Patients with paraosteal osteosarcoma generally have an excellent prognosis, but ingrowth into the medullary cavity may adversely affect the prognosis.

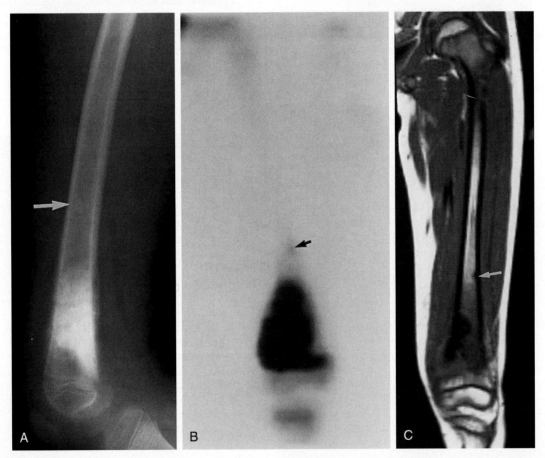

FIGURE 18. A, Lateral radiograph of the femur of a 9-year-old boy with osteosarcoma shows a sclerotic intramedullary distal femoral tumor with slight periosteal new bone formation. A small, dense skip metastasis *(arrow)* is seen proximal to the primary tumor of the main tumor mass. The skip metastasis *(arrow)* is also seen on a technetium-99m methylene diphosphonate bone scan **(B)** and is shown as a cortical-based intramedullary lesion *(arrow)* on a coronal T_1-weighted magnetic resonance image **(C).**

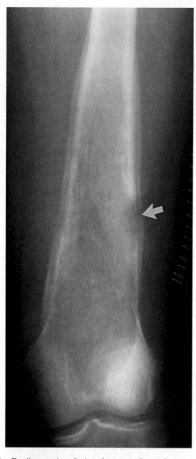

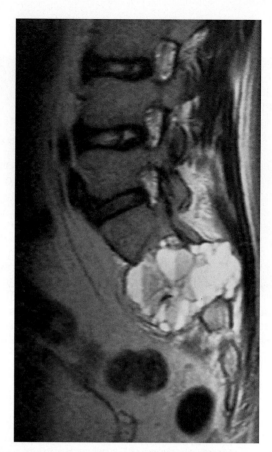

FIGURE 19. Radiograph of the femur of a 16-year-old boy with telangiectatic osteosarcoma shows a large lesion in the distal metadiaphysis extending into the epiphysis. The tumor is lytic rather than bone forming. There is mild periosteal reaction. There has been a recent incisional biopsy *(arrow)*.

FIGURE 20. Sagittal T_2-weighted magnetic resonance image of the sacrum of a 14-year-old girl with telangiectatic osteosarcoma shows a large, well-defined cystic lesion with fluid–fluid levels simulating an aneurysmal bone cyst (see also Figs. 8*B* and 9*C*).

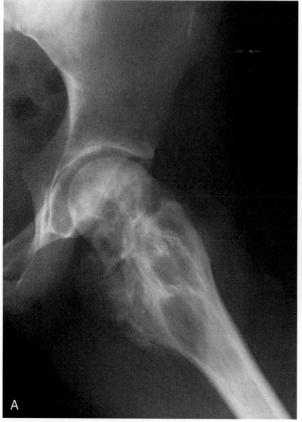

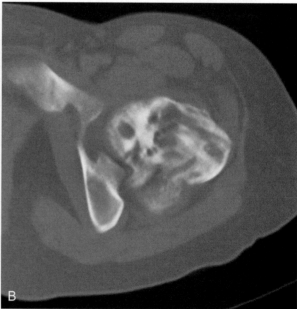

FIGURE 21. Radiographic **(A)** and computed tomography **(B)** images of the left hip of a 17-year-old girl show an expansile lesion of the proximal femur with osseous sclerosis. This patient had a 3-year history of hip pain. The resected specimen contained a mixture of low- and high-grade medullary osteo-sarcoma.

Parosteal osteosarcomas are composed of extensive osteoid tissue with a fibrous stroma and form a lobulated, ossified juxtacortical mass. Early lesions may have a radiologic cleavage plane between the cortex and the tumor. As growth progresses, the mass envelops the cortex. CT and axial MR images demonstrate the superficial nature of the mass: dense ossification is seen on CT images, and diminished signal as the result of bone formation is observed on T_1- and T_2-weighted MR images (Fig. 22). The tumor may also grow through the cortex into the medullary cavity.

The differential diagnosis includes myositis ossificans, which has a more heavily mineralized periphery than that of parosteal osteosarcoma (see Section IX, Part II, Chapter 1, Fig. 6, page 2002). Because parosteal osteosarcoma can also have a cartilaginous cap, it must be differentiated from osteochondroma (see Figs. 1 and 2).

The deeper origin of periosteal osteosarcoma within the cortex results in a fusiform mass with periosteal elevation and perpendicular spiculated periosteal new bone formation with Codman's triangles and a scalloped cortex (Fig. 23). Cartilaginous differentiation causes areas of low attenuation on CT images, low signal on T_1-weighted MR images, and very high signal on T_2-weighted images. Hypointense rays of periosteal new bone may be seen within the mass. Medullary invasion is rare, but signal abnormalities caused by reactive changes of the marrow are common. These tumors tend to occur in the diaphysis of the tibia and femur. Patients with these tumors have a less favorable prognosis than do those with parosteal osteosarcoma. The differential features of parosteal osteosarcoma, periosteal osteosarcoma, and the benign soft tissue lesion myositis ossificans are summarized in Table 6.

The least common surface osteosarcoma, high-grade surface osteosarcoma, is similar in appearance to periosteal osteosarcoma, but histologically it resembles conventional intramedullary osteosarcoma. Metastases are more common, and prognosis is consequently poorer than that associated with periosteal osteosarcoma.

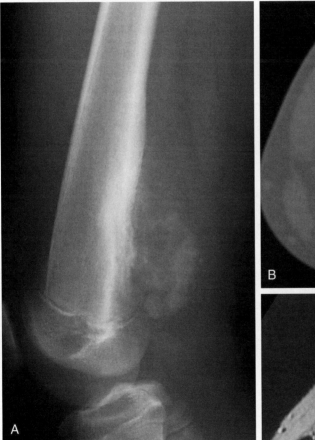
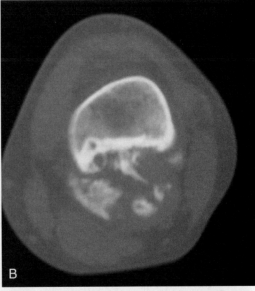
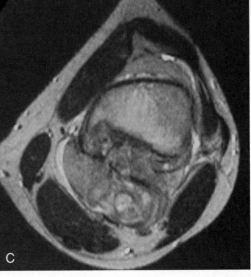

FIGURE 22. Parosteal osteosarcoma in a 13-year-old girl. **A,** Lateral radiograph of the femur shows a mineralized mass arising from the sclerotic posterior cortex of the distal metaphysis. Computed tomography scan **(B)** and transverse T_2-weighted magnetic resonance image **(C)** show sclerosis and irregular thickening of the affected cortex; no evidence of medullary involvement is observed.

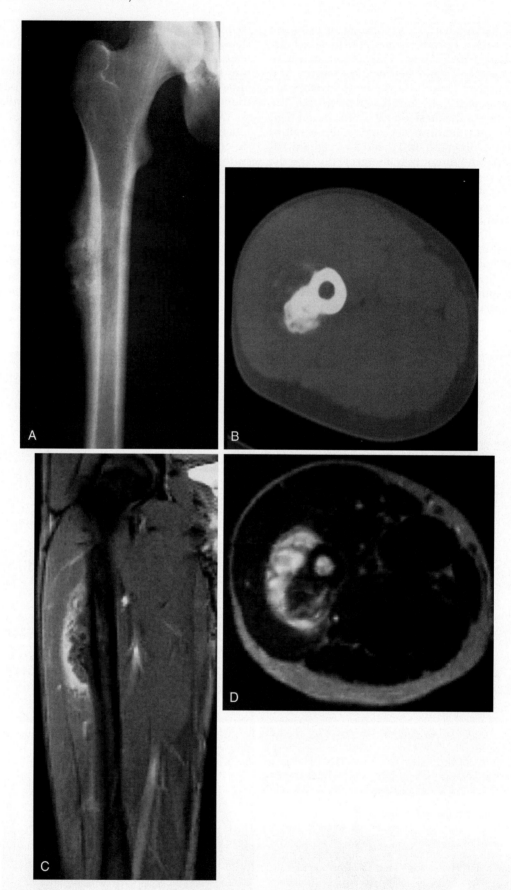

FIGURE 23. Periosteal osteosarcoma in a 15-year-old boy. **A,** Radiograph of the femur shows a fusiform ossified mass arising from the cortical surface of the diaphysis. Computed tomography scan **(B)** and contrast-enhanced coronal T_1-weighted gradient-echo **(C)** and axial T_2-weighted **(D)** magnetic resonance images show the close proximity of the mass to the periosteal surface of the cortex.

Table 6 ■ DIFFERENTIAL FEATURES OF MYOSITIS OSSIFICANS, PAROSTEAL OSTEOSARCOMA, AND PERIOSTEAL OSTEOSARCOMA

	MYOSITIS OSSIFICANS	PAROSTEAL OSTEOSARCOMA	PERIOSTEAL OSTEOSARCOMA
Origin	Soft tissue	Outer periosteum	Deep periosteum–cortex
Common location	Thigh or arm	Metaphysis of distal femur	Diaphysis of tibia or femur
Shape	Circular	Exophytic	Fusiform
Cleavage plane	Occurs late	Occurs early	Does not occur
Periosteal reaction	Occurs frequently	Does not occur	Occurs sometimes
Cortex	Intact	Intact	Scalloped
Site of mineralization	Peripheral rim	Center of tumor	Center of tumor
Prognosis	Benign	Good	Poor

Multifocal Osteosarcoma

There is considerable debate about whether simultaneously occurring osteosarcomas represent true multifocal disease or are manifestations of early metastatic spread. Some authors consider that synchronous occurrence of osteosarcomas in skeletally immature patients with symmetric skeletal involvement in the absence of a dominant mass and of early pulmonary metastases is characteristic of multifocal disease. In a review from the Armed Forces Institute of Pathology of patients with multifocal skeletal involvement, a dominant lesion was present in all patients younger than 18 years of age (Amstutz type I osteosarcomatosis); this dominant le-

sion almost always involved the metaphysis of the distal femur or proximal tibia. Histologic characteristics of the dominant tumors were similar to those of conventional solitary osteosarcomas. The secondary lesions were smaller, better defined, and more sclerotic, and they mainly involved the metaphyses of the long bones. Nearly 75% of the patients in this age range had pulmonary metastases that were detected by chest radiography. These investigators believed that the presence of a radiographically dominant tumor, the high incidence of pulmonary metastases, and the similar distributions of skeletal tumors and metastases indicate that this unusual presentation is due to widespread metastatic disease rather than multifocality (Fig. 24). In

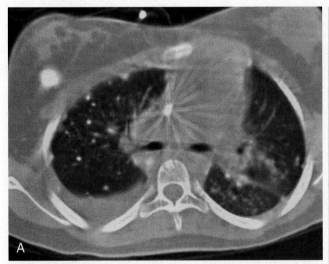

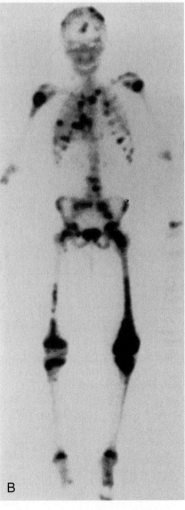

FIGURE 24. A, Computed tomography scan of a 9-year-old girl with osteosarcoma shows multiple calcified pulmonary metastases, a right pleural effusion, and a calcified metastasis in the right anterior chest wall. **B,** Anterior technetium-99m methylene diphosphonate bone scan shows multiple foci of abnormally increased radiotracer uptake in the soft tissues and bones. The primary tumor arose from the distal metaphysis of the left femur. This patient also had rare involvement of lymph nodes.

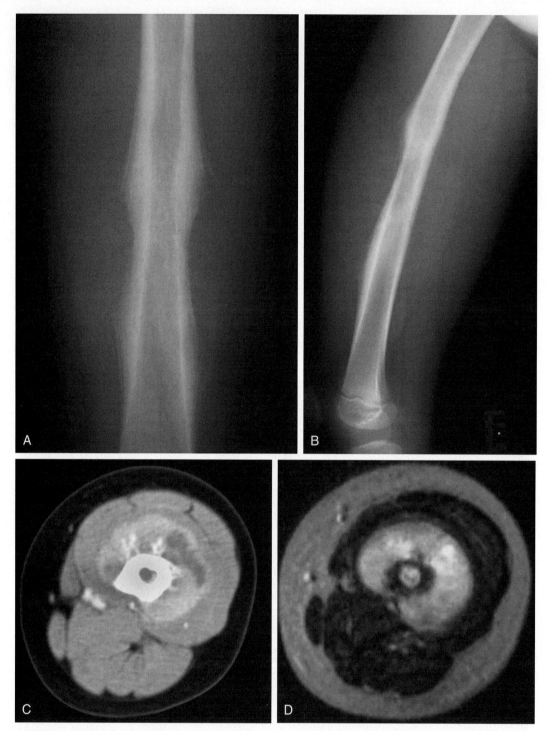

FIGURE 25. Anteroposterior **(A)** and lateral **(B)** radiographs of the femur of a 6-year-old girl show a Ewing's sarcoma arising from the mid-diaphysis. There is lamellar periosteal reaction and new bone formation with Codman's triangles at the proximal and distal ends of the tumor. Faint periosteal new bone extends perpendicularly into the soft tissue component of the tumor. The medulla is not expanded. Contrast-enhanced computed tomography scan **(C)** and T_2-weighted magnetic resonance image **(D)** show a large soft tissue mass.

any event, survival rates of pediatric patients with multiple osteosarcomas are very poor.

EWING'S SARCOMA

In 1921, James Ewing described a radium-sensitive bone tumor consisting of sheets of small polyhedral cells of probable endothelial origin that he called an endothelioma. Although the origin of this undifferentiated tumor has been debated since its initial description, Ewing's sarcoma has proved to be a distinct entity with characteristic histologic, radiologic, and cytogenetic features. The Ewing family of tumors includes Ewing's sarcoma of bone, extraosseous Ewing's sarcoma, and peripheral primitive neuroectodermal tumor (PPNET), which is also known as peripheral neuroepithelioma. PPNET exhibits neural differentiation and may arise from either bone or soft tissues. The Ewing family of tumors shares a distinctive cytogenetic feature: reciprocal translocation of chromosome bands q24 and q12 of chromosomes 11 and 22. This same translocation is also found in Askin's tumor of the thorax (see Section IV, Part V, page 857).

In younger patients, Ewing's sarcoma of bone occurs less frequently than osteosarcoma; most cases are detected in patients between 10 and 25 years of age. Like osteosarcoma, Ewing's sarcoma occurs mostly in males. However, Ewing's sarcoma and PPNET are rarely found in black patients. Fever, leukocytosis, and elevation of the erythrocyte sedimentation rate may accompany these neoplasms.

More than 50% of Ewing's sarcomas involve a single long bone (Fig. 25); Ewing's sarcoma involving the bones of the hands and feet, which is often initially diagnosed as an infection, is rare (Fig. 26). Within the long bones, the metaphysis and diaphysis are the usual locations for these types of malignancies. The flat bones, especially the ribs and pelvis, are also commonly involved. Most Ewing's sarcomas appear to arise from the medullary cavity. Multifocal osseous involvement at the time of diagnosis is rare.

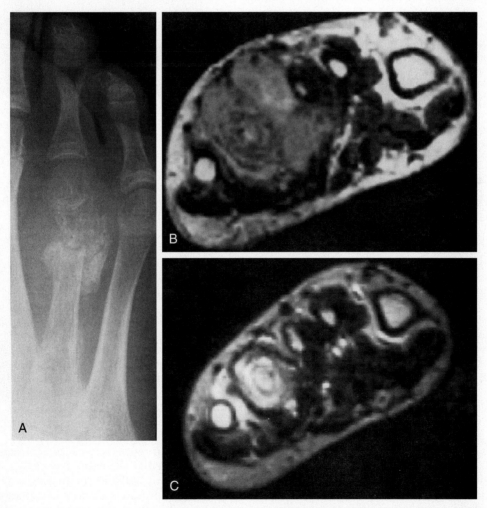

FIGURE 26. A 13-year-old boy with Ewing's sarcoma of the foot. **A,** Anteroposterior radiograph shows a destructive lesion of the fourth metatarsal with a pathologic fracture. **B,** Transverse T$_2$-weighted magnetic resonance (MR) image shows a large soft tissue mass. **C,** After completion of chemotherapy, a transverse T$_2$-weighted MR image shows high signal within the marrow cavity and a smaller periosseous soft tissue mass.

The typical radiographic appearance of Ewing's sarcoma in the long bones is that of a permeative lesion with a lamellar "onion-skin" periosteal reaction (Fig. 25A, B). However, nearly 40% of these tumors display diffuse sclerosis, sometimes with a mixed lytic–sclerotic pattern (Fig. 27). The sclerosis correlates histologically with the presence of dead bone.

Because Ewing's sarcomas do not ossify, soft tissue extension is often poorly detected by plain radiographs but is almost always apparent on contrast-enhanced CT images or on T_2-weighted or contrast-enhanced T_1-weighted MR images (Fig. 25C, D). Indeed, the soft tissue masses tend to be disproportionately large in comparison to the amount of bone destruction, and they are especially extensive in Ewing's sarcoma of the pelvis (Fig. 28). Cortical permeation and destruction may be visible on CT or MRI; however, these tumors can permeate haversian canals and grow into the soft tissues without causing large areas of cortical loss. Extensive marrow involvement is particularly well shown as nonspecific low signal, isointense to muscle on T_1-weighted images. We have observed that most Ewing's sarcomas found in the medullary cavity display intermediate signal that is isointense to that of fat on T_2-weighted images (Fig. 28C).

Rarely, Ewing's sarcoma can arise from the surface of the bone rather than from the medullary cavity. In this periosteal or subperiosteal location, Ewing's sarcoma resembles other surface malignancies, such as periosteal osteosarcoma with periosteal elevation and Codman's triangles. The affected cortex is typically excavated or saucerized (Fig. 29). Cross-sectional imaging is required to exclude medullary involvement. Patients with this form of Ewing's sarcoma are thought to have a relatively favorable prognosis.

With appropriate multimodality therapy, the long-term survival rate of patients with nonmetastatic medullary Ewing's sarcoma approaches that of patients with osteosarcoma (about 70%). In some series, tumor volume has been shown to influence prognosis. Survival of patients with pelvic tumors may be somewhat shortened and is much reduced in patients with metastatic disease. As many as 25% of patients with Ewing's sarcoma have detectable metastases at the time of diagnosis; most of these are found in the lung. Metastases in bone or bone marrow are less frequent. Skip metastases have been reported. In addition to MRI of the primary tumor, technetium-99m methylene diphosphonate (MDP) scintigraphy, thoracic CT scanning, and bone marrow examination should be performed to detect possible disseminated disease.

Most Ewing's sarcomas respond well to initial chemotherapy: increased bony sclerosis develops, and the soft tissue mass disappears (Fig. 30). Percentage change in size of the soft tissue mass appears to be an important prognostic indicator. T_2-weighted MR images show an increase in intensity of the treated medullary component because of serous atrophy, with increased interstitial fluid of the yellow marrow and replacement of cytoplasmic lipid with serous material (Fig. 26C). High T_2-weighted signal intensity caused by radiation-

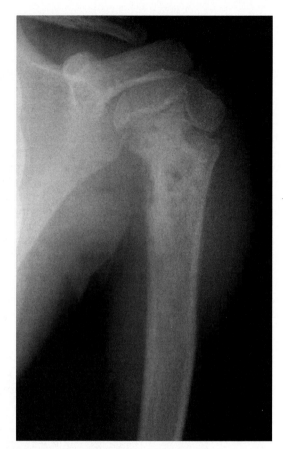

FIGURE 27. Ewing's sarcoma of the proximal humerus of a 5-year-old boy. The tumor is predominantly sclerotic with "moth-eaten" permeation. Little periosteal reaction is apparent.

induced inflammatory reactions may also be observed in those patients treated with radiation therapy.

CHONDROSARCOMA

Chondrosarcomas are rare in children, but their clinical, pathologic, and radiologic features have been described in two modern series comprising a total of 126 young patients. These neoplasms may be primary or, less commonly, may be caused by previous irradiation or by malignant transformation of benign cartilaginous lesions, namely solitary or multiple osteochondromas and enchondromas (see Cartilaginous Tumors earlier). Several histologic types of chondrosarcoma have been described: conventional, myxoid, mesenchymal, and spindle cell. Many chondrosarcomas have only low-grade malignant potential.

Primary chondrosarcoma most frequently involves the appendicular skeleton, especially the diaphysis or metaphysis (or both) of the humerus or femur. Nearly 15% of chondrosarcomas arise in the craniofacial bones. Radiographically, these tumors are similar to chondrosarcomas of adults in that they are central lesions that grow from cancellous bone into the medulla. They are usually elongated, poorly delineated lytic lesions with

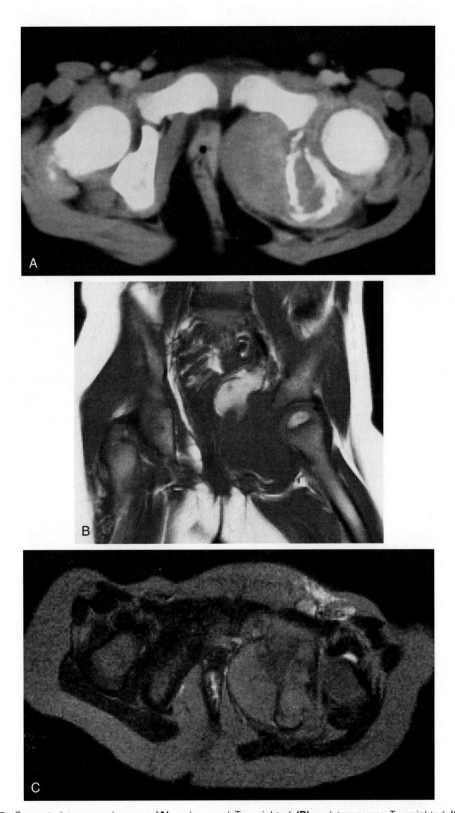

FIGURE 28. Computed tomography scan **(A)** and coronal T_1-weighted **(B)** and transverse T_2-weighted **(C)** magnetic resonance images of the pelvis of a 3-year-old girl with Ewing's sarcoma show an expansile tumor involving the medulla and cortex of the left ischium and a large soft tissue mass. In **C,** signal intensity of the tumor is similar to that of the subcutaneous fat. The high signal in the left groin is due to a recent biopsy. (**C** from Hanna SL, Fletcher BD, Kaste SC, et al: Increased confidence of diagnosis of Ewing sarcoma using T_2-weighted MR images. Magn Reson Imaging 1994;12:560, with permission.)

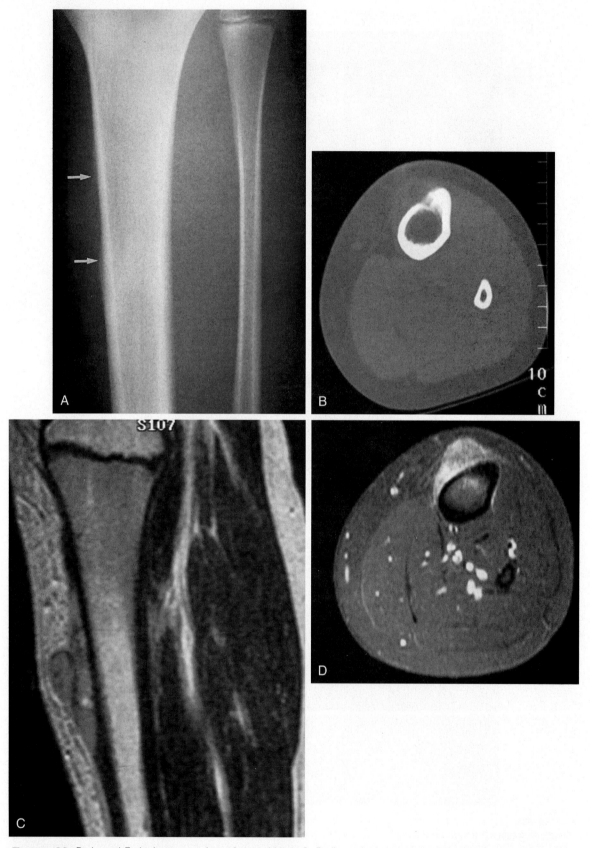

FIGURE 29. Periosteal Ewing's sarcoma in a 12-year-old-boy. **A,** Radiograph shows very subtle excavation of the cortex, Codman's triangles *(arrows)*, and a soft tissue mass. **B,** Computed tomography scan obtained without the administration of contrast shows a small cortical defect. A sagittal T_2-weighted magnetic resonance (MR) image **(C)** demonstrates a superficial soft tissue mass adjacent to the slightly thinned cortex that is also seen on a transverse contrast-enhanced, fat-saturated T_1-weighted MR image **(D).** The slight hyperintensity in the contiguous marrow suggests tumor extension into the medulla.

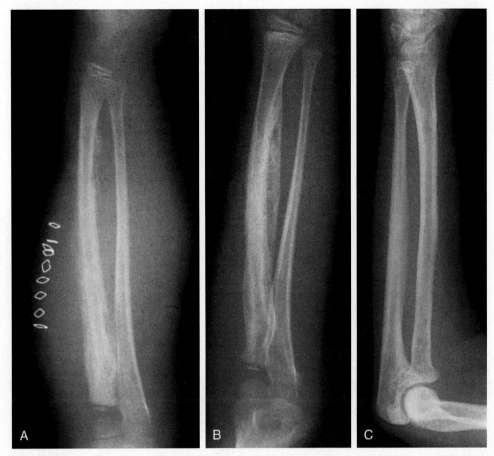

FIGURE 30. Ewing's sarcoma of the radius of a 7-year-old girl who received chemotherapy and radiation therapy. **A,** Radiograph of the forearm obtained after incisional biopsy and before the initiation of therapy shows a long, permeative lesion of the radius, periosteal reaction, and new bone formation. There is a large, ill-defined soft tissue mass. **B,** There is solidification of the periosteal reaction and reduction in the soft tissue mass after completion of initial chemotherapy. **C,** One year after diagnosis, and the completion of all chemotherapy and radiation therapy, the appearance of the radius is nearly normal.

variable matrix mineralization, endosteal scalloping, periosteal reaction, and soft tissue reaction (Fig. 31). Chondrosarcomas are capable of growing into draining veins. MRI is helpful in determining tumor extent before en bloc resection. Cartilaginous and myxoid tumor tissue is isointense to muscle on T_1-weighted images and markedly hyperintense on T_2-weighted images.

Secondary chondrosarcomas occur more frequently in the vertebrae than do primary tumors. In the long bones, they are most often on the periphery and may be identified by thickening of the cartilaginous cap of an osteochondroma or by the loss of the organized appearance of pre-existing benign exostotic lesions. Extraskeletal mesenchymal chondrosarcomas have also been identified in children.

PRIMARY OSSEOUS LYMPHOMA

Although secondary bone involvement in patients with non-Hodgkin's lymphoma is common, primary skeletal lymphoma (formerly called reticulum cell sarcoma) is rare. In adults, non-Hodgkin's lymphoma comprises 5% or fewer of all malignant bone tumors. Lymphoma can be primary in any part of the skeleton, but occurs most commonly in the lower extremities. Cases of multifocal bone lymphoma have been reported.

Both technetium-99m MDP bone scintigrams and gallium-67 scans are capable of detecting skeletal involvement. Nodal and extranodal spread from the primary lesion can occur. The image of the primary bone tumor is often quite subtle on radiographs: it can be either sclerotic or lytic or can display a mixture of these two features (Fig. 32). Periosteal reaction may be minimal or absent.

MRI, an important method of evaluating osseous non-Hodgkin's lymphoma, will often unexpectedly reveal extensive bone marrow involvement. Frequently, soft tissue extension is disproportionately extensive as compared with the relatively small amount of cortical destruction. The MR signal of lymphoma is nonspecific, heterogeneous, and somewhat variable. T_1-weighted signal intensity ranges from isointense to hypointense to muscle, and T_2-weighted intensities can be hypointense, isointense, or hyperintense to fat. Intermixed bone marrow fibrosis may contribute to the heterogeneity of MR signal characteristics.

DISSEMINATED SKELETAL MALIGNANCY

The skeleton is a frequent site of metastatic disease, leukemia, non-Hodgkin's lymphoma, and Hodgkin's disease in pediatric patients. Approximately 25% of children with leukemia exhibit bone lesions, and they are frequently symptomatic. However, radiographically evident bone involvement does not adversely affect prognosis. Submetaphyseal lucency is a classical radiographic presentation of leukemia (Fig. 33), but there are numerous other, less specific skeletal manifestations of the disease, including extensive skeletal permeation and destruction with periosteal new bone formation that primarily affects the metaphysis. Pathologic fractures can occur in the affected long bones; involvement of the axial skeleton, osteoporosis, and vertebral collapse are also seen in some patients (Fig. 34). Extensive bone marrow involvement may result in generalized

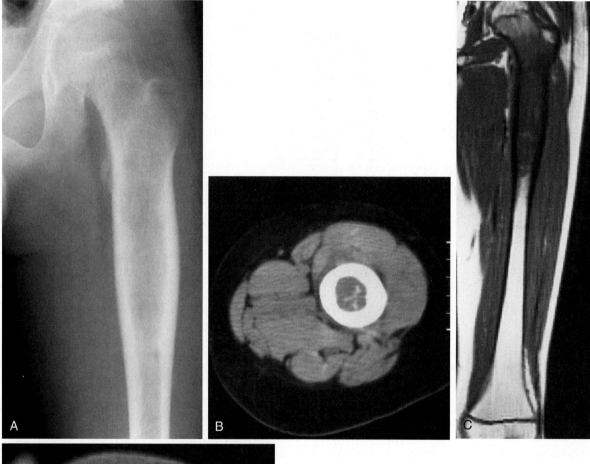

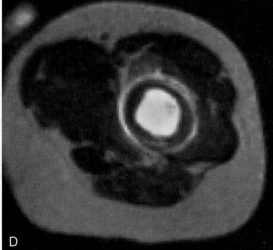

FIGURE 31. **A,** Radiograph of the femur of a 12-year-old boy with chondrosarcoma. The tumor has caused mild diaphyseal expansion and slight cortical thickening. **B,** Unenhanced computed tomography scan demonstrates slight calcification of the medullary tumor matrix. **C,** Coronal T$_1$-weighted magnetic resonance (MR) image shows the distal and proximal limits of the low-intensity tumor. **D,** Transverse T$_2$-weighted MR image shows uniform high signal of the mixed cartilaginous–myxoid tumor matrix. The peritumoral high signal was due to periosteal elevation and soft tissue edema. (**A, C** and **D** from Hanna SL, Magill HL, Parham DM, et al: Childhood sarcoma: MR imaging with Gadolinium-DTPA. Magn Reson Imaging 1990;8:670, with permission.)

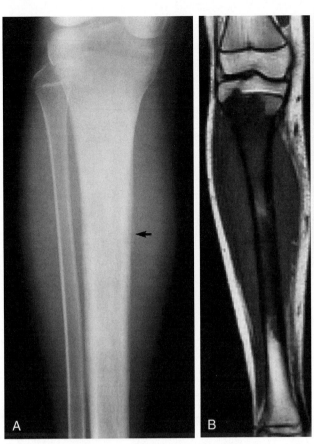
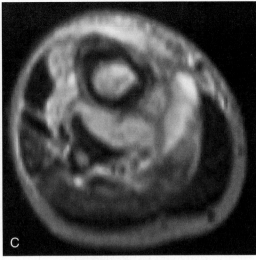

FIGURE 32. A, Radiograph of the tibia of a 15-year-old girl with a primary large cell lymphoma shows subtle sclerosis, medial periosteal new bone formation *(arrow),* and soft tissue swelling. **B,** Coronal T$_1$-weighted magnetic resonance (MR) image shows extensive marrow involvement of the tibial diame-taphysis with extension into the epiphysis. **C,** Trans-verse T$_2$-weighted MR image demonstrates abnor-mally high signal in the tibial medulla and a large, hyperintense soft tissue mass.

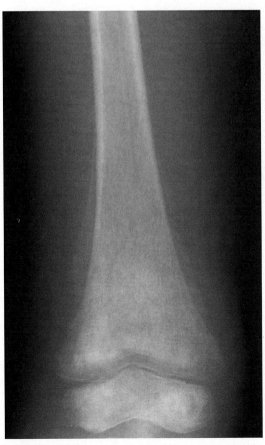

FIGURE 33. Radiograph of the femur of a 4-year-old girl with acute myeloblastic leukemia reveals a submetaphyseal lucent band, periosteal reaction, and metaphyseal and epiphyseal sclerosis.

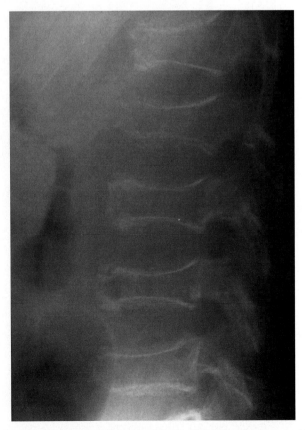

FIGURE 34. Lateral radiograph of the lumbar spine of a 14-year-old girl with acute lymphoblastic leukemia shows osteoporosis and collapse of the vertebral bodies.

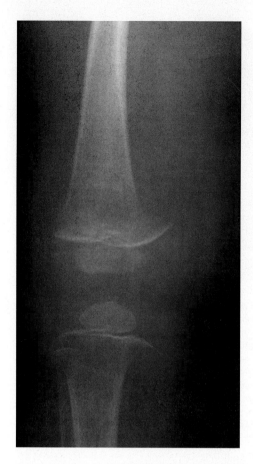

FIGURE 35. Radiograph of the knee of a 15-month-old girl with acute megakaryocytic leukemia shows marked metaphyseal involvement and pathologic fractures.

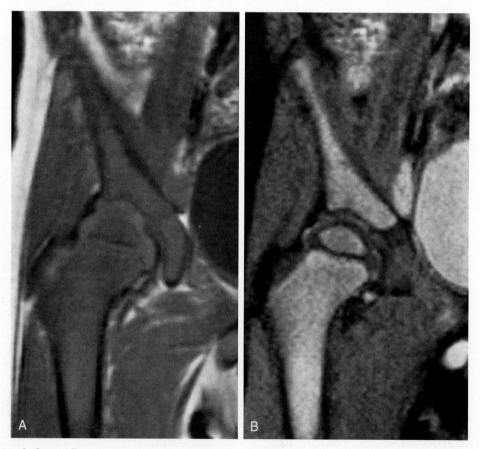

FIGURE 36. A, Coronal T$_1$-weighted magnetic resonance image of the right femur and hemipelvis of a 3-year-old girl with acute lymphoblastic leukemia shows homogeneously diminished signal intensity of the marrow. Even the normally nonhematopoietic, yellow marrow–containing proximal femoral epiphysis is involved. **B,** Coronal short tau inversion–recovery image shows reversal of the intensity of the marrow signal seen in **A.**

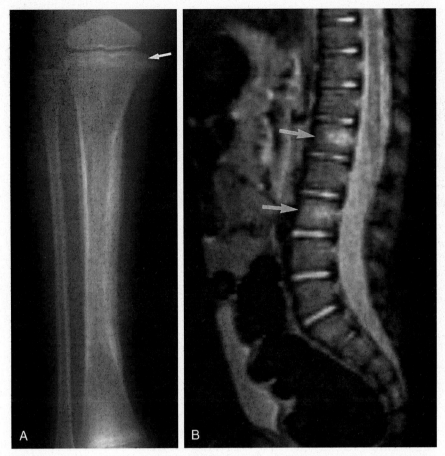

FIGURE 37. A, Radiograph of the lower leg of a 4-year-old boy with neuroblastoma shows an irregular proximal tibial submetaphyseal lucency *(arrow)* and extensive diaphyseal periosteal reaction. **B,** Sagittal short tau inversion–recovery image of the lower thoracic and lumbosacral spine shows abnormally high signal intensity in the bodies of L1 and L3, a finding consistent with metastases *(arrows).*

osteosclerosis, especially in patients with myelogenous leukemia (Fig. 33). Focal osteoblastic lesions are uncommon. Patients with megakaryocytic leukemia (French-American-British subtype M7) may present with aggressive bone destruction and marked periosteal reaction (Fig. 35).

Leukemic infiltration of the bone marrow can be detected by MRI as a patchy or diffuse decrease in signal in locations in which high-intensity fatty marrow normally appears, such as in the long bones (Fig. 36). In sites such as the vertebrae, in which red marrow is abundant and contrast between marrow and disease is therefore diminished, fat- and water-fraction images may be necessary to distinguish leukemic involvement. T_1 relaxation time measurements of marrow have been successful in distinguishing between relapse and remission states.

Granulocytic sarcoma, also known as chloroma, is a localized collection of granulocyte precursors that affects many tissues of patients with myelogenous leukemia. Less than 10% of chloromas involve bone. Found most frequently in the skull, spine, ribs, and sternum, chloromas cause localized expansion of bone with irregular margins. They are isointense to muscle and marrow on T_1- and T_2-weighted MR images and enhance homogeneously.

Many solid tumors that metastasize to bone or bone marrow are detected radiographically. Neuroblastoma is the most common source of metastatic bone disease. The lesions are usually osteolytic. Neuroblastoma typically metastasizes to the metaphysis of a long bone, where it produces a submetaphyseal lucency resembling leukemia (Fig. 37*A*). Vertebral collapse is common, and calvarial metastases appear as numerous small punctate areas of lucency. Metastases from medulloblastoma, osteosarcoma, and retinoblastoma are often blastic.

Technetium-99m MDP bone scintigraphy is the most effective way of detecting skeletal metastases, but, for patients with neuroblastoma, the results may be either false positive or false negative. Thus radiographic skeletal surveys should also be performed. Iodine-131 or Iodine-123 metaiodobenzylguanidine (MIBG) scintigraphy is a useful adjunct to bone scintigrams and skeletal surveys because it further characterizes the extent of skeletal involvement resulting from neuroblastoma. However, the effect of MIBG scintigraphy on tumor staging or therapy is questionable. Recent development of faster MRI techniques has led to investigations of the use of whole-body MRI to detect bone marrow metastases that may be applicable to pediatric patients. In studies of neuroblastoma, MR images have shown diffuse or multifocal nodular bone marrow

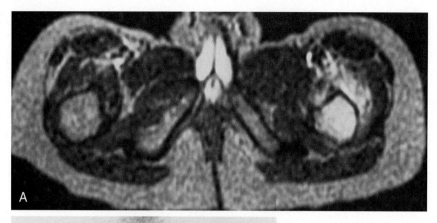

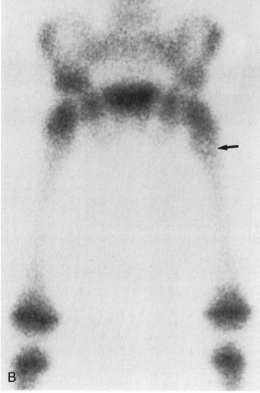

FIGURE 38. A, Transverse T₂-weighted magnetic resonance image of a 2-year-old boy with neuroblastoma demonstrates abnormally high signal in the proximal left femur and adjacent musculature. **B,** Anterior technetium-99m methylene diphosphonate bone scintigram of the pelvis shows a subtle increase in activity in the trochanteric region of the left femur *(arrow)*. No abnormalities were demonstrated on radiographs.

signal abnormalities in the spine, pelvis, and proximal long bones (Fig. 37*B*). Cortical bone metastases are almost always accompanied by marrow disease. In some cases, reactive changes with high T₂-weighted signal intensities are demonstrated in adjacent soft tissues (Fig. 38).

SUGGESTED READINGS

General

Dorfman HD, Czerniak B: Bone Tumors. St. Louis, Mosby, 1998

Mirra JM, Picci P, Gold RH: Bone Tumors: Clinical, Radiologic, and Pathologic Correlations. Philadelphia, Lea & Febiger, 1989

Pizzo PA, Poplack DG: Principles and Practice of Pediatric Oncology, 2nd ed. Philadelphia, JB Lippincott, 1993

Cartilaginous Tumors

Osteochondroma, Periosteal Chondroma, and Endochondroma

Aoki J, Sone S, Fujioka F, et al: MR of enchondroma and chondrosarcoma: rings and arcs of Gd-DTPA enhancement. J Comput Assist Tomogr 1991;15:1011–1016

Caballes RL: Enchondroma protuberans masquerading as osteochondroma. Hum Pathol 1982;13:734–739

Fletcher BD, Crom DB, Krance RA, et al: Radiation-induced bone abnormalities after bone marrow transplantation for childhood leukemia. Radiology 1994;191:231–235

Greenspan A, Unni K, Matthews J II: Periosteal chondroma masquerading as osteochondroma. Can Assoc Radiol J 1993;44: 205–208

Hisaoka M, Aoki T, Kouho H, et al: Maffucci's syndrome associated with spindle cell hemangioendothelioma. Skeletal Radiol 1997;26: 191–194

Jaffe N, Ried HL, Cohen M, et al: Radiation induced osteochondroma in long-term survivors of childhood cancer. Int J Radiat Oncol Biol Phys 1983;9:665–670

Karasick D, Schweitzer ME, Eschelman DJ: Symptomatic osteochondromas: imaging features. AJR Am J Roentgenol 1997;168:1507–1512

Lewis MM, Kenan S, Yabut SM, et al: Periosteal chondroma: a report of ten cases and review of the literature. Clin Orthop 1990;256: 185–192

Libshitz HI, Cohen MA: Radiation-induced osteochondromas. Radiology 1982;142:643–647

Mahboubi SM, Dormans JP, D'Angio G: Malignant degeneration of radiation-induced osteochondroma. Skeletal Radiol 1997;26: 195–198

Chondroblastoma and Chondromyxoid Fibroma

Bloem JL, Mulder JD: Chondroblastoma: a clinical and radiological study of 104 cases. Skeletal Radiol 1985;14:1–9

Brower AC, Moser RP, Kransdorf MJ: The frequency and diagnostic significance of periostitis in chondroblastoma. AJR Am J Roentgenol 1990;154:309–314

Ecklund K, Jaramillo D, Buonomo C: Pediatric case of the day. Radiographics 1996;16:979–982

Oxtoby JW, Davies AM: MRI characteristics of chondroblastoma. Clin Radiol 1996;51:22–26

Weatherall PT, Maale GE, Mendelsohn DB, et al: Chondroblastoma: classic and confusing appearance at MR imaging. Radiology 1994; 190:467–474

Wilson AJ, Kyriakos M, Ackerman LV: Chondromyxoid fibroma: radiographic appearance in 38 cases and in a review of the literature. Radiology 1991;179:513–518

White PG, Saunders L, Orr W, et al: Chondromyxoid fibroma. Skeletal Radiol 1996;25:79–81

Wu CT, Inwards CY, O'Laughlin S, et al: Chondromyxoid fibroma of bone: a clinicopathologic review of 278 cases. Hum Pathol 1998;29: 438–446

Yamamura S, Sato K, Sugiura H, et al: Inflammatory reaction in chondroblastoma. Skeletal Radiol 1996;25:371–376

Cysts

Solitary and Aneurysmal Bone Cysts

Baker DM: Benign unicameral bone cyst: a study of 45 cases with long-term follow-up. Clin Orthop 1970;71:140–151

Beltran J, Simon DC, Levy M, et al: Aneurysmal bone cysts: MR imaging at 1.5 T. Radiology 1986;158:689–690

Bertoni F, Bacchini P, Capanna R, et al: Solid variant of aneurysmal bone cyst. Cancer 1993;71:729–734

Bonakdarpour A, Levy WM, Aegerter E: Primary and secondary aneurysmal bone cyst: a radiological study of 75 cases. Radiology 1978;126:75–83

Burr BA, Resnick D, Syklawer R, et al: Fluid-fluid levels in a unicameral bone cyst: CT and MR findings. J Comput Assist Tomogr 1993;17: 134–136

Campanacci M, Capanna R, Picci P: Unicameral and aneurysmal bone cysts. Clin Orthop 1986;204:25–36

Capanna R, Dal Monte A, Gitelis S, et al: The natural history of unicameral bone cyst after steroid injection. Clin Orthop 1982;166: 204–211

Cohen J: Unicameral bone cysts: a current synthesis of reported cases. Orthop Clin North Am 1977;8:715–736

Jaffe HL, Lichtenstein L: Solitary unicameral bone cyst: with emphasis on the roentgen picture, the pathologic appearance and the pathogenesis. Arch Surg 1942;44:1004–1025

Kransdorf MJ, Sweet DE: Aneurysmal bone cyst: concept, controversy, clinical presentation, and imaging. AJR Am J Roentgenol 1995;164: 573–580

Munk PL, Helms CA, Holt RG, et al: MR imaging of aneurysmal bone cysts. AJR Am J Roentgenol 1989;153:99–101

Oda Y, Tsuneyoshi M, Shinohara N: "Solid" variant of aneurysmal bone cyst (extragnathic giant cell reparative granuloma) in the axial skeleton and long bones. Cancer 1992;70:2642–2649

Tsai JC, Dalinka MK, Fallon MD, et al: Fluid-fluid level: a nonspecific finding in tumors of bone and soft tissue. Radiology 1990;175: 779–782

Van Linthoudt D, Lagier R: Calcaneal cysts: a radiological and anatomical-pathological study. Acta Orthop Scand 1978;49:310–316

Giant Cell Tumor

Aoki J, Tanikawa H, Ishii K, et al: MR findings indicative of hemosiderin in giant-cell tumor of bone: frequency, cause, and diagnostic significance. AJR Am J Roentgenol 1996;166:145–148

Kransdorf MJ, Sweet DE, Buetow PC, et al: Giant cell tumor in skeletally immature patients. Radiology 1992;184:233–237

Martinez V, Sissons HA: Aneurysmal bone cyst: a review of 123 cases including primary lesions and those secondary to other bone pathology. Cancer 1988;61:2291–2304

McEnery KW, Raymond AK: Giant cell tumor of the fourth metacarpal. AJR Am J Roentgenol 1999;172:1092

Schajowicz G, Granato DB, McDonald DJ, et al: Clinical and radiological features of atypical giant cell tumours of bone. Br J Radiol 1991;64:877–889

Tehranzadeh J, Murphy BJ, Mnaymneh W: Giant cell tumor of the proximal tibia: MR and CT appearance. J Comput Assist Tomogr 1989;13:282–286

Fibrous Tumors

Nonossifying Fibroma and Fibrous Dysplasia

Cabral CEL, Guedes P, Fonseca T, et al: Polyostotic fibrous dysplasia associated with intramuscular myxomas: Mazabraud's syndrome. Skeletal Radiol 1998;27:278–282

Fisher AJ, Totty WG, Kyriakos M: MR appearance of cystic fibrous dysplasia. J Comput Assist Tomogr 1994;18:315–318

Jee W-H, Choe B-Y, Kang H-S, et al: Nonossifying fibroma: characteristics at MR imaging with pathologic correlation. Radiology 1998; 209:197–202

Jee W-H, Choi K-H, Choe B-Y, et al: Fibrous dysplasia: MR imaging characteristics with radiopathologic correlation. AJR Am J Roentgenol 1996;167:1523–1527

Mirra JM, Gold RH, Rand F: Disseminated nonossifying fibromas in association with café-au-lait spots (Jaffe-Campanacci syndrome). Clin Orthop 1982;168:192–205

Scully RE, Mark EJ, McNeely WF, et al: Case records of the Massachusetts General Hospital. Case 37-2000: an 11-day-old boy with an osteolytic tibial lesion. N Engl J Med 2000;343:1634–1638

Utz JA, Kransdorf MJ, Jelinek JS, et al: MR appearance of fibrous dysplasia. J Comput Assist Tomogr 1989;13:845–851

Yao L, Eckardt JJ, Seeger LL: Fibrous dysplasia associated with cortical bony destruction: CT and MR findings. J Comput Assist Tomogr 1994;18:91–94

Osteofibrous Dysplasia and Adamantinoma

Bloem JL, van der Heul RO, Schuttevaer HM, et al: Fibrous dysplasia vs adamantinoma of the tibia: differentiation based on discriminant analysis of clinical and plain film findings. AJR Am J Roentgenol 1991;156:1017–1023

Campanacci M, Laus M: Osteofibrous dysplasia of the tibia and fibula. J Bone Joint Surg Am 1981;63:367–375

Czerniak B, Rojas-Corona RR, Dorfman HD: Morphologic diversity of long bone adamantinoma: the concept of differentiated (regressing) adamantinoma and its relationship to osteofibrous dysplasia. Cancer 1989;64:2319–2334

Hindman BW, Bell S, Russo T, et al: Neonatal osteofibrous dysplasia: report of two cases. Pediatr Radiol 1996;26:303–306

Ishida T, Iijima T, Kikuchi F, et al: A clinicopathological and immunohistochemical study of osteofibrous dysplasia, differentiated adamantinoma, and adamantinoma of long bones. Skeletal Radiol 1992;21:493–502

Nakashima Y, Yamamuro T, Fujiwara Y, et al: Osteofibrous dysplasia (ossifying fibroma of long bones): a study of 12 cases. Cancer 1983;52:909–914

Zeanah WR, Hudson TM, Springfield DS: Computed tomography of ossifying fibroma of the tibia. J Comput Assist Tomogr 1983;7: 688–691

Langerhans' Cell Histiocytosis of Bone

Bar-Sever Z, Connolly LP, Jaramillo D, et al: Thallium-201 uptake in Langerhans cell histiocytosis of bone. Pediatr Radiol 1996;26:739–741

Beltran J, Aparisi F, Bonmati LM, et al: Eosinophilic granuloma: MRI manifestations. Skeletal Radiol 1993;22:157–161

DeSchepper AMA, Ramon F, Van Marck E: MR imaging of eosinophilic granuloma: report of 11 cases. Skeletal Radiol 1993;22:163–166

Doyle AJ, Christie M, French G: Bone surface lesions (Letter to the Editor). Radiology 1998;209:282

Hindman BW, Thomas RD, Young LW, et al: Langerhans cell histiocytosis: unusual skeletal manifestations observed in thirty-four cases. Skeletal Radiol 1998;27:177–181

Kilpatrick SE, Wenger DE, Gilchrist GS, et al: Langerhans' cell histiocytosis (histiocytosis X) of bone: a clinicopathologic analysis of 263 pediatric and adult cases. Cancer 1995;76:2471–2484

Senac MO Jr, Isaacs H, Gwinn JL: Primary lesions of bone in the 1st decade of life: retrospective survey of biopsy results. Radiology 1986;160:491–495

Siegelman SS: Taking the X out of histiocytosis X. Radiology 1997;204:322–324

Stull MA, Kransdorf MJ, Devaney KO: Langerhans cell histiocytosis of bone. Radiographics 1992;12:801–823

Van Nieuwenhuyse J-P, Clapuyt P, Malghem J, et al: Radiographic skeletal survey and radionuclide bone scan in Langerhans cell histiocytosis of bone. Pediatr Radiol 1996;26:734–738

Osseous Tumors

Osteoid Osteoma and Osteoblastoma

Azouz EM, Kozlowski K, Marton D, et al: Osteoid osteoma and osteoblastoma of the spine in children: report of 22 cases with brief literature review. Pediatr Radiol 1986;16:25–31

Gangi A, Dietemann JL, Gasser B, et al: Interstitial laser photocoagulation of osteoid osteomas with use of CT guidance. Radiology 1997;203:843–848

Kayser F, Resnick D, Haghighi P, et al: Evidence of the subperiosteal origin of osteoid osteomas in tubular bones: analysis by CT and MR imaging. AJR Am J Roentgenol 1998;170:609–614

Kransdorf MJ, Stull MA, Gilkey FW, et al: Osteoid osteoma. Radiographics 1991;11:671–696

Kroon HM, Schurmans J: Osteoblastoma: clinical and radiologic findings in 98 new cases. Radiology 1990;175:783–790

Lefton DR, Torrisi JM, Haller JO: Vertebral osteoid osteoma masquerading as malignant bone or soft-tissue tumor on MRI. Pediatr Radiol 2001;31:72–75

Lindbom A, Lindvall N, Söderberg G, et al: Angiography in osteoid osteoma. Acta Radiol 1960;54:327–333

McLeod RA, Dahlin DC, Beabout JW: The spectrum of osteoblastoma. Am J Roentgenol 1976;126:321–335

Orlowski JP, Mercer RD: Osteoid osteoma in children and young adults. Pediatrics 1977;59:526–532

Roach PJ, Connolly LP, Zurakowski D, et al: Osteoid osteoma: comparative utility of high-resolution planar and pinhole magnification scintigraphy. Pediatr Radiol 1996;26:222–225

Roger B, Bellin MF, Wioland M, et al: Osteoid osteoma: CT-guided percutaneous excision confirmed with immediate follow-up scintigraphy in 16 outpatients. Radiology 1996;210:239–242

Shankman S, Desai P, Beltran J: Subperiosteal osteoid osteoma: radiographic and pathologic manifestations. Skeletal Radiol 1997;26:457–462

Towbin R, Kaye R, Meza MP, et al: Osteoid osteoma: percutaneous excision using a CT-guided coaxial technique. AJR Am J Roentgenol 1995;164:945–949

Woods ER, Martel W, Mandell SH, et al: Reactive soft-tissue mass associated with osteoid osteoma: correlation of MR imaging features with pathologic findings. Radiology 1993;186:221–225

Yamamura S, Sato K, Sugiura H, et al: Magnetic resonance imaging of inflammatory reaction in osteoid osteoma. Arch Orthop Trauma Surg 1994;114:8–13

Osteosarcoma

Bloem JL, Taminiau AHM, Eulderink F, et al: Radiologic staging of primary bone sarcoma: MR imaging, scintigraphy, angiography, and CT correlated with pathologic examination. Radiology 1988;169:805–810

Brown ML: The role of radionuclides in the patient with osteogenic sarcoma. Semin Roentgenol 1989;24:185–192

Doud TM, Moser RP Jr, Giudici MAI, et al: Case report 704: extraskeletal osteosarcoma of the thigh with several suspected skeletal metastases and extensive metastases to the chest. Skeletal Radiol 1991;20:628–632

Ellis JH, Siegel CL, Martel W, et al: Radiologic features of well-differentiated osteosarcoma. AJR Am J Roentgenol 1988;151:739–742

Fletcher BD: Imaging pediatric bone sarcomas: diagnosis and treatment-related issues. Radiol Clin North Am 1997;35:1477–1494

Gomes H, Menanteau B, Gaillard D, et al: Telangiectatic osteosarcoma. Pediatr Radiol 1986;16:140–143

Goorin AM, Abelson HT, Frei E III: Osteosarcoma: fifteen years later. N Engl J Med 1985;313:1637–1643

Graham NJ, Cairns RA, Anderson RA: Osteosarcoma in a 19-month-old-girl. Can Assoc Radiol J 1996;47:33–35

Griffith JF, Kumta SM, Chow LTC, et al: Intracortical osteosarcoma. Skeletal Radiol 1998;27:228–232

Hanna SL, Fletcher BD, Parham DM, et al: Muscle edema in musculoskeletal tumors: MR imaging characteristics and clinical significance. J Magn Reson Imaging 1991;1:441–449

Hasegawa T, Shimoda T, Yokoyama R, et al: Intracortical osteoblastic osteosarcoma with oncogenic rickets. Skeletal Radiol 1999;28:41–45

Hopper KD, Moser RP, Haseman DB, et al: Osteosarcomatosis. Radiology 1990;175:233–239

Hudson TM, Schiebler M, Springfield DS, et al: Radiologic imaging of osteosarcoma: role in planning surgical treatment. Skeletal Radiol 1983;10:137–146

Iemoto Y, Ushigome S, Fukunaga M, et al: Case report 679: central low-grade osteosarcoma with foci of dedifferentiation. Skeletal Radiol 1991;20:379–382

Kaufman RA, Towbin RB: Telangiectatic osteosarcoma simulating the appearance of an aneurysmal bone cyst. Pediatr Radiol 1981;11:102–104

Murphey MD, Robbin MR, McRae GA, et al: The many faces of osteosarcoma. Radiographics 1997;17:1205–1231

Olson PN, Prewitt L, Griffiths HJ, Cherkna B: Case report 703: multifocal osteosarcoma. Skeletal Radiol 1991;20:624–627

Onikul E, Fletcher BD, Parham DM, et al: Accuracy of MR imaging for estimating intraosseous extent of osteosarcoma. AJR Am J Roentgenol 1996;167:1211–1215

Panicek DM, Gatsonis C, Rosenthal DI, et al: CT and MR imaging in the local staging of primary malignant musculoskeletal neoplasms: report of the Radiology Diagnostic Oncology Group. Radiology 1997;202:237–246

Panuel M, Gentet JC, Scheiner C, et al: Physeal and epiphyseal extent of primary malignant bone tumors in childhood: correlation of preoperative MRI and the pathologic examination. Pediatr Radiol 1993;23:421–424

Schima W, Amann G, Stiglbauer R, et al: Preoperative staging of osteosarcoma: efficacy of MR imaging in detecting joint involvement. AJR Am J Roentgenol 1994;163:1171–1175

Sim FH, Kurt A-M, McLeod RA, Unni KK: Case report 628: low-grade central osteosarcoma. Skeletal Radiol 1990;19:457–460

Sundaram M, McGuire MH, Herbold DR: Magnetic resonance imaging of osteosarcoma. Skeletal Radiol 1987;16:23–29

Sundaram M, Totty WG, Kyriakos M, et al: Imaging findings in pseudocystic osteosarcoma. AJR Am J Roentgenol 2001;176:783–788

Tsuneyoshi M, Dorfman HD: Epiphyseal osteosarcoma: distinguishing features from clear cell chondrosarcoma, chondroblastoma and epiphyseal enchondroma. Am J Surg Pathol 1986;10:754–764

van Zanten TEG, Golding RP, Taets ven Amerongen AHM: Osteosarcoma with calcific mediastinal lymphadenopathy. Pediatr Radiol 1987;17:258–259

Vanel D, Picci P, De Paolis M, Mercuri M: Osteosarcoma arising in an exostosis: CT and MRI imaging [Letter to the Editor]. AJR Am J Roentgenol 2001;176:259–260

Wetzel LH, Schweiger GD, Levine E: MR imaging of transarticular skip metastases from distal femoral osteosarcoma. J Comput Assist Tomogr 1990;14:315–317

Ewing's Sarcoma

Coombs RJ, Zeiss J, McCann K, Phillips E: Case report 360: multifocal Ewing tumor of the skeletal system. Skeletal Radiol 1986;15:254–257

Coombs RJ, Zeiss J, Paley KJ, Kini J: Case report 802: Ewing's tumor of the proximal phalanx of third finger with radiographic progression documented over a 6-year-period. Skeletal Radiol 1993;22:460–463

Daugaard S, Sunda LM, Kamby C, et al: Ewing's sarcoma: a retrospective study of prognostic factors and treatment results. Acta Oncol 1987;26:281–287

Davies AM, Makwana NK, Grimer RJ, et al: Skip metastases in Ewing's sarcoma: a report of three cases. Skeletal Radiol 1997;26:379–384

Ewing J: Diffuse endothelioma of bone. Proc N Y Pathol Soc 1921;21:17; reprinted in Clin Orthop 1984;185:2–5

Hanna SL, Fletcher BD, Kaste SC, et al: Increased confidence of diagnosis of Ewing sarcoma using T_2-weighted MR images. Magn Reson Imaging 1994;12:559–568

Jaffe R, Santamaria M, Yunis EJ, et al: The neuroectodermal tumor of bone. Am J Surg Pathol 1984;8:885–898

Jürgens H, Exner U, Gadner H, et al: Multidisciplinary treatment of primary Ewing's sarcoma of bone: a 6-year experience of a European Cooperative Trial. Cancer 1988;61:23–32

Lemmi MA, Fletcher BD, Marina NM, et al: Use of MR imaging to assess results of chemotherapy for Ewing sarcoma. AJR Am J Roentgenol 1990;155:343–346

Kretschmar CS: Ewing's sarcoma and the "peanut" tumors. N Engl J Med 1994;331:325–327

Mueller DL, Grant RM, Riding MD, et al: Cortical saucerization: an unusual imaging finding of Ewing sarcoma. AJR Am J Roentgenol 1994;163:401–403

Reinus WR, Gilula LA, Donaldson S, et al: Prognostic features of Ewing sarcoma on plain radiograph and computed tomography scan after initial treatment: a Pediatric Oncology Group Study (8346). Cancer 1993;72:2503–2510

Shapeero LG, Vanel D, Sundaram M, et al: Periosteal Ewing sarcoma. Radiology 1994;191:825–831

Shirley SK, Gilula LA, Siegal GP, et al: Roentgenographic-pathologic correlation of diffuse sclerosis in Ewing sarcoma of bone. Skeletal Radiol 1984;12:69–78

Taber DS, Libshitz HI, Cohen MA: Treated Ewing sarcoma: radiographic appearance in response, recurrence, and new primaries. AJR Am J Roentgenol 1983;140:753–758

Vanel D, Lacombe M-J, Couanet D, et al: Musculoskeletal tumors: follow-up with MR imaging after treatment with surgery and radiation therapy. Radiology 1987;164:243–245

Wuisman P, Roessner A, Blasius S, et al: (Sub)periosteal Ewing's sarcoma of bone. J Cancer Res Clin Oncol 1992;118:72–74

Chondrosarcoma

Giuliano C, Kauffman WM, Haller JO, et al: Inferior vena cava–right atrial tumor thrombus in malignant pelvic bone tumors in children. Pediatr Radiol 1992;22:206–208

Hanna SL, Magill HL, Parham DM, et al: Childhood chondrosarcoma: MR imaging with gadolinium-DTPA. Magn Reson Imaging 1990;8:669–672

Huvos AG, Marcove RC: Chondrosarcoma in the young: a clinicopathologic analysis of 79 patients younger than 21 years of age. Am J Surg Pathol 1987;11:930–942

Shapeero LG, Vanel D, Couanet D, et al: Extraskeletal mesenchymal chondrosarcoma. Radiology 1993;186:819–826

Young CL, Sim FH, Unni KK, et al: Chondrosarcoma of bone in children. Cancer 1990;66:1641–1648

Primary Osseous Lymphoma

Häussler MD, Fenstermacher MJ, Johnston DA, et al: MRI of primary lymphoma of bone: cortical disorder as a criterion for differential diagnosis. J Magn Reson Imaging 1999;9:93–100

Hicks DG, Gokan T, O'Keefe RJ, et al: Primary lymphoma of bone: correlation of magnetic resonance imaging features with cytokine production by tumor cells. Cancer 1995;75:973–980

Melamed JW, Martinez S, Hoffman CJ: Imaging of primary multifocal osseous lymphoma. Skeletal Radiol 1997;26:35–41

Mouratidis B, Gilday DL, Ash JM: Comparison of bone and ^{67}Ga scintigraphy in the initial diagnosis of bone involvement in children with malignant lymphoma. Nucl Med Commun 1994;15:144–147

Schmidt A-G, Kohn D, Bernhards J, et al: Solitary skeletal lesions as primary manifestations of non-Hodgkin's lymphoma: report of two cases and review of the literature. Arch Orthop Trauma Surg 1994;113:121–128

Stiglbauer S, Augustin I, Kramer J, et al: MRI in the diagnosis of primary lymphoma of bone: correlation with histopathology. J Comput Assist Tomogr 1992;16:248–253

White LM, Schweitzer ME, Khalili K, et al: MR imaging of primary lymphoma of bone: variability of T_2-weighted signal intensity. AJR Am J Roentgenol 1998;170:1243–1247

Disseminated Skeletal Malignancy

Andrich MP, Shalaby-Rana E, Movassaghi N, et al: The role of 131 iodine-metaiodobenzylguanidine scanning in the correlative imaging of patients with neuroblastoma. Pediatrics 1996;97:246–250

Bohndorf K, Benz-Bohm G, Gross-Fengels W, et al: MRI of the knee region in leukemic children: Part I. Initial pattern in patients with untreated disease. Pediatr Radiol 1990;20:179–183

Cohen MD: Imaging of Children with Cancer. St. Louis, Mosby–Year Book, 1992:254

Fisher D, Ruchlemer R, Hiller N, et al: Aggressive bone destruction in acute megakaryocytic leukemia: a rare presentation. Pediatr Radiol 1997;27:20–22

Fletcher BD, Miraldi FD, Cheung N-KV: Comparison of radiolabeled monoclonal antibody and magnetic resonance imaging in the detection of metastatic neuroblastoma in bone marrow: preliminary results. Pediatr Radiol 1989;20:72–75

Kaufman RA, Thrall JH, Keyes JW, et al: False negative bone scans in neuroblastoma metastatic to the ends of long bones. AJR Am J Roentgenol 1978;130:131–135

McKinstry SC, Steiner RE, Young AT, et al: Bone marrow in leukemia and aplastic anemia: MR imaging before, during and after treatment. Radiology 1987;162:701–707

Moody A, Simpson E, Shaw D: Florid radiological appearance of megakaryoblastic leukaemia—an aid to earlier diagnosis. Pediatr Radiol 1989;19:486–488

Moore SG, Gooding CA, Brasch RC, et al: Bone marrow in children with acute lymphocytic leukemia: MR relaxation times. Radiology 1986;160:237–240

Newman AJ, Melhorn DK: Vertebral compression in childhood leukemia. Am J Dis Child 1973;125:863–865

Parker BR, Marglin S, Castellino RA: Skeletal manifestations of leukemia, Hodgkin disease, and non-Hodgkin lymphoma. Semin Roentgenol 1980;15:302–315

Pui MH, Fletcher BD, Langston JW: Granulocytic sarcoma in childhood leukemia: imaging features. Radiology 1994;190:698–702

Shulkin BL, Shapiro B, Hutchinson RJ: Iodine-131-metaiodobenzylguanidine and bone scintigraphy for the detection of neuroblastoma. J Nucl Med 1992;33:1735–1740

Steinbron MM, Heuck AF, Tiling R, et al: Whole-body bone marrow MRI in patients with metastatic disease to the skeletal system. J Comput Assist Tomogr 1999;23:123–129

Tanabe M, Ohnuma N, Iwai J, et al: Bone marrow metastasis of neuroblastoma analyzed by MRI and its influence on prognosis. Med Pediatr Oncol 1995;24:292–299

PART XIII

BONE CHANGES ASSOCIATED WITH SYSTEMIC DISEASES

SAMBASIVA R. KOTTAMASU

■ C h a p t e r   1

BONE CHANGES IN DISEASES OF THE BLOOD AND BLOOD-FORMING ORGANS

SAMBASIVA R. KOTTAMASU

ERYTHROBLASTOSIS FETALIS

This disorder usually results from immunization of a pregnant woman of one blood type by fetal erythrocytes of another type. The Rh blood factors are most frequently involved, but the major ABO blood factors may also cause a rise in maternal antibodies to the specific factor. The antibodies cross the placenta to the fetal circulation and cause hemolysis of the fetal red blood cells. The hemolysis is responsible for icterus, anemia, edema, erythroblastemia, splenomegaly, and hepatomegaly in the newborn infant. In many cases, mild and severe, there are no radiographic changes in the skeleton. Diffuse sclerosis of the bones may be observed but is indistinguishable from physiologic osteosclerosis of the newborn. In some cases, interference with prenatal endochondral bone formation causes nonspecific transverse bands of increased and diminished density to develop in the ends of the shafts of tubular bones (Fig. 1). The almost universal monitoring of blood types and antibody levels, as well as the prophylactic administration of specific antibody to mothers following the birth of an infant with the potential for having sensitized her, has practically eliminated this disease for subsequent pregnancies.

FANCONI'S ANEMIA

This is a congenital hypoplastic anemia with multiple anomalies. There is pancytopenia, with hypoplastic changes in the bone marrow and peripheral blood. The onset of the disease usually is in the second half of the first decade or even later. Congenital malformations that indicate the patient may be at risk for the hematologic abnormality include aplasia and hypoplasia of the bones of the thumb, first metacarpal, and radius; syndactyly; congenital dislocation of the hip; and occasionally deformities of some of the large tubular bones (see Section IX, Part VI, Fig. 16, page 2193). Glycosuria, various aminoacidurias, phosphaturia, and hypophosphatemic rickets and osteomalacia are associated manifestations.

CHRONIC HEMOLYTIC ANEMIAS

Heritable hemoglobinopathies comprise a group of important clinical diseases characterized by excessive amounts of abnormal hemoglobins or fetal hemoglobin. They are all determined genetically and tend to be limited to specific racial groups. The abnormality resides in the polypeptide chains that make up the globin moiety of hemoglobin. Combinations of these hemoglobin variants give rise to different disorders that are identified by electrophoretic mobility, which in turn depends on the chemical differences and the electrical charges they produce.

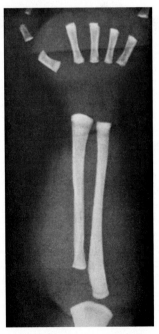

FIGURE 1. Radiographic appearance of erythroblastosis fetalis 4 hours after birth. Note the deep transverse bands of increased density in the distal ends of the radius and ulna. The depth of these bands suggests that endochondral bone formation had been disturbed for several weeks prior to birth.

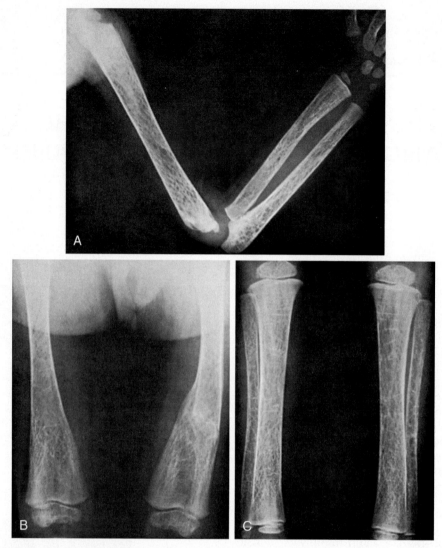

FIGURE 2. Mediterranean (Cooley's) anemia (thalassemia major) in an Italian boy 3 years of age. In radiographs of the upper extremity **(A)**, thighs **(B)**, and lower legs **(C)**, the medullary cavities are widened, the shafts are rectangular in outline, and the cortex is thin. All of the bones are osteoporotic and present a bizarre trabeculated appearance resulting from irregular destruction of the spongiosa and irregular endosteal erosion of the cortex. Multiple transverse lines mark the tibias. The deformity of the left femur is secondary to an old pathologic fracture.

THALASSEMIA

Thalassemia, or Cooley's (erythroblastic) anemia, has strong familial and racial characteristics. It occurs with high frequency in the central and eastern Mediterranean regions and in parts of North Africa; this geographic predominance gave rise to its earlier designation as Mediterranean anemia (Greek *thalassa*, the sea). It is now recognized to be a common disorder of extensive distribution involving the Middle East and Southeast Asia, as well as American Indians and blacks. Clinically, thalassemia occurs in two main forms. The severe cases present a uniform clinical picture of progressive anemia and jaundice that begin during the first 2 years; death usually occurs before adolescence. Splenomegaly is invariably present and is usually accompanied by hepatomegaly. In the most severe cases of thalassemia major, a peculiar facies occurs as a result of

marrow hyperplasia involving the facial bones. Some patients also have hypogonadism. The blood is characterized by erythroblastemia and marked changes in size and shape of the red blood cells. Showers of nucleated red cells appear, a feature that is aggravated by splenectomy, and these cells may persist for many months. In milder cases (thalassemia minor), the clinical and hematologic manifestations are less conspicuous, and in some cases only the laboratory features of hemoglobinopathy are found.

The radiographic findings are diagnostic in severe cases. The shafts of the long bones are osteopenic and undertubulated; the spongiosa is partially destroyed and deformed and the cortex is thin (Fig. 2). The entire skeleton is affected, but the changes are usually most conspicuous in both short and long tubular bones. The hyperplastic marrow distends the medullary cavity and interferes with normal tubulation of the bones. In some cases, the spongiosa is almost completely destroyed and the bones have a widened and featureless appearance, in contrast with the usually coarse trabeculated spongiosal pattern. The skeletal changes are indistinct during the first year of life but become more clearly defined as age advances. During late childhood and early adult life there is a tendency to sclerosis in some cases (Fig. 3); this is apparently due to the increased formation of cortical bone. Caffey has shown that the bone lesions in the limbs begin to involute during early adolescence and may then disappear, while the lesions in the bones of the trunk persist into adult life. The bone lesions disappear in the peripheral segments of the skeleton, where normally red marrow is converted to yellow marrow with advancing age, but they persist in the central skeletal segments, where the bone marrow normally remains red throughout life.

In longstanding severe cases, both maturation and growth of the skeleton are retarded. In the study of Currarino and Erlandson, premature fusion of the epiphyseal ossification centers with their shafts occurred in 23% of children older than 10 years. The proximal end of the humerus and the distal end of the femur were the only sites of these early fusions, excepting one tibia at its proximal end. Thus Cooley's anemia presents the paradox of delayed appearance of the secondary centers in the epiphyseal cartilages and subsequent premature fusion of these secondary centers with the shafts. Pathologic fractures of the femur have been serious complications in several patients; in view of the fre-

quency of extreme cortical atrophy, it is surprising that pathologic fractures are not more common. The classical cranial findings in children with thalassemia major include marked widening of the diploic space, thinning of inner and outer tables, and "hair on end" appearance.

The major form of thalassemia results from a homozygous state for the gene causing the hemoglobin abnormality. Thalassemia variants result from the heterozygous state of the gene. In general, the skeletal abnormalities, when present, are much less marked in the variants than in thalassemia major. The thalassemia–sickle cell combination may have moderately severe bone changes that resemble those in sickle cell anemia more than those in thalassemia. Instances of thalassemia–hemoglobin E disease have been reported with bone changes similar to those in thalassemia major, but those cases involving combination with hemoglobin C and other forms of deviant hemoglobin demonstrate few or no skeletal abnormalities.

Bone mineral density (BMD) is an important indicator of osteoporosis and gonadal function in patients with thalassemia major. Voskaridou et al. evaluated BMD in 45 thalassaemic patients using dual X-ray absorptiometry. Their results showed that patients on regular transfusions had a markedly low BMD in contrast to those not requiring blood support and that this finding was more pronounced in patients of both sexes with associated hypogonadism. Bone formation, as evidenced by the levels of serum alkaline phosphatase

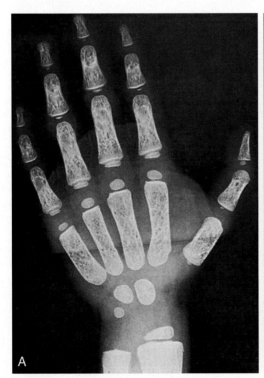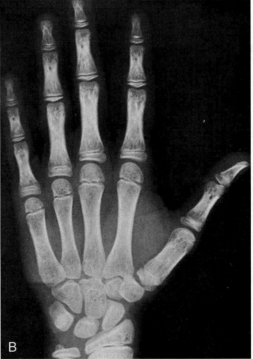

FIGURE 3. Radiographic changes in the hands with advancing age in Mediterranean (Cooley's) anemia in a Greek girl. **A,** In the third year, all of the characteristic changes are present: cortical atrophy and widened external contours, rarefaction, and coarse reticulation. **B,** In the 12th year, all the characteristic changes have disappeared despite the fact that severe hemolytic anemia persisted. In our experience, the characteristic infantile changes always disappear completely or partially in the long bones if the patient survives late childhood.

and osteocalcin, was not impaired, while bone resorption was grossly increased in all patients.

Molyvda-Athanasopoulou et al. evaluated the BMD of 50 patients with thalassemia major to assess the alterations in bone density over a 4-year period. All 50 patients received calcium and vitamin D supplements, and 8 received gonadal hormone replacement therapy (HRT). All patients had a significantly lower BMD compared with healthy subjects. All adolescent patients with normal gonadal function and those who received HRT showed an increase in BMD during the period of the study. However, adolescent and adult patients who had hypogonadotropic hypogonadism but did not receive HRT demonstrated a decrease in bone density.

Extramedullary hematopoiesis (EMH) refers to the production of blood cells outside the bone marrow; and is a common finding in patients with chronic severe anemia, such as thalassemia major. EMH should be suspected when lobulated or rounded masses of soft tissue density are found in the mediastinum contiguous to the spine. The vertebrae are usually not eroded by the mediastinal masses. "Prophylactic" transfusions to young children with thalassemia major have tended to delay the development of skeletal signs of the disease. Nevertheless, marked accumulation of hemosiderin in lymph nodes, spleen, bone marrow, and liver is a frequent manifestation. The spleen is usually enlarged. Hemosiderin deposits in the paravertebral lower thoracic and lumbar nodes and liver manifest as areas of increased opacity on radiographs and computed tomographic (CT) images. These features are clearly defined by magnetic resonance imaging (MRI) when the areas of iron deposition lead to a marked signal void on both T_1- and T_2-weighted sequences. Bone marrow scintigraphy with ^{99m}Tc sulfur colloid demonstrates intense uptake in the areas of EMH and confirms the diagnosis. Tsitouridis et al. presented a comparative CT and MRI study of the paraspinal EMH in 32 thalassemic patients. Active paraspinal EMH masses showed soft tissue characterics in both CT and MRI. Older inactive masses revealed iron deposition or fatty replacement.

EMH rarely produces neurologic manifestations. Aliberti et al., however, presented two patients suffering from thalassaemia (intermedia and β homozygous) and paraparesis resulting from spinal cord compression by intrathoracic EMH masses. Diagnosis was based on MRI findings. Treatment consisted of blood hypertransfusions, and both patients recovered completely. An unusual gastrointestinal manifestation of EMH was reported by Wongwaisayawan et al. in a 7-year-old boy with β-thalassemia–hemoglobin E disease. The patient presented with an ileoileal intussusception, the lead point of which was an EMH mass.

Some patients affected by thalassemia major and treated with an iron-chelating drug such as deferoxamine to reduce transfusional iron overload can suffer from severe osteochondrodystrophic lesions of the long bones. de Sanctis et al. concluded that, in patients with thalassemia major on chelation therapy, even without radiographic abnormalities, seriously damaged columnar cartilage, altered bone mineralization, and microfractures are common. High-dose deferoxamine chelation therapy begun early in life has been implicated in the production of radiographically evident rickets-like abnormalities of the long bones and platyspondyly.

SICKLE CELL ANEMIA

In sickle cell anemia, affected persons are homozygous for S hemoglobin (SS), which causes the red cell to assume an elongated, curved sickle configuration under conditions of reduced oxygen tension. The disease is most common in blacks but has been found in other races as well. It is characterized by an anemia associated with acute painful crises affecting the bones and joints of the limbs, usually beginning during the second or third year of life. Up to that age, residual fetal hemoglobin (F) apparently protects the child from the usual manifestations of the disease. The crises are associated with fever, increasing anemia, nausea, vomiting, abdominal pain, severe bone and joint pain and prostration. The anemia frequently results in cardiomegaly and heart murmurs, findings that are frequently confused with rheumatic fever. These crises usually resolve after a period of time, following which the patient may be well until another crisis supervenes. The abnormal shape of the red cells as a result of hypoxic stimuli (pulmonary infection, hypoxia of high altitudes or its equivalent during air travel, etc.) results in mechanical capillary stasis rather than thrombosis when the deformed red cells are unable to traverse the small vessels. This obstruction leads in turn to hypoxic damage of tissues distal to the obstruction, primarily bone marrow and bone, which undergo necrosis. The skeletal changes reflect infarction with focal destruction and sclerosis of medullary and cortical bone and secondary periosteal new bone formation (Figs. 4 and 5). Comparable changes in the epiphyseal ossification centers are less common in younger than in

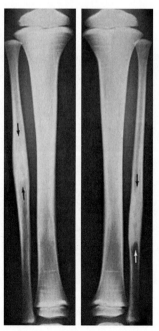

FIGURE 4. Sickle cell anemia in a black girl 4 years of age. The medullary canals of both fibulas are obliterated in their middle thirds by endosteal thickening and sclerosis *(arrows)*.

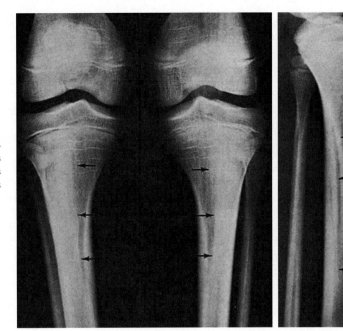

FIGURE 5. Radiograph of same patient as in Figure 4 showing endosteal cortical thickenings and sclerosis *(arrows)* at 7 years of age. The distal portions of the tibias were not affected, and the rest of the skeleton was normal radiographically.

older children but may lead to radiographic features resembling Legg-Perthes disease and to metaphyseal irregularities (Fig. 6).

The skeletal complications in patients with sickle cell disease include aseptic necrosis, bone infarcts, and osteomyelitis (Table 1). Patients with sickle cell disease appear to have a diminished resistance to infections that probably relates to tissue injury from the infarcts, diminished phagocytosis with the lowered oxygen tension in the area of involvement, and diminished splenic function. In some series of children with sickle cell anemia and osteomyelitis, salmonella infection is encountered in over 50% of cases.

The destructive and productive changes associated with osteomyelitis can be indistinguishable clinically from those of osteonecrosis after infarction, and both may be present simultaneously (Fig. 7). However, combined bone marrow scintigraphy with ^{99m}Tc sulfur colloid and gallium scintigraphy or gadolinium-enhanced MRI is useful in differentiating osteomyelitis and osteonecrosis. Rao, Solomon, et al. reviewed bone marrow scans and bone scans obtained during episodes of bone pain in children with sickle cell disease. On the basis of the subsequent clinical course, a diagnosis of bone infarction or osteomyelitis was made. They concluded that decreased uptake on bone marrow scan in a

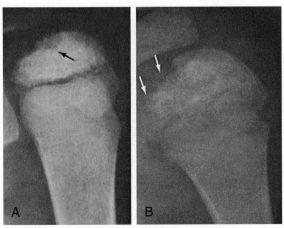

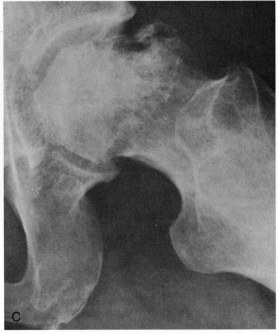

FIGURE 6. Radiographic appearance of lesions of sickle cell anemia in the epiphyseal ossification centers. **A,** Irregularity and sclerosis of the proximal epiphysis of the humerus *(arrow)* in a black boy 6 years of age. **B,** Similar changes in the same site in another black boy 7 years of age *(arrows)*. **C,** Destruction, fragmentation, flattening, and sclerosis of the femoral head in a black girl 22 years of age.

Table 1 ■ CONDITIONS ASSOCIATED WITH BONE INFARCTION

Idiopathic
Sickle cell disease
Pancreatitis
Osteomyelitis
Caisson disease
Fat embolism (trauma, alcoholism)
Gaucher's disease
Connective tissue disorders (e.g., lupus, polyarteritis nodosa)
Radiation therapy

patient with sickle cell disease and bone pain almost invariably indicates infarction, whereas normal uptake strongly suggests a diagnosis of osteomyelitis. The bone marrow scans were considered to be more useful than bone scans in differentiating bone infarction and osteomyelitis.

Other imaging techniques, including white cell scintigraphy, ultrasound, and MRI, play a valuable role in difficult cases. MRI of bone marrow demonstrates low-intensity T_1-weighted signal from hyperplastic marrow in comparison with marrow signal from normal children (Fig. 8). In sickle cell disease, focal areas of further decreased intensity on short repetition time–echo time (TR-TE) images indicate areas of recent or remote infarction whether or not pain is present. On long TR-TE images, however, high-intensity signals are observed in these areas in most patients with pain, but not in those without pain. It is believed that the high-intensity signals result from edema in areas of acute infarction, whereas the persisting low-intensity signals arise from areas of old infarction or fibrosis.

In infants between 6 months and 2 years, a special form of infarction takes place with some frequency in the small bones of the hand and foot that has given rise to the term *hand–foot syndrome.* In this condition, painful soft tissue swelling of the hands and feet is usually present 1 to 2 weeks prior to the development of patchy radiolucency of the shafts of the short tubular bones associated with periosteal new bone formation (Fig. 9). Clinical differentiation from osteomyelitis is difficult (Fig. 10), but reconstitution of bone generally takes place after a period of several months without any deformity.

In addition, cranial changes similar to, but much less severe than, those in thalassemia can be observed. The facial bones are generally not affected as they are in thalassemia major. However, there are a few exceptions. Fernandez et al. reported extensive maxillary sinus marrow hyperplasia in a 28-month-old child with sickle cell anemia. Compression fractures are frequently observed in vertebrae, owing partly to the loss of bony support resulting from marrow hypertrophy and partly to infarcts involving the vessels supplying the central portions of the superior and inferior vertebral plates (Fig. 11). A depression of the central portion of the vertebral plate, presumably as a result of growth disturbance from vascular compromise, has been advanced as a pathognomonic sign of the disease, but similar changes have been observed in patients with other

hemoglobinopathies. Cupping of the ends of the shafts of the long bones has been observed in children suffering from sickle cell anemia (Fig. 12).

The sickle cell trait is found in persons who are heterozygous for hemoglobin S. Bone disease is very rare in persons with the trait, and the clinical signs and symptoms are very mild if they occur at all. Combinations of sickle hemoglobin (HbS) and other abnormal hemoglobins occur. Patients with the combination of sickle hemoglobin and hemoglobin C demonstrate clinical and radiographic changes similar to, but less severe than, those in the homozygous sickle cell disease. They usually have large spleens, in contrast to the small infarcted spleens (or functional asplenia) in homozygous sickle cell anemia. As noted previously, patients with the thalassemia gene and the sickle cell gene present with clinical signs and symptoms reflecting sickle cell disease more than thalassemia.

OTHER ANEMIAS

Other anemias may have associated skeletal changes, but none so severe as those in the hemoglobinopathies. In *familial hemolytic (spherocytic) anemia,* also known as

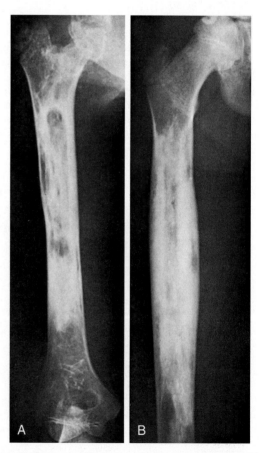

FIGURE 7. Osteomyelitis in the shafts of the humerus **(A)** and femur **(B)** of a black girl 9 years of age who had sickle cell anemia. Salmonella was probably the causal agent, judging from the clinical course; it was not proved bacteriologically. (Courtesy of Drs. F. J. Hodges and J. F. Holt, University of Michigan, Ann Arbor, MI.)

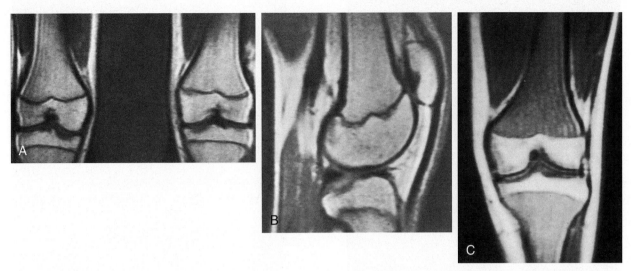

FIGURE 8. Coronal **(A)** and sagittal **(B)** T$_1$-weighted MR images of normal marrow in a 15-year-old child. Signal intensity of the marrow is uniform. **C,** Coronal T$_1$-weighted image in a child with sickle cell anemia. The signal from the diaphyses and metaphyses is significantly less compared to the epiphyses, consistent with active hematopoiesis in the shaft. (From Kangerloo H, Dietrich RB, Taira RT, et al: MR imaging of bone marrow in children. J Comput Assist Tomogr 1986;10:205-209, with permission.)

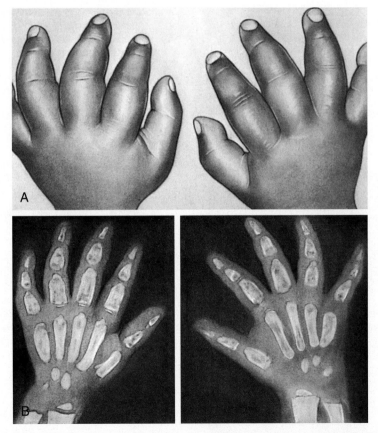

FIGURE 9. Multiple lesions of the "hand–foot syndrome" in the tubular bones of the hands and swellings of the fingers in a girl 12 months of age who had sickle cell anemia and probably shigellosis. **A,** Diffuse swelling of the soft tissues. **B,** Drawing of a radiograph showing destructive and productive osteitis of the phalanges and metacarpals. (**B** redrawn from Ivey RE, Howard FH: J Pediatr 1953;43:312-315.)

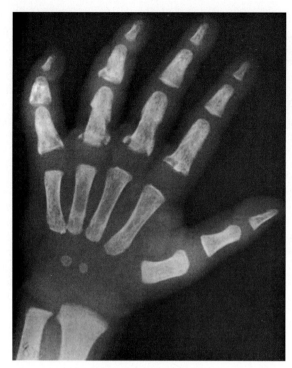

FIGURE 10. Polyphalangeal osteomyelitis that resembles the phalangeal radiographic changes of sickle cell anemia. This black girl, 10 months of age, had neither active nor latent sickle cell anemia in several tests. The soft tissues of the affected fingers are swollen and the phalanges are generally sclerotic, with sequestra at their bases. Similar changes were present in the other hand and both feet. Streptococcus A was cultured several times directly from the bone lesions. (Courtesy of Drs. Kenneth Haltalin and John Nelson, Dallas, TX.)

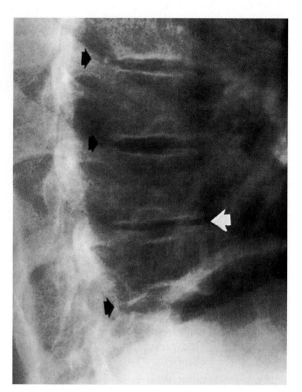

FIGURE 11. Radiographic spine changes in sickle cell anemia. The smooth concavity of several end plates *(black arrows)* results from osteopenia secondary to marrow hyperplasia. The opposing central end plate depressions *(white arrow)* are believed to result from local vascular occlusion and focal fracture. (Courtesy of Dr. Henry Jones, Stanford, CA.)

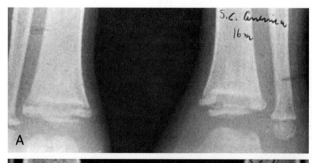

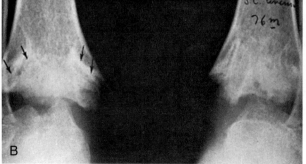

FIGURE 12. Cupping of the distal end of the shaft in sickle cell anemia. **A,** At 16 months of age, the central segment of the end of the shaft is partially destroyed, but there is no cupping. **B,** At 76 months, the sclerotic, enlarged epiphyseal ossification center has fused with the cupped central segment of the shaft, and the peripheral segments of the shaft have grown caudad around the ossification center to produce the central depression or cup *(arrows)*. The epiphyseal ossification center and shaft have fused over a long segment at the base of the cup.

hereditary spherocytosis, the abnormality is in the cell membrane of the red cell, allowing it to become spherical and, as a consequence, easily hemolyzed. The hemoglobin itself is not abnormal. Patients are anemic and have mild to moderate jaundice with splenomegaly. Gallstones are a frequent complication. Although compensatory hyperplasia of the bone marrow occurs as in other forms of anemia, only the mildest changes are recognized in the cranial vault, with diploic widening and thinning of the outer table. Snelling and Brown described a case in which the skeletal lesions improved following splenectomy.

Other hemolytic anemias occur without alteration in the shape of the red blood cell and are associated with enzyme deficiencies that predispose the red cell to hemolysis under certain special conditions. *Pyruvate kinase–deficiency hemolytic anemia,* according to Becker and associates, has bone changes similar to thalassemia major except that the maxillary sinuses pneumatize normally. In *glucose-6-phosphate dehydrogenase deficiency,* the red blood cells undergo hemolysis following exposure to various drugs and even foods, such as the fava bean. In general, radiologic signs are lacking in this condition.

LEUKEMIA

The growing skeleton is an important site of proliferation of leukemic cells. In the course of the disease, multiple areas of destruction and production may appear in the bones. The recognition of bone lesions caused by leukemia is much less frequent currently than in past years because of earlier recognition of the disease and prompt effective treatment. Nevertheless, the radiographic examination can be useful in suggesting the diagnosis and, occasionally, in assisting in the long-term management of the disease (see Section IX, Part XII, Figs. 33 through 35, pages 2409 and 2410).

The spectrum of radiographic bony changes in patients with chronic myelogenous leukemia include diffuse osteoporosis, focal osteolytic and osteoblastic lesions, chloroma, and arthritis. Four types of bone lesions have been traditionally described. Transverse bands of diminished density at the ends of the major long bones are the most frequent finding (see Section IX, Part VII, Chapter 2, Table 2, page 2255). These may merely indicate the response of growing bone to the stress of a severe disease, but may also indicate sites of rapidly proliferating leukemic cells in the metaphyses. Subperiosteal new bone formation along the shafts results from extension of proliferating cells from the marrow to the cortex, presumably through haversian canals, and bone production by the elevated periosteum. Subperiosteal hemorrhage may also contribute to some of these periosteal reactions. Focal destructive lesions are caused by accumulations of leukemic cells and can occur in any portion of the bones. Diffuse sclerosis, associated most frequently with myelogenous leukemia, may result from osteoblastic stimulation and

may also reflect the origin of osteoblasts from marrow cells. These four types of lesions occur singly or in combination (Figs. 13 through 15). None is specific for leukemia, but all generally resolve following successful therapy.

Chloroma, also known as myeloblastoma or granulocytic sarcoma (GS), is a localized tumor consisting of immature myeloid cells. It is an uncommon tumor that occurs in 2.5% to 8% patients with leukemia, mostly the myeloid type. The greenish color of the majority of these tumors has been attributed to the presence of myeloperoxidase and degeneration of hemoglobin. The presence of a mass together with destruction and production of bone in a patient with known or suspected diagnosis of leukemia should suggest the possibility of chloroma. GS may occur concurrently with or present as a first manifestation of acute myeloid leukemia (AML) but may also occur during remission or relapse. Occasionally, it presents as a first sign of a blastic crisis of chronic myeloid leukemia. The prognosis is generally poor.

GS can involve several different organ systems, including bone, and is especially likely to occur in the cranium and facial bones. It is important to include GS in the differential diagnosis of lesions in patients with AML. Hermann et al. reviewed findings in skeletal GS proven by biopsy in five patients. In four cases, it was the initial manifestation of AML. Two patients presented with lytic lesions of the ribs, two with lytic lesions of the femur, and one with a predominantly sclerotic lesion of the scapula. Novick et al. reported a case of GS (chloroma) of the sacrum that predated the initial clinical manifestation of AML. Libson et al. described a mixed sclerotic and lytic pattern in a skeletal chloroma on CT. Bassichis et al. reported a case of GS involving the masseter muscle in an 8-month-old white male with AML.

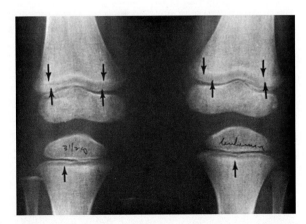

FIGURE 13. Leukemia in a girl 3 years of age, with terminal transverse striping of the shafts *(arrows)*. These transverse lines of both increased and diminished density are the most common and the earliest radiographic bone changes and may persist for weeks or months as the only changes in leukemia. The lines are usually best developed in the large metaphyses at the knees.

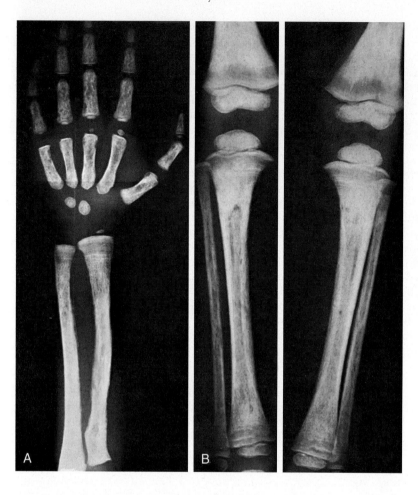

FIGURE 14. Acute lymphoblastic leukemia in a boy 2 years of age. On radiographs of the hand and forearm **(A)** and lower limbs **(B)**, irregular destruction of all the bones is evident. Deep transverse zones of diminished density occupy the ends of the shafts. In addition to these destructive features, there are numerous large and small irregular patches of sclerosis indicative of massive osteoblastic reaction.

The appearance of extracranial GS on CT is that of nodular densities that resemble lymphoma. On MRI, most granulocytic sarcomas are isointense to muscle and marrow on both T_1- and T_2-weighted images, and they enhance homogeneously with gadolinium. These features may help differentiate GS from other complications of leukemia such as hematoma and abscess. There are no radiographic, scintigraphic or ultrasonographic features that are diagnostic of GS.

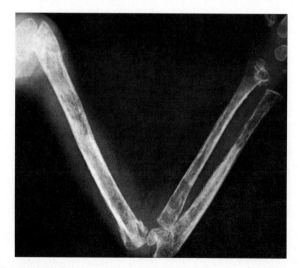

FIGURE 15. Acute lymphoblastic leukemia in a girl 3 years of age. Moth-eaten areas of lytic rarefaction are scattered in the long tubular bones on this radiograph. Leukopenia persisted until death; the diagnosis of leukemia was proved at necropsy.

HEMOPHILIA

Hemophilia is a bleeding diathesis caused by a genetic deficiency of factor VIII (hemophilia A) or factor IX (hemophilia B). The more common hemophilia A occurs in 1 of every 10,000 live male births and hemophilia B in 1 of every 40,000 live male births. Most patients exhibit a family history pointing to a bleeding disorder, although spontaneous mutations are responsible for about 30% of cases. In addition to intracranial hemorrhage, hemarthrosis, arthropathy, intramuscular bleeding, and pseudotumors are common manifestations of hemophilia.

Hemophilic arthropathy is an incapacitating complication of severe hemophilia resulting from recurrent bleeding in the same joint. Skeletal lesions in patients with hemophilia may be due to bleeding directly into the bones (Fig. 16) or to secondary changes in the bones that result from recurrent hemorrhages into adjacent joints (Fig. 17). Subperiosteal hemorrhages in hemophilia are rare, but can result in new bone formation and pressure erosion of the underlying cortex (Fig. 18).

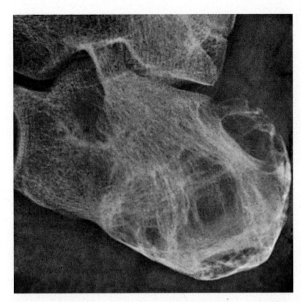

FIGURE 16. Radiograph of hemophilic intraosseous hemorrhages into the medullary cavity of the calcaneus of a young adult. The large radiolucent areas represent intramedullary hematomas in different stages of organization. (Courtesy of Dr. Bruce Ward, Grand Junction, CO.)

Subchondral hemorrhages may be responsible for marginal bony defects on the juxta-articular borders of epiphyseal ossification centers (Fig. 19); they may also be produced by synovial intrusion in cases of chronic, recurrent hemarthroses. In this very common manifestation of the disease, there arises a chronic inflammatory reaction with accelerated maturation and hypertrophy of adjacent epiphyses as well as of the synovium (Table 2). Hypertrophied synovium encroaches on the cartilaginous margins which are invaded and destroyed, producing irregular marginal bony defects. The space between cartilaginous surfaces of an affected joint is decreased, the soft tissues are swollen, and muscular atrophy and contractures supervene (Fig. 20).

Hemophilic pseudotumors are well-defined masses containing blood and blood clots in various stages of organization surrounded by a fibrous capsule in subcutaneous fat or in intramuscular, interfascial, subperiosteal, or intraosseous locations. Intramuscular pseudotumors frequently have mural nodules. Intraosseous pseudotumors may heal spontaneously

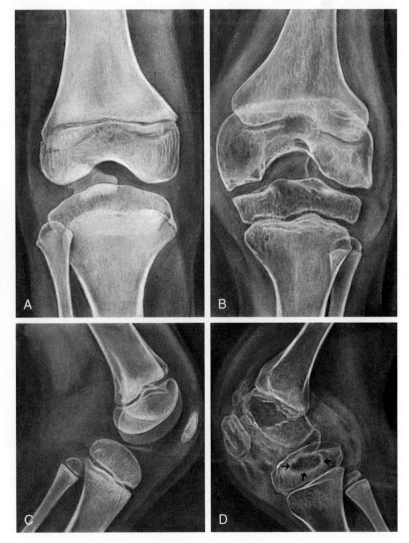

FIGURE 17. Hemophilic arthropathy of the left knee in a boy 7 years of age. Frontal **(A)** and lateral **(C)** projections show his normal right knee. On frontal **(B)** and lateral **(D)** projections of the left knee, the soft tissues are swollen and increased in density. In addition, there is marked generalized rarefaction of the epiphyses and shafts. The epiphyseal centers and patella are enlarged on the left side; the intercondyloid notch is deepened, and the juxta-articular surfaces of the bones are ragged. In **D,** a large intraosseous hematoma is visible in the tibial epiphysis *(arrows).*

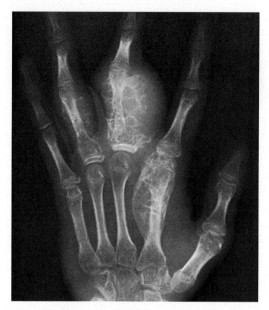

FIGURE 18. Radiographic evidence of hemophilia in a boy 14 years of age. Old and recent subperiosteal hemorrhages have swollen the soft tissues and destroyed the cortex of the proximal phalanx of the third and fourth digits. The old cortical walls are still visible, and are surrounded by partly ossified subperiosteal hematomas. The epiphyseal ossification center at the proximal end of the proximal phalanx of the third digit is slightly displaced.

Table 2 ■ LOCALIZED OVERGROWTH OF BONE
Arteriovenous fistula
Chronic arthritis (juvenile rheumatoid arthritis)
Hemangioma
Lymphangioma
Neurofibromatosis
Fibromatosis
Hemophilic arthropathy
Macrodystrophia lipomatosa

with sclerosis (Fig. 21). MRI allows determination of number, size, and extent of the lesions, evidence of neurovascular involvement, and accompanying musculoskeletal alterations. MRI is not only a sensitive and accurate method for diagnosing hemophiliac pseudotumor and providing useful information for therapeutic

decision making, but can also be used to assess results of treatment of lesions in regions difficult to access by physical examination, and recurrent bleeding within a chronic lesion.

Hermann et al. evaluated musculoskeletal involvement in hemophiliac patients with CT, sonography, and MRI. MRI imaging can exquisitely demonstrate joint effusions, synovial proliferation, articular cartilage abnormalities, subchondral bone erosions, hemosiderin deposition (manifested by dark signal on T_1- and T_2-weighted images), and associated abnormalities of the menisci, ligaments, muscles, and juxta-articular soft tissues (Fig. 22). MRI can be used to detect early synovial and cartilaginous changes that may not be evident on conventional radiography and to differentiate between acute and chronic bleeding. CT is useful in evaluating subtle bony erosions and intra- and extraosseous pseudotumors, and sonography is valuable in following progression and regression of soft tissue hematomas. Hemophilic arthropathy is discussed in Section IX, Part XIV, page 2455.

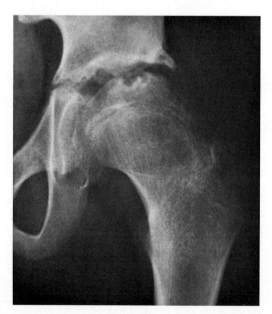

FIGURE 19. Radiograph showing hemophilic subchondral hemorrhages in the proximal epiphysis of the femur that may be responsible for the marginal defects. The epiphysis is flattened in its longitudinal axis, and the neck of the femur is broadened. A large bony spur protrudes laterally from the roof of the acetabulum.

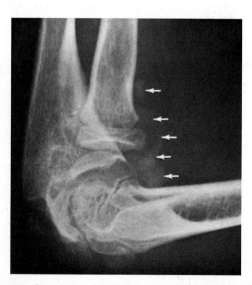

FIGURE 20. Chronic hemophilic hemarthrosis of the right elbow in a boy 10 years of age. The *arrows* on this radiograph are directed at increased density of the periarticular soft tissues, which is related to the high iron content of these tissues. Acceleration of maturation and overgrowth of the bones as a result of chronic regional hyperemia are also evident.

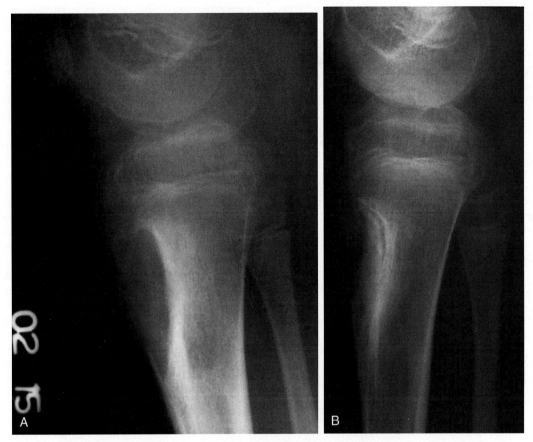

FIGURE 21. Healing of pseudotumor in a patient with hemophilia. **A,** Lytic lesion with surrounding sclerosis in anterior aspect of the proximal tibia is consistent with a subperiosteal intraosseous hemorrhage. **B,** Healing with sclerosis of the lesion is demonstrated 3 months later.

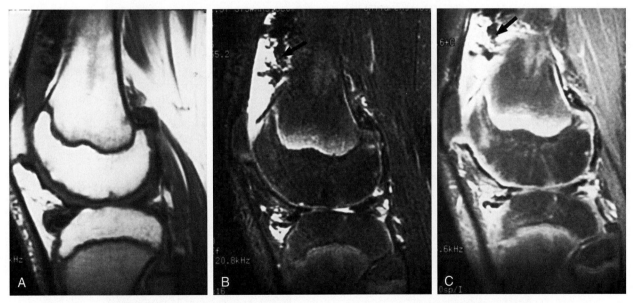

FIGURE 22. Magnetic resonance imaging T_1-weighted **(A),** T_1-weighted postgadolinium fat saturation **(B),** and fast spin-echo T_2-weighted **(C)** sagittal images of the knee in a patient with chronic hemophilic arthropathy. Synovial hypertrophy and enhancement associated with joint effusion, blood products, and hemosiderin deposition are manifested by low signal on T_1- and T_2-weighted images *(arrows),* as are loss of cartilage and irregularity of the subchondral bone, which are characteristic of hemophilic arthropathy.

CLASS I LANGERHANS' CELL HISTIOCYTOSIS

New terminology has been applied to this disorder, also known as reticuloendotheliosis, based on recent studies of mononuclear phagocytes (histiocytes). The conditions identified by the former terms *Letterer-Siwe disease, Hand-Schuller-Christian disease,* and *eosinophilic granuloma of bone* are now known to share a common, chemically and electron microscopically distinct histiocyte called the Langerhans' cell that characterizes the class I type of histiocytosis. It has been suggested that the disorder be called class I Langerhans' cell histiocytosis (LCH). Infants, children, adolescents, and young adults may be affected by class I LCH. Class II histiocytosis (hemophagocytic lymphohistiocytosis, sinus histiocytosis, etc.) and class III histiocytosis (malignant histiocytic disorders) do not involve the Langerhans' cell and are rare in children.

Class I LCH is characterized by granulomatous proliferation of the specific cells at one or several sites in the body. Focal hemorrhage frequently accompanies the proliferation. The cause of the proliferation is not established; infection may play a causal role in some cases.

Early reports of Hand-Schüller-Christian disease emphasized exophthalmos, diabetes insipidus, and lytic lesions involving the orbits, base of the skull, and calvaria; this triad is now recognized as rare. In older children and young adults, the condition may be limited to a single lesion in bone with the same radiographic characteristics, commonly referred to as eosinophilic granuloma. If a lesion in a tubular bone erodes to the periosteum, subperiosteal new bone formation occurs. Pathologic fracture may occur at the site of large lesions. Osseous lesions are generally lytic, involving flat and long bones (Fig. 23), and may be absent in some patients with cutaneous lesions. Reactive sclerosis may be seen around the lytic lesions. Healing of the bony lesions spontaneously or following radiation therapy may be associated with sclerosis. Orbital sclerosis resulting from healed lesions of histiocytosis has been described. MRI is considered to be the procedure of choice for defining multifocal lesions in the central nervous system and skull; it is also considered useful for monitoring response to therapy.

Hindman et al. retrospectively reviewed 262 skeletal lesions in 34 children with biopsy-proven LCH. They found 24 lesions that were in an atypical location or manifested an atypical radiographic appearance. These

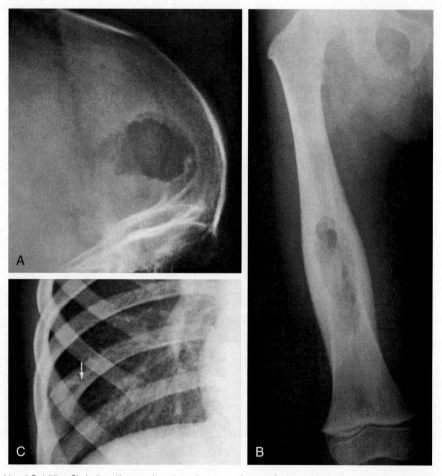

FIGURE 23. Hand-Schüller-Christian disease in a boy 3 years of age. **A,** Large lytic lesion in the frontal bone. **B,** Lytic rarefaction with regional cortical thickening of the femur. The cortical thickening is unusual. There was no clinical or radiographic evidence of pathologic fracture. **C,** Expansion, destruction, and thickening of the eighth rib *(arrow).*

included epiphyseal lesions, transphyseal lesions, involvement of small bones of the hands and feet, extracranial "button" sequestra, posterior vertebral arch lesions, dural extension of vertebral lesions, and fluid–fluid levels within the lesions.

The clinical and radiographic findings of class I LCH vary somewhat depending on the age at onset. The predominant clinical manifestations of the infantile form include purpuric rash, progressive anemia, hepatomegaly, splenomegaly, and focal skeletal lesions. In the first year of life, the skin and viscera, as well as skeletal structures, are affected, and the course is rapid and usually fatal (Letterer-Siwe disease). These patients have multifocal LCH together with dysfunction of liver and/or lungs, and abnormal blood counts. The bone lesions may be single, few, or widespread and demonstrate focal destructive lesions that are punched out and show little or no surrounding reaction. These are indistinguishable from the multiple bone lesions (Fig. 23) found in slightly older children in whom cutaneous and visceral manifestations are meager or absent (Hand-Schüller-Christian disease). LCH lesions can be very extensive and yet have a good response to therapy, whereas less extensive lesions may not respond or respond only partially to therapy. Thus an important factor in establishing prognosis is the presence of multisystem involvement at diagnosis.

In rare instances, especially when there is an element of hypersensitization, the cutaneous lesions of scabies can be confused with those of Letterer-Siwe disease in infants. Granulomatous changes in the lungs are common in the systemic forms of Letterer-Siwe disease; initially, the lesions may simulate those of miliary tuberculosis. Pleural granulomas may result in changes suggesting suppurative pleurisy.

Vesiculopustular lesions are common in congenital/neonatal LCH, but the morphologic characteristics of lesions are not helpful in predicting the extent of extracutaneous disease. Disease may be limited to the skin and/or mucous membranes, but more commonly there is multisystem involvement, and diabetes insipidus may be present in over 20% of these patients. Therefore, multisystem evaluation is recommended at the time of diagnosis for detection of multiorgan involvement.

Vertebra plana is the most common spinal manifestation of LCH. LCH can also manifest as a lytic lesion of the posterior vertebral arches, with or without involvement of the vertebral body. Damry et al. reported unusual findings in two patients with LCH, namely a cervical mass lesion with extensive destruction of the posterior elements of a cervical vertebra and gastrointestinal lesions and protein-losing gastroenteropathy as part of multisystem involvement.

Bodart et al. reported an isolated eosinophilic granuloma involving the posterior elements of a lumbar vertebra in a 3-year-old boy presenting with progressive limp. Radiologic investigations revealed a lytic lesion involving the L5 right pedicle. MRI showed a well-defined homogeneous mass that extended to involve paravertebral muscles.

MRI of LCH lesions can be very informative. An active lesion of LCH manifests as low signal intensity on T_1-weighted sequences and high signal intensity on T_2-weighted sequences in the marrow of the vertebral body, whereas an old lesion of LCH demonstrates low signal on T_1- and T_2-weighted sequences. This distinction cannot be made by plain radiography or bone scintigraphy. In cases where biopsy is required for diagnosis, MRI is recommended to guide the biopsy toward levels suggestive of active involvement. Typically, soft tissue involvement with LCH is the result of extension from adjacent bone marrow. Henck et al. presented a patient who developed soft tissue masses of LCH that did not arise as a result of extension from bone marrow, but instead produced extrinsic cortical erosion, preserving the marrow signal on MRI.

MASTOCYTOSIS

Mastocytosis is characterized by abnormal proliferation of tissue mast cells that produce histamine. Mast cell disease or mastocytosis occurs in two main forms. The *cutaneous* form is primarily a childhood disease associated with pigmented skin lesions called urticaria pigmentosa that spontaneously resolve by adolescence in 90% of instances but in about 10% of patients progress to systemic form. The adult form, with skin involvement, has an onset around puberty and manifests systemic progression in about 50% of patients. *Systemic* mastocytosis constitutes about 10% of all cases of mast cell disease. In about 90% of patients with systemic mastocytosis, the bone marrow is infiltrated by mast cells. Skeletal lesions include widespread osteosclerosis mixed with osteolytic lesions, generalized osteoporosis, and poorly defined focal lytic and sclerotic lesions involving the axial and appendicular skeleton (Fig. 24). MRI is a sensitive method of detecting bone marrow involvement in these patients.

The pathogenesis of osteosclerosis in mastocytosis is not well understood. Ischemic injury resulting from occlusion of vascular channels by mast cells may cause reactive fibrous tissue formation and osteogenesis. The various biogenic amines secreted by mast cells, such as histamine, heparin, serotonin, and prostaglandins, have been demonstrated to have a bone-resorbing effect and are considered to have a pathogenic role in the manifestation of osteoporosis. Prostaglandins have also been known to stimulate bone formation in low concentrations.

Proliferation of mast cells may also occur in other organs such as liver, spleen, gastrointestinal tract, and lymph nodes. Clinical signs of vomiting, diarrhea, hepatosplenomegaly, and urticarial skin lesions may provide a clue to diagnosis when these bizarre skeletal features are noted on radiographs. Diagnosis is by biopsy and histochemical evaluation for histamine.

Abdominal findings at CT and ultrasound are common in patients with systemic mastocytosis. These findings include hepatosplenomegaly, retroperitoneal adenopathy, periportal adenopathy, mesenteric adenopathy, thickening of the omentum and the mesentery, and ascites. Less common findings include

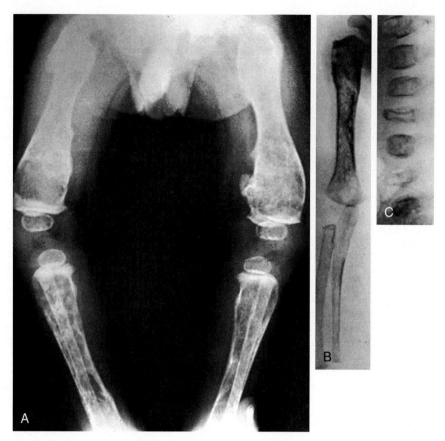

FIGURE 24. Radiographic evidence of mastocytosis (urticaria pigmentosa) in a boy 6 months of age who had been irritable since birth with "constant crying, vomiting, and diarrhea." Scattered urticarial pruritic skin lesions were relieved by antihistaminic medication. In several tests, histamine levels in the blood had been increased. The liver and spleen were enlarged, and the left leg and foot were paralyzed. The diagnosis was based on a biopsy study of one femur. **A,** All long bones in the legs are widened as a result of failure of normal constriction of the shafts, and hypertrophy of the marrow resulting from hyperplasia of mast cells. The cortical walls are thin, and the bones demonstrate patchy lytic and sclerotic areas. The irregular bony projections on the medial aspects of the femora are not satisfactorily explained. **B,** Similar but less marked changes in the bones of the arm. **C,** Compression fractures have flattened the L3 and L5 vertebral bodies. (Courtesy of Dr. Edward B. Singleton, Houston, TX.)

hepatofugal portal venous flow, Budd-Chiari syndrome, cavernous transformation of the portal vein, and ovarian mass.

SUGGESTED READINGS

Erythroblastosis and Fanconi's Anemia

Bishop PA: The roentgenologic diagnosis of fetal hydrops. Am J Roentgenal Radium Ther Nucl Med 1961;86:415–424

Brenner G, Allen RP: Skeletal changes in erythroblastosis foetalis. Radiology 1963;80:427–429

Follis RH Jr, Jackson D, Carnes WH: Skeletal changes associated with erythroblastosis fetalis. J Pediatr 1942;21:80–92

Glanz A, Fraser FC: Spectrum of anomalies in Fanconi anemia. J Med Genet 1982;18:412–416

Juhl JH, Wesenberg RL, Gwinn JL: Roentgenographic findings in Fanconi's anemia. Radiology 1967;89:646–653

Minagi H, Steinbach HL: Roentgen appearance of anomalies associated with hypoplastic anemias of childhood: Fanconi's anemia and congenital hypoplastic anemia (erythrogenesis imperfecta). Am J Roentgenol Radium Ther Nucl Med 1966;97:100–109

Thalassemia

Alam R, Padmanabhan K, Rao H: Paravertebral mass in a patient with thalassemia intermedia. Chest 1997;112:265–267

Aliberti B, Patrikiou A, Terentiou A, et al: Spinal cord compression due to extramedullary haematopoiesis in two patients with thalassaemia: complete regression with blood transfusion therapy. J Neurol 2001;248:18–22

Bruneteau G, Fenelon G, Khalil A, et al: Spinal cord compression secondary to extramedullary hematopoiesis in a patient with thalassemia. Rev Neurol (Paris) 2000;156:510–513

Caffey J: Cooley's anemia: a review of the roentgenographic findings in the skeleton. Am J Roentgenol Radium Ther Nucl Med 1957;78:381–391

Chan Y, Li C, Chu WC, et al: Deferoxamine-induced bone dysplasia in the distal femur and patella of pediatric patients and young adults: MR imaging appearance. AJR Am J Roentgenol 2000;175:1561–1566

Currarino G, Erlandson ME: Premature fusion of epiphyses in Cooley's anemia. Radiology 1964;83:656–664

de Sanctis V, Stea S, Savarino L, et al: Osteochondrodystrophic lesions in chelated thalassemic patients: an histological analysis. Calcif Tissue Int 2000;67:134–140

Dines DM, Canale VC, Arnold WD: Fractures in thalassemia. J Bone Joint Surg Am 1976;58:662–666

Emery JL, Follett GF: Regression of bone-marrow haemopoiesis from terminal digits in the foetus and infant. Br J Haematol 1964;10:485–489

Images in clinical medicine: A hair-on-end skull. N Engl J Med 2001;345:e1

Kangarloo H, Dietrich RB, Taira RT, et al: MR imaging of bone marrow in children. J Comput Assist Tomogr 1986;10:205–209

Korsten J, Grossman H, Winchester PH, et al: Extramedullary hematopoiesis in patients with thalassemia anemia. Radiology 1970;95:257–263

Lala R, Chiabotto P, Di Stefano M, et al: Bone density and metabolism in thalassaemia. J Pediatr Endocrinol Metab 1998;11 (Suppl 3):785–790

Lawson JP, Ablow RC, Pearson HA: The ribs in thalassemia. 1. The relationship to therapy. Radiology 1981;140:663–672

Levin TL, Sheth S, Berdon WE, et al: Deferoxamine-induced platyspondyly in hypertransfused thalassemic patients. Pediatr Radiol 1995;25(Suppl 1):S122–S124

Long JA Jr, Doppman JL, Nienhuis AW: Computed tomographic studies of thoracic extramedullary hematopoiesis. J Comput Assist Tomogr 1980;4:67–70

Molyvda-Athanasopoulou E, Sioundas A, Karatzas N, et al: Bone mineral density of patients with thalassemia major: four-year follow-up. Calcif Tissue Int 1999;64:481–484

Moseley JR: Skeletal changes in the anemias. Semin Roentgenol 1974;9:169–184

Ozdemir A, Gungor F, Tuncdemir F, et al: Scintigraphic diagnosis of intrathoracic extramedullary hematopoiesis in a patient with beta-thalassemia. Ann Nucl Med 1998;12:149–155

Reynolds J, Pritchard JA, Ludders D, et al: Roentgenographic and clinical appraisal of sickle cell beta-thalassemia disease. Am J Roentgenol Radium Ther Nucl Med 1973;118:378–400

Ross P, Logan W: Roentgen findings in extramedullary hematopoiesis. Am J Roentgenol Radium Ther Nucl Med 1969;106:604–613

Sfikakis P, Stamatoyannopoulos G: Bone changes in thalassemia trait. Acta Haematol 1963;29:193–201

Tchang S, Tyrrell MJ, Bharadwaj B: Skeletal changes in cyanotic heart diseases simulating Cooley's anemia: report of a case with regression of the bone changes following palliative cardiac surgery. J Can Assoc Radiol 1973;24:274–279

Tsitouridis J, Stamos S, Hassapopoulou E, et al: Extramedullary paraspinal hematopoiesis in thalassemia: CT and MRI evaluation. Eur J Radiol 1999;30:33–38

Tunaci M, Tunaci A, Engin G, et al: Imaging features of thalassemia. Eur Radiol 1999;9:1804–1809

Valdez VA, Jacobstein JG: Decreased bone uptake of technetium-99m polyphosphate in thalassemia major. J Nucl Med 1980;21:47–49

Voskaridou E, Kyrtsonis MC, Terpos E, et al: Bone resorption is increased in young adults with thalassaemia major. Br J Haematol 2001;112:36–41

Wongwaisayawan S, Pornkul R, Teeraratkul S, et al: Extramedullary haematopoietic tumor producing small intestinal intussusception in a beta-thalassemia/hemoglobin E Thai boy: a case report. J Med Assoc Thai 2000;83 (Suppl 1):S17–S22

Winchester PH, Cerwin R, Dische R, et al: Hemosiderin laden lymph nodes: an unusual roentgenographic manifestation of homozygous thalassemia. Am J Roentgenol Radium Ther Nucl Med 1973;118:222–226

Sickle Cell Disease and Other Anemias

Becker MH, Genieser NB, Piomelli S, et al: Roentgenographic manifestations of pyruvate-kinase-deficiency hemolytic anemia. Am J Roentgenol Radium Ther Nucl Med 1971;113:491–498

Ben Dridi MF, Oumaya A, Gastli H, et al: Radiological abnormalities in the skeleton in patients with sickle-cell anemia: a study of 222 cases in Tunisia. Pediatr Radiol 1987;17:296–302

Bennett OM, Namnyak SS: Bone and joint manifestations of sickle cell anemia. J Bone Joint Surg Br 1990;72:494–499

Burke TS, Tatum JL, Fratkin MJ, Baker K: Radionuclide bone imaging findings in recurrent calvarial infarction in sickle cell disease. J Nucl Med 1988;29:411–413

Burko H, Watson J, Robinson M: Unusual bone changes in sickle cell disease in childhood. Radiology 1963;80:957–962

Cassady JR, Berdon WE, Baker DH: The "typical" spine changes of sickle cell anemia in a patient with thalassemia major (Cooley's anemia). Radiology 1967;89:1065–1068

Dennis GJ, Keating RM: Muscle infarction in sickle cell anemia. Ann Intern Med 1991;115:831–832

Dhekne RD: Splenic concentration of bone imaging agents in functional asplenia. Clin Nucl Med 1981;6:313–317

Ebong WW, Kolawole TM: Aseptic necrosis of the femoral head in sickle-cell disease. Br J Rheumatol 1986;25:34–39

Erenberg G, Rinsier SS, Fish BG: Lead neuropathy in sickle cell disease. Pediatrics 1974;54:438–441

Fernandez M, Slovis TL, Whitten-Shurney W: Maxillary sinus marrow hyperplasia in sickle cell anemia. Pediatr Radiol 1995;25 (Suppl 1):S209–S211

Gellett LR, Williams MP, Vivian GC: Focal intrasplenic extramedullary hematopoiesis mimicking lymphoma: diagnosis made using liver-spleen scintigraphy. Clin Nucl Med 2001;26:145–146

Heck LL, Brittin GM: Splenic uptake of both technetium-99m diphosphonate and technetium-99m sulfur colloid in sickle cell beta (0) thalassemia. Clin Nucl Med 1989;14:557–563

Honasoge M, Kottamasu SR, Frame B: Vascular insufficiency: osteonecrosis. In Frame B, Honasoge M, Kottamasu SR (eds): Osteosclerosis, Hyperostosis and Related Disorders. New York, Elsevier Science Publishing Company, 1987:214–239

Hung GL, Stewart CA, Yeo E, et al: Incidental demonstration of cerebral infarction on bone scintigraphy in sickle cell disease. Clin Nucl Med 1990;15:671–672

Kahn CE Jr, Ryan JW, Hatfield MK, Martin WB: Combined bone marrow and gallium imaging: differentiation of osteomyelitis and infarction in sickle hemoglobinopathy. Clin Nucl Med 1988;13:443–449

Kangarloo H, Dietrich RB, Taira RT, et al: MR imaging of bone marrow in children. J Comput Assist Tomogr 1986;10:205–209

Levin TL, Berdon WE, Haller JO, et al: Intrasplenic masses of "preserved" functioning splenic tissue in sickle cell disease: correlation of imaging findings (CT, ultrasound, MRI, and nuclear scintigraphy). Pediatr Radiol 1996;26:646–649

Mallouh A: Acute splenic sequestration in sickle cell disease. J Pediatr 1986;108:1035–1036

Milner PF: Bone marrow infarction in sickle cell anemia. Blood 1984;63:490

Moore SG: Pediatric bone marrow and musculoskeletal imaging. In Stark DD, Bradley WG (eds): Magnetic Resonance Imaging. St Louis, Mosby–Year Book, 1991:145–157

Murphy KJ: Skull abnormalities on MR of children with sickle cell disease. AJNR Am J Neuroradiol 1997;18:596

Paknikar S, Singh A: Nonvisualization of spleen on sulfur colloid images: a sequel of massive infarction. Semin Nucl Med 1998;28:188–191

Pardoll DM, Rodeheffer RJ, Smith RR, Charache S: Aplastic crisis due to extensive bone marrow necrosis in sickle cell disease. Arch Intern Med 1982;142:2223–2225

Rao S, Solomon N, Miller S, Dunn E: Scintigraphic differentiation of bone infarction from osteomyelitis in children with sickle cell disease. J Pediatr 1985;107:685–688

Rao VM, Fishman M, Mitchell DG, et al: Painful sickle cell crisis: bone marrow patterns observed with MR imaging. Radiology 1986;161:211–215

Reynolds J: A re-evaluation of the "fish vertebrae" sign in sickle cell hemoglobinopathy. Am J Roentgenol Radium Ther Nucl Med 1966;97:693–707

Rosner F: Hand-foot syndrome in sickle cell disease. J Clin Oncol 1998;16:808–809

Sarton CJ, Cockshott WP: Bone changes in hemoglobin SC disease. Am J Roentgenol Radium Ther Nucl Med 1962;88:523–532

Saywell WR: Bone marrow MRI in sickle cell disease. Clin Radiol 1990;41:364

Sebes JI, Massie JD, White TJ 3rd, Kraus AP: Pelvic extramedullary hematopoiesis. J Nucl Med 1984;25:209–210

Silberstein EB, DeLong S, Cline J: Tc-99m diphosphonate and sulfur colloid uptake by the spleen in sickle disease: interrelationship and clinical correlates: concise communication. J Nucl Med 1984;25:1300–1303

Snelling CE, Brown A: A case of hemolytic jaundice with bone changes. J Pediatr 1936;8:330–337

Spencer RP, Sziklas JJ, Zubi SM: Disassociation of splenic accumulation of Tc-99m MDP and radiocolloid. Clin Nucl Med 1991;16:747–749

van Zanten TE, Statius van Eps LW, Golding RP, et al: Imaging the bone marrow with magnetic resonance during a crisis and in chronic forms of sickle cell disease. Clin Radiol 1989;40:486–489

Watson RJ, Burko H, Megas H, et al: The hand-foot syndrome in sickle cell disease in young children. Pediatrics 1963;31:975–982

Wolff MH, Sty JR: Orbital infarction in sickle cell disease. Pediatr Radiol 1985;15:50–52

Worrall VT, Butera V: Sickle cell dactylitis. J Bone Joint Surg Am 1976;58:1161–1163

Leukemia

Bassichis B, McClay J, Wiatrak B: Chloroma of the masseteric muscle. Int J Pediatr Otorhinolaryngol 2000;53:57–61

Benz G, Brandeis WE, Willich E: Radiological aspects of leukemia in childhood: an analysis of 89 children. Pediatr Radiol 1976;4:201–213

Capdeville R, Bertrand Y, Manel AM, et al: Granulocytic sarcoma (chloroma): rare extramedullary tumors associated with acute non-lymphoblastic leukemia. Pediatrie 1990;45:245–250

Crain SM, Choudhury AM, Molnar Z, Jablokow VR: Destructive osteolytic bone lesions in chronic granulocytic leukemia. Ill Med J 1982;162:213–217

Hermann G, Feldman F, Abdelwahab IF, Klein MJ: Skeletal manifestations of granulocytic sarcoma (chloroma). Skeletal Radiol 1991;20:509–512

Kozlowski K, Campbell JB, Leonidas JC, Stevens M: Unusual radiographic bone abnormalities in leukaemia: report of three cases. J Belge Radiol 1987;70:229–233

Libson E, Bloom RA, Galun E, Polliack A: Granulocytic sarcoma (chloroma) of bone: the CT appearance. Comput Radiol 1986;10:175–178

Nijland E, Wuisman P, van Royen B, et al: Vertebral chloroma in a 1½-year-old boy with no evidence of leukemia. Med Pediatr Oncol 2001;36:341–342

Novick SL, Nicol TL, Fishman EK: Granulocytic sarcoma (chloroma) of the sacrum: initial manifestation of leukemia. Skeletal Radiol 1998;27:112–114

Pomeranz SJ, Hawkins HH, Towbin R, et al: Granulocytic sarcoma (chloroma): CT manifestations. Radiology 1985;155:167–170

Pui MH, Fletcher BD, Langston JW: Gransulocytic sarcoma in childhood leukemia: imaging features. Radiology 1994;190:698–702

Rosenfield NS, McIntosh S: Prospective analysis of bone changes in treated childhood leukemia. Radiology 1977;123:413–415

Schabel SI, Tyminski L, Holland RD, Rittenberg GM: The skeletal manifestations of chronic myelogenous leukemia. Skeletal Radiol 1980;5:145–149

Hemophilia

Brant EE, Jordan HH: Radiologic aspects of hemophilic pseudotumors of bone. Am J Roentgenol Radium Ther Nucl Med 1972;115:525–539

Hennes H, Losek JD, Sty JR, et al: Computerized tomography in hemophiliacs with head trauma. Pediatr Emerg Care 1987;3:147–149

Hermann G, Gilbert MS, Abdelwahab IF: Hemophilia: evaluation of musculoskeletal involvement with CT, sonography, and MR imaging. AJR Am J Roentgenol 1992;158:119–123

Horton DD, Pollay M, Wilson DA, et al: Cranial hemophilic pseudotumor: Case report. J Neurosurg 1993;79:936–938

Jaovisidha S, Ryu KN, Hodler J, et al: Hemophilic pseudotumor: spectrum of MR findings. Skeletal Radiol 1997;26:468–474

Kulkarni MV, Drolshagen LF, Kaye JJ, et al: MR imaging of hemophilic arthropathy. J Comput Assist Tomogr 1985;10:445–449

Lan HH, Eustace SJ, Dorfman D: Hemophilic arthropathy. Radiol Clin North Am 1996;34:446–450

Llauger J, Palmer J, Roson N, et al: Nonseptic monoarthritis: imaging features with clinical and histopathologic correlation. Radiographics 2000;20(Suppl):263–278

Mathew P, Talbut DC, Frogameni A, et al: Isotopic synovectomy with P-32 in paediatric patients with haemophilia. Haemophilia 2000;6:547–555

Nuss R, Kilcoyne RF, Geraghty S, et al: MRI findings in haemophilic joints treated with radiosynoviorthesis with development of an MRI scale of joint damage. Haemophilia 2000;6:162–169

Nuss R, Kilcoyne RF, Geraghty S, et al: Utility of magnetic resonance imaging for management of hemophilic arthropathy in children. J Pediatr 1993;123:388–392

Pettersson H, Ahlberg A, Nillson IM: A radiologic classification of hemophilic arthropathy. Clin Orthop 1980;149:153–159

Pettersson H, Gillespy T, Kitchens C, et al: Magnetic resonance imaging in hemophilic arthropathy of the knee. Acta Radiol 1987;28:621–625

Plazanet F, du Boullay C, Defaux F, et al: Open synovectomy for the prevention of recurrent hemarthrosis of the ankle in patients with hemophilia: a report of five cases with magnetic resonance imaging documentation. Rev Rhum Engl Ed 1997;64:166–171

Rand T, Trattnig S, Male C, et al: Magnetic resonance imaging in hemophilic children: value of gradient echo and contrast-enhanced imaging. Magn Reson Imaging 1999;17:199–205

Reeves A, Edwards-Brown M: Intraosseous hematoma in a newborn with factor VIII deficiency. AJNR Am J Neuroradiol 2000;21:308–309

Langerhans' Cell Histiocytosis

Arico M, Haupt R, Russotto VS, et al: Langerhans cell histiocytosis in two generations: a new family and review of the literature. Med Pediatr Oncol 2001;36:314–316

Aterman K, Krause VW, Ross JB: Scabies masquerading as Letterer-Siwe's disease. Can Med Assoc J 1976;115:443–444

Bodart E, Nisolle JF, Maton P, et al: Limp as unusual presentation of Langerhans' cell histiocytosis. Eur J Pediatr 1999;158:384–386

Broker LE, van den Berg H, van Groningen K, et al: Juvenile xanthogranuloma: a form of histiocytosis with an excellent prognosis. Ned Tijdschr Geneeskd 2001;145:635–639

Chu T, D'Angio GJ, Favara B, et al, for the Writing Group of the Histiocyte Society: Histiocytosis syndromes in children. Lancet 1987;1:208–209

Damry N, Hottat N, Azzi N, et al: Unusual findings in two cases of Langerhans' cell histiocytosis. Pediatr Radiol 2000;30:196–199

Fischer A, Jones L, Lowis SP: Concurrent Langerhans cell histiocytosis and neuroblastoma. Med Pediatr Oncol 1999;32:223–224

Henck ME, Simpson EL, Ochs RH, Eremus JL: Extraskeletal soft tissue masses of Langerhans' cell histiocytosis. Skeletal Radiol 1996;25:409–412

Hindman BW, Thomas RD, Young LW, Yu L: Langerhans cell histiocytosis: unusual skeletal manifestations observed in thirty-four cases. Skeletal Radiol 1998;27:177–181

Kaplan GR, Saifuddin A, Pringle JA, et al: Langerhans' cell histiocytosis of the spine: use of MRI in guiding biopsy. Skeletal Radiol 1998;27:673–676

Kayser R, Mahlfeld K, Grasshoff H: Vertebral Langerhans-cell histiocytosis in childhood—a differential diagnosis of spinal osteomyelitis. Klin Padiatr 1999;211:399–402

Kraus MD, Haley JC, Ruiz R, et al: "Juvenile" xanthogranuloma: an immunophenotypic study with a reappraisal of histogenesis. Am J Dermatopathol 2001;23:104–111

Lahiri K, Dole M, Kamat J, et al: Letterer-Siwe disease (histiocytosis-X) (a case report). J Postgrad Med 1988;34:111–113

Lichtenstein L: Histiocytosis X (eosinophilic granuloma of bone, Letterer-Siwe disease, and Schuller-Christian disease): further observations of pathological and clinical importance. J Bone Joint Surg Am 1964;46:76–90

McCullough CJ: Eosinophilic granuloma of bone. Acta Orthop Scand 1980;51:389–398

Moore JB, Kulkarni R, Crutcher DC, et al: MRI in multifocal eosinophilic granuloma: Staging disease and monitoring response to therapy. Am J Pediatr Hematol Oncol 1989;11:174–177

Raney RB Jr, D'Angio GJ: Langerhans' cell histiocytosis (histiocytosis-X): experience at the Children's Hospital of Philadelphia, Pennsylvania. Med Pediatr Oncol 1989;17:20–28

Rose PS, Lietman SA, McCarthy EF, Frassica FJ: Destructive scapular lesion in an infant [review]. Clin Orthop 2001;386:260–262, 264–267

Schroers C, Donauer E, Laudan M, et al: Symptomatic Langerhans-cell-histiocytosis of the cervical spine in a child: case report. Klin Padiatr 2000;212:121–125

Stein SL, Paller AS, Haut PR, Mancini AJ: Langerhans cell histiocytosis presenting in the neonatal period: a retrospective case series. Arch Pediatr Adolesc Med 2001;155:778–783

Tordeur M, Wybier M, Laporte JL, et al: Button sequestrum in a case of localized Langerhans' cell histiocytosis of the ilium: case report. Can Assoc Radiol J 2000;51:90–92

Vanel D, Cousnest D, Piekarski JD, et al: Radiological findings on 23 pediatric cases of malignant histiocytosis. Eur J Radiol 1983;3:60–62

Yeom JS, Lee CK, Shin HY, et al: Langerhans' cell histiocytosis of the spine: analysis of twenty-three cases. Spine 1999;24:1740–1749

Mastocytosis

Avila NA, Ling A, Metcalfe DD, Worobec AS: Mastocytosis: magnetic resonance imaging patterns of marrow disease. Skeletal Radiol 1998;27:119–126

Avila NA, Ling A, Worobec AS, et al: Systemic mastocytosis: CT and US features of abdominal manifestations. Radiology 1997;202: 367–372

Gagnon JH, Kalz F, Kadri AM, Graefe IV: Mastocytosis: unusual manifestations; clinical and radiologic changes. Can Med Assoc Journal 1975;112:1328–1332

Korenblat PE, Wedner J, Whyte MP, et al: Systemic mastocytosis. Arch Intern Med 1984;144:2249–2253

Lucaya J, Perez-Candela V, Aso C, et al: Mastocytosis with skeletal and gastrointestinal involvement in infancy: two case reports and review of the literature. Radiology 1979;131:363–366

C h a p t e r   2

BONE CHANGES IN ENDOCRINOPATHIES

SAMBASIVA R. KOTTAMASU

Several endocrine glands play a significant role in the normal modeling and remodeling of the skeleton during growth and maturation. Skeletal abnormalities are encountered in a number of endocrine disorders. The hormonal effects on the bone manifest themselves in the size of skeletal structures, degree of mineralization, and growth and maturation of ossification centers. Although interrelations are common among the endocrine glands, the following discussion focuses on features that indicate major roles for specific glands.

GROWTH HORMONE EXCESS

An excess of growth hormone (GH) in a skeletally immature individual results in increased endochondral bone formation and gigantism. After epiphyseal fusion, hypersecretion of GH stimulates endosteal and periosteal new bone formation, resulting in acromegaly.

GIGANTISM

Patients with gigantism have extreme height with normal body proportions. Gigantism is much rarer than acromegaly. Most children with gigantism secondary to a pituitary eosinophilic adenoma have normal skeletal maturation. Therefore, when bone age is advanced in a child with gigantism, a cause other than pituitary overactivity should be considered. Iwatani et al. de-

scribed a female child with pituitary gigantism and precocious adrenarche. They also reviewed nine previous reports of gigantism in children under 10 years of age, eight of whom had an associated manifestation of precocious adrenarche.

ACROMEGALY

Acromegaly is characterized by GH hypersecretion and insulin-like growth factor excess, both of which stimulate osteoblast proliferation. At diagnosis, GH excess has usually been present for years. The effects of chronic elevation of GH on bony structures after fusion of the physes produce the typical physical changes associated with acromegaly, whereas the effects on cartilage result in arthropathy, which is usually degenerative. Furthermore, impaired gonadotropin secretion with hypogonadism is frequent.

One of the well-recognized skeletal findings in acromegaly is widening of the tufts of the distal phalanges. The sesamoid bones, particularly around the first metacarpophalangeal joint, are enlarged. The greatest soft tissue thickening in the hand appears to be in the region of the proximal and middle phalanges. The heel pad thickness is characteristically increased in association with prominent calcaneal spurs. Bony excrescences arising from tuberosities, trochanters, and the patella are frequent manifestations. The tubular bones demonstrate cortical thickening. The vertebrae manifest increased transverse and longitudinal diameter as a result of increased periosteal new bone apposition. Posterior vertebral margins may be concave. Prominent osteophytes are noted in the spine and bones of the larger joints.

Ho et al. investigated proximal femur and lumbar spine bone mineral density (BMD) using dual-photon absorptiometry in 25 patients with acromegaly (8 eugonadal, 17 hypogonadal). They concluded that BMD is normal in these regions in most patients with acromegaly, including those who are hypogonadal.

THYROID GLAND DISORDERS

HYPERTHYROIDISM

Hyperthyroidism is extremely rare in infancy and uncommon, and usually not severe, during childhood. In pediatric practice, toxic goiter is encountered most frequently in preadolescent and adolescent females; skeletal maturation may be normal or advanced (Table 1) depending on the duration of the disturbance. Hyperthyroidism is observed in some children with McCune-Albright syndrome (polyostotic fibrous dysplasia). Thyrotoxicosis and accelerated development of the skeleton may also result from excessive treatment with thyroid extract.

Acceleration of skeletal maturation may occur in infants born to mothers suffering from severe thyrotoxicosis, especially if it is uncontrolled during the last trimester of pregnancy. In neonatal and early infantile hyperthyroidism, there is marked acceleration of skeletal maturation. Premature craniosynostosis may be associated with hyperthyroidism in the neonate and young child. Brachydactyly secondary to premature epiphyseal fusion, and cardiomegaly may occur. Calcification of the costal cartilages and signs of increased bone turnover, such as intracortical striations in tubular bones, may be observed.

HYPOTHYROIDISM

Thyroid hormone is essential for normal brain development and skeletal growth and maturation. In hypothy-

Table 1 ■ CAUSES OF GENERALIZED ADVANCED SKELETAL AGE

Hyperthyroidism (maternal or acquired)
McCune-Albright syndrome (polyostotic fibrous dysplasia)
Idiopathic isosexual precocious puberty
Premature thelarche
Premature adrenarche
Hypothalamic tumors
Pinealoma
Liver tumors (choriocarcinoma, hepatoma)
Adrenogenital syndrome (adrenocortical tumor or hyperplasia)
Gonadal tumors (androgen or estrogen secreting)
Medication with sex hormones
Acrodysostosis
Cerebral gigantism (Soto's syndrome)
Pseudohypoparathyroidism
Lipodystrophy
Weaver syndrome

Table 2 ■ CAUSES OF GENERALIZED DECREASED SKELETAL AGE

Hypothyroidism
Chronic severe anemia (e.g., Sickle cell anemia, thalassemia)
Constitutional
Addison's disease
Cushing's syndrome
Steroid therapy
Hypogonadism (e.g., Turner's syndrome)
Panhypopituitarism
Growth hormone deficiency
Chromosomal disorders (e.g., trisomy 21, trisomy 18)
Most skeletal dysplasias
Congenital malformation syndromes
Congenital heart disease (especially cyanotic)
Juvenile diabetes mellitus
Chronic illness
Inflammatory bowel disease
Intrauterine growth retardation
Legg-Perthes disease
Malnutrition
Malabsorption syndromes (e.g., celiac disease)
Neurologic disorders
Chronic renal disease
Rickets
Idiopathic

roidism, skeletal maturation is retarded; although retardation of skeletal maturation is noted in several other conditions, very rarely is the retardation as severe as in longstanding hypothyroidism (Table 2). Before the onset of puberty, the progress of skeletal maturation is one of the most sensitive indices of thyroid function. The development of the secondary ossification centers is grossly retarded in hypothyroidism. The growth plates may remain open in some patients with hypothyroidism who reach adulthood. The medullary cavities in the tubular and flat bones are characteristically narrow and small, with corresponding thickening of the overlying cortex. These features disappear with treatment. Dental development is consistently delayed but not to the degree that occurs in skeletal maturation. Maldevelopment of the ossification centers in hypothyroid children can reflect equivalent maldevelopment of the brain, which unlike that of the skeletal structures, is not reversible. Hypothyroidism and Down syndrome may coexist.

Athyrotic newborn infants may appear normal in size for several months. Subsequently, the skeleton grows slowly and delay in development of ossification centers becomes progressively greater. Pseudoepiphyseal centers in the metacarpal bones are more frequent in children with congenital hypothyroidism than in the normal population but are not in themselves diagnostic of the condition. Smith and Popich suggested that a large anterior fontanelle and an open posterior fontanelle of unexplained cause in a neonate could be the initial clue to suspect hypothyroidism.

Ossification of the epiphyseal centers is frequently fragmented and irregular as well as delayed in hypothyroid infants (Table 3). Instead of developing from a single focus of ossification followed by uniform marginal extension as in the normal infant, ossification centers in children with hypothyroidism may begin in numerous small foci in the cartilage; these grow larger and coalesce

Table 3 ■ CONDITIONS ASSOCIATED WITH STIPPLING OF EPIPHYSEAL OSSIFICATION CENTERS

Congenital hypothyroidism
Spondyloepiphyseal dysplasia
Multiple epiphyseal dysplasia (Fairbank's disease)
Legg-Perthes disease
Aseptic necrosis
Normal variant
Endemic cretinism
Down syndrome
Mucopolysaccharidosis (e.g., Morquio's syndrome)
Stickler's syndrome (hereditary arthro-ophthalmopathy)
Osteopoikilosis
Osteopathia striata
Dysplasia epiphysialis hemimelica (Trevor's disease)

to form a single center of uneven density with irregular margins (Fig. 1). This phenomenon has been called *hypothyroid epiphyseal dysgenesis*. Epiphyseal dysgenesis is more common in the hips than in the hands and feet. In older untreated hypothyroid patients, the metaphyses are sometimes irregularly mineralized. The proximal femoral epiphyses may be flattened as well as irregularly mineralized, the neck of the femur may be broadened, and coxa vara deformity may be observed in hypothyroid children; the delay in ossification of cartilage may result in features resembling congenital hip dislocation (Fig. 2). Slipped femoral capital epiphysis seems to occur in juvenile hypothyroid children with a somewhat greater frequency than in normal children.

Newborn screening programs for the detection of congenital hypothyroidism have provided a means to early diagnosis. Scintigraphy and postnatal ultrasound have improved the ability to identify or exclude abnormalities of structure, location, and function of the thyroid gland at an early date.

In primary hypothyroidism, in particular when the endocrine deficiency has persisted unrecognized for sometime, hyperplasia of the pituitary gland resulting from inadequate feedback from the hypofunctioning thyroid gland can be associated with radiologically demonstrable enlargement of the pituitary fossa. The sellar area may be increased in relation to bone age. Because of associated growth disturbances, pituitary tumor may be erroneously suspected from the radiographic findings.

ENDEMIC CRETINISM

Endemic cretinism, caused by severe iodine deficiency during pregnancy, is the world's most common preventable cause of mental retardation. Endemic cretinism has been classified into neurologic and myxedematous types. Profound mental deficiency, deaf-mutism, and cerebral diplegia are found in both types. In addition, the latter demonstrates severe growth retardation, myxedematous features, and delayed sexual maturation. Boyages and Halpern postulated that the clinical picture of endemic cretinism results from two pathophysiologic events which share a common feature—iodine deficiency. The first event occurs in all cretins and represents the effect of prenatal thyroid hormone deficiency on brain development, transmitted from mother to fetus, resulting in the neurologic disorder of endemic cretinism.

The nature of the deficits points to an intrauterine insult to the developing fetal nervous system around the time of the mid-trimester. The second event represents

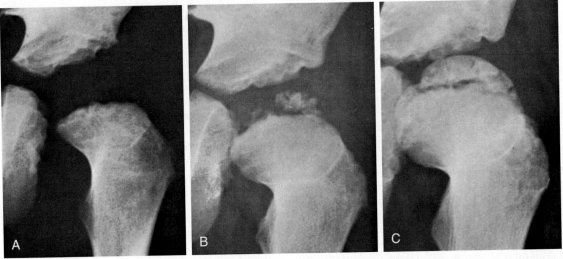

FIGURE 1. Epiphyseal dysgenesis in a hypothyroid girl 8 years of age. **A,** Before treatment, the proximal femoral epiphyseal center is not visible radiographically. **B,** After 1 year of treatment, at 9 years of age, an irregularly mineralized, fragmented, small femoral head has appeared. **C,** After 3 years of treatment, at 11 years of age, the femoral epiphyseal center is flattened and the femoral neck broadened into a coxa plana deformity. A narrow irregular strip of ossification is evident in the medial segment of the epiphyseal center. Similar changes were present in the other femur. In serial examinations, similar dysgenesis was also demonstrated in the proximal and distal epiphyses of the humeri, distal epiphyses of the femora, and both ends of the tibias.

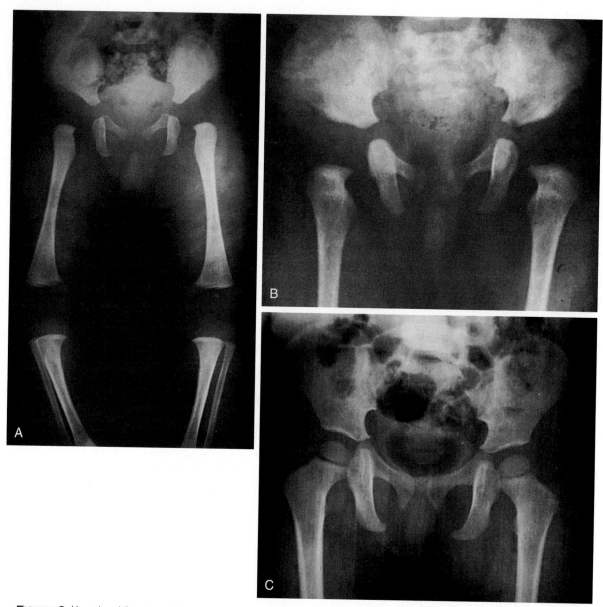

FIGURE 2. Hypothyroidism simulating congenital dislocation of the hips on radiographs. **A,** Apparent dislocation at the time of diagnosis at 4 months. Delayed ossification of the acetabular roofs accounts for the resemblance to acetabular dysplasia. **B** and **C,** "Spontaneous recovery" with thyroid medication alone at 9 and 30 months, respectively. (From Silverman FN, Currarino G: Metabolism 1960;9:248–283, with permission.)

the effect of postnatal thyroid hormone deficiency on somatic as well as brain development. The type of endemic cretin can be distinguished by the length and severity of postnatal thyroid hormone deficiency. Endemic cretins with predominantly neurologic features have had only transient hypothyroidism in the postnatal period, evidenced by near-normal thyroid function and a lack of hypothyroid clinical features. By contrast, cretins with marked myxedematous features are characterized by severe postnatal thyroid hormone deficiency. Delayed skeletal maturation and irregular epiphyses are present in both types of cretins.

The nature and extent of the neurologic deficit found in endemic cretinism was investigated by Halpern et al. in cretins from western China and central Java, Indonesia. They found a similar pattern of neurologic involvement in nearly all cretins, regardless of type (myxedematous or neurologic), and of current thyroid function. Patients with severe hypothyroidism had basal ganglia calcification on cranial computed tomography (CT). No other significant abnormalites were noted on cranial CT.

In another study of cretins in Asia, Boyages et al. (1989) found that severe protracted thyroid hormone deficiency may result in thyrotropin adenomas of the pituitary gland. Disturbances of growth, puberty, and sexual function in endemic cretins are explained by the secondary effects of thyroid hormone deficiency on pituitary function.

Magnetic resonance imaging (MRI) findings include abnormal signal in the globus pallidus and substantia nigra, with hyperintensity on T_1-weighted and hypointensity on T_2-weighted images. The motor abnormality, characterized by truncal and proximal limb spasticity, with relative sparing of the hands and feet, is analogous to that of other extrapyramidal disorders.

PARATHYROID GLAND DISORDERS

HYPERPARATHYROIDISM

Hyperparathyroidism may be primary, secondary, or tertiary. Increased serum levels of parathyroid hormone (PTH) and skeletal manifestations of hyperparathyroidism are common to all three forms of hyperparathyroidism.

Primary Hyperparathyroidism

Primary hyperparathyroidism (PHPT) in children is associated with an abnormality within the parathyroid glands, such as an adenoma. Excess PTH affects growing bones in two ways: (1) it promotes abnormally rapid urinary excretion of phosphate by lowering the threshold for tubular excretion of phosphate and raising the threshold for tubular reabsorption; and (2) it mobilizes calcium from the skeleton largely through osteocytic osteolysis, often associated with bone remodeling as a result of osteoblast and osteoclast stimulation. The bones lose radiographic density in a variety of patterns, and the blood shows decreased inorganic phosphate levels and reciprocal hypercalcemia while the urine exhibits an excess of calcium and phosphate.

Osteitis fibrosa is the term used to describe the histologic alterations of chronic PTH excess on the skeleton. The typical radiographic features in PHPT include subperiosteal bone resorption, generalized osteopenia, brown tumors, and cysts (Fig. 3), but in some cases the skeleton is radiographically normal. The degree of skeletal change depends on the severity and duration of the disease. Subperiosteal resorption of cortical bone is

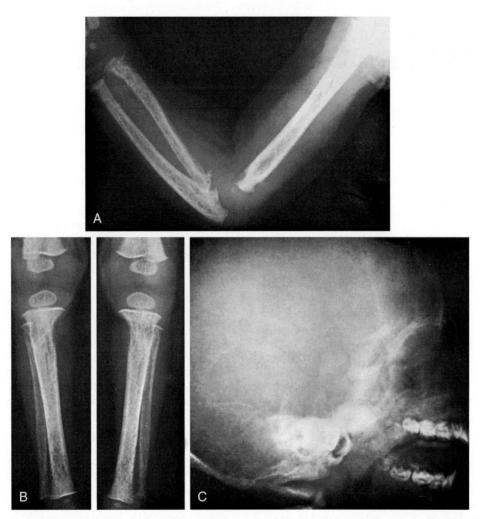

FIGURE 3. Fatal hyperparathyroidism in an infant 12 months of age. On necropsy radiographs of an upper extremity **(A)** and legs **(B)**, the tubular bones show extreme coarse rarefaction of the cortices and the spongiosa, but the provisional zones of calcification are surprisingly well mineralized. Active rickets could not be diagnosed according to the usual criteria. **C,** On a lateral projection of the skull, there is extreme generalized osteopenia of all bones. The walls of the semicircular canals are conspicuous in the petrous pyramids. The well-calcified teeth stand out in the severely osteopenic maxillas. The lamina dura in the maxilla and mandible is invisible radiographically.

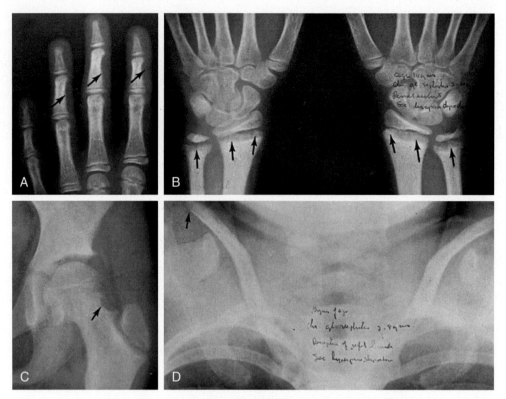

FIGURE 4. Radiographic evidence of secondary hyperparathyroidism in a 10-year-old girl with renal rickets. **A,** Subperiosteal bone resorption on the radial side of the phalanges *(arrows).* **B,** Severe rickets in the metaphyses of the radius and ulna *(arrows).* **C,** Subperiosteal bone resorption on the lateral edge of the femoral neck *(arrow);* a similar lesion was present in the other femoral neck. **D,** Resorption of the lateral end of the clavicle *(arrow).* The patient was suffering from renal obstructive disease.

pathognomonic of hyperparathyroidism (Fig. 4). The subperiosteal resorption is most prominent on the radial side of the middle phalanges of the middle and index fingers, on the tufts of the terminal phalanges, and on the medial aspects of the proximal tibial, humeral, and femoral shafts. Intracortical, endosteal, subchondral, periarticular, and metaphyseal bone resorption is frequently observed in patients with hyperparathyroidism. Localized accumulation of fibrous tissue and giant cells replacing or expanding bone, known as brown tumors, and associated pathologic fractures are additional diagnostic features. Brown tumors and cystic rarefactions are less frequent in pediatric than in adult patients. On scintigraphic blood flow studies, brown tumors demonstrate evidence of blood flow, while cysts are visualized as photopenic areas. Brown tumors heal with sclerosis following parathyroidectomy.

All parts of the long bones including the epiphyseal ossification centers and the shafts, manifest osteopenia. The trabecular pattern is coarse owing to the disappearance of the smaller secondary trabeculae. Slipped capital femoral epiphysis is observed more frequently in children with various forms of hyperparathyroidism and may be bilateral. The calvaria may be normal or exhibit a granular rarefaction. The lamina dura gradually loses its sclerotic density and disappears in severe cases. Vertebral bodies become more radiolucent and are weakened so that the nuclei pulposi dilate against them and compress them into biconcave shapes. In longstand-ing cases, kyphosis, scoliosis, and loss of stature from spinal deformity are common. Bony resorption is frequently noted at both ends of the clavicles. Patchy osteosclerosis involving metaphyseal regions has been reported in some children with PHPT (Fig. 5). Important radiologic findings in the abdomen and pelvis include calculi in the kidneys, renal pelves, ureters, and urinary bladder. Calcification may also develop in the renal parenchyma and the walls of arteries. In the case of large, medially placed parathyroid tumors, indentation on the contiguous barium-filled esophagus has been demonstrated. Ultrasound, radionuclide scintigraphy, and MRI have been useful in preoperative localization and evaluation of morphologic abnormalities of parathyroid glands, particularly in patients with recurrent hyperparathyroidism after parathyroidectomy.

Secondary Hyperparathyroidism

Hyperparathyroidism may be secondary to hypocalcemia of various etiologies, such as chronic renal insufficiency, intestinal malabsorption, and vitamin D deficiency. Chronic renal insufficiency with rickets and osteomalacia is a frequent cause of secondary hyperparathyroidism; this manifestation is often referred to as renal osteodystrophy (ROD). The biochemical abnormalities and skeletal manifestations of ROD are a consequence of two major hormonal changes: a deficiency of 1,25-dihydroxyvitamin D and an excess of

PTH. Radiographic manifestations include evidence of rickets and osteomalacia, osteopenia, subperiosteal bone resorption, brown tumors, cystic areas of rarefaction, and focal and generalized osteosclerosis. In many instances, the skeletal structures become recognizably dense to the point of being confused with osteosclerotic disorders. Skeletal findings in ROD are discussed in detail in Section IX, Part VII, Chapter 2, page 2242.

Osteosclerosis is rare in patients with intestinal malabsorption, osteomalacia and biochemical evidence of secondary hyperparathyroidism.

Tertiary Hyperparathyroidism

In some patients with improved renal function following renal transplantaion for chronic renal insufficiency, hyperparathyroidism may persist as a result of autonomous hyperfunction of the parathyroid glands. This condition is called tertiary hyperparathyroidism. Skeletal findings in this entity are similar to those described in ROD. In severe cases, parathyroidectomy is the treatment of choice. Parathyroid single-photon emission computed tomography (SPECT), ultrasound, and MRI play a significant role in preoperative localization and demonstration of morphologic abnormalities of parathyroid glands.

Neonatal and Infantile Hyperparathyroidism

Neonatal and infantile hyperparathyroidism can also be primary or secondary. In primary cases, there is generalized hyperplasia of the glands or an adenoma in infants of normocalcemic mothers. In secondary cases, the parathyroid hyperplasia of the infant is a response to maternal hypoparathyroidism. The primary form, which can be hereditary, carries a grave prognosis if not diagnosed promptly and treated by subtotal parathyroidectomy. Some cases, however, may resolve spontaneously. In most instances of both types, the diagnosis can be suspected by radiographic identification of marked osteopenia with coarse trabecular markings and subperiosteal bone resorption. The ribs are especially prone to involvement and may demonstrate multiple fractures. Subperiosteal resorption along the long tubular bones is frequently more striking than along the short tubular bones. Eftekhari and Yousefzadeh, emphasized hypotonicity, respiratory symptoms, and constipation in conjunction with osteopenia as important clues to the diagnosis. Bronsky and associates described two newborn infants with intrauterine hyperparathyroidism secondary to maternal hypoparathyroidism. In one of the babies, rarefaction of the bones was demonstrated on the seventh postnatal day (Fig. 6); the bones of the other patient were normal. The productive and destructive changes in the bones can simulate syphilis. Ultrasound, parathyroid SPECT, and MRI are useful imaging methods for demonstration of morphologic abnormalities of parathyroid glands associated with neonatal and infantile hyperparathyroidism.

FAMILIAL HYPOCALCIURIC HYPERCALCEMIA

Familial hypocalciuric hypercalcemia can be confused with hyperparathyroidism. It usually begins before 10

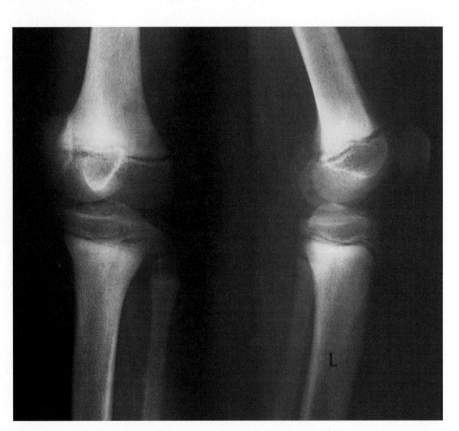

FIGURE 5. Metaphyseal sclerosis in primary hyperparathyroidism: Sclerosis of distal femoral and proximal tibial metaphyses observed in a 12-year-old girl with primary hyperparathyroidism.

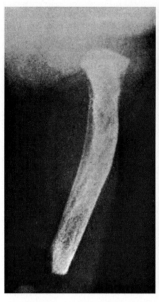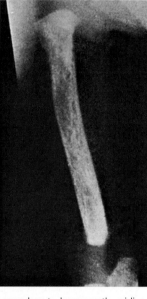

FIGURE 6. Hyperparathyroidism secondary to hypoparathyroidism of the pregnant mother. Coarse rarefaction and subperiosteal resorption of cortical bone are clearly visible in the humeral shafts. These radiographs were made 7 days after birth. (From Bronsky D, Kiamko RT, Moncala R, et al: Intrauterine hyperparathyroidism secondary to maternal hypoparathyroidism. Pediatrics 1968;42:606–613, with permission.)

years of age and is not accompanied by renal stones or damage; it does not respond to parathyroidectomy. Its complications include pancreatitis and chondrocalcinosis.

HYPOPARATHYROIDISM

Idiopathic (Hormonopenic) Hypoparathyroidism

Hypoparathyroidism may result from congenital absence of the parathyroid glands or from atrophy of the parathyroid glands in infants born to mothers with hyperparathyroidism. An idiopathic form that is familial has been observed in some children. It is probably an autoimmune disorder and is often associated with other endocrine, particularly adrenal, disturbances. Sometimes the only clue to the existence of the condition in a newborn infant is the recognition of hyperparathyroidism in the mother.

Significant skeletal changes have not been emphasized in the few authentic cases of chronic hypoparathyroidism reported in infants and younger children. In older children and adults, radiographic manifestations include osteosclerosis and cranial vault thickening; in addition, there may be intracranial calcifications, dental abnormalities, and a "bone within bone" appearance of the vertebrae (Fig. 7). The differences in the two age groups probably reflect the duration of the disease as well as its severity. Emerson and colleagues described osteosclerosis in a boy 15 years of age who had congenital absence of the parathyroids.

A special form of hypoparathyroidism occurs in

DiGeorge syndrome, in which congenital absence of the parathyroid glands and the thymus results in hypocalcemic tetany and frequent infections secondary to absent or depressed cellular immunity. Associated cardiovascular abnormalities, especially aortic arch anomalies, are common, reflecting maldevelopment of the third and fourth pharyngeal pouches. The hyoid bone may be uncalcified and radiologically invisible in early life.

Of 13 hypoparathyroid patients studied by Miller and associates, 4 had associated anomalies of branchial cleft origin. One had cleft palate and two had functional and structural anomalies of the muscles of the pharynx and soft palate. In the fourth patient, the thymus and parathyroid glands were absent, the ears were set low with their pinnas folded ventrad, and the mandible was small. This case was an example of DiGeorge syndrome.

Pseudohypoparathyroidism

Pseudohypoparathyroidism is a disorder characterized by end organ resistance to the effects of PTH in which serum calcium and phosphorus are decreased as in idiopathic (hormonopenic) hypoparathyroidism but PTH levels are elevated. Many, but not all, patients have characteristic somatic features known as Albright's hereditary osteodystrophy (AHO), which include short

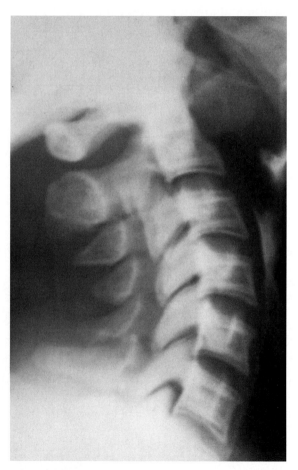

FIGURE 7. Idiopathic hypoparathyroidism. Bone-within-bone appearance and patchy osteosclerosis of cervical vertebrae are observed in a patient with idiopathic hypoparathyroidism.

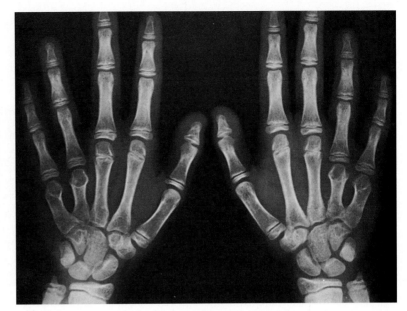

FIGURE 8. Radiograph of the hands of a patient with pseudopseudohypoparathyroidism. The patient was short but of normal proportions and had no clinical or biochemical evidence of hypoparathyroidism. The shortening of the metacarpal bones in this condition cannot be differentiated from that in other conditions associated with brachymetacarpia.

stature, obesity, brachydactyly, subcutaneous calcifications and ossifications, and subnormal intelligence. The diagnosis is often suggested by radiographic findings in the hands, which are short with disproportionate shortening of the fourth and fifth metacarpals and distal phalanges (Fig. 8), as well as widespread punctate soft tissue calcifications/ossifications. The skeletal findings in the hands and feet may resemble those of acrodysostosis. Patients with end organ resistance to PTH, but who lack the somatic features of AHO, have also been reported.

End organ resistance at the renal tubule site of action of PTH is clinically confirmed by impaired renal excretion of cyclic AMP and phosphorus following exogenous administration of PTH intravenously (pseudohypoparathyroidism type I). Patients have been described in whom the nephrogenous cyclic AMP response to exogenous PTH is intact but the phosphaturic response is blunted; this group of patients has been categorized as pseudohypoparathyroidism type II. Hormone resistance at the skeletal level is usually inferred, based on a blunted calcemic response to exogenous PTH. The blunted calcemic response, however, does not reflect absence of a bone-remodeling effect of PTH in all patients. In fact, some patients with renal resistance to PTH may demonstrate extensive skeletal findings of hyperparathyroidism, including subperiosteal bone resorption and multiple brown tumors. These manifestations reflect variable PTH resistance at separate end organ sites. We reported a series of patients in whom biochemical, radiographic, and bone histomorphometry suggested that the resistance can be complete or occur at only one or two of the sites of PTH resistance in the kidneys and skeleton. This latter entity is known as renal resistance to PTH with skeletal hyperparathyroidism or pseudohypohyperparathyroidism (Fig. 9).

Pseudopseudohypoparathyroidism

Pseudopseudohypoparathyroidism is characterized by somatic features of AHO but without clinical or biochemical evidence of hypoparathyroidism. Serum calcium, phosphorus, and PTH levels are normal. Pseudohypoparathyroidism and pseudopseudohypoparathyroidism may occur in the same family.

ADRENAL GLAND DISORDERS

Radiographic abnormalities are observed in Cushing's syndrome, Addison's disease, adrenogenital syndrome, and pheochromocytoma.

Cushing's syndrome in infants and children is most commonly the result of a malignant adrenal tumor or an adrenal adenoma rather than being of pituitary origin, as in adults. Levy et al. reported an 11-month-old boy with Cushing's syndrome who had a sellar mass demonstrated by CT, as well as skull erosion on conventional radiographs. In the literature they found more than 60 infants with Cushing's syndrome of adrenal origin and only 2 with pituitary tumors.

Cushing's syndrome is more often observed in children treated with adrenocorticosteroids for a variety of diseases, often immunologic disorders. It is well recognized that administration of pharmacologic doses of glucocorticoids over a prolonged period results in severe bone loss. The effects of glucocorticoids on bone formation are complex and result in increased resorption and decreased formation of bone. The increased bone resorption appears to be mediated indirectly by secondary hyperparathyroidism caused by a decrease in intestinal absorption of calcium. Glucocorticoids may also stimulate the release of PTH by a direct action on the parathyroid glands. In addition, glucocorticoids are

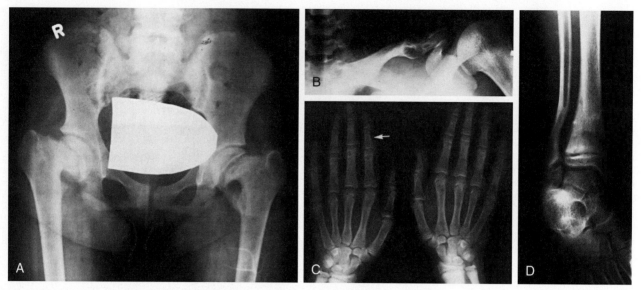

FIGURE 9. Pseudohypoparathyroidism with radiographic skeletal changes of hyperparathyroidism. **A,** Bilateral slipped capital femoral epiphyses and erosive changes involving the sacroiliac joints. **B,** Focal expansile lytic lesion in lateral aspect of the clavicle, consistent with a brown tumor. **C,** Subperiosteal bone resorption in the middle phalanges *(arrow)*. **D,** Metaphyseal irregularity. All of these findings are manifestations of hyperparathyroidism in this patient with pseudohypoparathyroidism characterized by hypocalcemia, elevated serum parathyroid hormone levels, and renal resistance to parathyroid hormone demonstrated by lack of normal cyclic AMP and reduced phosphaturic response to exogenous parathyroid hormone.

known to interfere with the action of somatomedin on cartilage growth.

The skeletal findings are similar in endogenous or exogenous corticosteroid excess. They include generalized osteopenia and compression fractures of vertebral bodies associated with characteristic sclerosis of their end plates, osteonecrosis, and abundant callus formation at fracture sites (Fig. 10). Excessive callus formation associated with compression fractures of the vertebral bodies probably accounts for sclerosis along their end plates and is an important clue in diagnosing Cushing's syndrome in a patient with osteopenia. Osteonecrosis, particularly of the femoral head, is a well-recognized complication of exogenous corticosteroid administration as well as spontaneous Cushing's syndrome. The characteristic findings include subchondral fracture, bone collapse, fragmentation, and patchy osteosclerosis. Occasionally, osteonecrosis may be a presenting feature of Cushing's syndrome.

In *Addison's disease* (adrenal cortical insufficiency), there are no specific skeletal changes unless the features of associated hypoparathyroidism are present. Adrenal calcification may be noted on radiographs of the abdomen.

In the *adrenogenital syndrome,* more obvious in girls than in boys, in addition to virilization, accelerated skeletal maturation and increased size of the bones are noted. The salt-losing form manifests itself, in addition, by microcardia because of severe water loss and dehydration. Premature fusion of ossification centers may lead to shortness of stature.

Becker and associates have described changes in the long bones in a child with benign *pheochromocytoma* that resemble infarcts radiographically. These were explained by microthrombi from hemoconcentration

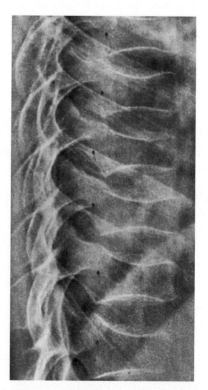

FIGURE 10. Diffuse severe rarefaction of the vertebral bodies on radiographs in a 13-year-old girl, similar to that seen in some instances of Cushing's syndrome, after prolonged high-dosage treatment with adrenal cortical steroids for rheumatoid arthritis. This is an example of pharmacologically induced Cushing's syndrome. The nuclei pulposi have expanded against the weakened endplates of the vertebral bodies and compressed each into a biconcave disk.

and increased viscosity of blood as a result of the excess epinephrine formed by the tumor.

PROSTAGLANDINS AND BONE REMODELING

In general, prostaglandins have a resorptive effect on bone. However, prostaglandins stimulate bone formation at lower concentrations. Infants treated with prostaglandin E to maintain patency of the ductus arteriosus may manifest extensive periosteal new bone formation, predominantly along long tubular bones.

GONADAL DYSGENESIS (TURNER'S SYNDROME)

Turner's syndrome (TS) is a chromosomal disease frequently associated with autoimmune conditions, including thyroid disease, inflammatory bowel disease, and diabetes. Recent reports have described an association with juvenile rheumatoid arthritis (JRA) and psoriatic arthritis. Wihlborg et al. described three cases of TS associated with JRA. It is important to consider the diagnosis of TS in girls with JRA, recognizing that characteristic radiographic findings such as metacarpal shortening are usually present in Turner's syndrome (see Section IX, Part VI, Fig. 56, page 2222). Conversely, suspicion of an underlying inflammatory arthritis is warranted in the search for radiologic findings consistent with JRA in girls with TS and joint symptoms.

DIABETES MELLITUS

The osseous changes in diabetes mellitus (DM) may include growth retardation, osteopenia, and neuropathic joint disease. The fracture rates in diabetic patients have been reported to be no different from those in the nondiabetic population. Vascular calcification is more frequent in diabetics than in nondiabetics. Contractures of the hand, more frequently involving the fifth digit, have been described in children with diabetes mellitus. A majority of investigators support the roles of loss of pain sensation and recurrent micro- or macrotrauma in the pathogenesis of neuroarthropathy associated with DM. The unusual mechanical stresses on joints with decreased pain sensation result in recurrent trauma and progressive disorganization of the joints. Vascular compromise secondary to osseous fragmentation may also lead to osteonecrosis.

Early radiographic findings include joint space narrowing, sclerosis, and marginal hypertrophic changes resembling degenerative joint disease. The presence of minimal fragmentation, subluxation, and persistent joint effusion should suggest the possibility of neuroarthropathy. Superimposed infection is a common complication and may accentuate the osseous and articular destruction. The subtalar, intertarsal, and tarsometatarsal joints are frequently involved, although the ankle, knee, and spine may also be affected.

SUGGESTED READINGS

Gigantism and Acromegaly

Anton HC: Hand measurements in acromegaly. Clin Radiol 1972; 23:445

Chew FS: Radiologic manifestations in the musculoskeletal system of miscellaneous endocrine disorders. Radiol Clin North Am 1991;29: 135–147

Gertner JM, Tamborlane WV, Gianfredi SP, Genel M: Renewed catch-up growth with increased replacement doses of human growth hormone. J Pediatr 1987;110:25–28

Ho PJ, Fig LM, Barkan AL, Shapiro B: Bone mineral density of the axial skeleton in acromegaly. J Nucl Med 1992;33:1608–1612

Honasoge M, Frame B, Kottamasu SR: Endocrine disorders. In Frame B, Honasoge M, Kottamsu SR (eds): Osteosclerosis, Hyperostosis and Related Disorders. New York, Elsevier Science Publishing Company, 1987:95–145

Iwatani N, Kodama M, Seto H: A child with pituitary gigantism and precocious adrenarche: does GH and/or PRL advance the onset of adrenarche? Endocrinol Jpn 1992;39:251–257

Lang EK, Bessler WT: The roentgenologic features of acromegaly. Am J Roentgenol Radium Ther Nucl Med 1961;86;321–1961

Lieberman SA, Bjorkengren AG, Hoffman AR: Rheumatologic and skeletal changes in acromegaly. Endocrinol Metab Clin North Am 1992;21:615–631

Mann DC: Endocrine disorders and orthopedic problems in children. Curr Opin Pediatr 1996;8:68–70

Pellini C, di Natale B, De Angeiis R, et al: Growth hormone deficiency in children: role of magnetic resonance imaging in assessing aetiopathogenesis and prognosis in idiopathic hypopituitarism. Eur J Pediatr 1990;149:536–541

Shimizu C, Kubo M, Kijima H, et al: A rare case of acromegaly associated with pachydermoperiostosis. J Endocrinol Invest 1999; 22:386–389

Whyte MP: Heritable metabolic and dysplastic bone diseases. Endocrinol Metab Clin North Am 1990;19:133–173

Thyroid Gland Disorders

Hyperthyroidism and Hypothyroidism

Bonakdarpour A, Kirkpatrick JA, Renzi A, et al: Skeletal changes in neonatal thyrotoxicosis. Radiology 1972;102:149–150

Brooks PT, Archard ND, Carty HM: Thyroid screening in congenital hypothyroidism: a review of cases. Nucl Med Commun 1988; 9:613–617

Chanoine JP, Toppet V, Body JJ, et al: Contribution of thyroid ultrasound and serum calcitonin to the diagnosis of congenital hypothyroidism. J Endocrinol Invest 1990;13:103–109

Farley JD, Toth EL, Ryan EA: Primary hypothyroidism presenting as growth delay and pituitary enlargement. Can J Neurol Sci 1988;15: 35–37

Heyerman W, Weiner D: Slipped epiphysis associated with hypothyroidism. J Pediatr Orthop 1984;4:569–573

Hollingsworth DR, Mabry CH: Congenital Graves' disease: four familial cases with long-term follow-up and perspective. Am J Dis Child 1976;130:148–155

Lusted LB, Pickering DE, Fisher DA, et al: Growth and metabolism in normal and thyroid-ablated infant rhesus monkeys (Macaca mulatta): roentgenographic features of skeletal development in normal and thyroid-ablated infant rhesus monkeys (Macaca mulatta). Am J Dis Child 1953;86:426–435

McCarten KM, Kuhns LR: The area and volume of the sella turcica in childhood primary hypothyroidism. Radiology 1976;119:645–650

Riggs W Jr, Wilroy RS Jr, Etteldorf JN: Neonatal hyperthyroidism with accelerated skeletal maturation, craniostenosis and brachydactyly. Radiology 1972;105:621–625

Schlesinger B, Fisher OD: Accelerated skeletal development from thyrotoxicosis and thyroid overdosage in childhood. Lancet 1951;2: 289–290

Schoen EJ, dos Remedios LV, Backstrom M: Heterogeneity of congenital primary hypothyroidism: the importance of thyroid scintigraphy. J Perinat Med 1987;15:137–142

Smith DW, Popich G: Large fontanels in congenital hypothyroidism: A potential clue toward earlier recognition. J Pediatr 1976;80:753–756

Van Wyck JJ, Grumbach MM: Syndrome of precocious menstruation and galactorrhea in juvenile hypothyroidism: an example of hormonal overlap in pituitary feedback. J Pediatr 1960;57:416–435

Endemic Cretinism

Boyages SC, Halpern JP: Endemic cretinism: toward a unifying hypothesis. Thyroid 1993;3:59–69

Boyages S, Halpern JP, Maberly GF, et al: Effects of protracted hypothyroidism on pituitary function and structure in endemic cretinism. Clin Endocrinol (Oxf) 1989;30:1–12

Boyages SC, Halpern JP, Maberly GF, et al: Supplementary iodine fails to reverse hypothyroidism in adolescents and adults with endemic cretinism. J Clin Endocrinol Metab 1990;70:336–341

Cao XY, Jiang XM, Dou ZH, et al: Timing of vulnerability of the brain to iodine deficiency in endemic cretinism. N Engl J Med 1994;331:1770–1771

Halpern JP, Boyages SC, Maberly GF, et al: The neurology of endemic cretinism: a study of two endemias. Brain 1991;114:825–841

Held KR, Cruz ME, Moncayo F: Clinical pattern and the genetics of the fetal iodine deficiency disorder (endemic cretinism): results of a field study in Highland Ecuador. Am J Med Genet 1990;35:85–90

Ma T, Lian ZC, Qi SP, et al: Magnetic resonance imaging of brain and the neuromotor disorder in endemic cretinism. Ann Neurol 1993;34:91–94

Rajatanavin R, Chailurkit L, Winichakoon P, et al: Endemic cretinism in Thailand: a multidisciplinary survey. Eur J Endocrinol 1997;137:336–337

Squatrito S, Delange F, Trimarchi F, et al: Endemic cretinism in Sicily. J Endocrinol Invest 1981;4:295–302

Parathyroid Gland Disorders

Ablow RC, Hsia YE, Brandt IK: Acrodysostosis coinciding with pseudohypoparathyroidism and pseudopseudohypoparathyroidism. AJR Am J Roentgenol 1977;128:95–99

Aceto T Jr, Ball RE, Bruck ER, et al: Intra-uterine fetal hyperparathyroidism: a complication of untreated maternal hypoparathyroidism. J Clin Endocrinol 1966;26:487–492

Bronsky D, Kiamko RT, Moncada R, et al: Intrauterine hyperparathyroidism secondary to maternal hypoparathyroidism. Pediatrics 1968;42:606–613

Burnstein MI, Kottamasu SR, Peffifor JM, et al: Metabolic bone disease in pseudohypoparathyroidism: radiologic features. Radiology 1985;155:351–356

DiGeorge AM: Congenital absence of the thymus and its immunologic consequences: Concurrence with congenital hypoparathyroidism. Birth Defects 1968;4:116–123

Eftekhari F, Yousefzadeh DK: Primary infantile hyperparathyroidism: clinical, laboratory and radiographic features in 21 cases. Skeletal Radiol 1982;8:201–208

Emerson K Jr, Walsh FB, Howard JE: Idiopathic hypoparathyroidism: report of two cases. Ann Intern Med 1941;14:1256–1270

Frame B, Hanson CA, Frost HM, et al: Renal resistance to parathyroid hormone with osteitis fibrosa: pseudohypohyperparathyroidism. Am J Med 1972;52:311–321

Honasoge M, Frame B, Kottamasu SR: Endocrine disorders. In Frame B, Honasoge M, Kottamasu SR (eds): Osteosclerosis, Hyperostosis and Related Disorders. New York, Elsevier Science Publishing Company, 1987:95–145

Kidd GS, Schaaf M, Adler RA, et al: Skeletal responsiveness in pseudohypoparathyroidism: a spectrum of clinical disease. Am J Med 1980;68:772–780

Marx SJ, Speigel AM, Levine MA, et al: Familial hypocalciuric hypercalcemia: the relation to primary parathyroid hyperplasia. N Engl J Med 1982;307:416–426

Miller MJ, Frame B, Poznanski AK, et al: Branchial anomalies in idiopathic hypoparathyroidism: branchial dysembryogenesis. Henry Ford Hosp Med J 1972;20:3–14

Potter DE, Wilson CJ, Ozonoff MB: Hyperparathyroid disease in children undergoing long-term dialysis: treatment with vitamin D. J Pediatr 1974;85:60–66

Pugh DG: Subperiosteal resorption of bone: roentgenologic manifestation of primary hyperparathyroidism and renal osteodystrophy. Am J Roentgenol Radium Ther Nucl Med 1951;66:577–586

Steinbach HL, Rudhe U, Jonsson M, et al: Evolution of skeletal lesions in pseudohypoparathyroidism. Radiology 1965;85:670–676

Taybi H, Keele D: Hypoparathyroidism: review of the literature and review of 2 cases in sisters, 1 with steatorrhea and intestinal pseudo-obstruction. Am J Roentgenol Radium Ther Nucl Med 1962;88:432–442

Teplick JG, Eftekhari F, Haskin ME: Erosion of the sternal ends of the clavicles: a new sign of primary and secondary hyperparathyroidism. Radiology 1974;113:323–326

Wells TR, Gilsanz V, Senac MO Jr, et al: Ossification centre of the hyoid bone in DiGeorge syndrome and tetralogy of Fallot. Br J Radiol 1986;59:1065–1068

Adrenal Gland Disorders

Becker MH, Redisch W, Messina EJ: Bone and microcirculatory changes in a child with benign pheochromocytoma. Radiology 1967;88:487–490

Canalis E: Clinical Review 83: Mechanisms of glucocorticoid action in bone: implications to glucocorticoid-induced osteoporosis. J Clin Endocrinol Metab 1996;81:3441–3447

Hermus AR, Huysmans DA, Smals AG, et al: Remarkable improvement of osteopenia after cure of Cushing's syndrome. Horm Metab Res 1994;26:209–210

Levy SR, Wynne V Jr, Lorentz WB Jr: Cushing's syndrome in infancy secondary to pituitary adenoma. Am J Dis Child 1982;136:605–607

Murray RO: Steroids and the skeleton. Radiology 1961;77:729

Gonadal Dysgenesis (Turner's syndrome)

Wihlborg CE, Babyn PS, Schneider R: The association between Turner's syndrome and juvenile rheumatoid arthritis. Pediatr Radiol 1999;29:676–681

Chapter 3

BONE CHANGES IN OTHER SYSTEMIC DISORDERS

SAMBASIVA R. KOTTAMASU

RENAL DISEASES

The growing skeleton is usually profoundly affected by chronic renal insufficiency. Renal rickets and osteomalacia are associated with various conditions causing chronic renal failure: renal hypoplasia, congenital polycystic disease, prune-belly syndrome, bilateral renal atrophy secondary to distal obstructive lesions in the urinary tract, and others. The bone changes of secondary hyperparathyroidism are also associated with chronic renal failure. Disorders associated with renal disease include asphyxiating thoracic dystrophy, nail–patella syndrome (osteo-onychodysplasia), cerebrohepatorenal syndrome, and Saldino-Mainzer syndrome, among others. Skeletal findings in renal osteodystrophy are discussed in Section IX, Part VII, Chapter 2, page 2242.

CENTRAL NERVOUS SYSTEM DISEASES

Growth and maturation of the skeleton may be retarded or normal in cerebral hypoplasia. In the extreme cases of microcephaly, skeletal growth and maturation are retarded. In all of the chronic paralytic diseases of neural origin, regional bone atrophy develops shortly after onset of the paralysis, and may result in flexion deformities despite vigorous physiotherapy.

Maturation of the skeleton may be delayed, normal, or (rarely) advanced in Down syndrome. The slow growth in Down syndrome is due to premature degeneration of the cartilage columns in the metaphyses of the tubular bones. The most valuable diagnostic changes in the skeleton in Down syndrome are noted in the pelvic bones, where they are most significant during the first weeks and months of life when clinical diagnosis may be equivocal. The acetabular angles are decreased, and the iliac wings are relatively large and flare laterally (see Section IX, Part VI, Fig. 55, page 2221).

TUBEROUS SCLEROSIS

Tuberous sclerosis is a congenital malformation syndrome, probably with an autosomal dominant inheri-

tance, that consists of a classical clinical triad of epilepsy, mental retardation, and skin lesions of adenoma sebaceum. Widespread hamartomas are noted in the skin, brain, eyes, kidneys, heart, lungs, liver, and bones. Pituitary, thyroid, and adrenal dysfunction as well as abnormal glucose tolerance and elevated alkaline phosphatase levels have been noted in patients with tuberous sclerosis. Calcified subependymal nodules around the lateral ventricles and scattered intracerebral calcifications of varying size are frequent manifestations. Bone changes in tuberous sclerosis are asymptomatic and present in up to 50% of patients. The findings may be mistaken for osteoblastic metastases. Patchy sclerotic areas involving the calvarium, spine, and pelvis; lytic lesions in the phalanges; and wavy cortical hyperostosis of the metacarpals and metatarsals can be observed. Occasionally, diffuse sclerosis of a single rib may develop (Fig. 1).

NEUROFIBROMATOSIS

Neurofibromatosis (NF) is a relatively common disease with an autosomal dominant inheritance. Neurofibromatosis types 1 and 2 are multisystem disorders associated with a variety of neoplastic and non-neoplastic manifestations that typically progress in severity during the lifetime of the affected patient. The cutaneous abnormalities consist of café au lait spots ("coast of California" type with smooth margins), neurofibromas, plexiform neurofibromas, schwannomas, and lipomas. Plexiform neurofibromas may be associated with massive enlargement of the skin, soft tissues, and underlying skeleton (see Section IX, Part XIII, Chapter 1, Table 2, page 2428). Macrocranium, spinal cord and cerebral tumors, optic gliomas, and meningiomas are frequently associated with NF. There is an increased incidence of intracranial aneurysms. The endocrine abnormalities include multiple endocrine adenomatosis, hyperparathyroidism, pheochromocytoma, carcinoid tumor, and sexual precocity. Hypertension in this disorder may be idiopathic, secondary to associated renal artery stenosis or to pheochromocytoma.

NF1 is the most common of the phakomatoses and has a variety of localized or, more frequently, systemic manifestations throughout the thorax, abdomen, pelvis, and extremities, whereas NF2 is characterized by eighth nerve acoustic neuromas and other central nervous system tumors. Classical computed tomographic findings in NF1 with thoracic involvement include small, well-defined subcutaneous neurofibromas, focal thoracic scoliosis, posterior vertebral scalloping, enlarged neural foramina, and characteristic rib abnormalities caused by mesenchymal dysplasia or erosion from adjacent neurofibromas. Abdominopelvic involvement includes desmoid tumors that arise in the retroperitoneal, mesenteric, and paraspinal regions of older children and adults. Magnetic resonance imaging is the modality of choice in evaluating affected patients (see Section IX, Part II, Chapter 2, Fig. 10, page 2027 and Section IX, Part IV, Fig. 18, page 2110). The classical peripheral manifestations of NF1 include limb hemihypertrophy, pseudarthrosis, peripheral nerve neurofibromas, and subcutaneous and plexiform neurofibromas. Steenbrugge et al. reported a 13-year-old child with NF1 who manifested recurrent massive subperiosteal hematoma following a blunt trauma. Gonzalez-Martin et al. reported a patient with both NF1 and McCune-Albright syndrome.

Other skeletal manifestations in NF include osseous lytic lesions, many of which are due to mesodermal dysplasia, gigantism, pseudoarthrosis of long bones, and

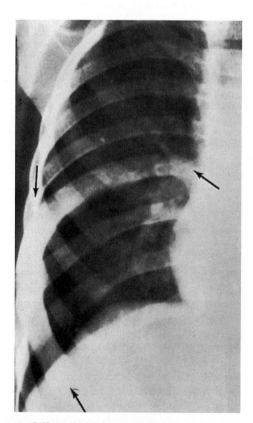

FIGURE 1. Diffuse thickening and sclerosis of the sixth right rib *(arrows)* of a child of 3 years who suffered from convulsions and adenoma sebaceum, characteristic of tuberous sclerosis. The rest of the skeleton was normal. There were also numerous intracranial patches of calcium density. (Courtesy of Dr. Harold G. Jacobson, New York City, NY.)

hypoplasia of the posterosuperior orbital wall resulting from agenesis of the greater wing of the sphenoid. Congenital pseudoarthrosis of the tibia is a difficult orthopedic problem in patients with NF1. Boero et al. retrospectively reviewed results of surgery for congenital pseudarthrosis of the tibia (CPT) using Ilizarov's external fixator. Of the 21 tibias operated on, 17 healed after the first treatment and 4 did not. Of the 17 healed tibias, 4 re-fractured and were retreated by using a variety of methods; only 1 healed. Patients who were 5 years or older at operation had better results. Their results showed that treatment with Ilizarov's fixator allows healing over time in 66.7% of cases of CPT associated with NF1.

WILSON'S DISEASE

Wilson's disease (hepatolenticular degeneration) is a rare autosomal recessive disorder of copper metabolism characterized by an increased absorption of copper from the gastrointestinal tract; an increased concentration of copper in liver, kidney, brain, and other organs; and elevated urinary copper excretion. Serum copper is normally bound to ceruloplasmin. Serum levels of ceruloplasmin and copper are generally decreased in patients with Wilson's disease. Major manifestations include deranged basal ganglia function and irreversible hepatic cirrhosis.

The renal tubular abnormalities consist of aminoaciduria and phosphaturia, with resultant hypophosphatemia, which contribute to metabolic bone disease. The skeletal findings include generalized bone rarefaction, evidence of rickets and osteomalacia, irregular fragmentation of subchondral bone, chondrocalcinosis, and osteosclerosis near the larger joints. Patellofemoral involvement is often present. Irregularities of the vertebral margins resemble Schmorl's nodes and Scheuermann's disease (juvenile kyphosis). Among 38 patients, Mindelzun and associates found normal skeleton in only 5; 9 had subarticular cysts. The bones near the joints were "fragmented" in 6 patients.

PHENYLKETONURIA

Phenylketonuria, the result of a failure of conversion of phenylalanine to tyrosine, is a hereditary condition in which mental retardation can be severe if diagnosis is not made in the newborn period and appropriate therapy instituted. In 5 of 10 patients younger than 13 months, Feinberg and Fisch (1962) found cupping and fraying of the distal ends of the radius and ulna but without demineralization of the zone of provisional calcification as in rickets (Fig. 2). Fisch et al. found bone abnormalities on wrist radiographs in 56 of 73 infants between 6 and 57 days old. Murdoch and Holman found similar bone changes in two patients who had been fed low-phenylalanine diets since infancy. The skeletal lesions have been found in patients prior to the beginning of dietary treatment, suggesting that they do not result from the treatment.

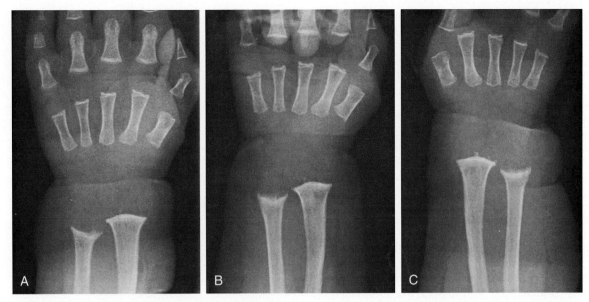

FIGURE 2. Radiograph showing opaque longitudinal spiculation of the metaphysis of the radius and, to a lesser degree, of the ulna of a boy 2 months of age who had chemically proven phenylketonuria. **A,** At 2 months, the spicules project beyond the provisional zone of calcification into the contiguous epiphyseal cartilage. **B** and **C,** At 4 and 5 months of age, respectively, the spiculations are buried into the shaft as the bone grows distalward. The cupping of the ulna and slightly frayed appearance of the metaphyses are both suggestive of rickets, but the intact provisional zones of calcification negate this diagnosis. (From Feinberg SB, Fisch RO: Roentgenologic findings in growing long bones in phenylketonuria. Radiology 1962;78:394–398, with permission.)

CARDIOVASCULAR DISEASES

Patients with poorly compensated cardiovascular disease, particularly cyanotic heart disease, exhibit retardation of growth and skeletal maturation. Berdah et al. described hypertrophic osteoarthropathy (HOA) in two patients with tetralogy of Fallot. However, although clubbing is frequently seen in these patients, HOA is an uncommon manifestation of congenital heart disease. Cranial changes similar to those seen in chronic hemolytic anemia have been described only rarely.

The skeletal changes associated with congenital heart disease were studied by White and associates in 126 adolescents and young adults. Thoracic scoliosis was present in 44% of the patients, none of whom had congenital vertebral anomalies. Sixty percent of patients with cyanotic heart disease had scoliosis, compared to 24% of acyanotic patients. The scoliosis of congenital heart disease differed from idiopathic scoliosis primarily in the more nearly equal female:male ratio; females outnumber males three to one in patients with idiopathic scoliosis without heart disease. Furthermore, patients with cyanotic heart disease suffered much more severe deformity than those with acyanotic disease. Spinal malformations are frequent in children with congenital heart disease. Forney and associates reported a mother and two daughters with mitral insufficiency, conductive deafness, short stature, and skeletal anomalies. These included fused cervical vertebrae and carpal fusion in all three patients and tarsal fusion in only one. Sternal anomalies with premature fusion of the chondromanubrial joint and pigeon-breast deformity

are frequently associated with congenital heart disease. Premature narrowing of the cartilage between adjacent centers seen in lateral projections of very young infants may precede protrusion of the sternum. The observation of premature fusion of sternal ossification centers in lateral chest radiographs may serve as a marker for possible congenital heart disease. Sanchez-Cascos studied the association between cardiac and sternal anomalies in a series of 2000 cases of congenital heart disease and reported an incidence of pectus excavatum of 2.5% and of pectus carinatum of 3%.

HOLT-ORAM SYNDROME

Among the many syndromes associated with congenital cardiac disease, Holt-Oram syndrome is one of the most commonly mentioned. This autosomal dominant condition presents with intracardiac shunts, conduction disturbances, pulmonary hypertension, or a combination of these, and skeletal abnormalities of the upper limbs. The radial rays are most conspicuously involved in the forearm, wrist, and hand. The thumb is missing or hypoplastic, or has three phalanges and looks like a finger (see Section IX, Part VI, Fig. 22, page 2114). The first metacarpal may be absent or may appear thin, but its length is actually increased in relation to normal standards; this is shown clearly in a metacarpophalangeal profile-pattern analysis described by Poznanski and associates. Abnormalities of the carpal bones are very common, especially deformity of the scaphoid bone and extra carpal bones.

Other skeletal anomalies include scapular tilt, coraco-clavicular fusions, and medial humeral epicondyle and sternal deformity. Abnormalities of the radial side of the forearm and hand can occur in association with heart disease but do not qualify as examples of the Holt-Oram syndrome when they are not bilateral, lack the carpal changes, and are associated with other visceral malformations and cardiac malformations different from the intracardiac shunts, conduction disturbances, or pulmonary hypertension characteristic of Holt-Oram syndrome. These are referred to as "other cardiomelic syndromes" and include a wide variety of disorders.

OTHER CARDIOVASCULAR DISEASES

Osteosclerosis is seen in association with supravalvular aortic stenosis and peripheral pulmonary stenoses in the syndrome of *idiopathic hypercalcemia (Williams syndrome)*. A positive metacarpal sign (short third metacarpal) occurs in *Turner's syndrome*, which has a high incidence of coarctation of the aorta. These subjects are discussed in Section IX, Part VI, page 2181.

ALIMENTARY TRACT DISEASES

In patients with *biliary atresia*, rachitic changes in the growing bones were common prior to the commercial

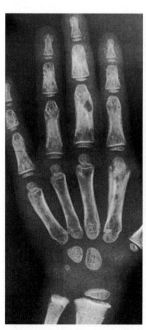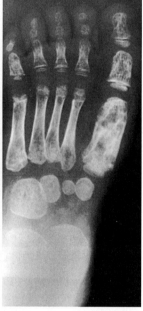

FIGURE 3. Patchy rarefaction and sclerosis of the tubular bones of the hand and foot of a 3-year-old girl who had clinical and radiographic findings typical of acute pancreatitis 6 weeks earlier. These radiographic changes represent the lesions 2 weeks after clinical recovery. Aspiration biopsy of the bone lesions disclosed a cellular debris that lacked bacteria, fungi, and leukocytes. Results of cultures were also negative. (Courtesy of Dr. Patrick Lester, Salt Lake City, UT. From Keating JP, Shackelford GD, Shackelford PG, et al: Pancreatitis and osteolytic lesions. J Pediatr 1972;81:350–353, with permission.)

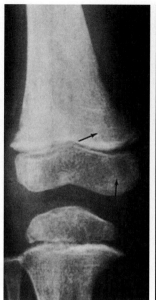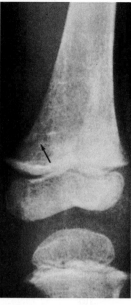

FIGURE 4. Less marked destructive lesions are seen in the metaphyses of the femur *(arrows)* and in the epiphyseal ossification center of the right femur *(arrow, right)* of the patient in Figure 3. (Courtesy of Dr. Patrick Lester, Salt Lake City, UT. From Keating JP, Shackelford GD, Shackelford PG, et al: Pancreatitis and osteolytic lesions. J Pediatr 1972;81:350–353, with permission.)

availability of hydroxylated compounds of vitamin D. Skeletal changes in hepatic rickets are discussed in Section IX, Part VII, Chapter 2, page 2242.

Focal destructive and productive changes, particularly in the tubular bones of the hands and feet (Figs. 3 and 4), have been associated with *acute pancreatitis*. Lesions occur in the skin and in the long bones as well. Characteristically, the lesions do not appear until 3 to 6 weeks after the peak of the pancreatic disease, when the patients are actually improving clinically. The bone lesions appear, enlarge, and become numerous during vigorous antibiotic treatment. They persist for months in some cases and may mimic skeletal abnormalities noted with nonaccidental trauma.

Crohn's regional enteritis has been associated with several skeletal and articular lesions. These include ankylosing granulomatous synovitis, HOA, aseptic necrosis, and granulomatous synovitis. These abnormalities are much more common in adults than in children.

Compton et al. described a new syndrome of Crohn's disease and pachydermoperiostosis associated with antineutrophil cytoplasmic antibodies in three brothers. All of them developed pachydermoperiostosis between ages 14 and 17 years. Pachydermoperiostosis preceded Crohn's ileocolitis by 6 and 20 years in two probands. Inheritance is most likely autosomal recessive.

Shwachman syndrome includes pancreatic exocrine insufficiency, dysfunction of the bone marrow, and a special form of metaphyseal chondrodysplasia (see Section IX, Part V, Fig. 27, page 2154). Cystic fibrosis (CF) is excluded by a negative sweat test. Rickets associated with gastrointestinal disease in a patient with *chronic granulomatous disease* has been reported. None of the skeletal changes in association with gastrointestinal disease are particularly diagnostic other than the bizarre changes of acute pancreatitis and the metaphyseal lesions of the Schwachman syndrome.

Erkul et al. reported a 7-year-old girl with multiple hamartomatous polyps of the colon and bilateral and symmetric lamellar periosteal reaction and osteopenia in her extremity bones. The authors' review of the literature revealed previous reports of association of generalized juvenile polyposis and HOA in five cases; arteriovenous malformations were present in four of them. In the case described by Erkul et al., the polyps were localized in the colon, without associated arteriovenous malformation.

RESPIRATORY DISEASES

CYSTIC FIBROSIS

Growth and development of the skeleton may be retarded in severe, longstanding diseases of the lungs and bronchi, especially CF. Some patients also develop arthropathy. Dixey et al. reviewed the clinical features in 29 patients with CF who had significant arthropathy. Twelve had episodic arthritis characterized by repeated short attacks of severe, incapacitating polyarthritis, which in seven was associated with fever and erythema nodosum. Ten patients also had hypertrophic pulmonary osteoarthropathy (HPOA) (Fig. 5). Rush et al. reviewed clinical and radiographic manifestations in 27 patients with CF and joint complaints. Twelve patients had arthritis, 11 had HPOA, and 4 had neck and back pain. A subgroup of these patients later developed persistent synovitis with progressive asymmetric osseous erosive changes. The etiology of CF arthritis is unclear; some investigators postulate that it may relate to chronic infection and immune complex mechanisms. CF arthritis can be contrasted with CF-induced HPOA, which is associated with worse lung disease, a male predominance, and an older age (mean age 20 years) of onset of symptoms. The neck and back pain may relate to an associated scoliosis or kyphosis in CF. Lipnick and Glass reviewed radiographs of the hands and wrists and of the tibias and fibulas in 56 patients with CF. The fourth metacarpal was shortened in 5 of 56 patients (9%). HPOA was present in three patients (5.5%).

Massie et al. reviewed bone scans in 125 patients with CF; 17 had musculoskeletal complications, including HPOA in 11, kyphosis in 4, and thoracic deformity in 2 children. Three patients with HPOA died within 12 months of reporting symptoms. Increasing age with deteriorating clinical and pulmonary function were associated with a higher incidence of musculoskeletal involvement. The development of symptomatic HPOA is a marker of poor prognosis.

HYPERTROPHIC OSTEOARTHROPATHY

HOA, well known in adults, is rarely encountered in children. The clinical features include clubbing of the

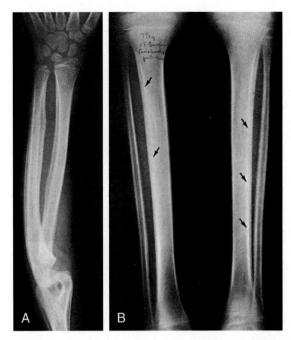

FIGURE 5. Radiographs of the left forearm **(A)** and lower legs **(B)** showing generalized lamellated cortical hyperostosis (hypertrophic pulmonary osteoarthropathy) *(arrows)* in a girl 7 years of age who had had cystic fibrosis of the pancreas with severe obstructive emphysema, recurrent bronchopneumonia, and cor pulmonale since the second half of her first year. On both sides, the femur, humerus, tibia, fibula, radius, and ulna were affected.

fingers and toes, arthritis, and a sometimes painful periosteal new bone formation along the tubular bones. Ansell et al. suggested that HOA should be considered in any child who presents with a synovitis of the knees, ankles, and wrists associated with clubbing of the fingers. Apart from a hereditary form (primary HOA), most of the cases encountered in children are secondary and associated with conditions such as chronic pulmonary disease (e.g., cystic fibrosis, tuberculosis), congenital heart disease, biliary atresia, and polyposis coli (Table 1).

Wadhwa et al. reported a case of HOA in a 14-month-old girl with adult respiratory distress syndrome secondary to severe burn injury. Hugosson et al. described typical radiographic findings of HPOA in a 5-year-old Saudi boy who presented with clubbing of fingers and

Table 1 ■ CONDITIONS ASSOCIATED WITH HYPERTROPHIC OSTEOARTHROPATHY
Cyanotic congenital heart disease
Chronic pulmonary infection (e.g., bronchiectasis, empyema, lung abscess)
Cystic fibrosis
Cirrhosis of the liver
Chronic ulcerative colitis
Prostaglandin therapy
Nasopharyngeal carcinoma
Lymphoma
Pachydermoperiostosis
Polyposis coli

painful joints. The underlying cause of the condition was a chronic lung inflammation resulting from lipoid pneumonia caused by aspiration of ingested animal fat in infancy.

CUTANEOUS DISEASES

PACHYDERMOPERIOSTOSIS

In addition to the secondary type of HOA, a rare idiopathic type exists that occurs predominantly in males and is not associated with any known disease process. When idiopathic hypertrophic osteoarthropathy (IHOA) is associated with pachyderma, it is called pachydermoperiostosis. In extremely rare instances, IHOA may occur without pachyderma. Bartolozzi et al. reported a 3-year-old boy with primary hypertrophic osteoarthropathy without pachydermia. Jajic et al. reported clinical, radiologic, scintigraphic, and histologic findings in 76 patients with primary HOA. Family history was positive, and clubbing of the digits and toes was found in all patients, while hyperhydrosis was found in 85%, and swollen and painful joints were noted in 68% of patients. Histologic evaluation in 18 patients showed periarticular edema and moderate cellular activity. Periosteal new bone formation along the long bones was also found in all patients, while scintigraphy, performed in 44 patients, was positive in 18 (33.5%) patients in the active phase of the disease. Diren et al. reported a family with five members suffering from primary HOA, characterized by swollen and painful joints and clubbing of distal phalanges of hands and feet. Other conditions associated with periosteal new bone formation are listed in Table 2.

OTHER CUTANEOUS DISEASES

Several congenital disorders have been described in which lesions of the skeleton and the skin and its appendages—the hair, nails, and teeth—are associated. *Polyostotic fibrous dysplasia (McCune-Albright syndrome)* is characterized by patchy areas of excessive skin pigmentation (café au lait spots), disseminated fibro-osseous lesions, and precocious puberty in females. The nails and teeth are hypoplastic in the *Ellis-van Creveld syndrome* (chondroectodermal dysplasia), and *osteopoikilosis* may be complicated by dermatofibrosis lenticularis. The combination of dysplastic nails, hypoplasia of the radial head, bilateral iliac horns and absence, hypoplasia, or dislocation of the patella is a distinct clinical entity that has been called the *nail–patella syndrome* or osteo-onychodysplasia.

Follicular atrophy of the skin may be an important diagnostic feature of *chondrodysplasia punctata (Conradi-Hünermann type)*, and focal dermal hypoplasia is frequently associated with *osteopathia striata*. Scleroderma-like changes and melorheostosis have been found in conjunction in several patients; the lesions are usually regional, overlying the sites of melorheostosis. Urticaria pigmentosa may be the clue that permits a

Table 2 ■ CONDITIONS ASSOCIATED WITH SYMMETRIC PERIOSTEAL NEW BONE FORMATION
Hypertrophic osteoarthropathy (see Table 1)
Leukemia
Metastatic neuroblastoma
Physiologic in early infancy
Healing rickets
Juvenile rheumatoid arthritis
Battered child syndrome
Venous or lymphatic stasis
Congenital syphilis
Acromegaly
Engelmann's disease
Hypervitaminosis A
Hypervitaminosis D
Infantile cortical hyperostosis
Pachydermoperiostosis
Scurvy
Fluorosis
Congenital hyperphosphatasia
Tuberous sclerosis

diagnosis of *systemic mastocytosis* in a child with widespread skeletal lesions found incidentally in the course of a radiographic survey for gastrointestinal complaints. This subject is discussed in Section IX, Part XIII, Chapter 1, page 2417.

MALIGNANT DISEASES

HOA accompanying a malignant tumor, which is relatively common in adults, is very rare in children. Kebudi et al. reviewed from the literature four children with HOA and Hodgkin's disease. They also reported a 12-year-old boy with intrathoracic Hodgkin's disease and HOA in whom complete remission of Hodgkin's disease and regression of clinical signs and symptoms of HOA were observed after chemotherapy and radiotherapy. Ilhan et al. reported a case of intrathoracic undifferentiated carcinoma of the thymus with HPOA in a 13-year-old girl. Mas Estelles et al. reported three cases of pulmonary plasma cell granuloma in the pediatric age group. In one of the cases, plasma cell granuloma of the lung was seen in association with HOA, which resolved after excision of the mass. Flueckiger et al. reported HOA in a 14-year-old boy with osteosarcoma and pulmonary metastases; the HOA resolved following chemotherapy.

Staalman and Umans reported two children with carcinoma of the nasopharynx who developed HOA. In both, the appearance of HOA was associated with a very poor prognosis. In contrast to suppurative processes in the lungs, in patients with neoplastic disease involving the chest, HOA may precede pulmonary symptoms by 1 to 18 months. Liu et al. retrospectively investigated the incidence of HPOA in adolescent and adult patients with nasopharyngeal carcinoma. HPO was found in 6.6% of the patients, among whom 48% had pulmonary metastases. HPO preceded lung metastases by 7 to 22 months in 52% of these patients.

SUGGESTED READINGS

Renal Diseases

Davis JG: Osseous radiographic findings of chronic renal insufficiency. Radiology 1953;60:406–411

McAfee PC, Cady RB: Endocrinologic and metabolic factors in atypical presentations of slipped capital femoral epiphysis: report of four cases and review of the literature. Clin Orthop 1983;130: 188–197

Central Nervous System Diseases

Benda CE: Mongolism and Cretinism, 2nd ed. New York, Grune & Stratton, 1949

Kottamasu SR, Honasoge M, Frame B: Neuroectodermal and mesodermal dysplasias. In Frame B, Honsoge M, Kottamasu SR (eds): Osteosclerosis, Hyperostosis and Related Disorders. New York, Elsevier Science Publishing Company, 1987a:361–375

Kottamasu SR, Honasoge M, Frame B: Periosteal new bone rormation. In Frame B, Honasoge M, Kottamasu SR (eds): Osteosclerosis, Hyperostosis and Related Disorders. New York, Elsevier Science Publishing Company, 1987b:270–289

Tuberous Sclerosis

Fluckiger F, Kullnig P: Skeletal changes in tuberous sclerosis. Rontgenblatter 1988;41:246–250

Holt JF, Dickerson WW: Osseous lesions of tuberous sclerosis. Radiology 1952;58:1–7

Kreuzberg B, Koudelkova J: Bone changes in tuberous sclerosis (Bourneville-Pringle disease). Cesk Radiol 1989;43:332–338

Neurofibromatosis

Boero S, Catagni M, Donzelli O, et al: Congenital pseudarthrosis of the tibia associated with neurofibromatosis-1: treatment with Ilizarov's device. J Pediatr Orthop 1997;17:675–684

Elster AD: Radiologic screening in the neurocutaneous syndromes: strategies and controversies. AJNR Am J Neuroradiol 1992;13:1071–1077

Flexon PB, Nadol JB Jr, Schuknecht HF, et al: Bilateral acoustic neurofibromatosis (neurofibromatosis 2): a disorder distinct from von Recklinghausen's neurofibromatosis (neurofibromatosis 1). Ann Otol Rhinol Laryngol 1991;100:830–834

Fortman BJ, Kuszyk BS, Urban BA, Fishman EK: Neurofibromatosis type 1: a diagnostic mimicker at CT. Radiographics 2001;21:601–612

Gillespie JE: Imaging in neurofibromatosis type 2: screening using magnetic resonance imaging. Ear Nose Throat J 1999;78:102–109

Gonzalez-Martin J, Glover S, Dixon S, et al: Neurofibromatosis type 1 and McCune-Albright syndrome occurring in the same patient. Br J Dermatol 2000;143:1288–1291

Gutmann DH, Aylsworth A, Carey JC, et al: The diagnostic evaluation and multidisciplinary management of neurofibromatosis 1 and neurofibromatosis 2. JAMA 1997;278:1493–1494

Pollack IF, Mulvihill JJ: Neurofibromatosis 1 and 2. Brain Pathol 1997;7:823–836

Steenbrugge F, Verstraete K, Poffyn B, et al: Recurrent massive subperiosteal hematoma in a patient with neurofibromatosis. Eur Radiol 2001;11:480–483

von Zitzewitz H, Kreitner KF, Kohler H: Osseous manifestations of Bourneville-Pringle disease. Aktuelle Radiol 1995;5:53–55

Wilson's Disease

Cavallino R, Grossman H: Wilson's disease presenting with rickets. Radiology 1968;90:493–494

Gow PJ, Smallwood RA, Angus PW, et al: Diagnosis of Wilson's disease: an experience over three decades. Gut 2000;46:415

Mindelzun RR, Elkin M, Scheinberg IH, et al: Skeletal changes in Wilson's disease: a radiological study. Radiology 1970;94:127–132

Pilloni L, Lecca S, Coni P, et al: Wilson's disease with late onset. Dig Liver Dis 2000;32:180

Riley D, Wiznitzer M, Schwartz S, Zinn AB: A 13-year-old boy with cognitive impairment, retinoblastoma, and Wilson disease. Neurology 2001;57:141–143

Robertson WM: Wilson's disease [review]. Arch Neurol 2000;57: 276–277

Rosenoer VM, Michell AC: Skeletal changes in Wilson's disease (hepato-lenticular degeneration). Br J Radiol 1959;32:805–809

Svetel M, Kozic D, Stefanova E, et al: Dystonia in Wilson's disease. Mov Disord 2001;16:719–723

Wu JC, Huang CC, Jeng LB, Chu NS: Correlation of neurological manifestations and MR images in a patient with Wilson's disease after liver transplantation. Acta Neurol Scand 2000;102:135–139

Yuce A, Kocak N, Gurakan F, Ozen H: Wilson's disease presented with fulminating hepatic failure in children. Dig Dis Sci 2000; 45:704

Phenylketonuria

Feinberg SB, Fisch RC: Roentgenologic findings in growing long bones in phenylketonuria. Radiology 1962;78:394–398

Feinberg SB, Fisch RO: Bone changes in untreated neonatal phenylketonuric patients: a new radiographic observation and interpretation. J Pediatr 1972;81:540–543

Fisch RO, Feinberg SB, Weisberg S, Day D: Bony changes of PKU in neonates unrelated to phenylalanine levels. J Inherit Metab Dis 1991;14:890–895

Hillman L, Schlotzhauer C, Lee D, et al: Decreased bone mineralization in children with phenylketonuria under treatment. Eur J Pediatr 1996;155(Suppl 1):S148–S152

Murdoch MM, Holman GH: Roentgenologic bone changes in phenylketonuria: relation to dietary phenylalanine and serum alkaline phosphatase. Am J Dis Child 1964;107:523–532

Schwahn B, Mokov E, Scheidhauer K, et al: Decreased trabecular bone mineral density in patients with phenylketonuria measured by peripheral quantitative computed tomography. Acta Paediatr 1998; 87:61–63

Woodring JH, Rosenbaum HD: Bone changes in phenylketonuria reassessed. AJR Am J Roentgenol 1981;137:241–243

Cardiovascular Diseases

Berdah C, Girardet JP, Silberman B, et al: Hypertrophic osteoarthropathy and congenital cyanotic heart defects. Arch Fr Pediatr 1989;46:31–33

Chang CH: Holt-Oram syndrome. Radiology 1967;88:479–483

Currarino G, Silverman FN: Premature obliteration of the sternal sutures and pigeon-breast deformity. Radiology 1958;70: 532–540

Forney WR, Robinson SJ, Pascoe DJ: Congenital heart disease, deafness and skeletal malformations: a new syndrome? J Pediatr 1966;68:14–26

Holt M, Oram S: Familial heart disease with skeletal malformation. Br Heart J 1965;22:236–242

Poznanski AK, Stern AM, Gall JC Jr: Skeletal anomalies in genetically determined congenital heart disease. Radiol Clin North Am 1971; 9:435–458

Sanchez-Cascos A: Association of cardiac and sternal malformations. An Esp Pediatr 1989;30:272–274

Sanchez-Cascos A, Sanchez-Harguinday L, De Rabago P: Cardioauditory syndromes: cardiac and genetic study of 511 deaf-mute children. Br Heart J 1969;31:26–33

Shamberger RC, Welch KJ: Surgical correction of chondromanubrial deformity (Currarino-Silverman syndrome). J Pediatr Surg 1988;23: 319–322

White RI Jr, Jordan CE, Fischer KC, et al: Skeletal changes associated with adolescent congenital heart disease. Am J Roentgenol Radium Ther Nucl Med 1972;116:531–538

Alimentary Tract Diseases

Baker DH, Harris RC: Congenital absence of the intrahepatic bile ducts. Am J Roentgenol Radium Ther Nucl Med 1964;91:875–884

Compton RF, Sandborn WJ, Yang H, et al: A new syndrome of Crohn's disease and pachydermoperiostosis in a family. Gastroenterology 1997;112:241–249

Erkul PE, Ariyurek OM, Altinok D, et al: Colonic hamartomatous polyposis associated with hypertrophic osteoarthropathy. Pediatr Radiol 1994;24:145–146

Greenwald M, Couper R, Laxer R, et al: Gastroesophageal reflux and esophagitis-associated hypertrophic osteoarthropathy. J Pediatr Gastroenterol Nutr 1996;23:178–181

Hogan MB, Millman E, Jones E, Wilson NW: Rickets associated with gastrointestinal disease in a patient with chronic granulomatous disease. J Allergy Clin Immunol 1998;101:851–853

Keating JP, Shackelford GD, Shackelford PG, et al: Pancreatitis and osteolytic lesions. J Pediatr 1972;81:350–353

Nugent FW, Glazer D, Fernandez-Herlihy L: Crohn's colitis associated with granulomatous bone disease. N Engl J Med 1976;294:262–263.

Rosario N, Farias L: Gastroesophageal reflux and esophagitis-associated hypertrophic osteoarthropathy. J Pediatr Gastroenterol Nutr 1996;23:178–181

Schutte HE, Wackwitz JD: Case Report 171: Metastatic fat necrosis involving the tubular bones of the hands (and probably the feet) secondary to traumatic pancreatitis. Skeletal Radiol 1981;7:147–149

Sty JR, Krecak J, Gregg DC: Bone scintigraphy: hypertrophic osteoarthropathy in biliary atresia. Clin Nucl Med 1987;12:657–658

Sutcliffe J, Stanley P: Metaphyseal chondrodysplasia with dwarfism, pancreatic insufficiency and neutropenia. Pediatr Radiol 1973;1:119–126

Respiratory Diseases

Ansell BM: Hypertrophic osteoarthropathy in the paediatric age. Clin Exp Rheumatol 1992;10:15–18

Dixey J, Redington AN, Butler RC, et al: The arthropathy of cystic fibrosis. Ann Rheum Dis 1988;47:218–223

Gervais DA, Bagley L, Connolly S: Neonate with respiratory distress and diffuse skeletal abnormalities. Acad Radiol 1995;2:83–85

Gottlieb C, Sharlin HS, Feld H: Hypertrophic pulmonary osteoarthropathy. J Pediatr 1947;30:462–467

Grossman H, Denning CR, Baker DH: Hypertrophic osteoarthropathy in cystic fibrosis. Am J Dis Child 1964;107:1–6

Gutowska-Grzegorczyk G, Michalak-Wiejak H: Hypertrophic osteoarthropathy of cystic fibrosis. Pediatr Pol 1995;70:263–267

Hugosson C, Bahabri S, Rifai A, al-Dalaan A: Hypertrophic osteoarthropathy caused by lipoid pneumonia. Pediatr Radiol 1995;25:482–483

Lipnick RN, Glass RB: Bone changes associated with cystic fibrosis. Skeletal Radiol 1992;21:115–116

Massie RJ, Towns SJ, Bernard E, et al: The musculoskeletal complications of cystic fibrosis. J Paediatr Child Health 1998;34:467–470

Rush PJ, Shore A, Coblentz C, et al: The musculoskeletal manifestations of cystic fibrosis. Semin Arthritis Rheum 1986;15:213–225

Sehgal SK, Prasad SR, Wadhwa A: Hypertrophic osteoarthropathy in pulmonary tuberculosis. Indian Pediatr 1987;24:1161

Wadhwa N, Balsam D, Ciminera P: Hypertrophic osteoarthropathy in a young child with adult respiratory distress syndrome (ARDS) secondary to burns. Pediatr Radiol 1992;22:539–540

Pachydermoperiostosis

Bartolozzi G, Bernini G, Maggini M: Hypertrophic osteoarthropathy without pachydermia: idiopathic form. Am J Dis Child 1975;129:849–851

Bhate DV, Pizarro AJ, Greenfield GB: Idiopathic hypertrophic osteoarthropathy without pachyderma. Radiology 1978;129:379–381

Diren HB, Kutluk MT, Karabent A, et al: Primary hypertrophic osteoarthropathy. Pediatr Radiol 1986;16:231–234

Gomez Rodriguez N, Atanes Sandoval A, Grana Gil J, et al: Pachydermoperiostosis (primary hypertrophic osteoarthropathy). An Med Interna 1990;7:80–82

Jajic Z, Jajic I, Nemcic T: Primary hypertrophic osteoarthropathy: clinical, radiologic, and scintigraphic characteristics. Arch Med Res 2001;32:136–142

Schumacher HR Jr: Hypertrophic osteoarthropathy: rheumatologic manifestations. Clin Exp Rheumatol 1992;10(Suppl 7):35–40

Cutaneous Diseases

Other Cutaneous Diseases

Kottamasu SR, Honasoge M, Frame B: Neuroectodermal and mesodermal dysplasias. In Osteosclerosis, Hyperostosis and Related Disorders. New York, Elsevier Science Publishing Company, 1987:361–375

Silengo M, Luzzatti L, Silverman FN: Clinical and genetic aspects of Conradi-Hunermann disease: a report of 3 familial cases and review of the literature. J Pediatr 1980;97:911–917

Thompson NM, Allen CEL, Andrews GS, et al: Scleroderma and melorheostosis: report of a case. J Bone Joint Surg Br 1951;33:430–433

Williams HJ, Hoyer JP: Radiographic diagnosis of osteoonychodysostosis in infancy. Radiology 1973;109:151 154

Malignant Diseases

Desnoulez L, Nelken B, Lambilliotte A, Robert Y: Radiology case of the month: Pulmonary hypertrophic osteoarthropathy in the course of Hodgkin's disease. Arch Pediatr 1998;5:1253–1255

Flueckiger F, Fotter R, Hausegger K, Urban C: Hypertrophic osteoarthropathy caused by lung metastasis of an osteosarcoma. Pediatr Radiol 1989;20:128–130

Gharbi A, Benjelloun A, Ouzidane L, Ksiyer M: Hypertrophic osteoarthropathy associated with malignant thymoma in a child. J Radiol 1997;78:303–304

Ilhan I, Kutluk T, Gogus S, et al: Hypertrophic pulmonary osteoarthropathy in a child with thymic carcinoma: an unusual presentation in childhood. Med Pediatr Oncol 1994;23:140–143

Kebudi R, Ayan I, Erseven G, et al: Hypertrophic osteoarthropathy and intrathoracic Hodgkin disease of childhood. Med Pediatr Oncol 1997;29:578–581

Ladeb MF, Chaabane M, Gannouni A: Hypertrophic osteoarthropathy in nasopharyngeal carcinoma of a child. Pediatr Radiol 1988;18:339

Liu RS, Chen YK, Yen SH, et al: Hypertrophic pulmonary osteoarthropathy in nasopharyngeal carcinoma: an early sign of pulmonary metastasis. Nucl Med Commun 1995;16:785–789

Mas Estelles F, Andres V, Vallcanera A, et al: Plasma cell granuloma of the lung in childhood: atypical radiologic findings and association with hypertrophic osteoarthropathy. Pediatr Radiol 1995;25:369–372

Staalman CR, Umans U: Hypertrophic osteoarthropathy in childhood malignancy. Med Pediatr Oncol 1993;21:676–679

PART XIV

THE JOINTS

PAUL S. BABYN
MARILYN D. RANSON

NORMAL ANATOMY

Joints comprise the tissues that allow normal motion between articulating bones. Depending on the type of interposed tissue, joints may be classified into fibrous, cartilaginous, or synovial articulations. Fibrous joints include the cranial sutures and syndesmoses where the articulating bones are bound together either by a fibrous interosseous ligament or fibrous membrane. Cartilaginous joints have interposed cartilage connecting adjacent bones. These joints may be temporary, as in the synchondroses or growth plates between the primary and secondary ossification centers of the tubular bones, or permanent, as in the symphysis pubis. Most common are synovial joints, where the joint cavity contains synovial fluid and articular cartilage covers the opposing ends of the articulating bones (Fig. 1).

Synovial joints are contained within a joint capsule that arises from the periosteum near the ends of the opposing bones. The joint capsule usually originates near the epiphyseal plate to encompass the epiphysis; however, for some joints, it also contains a portion of the metaphysis (as in the hip joint), making these joints more susceptible to infection arising from the metaphysis. The outer layer of the joint capsule is fibrous tissue that develops variable thickness as surrounding capsular ligaments thicken and reinforce the capsule. The synovial membrane lies along the inner aspect of the capsule and lines the nonarticular portion of the joint. Composed of two layers, a thin cellular intima and a vascular subintima containing blood vessels and lymphatics, the synovial membrane secretes synovial fluid to both lubricate and nourish articular cartilage. Normally, the articular cartilage surfaces are in close apposition; however, in some synovial joints, an intervening disk of fibrocartilage is present (e.g., the menisci of the knee) that separates the apposing articular cartilage. The normal amount of synovial fluid is usually slight but varies with each individual joint.

Articular cartilage is derived from the immature articular epiphyseal cartilage complex. During infancy and childhood, epiphyseal and articular cartilage are directly continuous with each other. With maturation, the underlying epiphyseal cartilage is progressively ossified until only the covering articular cartilage remains when growth is completed.

Fat pads may also be present within the joint capsule. Bursae are fluid-filled spaces in the periarticular connective space. They are lined with a cellular membrane similar to the synovial covering of the articular spaces and are located at sites of maximal frictional impact between neighboring movable structures. Variable in number, bursae may be multilocular and often communicate with one another and the adjacent joint space. For example, the multiple bursae around the knee are shown in Figure 2.

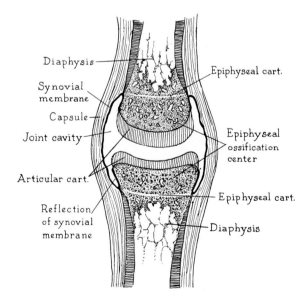

FIGURE 1. Schematic representation of the principal structures in a typical joint. The synovial membrane is the inner aspect of the articular capsule; it does not extend onto the articular cartilages. The joint cavity is artificially dilated to many times its normal depth.

2455

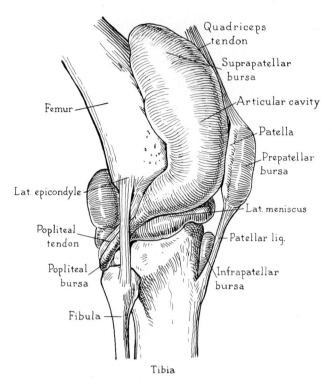

FIGURE 2. Normal bursae around the knee joint.

NORMAL IMAGING APPEARANCE

Composed almost entirely of tissues of water density, normal articular components are all of a similar radiographic density. Thus the individual components of the normal joint cannot be clearly differentiated from each other or from neighboring muscles, fascia, tendons, ligaments, nerves, or vessels by conventional radiography. Displacement of fat deposits in fascial and intermuscular planes readily demonstrates abnormal intraarticular content, including joint effusions in the elbow and ankle. However, around the hip, the shape of these radiolucent stripes and their relationship to the underlying joint is complex (Fig. 3), making accurate determi-

nation of hip joint effusions difficult because they are modified by slight changes of femoral rotation and abduction.

In the newborn, radiography demonstrates wide areas between the bony structures on the two sides of the joints (Fig. 4). These are filled with the unossified epiphyseal cartilage that, as it ossifies, ultimately narrows the separation to the thickness of the opposing layers of articular cartilage. A vacuum phenomenon caused by the presence of gas within a joint can occur normally and appear radiographically as a crescentic lucency. This may follow a sudden lowering of intra-articular pressure by endogenous muscle pulls or from external traction. The gases move from contiguous structures to the lowered pressure in the suddenly expanded joint space. Vacuum phenomena are most frequently evident in the shoulders and hips of infants when the extremities are suddenly abducted during positioning for a radiographic study (Fig. 5). The gas is rapidly absorbed or replaced by fluid even if the distraction force is maintained. In the presence of a significant joint effusion, the vacuum phenomenon cannot normally be produced, and its presence has been relied on to exclude a significant effusion. However, a recent case report has demonstrated a significant effusion sonographically following a positive traction sign. Vacuum phenomena can be seen on sonography and magnetic resonance imaging (MRI). On MRI, intra-articular gas may simulate meniscal tears, intra-articular loose bodies, or chondrocalcinosis.

Although plain films should almost always be used initially to evaluate joints, the introduction of cross-sectional imaging techniques has provided a significant improvement in anatomic delineation and diagnosis. Sonography is ideal for assessing the pediatric musculoskeletal system largely because of its ability to visualize cartilage, which is abundant in the immature skeleton. Hyaline cartilage is hypoechoic and allows through-transmission of the sound beam because of its homogeneous structure. Tiny specular echoes, which represent vascular cartilage canals, help differentiate cartilage from fluid. Cartilage canals are prominent in infancy and early childhood and diminish with advancing age.

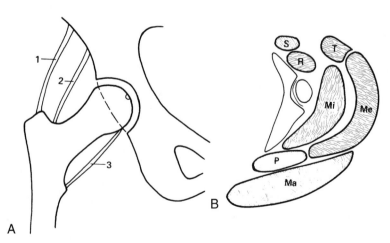

FIGURE 3. Diagrams of fat planes adjacent to the hip. **A,** Frontal plane. *1,* More superficial of the two lateral fat planes. *2,* More medial lateral fat plane. *3,* Fat plane medial to the hip. Plane 1 is cast by fat between the gluteus medius and minimus muscles and 2, by the fat anteriorly between the rectus femoris muscle and the tensor fasciae latae muscle and is continuous with the more narrow fat plane that overlies the capsule; plane 3 derives from fat along the medial border of the iliopsoas muscle. **B,** Horizontal section. *S* = sartorius; *R* = rectus femoris; *T* = tensor fasciae latae; *Mi, Me, Ma* = gluteus minimus, medius, and maximus, respectively; *P* = piriformis. (Modified from Reichmann S: Roentgenologic soft tissue appearances in hip joint disease. Acta Radiol 1967;6:167–176.)

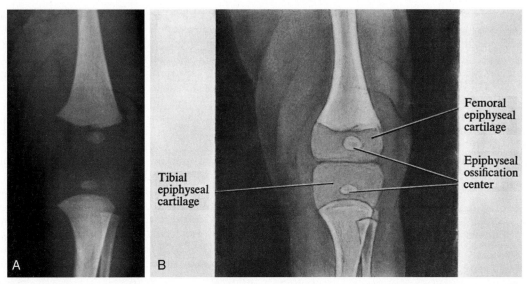

FIGURE 4. Cartilage space between the ends of the opposing bones at the knee joint of a newborn infant. **A,** Radiograph. **B,** Schematic drawing of **A.** The space between the ends of the opposing bones is occupied by a shadow of water density in the radiograph. In the drawing, this space is filled completely by the epiphyseal cartilages and their overlaying articular cartilages. In the normal living joint, the joint cleft is exceedingly narrow and casts an insignificant shadow in the radiograph.

Fibrocartilage is echogenic, especially within the acetabular labrum and menisci. Sonography is sensitive in detecting joint effusion, particularly in the hip and shoulder, where plain films are insensitive. It can demonstrate synovial thickening, which may be hypervascular with color Doppler examination. Intra-articular masses may also be detected with sonography, although the appearance is often nonspecific. Ultrasound can also be used to assess tendons and ligaments with higher frequency transducers. Tendons normally have an echogenic fibrillar appearance on ultrasound. Fluid or synovial thickening within the tendon sheath appears as an anechoic or hypoechoic halo surrounding the tendon.

Computed tomography (CT) can be used to evaluate the joint space and detect adjacent bone abnormalities, including coalitions, erosions, and subchondral cysts. CT is primarily used to assess osseous structures because

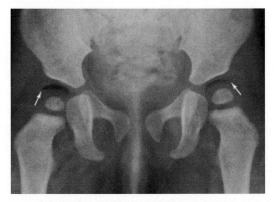

FIGURE 5. Bilateral natural pneumograms of the hips of a normal infant 12 months of age. The radiolucent strips *(arrows)* represent intra-articular gas between the cartilaginous edge of the acetabulum and the epiphyseal cartilage of the femoral head.

MRI now provides better tissue contrast with multiplanar imaging capability.

MRI has had a dramatic impact on the evaluation of joint disease. It can provide multiplanar images without radiation, achieve superb tissue contrast, and define vascular anatomy with or without contrast. However high cost, limited availability, and frequent need for sedation limit its more widespread use. It is the best modality to examine all the components of the joints, including bone marrow, cortical bone, hyaline and fibrocartilage, ligaments, menisci, synovium and joint capsule, joint fluid, and the unossified cartilaginous skeleton.

MRI technique should include multiplanar evaluation with a combination of T_1- and T_2-weighted sequences, fast spin-echo, and postcontrast studies tailored to the specific clinical problem. Appropriate field of view depends on the age and size of the child and the joint and structures needing to be visualized. Cartilaginous structures, including the physis, are well seen with gradient-recalled echo techniques or fat-suppressed fast proton-density sequences. Gadolinium-enhanced MRI can differentiate physeal from epiphyseal cartilage and can visualize normal vessels present within the chondroepiphysis. MRI is useful in detecting synovial abnormalities within the joint and associated changes affecting the articular cartilage and osseous structures. The normal synovium is virtually imperceptible on MRI and enhances only minimally. Slight enhancement may be seen in richly vascularized areas such as the tissues adjacent to the posterior attachment of the temporomandibular joint. A small amount of joint fluid may normally be seen with MRI.

Multiphase bone scintigraphy can help differentiate osseous causes of pain from other causes of joint pain, including synovial, neuromuscular, or periarticular soft tissue disorders. Bone scintigraphy is helpful to establish whether an osseous lesion is solitary or multifocal and can reveal increased activity across the joint in arthritis or infection. Specialized adjuncts to routine scintigraphic imaging include magnification scintigraphy and single-photon emission CT, while dual-energy x-ray absorptiometry is often used in assessment of bone density.

Currently, arthrography is rarely indicated. However, intra-articular contrast injection may be combined with CT, or now more frequently with MRI, to better delineate joint detail, including the evaluation of labral tears within the shoulder or hip joint.

DISEASES OF THE JOINTS

Joint abnormalities may be caused by a wide variety of disorders, including congenital abnormalities, trauma, infection, juvenile rheumatoid arthritis (JRA) and other inflammatory arthritides, synovial disease, malignancy, and numerous noninflammatory mechanical joint lesions. A number of significant joint disorders are discussed in detail elsewhere and are not addressed here, including Legg-Calvé-Perthes disease (see Section IX, Part X, page 2319), slipped capital femoral epiphysis (see Section IX, Part VIII, page 2269), developmental hip dysplasia (see Section IX, Part XV, page 2494) and joint disease related to metabolic disorders (see Section IX, Part VII, page 2232).

CONGENITAL MALFORMATIONS

Many congenital anomalies of the joints can be encountered, including congenital dislocations, subluxation, ankylosis, and other deformities. Usually plain films suffice, but MRI may be of benefit if surgery is planned and better definition of cartilaginous structures or ligaments is needed. These anomalies are not discussed further here because they are discussed elsewhere (see Section IX, Part IV, page 2099). Contractures of one or more joints may be present at birth in a wide variety of syndromes, including arthrogryposis multiplex, fetal alcohol syndrome, chromosomal abnormalities, and nail–patella syndrome. In congenital lateral dislocation of the patella, there is typically a persistent flexion contracture with limited extension. Malposition of the patellar cartilaginous shadow may be overlooked on lateral radiographs unless specifically considered. Larsen's syndrome is commonly associated with multiple congenital dislocations, particularly of the knees, hips, elbows, and feet (see Section IX, Part VI, Figs. 25 and 26, pages 2200 and 2201).

TRAUMA

Injury to joints may occur at birth or following sports injuries or other accidents and abuse. *Hemarthrosis* and *articular fractures* are usually readily recognized with conventional radiography. Occasionally further imaging with CT or MRI is needed to demonstrate undisplaced fractures, osteochondral injury, or bone contusions, especially around the knee. In hemarthrosis, MRI may show fluid–fluid levels from layering of blood components. With osteochondral injury, particularly around the knee or ankle, MRI can demonstrate displacement of bone and cartilaginous fragments and identify loose bodies. Occult purely chondral fractures can occur and may mimic meniscal injury with knee pain. Bone contusions probably represent trabecular microfractures and may be associated with soft tissue damage, including tears of the collateral and cruciate ligaments. Bone contusions are well seen as subchondral high-signal-intensity areas on T_2-weighted MRI sequences with fat suppression. MRI can also show post-traumatic synovitis, especially with gadolinium enhancement.

Cartilaginous injury, as in chondromalacia of the patella, may be noted with cartilage swelling and edema, cartilage surface irregularity, and later thinning, all of which can be appreciated on MRI. Imaging of the menisci, ligaments, and tendons is generally similar to that of adults, with MRI being the most effective imaging modality. Menisci are typically of uniformly low signal on MRI because of their fibrocartilaginous nature. Unlike in adults, normal menisci in childhood often show a triangular higher signal region peripherally as a result of intrameniscal vasculature. This normal finding should not be mistaken for a horizontal tear. Meniscal injuries are not uncommon, especially in active adolescents, and may be associated with injuries to the anterior cruciate or collateral ligaments. In childhood, the posterior horn of the medial meniscus is the most frequent site for a tear, while the anterior cruciate ligament is the most frequently injured knee ligament. High signal may be seen centrally or less frequently along the periphery of the anterior cruciate ligament from intrasubstance tears. MRI and high-frequency sonography may be used in assessment of other tendon and ligamentous injuries, including the patellar tendon for evaluation of Osgood–Schlatter disease at the tibial tuberosity or Sinding-Larsen–Johansson disease at the inferior patella.

Discoid menisci are abnormally thickened and elongated. They most commonly involve the lateral meniscus and may be bilateral in 5% to 20% of patients. Because of their abnormal structure, discoid menisci are susceptible to degeneration or tears (Fig. 6). Patients may present with knee pain, locking, or a clunking sensation. Children with discoid menisci are more commonly symptomatic, and the incidence of tears appears to be higher compared with adults. Symptoms may be secondary to the abnormal thickness interfering with movement, abnormal attachments, or an associated tear. Although its etiology is unknown, Kaplan theorized that the discoid meniscus develops after birth because of the absence of an attachment to the tibia, resulting in abnormal motion.

Plain radiographs are insensitive but may show widening of the lateral joint compartment on a standing frontal view. On MRI, a discoid meniscus is present if there is a transverse width of greater than 14 mm, or if three or more 5-mm-thick contiguous sagittal images reveal continuity of the anterior and posterior horns of

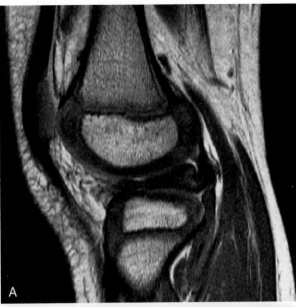

FIGURE 6. Discoid meniscus in 5-year-old male with clunk within left knee. **A,** Sagittal proton-density magnetic resonance image of left knee demonstrates discoid lateral meniscus with increased signal and displaced anterior horn consistent with a tear. Coronal T$_1$-weighted **(B)** and sagittal proton-density images **(C)** show a discoid lateral meniscus that is of normal signal intensity.

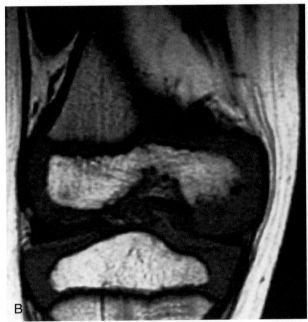

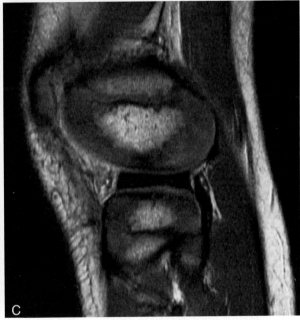

the lateral meniscus. Commonly there is a band of increased signal with or without extension to the joint surface, and tears can be difficult to grade or differentiate from mucoid degeneration on MRI. Tears involving the discoid meniscus usually occur at the posterior and middle segments, are often horizontal and peripheral, and may be associated with meniscal cysts. Frequently there may be a displaced meniscal segment. A discoid meniscus should be suspected in any child with a lateral meniscal tear because such tears are otherwise relatively uncommon in pediatric patients.

Osteochondritis dissecans (OCD) is a form of osteonecrosis that may be due to acute or repetitive injury or ischemia (see Section IX, Part X, page 2319). Clinical symptoms include pain, effusion, swelling, and decreased range of movement. Cartilaginous and bone fragments may be present. OCD most commonly involves the lateral aspect of the medial femoral condyle but can also involve the lateral femoral condyle, talus, and capitellum. Plain films may demonstrate irregularity of cortical bone outline. MRI can be used to assess the extent of disease, especially of the articular cartilage, and evaluate for fragment loosening. Signs of loosening include abnormal low signal within the subarticular bone with surrounding high-signal rim, cystic lesions in surrounding bone, or direct visualization of fragment displacement. Thickening and abnormal signal of overlying cartilage may be noted.

Birth trauma may lead to joint abnormalities, particularly with brachial plexus injury. With Erb-Duchenne palsy, shoulder deformities including subluxation or dislocation, marked humeral rotation, hypoplastic humeral heads, and shallow glenoid fossa are not uncommon. With MRI, additional abnormalities of the posterior and anterior labrum with tears, labral signal abnormalities, and blunting can be appreciated.

ARTHRITIS

Arthritis is commonly encountered in childhood and may be defined as joint swelling and/or joint pain associated with limitation of joint motion in at least one joint. Arthritis may arise from a wide variety of inflammatory and noninflammatory joint disorders. The synovium is often involved, with diffuse synovitis, focal synovial proliferation, synovial infiltration, and synovial masses. Arthritis may be subdivided into acute or chronic. Acute arthritis is a potential medical emergency that must be investigated and treated promptly. Imaging often plays a key role in establishing the presence of disease, determining its extent, and defining the specific diagnosis. In this section, we review common and important causes of acute and chronic arthritis.

JUVENILE RHEUMATOID ARTHRITIS

Clinically diagnosed, JRA is an idiopathic arthritis that begins under age 16 years and that persists for greater than 6 weeks. All other diseases that can cause arthritis need to be considered and excluded (both common and unusual) before the diagnosis of JRA is made. An approach to the significant differential diagnostic considerations of JRA is shown in Table 1. Chronic inflammatory arthritis is the most important rheumatic disease affecting children and one of the most common chronic diseases of childhood. Although JRA may be self-limited, with a majority of patients having no active synovitis in adulthood, many children have significant joint complications.

Several terms are in common use to describe chronic idiopathic synovitis in children, including *juvenile rheumatoid arthritis, juvenile chronic polyarthritis, juvenile chronic arthritis* (especially in Europe), *chronic childhood arthritis,* and *Still's disease.* However, they are not completely synonymous in their classification, with different inclusion and exclusion criteria. This multiplicity of terms makes review of the current and historical literature difficult. In an attempt to unify diagnostic criteria, the International League of Associations for Rheumatology (ILAR) has recently proposed a new classification scheme. Because the ILAR classification has not yet received broad currency, we shall continue to use the term *JRA* and the recognized subgroups previously established by the American College of Rheumatology while introducing the ILAR terminology. The subgroups of JRA include systemic-onset disease, pauciarticular disease (four or fewer joints involved), and polyarticular disease (greater than four joints) as determined by their clinical features, disease onset, and response to therapy. Disease onset is characterized by the pattern of disease during the first 6 months, including number of involved joints and the nature and prominence of extra-articular manifestations. An overview of the current classification schemes is provided in Table 2.

Table 1 ■ DIFFERENTIAL DIAGNOSIS OF JUVENILE RHEUMATOID ARTHRITIS

Synovial Disorders

Pauciarticular

Acute
- Infectious arthritis
  - Septic arthritis
  - Reactive arthritis
  - Tuberculous arthritis
  - Postinfectious arthritis
- Early rheumatic disease
  - Arthritis associated with chromosomal abnormalities—Down's, Turner's syndromes
  - Seronegative spondyloarthropathy
  - Acute transient arthritis
- Other
  - Foreign body arthritis
  - Hemophilic arthropathy

Chronic
- Rheumatic diseases
  - Arthritis associated with chromosomal abnormalities—Down's, Turner's syndromes
- Synovial masses
  - Nodular synovitis
  - Pigmented villonodular synovitis
  - Synovial hemangioma
  - Lipoma arborescens
  - Synovial osteochondromatosis
- Other
  - Hemophilic arthropathy
  - Sarcoidosis
  - Intra-articular osteoid osteoma

Polyarticular
- Seronegative spondyloarthropathies
- Infectious arthritis
  - Lyme disease
  - Reactive arthritis
  - Arthritis associated with chromosomal abnormalities—Down's, Turner's syndromes
- Connective tissue disorders
  - Systemic lupus erythematosus
  - Sarcoidosis
- Inherited disorders
  - Familial hypertrophic synovitis
  - Hemophilic arthropathy
  - Immunodeficiency

Nonsynovial Disorders

Pauciarticular

Acute
- Malignancy
  - Leukemia
  - Neuroblastoma

Chronic
- Noninflammatory disorders
  - Avascular necrosis
  - Slipped epiphyses and dysplasias
- Other
  - Juvenile osteoporosis
  - Multifocal osteolysis

Polyarticular
- Metabolic or inherited disorders
  - Diabetic cheiroarthropathy
  - Turner's syndrome
  - Lysosomal storage disease
- Others
  - Kniest syndrome, Winchester syndrome, chondrodysplasias
  - Frostbite
  - Goldbloom disease

Management of JRA includes use of nonsteroidal anti-inflammatory drugs for relief of pain and inflammation and to allow continued joint function; however, these drugs do not prevent radiographic progression. Joint injections with corticosteroids can be used for patients with pauciarticular joint involvement. Patients with polyarticular disease often need methotrexate, sulfasalazine, or other second-line therapy.

Subtypes

Systemic-Onset Arthritis

Systemic-onset JRA (SoJRA) accounts for 10% to 20% of all JRA cases, affecting males and females almost equally. It is most frequently seen under the age of 5 years, although it may occur at any age. SoJRA is characterized by its prominent extra-articular manifestations, including daily spiking fever (an essential diagnostic criterion), an evanescent rash, serositis, and other features, including lymphadenopathy and reticuloendothelial involvement. Although SoJRA accounts for a minority of JRA cases, there is disproportionate morbidity and mortality associated with this subtype. In SoJRA, the fever is almost always present at disease onset but

infrequently may appear only after onset of arthritis. Serositis, most often pericarditis, is a classical feature, but pleuritis and peritonitis with sizable fluid collections can occur. In SoJRA, there may be hepatosplenomegaly and reticuloendothelial involvement with generalized lymphadenopathy, including para-aortic mesenteric and more peripheral nodes. Macrophage activation syndrome is a potentially fatal complication resulting from uncontrolled macrophage activation and cytokine effects on various organs.

Arthritis in SoJRA usually develops within the first few months of disease onset; however, it may be delayed for years. Chronic destructive arthritis eventually develops in one third to 50% of cases, and the course is typically polyarticular, although the onset is usually pauciarticular. The most commonly involved joints are the knees, wrists, and ankles, but cervical spine disease and hip involvement are also common.

Pauciarticular Disease

Pauciarticular disease is the most common form of JRA, with a peak age of incidence in young childhood. Two main groups of pauciarticular disease are encountered; both have four joints or fewer involved within the first 6

Table 2 ■ CLASSIFICATION SCHEMES: AMERICAN COLLEGE OF RHEUMATOLOGY (ACR), EUROPEAN LEAGUE AGAINST RHEUMATISM (EULAR), AND INTERNATIONAL LEAGUE OF ASSOCIATION FOR RHEUMATOLOGY (ILAR)

ACR	EULAR	ILAR
Juvenile Rheumatoid Arthritis Subtypes	**Juvenile Chronic Arthritis** Subtypes	**Juvenile Idiopathic Arthritis** Subtypes
Systemic arthritis	*Systemic arthritis*	*Systemic arthritis*—associated with fever of 2 weeks' duration and one or more of rash, generalized lymphadenopathy, hepatosplenomegaly, or serositis
Pauciarticular arthritis	*Pauciarticular disease*	*Polyarthritis (RF positive)*—polyarticular disease, RF positive
Polyarticular arthritis Excludes spondyloarthritis Arthritis must be present for at least 6 weeks	*Polyarticular arthritis* *Juvenile rheumatoid arthritis (RF positive only)*	*Polyarthritis (RF negative)*—polyarticular disease, RF negative
	Spondyloarthritis Arthritis must be present for 3 months	*Oligoarthritis*—less than five joints involved
		Extended oligoarthritis—initially oligoarthritis but develops polyarticular disease
		Psoriatic arthritis—arthritis and psoriasis or arthritis with two of the following: dactylitis, nail abnormalities, positive family history
		Enthesitis-related arthritis—arthritis and enthesitis or arthritis or enthesitis with two of the following: sacroiliac joint tenderness and/or inflammatory spinal pain, presence of HLA-B27, family history of HLA-B27–associated disease, anterior uveitis, onset of arthritis in a boy after the age of 8 years
		Other arthritis—idiopathic arthritis that does not fulfill other criteria or fulfills more than one set of criteria *Arthritis must be present for at least 6 weeks*

From Petty RE: Classification of childhood arthritis: a work in progress. Baillieres Clin Rheumatol 1998;12:181–190, with permission.

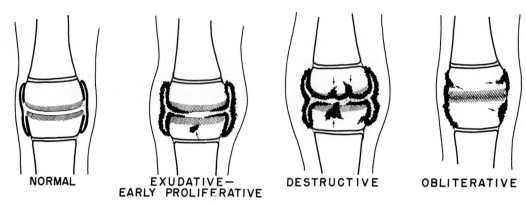

NORMAL   EXUDATIVE—
EARLY PROLIFERATIVE   DESTRUCTIVE   OBLITERATIVE

FIGURE 7. Gross progressive structural changes responsible for the radiographic findings in rheumatoid arthritis. The synovial layer is drawn in *heavy black.* In the *normal joint,* the synovium stops at the edges of the articular cartilages, which are uncovered and exposed directly to the synovial fluid and to the opposing articular cartilage. In the *early exudative and proliferative stage,* the synovial layer is thickened and the articular space laterally and medially, beyond the articular cartilages, is dilated, but the space between the cartilages themselves is not deepened. The synovium is beginning to grow over the articular cartilages from their edges and to abrade the cartilage edge on which they grow. Deep in the tibial ossification center and unrelated to the overgrowth of synovium, a patch of necrosis *(arrow)* has appeared that represents the overgrowth of mesenchymal elements in the marrow. At this time, radiographic findings include regional swelling of soft parts and beginning rarefaction of bones with destruction in the tibial epiphyseal center. In the *destructive phase,* the edges of the articular cartilages *(arrows)* are deeply abraded, with beginning destruction of subchondral bone and extension of the marrow overgrowth in the tibial center through the bone and cartilage into the joint space *(arrow).* In the *obliterative phase,* most of the articular cartilages have disappeared, and there is junction by bony union. Hypertrophic synovium is present on the sides *(arrows)* of the condyles and is growing into them and destroying them.

months but may later develop more joint involvement. Joints involved include knee, ankle, elbow, and wrist. The first type is rheumatoid factor (RF) negative in 30% to 40% of cases; the hips and sacroiliac joints are spared. This type is predominantly seen in females, with late childhood onset. Typically these patients have mild arthritis. Iridocyclitis or anterior uveitis will be present in 20% to 30%.

The second type is seen in males with late childhood onset. The hips and sacroiliac joints are often afflicted, and these patients likely have early undifferentiated spondyloarthropathy.

Polyarticular Disease

Patients with polyarticular disease are commonly divided into two groups: those who are RF positive and those who are RF negative. RF-negative disease is the most common form of polyarticular disease. There is often symmetric polyarthritis of small joints and large joints, and female preponderance with early or late childhood onset. Severe arthritis is present in 10% to 15% of patients.

RF-positive disease shows features and extra-articular manifestations similar to adult rheumatoid arthritis, with rheumatoid nodules and early erosive and symmetric polyarthritis. Arthritis involves the small joints of the hand and feet, including proximal interphalangeal joints, metacarpophalangeal joints, tarsus, and large joints, including the knees and ankles. There is female preponderance, with typically late childhood onset and severe arthritis in more than 50%.

Imaging

Imaging can be used to determine whether arthritis is indeed present, establish a specific diagnosis, and determine extent of disease. It may also be used to determine disease activity, detect disease complications, evaluate disease progression, and judge efficacy of drug treatment.

In JRA, the synovium is the target tissue for inflammation. Early in the disease course, the affected joints are clinically swollen, stiff, painful, and warm and show limited motion. There is synovial proliferation and infiltration by inflammatory cells, including polymorphonuclear leukocytes, lymphocytes, and plasma cells, and increased secretion of synovial fluid. With larger areas of infiltration, lymphoid follicles and granulation tissue form, leading to synovial thickening and pannus formation. Inflammation of synovial coverings of tendons and bursae, which can also be affected, can lead to periostitis. With prolonged inflammation, destruction of cartilage, adjacent bone erosions, and even joint ankylosis may be seen (Fig. 7).

Radiography

Plain films of symptomatic areas are usually obtained at initial presentation. The purpose is as much to exclude other differential diagnoses as it is to make a diagnosis of arthritis. Plain radiography in evaluation of early arthritis is of limited utility because the inflamed synovium, soft tissue changes, and cartilage erosion that precede bone erosions are not well seen. Initial radiographs are often nonspecific, reflecting early response of the soft

Table 3 ■ RADIOGRAPHIC FEATURES OF JUVENILE RHEUMATOID ARTHRITIS

Early Findings
Joint effusion
Soft tissue swelling
Osteoporosis—may be juxta-articular or diffuse, may lead to insufficiency fractures, rarely metaphyseal lucent bands
Periostitis—typically in periarticular regions of phalanges, metacarpals, metatarsals; rarely metaphyses or diaphyses of long bones
Tendinitis

Late Findings
Joint space loss—reflects underlying cartilage loss
Joint malalignment—subluxation, dislocations, protrusio acetabuli; common in the wrist, hip
Bony erosions—typically late manifestation if not seropositive or systemic-onset arthritis at the margins or along the articular surface
Growth disturbances—includes epiphyseal overgrowth, premature physeal closure, short broad phalanges/metacarpals/metatarsals,
    temporomandibular hypoplasia, leg length discrepancy
Ankylosis—intra-articular bone ankylosis; small joints of hand and wrist, cervical spine
Hypertrophic bursopathy
Synovial cysts—popliteal, subchondral, bicipital
Compression fractures—especially of weight-bearing epiphyses

Systemic Findings
Serositis
Generalized lymphadenopathy
Macrophage activation syndrome
Hepatosplenomegaly
Interstitial lung disease
Growth retardation
Amyloidosis
Rheumatoid vasculitis
Lymphedema

tissues and bones to inflammation, with soft tissue swelling, osteopenia, joint effusions, and periosteal reaction (Tables 3 and 4). The osteopenia is initially periarticular, with time becoming more diffuse. Rarely one sees the band-like pattern observed in leukemia. Periosteal reaction is commonly seen in the phalanges, metacarpals (Fig. 8), and metatarsals but can occur in the long bones (Fig. 9).

Soft tissue nodules can be noted, as may periarticular calcification, although this usually is a consequence of prior intra-articular therapy. Joint space narrowing and erosions are usually seen radiographically only 2 years or so after disease onset (Fig. 10). However in polyarticular RF-positive disease and in up to one third of patients with SoJRA, early erosive disease can occur. Abnormalities in growth and maturation may be present, including accelerated osseous growth and altered maturation, leading to enlarged epiphyses (Fig. 11).

Late sequela of JRA are not uncommon and include deformity of epiphyses, abnormal angular carpal bones, and premature fusion of the growth plate with brachydactyly (Fig. 12). Other changes include large, cyst-like, well-corticated erosions (Figs. 13 and 14) that may be lobulated. At the hip, protrusio acetabuli, premature

Table 4 ■ IMAGING MIMICS OF JUVENILE RHEUMATOID ARTHRITIS

IMAGING FINDINGS	DIFFERENTIAL DIAGNOSIS*
Joint effusion	Traumatic synovitis, infectious/septic arthritis, hemophilic arthropathy, acute transient synovitis, acute rheumatic fever, intra-articular tumors, connective tissue disorders, spondyloarthropathies
Soft tissue swelling	Infectious/septic arthritis, synovial hemangioma, hemophilic arthropathy, diabetic cheiroarthropathy, NOMID, sarcoidosis, PVNS, CAP syndrome
Osteoporosis	Juvenile osteoporosis, multifocal osteolysis, leukemia, collagen–vascular disease, hemophilic arthropathy, infectious arthritis
Joint space loss	Traumatic joint dislocation, septic arthritis, hemophilic arthropathy, avascular necrosis, Kniest syndrome, idiopathic chondrolysis, progressive pseudorheumatoid chondrodysplasia, slipped capital femoral epiphyses, osteoid osteoma
Ankylosis	Spondyloarthropathies, traumatic arthritis, infectious arthritis, iatrogenic
Bony erosions	Hemophilic arthropathy, septic arthritis, spondyloarthropathies, carpal osteolysis, CAP syndrome, PVNS, synovial osteochondromatosis
Periostitis	Trauma including abuse, osteomyelitis, spondyloarthropathies, osteoid osteoma, Goldbloom disease, hypertrophic osteoarthropathy, leukemia, sickle cell dactylitis
Growth disturbances	
Epiphyseal overgrowth	Hemophilic arthropathy, NOMID, trauma, tuberculous/fungal disease, spondyloarthropathies, Legg-Calvé-Perthes disease, skeletal dysplasias, Turner's syndrome
Growth arrest	Turner's syndrome, frostbite damage, infection
Dysplastic changes	CAP syndrome, mucopolysaccaridosis, mucolipidosis, Kniest syndrome

*CAP = camptodactyly–arthropathy–pericarditis; NOMID = neonatal-onset multisystem inflammatory disease; PVNS = pigmented villonodular synovitis.

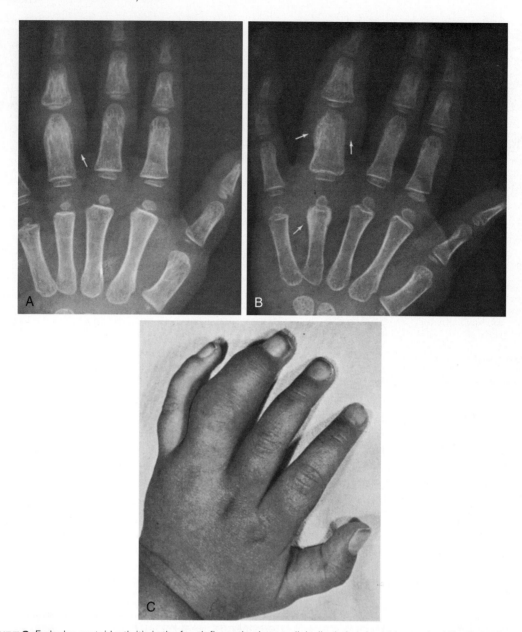

FIGURE 8. Early rheumatoid arthritis in the fourth finger that began clinically during the 14th month of life. **A,** At 20 months, the soft tissues overlying the basal and middle phalanges are swollen and have a fusiform external contour, and these two phalanges are swollen by periosteal thickening and cortical thickening. **B,** At 30 months, the soft tissues are more swollen, as are the phalanges; external cortical thickening has now begun in the distal end of the fourth metacarpal. **C,** Swelling of the fourth finger and in the hand at the distal end of the fourth metacarpal at 30 months. (Courtesy of Dr. Sigurd Eek, Oslo, Norway.)

degenerative changes, coxa magna, and coxa valga can be seen (Fig. 15). Joint space loss can progress to ankylosis, particularly in the apophyseal joints of the cervical spine (Fig. 16) and wrist. Subluxation of the joints, especially at the wrist, may also be evident, and atlantoaxial subluxation may also occur. Growth disturbance of the temporomandibular joint may lead to micrognathia and abnormalities of the temporomandibular disk.

Bone Densitometry

Osteopenia is often present in JRA even in those patients not taking systemic steroids. Global effects on minerali-

zation have been suspected because of overall poor linear and skeletal growth and an increased incidence of fractures. Bone densitometry may be used to help manage children with significantly decreased bone density.

Sonography

Sonography is gaining increasing utility in joint evaluation, especially with high-frequency transducers. Although total joint assessment is often hindered by acoustic barriers, sonography can be used to assess articular cartilage thickness and to detect synovial thickening, joint effusions, and associated synovial cysts.

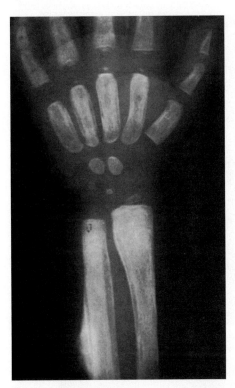

FIGURE 9. Radiograph showing external cortical thickenings of the tubular bones in the hands, radius, and ulna of an infant of 21 months who was reported to have had swelling periarticular soft tissues since the seventh month. Clinical and laboratory findings indicated rheumatoid arthritis. The patient did not have sickle cell anemia or familial hyperphosphatasemia. The preponderance of the evidence suggested that these changes represent the periosteal thickening of early rheumatoid arthritis. (Courtesy of La Rabida Children's Hospital and Research Center, Chicago, IL.)

Sonography can also be used to assess tendon sheath synovial proliferation and bursal hypertrophy and to guide joint aspiration or injection (Fig. 17). Power Doppler shows promise in evaluating the amount and activity of pannus. Sonography may also be used to identify extra-articular complications such as hepatosplenomegaly or serositis.

Magnetic Resonance Imaging

With MRI, one can directly image synovial proliferation, joint fluid, pannus formation, and erosion of cartilage and bone (Fig. 17). MRI is suitable to assess disease severity or progression and is playing an increasing role in diagnosis and outcome assessment. Uncomplicated joint fluid is usually of low signal on T_1- and hyperintense on T_2-weighted images. Other findings in JRA include popliteal cysts and meniscal hypoplasia or atrophy. MRI is more sensitive for detection of bone erosions than plain films.

MRI enhancement of the synovium can be used to detect early synovial proliferation, which precedes destructive changes. Normal synovium is thin and shows slight enhancement. Proliferating synovium on MRI without contrast appears as intermediate soft tissue density on T_1- and T_2-weighted sequences. It may have slightly higher signal than adjacent fluid on unenhanced T_1-weighted images. Pannus appears as thickened intermediate to low signal intensity on T_2-weighted images, best seen when outlined by high-signal joint fluid. Its variable signal intensity reflects its different amounts of fibrous tissue and hemosiderin.

Synovial thickening and effusion may be difficult to distinguish unless intravenous gadolinium is used to

FIGURE 10. Rheumatoid arthritis in a girl 6 years of age. **A,** Four weeks after onset of vague pains, the radiographic findings are normal. **B,** Fifteen months later, all of the bony tissues are rarefied and the tubular bones overconstricted. The latter is best seen in the flares at the ends of the radius and ulna, with marked constriction just proximal to the flares. All of the fingers show fusiform swelling owing to the swelling of soft parts at the interphalangeal joints. The most striking change is the loss of spaces between the carpal bones owing to destruction of the articular cartilages of the intercarpal joints and the carpal–radial joint as well. The same loss of cartilage is evident at the carpometacarpal joints.

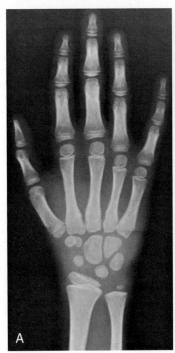
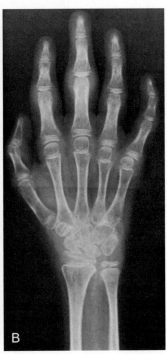

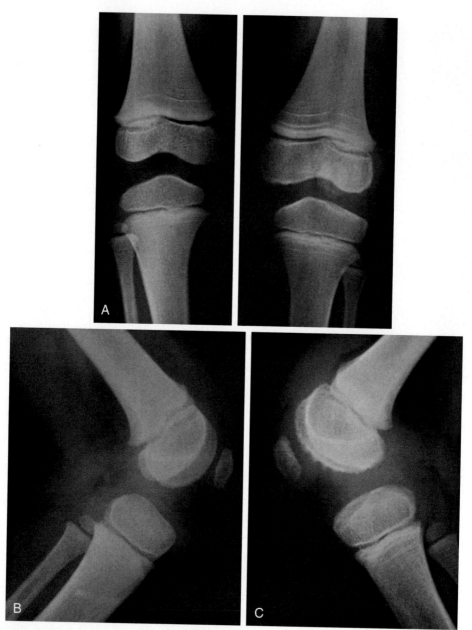

FIGURE 11. Radiographs showing rheumatoid arthritis in the left knee of a girl 3 years of age; the knees are in frontal **(A)** and lateral **(B** and **C)** projections. The swelling of the soft tissues at the left knee and atrophy of the muscles in the left thigh and shank are not visible in these films. The bones at the left knee are all diffusely rarefied, but there is no evidence of loss of articular cartilage or destruction of subchrondral bone. The femoral and tibial epiphyseal ossification centers and the patella on the left side are enlarged, owing presumably to the longstanding regional hyperemia induced by the chronic arthritis. Symmetric series of transverse lines have formed in the femoral and tibial metaphyses on both sides; the spaces between the transverse lines are deeper on the affected side, which indicates accelerated growth on that side as a result of chronic hyperemia.

demonstrate enhancement of hypervascular synovium (Fig. 17). Images should be obtained immediately after contrast injection because diffusion of contrast from the synovium into the joint fluid occurs over time. Contrast enhancement improves visualization of the thickened synovium dramatically, especially with use of fat suppression, allowing the proliferating synovium to be seen in regions normally devoid of synovium as enhancing linear, villous, or nodular tissue. Hypervascular in-

flamed pannus enhances significantly, while fibrous inactive pannus shows much less enhancement. Quantitative techniques may be used to determine synovial volume.

Hemosiderin deposition can occur in JRA, but more frequently is seen in disorders that are accompanied by hemarthrosis, including pigmented villonodular synovitis (PVNS), hemophilic arthropathy, synovial hemangioma, and post-traumatic synovitis. Gradient-echo se-

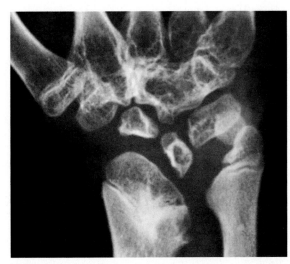

FIGURE 12. Radiograph showing severe rheumatoid arthritis of the left wrist of a girl 15 years of age with extensive destruction and ankylosis of carpometacarpal joints 2 through 5. Premature union of the central portion of the distal radial epiphysis with its shaft has occurred. The ends of the radius and ulna are tipped toward each other owing to slowed longitudinal growth in the medial and lateral segments of their respective cartilage plates. (Courtesy of Dr. Fred A. Lee, Pasadena, CA.)

quences are most sensitive in detecting hemosiderin deposition within the synovium as signal loss resulting from increased magnetic susceptibility.

With prolonged synovial inflammation, as in JRA and tuberculosis, well-defined intra-articular nodules termed *rice bodies* (because of their characteristic macroscopic appearance) can be noted. Rice bodies likely arise from detached fragments of hypertrophied synovial villi and may lead to painless swelling of the joint. On MRI, rice bodies are of low signal on T$_2$-weighted images. They are associated with joint effusion and synovial hypertrophy and may demonstrate synovial enhancement after gadolinium administration. Removal leads to symptomatic relief.

Response to Therapy

Assessment of disease activity is important for monitoring treatment efficacy and predicting outcome. Histopathologic evidence of persistent synovitis and radiologic deterioration has been observed in patients assumed clinically and biochemically to have inactive disease.

Radiography can be used to quantify joint destruction and assess disease treatment, with absence of change and lack of progression implying treatment success. In children who received methotrexate, Harel et al. found no interval intercarpal joint narrowing as measured by carpal length in responders versus the progressive worsening seen in nonresponders. Although joint space narrowing and erosion scores did not improve, some patients did show improvement in carpal length.

Intra-articular corticosteroids can be used to temporarily suppress local joint inflammation. Following injection of intra-articular corticosteroids, periarticular calcification can be noted. Other changes related to intra-articular therapy seem uncommon even with repeated joint injections.

Sonography may also be a useful means to noninvasively follow changes in synovitis with therapy. It may play a role in supporting clinical suspicion of disease activity in clinically mild or silent joints and in deciding on discontinuation of therapy. Increases in synovial thickening and synovial fluid accompany clinical worsening; however, the significance of residual synovial thickening and effusion seen on ultrasound in asymptomatic patients remains unclear. It may represent active silent disease or inactive fibrous pannus in a quiescent phase. Following intra-articular therapy for JRA in the hips and knees, decrease in synovial effusion, synovial proliferation, and adenopathy is noted on ultrasound.

Contrast-enhanced MRI can be used to quantitatively monitor synovial membrane volumes, effusion volumes, and cartilage and bone erosion scores. Synovial membrane volume may reflect degree of edema, dilated vessels, and cellular infiltration in the synovial membrane and may be a measure of synovial inflammatory

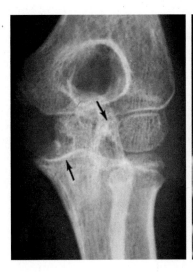
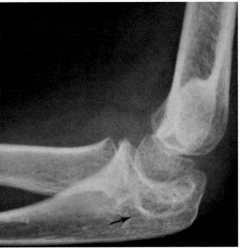

FIGURE 13. Radiograph showing large subchondral defects in the juxta-articular edges of the olecranon processes *(arrows)* in a girl with chronic rheumatoid arthritis of the elbow.

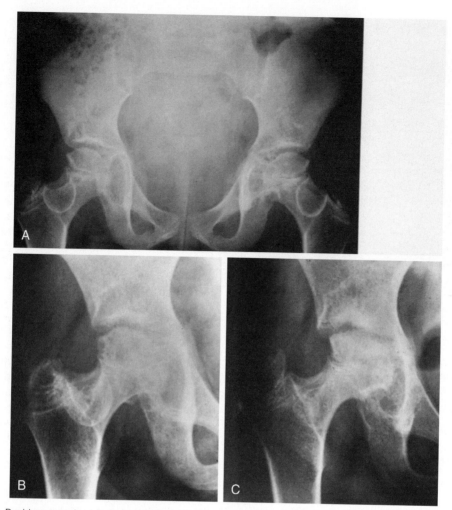

FIGURE 14. Rapid progression of erosive changes seen radiographically in the hips of a girl with systemic-onset juvenile arthritis beginning at 3½ years of age. **A,** Pelvis at 6 years 8 months. Cystic erosions appear to straddle both femoral necks. Mild to moderate irregularities of ossification centers for the femoral heads and in the acetabular roofs are apparent. **B,** At 7 years 10 months of age, there is progression of the erosions of the femoral necks from above and in front or in back. The femoral head and acetabular roof show more evidence of subchondral erosions that almost reach the medial cortex of the neck. **C,** At 8 years 9 months, the neck has become more attenuated at the site of the enlarging erosion, and there is further progression of disease in the head and acetabulum. The patient had had multiple exacerbations and recurrences of symptoms, but her hips had been less severely affected clinically than were the small joints.

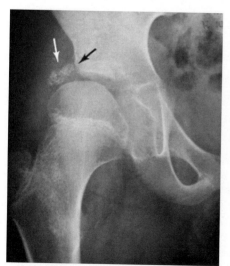

FIGURE 15. Radiograph showing rheumatoid arthritis with juxta-articular calcification in the soft tissues of the right hip *(arrows)* of a boy of 9½ years. The coxa valga is noteworthy; this lesion is common in rheumatoid arthritis of the pelvis and legs and is probably due to reduced use.

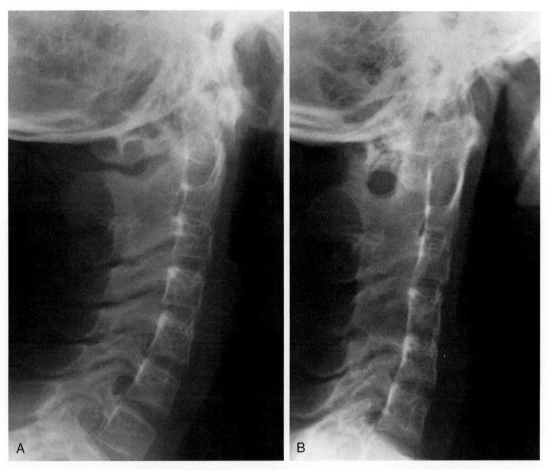

FIGURE 16. A, Lateral radiograph of the cervical spine of a 10-year-old girl with juvenile rheumatoid arthritis for several years shows ankylosis of C2–C3 facet joints. **B,** Subsequent radiograph 2 years later reveals progressive ankylosis at C4–C5.

activity. Synovial volume, however, may also reflect the cumulative synovial proliferative disease activity and appears to correlate with duration of clinical remission. Several studies have indicated a close relationship between the rate of contrast enhancement and inflammatory activity, with the enhancement rate apparently decreasing after intra-articular steroid administration, remaining low during clinical remissions, and increasing prior to the return of symptoms, indicating subclinical increase in synovial inflammatory activity. There may be regions of marked heterogeneity in rate of enhancement, so use of small regions of interest may be a limitation, with cases of clinical relapse showing increased enhancement back to pretreatment levels.

AUTOIMMUNE CONNECTIVE TISSUE DISEASES

Joint findings are generally limited in connective tissue disorders. In scleroderma, which can be localized or systemic, joint changes are generally mild, with osteopenia and joint contractures seen. Similarly, in juvenile dermatomyositis, a multisystem disorder primarily affecting blood vessels, there may be joint effusions but erosions are not typically found (Fig. 18). In systemic lupus erythematosus, an inflammatory polyarthritis

may be noted, typically without erosions being present. Subluxation may also occur.

OTHER RHEUMATIC OR INFLAMMATORY DISEASES

Conditions with prolonged synovial inflammation may mimic JRA, and often show signs of demineralization, soft tissue swelling, joint space narrowing, and erosions.

CHROMOSOMAL DISORDERS

Arthritis may be associated with chromosomal disorders. There is an increased incidence of arthritis associated with both Down and Turner's syndromes. Because patients with Down syndrome have various immunologic abnormalities, arthritis in these children is classified as a separate disease from JRA. It is important to be aware of the association of arthropathy with these syndromes because there is often a delay in making the diagnosis. Patients with Down syndrome usually present with polyarticular disease involving both large and small joints in a symmetric distribution, most commonly the proximal interphalangeal and metacarpophalangeal joints of the hands, wrists, and knees. Joint hypermobility and subluxations occur and are most common in the cervical spine. In Turner's syndrome, patients may have both radiographic bony changes of chronic inflammatory joint disease and the bony changes of Turner's syndrome, including short fourth metacarpals, Madelung's deformity, delayed maturation with flattening of the medial tibial plateau, and enlargement of the femoral condyle. These conditions often have overlapping features with JRA, including osteoporosis, premature fusion of bones, and metacarpal shortening. Patients with the chromosome 22q11.2 deletion syndrome (formerly known as DiGeorge syndrome or conotruncal-facial anomaly) and other immunodeficiencies also have a higher than chance probability of developing chronic polyarthritis.

JUVENILE SPONDYLOARTHROPATHIES

The juvenile spondyloarthropathies represent a group of disorders that affect the axial and extra-axial joints. They include juvenile ankylosing spondylitis (JAS), reactive arthritis or Reiter's syndrome, juvenile psoriatic arthritis (JPsA), and arthritis associated with inflamma-

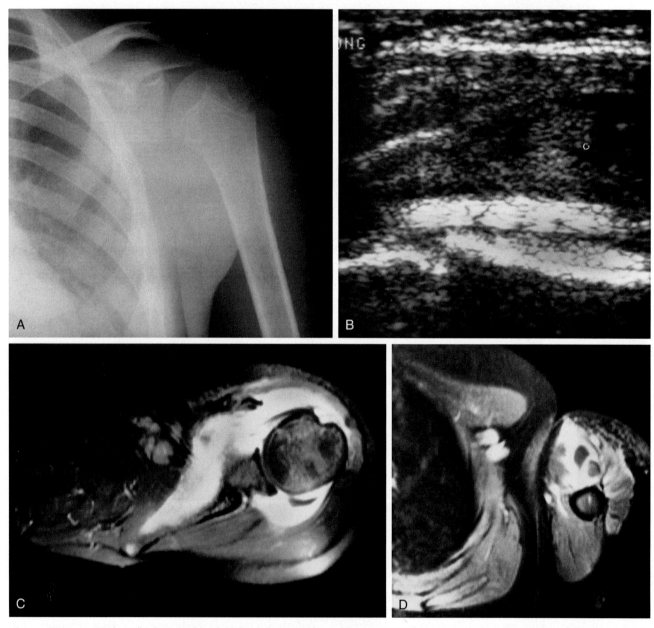

FIGURE 17. Juvenile rheumatoid arthritis in an 8-year-old boy with new onset of prominent soft tissue swelling of midarm. **A,** Frontal radiograph shows increased soft tissue density medial to upper arm. **B,** Longitudinal sonogram of upper arm shows hyperechoic fluid and synovium superior to highly echogenic bicipital tendon. **C** and **D,** Axial magnetic resonance (MR) T_1-weighted fat-suppressed images following gadolinium administration. **C,** Extensive enhancing thickened synovium within the glenohumeral joint, with enhancement seen extending medially subjacent to the scapula. Axillary lymph nodes are noted medial to the joint. **D,** More inferior image shows extensive enhancement with biceps from tenosynovitis anteriorly.

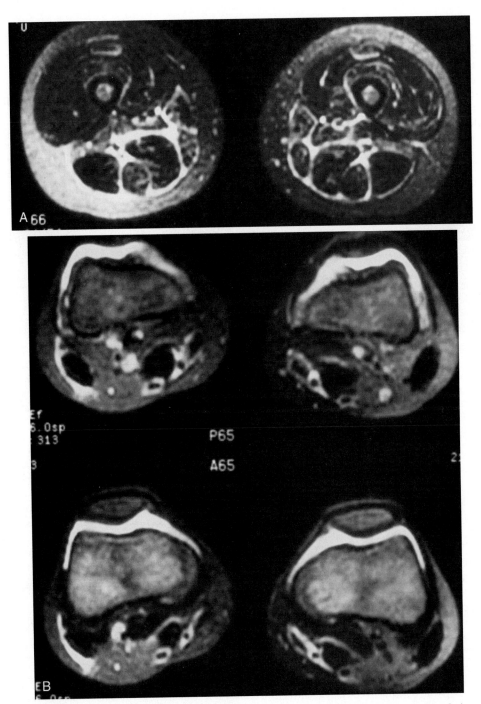

FIGURE 18. Axial fat-suppressed fast T_2-weighted magnetic resonance imaging of dermatomyositis. **A,** Image showing typical high signal within and around thigh muscles bilaterally. **B,** Images at the level of the knee joints shows bilateral effusions.

tory bowel disease, all occurring under the age of 16 years. The spondyloarthropathies share many common clinical and genetic characteristics, including positive family history, absence of subcutaneous nodules, presence of enthesitis and later sacroiliitis, and absence of RF and antinuclear antibody. Synovitis and enthesitis (inflammation at the site of attachment of ligaments or tendons to bone) are recognized as major target areas of inflammation. Enthesitis is commonly present, especially at the insertions of the Achilles tendon, plantar fascia, and patellar and quadriceps tendons. The clinical spectrum of juvenile spondyloarthropathies is broad and includes patients with undifferentiated manifestations that do not allow specific categorization, including peripheral arthritis, enthesitis, tendinitis, dactylitis, and uveitis and patients with more characteristic features such as sacroiliitis, spinal involvement, or extra-articular manifestations, including psoriasis or gut involvement. Often specific diagnostic criteria are not initially present in children, and most will be diagnosed as having

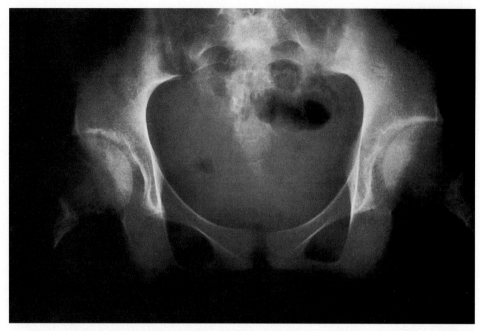

FIGURE 19. In a 13-year-old boy with juvenile ankylosing arthritis, frontal radiograph of the pelvis shows bilateral sacroiliitis with bilateral sclerosis and irregularity of the sacroiliac joints and bilateral hip joint space narrowing superiorly, greater on the left.

undifferentiated spondyloarthropathy. Although the juvenile spondyloarthropathies are considered separately from JRA, they can be difficult to clinically distinguish, especially early on. The term *seronegative enthesopathy arthropathy* syndrome has been proposed to separate children, typically boys, in their early teens who present with enthesitis and peripheral asymmetric, often lower limb arthritis from those with JRA. Other entities related to the seronegative spondyloarthropathies include the arthritis associated with hyperostosis, acne and/or palmar pustulosis, Whipple's disease, and Behçet's disease.

Juvenile Ankylosing Spondylitis

Despite the fact that children with JAS rarely have the classical adult presentation of bilateral sacroiliitis and spondylitis, radiologic evidence of inflammation of these joints is required for definitive diagnosis. Asymmetric extra-axial arthritis is common in JAS, commonly affecting the large joints of the lower extremity, including the hips, knees, and ankles (Fig. 19). Dactylitis with finger or toe involvement may manifest as swollen red digits with painful small joints, and enthesitis is commonly found (Fig. 20). Sacroiliitis is usually bilateral but asymmetric when present.

Reactive Arthritis and Reiter's Syndrome

Reactive arthritis is distinguished from the other spondyloarthropathies by its clear relationship to a precipitating infection, which may be asymptomatic. Susceptibility to reactive arthritis is closely linked to the presence of human leukocyte antigen allele B27. Infections of the gastrointestinal, genitourinary, and respiratory tract can provoke reactive arthritis, and a wide range of pathogens has been implicated. Both antigens and DNA of several microorganisms have been detected in joint material from patients with reactive arthritis. The role of these disseminated microbial elements in the provocation or maintenance of arthritis and the need for antibiotic therapy in the treatment of reactive arthritis remains unclear. Reiter's syndrome is the association of reactive arthritis with conjunctivitis and urethritis. Although several forms of joint disease could be consid-

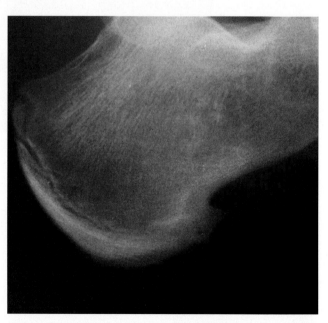

FIGURE 20. Radiograph of a 12-year-old boy with juvenile ankylosing spondylitis shows a prominent calcaneal spur extending anteriorly from the plantar aspect of the bone.

ered as reactive, particularly acute rheumatic fever, post–meningococcal septicemia arthritis, and Lyme disease, reactive arthritis is often restricted to an acute spondyloarthropathy, usually but not exclusively linked to an acute genitourinary or gastrointestinal infection. Reactive arthritis is usually self-limited and self-resolving. The arthritis is typically peripheral, monoarticular, or pauciarticular, but axial involvement with unilateral or bilateral sacroiliitis, enthesitis, and dactylitis can be seen.

Arthritis Associated with Inflammatory Bowel Disease

Approximately 15% of children with inflammatory bowel disease will develop a noninfectious arthritis, which typically is pauciarticular, involving the peripheral, large joints of the lower extremity.

Juvenile Psoriatic Disease

As opposed to the other spondyloarthropathies, JPsA is more common in girls than boys, especially in childhood. It can be definitively diagnosed when patients with psoriasis have arthritis or when arthritis and three of the following—dactylitis, nail pitting, or onycholysis or family history of psoriasis—are present. The arthritis not uncommonly may precede the development of psoriasis. The arthritis most commonly is asymmetric, is pauciarticular initially, and can involve the large and small joints, including the proximal and distal interphalangeal joints. Tendon sheath involvement is common, while enthesitis seems less common than in JAS.

Imaging in Juvenile Spondyloarthropathies

Radiographic findings are common among all the spondyloarthropathies and similar to those of JRA with the exception of sacroiliitis and enthesitis, which are more specific for spondyloarthropathy (Figs. 19 through 22). Plain films are usually normal initially but later on may demonstrate soft tissue swelling, effusion, osteopenia, joint space narrowing, or erosion and rarely fusion. Erosions are typically associated with irregular bone apposition at joint margins, referred to as "whiskering" spondyloarthropathy (Fig. 22). Rapid joint destruction can be noted. With hip involvement, these proliferative changes are noted at the junction of the femoral head and neck. Dactylitis may be seen with soft tissue swelling and periosteal reaction along the shaft of metacarpals, metatarsals, or phalanges (Table 5). In JAS, extra-axial arthritis usually involves one or more large joints of the lower extremities (e.g., hips, knees, and ankles). In JPsA, severe erosions can be seen, particularly in the digits (Fig. 22).

Enthesitis may be revealed by soft tissue swelling, localized osteopenia, or bone erosion and/or spur formation, particularly at the site of insertion of the Achilles tendon into the calcaneus (Fig. 20), plantar aponeurosis, or patella. With MRI one may see bone marrow edema, granulation tissue, or cortical erosion.

Plain films may demonstrate unilateral or bilateral

Table 5 ■ RADIOGRAPHIC FEATURES OF THE JUVENILE SPONDYLOARTHROPATHIES
Axial Skeleton
Sacroiliac joint
Sacroiliitis—unilateral or bilateral
Indistinct articular margins
Erosions
Reactive sclerosis
Joint space narrowing
Joint fusion
Adjacent bone marrow edema and enhancement on magnetic resonance imaging
Vertebrae
Apophysitis (shining corners)
Anterior vertebral squaring
Anterior ligament calcification
Appendicular Skeleton
Enthesitis
Soft tissue swelling
Erosions at insertions
Spur formation
Bone edema
Localized bone overgrowth
Periostitis
Tenosynovitis
Arthritis
Synovitis
Joint fluid
Soft tissue swelling
Accelerated ossification and epiphyseal overgrowth
Joint space narrowing
Erosions
Demineralization
Joint fusion
Protrusio acetabuli

sacroiliitis with indistinct articular margins, pseudowidening, erosions, and reactive sclerosis, particularly on the iliac side of the joint (Figs. 19 and 21). CT or MRI can be used if necessary to diagnose sacroiliitis earlier than radiographically present. On CT, angled scans through the sacroiliac joint should be used to lower radiation dose. On MRI, periarticular low signal may be seen on T_1-weighted images with high signal on T_2-weighted images from inflammatory changes in bone marrow, while low signal will be seen with bone sclerosis (Fig. 21). MRI may also demonstrate changes in articular cartilage with erosions. MRI evaluation, particularly with gadolinium enhancement, may allow earlier diagnosis of back pain caused by acute sacroiliitis than will conventional radiography.

In juvenile spondyloarthropathy, vertebral involvement is not usually present because it develops quite late. Occasionally there may be localized osteitis, erosions, and sclerosis, particularly at vertebral margins. Syndesmophytes are rarely seen in children. Rarely atlantoaxial subluxation can be present.

INFECTIOUS ARTHRITIS

Arthritis caused by infectious agents can be due to direct invasion by viable microorganisms (septic arthritis) or due to a variety of immune mechanisms (postinfectious arthritis) (Table 6). Infectious synovitis can be caused by various pathogens, including bacteria, viruses, and fungi. The term *septic arthritis* is reserved for bacterial infections in which bacteria are recovered from the synovial fluid with the use of standard microbiologic techniques. If the synovial fluid is "sterile," the condition is termed *postinfectious arthritis* even though the triggering infection can precede (acute rheumatic fever, post-*Yersinia* arthritis) or coexist with (brucellosis, rat-bite fever) the articular symptoms. Reactive arthritides are generally defined as sterile arthritides following remote infections of the urogenital or intestinal tracts.

Septic Arthritis

Identification of the obvious septic joint is not much of a diagnostic challenge, although time to diagnosis is critical to avoid a poor outcome such as destruction of the femoral head, degenerative arthritis, or permanent deformity. Much more of a challenge is the diagnosis of

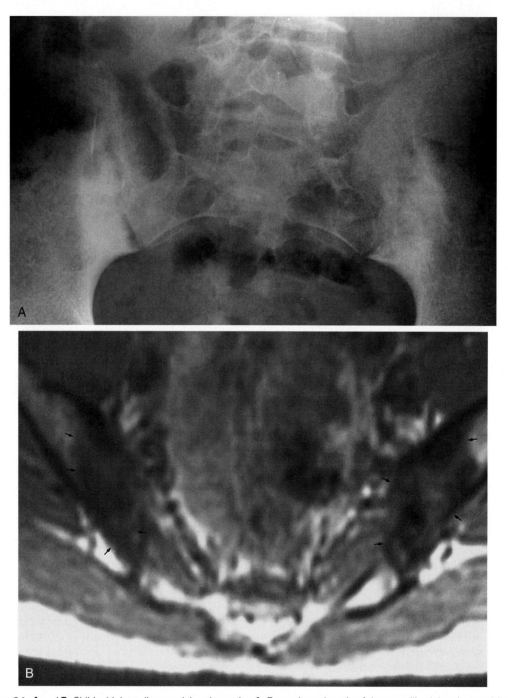

FIGURE 21. **A** and **B,** Child with juvenile spondyloarthropathy. **A,** Extensive sclerosis of the sacroiliac joints is seen bilaterally on frontal radiograph. **B,** Corresponding axial T₁-weighted magnetic resonance (MR) image showing low signal *(arrows)* that remained low on T₂-weighted images (not shown).

Illustration continued on opposite page

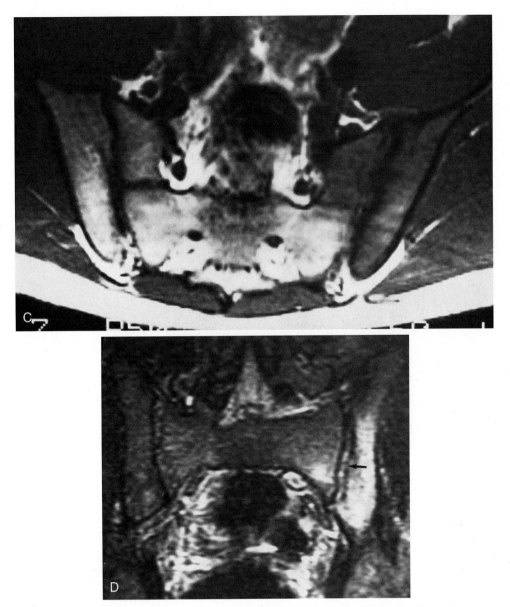

FIGURE 21. *Continued.* **C** and **D,** MR images in another child with juvenile spondyloarthropathy. **C,** Axial T₁-weighted image shows periarticular low signal on the left and irregular joint subchondral bone. **D,** Coronal T₂-weighted image shows corresponding high signal, and high signal within the sacroiliac joint *(arrow).*

musculoskeletal infections caused by unusual organisms or in unusual locations. Infection in the bones and joints of the back and pelvis is often difficult to diagnose because the physical examination may suggest a knee, hip, or abdominal problem, and tuberculous infections may simulate juvenile arthritis with subacute symptoms.

Acute purulent infection of the joints is more common in infancy and early childhood because of the greater blood flow to the joints during the active stages of growth. The usual cause is hematogenous dissemination related to an upper respiratory infection or pyoderma. Infection may also spread from adjacent osteomyelitis, cellulitis, abscess, or traumatic joint invasion (Fig. 23). In children, septic arthritis develops commonly from osteomyelitis in metaphyses that are intraarticular, such as the hip. During infancy, septic arthritis frequently is associated with osteomyelitis because cap-

illaries from the metaphysis traverse the physis into the epiphysis. Infants with immune dysfunction, with indwelling vascular lines, or undergoing invasive procedures are at increased risk. Neonatal septic arthritis represents a different spectrum of disease than septic arthritis of childhood. A high clinical index of suspicion is necessary because signs and symptoms may be subtle. Early signs include failure to move a limb spontaneously, while swelling, erythema, and warmth are late findings.

Staphylococcus aureus is the most common cause of bacterial arthritis, with group B streptococcus commonly seen in the neonate and *Haemophilus influenzae* in the 1- to 4-year age range. Children with varicella infection (chicken pox) are at increased risk of developing septic arthritis and other musculoskeletal infections secondary to group A streptococcus. Pneumococcal joint infection may be seen in children with splenic

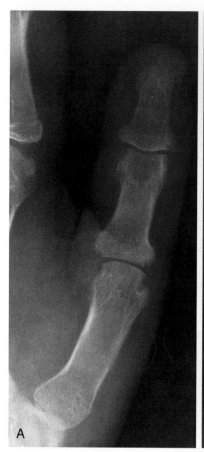
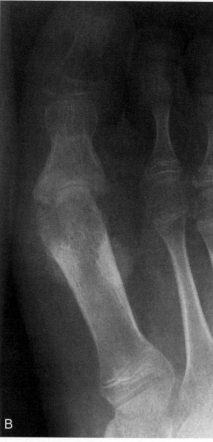

FIGURE 22. Radiographs of the hand and foot of a 14-year-old boy with psoriatic arthritis. **A,** Soft tissue swelling of the first digit with narrowing of the first metacarpal–phalangeal joint with marginal erosions and proliferative periostitis. **B,** Similar changes are seen at the first metatarsal-phalangeal joint.

Table 6 ■ INFECTION-RELATED ARTHRITIS

Infectious Arthritis
Viral
   Parvovirus
   Rubella
   Epstein-Barr
   Hepatitis B
   Varicella-zoster
   Coxsackie
Bacterial
   Staphylococcus aureus
   Group B hemolytic streptococcus
   Haemophilus influenzae
   Streptococcus pneumoniae
   Streptococcus pyogenes
   Pneumococcal pneumonia
   Klebsiella pneumoniae
   Pseudomonas aeruginosa
   Neisseria meningitidis
   Neisseria gonorrhoea
Fungal
   Candida albicans
   Coccidiomycosis
Myocobacterium tuberculosis

Reactive Arthritis (Postinfectious)
Tuberculosis (Poncet's disease)
Acute rheumatic fever (poststreptococcal)
Yersinia
Brucellosis
Rat-bite fever *(Streptobacillus moniliformis)*
Lyme borreliosis
Mycoplasma pneumonia

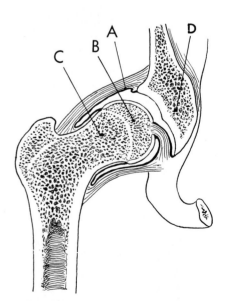

FIGURE 23. Primary sites of origin from which infection may extend secondarily into the hip joint. The initial focus may be in the femoral epiphysis *(A)*, in the synovium itself *(B)*, in the femoral metaphysis *(C)*, or in the innominate bone *(D)*. In some cases, the hip joint may be infected by extension from more than one of these neighboring primary foci.

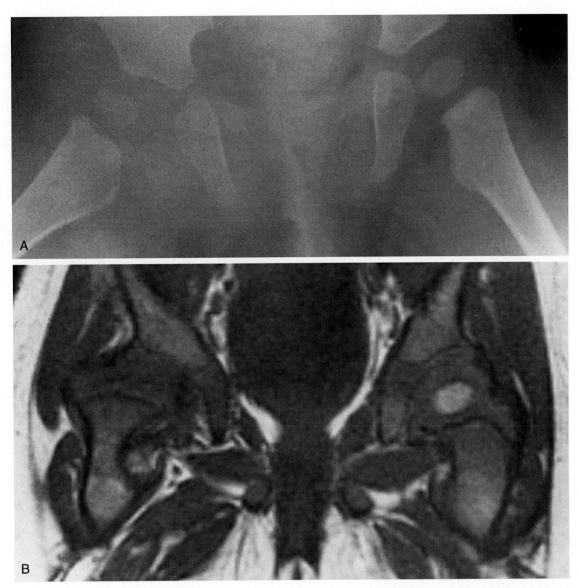

FIGURE 24. Septic arthritis in a 7-month-old female. **A,** Frontal radiograph demonstrates osteopenia of the right femur, increased soft tissue density, and subluxation of the right hip. **B,** On follow-up magnetic resonance imaging at 1 year of age, coronal T_1-weighted image of the pelvis shows irregular delayed ossification of the right femoral epiphysis related to complications of infection with necrosis and persistent subluxation.

dysfunction from hemoglobinopathy or immune deficiency.

The vast majority of septic arthritides are monoarticular, with the most commonly affected joints being the knee, hip, and ankle. In septic arthritis, bacterial contamination causes hypertrophy and edema of the synovium. In infants with septic arthritis, distention of the joint capsule may result in pathologic dislocation, particularly in the hip or shoulder (Fig. 24). Joint space narrowing results from cartilage destruction by proteolytic enzymes. There may be associated bone erosion and destruction or periosteal reaction. Pus in the joint increases intra-articular pressure and may result in osteonecrosis of the epiphysis (Fig. 24). Other sequelae include angular deformities, leg length discrepancy, and ankylosis. Prompt diagnosis of septic arthritis is essential in infants and children to prevent complications.

The classical radiographic findings of acute septic arthritis are rapid joint space loss and erosions with relative preservation of mineralization (Fig. 25). These findings indicate advanced irreversible destruction of the joint but are not specific for infection. Early findings of joint effusion may be detected in the knee, ankle, or elbow, but radiographs are insensitive for detecting effusion in the shoulder, hip, or sacroiliac joints. Ultrasound, CT, and MRI are sensitive in demonstrating joint effusion but cannot distinguish infected from noninfected joint effusion, and aspiration is still necessary for diagnosis. CT is useful for guiding diagnostic aspiration or drainage of the joint and may be the best modality for evaluating certain joints such as the sternoclavicular joint. MRI may be used to demonstrate early bone erosions and cartilage destruction. In addition to joint effusions, associated findings include synovial thickening and enhancement, septations, and debris within the joint. Uncomplicated septic arthritis may cause abnormal signal within the marrow on both sides of the joint secondary to reactive edema, which may be difficult to differentiate from osteomyelitis. A secondary complication of septic arthritis is soft tissue abscess, which demonstrates localized fluid collection with peripheral enhancement following gadolinium enhancement. Edema within periarticular structures or fluid collections in tendon sheaths will also show increased signal on T_2-weighted images.

Radionuclide imaging is more sensitive than radiographs in supporting the diagnosis of arthritis and may be used to screen the entire skeleton. A bone scan localizes the site of infection and is positive as early as 2 days after the onset of symptoms. In septic arthritis, there is increased articular activity in the blood flow and blood pool phases, and there may be uptake in the juxta-articular bones on the delayed phase as a result of hyperemia. Increased intra-articular pressure from joint effusion may result in reduced radionuclide uptake within the epiphysis as a result of ischemia.

Other Causes of Infectious Arthritis

In viral arthritis, the virus may actually invade synovial tissues, causing local inflammation and cell necrosis. Commonly encountered viruses include parvovirus,

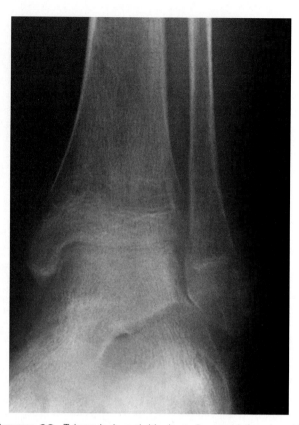

FIGURE 26. Tuberculosis arthritis in a 9-year-old female with 6-month history of monoarticular arthritis of the left ankle, presumed to be juvenile rheumatoid arthritis, treated with steroid injections. Patient was lost to follow-up and returned 4 months later with marked worsening of arthritis. Radiograph of the left ankle shows soft tissue swelling, periarticular osteopenia, and severe joint space narrowing. She also had a cough, and chest radiograph showed miliary tuberculosis.

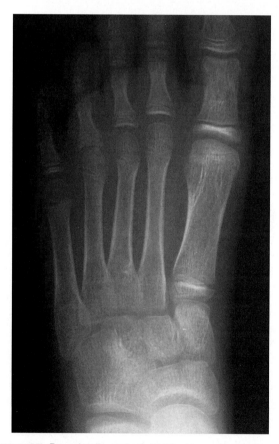

FIGURE 25. Frontal radiograph of right foot in a patient with septic arthritis shows joint space narrowing of the fourth metatarsal-phalangeal joint.

rubella, Epstein-Barr and coxsackie. Most viral arthritides generally resolve within 6 weeks without specific therapy. Viral arthritis may also result from local host immune responses to the virus or viral products. In most cases it is probably a systemic serum sickness type of reaction with formation of immune complexes that are demonstrable in both serum and synovial fluid. Viral arthritides may be monoarticular, pauciarticular, or polyarticular and can resemble septic arthritis or JRA.

Mycobacterium tuberculosis has made a resurgence, and in children the frequency of bone or joint infection may be as high as 6%. Tuberculous infection usually begins as an insidious monoarticular arthritis and commonly involves the spine, hip, and knee (see Section IX, Part XI, page 2343). In children, extrapulmonary tuberculosis usually results from lymphohematogenous dissemination during a primary infection. *Mycobacterium tuberculosis* may also cause postinfectious polyarthritis or Poncet's disease. Radiographs in tuberculous arthritis classically show osteopenia and periarticular erosions with relative preservation of the joint space. With chronic infection there may be joint space narrowing (Fig. 26), abscess formation, and draining sinuses. Tuberculous arthritis frequently causes extensive fibrous bridging and obliteration of the joint space.

Postinfectious arthritis resulting from an immune response is usually self-limited with the exception of acute rheumatic fever and Lyme disease, where there may be significant morbidity. Rheumatic fever is secondary to group A streptococci. It usually presents as a migratory arthritis involving the large joints of the extremities, with the exception of the hip. Lyme disease is caused by *Borrelia burgdorferi*, which is a tick-transmitted spirochete. It usually presents with intermittent monoarthritis most commonly in the knee. The radiologic findings may be similar to those of pauciarticular JRA. The diagnosis is confirmed with serology demonstrating antibodies to the infectious agent.

OTHER INFLAMMATORY ARTHRITIDES

Transient Synovitis of the Hip

Transient synovitis is a self-limited inflammatory condition specific to the hip. It affects boys more commonly than girls in all age ranges but is most common between 3 and 6 years. Its etiology is unknown, but some children have a preceding history of upper respiratory infection or trauma. Patients present with acute onset of pain and limp that generally lasts less than 2 weeks. Only 1% have bilateral disease, while a small number of patients have a second episode, which usually occurs within the first 6 months after the initial symptoms. Transient synovitis is a diagnosis of exclusion, with the most common disorders in the differential including traumatic synovitis, septic arthritis, JRA, and Legg-Calvé-Perthes disease.

Long-term sequelae are rare. Avascular necrosis has been described as a complication in a few patients, but it is uncertain whether these cases actually represent Legg-Calvé-Perthes disease that was initially undetectable on radiographs. Treatment consists of bed rest and nonsteroidal anti-inflammatory medications.

Radiographs are usually normal but may demonstrate evidence of a joint effusion with mild widening of the medial joint space. Scintigraphy often shows slight increase in isotope uptake in the affected hip. In approximately 25% of patients there may be a transient decrease in uptake in the first week or two, followed by evidence of rebound hyperemia within 1 month. These findings suggest that some patients develop transient ischemia of the capital femoral epiphysis that may be secondary to the increased intracapsular pressure caused by the effusion. Sonography is a sensitive and noninvasive method of detecting joint effusion. It is performed by scanning along the anterior aspect of the femoral neck because this is where fluid tends to accumulate within the hip joint (Fig. 27). However, joint effusion is not specific, and aspiration is required if infection is a consideration. On MRI, there is evidence of joint effusion but no evidence of bone abnormality.

Hemophilic Arthropathy

Hemophilia is an X-linked recessive disorder characterized by abnormality of the coagulation mechanism. It may be secondary to a deficiency in factor VIII, as in classical hemophilia (hemophilia A), or secondary to a

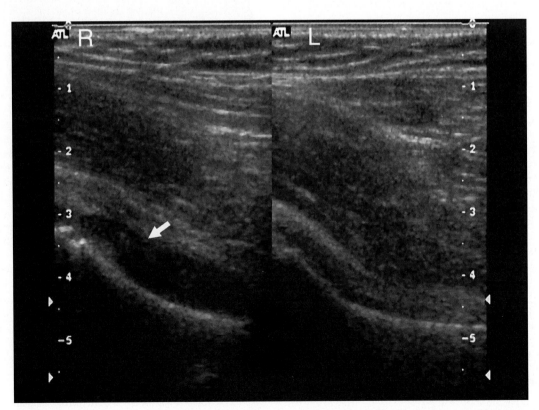

FIGURE 27. Sagittal sonographic images along the anterior aspect of the hips in a child with transient synovitis demonstrate a right hip joint effusion with bulging of the joint capsule *(arrow)* compared to the normal left hip.

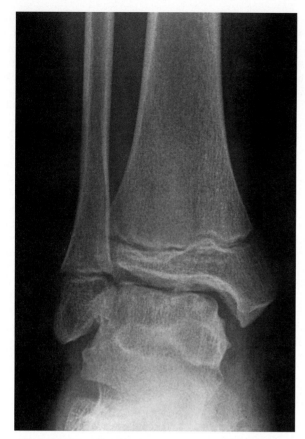

FIGURE 28. Ten-year-old male with hemophilia and recurrent hemarthrosis, frontal radiograph of the right ankle demonstrates joint narrowing and slight overgrowth of the distal tibial epiphysis. There is irregularity of the talar articular surface and subchondral cyst formation.

deficiency of factor IX, as in Christmas disease (hemophilia B). Hemarthrosis occurs in approximately 75% to 90% of patients with hemophilia. The most commonly affected joints include the knee, elbow, and ankle. Hemorrhage may be secondary to trauma or may occur spontaneously. Recurrent hemarthrosis leads to synovial inflammation and proliferation associated with absorption of hemosiderin and red cell products. With synovial inflammation, cartilage destruction and subchondral bone damage lead to joint space narrowing. With hyperemia and prolonged inflammation, epiphyseal overgrowth, early growth plate fusion, and fibrosis of ligaments can be seen.

The radiographic changes may be identical to those of JRA, but clinical findings and typical joint involvement help distinguish these entities. Radiodense joint effusions and subchondral changes are more common in hemophilic arthropathy (Fig. 28). In the knee, the classical radiographic findings include squaring of the femoral condyles, a widened intercondylar notch, and squaring of the patella (see Section IX, Part XIII, Chapter 1, Fig. 17, page 2427). In the elbow, enlargement of the radial head may result in limited movement, and there may be broadening of the distal humerus and enlargement of the olecranon fossa (Fig. 29).

MRI may be used to determine whether hemarthrosis

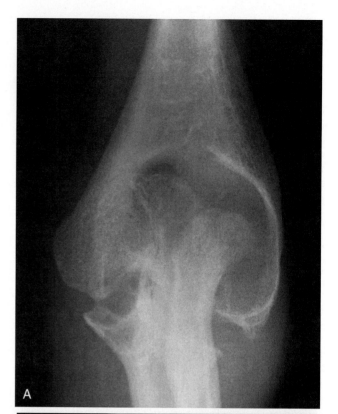

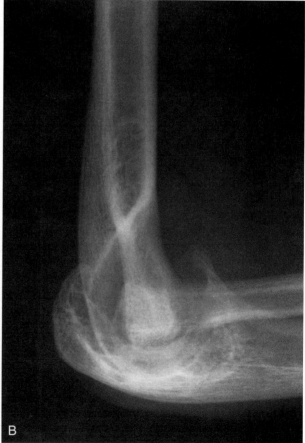

FIGURE 29. Hemophiliac arthropathy in a 15-year-old male with severe hemophilia. Frontal **(A)** and lateral **(B)** radiographs of the right elbow reveal marked joint space narrowing and pseudotumor of the distal humerus.

has occurred, so that therapy with factor VIII can be administered to prevent chronic joint damage. Acute hemarthrosis and chronic joint effusion may be indistinguishable, with low signal on T_1- and high signal on T_2-weighted images. Subacute hemarthrosis is usually of high signal on both T_1- and T_2-weighted images related to the presence of extracellular methemoglobin (Fig. 30). The synovial thickening often has areas of low signal on T_1- and T_2-weighted images related to fibrosis or hemosiderin deposition. Gadolinium better delineates the extent of synovial thickening, which shows less enhancement compared with rheumatoid arthritis. This is likely secondary to hypovascular connective tissue and hemosiderin deposition within the synovium. MRI de-

tects early changes within the cartilage, which may be localized or diffuse. Gradient-echo MR imaging is helpful for evaluation of hemosiderin and cartilage abnormalities. Subchondral cysts may result from intraosseous bleeding, and rarely pseudotumours may develop secondary to hemorrhage in the periarticular soft tissues. Signal characteristics are variable depending on the age of the hematoma.

Neuropathic Joint

Neuropathic arthritis is a destructive arthropathy secondary to longstanding repetitive trauma, frequently associated with loss of proprioception. In children, this

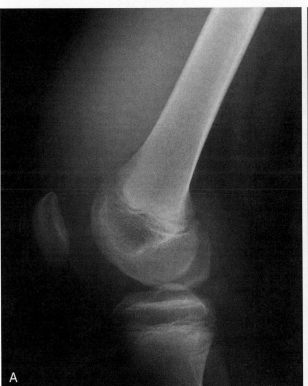

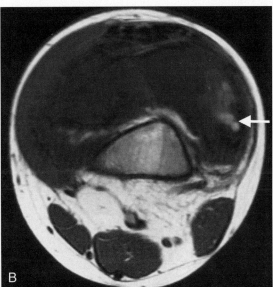

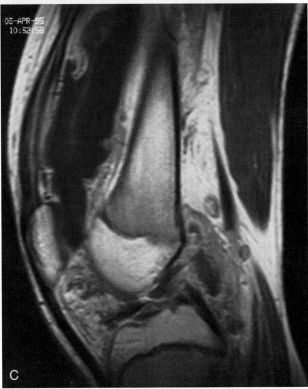

FIGURE 30. Twelve-year-old male with chronic hemophiliac arthropathy. **A,** On lateral radiograph of the left knee, there is marked soft tissue swelling in the suprapatellar bursa from extensive joint effusion. **B,** Axial T_1-weighted magnetic resonance image demonstrates low-signal chronic synovial thickening and heterogeneous signal of the joint effusion, with high-signal area laterally (arrow) consistent with subacute hemarthrosis. **C,** Sagittal T_1-weighted image following contrast enhancement shows irregular enhancing synovium in the popliteal region with several small enhancing popliteal lymph nodes.

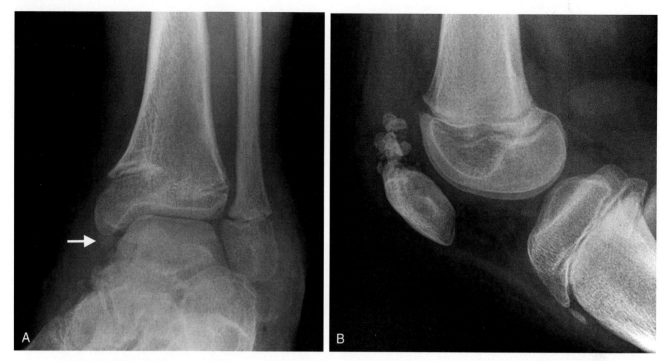

FIGURE 31. Neuropathic joints in a 10-year-old female with congenital insensitivity to pain. **A,** Frontal oblique radiograph of the ankle demonstrates soft tissue swelling, epiphyseal overgrowth, premature growth plate fusion, and loose bodies *(arrow).* **B,** Lateral radiograph of the knee shows joint effusion with multiple ossific loose bodies in the suprapatellar region.

may be related to myelomeningocele, syringomyelia, familial dysautonomia, or congenital insensitivity to pain. The most common radiographic findings include distention related to hypertrophic synovitis and effusion; degeneration of the articular surface, resulting in debris within the joint; and fracture or dislocation (Fig. 31). In children, there may be growth plate widening and metaphyseal fragmentation related to growth plate injury. MRI findings of neuropathic joint include fragmentation of areas of articular cartilage and subchondral bone, which are embedded in the synovium. In addition to synovial thickening and effusion, there may be associated tears of the menisci and ligaments. The periarticular bone is generally devoid of inflammation, but there may be inflammatory masses in the periarticular soft tissues that have heterogeneous signal intensity. MRI may help to distinguish infection from neuropathic destruction.

Foreign Body Synovitis

Foreign body synovitis usually presents with a monoarticular synovitis and may be suggested by the presence of a puncture wound. There is often a delay in diagnosis, especially if there is no history of injury and the foreign body is nonradiopaque and difficult to detect. Wood splinters, especially plant thorns such as palm or blackthorn, may dissect in from the surface and produce a chronic synovitis or tendonitis. Foreign body synovitis can simulate osteomyelitis or, rarely, primary bone tumors. Extraction of the foreign body is essential for recovery, and identification of the foreign body by imaging will allow a localized synovectomy. Plant thorns

have slightly higher density than soft tissue and may be detected on CT. Nonradiopaque foreign bodies may also be identified with ultrasound or MRI.

MISCELLANEOUS DISORDERS

INTRA-ARTICULAR MASSES

A number of articular masses arise from either the synovium or capsule of a joint and lead to joint dysfunction (Table 7). Imaging findings may be diagnostic.

Vascular Malformations

Vascular malformations are benign lesions, usually diagnosed in childhood or young adulthood. Clinically they mimic chronic arthritis, and not uncommonly there is a delay in diagnosis. They may have associated cutaneous lesions, recurrent hemarthrosis, and arthropathy. The knee is the most commonly involved joint and the suprapatellar region is the most common location. Most commonly they are venous, and rarely arteriovenous

Table 7 ■ INTRA-ARTICULAR MASSES
Synovial hemangioma
Pigmented villonodular synovitis
Synovial osteochondromatosis
Lipoma arborescens

malformations. Radiographs are normal in over half of patients; however, they may demonstrate a soft tissue mass or joint effusion. Occasionally osteoporosis, erosions, and epiphyseal overgrowth are present, and the presence of phleboliths suggests the diagnosis. MRI findings are usually diagnostic and help in defining the extent of disease. The typical MRI appearance is of a slightly lobulated, nonencapsulated mass without significant displacement of surrounding structures. It is of low or intermediate signal, similar to muscle, on T_1-weighted images and of high signal on T_2-weighted images, with low-signal septa, phleboliths, or vascular channels. There may be fluid levels, low-signal hemosiderin, or bone erosions related to hemarthrosis. Vascular malformations demonstrate extensive enhance-

ment after the administration of gadolinium (Figs. 32 and 33).

Nodular and Pigmented Villonodular Synovitis

Nodular synovitis and PVNS are uncommon proliferative disorders of the synovium of unknown etiology that may be post-traumatic or may represent benign synovial neoplasms. Although PVNS is more common in adults, 15% of cases will occur in children between 10 and 20 years of age. PVNS is usually monoarticular and only rarely polyarticular. Children may be more likely to have polyarticular involvement, and PVNS has been associ-

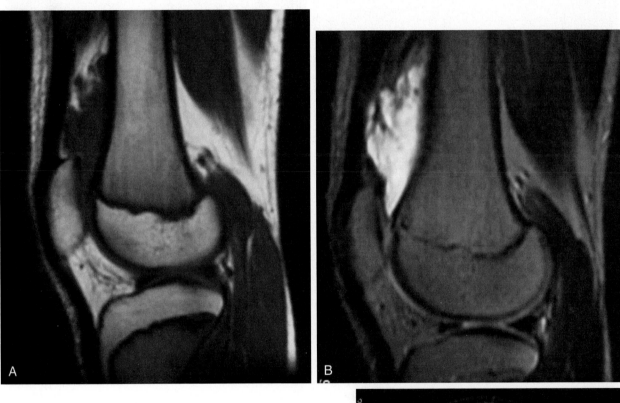

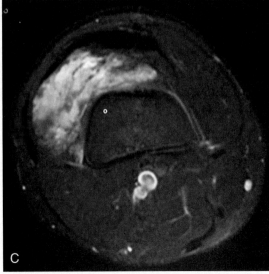

FIGURE 32. Magnetic resonance imaging of a vascular malformation in a 2-year-old female presenting with limp and swelling in the right knee. Sagittal T_1-weighted **(A)** and T_2-weighted **(B)** images and axial T_1-weighted image **(C)** with fat saturation postgadolinium demonstrate lobulated suprapatellar bursal mass, which is intermediate on T_1- and hyperintense on T_2-weighted images, with marked heterogeneous enhancement.

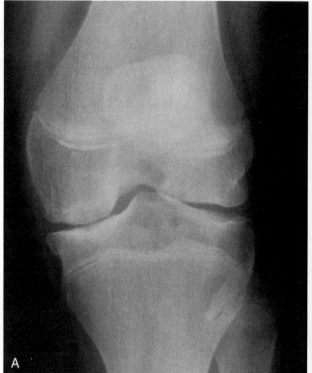

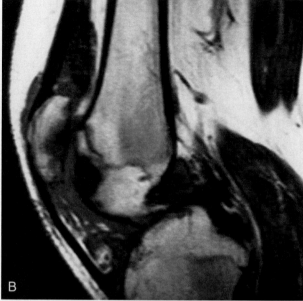

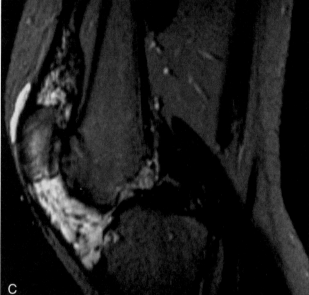

FIGURE 33. Vascular malformation with associated arthropathy related to recurrent hemarthrosis in a 16-year-old female with right knee monoarthritis for 12 years. **A,** Frontal radiograph of right knee shows irregular joint space narrowing, erosions, and early osteophyte formation. **B,** On sagittal T_1-weighted magnetic resonance (MR) image through lateral aspect of knee, there is marked joint destruction with erosions and posterior subluxation of the tibia secondary to disruption of the cruciate ligaments. **C,** Sagittal fast T_2-weighted MR image with fat saturation shows large, lobulated high-signal mass involving suprapatellar bursa, Hoffa's fat pad, and the intercondylar region.

ated with congenital anomalies of the genitourinary, cardiac, musculoskeletal, and neurologic systems. There are two forms: a nodular type that usually involves the tendon sheath of the hand and wrist, and a less common diffuse form that involves a joint, most commonly the knee. Other joints that may be affected in the diffuse form include the hip, ankle, shoulder, and elbow in decreasing order of frequency. The histology is identical in both types of PVNS and is characterized by synovial proliferation with an infiltrate of inflammatory cells with macrophages containing lipid and hemosiderin.

Radiographic findings are usually normal. Occasionally there are bone erosions or cysts with preservation of the joint space and bone density. There may be a joint effusion or mass of increased radiodensity on plain film or CT resulting from iron deposition, but calcification is rare. MRI demonstrates multinodular synovial masses with variable amounts of hemosiderin, which causes marked signal dropout on T_2-weighted and particularly gradient-echo images. Regions of increased signal on T_1-weighted images related to lipid deposition or increased signal on T_2-weighted images secondary to edema may be seen. The synovial masses show prominent contrast enhancement after gadolinium administration (Fig. 34). If the typical features are present, the MRI appearance is diagnostic. PVNS may invade into the bone and periarticular soft tissues and extend around neurovascular structures. MRI is useful in determining the extent of disease for surgical planning. In villonodular synovitis, a synovial mass will be seen that does not have the low MRI signal associated with hemosiderin.

Synovial Osteochondromatosis

This is a rare benign disorder characterized by metaplastic transformation of the synovium with the formation of osteocartilaginous foci. These foci may become calcified or ossified and can detach from the synovium to become loose bodies within the joint. They are usually similar in size and may enlarge with continuing nourishment from synovial fluid. Synovial osteochondromatosis is usually monoarticular and occurs most commonly in large joints. Up to 50% of cases occur in the knee, followed in decreasing frequency by the elbow, hip, and shoulder. Less commonly, small joints such as the

temporomandibular, acromioclavicular, and interphalangeal joints may be involved. Degenerative changes may occur as a late sequela, and rarely there is transformation to chondrosarcoma. Secondary osteochondromatosis may result from underlying disorders such as osteoarthritis, OCD, avascular necrosis, neuropathic osteoarthropathy, and trauma.

The radiographic finding of multiple calcified or ossified loose bodies of uniform size in a joint free of

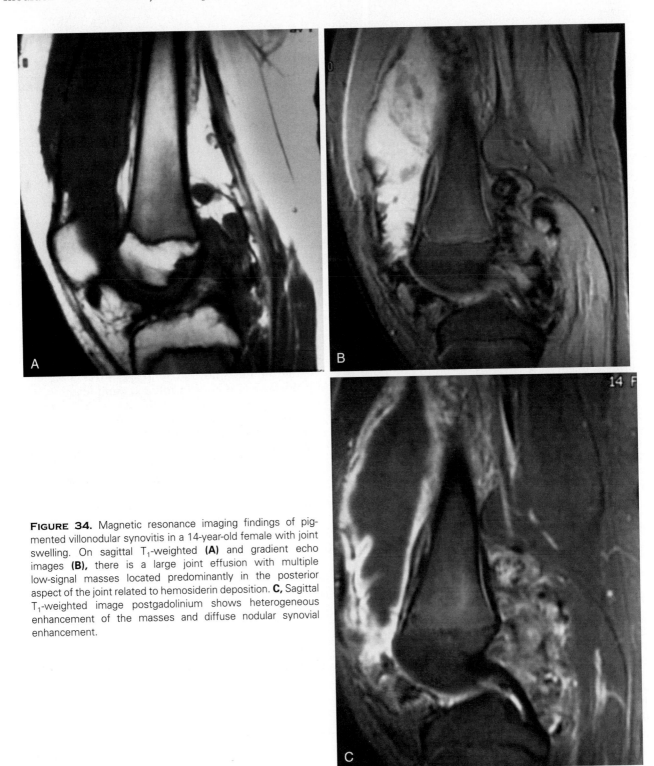

FIGURE 34. Magnetic resonance imaging findings of pigmented villonodular synovitis in a 14-year-old female with joint swelling. On sagittal T_1-weighted **(A)** and gradient echo images **(B)**, there is a large joint effusion with multiple low-signal masses located predominantly in the posterior aspect of the joint related to hemosiderin deposition. **C,** Sagittal T_1-weighted image postgadolinium shows heterogeneous enhancement of the masses and diffuse nodular synovial enhancement.

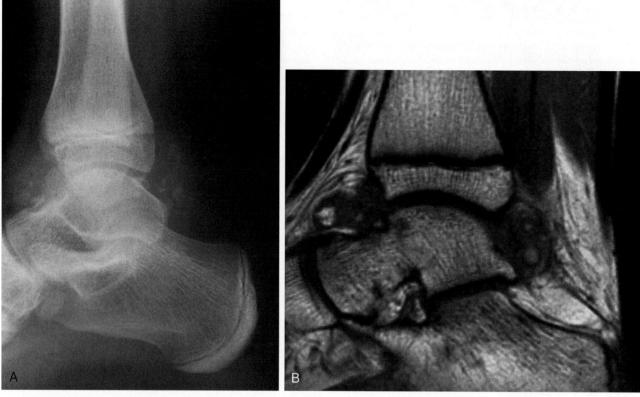

FIGURE 35. Synovial osteochondromatosis in an 11-year-old male with persistent right ankle swelling. **A,** On lateral radiograph of the right ankle, there are multiple radiopaque ossific loose bodies around the ankle joint with joint space preservation. **B,** On sagittal T_1-weighted magnetic resonance image of the ankle, multiple ossific foci are embedded in thickened synovium and have high signal intensity similar to adjacent marrow fat, with low-signal cortical rim.

arthritis is diagnostic. However, in up to one third of patients no calcification is present. CT may be helpful in detecting faintly calcified loose bodies. The MRI appearance depends on the composition of the foci. MRI can better demonstrate the noncalcified cartilaginous loose bodies. Hyaline cartilaginous foci are of low to intermediate signal on T_1- and high signal on T_2-weighted images. With calcification, low signal on T_1- and T_2-weighted images is evident. Ossific foci have internal signal similar to marrow, being hyperintense on T_1- and of intermediate signal on T_2-weighted images, with a peripheral rim of low-signal cortical bone (Fig. 35). Patients usually have associated joint effusion and synovial thickening.

Lipoma Arborescens

Lipoma arborescens is a rare benign intra-articular lesion consisting of villous lipomatous proliferation of the synovium. It usually is monoarticular, but 20% of the time the presentation is bilateral. Infrequent in children, it most commonly involves the knee joint but can be seen elsewhere, including in the glenohumeral joint, subdeltoid bursa, hip, elbow, ankle, and wrist joints. Most cases arise in an otherwise normal joint, but they may be associated with osteoarthritis, rheumatoid arthritis, Turner's syndrome, or internal derangement. Of unknown etiology, it may be a nonspecific reactive

change of the synovium in response to a variety of insults, such as trauma or inflammation. Pathologically, there is marked villous proliferation of the synovial membrane with hyperplasia of the subsynovial fat.

Radiographs may demonstrate a joint effusion and mass that is of fat density, but the fat content is more easily detected with cross-sectional imaging with CT or MRI. The MRI findings are pathognomonic, with frond-like synovial masses with signal characteristics paralleling fat on all pulse sequences, with high signal on T_1- and intermediate signal on T_2-weighted images (Fig. 36) and suppression of signal with fat saturation techniques.

ARTHRITIS RELATED TO CHILDHOOD MALIGNANCIES

Any of the childhood malignancies can cause musculoskeletal complaints that mimic rheumatic disease, including the leukemias, neuroblastoma, lymphoma, Hodgkin's disease, malignant histiocytosis, rhabdomyosarcoma, and the primary bone tumors, including osteosarcoma and Ewing's sarcoma.

Acute Leukemia

Leukemic arthritis typically presents with transient arthralgias and joint pain that is out of proportion to

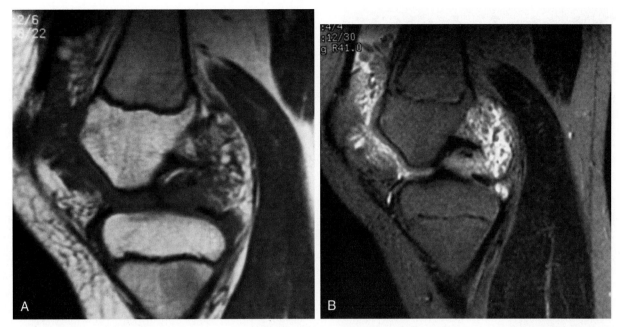

FIGURE 36. Magnetic resonance imaging findings of lipoma arborescens in an 11-year-old male with chronic right knee swelling for 4 years. Sagittal T$_1$-weighted **(A)** and sagittal T$_2$-weighted **(B)** images demonstrate a lobulated soft tissue mass within the suprapatellar bursae and posterior joint space. It has high signal foci on T$_1$ and intermediate signal on T$_2$-weighting identical to subcutaneous fat with associated joint effusion.

physical findings. Leukemic arthritis is much more common in children than adults, occurring in 12% to 65% of childhood leukemia cases. It is often polyarticular, with a predilection for large joints such as the knees, shoulders, and ankles. Arthritic symptoms may be related to metaphyseal periostitis, hemorrhage, or leukemic infiltration of the synovium. Hematologic abnormalities may be absent in 5% of children, and, if the incorrect diagnosis of rheumatologic arthritis is made and steroids are instituted, there is a worse prognosis. Plain films, bone scan, and MRI may clarify the diagnosis. Although often normal, radiologic findings include joint effusion, osteopenia, periostitis, lytic or sclerotic bone lesions, and metaphyseal radiolucent bands (Fig. 37). Diffuse abnormal signal intensity of bone marrow, which is low on T$_1$- and high on T$_2$-weighted sequences, can be seen on MRI (see Section IX, Part XII, page 2374).

SYSTEMIC DISORDERS

Sarcoidosis

Sarcoidosis is a chronic granulomatous disease that is rare in children; the early symptoms may simulate JRA. Common manifestations include rash, ocular disease, and chronic arthritis. Pulmonary findings are uncommon in children, and other organs that may be involved include the liver, spleen, lymph nodes, and parotid gland. The arthritis in childhood appears to be divided into two phases: an insidious pauciarticular arthritis in children younger than 4 to 5 years and a second phase

that develops into polyarticular arthritis in older children.

Radiographs may show bone changes that include acro-osteolysis, honeycombing, or small lytic areas in the phalanges, metacarpals, and metatarsals (Fig. 38). In young children, sarcoidosis may result in synovial thickening that predominantly affects the large joints and

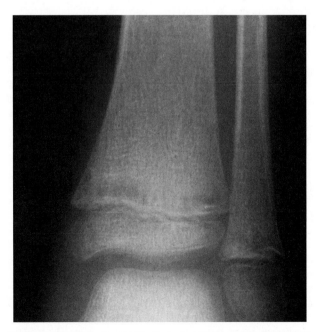

FIGURE 37. Acute lymphoblastic leukemia in a 5-year-old female with 4-month history of fever and right ankle pain. Radiograph of ankle shows metaphyseal tibial lucent band and normal joint space.

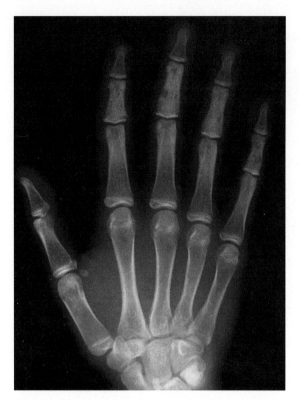

FIGURE 38. Sarcoidosis in a 15-year-old female with weight loss, hypothalamic dysfunction, joint pain, and swelling in fingers for 2 years. Radiograph of left hand demonstrates soft tissue swelling of several digits and multiple small lytic lesions predominantly in the middle phalanges, which were bilateral.

tendon sheaths. Other than soft tissue swelling, radiographic findings related to the joint, including erosions, are rare (see Section IX, Part XI, page 2343).

Storage Disorders, Skeletal Dysplasias, and Syndromes

Mucopolysaccharidosis I S (Scheie's syndrome) is a lysosomal storage disease related to a deficiency of α-L-iduronidase with excessive urinary excretion of dermatan sulfate and heparan sulfate. The biochemical abnormality is identical to Hurler's syndrome (mucopolysaccharidosis I), but manifestations are less severe. Abnormalities usually appear in childhood, including corneal clouding and cardiovascular disease such as aortic valve stenosis (see Section IX, Part V, page 2122). Joint abnormalities include stiffness with claw hand deformity and cystic changes in the carpals, metacarpals, tarsals, metatarsals, and femoral heads (Fig. 39). Other bone abnormalities include widening of the clavicles and ribs, which is characteristically seen in storage disorders. Inheritance is autosomal recessive, and patients have normal intelligence or mild mental retardation. Other storage disorders associated with joint abnormalities include mucolipidosis III and hyaluronidase deficiency. Abnormal low signal around affected joints can be in patients with mucolipidosis III on MRI.

Progressive pseudorheumatoid arthritis of childhood (PPAC) is an autosomal recessive noninflammatory

chondrodysplasia. Initial symptoms of difficulty walking and muscular weakness develop between 3 and 8 years of age. The main clinical features are generalized, progressive joint stiffness and swelling related to osseous enlargement, which is most marked in the hands. There are characteristic dysplastic skeletal abnormalities, particularly in the spine with platyspondyly, that distinguish this disorder from JRA. Other skeletal dysplasias associated with joint symptoms include Kniest syndrome, multiple epiphyseal dysplasia, and spondyloepiphyseal dysplasia tarda with progressive arthropathy, which may represent the same disorder as PPAC.

Camptodactyly–arthropathy syndrome is a rare autosomal recessive disorder consisting of congenital camptodactyly, arthropathy, and pericarditis. The lack of inflammation and absence of joint narrowing with chronic disease help differentiate this disorder from JRA. Flexion deformities are symmetric, involving the proximal interphalangeal joint of the hands. Arthropathy predominantly affects large joints, and radiographic findings are most marked in the hips, where there is coxa vara, short broad femoral necks, and intraosseous cysts (Fig. 40).

Neonatal-onset multisystem inflammatory disease is a rare systemic disease characterized by arthropathy with rash,

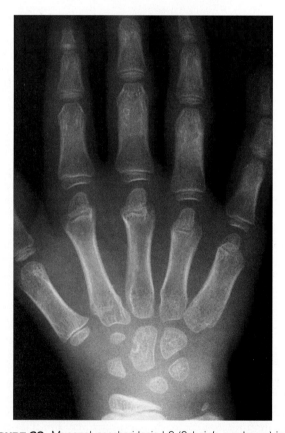

FIGURE 39. Mucopolysaccharidosis I S (Scheie's syndrome) in an 11-year-old male with history of chronic arthritis with multiple joint contractures treated initially as juvenile rheumatoid arthritis. Patient was noted to have corneal clouding, glaucoma, and more recently aortic insufficiency. Chest radiograph demonstrated short, broad clavicles. Hand radiograph shows short metacarpals and small carpal bones with an intraosseous cyst in the capitate, as well as soft tissue swelling and joint space narrowing.

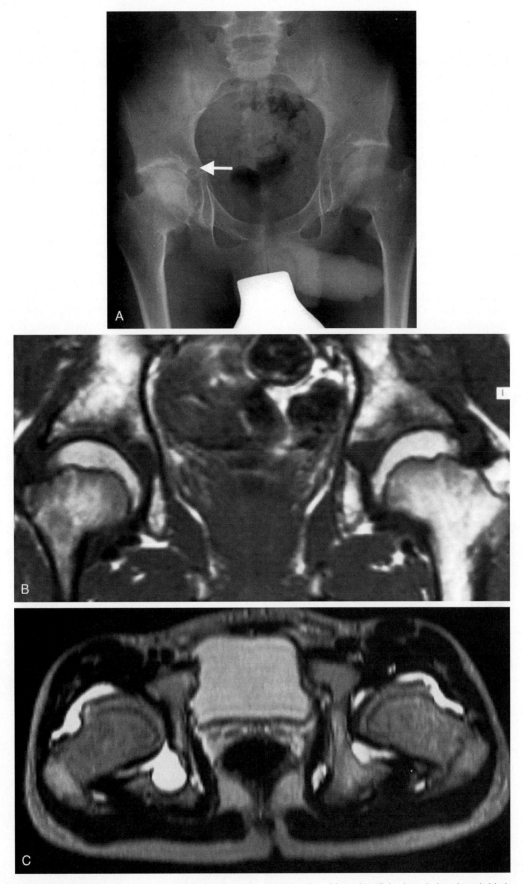

FIGURE 40. Camptodactyly–arthropathy syndrome in a 15-year-old male with pericardial rub and chronic arthritis involving hips, knees, and ankles and history of flexion deformities of fingers since birth. Chest radiograph showed enlargement of pericardial silhouette secondary to pericardial effusion. **A,** Radiograph of the pelvis shows short broad femoral necks, coxa magna and varus deformity with symmetric narrowing of hip joints, and intraosseous cysts within the acetabulum *(arrow)* better seen on magnetic resonance (MR) images. Coronal T_1-weighted **(B)** and axial T_2-weighted **(C)** MR images demonstrate bilateral joint effusions with intraosseous cysts that are of intermediate signal on T_1- and high signal on T_2-weighted sequences.

fever, hepatosplenomegaly, central nervous system and eye involvement, and deforming arthropathy of mainly large joints distinct from JRA. The typical radiographic appearance includes periarticular soft tissue swelling; enlarged, irregularly ossified epiphyses, especially around the knee; and metaphyseal splaying, osteoporosis, and metadiaphyseal periosteal new bone formation.

Goldbloom's disease is a rare disorder consisting of idiopathic periosteal hyperostosis and dysproteinemia (see Section IX, Part XI, page 2343). It usually presents after infancy with an upper respiratory infection, limb pain, and joint swelling. Radiographs show lamellar periosteal reaction predominantly involving long bones but also the mandible, facial bones, metacarpals, and metatarsals. One of the distinguishing features is an abnormality of serum proteins with hypergammaglobulinemia and hypoalbuminemia. Other disorders associated with periostitis and joint swelling, such as hypertrophic osteoarthropathy, must be excluded. Treatment is symptomatic with salicylates, and recovery is complete after weeks or months.

BAKER'S CYST

Synovial cysts are fluid collections resulting from herniation of synovium through the joint capsule. The most common is the popliteal or Baker's cyst, located within the gastrocnemius–semimembranosus bursa. Popliteal cysts may develop at any age, but up to 33% occur in children 15 years or younger and they are slightly more common in boys than in girls. They may be associated with previous injury or arthritis, but, in children, the majority (95%) of popliteal cysts are isolated. In contrast to adults, popliteal cysts in children usually resolve spontaneously, and surgery is only indicated when there is associated pain or restriction of movement. Synovial cysts may simulate hematoma or tumor clinically, and, with rupture into the soft tissues of the calf, they can be confused with thrombophlebitis. Other intra-articular cysts that are not synovial in origin include ganglia and meniscal cysts. Ganglia result from myxomatous degeneration of connective tissue and are usually associated with tendons or ligaments. Meniscal cysts are associated with horizontal tears of the menisci.

On lateral radiographs of the knee, Baker's cysts may be seen as a well-defined soft tissue mass in the popliteal fossa. They are located along the posteromedial aspect of the knee joint, and can be seen extending between the head of the medial gastrocnemius and the semimembranous muscles on cross-sectional imaging. On sonography, popliteal cysts are seen as well-encapsulated, anechoic fluid collections. On MRI, they are usually homogeneous, with signal intensity identical to joint fluid, low on T_1- and high on T_2-weighted images (Fig. 41). Occasionally, they can be infected, demonstrate wall thickening or septations, or contain debris.

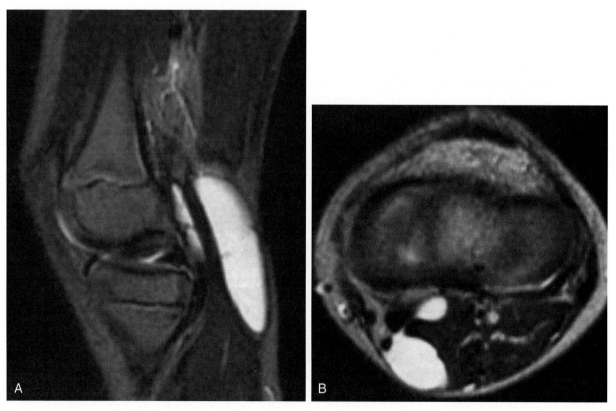

FIGURE 41. Magnetic resonance imaging findings with Baker's cyst. Sagittal **(A)** and axial **(B)** T_2-weighted images with well-defined encapsulated fluid collection with homogeneous high signal intensity on T_2-weighted image.

SUGGESTED READINGS

Normal Anatomy and Imaging Appearance

Balkissoon AR: Radiologic interpretation of vacuum phenomena. Crit Rev Diagn Imaging 1996;37:435–460

Gylys-Morin VM: MR imaging of pediatric musculoskeletal inflammatory and infectious disorders. Magn Reson Imaging Clin N Am 1998;6:537–559

Smith HJ: Contrast-enhanced MRI of rheumatic joint disease. Br J Rheumatol 1996;3:45–47

Congenital Malformations and Trauma

Aichroth PM, Patel DV, Marx CI: Congenital discoid lateral meniscus in children: a follow-up study and evolution of management. J Bone Joint Surg Br 1991;73:932

Al-Otaibi L, Siegel MJ: The pediatric knee. Magn Reson Imaging Clin N Am 1998;6:643–660

Azouz EM, Babyn P, Chhem RK: MRI of the pediatric knee. *In* Munk PL, Helms CA (eds): MRI of the Knee. Philadelphia, Lippincott–Raven, 1995:281-314

Bellier G, Dupont J, Larrain M, et al: Lateral discoid menisci in children. J Arthrosc Rel Surg 1989;5:52–56

Bohordorf K: Osteochondritis (osteochondrosis) dissecans: a review and new MRI classification. Eur Radiol 1998;8:103–112

Connolly B, Babyn PS, Wright JG, Thorner PS: Discoid meniscus in children: magnetic resonance imaging characteristics. Can Assoc Radiol J 1996;47:347–354

Gudinchet F, Maeder P, Oberson JC, Schnyder P: Magnetic resonance imaging of the shoulder in children with brachial plexus birth palsy. Pediatr Radiol 1995;25:S125–S128

Hayashi LK, Yamaga H, Ida K, et al: Arthroscopic meniscectomy for discoid lateral meniscus in children. J Bone Joint Surg Am 1989;70:1495

Kaplan EB: Discoid lateral meniscus of the knee joint. J B J Surg 1957;39:77–87

Raber DA, Friederich NF, Hefti F: Discoid lateral meniscus in children: long-term follow-up after total meniscectomy. J Bone Joint Surg Am 1998;80:1579–1586

Ryu KN, Kim IS, Kim EJ, et al: MR imaging of tears of discoid lateral menisci. AJR Am J Roentgenol 1998;171:963–967

Silverman JM, Mink JH, Deutsch AL: Discoid menisci of the knee: MR imaging appearance. Radiology 1989;173:351–354

Stark JE, Siegel MJ, Weinberger EW, Shaw DW: Discoid menisci in children: MR features. J Comput Assist Tomogr 1995;19:608–611

Arthritis

Juvenile Rheumatoid Arthritis, Autoimmune Connective Tissue Disease, and Chromosomal Disorders

Balestrazzi P, Ferraccioli GF, Ambanelli U, Giovannelli G: Juvenile rheumatoid arthritis in Turner's syndrome. Clin Exp Rheumatol 1986;4:61–62

Cellerini M, Salti S, Trapani S, et al: Correlation between clinical and ultrasound assessment of the knee in children with mono-articular or pauci-articular juvenile rheumatoid arthritis. Pediatr Radiol 1999;29:117–123

Chung C, Coley BD, Martin LC: Rice bodies in juvenile rheumatoid arthritis. AJR Am J Roentgenol 1998;170:698–700

Dressler F: Juvenile rheumatoid arthritis and spondyloarthropathies. Curr Opin Rheumatol 1998;10:468–474

Eich GF, Halle F, Hodler J, et al: Juvenile chronic arthritis: imaging of the knees and hips before and after intraarticular steroid injection. Pediatr Radiol 1994;24:558–563

Gylys-Morin VM: MR imaging of pediatric musculoskeletal inflammatory and infectious disorders. Magn Reson Imaging Clin N Am 1998;6:537–559

Harel L, Wagner-Weiner L, Poznanski AK, et al: Effects of methotrexate on radiologic progression in juvenile rheumatoid arthritis. Arthritis Rheum 1993;36:1370–1374

Kaye J: Arthritis: roles of radiography and other imaging techniques in evaluation. Radiology 1990;177:601–608

Lamer S, Sebag GH: MRI and ultrasound in children with juvenile chronic arthritis. Eur J Radiol 2000;33:85–93

Lang BA, Schneider R, Reilly BJ, et al: Radiologic features of systemic onset juvenile rheumatoid arthritis. J Rheumatol 1995;22:168–173

Laxer RM, Clarke HM: Rheumatic disorders of the hand and wrist in childhood and adolescence. Hand Clin 2000;16:659–671

Olson JC, Bender JC, Levinson JE, et al: Arthropathy of Down syndrome. Pediatrics 1990;86:931–936

Ostergaard M, Stoltenberg M, Gideon P, et al: Changes in synovial membrane and joint effusion volumes after intraarticular methylprednisolone: quantitative assessment of inflammatory and destructive changes in arthritis by MRI. J Rheumatol 1996;23:1151–1156

Patriquin HB, Camerlain M, Trias A: Late sequelae of juvenile rheumatoid arthritis of the hip: a follow-up study into adulthood. Pediatr Radiol 1984;14:151–157

Pettersson H, Rydholm U: Radiologic classification of knee joint destruction in juvenile chronic arthritis. Pediatr Radiol 1984;14: 419–421

Poznanski AK: Radiological approaches to pediatric joint disease. J Rheumatol 1992;19:78–93.

Reed MH, Wilmot DM: The radiology of juvenile rheumatoid arthritis: a review of the English language literature. J Rheumatol Suppl 1991;31:2–22

Rothschild BM: Recognition and treatment of arthritis in children. Compr Ther 1999;25:347–359

Ruhoy MK, Tucker L, McCauley RG: Hypertrophic bursopathy of the subacromial-subdeltoid bursa in juvenile rheumatoid arthritis: sonographic appearance. Pediatr Radiol 1996;26:353–355

Schanberg LE, Sandstrom MJ: Causes of pain in children with arthritis. Rheum Dis Clin North Am 1998;25:31–53, vi

Schneider R, Laxer RM: Systemic onset juvenile rheumatoid arthritis. Bailliers Clin Rheumatol 1998;12:245–271

Smith HJ: Contrast-enhanced MRI of rheumatic joint disease. Br J Rheumatol 1996;3:45–47

Sparling M, Malleson P, Wood B, Petty R: Radiographic follow-up of joints injected with triamcinolone hexacetonide for the management of childhood arthritis. Arthritis Rheum 1990;33:821–826

Sureda D, Quiroga S, Arnal C, et al: Juvenile rheumatoid arthritis of the knee: evaluation with US. Radiology 1994;190:403–406

White EM: Magnetic resonance imaging in synovial disorders and arthropathy of the knee. Magn Reson Imaging Clin N Am 1994;2: 451–461

Wihlborg CE, Babyn PS, Schneider R: The association between Turner's syndrome and juvenile rheumatoid arthritis. Pediatr Radiol 1999;29:676–681

Yancey CL, Zmijewski C, Athreya BH, Doughty RA: Arthropathy of Down's syndrome. Arthritis Rheum 1984;27:929–934

Juvenile Spondyloarthropathies

Azouz EM, Duffy CM: Juvenile spondyloarthropathies: clinical manifestations and medical imaging. Skeletal Radiol 1995;24:399–408

Cabral DA, Malleson PN, Petty RE: Spondyloarthropathies of childhood. Pediatr Clin North Am 1995;42:1051–1070

Foster HE, Cairns RA, Burnell RH, et al: Atlantoaxial subluxation in children with seronegative enthesopathy and arthropathy syndrome: 2 case reports and a review of the literature. J Rheumatol 1995;22:548–551

Jacobs JC: Juvenile arthritis. Am J Dis Child 1982;136:81–82

Keat A: Reactive arthritis. Adv Exp Med Biol 1999;455:201–206

Prieur AM: Spondyloarthropathies in childhood. Baillieres Clin Rheumatol 1998;12:287–307

Infectious Arthritis

Bettencourtt HL: A preterm infant with knee swelling. Clin Pediatr (Phila) 1999;38:45–47

Bradley JS, Kaplan SL, Tan TQ, et al: Pediatric pneumococcal bone and joint infections. The Pediatric Multicenter Pneumococcal Surveillance Study Group (PMPSSG). Pediatrics 1998;102:1376–1382

Brower AC: Septic arthritis. Radiol Clin North Am 1996;34:293–309, x

Forrester DM, Feske WI: Imaging of infectious arthritis. Semin Roentgenol 1996;31:239–249

Goldenberg DL, Reed JI: Bacterial arthritis. N Engl J Med 1985;312: 764–771

Gylys-Morin VM: MR imaging of pediatric musculoskeletal inflammatory and infectious disorders. Magn Reson Imaging Clin N Am 1998;6:537–559

Jacobs JC, Li SC, Ruzal-Shapiro C, et al: Tuberculous arthritis in children: diagnosis by needle biopsy of the synovium. Clin Pediatr (Phila) 1994;33:344–348

Jaramillo D, Treves S, Kasser J, et al: Osteomyelitis and septic arthritis in children: appropriate use of imaging to guide treatment. AJR Am J Roentgenol 1995;165:399–403

Lawson J, Rahn D: Lyme disease and radiologic findings in Lyme arthritis. AJR Am J Roentgenol 1992;158:1065–1069

Lee SK, Suh KJ, Kim YW, et al: Septic arthritis versus transient synovitis at MR imaging: preliminary assessment with signal intensity alterations in bone marrow. Radiology 1999;211:459–465

Mitchell CS, Parisi MT: Pediatric acetabuloplasty procedures: radiologic evaluation. AJR Am J Roentgenol 1998;170:49–54

Poon AH, Terk MR, Colletti PM: The association of primary varicella infection and streptococcal infection of the cutaneous and musculoskeletal system: a case report. Magn Reson Imaging 1997;15:131–133

Rose C, Eppes S: Infection-related arthritis. Pediatr Rheumatol 1997;23:677–695

Rutten MJ, van den Berg JC, van den Hoogen FH, Lemmens JA: Nontuberculous mycobacterial bursitis and arthritis of the shoulder. Skeletal Radiol 1998;27:33–35

Spencer CH: Bone and joint infections in children. Curr Opin Rheumatol 1998;10:494–497

White EM: Magnetic resonance imaging in synovial disorders and arthropathy of the knee. Magn Reson Imaging Clin N Am 1994;2:451–461

Zahraa J, Johnson D, Lim-Dunham JE, Herold BC: Unusual features of osteoarticular tuberculosis in children. J Pediatr 1996;129:597–602

Other Inflammatory Arthritides

Baunin C, Railhac JJ, Younes I, et al: MR imaging in hemophilic arthropathy. Eur J Pediatr Surg 1991;1:358–363

Hermann G, Gilbert MS, Abdelwahab IF: Hemophilia: evaluation of musculoskeletal involvement with CT, sonography, and MR imaging. AJR Am J Roentgenol 1992;158:119–123

Koop S, Quanbeck D: Three common causes of childhood hip pain. Pediatr Clin North Am 1996;43:1053–1066

Lee SK, Suh KJ, Kim YW, et al: Septic arthritis versus transient synovitis at MR imaging: preliminary assessment with signal intensity alterations in bone marrow. Radiology 1999;211:459–465

Maillot F, Goupille P, Valat JP: Plant thorn synovitis diagnosed by magnetic resonance imaging. Scand J Rheumatol 1994;23:154–155

Marchal GJ, Van Holsbeeck MT, Raes M, et al: Transient synovitis of the hip in children: role of US. Radiology 1987;162:825–828

Nagele M, Bruning R, Kunze V, et al: Hemophilic arthropathy of the knee joint: static and dynamic Gd-DTPA-enhanced MRI. Eur Radiol 1995;5:547–552

Nuss R, Kilcoyne RF, Geraghty S, et al: Utility of magnetic resonance imaging for management of hemophilic arthropathy in children. J Pediatr 1993;123:388–392

Ozonoff MB: Pediatric Orthopedic Radiology. Philadelphia, WB Saunders, 1992

Rand T, Trattnig S, Male C, et al: Magnetic resonance imaging in hemophilic children: value of gradient echo and contrast-enhanced imaging. Magn Reson Imaging 1999;17:199–205

Ranner G, Ebner F, Fotter R, et al: Magnetic resonance imaging in children with acute hip pain. Pediatr Radiol 1989;20:67–71

Rawat B, Bell RS: Case report: rapidly progressive neuropathic arthropathy in syringohydromyelia—radiographic and magnetic resonance imaging findings. Clin Radiol 1994;49:504–507

Resnick D, Niwayama G: Diagnosis of Bone and Joint Disorders. Philadelphia, WB Saunders, 1995

Robben SG, Lequin MH, Diepstraten AF, et al: Anterior joint capsule of the normal hip in children with transient synovitis: US study with anatomic and histologic correlation. Radiology 1999;210:499–507

Rodriguez-Merchan EC: Effects of hemophilia on articulations of children and adults. Clin Orthop 1996;(328):7–13

Sequeira W: The neuropathic joint. Clin Exp Rheumatol 1994;12:325–337

Yulish B, Lieberman J, Strandjord S, et al: Hemophilic arthropathy: assessment with MR imaging. Radiology 1987;164:759–762

Miscellaneous Disorders

Bessette PR, Cooley PA, Johnson RP, Czarnecki DJ: Gadolinium-enhanced MRI of pigmented villonodular synovitis of the knee. J Comput Assist Tomogr 1992;16:992–994

Bravo SM, Winalski CS, Weissman BN: Pigmented villonodular synovitis. Radiol Clin North Am 1996;34:311–326, x–xi

Cameron BJ, Laxer RM, Wilmot DM, et al: Idiopathic periosteal hyperostosis with dysproteinemia (Goldbloom's syndrome): case report and review of the literature. Arthritis Rheum 1987;30:1307–1312

Cardinal E, Dussault RG, Kaplan PA: Imaging and differential diagnosis of masses within a joint. Can Assoc Radiol 1994;45:363–372

Coles MJ, Tara HH Jr: Synovial chondromatosis: a case study and brief review. Am J Orthop 1997;26:37–40

Cotten A, Flipo RM, Herbaux B, et al: Synovial haemangioma of the knee: a frequently misdiagnosed lesion. Skeletal Radiol 1995;24:257–261

Coumas JM, Palmer WE: Knee arthrography: Evolution and current status. Radiol Clin North Am 1998;36:703–728

De Maeseneer M, Debaere C, Desprechins B, Osteaux M: Popliteal cysts in children: prevalence, appearance and associated findings at MR imaging. Pediatr Radiol 1999;29:605–609

Donnelly LF, Bisset GS 3rd, Passo MH: MRI findings of lipoma arborescens of the knee in a child: case report. Pediatr Radiol 1994;24:258–259

Eustace S, Harrison M, Srinivasen U, Stack J: Magnetic resonance imaging in pigmented villonodular synovitis. Can Assoc Radiol J 1994;45:283–286

Evans T, Nercessian B, Sanders K: Leukemic arthritis. Semin Arthritis Rheum 1994;24:48–56

Feller JF, Rishi M, Hughes EC: Lipoma arborescens of the knee: MR demonstration. AJR Am J Roentgenol 1994;163:162–164

Gallagher D, Heinrich SD, Craver R, et al: Skeletal manifestations of acute leukemia in childhood [clinical conference]. Orthopedics 1991;14:485–492

Gerscovich EO, Greenspan A, Lehman WB: Idiopathic periosteal hyperostosis with dysproteinemia—Goldbloom's syndrome. Pediatr Radiol 1990;20:208–211

Goldbloom RB, Stein PB, Eisen A, et al: Idiopathic periosteal hyperostosis with dysproteinemia: a new clinical entity. N Engl J Med 1966;274:873–878

Goldman AB, DiCarlo EF: Pigmented villonodular synovitis: diagnosis and differential diagnosis. Radiol Clin North Am 1988;26:1327–1347

Greenspan A, Azouz EM, Matthews J 2nd, Decarie JC: Synovial hemangioma: imaging features in eight histologically proven cases, review of the literature, and differential diagnosis. Skeletal Radiol 1995;24:583–590

Grieten M, Buckwalter KA, Cardinal E, Rougraff B: Case report 873: lipoma arborescens (villous lipomatous proliferation of the synovial membrane). Skeletal Radiol 1994;23:652–655

Hallel T, Lew S, Bansal M: Villous lipomatous proliferation of the synovial membrane (lipoma arborescens). J Bone Joint Surg Am 1988;70:264–270

Hossien RD: Progressive pseudorheumatoid chondrodysplasia. Skeletal Radiol 1994;23:411–419

Hughes TH, Sartoris DJ, Schweitzer ME, Resnick DL: Pigmented villonodular synovitis: MRI characteristics. Skeletal Radiol 1995;24:7–12

Hugosson C, Bahabri S, McDonald P, et al: Radiological features in congenital camptodactyly, familial arthropathy and coxa vara syndrome. Pediatr Radiol 1994;24:523–526

Katz DS, Vaughn CJ, Goldschmidt AM, et al: A 15-year-old girl with a right leg mass. Clin Imaging 1995;19:65–68

Kramer J, Recht M, Deely DM, et al: MR appearance of idiopathic synovial osteochondromatosis. J Comput Assist Tomogr 1993;17:772–776

Lamon JM, Trojak JE, Abbott MA: Bone cysts in mucopolysaccharidosis I S (Scheie syndrome). Johns Hopkins Med J 1980;146:73–75

Lang IM, Hughes DG, Williamson JB, Gough SG: MRI appearance of popliteal cysts in childhood. Pediatr Radiol 1997;27:130–132

Laxer RM, Cameron BJ, Chaisson D, et al: The camptodactyly-arthropathy-pericarditis syndrome: case report and literature review. Arthritis Rheum 1986;29:439–444

Lin J, Jacobson JA, Jamadar DA, Ellis JH: Pigmented villonodular synovitis and related lesions: the spectrum of imaging findings. AJR Am J Roentgenol 1999;172:191–197

Lindsley CB, Godfrey WA: Childhood sarcoidosis manifesting as juvenile rheumatoid arthritis. Pediatrics 1985;76:765–768

Llauger J, Monill JM, Palmer J, Clotet M: Synovial hemangioma of the knee: MRI findings in two cases. Skeletal Radiol 1995;24:579–581

Martin S, Hernandez L, Romero J, et al: Diagnostic imaging of lipoma arborescens. Skeletal Radiol 1998;27:325–329

Natowicz MR, Short MP, Wang Y, et al: Clinical and biochemical manifestations of hyaluronidase deficiency. N Engl J Med 1996;335:1029–1033

Norman A, Steiner GC: Bone erosion in synovial chondromatosis. Radiology 1986;161:749–752

North AF, Fink CW, Gibson WM, et al: Sarcoid arthritis in children. Am J Med 1970;48:449–455

Ostrov BE, Goldsmith DP, Athreya BH: Differentiation of systemic juvenile rheumatoid arthritis from acute leukemia near the onset of disease. J Pediatr 1993;122:595–598

Ozonoff MB: Pediatric Orthopedic Radiology. Philadelphia, WB Saunders, 1992

Poznanski AK: Radiological approaches to pediatric joint disease. J Rheumatol Suppl 1992;33:78–93

Resnick D, Niwayama G: Diagnosis of Bone and Joint Disorders. Philadelphia, WB Saunders, 1995

Resnick D, Oliphant M: Hemophilia-like arthropathy of the knee associated with cutaneous and synovial hemangiomas: report of 3 cases and review of the literature. Radiology 1975;114:323–326

Ryu KN, Jaovisidha S, Schweitzer M, et al: MR imaging of lipoma arborescens of the knee joint. AJR Am J Roentgenol 1996;167:1229–1232

Sahn EE, Hampton MT, Garen PD, et al: Preschool sarcoidosis masquerading as juvenile rheumatoid arthritis: two case reports and a review of the literature. Pediatr Dermatol 1990;7:208–213

Sarigol SS, Hay MH, Wyllie R: Sarcoidosis in preschool children with hepatic involvement mimicking juvenile rheumatoid arthritis. J Pediatr Gastroenterol Nutr 1999;28:510–512

Spilberg I, Meyer GJ: The arthritis of leukemia. Arthritis Rheum 1972;15:630–635

Spranger J, Albert C, Schilling F, et al: Progressive pseudorheumatoid arthritis of childhood (PPAC): a hereditary disorder simulating rheumatoid arthritis. Eur J Pediatr 1983;140:34–40

Sundaram M, Chalk D, Merenda J, et al: Case report 563: pigmented villonodular synovitis (PVNS) of knee. Skeletal Radiol 1989;18:463–465

Tabyi H, Lachman RS: Radiology of Syndromes, Metabolic Disorders and Skeletal Dysplasias. St. Louis, Mosby–Year Book, 1996

Torbiak RP, Dent PB, Cockshott WP: NOMID—a neonatal syndrome of multisystem inflammation. Skeletal Radiol 1989;18:359–364

Vedantam R, Strecker W, Schoenecker P, Salinas-Madrigal L: Polyarticular pigmented villonodular synovitis in a child. Clin Orthop 1998;348:208–211

Wagner S, Bennek J, Grafe G, et al: Chondromatosis of the ankle joint (Reichel syndrome). Pediatr Surg Int 1999;15:437–439

Walls J, Nogi J: Multifocal pigmented villonodular synovitis in a child. J Pediatr Orthop 1985;5:229–231

Wihlborg CE, Babyn PS, Schneider R: The association between Turner's syndrome and juvenile rheumatoid arthritis. Pediatr Radiol 1999;29:676–681

Wong K, Sallomi D, Janzen DL, et al: Monoarticular synovial lesions: radiologic pictorial essay with pathologic illustration. Clin Radiol 1999;54:273–284

P A R T   X V

DEVELOPMENTAL DYSPLASIA OF THE HIP

PAUL S. BABYN

Developmental dysplasia of the hip (DDH) represents a spectrum of disorders with abnormal development of the growing acetabulum, femoral head, and adjacent soft tissues. DDH ranges from stable joints with abnormalities in acetabular slope and reduced femoral head coverage, termed *acetabular dysplasia,* to unstable joints, hip subluxation, and frank hip dislocation. Early diagnosis of DDH is necessary to favorably alter its natural history, improve treatment results, and decrease complications.

Until recently, infantile dislocation or dysplasia of the hip was referred to as *congenital dysplasia or dislocation of the hip.* However, it is now well recognized that subluxation and dislocation may occur in utero or perinatally and that not all instances of hip dysplasia are present or identifiable at birth. *Developmental dysplasia of the hip* is the preferred terminology because it better encompasses those cases that present later in infancy or childhood. DDH generally also includes those less common hip disorders, associated with childhood neurologic disorders such as myelodysplasia and myopathic disorders, including arthrogryposis and syndromic conditions such as Larsen's syndrome.

The hip is at risk for dislocation at several critical time periods during its in utero development, including shortly after its formation is complete at 12 weeks and at 18 weeks when the hip muscles develop. These early in utero dislocations are often associated with other anomalies or conditions and are termed *teratologic dislocations.* Teratologic dislocations are usually fixed and secondary to paralysis from myelodysplasia, arthrogryposis, or other neuromuscular disorder. However, the vast majority of cases of DDH result from forces acting on a vulnerable, unstable, but otherwise normal hip in the immediate prenatal and postnatal period. These forces alter the relative proportion of ossified to cartilaginous portions of the acetabular roof in favor of structurally weaker cartilage and predispose to subsequent dislocation. These are termed *typical dislocations.*

Commonly used terms in DDH include *hip instability,* defined as a lack of normal resistance to sudden change in femoral head position. *Unstable* hips have lost the normally tight fit between the femoral head and acetabulum and may be *subluxed,* wherein the hips demonstrate increased femoral head motion but the femoral head remains in contact with a portion of the acetabulum, or is *dislocated* out of the acetabulum. Both subluxed and dislocated hips remain intracapsular. With a *dislocatable hip,* the femoral head initially lies within the joint but can be dislocated out of the acetabulum by the application of gentle traction. Dislocated hips may be *reducible* with gentle traction back within the confines of the acetabulum, or fixed and *irreducible.*

ETIOLOGY AND EPIDEMIOLOGY

The etiology of DDH is uncertain but appears multifactorial, with genetic, mechanical, and hormonal factors. An elevated risk of DDH has been reported in those with a family history or a first-degree relative with DDH and with female gender, congenital deformities such as torticollis or metatarsus adductus, oligohydramnios, increased birth weight, and breech intrauterine position. However, more than 60% of infants with DDH have no identifiable risk factors.

Mechanical factors, involving in utero space and movement restriction, are thought to be causative in conditions such as oligohydramnios and breech presentation. Breech presentation leads to knee extension of the fetus, resulting in sustained hamstring forces about the hip and hip instability. The majority of breech presentations are found in first-born children, likely because of the unstretched uterus and tight abdominal structures. Normally seen in 2% to 4% of deliveries, breech presentation has a much higher incidence in DDH, roughly 20%. Twice as many girls are born with breech presentation as males. In DDH, the left hip is more frequently involved, likely because of its being more usually adducted against the mother's lumbosacral spine. In this position, the bone of the acetabulum covers less of the femoral cartilage and instability may be more likely to develop; however, bilateral involvement may be seen in up to 25%.

Females are likely more affected because of increased ligamentous laxity that transiently exists as a result of circulating maternal relaxin and their own circulating estrogen. The risk for DDH of a female fetus with breech presentation and a history of maternal DDH is 1 in 15.

The true incidence of DDH can only be presumed because no gold standard exists. The incidence of *hip dislocation* at birth is roughly 1 to 2 per 1000 newborns, while *hip dysplasia* is approximately 10 times more common. Certain ethnic and geographic populations are known to be at higher risk for DDH, especially those with a cultural tradition of positioning the infant with the hips in extension. Traditionally Aboriginal Canadians strapped their infants to cradle boards with their legs in extension, leading to increased incidence of postnatal DDH within the latter half of the first year of life. A significant reduction in the incidence of DDH occurred after the institution of a national program in Japan to discourage the use of swaddling infants in extension.

NATURAL HISTORY AND PATHOLOGY

The growth of the normal proximal femur and acetabulum are interdependent. The acetabulum and femoral head develop from the same primitive mesenchymal cells, with the joint cleft appearing at 7 weeks' gestation. The hip joint is fully formed by 11 weeks. Entirely cartilaginous at birth, the proximal femur has growth areas including the physeal plate, the growth plate of the greater trochanter, and along the isthmus of the femoral neck. Continued normal growth of the proximal femur is extremely important for development of the hip joint. The absence of the femoral head within the hip during growth, as in dislocation, causes the acetabulum to assume a flat shape, while the normal concave shape of the acetabulum develops in response to the presence of a spheric femoral head.

DDH should be considered as a dynamic chain of events with progressive deformity developing over time. At birth, a significant percentage of newborns will show some hip laxity, with a large majority of these cases resolving spontaneously by 2 months of age. However, some will stabilize with acetabular dysplasia, while others will progress to subluxation or dislocation. These pathologic changes may be arrested or even reversed if appropriate therapy is begun early enough. If treatment is delayed, then inevitably further pathologic deformity will occur that may become irreversible, with limited potential for normal joint function. In DDH, these abnormalities include alteration and replacement of the normal cup-shaped structure of the acetabulum by a shallow, saucer-shaped acetabulum that is not congruent with the femoral head and persistent femoral anteversion. The longer the head is displaced, the greater the degree of acetabular dysplasia and femoral head deformity.

Secondary changes can also be observed in the surrounding soft tissues, with contractures, thickening of the ligamentum teres and transverse acetabular ligament, increased pulvinar fat, and interposition of the iliopsoas tendon and hip joint capsule. With persistent femoral head dislocation, the ligamentum teres lengthens and hypertrophies. The pulvinar fat, which is fibrofatty tissue found in the depths of the acetabulum, may increase. In long-standing dislocation, the stretched hip capsule may also become constricted by the contracted iliopsoas tendon and assume an hourglass configuration that prevents reduction.

Soft tissue adaptations can develop at the acetabular labrum, with formation of a neolimbus. The acetabular *labrum* is a fibrocartilaginous structure located at the rim of the acetabulum, which contributes to acetabular growth. With superior migration of the femoral head, one gets gradual eversion of the labrum with capsular tissue interposed between it and the outer wall of the acetabulum. In the older infant with DDH, the labrum is deformed and elongated and appears inverted, and it may mechanically block concentric reduction. The *neolimbus* is frequently confused with the acetabular labrum and represents a pathologic response of the acetabulum. With abnormal pressure, there is formation of fibrous tissue that merges with the hyaline cartilage of the acetabulum along its rim to form the neolimbus. The size of the labrum and presence of a neolimbus is best evaluated with arthrographic techniques or magnetic resonance imaging (MRI). The neolimbus is a reversible change early on in the vast majority of patients with DDH.

The natural history of untreated DDH is variable. Abnormal gait and leg length discrepancy may be present. In some cases of complete bilateral dislocation, in adulthood there may be little or no functional disability, while in others, particularly with subluxation, severe disability may be found, with pain and premature osteoarthritis even in adolescence. DDH appears to be responsible for a significant percentage of adult hip osteoarthritis.

CLINICAL EVALUATION

Diagnosis of DDH may be made by clinical examination or by imaging. Extensive studies of DDH in the newborn by Andren and Von Rosen have demonstrated that physical examination is a reliable means of detecting dislocation in most patients. Range-of-motion and provocative tests are now fundamental examinations for all infants. The most reliable signs of DDH are the tests for instability, including the Ortolani and Barlow maneuvers. With the Ortolani maneuver, one tests to see whether the dislocated femoral head can be reduced. The flexed hip is gently reduced by slowly abducting with simultaneous exertion of an upward force on the greater trochanter. One gets the sensation of a palpable "clunk," which signifies the reduction of the femoral head into the joint, with a positive test. This indicates a defect in the superior aspect of the acetabulum. With the Barlow maneuver, one attempts to dislocate the femoral head by applying gentle downward force to the thigh; again, there is a "clunk" sensation when the test is positive. The use of the Ortolani and Barlow maneuvers becomes less reliable with increasing age of the infant as progressive soft tissue contractures develop. The palpable clunks of positive Barlow or Ortolani maneuvers must be distinguished from high-pitched clicks that are commonly found with hip motion in infants and are of no significance.

Subluxation is characterized by a feeling of looseness, a shifting in movement within the hip without the clunks of the Ortolani or Barlow maneuver. Acetabular dysplasia or maldevelopment of the acetabulum without instability can be determined only by imaging techniques because abnormal physical findings are absent.

Other physical signs are more equivocal for DDH because they may be seen in other orthopedic disorders and in normal infants. These include range-of-motion tests and asymmetry of inguinal or thigh skinfolds. Normally abduction should be symmetric for each hip. With DDH, limited abduction will eventually occur on the affected side but may not develop for several months. The older child who presents late may demonstrate an abnormal gait or leg length discrepancy.

Repeat hip examination during all well-baby visits is recommended to ensure that cases of DDH developing late are detected.

DIAGNOSIS

Radiologic evaluation with use of plain films, ultrasound, computed tomography (CT) and MRI may be of value at the time of diagnosis, during treatment, or in follow-up. The choice of study depends on the age of the child, information desired, and expertise of the radiologist. Generally CT and MRI are not needed for initial diagnosis.

RADIOLOGIC EVALUATION

Because the neonatal hip is composed almost entirely of cartilage, radiographs of the hip early on frequently are normal, especially if instability alone is present. It is difficult to evaluate femoral head and acetabular relationships on neonatal radiographs. Generally only an anteroposterior (AP) projection is obtained. Patient positioning is demanding; the infant must be placed so that the pelvis is in neutral position and not rotated with the hips slightly flexed. An AP radiograph of the hips is recommended in infants with fixed hip dislocation or limited abduction to evaluate for teratologic dislocations of the hips and congenital anomalies of the femur, pelvis, or caudal spine such as congenital coxa vara and proximal focal femoral deficiency. Because it is difficult to evaluate neonatal femoral head–acetabular relationships with radiography, sonography is generally preferred because it better assesses the cartilaginous structures and their relationship.

By 4 to 6 months, especially once the femoral head ossifies, radiographs become more reliable for evaluation of subluxation, dislocation, and acetabular dysplasia. Dislocation or subluxation is recognized by evaluating the relationship of the ossific nucleus and metaphysis to the acetabulum. Several reference lines and angles have been described that are helpful in evaluation of the infant pelvic radiograph. These include Hilgenreiner's line, Shenton's line, and Perkin's line as well as the acetabular index (Fig. 1). *Hilgenreiner's line* is a horizontal line connecting each triradiate cartilage of the pelvis at the depths of the acetabulum. *Perkin's line* is drawn perpendicular to Hilgenreiner's line downward from the lateralmost ossified margin of the acetabulum. The femoral head normally lies within the inferomedial quadrant that is created by Perkin's line, while the proximal femoral metaphysis does not project above Hilgenreiner's line or lie lateral to Perkin's line. *Shenton's line* is a continuous arc drawn along the medial border of the neck of the femur and superior border of the obturator foramen. In normal infants it should be continuous, but it is sensitive to rotation. Displacement of the femoral head or severe external rotation results in a break in continuity of Shenton's line. The *acetabular index* is the angle subtended by an oblique line drawn through the outer edge of the acetabulum, tangential to the acetabulum and Hilgenreiner's line. In the newborn this averages 28 degrees, with an upper limit of normal of 35 degrees. This angle reduces with increasing age.

In older children other radiographic measurements may be useful. These include the center-edge angle, which should be reserved for children older than 5 years. The center edge angle is obtained by drawing a vertical line through the center of the femoral head and

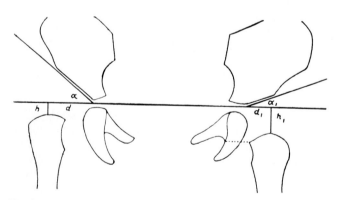

FIGURE 1. Hilgenreiner's method for measuring the acetabular index angles and degree of femoral dislocation before the femoral ossification centers appear. The horizontal line drawn through the triradiate cartilages is known as Hilgenreiner's line. The oblique line parallel to the acetabular roof is drawn to intersect the triradiate line; the angle between these lines is the acetabular index angle. Vertical lines (*h*) are dropped from Hilgenreiner's line to the middle of the superior edge of each femoral shaft; their lengths measure the cephalad displacement if any is present. The distance (*d*) between the intersections of the rooflines and the *h* lines measures the lateral displacement of the femur. In this figure, the right acetabular index angle is increased to 40 degrees and the right femur is dislocated cephalad and lateral.

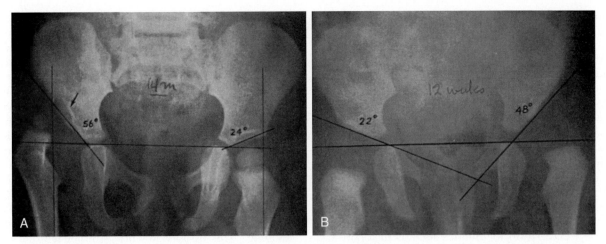

FIGURE 2. Developmental dysplasia of the hip. **A.** Unilateral DDH in a girl 14 months of age. On the right side there is (1) hypoplasia of the acetabular roof with increase in its pitch, (2) hypoplasia of the femoral ossification center, and (3) dislocation of the femur cephalad and laterad. The *arrow* points to a pseudoacetabulum. **B,** Dysplasia with dislocation of the hip at 3 months of age. The left acetabular index angle measures 48 degrees and the left femur is dislocated cephalad and laterad.

perpendicular to Hilgenreiner's line. A second line is drawn obliquely from the outer edge of the acetabulum through the center of the femoral head. The resulting angle reflects the degree of acetabular coverage in acetabular dysplasia and the degree of femoral head displacement in the unstable hip. The center edge angle of less than 20 degrees is abnormal and may be associated with acetabular dysplasia or femoral head subluxation.

In DDH, radiographic abnormalities will be seen in the proximal femur and acetabulum. Compared with the normal side, there is delayed growth of the ossific nucleus of the proximal femur and a characteristic increased slope of the ossified acetabulum (Figs. 2 and 3). A delay in appearance of the femoral ossific nucleus, however, can also be the result of an vascular insult following intervention. The acetabular sourcil, which is the curved line of dense bone representing the weight-bearing surface of the acetabulum, nor-

mally has a smooth configuration and a horizontal orientation. In the dysplastic hip, the sourcil is irregular and interrupted, with an upward slope that does not extend to the lateral bony margin. Absence of a sharply defined lateral edge of the acetabulum suggests dysplasia but also alters the lateral edge of the acetabulum, making reproducible determination of the acetabular index difficult. Changes of acetabular dysplasia or formation of a pseudoarticulation superiorly are late radiographic findings in DDH, typically not seen in neonates.

With subluxation or dislocation one sees widening of the acetabular teardrop. Widening of the teardrop may suggest low-grade instability not clinically apparent. The acetabular teardrop is not visible in the newborn, however, because it does not develop until after the first few months of life.

It has been recommended by some authors that all neonates suspected of having DDH have a subsequent

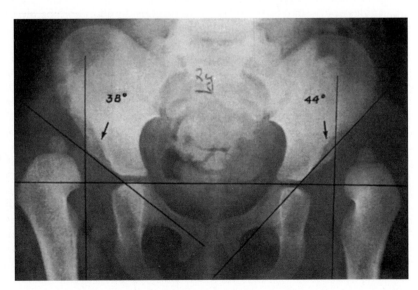

FIGURE 3. Bilateral DDH in a girl 2 years of age. The right acetabular index angle is increased to 38 degrees, and the left to 44 degrees. The *arrows* point to bilateral false acetabula.

radiographic examination at 4 to 6 months to verify the presence of normal hip development.

SONOGRAPHIC EVALUATION

Sonography has become the primary imaging technique for the initial radiologic evaluation of the neonate with suspected hip instability because of its ability to directly visualize cartilage, assess acetabular morphology, and document hip reducibility and stability. In 1980, Graf first described the sonographic anatomy of the normal and abnormal hip in static projections. Dynamic scanning of the hip as proposed by Grissom and Harcke incorporates motion and stress maneuvers based on clinical examination techniques such as Ortolani and Barlow maneuvers. A dynamic examination can be used to evaluate for stability of the hip. Stress maneuvers under sonographic guidance have shown that neonates may have up to 6 mm of physiologic laxity of the hip during the first few days of life, so care must be taken in diagnosing instability during this period.

To quantify acetabular maturity, Graf proposed the use of alpha and beta angles determined by the application of three lines drawn in the standard coronal plane. The standard coronal sectioning plane is defined as the deepest portion of the acetabulum, where the ilium appears as a straight line perpendicular to the femoral head and parallel to the surface of the transducer. One line, termed the *baseline,* passes through the plane of the ilium, where it connects to the osseous acetabular convexity. The *inclination line* passes from the lateral end of the acetabulum to the labrum, parallel to the cartilaginous roof. The *roofline* passes along the plane of the bony acetabular convexity. All measurements must be done within the standard plane.

The *alpha angle* is used most commonly as a measurement of acetabular concavity, and it is calculated as the angle between the baseline and the roofline. A normal alpha angle is 60 degrees or greater. Angles of 50 to 60 degrees may be physiologic in the immediate neonatal period, but hips with these angles are considered immature and require clinical and sonographic follow-up. Angles of less than 50 degrees are always considered abnormal and require treatment. The *beta angle* is measured between the baseline and the inclination line. It indicates the acetabular cartilaginous roof coverage. An angle of less than 55 degrees is considered normal. Beta angles have little clinical relevance.

The femoral head should be centered in the joint space, with 50% or more of the femoral head medial to the baseline in the coronal plane. The extent of maturity of the acetabulum also can be quantified by using angular measurements.

Not all hip imagers use these angles for the diagnosis and care of babies with DDH. Many use descriptive terms instead of numbers. With both sonographic techniques, considerable interobserver variability exists, especially within the first 3 weeks of life. With sonography, one has the ability to detect abnormal position of the hip, instability, and dysplasia that may not be evident clinically. However, early mild findings on sonography, including minor degrees of instability, may resolve spontaneously.

In 1993, a combined examination utilizing elements of both the Graf and dynamic techniques was recommended, with standardization adopted by the American College of Radiology (ACR) in 1999. The ACR standard ultrasound examination of the infant hip is performed in two planes—coronal and transverse—and includes stress maneuvers using a high-resolution linear array transducer. The infant may be examined in the supine or lateral decubitus position with the hip in a 90-degree flexed position. The operator uses one hand to hold the infant's knee at a right angle to the thigh. The palm of an open hand may be placed on the small of the infant's back. The thigh is held in the neutral position for imaging. The unossified cartilaginous femoral head appears as a ball within the acetabular fossa, with cartilage canals showing speckled increased echogenicity. With growth of the ossific nucleus, a central area of increased echogenicity develops in the center of the cartilaginous head (Fig. 4).

In a complementary method of assessing acetabular development, the distance between the medial aspect of the femoral head and the baseline (d) is compared with the maximum diameter of the femoral head (D); this $d{:}D$ ratio is expressed as a percentage. This ratio represents the coverage of the femoral head by the bony acetabulum in the standard coronal plane. Coverage of 58% or greater is considered normal. The smaller the degree of coverage, the greater the degree of acetabular immaturity.

Stress maneuvering (i.e., Barlow maneuver) with the femur in 90 degrees of flexion and maximum adduction is performed during transverse imaging to assess stability. The use of stress is optional in coronal imaging, which may be performed with the patient's leg in a flexed or neutral position. Stress is omitted if the infant is receiving treatment for DDH with a Pavlik harness. Stress maneuvering reveals the presence of instability, subluxation, or dislocation. In dislocated hips, the Ortolani maneuver should be performed to check for reducibility. An ancillary sign of instability is asymmetry in the degree of ossification of the femoral heads.

Not all sonographically abnormal hips need treatment, because spontaneous normalization of mild abnormalities is common in some infants by the time they are 4 weeks of age. Mild instability may be observed in healthy neonates in their first few days of life, when the typical femoral head has a laxity of 3 to 4 mm on average. This amount of motion should resolve spontaneously within the first few weeks of an infant's life, after maternal hormonal influences diminish. Therefore, the decision to treat is based not only on sonographic findings but also on clinical findings. Because many unstable hips may spontaneously normalize, delaying the first ultrasound study for 4 to 6 weeks is generally recommended unless dislocation is present.

Sonography is not indicated if the results of physical examination are reliably positive, with a positive Ortolani or Barlow maneuver, because treatment is based on the physical examination. Sonography is of value when the clinical examination is equivocal, or in high-risk

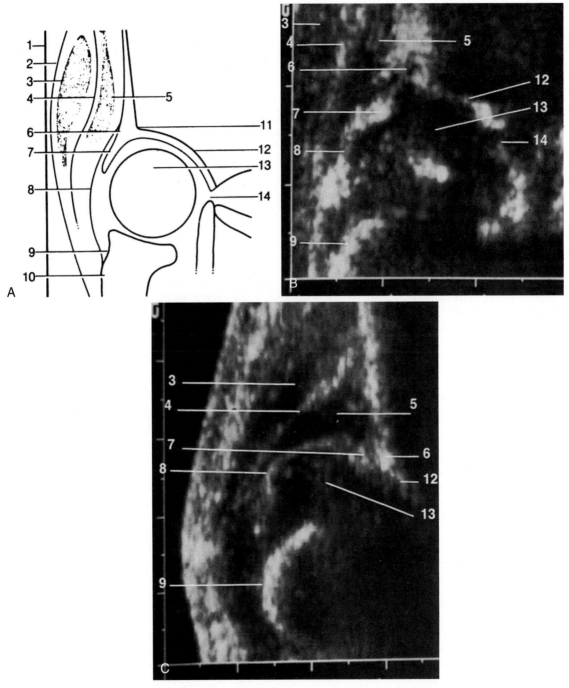

FIGURE 4. Sonographic features in the infant hip. **A,** Diagram of landmarks in coronal section of normal hip; *1,* skin; *2,* subcutaneous tissue; *3,* gluteus medius muscle; *4,* intermuscular septum; *5,* gluteus minimus muscle; *6,* cartilaginous rim; *7,* acetabular labrum; *8,* articular capsule; *9,* osteocartilaginous border of the femoral neck; *10,* greater trochanter; *11,* osseous rim of acetabulum; *12,* acetabular roof (ilium); *13,* cartilaginous head; *14,* triradiate cartilage. (From Schulz RD, Zieger M: Radiol Today 1987;4:103–105, with permission.) **B,** Sonogram of the hip in a normal 7-week-old boy with early ossification of the femoral head. **C,** Sonogram in a 4-day-old girl with complete dislocation of the right hip superolaterally. (**B** and **C** courtesy of Dr. R.D. Schulz, Stuttgart, Germany.)

groups when the physical examination is negative. Sonography is helpful in monitoring the hip that is being treated with a Pavlik harness, ensuring satisfactory relocation.

COMPUTED TOMOGRAPHY AND MAGNETIC RESONANCE IMAGING EVALUATION

Cross-sectional imaging with CT and MRI is not required for initial diagnosis but may be helpful in evaluation of complex cases preoperatively, or during treatment to assess concentric reduction or complications. Cross-sectional imaging to confirm adequate reduction is often obtained following intraoperative hip reduction and placement in a spica cast because conventional films are limited, especially in depicting posterior dislocation. CT with three-dimensional reconstruction may be used to evaluate the older child with complex hip deformity prior to surgery, allowing better depiction of acetabular deformity and degree of femoral anteversion. CT can also be used in evaluation of complications of therapy, including avascular necrosis.

MRI, with its inherent soft tissue contrast advantage and lack of ionizing radiation, may also be used in evaluation of the child with question of hip position postsurgery. MRI may supply useful information regarding vascular integrity or potential for avascular necrosis with various degrees of abduction. Limited evaluation with coronal and axial sequences depicting cartilage is usually all that is required to confirm satisfactory position postoperatively. When minor residual lateral subluxation is seen on CT or MRI as a result of increased pulvinar fat, the vast majority of cases will resolve without any further therapy once satisfactory repositioning of forces has been achieved. MRI may also be of value in assessment of the child or adolescent with associated abnormality, such as acetabular labral tear. Magnetic resonance arthrography may be needed to evaluate for labral tears or to better outline the intra-articular structures.

DIFFERENTIAL DIAGNOSIS

Radiographic features similar to those described for DDH, including shallow acetabula with highly angled roofs, lateral and cephalad displacement of the upper end of the femur, and small ossification center for the head, can be observed occasionally in congenital hypothyroidism. Following appropriate therapy, with improved tone and extension of ossification into the radiolucent cartilage of the acetabular roof, spontaneous resolution of the dislocation can occur.

Traumatic epiphyseal separation of the femoral neck in very young infants may simulate congenital dislocation, because the head and neck are still cartilaginous and not visible radiographically. The possibility of trauma must be entertained, especially when associated with a history of abnormal presentation, difficulty delivery, or other traumatic episode.

Acquired nontraumatic dislocation may develop rapidly in pyarthrosis of the hip; in such cases, clinical signs of infection and swelling of soft tissues may point to the proper diagnosis. Recurrent dislocation has also been observed in patients with congenital indifference to pain.

SCREENING

Screening programs have been established using clinical examination, radiography, and sonography. Universal clinical screening of the hips has been accepted as worthwhile and is now incorporated into all routine physical examinations of the infant and young child. Despite this, late presentations of DDH still occur, raising concerns regarding the accuracy of screening. Radiographic screening at 3 to 4 months of age has been implemented but requires exposure of a large number of normal children. Infants detected with radiography are also at the upper age range for early treatment with the Pavlik harness, and thus radiographic screening is not recommended currently. Although the use of sonography for universal screening has been implemented in several countries in central Europe, its use remains controversial. In North America, universal sonographic screening is not recommended because it may lead to increased false positives and consequent treatment-induced avascular necrosis and significantly increased costs.

Selective screening of children at high risk for DDH, including girls with positive family history and/or breech position and boys born breech, has been recommended by some but not all authors. Screening may be performed either by a radiograph of the pelvis at 4 to 6 months of age to confirm normal hip development or by a sonographic examination, obtained at 6 weeks of age. This allows those normal newborns with lax hips sufficient time to resolve spontaneously and avoid unneeded treatment. The hip abnormalities seen with breech presentation for the most part include inadequate development of the acetabulum, best found by a radiographic examination at 6 months of age or older.

TREATMENT

It is important to diagnose DDH early to favorably alter its natural history and improve the results. The treatment algorithm depends on the degree of abnormality and age of the patient. Treatment is easiest in the young infant and includes obtaining and maintaining concentric hip reduction until the hip is stable while avoiding complications such as avascular necrosis of the hip. Several devices, including the Pavlik harness and Frjka pillow, are used in younger infants in whom subluxation persists beyond 3 weeks after birth or with reducible hip dislocation. In North America, the Pavlik harness is most commonly used. This is a dynamic positioning device that achieves spontaneous reduction by positioning the hips in flexion, while allowing the child some movement within the confines of the harness. Radiographs are usually taken at the beginning and end of treatment with Pavlik harness.

Complications of Pavlik harness therapy, although infrequent, include avascular necrosis of the femoral head, femoral nerve palsy, and failure to reduce. Avascular necrosis of the femoral head may be noted in those who undergo extreme abduction, internal rotation, and flexion. Arterial compression of the medial circumflex artery against the labrum in the intertrochanteric fossa is the likely etiology. Satisfactory hip positioning with the Pavlik harness should be confirmed by sonography, but instability tests should not be performed. The use of power Doppler sonography or MRI has been suggested to better determine the safe zone of abduction possible without compromising femoral head arterial supply.

Pavlik harness therapy is successful in 95% of patients with acetabular dysplasia and subluxation but falls to 80% in those with dislocation. If the hip is not reduced by 3 weeks of harness therapy, harness therapy is discontinued and alternative therapy used. At age 6 months, treatment in a Pavlik harness is no longer effective because the child is too strong and redislocation is common.

When the hips are not reducible by Pavlik harness, closed reduction under anesthesia is attempted and, if successful, the child is placed in a hip spica cast. Percutaneous arthrography may be needed if closed reduction fails, to determine why the hip is not reducible. An inverted labrum, interpositioned iliopsoas tendon, or thickened ligamentum teres may be noted. Open reduction is usually required for those infants with teratologic and irreducible hip dislocations.

In almost all patients who present after the age of 6 months, treatment is generally more complicated. The success of closed reduction is markedly diminished, and open reduction is usually needed. Traction and percutaneous adductor tenotomy may be used, and capsulorrhaphy to remove the excess joint capsule may be needed. Femoral varus derotational osteotomy may be needed to correct excessive anteversion of the neck and valgus deformity often found in DDH. Often CT, or preferably now MRI, is needed to document satisfactory femoral head position postoperatively and exclude dislocation. Other complications of open therapy include increased leg length discrepancy, coxa vara deformity, and possible fracture and infection.

As a child gets older and the femoral head has spent more time outside the acetabulum, developmental abnormalities of the femoral head and acetabulum become more severe, making surgical treatment more complex and overall less successful. Older children have higher incidences of dysplasia and recurrent problems after open reduction that often lead to osteoarthritis, pain, stiffness, and disability.

In the older child who presents with acetabular dysplasia, the goal of treatment is to prevent or delay degeneration of the hip joint. This can be achieved by redirectional osteotomies such as the Salter osteotomy or reshaping osteotomies. Redirectional osteotomies are useful when the acetabular size and shape are adequate and the joint is spherical and congruent. These redirectional osteotomies allow the hip to become stable in normal weight bearing. Reshaping osteotomies are used in patients whose femoral heads are fairly spherical but articulate in an acetabulum that is much longer, with an upward shape. Imaging may be needed postoperatively to assess for satisfactory healing or to document complications such as Kirschner wire migration.

Patients with DDH should be followed until skeletal maturity because a substantial proportion will have radiographic evidence of acetabular dysplasia. Continued radiographic evaluation is needed every 1 to 2 years until skeletal maturity to ensure normal hip development.

SUGGESTED READING

Agus H, Omeroglu H, Ucar H, et al: Evaluation of the risk factors of avascular necrosis of the femoral head in developmental dysplasia of the hip in infants younger than 18 months of age. J Pediatr Orthop B 2002;11:41–46

American Academy of Pediatrics: Clinical practice guideline: early detection of developmental dysplasia of the hip. Committee on Quality Improvement, Subcommittee on Developmental Dysplasia of the Hip. Pediatrics 2000;105(4 pt 1):896–905

Andrew L, Von Rosen S: The diagnosis of dislocation of the hip in newborns and the primary results of immediate treatment. Acta Radiologica 1958;49:89

Babcock DS, Hernandez RJ, Kushner DC, et al: Developmental dysplasia of the hip. American College of Radiology ACR Appropriateness Criteria. Radiology 2000;215:819–827

Bellah R: Ultrasound in pediatric musculoskeletal disease. Radiol Clin North Am 2001;39:597–618

Bialik V, Eidelman M: At the crossroads—neonatal detection of developmental dysplasia of the hip. J Bone Joint Surg Br 2002;84:149

Brien EW, Randolph DA, Zahiri CA: Radiographic analysis to determine the treatment outcome in developmental dysplasia of the hip. Am J Orthop 2000;29:773–777

Cashman JP, Round J, Taylor G, Clarke NM: The natural history of developmental dysplasia of the hip after early supervised treatment in the Pavlik harness. J Bone Joint Surg Br 2002;84:418–425

Coleman SS: Diagnosis of congenital dysplasia of the hip in the newborn infant. JAMA 1956;72:548–554

Delaunay S, Dussault RG, Kaplan PA, Alford BA: Radiographic measurements of dysplastic adult hips. Skeletal Radiol 1997;26:75–81

Donaldson JS, Feinstein KA: Imaging of developmental dysplasia of the hip. Pediatr Radiol 1997;44:591–614

Duffy CM, Taylor FN, Coleman L, et al: Magnetic resonance imaging evaluation of surgical management in developmental dysplasia of the hip in childhood. J Pediatr Orthop 2002;22:92–100

French LM, Dietz FR: Screening for developmental dysplasia of the hip. Am Fam Physician 1999;60:177–184

Garvey M, Donoghue VB, Gorman WA, et al: Radiographic screening at four months of infants at risk for congenital hip dislocation. J Bone Joint Surg Br 1992;74:704–707

Gerscovich E: A radiologist's guide to the imaging in the diagnosis and treatment of developmental dysplasia of the hip, Part I. Skeletal Radiol 1997;26:386–397

Gerscovich E: A radiologist's guide to the imaging in the diagnosis and treatment of developmental dysplasia of the hip, Part II. Skeletal Radiol 1997;26:447–456

Gillingham BL, Sanchez AA, Wenger DR: Pelvic osteotomies for the treatment of hip dysplasia in children and young adults. Journal Am Acad Orthop Surg 1999;17:325–337

Goldbery MJ: Early detection of developmental hip dysplasia: synopsis of the AAP clinical practice guideline. Pediatr Rev 2001;22:131–134

Graf R: Guide to Sonography of the Infant Hip. New York, Thieme Medical, 1987

Grissom LE, Harcke HT: Developmental dysplasia of the pediatric hip with emphasis on sonographic evaluation. Semin Musculoskeletal Radiol 1999;4:359–369

Grissom LE, Harcke HT: Ultrasonography and developmental dysplasia of the infant hip. Curr Opin Pediatr 1999;11:66–69

Haynes RJ: Developmental dysplasia of the hip: etiology, pathogenesis, and examination and physical findings in the newborn. Instr Course Lect 2001;50:535–540

Hennrikus WL: Developmental dysplasia of the hip: diagnosis and treatment in children younger than 6 months. Pediatr Ann 1999;28: 740–746

Hickman JM, Peters CL: Hip pain in the young adult: diagnosis and treatment of disorders of the acetabular labrum and acetabular dysplasia. Am J Orthop 2001;30:459–467

Hubbard AM, Dormans JP: Evaluation of developmental dysplasia, Perthes disease, and neuromuscular dysplasia of the hip in children before and after surgery: an imaging update. AJR Am J Roentgenol 1995;164:1067–1073

Kim HT, Kim J II, Yoo C: Diagnosing childhood acetabular dysplasia using the lateral margin of the sourcil. J Pediatr Orthop 2000;20: 709–717

Kocher MS: Ultrasonographic screening of developmental dysplasia of the hip: an epidemiologic analysis. Am J Orthop 2000;29:929–933

Laor T, Roy DR, Mehlman C: Limited magnetic resonance imaging examination after surgical reduction of developmental dysplasia of the hip. J Pediatr Orthop 2000;20:572–574

Lin YK, Tien YC, Lin SY: Hip ganglion cyst associated with developmental dysplasia of hip in a child—a case report. Acta Orthop Scand 2002;73:109–110

Lotito F, Rabbaglietti G, Notarantonio M: The ultrasonographic image of the infant hip affected by developmental dysplasia with a positive Ortolani's sign. Pediatr Radiol 2002;32:418–422

Mooney JF III, Emans JB: Developmental dislocation of the hip: a clinical overview. Pediatr Rev 1995;16:299–303

Murray KA, Crim JR: Radiographic imaging for treatment and follow-up of developmental dysplasia of the hip. Semin Ultrasound CT MR 2001;22:306–340

Novacheck TF: Developmental dysplasia of the hip. Pediatr Clin North Am 1996;43:829–848

Ortolani M: The classic congenital hip dysplasia in the light of early and very early diagnosis. Clin Orthop Rel Res 1948;119:6–10

Ozonoff MB: Pediatric Orthopedic Radiology, 2nd ed. Philadelphia, WB Saunders, 1992

Patel H: Preventive health care, 2001 update: screening and management of developmental dyplasia of the hip in newborns. CMAJ 2001;164:1669–1677

Ponseti IV: Growth and development of the acetabulum in the normal child. J Bone Joint Surg 1978;60:575–585

Ponseti IV: Morphology of the acetabulum in congenital dislocation of the hip. J Bone Joint Surg 1978;60:586–599

Salter RB: Dislocation and subluxation of the hip (developmental displacement of the hip; developmental dysplasia of the hip. *In* Disorders and Injuries of the Musculoskeletal System, 3rd ed. Baltimore, Williams & Wilkins, 1999:146–156

Tan L, Aktas S, Copuroglu C, et al: Reliability of radiological parameters measured on anteroposterior pelvis radiographs of patients with developmental dysplasia of the hip. Acta Othop Belg 2001;67:374–379

Toma P, Valle M, Rossi U, Brunenghi GM: Paediatric hip—ultrasound screening for developmental dysplasia of the hip: a review. Eur J Ultrasound 2001;14:45–55

Von Rosen S: Diagnosis and treatment of congenital dislocation of the hip in the newborn. J Bone Joint Surg Br 1962;44:284–291

Weinstein SL: Natural history and treatment outcomes of childhood hip disorders. Clin Orthop Rel Res 1997;344:227–242

Weinstein SL: Developmental hip dysplasia and dislocation: normal growth and development of the hip joint. *In* Morrissy RT, Weinstein SL (eds): Lovell & Winter's Pediatric Orthopedics, 5th ed. Philadelphia, Lippincott Williams and Wilkins, 2001:905–956

Wientroub S: Current concepts review: ultrasonography in developmental dysplasia of the hip. J Bone Joint Surg Am 2000;82:1004–1018

Wientroub S, Grill F: Ultrasonography in developmental dysplasia of the hip. J Bone Joint Surg Am 2000;82:1004–1018

INDEX

Note: Page numbers followed by the letter f refer to figures and those followed by t refer to tables.